a LANGE medical book

CURRENT
Diagnosis & Treatment
Surgery

FOURTEENTH EDITION

Edited by

Gerard M. Doherty, MD
James Utley Professor of Surgery and Chair,
Department of Surgery
Boston University School of Medicine
Surgeon-in-Chief, Boston Medical Center
Boston, Massachusetts

Mc
Graw
Hill
Education

New York   Chicago   San Francisco   Athens   London   Madrid   Mexico City
Milan   New Delhi   Singapore   Sydney   Toronto

Current Diagnosis & Treatment: Surgery, Fourteenth Edition

1 2 3 4 5 6 7 8 9 10   DOC/DOC   19 18 17 16 15 14

ISBN 978-0-07-179211-0
MHID 0-07-179211-2
ISSN: 0894-227

Notice

Medicine is an ever-changing science. As new research and clinical experience broaden our knowledge, changes in treatment and drug therapy are required. The authors and the publisher of this work have checked with sources believed to be reliable in their efforts to provide information that is complete and generally in accord with the standards accepted at the time of publication. However, in view of the possibility of human error or changes in medical sciences, neither the authors nor the publisher nor any other party who has been involved in the preparation or publication of this work warrants that the information contained herein is in every respect accurate or complete, and they disclaim all responsibility for any errors or omissions or for the results obtained from use of the information contained in this work. Readers are encouraged to confirm the information contained herein with other sources. For example and in particular, readers are advised to check the product information sheet included in the package of each drug they plan to administer to be certain that the information contained in this work is accurate and that changes have not been made in the recommended dose or in the contraindications for administration. This recommendation is of particular importance in connection with new or infrequently used drugs.

This book was set in Minion by Cenveo® Publisher Services.
The editors were Brian Belval and Peter J. Boyle.
The production supervisor was Catherine H. Saggese.
Project management was provided by Vastavikta Sharma, Cenveo Publisher Services.
RR Donnelley was the printer and binder.

This book is printed on acid-free paper.

International Edition ISBN 978-1-25-925516-8; MHID 1-25-925516-6. Copyright © 2015. Exclusive rights by McGraw-Hill Education, for manufacture and export. This book cannot be re-exported from the country to which it is consigned by McGraw-Hill Education. The International Edition is not available in North America.

McGraw-Hill Education books are available at special quantity discounts to use as premiums and sales promotions, or for use in corporate training programs. To contact a representative, please visit the Contact Us pages at www.mhprofessional.com.

Contents

Authors

Cary B. Aarons, MD
Assistant Professor of Surgery
University of Pennsylvania
Philadelphia, Pennsylvania
Chapter 31: Anorectum

Suresh Agarwal, MD
Associate Professor of Surgery
University of Wisconsin
Madison, Wisconsin
Chapter 5: Postoperative Complications

Craig T. Albanese, MD, MBA
Professor of Surgery and Pediatrics
Department of Surgery
Vice President of Quality and Performance Improvement
John A. and Cynthia Fry Gunn Director of Surgical Services
Stanford Children's Health
Stanford, California
Chapter 43: Pediatric Surgery

Marco E. Allaix, MD
Department of Surgery
University of Chicago Pritzker School of Medicine
Chicago, Illinois
Chapter 20: Esophagus & Diaphragm
Chapter 29: Small Bowel

John T. Anderson, MD
Associate Professor
Department of Surgery
Division of Trauma and Emergency Surgery
University of California, Davis
Davis, California
Chapter 12: Shock & Acute Pulmonary Failure in Surgical Patients

Edward L. Bove, MD
Professor
Pediatric Cardiac Surgery, Section of Cardiac Surgery
University of Michigan
Ann Arbor, Michigan
Chapter 19: The Heart: Part II. Congenital Heart Disease

Matthew Brady, MD
Resident in Surgery
Boston Medical Center
Boston, Massachusetts
Chapter 22: Peritoneal Cavity

Elisha G. Brownson, MD
Resident in Surgery
Boston Medical Center
Boston, Massachusetts
Chapter 21: The Acute Abdomen

Peter A. Burke, MD
Professor of Surgery
Boston University
Chief, Section of Acute Care and Trauma Surgery
Boston Medical Center
Boston, Massachusetts
Chapter 28: Appendix

Jason Buseman, MD
Aesthetic Plastic Surgery Center
Thomasville, Georgia
Chapter 41: Plastic & Reconstructive Surgery

Andrew C. Chang, MD
Associate Professor and Head
Section of Thoracic Surgery
John Alexander Distinguished Professor
University of Michigan
Ann Arbor, Michigan
Chapter 18: Thoracic Wall, Pleura, Mediastinum, & Lung

Emily A. Chapman, RD, LD, CNSC
Adult Nutrition Service
University Hospital
Medical University of South Carolina
Charleston, South Carolina
Chapter 10: Surgical Metabolism & Nutrition

Huiting Chen, MD
Resident in Surgery
Department of Surgery
University of Michigan
Ann Arbor, Michigan
Chapter 35: Veins & Lymphatics

Daniel I. Chu, MD
Assistant Professor of Surgery
University of Alabama, Birmingham
Birmingham, Alabama
Chapter 5: Postoperative Complications

Jessica Cohan, MD
General Surgery Resident
Department of Surgery
University of California, San Francisco
Chapter 30: Large Intestine

Christopher S. Cooper, MD
Associate Professor of Pediatric Urology
Department of Urology
University of Iowa College of Medicine and Children's
    Hospital of Iowa
Iowa City, Iowa
Chapter 38: Urology

K. Barrett Deatrick, MD
Resident in Surgery
University of Michigan
Ann Arbor, Michigan
Chapter 7: Power Sources in Surgery
Chapter 18: Thoracic Wall, Pleura, Mediastinum, & Lung

Tracey Dechert, MD
Assistant Professor of Surgery
Boston University School of Medicine
Division of Trauma and Surgical Critical Care
Associate Program Director, General Surgery Residency
Boston Medical Center
Boston, Massachusetts
Chapter 9: Fluid, Electrolyte, & Acid-Base Disorders

Robert H. Demling, MD
Professor
Department of Surgery
Harvard Medical
Boston, Massachusetts
Chapter 14: Burns & Other Thermal Injuries

Karen E. Deveney, MD
Professor
Department of Surgery
Oregon Health & Science University
Portland, Oregon
Chapter 32: Hernias & Other Lesions of the Abdominal Wall

Gerard M. Doherty, MD
James Utley Professor of Surgery and Chair, Department of
    Surgery
Boston University School of Medicine
Surgeon-in-Chief, Boston Medical Center
Boston, Massachusetts
Chapter 2: Training, Communication, Professionalism, &
    Systems-Based Practice
Chapter 7: Power Sources in Surgery
Chapter 16: Thyroid & Parathyroid
Chapter 23: Stomach & Duodenum
Chapter 25: Biliary Tract
Chapter 26: Pancreas
Chapter 27: Spleen

Quan-Yang Duh, MD
Professor
Department of Surgery
University of California, San Francisco
San Francisco, California
Chapter 33: Adrenals

J. Englebert Dunphy, MD*
Formerly Professor of Surgery Emeritus
University of California, San Francisco
Chapter 1: Approach to the Surgical Patient

Alessandro Fichera, MD
Professor, Department of Surgery
University of Washington Medical Center
Seattle, Washington
Chapter 29: Small Bowel

Michael G. Franz, MD
Director of Surgical Research
Saint Joseph's Mercy Health System
Ypsilanti, Michigan
Chapter 6: Wound Healing

Warren Gasper, MD
Assistant Professor of Clinical Surgery
Vascular and Endovascular Surgery
University of California, San Francisco
San Francisco, California
Chapter 34: Arteries

Armando E. Giuliano, MD
Executive Vice Chair, Surgery
Associate Director, Surgical Oncology
Samuel Oschin Comprehensive Cancer Institute
Cedars-Sinai Medical Center
Los Angeles, California
Chapter 17: Breast Disorders

Jonathan W. Haft, MD
Associate Professor
Department of Cardiac Surgery
University of Michigan
Ann Arbor, Michigan
Chapter 19: The Heart: Part I. Surgical Treatment of Acquired
    Cardiac Disease

Scott L. Hansen, MD
Assistant Professor of Surgery
Department of Surgery
University of California, San Francisco
San Francisco, California
Chapter 42: Hand Surgery

Mark R. Hemmila, MD
Associate Professor
Department of Surgery
University of Michigan
Ann Arbor, Michigan
Chapter 13: Management of the Injured Patient

Virginia M. Hermann, MD
Professor
Department of Surgery
Medical University of South Carolina
Charleston, South Carolina
Chapter 10: Surgical Metabolism & Nutrition

*Deceased.

Jennifer C. Hirsch-Romano, MD
Assistant Professor
Department of Surgery
University of Michigan
Ann Arbor, Michigan
Chapter 19: The Heart: Part II. Congenital Heart Disease

James W. Holcroft, MD
Professor
Department of Surgery
University of California, Davis
Davis, California
*Chapter 12: Shock & Acute Pulmonary Failure in Surgical
    Patients*

Sara A. Hurvitz, MD
Associate Professor of Medicine
Department of Medicine, Division of Hematology Oncology
University of California, Los Angeles
Los Angeles, California
Chapter 17: Breast Disorders

Kamal M. F. Itani, MD
VA Boston Healthcare System
West Roxbury, Massachusetts
Boston University School of Medicine
Harvard Medical School
Boston, Massachusetts
*Chapter 8: Inflammation, Infection, & Antimicrobial Therapy in
    Surgery*

William R. Jarnagin, MD
Professor of Surgery, Chief HPB Service
Department of Surgery
Memorial Sloan-Kettering Cancer Center, Weill Medical
    College of Cornell University
New York, New York
Chapter 24: Liver & Portal Venous System

Fadi N. Joudi, MD
Assistant Professor
Department of Urology
University of Iowa
Iowa City, Iowa
Chapter 38: Urology

Haytham M. A. Kaafarani, MD, MPH
Assistant Professor of Surgery
Harvard Medical School
Boston, Massachusetts
Department of Surgery
Massachusetts General Hospital
Boston, Massachusetts
*Chapter 8: Inflammation, Infection, & Antimicrobial Therapy in
    Surgery*

Stephen A. Kamenetzky, MD
Clinical Professor
Department of Ophthalmology and Visual Science
Washington University School of Medicine
St. Louis, Missouri
Chapter 37: The Eye & Ocular Adnexa

Mark H. Katz, MD
Assistant Professor of Urology
Boston University School of Medicine
Boston, Massachusetts
Chapter 38: Urology

Mukta Krane, MD
Department of Surgery
University of Chicago Pritzker School of Medicine
Chicago, Illinois
Chapter 29: Small Bowel

Chienying Liu, MD
Associated Clinical Professor of Medicine
University of California, San Francisco
San Francisco, California
Chapter 33: Adrenals

Jason Long, MD, MPH
Assistant Professor of Surgery
Division of Cardiothoracic Surgery
UNC School of Medicine
The University of North Carolina at Chapel Hill
Chapel Hill, North Carolina
Chapter 18: Thoracic Wall, Pleura, Mediastinum, & Lung

Jason MacTaggart, MD
Clinical Instructor
Division of Vascular Surgery
University of California, San Francisco
School of Medicine
San Francisco, California
Chapter 34: Arteries

Eric Mahoney, MD
Walden Surgical Associates
Emerson, Massachusetts
Chapter 22: Peritoneal Cavity

Katherine Mandell, MD
Swedish Medical Center
Seattle, Washington
Chapter 21: The Acute Abdomen

David McAneny, MD
Associate Professor of Surgery
Boston University School of Medicine
Boston, Massachusetts
Chapter 3: Preoperative Preparation

Satish N. Nadig, MD, PhD
Assistant Professor of Surgery
Microbiology and Immunology
Medical University of South Carolina
Charleston, South Carolina
Chapter 45: Organ Transplantation

Jennifer S. Nelson, MD
Assistant Professor of Surgery
University of North Carolina
Chapel Hill, North Carolina
Chapter 19: The Heart: Part II. Congenital Heart Disease

Richard G. Ohye, MD
Associate Professor
Department of Surgery
University of Michigan
Ann Arbor, Michigan
Chapter 19: The Heart: Part II. Congenital Heart Disease

Aditya S. Pandey, MD
Assitant Professor of Neurosurgery
University of Michigan
Ann Arbor, Michigan
Chapter 36: Neurosurgery

Marco G. Patti, MD
Professor
Department of Surgery
University of Chicago Pritzker School of Medicine
Chicago, Illinois
Chapter 20: Esophagus & Diaphragm

Elliot C. Pennington, MD
Resident in Surgery
Boston Medical Center and Boston University
Boston, Massachusetts
Chapter 28: Appendix

Ian Pitha, MD, PhD
Wilmer Eye Institute
Glaucoma Center of Excellence
Johns Hopkins University
Baltimore, Maryland
Chapter 37: The Eye & Ocular Adnexa

Jeffrey D. Punch, MD
Professor of Surgery
University of Michigan
Ann Arbor, Michigan
Chapter 45: Organ Transplantation

Joseph H. Rapp, MD
Professor of Surgery in Residence
University of California, San Francisco
Chief, Vascular Surgery Service
San Francisco Veterans Administration Medical Center
San Francisco, California
Chapter 34: Arteries

John R. Rectenwald, MD
Assistant Professor
Department of Surgery
University of Michigan
Ann Arbor, Michigan
Chapter 35: Veins & Lymphatics

R. Kevin Reynolds, MD
The George W. Morley Professor and Chief, Division of
  Gyn Oncology
Director, Gynecologic Oncology Fellowship
Department of Obstetrics and Gynecology
The University of Michigan
Ann Arbor, Michigan
Chapter 39: Gynecology

Jennifer E. Rosen, MD
Chief of Endocrine Surgery
Vice Chair for Research
MedSTAR Washington Hospital Center
Washington, DC
Chapter 4: Postoperative Care

Michael S. Sabel, MD
Associate Professor
Department of Surgery
University of Michigan
Ann Arbor, Michigan
Chapter 44: Oncology

Theodore J. Sanford Jr., MD
Professor of Clinical Anesthesiology
University of Michigan
Ann Arbor, Michigan
Chapter 11: Anesthesia

Matthew J. Sena, MD
Assistant Professor
Division of Trauma and Emergency Surgery
University of California, Davis Medical Center
Sacramento, California
*Chapter 12: Shock & Acute Pulmonary Failure in Surgical
  Patients*

Stephen M. Sentovich, MD
Clinical Professor of Surgery
City of Hope Cancer Center
Duarte, California
Chapter 31: Anorectum

Thomas M. Shary, MD
General Surgery Associates
San Antonio, Texas
Chapter 10: Surgical Metabolism & Nutrition

David J. Terris, MD
Porubsky Distinguished Professor and Chairman
Department of Otolaryngology—Head and Neck Surgery
Medical College of Georgia
Augusta, Georgia
Chapter 15: Otolaryngology—Head & Neck Surgery

B. Gregory Thompson, MD
Professor of Neurosurgery, Otolaryngology and Radiology
Department of Neurosurgery
University of Michigan
Ann Arbor, Michigan
Chapter 36: Neurosurgery

Linda M. Tsai, MD
Associate Professor
Department of Ophthalmology and Visual Sciences
Washington University
St. Louis, Missouri
Chapter 37: The Eye & Ocular Adnexa

Simon Turcotte, MD, MSc
Assistant Professor
Hepatopancreatobiliary Surgery
University of Montreal
Montreal, Quebec, Canada
Chapter 24: Liver & Portal Venous System

J. Blake Tyrrell, MD
Clinical Professor
Division of Endocrinology and Metabolism
University of California
San Francisco, California
Chapter 33: Adrenals

Kelly L. Vanderhave, MD
Assistant Professor
Pediatric Orthopedic Surgery
Carolinas Healthcare System
Charlotte, North Carolina
Chapter 40: Orthopedic Surgery

Madhulika G. Varma, MD
Professor and Chief
Section of Colorectal Surgery
University of California, San Francisco
San Francisco, California
Chapter 30: Large Intestine

Henry C. Vasconez, MD
Professor of Surgery and Pediatrics, William S. Farish Endowed
    Chair of Plastic Surgery
Department of Surgery—Division of Plastic Surgery
University of Kentucky
Lexington, Kentucky
Chapter 41: Plastic & Reconstructive Surgery

Wendy L. Wahl, MD
Associate Professor of Surgery
St. Joseph's Mercy Healthcare
Ypsilanti, Michigan
Chapter 13: Management of the Injured Patient

Thomas W. Wakefield, MD
Stanley Professor of Surgery
Head, Section of Vascular Surgery
Department of Surgery
Director, Samuel and Jean Frankel Cardiovascular Center
University of Michigan
Ann Arbor, Michigan
Chapter 35: Veins & Lymphatics

James Wall, MD
Assistant Professor of Pediatric Surgery
Assistant Professor of Bioengineering by courtesy
Lucile Packard Children's Hospital Stanford
Palo Alto, California
Chapter 43: Pediatric Surgery

Lawrence W. Way, MD
Professor
Department of Surgery
University of California, San Francisco
San Francisco, California
Chapter 1: Approach to the Surgical Patient

Paul M. Weinberger, MD
Resident
Otolaryngology/Head and Neck Surgery
Medical College of Georgia
Augusta, Georgia
Chapter 15: Otolaryngology—Head & Neck Surgery

David M. Young, MD
Professor, Plastic Surgery
University of California, San Francisco
San Francisco, California
Chapter 42: Hand Surgery

Preface

Current Diagnosis & Treatment: Surgery is a ready source of information about diseases managed by surgeons. Like other books in the Lange series, it emphasizes quick recall of major diagnostic features and brief descriptions of disease processes, followed by approaches for definitive diagnosis and treatment. Epidemiology, pathophysiology, and pathology are discussed to the extent that they contribute to the ultimate purpose of the book, which is guidance for patient care. About one-third of the book is focused on general medical and surgical topics important in the management of all patients.

The book also includes limited current references to journal literature for the reader who wishes to pursue specific additional detail. Because of the concise nature of this text, more focused exploration may be useful to gain detail in specific areas.

OUTSTANDING FEATURES

To maintain currency of the information, this text is revised and updated frequently. The most recent edition was published in 2010. With each revision, particular subjects are completely, substantially, partially, or minimally rewritten as indicated by the progress in each field. New authors and chapters are introduced for the text as needed.

This edition includes major revisions of many chapters, and entirely new chapters on:

- Infection, Inflammation, & Antibiotics
- Thoracic Wall, Pleura, Mediastinum, & Lung
- Pancreas
- Large Intestine
- Small Intestine

INTENDED AUDIENCE

- Students: This is an authoritative introduction to surgery as the discipline is taught and practiced at major teaching institutions.
- Residents: This is a ready reference for concise discussions of the diseases faced each day, as well as the less common ones calling for quick study.
- Medical practitioners: Those who have occasion to counsel patients needing surgical referrals appreciate the concise readability of this book.
- Practicing surgeons: A most useful guide to current management strategies.

ORGANIZATION

This book is arranged chiefly by organ system. Early chapters provide general information about the relationship between surgeons and their patients (Chapter 1), training and professionalism (Chapter 2), preoperative care (Chapter 3), postoperative care (Chapter 4), and surgical complications (Chapter 5). Subsequent chapters deal with wound healing, inflammation, infection, antibiotics, fluid and electrolyte management, and surgical metabolism and nutrition. The main series of body systems topics begins with the chapter on head and neck tumors and ends with the chapter on hand surgery. Further chapters on pediatric surgery, oncology, and organ transplantation complete the coverage.

MULTIPLE CHOICE QUESTIONS

Along with the customary revision of all sections as called for by changing concepts in each field covered, in this edition, multiple choice questions and answers have been added to supplement each chapter.

ACKNOWLEDGMENTS

The editor and contributors continue to acknowledge their gratitude to J. Englebert Dunphy, MD, for the inspiration to begin the first edition of this text, and his lifetime of service to the practice and teaching of surgery, and to Lawrence W. Way, the long-time editor of editions 2 through 12, and conscience of the UCSF surgical training program. I have witnessed that same dedication to surgical students and trainees from faculty members at Washington University in St. Louis, the University of Michigan, and now at Boston University and Boston Medical Center, as well as at dozens of other universities and hospitals that I have visited. At each institution, I have appreciated the diligence and curiosity of our trainees, but I have admired none more than our present group at Boston Medical Center.

I am particularly grateful for the important contributions that the staff at McGraw-Hill has made to ensuring an accurate, high-quality text. In particular, Brian Belval has been extremely supportive and helpful. I am also grateful to colleagues and readers who have offered comments and criticisms to guide preparation for future editions. I hope that anyone with an idea, suggestion, or criticism regarding this book will contact me.

Finally, I thank my wife, Faith Cuenin, and our children Kevin and Megan for their constant love and support.

Gerard M. Doherty, MD
Boston, Massachusetts
November 2014

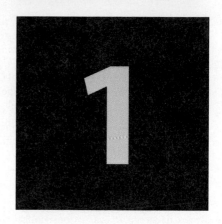

Approach to the Surgical Patient

J. Englebert Dunphy, MD[*]
Lawrence W. Way, MD

The management of surgical disorders requires not only the application of technical skills and training in the basic sciences to the problems of diagnosis and treatment but also a genuine sympathy and indeed love for the patient. The surgeon must be a doctor in the old-fashioned sense, an applied scientist, an engineer, an artist, and a minister to his or her fellow human beings. Because life or death often depends upon the validity of surgical decisions, the surgeon's judgment must be matched by courage in action and by a high degree of technical proficiency.

THE HISTORY

At their first contact, the surgeon must gain the patient's confidence and convey the assurance that help is available and will be provided. The surgeon must demonstrate concern for the patient as a person who needs help and not just as a "case" to be processed. This is not always easy to do, and there are no rules of conduct except to be gentle and considerate. Most patients are eager to like and trust their doctors and respond gratefully to a sympathetic and understanding person. Some surgeons are able to establish a confident relationship with the first few words of greeting; others can only do so by means of a stylized and carefully acquired bedside manner. It does not matter how it is done, so long as an atmosphere of sympathy, personal interest, and understanding is created. Even under emergency circumstances, this subtle message of sympathetic concern must be conveyed.

Eventually, all histories must be formally structured, but much can be learned by letting the patient ramble a little. Discrepancies and omissions in the history are often due as much to overstructuring and leading questions as to the unreliability of the patient. The enthusiastic novice asks leading questions; the cooperative patient gives the answer

that seems to be wanted; and the interview concludes on a note of mutual satisfaction with the wrong answer thus developed.

BUILDING THE HISTORY

History taking is detective work. Preconceived ideas, snap judgments, and hasty conclusions have no place in this process. The diagnosis must be established by inductive reasoning. The interviewer must first determine the facts and then search for essential clues, realizing that the patient may conceal the most important symptom—for example, the passage of blood by rectum—in the hope (born of fear) that if it is not specifically inquired about or if nothing is found to account for it in the physical examination, it cannot be very serious.

Common symptoms of surgical conditions that require special emphasis in the history taking are discussed in the following paragraphs.

▶ Pain

A careful analysis of the nature of pain is one of the most important features of a surgical history. The examiner must first ascertain how the pain began. Was it explosive in onset, rapid, or gradual? What is the precise character of the pain? Is it so severe that it cannot be relieved by medication? Is it constant or intermittent? Are there classic associations, such as the rhythmic pattern of small bowel obstruction or the onset of pain preceding the limp of intermittent claudication?

One of the most important aspects of pain is the patient's reaction to it. The overreactor's description of pain is often obviously inappropriate, and so is a description of "excruciating" pain offered in a casual or jovial manner. A patient who shrieks and thrashes about is either grossly overreacting or suffering from renal or biliary colic. Very severe pain—due to infection, inflammation, or vascular disease—usually forces the patient to restrict all movement as much as possible.

[*]Deceased

Moderate pain is made agonizing by fear and anxiety. Reassurance of a sort calculated to restore the patient's confidence in the care being given is often a more effective analgesic than an injection of morphine.

Vomiting

What did the patient vomit? How much? How often? What did the vomitus look like? Was vomiting projectile? It is especially helpful for the examiner to see the vomitus.

Change in Bowel Habits

A change in bowel habits is a common complaint that is often of no significance. However, when a person who has always had regular evacuations notices a distinct change, particularly toward intermittent alternations of constipation and diarrhea; colon cancer must be suspected. Too much emphasis is placed upon the size and shape of the stool—for example, many patients who normally have well-formed stools may complain of irregular small stools when their routine is disturbed by travel or a change in diet.

Hematemesis or Hematochezia

Bleeding from any orifice demands the most critical analysis and can never be dismissed as due to some immediately obvious cause. The most common error is to assume that bleeding from the rectum is attributable to hemorrhoids. The character of the blood can be of great significance. Does it clot? Is it bright or dark red? Is it changed in any way, as in the coffee-ground vomitus of slow gastric bleeding or the dark, tarry stool of upper gastrointestinal bleeding? The full details and variations cannot be included here but will be emphasized under separate headings elsewhere.

Trauma

Trauma occurs so commonly that it is often difficult to establish a relationship between the chief complaint and an episode of trauma. Children in particular are subject to all kinds of minor trauma, and the family may attribute the onset of an illness to a specific recent injury. On the other hand, children may be subjected to severe trauma though their parents are unaware of it. The possibility of trauma having been inflicted by a parent must not be overlooked.

When there is a history of trauma, the details must be established as precisely as possible. What was the patient's position when the accident occurred? Was consciousness lost? Retrograde amnesia (inability to remember events just preceding the accident) always indicates some degree of cerebral damage. If a patient can remember every detail of an accident, has not lost consciousness, and has no evidence of external injury to the head, brain damage can be excluded.

In the case of gunshot wounds and stab wounds, knowing the nature of the weapon, its size and shape, the probable trajectory, and the position of the patient when hit may be very helpful in evaluating the nature of the resultant injury.

The possibility that an accident might have been caused by preexisting disease such as epilepsy, diabetes, coronary artery disease, or hypoglycemia must be explored.

When all of the facts and essential clues have been gathered, the examiner is in a position to complete the study of the present illness. By this time, it may be possible to rule out (by inductive reasoning) all but a few diagnoses. A novice diagnostician asked to evaluate the causes of shoulder pain in a given patient might include ruptured ectopic pregnancy in the list of possibilities. The experienced physician will automatically exclude that possibility on the basis of gender or age.

Family History

The family history is of great significance in a number of surgical conditions. Polyposis of the colon is a classic example, but diabetes, Peutz-Jeghers syndrome, chronic pancreatitis, multiglandular syndromes, other endocrine abnormalities, and cancer are often better understood and better evaluated in the light of a careful family history.

Past History

The details of the past history may illuminate obscure areas of the present illness. It has been said that people who are well are almost never sick, and people who are sick are almost never well. It is true that a patient with a long and complicated history of diseases and injuries is likely to be a much poorer risk than even a very old patient experiencing a major surgical illness for the first time.

In order to make certain that important details of the past history will not be overlooked, the system review must be formalized and thorough. By always reviewing the past history in the same way, the experienced examiner never omits significant details. Many skilled examiners find it easy to review the past history by inquiring about each system as they perform the physical examination on that part of the body.

In reviewing the past history, it is important to consider the nutritional background of the patient. There is a clear awareness throughout the world that the underprivileged malnourished patient responds poorly to disease, injury, and operation. Malnourishment may not be obvious on physical examination and must be elicited by questioning.

Acute nutritional deficiencies, particularly fluid and electrolyte losses, can be understood only in the light of the total (including nutritional) history. For example, low serum sodium may be due to the use of diuretics or a sodium-restricted diet rather than to acute loss. In this connection, the use of any medications must be carefully recorded and interpreted.

A detailed history of acute losses by vomiting and diarrhea—and the nature of the losses—is helpful in estimating the probable trends in serum electrolytes. Thus, the patient who has been vomiting persistently with no evidence of bile in the vomitus is likely to have acute pyloric stenosis associated with benign ulcer, and hypochloremic alkalosis must be anticipated. Chronic vomiting without bile—and particularly with evidence of changed and previously digested food—is suggestive of chronic obstruction, and the possibility of carcinoma should be considered.

It is essential for the surgeon to think in terms of nutritional balance. It is often possible to begin therapy before the results of laboratory tests have been obtained, because the specific nature and probable extent of fluid and electrolyte losses can often be estimated on the basis of the history and the physician's clinical experience. Laboratory data should be obtained as soon as possible, but knowledge of the probable level of the obstruction and of the concentration of the electrolytes in the gastrointestinal fluids will provide sufficient grounds for the institution of appropriate immediate therapy.

▶ The Patient's Emotional Background

Psychiatric consultation is seldom required in the management of surgical patients, but there are times when it is of great help. Emotionally and mentally disturbed patients require surgical operations as often as others, and full cooperation between psychiatrist and surgeon is essential. Furthermore, either before or after an operation, a patient may develop a major psychotic disturbance that is beyond the ability of the surgeon to appraise or manage. Prognosis, drug therapy, and overall management require the participation of a psychiatrist.

On the other hand, there are many situations in which the surgeon can and should deal with the emotional aspects of the patient's illness rather than resorting to psychiatric assistance. Most psychiatrists prefer not to be brought in to deal with minor anxiety states. As long as the surgeon accepts the responsibility for the care of the whole patient, such services are superfluous.

This is particularly true in the care of patients with malignant disease or those who must undergo mutilating operations such as amputation of an extremity, ileostomy, or colostomy. In these situations, the patient can be supported far more effectively by the surgeon and the surgical team than by a consulting psychiatrist.

Surgeons are increasingly aware of the importance of psychosocial factors in surgical convalescence. Recovery from a major operation is greatly enhanced if the patient is not worn down with worry about emotional, social, and economic problems that have nothing to do with the illness itself. Incorporation of these factors into the record contributes to better total care of the surgical patient.

▼ THE PHYSICAL EXAMINATION

The complete examination of the surgical patient includes the physical examination, certain special procedures such as gastroscopy and esophagoscopy, laboratory tests, x-ray examination, and follow-up examination. In some cases, all of these may be necessary; in others, special examinations and laboratory tests can be kept to a minimum. It is just as poor practice to insist on unnecessary thoroughness as it is to overlook procedures that may contribute to the diagnosis. Painful, inconvenient, and costly procedures should not be ordered unless there is a reasonable chance that the information gained will be useful in making clinical decisions.

THE ELECTIVE PHYSICAL EXAMINATION

The elective physical examination should be done in an orderly and detailed fashion. One should acquire the habit of performing a complete examination in exactly the same sequence, so that no step is omitted. When the routine must be modified, as in an emergency, the examiner recalls without conscious effort what must be done to complete the examination later. The regular performance of complete examinations has the added advantage of familiarizing the beginner with what is normal so that what is abnormal can be more readily recognized.

All patients are sensitive and somewhat embarrassed at being examined. It is both courteous and clinically useful to put the patient at ease. The examining room and table should be comfortable, and drapes should be used if the patient is required to strip for the examination. Most patients will relax if they are allowed to talk a bit during the examination, which is another reason for taking the past history while the examination is being done.

A useful rule is to first observe the patient's general physique and habitus and then to carefully inspect the hands. Many systemic diseases show themselves in the hands (cirrhosis of the liver, hyperthyroidism, Raynaud disease, pulmonary insufficiency, heart disease, and nutritional disorders).

Details of the examination cannot be included here. The beginner is urged to consult special texts.

Inspection, palpation, and auscultation are the time-honored essential steps in appraising both the normal and the abnormal. Comparison of the two sides of the body often suggests a specific abnormality. The slight droop of one eyelid characteristic of Horner syndrome can only be recognized by comparison with the opposite side. Inspection of the female breasts, particularly as the patient raises and lowers her arms, will often reveal slight dimpling indicative of an infiltrating carcinoma barely detectable on palpation.

Successful palpation requires skill and gentleness. Spasm, tension, and anxiety caused by painful examination procedures may make an adequate examination almost impossible, particularly in children.

Another important feature of palpation is the laying on of hands that has been called part of the ministry of medicine. A disappointed and critical patient often will say of a doctor, "He hardly touched me." Careful, precise, and gentle palpation not only gives the physician the information being sought but also inspires confidence and trust.

When examining for areas of tenderness, it may be necessary to use only one finger in order to precisely localize the extent of the tenderness. This is of particular importance in examination of the acute abdomen.

Auscultation, once thought to be the exclusive province of the physician, is now more important in surgery than it is in medicine. Radiologic examinations, including cardiac catheterization, have relegated auscultation of the heart and lungs to the status of preliminary scanning procedures in medicine. In surgery, however, auscultation of the abdomen and peripheral vessels has become absolutely essential. The nature of ileus and the presence of a variety of vascular lesions are revealed by auscultation. Bizarre abdominal pain in a young woman can easily be ascribed to hysteria or anxiety on the basis of a negative physical examination and x-rays of the gastrointestinal tract. Auscultation of the epigastrium, however, may reveal a murmur due to obstruction of the celiac artery.

▶ Examination of the Body Orifices

Complete examination of the ears, mouth, rectum, and pelvis is accepted as part of a complete examination. Palpation of the mouth and tongue is as essential as inspection. Every surgeon should acquire familiarity with the use of the ophthalmoscope and sigmoidoscope and should use them regularly in doing complete physical examinations.

THE EMERGENCY PHYSICAL EXAMINATION

In an emergency, the routine of the physical examination must be altered to fit the circumstances. The history may be limited to a single sentence, or there may be no history if the patient is unconscious and there are no other informants. Although the details of an accident or injury may be very useful in the total appraisal of the patient, they must be left for later consideration. The primary considerations are the following: Is the patient breathing? Is the airway open? Is there a palpable pulse? Is the heart beating? Is massive bleeding occurring?

If the patient is not breathing, airway obstruction must be ruled out by thrusting the fingers into the mouth and pulling the tongue forward. If the patient is unconscious, the respiratory tract should be intubated and mouth-to-mouth respiration started. If there is no pulse or heartbeat, start cardiac resuscitation.

Serious external loss of blood from an extremity can be controlled by elevation and pressure. Tourniquets are rarely required.

Every victim of major blunt trauma should be suspected of having a vertebral injury capable of causing damage to the spinal cord unless rough handling is avoided.

Some injuries are so life threatening that action must be taken before even a limited physical examination is done. Penetrating wounds of the heart, large open sucking wounds of the chest, massive crush injuries with flail chest, and massive external bleeding all require emergency treatment before any further examination can be done.

In most emergencies, however, after it has been established that the airway is open, the heart is beating, and there is no massive external hemorrhage—and after antishock measures have been instituted, if necessary—a rapid survey examination must be done. Failure to perform such an examination can lead to serious mistakes in the care of the patient. It takes no more than 2 or 3 minutes to carefully examine the head, thorax, abdomen, extremities, genitalia (particularly in females), and back. If cervical cord damage has been ruled out, it is essential to turn the injured patient and carefully inspect the back, buttocks, and perineum.

Tension pneumothorax and cardiac tamponade may easily be overlooked if there are multiple injuries.

Upon completion of the survey examination, control of pain, splinting of fractured limbs, suturing of lacerations, and other types of emergency treatment can be started.

▼ LABORATORY & OTHER EXAMINATIONS

▶ Laboratory Examination

Laboratory examinations in surgical patients have the following objectives:

1. Screening for asymptomatic disease that may affect the surgical result (eg, unsuspected anemia or diabetes)

2. Appraisal of diseases that may contraindicate elective surgery or require treatment before surgery (eg, diabetes, heart failure)

3. Diagnosis of disorders that require surgery (eg, hyperparathyroidism, pheochromocytoma)

4. Evaluation of the nature and extent of metabolic or septic complications

Patients undergoing major surgery, even though they seem to be in excellent health except for their surgical disease, should have age-appropriate laboratory examination. A history of renal, hepatic, or heart disease requires detailed studies. Medical consultation may be helpful in the total preoperative appraisal of the surgical patient. It is essential, however, that the surgeon not become totally dependent upon a medical consultant for the preoperative evaluation and management of the patient. The total management must be the surgeon's responsibility and is not to be delegated. Moreover, the surgeon is the only one with the experience and background to interpret the meaning of laboratory tests in the light of other features of the case—particularly the history and physical findings.

▶ Imaging Studies

Modern patient care calls for a variety of critical radiologic examinations. The closest cooperation between the radiologist and the surgeon is essential if serious mistakes are to be avoided. This means that the surgeon must not refer the patient to the radiologist, requesting a particular examination, without providing an adequate account of the history and physical findings. Particularly in emergency situations, review of the films and consultation are needed.

When the radiologic diagnosis is not definitive, the examinations must be repeated in the light of the history and physical examination. Despite the great accuracy of x-ray diagnosis, a negative gastrointestinal study still does not exclude either ulcer or a neoplasm; particularly in the right colon, small lesions are easily overlooked. At times, the history and physical findings are so clearly diagnostic that operation is justifiable despite negative imaging studies.

▶ Special Examinations

Special examinations such as cystoscopy, gastroscopy, esophagoscopy, colonoscopy, angiography, and bronchoscopy are often required in the diagnostic appraisal of surgical disorders. The surgeon must be familiar with the indications and limitations of these procedures and be prepared to consult with colleagues in medicine and the surgical specialties as required.

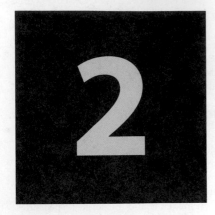

Training, Communication, Professionalism, & Systems-Based Practice

Gerard M. Doherty, MD

TRAINING

The process of medical education and surgical training in the United States is overseen by an interconnected group of organizations. Each of these organizations has their specific focus; however, the common theme is continuous process improvement encouraged by intermittent external review (Table 2–1). The ultimate goal is the provision of a consistent, qualified, and professional workforce for medical care in the United States.

Medical Student Education

The Liaison Committee on Medical Education (LCME) is the group that provides accreditation for medical schools in the United States and Canada. *Accreditation* is the process of quality assurance in postsecondary education that assesses whether an institution meets established standards. Accreditation by the LCME is effectively necessary for schools to function in the United States. Without accreditation, the schools cannot receive federal grants for medical education or participate in federal loan programs. Graduation from an LCME-accredited school enables students to sit for medical licensing examinations (the USMLE) and to achieve licensure in most states around the country. Graduation from an LCME-accredited medical school is also necessary for acceptance into an ACGME-accredited residency program (see below) for graduates of US medical schools. The authority for the LCME to provide this accreditation is delegated by the United States Department of Education in the United States and the Committee on Accreditation of Canadian Medical Schools (CACMS) in Canada.

Each accredited medical school is reviewed annually for appropriateness of their function, structure, and performance. Formal site visits are conducted periodically with more in-depth review and reaccreditation at that time.

The usual period of full accreditation is 8 years. At the time of this in-depth accreditation visit, and in the intervals between, the LCME works to disseminate best practices and approve the overall quality of education leading to the MD degree.

Graduate Medical Education

The Accreditation Council for Graduate Medical Education (ACGME) is responsible for the accreditation of post MD medical training programs within the United States. Accreditation is accomplished through a peer review process based on established standards and guidelines. The member organizations of the ACGME as an accrediting group are the American Board of Medical Specialties (ABMS), the American Hospital Association (AHA), the American Medical Association (AMA), the Association of American Medical Colleges (AAMC), and the Council of Medical Specialty Societies. The ACGME oversees a variety of graduate medical education programs in specific specialties. These ACGME-accredited residency programs must adhere to the ACGME common program requirements that apply to all residencies, as well as specific program requirements that apply to each training program. The ACGME also accredits institutions to house the residency training programs. There are thus also institutional requirements that must be met for overall accreditation of the institution to house training programs.

The ACGME has identified six general competency areas that must be addressed during every graduate residency training program (Table 2–2). The specific application of these competency areas varies widely among training programs. However, each rotation of each residency must include attention to, and assessment of, progress in fulfilling the general competency requirements.

The review and accreditation of specialty residency programs is undertaken by a committee specific for that field. In surgery, the group is the Residency Review Committee

Table 2–1. US organizations with medical education oversight.

Organization	Acronym and Website	Purpose
Liaison Committee on Medical Education	LCME www.LCME.org	Accreditation of medical schools in the United States and Canada
Accreditation Council for Graduate Medical Education	ACGME www.ACGME.org	Accreditation of post-MD training programs in some specialties
American Board of Surgery	ABS www.absurgery.org	Certifies and recertifies individual surgeons who have met standards of education, training, and knowledge
American College of Surgeons	ACS www.facs.org	Scientific and educational association of surgeons to improve the quality of care for the surgical patient

for Surgery (RRC-S). The RRC-S assesses program compliance with accreditation standards both at the common program requirement level, and at the program specific level. Programs are typically fully accredited on a five year cycle, with annual updates and questionnaires in the interim. Early site visits can be triggered by a variety of events including significant changes in the program or its leadership. The Residency Review Committees also control the number of positions that each program is accredited to have. This effectively sets the maximum number of graduates that can finish from a given training program in any given year.

▶ American Board of Surgery

The American Board of Surgery (ABS) is an independent, non-profit organization with the purpose of certifying individual surgeons who have met defined standards of education, training, and knowledge. The distinction between the ACGME and the ABS is that the ACGME accredits training programs, while the ABS certifies individuals. This distinction is similar for specialty boards in other disciplines as well. The ABS also recertifies practicing surgeons, and is making a fundamental philosophical change from periodic retesting for recertification to a more continuous maintenance of certification (MOC) plan.

The ACGME and the specialty boards interact. The success of individuals in achieving board certification is

considered an important measure of graduate medical education program success, and the measures that can be required of an individual for board certification must somehow also reflect the education that is offered to them through their graduate medical education. Thus though these entities have different purposes, they must, optimally, mesh their efforts constructively.

Board certification within a defined period after completing residency is necessary for privileging to perform surgery in many hospitals in the United States. Thus the most straightforward route into surgical practice in the United States includes graduation from an LCME-accredited medical school, completion of an ACGME-accredited residency training program, and satisfactory completion of the Qualifying Examination (written boards), and Certifying Examination (oral boards) of the American Board of Surgery.

There are other entry points into surgical practice in the United States, most prominently by physicians who have graduated from medical schools in countries outside the United States and Canada. These graduates can be certified by the Educational Commission for Foreign Medical Graduates (ECFMG). Once an individual graduate has been certified by the ECFMG, then he or she is eligible to train in an ACGME-approved residency training program, and can thus be eligible for board certification.

▶ American College of Surgeons

The American College of Surgeons (ACS) is a scientific and educational association of surgeons whose mission is to improve the quality of care for the surgical patient by setting high standards for surgical education and practice. The ACS has members, known as fellows, who are entitled to use the letters FACS after their name. Membership as a fellow implies that the surgeon has met standards of education, training, professional qualifications, surgical competence, and ethical conduct. However, despite these requirements, the ACS is a voluntary professional membership group,

Table 2–2. ACGME general competencies for graduate medical education.

General Competency
- Patient care
- Medical knowledge
- Interpersonal and communication skills
- Professionalism
- Practice-based learning
- Systems-based practice

and does not certify individuals for practice. The ACS does sponsor a wide variety of educational and professional support programs both for practicing surgeons and trainees. In addition, they have membership categories for surgeons in training (Resident Membership) and students (Medical Student Membership), and for those surgeons who have completed training but have not yet met all the requirements for fellowship (Associate Fellow). The ACS also engages in important advocacy roles on behalf of patients and the surgeon members.

COMMUNICATION

Efficient and effective communication skills are a critical resource for all clinicians including surgeons. A surgeon must be capable of establishing a rapport with the patient and family quickly and reliably. This mutual respect is critical to a therapeutic relationship. The patient and family must be confident of the competence of the surgeon in order to participate in the recommended management and recovery. Judgments about surgeon competence frequently come within the first few moments of interaction based on the surgeon's ability to communicate. In addition to communicating with patients, clinicians must communicate with referring and collaborating physicians, and also within their own health care teams.

▶ Communicating With Patients

Communication with patients requires attention to several aspects. First, the clinician must demonstrate respect for the patient as a person. Second, the clinician must display effective listening to the patient's message, followed by demonstrated empathy to their situation or concerns. Finally, the clinician must have clarity in the response. If any of these items are omitted, then the interaction will be less effective than it could be. Many surgeons try to jump straight to a very clear concise statement of the plan; however, unless the first three steps have occurred, the patient may not listen to the plan at all.

Respect

It is critically important to show respect for the patient and family as persons. The health care environment is often inconvenient and encountered during a time of stress. The patients are out of their normal venue and zone of comfort. They are often frightened by the prospect of what they may learn. Showing respect for their identity will place the patient at more ease and encourage their trusting communication with the clinician. Failing to show respect will have the contrary effect. Thus meeting an adult for the first time and addressing them by their first name can immediately put many patients on guard with respect to their personal independence and control. Similarly, referring to the mother

of a pediatric patient as "Mom" rather than using her name implies lack of attention to her as an individual worthy of learning her identity. On initial meetings, the clinician should use the patient's last name preceded by an honorific title (Mr. Smith, or Ms. Jones). If you are not certain if a woman prefers Mrs. or Ms, then ask her. In contemporary US society, a woman over 18 years of age is never referred to as Miss.

In addition, engaging in brief small talk regarding some aspect of a patient's life other than the medical matter at hand can additionally put them at ease ("It must be interesting to be a dog trainer. What is your favorite breed?"). These efforts will be rewarded by a more trusting patient and a more efficient interview, with a better therapeutic relationship over the long term.

Listening

Listening to the patient is critical to establishing a correct diagnosis and appropriate therapeutic plan for the individual. Every patient who comes to the medical system with a problem has a story that they have thought through and decided to tell. It is important to let them do so. Not only is the patient likely to reveal critical issues regarding the clinical matter, but they are also often determined to tell the story eventually, whether they are allowed to do so at the outset or not. Allowing, and in fact encouraging them, to tell the story at the beginning of the interview relieves them of this burden of information, and allows the clinician to move on to interpretation.

Listening should be an active, engaged activity. The clinician should appear comfortable, settled, and upon as much of an even eye level with the patient as possible. It is important not to appear rushed, inattentive, or bored by their account. Interjecting questions for clarity or intermittent, brief verbal encouragements will let the patient know that the clinician is engaged with the problem.

It may be helpful at the outset of the listening phase to let the patient know what materials have been reviewed; for example, telling the patient that the clinician has reviewed the referral letter from the primary physician, the results of the last two operations, and their recent laboratory work may help the patient to be more concise in their discussion.

Empathy

Once the patient has recounted their history and the other aspects of examination and data review have been completed, it is important to review this material with the patient in a way that demonstrates empathy with their situation. A surgeon's understanding of the problem is important for the patient, but the problem is not confined to the medical issue, the problem must be understood in the context of the patient. For this reason demonstration of empathy is important to the patient's trust of the physician. Establishing this connection with the patient is crucial to their engagement in the process of care.

Clarity

Having established respect for the patient, heard and understood their story, and empathized with their situation, the physician must speak clearly and in a vocabulary understood by the individual, about the recommendations for further evaluation or care. This portion of the conversation should include a clear distinction between what is known about the patient's diagnosis or condition and what is not known but might be anticipated. When appropriate, likelihoods of various outcomes should be estimated in a way that the patient can grasp. The recommended approach to next steps should be listed clearly, along with alternative approaches. Patients always have at least one alternative to the recommended choice, even if this is only to decide not to have further medical care. This portion of the conversation can be augmented with illustrations or models that may improve the patient's understanding. Often reviewing radiological studies directly with the patient or family at this time can help their understanding.

The risk taken by failing to establish this relationship with the patient is great. This can lead to errors in judgment about diagnosis or management. It also precludes the opportunity to engage the patient as an ally in his or her care. If things go badly, it also can make subsequent communication about problems or complications difficult or impossible. Finally, the surgeon who communicates poorly excludes him- or herself from enjoying a personally and professionally satisfying physician-patient relationship.

▶ Communication With Collaborating Physicians

Surgeons often work with other physicians in collaboration of care for patients. Communication in these settings is important to the overall patient outcome, particularly when the surgeon will be involved in the patient's care for some defined interval which has been preceded and will be followed by the ongoing care provided by the primary care physician. The communication in these settings can be separated into two basic types: routine and urgent. Routine communication can take place in a variety of ways depending on the health care setting. This communication is typically asynchronous and written. It may take the form of a note in the patient's electronic medical record, or a letter sent to the physician's office. This is an appropriate way to communicate reasonably expected information that does not need to be acted on urgently. For example, a patient who is referred to a surgeon for cholecystectomy and who has a plan made for cholecystectomy can have routine communication back to the referring physician.

Urgent communication should occur to the collaborating physicians when there are unexpected or adverse outcomes. Again, there are a variety of communication modes that may be utilized for this, but the communication is more often synchronous via a direct conversation either in person or by telephone. The communication is more than courtesy to the collaborating physician, as knowledge of these events allows them to participate constructively on behalf of the patient. Examples of situations that warrant more urgent communication include new diagnosis of significant cancers, life-altering complications from interventions, and certainly death of the patient.

Clarity in transfer of care responsibility is critical to the continuous optimal care of the patient. For that reason, any communication with the collaborating physicians should indicate either the ongoing role of the surgeon in the patient's care, or the deliberate transfer of responsibility for ongoing care issues back to other collaborating physicians.

▶ Communications Within Teams

Surgical care is often provided in a team setting. Current surgical teams typically include physicians, nonphysician mid-level providers (often physician assistants or nurse practitioners), and a variety of students. The student trainees may include students in medical school, physician assistant programs, or nursing school. These teams have become increasingly complex, and the information that they manipulate as a team to provide patient care is voluminous. In addition, the transfer of information from one provider to another as shifts or rotations change is recognized as a weak point in the patient care continuum.

With these complex teams and extensive information, the keys to efficient and effective team processes appear to be clarity of roles and designing processes that involve only writing things down once. The advent of electronic medical records has allowed the generation of electronic tools to transfer information from team member to team member. This may be useful to facilitate this process. Careful attention to transfers of care from one provider to another and explicit recognition that this is a potential time for errors is important.

PROFESSIONALISM

Professionalism denotes a series or group of behaviors that demonstrates that a person has achieved status as a professional. A *professional* in this context is implied to possess the specialized knowledge and have gone through long and intensive academic preparation for their vocation. These behaviors affect the interactions that professionals have both with patients and with other health care professionals. For optimal effectiveness, the surgeon should behave in a professional way both with patients and within their health

Table 2–3. AMA principles of medical ethics.

1. A physician shall be dedicated to providing competent medical care, with compassion and respect for human dignity and rights.
2. A physician shall uphold the standards of professionalism, be honest in all professional interactions, and strive to report physicians deficient in character or competence, or engaging in fraud or deception, to appropriate entities.
3. A physician shall respect the law and also recognize a responsibility to seek changes in those requirements which are contrary to the best interests of the patient.
4. A physician shall respect the rights of patients, colleagues, and other health professionals, and shall safeguard patient confidences and privacy within the constraints of the law.
5. A physician shall continue to study, apply, and advance scientific knowledge, maintain a commitment to medical education, make relevant information available to patients, colleagues, and the public, obtain consultation, and use the talents of other health professionals when indicated.
6. A physician shall, in the provision of appropriate patient care, except in emergencies, be free to choose whom to serve, with whom to associate, and the environment in which to provide medical care.
7. A physician shall recognize a responsibility to participate in activities contributing to the improvement of the community and the betterment of public health.
8. A physician shall, while caring for a patient, regard responsibility to the patient as paramount.
9. A physician shall support access to medical care for all people.

Available at http://www.ama-assn.org/ama/pub/category/2512.html

Table 2–4. Principles of medical ethics: "The Principles Approach."

Principle	Definition
Autonomy	Deliberated self-rule; the patient has the right to choose or refuse their treatments; requires physicians to consult and obtain patient agreement before doing things to them
Beneficence	A practitioner should act in the best interest of the patient, without regard to physician's self-interest
Nonmaleficence	Do no harm; the practitioner should avoid treatments that harm the patient
Justice	Rendering what is due to others; affects the distribution of medical care among patients and populations

care institutions. The American Medical Association has promulgated a set of medical ethical principles that apply equally well to surgical practice, and that can help to guide professional behavior (Table 2–3).

The ethics of surgical practice are complex, and can be approached from a variety of theoretical frameworks. The most commonly applied framework for the evaluation of ethical dilemmas for individual patient decisions in medicine, known as "The Principles Approach," involves four principles: Autonomy, Beneficence, Nonmaleficence, and Justice, as promulgated by Beauchamp and Childress (Table 2–4). A detailed analysis of these principles is beyond the scope here; however, the need for a code of medical ethics that is distinct from general societal ethics is the basis for medical professionalism. The following are five features of medical relationships that provide the moral imperatives underlying the profession and the requirement for a separate ethical code from other forms of business.

1. The inequality in medical knowledge, and attendant vulnerability, of the patient
2. The requirement for the patient to trust the physician, known as the fiduciary nature of the relationship
3. The moral nature of medical decisions that encompass both the technical aspects of health management and the ultimate effect on the patient's life
4. The nature of medical knowledge as a public property that physicians receive in order to apply to the practical improvement of patients' lives
5. The moral complicity of the physician in the outcome of the prescribed care, in that no formal medical care can take place without the physician's collusion

Because of these characteristics of the relationship between physicians and their patients, physicians must adhere to a set of ethical constraints specific to their profession.

While these imperatives are not generally understood explicitly by patients, patients can clearly grasp when these principles are in danger. They may even be suspicious that their physician or surgeon has competing motives to the patient's best interest. One of the goals of the physician-patient interaction is to allay these fears, and construct a trusting relationship based on the patient's needs, within the principles noted above.

▶ Interaction With Patients

The interactions with patients should be characterized by polite and possibly somewhat formal manners. These manners will aid the professional in their communication efforts as noted above. In order to meet the patient's expectations of what the physician or surgeon should be, proper socially acceptable manners should be observed. The purpose of these manners is to put the patient at ease that the physician is an empathetic person with the self-awareness to recognize the way that he or she appears to other people. The manners that the physician projects affect the credibility of the subsequent interactions. These conventions extend to the type of dress that is worn in a professional setting. The details of whether a physician wears a white coat or formal business clothing (suits, ties, pantsuits, blouses, skirts, etc) are best left to local custom and practice. However, the mode of dress in general should be neat, clean, and formal rather than casual, and not distracting to the interaction.

Another aspect to professionalism is the capability of the physician to do the right thing for the patient and the family even when that course is difficult or unpleasant. This includes such situations as frankly and openly disclosing errors made during care, or delivering bad news about new or unexpected diagnoses. While human nature can make these interactions difficult, the professional must rise to the task and perform it well. Avoiding the opportunity to do so not only obviates the professional's role as advisor on the issue at hand, but affects the physician's credibility in the remainder of that therapeutic relationship.

▶ Interactions With Health Care Personnel

Surgeons frequently work in complex, multilayered organizations. The behavior of the surgeon within this group should always remain productive and patient-centered. In any complex organization with multiple people and personalities, conflicts arise. In that context, it is not appropriate for the surgeon to necessarily shrink from the conflict, but rather the surgeon should take up the role of constructive evaluator and team builder to resolve the issue. At all times, the surgeon must avoid personal attacks on people based upon their personal characteristics but may legitimately criticize behavior. Professional comportment in these matters will be rewarded with progress in resolving the issue.

Reputation is a fragile and valuable commodity. All health care professionals have a reputation, and it works either for or against them in achieving their patient care and professional goals. Careful adherence to professional behavior in dress, speech, manners, and conflict resolution will create the professional reputation that is most advantageous for the surgeon. With a positive reputation, the surgeon's behavior in ambiguous situations will be interpreted in a benevolent way. The reputation of any clinician is as valuable as their education or certification.

▼ SYSTEMS-BASED PRACTICE

Systems-based practice is one of the core competencies defined by the ACGME as a necessary skill to be developed by graduate medical trainees. These residents must demonstrate an awareness of and responsiveness to the larger context and system of health care and the ability to effectively call on system resources to provide care that is of optimal value. The process of teaching and learning, systems-based practice has been in place for many years. This is what might be considered the practical part of graduate medical training.

However, it is only more recently that it has become a focus and metric for performance by training programs.

As a part of training then, residents must learn how different types of medical practice and health care delivery systems differ from one another, including methods that they use to control health care costs and allocate resources. They must use this knowledge to practice cost-effective health care and resource allocation that limits the compromise of quality of care. They must advocate for quality patient care and assist patients in dealing with complexities of the health care delivery system. They must also understand how to work with health care managers and other collaborating health care providers to assess, coordinate, and improve health care for patients.

In practice, this is easier to understand. The role of the resident in identifying both the health care needs of the patient and the capability of the system to meet those needs is well-established. Surgery residents in their senior years are often important resources for hospital systems by understanding how to manipulate the system to meet the needs of the patient. Medical students and surgical trainees must also recognize their role as a part of these complex systems.

▶ Reference

Rowland PA, Lang NP. *Communication & Professionalism Competencies: A Guide for Surgeons.* Woodbury CT: Cine-Med; 2007.

MULTIPLE CHOICE QUESTIONS

1. All of the following are true of the Principles of Medical Ethics, except

    A. Beneficence and nonmaleficence are synonyms
    B. Justice addresses the distribution of medical care among patients and populations
    C. Autonomy includes the concept that the patient has the right to choose or refuse their treatments.
    D. Beneficence asserts that a practitioner should act in the best interest of the patient, without regard to physician's self-interest
    E. Autonomy requires physicians to consult and obtain patient agreement before doing things to them

2. The LCME and the ACGME

    A. Both accredit institutions to provide education or training
    B. Provide diplomas and credentialing to individual practitioners
    C. Conduct periodic reviews to ensure that institutions maintain their programs
    D. Are units of the US Department of Commerce
    E. Both A and C are true

3. ACGME general competencies include all of the following except

   A. Interpersonal and communication skills
   B. Professionalism
   C. Technical skills
   D. Practice-based learning
   E. Systems-based practice

4. The American Board of Surgery and the American College of Surgeons

   A. Are both part of the American Medical Association
   B. Both report directly to the Surgery RRC of the ACGME
   C. Work together to accredit individuals to practice general surgery
   D. Are separate organizations that credential surgeons, and educate surgeons, respectively, as primary parts of their missions
   E. A and C

5. Effective communication with patients requires

   A. Demonstrated respect for the patient as a person
   B. Effective listening to the patient's message
   C. Clarity in the physician's response to the patient
   D. Family members who can reinforce the messages
   E. A, B, and C

Preoperative Preparation

David McAneny, MD

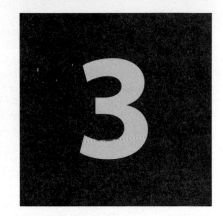

INTRODUCTION

The preoperative management of any patient is part of a continuum of care that extends from the surgeon's initial consultation through the patient's full recovery. While this ideally involves a multidisciplinary collaboration, surgeons lead the effort to assure that correct care is provided to all patients. This involves the establishment of a culture of quality care and patient safety with high, uniform standards. In addition, the surgeon is responsible for balancing the hazards of the natural history of the condition if left untreated versus the risks of an operation. A successful operation depends upon the surgeon's comprehension of the biology of the patient's disease and keen patient selection.

This chapter will consider preoperative preparation from the perspectives of the patient, the operating room facility and equipment, the operating room staff, and the surgeon.

PREPARATION OF THE PATIENT

▶ History & Physical Examination

The surgeon and team should obtain a proper history from each patient. The history of present illness includes details about the presenting condition, including establishing the acuity, urgency, or chronic nature of the problem. Inquiries will certainly focus on the specific disease and related organ system. Questions regarding pain can be guided by the acronym OPQRST, relating to Onset (sudden or gradual), Precipitant (eg, fatty foods, movement, etc), Quality (eg, sharp, dull, or cramps), Radiation (eg, to the back or shoulder), Stop (what offers relief?), and Temporal (eg, duration, frequency, crescendo-decrescendo, etc). The presence of fevers, sweats, or chills suggests the possibility of an acute infection, whereas significant weight loss may imply a chronic condition such as a tumor. The history of present illness is not necessarily confined to the patient interview. Family members or guardians provide useful information,

and outside records can be indispensable. Documents might include recent laboratory or imaging results that preclude the need for repetitive, costly testing. The surgeon should request CD-ROM disks of outside imaging, if appropriate. In the case of reoperative surgery, prior operative reports and pathology reports are essential (eg, when searching for a missing adenoma in recurrent primary hyperparathyroidism).

The past medical history should include prior operations, especially when germane to the current situation, medical conditions, prior venous thromboembolism (VTE) events such as deep vein thromboses (DVT) or pulmonary emboli (PE), bleeding diatheses, prolonged bleeding with prior operations or modest injuries (eg, epistaxis, gingival bleeding, or ecchymoses), and untoward events during surgery or anesthesia, including airway problems. One must secure a list of active medications, with dosages and schedule. Moreover, it is beneficial to inquire about corticosteroid usage within the past 6 months, even if not current, to avoid perioperative adrenal insufficiency. Medication allergies and adverse reactions should be elicited, although knowledge about environmental and food allergies is also valuable and should be recorded so that these exposures are avoided during the hospital stay. Some anesthesiologists are reluctant to use propofol in patients with egg allergies, and reactions to shellfish suggest the possibility of intolerance of intravenous iodinated contrast agents.

The social history classically involves inquiries into tobacco, alcohol, and illicit drug usage, but this moment also offers the opportunity to establish a personal relationship with patients (and their loved ones). It is fun and often stimulating to learn about patients' occupations, avocations, exercise, interests and accomplishments, fears and expectations, and family lives. Patients' regular activities offer insight into physiologic reserve; an elite athlete should tolerate nearly any major operation, whereas a frail, sedentary patient can be a poor candidate for even relatively minor operations.

A family history includes queries pertinent to the patient's presenting condition. For example, if a patient with a colorectal cancer has relatives with similar or other malignancies, genetic conditions such as familial adenomatous polyposis or hereditary nonpolyposis colorectal cancer could be indicted. This scenario would have screening implications for both the patient and family members. In addition, one should also elicit a family history of VTE complications, bleeding disorders, and anesthesia complications. For example, a sudden and unexpected death of a relatively young family member during an operation could suggest the possibility of a pheochromocytoma, particularly in the setting of a medullary cancer or related endocrine disorder. A strong family history of allergic reactions might imply hypersensitivity to medications.

A review of systems assesses the patient's cardiovascular, pulmonary, and neurologic status, including questions about exertional chest pain or dyspnea, palpitations, syncope, productive cough, or central nervous symptoms. It is also important to have a basic understanding of the patient's symptoms relative to other major organ systems. For example, while one might not necessarily expect an orthopedic surgeon to have an interest in a patient's gastrointestinal or genitourinary habits or problems, these issues may bear grave consequences if a patient experiences postoperative incontinence following joint replacement. Regardless of degree of specialization, surgeons and their designated teams are capable of identifying and investigating potentially confounding conditions.

A thorough physical examination is also an essential part of the patient assessment. Even if the surgeon already knows from imaging that there will be no pertinent physical findings, human touch and contact are fundamental to the development of a trusting physician-patient relationship. In addition to the traditional vital signs of pulse, blood pressure, respiratory rate, and temperature, for many operations it is also important to record the patient's baseline oxygen saturation on room air, weight, height, and body mass index (BMI). The physical examination includes an assessment of general fitness, exercise tolerance, cachexia, or obesity, as well as focusing on the patient's condition. Additional observations may detect findings such as cardiopulmonary abnormalities, bruits, absent peripheral pulses or bruits, adenopathy, skin integrity, incidental masses, hand dominance, neurologic deficits, or deformities. A thorough abdominal examination may include digital anorectal and pelvic examinations. The surgeon should also appreciate potential airway problems, particularly if general anesthesia is anticipated.

▶ Preoperative Testing

Laboratory and imaging investigations are tailored to the individual patient's presenting condition, as discussed in later chapters. However, there should be no "routine" battery of preoperative laboratory studies for all patients. In fact, published data do not support an association between routine studies and outcome. In addition, laboratory tests are costly and may result in harm due to false-positive and fortuitous findings. Instead, tests should be selected based upon the patient's age, comorbidities, cardiac risk factors, medications, and general health, as well as the complexity of the underlying condition and proposed operation. For example, children uncommonly require preoperative laboratory tests for most operations. On the other hand, a complete blood count, chemistries, and an electrocardiogram are proper for high-risk patients before complex operations. Algorithms and grid matrices are available to individualize the selection of preoperative tests (Table 3–1). Importantly, each system should establish a practice for managing abnormal test results, whether germane to the patient's active condition or a serendipitous finding.

A complete blood cell count and basic chemistries are reasonable for some operations, but their likelihood of predicting abnormal or meaningful results should be considered. Coagulation factors such as prothrombin time (PT), international normalized ratio (INR), and partial thromboplastin time (PTT) are not routinely indicated but should be pursued when patients report prolonged bleeding or the usage of anticoagulants. Moreover, INR and PTT may be warranted for operations that have little threshold for intraoperative or postoperative bleeding, such as those on the brain, spine, or neck. Bile duct obstruction, malnutrition, or an absent terminal ileum can affect vitamin K absorption, and a preoperative assessment of INR is important in those instances as well. A pregnancy test (eg, urine beta-human chorionic gonadotropin [beta-HCG]) should be performed shortly before surgery on women with childbearing potential. Other laboratory testing will be dictated by specific conditions, including liver chemistries, tumor markers, and hormone levels. A blood bank specimen should be selectively submitted in advance of operations that are associated with significant hemorrhage or in the setting of anemia with prospects for further blood loss. The preparation of blood for transfusion is costly, so blood-typing alone may suffice without actual cross-matching.

Routine preoperative testing of blood glucose is an intriguing concept, given the relationship between elevated blood sugars and surgical site infections (SSIs), although hemoglobin A_{1C} levels have not correlated with postoperative infections. Some reckon that nondiabetic patients comprise 30%-50% of cases with perioperative hyperglycemia, perhaps constituting an argument for measuring preoperative glucose levels in all candidates for major operations. While it is accepted that diabetic patients require close monitoring of perioperative glucose levels, including immediately before the operation, the value of doing this for all patients is evolving and warrants thoughtful investigation.

Table 3–1. Sample preoperative testing grid.

	CBC	Basic Chemistries	INR or PT	PTT	Liver Chemistries	Urinalysis	EKG	CXR	Urine Pregnancy Test
Cardiac disease (MI, CHF, pacemaker/AICD, coronary stents)	X						X		
Pulmonary disease (COPD, active asthma)	X						X	X	
End-stage renal disease on dialysis	X	X					X		
Renal insufficiency	X	X							
Liver disease	X	X	X		X				
Hypertension							X		
Diabetes		X					X		
Vascular disease	X						X		
Symptoms of urinary tract infection						X			
Chemotherapy	X	X							
Diuretics		X							
Anticoagulants			X	X					
Major operation (eg, cardiac, thoracic, vascular, or abdominal)	X	X					X	X	
Menstruating women									X

AICD, automated implantable cardioverter-defibrillator; CBC, complete blood count; CHF, congestive heart failure; COPD, chronic obstructive pulmonary disease; CXR, chest radiograph; EKG, electrocardiogram; INR, international normalized ratio; MI, myocardial infarction; PT, prothrombin time; PTT, partial thromboplastin time.
Adapted from Surgical Directions LLC © 2009-2010, with permission.

Some investigators have advocated routine nasal swab screening to identify carriers of *Staphylococcus aureus*. The results can guide decontamination measures such as intranasal application of antibiotic ointment (eg, mupirocin) and local hygiene with 2% chlorhexidine showers for 5 days before surgery. Patients with methicillin-resistant *S aureus* (MRSA) receive appropriate antibiotic prophylaxis and contact precautions. Although the issue of routine MRSA screening is not fully resolved, this practice may be ideal at least for immunocompromised patients and for those undergoing open cardiac operations and implantations of foreign bodies, particularly in orthopedics and neurosurgery. Prospective wound or abscess culture results should also influence decisions about perioperative antibiotics.

Electrocardiograms are not routinely performed but are justified for patients older than 50 years; those having vascular operations; and those with a history of hypertension, cardiac disease, significant respiratory disease, renal

dysfunction, and diabetes mellitus. Chest radiographs are no longer performed on a regular basis but are primarily reserved for patients with malignancies or perhaps with significant pulmonary disease. Further special tests are selectively obtained when clinically indicated and often with guidance from consultants; these tests may include echocardiography, cardiac stress testing, baseline arterial blood gases, and pulmonary function tests. Carotid ultrasonography may be valuable in patients with carotid bruits or histories of cerebrovascular accidents or transient ischemia attacks. Noninvasive venous studies may be considered in patients who have had prolonged immobility and/or hospital stays before surgery.

PREOPERATIVE PROCESS

At its simplest, the process of preparing a patient for an operation can involve a rapid assessment in the clinic or emergency room followed by an expeditious trip to the operating room. However, like most care in the contemporary health care system, the process is more commonly complex and involves a formal series of integrated steps to assure best outcomes. It is incumbent upon the surgery team to create an efficient and cost-effective preoperative system and scheduling protocol that result in optimally prepared patients, rare cancellations of operations, and few disruptions of the operating room schedule. A systemic approach to patient preparation focuses upon risk assessment and reduction, as well as education of the patient and family. This effort begins during the first encounter with the surgeon and continues through the moments before the operation. Ideal preoperative systems assign risk based upon evaluations that are derived from sound published evidence and best practices and driven by standardized algorithms to identify and then modify hazards before operations.

▶ Risk Assessment & Reduction

Overview

The essence of preparing a patient for an operation regards considering whether the benefits of the operation justify the risks of doing harm, along with deciding how to minimize or eliminate those hazards. The American Society of Anesthesiologists (ASA) classification system (Table 3–2) stratifies the degree of perioperative risk for patients. While somewhat rudimentary, this system has faithfully served anesthesiologists and surgeons in predicting how well patients might tolerate operations, and the scores have been validated by several recent publications. The Acute Physiology and Chronic Health Evaluation (APACHE II and III) is an example of a severity of illness scoring system that may be applied to intensive care unit patients to predict mortality. The value of such assessments lies in numerically designating the severities of patients' conditions, permitting comparisons of outcomes.

The University Health Systems Consortium (UHC) analyses derive from inpatient administrative and financial datasets to predict risk-adjusted outcomes for mortality, lengths of stay, and cost of care. The vagaries of medical coding can result in discrepancies, and the UHC system does not monitor patients after hospital discharge. Nevertheless, UHC data can identify deficiencies in practice. Although clinical databases are more costly and challenging to implement than commercially available products such as the UHC program, they provide more robust risk-adjusted outcomes data. Examples of clinical databases include those from the Society of Thoracic Surgeons (STS) and the National Surgical Quality Improvement Program (NSQIP). In NSQIP, dedicated nurses prospectively collect and validate an established panel of defined patient variables, comorbidities, and outcomes, and they pursue surveillance for 30 days after hospital discharge. The NSQIP analysis considers patient

Table 3–2. American Society of Anesthesiologists (ASA) classification system.

ASA Classification	Preoperative Health Status	Example
ASA 1	Normal healthy patient	No organic, physiologic, or psychiatric disturbance; excludes the very young and very old; healthy with good exercise tolerance
ASA 2	Patients with mild systemic disease	No functional limitations; has a well-controlled disease of one body system; controlled hypertension or diabetes without systemic effects, cigarette smoking without chronic obstructive pulmonary disease (COPD); mild obesity, pregnancy
ASA 3	Patients with severe systemic disease	Some functional limitation; has a controlled disease of more than one body system or one major system; no immediate danger of death; controlled congestive heart failure (CHF), stable angina, former heart attack, poorly controlled hypertension, morbid obesity, chronic renal failure; bronchospastic disease with intermittent symptoms
ASA 4	Patients with severe systemic disease that is a constant threat to life	Has at least one severe disease that is poorly controlled or at end stage; possible risk of death; unstable angina, symptomatic COPD, symptomatic CHF, hepatorenal failure
ASA 5	Moribund patients who are not expected to survive without the operation	Not expected to survive > 24 h without surgery; imminent risk of death; multiorgan failure, sepsis syndrome with hemodynamic instability, hypothermia, poorly controlled coagulopathy
ASA 6	A declared brain-dead patient whose organs are being removed for donor purposes	

factors, effectiveness of care, and random variation, and logistic regression models calculate risk-adjusted 30-day morbidity and mortality. These data are reported as odds ratios for comparison with expected outcomes, allowing for the severity of the patients' illnesses. Immediate benefits of NSQIP present the ability to identify true risk-adjusted data and local opportunities for improvement. For example, Veterans Administration (VA) surgeons reduced postoperative mortality from 3.2% in 2003 to 1.7% in 2005, while the complication rate declined from 17% to 10% ($p < 0.0001$). This effort focuses upon systems of care, providing reliable data to assess and reduce risks associated with operations. When compared to UHC, NSQIP is much more likely to identify complications because of its surveillance of patients 30 days beyond their hospitalizations.

The NSQIP program has also generated a tremendous repository of data to develop "risk calculators" for a variety of operations and conditions, allowing preoperative risk assessments and hopefully facilitating significant reductions of preoperative hazards. Finally, NSQIP participants have fostered a culture of sharing best practices and processes, both within the published literature and through formal and personal collaborations.

Beyond the obvious physical and emotional implications of adverse outcomes for patients and their families, the financial costs of postoperative complications to the health care system are staggering. It has been postulated that a major postoperative complication adds over $11,000 to the cost of the hospital care of an affected individual and significantly extends the duration of the inpatient confinement. In fact, the total cost of care increases by more than half when a complication develops. Notably, respiratory complications may increase the cost of care by more than $52,000 per patient. Strikingly, data from NSQIP have demonstrated that the occurrence of a serious complication (excluding superficial wound infections) after major operations is an independent risk factor for decreased long-term survival. Therefore, it is crucial that efforts focus upon reducing and eliminating postoperative complications.

Well-designed, systematic preoperative assessment programs can prospectively identify predictors of various complications and drive the ability to attenuate risks and improve outcomes. The perspective of teams of surgeons, physicians, nurses, and others with expertise managing standardized, algorithm-driven preoperative evaluations, often with checklists, is a departure from traditional care that primarily involved solitary surgeons with disparate practices. The new paradigm recognizes that variability in practice is the enemy of efficiency.

The financial dividends appreciated from enhanced results and diminished death and complication rates more than compensate for the expenditures associated with quality improvement efforts and participation in auditing programs such as NSQIP. It is essential that surgeons monitor

their patients' outcomes, preferably in a risk-adjusted fashion, to understand their practices and to demonstrate opportunities for improvement.

Cardiovascular

In 1977, Goldman published a multifactorial index for assessing cardiac hazards among patients undergoing noncardiac operations. The same group issued a Revised Cardiac Risk Index (RCRI) in 1999, reporting six independent predictors of cardiac complications. These include a history of ischemic heart disease, congestive heart failure, cerebrovascular disease, a high-risk operation, preoperative treatment with insulin, and a preoperative serum creatinine greater than 2.0 mg/dL. The likelihood of major cardiac complications increases incrementally with the number of factors present. Contemporary NSQIP data have led to the development of a risk calculator to predict postoperative cardiac complications. A multivariate logistic regression analysis demonstrated five prognostic factors for perioperative myocardial infarction (MI) or cardiac arrest: the type of operation, dependent functional status, abnormal creatinine, ASA class, and increasing age. The analysis has been validated and has led to the composition of an interactive risk calculator. Another multivariate model demonstrated criteria that predict adverse cardiac events among patients who have had elective vascular operations, and it also suggests improved predictive accuracy among these patients compared to the RCRI. Independent hazards include increasing age, smoking, insulin-dependent diabetes, coronary artery disease, congestive heart failure (CHF), abnormal cardiac stress test, long-term beta-blocker therapy, chronic obstructive pulmonary disease, and creatinine ≥1.8 mg/dL. Conversely, the analysis demonstrated a beneficial effect of prior cardiac revascularization. There is obviously overlap among the factors identified in these models.

The determination of an increased chance of a patient developing postoperative cardiac complications will certainly influence the tenor of preoperative discussions with patients and their family members, especially if the surgeon can present validated data regarding the actual likelihood of a cardiac complication or death. In addition, correctable hazards may be addressed, including smoking cessation, optimal control of diabetes, hypertension, and fluid status, and assurance of compliance with medical measures. Finally, formal risk assessments guide cardiologists with respect to cardiac stress testing, echocardiography, and coronary catheterization among higher-risk patients. Selected patients may be candidates for preoperative revascularization, either with coronary artery stent placement or surgical bypass.

The American College of Cardiology (ACC) Foundation and the American Heart Association (AHA) periodically issue joint recommendations about the cardiac evaluation and preparation of patients in advance of noncardiac operations. These guidelines are evidence based, include an explanation of the quality of the data, and provide comprehensive algorithms for the propriety of testing, medications, and revascularization to assure cardiac fitness for operations. As important as preoperative cardiac risk stratification is, a cardiology consultation also lays the groundwork for postoperative risk assessment and later modifications of coronary risk factors.

Noninvasive and invasive preoperative testing should be performed only when the results will influence patient care. Noninvasive stress testing before noncardiac operations is indicated in patients with active cardiac conditions (eg, unstable angina, recent MI, significant arrhythmias, or severe valvular disease), or in patients who require vascular operations and have clinical risk factors and poor functional capacity. Good data support coronary revascularization before noncardiac operations in patients who have significant left main coronary artery stenosis, stable angina with three-vessel coronary disease, stable angina with two-vessel disease and significant proximal left anterior descending coronary artery stenosis with either an ejection fraction < 50% or ischemia on noninvasive testing, high-risk unstable angina or non–ST-segment elevation MI, or acute ST-elevation MI. However, current data do not support routine preoperative percutaneous revascularization among patients with asymptomatic coronary ischemia or stable angina.

The role of beta-blockers for cardiac protection is evolving, and these agents are no longer empirically advised for all high-risk patients due to potential adverse consequences. Beta-blockers should be continued perioperatively among those patients who are already taking them and among those having vascular operations and at high cardiac risk, including known coronary heart disease or the presence of ischemia on preoperative testing. The role of beta-blockers is uncertain for patients with just a single clinical risk factor for coronary artery disease. Cardiac complication risk calculators may become beneficial in the stratification of patients who should receive beta-blockers to reduce perioperative cardiac complications.

Preoperative aspirin usage should continue among patients at moderate to high risk for coronary artery disease, unless the risk of resultant hemorrhage definitely outweighs the likelihood of an atherothrombotic event. Thienopyridines, such as ticlopidine or clopidogrel, are administered in concert with aspirin as dual antiplatelet therapy following placement of coronary artery stents. They are intended to inhibit platelet aggregation and resultant stent thrombosis, although they certainly increase the risk of hemorrhage. Therefore, if an operation can be anticipated, the surgeon and cardiologist must coordinate efforts regarding the sequence of the proposed operation and coronary stenting, weighing the hazards of operative bleeding while on antiplatelet therapy for a stent versus potential postoperative coronary ischemia. Elective operations with a significant risk of bleeding should be delayed 12 months before the discontinuation of the thienopyridine in the presence of a drug-eluting stent, at least 4-6 weeks for bare-metal stents, and 4 weeks after balloon angioplasty. Therefore, if a patient requires percutaneous coronary artery intervention prior to noncardiac surgery, bare-metal stents or balloon angioplasty should be employed rather than drug-eluting stents. Even when thienopyridines are withheld, aspirin should be continued, and the thienopyridine is to be resumed as soon as possible after the operation. In circumstances such as cardiovascular surgery, the dual antiplatelet agents are continued throughout the perioperative course to minimize the likelihood of vascular thrombosis.

Pulmonary

Postoperative pulmonary complications (PPC), such as the development of pneumonia and ventilator dependency, are debilitating and costly. They are associated with prolonged lengths of hospital stay, an increased likelihood of readmission, and increased 30-day mortality. Therefore, it is critical to identify patients at greatest risk for PPC. Established risk factors for PPC include advanced age, elevated ASA class, congestive heart failure, functional dependence, known chronic obstructive pulmonary disease, and perhaps malnutrition, alcohol abuse, and altered mental status. In addition, hazards are greater for certain operations (eg, aortic aneurysm repair, thoracic or abdominal, neurosurgery, head and neck, and vascular), prolonged or emergency operations, and those done under general anesthesia. A risk calculator was devised to predict the likelihood of PPC occurrence, indicating seven independent risk factors. These include low preoperative arterial oxygen saturation, recent acute respiratory infection, age, preoperative anemia, upper abdominal or thoracic operations, duration of operation over 2 hours, and emergency surgery.

A multivariable logistic regression has affirmed that active smoking is significantly associated with postoperative pneumonia, SSI, and death, when compared to nonsmokers or those who have quit smoking. Moreover, this is a dose-dependent phenomenon, predicated upon the volume and duration of tobacco consumption. The benefits of preoperative smoking cessation seem to be conferred after an interval of at least 4 weeks. Conversely, the risk of developing PPC is the same for current smokers versus those who quit smoking for less than 4 weeks before an operation. Smoking cessation also confers favorable effects on wound healing. Therefore, patients should be encouraged to stop smoking at least 1 month before operations, ideally with programmatic support through formal counseling programs and possibly smoking cessation aids such as varenicline or transdermal nicotine.

A recent analysis of patients having general surgery and orthopedic operations demonstrated that sleep apnea is an independent risk factor for the development of PPC. A simple "STOP BANG" questionnaire can screen patients for sleep apnea. The acronym queries Snoring, Tired during day, Obstructed breathing pattern during sleep, high blood Pressure, BMI, Age over 50 years, Neck circumference, and male Gender. Patients with sleep apnea may be managed with continuous positive pressure (CPAP) or bilevel positive airway pressure (BiPAP) devices, both before and after operations. The presence of sleep apnea may also influence anesthesia techniques.

Patients identified as being at highest risk for the development of PPC may benefit from preoperative consultations with respiratory therapy and pulmonary medicine experts. Pulmonary function tests and baseline arterial blood gas tests guide the care of select patients, especially those anticipating lung resections. In addition to smoking cessation, asthma should be medically controlled. Patient education focuses upon inspiratory muscle training (including the usage of incentive spirometry), the concepts of postoperative mobilization, deep inspiration, and coughing, along with oral hygiene (tooth brushing and mouth washes). Respiratory therapists can provide expertise with CPAP and BiPAP systems for patients with sleep apnea. Surgeons and anesthesiologists should collaborate regarding plans for neuromuscular blocking agents and strategies to reduce pain, including the administration of epidural analgesics and the consideration of minimally invasive techniques to avoid large abdominal or thoracic incisions. Finally, formal intensive care unit protocols can promote liberation from ventilator support.

Venous Thromboembolism

Venous thromboembolism (VTE) events such as DVT or PE are major complications that can lead to death or serious long-term morbidity, including chronic pulmonary hypertension and postthrombotic limb sequelae. Scoring systems stratify patients by their probability of developing a postoperative VTE to guide preventative measures. In the 2012 American College of Chest Physicians (ACCP) recommendations, the patient's score selects the alternatives of early ambulation alone (very low risk), mechanical prophylaxis with intermittent pneumatic compression (IPC) devices (low risk), options of low-molecular-weight heparin (LMWH) or low-dose unfractionated heparin or IPC (moderate risk), and IPC in addition to either LMWH or low-dose heparin (high risk). Furthermore, an extended course (4 weeks) of LMWH may be indicated among patients undergoing resections of abdominal or pelvic malignancies. Of course, the surgeon must entertain the hazards of pharmacologic prophylaxis when bleeding poses even greater harm than VTE, in which case IPC alone may suffice. Heparin prophylaxis is associated with a 4%-5% chance of wound hematomas, 2%-3% incidence of mucosal bleeding and the need to stop

the anticoagulation, and a 1%-2% risk of reoperation. The ACCP 2012 guidelines do not advocate routine vein surveillance with ultrasonography or the insertion of inferior vena cava filters for primary VTE prevention. Notably, antiembolism graduated compression stockings (GCS) do not promote venous blood flow from the leg and can violate skin integrity and result in the accumulation of edema. The efficacy of stocking for VTE prevention is unproven.

Caprini has developed a more elaborate risk calculation that has been validated in a variety of clinical settings and specialties, and is adaptable to standardized order sets (Figure 3–1). This scoring system acknowledges the gravity of individual hazards, including personal and family histories of VTE, the diagnosis of a malignancy, a history of obstetrical complications or known procoagulants, and prolonged operations, among several other factors. It also identifies patients who may either entirely avoid anticoagulation or benefit from an extended duration of LMWH. There is no doubt that the cumulative incidence of VTE extends many weeks after operations, particularly for malignancies and in an era when the duration of hospital stays (and inpatient prophylaxis) has declined. In fact, about one-third to half of patients who manifest a postoperative VTE after cancer surgery do so following hospital discharge. Therefore, regimens of pharmacologic prophylaxis should be maintained after the discharge of patients who have elevated risk scores. The ACCP and Caprini systems are two among several VTE risk assessment tools, each of which has advantages and disadvantages. The system adopted in any hospital or surgery center will be a function of local resources and culture, but it is ideal that surgeons develop and maintain a local standard to minimize the threat of postoperative VTE.

Diabetes Mellitus

Patients with diabetes mellitus are more likely to undergo operations than are those without diabetes, and their care is associated with longer lengths of hospital stay, increased rates of postoperative death and complications, and relatively greater utilization of health care resources. It has been established that elevated postoperative blood glucose levels in diabetic patients translate to progressively greater chances of SSIs following cardiac operations, as well as a greater likelihood of postoperative infections and prolonged hospital stays in patients with noncardiac operations. In fact, increased perioperative glucose levels have correlated with a higher risk of SSIs in general surgery, cardiac surgery, colorectal surgery, vascular surgery, breast surgery, hepatobiliary and pancreas surgery, orthopedic surgery, and trauma surgery. The relative risk of an SSI seems to incrementally increase in a linear pattern with the degree of hyperglycemia, with levels greater than 140 mg/dL being the sole predictor of SSI upon multivariate analysis. In one study, the likelihood of an adverse postoperative outcome increased by

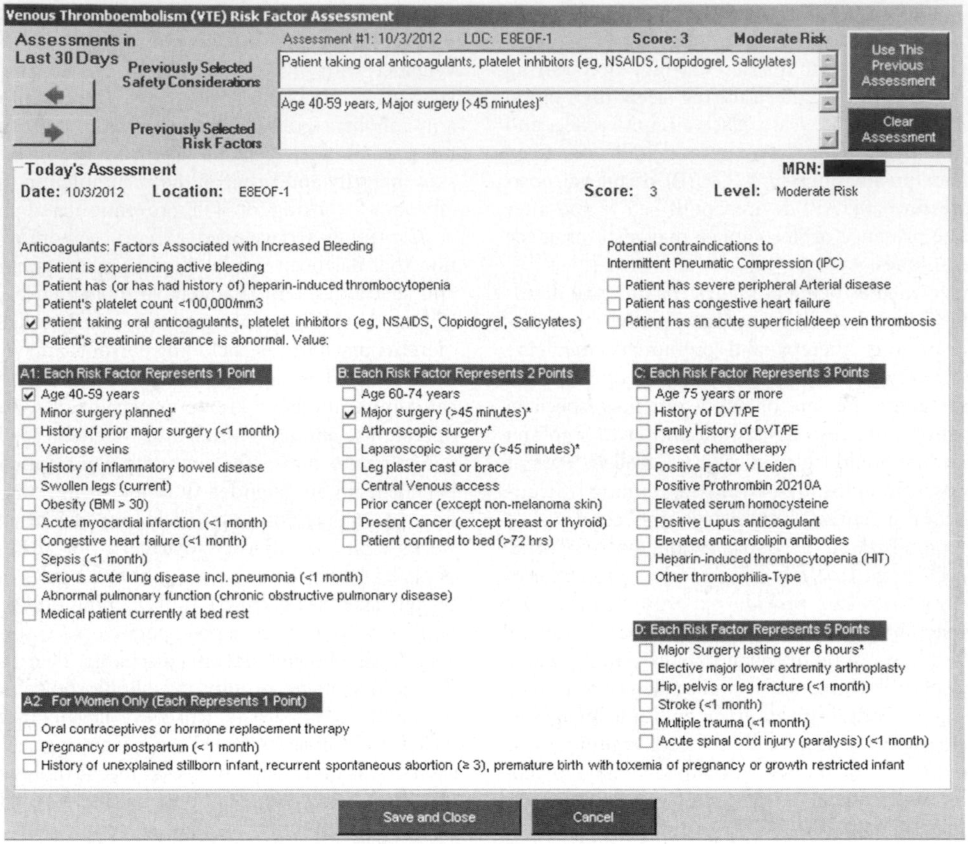

Venous Thromboembolism (VTE) Risk Factor Assessment

Assessments in Last 30 Days   Previously Selected Safety Considerations   Assessment #1: 10/3/2012   LOC: E8EOF-1   Score: 3   Moderate Risk   Use This Previous Assessment

Patient taking oral anticoagulants, platelet inhibitors (eg, NSAIDS, Clopidogrel, Salicylates)

Age 40-59 years, Major surgery (>45 minutes)"

Previously Selected Risk Factors   Clear Assessment

Today's Assessment   MRN:
Date: 10/3/2012   Location: E8EOF-1   Score: 3   Level: Moderate Risk

Anticoagulants: Factors Associated with Increased Bleeding
☐ Patient is experiencing active bleeding
☐ Patient has (or has had history of) heparin-induced thrombocytopenia
☐ Patient's platelet count <100,000/mm3
☑ Patient taking oral anticoagulants, platelet inhibitors (eg, NSAIDS, Clopidogrel, Salicylates)
☐ Patient's creatinine clearance is abnormal. Value:

Potential contraindications to Intermittent Pneumatic Compression (IPC)
☐ Patient has severe peripheral Arterial disease
☐ Patient has congestive heart failure
☐ Patient has an acute superficial/deep vein thrombosis

A1: Each Risk Factor Represents 1 Point
☑ Age 40-59 years
☐ Minor surgery planned*
☐ History of prior major surgery (<1 month)
☐ Varicose veins
☐ History of inflammatory bowel disease
☐ Swollen legs (current)
☐ Obesity (BMI > 30)
☐ Acute myocardial infarction (<1 month)
☐ Congestive heart failure (<1 month)
☐ Sepsis (<1 month)
☐ Serious acute lung disease incl. pneumonia (<1 month)
☐ Abnormal pulmonary function (chronic obstructive pulmonary disease)
☐ Medical patient currently at bed rest

B: Each Risk Factor Represents 2 Points
☐ Age 60-74 years
☑ Major surgery (>45 minutes)*
☐ Arthroscopic surgery*
☐ Laparoscopic surgery (>45 minutes)*
☐ Leg plaster cast or brace
☐ Central Venous access
☐ Prior cancer (except non-melanoma skin)
☐ Present Cancer (except breast or thyroid)
☐ Patient confined to bed (>72 hrs)

C: Each Risk Factor Represents 3 Points
☐ Age 75 years or more
☐ History of DVT/PE
☐ Family History of DVT/PE
☐ Present chemotherapy
☐ Positive Factor V Leiden
☐ Positive Prothrombin 20210A
☐ Elevated serum homocysteine
☐ Positive Lupus anticoagulant
☐ Elevated anticardiolipin antibodies
☐ Heparin-induced thrombocytopenia (HIT)
☐ Other thrombophilia-Type

D: Each Risk Factor Represents 5 Points
☐ Major Surgery lasting over 6 hours*
☐ Elective major lower extremity arthroplasty
☐ Hip, pelvis or leg fracture (<1 month)
☐ Stroke (<1 month)
☐ Multiple trauma (<1 month)
☐ Acute spinal cord injury (paralysis) (<1 month)

A2: For Women Only (Each Represents 1 Point)
☐ Oral contraceptives or hormone replacement therapy
☐ Pregnancy or postpartum (< 1 month)
☐ History of unexplained stillborn infant, recurrent spontaneous abortion (≥ 3), premature birth with toxemia of pregnancy or growth restricted infant

Save and Close   Cancel

▲ **Figure 3–1.** Sample order set page with "Caprini" calculation of venous thromboembolism risk. The total value of checked-off factors indicates the proper preoperative and postoperative prophylaxis regimens, including upon discharge from hospital. (© Boston Medical Center Corporation 2012.)

30% for every 20 mg/dL increase in the mean intraoperative glucose level. Interestingly, about one-third of patients with perioperative hyperglycemia are not diabetics. Furthermore, the risk of death relative to perioperative hyperglycemia among patients undergoing noncardiac operations has been shown to be greater for those without a history of diabetes than for those with known diabetes. Nevertheless, these data pertain to intraoperative and postoperative blood sugars, not preoperative values.

Current recommendations for desirable glucose ranges in critically ill patients are commonly about 120-180 mg/dL, but the best range for perioperative glucose levels is not yet established, and low levels may result in harm when clinicians try to achieve "tight" control of blood sugars. In fact, trials and meta-analyses have failed to prove a clinical benefit of maintaining glucose levels in the normal laboratory reference range (80-110 mg/dL). Although preoperative blood sugar and hemoglobin A_{1C} levels have not clearly

correlated with adverse outcomes, good control of glucose before operations likely facilitates blood sugar management during and after operations. An abundance of data support postoperative glucose control as a major determinant of postoperative complications, with emerging data also indicating an adverse effect of intraoperative hyperglycemia. Interestingly, surgeons may actually be more influential than are patients' primary care physicians in terms of encouraging preoperative compliance with diabetes medications, at least in the short term. Patients are commonly motivated to attend to medical conditions such as diabetes to enhance chances of postoperative success.

Patients having operations that require fasting status are advised about oral antihyperglycemic medications on the day of surgery in accordance to Table 3–3. Injectable medications such as exenatide and pramlintide are not administered on the day of surgery, and insulin therapy is determined by the duration of action of the particular

Table 3–3. Instructions for preoperative management of oral antihyperglycemic medications.

Medication	Prior to Procedure	After Procedure
Short-acting sulfo-nylureas: Glipizide (Glucotrol), gly-buride (DiaBeta, Glynase, Micronase)	Do not take the morn-ing of procedure	Resume when eating
Long-acting sulfonyl-ureas: ƒ Glimepiride (Amaryl), glipizide XL (Glucotrol XL)	Do not take the evening prior to or the morning of procedure	Resume when eating
Biguanides: ƒ Metformin (Glucophage), metformin ER (Glucophage XL)	Do not take the morn-ing of procedure; do not take the day prior to procedure if receiving contrast dye	Resume when eat-ing. After contrast dye wait 48 h and repeat creatinine prior to restarting
Thiazolidinediones: ƒ Pioglitazone (Actos), rosigli-tazone (Avandia)	Do not take the morn-ing of procedure	Resume when eating
Alpha-glucosidase inhibitors: Acarbose (Precose), miglitol (Glyset)	Do not take the morn-ing of procedure	Resume when eating
DPP-4 Inhibitors: ƒ Sitagliptin (Januvia)	Do not take the morn-ing of procedure	Resume when eating
Meglitinides: ƒ Nateglinide (Starlix), repa-glinide (Prandin)	Do not take the morn-ing of procedure	Resume when eating

© Boston Medical Center Corporation 2012.

Table 3–4. Instructions for preoperative management of injectable antihyperglycemic medications and insulin.

Medication	Prior to Procedure	After Procedure
Injectable Medications		
Exenatide (Byetta)	Do not take the morn-ing of procedure	Resume when eating
Symlin (Pramlintide)	Do not take the morn-ing of procedure	Resume when eating
Insulins		
Glargine (Lantus)	Take usual dose the night before or the morning of pro-cedure	Resume usual schedule after procedure
Detemir (Levemir)	Take usual dose the night before or the morning of pro-cedure	Resume usual schedule after procedure
NPH (Humulin N, Novolin N)	Take ½ of usual dose the morning of procedure	Resume usual schedule when eating, ½ dose while NPO
Humalog mix 70/30, 75/25, Humulin 70/30, 50/50 Novolin 70/30 (all mixed insulins)	Do not take the morn-ing of procedure	Resume usual schedule when eating
Regular insulin (Humulin R, Novolin R)	Do not take the morn-ing of procedure	Resume when eating
Lispro (Humalog), Aspart (Novolog), Glulisine (Apidra)	Do not take the morn-ing of procedure	Resume when eating
Subcutaneous insulin infusion pumps	Requires tailored recommendations. In general, most patients may continue their usual basal rate and correction doses, and resume meal-time boluses when eating again	

© Boston Medical Center Corporation 2012.

preparation, as outlined in Table 3–4. Patients with type 1 diabetes require basal insulin at all times. Patients with insulin pumps may continue their usual basal rates.

Multidisciplinary teams, including endocrinologists, surgeons, anesthesiologists, nurses, pharmacists, information technology experts, and others, have developed formal protocols and algorithms for perioperative glycemic control, and an example of a preoperative order set is illustrated in Table 3–5. A typical protocol is nurse-driven and involves checking glucose levels on all diabetic patients in the holding area shortly before an operation. As an example of one protocol, glucose values ≤180 mg/dL are satisfactory and require no treatment. Glucose levels of 181-300 mg/dL prompt the nurse to begin an infusion of intravenous (IV) insulin before

the operation, along with a 5% dextrose solution to minimize the chances of hypoglycemia. Endocrinologists are automatically consulted to assist with postoperative insulin management in these patients and in those with insulin pumps. In general, insulin pump therapy is continued along with the infusion of a dextrose solution. Patients with pumps may also require the addition of IV insulin, as per the protocol.

Patients with glucose levels > 300 mg/dL are assessed for ketones or for acidosis prior to starting an insulin infusion.

Table 3–5. Example of adult perioperative glycemic control protocol.

Adult 120-180 mg/dL
Perioperative Insulin
Infusion Guideline
*** Not to be used in patients with acute diabetic ketoacidosis or hyperglycemic hyperosmolar syndrome ***
Goal: The goal is to maintain whole blood glucose levels and/or fingersticks between 120 and 180 mg/dL.

Glucose Level	Below Desired Range			Desired Range		Above Desired Range			
	< 80 mg/dL	80-99 mg/dL	100-119[b] mg/dL	120-180 mg/dL [b]	181-220[b] mg/dL	221-250 mg/dL	251-300 mg/dL	301-350 mg/dL	> 350 mg/dL
Infusion rate of 1 U/h	Stop insulin infusion: give 25 mL of D50 IVP, maintain continuous dextrose source	Stop insulin infusion. Maintain continuous dextrose source		Once in range If glucose ↑over 2 consecutive checks, ↑Infusion by 0.5 U/h[a]	↑Infusion by 1 U/h	Give 2 units insulin IVP and ↑infusion by 1 U/h.	Give 3 units insulin IVP and ↑infusion by 1 U/h	Give 4 units insulin IVP and ↑infusion by 1 U/h	Give 5 units insulin IVP and ↑infusion by 1 U/h
Infusion rate of 2-5 U/h	Call MD			Once in range If glucose ↑over 2 consecutive checks, ↑Infusion by 0.5 U/h[a]	↑Infusion by 1 U/h	Give 2 units insulin IVP and ↑infusion by 1 U/h	Give 3 units insulin IVP and ↑infusion by 1 U/h	Give 6 units insulin IVP and ↑infusion by 1 U/h	Give 8 units insulin IVP and ↑infusion by 1 U/h
Infusion rate of 6-10 U/h	Glucose level in 15 min. If > 120 mg/dL, restart at ½ previous rate	glucose level in 15 min. If > 120 mg/dL, restart at ½ previous rate	Decrease infusion rate by 50%	Once in range If glucose ↑over 2 consecutive checks, ↑Infusion by 1 U/h[a]	↑Infusion by 1.5 U/h	Give 2 units insulin IVP and ↑infusion by 2 U/h	Give 3 units insulin IVP an ↑infusion by 2 U/h	Give 6 units insulin IVP and ↑infusion by 2 U/h	Give 8 units insulin IVP and ↑infusion by 2 U/h
Infusion rate of 11-16 U/h	Resume fingersticks every hour until stable. Restart drip as above any time glucose is > 120	Resume fingersticks every hour until stable. Restart drip as above any time glucose is > 120		Once in range If glucose ↑over 2 consecutive checks, ↑Infusion by 2 U/h[a]	↑Infusion by 2 U/h	Give 2 units insulin IVP and ↑infusion by 3 U/h	Give 3 units insulin IVP and ↑infusion by 3 U/h	Give 6 units insulin IVP and ↑infusion by 3 U/h	Give 8 units insulin IVP and ↑infusion by 3 U/h
Infusion rate of > 16 U/h					Call MD				

Monitoring: Check glucose every hour.

[a]"Once in range" example:

Glucose	190	140 (in range now)	130 (drop 1)	120 (drop 2)	130
U	4	4	4	↑3.5	3.5

[b]If the glucose drops by > 100 mg/dL/h, consider decreasing infusion rate or discontinuing infusion if BG is declining rapidly and < 150 mg/dL.

© Boston Medical Center Corporation 2012.

Markedly elevated preoperative blood sugars warrant special deliberation by all involved. Matters to be considered include the urgency of the operation, whether the underlying condition itself may be contributing to hyperglycemia, metabolic consequences such as the presence of ketoacidosis, the risks of proceeding with an operation at that moment, the likelihood of establishing better control at a later date, and the dangers imposed by postponing the operation. Dramatic elevations (eg, > 300 mg/dL) are typically indicative of chronic poor glucose control, but the clinician often does not have the luxury of perfectly managing diabetes before operations.

Intravenous insulin is best for perioperative glucose control due to its rapid onset of action, short half-life, and immediate availability (as opposed to subcutaneous absorption). Insulin may be administered with an IV bolus technique or via continuous IV infusion, but regular glucose monitoring (eg, hourly for continuous insulin infusions) is necessary in either system to assure adequate control and to avoid hypoglycemia. The insulin administration method before, during, and after an operation (infusion vs bolus) is a function of local resources (eg, glucose meters, blood sample processing, and staffing), as well as the patient's individual circumstances. After the operation, a patient should be assessed for an insulin infusion regimen if being transferred to a critical care setting, a basal-bolus insulin program, or the resumption of the patient's usual diabetes medications.

Surgical Site Infection

Surgical site infections (SSIs) are major contributors to postoperative morbidity and can be monitored and reduced by multiple complex interventions that are institution-specific. Excellent surgical technique is obviously a major factor in eliminating SSIs, and this involves limiting wound contamination, blood loss, the duration of the operation, and local tissue trauma and ischemia (eg, using sharp dissection rather than excessive electrocoagulation). However, a variety of adjuvant preoperative measures, beyond glycemic control described above, also contribute to the prevention of SSIs. Antibiotics should be administered within the 1-hour period before incision for certain clean operations and for all clean-contaminated, contaminated, and dirty operations. In addition, further dosages of the antibiotics should be infused about every two half-lives during the operation (eg, every 4 hours for cefazolin). Correct antibiotic selection is determined by several factors, such as the bacterial flora that are most likely to cause an infection, local bacterial sensitivities, medication allergies, the presence of MRSA, and the patient's overall health and ability to tolerate an infection. In clean operations with low rates of infections, the surgeon should contrast the cost and hazards of antibiotics with the likelihood, cost, and morbidity of a postoperative infection. Antibiotic choices for prophylaxis against SSIs are cited in

Table 3–6 for a variety of operations. Operations that involve bacteroides should prompt the addition of metronidazole to the regimen, and operations with a dirty wound classification may be guided by culture results and hospital-specific bacteria sensitivities. When antibiotics are administered for SSI prophylaxis rather than for treatment of an established or suspected infection, they are typically not continued after surgery, except in special circumstances such as vascular grafts, cardiac surgery, or joint replacements. Even then, prophylaxis should expire within one to two days. Order sets, automated reminders, and team vigilance are essential to assure the consistent usage of the correct antibiotics at the right time and for the proper duration.

Wound perfusion and oxygenation are also essential to minimize the likelihood of SSIs. A sufficient intravascular blood volume provides end-organ perfusion and oxygen delivery to the surgical site. The maintenance of perioperative normothermia also has salutary effects on wound oxygen tension levels and can consequently reduce the incidence of SSIs. Therefore, the application of warming blankets immediately prior to the operation may support the patient's temperature in the operating room, especially for high-risk operations such as bowel resections that often involved a prolonged interval of positioning and preparation when a broad surface area is exposed to room air. Similarly, some data support hyperoxygenation with FIO_2 ≥80% during the first 2 hours after a major colorectal operation.

Several other adjuvant measures are employed at the surgical site to reduce the incidence of SSIs. Protocols with mupirocin nasal ointment application and chlorhexidine soap showers have reduced the incidence of SSIs among patients colonized with methicillin-sensitive *S aureus*. During an operation, wound protectors may be deployed to minimize the chances of a superficial or deep SSI developing. Some surgeons (and their teams) change gloves and gowns, and may use a separate set of instruments (that have not come into contact with potential contaminants) for wound closure.

▶ Fluid & Blood Volume

Likely out of concerns about incurring renal insult, surgeons and anesthesiologists have traditionally advocated liberal perioperative fluid resuscitation during recent decades, often overestimating insensible and "third space" fluid losses. As a result, patients can develop significant volume overload that is associated with serious complications. Recent data instead support goal-directed (or protocol-based) fluid restriction as likely resulting in a decreased incidence of cardiac and renal events, pneumonia, pulmonary edema, ileus, wound infections, and anastomosis and wound healing problems, as well as shorter durations of hospital stay. Unfortunately, traditional vital signs, including even central venous pressure, do not reliably correlate with intravascular volume or

Table 3–6. Examples of prophylactic antibiotic selections for various operations.[a]

Operation	Standard Selection	Penicillin Allergy	MRSA Colonization
Clean			
Adrenalectomy	Cefazolin	Vancomycin	Vancomycin
Breast	Cefazolin	Vancomycin	Vancomycin
Cardiac surgery	Cefazolin/vancomycin	Vancomycin/gentamicin	Cefazolin/vancomycin
Distal pancreatectomy	Cefazolin	Vancomycin	Vancomycin
Hernia	Cefazolin	Gentamicin/clindamycin	Vancomycin/gentamicin
Neurosurgery	Cefazolin	Vancomycin	Vancomycin
Orthopedic Arthroscopy ORIF	Cefazolin	Vancomycin	Vancomycin
Plastic surgery	Cefazolin	Vancomycin	Vancomycin
Renal transplantation	Cefazolin	Vancomycin	Vancomycin
Soft tissue	Cefazolin	Vancomycin (foreign body) Clindamycin (no foreign body)	
Splenectomy	Cefazolin	Vancomycin	Vancomycin
Thoracotomy or laparotomy	Cefazolin	Vancomycin	Vancomycin
Thyroid/parathyroid	Cefazolin	Clindamycin	Cefazolin
Vascular (no foreign body)	Cefazolin	Vancomycin	Vancomycin
Vascular (with foreign body)	Cefazolin/vancomycin	Vancomycin/gentamicin	Cefazolin/vancomycin
Clean-contaminated			
Bariatric surgery	Cefazolin/metronidazole	Vancomycin/metronidazole	Vancomycin/metronidazole
Biliary (elective)	Cefazolin	Clindamycin/gentamicin	Cefazolin
Biliary (emergency)	Ceftriaxone	Gentamicin	
Colorectal surgery (elective)	Cefazolin/metronidazole	Clindamycin/gentamicin	Cefazolin/metronidazole
Esophageal resection	Cefazolin	Vancomycin	Vancomycin
Gastroduodenal resection	Cefazolin	Clindamycin/gentamicin	Cefazolin
Gynecology	Cefoxitin or cefazolin/metronidazole	Clindamycin/gentamicin	Cefoxitin or cefazolin/metronidazole
Head and neck (incision through the oral or pharyngeal mucosa)	Cefazolin or clindamycin	Clindamycin	Cefazolin or clindamycin
Lung resection	Cefazolin	Vancomycin	Vancomycin
Urology (no entry into urinary tract or intestine)	Cefazolin	Clindamycin	Cefazolin
Urology (entry into urinary tract or intestine)	Cefoxitin	Clindamycin/gentamicin	Cefoxitin
Whipple resection	Cefazolin/metronidazole	Clindamycin/gentamicin	Cefazolin/metronidazole
Contaminated or dirty			
Gastrointestinal (emergency)	Ceftriaxone/metronidazole	Clindamycin/gentamicin	

[a] These recommendations differ depending on local antibiotic resistance patterns.

cardiac output. Moreover, pulmonary artery catheterization has actually been associated with increased mortality, and its implementation for the optimization of hemodynamic status is rarely required. Pulmonary artery catheterization is valuable for few, highly selected patients who exhibit clinical cardiac instability along with multiple comorbid conditions. Newer, minimally invasive modalities for monitoring cardiac output offer promise to determine optimal preload volume and tissue oxygen delivery before and during operations, including esophageal Doppler and analyses of stroke volume variation and pulse pressure variation. The precise standards of goal-directed volume resuscitation remain elusive, but surgeons and anesthesiologists should prospectively collaborate regarding plans for both volume resuscitation and the selection of the type of anesthesia. This is especially so during the management of challenging problems such as pheochromocytomas, when patients require preoperative vasodilatation and then intravascular volume expansion. Another clinical dilemma involves patients with end-stage renal failure. Dialysis should be performed within about 24-36 hours before an operation to avoid electrolyte disturbances, but the surgeon should confer with the nephrologist to minimize intravascular blood volume depletion.

Blood transfusions may be necessary before operations, especially in the setting of active hemorrhage or profound anemia. However, transfusions have been associated with increased operative mortality and morbidity, decreased long-term survival, greater lengths of hospital stay, and higher chances of tumor recurrence due to immunosuppressive effects imparted by transfused blood. The benefits of transfusions must be balanced against their hazards. Of course, bleeding diatheses require preoperative correction, including transfusions of blood products such as fresh frozen plasma, specific clotting factors, or platelets. Hematology consultations are invaluable when blood incompatibilities or unusual factor deficiencies are present.

▶ Nutrition

Preoperative nutritional status bears a major impact on outcome, especially with respect to wound healing and immune status. A multivariate analysis recognizes hypoalbuminemia (albumin < 3.0 mg/dL) as an independent risk factor for the development of SSIs, with a fivefold increased incidence versus patients with normal albumin levels, corroborating the results of previous studies. Among moderately to severely malnourished patients, efforts may be focused upon preoperative feedings, ideally via the gut, although at least 1 week of the regimen is necessary to confer benefit. Total parenteral nutrition is an option for select patients in whom the gut cannot be used, but it conveys potential hazards. Immune modulating nutrition (IMN), with agents such as L-arginine, L-glutamine, ω-3 fatty acids, and nucleotides, can enhance immune and inflammatory responses. A recent meta-analysis of randomized controlled trials suggests that perioperative IMN with open, elective gastrointestinal operations is associated with fewer postoperative complications and shorter lengths of hospital stay compared to results for patients with standard enteral nutrition. However, the value of preoperative IMN is not firmly established.

At the other end of the spectrum, investigators have demonstrated that severe obesity is associated with increased rates of postoperative mortality, wound complications, renal failure, and pulmonary insufficiency, as well as greater durations of operative time and hospital stays. The AHA has issued guidelines for the assessment and management of morbidly obese patients, including an obesity surgery mortality score for gastric bypass. Unfavorable prognostic elements include BMI ≥50 kg/m², male sex, hypertension, PE risks (eg, presence of a VTE event, prior inferior vena cava filter placement, history of right heart failure or pulmonary hypertension, findings of venous stasis disease), and age ≥45 years. Bariatric surgeons typically enforce a preoperative regimen of weight reduction before proceeding with surgery to enhance outcomes and to assure the patient's commitment to the process.

▶ Endocrine

Endocrine deficiencies pose special problems. Patients may have either primary adrenal insufficiency or chronic adrenal suppression from chronic corticosteroid usage. Inadequate amounts of perioperative steroids can result in an Addisonian crisis, with hemodynamic instability and even death. The need for perioperative "stress" steroid administration is a function of the duration of steroid therapy and the degree of the physiologic stress imposed by the operation. Supplemental corticosteroids should definitely be administered for established primary or secondary adrenal insufficiency, for a current regimen of more than the daily equivalent of 20 mg of prednisone, or for those with a history of chronic steroid usage and a Cushingoid appearance. Perioperative steroids should be considered if the current regimen is 5 to 20 mg of prednisone for 3 weeks or longer, for a history of more than a 3-week course of at least 20 mg of prednisone during the past year, for chronic usage of oral and rectal steroid therapy for inflammatory bowel disease, or for a significant history of chronic topical steroid usage (> 2 g daily) on large areas of affected skin. Increased amounts of corticosteroids are not necessary for patients who have received less than a 3-week course of steroids. Patients having operations of moderate (eg, lower extremity revascularization or total joint replacement) and major (eg, cardiothoracic, abdominal, central nervous system) stress should receive additional corticosteroids as outlined in Table 3–7. Minor or ambulatory operations, including those under local anesthesia, do not require supplemental steroids. Excessive amounts of steroids can have adverse

Table 3–7. Recommendations for perioperative corticosteroid management.

Type of Operation	Corticosteroid Administration
Minor/ambulatory operation[a] Example: inguinal hernia repair or operation under local anesthesia	Take usual morning steroid dose; no supplementary steroids are needed.
Moderate surgical stress[a] Example: lower extremity revascularization, total joint replacement	Day of surgery: Take usual morning steroid dose. Just before induction of anesthesia: Hydrocortisone 50 mg IV, then hydrocortisone 25 mg IV every 8 h × 6 doses (or until able to take oral steroids). When able to take oral steroids, change to daily oral prednisone equivalent of hydrocortisone, or preoperative steroid dose if that dose was higher. On the second postoperative day: Resume prior outpatient dose, assuming the patient is in stable condition.[a]
Major surgical stress[a] Example: major cardiac, brain, abdominal, or thoracic surgery Inflammatory bowel disease[b]	Day of surgery: Take usual morning steroid dose. Just before induction of anesthesia: Hydrocortisone 100 mg IV, then hydrocortisone 50 mg every 8 h × 6 doses (or until able to take oral steroids). On the second postoperative day: Reduce to hydrocortisone 25 mg q8h if still fasting, or oral prednisone 15 mg daily (or preoperative steroid dose if that was higher). Postoperative day 3 or 4: Resume preoperative steroid dose if the patient is in stable condition.[a]

[a]For patients who have a complicated postoperative course or a prolonged illness, consider endocrinology consultation for dosing recommendations. If the steroid-requiring disease *may directly impact* the postoperative course (eg, autoimmune thrombocytopenia [ITP] or hemolytic anemia), specific dosing programs and tapers should be advised prior to surgery and in consultation with the appropriate service (eg, hematology for ITP patients) during hospital stay.

[b]For patients with inflammatory bowel disease in whom all affected bowel was resected, taper to prednisone 10 mg daily (or IV equivalent) by discharge (or no later than postoperative day 7), followed by an outpatient taper over the next 1-3 months, depending on the duration of prior steroid usage and assuming that there are no concurrent indications for steroids (eg, COPD). © Boston Medical Center Corporation 2012.

consequences, including increased rates of SSIs, so hydrocortisone should not be indiscriminately prescribed. Of course, glucose levels should be closely monitored while patients receive steroids. Conversely, patients with advanced Cushing syndrome require expeditious medical and perhaps surgical treatment due to the potential for rapid deterioration, including fungal sepsis. Cushing syndrome and pheochromocytomas are separately addressed in Chapter 33.

Thyrotoxicosis must be corrected to avoid perioperative thyroid storm. Management includes antithyroid medications (eg, methimazole or propylthiouracil) and beta-blockers; saturated solution of potassium iodide controls hyperthyroidism and reduces the vascularity of the gland in patients with Graves disease. On the other hand, significant hypothyroidism can progress to perioperative hypothermia and hemodynamic collapse and thus requires preoperative hormone replacement. This is normally accomplished with daily oral levothyroxine, but greater doses of IV thyroid hormone may be necessary to acutely reverse a significant deficit. Large goiters can affect the airway and require collaboration between surgeon and anesthesiologist, possibly including a review of imaging to demonstrate the extent and location (eg, substernal) of the goiter. When possible, computed tomography contrast should be avoided in patients with significant goiters as the iodine load may provoke thyrotoxicosis.

▶ Geriatric Patients

As the elderly demographic expands, surgeons are confronted with increasingly frail patients who have multiple comorbidities. Simple, noninvasive, yet focused elements from the patient's history and physical examination serve as prognostic factors based upon the patient's well-being or frailty. Makary has reported graded scores (allowing for BMI, height, and gender) that are predicated upon degree of weight loss, diminished dominant grip strength, self-reported description of exhaustion levels, and weekly energy expenditure in the course of routine activities, along with walking speed. Preoperative frailty is predictive of an increased chance of postoperative complications, prolonged lengths of hospital stay, and discharge to a skilled or assisted-living facility after having previously lived at home. A recent multivariate analysis demonstrated that among more than 58,000 patients undergoing colon resection, independent predictors of major complications were an elevated frailty index, an open (vs laparoscopic) operation, and ASA Class 4 or 5, but interestingly not wound classification or emergency status. The care of the elderly requires thoughtful considerations of their diminished physiologic reserve and tolerance of the insult of an operation. Interventions may include preoperative and early postoperative physical therapy, prospective discharge planning, and the introduction of elder-specific order sets. Simple scoring systems can provide valuable information for the surgeon to present to the patient and family so that they can anticipate the nature of the postoperative care and recovery, including potential transfer to a rehabilitation facility and long-term debility.

▶ Illicit Drug & Alcohol Usage

The value of routine testing for the presence of illicit drugs, at least among patients with suggestive histories, is uncertain. The presence of drugs in blood or urine might result in a cancellation of an operation, particularly if it is not immediately required. Conversely, some clinicians are not concerned about proving recent drug usage as long as the patient does not exhibit current evidence of toxicity or a hypermetabolic state. The confirmation of illicit drug usage obviously heightens awareness about the possibility of postoperative withdrawal. In general, patients should be advised to refrain from taking illicit drugs for at least a couple of weeks before an operation. Similarly, a history of heavy alcohol consumption raises the possibility of a postoperative withdrawal syndrome, which can be associated with significant morbidity and even death. It is ideal if patients can cease drinking alcohol for at least one week before an operation. Regardless of whether the patient can suspend alcohol consumption, the surgeon must closely monitor for symptoms of withdrawal among these patients and consider the regular administration of a benzodiazepine during recovery to prevent or treat acute withdrawal.

▶ Cancer Therapy

Many patients undergo neoadjuvant therapy for malignancies involving the breast, esophagus, stomach pancreas rectum, soft tissues, and other sites. The surgeon is responsible for restaging the tumor before proceeding with a resection. In general, the interval between the completion of the external beam radiation and the operation is commensurate with the duration of the radiation therapy. Similarly, a reasonable amount of time should elapse after systemic therapy to permit restoration of bone marrow capacity and nutrition, to the extent possible. Angiogenesis inhibitors such as bevacizumab disrupt normal wound perfusion and healing. The duration of time between biological therapy and an operation is not firmly established. However, it is probably best to allow 4 to 6 weeks to elapse after treating with bevacizumab before proceeding with an operation, and the therapy should not be resumed until the wound is fully healed, perhaps 1 month later.

▶ Emergency Operations

Emergency operations generally permit little time for risk reduction, although fluid and blood resuscitation can be instituted and antibiotics administered. Emergency operations among patients who have undergone chemotherapy within the past month are associated with increased rates of major complications and death. In patients with profound neutropenia, operations should be deferred to the extent possible due to severely impaired wound healing and the likelihood of irreversible postoperative sepsis.

INFORMED CONSENT

The informed consent process is far more that a signed document or "permission slip," Consent involves a conversation between the surgeon and patient (and perhaps family members or a legal guardian) that extends from the initial consultation through subsequent clinic visits or correspondence and into the preoperative holding area. The discussion addresses indications for the operation and its expected outcome, alternative treatments, the natural history of the underlying condition without intervention, the basic mechanics and details of the operation, potential risks, the impact of the operation on the patient's health and quality of life, the extent of hospitalization and recuperation (including possible rehabilitation care), the timing of resumption of normal activities, and residual effects. The informed consent process may also indicate that a resident will participate in the patient's care, under the supervision of the teaching surgeon and with the appropriate level of competence. Spouses and other family members should be included in the consent process for major operations that present chances of death or major debilitation.

In some circumstances, the patient may not be able to provide consent and no family members or guardians may be available. The surgeon should consider the acuity of the patient's condition and whether it requires an immediate operation. If emergency surgery is indicated, the surgeon should document the situation and advise a hospital administrator, if possible. Some unusual, nonacute scenarios may require seeking legal consent for an operation through the judicial process.

PREOPERATIVE INSTRUCTIONS

In some settings, all preoperative preparation is conducted through surgeons and their office staffs. Conversely, more robust systems may employ an elaborate process to prepare patients for operations. Regardless of the preoperative process, education constitutes a major component. In addition to learning about the actual operation, patients (and family members or caretakers) need to understand both preparation for and recovery from the operation.

Consistent information should be provided about how long a patient should fast and what medications are to be taken on the morning of the operation. The ASA has issued guidelines about preoperative fasting. To minimize retained gastric volume and maximize gastric pH, anesthesiologists advise adults and children to refrain from drinking clear liquids for at least 2 hours before general anesthesia, regional anesthesia, or sedation/analgesia (vs 4 hours for infants taking breast milk, or 6 hours for infant formula). Patients should avoid eating light meals for at least 6 hours and fatty meals for 8 hours before receiving anesthetics or sedatives.

In general, it is ideal for patients to continue to take their usual critical medications with a sip of water on the morning of an operation, including beta-blockers, calcium channel blockers, nitrates, and other hypertension control agents, alpha agonists or alpha antagonists, statins, hormones such as levothyroxine, psychotropic agents, oral contraceptives, and medications for cardiac rhythm problems, chronic obstructive pulmonary disease, gastroesophageal reflux, peptic diatheses, and neurologic disorders. Some surgeons and anesthesiologists advise patients to not take angiotensin-converting enzyme (ACE) inhibitors on the day of surgery due to the possibility of patients developing refractory hypotension during general anesthesia, although ACE inhibitors should be resumed shortly after the operation. Similarly, diuretics are commonly withheld on the morning of operations that involve potentially significant amounts of fluid losses and resuscitation. Of course, these recommendations are tempered by individual circumstances and clinical judgment; for example, patients probably should take their ACE inhibitors and diuretics before operations that do not require general anesthesia or involve much intravenous fluid, and when inadequately controlled hypertension could postpone the operation. Glucose and corticosteroid management have already been addressed.

Chronic narcotics (eg, methadone) are continued on the day of surgery to avoid possible withdrawal. Monoamine oxidase (MAO) inhibitors are associated with drug interactions with indirect sympathomimetics such as ephedrine (resulting in severe hypertension) or with phenylpiperidine opioids such as meperidine, tramadol, methadone, dextromethorphan, and propoxyphene (causing a serotonin syndrome with potential coma, seizures, or even death). Acute withdrawal of MAO inhibitors can provoke major depression, so they can be continued preoperatively, but without the concomitant usage of confounding medications.

The management of aspirin and thienopyridines for active coronary (or cerebrovascular) disease was reviewed earlier. Aspirin taken for other reasons, nonsteroidal anti-inflammatory agents, herbal preparations, and vitamin E can disrupt normal coagulation and should be stopped one week before an operation. Epoprostenol is a prostaglandin that is used to treat pulmonary hypertension; it also inhibits platelet aggregation and behaves like "liquid aspirin." The discontinuation of epoprostenol will provoke pulmonary hypertension, so it is best to continue the infusion, accepting possible oozing from surgical sites that can be controlled with standard measures. Estrogen receptor antagonists (eg, tamoxifen) can be associated with an increased risk of VTE. Therefore, the surgeon should consider stopping such medications 2-4 weeks before an operation and resuming them after a similar postoperative interval, especially in patients at a heightened risk of developing VTE.

Patients receiving anticoagulants require consideration of the indication for this therapy, the potential hazards of thrombosis developing while the anticoagulation is suspended, and the dangers of perioperative hemorrhage. Stopping warfarin 5 days before the operation will ordinarily allow normalization of INR, and the surgeon will determine if a "bridge" of a quickly reversible infusion of unfractionated heparin or LMWH injections is necessary to minimize the duration of time during which anticoagulation is withheld.

Patients should bring asthma inhalers to the hospital for usage shortly before being anesthetized. Similarly, eye drops, particularly those with beta-blockade properties, should be taken in accordance with their usual schedule.

Additional preoperative instructions include skin hygiene (eg, preoperative chlorhexidine showers, although their benefit is not absolutely proven), local care of preexisting wounds or ulcers, and discussions about tobacco, drug, or alcohol cessation, glucose management, and nutrition. Nurses may mark potential sites for bowel stomae. Some patients will require vaccinations when a splenectomy is possible.

Education also addresses what patients can expect during convalescence. This includes the importance of early postoperative mobilization and ambulation, pulmonary toilet, oral care, wound care, diet, physical therapy, rehabilitation, later adjuvant care, and even complementary or alternative options. Patients may be shown videos or provided brochures, which can be available in multiple languages. The team should definitely provide details about the logistics of the operation, including when and where the patient will report for preoperative visits and tests and for the operation itself. Finally, patients should know whom to contact with questions.

PREOPERATIVE HOLDING AREA

The time in the preoperative holding unit offers a final opportunity to educate the patient and family and to coordinate care before proceeding into the operating room. Patients (and their loved ones) are often anxious before operations and will be reassured by an organized, professional, and collegial environment. Members of the surgery team should introduce themselves and discuss the proposed operation and the anticipated postoperative care and recovery, including the possibilities of transfer to an intensive care unit or later to a rehabilitation facility. Traditional vital signs are recorded, ideally including baseline oxygen saturation. Special instructions address postoperative mobilization and pulmonary care for those patients undergoing general anesthesia or at high risk for PPC and might involve breathing exercises with incentive spirometry. This setting is definitely a good moment to formally mark the correct site and laterality of the operation, when pertinent, and to confirm fasting status, medications taken during the past 24 hours (especially beta-blockers), allergies, recent corticosteroid usage, and pregnancy status. Checklists (Figure 3–2) have become an important mechanism to assure the application of standard practices, and a section can be devoted to the preoperative unit. In addition, order sets greatly contribute to the delivery of consistent and correct care, including the administration of prophylactic antibiotics, adequate VTE prophylaxis (including the application of compression boots), and hydrocortisone for those patients with a recent history of significant corticosteroid usage. The infusion of antibiotics is not necessarily begun in the holding area, as it may still be more than 1 hour before the actual incision, but antibiotics can be secured for delivery to the operating room with the patient. Glycemic control protocols are begun in the holding area, as outlined earlier. For patients having bowel resections, the effectiveness of the mechanical prep may be investigated, and warming blankets can be applied. Finally, surgeons and anesthesiologists have the chance to discuss blood volume status and strategies for fluid administration, which may begin in the holding area.

OPERATING ROOM

Preparation of the patient continues in the operating room, up to the moment of the incision. When local hair removal is necessary for exposure, this should be done immediately before the operation, with electric clippers. Razors traumatize skin and have been associated with a greater chance of infection. Most surgical site skin preparations contain iodine-based compounds or chlorhexidine, but the addition of isopropyl alcohol to either of these agents seems to confer the best outcomes. Regardless of the agent selected, it is important that the skin prep be applied in a standard fashion—ideally by an assigned, trained individual to assure consistency—and that it dries prior to the application of the sterile drapes. Iodine-impregnated adherent drapes can also be used to cover the skin surrounding the surgical site. The role of mechanical bowel preparations and antibiotic prophylaxis (oral and/or parenteral) in colorectal operations is addressed in another chapter. The placement of urinary catheters in the operating room merits special comment. Urinary tract infections (UTI) are costly and can be reduced in frequency by sterile placement and prompt postoperative removal. The routine practice of two people (one for exposure and one for insertion) catheterizing obese women can decrease the incidence of UTI.

Proper positioning of the patient for an operation is critical to enhance exposure, to protect potential pressure points or muscle compartments, and to avoid traction injuries to nerves. Surgeons, nurses, and anesthesia staff share responsibility for patient safety during operations and should concur about how the patient is situated on the operating room table.

PREPARATION OF THE OPERATING ROOM FACILITY

Beyond the hazards for SSIs discussed earlier, wound sepsis is also related to the bacteriologic status of both the hospital setting in general and the operating room in particular. The entire hospital environment must be protected from undue contamination to avoid colonization and cross-infection of patients with virulent strains of microorganisms that could invade surgical sites despite the practice of asepsis, antisepsis, and sterile surgical technique. All staff should diligently wash their hands before and after contact with patients, regardless of location (ie, in the operating room or elsewhere in the facility). Patients with especially dangerous or resistant organisms (eg, *Clostridium difficile*, MRSA, and vancomycin-resistant *Enterococcus*) may warrant special precautions such as isolation and staff wearing gowns and gloves during direct contact with the patient and secretions. Notably, alcohol-based hand sanitizers are not effective against *C difficile*.

In the United States, it is standard for members of the operating room team to wear issued "scrub" clothes, caps, shoe covers, and masks, although this practice is less dogmatic in other countries. Surgeons and staff who perform the operation and handle sterile instruments wear sterile gowns, protective eye gear, and gloves. "Universal precautions" are practiced for the safety of the team, under the presumption that any patient's blood or fluids can convey communicable diseases such as human immunodeficiency virus (HIV) or hepatitis. Formal procedures and policies should be developed locally for injured staff or those exposed to blood or other potential hazards during operations.

▶ Sterilization

Items used during an operation are sterilized to destroy microorganisms on the surface of the instrument or in a fluid. Current sterilization methods include steam autoclave, hydrogen peroxide gas plasma, gamma irradiation, ethylene oxide gas, and dry heat. An autoclave system uses saturated steam under pressure. This is the most widely used method due to its ability to rapidly sterilize devices while being relatively inexpensive and nontoxic. The two most common types of steam autoclaves are gravity displacement, which must reach temperatures of 121°C, and prevacuum sterilizers, which must reach temperatures of 132°C. Minimum exposure periods for wrapped devices are 30 minutes for the former technique and 4 minutes for the latter system. Of course, the implementation of steam is limited by its corrosive effect on heat-sensitive items.

Before entering OR	Before inducing anesthesia	Final pause before incision	Before leaving OR	Postoperative destination
Patient check-in ☐ Patient states name and D.O.B. ☐ Patient confirms ID band/consent ☐ Patient states procedure, site, side ☐ Patient names his/her surgeon ☐ Patient asked when they last ate ☐ Determine need for interpreter ☐ Allergies reviewed/recorded ☐ Verify with or board ☐ Site marked if applicable and confirmed* ☐ H & P updated and in chart ☐ Consents up-to-date/signed ☐ Anesthesia preop/consent done ☐ ASA status verified/documented ☐ Antibiotic ordered if applicable ☐ VTE prophylaxis if applicable ☐ Precautions identified ☐ Preop RN/circulator briefing ☐ Implants, special equipment, blood and tissue available if applicable ☐ Determine potential need for unit bed ☐ Confirm B blocker usage and document if applicable ☐ Steroid protocol if applicable **Hand off** Preop RN: _____ Circulator: _____ Date: _____ Time: _____ (mm/dd/yyyy) *Attending surgeon's initials	**Upon entry** ☐ Stretcher/table locked for transfer ☐ Safety belt in place ☐ Team members introduced ☐ Patient identity confirmed ☐ Confirm record labeling ☐ Allergies verbalized ☐ Confirm procedure(s) being performed ☐ Patient positioning confirmed ☐ Emergency equipment available ☐ Special equipment available ☐ Imaging displayed and reviewed **Review prior to induction** ☐ Pulse oximeter on/functioning ☐ Risk of difficult airway/aspiration ☐ Surgeon reviews duration, irrigation fluids and risk of retained foreign body ☐ Blood available if applicable ☐ **All** drugs/solutions labeled ☐ Compression boots if applicable ☐ Antibiotics dose/redosing ☐ B-blocker/glucose control ☐ Temperature control measures ☐ Fluid management strategy **Perform or timeout** Patient, procedure, site, side, level, implants, structure, position and consents reviewed and verified Stop all activity Attending surgeon: _____ Attending anesthesiologist: _____ Circulator: _____ Time: _____	**All staff review critical events before incision** ☐ Attending surgeon reviews critical/additional steps and anticipated blood loss ☐ Anesthesia provider reviews patient specific concerns/issues ☐ Circulator reviews sterility and equipment issues ☐ Tissue and implants checked and verified ☐ Neutral zone established **Final pause** ☐ Stop all activity ☐ Attending surgeon present ☐ Prep dried ☐ Surgeon site marking visible and confirmed after prep and drape and prior to incision when applicable ☐ Remark site and redo timeout if initials not visible ☐ Incision time confirmed and recorded **For additional surgeons** **OR timeout** Patient, procedure, site, side, level, implants, structures, position and consents reviewed and verified Attending surgeon _____ Attending anesthesiologist _____ Circulator: _____ Time: _____ ☐ N/A	**Nurse verbally reviews with the team** **Final count pause** ☐ Instrument, sponge, needle counts performed per policy ☐ Specimens reconciled by RN ☐ Final diagnosis confirmed and recorded ☐ Name of procedures(s) ☐ Wound classification verified with surgeon **Attending surgeon** Date: _____ Time: _____ (mm/dd/yyyy) RN: _____ Date: _____ Time: _____ (mm/dd/yyyy) **Review critical events** ☐ Anesthesia provider, nurse and surgeon review the key concerns for recovery and management of the patient ☐ Discussion of post operative analgesia/block ☐ Procedure note by surgeon ☐ Determine if there were any equipment issues ☐ Steps to exit initiated ☐ Call postop destination with any precautions and equipment	**Upon arrival** ☐ O$_2$ saturation ☐ Team members introduced ☐ Vital signs and temperature ☐ Or nurse/surgeon review concerns for recovery ☐ Orders by surgeon **Anesthesia report** ☐ Allergies verbalized ☐ Patient history ☐ Last or vital signs ☐ Drugs administered ☐ Urine output/blood loss ☐ Fluids/blood products **Prior to final sign out** ☐ Procedure note in chart ☐ Anesthesia drug/discharge orders ☐ Need for consults/x-rays/labs ☐ Post anesthesia progress note ☐ Timing of antibiotics if applicable ☐ Final disposition RN: _____ Date: _____ Time: _____ (mm/dd/yyyy)

▲ **FIGURE 3–2.** Sample of Universal Checklist for perioperative care. © Boston Medical Center Corporation 2012.

Liquid hydrogen peroxide is a nontoxic sterilizing agent that initiates the inactivation of microorganisms on a heat-sensitive device within 75 minutes. Liquid hydrogen peroxide is vaporized and diffused through the sterilization chamber to contact the surfaces of the device. An electrical field is created within the chamber, changing the vapor to gas plasma. Microbicidal free radicals are generated in the plasma, rendering the device sterile.

Gamma sterilization utilizes Cobalt-60 radiation to inactivate microorganisms on single-use medical supplies, pharmaceuticals, and biological-based products, although the US Food and Drug Administration does not approve gamma irradiation in health care facilities. Liquid and gaseous ethylene oxide is a toxic, flammable sterilizing agent that initiates the inactivation of microorganisms on a heat-sensitive device within 1-6 hours, with 8-12 hours required for aeration. Ethylene oxide gas is diffused through the sterilization chamber at temperatures between 37°C and 63°C and a relative humidity of 40%-80%. The gas bonds with water molecules to reach the device surfaces and render the device sterile. Due to the extended aeration time requirement and high level of toxicity, ethylene oxide gas sterilization is being replaced with nontoxic processes that have shorter process times.

Dry heat sterilization utilizes heating coils to raise the temperature of the air inside the sterilization chamber to sterilize surfaces of devices. It is appropriate only for items that have a low moist heat tolerance but high temperature tolerance. The most common time-temperature relationships for dry heat sterilization are 170°C for 1 hour, 160°C for 2 hours, and 150°C for 2.5 hours.

Operating Room Plans

Surgeons should prospectively communicate with the operating room staff about what operation will be performed, including its anticipated duration and all necessary items, to enhance efficiency and avoid delays. "Case cards" contain information about standard equipment, devices, and sutures. Surgeons must also anticipate special needs such as unusual instruments or hardware, prosthetic materials for implantation, coagulation devices (eg, electrocautery, ultrasound or radiofrequency energy devices, lasers), intraoperative laboratory testing (eg, glucose, hematocrit, parathyroid hormone), imaging (eg, fluoroscopy, ultrasonography), nerve monitoring, and any other details specific to the operation. The primary surgeon is responsible for coordinating surgery teams when multiple consultants and allied professionals collaborate in a patient's care, including surgeons, anesthesiologists, nurses, technicians, and others. A checklist hopefully promotes communication about these matters to assure that it is safe to proceed with an operation.

Preparations also include the development of contingency plans for a variety of dangerous scenarios. These could include environmental problems in the operating room (eg, a fire, the loss of humidity control or power, or computer failure), or threatening clinical conditions (eg, massive hemorrhage, cardiac arrest, air embolus, malignant hyperthermia, etc). Plans can be composed as algorithms and documented on paper or online and even projected on monitors for the entire team to review.

Preparation of the Surgery Team

Attention is being increasingly focused upon the development of teams in the operating room. Much of this work has been modeled upon the concepts of crew resource management (CRM), as promulgated by the aviation profession. Psychologists analyzed behaviors of flight crews in the 1970s and proposed measures to improve safety, including reducing the hierarchy of that time, empowering junior team members to express concerns about potential problems, and training senior crew members to listen to the perspectives of other team members while accepting questions as honest communication rather than insubordination. This approach encourages the crew to participate in the enterprise and offer their expertise and talents, while the captain remains the ultimate authority.

As in the airline industry, the implementation of CRM in the operating room is supported by a series of activities before the main event. The ideal preoperative briefing establishes the team leader, facilitates communication, outlines the team's work, and specifies protocols, responsibilities, expectations, and contingency plans. This collaboration can result in improved outcomes, greater patient satisfaction, and better morale among team members. Checklists should not merely be perfunctory recitations of goals; they should promote a culture of teamwork. These checklists can be modified to suit local circumstances, resources, and cultures, and they codify critical steps, such as having necessary materials and medications on hand as well as indicating the appropriate location and side of the operation in instances when wrong-site mistakes could be made. Simulation training is also becoming more readily available, particularly regarding rare, complex, or high-risk scenarios, as well as the introduction of new members to teams.

Preparation of the Surgeon

The professional development of a surgeon is a privilege and an enduring pursuit involving emotional and intellectual growth, discipline, creativity, dedication, equanimity, technical talent, and formal education. College, postgraduate, and medical school curricula are certainly preludes to accredited surgery residencies and fellowships. That certain personalities are drawn to different surgical specialties is part of the joy and diversity of the profession.

Board certification confirms that a surgeon has completed the requisite years of residency and passed a rigorous examination to indicate competence. Learning continues well beyond formal training, as exemplified by specialty board certification and the recent Maintenance of Certification program, instituted by the American Board of Surgery and 23 other member boards of the American Board of Medical Specialties to assure lifelong professional development. The surgeon must be familiar with contemporary literature and adapt to emerging technologies and operative techniques, building upon established knowledge and skills. Moreover, the surgeon critically assesses data to decide the wisdom and value of new developments for the individual patient, the surgeon, and the prevailing health care system. Fellowship in the American College of Surgeons (or comparable organizations outside the United States and Canada) endorses that the surgeon has successfully completed a thorough evaluation of professional competence and ethical fitness. The qualifications include board certification, commitment to the welfare of patients above all else, and pledges regarding appropriate compensation and the avoidance of unjustified operations.

The surgeon must also be versed in and a leader of quality improvement within the process of caring for patients. Naturally, the proficiency provided by performing large numbers of certain high-risk operations results in improved outcomes. This is a matter of designing excellent systems that support surgical care, rather than the exclusive talents of a solitary surgeon. Ideal care involves a coordinated series of steps and collaborations—bundles of care—among teams of professionals so that the system and culture are sustained despite the loss of any individual, and the surgeon is the leader of that team. Crew Resource Management, as described earlier, has defined seven characteristics of leaders of high-performance teams:

1. **Command:** One person retains the ultimate authority and responsibility for the team and outcomes.

2. **Leadership:** The leader establishes a culture of open communication, accountability, and teamwork, serves as a mentor, manages conflict, and establishes high standards of excellence and professionalism. An effective leader inspires the team with strength and humanity.

3. **Communication:** A work environment thrives upon an effective and timely exchange of ideas among professionals to create the essential bond within the team. Members of the team should be empowered to raise concerns and to ask questions, particularly when doing so might prevent harm to a patient.

4. **Situational Awareness:** This involves a comprehension of the present circumstances through active communication with team members and knowledge of preceding events.

5. **Workload Management:** Tasks are delegated among team members commensurate with their skills and training so that everybody is doing the right job in synergy with others.

6. **Resource Management:** This trait prospectively identifies the local resources to result in optimal outcomes.

7. **Decision Making:** This process includes collecting data from the environment and soliciting opinions from team members to permit informed judgments.

Leadership traits are not necessarily intuitive, and they require introspection, training, and practice. The surgeon remains the proverbial captain of the ship regarding the care of patients having operations, but as a consultative leader among trusted colleagues.

▶ References

American Society of Anesthesiologists Committee. Practice guidelines for preoperative fasting and the use of pharmacologic agents to reduce the risk of pulmonary aspiration: application to healthy patients undergoing elective procedures. An updated report by the American Society of Anesthesiologists Committee on Standards and Practice Parameters. *Anesthesiology*. 2011;114:495-511.

Ata A, Lee J, Bestle SL, et al. Postoperative hyperglycemia and surgical site infection in general surgery patients. *Arch Surg*. 2010;145:858-864.

Bahl V, Hu HM, Henke PK, et al. A validation study of a retrospective venous thromboembolism risk scoring method. *Ann Surg*. 2010;251:344-350.

Bertges DJ, Goodney PP, Zhao Y, et al. The Vascular Study Group of New England Cardiac Risk Index (VSG-CRI) predicts cardiac complications more accurately than the Revised Cardiac Risk Index in vascular surgery patients. *J Vasc Surg*. 2010;52:674-683.

Bode LG, Kluytmans JA, Wertheim HF, et al. Preventing surgical-site infections in nasal carriers of *Staphylococcus aureus*. *N Engl J Med*. 2010;362:9-17.

Canet J, Gallart L, Gomar C, et al. Prediction of postoperative pulmonary complications in a population-based surgical cohort. *Anesthesiology*. 2010;113:1338-1350.

Corcoran T, Rhodes JEJ, Clarke S, et al. Perioperative fluid management strategies in major surgery: a stratified meta-analysis. *Anesth Analg*. 2012;114:640-651.

Darouiche RO, Wall MJ, Itani KMF, et al. Chlorhexidine-alcohol versus povidone-iodine for surgical-site antisepsis. *N Engl J Med*. 2010;362:18-26.

Frisch A, Chandra P, Smiley D, et al. Prevalence and clinical outcome of hyperglycemia in the perioperative period in noncardiac surgery. *Diabetes Care*. 2010;33:1783-1788.

Gould MK, Garcia DA, Wren SM, et al. Prevention of VTE in nonorthopedic surgical patients: antithrombotic therapy and prevention of thrombosis, 9th ed. American College of Chest Physicians evidence-based clinical practice guidelines. *Chest*. 2012; 141(suppl 2): e227S-e277S.

Gupta PK, Gupta H, Sundaram A, et al. Development and validation of a risk calculator for prediction of cardiac risk after surgery. *Circulation*. 2011;124:381-387.

Hawn MT, Houston TK, Campagna EJ, et al. The attributable risk of smoking on surgical complications. *Ann Surg.* 2011;254:914-920.

Hennessey DB, Burke JP, Ni-Dhonochu T, et al. Preoperative hypoalbuminemia is an independent risk factor for the development of surgical site infection following gastrointestinal surgery: a multi-institutional study. *Ann Surg.* 2010;252:325-320.

Makary MA, Segev DL, Pronovost PJ, et al. Frailty as a predictor of surgical outcomes in older patients. *J Am Coll Surg.* 2010;210:901-908.

Marimuthu K, Varadhan KK, Ljungqvist O, et al. A meta-analysis of the effect of combinations of immune modulating nutrients on outcome in patients undergoing major open gastrointestinal surgery. *Ann Surg.* 2012;255:1060-1068.

Memtsoudis S, Liu SS, Ma Y, et al. Perioperative pulmonary outcomes in patients with sleep apnea after noncardiac surgery. *Anesth Analg.* 2011;112:113-121.

Merkow RP, Bilimoria KY, McCarter MD, et al. Post-discharge venous thromboembolism after cancer surgery. *Ann Surg.* 2011;254:131-137.

Pannucci CJ, Bailey SH, Dreszer G, et al. Validation of the Caprini risk assessment model in plastic and reconstructive surgery patient. *J Am Coll Surg.* 2011;212:105-112.

Obeid NM, Azuh O, Reddy S, et al. Predictors of critical care-related complications in colectomy patients using the National Surgical Quality Improvement Program: exploring frailty and aggressive laparoscopic approaches. *J Trauma Acute Care Surg.* 2012;72:878-883.

Pannucci CJ, Bailey SH, Dreszer G, et al. Validation of the Caprini risk assessment model in plastic and reconstructive surgery patient. *J Am Coll Surg.* 2011;212:105-112.

Poirier P, Alpert MA, Fleisher LA, et al. Cardiovascular evaluation and management of severely obese patients undergoing surgery: a science advisory from the American Heart Association. *Circulation.* 2009;120:86-95.

Rutala WA, Weber DJ, the Healthcare Infection Control Practices Advisory Committee. Guideline for disinfection and sterilization in healthcare facilities, 2008. http://www.cdc.gov/hicpac/pdf/guidelines/disinfection_nov_2008.pdf.

Shuman AG, Hu HM, Pannucci CJ, et al. Stratifying the risk of venous thromboembolism in otolaryngology. *Otolaryngol Head Neck Surg.* 2012;146:719-724.

Swenson BR, Hedrick TL, Metzger R, et al. Effects of preoperative skin preparation on postoperative wound infection rates: a prospective study of 3 skin preparation protocols. *Infect Control Hosp Epidemiol.* 2009;30:964-971.

Wong J, Lam DP, Abrishami A. Short-term preoperative smoking cessation and postoperative complications: a systematic review and meta-analysis. *Can J Anaesth.* 2012; 59:268-279.

MULTIPLE CHOICE QUESTIONS

1. The American Society of Anesthesiologists (ASA) patient classification system

   A. Is an approach to categorizing patients preoperatively to assess their risk for an operative procedure
   B. Requires specific measures of certain laboratory values in order to complete the scoring system
   C. Can be used to determine who not to operate on, for example, no ASA 5 patients should undergo operation
   D. Includes categories ASA 1 through ASA 5
   E. Both A and C are true

2. The perioperative process, including the workup regarding safety for anesthetic, after the decision to operate has been made

   A. Is the sole province of the anesthesiology specialists
   B. Should not take into account the planned operation
   C. Is best performed by specialists not directly invested in the planned operation
   D. Should include a pain assessment to aid in the management of postoperative pain
   E. Both A and C are true

3. Venous thromboembolism (VTE) risk

   A. Has no relationship to the family history
   B. Is assessed using the RCRI score
   C. Can be modified by risk-based interventions
   D. Has few long-term consequences as long as a pulmonary embolus is not fatal
   E. Frequently should be modified by placement of an inferior vena cava filter preoperatively

4. Patients with diabetes mellitus require more operations than their nonaffected counterparts, and if diabetes mellitus is not carefully controlled, they have increased risk of

   A. Surgical site infection (SSI)
   B. Perioperative adrenal insufficiency
   C. Perioperative hypoglycemia
   D. A, B, and C are all true
   E. Both A and C are true

5. Geriatric patients

   A. Are a limited portion of a general surgery practice now and in the future
   B. Can have their perioperative risk very closely estimated by their chronological age
   C. Can have frailty measured by a variety of means that predict the risk of complications
   D. Require limited special assessment other than modification of drug dosages
   E. Both A and C are true

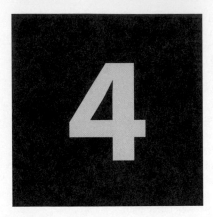

Postoperative Care

Jennifer E. Rosen, MD

The modern surgeon is involved with the management of a patient from preoperative evaluation, through the conduct of the operation into the postoperative care period and often into generating a long-term plan. As the operating surgeon, he/she is best situated to apply evidence-based scientific knowledge and a deep understanding of potential complications to that patient's care. The recovery from major surgery can be divided into three phases:

1. An immediate, or postanesthetic phase
2. An intermediate phase, encompassing the hospitalization period
3. A convalescent phase

During the first two phases, care is principally directed at maintenance of homeostasis, treatment of pain, and prevention and early detection of complications. The convalescent phase is a transition period from the time of hospital discharge to full recovery. The trend toward earlier postoperative discharge after major surgery has shifted the venue of this period.

THE IMMEDIATE POSTOPERATIVE PERIOD

The primary causes of early complications and death following major surgery are acute pulmonary, cardiovascular, and fluid derangements. The postanesthesia care unit (PACU) is staffed by specially trained personnel and provided with equipment for early detection and treatment of these problems. All patients should be monitored in this specialized unit initially following major procedures unless they are transported directly to an intensive care unit. While en route from the operating room to the PACU, the patient should be accompanied by a physician and other qualified attendants. In the PACU, the anesthesiology service generally exercises primary responsibility for cardiopulmonary function. The surgeon is responsible for the operative site

and all other aspects of the care not directly related to the effects of anesthesia. The patient can be discharged from the recovery room when cardiovascular, pulmonary, and neurologic functions have returned to baseline, which usually occurs 1-3 hours following operation. Patients who require continuing ventilatory or circulatory support or who have other conditions that require frequent monitoring are transferred to an intensive care unit. In this setting, nursing personnel specially trained in the management of respiratory and cardiovascular emergencies are available, and the staff-to-patient ratio is higher than it is on the wards. Monitoring equipment is available to enable early detection of cardiorespiratory derangements.

► Postoperative Orders

Detailed treatment orders are necessary to direct postoperative care. The transfer of the patient from OR to PACU requires reiteration of any patient care orders. Unusual or particularly important orders should also be communicated to the nursing team orally. The nursing team must also be advised of the nature of the operation and the patient's condition. Errors in postoperative orders, including medication errors and omission of important orders, are diminished by electronic order entry systems that can contain postoperative order sets. Careful review of order sets is still warranted, as individual patients require specialized attention. Postoperative orders should cover the following.

A. Monitoring

1. Vital signs—Blood pressure, pulse, and respiration should be recorded frequently until stable and then regularly until the patient is discharged from the recovery room. The frequency of vital sign measurements thereafter depends upon the nature of the operation and the course in the PACU. When an arterial catheter is in place, blood pressure and pulse should be monitored continuously. Continuous electrocardiographic monitoring is indicated for most patients in the PACU. Any major changes in vital signs should be communicated to the anesthesiologist and attending surgeon immediately.

2. Central venous pressure—Central venous pressure should be recorded periodically in the early postoperative period if the operation has entailed large blood losses or fluid shifts, and invasive monitoring is available. A Swan-Ganz catheter for measurement of pulmonary artery wedge pressure is indicated under these conditions if the patient has compromised cardiac or respiratory function.

3. Fluid balance—The anesthetic record includes all fluid administered as well as blood loss and urine output during the operation. This record should be continued in the postoperative period and should also include fluid losses from drains and stomas. This aids in assessing hydration and helps to guide intravenous fluid replacement. A bladder catheter can be placed for frequent measurement of urine output. In the absence of a bladder catheter, the surgeon should be notified if the patient is unable to void within 6-8 hours after operation to determine whether intermittent catheterization may be warranted.

4. Other types of monitoring—Depending on the nature of the operation and the patient's preexisting conditions, other types of monitoring may be necessary. Examples include measurement of intracranial pressure and level of consciousness following cranial surgery and monitoring of distal pulses following vascular surgery or in patients with casts, evaluating for expanding hematoma in patients after thyroid surgery et cetera.

5. The "postoperative check"—Most patients who remain in the hospital beyond the immediate postoperative period require an evaluation by a physician or adjunct during the 4-6 hours following surgery. This evaluation should include a review of the patient's overall subjective status, any objective alterations during that time period, an assessment of whether the postoperative orders are appropriate and adequate and if the patient has developed any signs or symptoms indicative of a complication related to their particular procedure or the anesthesia and medications administered since that time. A thorough understanding of the patient's history and surgical course will help in anticipating, preventing, and identifying any complications. Any worrisome findings should be directly and quickly communicated to the attending surgeon, who is in the best position to determine if an intervention is warranted.

B. Respiratory Care

In the early postoperative period, the patient may remain mechanically ventilated or be treated with supplemental oxygen by mask or nasal prongs, preferably with humidification. These orders should be specified. For intubated patients, tracheal suctioning or other forms of respiratory therapy must be specified as required. Patients who are not intubated should be instructed on how to cough and do deep breathing exercises frequently to prevent atelectasis.

C. Position in Bed and Mobilization

The postoperative orders should describe any required special positioning of the patient. Unless doing so is contraindicated, the patient should be turned from side to side every 30 minutes until conscious and then hourly for the first 8-12 hours to minimize atelectasis. Early ambulation is encouraged to reduce venous stasis; the upright position helps to increase diaphragmatic excursion. Venous stasis may also be minimized by intermittent compression of the calf by pneumatic stockings. Safety considerations are paramount, including special alerts to fall risk (such as using red socks and bed rails), one-on-one monitoring, and assistance with all transfers. Support under the knees and heels can help reduce back pain and tension from immobility during surgery.

D. Diet

Patients at risk for emesis and pulmonary aspiration should have nothing by mouth until some gastrointestinal function has returned (usually within 4 days). Most patients can tolerate liquids by mouth shortly after return to full consciousness.

E. Administration of Fluid and Electrolytes

Orders for postoperative intravenous fluids should be based on maintenance needs, operative losses, and the replacement of gastrointestinal losses from drains, fistulas, or stomas.

F. Drainage Tubes

Drain care instructions should be included in the postoperative orders. Details such as type and pressure of suction, irrigation fluid and frequency, skin exit site care and support during ambulation or showering should be specified. The surgeon should examine drains frequently, since the character or quantity of drain output may herald the development of postoperative complications such as bleeding or fistulas. Careful positioning and reinforcement of anchors can prevent the dreaded early loss of key placement of nasogastric tubes, chest tubes, and drains.

G. Medications

Orders should be written for antibiotics, analgesics, gastric acid suppression, deep vein thrombosis prophylaxis, and sedatives. If appropriate, preoperative medications should be reinstituted. Medication reconciliation is important, as interactions are possible and potentially harmful. Route of administration of medications and medication substitution should be discussed with the pharmacy when necessary. Careful attention should be paid to replacement of corticosteroids in patients at risk, since postoperative adrenal insufficiency may be life threatening, but over-supplementation can affect wound healing. Other medications such as antipyretics, laxatives, and stool softeners should be used selectively as indicated. Prophylaxis for postoperative nausea and vomiting can be useful; the type and route of medication remains controversial and should be tailored to the patient.

H. Laboratory Examinations and Imaging

Postoperative laboratory and radiographic examinations should be used to detect specific abnormalities in high-risk groups. The routine use of daily chest radiographs, blood counts, electrolytes, and renal or liver function panels is not useful. Identification and treatment of hyperglycemia should be instituted in patients who require management.

THE INTERMEDIATE POSTOPERATIVE PERIOD

The intermediate phase begins with complete recovery from anesthesia and lasts for the rest of the hospital stay. During this time, the patient recovers most basic functions and becomes self-sufficient and ready to continue convalescence at home. Transfer from the PACU/SICU to a less monitored setting usually occurs at the start of this period. Communication within the care team is important during this transition; this team can include surgeons, nurses, nutritionists, social workers and case managers, respiratory, physical and occupational therapists, residents and consulting physicians. Isolation and specialized management of patients colonized or infected with drug-resistant organisms or highly contagious infectious agents continues from the OR through stay in the PACU and then with appropriate barrier devices and room determination throughout the hospital stay.

▶ Care of the Wound

Within hours after a wound is closed, the wound space fills with an inflammatory exudate. Epidermal cells at the edges of the wound begin to divide and migrate across the wound surface. By 48 hours after closure, deeper structures are completely sealed off from the external environment. Sterile dressings applied in the operating room provide protection during this period.

Removal of the dressing and handling of the wound during the first 24 hours should be done with aseptic technique. Medical personnel should wash their hands before and after caring for any surgical wound. Gloves should always be used when there is contact with open wounds or fresh wounds.

Dressings over closed wounds should be removed by the third or fourth postoperative day. If the wound is dry, dressings need not be reapplied; this simplifies periodic inspection. Dressings should be removed earlier if they are wet or placed in a contaminated setting, because soaked dressings increase bacterial contamination of the wound. Dressings should also be removed if the patient has new manifestations of infection (such as fever or increasing wound pain). The wound should then be inspected and the adjacent area gently compressed. Any drainage from the wound should be examined by culture and Gram-stained smear.

Vacuum dressings should usually be replaced within 24-72 hours. Pain management around the time of dressing change is important to consider, as proper prophylaxis can make the procedure less difficult for both the patient and the surgical team.

Generally, skin sutures or skin staples may be removed by the fifth postoperative day and replaced by tapes. Sutures should be left in longer (eg, for 2 weeks) for incisions that cross creases (eg, groin, popliteal area), for incisions closed under tension, for some incisions in the extremities (eg, the hand), and for incisions of any kind in debilitated patients. Sutures should be removed if suture tracts show signs of infection. If the incision is healing normally, the patient may be allowed to shower or bathe by the seventh postoperative day (and often sooner, depending on the incision).

▶ Management of Drains

Drains are used either to prevent or to treat an unwanted accumulation of fluid such as pus, blood, or serum. Drains are also used to evacuate air from the pleural cavity so that the lungs can re-expand. When used prophylactically, drains are usually placed in a sterile location. Strict precautions must be taken to prevent bacteria from entering the body through the drainage tract in these situations. The external portion of the drain must be handled with aseptic technique, and the drain must be removed as soon as it is no longer useful. When drains have been placed in an infected area, there is a smaller risk of retrograde infection of the peritoneal cavity, since the infected area is usually walled off. Drains should usually be brought out through a separate incision, because drains through the operative wound increase the risk of wound infection. Closed drains connected to suction devices (Jackson-Pratt or Blake drains are two examples) are preferable to open drains (such as Penrose) that predispose to wound contamination. The quantity and quality of drainage should be recorded and contamination minimized. When drains are no longer needed, they may be withdrawn entirely at one time if there has been little or no drainage or may be progressively withdrawn over a period of a few days.

Sump drains (such as Davol drains) have an airflow system that keeps the lumen of the drain open when fluid is not passing through it, and they must be attached to a continuous suction device. Sump drains are especially useful when the amount of drainage is large or when drainage is likely to plug other kinds of drains. Some sump drains have an extra lumen through which saline solution can be infused to aid in keeping the tube clear. After infection has been controlled and the discharge is no longer purulent, the large-bore catheter may be progressively replaced with smaller catheters as the cavity closes.

Drains that have clot or thick material within them or that have lost their drainage capacity can be stripped or flushed to restore function; this should be performed only under the supervision and approval of the attending surgeon as doing so could disrupt the operative bed in some circumstances.

Postoperative Pulmonary Care

The changes in pulmonary function observed following anesthesia and surgery are principally the result of decreased vital capacity, functional residual capacity (FRC), and pulmonary edema. Vital capacity decreases to about 40% of the preoperative level within 1-4 hours after major intra-abdominal surgery. It remains at this level for 12-14 hours, slowly increases to 60%-70% of the preoperative value by 7 days, and returns to the baseline level during the ensuing week. FRC is affected to a lesser extent. Immediately after surgery, FRC is near the preoperative level, but by 24 hours postoperatively, it has decreased to about 70% of the preoperative level. It remains depressed for several days and then gradually returns to its preoperative value by the tenth day. These changes are accentuated in patients who are obese, who smoke heavily, or who have preexisting lung disease. Elderly patients are particularly vulnerable because they have decreased compliance, increased closing volume, increased residual volume, and increased dead space, all of which enhance the risk of postoperative atelectasis. In addition, reduced forced expiratory volume in 1 second (FEV_1) impairs the aged patient's ability to clear secretions and increases the chance of infection postoperatively.

The postoperative decrease in FRC is caused by a breathing pattern consisting of shallow tidal breaths without periodic maximal inflation. Normal human respiration includes inspiration to total lung capacity several times each hour. If these maximal inflations are eliminated, alveolar collapse begins to occur within a few hours, and atelectasis with transpulmonary shunting is evident shortly thereafter. Pain is thought to be one of the main causes of shallow breathing postoperatively. Complete abolition of pain, however, does not completely restore pulmonary function. Neural reflexes, abdominal distention, obesity, and other factors that limit diaphragmatic excursion appear to be as important.

The principal means of minimizing atelectasis is deep inspiration and cough. Using an incentive spirometer can facilitate periodic hyperinflation. This is particularly useful in patients with a higher risk of pulmonary complications (eg, elderly, debilitated, or markedly obese patients). Early mobilization, encouragement to take deep breaths (especially when standing), and good coaching by the nursing staff suffice for most patients.

Postoperative pulmonary edema is caused by high hydrostatic pressures (due to left ventricular failure, fluid overload, decreased oncotic pressure, etc), increased capillary permeability, or both. Edema of the lung parenchyma narrows small bronchi and increases resistance in the pulmonary vasculature. In addition, pulmonary edema may increase the risk of pulmonary infection. Adequate management of fluids postoperatively and early treatment of cardiac failure are important preventive measures.

Systemic sepsis increases capillary permeability and can lead to pulmonary edema. In the absence of deranged cardiac function or fluid overload, the development of pulmonary edema postoperatively should be regarded as evidence of sepsis. Signs and symptoms of pulmonary complications include fever, tachypnea, tachycardia, and an alteration in mental status. Development of atrial fibrillation or an abnormal cardiac rhythm can often precede identification of pulmonary complications.

Patients who smoked tobacco up until the time of surgery should be considered at higher risk for postoperative pulmonary complications. Symptoms of withdrawal from nicotine can be managed with a nicotine patch or gum.

Many patients undergoing surgery are offered vaccination against pneumococcal or influenza infection during their hospital stay; these should be considered where there are no contraindications.

RESPIRATORY FAILURE

Most patients tolerate the postoperative changes in pulmonary function described above and recover from them without difficulty. Patients who have marginal preoperative pulmonary function may be unable to maintain adequate ventilation in the immediate postoperative period and may develop respiratory failure. In these patients, the operative trauma and the effects of anesthesia reduce respiratory reserve below levels that can provide adequate gas exchange. In contrast to acute respiratory distress syndrome (see Chapter 12), early postoperative respiratory failure (which develops within 48 hours after the operation) is usually only a mechanical problem; that is, there are minimal alterations of the lung parenchyma. However, this problem is life threatening and requires immediate attention.

Early respiratory failure develops most commonly in association with major operations (especially on the chest or upper abdomen), severe trauma, and preexisting lung disease. In most of these patients, respiratory failure develops over a short period (minutes to 1-2 hours) without evidence of a precipitating cause. By contrast, late postoperative respiratory failure (which develops beyond 48 hours after the operation) is usually triggered by an intercurrent event such as pulmonary embolism, abdominal distention, or opioid overdose.

Respiratory failure is manifested by tachypnea of 25-30 breaths per minute with a low tidal volume of less than 4 mL/kg. Laboratory indications are acute elevation of P_{CO_2} above 45 mm Hg, depression of P_{O_2} below 60 mm Hg, or evidence of low cardiac output. Treatment consists of immediate endotracheal intubation and ventilatory support to ensure adequate alveolar ventilation. As soon as the patient is intubated, it is important to determine whether there are any associated pulmonary problems such as atelectasis, pneumonia, or pneumothorax that require immediate treatment.

Prevention of respiratory failure requires careful postoperative pulmonary care. Atelectasis must be minimized using the techniques described above. Patients with preexisting pulmonary disease must be hydrated carefully to avoid hypovolemia or hypervolemia. These patients must hyperventilate in order to compensate for the inefficiency of the lungs. This extra work causes greater evaporation of water and dehydration. Hypovolemia leads to dry secretions and thick sputum, which are difficult to clear from the airway. High fraction of inspired oxygen (F_{IO_2}) in these patients removes the stabilizing gas nitrogen from the alveoli, predisposing to alveolar collapse. In addition, it may impair the function of the respiratory center, which is driven by the relative hypoxemia, and thus further decrease ventilation. The use of epidural blocks or other methods of local analgesia in patients with chronic obstructive pulmonary disease (COPD) may prevent respiratory failure by relieving pain and permitting effective respiratory muscle function.

▶ Postoperative Fluid & Electrolyte Management

Postoperative fluid replacement should be based on the following considerations:

1. Maintenance requirements
2. Extra needs resulting from systemic factors (eg, fever, burns, loss during surgery)
3. Losses from drains
4. Requirements resulting from tissue edema and ileus (third space losses)

Daily maintenance requirements for sensible and insensible loss in the adult are about 1500-2500 mL depending on the patient's age, gender, weight, and body surface area. A rough estimate can be obtained by multiplying the patient's weight in kilograms times 30 (eg, 1800 mL/24 h in a 60-kg patient). Maintenance requirements are increased by fever, hyperventilation, and conditions that increase the catabolic rate.

For patients requiring intravenous fluid replacement for a short period (most postoperative patients), it is not necessary to measure serum electrolytes at any time during the postoperative period, but measurement is indicated in patients with extra fluid losses, sepsis, preexisting electrolyte abnormalities, renal insufficiency or other factors. Assessment of the status of fluid balance requires accurate records of fluid intake and output and is aided by obtaining the patient's body weight prior to surgery and weighing the patient daily.

As a rule, 2000-2500 mL of 5% dextrose in normal saline or in lactated Ringer solution is delivered daily (Table 4–1). Potassium should usually not be added during the first 24 hours after surgery, because increased amounts of potassium enter the circulation during this time as a result of operative trauma and increased aldosterone activity.

In most patients, fluid loss through a nasogastric tube is less than 500 mL/d and can be replaced by increasing the infusion used for maintenance by a similar amount. About 20 mEq of potassium should be added to every liter of fluid used to replace these losses. However, with the exception of urine, body fluids are isosmolar, and if large volumes of gastric or intestinal juice are replaced with normal saline solution, electrolyte imbalance will eventually result. Whenever external losses from any site amount to 1500 mL/d or more, electrolyte concentrations in the fluid should be measured periodically, and the amount of replacement fluids should be adjusted to equal the amount lost. Table 4–1 lists the compositions of the most frequently used solutions.

Losses that result from fluid sequestration at the operative site are usually adequately replaced during operation, but in a patient with a large retroperitoneal dissection, severe pancreatitis, etc, third space losses may be substantial and should be considered when postoperative fluid needs are assessed.

Fluid requirements must be evaluated frequently. Intravenous orders should be evaluated every 24 hours or more often if indicated by special circumstances. Following an extensive operation, fluid needs on the first day should be reevaluated every 4-6 hours. Potassium administration can be added to the intravenous infusion only if the patient has good urine flow, has a demonstrated deficiency after significant pathologic fluid losses, and is not anticipated to start enteral feedings shortly. Postoperative ionized serum calcium in patients who have undergone thyroid or parathyroid surgery should be monitored and replaced as per the operating surgeon.

▶ Postoperative Care of the Gastrointestinal Tract

Following laparotomy, gastrointestinal peristalsis temporarily decreases. Peristalsis returns in the small intestine within 24 hours, but gastric peristalsis may return more slowly.

Table 4–1 Composition of frequently used intravenous solutions.

Solution	Glucose (g/dL)	Na$^+$ (mEq/L)	C$\tilde{l}$ (mEq/L)	HCO$_3^-$ (mEq/L)	K$^+$ (mEq/L)
Dextrose 5% in water	50	...	...	...	...
Dextrose 5% and sodium chloride 0.45%	50	77	77	...	...
Sodium chloride 0.9%	...	154	154	...	...
Sodium chloride 0.45%	...	77	77	...	...
Lactated Ringer solution	...	130	109	28	4
Sodium chloride 3%	...	513	513	...	...

Function returns in the right colon by 48 hours and in the left colon by 72 hours. After operations on the stomach and upper intestine, propulsive activity of the upper gut can remain disorganized for 3-4 days. In the immediate postoperative period, the stomach may be decompressed with a nasogastric tube. Nasogastric intubation was once used in almost all patients undergoing laparotomy to avoid gastric distention and vomiting, but it is now recognized that routine nasogastric intubation is unnecessary and may contribute to the occurrence of postoperative atelectasis and pneumonia. For example, following cholecystectomy, pelvic operations, and colonic resections, nasogastric intubation is not needed in the average patient and it is probably of marginal benefit following operations on the small bowel. On the other hand, nasogastric intubation is probably useful after esophageal and gastric resections and should always be used in patients with marked ileus or a very low level of consciousness (to avoid aspiration) and in patients who manifest acute gastric distention or vomiting postoperatively.

The nasogastric tube should be connected to low intermittent suction and assessed frequently to ensure patency. The tube should be left in place for 2-3 days or until there is evidence that normal peristalsis has returned (eg, return of appetite, audible peristalsis, or passage of flatus). Suture placement is usually unnecessary but careful placement of the tube and tape fixation in a natural curve can enable the patient to move their head without risk of inadvertent removal. The nasogastric tube enhances gastroesophageal reflux, and if it is clamped for a period to assess residual volume, there is a slight risk of aspiration. Most tubes are used as a "sump" where one port is for suction and the other left open to air to allow for continuous flow. This sump port should not be clamped, tied, or flushed with saline unless clogged with material.

Once the nasogastric tube has been withdrawn, fasting is usually continued for another 24 hours, and the patient is then started on a liquid diet. Opioids may interfere with gastric motility and should be limited if possible for patients who have slow gastric emptying beyond the first postoperative week. Routine use of promotility agents or chewing gum has not demonstrated benefit in terms of quicker return to GI function.

Gastrostomy and jejunostomy tubes should be connected to low intermittent suction or dependent drainage for the first 24 hours after surgery. Absorption of nutrients and fluids by the small intestine is not affected by laparotomy, and enteral nutrition through a jejunostomy feeding tube may be started on the second postoperative day even if motility is not entirely normal. Gastrostomy or jejunostomy tubes should not be removed before the third postoperative week once firm adhesions have developed between the viscera and the parietal peritoneum. The length of tube from its point of entry into the abdominal cavity should be measured and similar between the time of insertion and the time of use; dislodgement of the tubes can be catastrophic if unrecognized before use. Any pills or medication used through the tube should be crushed (and crushable) and flushed carefully to ensure that the tube is not clogged and rendered unusable.

After most operations in areas other than the peritoneal cavity, the patient may be allowed to resume a regular diet as soon as the effects of anesthesia have completely resolved. Short-term use of parenteral nutrition in patients with good preoperative nitrogen balance and caloric intake is ill-advised; patients with preoperative catabolic states may benefit from longer-term nutritional support.

IDENTIFICATION & MANAGEMENT OF PERIOPERATIVE HYPERGLYCEMIA

Patients should be assessed at admission for history of diabetes and should undergo blood glucose testing on admission. Point of care assessment should be made in cases of elevated blood glucose for patients with known diabetes regarding monitoring, testing schedules, and glycemic targets to allow for careful coordination of blood glucose control and return to reinstitution of preadmission regimens. For patients not previously known to have diabetes or those who may have new glucocorticoid- or surgery-induced diabetes, discharge planning may need to include management of this new diagnosis.

TRANSFUSION THERAPY

Determination of the need for transfusion and what type of transfusion is necessary can do much to improve patient outcome or can obfuscate a complication when performed without consideration of the underlying etiology of the patient's need. Knowledge of the patient's preoperative status, the course of the operation and any complications, and proper preparation for potential complications should help the physician who is considering transfusion. Restrictive transfusion thresholds may minimize patient exposure to adverse outcomes. Ultimately, the attending surgeon should determine the need for transfusion, as patients can have deficits even when laboratory values appear transiently normal.

▶ Whole Blood

Whole blood is composed of 450-500 mL of donor blood, containing RBCs (hematocrit, 35%-45%), plasma, clotting factors (reduced levels of labile factors V and VIII), and anticoagulant. Platelets and granulocytes are not functional. It is indicated for red cell replacement in massive blood loss with pronounced hypovolemia. However, whole blood for transfusion is not routinely available.

▶ Red Blood Cells

Red blood cells (RBCs) are obtained by apheresis collection or prepared from whole blood by centrifugation and removal of plasma, followed by supplementation with 100 mL of adenine-containing red cell nutrient solution. The hematocrit is 55%-60%, and the volume is 300-350 mL. RBCs collected in CPDA-1 anticoagulant have a hematocrit of 65%-80% and a storage volume of 250-300 mL. RBC transfusions are indicated to increase oxygen-carrying capacity in anemic patients. Hemoglobin levels of 7-9 g/dL are well tolerated by most asymptomatic patients. A transfusion trigger of 7 g/dL is commonly used in most stable patients. Symptomatic patients with cardiac, pulmonary, or cerebrovascular disease may require RBC transfusions to achieve higher hemoglobin levels. In a nonbleeding 70-kg recipient, transfusion of 1 unit of RBCs should increase hemoglobin level by 1 g/dL and the hematocrit by 3%. Patients can donate autologous blood in the month before surgery when appropriate; directed donors do not necessarily reduce the risk of transfusion or transfusion reaction.

▶ Washed Red Blood Cells

RBCs are washed with saline to remove more than 98% of plasma proteins and resuspended in approximately 180 mL

of saline, at an approximate hematocrit of 75%. Anemic patients with recurrent or severe allergic reactions benefit from washed RBCs. Patients with severe IgA deficiency who test positive for anti-IgA antibodies should receive RBCs washed with 2-3 L of saline or receive blood collected from IgA-deficient donors.

▶ Leukocyte-Reduced Red Blood Cells

Third-generation leukocyte reduction filters remove more than 99.9% of the contaminating leukocytes, leaving less than 5×10^6 white blood cells (WBCs) per unit. Filtration done soon after collection (prestorage leukoreduction) is more effective than bedside filtration. Patients experiencing recurrent febrile nonhemolytic transfusion reactions (FNHTRs) to RBCs or platelets should receive leukocyte-reduced products. The prophylactic use of leukoreduced RBCs and platelets in patients with long-term transfusion needs decreases the likelihood of human leukocyte antigens (HLA) alloimmunization and protects from immune platelet refractoriness and recurrent FNHTRs. Leukoreduction also decreases the risk of transmission of cytomegalovirus (CMV) infection in immunosuppressed CMV-seronegative patients.

▶ Irradiated Red Blood Cells

RBCs are irradiated with 25 Gy of gamma irradiation. All cellular products should be irradiated for patients who are at risk for transfusion-associated graft-versus-host disease (TA-GVHD). Adult patients at risk for TA-GVHD include, but are not limited to, the following: those with congenital severe immunodeficiency, hematological malignancy receiving intensive chemoradiotherapy, Hodgkin and non-Hodgkin lymphoma, certain solid tumors (neuroblastoma and sarcoma), peripheral blood stem cell and marrow transplants, or recipients of fludarabine-based chemotherapy, and those receiving directed donations from blood relatives or HLA-matched platelets. Acellular products such as fresh frozen plasma (FFP) and cryoprecipitate are not irradiated. Leukoreduction is not an acceptable substitute for irradiation.

▶ Frozen-Deglycerolized Red Blood Cells

RBCs frozen in glycerol are washed extensively in normal saline to remove the cryoprotectant and then resuspended in saline at a hematocrit of approximately 75%. More than 99.9% of the plasma is removed, and few leukocytes remain in the product. Patients who are alloimmunized to multiple antigens or those with antibodies against high-frequency antigens are supported with blood collected from donors with rare phenotypes. Most patients with severe IgA deficiency can safely receive RBCs washed with 2 L or more of saline. Frozen-deglycerolized RBCs are an equally safe and effective, albeit more cumbersome, alternative for these patients. Rarely, patients may require RBCs collected from IgA-deficient donors. A national rare donor program facilitates the collection and storage of rare blood types.

Platelets

Apheresis platelets are collected from single donors by apheresis and contain at least 3×10^{11} platelets in 250-300 mL plasma. Random-donor platelets (RDP) are platelet concentrates prepared from whole blood and contain 5.5×10^{10} platelets suspended in approximately 50 mL of plasma. To provide an adult dose, 5-6 units of RDP are pooled into a single pack. Platelet transfusions are indicated for the management of active bleeding in thrombocytopenic patients. Nonthrombocytopenic patients with congenital or acquired disorders of platelet function may also require platelets to stop bleeding. Platelet transfusions are also indicated prophylactically in patients requiring line placement or minor surgery when the platelet counts are less than $50,000/\mu L$ and in patients undergoing major surgical procedures when the count falls below $50-75,000/\mu L$. Patients scheduled for ophthalmic, upper airway, or neurosurgical procedures should have platelet counts above $100,000/\mu L$. Platelets are not usually recommended for the correction of thrombocytopenia in patients with heparin-induced thrombocytopenia (HIT), type IIB von Willebrand disease (vWD), idiopathic thrombocytopenic purpura (ITP), or thrombotic thrombocytopenic purpura (TTP). The clinical indications for the use of washed, irradiated, and leukoreduced platelets are analogous to those described in the section on RBCs. Patients with platelet refractoriness secondary to HLA alloimmunization should be supported with HLA-matched platelets.

Fresh Frozen Plasma

Fresh frozen plasma (FFP) is obtained by apheresis or prepared by centrifugation of whole blood and frozen within 8 hours of collection. It contains normal levels of all clotting factors, albumin, and fibrinogen. FFP is indicated for the replacement of coagulation factors in patients with deficiencies of multiple clotting factors as occurs in the coagulopathy of liver disease, disseminated intravascular coagulation (DIC), warfarin overdose, and massive transfusions. One mL of FFP contains 1 unit of coagulation factor activity; soon after the infusion of a 10-15 mL/kg dose, the activity of all coagulation factors is increased by 20%-30%. Coagulation tests should be monitored to determine efficacy and appropriate dosing intervals. FFP should be used only if the INR is greater than 1.5 or the PT/aPTT are elevated more than 1.5 times the normal. Patients with liver disease who have minimally altered PT/aPTT and nominal bleeding should initially be managed with vitamin K replacement. Similarly, most patients with warfarin overdose can be managed by stopping warfarin for 48 hours and monitoring coagulation tests until they return to baseline levels. FFP is indicated only for active bleeding or if there is a risk for bleeding from an emergent procedure. FFP is the only replacement product currently available for patients with rare disorders such as isolated factor deficiencies (V, X, XI) or C-1 esterase inhibitor deficiency. Patients with severe IgA deficiency should be supported with IgA-deficient plasma. FFP is the first choice for fluid replacement in patients with TTP undergoing therapeutic plasma exchange. FFP is not indicated for volume replacement, nutritional support, or replacement of immunoglobulins.

Cryoprecipitate

Cryoprecipitate is the cold-insoluble precipitate formed when FFP is thawed at 1-6°C. This is then resuspended in 10-15 mL plasma. It contains 150 mg or more of fibrinogen, 80 IU or more of factor VIII, 40%-70% of vWF and 20%-30% of factor XIII present in the initial unit of FFP, and 30-60 mg of fibronectin. Each unit (bag) of cryoprecipitate increases fibrinogen level by 5-10 mg/dL. Eight to 10 bags are pooled and infused as a single dose in a 70-kg adult. Cryoprecipitate is indicated for the correction of hypofibrinogenemia in dilutional coagulopathy and the hypofibrinogenemia/dysfibrinogenemias of liver disease and DIC. Cryoprecipitate improves platelet aggregation and adhesion and decreases bleeding in uremic patients. It has been used for the correction of factor XIII deficiency, and it is the source of fibrinogen in the two-component fibrin sealant (Tisseel). Cryoprecipitate is no longer used to treat patients with hemophilia A or vWD.

Granulocyte Transfusions

Granulocytes are collected by leukapheresis from donors stimulated with granulocyte colony-stimulating factor (G-CSF) and steroids to mobilize neutrophils from the marrow storage pool into peripheral blood. On average they contain 1×10^{10} or more granulocytes suspended in 200-300 mL plasma. About $1-3 \times 10^{11}$ platelets and 10-30 mL RBCs are also present in the product. Granulocyte transfusions are indicated in severely neutropenic (absolute neutrophil count $< 0.5 \times 10^3/\mu L$) patients with bacterial sepsis who have not responded to optimum antibiotic therapy after 48-72 hours, provided there is a reasonable expectation of recovery of bone marrow function. Transfusions are given daily until clinical improvement or neutrophil recovery occurs.

Erythropoietin Stimulating Agents & Other Blood Substitutes

Routine use of erythropoietin stimulating agents for patients undergoing surgery is not recommended. Selective use in patients with anemia undergoing major elective surgery is under investigation. Likewise, the effectiveness of recombinant human factor VIIa and other coagulation factor replacement for routine prophylactic use in general surgery in patients without hemophilia remains unproven.

POSTOPERATIVE PAIN

Severe pain is a common sequela of intrathoracic, intra-abdominal, and major bone or joint procedures. About 60% of such patients perceive their pain to be severe, 25% moderate, and 15% mild. In contrast, following superficial operations on the head and neck, limbs, or abdominal wall, less than 15% of patients characterize their pain as severe. The factors responsible for these differences include duration of operation, degree of operative trauma, type of incision, and magnitude of intraoperative retraction. Gentle handling of tissues, expedient operations, and good muscle relaxation help lessen the severity of postoperative pain. Objective measures of pain remain elusive.

While factors related to the nature of the operation influence postoperative pain, it is also true that the same operation produces different amounts of pain in different patients. This varies according to individual physical, emotional, and cultural characteristics. Much of the emotional aspect of pain can be traced to anxiety. Feelings such as helplessness, fear, and uncertainty contribute to anxiety and may heighten the patient's perception of pain.

It was once thought that anesthesia and analgesia in neonates and infants was too risky and that these young patients did not perceive pain. It is now known that reduction of pain with appropriate techniques actually decreases morbidity from major surgery in this age group.

The physiology of postoperative pain involves transmission of pain impulses via splanchnic (not vagal) afferent fibers to the central nervous system, where they initiate spinal, brain stem, and cortical reflexes. Spinal responses result from stimulation of neurons in the anterior horn, resulting in skeletal muscle spasm, vasospasm, and gastrointestinal ileus. Brain stem responses to pain include alterations in ventilation, blood pressure, and endocrine function. Cortical responses include voluntary movements and psychologic changes, such as fear and apprehension. These emotional responses facilitate nociceptive spinal transmission, lower the threshold for pain perception, and perpetuate the pain experience.

Postoperative pain serves no useful purpose and may cause alterations in pulmonary, circulatory, gastrointestinal, and skeletal muscle function that contribute to postoperative complications. Pain following thoracic and upper abdominal operations, for example, causes voluntary and involuntary splinting of thoracic and abdominal muscles and the diaphragm. The patient may be reluctant to breathe deeply, promoting atelectasis. The limitation in motion due to pain predisposes to venous stasis, thrombosis, and embolism. Release of catecholamines and other stress hormones by postoperative pain causes vasospasm and hypertension, which may in turn lead to complications such as stroke, myocardial infarction, and bleeding. Prevention of postoperative pain is thus important for reasons other than the pain itself. Effective pain control may improve the outcome of major operations.

▶ A. Communication

Close attention to the patient's needs, frequent reassurance, and genuine concern help to minimize postoperative pain. Spending a few minutes with the patient every day in frank discussions of progress and any complications does more to relieve pain than many physicians realize. Patients with preoperative drug and substance abuse still have postoperative pain needs and may require more medication than others. Communication among the patient care team can help in the understanding of specific pain-control needs.

▶ B. Parenteral Opioids

Opioids are the mainstay of therapy for postoperative pain. Their analgesic effect is via two mechanisms:

1. A direct effect on opioid receptors
2. Stimulation of a descending brain stem system that contributes to pain inhibition

Although substantial relief of pain may be achieved with opioids, they do not modify reflex phenomena associated with pain, such as muscle spasm. Opioids administered intramuscularly, while convenient, result in wide variations in plasma concentrations. This, as well as the wide variations in dosage required for analgesia among patients, reduces analgesic efficacy. Physician and nurse attitudes reflect a persistent misunderstanding of the pharmacology and psychology of pain control. Frequently, the dose of opioid prescribed or administered is too small and too infrequent. When opioid usage is limited to temporary treatment of postoperative pain, drug addiction is extremely rare.

Morphine is the most widely used opioid for treatment of postoperative pain. Morphine may be administered intravenously, either intermittently or continuously. Except as discussed below in the section on patient-controlled analgesia (PCA), continuous intravenous administration requires close supervision and is impractical except in the PACU or intensive care unit. Side effects of morphine include respiratory depression, nausea and vomiting, and clouded sensorium. In the setting of severe postoperative pain, however, respiratory depression is rare, because pain itself is a powerful respiratory stimulant.

Meperidine is an opioid with about one-eighth the potency of morphine. It provides a similar quality of pain control with similar side effects. The duration of pain relief is somewhat shorter than with morphine. Like morphine, meperidine may be given intravenously, but the same requirements for monitoring apply.

Other opioids useful for postoperative analgesia include hydromorphone and methadone. Hydromorphone is usually administered in a dose of 1-2 mg intramuscularly every 2-3 hours. Methadone is given intramuscularly or orally in an average dose of 10 mg every 4-6 hours. The main advantage of methadone is its long half-life (6-10 hours) and its ability to prevent withdrawal symptoms in patients with morphine dependence. Patients who use methadone preoperatively should be continued postoperatively on their usual dose to avoid withdrawal; most clinics maintain records on their patients and should be consulted to confirm the appropriate replacement.

C. Nonopioid Parenteral Analgesics

Ketorolac tromethamine is a nonsteroidal anti-inflammatory drug (NSAID) with potent analgesic and moderate anti-inflammatory activities. It is available in injectable form suitable for postoperative use. In controlled trials, ketorolac (30 mg) demonstrated analgesic efficacy roughly equivalent to that of morphine (10 mg). A potential advantage over morphine is its lack of respiratory depression. Gastrointestinal ulceration, impaired coagulation, and reduced renal function—all potential complications of NSAID use—have not yet been reported with short-term perioperative use of ketorolac.

D. Oral Analgesics

Within several days following most abdominal surgical procedures, the severity of pain decreases and oral analgesics suffice for control. Aspirin is often avoided as an analgesic postoperatively, since it interferes with platelet function, prolongs bleeding time, and interferes with the effects of anticoagulants; however, in some settings aspirin is used to diminish the risk of cardiovascular complications by these mechanisms. For most patients, a combination of acetaminophen with codeine (eg, Tylenol No. 3) or propoxyphene (Darvocet-N 50 or -N 100) suffices. Hydrocodone with acetaminophen (Vicodin) is a synthetic opioid with properties similar to those of codeine. For more severe pain, oxycodone is available in combination with aspirin (Percodan) or acetaminophen (Percocet, Tylox). Oxycodone is an opioid with slightly less potency than morphine. As with all opioids, tolerance develops with long-term use.

E. Patient-Controlled Analgesia

Patient-controlled analgesia puts the frequency of analgesic administration under the patient's control but within safe limits. A device containing a timing unit, a pump, and the analgesic medication is connected to an intravenous line. By pressing a button, the patient delivers a predetermined dose of analgesic (usually morphine, 1-3 mg). The timing unit prevents overdosage by interposing an inactivation period

(usually 6-8 minutes) between patient-initiated doses. The possibility of overdosage is also limited by the fact that the patient must be awake in order to search for and push the button that delivers the morphine. The dose and timing can be changed by medical personnel to accommodate the needs of the patient. This method appears to improve pain control and even reduces the total dose of opioid given in a 24-hour period. The addition of a background continuous infusion to the patient-directed administration of analgesic appears to offer no advantage over PCA alone.

F. Continuous Epidural Analgesia

Opioids are also effective when administered directly into the epidural space. Topical morphine does not depress proprioceptive pathways in the dorsal horn, but it does affect nociceptive pathways by interacting with opioid receptors. Therefore, epidural opioids produce intense, prolonged segmental analgesia with relatively less respiratory depression or sympathetic, motor, or other sensory disturbances. In comparison with parenteral administration, epidural administration requires similar dosage for control of pain, has a slightly delayed onset of action, provides substantially longer pain relief, and is associated with better preservation of pulmonary function. Epidural morphine is usually administered as a continuous infusion at a rate of 0.2-0.8 mg/h with or without the addition of 0.25% bupivacaine. Analgesia produced by this technique is superior to that of intravenous or intramuscular opioids. Patients managed in this way are more alert and have better gastrointestinal function. Side effects of continuous epidural administration of morphine include pruritus, nausea, and urinary retention. Respiratory depression may occur.

G. Intercostal Block

Intercostal block may be used to decrease pain following thoracic and abdominal operations. Since the block does not include the visceral afferent nerve fibers, it does not relieve pain completely, but it does eliminate muscle spasm induced by cutaneous pain and helps to restore respiratory function. It does not carry the risk of hypotension—as does continuous epidural analgesia—and it produces analgesia for periods of 3-12 hours. The main disadvantage of intercostal blocks is the risk of pneumothorax and the need for repeated injections. These problems can be minimized by placing a catheter in the intercostal space or in the pleura through which a continuous infusion of bupivacaine 0.5% is delivered at a rate of 3-8 mL/h.

H. Direct Infiltration

Direct administration of a combination of short- and long-acting local anesthetics can help significantly in management of postoperative pain in a variety of settings. Optimally, wound infiltration or local nerve block should occur following the induction of intravenous anesthesia and prior to skin incision but may still be beneficial after incision.

► Special Considerations

Patients at the extreme of ages, who underwent acute/emergency surgery or had a poor preoperative functional and nutritional status require special postoperative consideration.

Infants and children can be both more easily taken out of equilibrium and yet can return to health more quickly. Reassessment should occur more frequently with calculation of fluid needs tailored to their body surface area and losses. The nursing ratio is expected to be higher for more critically ill children. Elderly patients tend to have more complex preoperative medical issues, require a careful preoperative functional assessment of their nutritional reserve, and may have a more sensitive response to sedatives and other medications with a prolonged return to full mental function. Careful attention to even small changes in status should trigger thoughtful appraisal of the patient.

THE CONVALESCENT PHASE

Determination and planning for discharge should start even before the operation and should be modified accordingly. It is not uncommon for patients to be discharged to a setting other than home; emergency or acute care surgery is more likely to lend itself to a change in disposition of the patient. Plans should be made early for home assistance in the activities of daily living and in assisting recovery from surgery including education on the care of ostomies, new tubes/drains, intravenous or intramuscular medications.

Daily rounds should include a plan for discontinuation of drains, supplemental oxygen, nasogastric tubes, indwelling urinary catheters, medications including antibiotics, and the need for ongoing antithrombotic therapy. Transition of medication to oral route where possible should occur early; otherwise, preparation for home administration of IV or SQ/IM medication should be made.

► References

Postoperative Outcomes

Cronin J, Livhits M, Mercado C, et al. Quality improvement pilot program for vulnerable elderly surgical patients. *Am Surg.* 2011 Oct;77(10):1305-1308.

Guillamondegui OD, Gunter OL, Hines L, et al. Using the National Surgical Quality Improvement Program and the Tennessee Surgical Quality Collaborative to improve surgical outcomes. *J Am Coll Surg.* 2012 Apr;214(4):709-714; discussion 714-716.

Ingraham AM, Richards KE, Hall BL, Ko CY. Quality improvement in surgery: the American College of Surgeons National Surgical Quality Improvement Program Approach. *Adv Surg.* 2010 Oct;44:251-267.

Vonlanthen R, Slankamenac K, Breitenstein S, et al. The impact of complications on costs of major surgical procedures. *Ann Surg.* 2011;254:907-913.

Fluid Therapy

Pearse RM, Ackland GL. Perioperative fluid therapy. *BMJ.* 2012 Apr 26;344:e2865.

Transfusion Therapy

Society of Thoracic Surgeons Blood Conservation Guideline Task Force, International Consortium for Evidence Based Perfusion; Ferraris VA, Brown JR, Despotis GJ, et al. 2011 update to the Society of Thoracic Surgeons and the Society of Cardiovascular Anesthesiologists blood conservation clinical practice guidelines. *Ann Thorac Surg.* 2011 Mar;91(3):944-982.

Postoperative Analgesia

Practice guidelines for acute pain management in the perioperative setting: an updated report by the American Society of Anesthesiologists Task Force on Acute Pain Management. *Anesthesiology.* 2012 Feb;116(2):248-273.

Hyperglycemia

Umpierrez GE, Hellman R, Korytkowski MT, et al. Management of hyperglycemia in hospitalized patients in non-critical care setting: an Endocrine Society clinical practice guideline. *J Clin Endocrinol Metab.* 2012 Jan;97(1):16-38.

MULTIPLE CHOICE QUESTIONS

1. A 65-year-old woman undergoes a thyroid lobectomy for a follicular neoplasm. She has a history of coronary artery disease, hypertension, insulin-dependent diabetes, and stroke. The procedure lasted 2 hours during which the patient required occasional Neo-Synephrine for brief interoperative hypotension. Two hours after the procedure, the nurse calls from the PACU to report that the patient is agitated and hypertensive. Which of the following is unlikely to be the cause for her agitation?

   A. Hypoxia
   B. Stroke
   C. "Unmasking" of cognitive dysfunction
   D. Hyperglycemia
   E. Hypocalcemia

2. A 43-year-old man with a distant history of intravenous drug use is now status post a right inguinal hernia

repair and is complaining of severe groin pain on the side of the operation. All of the following are appropriate maneuvers except

A. Evaluate the patient for necrotizing fasciitis
B. Reassure the patient that his use of preoperative suboxone that morning may have blocked his postoperative response to narcotics
C. Allow the nurse to administer a postoperative parenteral nonopioid analgesic
D. Discharge the patient with a prescription for pain medication and a plan for follow-up in 2 weeks
E. Perform a nerve block with local anesthetics

3. A 56 year-old woman is being prepared for an elective ventral hernia repair in the preoperative care unit. She is overweight, with a history of non–insulin-dependent diabetes, hypertension, and smoking. Her fingerstick glucose is 326, and you note that her most recent HgA_{1C} is 8.4%. She wants to proceed with the operation and has traveled a long distance to see you and has taken the day off from work. The most appropriate choice of management is

A. Proceed with the operation and plan for an intraoperative insulin drip
B. Repeat the fingerstick after insulin administration and proceed with the operation if the glucose is improved with the plan for consultation of the diabetes team postoperatively for management
C. Cancel the operation with the plan for improved preoperative preparation
D. Admit the patient for preoperative glucose management and reschedule the operation for several days from now

4. Which of the following are routine components of the first 24-hour postoperative check in patients who have undergone colon resection?

A. Vital signs including heart rate, blood pressure, oxygen saturation

B. Wound evaluation including assessment of drain output and content
C. Assessment of the adequacy of pain management
D. Plan for removal of the nasogastric tube, Foley catheter, and advancement of diet
E. All of the above except for D

5. A 72-year-old man underwent resection of hepatic segments 5/6 for a hepatoma in the setting of hepatocellular carcinoma 2 days ago and was recently discharged to the floor. Perioperatively, he required a large volume of fluid resuscitation. He now has bloody output from his two Jackson-Pratt drains that are seated in the liver bed, his hematocrit has fallen 7 points to 23 and his INR is 2.7, and he is febrile to 102.8°F and confused. Which of the following is the most appropriate order and choice of management?

A. Evaluation of the patient, transfer to higher level of care, transfusion with 2 units of unmatched packed RBCs, return to the operating room for surgical control of bleeding
B. Evaluation of the patient, transfusion with two packs of FFP and 2 units of matched packed RBCs, computed tomography with angiography for possible embolization
C. Evaluation of the patient, intubation for protection of airway, transfer to higher level of care, transfusion with cryoprecipitate, antibiotic administration, return to the operating room for surgical control of bleeding.
D. Evaluation of the patient, intubation for protection of airway, transfer to a higher level of care, transfusion with 2 units of FFP and 2 units of matched packed RBCs, antibiotic administration, and computed tomography of the abdomen.

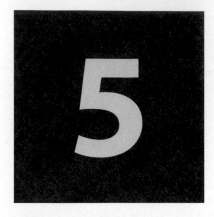

Postoperative Complications

Daniel I. Chu, MD

Suresh Agarwal, MD

INTRODUCTION

Complications occur after operations and surgeons must be versed in anticipating, recognizing, and managing them. The spectrum of these complications ranges from the relatively minor, such as a small postoperative seroma, to the catastrophic, such as postoperative myocardial infarction or anastomotic leak. The management of these complications also spans a spectrum from nonoperative strategies to those requiring an emergent return to the operating room.

When considering postoperative complications, it is helpful to categorize them in a system-based method that has additional usefulness in clinical research.

MECHANICAL COMPLICATIONS

Mechanical complications are defined as those that occur as a direct result of technical failure from a procedure or operation. These complications include postoperative hematoma and hemoperitoneum, seroma, wound dehiscence, anastomotic leak, and those related to lines, drains, and retained foreign bodies.

► Hematoma

Wound hematoma, a collection of blood and clot in the wound, is a common wound complication and is usually caused by inadequate hemostasis. The risk is much higher in patients who have been systemically anticoagulated and in those with preexisting coagulopathies. However, patients receiving aspirin or low-dose heparin also have a slightly higher risk of developing this complication. Vigorous coughing or marked arterial hypertension immediately after surgery may contribute to the formation of a wound hematoma.

Hematoma produces elevation and discoloration of the wound edges, discomfort, and swelling. Blood sometimes leaks between skin sutures. Neck hematoma following operation on the thyroid, parathyroid, or carotid artery are particularly dangerous, because it may expand rapidly and compromise the airway. Small hematomas may resorb, but they increase the incidence of wound infection. Treatment in most cases consists of evacuation of the clot under sterile conditions, ligation of bleeding vessels, and reclosure of the wound.

► Hemoperitoneum

Bleeding is the most common cause of shock in the first 24 hours after abdominal surgery. Postoperative hemoperitoneum—a rapidly evolving, life-threatening complication—is usually the result of a technical problem with hemostasis, but coagulation disorders may play a role. Causes of coagulopathy, such as dilution of hemostatic factors after massive blood loss and resuscitation, mismatched transfusion, or administration of heparin, should also be considered. In these cases, bleeding tends to be more generalized, occurring in the wound, venipuncture sites, etc.

Hemoperitoneum usually becomes apparent within 24 hours after the operation. It manifests as intravascular hypovolemia: tachycardia, hypotension, decreased urine output, and peripheral vasoconstriction. If bleeding continues, abdominal girth may increase and intra-abdominal hypertension or abdominal compartment syndrome may ensue. Changes in the hematocrit are usually not obvious for 4-6 hours and are of limited diagnostic help in patients who sustain rapid blood loss.

Manifestations may be so subtle that the diagnosis is initially overlooked. Only a high index of suspicion, frequent examination of patients at risk, and systematic investigation of patients with postoperative hypotension will reliably result in early recognition. Preexisting disease and drugs taken before surgery as well as those administered during the operation may cause hypotension. The differential diagnosis of immediate postoperative circulatory collapse also includes pulmonary embolism, cardiac dysrhythmias, pneumothorax, myocardial infarction, and severe allergic reactions. Infusions to expand the intravascular volume should be started as soon as other diseases have been ruled out. If hypotension or other signs of hypovolemia persist, one usually must reoperate promptly. At operation, bleeding should be stopped, clots evacuated, and the peritoneal cavity rinsed with saline solution.

▶ Seroma

A seroma is a fluid collection in the wound other than pus or blood. Seromas often follow operations that involve elevation of skin flaps and transection of numerous lymphatic channels (eg, mastectomy, operations in the groin). Seromas delay healing and increase the risk of wound infection. Those located under skin flaps can usually be evacuated by needle aspiration if necessary. Compression dressings can then occlude lymphatic leaks and limit reaccumulation. Small seromas that recur may be treated by repeated evacuation. Seromas of the groin, which are common after vascular operations, are best left to resorb without aspiration, since the risks of introducing a needle (infection, disruption of vascular structures, etc) are greater than the risk associated with the seroma itself. If seromas persist—or if they leak through the wound—the wound should be explored in the operating room and the draining sites oversewn. Open wounds with persistent lymph leaks can be treated with wound vacuum devices.

▶ Wound Dehiscence

Wound dehiscence is partial or total disruption of any or all layers of the operative wound. Rupture of all layers of the abdominal wall and extrusion of abdominal viscera is evisceration. Wound dehiscence occurs in 1%-3% of abdominal surgical procedures. Systemic and local factors contribute to the development of this complication.

Systemic Risk Factors

Dehiscence after laparotomy is rare in patients younger than 30 years but affects about 5% of patients older than 60 years. It is more common in patients with diabetes mellitus, uremia, immunosuppression, jaundice, sepsis, hypoalbuminemia, cancer, obesity, and in those receiving corticosteroids.

Local Risk Factors

The three most important local factors predisposing to wound dehiscence are inadequate closure, increased intra-abdominal pressure, and deficient wound healing. Dehiscence often results from a combination of these factors rather than from a single one. The type of incision (transverse, midline, etc) does not influence the incidence of dehiscence.

1. Closure—This is the single most important factor. The fascial layers give strength to a closure, and when fascia disrupts, the wound separates. Accurate approximation of anatomic layers is essential for adequate wound closure.

Most wounds that dehisce do so because the sutures tear through the fascia. Prevention of this problem includes performing a neat incision, avoiding devitalization of the fascial edges by careful handling of tissues during the operation, placing and tying sutures correctly, and selecting the proper suture material. Sutures must be placed 2-3 cm from the wound edge and about 1 cm apart. *Dehiscence is often the result of using too few stitches and placing them too close to the edge of the fascia.* It is unusual for dehiscence to recur following reclosure, implying that adequate closure was technically possible at the initial procedure. In patients with risk factors for dehiscence, the surgeon should "do the second closure at the first operation"; that is, take extra care to prevent dehiscence. Modern synthetic suture materials (polyglycolic acid, polypropylene, and others) are clearly superior to catgut for fascial closure. In infected wounds, polypropylene sutures are more resistant to degradation than polyglycolic acid sutures and have lower rates of wound disruption. Wound complications are decreased by obliteration of dead space. Stomas and drains should be brought out through separate incisions to reduce the rate of wound infection and disruption.

2. Intra-abdominal pressure—After most intra-abdominal operations, some degree of ileus exists, which may increase pressure by causing distention of the bowel. High abdominal pressure can also occur in patients with chronic obstructive pulmonary disease who use their abdominal muscles as accessory muscles of respiration. In addition, coughing produces sudden increases in intra-abdominal pressure. Other factors contributing to increased abdominal pressure are postoperative bowel obstruction, obesity, and cirrhosis with ascites formation. Extra precautions are necessary to avoid dehiscence in such patients.

3. Poor wound healing—Infection is an associated factor in more than half of wounds that rupture. The presence of drains, seromas, and wound hematomas also delays healing. Normally, a "healing ridge" (a palpable thickening extending about 0.5 cm on each side of the incision) appears near the end of the first week after operation. The presence of this ridge is clinical evidence that healing is adequate, and it is invariably absent from wounds that rupture.

Diagnosis and Management

Although wound dehiscence may occur at any time following wound closure, it is most commonly observed between the fifth and eighth postoperative days, when the strength of the wound is at a minimum. Wound dehiscence may occasionally be the first manifestation of intra-abdominal sepsis. The earliest sign of dehiscence is often discharge of serosanguineous fluid from the wound or, in some cases, sudden evisceration. The patient may describe a popping sensation associated with severe coughing or retching.

Thoracic wounds, with the exception of sternal wounds, are much less prone to dehiscence than are abdominal wounds.

When a thoracotomy closure ruptures, it is heralded by leakage of pleural fluid or air and paradoxic motion of the chest wall. Sternal dehiscence, which is almost always associated with infection, produces an unstable chest and requires early treatment. If infection is not overwhelming and there is minimal osteomyelitis of the adjacent sternum, the patient may be returned to the operating room for reclosure. Continuous mediastinal irrigation through small tubes left at the time of closure appears to reduce the failure rate. In cases of overwhelming infection, the wound is best treated by debridement and closure with a pectoralis major muscle flap, which resists further infection by increasing vascular supply to the area.

Patients with dehiscence of a laparotomy wound and evisceration should be returned to bed and the wound covered with moist towels. With the patient under general anesthesia, any exposed bowel or omentum should be rinsed with lactated Ringer solution containing antibiotics and then returned to the abdomen. After mechanical cleansing and copious irrigation of the wound, the previous sutures should be removed and the wound reclosed using additional measures to prevent recurrent dehiscence, such as full-thickness retention sutures of no. 22 wire or heavy nylon. Evisceration carries a 10% mortality rate due both to contributing factors (eg, sepsis and cancer) and to resulting local infection.

Wound dehiscence without evisceration is best managed by prompt elective reclosure of the incision. If a partial disruption is stable and the patient is a poor operative risk, treatment may be delayed and the resulting incisional hernia accepted. It is important in these patients that skin stitches, if present, not be removed before the end of the second postoperative week and that the abdomen be wrapped with a binder or corset to limit further enlargement of the fascial defect or sudden disruption of the covering skin. When partial dehiscence is discovered during treatment of a wound infection, repair should be delayed if possible until the infection has been controlled, the wound has healed, and 6-7 months have elapsed. In these cases, antibiotics specific for the organisms isolated from the previous wound infection must be given at the time of hernia repair.

Recurrence of evisceration after reclosure of disrupted wounds is rare, though incisional hernias are later found in about 20% of such patients—usually those with wound infection in addition to dehiscence.

Of special circumstance, patients with ascites are at risk of fluid leak through the wound. Left untreated, ascitic leaks increase the incidence of wound infection and, through retrograde contamination, may result in peritonitis. Prevention in susceptible patients involves closing at least one layer of the wound with a continuous suture and taking measures to avoid the accumulation of ascites postoperatively. If an ascitic leak develops, the wound should be explored and the fascial defect closed. The rest of the wound, including the skin, should also be closed.

In patients at high risk for wound dehiscence, placement of retention stitches at the initial operation should be considered. Although these do not prevent dehiscence, they may prevent evisceration and the morbidity and mortality that are associated with it.

▶ Anastomotic Leak

Anastomotic leaks are reported in 1%-24% of anastomoses with higher frequencies in low pelvic anastomoses compared to more proximal ones. The morbidity and mortality for a patient with an anastomotic leak is significantly increased with a reportedly threefold increase in mortality.

Anastomotic healing follows the same principles of normal wound healing, and the risk factors for developing an anastomotic leak are identical to those that predict wound dehiscence. Systemic risk factors include age, malnutrition, vitamin deficiencies, and comorbid conditions such as diabetes, smoking, inflammatory bowel disease such as regional enteritis, previous radiation/chemotherapy and anemia. Local risk factors include tension, poor blood flow, hypotension, radiation, and contamination.

Technical considerations such as hand-sewn versus stapled anastomoses, continuous versus interrupted sutures, and single versus double-layer hand-sewn anastomoses have been extensively studied. While such topics generate much discussion and controversy, the technique chosen has less to do with anastomotic leaks than systemic and local factors. Stapled end-to-end anastomoses, however, may lead to higher rates of anastomotic strictures in long-term follow-up.

The diagnosis of an anastomotic leak can be made clinically, radiographically, and intraoperatively. Clinical signs include pain, fever, peritonitis, and drainage of purulent material, bilious succus, or fecal material. Radiographic signs include fluid and gas-containing collections tracking to an anastomosis. Intraoperative findings include gross contamination from gastrointestinal contents and evidence of anastomotic disruption.

The management of an anastomotic leak depends on several factors, including the patient's clinical status, the time from initial operation, and the location and severity of the leak. The management strategies can range from nonoperative (observation, bowel rest, antibiotics, and percutaneous drainage of abscesses) to the operative (open drainage, proximal diversion, and revision of anastomosis).

▶ Complications of Lines, Drains, & Retained Foreign Bodies

Lines

Complications due to central line placement and maintenance are preventable with adequate experience, preparation, and technique. Choice of site, utilization of ultrasound, and assiduous adherence to sterile technique decrease infection, as well as mechanical complications such as pneumothorax and arterial injury.

Phlebitis—A needle or a catheter inserted into a vein and left in place will in time cause inflammation at the entry site. When this process involves the vein wall, it is called *phlebitis*. Factors determining the degree of inflammation are the nature of the cannula, the solution infused, bacterial infection, and venous thrombosis. Phlebitis is one of the most common causes of fever after the third postoperative day. The symptomatic triad of induration, edema, and tenderness is characteristic. Visible signs may be minimal. Prevention of phlebitis is best accomplished by observance of aseptic techniques during insertion of venous catheters, frequent change of tubing (ie, every 48-72 hours), and rotation of insertion sites (ie, every 4 days). Silastic catheters, which are the least reactive, should be used when the line must be left in for a long time. Hypertonic solutions should be infused only into veins with substantial flow, such as the subclavian, jugular, or vena cava. Venous catheters should be removed at the first sign of redness, induration, or edema. Because phlebitis is most frequent with cannulation of veins in the lower extremities, this route should be used only when upper extremity veins are unavailable. Removal of the catheter is adequate treatment.

Suppurative phlebitis—Suppurative phlebitis may result from the presence of an infected thrombus around the indwelling catheter. Staphylococci are the most common causative organisms. Local signs of inflammation are present, and pus may be expressed from the venipuncture site. High fever and positive blood cultures are common. Treatment consists of excising the affected vein, extending the incision proximally to the first open collateral, and leaving the wound open.

Cardiopulmonary complications—Pneumothorax after placement of a central catheter into either the subclavian or internal jugular veins occurs with an incidence approaching 1%. Chances for occurrence may be minimized by proper positioning, use of ultrasound, and experience. Ultrasound, in general, has markedly decreased the complication rate of central line placement. By adequately imaging the vein prior to venipuncture, the rate of arterial injury has markedly decreased. Injury to arteries can lead to pseudoaneurysm formation, continuous bleeding, or stroke, depending upon the vessel injured, size of arteriotomy, and presence of coagulopathy. Perforation of the right atrium with cardiac tamponade can occur due to central venous lines. This complication can be avoided by checking the position of the tip of the line, which should be in the superior vena cava, not the right atrium. Complications associated with the use of the flow-directed balloon-tipped (Swan-Ganz) catheter include cardiac perforation (usually of the right atrium),

intracardiac knotting of the catheter, and cardiac dysrhythmias. Pulmonary hemorrhage may result from disruption of a branch of the pulmonary artery during balloon inflation and may be fatal in patients with pulmonary hypertension. Steps in prevention include careful placement, advancement under continuous pressure monitoring, and checking the position of the tip before inflating the balloon.

Air embolism—Air embolism may occur during or after insertion of a venous catheter or as a result of accidental introduction of air into the line. Intravenous air lodges in the right atrium, preventing adequate filling of the right heart. This is manifested by hypotension, jugular venous distention, and tachycardia. This complication can be avoided by placing the patient in the Trendelenburg position when a central venous line is inserted. Emergency treatment consists of aspiration of the air with a syringe. If this is unsuccessful, the patient should be positioned right side up and head down, which will help dislodge the air from the right atrium and return circulatory dynamics to normal.

Ischemic necrosis of the finger—Continuous monitoring of arterial blood pressure during the operation and in the intensive care unit requires insertion of a radial or femoral arterial line. The hand receives its blood supply from the radial and ulnar arteries, and because of the anatomy of the palmar arches, patency of one of these vessels is usually enough to provide adequate blood flow through the hand. Occasionally, ischemic necrosis of the finger follows use of an indwelling catheter in the radial artery. This serious complication may be limited by evaluating the patency of the ulnar artery (Allen test) before establishing the radial line and by changing arterial line sites every 3-4 days. After an arterial catheter is withdrawn, a pressure dressing should be applied to avoid formation of an arterial pseudoaneurysm.

Drains

Postoperative drainage of the peritoneal cavity is indicated to prevent accumulation of fluid such as bile or pancreatic fluid, or to treat established abscess. Drains may be left to evacuate small amounts of blood, but drain output cannot be used to provide a reliable estimate of the rate of bleeding. The use of drains in operations not expected to have fluid leak (such as cholecystectomy, splenectomy, and colectomy) increases the rate of postoperative intra-abdominal and wound infection. Latex Penrose drains, which were used frequently in the past, should generally be avoided because of the risk of introducing infection. Large rigid drains may erode into adjacent viscera or vessels and cause fistula formation or bleeding. This risk is lessened with the use of softer Silastic drains, and removing them as early as possible. Drains should not be left in contact with intestinal anastomoses, as they may promote anastomotic leakage and fistula formation.

Retained Foreign Bodies

Studies based on hospital claims data estimate that cases of retained objects, which include sponges and instruments, occur at least once a year in those hospitals where 8000 to 18,000 major procedures are performed annually. While mortality is low, the morbidity is high due to the almost universal need for reoperation. The most common body cavity involved is the abdomen followed by the thoracic cavity. Improving communication within the operating room, formal sponge and instrument counts, and appropriate use of radiography all contribute to a decrease in this complication.

NEUROLOGICAL COMPLICATIONS

▶ Postoperative Cerebrovascular Accidents

Postoperative cerebrovascular accidents are almost always the result of ischemic neural damage due to poor perfusion. These often occur in elderly patients with atherosclerosis who become hypotensive during or after surgery (from sepsis, bleeding, cardiac arrest, or anesthetic effects). Normal regulatory mechanisms of the cerebral vasculature can maintain blood flow over a wide range of blood pressures down to a mean pressure of about 55 mm Hg. Abrupt hypotension, however, is less well tolerated than a more gradual pressure change. Irreversible brain damage occurs after about 4 minutes of total cerebral ischemia.

Strokes occur in 1%-5% of patients after carotid endarterectomy and other reconstructive operations of the extracranial portion of the carotid system. Rates of cerebrovascular accidents vary depending upon patient symptomatology, plaque anatomy, and degree of stenosis. Causative factors such as embolization from atherosclerotic plaques, ischemia during carotid clamping, postoperative thrombosis at the site of the arteriotomy, or intimal flap development are usually responsible. Aspirin, which inhibits platelet aggregation, may prevent immediate postoperative thrombosis.

Open heart surgery using extracorporeal circulation or deep cooling is also occasionally followed by stroke. The pathogenesis of stroke may be related to hypoxemia, emboli, or poor perfusion. The presence of a carotid bruit preoperatively increases the risk of postoperative stroke after coronary bypass by a factor of 4. Previous stroke or transient ischemic attacks and postoperative atrial fibrillation also increase the risk. For patients undergoing noncardiac, noncarotid surgery, the risk of stroke is about 0.2%. Predictors of risk in these patients are the presence of cerebrovascular, cardiac, or peripheral vascular disease and arterial hypertension.

▶ Seizures

Epilepsy, metabolic derangements, and medications may lead to seizures in the postoperative period. For unknown reasons, patients with ulcerative colitis and Crohn disease are peculiarly susceptible to seizures with loss of consciousness after surgery. Seizures should be treated rapidly to minimize their harmful effects.

PSYCHIATRIC COMPLICATIONS

Anxiety and fear are normal in patients undergoing surgery. The degree to which these emotions are experienced depends upon diverse cultural and psychological variables. Underlying depression or a history of chronic pain may serve to exaggerate the patient's response to surgery. The boundary between the normal manifestations of stress and postoperative psychosis is difficult to establish, since the latter is not really a distinct clinical entity.

Postoperative psychosis develops in about 0.5% of patients having abdominal operations. It is more common after thoracic surgery, in the elderly, and in those with chronic disease. About half of these patients suffer from mood disturbances (usually severe depression). Twenty percent have delirium. Drugs given in the postoperative period may play a role in the development of psychosis; meperidine, cimetidine, and corticosteroids are most commonly implicated. Patients who develop postoperative psychosis have higher plasma levels of β-endorphin and cortisol than those who do not. These patients also lose, temporarily, the normal circadian rhythms of β-endorphin and cortisol. Specific psychiatric syndromes may follow specific procedures, such as visual hallucinations and the "black patch syndrome" after ophthalmic surgery. Preexisting psychiatric disorders not apparent before the operation sometimes contribute to the motivation for surgery (eg, circumcision or cosmetic operations in schizophrenic patients).

Clinical manifestations are rare on the first postoperative day. During this period, patients appear emotionless and unconcerned about changes in the environment or in themselves. Most overt psychiatric derangements are observed after the third postoperative day. The symptoms are variable but often include confusion, fear, and disorientation as to time and place. Delirium presents as altered consciousness with cognitive impairment. These symptoms may not be readily apparent to the surgeon, as this problem usually occurs in sick patients whose other problems may mask the manifestations of psychosis. Early psychiatric consultation should be obtained when psychosis is suspected so that adequate and prompt assessment of consciousness and cognitive function can be done and treatment instituted. The earlier the psychosis is recognized, the easier it is to correct. Metabolic derangements or early sepsis (especially in burn patients) must be evaluated and treated if present. Severe postoperative emotional disturbances may be avoided by appropriate preoperative counseling of the patient by the surgeon. This includes a thorough discussion of the operation and the expected outcome, acquainting the patient with the intensive care unit, etc. Postoperatively, the surgeon must attend to the patient's emotional needs, offering frequent reassurance, explaining the postoperative course, and discussing the prognosis and the outcome of the operation.

▶ Special Psychiatric Problems

The ICU Syndrome

The continuous internal vigilance that results from pain and fear and the sleep deprivation from bright lights, monitoring equipment, and continuous noise can cause a psychologic disorganization known as ICU psychosis. The patient whose level of consciousness is already decreased by illness and drugs is more susceptible than a normal individual, and the result is decreased ability to think, perceive, and remember. When the cognitive processes are thoroughly disorganized, delirium occurs. The manifestations include distorted visual, auditory, and tactile perception; confusion and restlessness; and inability to differentiate reality from fantasy. Prevention includes isolation from the environment, decreased noise levels, adequate sleep, and removal from the intensive care unit as soon as possible.

Postcardiotomy Delirium

Mental changes that occasionally follow open heart surgery include impairment of memory, attention, cognition, and perception and occasionally hysteria, depressive reaction, and anxiety crisis. The symptoms most often appear after the third postoperative day. The type of operation, the presence of organic brain disease, prolonged medical illness, and the length of time on extracorporeal circulation are related to the development of postcardiotomy psychosis. Mild sedation and measures to prevent the ICU syndrome may prevent this complication. In more severe cases, haloperidol (Haldol) in doses of 1-5 mg given orally, intramuscularly, or intravenously may be required. Haloperidol is preferred over phenothiazines in these patients because it is associated with a lower incidence of cardiovascular side effects.

Delirium Tremens

Delirium tremens occurs in alcoholics who stop drinking suddenly. Hyperventilation and metabolic alkalosis contribute to the development of the full-blown syndrome. Hypomagnesemia and hypokalemia secondary to alkalosis or nutritional deficits may precipitate seizures. Readaptation to ethanol-free metabolism requires about 2 weeks, and it is during this period that alcoholics are at greatest risk of developing delirium tremens.

The prodrome includes personality changes, anxiety, and tremor. The complete syndrome is characterized by agitation, hallucinations, restlessness, confusion, overactivity, and occasionally seizures and hyperthermia. The syndrome also causes a hyperdynamic cardiorespiratory and metabolic state. For example, cardiac index, oxygen delivery, and oxygen consumption double during delirium tremens and

return to normal 24-48 hours after resolution. The wild behavior may precipitate dehiscence of a fresh laparotomy incision. Diaphoresis and dehydration are common, and exhaustion may herald death.

Withdrawal symptoms may be prevented by giving small amounts of alcohol, but benzodiazepines are the treatment of choice. Vitamin B_1 (thiamine) and magnesium sulfate should also be given.

The aims of treatment are to reduce agitation and anxiety as soon as possible and to prevent the development of other complications (eg, seizures, aspiration pneumonia). General measures should include frequent assessment of vital signs, restoration of nutrition, administration of vitamin B, correction of electrolyte imbalance or other metabolic derangements, and adequate hydration. Physical restraint, though necessary for seriously violent behavior, should be as limited as possible. With proper care, most patients improve within 72 hours.

SEXUAL DYSFUNCTION

Sexual problems commonly occur after certain kinds of operations, such as prostatectomy, heart surgery, and aortic reconstruction. The pathogenesis can be due to injury to nerves necessary for sexual function, though in other cases the etiology is unclear. After abdominoperineal resection, severance of the peripheral branches of the sacral plexus may cause impotence. It is important to discuss this possibility with the patient before any operation with a risk of impotence is performed. When sexual dysfunction is psychogenic, reassurance is usually all that is needed. If impotence persists beyond 4-6 weeks, appropriate consultation is indicated.

CARDIAC COMPLICATIONS

Cardiac complications following surgery may be life threatening. Their incidence is reduced by appropriate preoperative preparation.

Dysrhythmias, unstable angina, heart failure, or severe hypertension should be corrected before surgery whenever possible. Valvular disease—especially aortic stenosis—limits the ability of the heart to respond to increased demand during operation or in the immediate postoperative period. When aortic stenosis is recognized preoperatively—and assuming that the patient is monitored adequately—the incidence of major perioperative complications is small. Patients with preexisting heart disease should be evaluated by a cardiologist preoperatively. Determination of cardiac function, including indirect evaluation of the left ventricular ejection fraction, identifies patients at higher risk for cardiac complications. Continuous electrocardiographic monitoring during the first 3-4 postoperative days detects episodes of ischemia or dysrhythmia in about a third of these patients. Oral anticoagulant drugs should be stopped 3-5 days before surgery, and the prothrombin time should be allowed to return to normal. Patients at high risk of thromboembolic disease should receive heparin until approximately 6 hours before the operation, when heparin should be stopped. If needed, heparin can be restarted 36-48 hours after surgery along with oral anticoagulation.

General anesthesia depresses the myocardium, and some anesthetic agents predispose to dysrhythmias by sensitizing the myocardium to catecholamines. Monitoring of cardiac activity and blood pressure during the operation detects dysrhythmias and hypotension early. In patients with a high cardiac risk, regional anesthesia may be safer than general anesthesia for procedures below the umbilicus.

The duration and urgency of the operation and uncontrolled bleeding with hypotension have been individually shown to correlate positively with the development of serious postoperative cardiac problems. In patients with pacemakers, the electrocautery current may be sensed by the intracardiac electrode, causing inappropriate pacemaker function.

Noncardiac complications may affect the development of cardiac complications by increasing cardiac demands in patients with a limited reserve. Postoperative sepsis and hypoxemia are foremost. Fluid overload can produce acute left ventricular failure. Patients with coronary artery disease, dysrhythmias, or low cardiac output should be monitored postoperatively in an intensive care unit.

▶ Dysrhythmias

Most dysrhythmias appear during the operation or within the first 3 postoperative days. They are especially likely to occur after thoracic procedures.

Intraoperative Dysrhythmias

The overall incidence of intraoperative cardiac dysrhythmias is 20%; most are self-limited. The incidence is higher in patients with preexisting dysrhythmias and in those with known heart disease (35%). About one-third of dysrhythmias occur during induction of anesthesia. These dysrhythmias are usually related to anesthetic agents (eg, halothane, cyclopropane), sympathomimetic drugs, digitalis toxicity, and hypercapnia.

Postoperative Dysrhythmias

These dysrhythmias are generally related to reversible factors such as hypokalemia, hypoxemia, alkalosis, digitalis toxicity, and stress during emergence from anesthesia. Occasionally, postoperative dysrhythmias may be the first sign of myocardial infarction. Most postoperative dysrhythmias are asymptomatic, but occasionally the patient complains of chest pain, palpitations, or dyspnea.

Supraventricular dysrhythmias usually have few serious consequences but may decrease cardiac output and coronary blood flow. Patients with atrial flutter or fibrillation with a rapid ventricular response and who are in shock require cardioversion. If they are hemodynamically stable, they should have the heart rate controlled with digitalis, beta-blockers, or calcium channel blockers. Associated hypokalemia should be treated promptly.

Ventricular premature beats are often precipitated by hypercapnia, hypoxemia, pain, or fluid overload. They should be treated with oxygen, sedation, analgesia, and correction of fluid losses or electrolyte abnormalities. Ventricular dysrhythmias have a more profound effect on cardiac function than supraventricular dysrhythmias and may lead to fatal ventricular fibrillation. Immediate treatment is with lidocaine, 1 mg/kg intravenously as a bolus, repeated as necessary to a total dose of 250 mg, followed by a slow intravenous infusion at a rate of 1-2 mg/min. Higher doses of lidocaine may cause seizures.

Postoperative complete heart block is usually due to serious cardiac disease and calls for the immediate insertion of a pacemaker. First- or second-degree heart block is usually well tolerated.

▶ Postoperative Myocardial Infarction

Approximately 0.4% of all patients undergoing an operation in the United States experience a postoperative myocardial infarction. The incidence increases to 5%-12% in patients undergoing operations for other manifestations of atherosclerosis (eg, carotid endarterectomy, aortoiliac graft). Other important risk factors include preoperative congestive heart failure, ischemia identified on dipyridamole-thallium scan or treadmill exercise test, and age over 70 years. In selected patients with angina, consideration should be given to coronary revascularization before proceeding with a major elective operation on another organ.

Postoperative myocardial infarction may be precipitated by factors such as hypotension or hypoxemia. Clinical manifestations include chest pain, hypotension, and cardiac dysrhythmias. Over half of postoperative myocardial infarctions, however, are asymptomatic. The absence of symptoms is thought to be due to the residual effects of anesthesia and to analgesics administered postoperatively.

Diagnosis is substantiated by electrocardiographic changes, elevated serum creatine kinase levels—especially the MB isoenzyme—and serum troponin I levels. The mortality rate of postoperative myocardial infarction is as high as 67% in high-risk groups. The prognosis is better if it is the first infarction and worse if there have been previous infarctions. Prevention of this complication includes postponing elective operations for 3 months or preferably 6 months after myocardial infarction, treating congestive heart failure preoperatively, and controlling hypertension perioperatively.

Patients with postoperative myocardial infarction should be monitored in the intensive care unit and provided with adequate oxygenation and precise fluid and electrolyte replacement. Anticoagulation, though not always feasible after major surgery, limits the risk of mural thrombosis development and arterial embolism after myocardial infarction. Congestive heart failure should be treated with positive pressure ventilation, diuretics, and vasodilators as needed. Chronic management of congestive heart failure includes ACE inhibitors, diuretics, beta-blockers, and, in severe cases, ventricular assist devices and transplantation.

▶ Postoperative Cardiac Failure

Left ventricular failure and pulmonary edema appear in 4% of patients over age 40 undergoing general surgical procedures with general anesthesia. Fluid overload in patients with limited myocardial reserve is the most common cause. Postoperative myocardial infarction and dysrhythmias producing a high ventricular rate are other causes. Clinical manifestations are progressive dyspnea, hypoxemia with normal CO_2 tension, and diffuse congestion on chest x-ray.

Clinically unapparent ventricular failure is frequent, especially when other factors predisposing to pulmonary edema are present (massive trauma, multiple transfusions, sepsis, etc). The diagnosis may be suspected from a decreased Pao_2, abnormal chest x-ray, or elevated pulmonary artery wedge pressure. The treatment of left ventricular failure depends on the hemodynamic state of the patient. Those who are in shock require transfer to the intensive care unit, placement of a pulmonary artery line, monitoring of filling pressures, and immediate preload and afterload reduction. Preload reduction is achieved by diuretics (and nitroglycerin if needed); afterload reduction, by administration of sodium nitroprusside. ACE inhibitors and beta-blockers have been demonstrated to reduce mortality. Fluids should be restricted, and diuretics may be given. Respiratory insufficiency calls for ventilatory support either with noninvasive positive pressure ventilation or with endotracheal intubation and a mechanical respirator. Although pulmonary function may improve with the use of positive end-expiratory pressure, hemodynamic derangements and decreased myocardial reserve preclude it in most cases.

PULMONARY COMPLICATIONS

Respiratory complications are the most common single cause of morbidity after major surgical procedures and the second most common cause of postoperative deaths in patients older than 60 years. Patients undergoing chest and upper abdominal operations are particularly prone to pulmonary complications. The incidence is lower after pelvic surgery and even lower after extremity or head and neck procedures. Pulmonary complications are more common after emergency operations. Special hazards are posed by preexisting chronic obstructive pulmonary disease (chronic bronchitis, emphysema, asthma, pulmonary fibrosis). Elderly patients are at much higher risk because they have decreased compliance, increased closing and residual volumes, and increased dead space, all of which predispose to atelectasis.

▶ Atelectasis

Atelectasis, the most common pulmonary complication, affects 25% of patients who have abdominal surgery. It is more common in patients who are elderly or overweight and in those who smoke or have symptoms of respiratory disease. It appears most frequently in the first 48 hours after operation and is responsible for over 90% of febrile episodes during that period. In most cases, the course is self-limited and recovery uneventful.

The pathogenesis of atelectasis involves obstructive and nonobstructive factors. Obstruction may be caused by secretions resulting from chronic obstructive pulmonary disease, intubation, or anesthetic agents. Occasional cases may be due to blood clots or malposition of the endotracheal tube. In most instances, however, the cause is not obstruction but closure of the bronchioles. Small bronchioles (≤ 1 mm) are prone to close when lung volume reaches a critical point ("closing volume"). Portions of the lung that are dependent or compressed are the first to experience bronchiole closure, since their regional volume is less than that of nondependent portions. Shallow breathing and failure to periodically hyperinflate the lung result in small alveolar size and decreased volume. The closing volume is higher in older patients and in smokers owing to the loss of elastic recoil of the lung. Other nonobstructive factors contributing to atelectasis include decreased functional residual capacity and loss of pulmonary surfactant.

The air in the atelectatic portion of the lung is absorbed, and since there is minimal change in perfusion, a ventilation/perfusion mismatch results. The immediate effect of atelectasis is decreased oxygenation of blood; its clinical significance depends on the respiratory and cardiac reserve of the patient. A later effect is the propensity of the atelectatic segment to become infected. In general, if a pulmonary segment remains atelectatic for over 72 hours, pneumonia is almost certain to occur.

Atelectasis is usually manifested by fever (pathogenesis unknown), tachypnea, and tachycardia. Physical examination may show elevation of the diaphragm, scattered rales, and decreased breath sounds, but it is often normal. Postoperative atelectasis can be largely prevented by early mobilization, frequent changes in position, encouragement to cough, and use of an incentive spirometer. Preoperative teaching of respiratory exercises and postoperative execution of these exercises prevent atelectasis in patients without preexisting lung disease. Intermittent positive pressure breathing is expensive and less effective than these simpler exercises.

Treatment consists of clearing the airway by chest percussion, coughing, or nasotracheal suction. Bronchodilators and mucolytic agents given by nebulizer may help in patients with severe chronic obstructive pulmonary disease. Atelectasis from obstruction of a major airway may require intrabronchial suction through an endoscope, a procedure that can usually be performed at the bedside with mild sedation.

Pulmonary Aspiration

Aspiration of oropharyngeal and gastric contents is normally prevented by the gastroesophageal and pharyngoesophageal sphincters. Insertion of nasogastric and endotracheal tubes and depression of the central nervous system by drugs interfere with these defenses and predispose to aspiration. Other factors, such as gastroesophageal reflux, food in the stomach, or position of the patient, may play a role. Trauma victims are particularly likely to aspirate regurgitated gastric contents when consciousness is depressed. Patients with intestinal obstruction and pregnant women—who have increased intra-abdominal pressure and decreased gastric motility—are also at high risk of aspiration. Two-thirds of cases of aspiration follow thoracic or abdominal surgery, and of these, one-half result in pneumonia. The death rate for grossly evident aspiration and subsequent pneumonia is about 50%.

Minor amounts of aspiration are frequent during surgery and are apparently well tolerated. Methylene blue placed in the stomach of patients undergoing abdominal operations can be found in the trachea at completion of the procedure in 15% of cases. Radionuclide techniques have shown aspiration of gastric contents in 45% of normal volunteers during sleep.

The magnitude of pulmonary injury produced by aspiration of fluid, usually from gastric contents, is determined by the volume aspirated, its pH, and the frequency of the event. If the aspirate has a pH of 2.5 or less, it causes immediate chemical pneumonitis, which results in local edema and inflammation, changes that increase the risk of secondary infection. Aspiration of solid matter can produce airway obstruction. Obstruction of distal bronchi, though well tolerated initially, can lead to atelectasis and pulmonary abscess formation. The basal segments are affected most often. Tachypnea, rales, and hypoxia are usually present within hours; less frequently, cyanosis, wheezing, and apnea may appear. In patients with massive aspiration, hypovolemia caused by excessive fluid and colloid loss into the injured lung may lead to hypotension and shock.

Aspiration has been found in 80% of patients with tracheostomies and may account for the predisposition to pulmonary infection in this group. Patients who must remain intubated for long periods should have a low-pressure, high-volume cuff on their tube, which helps prevent aspiration and limits the risk of pressure necrosis of the trachea.

Aspiration can be limited by preoperative fasting, proper positioning of the patient, and careful intubation. A single dose of H_2-blocker or proton pump inhibitor before induction of anesthesia may have value when the risk of aspiration is high. Treatment of tracheobronchial aspiration involves reestablishing patency of the airway and preventing further damage to the lung. Endotracheal suction should be performed immediately, as this procedure confirms the diagnosis and stimulates coughing, which helps to clear the airway. Bronchoscopy may be required to remove solid matter. Fluid resuscitation should be undertaken concomitantly. Antibiotics are used initially when the aspirate is heavily contaminated; they are used later to treat pneumonia.

Postoperative Pneumonia

Pneumonia is the most common pulmonary complication among patients who die after surgery. It is directly responsible for death—or is a contributory factor—in more than half of these patients. Patients with peritoneal infection and those requiring prolonged ventilatory support are at highest risk for developing postoperative pneumonia. Atelectasis, aspiration, and copious secretions are important predisposing factors.

Host defenses against pneumonitis include the cough reflex, the mucociliary system, and the activity of alveolar macrophages. After surgery, cough is usually weak and may not effectively clear the bronchial tree. The mucociliary transport mechanism is damaged by endotracheal intubation, and the functional ability of the alveolar macrophage is compromised by a number of factors that may be present during and after surgery (oxygenation, pulmonary edema, tracheobronchial aspiration, corticosteroid therapy, etc). In addition, squamous metaplasia and loss of ciliary coordination further hamper antibacterial defenses. More than half of the pulmonary infections that follow surgery are caused by gram-negative bacilli. They are frequently polymicrobial and usually acquired by aspiration of oropharyngeal secretions. Although colonization of the oropharynx with gram-negative bacteria occurs in only 20% of normal individuals, it is frequent after major surgery as a result of impaired oropharyngeal clearing mechanisms. Aggravating factors are azotemia, prolonged endotracheal intubation, and severe associated infection.

Occasionally, infecting bacteria reach the lung by inhalation—for example, from respirators. *Pseudomonas aeruginosa* and *Klebsiella* can survive in the moist reservoirs of these machines, and these pathogens have been the source of epidemic infections in intensive care units. Rarely, contamination of the lung may result from direct hematogenous spread from distant septic foci.

The clinical manifestations of postoperative pneumonia are fever, tachypnea, increased secretions, and physical changes suggestive of pulmonary consolidation. A chest x-ray usually shows localized parenchymal consolidation. Overall mortality rates for postoperative pneumonia vary from 20% to 40%. Rates are higher when pneumonia develops in patients who had emergency operations, are on respirators, or develop remote organ failure, positive blood cultures, or infection of the second lung.

Maintaining the airway clear of secretions is of paramount concern in the prevention of postoperative pneumonia. Respiratory exercises, deep breathing, and coughing help prevent atelectasis, which is a precursor of pneumonia. Although postoperative pain is thought to contribute to shallow breathing, neither intercostal blocks nor epidural narcotics prevent atelectasis and pneumonia when compared with traditional methods of postoperative pain control. The prophylactic use of antibiotics does not decrease the incidence of gram-negative colonization of the oropharynx or that of pneumonia. Treatment consists of measures to aid the clearing of secretions and administration of antibiotics. Sputum obtained directly from the trachea, usually by endotracheal suctioning, is required for specific identification of the infecting organism.

▶ Postoperative Pleural Effusion & Pneumothorax

Formation of a very small pleural effusion is fairly common immediately after upper abdominal operations and is of no clinical significance. Patients with free peritoneal fluid at the time of surgery and those with postoperative atelectasis are more prone to develop effusions. In the absence of cardiac failure or a pulmonary lesion, appearance of a pleural effusion late in the postoperative course suggests the presence of subdiaphragmatic inflammation (subphrenic abscess, acute pancreatitis, etc). Effusions that do not compromise respiratory function should be left undisturbed. If there is a suspicion of infection, the effusion should be sampled by needle aspiration. When an effusion produces respiratory compromise, it should be drained with a thoracostomy tube.

Postoperative pneumothorax may follow insertion of a subclavian catheter or positive-pressure ventilation, but it sometimes appears after an operation during which the pleura has been injured (eg, nephrectomy or adrenalectomy). Pneumothorax should usually be treated with a thoracostomy tube, depending upon the size and etiology of the pneumothorax.

▶ Fat Embolism

Fat embolism is relatively common but only rarely causes symptoms. Fat particles can be found in the pulmonary vascular bed in 90% of patients who have had fractures of long bones or joint replacements. Fat embolism can also be caused by exogenous sources of fat, such as blood transfusions, intravenous fat emulsion, or bone marrow transplantation. *Fat embolism syndrome* consists of neurologic dysfunction, respiratory insufficiency, and petechiae of the axillae, chest, and proximal arms. It was originally described

in trauma victims—especially those with long bone fractures—and was thought to be a result of bone marrow embolization. However, the principal clinical manifestations of fat embolism are seen in other conditions. The existence of fat embolism as an entity distinct from posttraumatic pulmonary insufficiency has been questioned.

Fat embolism syndrome characteristically begins 12-72 hours after injury but may be delayed for several days. The diagnosis is clinical. The finding of fat droplets in sputum and urine is common after trauma and is not specific. Decreased hematocrit, thrombocytopenia, and other changes in coagulation parameters usually occur.

Once symptoms develop, supportive treatment should be provided until respiratory insufficiency and central nervous system manifestations subside. Respiratory insufficiency is treated with positive end-expiratory pressure ventilation and diuretics. The prognosis is related to the severity of the pulmonary insufficiency.

GI COMPLICATIONS

▶ Alterations in Gastrointestinal Motility

The presence, strength, and direction of normal peristalsis are governed by the enteric nervous system. Anesthesia and surgical manipulation result in a decrease of the normal propulsive activity of the gut, or postoperative ileus. Several factors worsen ileus or prolong its course. These include medications—especially opioids—electrolyte abnormalities, inflammatory conditions such as pancreatitis or peritonitis, and pain. The degree of ileus is related to the extent of operative manipulation.

Gastrointestinal peristalsis returns within 24 hours after most operations that do not involve the abdominal cavity. In general, laparoscopic approaches cause less ileus than open procedures. After laparotomy, gastric peristalsis returns in about 48 hours. Colonic activity returns after 48 hours, starting at the cecum and progressing caudally. The motility of the small intestine is affected to a lesser degree, except in patients who have had small bowel resection or who were operated on to relieve bowel obstruction. Normal postoperative ileus leads to slight abdominal distention and absent bowel sounds. Return of peristalsis is often noted by the patient as mild cramps, passage of flatus, and return of appetite. Feedings should be withheld until there is evidence of return of normal gastrointestinal motility. There is no specific therapy for postoperative ileus.

▶ Gastric Dilation

Gastric dilation, a rare life-threatening complication, consists of massive distention of the stomach by gas and fluid. Predisposing factors include asthma, recent surgery, gastric outlet obstruction, and absence of the spleen. Infants and children in whom oxygen masks are used in the immediate postoperative period and adults subjected to forceful assisted respiration during resuscitation are also at risk. Occasionally, gastric dilation develops in patients with anorexia nervosa or during serious illnesses without a specific intercurrent event.

As the air-filled stomach grows larger, it hangs down across the duodenum, producing a mechanical gastric outlet obstruction that contributes further to the problem. The increased intragastric pressure produces venous obstruction of the mucosa, causing mucosal engorgement and bleeding and, if allowed to continue, ischemic necrosis and perforation. The distended stomach pushes the diaphragm upward, which causes collapse of the lower lobe of the left lung, rotation of the heart, and obstruction of the inferior vena cava. The acutely dilated stomach is also prone to undergo volvulus.

The patient appears ill, with abdominal distention and hiccup. Hypochloremia, hypokalemia, and alkalosis may result from fluid and electrolyte losses. When the problem is recognized early, treatment consists of gastric decompression with a nasogastric tube. In the late stage, gastric necrosis may require gastrectomy.

► Bowel Obstruction

Failure of postoperative return of bowel function may be the result of paralytic ileus or mechanical obstruction. Mechanical obstruction is most often caused by postoperative adhesions or an internal (mesenteric) hernia. Most of these patients experience a short period of apparently normal intestinal function before manifestations of obstruction supervene. About half of cases of early postoperative small bowel obstruction follow colorectal surgery.

Diagnosis may be difficult because the symptoms are difficult to differentiate from those of paralytic ileus. If plain films of the abdomen show air-fluid levels in loops of small bowel, mechanical obstruction is a more likely diagnosis than ileus. Enteroclysis or an ordinary small bowel series with barium sulfate may aid diagnosis.

Strangulation is uncommon because the adhesive bands are broader and less rigid than is typical of late small bowel obstruction. The death rate is high (about 15%), however, probably because of delay in diagnosis and the postoperative state. Treatment consists of nasogastric suction for several days and, if the obstruction does not resolve spontaneously, laparotomy.

Small bowel intussusception is an uncommon cause of early postoperative obstruction in adults but accounts for 10% of cases in the pediatric age group. Ninety percent of postoperative intussusceptions occur during the first 2 postoperative weeks, and more than half in the first week. Unlike idiopathic ileocolic intussusception, most postoperative intussusceptions are ileoileal or jejunojejunal. They most often follow retroperitoneal and pelvic operations. The cause is unknown. The symptom complex is not typical, and x-ray studies are of limited help. The physician should be aware that intussusception is a possible explanation for vomiting, distention, and abdominal pain after laparotomy in children and that early reoperation will avoid the complications of perforation and peritonitis. Operation is the only treatment, and if the bowel is viable, reduction of the intussusception is all that is needed.

► Postoperative Fecal Impaction

Fecal impaction after operative procedures is the result of colonic ileus and impaired perception of rectal fullness. It is principally a disease of the elderly but may occur in younger patients who have predisposing conditions such as megacolon or paraplegia. Postoperative ileus and the use of opioid analgesics and anticholinergic drugs are aggravating factors. Early manifestations are anorexia and obstipation or diarrhea. In advanced cases, marked distention may cause colonic perforation. The diagnosis of postoperative fecal impaction is made by rectal examination. The impaction should be manually removed, enemas given, and digital examination then repeated.

Barium remaining in the colon from an examination done before surgery may harden and produce barium impaction. This usually occurs in the right colon, where most of the water is absorbed, and is a more difficult management problem than fecal impaction. The clinical manifestations are those of bowel obstruction. Treatment includes enemas and purgation with polyethylene glycol-electrolyte solution (eg, CoLyte, GoLYTELY). Diatrizoate sodium (Hypaque), a hyperosmolar solution that stimulates peristalsis and increases intraluminal fluid, may be effective by enema if other solutions fail. Operation is rarely necessary.

► Postoperative Pancreatitis

Postoperative pancreatitis accounts for 10% of all cases of acute pancreatitis. It occurs in 1%-3% of patients who have operations in the vicinity of the pancreas and with higher frequency after operations on the biliary tract. For example, pancreatitis occurs in about 1% of patients undergoing cholecystectomy and in 8% of patients undergoing common bile duct exploration. In the latter cases, it does not appear to be related to the performance of intraoperative cholangiograms or choledochoscopy. Postoperative pancreatitis after biliary surgery is worse in patients who have had biliary pancreatitis preoperatively. Pancreatitis occasionally occurs following cardiopulmonary bypass, parathyroid surgery, and renal transplantation. Postoperative pancreatitis is frequently of the necrotizing type. Infected pancreatic necrosis and other complications of pancreatitis develop with a frequency three to four times greater than in biliary and alcoholic pancreatitis. The reason postoperative pancreatitis is so severe is unknown, but the mortality rate is 30%-40%.

The pathogenesis in most cases appears to be mechanical trauma to the pancreas or its blood supply. Nevertheless, manipulation, biopsy, and partial resection of the pancreas are usually well tolerated, so the reasons that some patients develop pancreatitis are unclear. Prevention of this complication includes careful handling of the pancreas and avoidance of forceful dilation of the choledochal sphincter or obstruction of the pancreatic duct. The 2% incidence of pancreatitis following renal transplantation is probably related to special risk factors such as use of corticosteroids or azathioprine, secondary hyperparathyroidism, or viral infection. Acute changes in serum calcium are thought to be responsible for pancreatitis following parathyroid surgery. Serum amylase elevation develops in about half of patients undergoing heart surgery with extracorporeal bypass, but clinical evidence of pancreatitis is present in only 5% of these patients.

The diagnosis of postoperative pancreatitis may be difficult in patients who have recently had an abdominal operation. Serum amylase elevation may or may not be present. One must be alert to renal and respiratory complications and the consequences of necrotizing or hemorrhagic pancreatitis. Because of the high frequency with which complications develop, frequent monitoring of the pancreas and retroperitoneum with CT scans is useful.

▶ Postoperative Hepatic Dysfunction

Hepatic dysfunction, ranging from mild jaundice to life-threatening hepatic failure, follows 1% of surgical procedures performed under general anesthesia. The incidence is greater following pancreatectomy, biliary bypass operations, and portacaval shunt. Postoperative hyperbilirubinemia may be categorized as prehepatic jaundice, hepatocellular insufficiency, and posthepatic obstruction (Table 5–1).

Table 5–1 Causes of postoperative jaundice.

Prehepatic jaundice (bilirubin overload)
Hemolysis (drugs, transfusions, sickle cell crisis)
Reabsorption of hematomas
Hepatocellular insufficiency
Viral hepatitis
Drug-induced (anesthesia, others)
Ischemia (shock, hypoxia, low-output states)
Sepsis
Liver resection (loss of parenchyma)
Others (total parenteral nutrition, malnutrition)
Posthepatic obstruction (to bile flow)
Retained stones
Injury to ducts
Tumor (unrecognized or untreated)
Cholecystitis
Pancreatitis
Occlusion of biliary stents

Prehepatic Jaundice

Prehepatic jaundice is caused by bilirubin overload, most often from hemolysis or reabsorption of hematomas. Fasting, malnutrition, hepatotoxic drugs, and anesthesia are among the factors that impair the ability of the liver to excrete increased loads of bilirubin in the postoperative period.

Increased hemolysis may result from transfusion of incompatible blood but more often reflects destruction of fragile transfused red blood cells. Other causes include extracorporeal circulation, congenital hemolytic disease (eg, sickle cell disease), and effects of drugs.

Hepatocellular Insufficiency

Hepatocellular insufficiency, the most common cause of postoperative jaundice, occurs as a consequence of hepatic cell necrosis, inflammation, or massive hepatic resection. Drugs, hypotension, hypoxia, and sepsis are among the injurious factors. Although posttransfusion hepatitis is usually observed much later, this complication may occur as early as the third postoperative week.

Benign postoperative intrahepatic cholestasis is a vague term used to denote jaundice following operations that often involve hypotension and multiple transfusions. Serum bilirubin ranges from 2 to 20 mg/dL and serum alkaline phosphatase is usually high, but the patient is afebrile and postoperative convalescence is otherwise smooth. The diagnosis is one of exclusion. Jaundice clears by the third postoperative week.

Hepatocellular damage occasionally occurs after intestinal bypass procedures for morbid obesity. Cholestatic jaundice may develop in patients receiving total parenteral nutrition.

Posthepatic Obstruction

Posthepatic obstruction can be caused by direct surgical injury to the bile ducts, retained common duct stones, tumor obstruction of the bile duct, or pancreatitis. Acute postoperative cholecystitis is associated with jaundice in one-third of cases, though mechanical obstruction of the common duct is usually not apparent.

One must determine if a patient with postoperative jaundice has a correctable cause that requires treatment. This is particularly true for sepsis (when decreased liver function may sometimes be an early sign), lesions that obstruct the bile duct, and postoperative cholecystitis. Liver function tests are not helpful in determining the cause and do not usually reflect the severity of disease. Liver biopsy, ultrasound and CT scans, and transhepatic or endoscopic retrograde cholangiograms are the tests most likely to sort out the diagnostic possibilities. Renal function must be monitored closely, since renal failure may develop in these patients. Treatment is otherwise expectant.

Postoperative Cholecystitis

Acute postoperative cholecystitis may follow any kind of operation but is more common after gastrointestinal procedures. Acute cholecystitis develops shortly after endoscopic sphincterotomy in 3%-5% of patients. Chemical cholecystitis occurs in patients undergoing hepatic arterial chemotherapy with mitomycin and floxuridine with such frequency that cholecystectomy should always be performed before infusion of these agents is begun. Fulminant cholecystitis with gallbladder infarction may follow percutaneous embolization of the hepatic artery for malignant tumors of the liver or for arteriovenous malformation involving this artery.

Postoperative cholecystitis differs in several respects from the common form of acute cholecystitis: It is frequently acalculous (70%-80%), more common in males (75%), progresses rapidly to gallbladder necrosis, and is not likely to respond to conservative therapy. The cause is clear in cases of chemical or ischemic cholecystitis but not in other forms. Factors thought to play a role include biliary stasis (with formation of sludge), biliary infection, and ischemia.

Abdominal Compartment Syndrome

Aggressive resuscitation of patients, particularly those involved in trauma or requiring an emergent celiotomy, may result in increased abdominal pressure. Intra-abdominal hypertension, as measured by bladder pressure, is generally self-limiting; however, it can become dangerous when pressures exceed 30 mm Hg. In this scenario venous outflow from the bowel and kidney may become compromised. Furthermore, respiratory complications may ensue as the pressure exerted upon the diaphragm may decrease tidal volume and result in respiratory acidosis. In this situation, the abdominal compartment must be rapidly decompressed, usually by opening the abdomen, in order to reestablish flow from the viscera.

Similar to compartment syndrome of the extremities, the fascia resists stretch exerted by the muscle and other tissue after injury and resuscitation. Unlike the extremities, patients with abdominal compartment syndrome do not exhibit the five Ps (pain, paresthesia, pallor, paralysis, and pulselessness) that may be easily followed in the limb. However, a high index of suspicion, rapid diagnosis, and expeditious treatment result in restoration of flow and prevention of morbidity in both scenarios.

GENITOURINARY COMPLICATIONS

Postoperative Urinary Retention

Inability to void postoperatively is common, especially after pelvic and perineal operations or operations conducted under spinal anesthesia. Factors responsible for postoperative urinary retention are interference with the neural mechanisms responsible for normal emptying of the bladder and overdistention of the urinary bladder. When its normal capacity of approximately 500 mL is exceeded, bladder contraction is inhibited. Prophylactic bladder catheterization should be considered whenever an operation is likely to last 3 hours or longer or when large volumes of intravenous fluids are anticipated. The catheter can be removed at the end of the operation if the patient is expected to be able to ambulate within a few hours. When bladder catheterization is not performed, the patient should be encouraged to void immediately before coming to the operating room and as soon as possible after the operation. During abdominoperineal resection, operative trauma to the sacral plexus alters bladder function enough so that an indwelling catheter should be left in place for 4-5 days. Patients with inguinal hernia who strain to void as a manifestation of prostatic hypertrophy should have the prostate treated before the hernia.

The treatment of acute urinary retention is catheterization of the bladder. In the absence of factors that suggest the need for prolonged decompression, such as the presence of 1000 mL of urine or more, the catheter may be removed.

Urinary Tract Infection

Infection of the lower urinary tract is the most frequently acquired nosocomial infection. Preexisting contamination of the urinary tract, urinary retention, and instrumentation are the principal contributing factors. Bacteriuria is present in about 5% of patients who undergo short-term (< 48 hours) bladder catheterization, though clinical signs of urinary tract infection occur in only 1%. Cystitis is manifested by dysuria and mild fever and pyelonephritis by high fever, flank tenderness, and occasionally ileus. Diagnosis is made by examination of the urine and confirmed by cultures. Prevention involves treating urinary tract contamination before surgery, prevention or prompt treatment of urinary retention, and careful instrumentation when needed. Treatment includes adequate hydration, proper drainage of the bladder, and specific antibiotics.

INFECTIOUS COMPLICATIONS

Infectious complications are perhaps the most common postoperative complication and include those related directly to the surgical incision, termed *surgical site infection* (SSI), and those that involve other systems, such as *Clostridium difficile* colitis and parotitis. Certain infections such as a urinary tract infection and postoperative pneumonia have already been discussed and will not be noted in this section.

A wide range of organisms are involved in these infections, but what is very concerning is the increasing prevalence of antibiotic-resistant bacteria, such as methicillin-resistant *Staphylococcus aureus* (MRSA) and vancomycin-resistant *Enterococcus* (VRE).

Surgical Site Infection

The Center for Disease Control (CDC) classifies SSIs into three locations:

1. Superficial incisional
2. Deep incisional
3. Organ space

The risk for developing an SSI has been estimated at 4% rate in clean wounds and 35% in grossly contaminated wounds.

Risk factors for SSI include systemic factors (diabetes, immunosuppression, obesity, smoking malnutrition, and previous radiation) and local factors (surgical wound classification and surgical techniques).

Prevention of SSI includes meticulous surgical techniques (skin preparation, maintaining sterility, judicious use of cautery, respecting dissection planes, approximating tissue neatly, etc) and administration of appropriate preoperative antibiotics as determined by the type of operation being performed (see http://www.cdc.gov/hicpac/pdf/guidelines/SSI_1999.pdf). Clean cases such as an inguinal hernia repair, for instance, would necessitate administration of antibiotics that would target skin flora such as cefazolin. Contaminated cases that enter the gastrointestinal tract, on the other hand, would require antibiotics such as cefazolin and metronidazole that would target both skin flora and gastrointestinal bacteria such as anaerobes.

The diagnosis of SSI is primarily clinical. Common symptoms include pain, warmth, and erythema with drainage through the incision. Deep and organ space infections may be further diagnosed with radiographic imaging.

Treatment for an SSI emphasizes primary source control. Gaining such control may require an operative procedure such as an incision and drainage of the infectious source. For superficial infections, the treatment would simply include opening the incision, exploring the space, irrigating, debriding, and leaving the wound open with local wound care. Deep incisional and organ space infections may necessitate open operative drainage and debridement or percutaneous drainage procedures. Antibiotics by themselves do not usually address the underlying focus of infection.

Clostridium difficile Colitis

Postoperative diarrhea due to *C difficile* is a common nosocomial infection in surgical patients. The spectrum of illness ranges from asymptomatic colonization to—rarely—severe toxic colitis. Transmission from hospital personnel probably occurs. The main risk factor is perioperative antibiotic use. The diagnosis is established by identification of a specific cytopathic toxin in the stool or culture of the organism from stool samples or rectal swabs. In severely affected patients, colonoscopy reveals pseudomembranes.

Prevention is accomplished by strict handwashing, enteric precautions, and minimizing antibiotic use. Treatment of established infection is with intravenous metronidazole or, for infections with resistant pathogens, oral vancomycin.

Drug-Resistant Organisms

An increase in the prevalence of multidrug-resistant organisms has been noted over the past two decades, particularly MRSA and VRE. Although routine screening of patients has found the prevalence as high as 30% in the community, these organisms are much more frequently found in the hospital or other institutions (nursing homes, prisons, gymnasiums, etc). Increased antibiotic usage in the inpatient and outpatient settings has been speculated to be the cause of the drug resistance; however, the spread within institutions has been demonstrated to be due to direct patient contact. Continuous surface decontamination, utilization of barrier techniques when examining patients, and assiduous hand hygiene have been shown to decrease transmission. Furthermore, discontinuation of inappropriate antibiotics has been shown to limit the colonization of patients with most drug-resistant organisms, including *C difficile*.

HEMATOLOGIC COMPLICATIONS

Besides causing bleeding, major surgery such as abdominal and trauma operations alter the fine balance of the body's hematologic system especially with regards to the coagulation pathway.

Venous Thromboembolism

Rudolf Virchow first postulated the pathophysiology of thrombosis in 1846. The tenets of his triad: hypercoagulable state, stasis, and vessel damage, largely hold today. Patients involved in trauma, cancer operations, or dissections of the pelvis are particularly susceptible to the phenomenon. Postoperative patients should be carefully monitored for lower extremity swelling, hypoxia, or new-onset pleuritic chest pain, as these may be harbingers of the syndrome. Risk factors include those that are nonmodifiable (thrombophilia, prior VTE, congestive heart failure, chronic lung disease, paralytic stroke, malignancy, spinal cord injury, obesity, age > 40, varicosities) and modifiable (type of surgery: hip, lower extremity, major general surgery, mechanical ventilation, major trauma, central venous lines, chemotherapy, hormone replacement therapy, pregnancy, immobility). Outcomes from pulmonary embolism vary in severity from being relatively asymptomatic to resulting in cardiac arrest or sudden death. Long-term complications, such as pulmonary hypertension, may ensue in patients who are not adequately treated.

Prevention of VTE is much more effective than management of this complication. The CHEST guidelines are a useful adjunct to stratifying risk and assigning appropriate preventive therapy. This usually requires heparin therapy with regular or low-molecular-weight heparin, sequential compression stockings, and early ambulation. Inferior vena cava filters may be considered as a preventive method in patients who have contraindications to anticoagulation or have progression of disease despite adequate anticoagulation.

Diagnosis of deep vein thrombosis may be performed in a cost-effective manner by utilizing duplex ultrasonography. CT, MRI, or traditional venography are more expensive and more invasive methods for establishing disease occurrence. Pulmonary embolism can be diagnosed by echocardiography, ventilation/perfusion scan, and formal angiography; however, helical CT angiography is the most commonly utilized technique. Unfortunately, although physical examination leads to a high degree of suspicion, it alone remains neither specific nor sensitive.

The goals of treatment of VTE remain stabilization of clot, revasculature of affected vessels, and prevention of long-term complications. The majority of these patients respond to anticoagulation with intravenous heparin or higher doses of subcutaneous low-molecular-weight heparin and, subsequent, conversion to oral therapy with warfarin. In patients who have hemodynamic instability due to a pulmonary embolus, consideration to system thrombolysis, suction embolectomy, or a Trendelenburg procedure should be given.

▶ Heparin-Induced Thrombocytopenia

Thrombocytopenia is a commonly found finding in the postoperative period and its cause may be several. Postoperative thrombocytopenia is generally considered to be a 50% reduction in total platelet volume. The platelet reduction in HIT generally is seen 1 week after initial exposure to heparin. The incidence is greater with unfractionated heparin than low-molecular-weight heparin. Although generally associated with thrombocytopenia, the initial phase is a procoagulative and thrombotic with many patients experiencing VTE, myocardial infarction, or stroke. Thrombocytopenia is a late finding in patients. Once suspicious of HIT, all heparin, including flushes and coated catheters, should be discontinued and an antibody assay should be performed.

If the diagnosis of HIT is confirmed, the discontinuation of heparin and heparin-coated products should be maintained. If anticoagulation is necessary, use of Lepirudin or Argatroban should be considered. The choice of agent is generally made by patient factors: Lepirudin should be avoided in patients with renal failure and Argatroban should be avoided in patients with hepatic failure. Long-term anticoagulation may be transitioned to warfarin; however, warfarin must not be administered during the acute phase of HIT as this may lead to a pronounced procoagulant phase.

SYSTEMIC COMPLICATIONS

▶ Postoperative Fever

Fever occurs in about 40% of patients after major surgery. In most patients the temperature elevation resolves without specific treatment. However, postoperative fever may herald a serious infection, and it is therefore important to evaluate the patient clinically. Features often associated with an infectious origin of the fever include preoperative trauma, ASA class above 2, fever onset after the second postoperative day, an initial temperature elevation above 38.6°C, a postoperative white blood cell count greater than 10,000/L, and a postoperative serum urea nitrogen of 15 mg/dL or greater. If three or more of the above are present, the likelihood of associated bacterial infection is nearly 100%.

Fever within 48 hours after surgery is usually caused by atelectasis. Reexpansion of the lung causes body temperature to return to normal. Because laboratory and radiologic investigations are usually unrevealing, an extensive evaluation of early postoperative fever is rarely appropriate if the patient's convalescence is otherwise smooth.

When fever appears after the second postoperative day, atelectasis is a less likely explanation. The differential diagnosis of fever at this time includes catheter-related phlebitis, pneumonia, and urinary tract infection. A directed history and physical examination complemented by focused laboratory and radiologic studies usually determine the cause.

Patients without infection are rarely febrile after the fifth postoperative day. Fever this late suggests wound infection or, less often, anastomotic breakdown and intra-abdominal abscesses. A diagnostic workup directed to the detection of intra-abdominal sepsis is indicated in patients who have high temperatures (> 39°C) and wounds without evidence of infection 5 or more days postoperatively. CT scan of the abdomen and pelvis is the test of choice and should be performed early, before overt organ failure occurs.

Fever is rare after the first week in patients who had a normal convalescence. Allergy to drugs, transfusion-related fever, septic pelvic vein thrombosis, and intra-abdominal abscesses should be considered.

▶ References

Compoginis JM, Katz SG. American College of Surgeons National Surgical Quality Improvement Program as a quality improvement tool: a single institution's experience with vascular surgical site infections. *Am Surg.* 2013 Mar;79(3):274-278.

Koch CG, Li L, Hixson E, et al. What are the real rates of postoperative complications: elucidating inconsistencies between administrative and clinical data sources. *J Am Coll Surg.* 2012 May;214(5):798-805.

Lawson EH, Louie R, Zingmond DS, et al. A comparison of clinical registry versus administrative claims data for reporting of 30-day surgical complications. *Ann Surg.* 2012 Dec;256(6):973-981.

O'Doherty AF, West M, Jack S, Grocott MP. Preoperative aerobic exercise training in elective intra-cavity surgery: a systematic review. *Br J Anaesth.* 2013 May;110(5):679-689.

MULTIPLE CHOICE QUESTIONS

1. All of the following are true of respiratory complications, *except*
   A. They are common after chest procedures, but rare after abdominal operations
   B. They are the most common single cause of morbidity after major surgical procedures
   C. They occur more commonly in the elderly, smokers, and obese patients
   D. Predisposing factors can be moderated by preoperative and postoperative activities
   E. They include atelectasis, pneumonia, aspiration, and pulmonary emboli

2. A 64-year-old woman is 12 days after total abdominal hysterectomy for benign disease. She returns to the emergency room with nausea and vomiting, and has an abdominal examination that is distended, but not very tender, and her wound is clean. An abdominal series shows some dilated loops of small bowel but no free air.
   A. She should return to the operating room as soon as is practical for lysis of adhesions.
   B. The abdominal focus of her symptoms rules out chest problems such as pneumonia.
   C. Her initial management can include intravenous hydration and nasogastric suction.
   D. The presence of dilated loops of bowel on radiographs rules out the possibility of a benign ileus.
   E. Both A and C are true.

3. A 82-year-old woman underwent a laparoscopic hand-assisted sigmoid colectomy with diverting loop ileostomy 5 days ago for a rectal cancer after neoadjuvant radiation therapy. She is tolerating a regular diet and her ileostomy is healthy and functional. The nurses report that she is somewhat somnolent, and has not urinated during the past two shifts. Which is the most likely cause of her anuria?
   A. Acute renal failure
   B. Inadequate fluid resuscitation in the operating room
   C. High ileostomy output with inadequate postoperative replacement
   D. Low cardiac output
   E. Urinary retention

4. A 30-year-old man is 16 hours s/p emergency laparotomy for blunt abdominal trauma from a motor vehicle accident. His spleen was removed, a liver laceration was managed with sutures and topical procoagulants, and a segment of damaged jejunum was resected. His operation took 3 hours, and he received 12 units of crystalloid, 6 units of blood, 4 units of fresh frozen plasma, and 5 units of platelets. His abdominal wall was closed primarily. He remains intubated and ventilated in the SICU. His urine output was 55 mL over the last 6 hours. Further steps in his management should include the following:
   A. Early extubation is preferable to limit the risk of pneumonia, even if his mental status is not yet clear.
   B. Aggressive early diuresis can promote continued renal function.
   C. Further fluid resuscitation is rarely necessary after the bleeding is controlled.
   D. Bladder pressure measurement may be useful to determine the likelihood of abdominal compartment syndrome.
   E. A and C.

5. All of the following are true about surgical site infection, except
   A. Classified by the Centers for Disease Control into: (1) wound only, (2) organ space, and (3) involving organ parenchyma
   B. Risk varies based upon degree of wound contamination by bacteria
   C. Risk is modified by patient factors such as diabetes and ongoing immunosuppression
   D. May have reduced risk by the use of appropriately chosen and timed antibiotics
   E. Treatment emphasizes primary source control

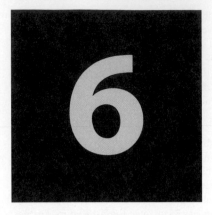

6

Wound Healing

Michael G. Franz, MD

Acute Wound

An acute wound results from the sudden loss of anatomic structure in tissue following the transfer of kinetic, chemical, or thermal energy. Functionally, an acute wound should pass predictably through the phases of wound healing to result in complete and sustained repair. Acute wounds typically occur in recently uninjured and otherwise normal tissue. Acute wound healing is timely and reliable, completing the entire process within 6-12 weeks. Most surgical wounds are acute wounds.

Chronic Wound

Wound healing fails in a chronic wound. The process of tissue repair is prolonged and pathologic. The usual mechanism is dysregulation of one of the phases of normal acute wound healing. Most often, healing arrest occurs in an inflammatory phase. This prolonged inflammatory phase may be due to wound infection or another form of chronic irritation. Tissue and wound hypoxia is the other important mechanism for the development of a chronic wound. Failed epithelialization due to repeat trauma or desiccation may also result in a chronic partial thickness wound. Surgeons may sharply convert a chronic wound into an acute wound.

GENERAL CONSIDERATIONS

Clinical Wound Healing

Surgeons often describe wound healing as primary or secondary. *Primary healing* occurs when tissue is cleanly incised and anatomically reapproximated. It is also referred to as healing by primary intention, and tissue repair usually proceeds without complication. *Secondary healing* occurs in wounds left open through the formation of granulation tissue and eventual coverage of the defect by migration of epithelial cells. Granulation tissue is composed of new capillaries, fibroblasts, and a provisional extracellular matrix that forms at the base of the early wound. This process is also referred to as healing by secondary intention. Most infected wounds and burns heal in this manner. Primary healing is simpler and requires less time and tissue synthesis than secondary healing. A wound healing primarily repairs a smaller volume than an open wound healing secondarily. The principles of primary and secondary healing are combined in *delayed primary closure*, when a wound is left open to heal under a carefully maintained, moist wound healing environment for approximately 5 days and is then closed as if primarily. Wounds treated with delayed primary closure are less likely to become infected than if closed immediately because bacterial balance is achieved and oxygen requirements are optimized through capillary formation in the granulation tissue.

The Mechanism of Wound Healing

The complex process of wound healing normally proceeds from coagulation and inflammation through fibroplasia, matrix deposition, angiogenesis, epithelialization, collagen maturation, and finally wound contraction (Figure 6–1). Wound healing signals include peptide growth factors, complement, cytokine inflammatory mediators, and metabolic signals such as hypoxia and accumulated lactate. Many of these cellular signaling pathways are redundant and pleiotropic.

A. Hemostasis and Inflammation

Following injury, a wound must stop bleeding in order to heal and for the injured host to survive. It is therefore not surprising that cellular and molecular elements involved in hemostasis also signal tissue repair. Immediately after injury, the coagulation products fibrin, fibrinopeptides,

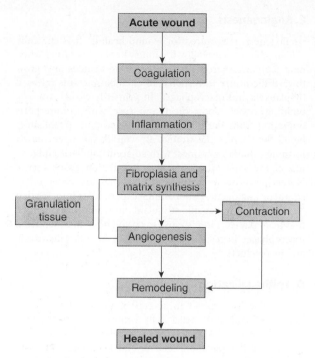

▲ Figure 6–1. Acute wound healing normally proceeds from coagulation and inflammation, through angiogenesis, fibroplasia, matrix deposition (granulation tissue formation), collagen maturation, epithelialization, and finally wound contraction. A chronic wound fails to heal anywhere along this wound healing pathway.

thrombin split products, and complement components attract inflammatory cells into the wound. Platelets activated by thrombin release insulinlike growth factor 1 (IGF-1), transforming growth factor α (TGF-α), transforming growth factor β (TGF-β), and platelet-derived growth factor (PDGF), which attract leukocytes, particularly macrophages, and fibroblasts into the wound. Damaged endothelial cells respond to a signal cascade involving the complement products C5a, tumor necrosis factor α (TNF-α), interleukin-1 (IL-1), and interleukin-8 (IL-8), and express receptors for integrin molecules on the cell membranes of leukocytes. Circulating leukocytes then adhere to the endothelium and migrate into the wounded tissue. Interleukins and other inflammatory components, such as histamine, serotonin, and bradykinin, cause vessels first to constrict for hemostasis and later to dilate, becoming porous so that blood plasma and leukocytes can migrate into the injured area.

The very early wound inflammatory cells increase metabolic demand. Since the local microvasculature is damaged, a local energy sink results, and Pao_2 falls while CO_2 accumulates. Lactate in particular plays a critical role, since its

source is mainly aerobic, and its level is tightly regulated by tissue oxygen levels. Oxidative stress is an important signal for tissue repair. These conditions trigger reparative processes and stimulate their propagation.

Macrophages assume a dominant role in the synthesis of wound healing molecules as coagulation-mediated tissue repair signals fall. Importantly, macrophages, stimulated by fibrin, continue to release large quantities of lactate. This process continues even as oxygen levels begin to rise, thereby maintaining the "environment of injury." Lactate alone stimulates angiogenesis and collagen deposition through the sustained production of growth factors. Unless the wound becomes infected, the granulocyte population that dominated the first days diminishes. Macrophages now cover the injured surface. Fibroblasts begin to organize, mixed with buds of new blood vessels. It has been shown that circulating stem cells, such as bone marrow–derived mesenchymal stem cells, contribute fibroblasts to the healing wound, but the extent of this process is as yet unknown.

B. Fibroplasia and Matrix Synthesis

Fibroplasia—Throughout wound healing, fibroplasia (the replication of fibroblasts) is stimulated by multiple mechanisms, starting with PDGF, IGF-1, and TGF-β released by platelets and later by the continual release of numerous peptide growth factors from macrophages and even fibroblasts within the wound. Growth factors and cytokines shown to stimulate fibroplasia and wound healing include fibroblast growth factor (FGF), IGF-1, vascular endothelial growth factor (VEGF), IL-1, IL-2, IL-8, PDGF, TGF-α, TGF-β, and TNF-α. Dividing fibroblasts localize near the wound edge, an active tissue repair environment with tissue oxygen tensions of approximately 40 mm Hg in normally healing wounds. In cell culture, this Pao_2 is optimum for fibroblast replication. Smooth muscle cells are also likely progenitors because fibroblasts seem to migrate from the adventitia and media of wound vessels. Lipocytes, pericytes, and other cell sources may exist for terminal differentiation into repair fibroblasts.

Matrix synthesis—Fibroblasts secrete the collagen and proteoglycans of the connective tissue matrix that hold wound edges together and embed cells of the healing wound matrix. These extracellular molecules assume polymeric forms and become the physical basis of wound strength (Figure 6–2). Collagen synthesis is not a constitutive property of fibroblasts but must be signaled. The mechanisms that regulate the stimulation and synthesis of collagen are multifactorial and include both growth factors and metabolic inputs such as lactate. The collagen gene promoter has regulatory binding sites to stress corticoids, the TGF-β signaling pathway, and retinoids, which control collagen gene expression. Other growth factors regulate glycosaminoglycans, tissue inhibitors of metalloproteinase (TIMP), and fibronectin synthesis.

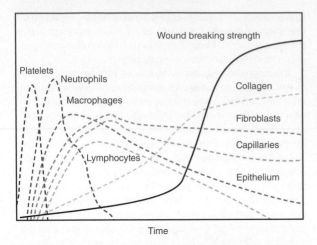

▲ Figure 6–2. The fundamental cellular and molecular elements activated during normal wound healing.

The accumulation of lactate in the extracellular environment is shown to directly stimulate transcription of collagen genes as well as posttranslational processing of collagen peptides. It is clear that the redox state and energy stores of repair cells occupying the wound regulate collagen synthesis.

The increase in collagen messenger RNA (mRNA) leads to an increased procollagen peptide. This, however, is not sufficient to increase collagen deposition because procollagen peptide cannot be transported from the cell to the extracellular space until, in a posttranslational step, a proportion of its proline amino acids are hydroxylated. In this reaction, catalyzed by prolyl hydroxylase, an oxygen atom derived from dissolved O_2 is inserted (as a hydroxyl group) into selected collagen prolines in the presence of the cofactors ascorbic acid, iron, and α-ketoglutarate. Thus, accumulation of lactate, or any other process that decreases the nicotinamide adenine dinucleotide (NAD^+) pool, leads to production of collagen mRNAs, increased collagen peptide synthesis, and (provided enough ascorbate and oxygen is present) increased posttranslational modification and secretion of collagen monomers into the extracellular space.

Another enzyme, lysyl hydroxylase, hydroxylates many of the procollagen lysines. A lysyl-to-lysyl covalent link then occurs between collagen molecules, maximizing mature collagen fiber strength. This process, too, requires adequate amounts of ascorbate and oxygen. These oxygenase reactions (and therefore collagen deposition) are rate limited by tissue oxygen level, Pao_2. The rates are half-maximal at about 20 mm Hg and maximal at about 200 mm Hg. Hydroxylation can be "forced" to supernormal rates by tissue hyperoxia. Collagen deposition, wound strength, and angiogenesis rates may be increased and accelerated as tissue Pao_2 is elevated.

C. Angiogenesis

Angiogenesis is required for wound healing. It is clinically evident about 4 days following injury but begins earlier when new capillaries sprout from preexisting venules and grow toward the injury in response to chemoattractants released by platelets and macrophages. In primarily closed wounds, budding vessels soon meet and fuse with counterparts migrating from the other side of the wound, establishing blood flow across the wound. In wounds left open, newly forming capillaries connect with adjacent capillaries migrating in the same direction, and granulation tissue forms. Numerous growth factors and cytokines are observed to stimulate angiogenesis, but animal experiments indicate that the dominant angiogenic stimulants in wounds are derived first from platelets in response to coagulation and then from macrophages in response to hypoxia or high lactate, fibrin, and its products.

D. Epithelialization

Epithelial cells respond to several of the same stimuli as fibroblasts and endothelial cells within the mesenchymal area of a wound. A variety of growth factors also regulate epithelial cell replication. TGF-α and keratinocyte growth factor (KGF), for instance, are potent epithelial cell mitogens. TGF-β tends to inhibit epithelial cells from differentiating and thus may potentiate and perpetuate mitogenesis, though it is itself not a mitogen for these cells. During wound healing, mitoses appear in the epithelium a few cells away from the wound edge. The new cells migrate over the cells at the edge and into the unhealed area and anchor to the first unepithelialized matrix position encountered. The Pao_2 on the underside of the cell at the anchor point is usually low. Low Pao_2 stimulates squamous epithelial cells to produce TGF-β, likely suppressing terminal differentiation and again supporting further mitosis. This process of epidermal-mesenchymal communication repeats itself until the wound is closed.

Squamous epithelialization and differentiation proceed maximally when surface wounds are kept moist. It is clear that even short periods of drying impair the process, and therefore wounds should not be allowed to desiccate. The exudates from acute, uninfected superficial wounds also contain growth factors and lactate, and therefore recapitulate the growth environment found at the base of the wound.

E. Collagen Fiber Remodeling and Wound Contraction

Remodeling of the wound extracellular matrix is also a well-regulated process. First, fibroblasts replace the provisional fibrin matrix with collagen monomers. Extracellular enzymes, some of which are Pao_2-dependent, quickly polymerize these monomers, initially in a pattern that is more random than in uninjured tissue, predisposing early

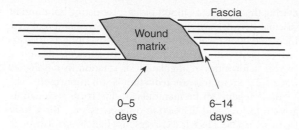

Figure 6–3. The very early wound matrix is weak and susceptible to mechanical failure, especially in load-bearing tissues like the abdominal wall. After 5 days, mechanical failure occurs at the interface of the wound matrix and the uninjured surrounding tissue.

wound to mechanical failure. Progressively, the very early provisional matrix is replaced with a more mature one by forming larger, better organized, stronger, and more durable collagen fibers. The very early wound provisional matrix usually mechanically fails within the matrix itself (days 0-5). Next, mechanical failure occurs at the matrix-tissue interface or fusion point (Figure 6–3). The mechanism for connecting the wound matrix to the uninjured tissue border is poorly understood.

Reorganization of the new matrix is an important feature of healing, and fibroblasts and leukocytes secrete collagenases that ensure the lytic component. Turnover occurs rapidly at first and then more slowly. Even in simple wounds, wound matrix turnover can be detected chemically for as long as 18 months. Healing is successful when a net excess of matrix is deposited despite concomitant lysis. Lysis, in contrast to anabolic synthesis, is less dependent upon energy and nutrition. If synthesis is impaired, however, lysis weakens wounds.

During rapid turnover, wounds normally gain strength and durability but are vulnerable to contraction or stretching. Fibroblasts exert the force for contraction. Fibroblasts attach to collagen and each other and pull the collagen network together when the cell membranes shorten as the fibroblasts migrate. The wound myofibroblast, a specialized phenotype, expresses intracellular actin filaments that also contribute force to fibroblast-mediated wound contraction. The collagen fibers are then fixed in the packed positions by a variety of cross-linking mechanisms. Both open and closed wounds tend to contract if not subjected to a superior counterforce. The phenomenon is best seen in surface wounds, which may close 90% or more by contraction alone in loose skin. For example, the residual of a large open wound on the back of the neck may be only a small area of epithelialization. On the back, the buttock, or the neck, this is often a beneficial process, whereas in the face

and around joints, the results may be disabling or disfiguring. Pathological wound contraction is usually termed a contracture or a stricture. Skin grafts, especially thick ones, may minimize or prevent disabling wound contractures. Dynamic splints, passive or active stretching, or insertion of flaps containing dermis and subdermis also counteract contraction. Prevention of a stricture often depends on ensuring that opposing tissue edges are well perfused so that healing can proceed quickly to completion and contraction stops. Healing wounds may also stretch during active turnover when tension overcomes contraction. This may account for the laxity of scars in ligaments of injured but unsplinted joints and the tendency for incisional hernia formation in abdominal wounds of obese patients.

F. Healing of Specialized Tissues

Tissue other than skin heals generally by the same fundamental pathways. Although tissue structure may be specialized, the initial repair processes are shared. It does appear that the rate and efficiency of wound healing in different tissue types depends in large part on total collagen content, collagen organization, and blood supply.

Gastrointestinal tract—The rate of repair varies from one part of the intestine to the other in proportion to blood supply. Anastomoses of the colon and esophagus heal least reliably and are most likely to leak, whereas failure of stomach or small intestine anastomoses is rare. Intestinal anastomoses regain strength rapidly when compared to skin wounds. After 1 week, bursting strength may exceed the uninjured surrounding intestine. However, the surrounding intestine also participates in the reaction to injury, initially losing collagen by lysis, and as a result may lose strength. For this reason, leakage can occur a few millimeters from the anastomosis. A tight suture line causing ischemia will exacerbate this surgical problem.

The mesothelial cell lining of the peritoneum also is important for healing in the abdomen and GI tract. The esophagus and retroperitoneal colon lack a serosal mesothelial lining, which may contribute to failed wound healing. There is evidence that mesothelial cells signal the repair of peritoneal linings and are a source of repair cells.

Comorbidities that delay collagen synthesis or stimulate collagen lysis are likely to increase the risk of perforation and leakage. The danger of leakage is greatest from the fourth to seventh days, when tensile strength normally would rise rapidly but may be impeded by impaired collagen deposition or increased lysis. Local infection, which most often occurs near esophageal and colonic anastomoses, promotes lysis and delays synthesis, thus increasing the likelihood of perforation.

Bone—Bone healing is controlled by many of the same mechanisms that control soft tissue healing. It too occurs in predictable, morphologic stages: inflammation, fibroplasia, and remodeling. The duration of each stage varies depending on the location and extent of the fracture.

Injury (fracture) causes hematoma formation from the damaged blood vessels of the periosteum, endosteum, and surrounding tissues. Within hours, an inflammatory infiltrate of neutrophils and macrophages is recruited into the hematoma as in soft tissue injuries. Monocytes and granulocytes debride and digest necrotic tissue and debris, including bone, on the fracture surface. This process continues for days to weeks depending on the amount of necrotic tissue. As inflammation progresses to fibroplasia, the hematoma is progressively replaced by granulation tissue that can form bone. This bone wound tissue, known as callus, develops from both sides of the fracture and is composed of fibroblasts, endothelial cells, and bone-forming cells (chondroblasts, osteoblasts). As macrophages (osteoclasts) phagocytose the hematoma and injured tissue, fibroblasts (osteocytes) deposit a collagenous matrix, and chondroblasts deposit proteoglycans in a process called enchondral bone formation. This step, prominent in some bones, is then converted to bone as osteoblasts condense hydroxyapatite crystals at specific points on the collagen fibers. Endothelial cells form a vasculature structure characteristic of uninjured bone. Eventually the fibrovascular callus is completely replaced by new bone. Unlike healing of soft tissue, bone healing has features of regeneration, and bone often heals without leaving a scar.

Bone healing also depends on blood supply. Following injury, the ends of fractured bone are avascular. Osteocyte and blood vessel lacunae become vacant for several millimeters from the fracture. New blood vessels must sprout from preexisting ones and migrate into the area of injury. As new blood vessels cross the bone ends, they are preceded by osteoclasts just as macrophages precede them in soft tissue repair. In bone, this unit is called the cutting cone because it bores its way through bone in the process of connecting with other vessels. Excessive movement of the bone ends during this revascularization stage will break the delicate new vessels and delay healing. Osteomyelitis originates most often in ischemic bone fragments. Hyperoxygenation optimizes fracture healing and aids in the cure (and potentially the prevention) of osteomyelitis. Acute or chronic hypoxia slows bone repair.

Bone repair may occur through primary or secondary intention. Primary repair can occur only when the fracture is stable and aligned, and its surfaces closely apposed. This is the goal of rigid plate fixation or rod fixation of fractures. When these conditions are met, capillaries can grow across the fracture and rapidly reestablish a vascular supply. Little or no callus forms. Secondary repair with callus formation is more common. Once the fracture has been bridged, the new bone remodels in response to the mechanical stresses upon it, with restoration to normal or near-normal strength.

During this process, as in soft tissue, preexisting bone and its vascular network are simultaneously removed and replaced. Increased bone turnover may be detected as long as 10 years after injury. Although remodeling is efficient, it cannot correct deformities of angulation or rotation in misaligned fractures. Careful fracture reduction is still important.

Bone repair can be manipulated. Electrical stimulation, growth factors, and distraction osteogenesis are three tools for this purpose. Electrical currents applied directly (through implanted electrodes) or induced by external alternating electromagnetic fields accelerate repair by inducing new bone formation in much the same way as small piezoelectric currents produced by mechanical deformation of intact bone controls remodeling along lines of stress. Electrical stimulation has been used successfully to treat nonunion of bone (where new bone formation between bone ends fails, often requiring long periods of bed rest). Bone morphogenetic protein (BMP)-impregnated implants have accelerated bone healing in animals and have been used with encouraging results to treat large bony defects and nonunions, including during spinal fusion.

The Ilizarov technique, linear distraction osteogenesis, can lengthen bones, stimulate bone growth across a defect, or correct defects of angulation. The Ilizarov device is an external fixator attached to the bones through metal pins or wires. A surgical break is created and then slowly pulled apart (1 mm/d) or slowly reangulated. The vascular supply and subsequent new bone formation migrate along with the moving segment of bone.

PATHOGENESIS

▶ Effect of Tissue Hypoxia

Impaired perfusion and inadequate oxygenation are the most frequent causes of healing failure. Oxygen is required for successful inflammation, bactericidal activity, angiogenesis, epithelialization, and matrix (collagen) deposition. The critical collagen oxygenases involved have Km values for oxygen of about 20 mm Hg and maximums of about 200 mm Hg, meaning that reaction rates are regulated by Pao_2 and blood perfusion throughout the entire physiologic range. The Pao_2 of wound fluid in human incisions is about 30-40 mm Hg, suggesting that these enzymes normally function just beyond half capacity. Wound Pao_2 is depressed by hypovolemia, catecholamine infusion, stress, fear, or cold. Under ideal conditions, wound fluid Pao_2 can be raised above 100 mm Hg by improved perfusion and breathing of oxygen. Human healing is profoundly influenced by local blood supply, vasoconstriction, and all other factors that govern perfusion and blood oxygenation. Wounds in well-vascularized tissues (eg, head, anus) heal rapidly and are remarkably resistant to infection (Figure 6–4).

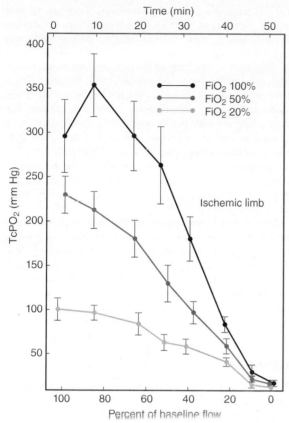

▲ Figure 6–4. Tissue oxygen concentration (TcPO₂) is a critical determinant of wound healing. Human healing is profoundly influenced by local blood supply, vasoconstriction, and all other factors that govern perfusion and blood oxygenation. Despite raising FIO₂ to 50% or 100%, the TcPO₂ remains in the ischemic range when flow is reduced to less than 25% of baseline. Supplementing the FIO₂ of oxygen will not benefit healing of ischemic ulcers. Flow must be increased to improve the TcPO₂.

▶ Dysregulated Inflammation During Impaired Wound Healing

Molecular growth signals and lytic enzymes released by inflammatory cells are necessary for repair. Inhibited or excessive inflammatory responses lead to wound complications. Failure to heal is common in patients taking anti-inflammatory corticosteroids, immune suppressants, or cancer chemotherapeutic agents that inhibit inflammatory cells. Open wounds are more effected than primarily repaired wounds. Anti-inflammatory drugs impair the wound less after the third day of healing, as the normal level of inflammation in wound healing is reduced. Inflammation may also be excessive. Increased wound inflammation (eg, in response

to infection and endotoxin or foreign bodies like mesh implants during hernia repair) can stimulate inflammatory cells to produce cytolytic cytokines and excessive proteases with the consequence of pathologic lysis of newly formed tissue. A pathological cycle of wound healing may ensue and result in an impaired quantity and quality of wound scar.

▶ Impaired Healing Due to Malnutrition

Malnutrition impairs healing, since healing depends on nucleic acid and protein synthesis, cell replication, specific organ function (liver, heart, lungs), and extracellular matrix production. Weight loss and protein depletion have been shown experimentally and clinically to be risk factors for poor healing. Deficient healing is seen mainly in patients with acute malnutrition (ie, in the weeks just before or after an injury or operation). Even a few days of starvation measurably impairs healing, and an equally short period of repletion can reverse the deficit. Wound complications increase in severe malnutrition. A period of preoperative corrective nutrition is generally helpful for patients who have recently lost 10% or more of their body weight.

▶ Scar Formation Versus Regeneration

In excessive healing or proliferative scarring, it is as if the equilibrium point between collagen deposition and collagen lysis is never reached. It is unclear why some wounds seem to continue in the dysregulated repair process. Upregulation of fibroplastic growth factors like TGF-β is implicated during hypertrophic or keloid scar formation. Because the mechanism of excessive scar formation is unknown, there is no universally accepted treatment regimen. In a recent meta-analysis of pathologic scar treatments, the mean amount of improvement to be expected was only 60%. Hypertrophic scars are generally self-limited, are related to residual inflammation, and may regress after a year or so. Keloids by definition extend beyond the borders of the wound and are most common in pigmented skin. The last areas of a burn to heal are the most often hypertrophic, possibly due to traction, reinjury, and tension. Immune mechanisms may also contribute to pathological scar. Prolonged inflammatory reactions potentiate scar. Therapy includes intralesional injection of anti-inflammatory steroids and dressing with Silastic sheets, which are shown to increase protease-based lytic activity in the scar. Excessive or hypertrophic scarring is rare in burn injuries that heal within 21 days. Pressure garments or compression dressings are effective in decreasing scarring in burn injuries that require more than 21 days to heal. The exact mechanism by which pressure is effective is unknown.

CLINICAL FINDINGS

Impediments to wound healing may be broadly categorized as those local to the wound, and those that are systemic comorbidities and diseases. Often, a clinical intervention is

Table 6–1. Local and systemic impediments to wound healing.

Systemic	Local
Malnutrition	Wound infection
Diabetes mellitus	Wound necrosis
Drugs (steroids, cytotoxins)	Foreign bodies
Obesity	Wound hypoperfusion and hypoxia
Shock	Repeat trauma
Immunodeficiency	Irradiated tissue
Renal failure	Neoplasm

possible to minimize or eliminate these obstacles to tissue repair (Table 6–1).

Acute Wounds

Acute wounds express normal wound healing pathways and are expected to heal. Over days and weeks, the undisturbed acute wound can be observed to progress reliably through the phases of hemostasis, normal inflammation, normal fibroplasia, and ultimately scar maturation with epithelialization. The most common acute wound complications are pain, infection, mechanical dehiscence, and hypertrophic scar.

Chronic Wounds & Decubiti

A. Chronic Wounds

Chronically unhealed wounds, especially on the lower extremity, are common in the setting of vascular, immunologic, and neurologic disease. Venous ulcers, largely of the lower leg, reflect poor perfusion and perivascular leakage of plasma into tissue. The extravasation of plasma proteins into the soft tissue stimulates chronic inflammation. This is the result of venous hypertension produced by incompetent venous valves. Most venous ulcers will heal if the venous congestion and edema are relieved by leg elevation, compression stockings, or surgical procedures that eliminate or repair incompetent veins or their valves.

Arterial or ischemic ulcers, which tend to occur on the lateral ankle or foot, are best treated by revascularization. Hyperbaric oxygen, which provides a temporary source of enhanced oxygenation that stimulates angiogenesis, is an effective though expensive alternative when revascularization is not possible. Useful information can be obtained by transcutaneous oximetry. Tissues with a low Pao_2

will not heal spontaneously. However, if oxygen tension can be raised into a relatively normal range by oxygen administration even intermittently, the wound may respond to oxygen therapy.

Sensory loss, especially of the feet, can lead to ulceration. Bony deformities due to chronic fractures, like the Charcot deformity, cause pathologic pressure on wounded tissue. Ulcers in patients with diabetes mellitus may have two causes. Patients with neuropathic ulcers usually have good circulation, and their lesions will heal if protected from trauma by off-loading, special shoes, or splints. Recurrences are common, however. Diabetics with ischemic disease, whether they have neuropathy or not, are at risk for gangrene, and they frequently require amputation when revascularization is not possible.

In pyoderma gangrenosum, granulomatous inflammation, with or without arteritis, causes skin necrosis, possibly by a mechanism involving excess cytokine release. These ulcers are associated with inflammatory bowel disease and certain types of arthritis and chondritis. Corticosteroids or other anti-inflammatory drugs are helpful. However, anti-inflammatory corticosteroids can also contribute to poor healing by inhibiting cytokine release and collagen synthesis.

B. Decubiti

Decubitus ulcers can be major complications of immobilization. The morbidity of decubitus ulcers lengthens hospital stays and increases health care costs. They result from prolonged pressure that reduces tissue blood supply, irritative or contaminated injections, and prolonged contact with moisture, urine, or feces. Most patients who develop decubitus ulcers are also poorly nourished. Pressure ulcers are common in paraplegics, immobile elderly patients following fractures, and intensive care unit patients. The ulcers vary in depth and often extend from skin to a bony pressure point such as the greater trochanter, the sacrum, the heels, or the head. Most decubitus ulcers are preventable. Hospital-acquired ulcers are nearly always the result of immobilization, unprotected positioning on operating tables, and ill-fitting casts or other orthopedic appliances.

COMPLICATIONS

Wound Infection

A wound infection results when bacterial proliferation and invasion overcomes wound immune defense mechanisms. When an imbalance in this quantitative equilibrium results in infection, a delay in wound healing occurs. Therefore, prevention and treatment of wound infection involves maintenance or reestablishment of the balanced equilibrium.

Wounds containing more than 10^5 bacteria/gram of tissue or any tissue level of β-hemolytic streptococci are at high risk for wound infection if closed by direct wound edge approximation, skin graft, pedicled, or free flap. Clean-contaminated and contaminated wounds result in high rates of postoperative infection (6%-15%), while clean cases have lower infection rates (1%-3%). When wounds are considered at risk for having a significant bacterial bioburden (clean-contaminated or contaminated cases), prophylactic operative antibiotics reduce wound infection rates. Wounds following clean cases with negligible bacterial bioburden do not clearly benefit from prophylactic antibiotics except when implanted prosthetic materials are used.

▶ Mechanical Wound Failure

Mechanical factors play an important and often underappreciated role in acute wound healing. Primary closure of an incision stabilizes distractive forces to allow wound healing and an optimized anatomic result (Figure 6–5). Cellular studies confirm that mechanical load forces are an important signal for acute wound repair. When anatomic stability of a wound is achieved, a particular suture material or suturing technique is of secondary importance. The increased use of foreign material implants, like meshes for hernia repair, are

suggested to manipulate the mechanical environment of the acute wound, even to the point of promoting "tension-free" wound healing. Negative pressure wound therapy is increasingly applied to stabilize acute wounds and to support acute wound healing. Mechanical microdeformation of repair cells in the wound bed is thought to stimulate acute wound healing.

Mechanical signaling pathways are important for the regulation of tissue repair, especially in load-bearing structures like the abdominal wall and Achilles tendon. From this perspective, the midline fascia behaves more like a ligament or tendon than skin, for example. It is observed that scars placed under mechanical loads ultimately will assume the morphology and function of tendons and, conversely, that incisions placed under "low" loads organize scars with reduced tensile strengths. The empiric observation that a suture length (SL)–wound length (WL) ratio of 4:1 results in the most reliable midline abdominal wall closure may reflect the technique resulting in establishing the optimal acute wound healing–load set point for the abdominal wall. When a laparotomy wound mechanically fails, a fundamental repair signal may be lost, contributing to the biology of hernia formation. Clinically, laparotomy dehiscence of only 12 mm on postoperative day 30 predicts a 94% incisional hernia rate after 3 years.

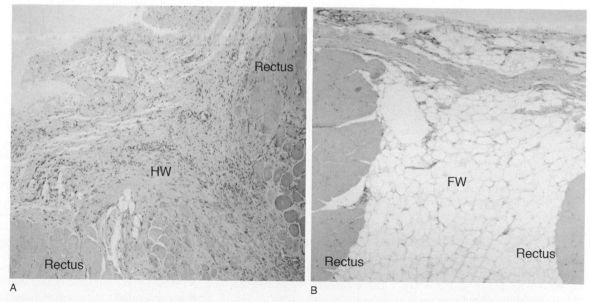

▲ Figure 6–5. A. In a healing laparotomy wound (HW), fibroplasia, matrix synthesis, and angiogenesis stabilize the rectus muscles at the wound edges until repair is complete. **B.** When laparotomy wounds fail to heal (FW), there is an absence of fibroplasia and herniated preperitoneal fat occupies the wound space.

TREETMENT

▶ Acute Wounds

A. Sutures

The ideal suture material is flexible, strong, easily tied, and securely knotted. It stimulates little tissue reaction and does not serve as a nidus for infection.

Silk is an animal protein but is relatively inert in human tissue. It is commonly used because of its track record and favorable handling characteristics. It loses strength over long periods and is unsuitable for suturing arteries to plastic grafts or for insertion of prosthetic cardiac valves. Silk sutures are multifilament, providing mechanical immune barriers for bacteria. Occasionally, silk sutures form a focus for small abscesses that migrate and "spit" through the skin, forming small sinuses that will not heal until the suture is removed.

Synthetic nonabsorbable sutures are generally inert polymers that retain strength. However, their handling characteristics are not as good as those of silk, and they must usually be knotted at least four times, resulting in increased amounts of retained foreign material. Multifilament plastic sutures may also become infected and migrate to the surface like silk sutures. Monofilament plastics will not harbor bacteria. Nylon monofilament is extremely nonreactive, but it is difficult to tie. Monofilament polypropylene is intermediate in these properties. Vascular anastomoses to prosthetic vascular grafts rely indefinitely on the strength of sutures; therefore, use of absorbable sutures may lead to aneurysm formation.

Synthetic absorbable sutures are strong, have predictable rates of loss of tensile strength, incite a minimal inflammatory reaction, and have special usefulness in gastrointestinal, urologic, and gynecologic operations that are contaminated. Polyglycolic acid and polyglactin retain tensile strength longer in gastrointestinal anastomoses. Polydioxanone sulfate and polyglycolate are monofilament and lose about half their strength in 50 days, thus solving the problem of premature breakage in fascial closures. Poliglecaprone monofilament synthetic sutures have faster reabsorption, retaining 50% tensile strength at 7 days and 0% at 21 days. This suture is suitable for low-load soft tissue approximation but is not intended for fascial closure.

Stainless steel wire is inert and maintains strength for a long time. It is difficult to tie and may have to be removed late postoperatively because of pain. It does not harbor bacteria, and it can be left in granulating wounds, when necessary, and will be covered by granulation tissue without causing abscesses. However, sinuses due to motion are fairly common.

Catgut (now made from the submucosa of bovine intestine) will eventually resorb, but the resorption time is highly variable. It stimulates a considerable inflammatory reaction and tends to potentiate infections. Catgut also loses strength rapidly and unpredictably in the intestine and in infected wounds as a consequence of acid and enzyme hydrolysis.

Staples, whether for internal use or skin closure, are mainly steel-tantalum alloys that incite a minimal tissue reaction. The technique of staple placement is different from that of sutures, but the same basic rules pertain. There are no real differences in the healing that follows sutured or stapled closures. Stapling devices tend to minimize errors in technique, but at the same time, they do not offer a feel for tissue and have limited ability to accommodate to exceptional circumstances. Staples are preferable to sutures for skin closure, since they do not provide a conduit for contaminating organisms. There is no reliable evidence that absorbable sutures lead to more incisional hernias or gastrointestinal anastomotic leaks.

Surgical glues or tissue adhesives are now established as safe and effective for the repair of small skin incisions. The most common forms are cyanoacrylate-based glues. Tissue adhesives are often less painful than sutures or staples, and the seal can serve as the wound dressing as well.

▶ Surgical Technique

Primarily closed wounds are of a smaller volume and heal mainly by the synthesis of a new matrix. Wound contraction and epithelialization, as in an open wound healing by secondary intent, contribute a small part to primary wound healing. An open wound, healing by secondary intent, must synthesize granulation tissue to fill in the wound bed, contract at the wound periphery, and cover the surface area with epithelial cells. Wounds heal faster following delayed primary closure than by secondary intent, as well. The mechanical load forces transmitted through a primarily reconstructed wound will stimulate repair. Successful delayed primary closure requires that the acute wound be in bacterial balance. Primary repair should approximate, but not strangulate, the incision. The type of suture material used does not matter, as long as the primary repair is anatomic and perfused.

The most important means of achieving optimal healing after operation is good surgical technique. Many cases of surgical wound failure are due to technical errors. Tissue should be protected from drying and contamination. The surgeon should use fine instruments; should perform clean, sharp dissection; and should make minimal, skillful use of electrocautery, ligatures, and sutures. All these precautions contribute to the most important goal of surgical technique, gentle handling of tissue. Anatomic tissue approximation should be achieved when possible but optimum tissue perfusion preserved.

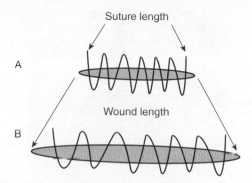

Suture length

A

Wound length

B

▲ **Figure 6–6.** The most reliable laparotomy closure uses a continuous technique at a suture length–wound length ratio of 4:1 (**A**). This allows for the normal 10% strain that occurs along the length of the incision, while maintaining mechanical integrity (**B**).

A. Wound Closure

As with many surgical techniques, the exact method of wound closure may be less important than how well it is performed. The tearing strength of sutures in fascia is no greater than 4 kg. There is little reason to use sutures of greater strength than this. Excessively tight closure strangulates tissue, likely leading to hernia formation or infection.

The most reliable laparotomy closure uses a continuous technique at SL-WL ratio of 4:1, which allows for the normal 10% strain that occurs along the length of the incision, while maintaining mechanical integrity. A 4:1 SL-WL ratio is achieved with suture placed 1-cm deep on normal fascia (the bite) followed by 1 cm of progress. The depth of the suture-line bite must extend beyond the wound lytic zone. Normal collagen lysis occurs for approximately 5 mm perpendicular to the incision, weakening the adjacent fascia. The most common technical causes of dehiscence are an SL-WL ratio less than 4:1, infection, and excessively tight sutures. Tight suture lines impair wound perfusion and oxygen delivery that is required for wound healing. If wound healing is impaired, wider, interrupted internal retention sutures may be added, although improved outcomes are not proven (Figure 6–6).

Delayed primary closure is a technique by which the subcutaneous portion of the wound is left open for 4-5 days prior to primary repair. During the delay period, angiogenesis and fibroplasia start, and bacteria are cleared from the wound. The success of this method depends on the ability of the surgeon to detect the signs of wound infection. Merely leaving the wound open for 4 days does not guarantee that it will not become infected. Some wounds (eg, fibrin-covered or inflamed wounds) should not be closed but should be left open for secondary closure. Quantitative

bacterial counts less than 10^5 non–β-hemolytic streptococcus organisms per gram of wound tissue predict successful healing after delayed primary closure. Any level of β-hemolytic streptococcal wound infection predicts delayed wound healing.

▶ Implantable Materials

Soft tissue prostheses reduce the incidence of wound failure and recurrence following hernia repair. The recurrence rate following inguinal hernia repairs using autologous tissues ranges from 5% to 25% in most series. The recurrence rate following primary incisional hernia repair using autologous tissues is even worse, ranging from 20% to 60%. The introduction of synthetic soft tissue prostheses to inguinal and incisional hernia repair has significantly reduced recurrence rates across general surgery. The prevailing view is that the mechanism for the reduced hernia recurrence rates is the reduction of tension along suture lines when using mesh and the replacement abnormal tissue.

No implantable prosthesis is ideal in regard to tissue compatibility, permanent fixation, and resistance to infection. Two principles are paramount: biocompatibility and a material that is incorporated into tissue. Both specific and nonspecific immune mechanisms are involved in the inflammatory reaction to foreign materials. Highly incompatible materials, such as wood splinters, elicit an acute inflammatory process that includes massive local release of proteolytic enzymes (inflammation). Consequently, the foreign body is never incorporated and instead is isolated loosely in a fibrous pocket. In less severe incompatibility, rejection is not so vigorous and proteolysis is not so prominent. Mononuclear cells and lymphocytes, the major components of wound inflammatory tissue, direct a response that creates a fibrous capsule that may be acceptable in a joint replacement but may distort a breast reconstruction (encapsulation). Newer biological prostheses are composed of acellularized tissue to abrogate the immune response. The expectation is that these materials recellularize with host cells and blood vessels during incorporation and assume a more physiological function (regeneration).

Most implants must become anchored to adjacent normal tissues through fibrous tissue ingrowth. This process requires biocompatibility and interstices large enough to permit repair fibroblast migration, just as in a wound, and to allow pedicles of vascularized tissue to enter and join similar units. In bone, this tissue incorporation imparts stability. In vascular grafts, the invading tissue supports neointima formation, which retards mural thrombosis and distal embolization. Soft tissue will grow into pores larger than about 50 μm in diameter. Of the vascular prostheses, woven Dacron is best for tissue incorporation. In bone, sintered, porous metallic surfaces are best. Large-screen polypropylene mesh can be used to support the abdominal wall or chest and is usually well incorporated into the granulation tissue that penetrates the mesh. Mesh porosity is increasingly recognized as an important design element for reliable implantation and wound healing. Microporous polytetrafluoroethylene (PTFE) sheets are often not well incorporated and are not suitable for use in infected tissues.

The implantation space remains vulnerable to infection for years and is a particular problem in implants that cross the body surface. Mesh cuffs around vascular access devices that incite incorporation have successfully forestalled infection for months, but infections that arise from bacteria entering the body along "permanently" implanted foreign bodies traversing the skin surface, such as ventricular assist devices, remain an unsolved problem.

▶ Negative Pressure Wound Therapy

Negative pressure wound therapy (NPWT) mechanically stabilizes the distractive forces of an open acute wound and supports healing. Distractive tissue forces keep a wound open with force vectors that oppose wound contraction, thereby delaying healing. NPWT also reduces periwound edema and improves wound perfusion. NPWT may directly stimulate repair fibroblast activity through mechanical microdeformation of the cell surface.

NPWT can also stabilize a therapeutically open abdomen (laparotomy), minimizing wound size and supporting closure of the abdominal wall. Distractive force from the rectus muscle components and lateral oblique muscles acts to keep the laparotomy open, leading to incisional hernia formation and potentially loss of abdominal, peritoneal volume (domain) (Figure 6–7).

A. Chronic Wounds

The first principle in managing chronic wounds is to diagnose and treat tissue hypoxia, such as underlying circulatory disease. The second principle is never to allow open wounds to dry—that is, use moist dressings, which may also relieve pain. A third principle is to control any infection with topical or systemic antibiotics. A fourth principle is to recognize that chronically scarred or necrotic tissue is usually poorly perfused. Debridement of unhealthy tissue, often followed by skin grafting, may be required for healing. A fifth principle is to reduce autonomic vasoconstriction by means of warmth, moisture, and pain relief.

A number of growth factors have been shown to accelerate healing of acute wounds in animals. They include FGFs, TGF-β, IGF-1, PDGF, and epidermal growth factor (EGF). However, in the setting of chronic human wounds, with the perfusion problems noted above and the hostile wound environment with elevated protease levels, proof of efficacy has been difficult to develop, and no clear-cut advantage to

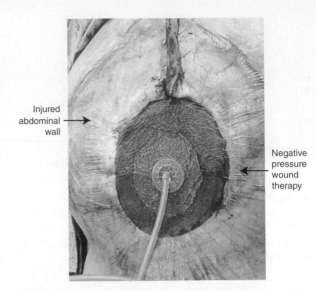

Injured abdominal wall

Negative pressure wound therapy

▲ **Figure 6–7.** Negative pressure dressings oppose distractive soft tissue vectors and mechanically stabilize a wound.

any formulation has yet been convincingly demonstrated. The one exception is the randomized, prospective, double-blind, placebo-controlled multicenter trial by the Diabetic Ulcer Study Group, which demonstrated that daily topical application of recombinant human PDGF-BB homodimer moderately accelerated healing and resulted in more wounds that healed completely.

B. Ducubiti

The first principle is to incise and drain any infected spaces or debride necrotic tissue. Dead tissue is debrided until the exposed surfaces are viable. Sources of pressure must again be unloaded. Many will then heal spontaneously. However, deep ulcers may require surgical closure, sometimes with removal of underlying bone. The defect may require closure by judicious movement of thick, well-vascularized tissue into the affected area. Musculocutaneous flaps are the treatment of choice when chronic infection and significant tissue loss are combined. However, recurrence is common because the flaps are usually insensate.

▶ Postoperative Care

Optimum postoperative care of the wound requires cleanliness, maintenance of a moist wound environment, protection from trauma, and support of the patient. Even closed wounds can be infected by surface contamination, particularly within the first 2-3 days. Bacteria gain entrance most easily through suture tracts. If a wound is likely to be traumatized or contaminated, it should be protected during this time. Such protection may require special dressings such as occlusive dressings or sprays and repeated cleansing.

Some mechanical stress enhances healing. Even fracture callus formation is greater if slight motion is allowed. Patients should move and stress their wounds a little. Early ambulation and return to normal activity are, in general, good for repair.

The appearance of delayed wound infections, weeks to years after operation, reinforces that all wounds are contaminated and may harbor bacteria. Most frequently, poor tissue perfusion and oxygenation of the wound during the postoperative period weakens host resistance. Regulation of perfusion is largely due to sympathetic nervous activity. The major stimuli of vasoconstriction are cold, pain, hypovolemia, cigarette smoking, and hypoxemia. Recent studies show that efforts to limit these impediments to wound healing reduce the wound infection rate by more than half. Maintenance of intraoperative normothermia and blood volume is particularly important. Appropriate assurance that peripheral perfusion is adequate is best obtained from peripheral tissues rather than urine output, central venous pressure, or wedge pressure, none of which correlate with peripheral wound tissue oxygenation. What does correlate with tissue oxygenation is the capillary refill time on the forehead or patella, which should be less than 2 and 5 seconds respectively. Collagen deposition is increased also by the addition of oxygen breathing (nasal prongs or light mask) but only in well-perfused patients.

The ideal care of the wound begins in the preoperative period and ends only months later. The patient must be prepared so that optimal conditions exist when the wound is made. Surgical technique must be clean, gentle, and skillful. Nutrition should be optimized preoperatively when possible. Cessation of cigarette smoking will improve wound outcomes. Postoperatively, wound care includes maintenance of nutrition, blood volume, oxygenation, and careful restriction of immunosuppressant drugs when possible. Although wound healing is in many ways a local phenomenon, ideal care of the wound is essentially ideal care of the patient.

▶ References

Franz MG. The biology of hernia formation. *Surg Clin N Am*. 2008;88:1.

Franz MG et al. Optimizing healing of the acute wound by minimizing complications. *Curr Prob Surg*. 2007;44:1.

Iorio ML, Shuck J, Attinger CE. Wound healing in the upper and lower extremities: a systematic review on the use of acellular dermal matrices. *Plast Reconstr Surg*. 2012 Nov;130(5 suppl 2):232S-241S.

Koh TJ, DiPietro LA. Inflammation and wound healing: the role of the macrophage. *Expert Rev Mol Med*. 2011 Jul 11;13: e23.

Park H, Copeland C, Henry S, Barbul A. Complex wounds and their management. *Surg Clin North Am*. 2010 Dec;90(6): 1181-1194.

Perez D et al. Prospective evaluation of vacuum-assisted closure in abdominal compartment syndrome and severe abdominal sepsis. *J Am Coll Surg*. 2007;205:586.

Rafehi H, El-Osta A, Karagiannis TC. Genetic and epigenetic events in diabetic wound healing. *Int Wound J*. 2011 Feb;8(1): 12-21.

Sanchez-Manuel FJ et al. Antibiotic prophylaxis for hernia repair. *Cochrane Database Syst Rev*. 2007;3: CD003769.

Sørensen LT. Wound healing and infection in surgery: the pathophysiological impact of smoking, smoking cessation, and nicotine replacement therapy: a systematic review. *Ann Surg*. 2012 Jun;255(6):1069-1079.

Velnar T, Bailey T, Smrkolj V. The wound healing process: an overview of the cellular and molecular mechanisms. *J Int Med Res*. 2009 Sep-Oct;37(5):1528-1542.

Wild T, Rahbarnia A, Kellner M, Sobotka L, Eberlein T. Basics in nutrition and wound healing. *Nutrition*. 2010 Sep;26(9): 862-866.

Wu SC, Marston W, Armstrong DG. Wound care: the role of advanced wound healing technologies. *J Vasc Surg*. 2010 Sep;52(3 suppl):59S-66S.

Young A, McNaught CE. The physiology of wound healing. *Surgery*. 2011;29(10):475-479.

MULTIPLE CHOICE QUESTIONS

1. Which phase of acute wound healing is prolonged during progression to a chronic wound?

   A. Coagulation
   B. Inflammation
   C. Fibroplasia
   D. Angiogenesis
   E. Remodeling

2. Which cell is most important for signaling wound healing?

   A. Platelet
   B. PMN
   C. Macrophage
   D. Fibroblast
   E. Endothelial cell

3. Which is the most predictive direct measure of impaired or delayed wound healing?

   A. Vitamin C deficiency
   B. Low serum albumin
   C. Irradiated tissue
   D. Smoking
   E. TcO_2 less than 30 mm Hg

4. Which of the following is not a clinical impediment to wound healing?

   A. Repeated trauma
   B. Wound infection
   C. A moist wound environment
   D. Foreign bodies
   E. Obesity

5. The fundamental mechanism for incisional hernia formation is

   A. Long-term fascial scar failure
   B. Suture failure
   C. Suture pulling through the fascia
   D. Early fascial dehiscence and wound failure
   E. Poor technique

Power Sources in Surgery

K. Barrett Deatrick, MD
Gerard M. Doherty, MD

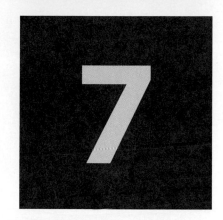

INTRODUCTION

Modern surgery has been redefined by powered instruments, technological tools that in many ways have revolutionized the delicacy, precision, and accuracy of the various operations performed. Yet many people who use these implements every day have very little understanding of the technology behind these tools. Although a complete treatise on electromagnetic generation of heat and the physics of current generation are beyond the scope of this chapter (and are available elsewhere), understanding some fundamental rules governing the behavior of electrical currents and some relatively straightforward principles helps guide the use of these technologies.

ELECTROSURGERY

Principles of Electricity

An electrical **circuit** is any pathway that allows the uninterrupted flow of electrons. Electrical **current** is the flow of electricity (the number of electrons) in a given circuit over a constant period of time and is measured in **amperes** (A). Current can be supplied either as direct current (DC) with constant positive and negative terminals or as alternating current (AC) with constantly reversing poles. The electromotive force, or **voltage,** is a measurement of the force that propels the current of electrons and is related to the difference in potential energy between two terminals. The **resistance** is the tendency of any component of a circuit to resist the flow of electrons and applies to DC circuits. The equivalent of this tendency in an AC circuit is known as impedance. Any electromagnetic wave, from household electricity to radio broadcasts to visible light, can be described by three components: speed, frequency, and wavelength. Because all electromagnetic waves travel at the speed of light, which is a constant, these waves depend on the relationship between

their frequency and wavelength. Since these three characteristics are defined by the equation:

$$c = f\lambda$$
(where c is the speed of light, 2.998×10^8 m/s)

frequency (f) and wavelength (λ) are inversely related; that is, as frequency increases, wavelength decreases, and vice versa. The ability to pass high-frequency current through the human body without causing excess damage makes electrosurgery possible.

Electrocautery

Electrosurgery is often incorrectly termed electrocautery, which is a separate technique. Electrocautery is a closed-circuit DC device in which current is passed through an exposed wire offering resistance to the current (Figure 7–1). The resistance causes some of the electrical energy to be dissipated as heat, increasing the temperature of the wire, which then heats tissue. In true electrocautery, *no current passes through the patient*. Electrocautery is primarily applied for microsurgery, such as ophthalmologic procedures, where a very small amount of heat will produce the desired effect or where more heat or current may be dangerous.

Principles of Electrosurgery

True electrosurgery, colloquially referred to as the "Bovie" (following its inventor, William T. Bovie, engineer and collaborator of Harvey Cushing), is perhaps the most ubiquitous power source in surgery. While the principle of using heat to cauterize bleeding wounds dates back to the third millennium BC, the directed use of electrical current to produce these effects is a far more recent development. While other scientists and engineers made significant contributions to the development of this new technology, it was Bovie who refined the electrical generator and made it practical

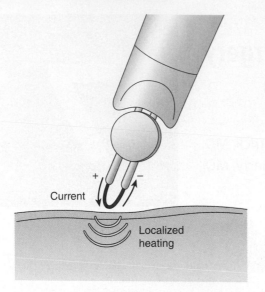

+

−

Current

Localized
heating

▲ **Figure 7–1.** In electrocautery, current passes through a wire loop and heats it. This heat cauterizes tissue. No current passes through the patient.

and applicable to everyday surgery. At the most fundamental level, electrosurgery uses high-frequency (radiofrequency) electromagnetic waves to produce a localized heating of tissues, leading to localized tissue destruction. The effect produced (cutting vs coagulation) depends on how this energy is supplied.

A useful exercise to understand the way electrosurgery works is to follow the flow of current from the power outlet as it travels through the patient and returns to the wall outlet. By convention, charge is depicted as moving from positive (cathode) to negative (anode) despite that the particles that are actually moving are electrons, which have a negative charge. These descriptions are based on that convention, following the flow of positive charge.

A. Monopolar Circuits

The electrosurgical circuit consists of four primary parts: the electrosurgical generator, the active electrode, the patient, and the return electrode. Current flows from the electrosurgical generator after it is modulated to a high-frequency, short wavelength current and where multiple waveforms can be produced. (The importance of the waveform is discussed in later sections.) The current flows from the machine, through the handpiece, out the tip of the device, to the patient. If the patient were not connected in some way either to a negative terminal or to ground, no current would flow, as there would be no way to complete the circuit, hence nowhere for the charge to go. However, the patient is always connected to the electrosurgical generator by a return electrode, which allows

the charge delivered by the electrosurgical probe to pass through the patient, exerting its effect, and back to the generator, completing the circuit. In reality, the term *monopolar circuit* is incorrect, as there are in fact two poles (the active and return electrodes); it is distinguished from bipolar electrosurgery in which both electrodes are under the surgeon's direct control (Figure 7–2A).

B. Bipolar Circuits

The essential components of the bipolar electrosurgical circuit are the same as those in the monopolar circuit; however, in this system, the active and return electrodes are in the same surgical instrument. In this technique, high-frequency current is passed through the active electrode and through the patient to heat and disrupt tissue. In this arrangement, however, the return electrode is in the handpiece, as the opposite pole of the active electrode. This method enables the surgeon to heat only a discrete amount of tissue (Figure 7–2B).

▶ The Electromagnetic Spectrum & Tissue Effects

The current that powers the electrosurgical generator is supplied at a frequency of 60 Hz. This type of electromagnetic energy can indeed cause very strong (potentially lethal) neuromuscular stimulation, making it unsuitable for use in its pure form. Muscle and nerve stimulation, however, ceases at around 100 kHz. Current with a frequency above this threshold can be delivered safely, without the risk of electrocution. The outputs of electrosurgical generators deliver current with a frequency greater than 200 kHz. Current at this frequency is known as **radiofrequency** (RF); it is in the same portion of the spectrum as some radio transmitters. This level of RF, released from a radio antenna, can produce serious RF burns if the proper precautions are not taken.

Applying electrosurgical current to a patient produces localized tissue destruction via intense heat production, yet barring a mishap, no other lesions are produced during application of this technique. The reason the effect is exerted only at the site where the surgeon is operating, and not at the site of the return electrode, is that the surface area by which the charge is delivered is much smaller than that to which it returns. Thus, there is a far greater density of charge at the site of the handpiece ("active" electrode) contact than there is at the site of return. If there is another connection between the patient and ground that offers less resistance to the flow of current, and if it also comprises a relatively small surface area, then the patient could be in danger of suffering an electrosurgical burn. Similarly, it is possible that if the return electrode were to be damaged, or if contact was not maintained, a burn could occur in this area. The possibility of a burn at the site of the return electrode is eliminated in most

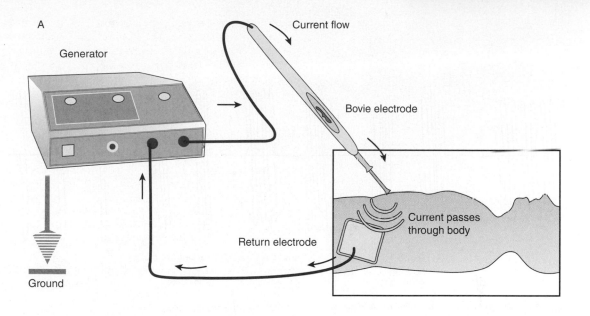

A

Generator

Current flow

Bovie electrode

Current passes through body

Return electrode

Ground

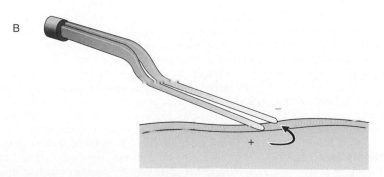

B

▲ **Figure 7–2.** **A.** In monopolar electrosurgery, current from an electrosurgical generator passes from an active electrode (the "Bovie" tip) through the patient to a return electrode of greater area. **B.** In bipolar electrosurgery, the active and return electrodes are in the handpiece, and current only flows through the surgical site.

modern machines by the presence of a monitoring system that assesses the completeness of contact (by maintaining a smaller, secondary circuit) and automatically disables power if full contact of the pad is lost (as could be caused by tripping over a wire and tearing the return pad).

▶ Types of Electrosurgery

All types of electrosurgery exert their effects via the localized production of heat and the subsequent changes in the heated tissue. Therefore, the different effects produced by electrosurgical instruments are created by altering the manner in which this heat is produced and delivered.

Adjustment is made possible by altering the wave pattern of the current.

A. Cutting

Cutting depends on the production of a continuous sine wave of current (Figure 7–3A). Compared with coagulation current (discussed later), cutting current has a relatively low voltage and a relatively high crest factor, which is the ratio of the peak voltage to the mean (root mean square) voltage of the current. Additionally, it has a relatively high "duty cycle"—that is, once the current is applied, the current is actively flowing during the entire application. In this

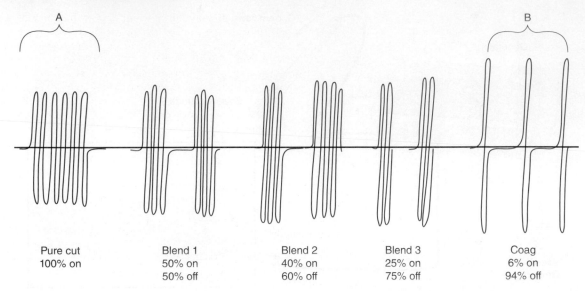

▲ **Figure 7–3.** Electrosurgical waveforms. **A.** Cutting current. **B.** Coagulation current.

technique, the tip of the electrode is held just slightly off the surface of the tissue. The flow of the high-frequency current through the resistance of the patient's tissue at a very small site produces intense heat, vaporizing water and exploding the cells in the immediate vicinity of the current. Thus, cutting occurs with minimal coagulum production and consequently minimal hemostasis. A combination of coagulation and cutting can be produced by setting the electrosurgical generator to blend, which damps down a portion of the waveform, allowing greater formation of a coagulum and consequently more control of local bleeding.

B. Coagulation: Desiccation and Fulguration

In contrast with cutting currents, **coagulation** currents do not produce a constant waveform. Rather, they rely on spikes of electric wave activity (Figure 7–3B). Although these currents produce less heat overall than the direct sine wave, enough heat is produced to disrupt the normal cellular architecture. Because the cells are not instantly vaporized, however, the cellular debris remains associated with the edge of the wound, and the heat produced is enough to denature the cellular protein. This accounts for the formation of a coagulum, a protein-rich mixture that allows sealing of smaller blood vessels and control of local bleeding. Compared to cutting, coagulation currents have a higher crest factor and a shorter duty cycle (94% off, 6% on). In part, the increased voltage is necessary to overcome the impedance of air during the process of arcing current to the tissues. Coagulation can be accomplished in one of two ways. With **desiccation**, the conductive tip is placed in direct contact with the tissue. Direct contact of the electrode with tissue

reduces the concentration of the current; less heat is generated, and no cutting action occurs. A relatively low power setting is used, resulting in a limited area of tissue ablation with coagulation. Desiccation is achieved most efficiently with the cutting current. The cells dry out and form a coagulum rather than vaporize and explode.

In **fulguration**, the tip of the active electrode is not actually brought into contact with the tissues but rather is held just off the surface, and following activation, the current arcs through the air to the target. Again, this process disrupts normal cellular protein to form a coagulum; the tissue is charred, and a black eschar forms at the site of operation. It is possible to cut with the coagulation current and, conversely, to coagulate with the cutting current by holding the electrode in direct contact with tissue. It may be necessary to adjust power settings and electrode size to achieve the desired surgical effect. The benefit of using the cutting current is that far less voltage is needed, an important consideration during minimally invasive procedures.

C. Variables

Just as the power setting and the waveform affect the results of the current application, any change in the circuit that influences the impedance of the system will influence the tissue effect. These include the size of the electrode, the position of the electrode, the type of tissue, and the formation of eschar.

Size of the electrode—The smaller the electrode, the higher the current concentration. Consequently, the same tissue effect can be achieved with a smaller electrode, even though

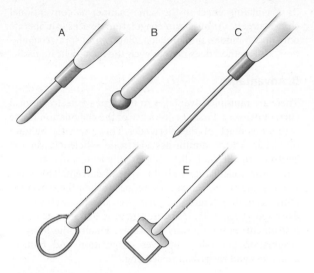

▲ **Figure 7–4.** **A.** Knife electrode. **B.** Ball electrode. **C.** Needle electrode. **D.** Loop electrode. **E.** Wire electrode.

the power setting is reduced. At any given setting, the longer the generator is activated, the more heat is produced. The greater the heat, the farther it will travel to adjacent tissue (thermal spread). (See various electrodes, Figure 7–4.)

Placement of the electrode—Placement can determine whether vaporization or coagulation occurs. Which one occurs is a function of current density and the heat produced while sparking to tissue versus holding the electrode in direct contact.

Type of tissue—Tissues vary widely in resistance.

Eschar—Eschar is relatively high in resistance to current. Electrodes should be kept clean and free of eschar, maintaining lower resistance within the surgical circuit.

D. Disadvantages and Potential Hazards

Alternate site burns—Early electrosurgical generators used a **ground referenced** circuit design. In this type of construction, grounded current from the wall outlet was directly modulated, and it was assumed that it would return to the generator via the return electrode. With this type of system, however, any path of low resistance to ground, including metal instruments, EKG leads, and other wire and conductive surfaces, can complete the circuit. The ground referenced circuit design presented a relatively high hazard for alternate site burns when current was not distributed over a great enough area to dissipate the current.

Modern electrosurgical units use isolated generator technology. The isolated generator separates the therapeutic current from ground by referencing it within the generator circuitry. In an isolated electrosurgical system, the circuit is completed by the generator, and electrosurgical current from isolated generators will not recognize grounded objects as pathways to complete the circuit. Isolated electrosurgical energy recognizes the patient return electrode as the preferred pathway back to the generator. Since the ground is not the reference for completion of the circuit, the potential for alternate site burns is greatly reduced. However, if the return electrode were to become partially disconnected, a burn could occur at the site of the return electrode if the area was too small to distribute the current widely enough to prevent heating of the tissue or if the impedance was too high. It is important to place the return electrode over a well-vascularized tissue mass, not over areas of vascular insufficiency or over bony prominences where contact might be compromised. Therefore, some electrosurgical generators use a monitoring system that assesses the quality of the contact between the return electrode and the patient by monitoring impedance, which is related to surface area. Any loss of contact between the electrode and the generator results in interruption of the circuit and deactivation of the system.

Surgical fires—In any setting with high heat sources and an ample supply of oxygen, vigilance against combustion is essential. Drapes, gowns, gas (particularly in bowel surgery and cases involving the upper airway), and hair, for example, are flammable and must be kept away from heat sources. Careful application of electrosurgery and use of a protective holster to store the electrode while not in use are important to minimize the risk of fire.

Minimally invasive surgery—Several safety concerns are unique to minimally invasive surgery, given the limited and relatively tight environment in which operations occur. One potential danger is that of direct coupling between the electrode and other conductive instruments, leading to inadvertent tissue damage. Another is the risk, with the use of high-voltage currents (especially those used for coagulation), of breakdown in the insulation, resulting in arcing from an exposed conductor to adjacent tissue, again, causing unwanted tissue damage. The risk can be reduced by using cutting current instead of coagulation current to lower the voltage used.

Yet another unique hazard is the potential for creating a capacitor with the cannula. A capacitor is any conductor separated from another conductor by a dielectric. The conductive electrode separated from either a metal cannula or the abdominal wall (both good conductors) can induce capacitance in either of these structures. For maximum safety, an all-metal cannula (by which current can escape to the rest of the body) rather than a combination of metal and plastic should be used, and vigilance must be maintained at all times.

E. Principal Applications for Electrosurgery

Electrosurgery is ubiquitous in its presence within the modern operating room. In its earliest use by Dr. Cushing, it allowed surgery on previously inoperable vascular tumors in neurosurgery. Today, electrosurgery is an essential component of all types of surgery. Applications include dissection in general and vascular surgery, allowing tissue to be resected with minimal blood loss. Additionally, use in urology facilitates transurethral prostatectomy (TURP) and other procedures. In gynecologic practice, electrosurgical instruments are essential in cervical resections and biopsies.

▶ Argon Beam Coagulation

A. Principles

Argon beam coagulation is closely related to basic electrosurgery. Argon beam coagulation uses a coaxial flow of argon gas to conduct monopolar RF current to the target tissue. Argon is an inert gas that is easily ionized by the application of an electrical current. When ionized, argon gas becomes far more conductive (has less impedance) than normal air and provides a more efficient pathway for transmitting current from the electrode to tissues (Figure 7–5). The current arcs along the pathway of the ionized gas, which is heavier than both oxygen and nitrogen, and thereby displaces air. Whereas current can sometimes follow unpredictable pathways while arcing through the air, the argon gas allows more accurate placement of current flow. Once the current arrives at the tissue, it produces

its coagulating effect in the same manner as conventional electrosurgery. Argon beam coagulation devices can operate only in two modes: pinpoint coagulation and spray coagulation. The method does not cut even the most delicate tissue.

B. Advantages

There are multiple advantages to this type of electrosurgical current delivery. First, it allows use of the coagulation mode without contact of the electrode. This prevents buildup of eschar, which diminishes electrode efficiency, on the electrode tip. Second, there is generally less smoke and less odor from coagulating with this type of current. Third, tissue loss and tissue damage are reduced when the current is more accurately targeted. Fourth, because the argon gas is delivered at room temperature, there is less danger of the instrument igniting gowns or drapes. Finally, the beam of coagulation generally improves coagulation and reduces blood loss and the risk of rebleeding.

C. Disadvantages

Argon beam coagulation cannot be used to produce a cutting effect in the same manner as other types of electrosurgical equipment. Also, the nozzle for gas delivery can become clogged, reducing its efficiency, and just as with other electrosurgical instruments, if it is used for a prolonged period of time, it may overheat and cause inadvertent damage when set aside.

D. Applications

Argon beam coagulation is especially useful for procedures in which the surgeon must rapidly and efficiently coagulate a wide area of tissue. It is especially suited to dissecting very vascular tissues and organs, such as the liver. Its efficient delivery of a consistent current load and its inability to become occluded with eschar are advantageous for operation with a significant risk of hemorrhage.

MECHANICAL (ULTRASONIC) TISSUE DISRUPTION

Apart from passing current through the patient to produce localized heating and tissue destruction (either cutting or coagulation), there are other means of transforming electrical potential energy into energy for surgery. Two of the most prominent technologies depend on the production of ultrasonic vibrations, although each produces its effect in a unique manner.

▶ Ultrasonic Scalpels & Clamps

A. Principles

Several types of ultrasonic "scalpels" and clamps allow cutting and coagulation of tissue in a technique completely

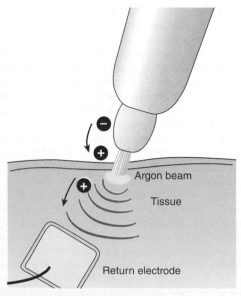

Argon beam

Tissue

Return electrode

▲ **Figure 7–5.** Ionized argon gas facilitates the flow of current from the handpiece to the tissue.

different from that employed in electrosurgery. In this type of an instrument, electrical energy from a power source is transformed into ultrasonic vibrations by a transducer, a unit that expands and contracts in response to electrical current at a frequency of up to 55.5 kHz/s. The vibration is amplified in the shaft of the instrument to magnify the vibrating distance of the blade, which moves longitudinally. The blade tip vibrates through an amplitude of around 200 μm. As the blade tip vibrates, it produces cellular friction and denatures proteins. The denatured proteins form a coagulum, which allows sealing of coapted blood vessels. With longer instrument applications, significant secondary heat is produced, and larger blood vessels may be sealed by coagulation of tissue at a small distance from the instrument. By producing cellular disruption in this fashion, the temperatures achieved are between 50°C and 100°C. In contrast, in conventional electrosurgery, tissues are subjected to temperatures between 150°C and 400°C. Thus, with an ultrasonic device, tissues can be dissected without burning or oxidizing tissues and without producing an eschar; there is also less potential to disrupt the coagulum when removing the instrument. When cutting using the clamp portion of the instrument, energy is transferred to the tissue through the active blade under applied force, minimizing lateral spread. Additionally, the motion of the blade induces cavitation along the cell surfaces, whereby low pressure causes cell fluid to vaporize and rupture (Figure 7–6).

B. Advantages

The advantages of an ultrasonic scalpel system are clearest when operating in tight spaces with the attendant risks of damage to adjacent structures. Ultrasonic instruments are especially suited for laparoscopic and other types of minimally invasive procedures. While the potential still exists for damaging adjacent tissue by inadvertently touching it with an active tip, there is no risk of current inadvertently arcing to adjacent structures, since the current is converted into mechanical energy in the handpiece. Further, there is no neuromuscular stimulation produced, since no current passes through the patient. Because the tissue effects are exerted through mechanical disruption of the cells, and coagulation occurs at much lower temperatures than used in conventional electrosurgery, lateral thermal tissue damage is minimized. And because tissue is not heated to the point of

combustion or carbonization of proteins, there is no eschar formation on the blade, and less smoke is produced.

C. Disadvantages

A primary disadvantage of ultrasonic scalpels and clamps is that the components are more expensive than those used for conventional electrosurgery, and with more mechanical parts, there are more potential points of equipment failure. Further, whereas electrosurgery can be applied throughout an operation, ultrasonic scalpels are typically used for more controlled dissection around the site of interest.

D. Applications

The primary applications of ultrasonic instruments are found when traditional electrosurgery is unsuitable or undesirable. As mentioned, they are particularly useful during minimally invasive procedures because they mitigate the risk of running an active electrode through a cannula and into a body cavity. Additionally, the reduced smoke production by instruments of this type is advantageous in this setting. When electrophysiology is involved (such as in patients with implantable cardiac defibrillators or pacemakers), ultrasonic instruments eliminate a source of concern by avoiding the hazard of passing current through the patient's body.

▶ Cavitational Ultrasonic Surgical Aspiration

A. Principles

Cavitational ultrasonic surgical aspirators work on many of the same principles as ultrasonic scalpels. In the handpiece, current passes through a coil and induces a magnetic field. The magnetic field excites a transducer of a nickel alloy (either a piezoelectric or magnetostrictive device), expanding and contracting to produce an oscillating motion (vibration) in the longitudinal axis with a frequency of 23 or 36 kHz. These ultrasonic mechanical vibrations are magnified over the length of the handpiece. The amount of oscillation varies: with low frequency, there is greater amplitude; with high frequency, there is lower amplitude. The oscillating tip, when brought into contact with tissue, causes fragmentation of tissue by producing cavitation at the cell surface, with low pressure outside the cell leading to cellular disruption. This high-frequency vibration produces heat, which is reduced via a closed, recirculating cooling-water system. This system maintains the temperature of the tip at approximately 40°C. As tissue is fragmented, the debris must be carried away, which is another function of the cavitational ultrasonic surgical aspirator, as its name implies. For irrigation, IV fluid (water or saline) is fed through tubing to the handpiece, where it irrigates the surgical site and suspends the fragmented tissue debris. Removal of this debris is possible because the instrument contains a vacuum pump that provides suction. Suction pulls irrigation fluid, fragmented

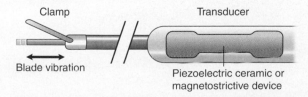

▲ **Figure 7–6.** Ultrasonic scalpel.

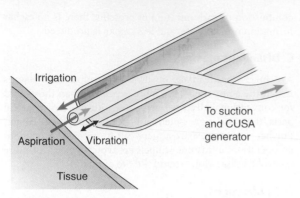

Irrigation

Aspiration   Vibration

To suction
and CUSA
generator

Tissue

▲ **Figure 7–7.** Cavitational ultrasonic surgical aspirator.

tissue, and other material through the distal tip of the handpiece. The material is contained in a separate canister.

Some ultrasonic surgical aspirator instruments enable the surgeon to influence the selectivity of the disruption induced by the instrument itself. Some surgeons attempt to gain extra control by lowering the amplitude of the tip oscillations. Lowering amplitude to gain greater selectivity when fragmenting tissue near critical structures, however, only results in reduced speed of tissue removal. By using a mode in which on/off power intervals are supplied, the reserve power (which governs the tip response when encountering tissue) is reduced. The total amount of power in the oscillating hollow tip is determined by the amount of reserve power available. Reserve power maintains tip oscillation when a resistive load is placed on the tip, as occurs when it contacts tissue. As the resistance increases, more power is supplied to the tip (Figure 7–7).

B. Applications

Ultrasonic surgical aspirator systems are primarily applicable in situations where fragmentation, emulsification, and aspiration of a significant amount of tissue are desirable. Since minimal additional hemostasis is provided, this instrument is not as versatile in its application to general surgery

as electrosurgery or the more high-power ultrasonic scalpel. In general surgery, its primary application is in liver resection, where it can disrupt parenchyma while leaving major vasculature and the biliary ducts intact.

▶ References

Duffy S, Cobb GV. *Practical Electrosurgery.* Chapman & Hall Medical, 1995.
Pearce JA. *Electrosurgery.* Chapman & Hall, 1986.
Valleylab. Principles of Electrosurgery Online. 2013. Available at http://valleylab.com/education/poes/index.html. Accessed May 1, 2013.

MULTIPLE CHOICE QUESTIONS

1. All of the following are true about electrosurgery, except

   A. In monopolar electrosurgery, the current flows through the patient from the active electrode to the return electrode
   B. In bipolar electrosurgery, the current flows from the handpiece to the return electrode
   C. The cutting mode of monopolar electrosurgery utilizes a continuous sine wave of current
   D. The coagulation mode of monopolar electrosurgery relies on spikes of electric wave activity
   E. The resistance of the tissue influences the effect of the electrosurgery

2. Fire in the operating room

   A. Is preventable by keeping the oxygen levels used for ventilation low
   B. Depends upon the presence of an oxygen source, an ignition source, and fuel
   C. Cannot be fed by alcohol from skin prep solutions because this is not flammable
   D. Cannot be ignited by electrosurgical instruments
   E. Has been eliminated by the abandonment of flammable anesthetic agents

Inflammation, Infection, & Antimicrobial Therapy in Surgery

Haytham M.A. Kaafarani, MD, MPH

Kamal M.F. Itani, MD

▼ INTRODUCTION

TERMINOLOGY

Surgery and infection are unfortunately intimately intertwined. For the purpose of this chapter, we will differentiate between infections resulting from surgery (*surgical site infections*) and those resulting from other disease processes but *requiring surgical management*. Surgical incisions involve a breach of the skin and immune barriers, and can thus be complicated by infection. The term "wound infection" has been replaced by the more accurate term "surgical site infection" (SSI), to emphasize that the infection can occur anywhere within any of the areas accessed surgically (not exclusively at the skin level) and to differentiate it from "traumatic wound infection."

As opposed to SSI, the term "surgical infection" is used to indicate infections that are unlikely to respond to medical and antimicrobial treatments, and require surgical intervention or management. Common examples include abscesses, empyema, intra-abdominal infections, and necrotizing skin and soft tissue infections. Surgical decision making involves, at its core, the knowledge and experience to determine the timing of surgery and a right balance between surgery and other adjunct therapy such as antibiotic therapy, resuscitative efforts, and nutritional optimization, in order to provide the patient with the best chances to cure the infection with the best overall outcomes.

▶ Pathogenesis

The development of a surgical infection involves a close interplay between three elements:

1. A susceptible host
2. An infectious agent
3. A suitable medium or environment (Figure 8–1).

The degree of contribution of each of these three factors to the eventual occurrence of the infection depends on the individual patient and the specific nature and site of the infection. Whether a given inoculum of bacteria results in an established infection or not depends on the virulence of the bacteria, the strength of the immune and inflammatory host response (eg, chemotaxis, phagocytosis, B- and T-lymphocyte activation), and the amount of blood perfusion and oxygen tension in the medium where the inoculum resides.

A. The Susceptible Host

Many surgical infections occur in patients with no evidence of decreased immune defenses. However, with the major advances in medicine and health care services over the last century, more immunocompromised patients (eg, transplant, HIV, and diabetic patients) are presenting with infections requiring surgical management or with SSIs following surgical interventions. Table 8–1 delineates a list of patient-related conditions associated with decreased immunity and potential predisposition to surgical infections. The mechanisms by which the listed conditions affect a host's immunity are diverse in nature. For example, diabetic patients have suboptimal neutrophil adherence, migration and anti-bacterial functions, making them less able to fight an occult infection. Such effect of diabetes on immunity is much more pronounced in patients whose glucose levels are poorly controlled than in those with appropriate and consistent management of their diabetes.

B. The Infectious Agent

Identification of the organism causing the infection is crucial. This is often achieved through the use of Gram stains and cultures of the tissue or purulent material at the site of infection. *Staphylococcus aureus* is the most common pathogen in SSIs, and its ability to develop resistance to antimicrobial therapy continues to be one of the biggest challenges currently faced

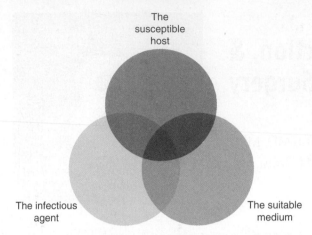

The susceptible host

The infectious agent

The suitable medium

▲ **Figure 8–1.** The interaction between susceptible host, infectious agent, and suitable medium to result in infection.

by the medical community. *Staphylococcus epidermidis* is one of the other 33 known species of the genus *Staphylococcus*, and is usually a skin and mucous membrane nonpathogenic colonizer. Nonetheless, in immunosuppressed individuals and those with indwelling surgical catheters or implants, *S epidermidis* can cause serious infections requiring treatment. In necrotizing skin and soft tissue infections, the etiology

Table 8–1. Patient-related conditions associated with decreased immunity and a higher risk for surgical infections.

Advanced age
Diabetes mellitus
Malnutrition
Smoking
Obesity
Immunosuppressive therapy (eg, posttransplant)
Systemic corticosteroid use
Peripheral vascular disease
Malignancy and anti-neoplastic treatment
Concomitant remote site infection
Human immunodeficiency virus/acquired immunodeficiency syndrome (HIV/AIDS)
Liver failure
Renal failure

is often polymicrobial with gram-positive, gram-negative, and anaerobic bacteria involved. Monobacterial necrotizing infections can result from either clostridial species (especially *Clostridium perfringens*) or *Streptococcus pyogenes*. Streptococci are well known for their ability to invade even minor breaks in the skin and to cause superficial skin and skin structure infections by spreading through connective tissue planes and lymphatic channels. When surgical procedures involve the small or large intestines, gram-negative and anaerobic bacteria are implicated in a significant proportion of the SSIs in addition to the regular gram-positive colonizers. Among these, *Escherichia coli, Klebsiella pneumoniae, Enterobacter,* and *Bacteroides* species are the most commonly isolated pathogens. In immunocompromised or critically ill patients, fungi (eg, *Candida, Aspergillus, Histoplasma*) may result in localized or systemic life-threatening infections. Parasites such as amebas and echinococcus may also cause abscesses in internal organs, especially the liver.

C. The Suitable Medium

A suitable medium for bacteria consists of a closed space with poor vascular perfusion, low oxygen tension, and low pH. Ischemic and necrotic tissues are perfect examples of such a medium where microorganisms can thrive. The appendix, with its narrow orifice presents a classical example. When an appendicolith blocks the orifice of the appendix, the intraluminal pressure increases and eventually blocks lymphatic and venous outflow. As the vascular perfusion of the appendix diminishes, the tissue oxygen tension decreases, the milieu becomes acidotic, and the appendix becomes ischemic and necrotic. Unless removed, the inflamed appendix and its blocked lumen contain colonic bacteria that will result in an appendiceal infection followed by perforation and a periappendiceal abscess and/or peritonitis.

A foreign body such as a joint prosthesis can become seeded in the event of a systemic infection. As with necrotic tissue, the lack of vascularity decreases the formation of free oxygen radicals within prosthesis and prevents the immune system from readily fighting microorganisms in that area.

SURGICAL SITE INFECTION

▶ Definition

The Centers for Disease Control and Prevention (CDC) define SSI as an infection that occurs at or near the surgical incision within 30 postoperative days of the surgical procedure, or within 1 year if an implant is left in place (eg, mesh, heart valve [www.cdc.gov]). The CDC further classifies SSI as

1. Superficial incisional
2. Deep incisional
3. Organ/space SSI

Table 8–2. Criteria and definitions of surgical site infection.

Superficial incisional SSI

Infection occurs *within 30 d* after the operative procedure

and

Involves only skin and subcutaneous tissue of the incision

and

Patient has at least one of the following:

- Purulent drainage from the superficial incision.
- Organisms isolated from an aseptically obtained culture of fluid or tissue from the superficial incision.
- At least one of the following signs or symptoms of infection: pain or tenderness, localized swelling, redness, or heat, and superficial incision are deliberately opened by surgeon, and are culture-positive or not cultured. A culture-negative finding does not meet this criterion.
- Diagnosis of superficial incisional SSI by the surgeon or attending physician.

Deep incisional SSI

Infection occurs *within 30 d* after the operative procedure if no implant is left in place or *within 1 y if implant* is in place and the infection appears to be related to the operative procedure

and

Involves deep soft tissues (eg, fascial and muscle layers) of the incision

and

Patient has at least one of the following:

- Purulent drainage from the deep incision but not from the organ/space component of the surgical site.
- A deep incision spontaneously dehisces or is deliberately opened by a surgeon and is culture-positive or not cultured and the patient has at least one of the following signs or symptoms: fever (> 38°C), or localized pain or tenderness. A culture-negative finding does not meet this criterion.
- An abscess or other evidence of infection involving the deep incision is found on direct examination, during reoperation, or by histopathologic or radiologic examination.
- Diagnosis of a deep incisional SSI by a surgeon or attending physician.

Organ/space SSI

Infection occurs *within 30 d* after the operative procedure if no implant is left in place or *within 1 y if implant* is in place and the infection appears to be related to the operative procedure

and

Infection involves any part of the body, excluding the skin incision, fascia, or muscle layers, that is *opened or manipulated* during the operative procedure

and

Patient has at least one of the following:

- Purulent drainage from a drain that is placed through a stab wound into the organ/space.
- Organisms isolated from an aseptically obtained culture of fluid or tissue in the organ/space.
- An abscess or other evidence of infection involving the organ/space that is found on direct examination, during reoperation, or by histopathologic or radiologic examination.
- Diagnosis of an organ/space SSI by a surgeon or attending physician.

CDC definition of an implant:
A nonhuman-derived object, material, or tissue that is placed in a patient during an operative procedure. Examples include porcine or synthetic heart valves, mechanical heart, metal rods, mesh, sternal wires, screws, cements, internal staples, hemoclips, and other devices. Nonabsorbable sutures are excluded because infection preventionists may not easily identify and/or differentiate the soluble nature of suture material used.

Table 8–2 illustrates the criteria that define each of these three classes of SSIs. It is noteworthy that a skin infection at or around the site of a traumatic wound is classified as a skin and skin structure infection.

▶ Epidemiology

At least 234 million surgical procedures are performed globally each year, including more than 16 million in the United States alone; SSIs develop in 2%-5% of these patients.

In this surgical patient population, SSI accounts for up to 38% of nosocomial infections, and as such is considered the most common nosocomial infection in surgical patients. If asymptomatic bacteriuria is excluded, SSI is arguably the most common nosocomial infection overall. The rate of SSI depends on the nature of the surgical procedure performed and the extent of concomitant intraoperative contamination. In an attempt to quantify the inoculum of bacteria typical of certain surgical procedures, a wound classification was developed in 1964 by the National Academy of Sciences (Table 8–3). This classification divides wounds into clean (eg, inguinal hernia repair), clean-contaminated (eg, right hemicolectomy), contaminated (eg, laparotomy for penetrating injury to small intestines), and dirty (eg, laparotomy for peritonitis and intra-abdominal abscesses) wounds. Several studies have emerged since the conception of the classification confirming that, with reasonable risk adjustment, the classes of contamination correlate well with the incidence of postoperative SSI. A more recent 2012 American College of Surgeons-National Surgical Quality Improvement (ACS-NSQIP) study of more than 600,000 patients, suggested that the rates of SSI increases as the degree of contamination increases: 2.58% for clean wounds, 6.67% for clean-contaminated wounds, 8.61% for contaminated wounds, and 11.80% for dirty wounds.

Table 8–3. Wound classification.

Clean	These are uninfected operative wounds in which no inflammation is encountered and the respiratory, alimentary, genital, or uninfected urinary tracts are not entered.
Clean/ contaminated	These are operative wounds in which the respiratory, alimentary, genital, or urinary tract is entered under controlled conditions and without unusual contamination.
Contaminated	These include open, fresh, accidental wounds, operations with major breaks in sterile technique or gross spillage from the gastrointestinal tract, and incisions in which acute, nonpurulent inflammation is encountered.
Dirty	These include old traumatic wounds with retained devitalized tissue and those that involve existing clinical infection or perforated viscera.

User Guide for the 2008 Participant Use Data File American College of Surgeons National Surgical Quality Improvement Program.

Attributable Cost & Impact

In addition to the morbidity incurred by patients, the health care and economic burden of SSIs is significant. Multiple studies have consistently documented that SSIs lead to a considerable increase in length of hospital stay (LOS), hospital charges, and societal health services cost. In a 2012 study, SSI occurring after colorectal surgery increased the LOS by 2.8-23.9 days, depending on the nature of the procedure (colon vs rectum resection), the operative approach (open vs laparoscopic), and the depth of the SSI. In another study of cardiac surgery, it was estimated that the total excess cost attributable to SSI is more than $12,000 per patient. This excess cost resulted from the additional procedures (eg, incision and drainage, wound washout, skin grafts), antibiotics and increased hospital LOS. Another study in general and vascular surgery patients estimated the excess cost and LOS at $10,497 and 4.3 days, respectively. In addition, even when SSI patients are successfully discharged, their rate of hospital readmission is at least doubled. Another study using patient-centered surveys and large administrative databases suggested almost a threefold increase in the total cost for patients diagnosed with SSI following discharge from the hospital compared to those who do not develop SSI. The increased costs were accounted for by a significant increase in the use of visiting nurses for wound care, diagnostic imaging, as well as an increase in readmissions to emergency departments and to the hospital.

Pathophysiology

The etiology of SSI is multifactorial; patient's comorbidities, the nature of the surgical procedure and technique, and the perioperative environment including infrastructure and processes of care all interact in SSI. It is thought that most SSIs are directly caused by the patient's endogenous flora at the time of surgery. This is further supported by the fact that, in clean wounds, SSIs are most commonly caused by *S aureus* or coagulase negative *Staphylococcus*, both abundantly present on patient's skin. On the other hand, SSIs following bowel surgery are usually caused by endogenous intestinal flora. When a surgical device or implant is left in place, bacteria can secrete special glycocalyx-based biofilms that shield the offending bacteria from the body's immune defenses. One of the immediate sequelae of such a phenomenon is the fact that the inoculums needed to cause a SSI in the presence of a foreign body such as a surgical implant or device is typically smaller than the inoculum needed to cause the same infection in the absence of a foreign body.

Despite the belief that most SSIs originate from endogenous microbes, there is convincing literature suggesting that nonendogenous sources are implicated in the occurrence of SSIs as well. Breach of the strict sterile surgical field, undetected surgical gloves' perforations, increased personnel traffic through the operating room, suboptimal air flow and ventilation in the operating room, and poor surgical technique with excessive tissue injury or tension are some of the many factors implicated in SSI that will be discussed further in the next few sections.

Risk Factors

Many risk factors have been implicated as predictors of SSI. Some are directly related to the patient's health status, immune system, and comorbidities, while others are inherent to the nature of the procedure being performed and therefore are not easily modifiable. A few risk factors reflect suboptimal health care systems' design and less than reliable processes of care delivery, and their importance relies in the possibility of subjecting them to improvement and optimization strategies.

A. Patient-Related Risk Factors

Several studies have shown that advanced age, diabetes mellitus, obesity, smoking, malnutrition, and immunosuppression (eg, chronic steroid use, HIV/AIDS, posttransplant) are all risk factors for the development of SSI (Table 8–1). Most of these factors are not amenable to immediate preoperative modification or prevention, although long-term control of glucose levels (reflected in better HBA1C levels), smoking cessation, and attempts to improve nutrition may help in the overall performance of the patient perioperatively and may also decrease complications, including SSI.

B. Procedure Related Risk Factors

The nature of the procedure, especially the wound classification (Table 8–3) and the expected inoculum of bacteria into the surgical site are key factors that influence the risk of developing a SSI. For example, the rate of SSIs complicating eye surgery, where the inoculum of bacterial contamination is minimal, is almost non-existent. In comparison, the rate of SSI complicating colorectal surgery remains closer to 20% despite strategies and efforts aimed at prevention. In the early 1990s, the National Healthcare Safety Network (NHSN) risk index, previously called the National Nosocomial Infections Surveillance System (NNIS), was developed in an attempt to better define a priori, a patient's risk of developing SSI. This index considered the following three factors:

1. An American Society of Anesthesiologists (ASA) score ≥ 3

2. A surgical wound classification as either contaminated or dirty

3. A prolonged duration of procedure over a certain number of hours T, where T depends on the nature of the procedure being performed

The analysis of the CDC data by Culver and colleagues revealed that the rates of SSIs are 1.5%, 2.9%, 6.8%, and 13%

in the presence of none, 1, 2, or 3 of the above risk index factors, respectively. More recently, The NHSN has introduced improved SSI risk adjustment models for specific operations based on easily tractable patient risk factors.

C. Process- and System-Related Risk Factors

Several process- and system-related risk factors have been identified over the years as potential factors contributing for a higher rate of SSI.

Suboptimal choice and timing of perioperative antibiotics—In a systematic review of more than 30,000 Medicare patients, Bratzler and colleagues found that less than 56% of patients undergoing surgery received their perioperative antibiotics within the recommended 60-minutes window before incision. In the same study, up to 10% of patients did not receive the appropriate antibiotic regimen that would cover the type of pathogens specific to the procedures the patients were undergoing. The two main components of prophylactic perioperative antibiotics, namely, choice and timing, will be discussed in further detail in the SSI prevention section below.

Unrecognized breach of asepsis—Operating room staff, including nursing, anesthesia and surgical personnel, are strongly encouraged to immediately report to the surgeon when suspecting a potential breach of the sterile field (eg, inadequate skin preparation, soiled clothes or equipment, glove perforation). In a study of gynecological laparotomies, glove perforations were found to occur in 27 out of 29 laparotomies. The relationship between the rates of SSIs and glove perforation is less than evident when the data is analyzed. In a study of more than 4000 procedures, the rates of SSIs increased with glove perforation only in the absence of appropriate antibiotic prophylaxis.

Preoperative hair removal—Preoperative hair removal has been correlated in several studies with a higher rate of SSI, even when the procedure involves the scalp or the patient has abundant hair at the surgical site. A 2006 Cochrane database systematic review and meta-analysis concluded that preoperative shaving increases the rate of SSI by at least twofold; it is noteworthy that there was no difference in the rates of SSI when hair clipping was compared to no hair removal. Therefore, if hair removal is deemed necessary, preoperative hair clipping is preferred to shaving.

Surgical technique—The use of "rough" surgical techniques with unnecessary or excessive tissue disruption and trauma, whether resulting from electrocautery, traction or blunt dissection, is believed to lead to higher rates of SSI. Even though most surgeons and common sense suggest the above correlation, strong evidence supporting a cause-effect relationship has not been demonstrated.

Operating room traffic—It is well established that the burden of airborne bacteria in a closed space is directly related to the number of people in the space, as well as to the number of people entering and exiting a closed space such as the OR. The link between increased traffic through the OR doors and SSIs has been studied mostly in the orthopedic literature, but has not been clearly established. Nonetheless, the CDC has issued guidelines that include a decrease in OR traffic.

Perioperative hypothermia—Even though hypothermia may protect tissue from ischemia and necrosis by decreasing cellular oxygen consumption, perioperative hypothermia may cause vasoconstriction at the skin level, and therefore decrease oxygen delivery. Two randomized trials attempted to study the effect of hypothermia on the incidence of SSI. The first one found an increased SSI risk with hypothermia in colorectal surgery, while the second failed to find any correlation in cardiac surgery. At present, maintenance of perioperative normothermia is recommended.

▶ Prevention Strategies

Prevention of SSI relies primarily on optimizing the patient's comorbidities and creating a systematic method to ensure that all modifiable risk factors are addressed. All processes of care proven or arguably thought to prevent SSIs should be executed in all patients at all times. Table 8–4 lists potential measures to minimize the risk of SSI. Although level-one evidence is lacking for many of those measures, inclusion of some or all in a bundle might prove to be a beneficial strategy. The surgical improvement project (SIP) established in 2004 and folded within the surgical care improvement program in 2006 (SCIP) created performance measures out of several of these preventative measures based on best evidence in literature (Table 8–5). A detailed discussion of SCIP is beyond the scope of this text and the reader is referred to the CDC and CMS websites for more details. Perioperative antibiotics and the choice of the skin preparation solution are discussed below.

A. Perioperative Antibiotics

The timing of prophylactic antibiotic administration (SCIP 1) and the choice of the appropriate perioperative antibiotic (SCIP 2) are key components in the strategy to prevent SSI. Prophylaxis implies discontinuation of the antibiotic within 24 hours in noncardiac surgery and within 48 hours in cardiac surgery (SCIP 3); this will also prevent side effects of the antibiotic and the emergence of drug resistance. Proper antibiotic dosing based on the patient's weight and manufacturer's recommendation for the antibiotic is an important consideration in prophylaxis. In addition, redosing of the antibiotic during surgery based on the antibiotic

Table 8–4. Potential[a] measures to prevent surgical site infections.

Optimizing the patient's nutritional status
Appropriate perioperative antibiotic prophylaxis (choice, dosing, and timing)
Adequate glucose level control in diabetic patients
Maintenance of perioperative normoglycemia in all patients
Maintenance of strict asepsis
Preoperative skin preparation with alcohol-based solutions
Gentle skin handling and minimization of cautery-related tissue damage
Improving ventilation and laminar air flow in the OR
Maintenance of perioperative normothermia
Avoiding hair removal; clipping instead of shaving, if necessary
Perioperative oxygen supplementation
Preoperative antibacterial soap showers
Antibacterial coated sutures
Antibacterial irrigation solutions
Operative wound barriers
Antibacterial dressings

[a]Many of these measures have shown controversial and nondefinitive results in the prevention of SSI.

Table 8–5. Surgical Care Improvement Project (SCIP) measures aimed at prevention of surgical site infections.

SCIP Infection Measure 1	Prophylactic antibiotic received within 1 h prior to surgical incision
SCIP Infection Measure 2	Appropriate prophylactic antibiotic selection for the surgical patient
SCIP Infection Measure 3	Prophylactic antibiotic discontinued within 24 h after surgery end time (within 48 h after cardiac surgery end time)
SCIP Infection Measure 4	Blood glucose level at 6 AM < 200 mg/dL on postoperative days 1 and 2 in cardiac surgery
SCIP Infection Measure 6	No or appropriate hair removal (clippers not shaving)
SCIP Infection Measure 7	Immediate postoperative normothermia (temperature > 96.8°F within 15 min postoperatively) in colorectal surgery

Table 8–6. Suggested initial dose and time to redosing for antimicrobial drugs commonly utilized for surgical prophylaxis.

| Antimicrobial | Renal Half-Life (h) | | Recommended Infusion Duration | Standard Dose | Weight-Based Dose Recommendation[a] | Recommended Redosing Interval,[b] (h) |
	Patients With Normal Renal Function	Patients With End-Stage Renal Disease				
Aztreonam	1.5-2	6	3-5 min,[c] 20-60 min[d]	1-2 g iv	2 g maximum (adults)	3-5
Ciprofloxacin	3.5-5	5-9	60 min	400 mg iv	400 mg	4-10
Cefazolin	1.2-2.5	40-70	3-5 min,[c] 15 60 min[d]	1-2 g iv	20-30 mg/kg (if < 80 kg, use 1 g; if > 80 kg, use 2 g)	2-5
Cefuroxime	1-2	15-22	3 5 min,[c] 15-60 min[d]	1.5 g iv	50 mg/kg	3-4
Cefamandole	0.5-2.1	12.3-18	3-5 min,[c] 15-60 min[d]	1 g iv		3-4
Cefoxitin	0.5-1.1	6.5-23	3-5 min,[c] 15-60 min[d]	1-2 g iv	20-40 mg/kg	2-3
Cefotetan	2.8-4.6	13-25	3-5 min,[c] 20-60 min[d]	1-2 g iv	20-40 mg/kg	3-6
Clindamycin	2-5.1	3.5-5[f]	10-60 min (do not exceed 30 mg/min)	600-900 mg iv	If < 10 kg, use at least 37.5 mg; if > 10 kg, use 3-6 mg/kg	3-6
Erythromycin base	0.8-3	5-6	NA	1 g po 19, 18, and 9 h before surgery	9-13 mg/kg	NA
Gentamicin	2-3	50-70	30-60 min	1.5 mg/kg iv[g]	...[g]	3-6
Neomycin	2-3 (3% absorbed orally)	12-24 or longer	NA	1g po 19, 18, and 9 h before surgery	20 mg/kg	NA
Metronidazole	6-14	7-21; no change	30-60 min	0.5-1 g iv	15 mg/kg initial dose (adult); 7.5 mg/kg on subsequent doses	6-8
Vancomycin	4-6	44.1-406.4 (CCl < 10 mL/min)	1 g over 60 min (use longer infusion time if dose > 1 g)	1 g iv	10-15 mg/kg (adult)	6-12

CCl, creatinine clearance.

[a]Data are primarily from published pediatric recommendations.

[b]For procedures of long duration, antimicrobials should be readministered at intervals of one to two times the half-life of the drug. The intervals in this table were calculated for patients with normal renal function.

[c]Dose injected directly into vein or via running intravenous fluids.

[d]Intermittent intravenous infusion.

[e]In patients with a serum creatinine level of 5-9 mg/dL.

[f]The half-life of clindamycin is the same or slightly increased in patients with end-stage renal disease, compared with patients with normal renal function.

[g]If the patient's body weight is > 30% higher than their ideal body weight (IBW), the dosing weight (DW) can be determined as follows: DW = IBW + (0.4 × [total body weight − IBW]).

Reproduced, with permission, from Bratzler DW, Houck PM: Antimicrobial prophylaxis for surgery: an advisory statement from the National Surgical Infection Prevention Project, *Clin Infect Dis.* 2004 Jun 15;38(12):1706–1715.

half-life, amount of fluid administration and blood loss is more important than the continuation of the antibiotic after the wound is closed. Table 8–6 is a practical guide to dosing and time for redosing for commonly used prophylactic antibiotics.

B. Antiseptic Skin Preparation

Based on a prospective randomized trial and an observational study, the National Quality Forum has recommended the use of alcohol-containing solutions for the preparation of patient's skin prior to surgery.

C. Additional Preventative Measures

Maintenance of perioperative normoglycemia (SCIP 4), normothermia (SCIP 7), and hair clipping or avoiding hair removal (SCIP 6) are definitely advocated and monitored as performance measures for certain operations. The use of preoperative antibacterial soap showers, perioperative oxygen administration, the use of antibacterial coated sutures, wound barriers, antimicrobial irrigants, and antibacterial dressings are additional measures that remain controversial in the prevention of SSI (Table 8–4). Mechanical bowel preparation and oral antibiotics in patients undergoing colorectal surgery are the subjects of renewed controversy and discussion but remain an important strategy in the prevention of SSI in this field.

▶ Treatment

The treatment of an established SSI consists of opening the incision, draining the purulent material, and debridement of any necrotic tissue. Adjunctive antimicrobial treatment is given when the patient has systemic symptoms, associated cellulitis or a deep SSI with risk for fascial and subcutaneous spread. Cultures are important to track emergence of resistant organisms, to de-escalate from broad-spectrum empiric antibiotics, and for epidemiological surveillance. In the case of an organ/space SSI, percutaneous drainage using radiological guidance, along with adequate antibiotic coverage, is the preferred approach.

INFECTIONS NEEDING SURGICAL MANAGEMENT

When infections fail to respond or are deemed unlikely to respond to medical and antimicrobial treatments alone, surgical intervention might be needed. The list of surgical infections necessitating surgical management is long, but the most common ones include abscesses, empyema, necrotizing skin and soft tissue infections (NSSTIs), intra-abdominal infections, and *Clostridium difficile* (*C difficile*) colitis. Many of these surgical infections can become life threatening by causing sepsis, septic shock, and multiple organ dysfunction syndrome (MODS) if not controlled and treated promptly. Spreading can occur through tissue planes (necrotizing infections), abscess/fistulae formation, or through the lymphatic system and the bloodstream. Spread of an infection through the bloodstream (bacteremia) can lead to distant seeding of bacteria and subsequent abscess formation (eg, brain, liver, adrenal glands, heart valves).

INFLAMMATION, SEPSIS, THE SYSTEMIC INFLAMMATORY RESPONSE SYNDROME, BACTEREMIA, & MULTIPLE ORGAN DYSFUNCTION SYNDROME

Microbial infection results in tissue damage that leads to an inflammatory response at the local tissue level in an effort by the patient's immune system to overcome the infection. At the site of injury, endothelial cells and leukocytes coordinate the local release of mediators of the inflammatory response, including cytokines (tumor necrosis factor-α), interleukins, interferons, leukotrienes, prostaglandins, nitric oxide, reactive oxygen species, and products of the classic inflammatory pathway (complement, histamine, and bradykinin) (Table 8–7). Once these mediators reach the infected site, they are extremely effective at recruiting and priming cells of both the innate and adaptive immune systems to identify and attack invading pathogens. In addition, these inflammatory mediators initiate the damaged tissue healing processes. However, if the degree of the infectious or traumatic insult overwhelms the ability of the body to control it, the inflammatory mediators might trigger a systemic inflammatory reaction of serious damaging consequences. Such a quasi-maladaptive systemic response can disrupt normal cellular metabolism and jeopardize tissue perfusion at the cellular level. From a terminology perspective, when the systemic response occurs in the absence of a documented infection (eg, burns, trauma, pancreatitis), it is called *systemic inflammatory response syndrome* (SIRS). The term sepsis is used when the systemic response results from a documented infection rather than systemic inflammation alone. Severe sepsis is reported when sepsis is associated with at least one sign of tissue or organ hypoperfusion. Septic shock occurs when severe sepsis is associated with hypotension or hemodynamic instability. When septic shock leads to progressive dysfunction of multiple organs such as the brain (delirium), lungs (hypoxia and respiratory failure), heart (hypotension, pulmonary edema), and kidneys (oliguria and renal failure), it is referred to as *multiple organ dysfunction syndrome* (MODS). Bacteremia is the presence of viable bacteria in blood, often documented through blood cultures. Transient bacteremia (eg, following dental work) is common, benign, and self-limited. It usually has no clinical implications except in patients with damaged heart valves; cardiac, vascular, or orthopedic implants; or impaired immunity. Bacteremia happening in a patient with an uncontrolled source of infection can be devastating and may result in severe sepsis, septic shock, and MODS. The interrelationships among infection, bacteremia, sepsis, and SIRS are depicted in Figure 8–2, and the detailed clinical definitions of sepsis, severe sepsis, septic shock, SIRS, and MODS are presented in Table 8–8.

▶ Diagnosis

Localizing the source of the suspected infection or sepsis is crucial, and a good and thorough physical examination is indispensable. Laboratory evaluation often shows leukocytosis, but leukopenia is not infrequent in cases of severe infection or sepsis. Acidosis is occasionally present and might be helpful in making the diagnosis. Radiologic examinations, including plain films for suspected pneumonia, computed

Table 8–7. Cytokines and growth factors.

Peptide	Site of Synthesis	Regulation	Target Cells	Effects
G-CSF	Fibroblasts, monocytes	Induced by IL-1, LPS, IFN-α	Committed neutrophil progenitors (CFU-G, Gran)	Supports the proliferation of neutrophil-forming colonies. Stimulates respiratory burst.
GM-CSF (IL-3 has almost identical effects)	Endothelial cells, fibroblasts, macrophages, T lymphocytes, bone marrow	Induced by IL-1, TNF	Granulocyte-erythrocyte-monocyte-megakaryocyte progenitor cells (CFU-GEMM, CFU-MEG, CFU-Eo, CFU-GM)	Supports the proliferation of macrophage-, eosinophil-, neutrophil-, and monocyte-containing colonies.
IFN-α, IFN-β, IFN γ	Epithelial cells, fibroblasts, lymphocytes, macrophages, neutrophils	Induced by viruses (foreign nucleic acids), microbes, microbial foreign antigens, cancer cells	Lymphocytes, macrophages, infected cells, cancer cells	Inhibits viral multiplication. Activates defective phagocytes, direct inhibition of cancer cell multiplication, activation of killer leukocytes, inhibition of collagen synthesis.
IL-1	Endothelial cells, keratinocytes, lymphocytes, macrophages	Induced by TNF-α, IL-1, IL-2, C5a; suppressed by IL-4, TGF-β	Monocytes, macrophages, T cells, B cells, NK cells, LAK cells	Stimulates T cells, B cells, NK cells, LAK cells. Induces tumoricidal activity and production to other cytokines, endogenous pyrogen (via PGE$_2$ release). Induces steroidogenesis, acute phase proteins, hypotension; chemotactic neutrophils. Stimulates respiratory burst.
IL-1ra	Monocytes	Induced by GM-CSF, LPS, IgG	Blocks type 1 IL-1 receptors on T cells, fibroblasts, chondrocytes, endothelial cells	Blocks type 1 IL-1 receptors on T cells, chondrocytes, endothelial cells. Ameliorates animal models of arthritis, septic shock, and inflammatory bowel disease.
IL-2	Lymphocytes	Induced by IL-1, IL-6	T cells, NK cells, B cells, activated monocytes	Stimulates growth of T cells, NK cells, and B cells
IL-4	T cells, NK cells, mast cells	Induced by cell activation, IL-1	All hematopoietic cells and many others express receptors	Stimulates B-cell and T-cell growth. Induces HLA class II molecules.
IL-6	Endothelial cells, fibroblasts, lymphocytes, some tumors	Induced by IL-1, TNF-α	T cells, B cells, plasma cells, keratinocytes, hepatocytes, stem cells	B-cell differentiation. Induction of acute phase proteins, growth of keratinocytes. Stimulates growth of T cells and hematopoietic stem cells.
IL-8	Endothelial cells, fibroblasts, lymphocytes, monocytes	Induced by TNF, IL-1, LPS, cell adherence (monocytes)	Basophils, neutrophils, T cells	Induces expression of endothelial cell LECAM-1 receptors, β$_2$ integrins, and neutrophil transmigration. Stimulates respiratory burst.
M-CSF	Endothelial cells, fibroblasts, monocytes	Induced by IL-1, LPS, IFN-α	Committed monocyte progenitors (CFU-M, mono)	Supports the proliferation of monocyte-forming colonies. Activates macrophages.
MCP-1, MCAF	Monocytes; some tumors secrete a similar peptide	Induced by IL-1, LPS, PHA	Unstimulated monocytes	Chemoattractant specific for monocytes
TNF-α (LT has almost identical effects)	Macrophages, NK cells, T cells, transformed cell lines, B cells (LT)	Suppressed by PGE$_2$, TGF-β, IL-4; induced by LPS	Endothelial cells, monocytes, neutrophils	Stimulates T-cell growth. Direct cytotoxin to some tumor cells. Profound proinflammatory effect via induction of IL-1 and PGE$_2$. Systemic administration produces many symptoms of sepsis. Stimulates respiratory burst and phagocytosis.

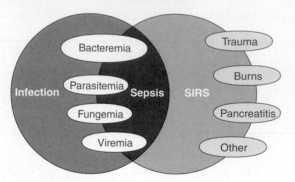

▲ **Figure 8–2.** The interplay between infection, sepsis, and systemic inflammatory response syndrome (SIRS).

Table 8–8. Definitions of sepsis, severe sepsis, septic shock, and systemic inflammatory response syndrome (SIRS).

SIRS

Two or more of the following:
Temperature > 38.3°C or < 36°C
Heart rate > 90 beats/min
Respiratory rate > 20 breaths/min or $Paco_2$ < 32 mmHg
WBC > 12,000 cells/mm³, < 4000 cells/mm³, or > 10% immature (band) forms

Sepsis

SIRS *and* a culture-proven or clinically evident infection

Severe sepsis

Sepsis *and* at least one of the following:
Areas of mottled skin
Capillary refilling requires three seconds or longer
Urine output < 0.5 mL/kg for at least 1 h, or renal replacement therapy
Lactate > 2 mmol/L
Abrupt change in mental status
Abnormal electroencephalographic (EEG) findings
Platelet count < 100,000 platelets/mcL
Disseminated intravascular coagulation
Acute respiratory distress syndrome (ARDS)
Cardiac dysfunction (ie, left ventricular systolic dysfunction)

Septic shock

Severe sepsis *and* at least one of the following:
MAP < 60 mm Hg despite adequate fluid resuscitation
Hemodynamic pressor agents requirement to maintain MAP > 60 mm Hg despite adequate fluid resuscitation

MAP, mean arterial pressure.
Adequate fluid resuscitation is defined by one of the three following parameters:
• Infusion of at least 40-60 mL/kg of saline solution
• Pulmonary capillary wedge pressure of 12-20 mm Hg
• A central venous pressure of 8-12 mm Hg

tomography or ultrasound for suspected intra-abdominal or intrathoracic abscesses, and bone scans or magnetic resonance imaging (MRI) for suspected osteomyelitis, are often essential for making the diagnosis and establishing the source of infection.

Identifying the causative organism by culturing the infected site, followed by testing the implicated pathogen's sensitivity to diverse antimicrobial agents are the two next key steps. If infection is suspected but the source remains unclear, cultures of blood, sputum, and urine should be performed. Culturing other body fluids (eg, cerebrospinal fluid, pleural and joint effusions, ascites) can be performed if warranted based on the patient's history, physical examination, and the degree of clinical suspicion.

▶ Treatment

Infectious source control and antibiotics constitute the mainstay of surgical infection treatment. When patients are septic with or without shock, "goal-directed" management of the sepsis with prompt patient resuscitation and immediate initiation of the appropriate empiric antibiotics are of ultimate importance, and have been shown by high-level evidence to improve patient survival. The *Surviving Sepsis Guidelines* emphasize the systematic and evidence-based approach to treating sepsis and septic shock patients. These guidelines are available at www.survivingsepsis.org.

▼ SURGICAL SKIN & SKIN STRUCTURE INFECTIONS

Surgical cutaneous infections span the spectrum of the superficial skin abscesses such as furuncles and carbuncles to the devastating and often fatal necrotizing deeper soft tissue infections.

FURUNCLE

▶ Pathophysiology

A furuncle (boil) is a superficial skin abscess usually caused by *S aureus* infection at the level of the hair follicle. Bacteria asymptomatically inhabit most hair follicles, but it is thought that obstruction of the pilosebaceous apparatus is the triggering event for the formation of furuncles.

▶ Risk Factors

Some of the identified risk factors include puberty, male gender, obesity, diabetes, poor hygiene, as well as living in weathers characterized by a high level of humidity.

▶ Causative Organisms

Even though staphylococci are the most common causative organisms, streptococci, gram-negative organisms, and anaerobic diphtheroids can also cause furuncles.

Clinical Presentation

Furuncles present as itchy indurated small abscesses, surrounded by skin erythema. A small white area of skin necrosis is often notable at the top of the abscess.

Treatment

Most furuncles resolve spontaneously, although larger lesions require incision and drainage. The use of antibiotics following incision and drainage is not routinely needed and is controversial. We recommend antibiotics only in the presence of concomitant extensive surrounding cellulitis. When antibiotics are prescribed, they should be stopped with resolution of the local and systemic symptoms. Antibacterial soap showers might be helpful in both treatment and prevention of recurrence.

CARBUNCLE

Pathophysiology

Carbuncles are rare and result when several furuncles coalesce, extend to the subcutaneous tissue, and/or form a "network" of multilocular interconnected abscesses and tracts.

Risk Factors

Carbuncles on the back of the neck are seen almost exclusively in diabetic or relatively immunocompromised patients. In addition to obesity and diabetes, chronic steroid intake and malnutrition are potential risk factors for carbuncles.

Causative Organism

Similar to furuncles, S aureus remains the most common organism involved in carbuncles.

Clinical Presentation

Carbuncles often have the appearance of multiple large furuncles with several openings draining pus. As carbuncles enlarge, the blood supply to the skin is destroyed and the tissue over the top of the abscess becomes white in color and necrotic in appearance. Patients might show some systemic signs such as fever and malaise.

Treatment

Carbuncles often require incision and drainage; occasionally, a more extensive excision is required. When appropriate, the excision is continued until the many associated deep sinus tracts are removed. Antibiotics are usually needed in view of the associated extensive skin cellulitis and induration.

HIDRADINITIS SUPPURATIVA

Pathophysiology

Hidradenitis suppurativa is a serious skin condition characterized by blockage and infection of the apocrine sweat glands. Hidradenitis most commonly involves the axilla or the groin. Since apocrine glands develop postpuberty, prepubertal disease is very rare. Even though hidradenitis often becomes chronic with serious patient morbidity and disability, systemic complications, and constitutional signs and symptoms are uncommon.

Risk Factors

Obesity, puberty, female gender, and smoking are some of the identified risk factors associated with hidradenitis.

Causative Agents

Hidradenitis is a polymicrobial infection involving grampositive, gram-negative, and anaerobic organisms. Superinfection with fungal organisms is not uncommon, especially in the patient with chronic or recurrent hidradenitis.

Clinical Presentation

Hidradenitis can affect any area where apocrine glands exist, most commonly the axilla and groin, but also the perineum, inframammary folds, gluteal folds, areola, and scrotum. On examination, erythematous tender skin nodules characterize early stages. This can quickly progress to deeper indurated abscesses with interconnected sinuses, purulent drainage, and associated regional lymphadenopathy.

Treatment

Drainage of the individual abscesses and their associated sinuses is needed. If healing is delayed, fungal superinfections should be suspected and, if confirmed, should be treated as well. With chronic and recurrent infections, the involved skin and apocrine glands can be excised, and the underlying soft tissue left to heal by secondary intention. Skin flaps and grafts might be needed in later stages, as the resultant scarring can be severe. Topical clindamycin, systemic tetracycline, and isotretinoin are potential adjunctive therapies. Weight loss and hygiene-focused interventions should be encouraged to decrease the risk of recurrence.

NECROTIZING SKIN & SKIN STRUCTURE INFECTIONS

Introduction

Accurate data on the incidence of necrotizing skin and skin structure infections (NSSSIs) is lacking, and most existing data are based on single institutions' experiences, suggesting a large variability in clinical presentation, severity as well as outcome. NSSSIs are skin and soft tissue infections characterized by widespread and severe tissue necrosis resulting from aggressive and life-threatening bacteria that are often able to secrete toxins. NSSSIs are also known as gas gangrene, necrotizing fasciitis (when involving fascial layers), Fournier gangrene (when involving the perineum and genitalia), and Ludwig angina (when involving the floor of the mouth).

Pathophysiology

NSSSIs can be caused by single agents such as clostridia or streptococci species, but most are polymicrobial in etiology. An inciting site (eg, puncture wound, insect bite) can occasionally be discovered by history or physical examination. In the perineum, manipulation of the urogenital tract and diabetes are known to be associated with NSSTI. The infection is classically one of sudden onset and rapid progression through ischemic tissue planes, occasionally with air formation at deeper layers. Small vessel thrombosis occurs along the infection progression pathway, and thus, the underlying deeper tissue damage is almost always much more pronounced than what the overlying skin appearance suggests.

Causative Agents

By definition, type I NSSSIs are polymicrobial (eg, streptococci, clostridia), while type II NSSSIs are monomicrobial. *C perfringens* secretes exotoxins (eg, lecithinases, collagenases, proteases, hemolysins) that lead to small vessel thrombosis and allow for rapid progression and aggressive invasion of fascial and muscle planes. These toxins contribute to the serious deep tissue destruction and the overlying skin grayish discoloration. The alpha toxin (a lecithinase) is believed to be an essential contributor to clostridial virulence. In addition to their local effect, these toxins may lead to severe sepsis, pronounced SIRS, and not uncommonly MODS. Streptococci can also secrete several exotoxins with similar virulence leading to fascial and deeper plane disruptions. *S pyogenes* (group A strep), although rare, is classically described to secrete a superantigen toxin that can result in toxic shock syndrome with resultant organ failure. NSSSIs are often caused by mixed nonclostridial, nonstreptococcal bacteria, including staphylococci, gram negatives, and anaerobes.

Risk Factors

Immunocompromised (eg, HIV, diabetes), intravenous drug abuse, and cancer patients are at a particularly higher risk of developing NSSSIs, as well as malnourished and obese patients.

Clinical Presentation

Prompt suspicion and early diagnosis of NSSSIs are essential. In early stages, patients often have fever and pain out of proportion to physical examination findings. Erythema, induration, hemorrhagic skin bulla, blisters, and vesicles are occasionally present. Grayish discoloration of the underlying skin and pain beyond the affected skin area are especially suggestive of deeper underlying tissue involvement. "Dishwasher-like" gray discharge might be seen and should raise suspicion of NSSSIs. Patients can quickly develop systemic signs of toxicity with hypotension, tachycardia, electrolyte imbalances, lethargy, and even organ failure. Laboratory workup typically shows leukocytosis (with or without bandemia) or leucopenia, hyponatremia, and acidosis. Several models have been developed over the years in an attempt to predict the probability of a skin infection being a NSSTI versus a more benign superficial skin infection. The Laboratory Risk Indicator for Necrotizing Fasciitis (LRINEC) score assigns different point scores to each of six laboratory values (Table 8–9). A LRINEC score of six or more was found in a study of 89 NSSSIs to have a positive predictive value of 92% and a negative predictive of 96% for NSSTI. Radiologically, plain films showing deep soft tissue air are pathognomonic. Computed tomography (CT) scan is the standard of care when difficulty arises in differentiating between "benign" skin or soft tissue infection and NSSSIs. CT images often show inflammation and edema at the deeper fascial or muscular layers, and occasionally will show gas between these tissue layers. Although crepitus as felt on physical examination and/or deep tissue air as diagnosed by plain radiography or CT imaging have been classically described with several (but not all) clostridial species, they

Table 8–9. The Laboratory Risk Indicator for Necrotizing Fasciitis (LRINEC) Score.

Variable	Points
C-reactive protein (mg/L) > 150	4
WBC count (× 103 cells/mcL)	
< 15	0
15-25	1
> 25	0
Hemoglobin (g/dL)	
> 13.5	0
11-13.5	1
< 11	2
Sodium (mmol/L) < 135	2
Creatinine (μmol/L) > 141	2
Glucose (mmol/L) > 10	1

may occur with nonclostridial infections as well. When the clinical picture and the radiological imaging fail to differentiate between benign soft tissue infection and NSSSIs, diagnostic surgical exploration of the area in question is needed. Operative findings suggestive of NSSSIs include pale and/or necrotic deep tissue, "dishwasher" nonpurulent gray discharge, nonbleeding soft tissue, and thrombosed microvessels. Easy separation with unopposed finger "sliding" between the tissue planes (the "finger test") is highly suggestive of NSSSIs. Pathologic examination will reveal severe inflammation and tissue necrosis.

▶ Treatment

A NSSSI is a surgical emergency and requires immediate

1. Wide surgical debridement
2. Broad-spectrum antibiotics
3. Hemodynamic and fluid resuscitation

Wide Surgical Debridement

All tissue that appears pale, ischemic, or necrotic, "lifts off" easily, or does not bleed appropriately needs to be removed. This should include the overlying skin, even when it appears viable, as studies have documented severe vasculitis and microvessel thrombosis that eventually lead to loss of skin, if not adequately debrided. Extensive debridement is usually needed, with one or more repeat trips to the operating room, until viable tissue is ensured. When an extremity is involved, amputation might be required, although attempts at debridement and limb salvage, with a planned "second look" are reasonable and might be preferred. Perirectal NSSSI and Fournier gangrene occasionally necessitate creation of an ostomy and/or urinary diversion. Depending on the extent and location of debridement, many patients, if they survive and recover, are disfigured and will need reconstructive surgery ranging from simple split thickness skin grafts to major flap reconstructions.

A. Antibiotics

As soon as a NSSSI is suspected, broad-spectrum antibiotics should be initiated. Gram-positive, gram-negative, and anaerobic organisms need to be covered. A combination of a penicillin-based agent or cephalosporin with an aminoglycoside or fluoroquinolone and an anti-anaerobic agent (eg, metronidazole or clindamycin) is a reasonable starting empiric regimen. Clindamycin has been shown by in vitro studies to have anti-inflammatory and toxin-neutralizing effects, in addition to its antibacterial effects. If methicillin-resistant *S aureus* is suspected, penicillins can be replaced by vancomycin or linezolid. Aminoglycosides can be replaced by third- or fourth-generation cephalosporins (eg, cefepime, cefotaxime) or by carbapenems (eg, imipenem, meropenem, ertapenem), if indicated (eg, in patients with acute

renal failure). The Infectious Diseases Society of America (IDSA) published guidelines for the antibiotic choices in NSSSIs are reported in Table 8–10.

B. Hyperbaric Oxygen

The usefulness of hyperbaric oxygen in the treatment of NSSTI is controversial. Several small retrospective studies have suggested decreased mortality with hyperbaric therapy, but the absence of supportive level one evidence, combined with the logistical difficulties in critically ill patients remain the main obstacles to recommend its routine utilization.

▶ Prognosis

NSSSI has a poor prognosis with reported mortality as high as 20%-50%, and an even higher morbidity rate. Diabetic patients and/or those presenting with septic shock and/or multisystem organ failure are at a particularly higher risk of mortality. Shorter time from onset of infection to operative debridement has been shown consistently to correlate with better survival.

ORGAN/SPACE INFECTIONS

Organ/space infections are often deep infections resulting from uncontrolled infection or perforation of an internal organ. Internal postoperative abscesses are termed organ/space SSIs, and have been discussed previously. In addition to antibiotic treatment, many of these organ/space infections will need drainage.

▶ Intra-Abdominal Abscesses and Infections

In the era of high-resolution CT imaging, diseases like acute diverticulitis and acute perforated appendicitis are more likely to be successfully managed nonoperatively in the acute clinical setting. When patients have no signs of diffuse peritonitis, periappendiceal, pericolonic abscesses, and other contained intraperitoneal abscesses may be drained percutaneously under radiological guidance when accessible. With the combination of percutaneous drainage and adequate antibiotic coverage, patients' intra-abdominal infections can be treated adequately, allowing for the inflammation to resolve with potentially one-stage and less complicated surgical intervention at a later time to address the diseased organ. When percutaneous drainage is not possible, usually because of the abscess location and its inaccessibility to radiological interventions, surgical drainage with removal of the infected organ (eg, appendectomy, colectomy) is warranted. If the abscess is less than 3-4 cm in diameter, an attempt at treatment with antibiotics alone without percutaneous or surgical drainage is a reasonable option in the stable patient without peritoneal signs. The management of complicated intra-abdominal infections, whether community acquired or health care associated,

Table 8–10. The Infectious Diseases Society of America guidelines for antibiotic treatment of NSSTIs.

First-Line Antimicrobial Agent, by Infection Type	Adult Dosage	Antimicrobial Agent(s) for Patients With Severe Penicillin Hypersensitivity
Mixed infection		
Ampicillin-sulbactam	1.5–3.0 g every 6–8 h iv	Clindamycin or metronidazole[a] with an aminoglycoside or fluoroquinolone
or		
piperacillin-tazobactam	3.37 g every 6–8 h iv	
plus		
clindamycin	600–900 mg/kg every 8 h iv	
plus		
ciprofloxacin	400 mg every 12 h iv	
Imipenem/cilastatin	1 g every 6–8 h iv	…
Meropenem	1 g every 8 h iv	…
Ertapenem	1 g every day iv	…
Cefotaxime	2 g every 6 h iv	…
plus		
metronidazole	500 mg every 6 h iv	
or		
clindamycin	600–900 mg/kg every 8 h iv	
Streptococcus infection		
Penicillin	2–4 MU every 4–6 h iv (adults)	Vancomycin, linezolid, quinupristin/dalfopristin, or daptomycin
plus		
clindamycin	600–900 mg/kg every 8 h iv	
S aureus infection		
Nafcillin	1–2 g every 4 h iv	Vancomycin, linezolid, quinupristin/dalfopristin, daptomycin
Oxacillin	1–2 g every 4 h iv	…
Cefazolin	1 g every 8 h iv	…
Vancomycin (for resistant strains)	30 mg/kg/day in 2 divided doses iv	…
Clindamycin	600–900 mg/kg every 8 h iv	Bacteriostatic; potential of cross-resistance and emergence of resistance in erythromycin-resistant strains; inducible resistance in methicillin-resistant *S aureus*
Clostridium infection		
Clindamycin	600–900 mg/kg every 8 h iv	…
Penicillin	2–4 MU every 4–6 h iv	…

iv, intravenously.
[a]If *Staphylococcus* infection is present or suspected, add an appropriate agent.

whether originating from the hepatobiliary system or the gastrointestinal system, is beyond the scope and goal of this chapter. The IDSA has recently published useful guidelines for diagnosis and treatment of intra-abdominal infections that emphasize

1. Source control (surgical or percutaneous drainage)
2. Early and appropriate antibiotics coverage
3. Fluid resuscitation
4. Microbiological evaluation, when feasible

These guidelines can be accessed at www.idsociety.org.

▶ Empyema

Empyema is a collection of pus in the pleural cavity, most commonly related to bacterial pneumonia and resulting parapneumonic effusions. Occasionally, empyemas occur postprocedurally, such as following thoracentesis, chest tube placement, or lung resection. When empyema occurs, drainage is needed. In addition to antibiotics, tube thoracostomy is the recommended initial management. Unfortunately, chest tubes lumens often get clogged with thick pus, leading to placement of additional tubes, and not infrequently, failure to completely drain the pleural cavity and re-expand the lung. When that occurs, surgical drainage with decortication using a video-assisted thoracoscopic approach or an open thoracotomy is indicated. In cases of recurrent or persistent empyema despite surgical management, creation of an Eloesser flap or window with an open track between the pleural cavity and the outside skin might be needed to allow adequate and definitive drainage of the empyema.

CLOSTRIDIUM DIFFICILE COLITIS

Clostridium difficile as an organism can be recovered in the feces of 5% of healthy individuals. The use of antibiotics can alter the colonic flora allowing for *C difficile* overgrowth and colonization of the colon. The result is *C difficile* colitis with severity ranging from simple watery diarrhea to life-threatening sepsis. *C difficile* is currently considered one of the most common and most serious health care–associated infections.

▶ Risk Factors

Antibiotic intake is the single most important risk factor for *C difficile* colitis and has been described even following a single antibiotic dose administration as with SSI prophylaxis. Although all antibiotics can be implicated, fluoroquinolones, clindamycin, penicillins, and cephalosporins are the most frequently encountered culprits, partly because of their widespread utilization. A Canadian study conducted during a relatively recent *C difficile* outbreak in Quebec strongly suggested that fluoroquinolones are currently the antibiotics most commonly associated with *C difficile* infections rather than clindamycin as classically and historically described. Table 8–11 lists the different antibiotics classified into those with high, moderate, and small risk of *C difficile* infection.

Transmission of *C difficile* by health care providers caring for patients with *C difficile* colitis has resulted in outbreaks of *C difficile* among patients within hospitals and the emergence of multidrug-resistant organisms. These epidemics are addressed and prevented by proper hand hygiene among health care providers and the isolation of patients with *C difficile* colitis.

▶ Clinical Presentation

The presentation of *C difficile* colitis can range from the asymptomatic carrier state that requires no treatment, and the mild diarrhea state that can easily be treated with oral antibiotics as an outpatient, to the severely toxic, septic, and MODS patient presentation. Across all the severity range, watery diarrhea, and abdominal distention remain the sine-qua-non of *C difficile* colitis. Lower abdominal pain may also be present, and is usually of a crampy nonspecific nature. Constitutional symptoms such as fever and malaise are also frequently reported. The presence of peritoneal signs such as rebound tenderness or guarding may be indicative of colonic perforation (rare) or severe and/or fulminant *C difficile* colitis. Leukocytosis is often present and not infrequently elevated above 20K cells/mcL. In fact, it is not unreasonable to test the hospitalized patient with unclear etiology of leukocytosis for occult *C difficile* infection, even in the absence of diarrhea. In a small study of inpatients with white blood cell counts above 15K cells/mcL, and without a clear etiology of the leukocytosis, Wanahita et al found that 58% of the patients tested positive for *C difficile*. Fecal leukocytes are also often present, but nonspecific. On colonoscopy, when performed, patients with *C difficile* colitis frequently show mucosal ulcerations with the pathognomonic pseudomembranes, often described as raised yellow plaques composed of fibrinous exudates. Abdominal x-rays may show "thumb printing" suggestive of colonic inflammation, but are often nonspecific. CT examination of the abdomen shows thickening of the colonic wall. In fulminant *C difficile* colitis, the abdominal x-rays and CT may show toxic megacolon with a diffusely dilated colon.

▶ Diagnosis

In addition to the clinical patient presentation described above, diagnostic tests for *C difficile* currently consist of either *C difficile* organism detection (eg, anaerobic stool culture, antigen testing) or toxin A or B detection tools (eg, cytotoxin assays, enzyme immunoassays, or polymerase chain reaction [PCR] testing). The best approach to diagnose

Table 8–11. Antibiotics associated with *Clostridium difficile* colitis.

Association With *C Difficile*	Very Strong	Strong	Moderate	Weak/Rare
Antibiotic class	Fluoroquinolones Lincosamides	Cephalosporins Penicillins Carbapenems	Sulfonamides Macrolides	Aminoglycosides Nitroimidazoles Glycopeptides
Common examples	Ciprofloxacin Levofloxacin Clindamycin	Ceftriaxone Cefoxitin Imipenem Amoxicillin	Trimethoprim- sulfamethoxazole Erythromycin Azithromycin	Gentamicin Amikacin Vancomycin (IV) Metronidazole

C difficile remains controversial and institution-dependent. The stool culture is a sensitive test, but has a long turnover time (2-3 days) that is suboptimal in the critically ill patient who needs a fast and accurate diagnosis. Antigen detection is a reasonable screening test, but needs further confirmation when positive. The most sensitive test (considered standard by many) is the cytotoxin assay. Its sensitivity is above 95%, and its specificity approaches 100%, but it is an expensive test with 24-48 hours turnover time.

Treatment

Treatment of asymptomatic patients is not indicated. On the other hand, the clinical, laboratory, and radiological presentation of the patient might carry a sufficient suspicion for *C difficile* infection that empiric antibiotics are justified pending *C difficile* organism or toxin detection tests. For patients with mild disease, level 1 evidence suggests the safety and equivalency of single-agent oral antibiotic treatment with PO metronidazole (500 mg every 8 hours) or PO vancomycin (125 mg every 6 hours). PO vancomycin is not systemically absorbed and is thus wholly available in the colonic lumen where the *C difficile* infection exists. A 2-week course of either antibiotics is recommended. Patients might still test positive for *C difficile* for many weeks despite treatment, and therefore retesting these patients for *C difficile* when the antibiotic course is done and the patient's signs and symptoms resolved, is not recommended. Adjunct therapies for *C difficile* such as probiotics, toxin-binding resins, and immunoglobulins have been used, but the evidence for their utility is still controversial.

Treatment of Severe C difficile Colitis

The definition of severe *C difficile* infection varies, but the IDSA 2010 guidelines define it as leukocytosis above 15K cells/mcL or a creatinine 1.5 times higher than the patient's predisease baseline. For severe *C difficile* colitis, these same guidelines recommend PO vancomycin rather than metronidazole as a first-line agent. Combination therapy with PO vancomycin, intravenous metronidazole +/– vancomycin enemas might be indicated in case of failure of single-agent therapy. Vancomycin enemas are particularly useful in patients with ileus (questionable adequate intracolonic concentration from PO vancomycin alone), those with PO intolerance, and possibly those with severe distal colonic inflammation (rectosigmoid colon). Fidaxomicin (200 mg every 12 hours) is a relatively new bactericidal antibiotic with promising results as an alternative therapy. In a randomized clinical trial comparing fidaxomicin and vancomycin, the cure rates were equivalent. Patients with refractory severe *C difficile* colitis, those who progress to toxic megacolon, or those with hemodynamic instability or showing signs of early MODS should be considered for prompt surgical intervention. The timing and decision to operate are controversial, but there is certainly value in earlier intervention in critically ill patients, as the mortality of fulminant *C difficile* infection remains as high as 30%-50%. Independent predictors of mortality include age more than 70 years, leukocytosis more than 35K cells/mcL, leucopenia less than 4K cells/mcL, hemodynamic instability and respiratory failure. When surgery is indicated, the procedure of choice is a subtotal colectomy with end ileostomy. A single-center study has recently demonstrated improved outcomes in severe *C difficile* colitis using an alternative approach where a loop ileostomy is created and subsequent intraoperative colonic washout was performed with polyethelene glycol solution. In this small study of fewer than 50 patients, the new approach was associated with decreased mortality and more than 90% colon preservation, when compared to the traditional subtotal colectomy approach.

ANTIMICROBIAL MANAGEMENT

General Principles

Antibiotic optimal management includes the following guiding principles:

1. Establishing a clinical diagnosis of infection and/or sepsis
2. Establishing an "evidence-based-guess" of the likely nature of the involved pathogen(s)
3. Attempting to obtain microbiological data (Gram stain and culture), when possible
4. Prompt initiation of broad-spectrum empiric antibiotics likely to cover the culprit pathogen(s)
5. Selectively narrowing the antibiotic regimen to cover the pathogen recovered in microbiological testing

The decisions to initiate, continue, or tailor the antibiotic choices for each patient should be carefully balanced against the increasingly serious challenge facing health care, namely, the epidemic emergence of multidrug-resistant organisms such as methicillin-resistant *S aureus* (MRSA), vancomycin-resistant **Enterococcus** (VRE), and multidrug-resistant gram-negative organisms.

EMPIRIC & PATHOGEN-DIRECTED ANTIBIOTIC SELECTION

Selecting the appropriate empiric antibiotics entails an understanding of the nature of the infectious process affecting the patient, the most likely organisms causing the infection, as well as awareness of the antibiotic resistance map at the local health care institution level. For example, simple skin infections are most likely caused by skin flora such as **staphylococci** and **streptococci**, and therefore an appropriate empiric treatment should at least cover gram-positive organisms. Acute diverticulitis with a pericolonic abscess is more likely to be caused by colonic flora, such as gram-negative and anaerobic bacteria, and therefore empiric treatment should focus on covering these pathogens. Once a specific organism has been recovered from the tested microbiological specimen, it is often possible to narrow the antibiotic regimen, even before the specific data on antibacterial susceptibilities is available using the microbiological properties of antibiotics and the currently available clinical experience. The use of local antibiograms is crucial and highly encouraged, as the patterns of bacterial susceptibilities and resistance vary not only from a region to the other but also from one institution to the other. Susceptibility testing methods include disk diffusion and dilution (broth microdilution, plates, and E-tests) procedures. Disk diffusion tests indicate whether a microbial culture is susceptible or resistant to serum-achievable, in vivo drug concentrations with conventional dosage regimens. In contrast, dilution procedures allow report of the minimal inhibitory concentration (MIC) and minimal bactericidal concentration (MBC). The MIC is the lowest concentration of a specific antimicrobial agent that inhibits the test organism, while the MBC is the lowest concentration of a specific antimicrobial agent that kills the test organism. Tailoring therapy based on reported of susceptibility via disk diffusion or MIC is recommended.

Antibiotic Duration of Therapy

If all the sent cultures were found to be negative, and the suspicion for continuing infection is low, empiric antibiotics should be discontinued, as unnecessary antibiotic therapy clearly increases the risk of multidrug-resistant bacteria, C difficile colitis, and other side effects. The duration of antibiotic treatment depends on the nature of the infection and the severity of the clinical presentation. Treatment of acute uncomplicated infections should be continued at least until the patient is afebrile, the white blood cell count is normal, and the patient looks clinically well. Evidence-based guidelines for type of antibiotics and duration in the treatment of various infections have been developed and should be followed when possible. Most antibiotic regimens are now limited, although more difficult infections such as liver abscesses, brain abscesses, endocarditis, septic arthritis, or osteomyelitis require prolonged antibiotic therapy.

Failure of Clinical Response

Upon failure of clinical response to initial surgical intervention and antibiotic therapy, the clinician is encouraged to think of all the possible following explanations of failure of therapy:

1. The existence of another organism
2. The presence of an uncontrolled source of infection needing additional interventions

3. The presence of a concomitant super-infection (eg, with fungal organisms)
4. The development of a new drug resistance by the same isolated organism
5. Failure of the chosen antibiotic medication (despite favorable susceptibility data) to penetrate the site of infection

The latter may be due to the properties of the antibiotic itself, the chosen route of administration, or the specific physiology and morbidity of the patients themselves.

Antibiotics' Side Effects

Adverse antibiotic reactions may occasionally mimic infection by causing fever, skin rashes, and mental status changes. Clinicians should consider this possibility in patients with persistent fevers despite appropriate antibiotic coverage and seeming resolution of the infectious process. In addition, antibiotics can result in microbial superinfections (eg, fungi, C difficile), emergence of new bacterial drug resistance, or organ toxicity.

Antibiotics in Renal or Hepatic Failure

Several antibiotics may induce or exacerbate existing organ dysfunction, most commonly renal or hepatic, and thus require intermittent assessment of kidney and liver function. Aminoglycosides and renal failure is a classic example.

In addition, decreased creatinine clearance at baseline or due to critical illness has an important influence on antimicrobial drug dosage, since most of these drugs are excreted, at least partially, by the kidneys. Therefore, many of these medications, such as vancomycin, penicillins, and aminoglycosides require adjustments in dosage or frequency of administration in the presence of renal insufficiency to prevent toxicity. Table 8–12 provides practical guidance into adjusting diverse antibiotic dosage and frequency for patients with hepatic or renal insufficiency, although additional assistance from the pharmacy department in these cases is universally advisable.

CONCLUSION

In conclusion, surgery can result in infection (such as SSI), but may also be the adjunct treatment to obtain source control in many infectious processes (ie, surgical infections). In the former, prevention by implementing processes of care (eg, timely provision of perioperative antibiotics, maintenance of strict sterile techniques) and patient risk factors optimization prior to surgery should be the goal of every surgeon, as SSI remains one of the biggest health care-associated perioperative challenges. For the latter (surgical infections), source control is the cornerstone in the prevention of systemic progression of the infection into sepsis, septic shock,

Table 8–12. Use of antibiotics in patients with renal failure and hepatic failure.

	Principal Mode of Excretion or Detoxification	Approximate Half-Life in Serum		Proposed Dosage Regimen in Renal Failure		Removal of Drugs by Dialysis	Dose After Dialysis	Dosage in Hepatic Failure
		Normal	Renal Failure[a]	Initial Dose[b]	Maintenance Dose			
Acyclovir	Renal	2.5-3.5 h	20 h	2.5 mg/kg	2.5 mg/kg q24h	Yes	2.5 mg/kg	NC
Ampicillin	Tubular secretion	0.5-1 h	8-12 h	1 g	1 g q8-12h	Yes	1 g	NC
Azlo-, mezlo-, piperacillin	Renal 50%-70%; biliary 20%-30%	1 h	3-6 h	3 g	2 g q6-8h	Yes	1 g	1-2 g q8h
Azithromycin	Mainly liver/biliary	> 24 h	> 24 h	500 mg	250 mg/d	No	No	NC
Carbenicillin	Tubular secretion	1 h	16 h	4 g	2 g q12h	Yes	2 g	NC
Ciprofloxacin	Renal and hepatic	4 h	8.5 h	0.5 g	0.25-0.75 g q24h	No	None	NC
Clindamycin	Hepatic	2-4 h	2.4 h	0.6 g IV	0.6 g q8h	No	None	0.3-0.6 g q8h
Erythromycin	Mainly hepatic	1.5 h	1.5 h	0.5-1 g	0.5-1 g q6h	No	None	0.25-0.5 g q6h
Fluconazole	Renal	30 h	98 h	0.2 g	0.1 g q24h	Yes	Give q24h dose	NC
Ganciclovir	Renal	3 h	11-28 h	1.25 mg/kg	1.25 mg/kg q24h	Yes	Give q24h dose	NC
Imipenem	Glomerular filtration	1 h	3 h	0.5 g	0.25-0.5 g q12h	Yes	0.25-0.5 g	NC
Levofloxacin		360-480 min	360-480 min	250-500 mg	250-500 mg/d	No	No	Avoid use
Meropenem		60 min	180 min	1000 mg	1000 mg q8h	Yes	500 mg q4h	NC
Metronidazole	Hepatic	6-10 h	6-10 h	0.5 g IV	0.5 g qh	Yes	0.25 g	0.25 g q12h
Moxifloxacin	Renal	720 min	720 min	400 mg	400 mg	No	No	Avoid use
Nafcillin	Hepatic 80%, kidney 20%	0.75 h	1.5 h	1.5 g	1.5 g q5h	No	None	2-3 g q12h
Penicillin G	Tubular secretion	0.5 h	7-10 h	1-2 million units	1 million units q8h	Yes	500,000 units	NC
Ticarcillin	Tubular secretion	1.1 h	15-20 h	3 g	2 g q6-8h	Yes	1 g	NC

Trimethoprim-sulfamethoxazole	Some hepatic	TMP 10-12 h; SMZ 8-10 h	TMP 24-48 h; SMZ 18-24 h	320 mg TMP + 1600 mg SMZ	80 mg TMP + 400 mg SMZ q12h	Yes	80 mg TMP + 400 mg SMZ	NC
Vancomycin	Glomerular filtration	6 h	6-10 d	1 g	1 g q6-10d based on serum levels	None	None	NC
Voriconazole	Hepatic	360 min	360 min	6 mg/kg IV × 2 doses	100-200 mg oral q12h	No	None	Normal load and ½ maintenance
Cefazolin	Renal	90 min		0.5 g	0.5 g qd	Yes	0.5 g	NC
Cefuroxime	Renal	80 min		1-2 g	1-2 g qd	Yes	0.5 g	NC
Cefotetan	Renal	150 min		0.5-1 g	0.5-1 g qd	Yes	0.5 g	NC
Cefoxitin	Renal	60 min		1-2 g	1-2 g qd	Yes	0.5 g	NC
Ceftriaxone	Renal and hepatic	480 min		1-2 g	1-2 g qd	No		NC
Ceftazidime	Renal	120 min		0.5-1 g	0.5-1 g qd	Yes	0.5 g	NC
Cefepime	Renal	120 min	600 min	1-2 g IV	1-2 g IV q12h	Yes	1 g q48h	NC

and/or MODS. Alongside surgical treatment of infections, antibiotic stewardship with appropriate timing, duration, and choice of antibiotics are needed now more than ever to prevent the emergence of resistant organisms as well as *C difficile* infection.

► References

Boltz MM, Hollenbeak CS, Julian KG, Ortenzi G, Dillon PW. Hospital costs associated with surgical site infections in general and vascular surgery patients. *Surgery.* 2011 Nov;150(5): 934-942.

Bratzler DW, Houck PM, Richards C, et al. Use of antimicrobial prophylaxis for major surgery: baseline results from the National Surgical Infection Prevention Project. *Arch Surg.* 2005 Feb;140(2):174-182.

Cohen SH, Gerding DN, Johnson S, et al. Clinical practice guidelines for Clostridium difficile infection in adults: 2010 update by the society for healthcare epidemiology of America (SHEA) and the infectious diseases society of America (IDSA). *Infect Control Hosp Epidemiol.* 2010 May;31(5):431-455.

Darouiche RO, Wall MJ Jr, Itani KM, et al. Chlorhexidine-alcohol versus povidone-iodine for surgical-site antisepsis. *N Engl J Med.* 2010 Jan 7;362(1):18-26.

Edwards JR, Peterson KD, Mu Y, et al. National Healthcare Safety Network (NHSN) report: data summary for 2006 through 2008, issued December 2009. *Am J Infect Control.* 2009 Dec;37(10):783-805.

Fry DE. Colon preparation and surgical site infection. *Am J Surg.* 2011 Aug;202(2):225-232.

Fukuda H, Morikane K, Kuroki M, et al. Impact of surgical site infections after open and laparoscopic colon and rectal surgeries on postoperative resource consumption. *Infection.* 2012 Aug 23. [Epub ahead of print]

Hospital acquired infections. The Centers for Disease Control (CDC). Available at http://www.cdc.gov/HAI/pdfs/toolkits/ SSI_toolkit021710SIBT_revised.pdf. Accessed November 3, 2012.

Louie TJ, Miller MA, Mullane KM, et al. Fidaxomicin versus vancomycin for Clostridium difficile infection. *N Engl J Med.* 2011 Feb 3;364(5):422-431.

Manjunath AP, Shepherd JH, Barton DP, Bridges JE, Ind TE. Glove perforations during open surgery for gynaecological malignancies. *BJOG.* 2008 Jul;115(8):1015-1019.

Misteli H, Weber WP, Reck S, et al. Surgical glove perforation and the risk of surgical site infection. *Arch Surg.* 2009 Jun;144(6):553-558; discussion 558.

Mu Y, Edwards JR, Horan TC, Berrios-Torres SI, Fridkin SK. Improving risk-adjusted measures of surgical site infection for the national healthcare safety network. *Infect Control Hosp Epidemiol.* 2011 Oct;32(10):970-986.

Neal MD, Alverdy JC, Hall DE, Simmons RL, Zuckerbraun BS. Diverting loop ileostomy and colonic lavage: an alternative to total abdominal colectomy for the treatment of severe, complicated Clostridium difficile associated disease. *Ann Surg.* 2011 Sep;254(3):423-427; discussion 427-429.

Ortega G, Rhee DS, Papandria DJ, et al. An evaluation of surgical site infections by wound classification system using the ACS-NSQIP. *J Surg Res.* 2012 May 1;174(1):33-38.

Panahi P, Stroh M, Casper DS, Parvizi J, Austin MS. Operating room traffic is a major concern during total joint arthroplasty. *Clin Orthop Relat Res.* 2012 Feb 3. [Epub ahead of print]

Sailhamer EA, Carson K, Chang Y, et al. Fulminant Clostridium difficile colitis: patterns of care and predictors of mortality. *Arch Surg.* 2009 May;144(5):433-439; discussion 439-440.

Solomkin JS, Mazuski JE, Bradley JS, et al. Diagnosis and management of complicated intra-abdominal infection in adults and children: guidelines by the Surgical Infection Society and the Infectious Diseases Society of America. *Surg Infect (Larchmt).* 2010 Feb;11(1):79-109.

Swenson BR, Hedrick TL, Metzger R, et al. Effects of preoperative skin preparation on postoperative wound infection rates: a prospective study of 3 skin preparation protocols. *Infect Control Hosp Epidemiol.* 2009 Oct;30(10):964-971.

The Surviving Sepsis Guidelines. Available at www.survivingsepsis.org. Accessed November 3, 2012.

Wanahita A, Goldsmith EA, Marino BJ, Musher DM. Clostridium difficile infection in patients with unexplained leukocytosis. *Am J Med.* 2003 Nov;115(7):543-546.

Weiser TG, Regenbogen SE, Thompson KD, et al. An estimation of the global volume of surgery: a modelling strategy based on available data. *Lancet.* 2008 Jul 12;372(9633):139-144.

MULTIPLE CHOICE QUESTIONS

1. Development of a SSI requires

   A. A susceptible host
   B. An infectious agent
   C. As suitable medium or environment
   D. Both A and C
   E. All of A, B, and C

2. The Centers for Disease Control classification of SSIs includes

   A. Infection at or near the surgical incision within 30 days of the procedure
   B. Infection at or near the surgical site within 2 months if an implant is left in place
   C. Subcategories of infection including deep incisional and organ/space
   D. Excludes superficial infections that involve only the skin.
   E. Both A and C are true

3. The efficacy of efforts to prevent SSI

   A. Is not affected by the timing of antibiotic dosing as long delivery occurs by the time of skin closure
   B. Is independent of the choice of antibiotic
   C. Can be improved by the use of alcohol-containing skin preparation solutions
   D. Is very similar at hospitals around the world
   E. Is currently well-known, and best practices are no longer controversial

4. The treatment of SSI includes

   A. Opening the incision for superficial SSI
   B. Antibiotics in every case
   C. Debridement of necrotic tissue if present
   D. Avoidance of wound cultures as this is expensive and unnecessary
   E. Both A and C

5. All of the following are true about necrotizing skin and skin structure infections (NSSSIs), except

   A. NSSSIs are generally self-limited and non-threatening
   B. Can be caused by single or polymicrobial infections
   C. Small vessel thrombosis occurs along the infection progression pathway
   D. Immunocompromised (eg, HIV, diabetes), intravenous drug abuse, and cancer patients are at a particularly higher risk of developing NSSSIs
   E. Grayish discoloration of the underlying skin and pain beyond the affected skin area are especially suggestive of deeper underlying tissue involvement

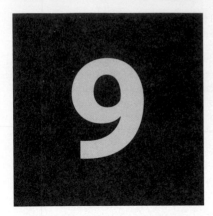

Fluid, Electrolyte, & Acid-Base Disorders

Tracey Dechert, MD

Fluid status, electrolyte homeostasis, and acid-base balance are clinical parameters of critical significance in surgical patients. Understanding normal physiology and pathophysiology related to these parameters is crucial.

▼ FLUIDS & ELECTROLYTES

Surgical patients are at high risk for derangements of body water distribution, electrolyte homeostasis, and acid-base physiology. These disturbances may be secondary to trauma, preexisting medical conditions which alter normal physiology, or the nature of the surgery.

BODY WATER DISTRIBUTION & COMPOSITION

Total body mass is 45%-60% water. The percentage in any individual is influenced by age and lean body mass, therefore the percentage is higher in men compared to women, in children compared to adults, and in people of normal body habitus compared to the obese (Table 9–1). Two-thirds of total body water (TBW), 30%-40% of body mass, is intracellular; one-third, 15%-20% of total body mass, is extracellular. The extracellular fluid is divided into two compartments, with 80% (12%-16% of total body mass) in the interstitial compartment, and 20% (3%-4%) in the intravascular compartment. One-fifth of intravascular fluid is proximal to the arterioles, the remaining four-fifths is distal to the arterioles.

The intracellular, interstitial, and intravascular compartments each hold fluid characterized by markedly different electrolyte profiles (Figure 9–1). The main intracellular cation is the potassium ion (K^+), while the main extracellular cation is the sodium ion (Na^+). Not only the electrolyte profile, but also the protein composition of the fluids differs: intracellular cations are electrically balanced mainly by the polyatomic ion phosphate (PO_4^{3-}) and negatively charged proteins, while extracellular cations are balanced mainly by the chloride ion (Cl^-). The intravascular fluid has a relatively higher concentration of protein and lower concentration of organic acids than the interstitial fluid. This higher concentration of protein, chiefly albumin, is the main cause of the high colloid osmotic pressure of serum, which in turn is the chief regulator of the fluid distribution between the two extracellular compartments. The relationship between colloid osmotic pressure and hydrostatic pressure governs the movement of water across the capillary membrane, and is modeled by the Starling equation.

The body's volume status and electrolyte composition are determined largely by the kidneys. The kidneys maintain a constant volume and osmolality by modulating how much free water and Na^+ is reabsorbed from the renal filtrate. Antidiuretic hormone (ADH), also known as arginine vasopressin, is the chief regulator of osmolality. The peptide hormone is released from the posterior pituitary in response to increased serum osmolality. ADH induces translocation of aquaporin channels to the collecting duct epithelium, increasing permeability to water and causing reabsorption of free water from the renal filtrate. Thus water is retained, and the urine concentrated. In the absence of ADH, the collecting duct is impermeable to water, leading to water loss and production of dilute urine. At high physiologic levels ADH has a direct vasoconstrictive effect on arterioles.

The main determinant of Na^+ reabsorption is the Na^+ load in the renal filtrate. Most filtered Na^+ (60%-70%) is reabsorbed in the proximal tubule. A further 20%-30% of filtered Na^+ is reabsorbed in the thick ascending limb of the loop of Henle; reabsorption here is determined by the Na^+ load delivered to the loop and a variety of hormones. The remaining distal tubule reabsorbs 5%-10% of filtered Na^+; again, the exact percentage is determined by the Na^+ load and a variety of hormonal factors, particularly aldosterone. The collecting duct reabsorbs a small percentage of filtered

Table 9–1. Approximate percentage water of total body mass.

Patient	%
Children	60
Nonelderly males	60
Nonelderly females	50
Elderly males	50
Elderly females	45

Na^+ under the influence of aldosterone and natriuretic hormone. Under normal circumstances the kidneys will adjust excreted water and Na^+ to match a wide spectrum of dietary intake.

Although the movement of ions and proteins between the different fluid compartments is normally restricted, water itself is freely diffusible between them. Consequently the osmolality of the different fluid compartments is identical, normally approximately 290 mOsm/kg. Control of osmolality occurs through regulation of water intake through diet and excretion through urine and insensible loses.

VOLUME DISORDERS

Hypo- and hypervolemia commonly occur in surgical patients, both following elective surgery and in the setting of trauma and acute care surgery. Volume disturbances run the gamut from being clinically insignificant to being immediately life threatening. The underlying cause of any volume disorder must be sought and addressed while the volume disorder itself is managed.

- Hypovolemia
  - Etiology: Hypovolemia is common in surgical patients. It is typically caused by loss of isotonic fluids in the setting of hemorrhage, gastrointestinal losses (eg, gastric suctioning, emesis, and diarrhea), sequestration of fluids in the gut lumen (eg, bowel obstruction, ileus, and enteric fistulas), burns, and excessive diuretic therapy. In resource poor settings sweat is often an additional important fluid loss, for example, in a non–air-conditioned operating room. In all of these cases, loss of isotonic fluid results in loss of Na^+ and water without significantly affecting the osmolality of the extracellular fluid compartment, thus there is very little shift of water into or out of the intracellular compartment. Hypovolemia stimulates aldosterone secretion from the zona glomerulosa of

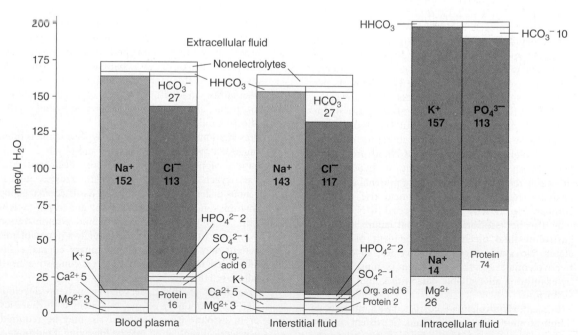

▲ **Figure 9–1.** Electrolyte composition of human body fluids. Note that the values are in mEq/L of water, not of body fluid. (From Leaf A, Newburgh LH: *Significance of the Body Fluids in Clinical Medicine*, 2nd ed. Thomas, 1955.)

the adrenal cortex, leading to increased reabsorption of Na^+ and water from the renal filtrate and excretion of low volumes (oliguria) of hypertonic urine with a low Na^+ concentration.

Fractional excretion of Na^+ (FENa) is a useful tool for differentiating causes of oliguria:

$$FENa = 100 \times \frac{(Na_u * Cr_p)}{(Cr_u * Na_p)}$$

where U: urine, P: plasma, Na: sodium, Cr: creatinine. FENa $\leq 1\%$ usually indicates prerenal azotemia. However, FENa $\leq 1\%$ may be found in patients with oliguria secondary to hepatorenal syndrome, as the liver does not effectively metabolize aldosterone. In patients already receiving diuretic therapy, fractional excretion of urea nitrogen (FEUN) is more helpful than FENa. FEUN is calculated analogously; FEUN $\leq 35\%$ indicates prerenal azotemia.

○ Presentation: Hypovolemia is suggested by a patient's history, physical examination, and laboratory data. Diagnosis by physical examination alone in the immediate postoperative setting is difficult, especially when volume loss is mild to moderate, and especially in very old and very young patients. One review found that longitudinal furrows on a patient's tongue and dry oral and nasal mucous membranes are 85% sensitive for hypovolemia; increased capillary refill time, unclear speech, upper or lower extremity weakness, a dry axilla, and postural hypotension were all relatively specific indicators of hypovolemia. The same review found that a postural (supine to standing) increase in heart rate of at least 30 beats per minute or severe postural dizziness which prevented the patient from standing had 6%-48% sensitivity for mild to moderate hypovolemia but 91%-100% sensitivity for severe hypovolemia. Laboratory evidence of hypovolemia includes elevated blood urea nitrogen (BUN): creatinine (Cr) ratio, as hypovolemia decreases renal perfusion, causing prerenal azotemia characterized by a disproportionate rise in BUN compared to Cr. However, an elevated BUN: Cr ratio may also be associated with renal failure and with gastrointestinal bleeding, independent of volume status. No single highly sensitive test to diagnose hypovolemia exists, thus the diagnosis must be made by examining all available data with a high index of suspicion.

○ Treatment: Hypovolemia is corrected with intravenous administration of an isotonic fluid. Coexistent electrolyte abnormalities should be addressed simultaneously. Care must be taken in patients in renal or heart failure not to exacerbate these conditions. If hypovolemia is allowed to worsen unimpeded it will eventually lead to circulatory collapse and shock, which is covered elsewhere.

• Hypervolemia
  ○ Etiology: Hypervolemia is also common in surgical patients. It often occurs after treatment of shock with colloid and crystalloid fluids, with or without attendant renal failure. It also occurs in the postoperative period as ADH is secreted in response to nonphysiologic stimuli, disrupting its role in regulation of osmolality. High physiologic levels of ADH have a vasoconstrictive effect, leading to a decreased filtered Na^+ load and thus greater Na^+ and water retention. This secretion of ADH typically ceases 2-3 days after the surgical insult, after which ADH levels return to an appropriate level and patients experience a so-called "autodiuresis." Heart failure, liver disease, renal disease, and malnutrition all exacerbate hypervolemia in the surgical patient. Preexisting heart failure decreases the range across which a patient will adequately compensate for increased intravascular volume. Liver disease decreases metabolism of circulating ADH and aldosterone, increasing the homeostatic set point for intravascular volume and thus decreasing the physiologic reserve remaining to respond to surgical insults. Renal disease disrupts all aspects of volume regulation. Syndrome of inappropriate ADH hypersecretion (SIADH) causes hypervolemia secondary to a sustained ADH release independent of the normal physiologic triggers. SIADH typically occurs in the setting of traumatic brain injury, brain tumors and abscesses, pneumonia and lung abscesses, as a paraneoplastic syndrome associated with small cell lung cancer and other neoplasias, and with a variety of drugs including morphine and the chemotherapeutic agents cyclophosphamide and vincristine.
  ○ Presentation: Like hypovolemia, hypervolemia is often suggested by the patient's history and physical examination. Signs include hypertension, decreased arterial oxygen saturation and basilar crackles, jugular venous distention, dependent soft tissue edema, gallop rhythms on cardiac auscultation, and rapid weight gain. Examination of recorded fluid administration may assist in the diagnosis. Eventually a hypervolemic patient may show signs of pulmonary edema, easily diagnosed on chest x-ray, or even congestive heart failure (CHF).
  ○ Treatment: If the hypervolemic patient develops CHF or pulmonary edema, treatment with diuretics, or in extreme cases hemodialysis, may be required. Mechanical ventilation may be lifesaving if pulmonary edema and/or CHF have progressed to the point of respiratory failure.

ELECTROLYTE DISORDERS

Electrolyte derangements may occur independently of each other, but are often closely linked. Like volume disorders, disturbances of electrolyte homeostasis run the gamut from mild and inconsequential to severe and immediately life threatening.

The underlying cause of any electrolyte disorder must be sought while the electrolyte disorder itself is managed. Special care must always be taken when repleting electrolytes in patients with renal insufficiency. These patients require slower repletion and more frequent monitoring of electrolyte levels.

- Sodium: Hypo- and hypernatremia reflect excessive gain or loss of TBW, respectively. Significant derangements of Na^+ homeostasis result in significant changes to plasma tonicity and eventually whole body osmolality, with potentially devastating consequences for the central nervous system (CNS).
  - Hyponatremia
    - Etiology: Hyponatremia is a sign of relative water gain; total body Na^+ may be decreased, normal or even increased. Hyponatremia is common in surgical patients postoperatively, as ADH is secreted in response to pain, nausea and vomiting, opiate administration, and positive-pressure ventilation. Typically, this hyponatremia is mild and inconsequential; however, it may be exacerbated by rapid parenteral administration of hypotonic fluids. Hyponatremia may result from severe hyperglycemia, or any other condition in which an osmotically active solute draws water from the intracellular space to the extracellular space. In the setting of hyperglycemia, a corrected Na^+ is calculated as:

      $$Na^+_{corrected} = Na^+_{measured} + 0.016$$
      (plasma glucose in mg/dL − 100)

      The correction factor 0.016 accounts for the unit conversion from mg/dL to mmol/L. Some investigators believe a correction factor of 0.024 is more appropriate.

      Other causes of hyponatremia include cerebral salt-wasting syndrome, liver disease, congestive heart failure, and SIADH.
    - Presentation: The signs of hyponatremia are caused by CNS dysfunction, as brain cells swell in a fixed-volume space (the Monro-Kellie hypothesis). Mental status changes, obtundation, coma, and seizures typically are not seen until serum Na^+ is less than 120 mmol/L. Such hyponatremia is a medical emergency requiring immediate intervention.
    - Treatment: CNS signs and symptoms attributable to hyponatremia require administration of normal saline and free water restriction. In general,

hypertonic saline should not be used to correct hyponatremia. Unless serum Na^+ falls very rapidly, it should be corrected slowly, as too-rapid correction has the devastating complication of osmotic demyelination. No consensus exists on the appropriate rate of correction. One review recommended correction by no more than 8 mmol/L/d, starting with correction of 1-2 mmol/L/h in patients with severe manifestations. Sodium levels should not be corrected beyond what is needed to alleviate CNS disturbances. Correction of Na^+ does not replace pharmacologic intervention in a seizing patient.

One formula used to calculate the expected change in Na^+ from intravenous administration of 1 L of any fluid is:

$$\text{Change in serum } Na^+ = \frac{(\text{fluid } Na^+ + \text{fluid } K^+ \text{ in mmol/L}) - \text{serum } Na^+}{\text{TBW in L} + 1}$$

Total body water is estimated as a fraction of body mass (Table 9–1). Hyponatremia causing CNS disturbances should prompt admission to an intensive care unit given the close monitoring needed in such patients, the need for rapid intervention, and the potentially devastating consequences of delays in management.

  - Hypernatremia
    - Etiology: Loss of free water alone occurs when patients do not have access to water (eg, preverbal, bed-bound or otherwise incapacitated patients), in diabetes insipidus, in the setting of high fevers, and in patients in whom enteral feeds do not contain adequate water. Hypernatremia typically occurs simultaneously with volume derangements, and total body Na^+ may be increased, normal or even decreased. Induced hypernatremia is a useful treatment modality in patients with traumatic brain injury to reduce cerebral edema, decrease intracranial pressure, and increase cerebral perfusion pressure.
    - Presentation: As with hyponatremia, the signs and symptoms of hypernatremia are caused by CNS dysfunction: lethargy, fatigue, hyperactive deep tendon reflexes, seizure, and coma may occur. Signs and symptoms are rare with Na^+ less than 158 mmol/L.
    - Treatment: Development of CNS symptoms requires parenteral administration of free water, typically as 5% dextrose in water. If the patient's hypernatremia developed over a period of hours it may safely be corrected at a rate of 1 mmol/L/h. In patients whose hypernatremia developed more slowly, a rate of 0.5 mmol/L/h is safe. As derangements in Na^+ are caused by derangements in TBW, the concept of a "water deficit" is a useful one in

treating hypernatremia. The free water deficit is calculated as:

water deficit = (TBW × (1 − [140/Na$^+$ in mmol/L])

This formula is accurate when calculating the water deficit in patients with pure water loss, but is inaccurate in patients with hypernatremia caused by loss of hypotonic fluid. Using the formula in the section on hyponatremia, one may calculate the estimated correction 1 L of any fluid will have on Na$^+$. As with hyponatremia, hypernatremia with clinical manifestations warrants admission to an intensive care unit so that correction may be achieved safely and effectively.

- Potassium: Potassium is the major intracellular cation. Plasma potassium ion (K$^+$) concentration is determined primarily by two factors. The first is acid-base homeostasis. Hydrogen ion (H$^+$) and K$^+$ are exchanged between the intracellular and extracellular spaces, thus disturbances of acid-base balance (see below) tend to cause disturbances in serum K$^+$. The second is the size of the total body K$^+$ pool. Intracellular stores of K$^+$ are large, but may be exhausted, especially in the setting of prolonged ketoacidosis.
  - Hypokalemia
    - Etiology: In the surgical setting, total body K$^+$ is typically decreased by gastrointestinal losses, excessive diuretic administration, and prolonged malnutrition, particularly in alcoholic patients. Prolonged alkalosis (see below) that also results in hypokalemia (eg, due to gastric losses of hydrochloric acid and K$^+$) results in a so-called "paradoxical aciduria" as the nephron conserves K$^+$ at the expense of H$^+$, which maintains the alkalosis instead of correcting it an attempt to prevent life-threatening hypokalemia (see below for details).
    - Presentation: The hallmark signs of hypokalemia are decreased muscle contractility eventually leading to diaphragmatic paralysis, EKG changes including a flattened or inverted T wave and a prominent U wave, and cardiac arrhythmias, which may present an immediate threat to life.
    - Treatment: When hypokalemia develops acutely it should be corrected with parenteral supplementation. Parenteral administration of K$^+$ must be done carefully so as not to cause iatrogenic hyperkalemia. Hypomagnesemia may cause hypokalemia refractory to parenteral administration. In such cases hypomagnesemia should be corrected along with hypokalemia (see below). In cases of chronic hypokalemia in which neuromuscular and cardiac manifestations are absent, oral supplementation (either through dietary changes or oral potassium chloride administration) should suffice.

  - Hyperkalemia
    - Etiology: In the surgical setting, hyperkalemia is often caused by crush injuries, burns and other catabolism-inducing events, renal insufficiency, adrenal insufficiency, and excessive K$^+$ administration. Acidosis may cause hyperkalemia as the intracellular space buffers acidemia by exchanging H$^+$ from the extracellular space for K$^+$ from within cells (see below).
    - Presentation: Hyperkalemia has few outward signs and symptoms until potentially lethal cardiac arrhythmias manifest. Initial EKG changes include flattened P waves and peaked T waves. Widening of the QRS complex is a later finding and demands immediate intervention, as it portends the imminent onset of ventricular fibrillation.
    - Treatment: A serum K$^+$ of 6.5 mmol/L or greater is a medical emergency and must prompt immediate intervention. The patient must be placed on continuous EKG monitoring. Initial treatment should consist of intravenous administration of 50% dextrose in water, 10 units of regular insulin, and calcium gluconate, as well as inhaled β-adrenergic agonists like albuterol. Insulin, glucose, and β-agonists drive K$^+$ from the extracellular space into the intracellular space, while calcium gluconate increases the excitability threshold of the myocardium, protecting against arrhythmias. If these measures are unsuccessful, hemodialysis may be required. Slowly developing hyperkalemia not severe enough to warrant intravenous interventions may be treated with oral sodium polystyrene sulfonate, which causes a slow enteral K$^+$ wasting.

- Magnesium: The magnesium ion (Mg^{2+}) is an essential cofactor in many of the most important biochemical reactions in the body. Adenosine triphosphate (ATP) must be bound to Mg^{2+} to be biologically active. Mg^{2+} is required for every step of DNA transcription and translation, nerve conduction, ion transport and Ca^{2+} channel activity. Approximately 50%-60% of total body magnesium is found in the bones. The large majority of the rest is intracellular, and approximately 1% is extracellular. A constant proportion of dietary Mg^{2+} is absorbed by the gut. If gut absorption exceeds Mg^{2+} needs, the excess is excreted by the kidneys. If dietary intake is insufficient the kidney retains Mg^{2+}, with urinary levels dropping to nearly zero.
  - Hypomagnesemia
    - Etiology: Hypomagnesemia occurs in the setting of malnutrition (especially malnutrition associated with alcoholism), gastrointestinal losses (especially prolonged diarrheal loses), diuretic or aminoglycoside use, hyper- or hypocalcemia, and hypophosphatemia.

- Presentation: In the surgical setting, hypomagnesemia most commonly presents as hypokalemia refractory to parenteral K^+ administration. Hypomagnesemia may cause sedation, muscle paralysis, tetany, seizures, and coma.
- Treatment: Parenteral administration of Mg^{2+} is generally preferred to oral supplementation, as orally-administered magnesium is a cathartic agent.

○ Hypermagnesemia
- Etiology: Hypermagnesemia is rare in the surgical setting, but may develop in acute renal failure.
- Presentation: At high concentrations, Mg^{2+} acts as a Ca^{2+} antagonist. Thus although hypermagnesemia may cause lethargy, weakness and diminished deep tendon reflexes, it most often presents as cardiac arrhythmias. Peaked T waves and widening of the QRS complex occur, which may progress to complete heart block, arrhythmias, and eventually asystole.
- Treatment: If hypermagnesemia is mild and caused by supplementation, withdrawal of supplementation, and close monitoring should be sufficient treatment. If hypermagnesemia is significant and causing EKG changes, calcium gluconate should be administered intravenously so as to overwhelm the Ca^{2+}-antagonizing effect of Mg^{2+} in neuromuscular function. Diuretic therapy may be required. In severe cases and in cases caused by renal failure, hemodialysis may be required.

- Calcium: Calcium (Ca^{2+}) is involved in a wide variety of physiologic processes, from maintenance of bone strength to neuromuscular function. Half of serum Ca^{2+} is protein-bound, chiefly to albumin. The unbound fraction is physiologically active, while the bound fraction is not; this unbound (or "ionized") fraction is normally held constant across a wide range of plasma Ca^{2+}. Ca^{2+} homeostasis is influenced by vitamin D, parathyroid hormone, calcitonin, acid-base balance, and PO_4^{3-} homeostasis.

Standard laboratory tests measure total serum Ca^{2+}, including the fraction bound to albumin. Thus, a low Ca^{2+} value on a serum chemistry may reflect hypoalbuminemia rather than true hypocalcemia. Many formulas exist to correct Ca^{2+} in the setting of hypoalbuminemia. The most commonly used is:

$$Ca^{2+}_{corrected} = 0.8(4 - \text{serum albumin in g/dL}) + Ca^{2+}_{measured}$$

This and other such formulas are inaccurate in the setting of hemodialysis. In dialyzed patients, the uncorrected Ca^{2+} should be used to determine if the patient is hypo- or hypercalcemic. If doubt exists, an ionized Ca^{2+} measurement should be obtained.

○ Hypocalcemia
- Etiology: Hypocalcemia in the surgical setting is often caused by hypothyroidism and hypoparathyroidism (either organic or iatrogenic after thyroid or parathyroid surgery), pancreatitis, renal insufficiency, crush injuries, severe soft tissue infections, and necrotizing infections like necrotizing fasciitis.
- Presentation: Hypocalcemia manifests as neuromuscular dysfunction, causing hyperactive deep tendon reflexes, Chvostek sign, muscle cramps, abdominal pain, and in severe cases tetany and cardiac arrhythmias.
- Treatment: In persistent hypocalcemia, whole blood pH must be determined, and any alkalosis corrected. Calcium supplementation, enterally if possible and parenterally if necessary, may be required. Chronic hypoparathyroidism and hypothyroidism require chronic vitamin D and Ca^{2+} supplementation, and may require aluminum hydroxide to decrease PO_4^{3-} absorption from the gut.

○ Hypercalcemia
- Etiology: Hypercalcemia in the surgical setting is often caused by primary or tertiary hyperparathyroidism, hyperthyroidism, bony cancer metastases, paraneoplastic syndromes in which parathyroid hormone-related peptide is elaborated, and as a complication of thiazide diuretic use.
- Presentation: Signs and symptoms of acute hypercalcemia include anorexia, nausea and vomiting, polydipsia, polyuria, depression, confusion, memory loss, stupor, coma, psychosis, and cardiac arrhythmias. Dyspepsia, constipation, acute pancreatitis, nephrolithiasis, osteoporosis, osteomalacia, and osteitis fibrosa cystica are indicative of chronic hypercalcemia. Untreated longstanding hypercalcemia, especially in conjunction with untreated hyperphosphatemia and especially in patients with chronic renal failure, may lead to calciphylaxis and high morbidity and mortality.
- Treatment: In a patient with healthy kidneys, administration of large volumes of normal saline over 1-3 days will often correct even a profound hypercalcemia. Treatment may be followed by targeting a urine output of 2-3 mL/kg/h and monitoring serum Ca^{2+} levels closely. Loop diuretics (eg, furosemide) inhibit Ca^{2+} reabsorption in the nephron, and will aid in calciuresis, but should not be used until the patient is clinically euvolemic. Calcitonin increases osteoblastic activity and inhibits osteoclastic activity, locking Ca^{2+} into the skeleton. In severe hypercalcemia or hypercalcemia secondary to renal failure, hemodialysis may be required. In patients whose hypercalcemia is caused by malignancy, bisphosphonates may provide a

means of controlling Ca^{2+} levels in the medium and long term. In hypercalcemia caused by hyperparathyroidism, parathyroidectomy is potentially curative, but is reserved for the elective setting unless the patient is in hypercalcemic crisis which is refractory to optimal medical management.

- Phosphate: Like Ca^{2+} and Mg^{2+}, the majority of PO_4^{3-} is found in the skeleton. The large majority of the remainder is found intracellularly, where it functions as a constituent of ATP. Like Mg^{2+}, it is essential to energy metabolism.
  - Hypophosphatemia
    - Etiology: As with hypomagnesemia, chronic hypophosphatemia is typically found in malnourished patients, especially alcoholic patients. It may also occur in patients who consume large amounts of antacids, and following liver resection. An important and often overlooked cause of hypophosphatemia is refeeding syndrome. This syndrome occurs after a patient who has been without significant caloric intake for at least 5 days begins to eat again. Severe hypophosphatemia may occur as phosphofructokinase binds PO_4^{3-} to glucose to begin glycolysis, and as PO_4^{3-} is consumed in production of large amounts of ATP. The syndrome usually manifests within 4 days of starting refeeding.
    - Presentation: Hypophosphatemia results in muscular and neurologic dysfunction. Muscle weakness, diplopia, depressed cardiac output, respiratory depression due to diaphragmatic weakness, confusion, delirium, coma, and death may all develop. An uncommon presentation is with rhabdomyolysis. Hypophosphatemia may leave a patient ventilator-dependent as they are unable to replenish ATP stores for proper functioning of the muscles of respiration.
    - Treatment: Severe hypophosphatemia is a medical emergency, requiring parenteral administration of Na_3PO_4 or K_3PO_4, depending on the patient's electrolyte profile. If hypophosphatemia is not severe it may be treated with oral supplementation, either with sodium phosphate/potassium phosphate or with high-phosphate foods like milk.
  - Hyperphosphatemia
    - Etiology: Hyperphosphatemia is unusual in the surgical setting, typically developing in the setting of severe renal disease or after severe trauma.
    - Presentation: Hyperphosphatemia is usually asymptomatic, but it may cause hypocalcemia as calcium phosphate precipitates and is deposited in tissues.
    - Treatment: Hyperphosphatemia is treated by diuresis, administration of phosphate-binders like aluminum hydroxide, or hemodialysis in the setting of renal failure.

ACID-BASE

The body's handling of hydrogen ion (H^+) is a particularly complex example of electrolyte management, as it involves not only dietary intake and renal clearance but also extracellular and intracellular buffer systems and respiratory as well as renal excretion.

NORMAL PHYSIOLOGY

An acid is a chemical that donates a H^+ in solution, for example, HCl or H_2CO_3. A base is a chemical that accepts H^+ in solution, for example, Cl^- or HCO_3^-. The concentration of H^+ in a solution determines the acidity of the solution. Acidity of a solution is measured by pH, which is the negative logarithm of H^+ concentration expressed in mol/L. The strength of an acid is determined by its degree of dissociation into H^+ and the corresponding base, as expressed in the Henderson-Hasselbalch (H-H) equation:

$$pH = pK \times \log [A^-]/[HA]$$

where K = dissociation constant, [A^-] = concentration of acid, [HA] = concentration of base. Stronger acids have a higher K than weaker acids.

The main buffer system in human blood is a carbonic acid/bicarbonate (H_2CO_3/HCO_3^-) system. Using the H-H equation, the pH of this buffer system is calculated as:

$$pH = pK \times \log [HCO_3^-]/[H_2CO_3]$$

H_2CO_3 in the blood exists mostly as CO_2 (the so-called "volatile acid"); conversion of one to the other is catalyzed by the enzyme carbonic anhydrase. The dissociation constant of CO_2 is 0.03. Making these substitutions into the equation, we have:

$$pH = pK \times \log [HCO_3^-]/[pCO_2 \times 0.03]$$

where Pco_2 is the partial pressure of CO_2. The pK for this buffer system is 6.1. In arterial blood, HCO_3^- normally ranges from 21 to 37 mmol/L, while Pco_2 ranges from 36 to 44 mm Hg. Thus, arterial pH normally ranges from 7.36 to 7.44. Venous blood is easier to sample than arterial blood (Table 9–2). Venous blood gas sampling varies significantly between institutions, and between central, mixed,

Table 9–2. Estimated arterial to venous blood gas conversions.

$pH_a = pH_v \times 1.005$
$Paco_2 = Pvco_2 \times 0.8$
$HCO_3{^-}_a = HCO_3{^-}_v \times 0.90$

a, arterial; p, partial pressure; v, venous.

and different peripheral sites of sampling, and thus must be interpreted with caution.

Acid-base homeostasis is maintained by pulmonary excretion of CO_2 and renal excretion of nonvolatile acids, which is discussed in further sections.

ACID-BASE DISORDERS

The fundamental acid-base disorders are:

- Acidemia: pH below the normal range
- Alkalemia: pH above the normal range
- Acidosis: a process that lowers the pH of the extracellular fluid
- Alkalosis: a process that raises the pH of the extracellular fluid

There are four primary or simple (as opposed to mixed) acid-base disorders:

- Metabolic acidosis: a disorder in which decreased HCO_3^- causes decreased pH
- Metabolic alkalosis: a disorder in which increased HCO_3^- causes increased pH
- Respiratory acidosis: a disorder in which increased PCO_2 causes decreased pH
- Respiratory alkalosis: a disorder in which decreased PCO_2 increased pH are found

Acid-base disorders are classified as simple or mixed. In a simple acid-base disorder, only one primary acid-base disorder is present, and the compensatory response is appropriate. In a mixed acid-base disorder, more than one primary acid-base disorder is present. Mixed acid-base disorders are suspected from a patient's history, from a lesser or greater than expected compensatory response, and from analysis of the serum electrolytes and anion gap (AG) (see below).

The use of a systematic approach to identifying and diagnosing acid-base disorders is essential. One must first determine alkalemia or academia based on pH. One must then determine whether a metabolic derangement with respiratory compensation or a respiratory derangement with metabolic compensation exists, based on the HCO_3^- and PCO_2 values (Table 9–3).

Whether the disturbance is primarily respiratory or metabolic, some degree of compensatory change occurs in an attempt to maintain normal pH. Changes in PCO_2 (respiratory disorders) are compensated for by changes in HCO_3^- (metabolic/renal compensation), and vice versa.

Acute respiratory disorders may develop in matter of moments. Such circumstances may not allow sufficient time for renal compensation, resulting in severe pH changes without significant compensatory changes. By contrast, chronic respiratory disturbances allow the full range of renal

Table 9–3. Changes in HCO_3^- and pCO_2 in primary acid-base disorders.

Disorder	pH	HCO_3^-	PCO_2
Metabolic acidosis	⇓	⇓	⇓ (compensatory)
Metabolic alkalosis	⇑	⇑	⇑ (compensatory)
Respiratory acidosis	⇓	⇑ (compensatory)	⇑
Respiratory alkalosis	⇑	⇓ (compensatory)	⇓

compensatory mechanisms to function. In these circumstances, pH may remain normal or nearly normal despite wide variations in PCO_2. By contrast, respiratory compensation for metabolic disorders occurs quickly. Thus there is little difference in respiratory compensation for acute and chronic metabolic disorders.

▶ Metabolic Acidosis

Metabolic acidosis is caused by increased production of H^+ or by excessive loss of HCO_3^-. In the surgical setting, metabolic acidosis is commonly encountered in trauma, critically ill, and postoperative patients, and especially in patients in shock.

A. The Anion Gap

The serum AG is vital to determining the cause of any metabolic acidosis. AG may help differentiate between metabolic acidosis caused by accumulation of acid and that caused by loss of HCO_3^-.

AG represents the difference between the primary measured serum cation, Na^+, and the primary measured serum anions, Cl^- and HCO_3^-:

$$AG = Na^+ - (Cl^- + HCO_3^-)$$

The AG is normally less than 12; however, the highest normal value varies by institution.

Increased acid production causes an increased AG, as unmeasured anions electrically neutralize Na^+. Thus metabolic acidosis caused by increased H^+ production is associated with a high AG. The most common causes of an AG metabolic acidosis include methanol ingestion, uremia/renal failure, diabetic ketoacidosis, polypropylene glycol ingestion, isoniazid ingestion, lactic acidosis, ethylene glycol ingestion, and salicylate poisoning. In the surgical setting lactic acidosis is by far the most common cause, seen in hypoperfused states like shock and sepsis.

A non-AG metabolic acidosis is caused by excessive HCO_3 loss. The nephron maintains electrical neutrality by reabsorbing Cl^- as HCO_3^- is lost, hence the normal AG. Non AG metabolic acidosis in the surgical setting typically results from diarrhea or high small bowel output, for example, from an ileostomy. Non-AG acidosis also occurs in renal tubular acidosis, as the nephron fails to reabsorb HCO_3^-. Iatrogenic hyperchloremia, especially from administration of large amounts of normal saline to trauma and postoperative patients, may induce a non-AG metabolic acidosis.

The AG may be influenced by phenomena unrelated to acid-base balance, which must be kept in mind. Hypoalbuminemia may lower AG, as Cl^- and HCO_3^- increase to electrically balance Na^+ which was previously balanced by albumin. Similarly, hyper- or hypostates of positively charged ions like calcium, magnesium, and potassium may affect the AG.

Treatment of metabolic acidosis involves identifying the underlying cause of the acidosis and correcting it. Often, this is sufficient. If this is not sufficient, correction may require administration of exogenous alkali in the form of $NaHCO_3^-$ to correct the derangement in pH. The degree of restoration is estimated by subtracting the plasma HCO_3^- from the normal value (24 mmol/L at our institution) and multiplying the resulting number by half TBW. This is a useful empiric formula, as in practice it is unwise (and unnecessary) to administer enough $NaHCO_3^-$ to completely correct pH. Doing so will likely cause fluid overload from the large Na^+ load delivered, and will likely overcorrect the acidosis. In patients with a chronic metabolic acidosis, often seen in chronic renal failure, alkali may be administered chronically as oral $NaHCO_3^-$. Efforts to minimize the magnitude of HCO_3^- loss in these patients must be undertaken as well.

B. Compensation

The body's response to metabolic acidosis is respiratory hyperventilation, "blowing off" H_2CO_3 as CO_2 and correcting the acidosis. This response is rapid, beginning within 30 minutes of the onset of acidosis and reaching full compensation within 24 hours. The adequacy of the respiratory response to metabolic acidosis is evaluated using Winter's formula:

$$P_{CO_2} = (1.5 \times HCO_3^- \text{ in mmol/L}) + (8 \pm 2)$$

If compensation is inadequate or excessive—that is, if P_{CO_2} is not within the range predicted by Winter's formula—one must evaluate for a mixed acid-base disorder (see below).

▶ Metabolic Alkalosis

Metabolic alkalosis is often encountered in surgical patients. The pathogenesis is complex, but often involves:

1. Loss of H^+, usually via gastric losses of HCl

2. Hypovolemia

3. Total body K^+ depletion

All three are commonly encountered with vomiting or gastric suctioning, diuretic use, and renal failure.

HCl is secreted by chief cells in the gastric mucosa; simultaneously, HCO_3^- is absorbed in the blood. $NaHCO_3$ is then secreted by the pancreas into the lumen of the duodenum, neutralizing the gastric acid, after which the neutralized acid and base are reabsorbed by the small intestine. Thus, under normal circumstances there is no net alteration of acid-base balance in the function of the gastrointestinal tract. However, when H^+ is lost from the gastric lumen, for example, through emesis, gastric suctioning or gastric drainage—the result is loss of H^+ from the gastric lumen and a corresponding gain of HCO_3^- in the blood, leading to metabolic alkalosis.

Normally, the kidneys excrete excess HCO_3^-; however, if volume depletion accompanies HCO_3^- excess, the kidneys attempt to maintain normovolemia by increasing tubular reabsorption of Na^+, which is reabsorbed in an electrically neutral fashion by increasing reabsorption of Cl^- and HCO_3^-. This impairs HCO_3^- excretion, perpetuating the metabolic alkalosis.

Severe K^+ depletion further exacerbates metabolic alkalosis. To preserve K^+, Na^+ is exchanged for H^+ in the kidney, through the Na^+-K^+ and Na^+-H^+ ATPases in the distal renal tubule. This explains why severe metabolic alkalosis with hypokalemia results in paradoxical aciduria. In such cases, urine Na^+, K^+, and Cl^- concentrations are low, and the urine is acidic. In simple volume depletion, urine Cl^- alone is low and the urine is alkaline. Severe metabolic alkalosis may lead to tetany and seizures, as seen in hypokalemia and hypocalcemia.

Treatment of metabolic alkalosis includes fluid administration, usually normal saline. With adequate fluid repletion, tubular reabsorption of Na^+ is diminished, and the kidneys will excrete excess HCO_3^-. K^+ must be repleted, both to allow for correction of the alkalosis and to prevent life-threatening hypokalemia. Repletion of volume with normal saline and of potassium with KCl also provides the nephron with needed Cl^-, allowing for reabsorption of K^+ and Na^+ with Cl^- instead of HCO_3^-. Acetazolamide, a carbonic anhydrase inhibitor diuretic, may also be used to treat metabolic alkalosis as long as the patient is euvolemic. Administration of exogenous acid in the form of HCl may be employed in the case of profound alkalosis.

A. Compensation

Adequate respiratory compensation for metabolic alkalosis should raise P_{CO_2} by 0.7 mm Hg for every 1 mmol/L elevation in HCO_3^-. Generally, respiratory compensation will not raise P_{CO_2} beyond 55 mm Hg. Thus a P_{CO_2} greater than 60 mm Hg in the setting of metabolic alkalosis suggests a mixed metabolic alkalosis and respiratory acidosis.

▶ Respiratory Acidosis

Acute respiratory acidosis occurs when ventilation suddenly becomes inadequate. CO_2 accumulates in the blood, and as carbonic anhydrase coverts it to H_2CO_3, acidosis develops.

Acute respiratory acidosis is most common in conditions where gas exchange is physically impaired, resulting in decreased ventilation. These conditions typically involve decreased oxygenation as well. They include respiratory arrest, acute airway obstruction, pulmonary edema, pneumonia, saddle pulmonary embolus, aspiration of intra-oral contents, and acute respiratory distress syndrome. Hypoventilation may occur in patients postoperatively who are oversedated (eg, from narcotics, benzodiazepines, or as they recover from general anesthesia). Pain, especially from large abdominal incisions or from rib fractures, leads to respiratory splinting and hypoventilation. Excess ethanol ingestion decreases respiratory drive, thereby impairing ventilation. Head trauma, either by direct damage to central nervous system respiratory centers or by global brain damage and brainstem herniation, may impair ventilation.

Patients with obesity hypoventilation syndrome and obstructive sleep apnea may develop a periodically recurring acute respiratory acidosis, leading eventually to some renal compensation. True chronic respiratory acidosis arises from chronic respiratory failure in which impaired ventilation leads to persistently elevated P_{CO_2}, for example, as seen in chronic obstructive pulmonary disease. Chronic respiratory acidosis is usually well tolerated with adequate renal compensation, thus pH may be normal or near normal.

Treatment of respiratory acidosis involves restoration of adequate ventilation by treating the underlying cause. Aggressive chest physical therapy and pulmonary toilet should be instituted on all postsurgical patients. Patients with pulmonary edema should receive appropriate diuretic therapy, and patients with pneumonia should receive appropriate antibiosis. Naloxone or flumazenil should be used as needed in the setting of narcotic or benzodiazepine overdose, respectively. If necessary, endotracheal intubation and mechanical ventilation should be employed in order to correct pCO_2.

Acute respiratory acidosis should be corrected rapidly. However, too rapid correction of chronic respiratory acidosis risks causing posthypercapnic metabolic alkalosis syndrome, characterized by muscle spasms and by potentially lethal cardiac arrhythmias.

A. Compensation

Over 80% of increased acid produced in respiratory acidosis is buffered by the body's tissues and intracellular hemoglobin. The remaining minority is buffered by HCO_3^- in the blood, which the kidney reclaims and reabsorbs. Thus, metabolic (renal) compensation for respiratory disorders is a much slower process than respiratory compensation for metabolic disorders. Furthermore, in acute respiratory acidosis renal mechanisms may not have had time to function at all, and HCO_3^- may be within normal limits.

Adequate renal compensation for respiratory acidosis involves an increase in HCO_3^- of 1 mmol/L for every 10 mm Hg increase in P_{CO_2}.

▶ Respiratory Alkalosis

Hyperventilation decreases P_{CO_2} (hypocapnia), leading to a respiratory alkalosis. In the surgical setting, anxiety, agitation, and pain are common causes of respiratory alkalosis. Hyperventilation and respiratory alkalosis may be an early sign of sepsis and of moderate pulmonary embolism. Chronic respiratory alkalosis occurs in chronic pulmonary and liver disease.

Acute respiratory alkalosis is treated by addressing the underlying cause. Patients may require pain control, sedation/anxiolytics, and even paralyzation and mechanical ventilation if necessary. Well-compensated chronic respiratory alkalosis does not require treatment. In these cases, rapid correction of pCO_2 leads to so-called posthypocapnic hyperchloremic metabolic acidosis, which is often severe.

A. Compensation

The renal response to respiratory alkalosis is decreased reabsorption of filtered HCO_3^- and increased urinary HCO_3^- excretion. HCO_3^- decreases as Cl^- increases, since Na^+ is reabsorbed with Cl^- instead of with HCO_3^-. This same pattern is seen in hyperchloremic metabolic acidosis; the two are distinguished only by pH measurements.

Adequate renal compensation for respiratory alkalosis involves a decrease in HCO_3^- of 2 mmol/L for every 10 mm Hg decrease in P_{CO_2}.

▶ Mixed Acid-Base Disorders

Many common pathophysiologic processes cause mixed acid-base disorders. In these situations, pH may be normal or near normal, but compensatory changes are either inadequate or exaggerated. One way of determining the presence of a simple versus mixed disorder is to plot the patient's acid-base disorder on a nomogram (Figure 9–2). If the set of data falls outside one of the confidence bands, then by definition the patient has a mixed disorder. If the acid-base data falls within one of the confidence bands, the patient more likely has a simple acid-base disorder.

As with simple acid-base disorders, a systematic approach to mixed acid-base disorders is essential. First, determine the primary acid-base disorder. Next, determine whether or not adequate compensation has occurred, using the equations and rules given above (Table 9–4). If compensation is "inadequate," meaning too little or too much, the patient has a mixed acid-base disorder.

An additional step is needed in the case of metabolic acidosis. After AG has been calculated, the "delta-delta" or

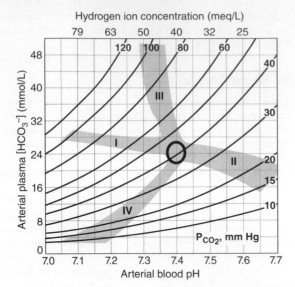

▲ Figure 9–2. Acid-base nomogram for use in evaluation of clinical acid-base disorders. Hydrogen ion concentration (top) or blood pH (bottom) is plotted against plasma HCO_3^- concentration; curved lines are isopleths of CO_2 tension ($Paco_2$, mm Hg). Knowing any two of these variables permits estimation of the third. The circle in the center represents the range of normal values; the shaded bands represent the 95% confidence limits of four common acid-base disturbances: I, acute respiratory acidosis; II, acute respiratory alkalosis; III, chronic respiratory acidosis; IV, sustained metabolic acidosis. Points lying outside these shaded areas are mixed disturbances and indicate two primary acid-base disorders.

"delta ratio" or "gap-gap" (three names for the same parameter) should be calculated:

$$\Delta\Delta = \Delta AG/\Delta HCO_3^-$$

where $\Delta\Delta$ = delta-delta, ΔAG = AG − maximum normal AG, ΔHCO_3^- = normal HCO_3^- − HCO_3^-.

Table 9–4. Expected compensation in primary acid-base disorders.

Metabolic acidosis	Winter's formula: $pCO_2 = 1.5 \times HCO_3^- + (8 \pm 2)$
Metabolic alkalosis	⇑ Pco_2 0.7 mm Hg for every 1 mmol/L increase in HCO_3^-
Respiratory acidosis	⇑ HCO_3^- 1 mmol/L for every 10 mm Hg increase in Pco_2
Respiratory alkalosis	⇓ HCO_3^- 2 mmol/L for every 10 mm Hg decrease in Pco_2

At our institution, maximum normal AG is 12 mmol/L and normal HCO_3^- concentration is 24 mmol/L, thus $\Delta\Delta$ = $(AG - 12)/(24 - HCO_3^-)$.

$\Delta\Delta$ < 1 indicates the coexistence of an AG and a non-AG metabolic acidosis, that is, a metabolic acidosis caused by increased production of acid and by renal loss of HCO_3^-. This may occur in the setting of diabetic ketoacidosis.

$\Delta\Delta$ > 1 indicates the coexistence of an AG metabolic acidosis and a metabolic alkalosis. This can occur in the intensive care unit in patients who have an underlying AG metabolic acidosis and are also undergoing diuresis or gastric suctioning, leading to the concurrent metabolic alkalosis.

The most common mixed acid-base disorder in surgical patients is a metabolic acidosis superimposed on a respiratory alkalosis. This occurs in patients with septic shock and hepatorenal syndrome, and also in the case of salicylate poisoning. Since the two acid-base disorders disrupt H^+ homeostasis in opposite directions, the patient's pH may be normal or near normal. Mixed respiratory acidosis and metabolic alkalosis is less common, occurring in the setting of cardiorespiratory arrest, which is a medical emergency.

▶ References

Adrogue H, Medias N: Secondary responses to altered mental status: the rules of engagement. *J Am Soc Nephrol.* 2010;21: 920-923.

Ayers P, Warrington L: Diagnosis and treatment of simple acid-base disorders. *Nutr Clin Pract.* 2008;2:122-127.

Bruno C, Valenti M: Acid-base disorders in patients with chronic obstructive pulmonary disease: a pathophysiological review. *J Biomed Biotechnol.* 2012;2012:1-8.

Calvi L, Bushinsky D: When is it appropriate to order an ionized calcium? *J Am Soc Nephrol.* 2008;19:1257-1260.

Cengiz M, Ulker P, Meiselman H, Baskurt O: Influence of tourniquet application on venous blood sampling for serum chemistry, hematological parameters, leukocyte activation and erythrocyte mechanical properties. *Clin Chem Lab Med.* 2009;6:769-776.

Gennari F: Pathophysiology of metabolic alkalosis: a new classification based on the centrality of stimulated collecting duct ion transport. *Am J Kidney Dis.* 2011;58:626-636.

Jung B, Rimmele T, Le Goff C, et al: Severe metabolic or mixed acidemia on intensive care unit admission: incidence, prognosis, and administration of buffer therapy. A prospective, multiple-center study. *Crit Care.* 2011;15:R238.

Kraut J, Madias N: Differential diagnosis of nongap metabolic acidosis: value of a systematic approach. *Clin J Am Soc Nephrol.* 2012;7:671-679.

Mortiz M, Ayus J: Water water everywhere. *Anesth Analg.* 2010 Feb;110(2):293-295.

Song Z, Gu W, Li H, Ge X: The incidence and types of acid-base imbalance for critically ill patients in emergency. *Hong Kong J Emerg Med.* 2012;19:13-17.

MULTIPLE CHOICE QUESTIONS

1. A 28-year-old man with history of depression is found down and brought to the emergency department. He responds to voice, moves his extremities spontaneously, and opens his eyes to pain only. Initial vital signs: T 98.0°F, P 72, BP 118/65 mm Hg, RR 28 breaths/min, O_2 saturation 99% on a non-rebreather mask. Primary survey is within normal limits, secondary survey reveals only superficial abrasions. Initial laboratory data include

   ABG: pH 7.36, Pco_2 38 mm Hg, Pao_2 173 mm Hg, HCO_3^- 20 mmol/L

$$\begin{matrix} & 14.1 & & & & \\ 13.2 & \times & 285 & \dfrac{145}{4.2} & \dfrac{102}{21} & \dfrac{18}{0.82} \diagdown 97 \\ & 41.1 & & & & \end{matrix}$$

   CPK 125
   Serum salicylate 824 mg/L (normal 30-300 mg/L)

   Based on this patient's history, examination findings and laboratory data, what is this patient's acid-base derangement?

   A. No disorder
   B. Respiratory acidosis with appropriate renal compensation
   C. Anion gap metabolic acidosis with appropriate respiratory compensation
   D. Nonanion gap metabolic acidosis with appropriate respiratory compensation
   E. Mixed metabolic acidosis and metabolic alkalosis

2. A 54-year-old alcoholic man is discovered to have a new gastric cancer. He reports 15 lb weight loss over the past month. Laboratory data includes an albumin of 2.4 g/dL, indicating significant longstanding malnutrition. Postoperatively, which of the following electrolyte derangements would be of initial concern, especially when he starts to eat or receive some other form of nutrition?

   A. Hypophosphatemia
   B. Hyperphosphatemia
   C. Hypermagnesemia
   D. Hyponatremia
   E. Hyperkalemia

3. A 70-year-old man undergoes a laparoscopic cholecystectomy for acute cholecystitis. On postoperative day 1 he complains of light-headedness while attempting to transfer from his bed to a chair. His vital signs include T 99.1°F, P 82, BP 109/63 mm Hg, RR 14 breaths/min, O_2 saturation 99% on room air. The nurse informs you that he has had poor enteral intake since the operation, and his urine output has diminished to 10 mL/h. She also informs you that his intravenous access was lost soon after his surgery and was never reestablished. His BUN and Cr preoperatively were 16 mg/dL and 0.8 mg/dL, respectively. Laboratory data include

   Urine Na 153 mmol/L Urine Cr 284 mg/dL

   You suspect the cause of his orthostasis and oliguria is hypovolemia. Which of the following findings would most strongly confirm your hypothesis?

$$\dfrac{139}{3.6} \mid \dfrac{99}{24} \mid \dfrac{32}{1.47} \diagdown 88$$

   A. BUN:Cr ratio < 20
   B. Fractional excretion of sodium (FENa) > 1%
   C. FENa < 1%
   D. Renal ultrasonography demonstrating normal kidney parenchyma and vasculature
   E. Fractional excretion of urea nitrogen (FEUN) > 35%

4. A 19-year-old woman arrives in the trauma bay after a helmeted motorcycle crash. She is hemodynamically unstable, and immediately taken to the operating room. Exploratory laparotomy reveals 3 L of hemoperitoneum, a grade 5 splenic laceration, and a grade 3 liver laceration. A splenectomy is performed and the liver laceration is packed. Inspection of the rest of the abdomen reveals no additional injuries. Two hours into the case anesthesia alerts you that her temperature is 93°F and her pH is 7.2; thus you decide to suspend the operation, leave her abdomen open, and admit her to the surgical intensive care unit (SICU) for resuscitation before returning to the operating room. Despite aggressive resuscitation with packed red blood cells (PRBCs) and other blood products, she remains hemodynamically unstable. Pelvic angiography reveals a bleeding right inferior gluteal artery, which is embolized. She is returned to the SICU for further resuscitation. You take over her care at this point, and notice that she has received 21 units of PRBCs, 19 units of fresh frozen plasma, and 20 units of platelets, but has not had her serum electrolytes checked in 5 hours. Which of the following electrolyte disorders is she most at risk for?

   A. Hypocalcemia
   B. Hypomagnesemia
   C. Hyperkalemia
   D. All of the above
   E. None of the above

5. A 61-year-old woman undergoes a sigmoid colectomy for perforated sigmoid diverticulitis. Postoperatively she is transferred to the surgical intensive care unit, still

intubated and mechanically ventilated. On postoperative day 3 she develops an ileus, and her orogastric tube is put to low wall suction. On postoperative day 8 she develops hypotension and tachycardia to 140 beats/min, and requires a norepinephrine infusion to maintain adequate mean arterial blood pressure. Laboratory data includes

$$\begin{array}{c} 8.1 \\ 13.4 \times 147 \\ 25.2 \end{array} \quad \begin{array}{c|c|c} 139 & 101 & 34 \\ \hline 3.4 & 22 & 1.2 \end{array} 88$$

ABG 7.32/40/154/20

What is the most likely explanation for her acid-base disorder?

A. AG metabolic acidosis with adequate respiratory compensation
B. Mixed metabolic alkalosis and AG metabolic acidosis
C. Metabolic alkalosis with respiratory compensation
D. Mixed metabolic alkalosis and respiratory acidosis
E. Mixed AG metabolic acidosis and respiratory alkalosis

Surgical Metabolism & Nutrition

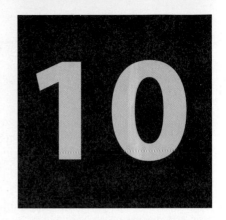

Thomas M. Shary, MD

Emily A. Chapman, RD, LD, CNSC

Virginia M. Herrmann, MD

The effects of malnutrition on the surgical patient are well characterized in the literature but are often overlooked in the clinical arena. Between 30% and 50% of hospitalized patients are malnourished. Protein-calorie malnutrition produces a reduction in lean muscle mass, alterations in respiratory mechanics, impaired immune function, and intestinal atrophy. These changes result in diminished wound healing, predisposition to infection, and increased postoperative morbidity. Although most healthy individuals can tolerate up to 7 days of starvation (with adequate glucose and fluid replacement), those subjected to major trauma, the physiologic stress of surgery, sepsis, or cancer-related cachexia require earlier nutritional intervention. Methods to identify those at greatest need for supplemental nutrition and to adequately address their needs are discussed in this chapter.

NUTRITIONAL ASSESSMENT

Nutrition screening is the process of identifying patients who are either malnourished or at risk for developing malnutrition. Major trauma and surgical stress alter the intake and absorption of nutrients, as well as their utilization and storage by the body. In select patients (eg, those with severe malnutrition as determined below), preoperative nutritional support has been shown to significantly reduce perioperative morbidity and mortality. Although most patients do not require this level of support, nutrition screening is imperative to identify the patient at high risk for malnutrition or its sequelae. A comprehensive nutritional assessment incorporates the initial history, physical examination, and laboratory testing to provide a snapshot of the patient's recent nutritional health.

▶ History & Physical Examination

The history and physical examination are the foundation of nutritional assessment. A complete medical history is essential to identify factors that predispose the patient to alterations in nutritional status (Table 10–1). Chronic illnesses such as alcoholism are commonly associated with protein-calorie malnutrition as well as vitamin and mineral deficiencies. Previous operative procedures such as gastrectomy or ileal resection may predispose to generalized malabsorption or isolated deficiency of iron, vitamin B_{12}, or folate. In most cases, the possibility of malnutrition is suggested by the underlying disease or by a history of recent weight loss. Patients with renal failure who require hemodialysis lose amino acids, vitamins, trace elements, and carnitine in the dialysate. Cirrhotics often suffer from whole-body sodium overload despite being hyponatremic, and they are typically protein-deficient. Patients with inflammatory bowel disease, particularly those with ileal involvement, may develop protein deficiency due to a combination of poor intake, chronic diarrhea, and treatment with corticosteroids. Furthermore, alterations in the enterohepatic circulation of bile salts lead to fat, vitamin, calcium, magnesium, and trace element deficiencies. Approximately 30% of patients with cancer have protein, calorie, and vitamin deficiencies due either to the underlying disease or to antimetabolite chemotherapy (eg, methotrexate). Patients infected with HIV are frequently malnourished and have protein, trace metal (selenium and zinc), mineral, and vitamin deficiencies.

A complete history of current medications is essential to alert caregivers to potential underlying deficiencies and drug-nutrient interactions. Although rarely the sole cause of malnutrition, certain over-the-counter herbal preparations can alter nutrient absorption. Agents containing ephedra and caffeine may be abused to induce excessive weight loss. Ginkgo and other preparations enhance cytochrome p450 metabolism of various drugs. Information about socioeconomic factors and a detailed dietary history may uncover other risk factors.

A careful physical examination begins with an overall assessment of the patient's appearance. Patients with severe malnutrition may appear frankly emaciated, but more subtle signs of malnutrition include temporal muscle wasting, skin pallor, edema, and generalized loss of body fat. Protein status

Table 10–1. Nutritional assessment.

History (Factors Predisposing to Malnutrition)

Absorption disorders (eg, celiac sprue)
AIDS
Alcoholism
Chronic renal insufficiency
Cirrhosis
Diabetes mellitus
Enteric obstruction
Inflammatory bowel disease
Malignancy
Past surgical history, especially involving gastrointestinal tract
Prolonged starvation
Psychiatric disorders (eg, anorexia nervosa)
Recent major surgery, trauma, or burn
Severe cardiopulmonary disease

Physical Examination

Skin: Quality, texture, rash, follicles, hyperkeratosis, nail deformities
Hair: Quality, texture, recent loss
Eyes: Keratoconjunctivitis, night blindness
Mouth: Cheilosis, glossitis, mucosal atrophy (eg, temporal wasting), dentition
Heart: Chamber enlargement, murmurs
Abdomen: Hepatomegaly, abdominal mass, ostomy, fistulas
Rectum: Stool color, perineal fistula, Guaiac test
Neurologic: Peripheral neuropathy, dorsolateral column deficit, mental status
Extremities: Muscle size and strength, pedal edema

Laboratory Tests

CBC: Hemoglobin, hematocrit, mean corpuscular volume (MCV), white blood cell count and differential, total lymphocyte count, platelet count
Electrolytes: Sodium, potassium, chloride, calcium, phosphate, magnesium
Liver function tests: AST (SGOT), ALT (SGPT), alkaline phosphatase, bilirubin, albumin, prealbumin, retinol-binding protein, prothrombin/INR
Miscellaneous: BUN, creatinine, triglycerides, cholesterol, free fatty acids, ketones, uric acid, calcium, copper, zinc, magnesium, transferrin

is evaluated from the bulk and strength of the extremity muscles and visible evidence of temporal and thenar muscle wasting. Cardiac flow murmurs may result from anemia. Vitamin deficiencies may be indicated by changes in skin texture, the presence of follicular plugging or a skin rash, corneal vascularization, cracks at the corners of the mouth (cheilosis), hyperemia of the oral mucosa (glossitis), cardiac enlargement, altered sensation in the hands and feet, absence of vibration and position sense (dorsal and lateral column deficits), or abnormal quality and texture of the hair. Trace metal deficiencies produce cutaneous and neurologic abnormalities similar to those associated with vitamin deficiency and may cause changes in the mental status of the patient.

▶ Anthropometric Measurements

Anthropometry is the science of assessing body size, weight, and proportions. Anthropometric measurements gauge body weight and composition with the intent of providing specific information about lean body mass and fat stores. Body composition studies may be used to determine total body water, fat, nitrogen, and potassium. Anthropometric measurements that can be easily performed in the clinic or at the bedside include determination of height and weight, with calculation of body mass index (BMI). Additional measurements such as arm span, body part summation, or knee-height measurement can also be used in nutrition assessment. More advanced techniques allow the clinician to assess the patient's visceral and somatic protein mass and fat reserve. Accurate weight is important, as is current weight expressed as a percentage of ideal body weight. Ideal body weight values are taken from the 1983 Metropolitan Height-Weight Tables.

The BMI is used to measure protein-calorie malnutrition as well as overnutrition (eg, obesity). A BMI between 18.5 and 24.9 is considered normal in most Western civilizations. Overweight is defined as a BMI from 25 to 29.9, and a BMI greater than 30 defines obesity. BMI is calculated as follows:

$$\mathrm{BMI} = \frac{\mathrm{Weight\,(kg)}}{\mathrm{Height\,(m)}^2} = 703 \times \frac{\mathrm{Weight\,(lb)}}{\mathrm{Height\,(in)}^2}$$

Dual-energy x-ray absorptiometry (DEXA) is increasingly available in hospitals and can be used to assess various body compartments (mineral, fat, lean muscle mass). Most protein resides in skeletal muscle. Somatic (skeletal) protein reserve is estimated by measuring the mid-humeral circumference. This measurement is corrected to account for subcutaneous tissue, yielding the mid-humeral muscle circumference (MHMC). The result is compared with normal values for the patient's age and gender to determine the extent of protein depletion. Fat reserve is commonly estimated from the thickness of the triceps skin fold (TSF). Reliability of anthropometric measurements is dependent on the skill of the person performing the measurement and is subject to error if performed by different caregivers on the same patient.

▶ Laboratory Data

The visceral protein reserve is estimated from various serum protein levels, total lymphocyte count, and antigen skin testing (Table 10–2). The serum albumin level provides a rough estimate of the patient's nutritional status but is a better prognostic indicator than tool for nutritional assessment. Serum albumin less than 3.5 mg/dL correlates with increased perioperative morbidity and mortality and increased length of hospital stay. Because albumin has a relatively long half-life (20 days), other serum proteins with shorter half-lives have greater utility for assessing response to nutritional repletion. Transferrin has a shorter half-life of 8-10 days and is a

Table 10–2. Staging of malnutrition.

Clinical & Laboratory Parameters	Extent of Malnutrition		
	Mild	Moderate[1]	Severe[1]
Albumin (g/dL)	2.8-3.5	2.1-2.7	< 2.1
Transferrin (mg/dL)	200-250	100-200	< 100
Prealbumin (mg/dL)	10-17	5-10	< 5
Retinol-binding protein (mg/dL)	4.1-6.1 (normal)	< 4.1	
Total lymphocyte count (cells/μL)	1200-2000	800-1200	< 800
Creatinine-height index (%)	60-80	40-60	< 40
Ideal body weight (%)	80-90	70-80	< 70
Weight loss/time	< 5%/month < 7.5%/3 months < 10%/6 months	< 2%/week > 7.5%/3 months > 10%/6 months	> 2%/week
Skin antigen testing (No. reactive/No. placed)	4/4 (normal)	1-2/4 (weak)	0/4 (anergic)
Anthropometric Measurements	**Male**	**Female**	
Triceps skin fold (mm)	≤ 12.5	≤ 16.5	
Mid-humeral circumference (cm)	> 29	> 28.5	

[1]Nutritional supplementation is indicated.

more sensitive indicator of adequate nutrition repletion than albumin. Prealbumin has a half-life of 2-3 days, and retinol-binding protein has a half-life of 12 hours. Unfortunately, their serum levels are also influenced by other factors, limiting their utility in assessing nutritional status or repletion.

Immune function may be assessed by hypersensitivity skin testing as well as total lymphocytic count, a reflection of T- and B-cell status. Subcutaneous injection of common antigens provides a semiobjective assessment of the antibody-mediated immune response, commonly impaired in malnourished patients. A low total lymphocyte count (TLC) correlates directly with the degree of malnutrition, though the count may be altered by infection, chemotherapy, and other factors, thus limiting its usefulness.

▶ Nutritional Indices

Indices provide a means of risk-stratification and objective comparison among patients (Table 10–3). Additionally, many nutritional indices have been prospectively validated and can provide prognostic information to further guide nutrition support services. Along with the BMI, these indices can assist surgeons in determining the correct timing for intervention and the progress being made toward the goal of adequate nourishment.

A. Creatinine-Height Index

Creatinine-height index (CHI) may be used to determine the degree of protein malnutrition, although it is less valid in patients who are severely catabolic or have chronic renal disease. A 24-hour urinary creatinine excretion is measured and compared with normal standards. CHI is calculated by the following equation:

$$CHI = \frac{Actual\ 24\text{-}hour\ urine\ creatine\ excretion}{Predicted\ creatine\ excretion}$$

The urinary excretion of 3-methylhistidine is a more precise measurement of lean body mass and associated protein stores. The amino acid histidine is irreversibly methylated in muscle. During protein turnover, 3-methylhistidine is not reutilized for synthesis, so the urinary excretion of this compound correlates well with muscle protein breakdown. Unfortunately, measurement of 3-methylhistidine is too expensive for use as a routine clinical test.

B. Prognostic Nutrition Index

The prognostic nutrition index (PNI) has been validated in patients undergoing either major cancer or gastrointestinal

Table 10–3. Nutritional indices.

Body Mass Index (BMI)	
BMI = weight (kg)/[height (m)]^2 = 703 × weight (lbs)/[height (in)]^2	
Normal	18.5-24.9
Overweight	25-29.9
Obese	30-40
Morbid obesity	> 40

Prognostic Nutritional Index (PNI)	
PNI = 158 - [16.6 × Alb[1]] − [0.78 × TSF[2]] − [0.2 × TFN[3]] − [5.8 × DH[4]]	
Note: for DH, > 5 mm induration = 2;	
1-5 mm induration = 1;	
anergy = 0	

Risk for complications:	
Low	< 40%
Intermediate	40-49%
High	> 50%

Nutrition Risk Index (NRI)	
NRI = [15.19 × Alb] + 41.7 × [actual weight (kg)/ideal weight (kg)]	
Well-nourished	> 100
Mild malnutrition	97.5-100
Moderate malnutrition	83.5-97.5
Severe malnutrition	< 83.5

Malnutrition Universal Screening Tool (MUST)
BMI score: weight loss score (unplanned weight loss):
BMI > 20 (> 30 obese) = 0; weight loss < 5% = 0
BMI 18.5-20 = 1; weight loss 5.10% = 1
BMI < 18.5 = 2; weight loss >10% = 2
Acute disease effect: add 2 if there has been or is likely to be no nutritional intake for > 5 days.
Risk of malnutrition: 0 = low risk; 1 = medium risk; ≥ 2 = high risk

Geriatric Nutrition Risk Index (GNRI)
GNRI = [1.489 × albumin (g/L)] + [41.7 × (weight/WLo)]
The GNRI results from replacement of ideal weight in the NRI formula by usual weight as calculated from the Lorentz formula (WLo). Four grades of nutrition-related risk: major risk (GNRI < 82), moderate risk (GNRI 82-91), low risk (GNRI 92 to ≤ 98), no risk (GNRI > 98).

Instant Nutritional Assessment Parameters (INA)
Parameter: abnormal if
Serum albumin < 3.5 g
Total lymphocyte count < 1500/mm^3

[1]Alb, albumin (g/dL).
[2]TSF, triceps skin fold (mm).
[3]TFN, transferrin (mg/dL).
[4]DH, delayed cutaneous hypersensitivity.

surgery and found to accurately identify a subset of patients at increased risk for complications. Furthermore, preoperative nutritional repletion has been shown to reduce postoperative morbidity in this patient group. The PNI has been widely adapted to identify patients at risk in nonsurgical populations, who may benefit from nutritional support.

C. Nutrition Risk Index

The nutrition risk index (NRI) was used by the VA TPN Cooperative Study Group for determining preoperative malnutrition, and it has since been prospectively cross-validated against other nutritional indices with good results. The index successfully stratifies perioperative morbidity and mortality using serum albumin and weight loss as predictors of malnutrition. Of note, the NRI is not a tool for tracking the adequacy of nutritional support, since supplemental nutrition often fails to improve serum albumin levels.

D. Subjective Global Assessment

Subjective global assessment (SGA) is a clinical method that has been validated as reproducible and that encompasses the patient's history and physical examination. It is based on five features of the medical history (weight loss in the past 6 months, dietary intake, gastrointestinal symptoms, functional status or energy level, and metabolic demands) along with four features of the physical examination (loss of subcutaneous fat, muscle wasting, edema, and ascites). Limitations of the SGA include its focus on chronic instead of acute nutritional changes and its enhanced specificity at the expense of sensitivity.

E. Mini-Nutritional Assessment

The mini-nutritional assessment (MNA) is a rapid and reliable tool for evaluating the nutritional status of the elderly. It is composed of 18 items and takes approximately 15 minutes to complete. The assessment includes an evaluation of a patient's health, mobility, diet, anthropometrics, and a subject self-assessment. An MNA score of 24 or higher indicates no nutritional risk, while a score of 17-23 indicates a potential risk of malnutrition and a score of less than 17 indicates definitive malnutrition.

F. Malnutrition Universal Screening Tool

The malnutrition universal screening tool (MUST) detects protein-energy malnutrition and identifies individuals at risk of developing malnutrition using three independent criteria: current weight status, unintentional weight loss, and acute disease effect. The patient's current body weight is determined by calculating the BMI (kg/m^2). Weight loss (over the past 3-6 months) is determined by looking at the individual's medical record. An acute disease factor is then included if the patient is currently affected by a pathophysiologic condition and there has been no nutritional intake for more than 5 days. A total score is calculated placing the patients in a low, medium, or high category for risk of malnutrition. A major advantage of this screening tool is its applicability to adults of all ages across all health care settings. Additionally, this method provides the user with management guidelines once an overall risk score has been determined. Studies have shown that MUST is quick and easy to use and has good concurrent validity with most other nutrition assessment tools tested.

G. Geriatric Nutritional Risk Index

The geriatric nutritional risk index (GNRI) is adapted from the NRI and is specifically designed to predict the risk of morbidity and mortality in hospitalized elderly patients. The GNRI is calculated using a formula incorporating both serum albumin and weight loss. After determining the GNRI score, patients are categorized into four grades of nutrition-related risk: major, moderate, low, and no risk. Finally, the GNRI scores are correlated with a severity score that takes into account nutritional status-related complications. The GNRI is not an index of malnutrition but rather a "nutrition-related" risk index.

H. Instant Nutritional Assessment

The quickest and simplest measure of nutritional status is the instant nutritional assessment (INA). Serum albumin level and the TLC form the basis of this evaluation. Significant correlations between depressed levels of these parameters and morbidity and mortality have been noted. Not surprisingly, abnormalities of these same parameters are even more significant in critically ill patients. Although not designed to replace more extensive assessment measures, this technique allows for quick identification and early intervention in those individuals in greatest danger of developing complications of malnutrition.

▶ Determining Energy Requirements

Adult basal energy expenditure (BEE) is calculated using a modification of the Harris-Benedict equation (Table 10–4). This calculation includes four variables: height (cm), weight (kg), gender, and age (y). Total energy expenditure (TEE) represents the caloric demands of the body under certain physiologic stresses. TEE is determined by multiplying BEE by a disease-specific stress factor. TEE should be used to guide nutritional supplementation.

Indirect calorimetry is the most accurate method for direct measurement of daily caloric requirements. Using a metabolic cart, oxygen consumption ($\dot{V}o_2$) and carbon dioxide production ($\dot{V}co_2$) are directly measured from the patient's pulmonary gas flow. Based on these measurements and the amount of nitrogen excreted in the urine, the resting

Table 10–4. Total energy expenditure equation for adults.

Basal energy expenditure (BEE) in kcal/day	
Male: 66.4 + [13.7 × weight (kg)] + [5.0 × height (cm)] − [6.8 × age (yrs)]	
Female: 655 + [9.6 × weight (kg)] + [1.7 × height (cm)] − [4.7 × age (yrs)]	
Stress factors	
Starvation	0.80–1.00
Elective surgery	1.00–1.10
Peritonitis	1.05–1.25
Adult respiratory distress syndrome (ARDS) or sepsis	1.30–1.35
Bone marrow transplant	1.20–1.30
Cardiopulmonary disease (uncomplicated)	0.80–1.00
Cardiopulmonary disease with dialysis or sepsis	1.20–1.30
Cardiopulmonary disease with major surgery	1.30–1.55
Acute renal failure	1.30
Liver failure	1.30–1.55
Liver transplantation	1.20–1.50
Pancreatitis or major burns	1.30–1.80
Total energy expenditure (TEE) in kcal/day	
TEE = BEE × stress factor	

energy expenditure (REE) can be derived using the Weir formula as follows:

$$\text{REE (Kcal/min)} = 3.9\ (\dot{V}o_2) + 1.1\ (\dot{V}co_2) - 2.2\ (\text{urine nitrogen})$$

where $\dot{V}o_2$ and $\dot{V}co_2$ are expressed in milliliters per minute and urine nitrogen is in grams per minute. The utility of this technique is limited by the expense and cumbersomeness of the metabolic cart.

The respiratory quotient (RQ) is the ratio of carbon dioxide production to oxygen consumption in the metabolism of fuels by the body. When the RQ is 1, pure carbohydrate is being oxidized. Patients metabolizing lipids only will have an RQ of 0.67. Lipogenesis occurs in patients with excess caloric intake (overfeeding). When excessive calories are ingested or administered, the RQ is greater than 1 and can theoretically approach 9. The excess production of CO_2 may impair ventilator weaning in patients, particularly those with intrinsic lung disease (eg, chronic obstructive pulmonary disease).

NUTRIENT REQUIREMENTS & SUBSTRATES

The body requires an energy source to remain in steady state. About 50% of the basal metabolic rate (BMR) reflects the work of ion pumping, 30% represents protein turnover, and the remainder is expended on recycling of amino acids, glucose, lactate, and pyruvate. Total energy expenditure is the sum of energy consumed by basal metabolic processes, physical activity, the specific dynamic action of protein, and extra requirements resulting from injury, sepsis, or burns.

Energy consumed in physical activity constitutes 10%-50% of the total in normal subjects but decreases to 10%-20% for hospitalized patients. Energy expenditure and requirements vary, depending on the illness or trauma. The increase in energy expenditure above basal needs is about 10% for elective operations, 10%-30% for trauma, 50%-80% for sepsis, and 100%-200% for burns (depending on the extent of the wound). Metabolic energy can be derived from carbohydrates, proteins, or fats.

Carbohydrate Metabolism

Carbohydrates are the body's primary fuel source, accounting for 35% of total caloric intake. Each gram of enteric carbohydrate provides 4.0 kilocalories (kcal) of energy. Parenterally administered carbohydrates (eg, intravenous dextrose) yield 3.4 kcal/g.

Carbohydrate digestion is initiated by salivary amylase, and absorption occurs within the first 150 cm of the small intestine. Salivary and pancreatic amylases cleave starches into oligosaccharides. Surface oligosaccharidases then hydrolyze and transport these molecules across the gastrointestinal tract mucosa. Deficiencies in carbohydrate digestion and absorption are rare in surgical patients. Pancreatic amylase is abundant, and maldigestion of starch is unusual, even in patients with limited pancreatic exocrine function. Patients with diseases such as celiac sprue, Whipple disease, and hypogammaglobulinemia often have generalized intestinal mucosal flattening leading to oligosaccharidase deficiency and diminished carbohydrate uptake.

More than 75% of ingested carbohydrate is broken down and absorbed as glucose. Hyperglycemia stimulates insulin secretion from pancreatic β cells, which stimulates protein synthesis. Intake of 400 kcal of carbohydrate per day minimizes protein breakdown, particularly after adaptation to starvation. Cellular uptake of glucose, stimulated by insulin, inhibits lipolysis and promotes glycogen formation. Conversely, pancreatic glucagon is released in response to starvation or stress; it promotes proteolysis, glycogenolysis, lipolysis, and increased serum glucose. Glucose is vital for wound repair, but excessive carbohydrate intake or repletion with excessive amounts of glucose can cause hepatic steatosis and neutrophil dysfunction.

Protein Metabolism

Proteins are composed of amino acids, and protein metabolism produces 4.0 kcal/g. Digestion of proteins yields single amino acids and dipeptides, which are actively absorbed by the gastrointestinal tract. Gastric pepsin initiates digestion. Pancreatic proteases, activated by enterokinase in the duodenum, are the principal effectors of protein degradation. Once digested, half of protein absorption occurs in the duodenum, and complete protein absorption is achieved by the mid-jejunum.

Table 10–5. Nitrogen balance.

$$Nitrogen_{(balance)} = Nitrogen_{(intake)} - Nitrogen_{(output)}$$
$$Nitrogen_{(intake)} = g \; protein_{(intake)} \, / \, 6.25$$
$$Nitrogen_{(output)} = (UUN \times Vol) \, + 3$$

UUN, urine urea nitrogen; Vol, volume of urine produced over the time of measurement.

Protein absorption occurs efficiently throughout the small intestine; therefore, protein malabsorption is relatively infrequent even after extensive intestinal resection. Protein balance reflects the sum of protein synthesis and degradation. Because protein turnover is dynamic, the published requirements for protein, amino acids, and nitrogen are only approximations.

Total body protein in a 70-kg person is approximately 10 kg, predominantly in skeletal muscle. Daily protein turnover is 300 g, or roughly 3% of total body protein. The daily protein requirement in healthy adults is 0.8 g/kg body weight. In the United States, the typical daily intake averages twice this amount. Protein synthesis or breakdown can be determined by measuring the nitrogen balance (Table 10–5). Protein intake of 6.25 g is equivalent to 1 g of nitrogen. Nitrogen intake is the sum of nitrogen delivered from enteric and parenteral feeding. Nitrogen output is the sum of nitrogen excreted in the urine and feces, plus losses from drainage (eg, exudative wounds, fistula). Urea nitrogen losses are determined from a 24-hour urine collection. Fecal nitrogen loss can be approximated by 1 g/d, and an additional 2-3 g/d of nonurea nitrogen loss occurs in the urine (eg, ammonia). The accuracy of nitrogen balance calculations can be improved through measurement over several weeks. When losses of nitrogen are large (eg, diarrhea, protein-losing enteropathy, fistula, or burn exudate), measurements of nitrogen balance lose accuracy because of the difficulty in collecting secretions for nitrogen measurement. Despite these shortcomings, 24-hour urine collection is the best practical means of measuring net protein synthesis and breakdown.

The 20 amino acids are divided into essential amino acids (EAAs) and nonessential amino acids (NEAAs) depending on whether they can be synthesized de novo in the body. They are further divided into aromatic (AAAs), branched chain (BCAAs), and sulfur-containing amino acids. Only the L-isotype of an amino acid is utilized in human protein. Certain amino acids have unique metabolic functions, particularly during starvation or stress. Alanine and glutamine preserve carbon during starvation, and leucine stimulates protein synthesis and inhibits catabolism. Specific amino acids are addressed below.

A. Glutamine

As the respiratory fuel for enterocytes, glutamine plays an important role in the metabolically stressed patient.

Following injury and other catabolic events, intracellular glutamine stores may decrease by over 50% and plasma levels by 25%. The decline of glutamine associated with injury or stress exceeds that of any other amino acid and persists during recovery after the concentrations of other amino acid have normalized. Supplementation with glutamine maintains intestinal cell integrity, villous height, and mucosal DNA activity and helps minimize reduction in numbers of T and B cells during stress.

Catabolic states are characterized by accelerated skeletal muscle proteolysis and translocation of amino acids from the periphery to the visceral organs. Glutamine accounts for a major portion of the amino acids released by muscle in these states. Intravenous supplementation with glutamine may improve neutrophil and macrophage function as well as decrease bacterial translocation across the intestinal mucosal barrier in burn and other critically ill patients. However, the utility of enteral supplementation remains controversial.

B. Arginine

Arginine is a substrate for the urea cycle and nitric oxide production and a secretagogue for growth hormone, prolactin, and insulin. Arginine has been identified as the sole precursor of nitric oxide (endothelial-derived relaxing factor). The effects of arginine on T cells may be very important in maintaining the gut barrier. Formulas supplemented with arginine have been shown to improve nitrogen balance and wound healing, promote T-cell proliferation, enhance neutrophil phagocytosis, and reduce production of inflammatory mediators and infectious complications.

Lipid Metabolism

Lipids comprise 25%-45% of caloric intake in the typical diet. Each gram of lipid provides 9.0 kcal of energy. The introduction of fat to the duodenum results in secretion of cholecystokinin and secretin, leading to gallbladder contraction and pancreatic enzyme release. Reabsorption of bile salts in the terminal ileum (eg, the enterohepatic circulation) is necessary to maintain the bile salt pool. The liver is able to compensate for moderate intestinal bile salt losses by increased synthesis from cholesterol. Ileal resection may lead to depletion of the bile salt pool and subsequent fat malabsorption. Lipolysis is stimulated by steroids, catecholamines, and glucagon but is inhibited by insulin.

The body can synthesize fats from other dietary substrates, but two of the long-chain fatty acids (linoleic and linolenic) are essential. Insufficient intake of these essential fats leads to fatty acid deficiency and can be prevented by supplying a minimum of 3% of the total caloric intake as essential fatty acids.

The polyunsaturated fatty acids (PUFAs) are grouped into two families: ω-6 and ω-3 fatty acids. Linoleic acid is an example of the ω-6 PUFAs; ω-linolenic acid of the ω-3 PUFAs. Both linoleic and linolenic acid can be processed into arachidonic acid, a precursor in the synthesis of eicosanoids.

Eicosanoids are potent biochemical mediators of cell-to-cell communication and are involved in inflammation, infection, tissue injury, and immune system modulation. They also modulate numerous events involving cell-mediated and humoral immunity and can be synthesized in varying amounts by immune cells, particularly macrophages and monocytes.

Medium-chain fatty acids are not components of most oral diets but are widely used in enteral tube feedings. They are easily digested, absorbed, and oxidized and are not precursors to the inflammatory or immunosuppressive eicosanoids. Short-chain fatty acids, such as butyrate and to a lesser extent propionate, are utilized by colonocytes and provide up to 70% of their energy requirements. Since butyrate is not synthesized endogenously, the colonic mucosa relies on intraluminal bacterial fermentation to obtain this fuel.

Nucleotides, Vitamins, & Trace Elements

In addition to the principal sources of metabolic energy (calories), many other substances are necessary to ensure adequate nutrition. Nucleotides are recognized as an important nutritional substrate in critically ill patients. Vitamins are essential for normal metabolism, wound healing and immune function, and cannot be synthesized de novo. The normal requirements for vitamins are shown in Table 10–6. Vitamin requirements may increase acutely in illness. Trace elements are integral cofactors for many enzymatic reactions and are generally not stored by the body in excess of requirements.

A. Nucleotides

Nucleic acids are precursors of DNA and RNA and are not normally considered essential for human growth and development. The need for dietary nucleotides increases in severe stress and critical illness. Nucleotides are formed from purines and pyrimidines, and their abundance is especially important for rapidly dividing cells such as enterocytes and immune cells. Immunosuppression has been reported in renal transplant patients being maintained on nucleotide-free diets. Dietary nucleotides are necessary for helper-inducer T-lymphocyte activity. Diets supplemented with RNA or the pyrimidine uracil have been shown to restore delayed hypersensitivity and augment both the lymphoproliferative response and IL-2 receptor expression. Nucleotides may facilitate recovery from infection. These substrates are often incorporated into enteral formulas as potential immunomodulators.

Table 10–6. Daily electrolyte, trace element, vitamin, and mineral requirements for adults.

	Enteral	Parenteral
Electrolytes		
Sodium	90–150 meq	90–150 meq
Potassium	60–90 meq	60–90 meq
Trace elements		
Chromium[1]	5–200 µg	10–15 µg
Copper[1]	2–3 mg	0.3–0.5 mg
Manganese[1]	2.5–5 mg	60–100 µg
Zinc	15 mg	2.5–5 mg
Iron	10 mg	2.5 mg
Iodine	150 µg	...
Fluoride[1]	3 mg	...
Selenium[1]	50–200 µg	20–60 µg
Molybdenum[1]	150–500 µg	20–120 µg
Tin[2]	...	...
Vanadium[2]	...	...
Nickel[2]	...	...
Arsenic[2]	...	...
Silicon[2]	...	...
Vitamins		
Ascorbic acid (C)	60 mg	200 mg
Retinol (A)	1000 µg	3300 IU
Vitamin D	5 µg	200 IU
Thiamin (B$_1$)	1.4 mg	6 mg
Riboflavin (B$_2$)	1.7 mg	3.6 mg
Pyridoxine (B$_6$)	2.2 mg	6 mg
Niacin	19 mg	40 mg
Pantothenic acid	4–7 mg	15 mg
Vitamin E	10 mg	10 IU
Biotin	100–200 µg	60 µg
Folic acid[1]	200 µg	600 µg
Cyanocobalamin (B$_{12}$)	2 µg	5.9 µg
Vitamin K[3]	70–149 mg	150 µg
Minerals		
Calcium	1300 mg	0.2–0.3 meq/kg
Phosphorus	800 mg	300–400 meq/kg
Magnesium	350 mg	0.34–0.45 meq/kg
Sulfur	2–3 g	...

[1]Estimated safe and adequate dose.
[2]No available data regarding human requirements.
[3]Weekly requirement.

B. Fat-Soluble Vitamins

Vitamins A, D, E, and K are fat soluble and are absorbed in the proximal small bowel in association with bile salt micelles and fatty acids. After absorption, they are delivered to the tissues in chylomicrons and stored in the liver (vitamins A and K) or subcutaneous tissue and skin (vitamins D and E). Although rare, there are reports of toxicity from excessive intake of fat-soluble vitamins (eg, hypervitaminosis A from consuming polar bear liver). Fat-soluble vitamins participate in immune function and wound healing. For example, intake of vitamin A 25,000 IU daily counteracts steroid-induced inhibition of wound healing, largely through increases in TBG-β.

C. Water-Soluble Vitamins

Vitamins B$_1$, B$_2$, B$_6$, and B$_{12}$, vitamin C, niacin, folate, biotin, and pantothenic acid are absorbed in the duodenum and proximal small bowel, transported in portal vein blood, and utilized in the liver and peripherally. Water-soluble vitamins serve as cofactors to facilitate reactions involved in the generation and transfer of energy and in amino acid and nucleic acid metabolism. Water-soluble vitamins have limited storage in the body. Because of their limited storage, water-soluble vitamin deficiencies are relatively common.

D. Trace Elements

The daily requirements for the trace elements (Table 10–6) vary geographically depending on differences in soil composition. There are currently nine identified essential trace minerals (Fe, Zn, Cu, Se, Mn, I, Mb, Cr, Co). Trace elements have important functions in metabolism, immunology, and wound healing. Subclinical trace element deficiencies occur commonly in hospitalized patients and various disease states.

Iron serves as the core of the heme prosthetic group in hemoglobin and in the mitochondrial cytochrome respiratory process. Impaired cerebral, muscular, and immunologic function can occur in patients with iron deficiency before anemia becomes clinically evident. Particular attention should be paid to assessing iron stores in pregnant and lactating women.

Zinc deficiency is characterized by a perioral pustular rash, darkening of skin creases, neuritis, cutaneous anergy, hair loss, and alterations in taste and smell. Copper deficiency is manifested by microcytic anemia (unresponsive to iron), defective keratinization, or pancytopenia. Chromium deficiency presents as glucose intolerance during prolonged parenteral nutrition administration without evidence of sepsis. Selenium deficiency, which can occur in patients receiving parenteral nutrition for a prolonged period, is manifested by proximal neuromuscular weakness or cardiac failure with electrocardiographic changes. Manganese deficiency is associated with weight loss, altered hair pigmentation, nausea, and low plasma levels of phospholipids and triglycerides. Molybdenum deficiency results in elevated plasma methionine levels and depressed uric acid concentrations, producing a syndrome consisting of nausea, vomiting, tachycardia, and central nervous system disturbances.

Iodine is a key component of thyroid hormone. Deficiency is rare in the United States because of the use of iodinated salt. Chronically malnourished patients can become iodine-deficient. Since thyroxine participates in the neuroendocrine response to trauma and sepsis, iodine should be included in parenteral nutrition solutions.

NUTRITIONAL PATHOPHYSIOLOGY

Physiologic processes, immunocompetence, wound healing, and recovery from critical illness all depend upon adequate nutrient intake. A working knowledge of nutritional pathophysiology is essential in planning nutritional regimens.

▶ Starvation

During an overnight fast, liver glycogen is rapidly depleted after a fall in insulin and parallel rise in plasma glucagon levels (Figure 10–1). Carbohydrate stores are depleted after a 24-hour fast. In the first few days of starvation, caloric needs are met by fat and protein degradation. There is an increase in hepatic gluconeogenesis from amino acids derived from the breakdown of muscle protein. Hepatic glucose production must satisfy the energy demands of the hematopoietic and the central nervous systems, particularly the brain, which is dependent on glucose oxidation during acute starvation. The release of amino acids from muscle is regulated

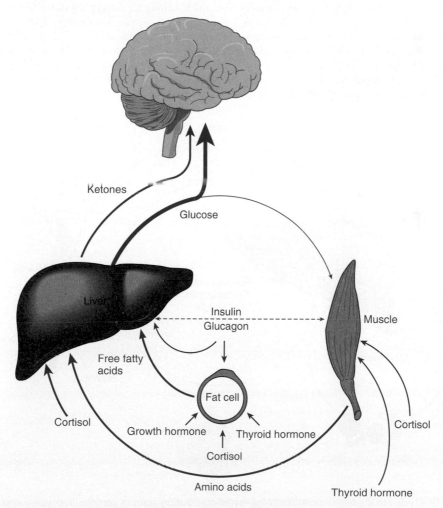

▲ **Figure 10–1.** The plasma substrate concentrations and hormone levels following an overnight fast. The brain is dependent on glucose, which is supplied predominantly by hepatic glycogenolysis until glycogen supplies are exhausted.

by insulin, which signals hepatic amino acid uptake, poly-ribosome formation, and protein synthesis. The periodic rise and fall of insulin associated with ingestion of nutrients stimulates muscle protein synthesis and breakdown. During starvation, chronically depressed insulin levels result in a net loss of amino acids from muscle. Protein synthesis drops while protein catabolism remains unchanged. Hepatic gluconeogenesis requires energy, which is supplied by the oxidation of unesterified free fatty acid (FFA). The fall in insulin along with a rise in plasma glucagon levels leads to an increase in the concentration of cyclic adenosine mono-phosphate (cAMP) in adipose tissue, stimulating hormone-sensitive lipase to hydrolyze triglycerides and release FFA. Gluconeogenesis and FFA mobilization require the presence of ambient cortisol and thyroid hormone (a permissive effect).

During starvation, the body attempts to conserve energy substrate by recycling metabolic intermediates. The hema-topoietic system utilizes glucose anaerobically, leading to lactate production. Lactate is recycled back to glucose in the liver via the glucogenic (not gluconeogenic) Cori cycle (Figure 10–2). The glycerol released during periph-eral triglyceride hydrolysis is converted into glucose via

gluconeogenesis. Alanine and glutamine are the preferred substrates for hepatic gluconeogenesis from amino acids and contribute 75% of the amino acid–derived carbon for glucose production.

BCAAs are unique because they are secreted rather than taken up by the liver during starvation; they are oxidized by skeletal and cardiac muscle to supply a portion of the energy requirements of these tissues; and they stimulate protein synthesis and inhibit catabolism. The amino groups derived from oxidation of BCAAs or transamination of other amino acids are donated to pyruvate or α-ketoglutarate to form alanine and glutamine. Glutamine is taken up by the small bowel, transaminated to form additional alanine, and released into the portal circulation. Along with glucose, these amino acids participate in the glucose-alanine/glutamine-BCAA cycle, which shuttles amino groups and carbon from muscle to liver for conversion into glucose.

Gluconeogenesis from amino acids results in a urinary nitrogen excretion of 8-12 g/d, predominantly as urea, which is equivalent to a loss of 340 g/d of lean tissue. At this rate, 35% of the lean body mass would be lost in 1 month, a uniformly fatal amount. However, starvation can be sur-vived for 2-3 months as long as water is available. The body

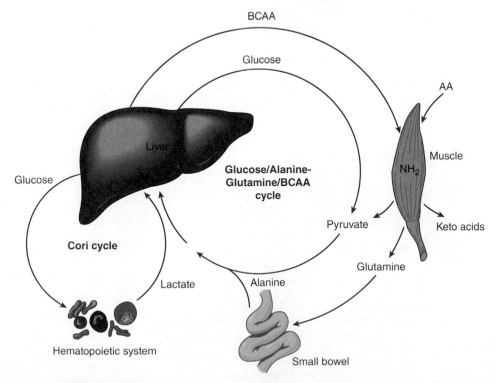

▲ **Figure 10–2.** The cycles that preserve metabolic intermediates during fasting. Lactate is recycled to glucose via the Cori cycle, while pyruvate is transaminated to alanine in skeletal muscle and converted to glucose by hepatic gluconeogenesis.

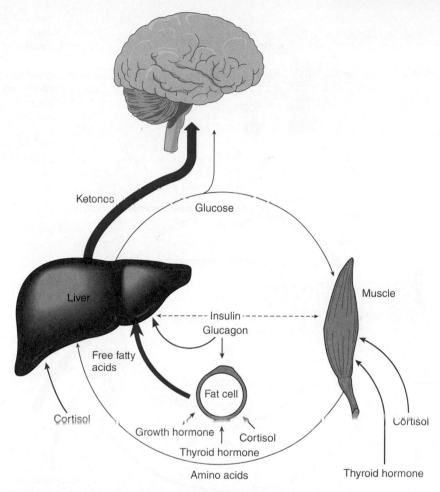

▲ **Figure 10–3.** The metabolic adaptation to chronic starvation whereby the brain shifts its substrate preference to ketones produced by the liver. Hepatic gluconeogenesis falls and protein breakdown is diminished, thus conserving lean tissue.

adapts to prolonged starvation by decreasing energy expenditures and shifting the substrate preference of the brain to ketones (Figure 10–3). After roughly 10 days of starvation, the brain adapts to use lipid as its primary fuel in the form of ketones. The BMR decreases by slowing the heart rate and reducing stroke work, while voluntary activity declines owing to weakness and fatigue. The RQ, which in early starvation is 0.85 (reflecting mixed carbohydrate and fat oxidation), falls to 0.70, indicating near-exclusive fatty acid utilization. Blood ketone levels rise sharply, accompanied by increased cerebral ketone oxidation. Brain glucose utilization drops from 140 g to 60-80 g/d, decreasing the demand for gluconeogenesis. Ketones also inhibit hepatic gluconeogenesis, and urinary nitrogen excretion falls to 2-3 g/d. The main component of urine nitrogen is now ammonia

(rather than urea), derived from renal transamination and gluconeogenesis from glutamine, and it buffers the acid urine that results from ketonuria. Acute or chronic starvation is characterized by hormone and fuel alterations orchestrated by changing blood substrate levels and can be conceptualized as a "substrate-driven" process. In summary, the adaptive changes in uncomplicated starvation are a decrease in energy expenditure (as much as a 30% reduction), a change in type of fuel consumed to maximize caloric potential, and preservation of protein.

▶ Elective Operation or Trauma

The metabolic effects of both surgical procedures and trauma (Figure 10–4) differ from those of starvation due

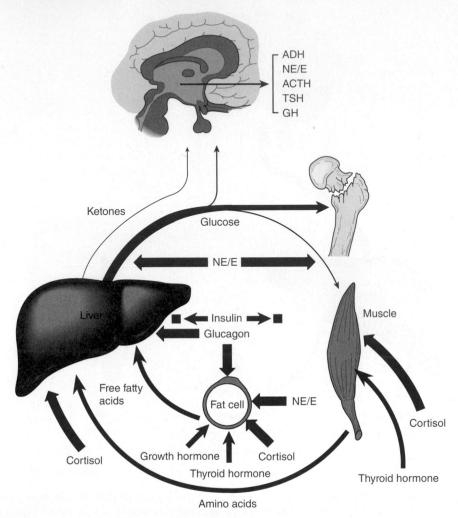

ADH
NE/E
ACTH
TSH
GH

Ketones

Glucose

NE/E

Liver

Insulin
Glucagon

Muscle

Free fatty
acids

Fat cell

NE/E

Cortisol

Cortisol

Growth hormone   Cortisol

Thyroid hormone

Thyroid hormone

Amino acids

▲ **Figure 10–4.** The metabolic response to trauma is a result of neuroendocrine stimulation, which accelerates protein breakdown, stimulates gluconeogenesis, and produces glucose intolerance.

to neurohormonal activation, accelerating the loss of lean tissue and inhibiting metabolic adaptation of starvation. Following injury, neural impulses stimulate the hypothalamus. Norepinephrine is released from sympathetic nerve endings, epinephrine from the adrenal medulla, aldosterone from the adrenal cortex, antidiuretic hormone (ADH) from the posterior pituitary, insulin and glucagon from the pancreas, and corticotropin, thyrotropin, and growth hormone from the anterior pituitary. This results in elevation of serum cortisol, thyroid hormone, and somatomedins. The effects of the heightened neuroendocrine secretion include peripheral lipolysis from activation of lipase by glucagon, epinephrine, cortisol, and thyroid hormone; accelerated catabolism, with a rise

in proteolysis stimulated by cortisol; decreased peripheral glucose uptake due to insulin antagonism by growth hormone and epinephrine.

These effects result in a rise in plasma FFA, glycerol, glucose, lactate, and amino acids. The liver subsequently increases glucose production, as a result of glucagon-stimulated glycogenolysis and enhanced gluconeogenesis induced by cortisol and glucagon.

Accelerated glucose production, along with inhibited peripheral uptake, produces the glucose intolerance commonly observed in traumatized patients. The kidney retains water and sodium due to increases in ADH and aldosterone. Urinary nitrogen excretion increases up to 15-20 g/d following severe trauma, equivalent to a daily lean tissue loss of

750 g. Without exogenous nutrients, the median survival under these circumstances is only 15 days.

In contrast to the substrate dependency of uncomplicated starvation, elective surgical procedures and trauma are "neuroendocrine-driven" processes. In contrast, however, metabolic responses observed following elective procedures are vastly different from those following major trauma. During general anesthesia, the neuroendocrine response is blunted in the operating room through the use of analgesics and immobilization. Sedated patients lack cortical stimulation to the hypothalamus. Careful intraoperative handling of tissues reduces proinflammatory cytokine release. The net result is that the REE rises only 10% in postoperative patients, compared with up to 30% following severe injury or trauma.

Sepsis

The metabolic changes during sepsis differ from those observed after acute injury (Figure 10–5). The REE may increase by 50%-80%, and urinary nitrogen excretion can reach up to 30 g/d, predominantly due to profound muscle catabolism and impaired synthesis. Catabolism at this rate results in a median survival of 10 days without nutritional input. The plasma glucose, amino acid, and FFA levels increase more than with trauma. Hepatic protein synthesis is

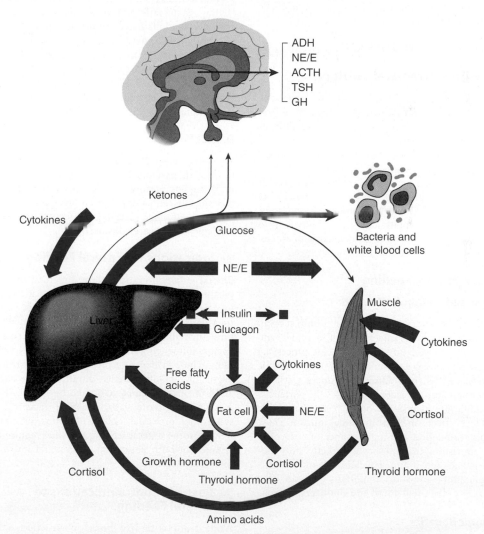

▲ **Figure 10–5.** During sepsis, cytokines (IL-1, IL-2, TNF) released by lymphocytes and macrophages contribute to catabolism of muscle and adipose tissue and amplify the neurohormonal response to antecedent trauma.

stimulated, with both enhanced secretion of export protein and accumulation of structural protein. The RQ falls to near 0.7, indicative of lipid oxidation. Lipolysis and gluconeogenesis continue despite supplementation with carbohydrate or fat, leading to the hyperglycemia and insulin resistance commonly observed in septic patients.

Sepsis results in elaboration of inflammatory cytokines, most notably TNF-α, IL-1, and IL-6. Alteration in hepatic protein synthesis toward production of acute-phase proteins is triggered by IL-6. Septic patients also develop an abnormal plasma amino acid pattern (increased levels of AAAs and decreased levels of BCAAs). In contrast to simple starvation, protein conservation does not occur in sepsis. Terminal sepsis results in further increases in plasma amino acids and a fall in glucose concentration, as hepatic amino acid clearance declines and gluconeogenesis ceases.

ENTERAL NUTRITIONAL THERAPY

▶ Enteral Versus Parenteral Nutrition

Enteral nutritional support is safer and less expensive than parenteral nutrition and has the added benefit of preserving gut functionality. Prospective, randomized trials have demonstrated the superiority of enteral nutrition in reducing postoperative complications and length of hospital stay. "Feeding the gut" also results in fewer septic complications. Parenteral nutrition has a role in the management of surgical patients, but utilizing the gastrointestinal tract should remain the preferred treatment option. Enteral supplementation is not risk-free; physicians must know how to prevent and treat the complications associated with enteral feedings to ensure safe and successful administration.

▶ Benefits of Enteral Feeding

A. Physiologic and Metabolic Benefits

The gastrointestinal tract can be used for administration of complex nutrients, such as intact protein, peptides, and fiber, that cannot be given intravenously. Gut processing of intact nutrients provides a stimulus for hepatic synthetic function of proteins, whereas administration of nutrients directly into the systemic circulation bypasses the portal circulation. In addition to its systemic benefits, enteral feeding has beneficial local effects on gastrointestinal mucosa. These include trophic stimulation and maintenance of absorptive structures by nourishing the enterocytes directly, thus supporting epithelial cell repair and replication. Luminal nutrients such as glutamine and short-chain fatty acids are used as fuel by the cells of the small bowel and colon, respectively.

B. Immunologic Benefits

The presence of food in the gut, particularly complex proteins and fats, triggers feeding-dependent neuroendocrine activity. This activity stimulates the transport of immunoglobulins into the gut, particularly secretory immunoglobulin A, which is important for preventing bacterial adherence to gut mucosa and bacterial translocation. Enteral feeds also prevent villus atrophy, minimizing subsequent loss of epithelial border function and help to maintain normal gut pH and flora, diminishing opportunistic bacterial overgrowth in the small bowel. In recent animal studies enteral nutrition has been shown to reverse the aberrant cytokine profile associated with parenteral nutrition that is believed to lead to enterocyte apoptosis.

C. Safety Benefits

Enteral feeding is generally considered safer than parenteral feeding. Systematic review of randomized trials involving critically ill adults has demonstrated fewer infectious complications with enteral nutrition compared with parenteral nutrition; however there was no significant difference in mortality. Hyperglycemia, and its resulting inhibition of neutrophil-mediated immunity, also occurs more frequently with parenteral feeding. Enteral nutrition has its own potential complications (discussed shortly).

D. Cost Benefits

The direct costs of enteral feeding are generally less than those with parenteral nutrition. Direct costs include formula, feeding pumps, and tube placement. The cost advantage for enteral feeding is even greater when indirect costs such as central line placement, infection or thrombosis, and home health care are considered.

▶ Indications for Enteral Feeding

Enteral nutrition is the preferred method of nutrition support for malnourished patients or those at risk for developing malnutrition and who have an intact gastrointestinal tract. Patients who are either unable or unwilling to eat to meet their daily needs are candidates for enteral support. Factors influencing the timing of initiation of enteral nutrition include evidence of preexisting malnutrition, expected degree of catabolic activity, duration of the current illness, and anticipated return to intake by mouth. Patients with partially functioning gastrointestinal tracts (eg, short bowel syndrome, proximal enterocutaneous fistula) often can tolerate some enteral feeding but may require a combined regimen of both parenteral and enteral nutrition to meet total caloric needs.

▶ Possible Contraindications to Enteral Feeding

Aside from complete bowel obstruction, contraindications to enteral feeding are relative or temporary rather than absolute. Patients with short bowel, gastrointestinal obstruction, gastrointestinal bleeding, protracted vomiting and diarrhea, fistulas, ileus, or active gastrointestinal ischemia may require a period of bowel rest. In times of physiologic stress, the body shunts blood away from the splanchnic circulation. Feeding a patient who is hemodynamically unstable or requires vasopressors may produce bowel ischemia in the setting of preexisting tenuous perfusion. The choice of an appropriate feeding site, administration technique, formula, and equipment may circumvent many of these contraindications.

▶ Implementing Enteral Supplementation

A. Delivery Methods

Prepyloric access via nasogastric tube is beneficial because it is less expensive, easier to secure and maintain, and less labor-intensive than small bowel access. Contraindications to delivery in the stomach are delayed gastric emptying, gastric outlet obstruction, and a history of repeated aspiration of tube feedings due to reflux. Some physicians consider the inability to protect the airway (eg, in comatose patients) a relative contraindication to gastric feeding. Diabetics and patients with severe head injuries may have profound gastroparesis. Postpyloric access via a duodenal or jejunal nasoenteric tube is preferred when gastric feedings are not tolerated, when patients are at risk for reflux or aspiration, or when early enteral nutrition is desired. A new feeding tube, guided in place by an external magnet, may provide ease of bedside placement of postpyloric tubes. Although a number of bedside methods (eg, auscultation, feeding tube aspirate pH measurements, observation for patient coughing) have been described to check tube placement, these methods can be unreliable. Therefore, tube position below the diaphragm should always be confirmed radiographically before initiating enteral feeding.

Permanent gastrostomy or jejunostomy tubes may be inserted when long-term enteral feeding is indicated. Placement of a feeding tube at the time of the initial operation requires forethought, with consideration given to the patient's expected postoperative course, anticipated ileus, and possible future need for supplementation (eg, during chemoradiation therapy).

B. Formulas

Currently available dietary formulations for enteral feedings may be divided into polymeric commercial formulas, chemically defined formulas, and modular formulas (Table 10–7). Selection of the correct formulation is predicated on patient need, cost, availability, and institutional custom.

Nutritionally complete commercial formulas or standard enteral diets vary in protein, carbohydrate, and fat composition. Most formulas use sucrose or glucose as the carbohydrate source and are suitable for lactose-deficient patients.

Commercial formulas are convenient, sterile, and affordable. They are recommended for patients experiencing minimal metabolic stress who have normal gut function.

Chemically defined formulas are commonly called *elemental diets*. The nutrients are provided in a predigested and readily absorbed form. They contain protein in the form of free amino acids or polypeptides. Amino acid (elemental) and polypeptide diets are efficiently absorbed in the presence of compromised gut function. However, they are more expensive than commercial formulas and are hyperosmolar, which may cause cramping, diarrhea, and fluid losses.

Modular formulations include special formulas used for specific clinical situations such as pulmonary, renal, or hepatic failure or immune dysfunction. The available preparations vary in (1) caloric and protein content; (2) protein, carbohydrate, and fat compositions; (3) nonprotein carbohydrate calorie-to-gram nitrogen ratio; (4) osmolality; (5) content of minor trace metals (selenium, chromium, and molybdenum); and (6) content of various amino acids (glutamine, glutamate, BCAAs).

C. Initiating Feedings

In the past, elaborate protocols for initiating tube feedings were used. It is currently recommended that feedings be started with full-strength formula at a slow rate and steadily advanced. This approach reduces the risk of microbial contamination and achieves full nutrient intake earlier. Formulas are often introduced at full strength at 10-40 mL/h initially and advanced to the goal rate in increments of 10-20 mL/h every 4-8 hours as tolerated. Conservative initiation and advancement rates are recommended for patients who are critically ill, those who have not been fed for some time, and those who are receiving high-osmolality or calorie-dense formula. In such patients, starting feeding at 10 mL/h yields the trophic benefit of enteral feeds without unduly stressing the gut. In patients with active lifestyles, gastric feeds can be provided as boluses of up to 400 mL each, delivered at intervals of 4-6 hours.

D. Monitoring Feedings

Assessing gastrointestinal tolerance to enteral feeding includes monitoring for abdominal discomfort, nausea and vomiting, abdominal distention, and abnormal bowel sounds or stool patterns. Gastric residual volumes are used to evaluate gastric emptying of enteral feedings. High residuals raise concerns about intolerance to gastric feedings and the potential risk for regurgitation and aspiration. While differences in the recommended threshold for gastric residual volume vary, a residual greater than 200-250 mL or associated signs or symptoms of intolerance should prompt holding of tube feeds. If the abdominal examination is unremarkable, feedings should be postponed for at least an hour and the residual volume rechecked. If high residuals persist without

Table 10–7. Enteral formulas.

Product Name	cal/mL	Pro g/L	CHO g/L	Fat g/L	Osmolality	mL to meet 100% RDI	Features
Osmolite 1 cal	1.06	44.3	143.9	34.7	300	1321	Isotonic, low residue
Jevity 1 cal	1.06	44.3	154.7	34.7	300	1321	14.4 g fiber/L
Jevity 1.5 cal	1.5	63.8	215.7	49.8	525	1000	22 g fiber/L
Promote	1.0	62.5	130	26	340	1000	High protein
Promote with Fiber	1.0	62.5	138.3	28.2	380	1000	14.4 g fiber/L, high protein
Oxepa	1.5	62.7	105.3	93.8	535	946	Elevated levels of antioxidants
Nepro with Carb Steady	1.8	81	166.8	96	600	948	15.6 g fiber/L; renal-appropriate electro-lytes for dialysis
TwoCal HN	2	83.5	218.5	90.5	725	948	Concentrated, low residue
Peptamen AF	1.2	75.6	107	54.8	390	1500	Elemental; high protein; 9.3 g fish oil/L, 5.2 g fiber/L, 50% fat as MCT
Crucial	1.5	94	134	67.6	490	1000	Peptide based; contains arginine, gluta-mine, DHA, and EPA
Portagen	1	35	115	48	350	Not applicable	87% fat as MCT
Oral Supplements							
Ensure Plus	8 fl oz	Concentrated calories	350	13	50	11	Lactose and gluten free, low residue
Glucerna Shake	8 fl oz	Diabetes	220	9.9	29.3	8.6	Lactose and gluten free
Juven	1 packet (23g)	Wound care	78	14	7.7	0	Contains arginine and glutamine; lactose and gluten free
Resource Healthshake	4 fl oz	Milk shake	200	6	45	4	Low residue
Resource Breeze	8 fl oz	Clear liquid	250	9	54	0	Fat free, lactose free, low residue
Modulars							
Pro-Stat 64	2 tbsp (30 mL)	Protein	60	15	0	0	Liquid protein supplement, sugar free
Resource Benefiber	1 tbsp	Fiber	16	0	4	0	3 g fiber per serving

All enteral products included are lactose and gluten free.

associated clinical signs and symptoms, a promotility agent (eg, erythromycin, metoclopramide) may be added to the feeding regimen.

▶ Complications of Enteral Feeding

Technical complications occur in about 5% of enterally fed patients and include clogging of the tube; esopha-geal, tracheal, bronchial, or duodenal perforation; and tracheobronchial intubation with tube feeding aspiration. Patients with decreased consciousness or impaired gag reflexes or those who have undergone endotracheal intuba-tion are at increased risk for technical complications. The tip of the feeding tube must be positioned and verified radiographically. Other methods to evaluate tube placement are not consistently reliable. Generally, the wire stylet used for positioning should not be reinserted once removed. The incidence of tube clogging can be reduced by periodic water flushes and avoiding administration of syrup-based medica-tions through the tube.

Functional complications occur in up to 25% of tube-fed patients and include nausea, vomiting, abdominal distention, constipation, and diarrhea. Feeding the small bowel instead of the stomach can diminish abdominal symptoms. In the critically injured patient, diarrhea is typically multifactorial; it results from polypharmacy (eg, multiple antibiotics), mechanical gut dysfunction (eg, partial small bowel obstruction), intestinal bacterial overgrowth (eg, *Clostridium difficile*), and protein content or osmolarity of the diet. Treatment consists of stopping any unnecessary medications, correcting gut dysfunction, changing enteral formulation (eg, intact protein vs amino acid or polypeptide formula), or reducing the osmolarity of the formula. In some circumstances, adding highly fermentable or viscous soluble fibers, such as guar gum, psyllium, pectin, or banana flakes have been shown to decrease diarrhea more than using fiber containing enteral formulas. Administering antidiarrheal agents can be beneficial after establishing that infection is not the source of diarrhea.

In the surgical population, *C difficile* is a common cause of diarrhea due to the routine use of perioperative antibiotics. The diagnosis of pseudomembranous colitis is confirmed by *C difficile* polymerase chain reaction or toxin assay, or sigmoidoscopy. The primary treatment is stopping unnecessary antibiotics. Additionally, either oral or intravenous metronidazole or vancomycin (oral or retention enema) can be started. Antimotility agents should be avoided.

Abnormalities in serum electrolytes, calcium, magnesium, and phosphorus can be minimized through vigilant monitoring. Hyperosmolarity (hypernatremia) may lead to mental lethargy or obtundation. The treatment of hypernatremia includes the administration of free water by giving either D_5W intravenously or additional water flushes. Volume overload and subsequent congestive heart failure may occur as a result of excess sodium administration and is typically observed in patients with impaired ventricular function or valvular heart disease. Hyperglycemia may occur in any patient but is particularly common in individuals with preexisting diabetes or sepsis. The serum glucose level should be determined frequently and regular insulin administered accordingly.

PARENTERAL NUTRITION THERAPY

The development of parenteral nutritional support in the late 1960s revolutionized care of the surgical patient, particularly those with permanent inability to obtain adequate enteral nourishment. Despite its utility in select patients and circumstances, overuse of parenteral nutrition not only is costly but also poses unnecessary risk to patients. In general, parenteral nutrition should be employed only when the gastrointestinal tract cannot be utilized. Parenteral formulas usually deliver 75-150 nonprotein carbohydrate kcal/g of nitrogen infused, a ratio that maximizes carbohydrate and protein assimilation and minimizes metabolic complications (aminoaciduria, hyperglycemia, and hepatic glycogenesis). Nonenteral nutrition can be given as peripheral parenteral nutrition (PPN) or total parenteral nutrition (TPN) via a central line. In addition to route of administration, the two differ in (1) dextrose and amino acid content of the parenteral solution, (2) primary caloric source (glucose vs fat), (3) frequency of fat administration, (4) infusion schedule, and (5) potential complications.

▶ Peripheral Parenteral Nutrition

Because peripheral parenteral nutrition (PPN) avoids the complications associated with central venous access, it is safer to administer than TPN. PPN is indicated for patients with compromised gut function who require supplemental nutrition for less than 14 days. It can be infused via an 18-gauge peripheral IV catheter or via a peripherally inserted central catheter (PICC line). Standard PPN therapy orders should include the administration schedule for the PPN solution and fat supplement, as well as explicit catheter care orders and monitoring guidelines.

A. PPN Formulation

The osmolarity of the PPN solution is limited to 900 mOsm to avoid phlebitis. Consequently, unacceptably large volumes of solution, greater than 2.5 L/d are needed to fulfill the typical patient's total nutritional requirements (Figure 10–6).

▶ Total Parenteral Nutrition

Total parenteral nutrition (TPN) via a central line is indicated for patients who cannot obtain adequate nourishment via the gastrointestinal tract or, very rarely, in patients with severe preoperative undernutrition who cannot tolerate adequate enteral nutrition. A minimum duration of treatment of 7-10 days of adequate TPN is needed for preoperative nutritional repletion. Likewise, the use of postoperative TPN for only 2-3 days (eg, while awaiting return of bowel function) is discouraged, as the risks outweigh the benefits incurred over this short a period of time.

A. TPN Formulation

TPN is typically formulated for patients on the basis of their individual nutritional assessment. Most frequently, TPN is prepared in the pharmacy and provided as a 3-in-1 admixture of protein, carbohydrates, and fat. Alternatively, the lipid emulsion can be administered as a separate intravenous piggyback infusion. Other additives, vitamins, and trace minerals are added to TPN formulations as required (Table 10–8).

1. TPN components:

Routine additives	Recommended dosage ranges per liter TPN	BAG #___	BAG #___	BAG #___
D$_{50}$W	500 mL	500 mL	500 mL	500 mL
AA 8.5%	500 mL	500 mL	500 mL	500 mL
NaCl	0–140 meq	meq	meq	meq
NaPO$_4$	0–20 mmol	mmol	mmol	mmol
K*Cl	0–40 meq	meq	meq	meq
MgSO$_4$	0–12 meq	meq	meq	meq
Ca gluconate	4.5 or 9 meq	meq	meq	meq
MVI-12®	10 mL/d	10 mL		
Multitrace®	5 mL/d	5mL		
Optional additives				
Na acetate	0–140 meq	meq	meq	meq
K* acetate	0–40 meq	meq	meq	meq
Regular insulin	0–40 units	units	units	units
H$_2$ antagonist**				
25% albumin***	25 g	g	g	g
Nurse's signature				

* Total potassium content per liter of TPN should not exceed 40 meq.
** Divide the daily dosage equally into each liter of TPN.
*** Only if the serum albumin < 2.5g/dl and enteral diet therapy is anticipated.

Rate: _____40_____ mL/h via pump.
Final dextrose concentration _25_ %   Final AA concentration _4.25_ %

2. Pharmacy to add vitamin K 10 mg to 1 L of TPN solution every Mon. and Thurs.
3. Fat emulsion 20% 500 mL every Mon., Wed., and Fri. IVPB per pump over 6-8 hours via at least an 18-gauge peripheral IV or via the subclavian catheter.
4. STAT upright and expirational portable chest x-ray to check the position of the subclavian catheter and to rule out a pneumothorax. Notify the physician when the chest x-ray is completed.
5. Heparin lock the TPN catheter with 2 mL of heparin (100 units/mL) until notified by the physician to start the first liter of TPN solution.
6. Strict I/O every shift. Total the I/O every 24 hours.
7. Record the daily weight in kilograms on the vital signs sheet.
8. Check the urine for sugar and acetone every shift and record on the vital signs sheet. If the urine sugar is 4+, request a STAT serum glucose measurement to be drawn by the physician. If the serum glucose is > 160 mg/dL, contact the physician for treatment orders.
9. Notify the physician if the oral temperature is >38C (>100.4F).
10. Routine TPN laboratory tests are to be drawn weekly on the days and times specified below:
    Sun. AM: CBC, SMAC-20
    Tues. AM: Electrolytes, BUN, creatinine, and glucose
    Thurs. AM: CBC, SMAC-20, copper, zinc, magnesium, transferrin, and triglycerides
11. Begin a 24-hour urine collection for urinary urea nitrogen (UUN) at 6:00 AM every Mon. and Thurs. for nitrogen balance determination.
12. TPN catheter dressing and tubing changes per the hospital TPN protocol.
13. Contact the physician for all problems related to TPN.
14. All changes in TPN therapy must be approved by the physician.

▲ **Figure 10–6.** TPN therapy orders.

B. Administration

The high osmolarity of TPN solutions necessitates administration via a central vein. The use of multilumen central venous catheters (CVCs) for TPN does not increase the risk of catheter infection; however, a port should be designated

Table 10–8. TPN solution formulation.

Components in 1 L of Standard TPN:	
Routine additives	
D$_{50}$W[1]	500 mL
8.5% amino acid[1]	500 mL
Sodium chloride[2]	0–140 meq
Sodium phosphate[3]	0–20 mmol
Potassium chloride[4]	0–40 meq
Magnesium sulfate[5]	0–12 meq
Calcium gluconate[5,6]	4.5–9.0 meq
Trace element-5[7]	1 mL
M.V.I.-13[7]	10 mL
Optional additives	
Sodium acetate[2]	0–140 meq
Potassium acetate[4]	0–40 meq
H$_2$ antagonist[8]	Variable
Regular insulin[9]	0–40 units
Vitamin K[10]	10 mg
Heparin[11]	Variable
Fat emulsion schedule:	
Infuse 20–25% fat emulsion intravenously via pump at least 3 times per week	

[1]The solution is formulated to deliver 125 nonprotein kcal/g of nitrogen infused.
[2]Add sodium chloride if the serum CO_2 > 25 meq/L. Add sodium acetate if the serum CO_2 ≤ 25 meq/L.
[3]The total phosphate dosage should not exceed 20 mmol/L or 60 mmol daily.
[4]Add potassium chloride if the serum CO_2 > 25 meq/L. Add potassium acetate if the serum CO_2 ≤ 25 meq/L. The potassium dosage should not exceed 40 meq/L.
[5]Added to each liter.
[6]Add calcium gluconate 9 meq to each liter if the serum calcium < 8.5 meq/L.
Add 4.5 meq if the serum calcium ≥ 8.5 meq/L.
[7]Administered in only 1 L per day.
[8]Dosage depends upon the H$_2$ antagonist selected. Divide the daily dosage equally in all liters of TPN administered.
[9]Total dosage should not exceed 40 units/L.
[10]Administered only once per week.
[11]Heparin administration in TPN is not required, but it may be added in place of subcutaneous dosing.

for exclusive use for TPN infusion to minimize handling of the line. CVC placement in the subclavian vein is ideal and well tolerated by the patient. Furthermore, the rate of catheter infection is lower for catheters placed in the subclavian compared to catheters placed in either the femoral or internal jugular vein. Femoral vein catheterization has the highest infectious rate and therefore should be avoided if possible.

The CVC should be dressed with a sterile, dry gauze, and transparent (nonocclusive) dressing; a chlorhexidine gluconate impregnated sponge may be used as well.

If refeeding syndrome is suspected, the introduction of TPN should be gradual, with approximately 10 kcal/kg/d for the first 3 days. This amount is increased 15-20 kcal/kg/d for days 4-10. For all patients, additional maintenance IV fluids should be tapered or discontinued accordingly to maintain an even fluid balance.

Standard TPN therapy orders (Figure 10–6) should include the administration schedule for the TPN solution and fat supplement as well as explicit catheter care orders and monitoring guidelines (Figure 10–7). For active patients on long-term TPN, cycling the intravenous nutrition therapy over 8-16 hours at night allows freedom from the infusion pump during the remainder of the day.

C. Special TPN Solutions

The TPN solution may be concentrated for patients who require fluid restriction (eg, those with pulmonary and cardiac failure). One liter of concentrated TPN solution usually contains a combination of $D_{60}W$ or $D_{70}W$, 500 mL, and 10% or 15% amino acids, 500 mL, plus additives.

Patients in renal failure who cannot be dialyzed and who require fluid restriction should receive low-nitrogen TPN solution. Patients in renal failure who can undergo dialysis may receive the standard or high-nitrogen TPN formulations, with special attention directed toward minimizing potassium and phosphate intake.

COMPLICATIONS OF PARENTERAL NUTRITION

▶ PPN Therapy

Technical complications of PPN are few. The most common problem is maintaining adequate venous access due to frequent incidence of phlebitis. The PPN infusion catheter must be moved frequently to other sites; therefore, prolonged PPN is rarely possible. Infectious complications such as catheter site skin infections and septic phlebitis develop in 5% of patients.

▶ TPN Therapy

Complications resulting from parenteral nutrition can be broken down into those of a technical, infectious, and metabolic nature (Table 10–9). Many of the complications originate from the CVC, with more than 15% of patients developing some line-related complication. Other morbidity is attributable to line infection (typically bacterial) or metabolic abnormalities.

A. Technical Complications

The risks of patient injury while placing a CVC are directly related to surgeon experience with the procedure.

Arterial puncture (more common in internal jugular or femoral attempts) can occur in up to 10% of patients, while pneumothorax (predominantly during subclavian insertion) can develop in 2%-5%. The risk for injury increases dramatically after three failed insertion attempts at the same site.

Air embolism occurs when negative intrathoracic pressure draws air into a catheter or needle into a central vein. This is particularly serious in the presence of pulmonary-systemic shunts (eg, patients with a patent foramen ovale). It is characterized by sudden, severe respiratory distress, hypotension, and a cogwheel cardiac murmur. To reduce this risk, the patient should be placed in the Trendelenburg position (head down) during line insertion. When suspicion of air embolism is high, treatment involves placing the patient in the Durant position (Trendelenburg and left lateral decubitus) to direct the embolus to the apex of the right ventricle. Catheter-based aspiration can then be attempted.

The use of peripherally introduced central catheters (PICCs) allows peripherally initiated solutions to be delivered to the central venous system. They are well tolerated and easy to care for because of their location in an upper extremity. PICCs may be preferable to CVCs because of lower cost and fewer mechanical complications at placement.

B. Infectious Complications

Infection of the catheter exit site is frequently characterized by mild fever (37.5°-38°C), purulent discharge around the catheter, and erythema/tenderness of the surrounding skin. Late changes include induration of the skin and systemic sepsis. Local wound care and sterile dressing changes every 3 days can reduce site infection rates.

Primary line (catheter) infection can occur in up to 15% of patients with CVCs. Line infection should be strongly considered in any patient with a CVC who develops fever, new-onset glucose intolerance, leukocytosis, or positive blood cultures. There may be a slight increase in infectious risk with multilumen catheters. The use of antibiotic-impregnated catheters has been shown to significantly reduce nosocomial bloodstream infections. As noted previously, insertion in the subclavian vein reduces the risk of infection. The most common offending organisms are skin flora (*Staphylococcus aureus, Staphylococcus epidermidis*), although gram-negative rods can also colonize an indwelling catheter. Table 10–10 depicts one treatment algorithm for treating suspected CVC infections. With documented positive blood cultures or more than 15 colony-forming units on catheter cultures, the catheter should be removed and a line holiday attempted with peripheral access. Insertion of a new CVC can then be performed at a separate site once bacteremia has resolved. Antibiotics should be started empirically in patients with sepsis.

NUTRITION GUIDELINES FOR THE ADULT PATIENT

ADULT PARENTERAL NUTRITION (PN) GUIDELINES

Table 1: INDICATIONS FOR PARENTERAL NUTRITION:

A. Patient has failed enteral nutrition (EN) trial with appropriate tube placement (post-pyloric).

B. Enteral nutrition is contraindicated. Examples include patients with a paralytic ileus, mesenteric ischemia, small bowel obstruction, or GI fistula, except when enterat access can be placed distal to the fistula or the volume of fistula output (< 230 mL/day) justifies a trial of EN.

C. Wound healing would be impaired if PN is not started within 5-10 days postoperatively unable to eat or tolerate EN.

Table 2: BODY WEIGHT CALCULATIONS

Actual body weight (ABW) = pt weight (kg) IF GREATER THAN 125% OF IDEAL. WEIGHT SEE**

Ideal body weight (IBW)   male = 50 kg + (2.3 × # inches > 5 ft)   OR   48 kg + (2 7 × # inches > 5 ft)

female = 45 kg + (2.3 × # inches > 5 ft)

**Dosing weight (DW) = IBW + 0.25 (ABW – IBW)

Table 3:

A. DAILY CALORIC NEEDS

		CONVERSIONS FOR KCAL TO GRAMS
Maintenance-mild stress:	20-25 kcal/kg/day (15-20 NPC*kg/day)	3.4 kcal = 1 gm dextrose
Mild-moderate stress (routine surgery, minor infection):	26-30 kcal/kg/day (21-25 NPC*/kg/day)	10 kcal = 1 gm lipid
Moderate-severe stress (major surgery, sepsis).	31-35 kcal/kg/day (26-30 NPC*/kg/day)	
	*NPC = nonprotein calories	

B. *HARRIS-BENEDICT (HB) ESTIMATE OF BASAL CALORIES   STRESS FACTOR

			STRESS FACTOR
Male:	66 + 13.8 (weight in kg) + 5 (height in cm**) – 6.8 (age in year	Maintenance-mild stress :	1-1.2
Female:	655 + 9.6 (weight in kg) + 1.8 (height in cm**) – 4.7 (age in years)	Moderate stress :	1.3 -1.4
		Severe stress:	1.5

*HB × stress factor = total coloric need/day ** height in cm = inches × 2.54

Table 4: DAILY PROTEIN NEEDS

		CONVERSIONS FOR KCAL TO GRAMS OF PROTEIN
Maintenance-Mild	0.8-1.2 gm/kg/day	4 kcal = 1 gm amino acid
Moderate stress	1.3-1.5 gm/kg/day	
Severe stress	1.6-2 gm/kg/day	
Very high stress	> 2 gm/kg/day	

SUGGESTED LABORATORY TESTS

Baseline: Finger stick blood glucose q 4 hours with correction insulin as written: basic metabolic panel (BMP), magnesium, phosphorus, trigleycerides, hepatic function panel, & prealbumin.

Daily: BMP, magnesium & phosphorus until stabilized, then as clinically indicated.

Weekly: Prealbumin. Triglycerides and hepatic function panel (if clinically indicated).

CALCULATION OF VOLUME OF MAXIMALLY CONCENTRATED PN

1. Amino acid (AA): _____ gm protein/day × 10mL/gm AA =_____ mL 10% AA solution

2. Carbohydrate (CHO): _____ gm/day × 1.43mL/gm = _____ mL 70% dextrose solution

3. Lipid: _____gm/day × 10 kcal/gm = _____ + 2kcal/mL = _____ mL 20% lipids

4. Maximally concentrated volume = _____ mL 10% AA + _____ mL 70% dextrose + _____ mL 20%
    (from 1 above)   (from 2 above)   (from 3 above)

    lipids + 150 mL for additives = _____ mL/day

5. Approximate infusion rate = _____ mL/day + 24 hr/day = _____ mL/hr

▲ **Figure 10–7.** TPN guidelines.

**CONTENT OF STANDARD
MULTIPLE VITAMINS (per 10 mL):**

Vitamin A	3300 international units
Vitamin D	200 international units
Vitamin E	10 international units
Vitamin B_1 (thiamine)	6 mg
Vitamin B_2	3.6 mg
Vitamin B_3	40 mg
Vitamin B_5	15 mg
Vitamin B_6 (pyridoxine HCl)	6 mg
Vitamin B_{12}	5 micrograms
Vitamin C (ascorbic acid)	200 mg
Biotin	60 micrograms
Folic acid	600 micrograms
Vitamin K	150 micrograms

**CONTENT OF STANDARD
TRACE ELEMENTS (per 1 mL):**

Chromium	10 micrograms
Copper	1 mg
Manganese	0.5 mg
Selenium	60 micrograms
Zinc	5 mg

▲ **Figure 10–7.** (Continued)

C. Metabolic Complications

The refeeding syndrome was first described in prisoners freed from concentration camps after World War II. Similar pathophysiology may develop when initiating TPN in patients with severe malnutrition and weight loss (> 30% of their usual weight). In starvation, energy is derived principally from fat metabolism. TPN results in a shift from fat to glucose as the predominant fuel, and rapid anabolism increases the production of phosphorylated intermediates of glycolysis. These intermediates trap phosphate, producing profound hypophosphatemia. Hypokalemia and hypomagnesemia also occur. The lack of phosphate and potassium lead to a relative adenosine triphosphate (ATP) deficiency, resulting in the insidious onset of respiratory failure and reduced cardiac stroke volume. Because of these risks, the rate of TPN administration in a severely malnourished patient should be slowly increased over several days. Twice-daily monitoring of electrolytes is also indicated, with repletion as appropriate.

Hepatic dysfunction is a common manifestation of long-term parenteral nutrition support. The exact etiology is unclear; however, in part it is related to the initial bypassing of the portal circulation when providing intravenous nutrition. Severe hepatic steatosis may progress to cirrhosis. Acalculous cholecystitis can also occur in these patients, likely from biliary stasis and lack of gallbladder contraction. Patients on TPN need weekly liver function tests and lipid panels.

▶ Home Nutrition Support

Patients requiring home nutrition support (HNS) present clinical challenges different from those in an acute care setting. Route of enteral or parenteral administration must be based on length of therapy, frequency of use, and caregiver/patient ability. Regular physical examinations and frequent laboratory monitoring (Figure 10–8) should continue as long as patients remain on HNS therapy. Home care services must be established prior to discharge and are vital to the success of these patients.

For patients requiring home parenteral nutrition, weekly laboratory monitoring continues until electrolytes stabilize. Once stable, laboratory values can often be checked on a monthly basis, and changes can be made to the TPN formula as needed. Electrolyte and hepatic enzymes must be followed to monitor for metabolic derangements and end-organ damage. Parenteral nutrition–associated liver disease is the most devastating complication of long-term parenteral nutrition therapy. Early clinical intervention with a combination of nutritional, medical, hormonal, and surgical therapies is potentially effective in preventing liver disease progression. However, as progression is frequently subtle, it is often not recognized until liver injury is irreversible. Although parenteral nutrition–associated liver failure is hypothesized to be multifactorial in origin, the etiology is poorly understood. When end-stage liver disease (ESLD) develops in these patients, multiorgan transplantation (liver and small bowel) is generally required.

DIETS

▶ Optimal Diet

The optimal diet should have the following distribution of energy sources: carbohydrate 55%-60%, fat 30%, and protein 10%-15%. Refined sugar should constitute less than 15% of dietary energy and saturated fats no more than 10%, the latter balanced by 10% monounsaturated and 10% polyunsaturated fats. Cholesterol intake should be limited to about 300 mg/d (one egg yolk contains 250 mg of cholesterol). The amount of salt in the average American diet, 10-18 g daily, far exceeds the recommended 3 g/d. For Western societies to meet the criteria for an optimal diet, consumption of fat must decrease (from 40%) and consumption of complex

Table 10–9. Complications of nutritional therapy.

Enteral Nutrition	Parenteral Nutrition
Technical	**Technical**
Abscess of nasal septum	Air embolus
Acute sinusitis	Arterial laceration
Aspiration pneumonitis	Arteriovenous fistula
Esophagitis (ulceration/stenosis)	Brachial plexus injury
Gastrointestinal perforation	Cardiac perforation
Hemorrhage (local erosion)	Catheter embolism
Hoarseness	Catheter malposition
Intestinal obstruction	Hemothorax
Intracranial passage	Pneumothorax
Knotting/clogging of tube	Subclavian vein thrombosis
Nasal/alar erosions	Thoracic duct injury
Otitis media	Thromboembolism
Pneumatosis intestinalis	Venous laceration
Skin excoriation	
Tracheoesophageal fistula	
Tube dislodgement	
Variceal rupture	
Functional	**Infectious**
Abdominal distention	Catheter-based bacteremia
Constipation	Catheter colonization
Diarrhea	Exit-site infection/cellulites
Nausea/vomiting	
Metabolic	**Metabolic**
Dehydration	Azotemia
Hypercalcemia	Essential fatty acid deficiency
Hyperglycemia	Fluid overload
Hyperkalemia	Hyperchloremic metabolic acidosis
Hypermagnesemia	Hypercalcemia
Hypernatremia	Hyperglycemia
Hyperphosphatemia	Hyperkalemia
Hypocalcemia	Hypermagnesemia
Hypokalemia	Hypernatremia
Hypomagnesemia	Hyperphosphatemia
Hyponatremia	Hypocalcemia
Hypophosphatemia	Hypokalemia
Hypozincemia	Hypomagnesemia
Overhydration	Hyponatremia
Vitamin deficiency	Hypophosphatemia
	Intrinsic liver disease
	Metabolic bone disease
	Trace element deficiency
	Ventilatory failure
	Vitamin deficiency

carbohydrate should increase. Meat is presently overemphasized as a protein source, at the expense of grain, legumes, and nuts. Diets that include substantial fish intake have been associated with a decrease in mortality from cardiovascular disease and are attributed to high concentrations of ω-3 fatty acids, principally eicosapentaenoic and docosahexaenoic acids.

Many adults, particularly those who do not drink milk, consume inadequate amounts of calcium. In women this may result in calcium deficiency and skeletal calcium depletion, predisposing women to osteoporosis and axial bony fractures. "Fiber" is the generic term for a chemically complex group of indigestible carbohydrate polymers, including cellulose, hemicellulose, lignins, pectins, gums, and mucilages. The amount of fiber in Western diets averages 25 g/d, but some people ingest as little as 10 g daily. Those who consume low-fiber diets are more likely to develop chronic constipation, appendicitis, diverticular disease, and possibly diabetes mellitus and colonic neoplasms. Bran cereals and bread, fruit, potatoes, rice, and leafy vegetables are rich sources of fiber.

▶ Regular Diets

Many concepts regarding diets are archaic and based on currently unaccepted views of illness. For example, the utility of a low-residue diet in diverticular disease is questionable. The "progressive diet," designed for postoperative feeding and consisting of a clear liquid (high in sodium), then a full liquid (high in sucrose), then a regular diet, is based on outmoded concepts. When peristalsis returns after operation, as evidenced by bowel sounds and ability to tolerate water, most patients are able to ingest a regular diet. Regular diets have an unrestricted spectrum of foods and are most attractive to the patient. An average regular hospital diet for 1 day contains 95-110 g of protein, with a total caloric content of 1800-2100 kcal. This composition reflects the nutritional needs of healthy persons of average height and weight and will not meet the increased demands imposed by malnutrition or disease.

▶ Lactose Intolerance & Lactose-Free Diets

A lactose-free diet is indicated for patients who have symptoms such as diarrhea, bloating, or flatulence after the ingestion of milk or milk products. Lactose intolerance is genetically determined and occurs in 5%-10% of European Caucasians, 60% of Ashkenazi Jews, and 70% of African Americans. Subclinical lactose intolerance may become unmasked following surgery on gastrointestinal tract (eg, gastrectomy). Similarly, avoidance of lactose-containing products is often beneficial advice for patients with Crohn disease, ulcerative colitis, and AIDS. The efficiency of lactose digestion and absorption can be measured by giving 100 g of oral lactose, then measuring the blood glucose concentration at 30-minute intervals over 2 hours.

Table 10–10. Complications of TPN.

Complication	Treatment
Catheter sepsis	**Algorithms:**
Incidence: 　Single-lumen catheter: 3.5% 　Triple-lumen catheter: 10%	*Negative blood cultures and no cardiovascular signs of sepsis:* (1) Aspirate a blood specimen via the TPN catheter and peripherally for bacterial and fungal culture and then sterilely exchange the preexisting TPN catheter for a new catheter over a guidewire; submit the previous catheter tip for bacterial and fungal culture and colony count; and continue the TPN infusion.
Diagnosis: 　• Unexplained hyperglycemia (> 160 mg/dL) 　• "Plateau" temperature elevation (> 38°C) for several hours or days. (***Note:*** *An isolated spike or "picket fence" temperature pattern is usually not indicative of an infected catheter.*) 　• Leukocytosis (> 10,000/μL) 　• Exclusion of other potential sources of infection, 　　*or* 　• A positive blood culture (> 15 colony count) aspirated via the TPN catheter or obtained peripherally, 　　*or* 　• Catheter site induration, erythema, or purulent drainage.	*then* (2) Monitor the patient's temperature closely. If the patient defervesces, no further therapy is necessary. If the fever continues or recurs, remove the catheter and insert a new one on the contralateral side and continue the TPN infusion. *Positive blood culture or cardiovascular signs of sepsis:* (1) Aspirate a blood specimen via the TPN catheter and peripherally for bacterial and fungal culture. Then remove the catheter immediately, and submit the catheter tip for bacterial and fungal culture and colony count. 　　*then* (2) Insert a new TPN infusion catheter on the contralateral side and continue the TPN infusion. 　　*then* (3) Initiate appropriate antibiotic therapy.
Hyperglycemia (> 160 mg/dL)	**Algorithms:** (1) Maintain the current TPN infusion rate. If the patient is critically ill, initiate intravenous regular insulin infusion. Otherwise initiate a sliding scale with regular insulin and add regular insulin in 10-unit increments to the TPN solution until the serum glucose is maintained at ≤ 140 mg/dL. (***Note:*** *The maximum allowable insulin dosage per liter of TPN is 10 units.*) 　　*then* (2) If blood glucose levels remain elevated, consider decreasing the dextrose concentration (eg, decrease the grams of carbohydrate) to 60.80% of the estimated needs until blood glucose levels are within goal range. In addition, either maintain regular insulin infusion or continue to adjust the amount of insulin in the TPN bag based on the amount taken via sliding scale. One-half to two-thirds of the previous day's regular insulin requirements can be added to the TPN bag. 　　*then* (3) Once goal blood glucose achieved, restart the original TPN solution as in (1) above with adequate insulin to maintain goal blood glucose range.
Hypoglycemia (< 65 mg/dL)	May occur with the sudden discontinuance of TPN infusion. If the TPN infusion administered to either an NPO patient or a patient consuming inadequate oral calories is suddenly discontinued, immediately begin an infusion of D_{10} NS at the previous TPN infusion rate via either the TPN catheter or a peripheral IV to prevent rebound hypoglycemia.
Hypernatremia (> 145 meq/L)	Determine the cause. Hypernatremia secondary to dehydration is treated by administering additional "free water" and providing only the daily maintenance sodium requirements (90-150 meq/L) via the TPN infusion. Hypernatremia secondary to increased sodium intake is treated by reducing or deleting sodium from the TPN solution until the serum sodium ≤ 145 meq/L.
Hyponatremia (< 135 meq/L)	Determine the cause. Hyponatremia secondary to dilution is treated by fluid restriction and by providing only the daily maintenance sodium requirements (90-150 meq/L). Hyponatremia secondary to inadequate sodium intake is treated by increasing the sodium content of the TPN solution until the serum sodium is ≥ 135 meq/L. (***Note:*** *The maximum sodium content per liter of TPN should not exceed 154 meq.*)

(continued)

Table 10–10. Complications of TPN. (*Continued*)

Complication	Treatment
Hyperkalemia (> 5 meq/L)	Immediately discontinue the current TPN infusion containing potassium and begin an infusion of $D_{10}NS$ at the previous TPN infusion rate. Then reorder a new TPN solution without potassium and continue to delete potassium from the TPN solution until the serum potassium ≤ 5 meq/L.
Hypokalemia (< 3.5 meq/L)	A TPN solution should not be utilized for the primary treatment of hypokalemia. The potassium content per liter of TPN solution should not exceed 40 meq. If additional potassium is necessary, it should be administered via another route, eg, IV interrupts.
Hyperphosphatemia (> 4.5 mg/dL)	Immediately discontinue the present phosphate-containing TPN infusion and begin an infusion of $D_{10}NS$ at the previous infusion rate. Then reorder a new TPN solution without phosphate and continue to delete phosphate from the TPN solution until the serum phosphate is ≤ 4.5 mg/dL.
Hypophosphatemia (< 2.5 mg/dL)	Increase the phosphate content of the TPN solution to a maximum of 20 mmol/L. (***Note:*** *The total daily phosphate dosage should not exceed 60 mmol.*) If severe hypophosphatemia exists, carbohydrate infusion or delivery should be restricted.
Hypermagnesemia (> 3 mg/dL)	Immediately discontinue the present magnesium-containing TPN infusion and begin an infusion of $D_{10}NS$ at the previous infusion rate.
Hypomagnesemia (< 1.6 mg/dL)	Increase the magnesium content of the TPN solution to a maximum of 12 meq/L. (***Note:*** *The total daily dosage of magnesium should not exceed 36 meq.*)
Hypercalcemia (> 10.5 mg/dL)	Immediately discontinue the present calcium-containing TPN infusion and begin an infusion of $D_{10}NS$ at the previous TPN infusion rate. Then reorder a new TPN solution without calcium and continue to delete calcium from the TPN dilution until the serum calcium is ≤ 10.5 mg/dL.
Hypocalcemia (< 8.5 mg/dL)	Increase the calcium content of the TPN solution to a maximum of 9 meq/L. (***Note:*** *The total daily calcium dosage should not exceed 27 meq.*)
High serum zinc (> 150 µg/L)	Discontinue the trace metal supplement (Multitrace 5 mL) in the TPN solution until the serum zinc is ≤ 150 µg/L.
Low serum zinc (< 55 µg/dL)	Add elemental zinc 2-5 mg daily to 1 L of TPN solution only until the serum zinc is ≥ 55 µg/dL. (***Note:*** *The elemental zinc is added in addition to the daily supplement.*)
High serum copper (> 140 µg/dL)	Discontinue the trace metal supplement in the TPN solution until the serum copper is ≤ 140 µg/dL.
Low serum copper (< 70 µg/dL)	Add elemental copper 2-5 mg daily to 1 L of TPN solution only until the serum copper is ≥ 70 µg/dL. (***Note:*** *The elemental copper is added in addition to the daily Multitrace 5 mL.*)
Hyperchloremic metabolic acidosis (CO_2 < 22 mmol/L and Cl^- > 110 meq/L)	Reduce the chloride intake by administering the Na^+ and K^+ in the acetate form as either sodium or potassium acetate (or both) until the acidosis resolves (serum CO_2 ≥ 22 mmol/L) and the serum chloride level returns to normal (< 110 meq/L).

Patients with lactose intolerance exhibit a rise in blood glucose of 20 mg/dL or less. A lactose-free diet may be deficient in calcium, vitamin D, and riboflavin.

▶ Postgastric Bypass Diet

The popularity of gastric bypass surgery for weight loss continues to increase. The diet changes that must occur to ensure safe and appropriate weight loss are quite specific after surgery. Immediately after surgery, only small amounts of liquids (eg, 30 mL q3h) should be consumed. After tolerance of liquids is established, pureed foods should be consumed for the 4 weeks after surgery. Food should be consumed as very small meals and snacks throughout the day. Choosing a variety of foods, avoiding concentrated sweets, and consuming adequate protein are essential to the success of these patients. Protein supplements are often required to ensure adequate protein consumption postoperatively. Particularly with gastric bypass procedures, patients are prone to deficiencies of the fat-soluble vitamins (A, D, E, and K), calcium, iron, vitamin B_{12}, and folate necessitating the indefinite supplementation of daily multivitamins.

Routine monitoring:

☐ Basic metabolic panel, Magnesium, and Phosphorus daily   Start date:_____   End date:_____

☐ Basic metabolic panel, Magnesium, Phosphorus and weight
     ☐ Weekly   ☐ Bimonthly ☐ Monthly ☐ Quarterly   Start date: _____

☐ Triglyceride
     ☐ Weekly   ☐ Monthly   ☐ Quarterly   Start date: _____

☐ Prealbumin
     ☐ Weekly   ☐ Monthly   ☐ Quarterly   Start date: _____

☐ CBS, AST, ALT, and total Bilirubin
     ☐ Weekly   ☐ Monthly   ☐ Quarterly   Start date: _____

☐ PT/INR, PTT if on Wartarin (Coumadin ®) or multi-vitamin contains Vitamin K
     ☐ Weekly   ☐ Monthly   ☐ Quarterly   Start date: _____

▲ **Figure 10–8.** Laboratory monitoring form for home nutrition support (HNS).

DISEASE-SPECIFIC NUTRITION SUPPORT

▶ Burns

Thermal injury has a tremendous impact on metabolism because of prolonged, intense neuroendocrine stimulation. Extensive burns can double or triple the REE and urinary nitrogen losses, producing a nitrogen loss of 20-25 g/m² TBSA/d. If left unattended, lethal cachexia becomes imminent in less than 30 days. The increase in metabolic demands following thermal injury is proportional to the extent of ungrafted body surface. The principal mediators of burn hypermetabolism are catecholamines, corticosteroids, and inflammatory cytokines, which return to baseline only after skin coverage is complete. Decreasing the intensity of neuroendocrine stimulation by providing adequate analgesia and a thermoneutral environment lowers the accelerated metabolic rate and helps to decrease catabolic protein loss until the burned surface can be grafted. Burned patients are prone to infection, and the cytokines activated by sepsis further augment catabolism.

Because infection often complicates the clinical course of patients with burn injury, and infectious complications are more likely with parenteral nutrition, the enteral route of feeding is preferred whenever tolerated. Enteral feeding may be started within the first 6-12 hours post burn to attenuate the hypermetabolic response and improve postburn survival. Gastric ileus can be avoided through the use of a nasojejunal tube.

Patients with burns have increased caloric requirements. In addition to estimated maintenance needs (females, 22 kcal/kg/d; males, 25 kcal/kg/d), these patients require an additional 40 kcal per percentage point of burned total body surface area (TBSA). A 70-kg man with 40% TBSA burns would require 48 kcal/kg/d. Protein requirements are also markedly increased from the normal 0.8 g/kg/d to approximately 1.5-2.5 g/kg/d in severely burned patients. Of course, these are initial estimates, and periodic reassessment of nutritional status (eg, prealbumin levels, nitrogen balance) is required in these patients. During the hypermetabolic phase of burn injury (0-14 days), the ability to metabolize fat is restricted, so a diet that derives calories primarily from carbohydrate is preferable. Following the hypermetabolic phase, the metabolism of fat becomes normal. The burn patient should also be given supplemental arginine, nucleotides, and ω-3 polyunsaturated fat to stimulate and maintain immunocompetence.

▶ Diabetes

Glucose intolerance often complicates nutritional supplementation, particularly with parenteral administration. Complications associated with TPN administration occur more frequently during prolonged hyperglycemia. Unopposed glycosuria may lead to osmotic diuresis, loss of electrolytes in the urine, and possibly nonketotic coma. Significant controversy exists, but the preponderance of available evidence suggests that intensive insulin therapy, as compared with standard therapy, does not provide an overall survival benefit, but instead may increase mortality, and is associated with a higher incidence of hypoglycemia. Factors that may aggravate hyperglycemia include the use of corticosteroids, certain vasopressors (eg, epinephrine), preexisting diabetes mellitus, and occult infection.

Maintaining normoglycemia in injured or postoperative patients may be challenging. Serial serum glucose levels should be monitored regularly. If hyperglycemia does not occur, these measurements can be obtained less frequently once the nutritional goal is reached. Patients may require subcutaneous insulin administered on a sliding scale or continuous intravenous insulin infusions to control their hyperglycemia. For patients who do not require an insulin infusion, the previous day's insulin total from a sliding scale may be determined and half to two-thirds of that amount added to the next TPN order to provide a more uniform administration.

▶ Cancer

Cancer is the second leading cause of death in the United States, and over two-thirds of patients with cancer will develop nutritional depletion and weight loss at some time during the course of the illness. Malnutrition and its sequelae are the direct cause of death in 20% of these patients. Weight loss is an ominous presenting sign in many malignancies. Furthermore, antineoplastic treatments, such as chemotherapy, radiation therapy, or operative extirpation, can worsen preexisting malnutrition. Cancer cachexia manifests as progressive involuntary weight loss, fatigue, anemia, wasting, and tissue depletion. It may occur at any stage of the disease. Nutrition support has become an essential adjunct in caring for the cancer patient.

Many studies have evaluated the effectiveness of nutrition support in patients with cancer, with varying results. Increasing efforts have been directed toward the use of enteral rather than parenteral nutrition because it is simpler, presumably safer, and less costly. Nutritional supplementation in cancer patients *may* reduce infectious complications or perioperative morbidity, but convincing evidence of improvement in overall survival is lacking.

Patients with cancer may have altered energy expenditure and abnormalities of protein and carbohydrate metabolism. REE increases by 20%-30% in certain malignant tumors. The increases in REE can occur even in patients with extreme cachexia in whom a similar degree of uncomplicated starvation would produce profound decreases in REE. Changes in carbohydrate metabolism consist of impaired glucose tolerance, elevated glucose turnover rates, and enhanced Cori cycle activity. Owing to the high rate of anaerobic glucose metabolism in neoplastic tissue, patients with extensive tumors are susceptible to lactic acidosis when given large glucose loads during TPN. These patients also exhibit increased lipolysis, elevated FFA and glycerol turnover, and hyperlipidemia.

Patients with cancer avidly retain nitrogen despite losses in most lean tissue. Animal carcass analysis has shown that the retained nitrogen resides in the tumor, which behaves as a nitrogen trap. Synthesis, catabolism, and turnover of body protein are all increased, but the change in catabolism is greatest.

The utility of enteral supplementation with immune-enhancing agents is unclear. These substances include arginine, glutamine, essential fatty acids, RNA, and BCAAs. Several studies have attempted to examine outcomes in patients with cancer who are fed with enteral formulas supplemented with immune-enhancing agents, compared to routine enteral feeding alone. The findings were summarized by Zhang and coworkers. Meta-analysis of 19 studies with a total of 2231 cancer patients demonstrated a significant decrease in overall postoperative infection complication risk, noninfection complication risk, and hospital stay when perioperative immunonutrition was compared to standard diet. Exactly which elements confer these benefits remains unknown.

▶ Renal Failure

Whether nutritional support improves the outcome from acute renal failure is difficult to determine because of the metabolic complexities of the disease. Patients with acute renal failure may have normal or increased metabolic rates. Renal failure precipitated by x-ray contrast agents, antibiotics, aortic or cardiac surgery, or periods of hypotension is associated with a normal or slightly elevated REE and a moderately negative nitrogen balance (4-8 g/d). When renal failure follows severe trauma, rhabdomyolysis, or sepsis, the REE may be markedly increased and the nitrogen balance sharply negative (15-25 g/d). When dialysis is frequent, losses into the dialysate of amino acids, vitamins, glucose, trace metals, and lipotrophic factors can be substantial.

Patients in renal failure (serum creatinine over 2 mg/dL) with a normal metabolic rate who cannot undergo dialysis should receive a concentrated (minimal volume) enteral or parenteral diet containing protein, fat, dextrose, and limited amounts of sodium, potassium, magnesium, and phosphate.

▶ Hepatic Failure

Most patients with hepatic failure present with acute decompensation superimposed on chronic hepatic insufficiency. Typically, a history of poor dietary intake contributes to the chronic depletion of protein, vitamins, and trace elements. Water-soluble vitamins, including folate, ascorbic acid, niacin, thiamin, and riboflavin, are especially likely to be deficient. Fat-soluble vitamin deficiency may be a result of malabsorption due to bile acid insufficiency (vitamins A, D, K, and E), deficient storage (vitamin A), inefficient utilization (vitamin K), or failure of conversion to active metabolites (vitamin D). Hepatic iron stores may be depleted either from poor intake or as a result of gastrointestinal blood loss. Total body zinc is decreased owing to the above factors plus increased urinary excretion.

The use of BCAA-enriched amino acid formulations for TPN in patients with liver disease is controversial because the results of controlled trials are inconclusive. The efficacy of BCAA-enriched amino acid formulations for TPN in patients with hepatic encephalopathy has been studied in numerous controlled trials that had contradicting results. Meta-analysis of these studies demonstrated an improvement in mental state by the BCAA-enriched solutions, however there was no definite benefit in survival.

Therefore, patients with hepatic failure should receive a concentrated enteral or parenteral diet with reduced carbohydrate content, a combination of EFAs and other lipids, a standard mixture of amino acids, and limited amounts of sodium and potassium.

Cardiopulmonary Disease

Malnutrition is associated with myocardial dysfunction, particularly in the late stages, and fatal cardiac failure can develop in extreme cachexia. Cardiac muscle uses FAAs and BCAAs as preferred metabolic fuels instead of glucose. During starvation, the heart rate slows, cardiac size decreases, and the stroke volume and cardiac output decrease. As starvation progresses, cardiac failure ensues, along with chamber enlargement and anasarca.

The profound nutritional depletion that may accompany chronic heart failure, particularly in valvular disease, results from anorexia of chronic disease, passive congestion of the liver, malabsorption due to venous engorgement of the small bowel mucosa, and enhanced peripheral proteolysis due to chronic neuroendocrine secretion. Attempts at aggressive nutritional repletion in patients with cardiac cachexia have produced inconclusive results. Concentrated dextrose and amino acid preparations should be used to avoid fluid overload. Nitrogen balance should be measured to ensure adequate nitrogen intake. Lipid emulsions must be administered cautiously because they can produce myocardial ischemia and negative inotropy. Feeding these patients with either enteral or parenteral nutrition should be undertaken cautiously to avoid refeeding syndrome and hypophosphatemia.

Patients with severe chronic obstructive pulmonary disease may have difficulty weaning from the ventilator if they are overfed. This relates to the RQ, a measure of oxygen consumption and carbon dioxide production by the body in metabolism. An RQ of 1 reflects pure carbohydrate utilization, while an RQ greater than 1 occurs during lipogenesis (energy storage). Although normal lungs can tolerate increased CO_2 production (RQ > 1) without adversely affecting respiration, patients with chronic obstructive pulmonary disease may experience CO_2 retention and inability to wean. The treatment is to increase the percentage of calories delivered as lipid and to avoid overfeeding at all costs.

Disease of the Gastrointestinal Tract

Benign gastrointestinal disease (eg, inflammatory bowel disease, fistula, pancreatitis) often leads to nutritional problems due to intestinal obstruction, malabsorption, or anorexia. Chronic involvement of the ileum in inflammatory bowel disease produces malabsorption of fat- and water-soluble vitamins, calcium and magnesium, anions (phosphate), and the trace elements iron, zinc, chromium, and selenium. Protein-losing enteropathy, accentuated by

transmural destruction of lymphatics, can add to protein depletion. Treatment with sulfasalazine can produce folate deficiency, and glucocorticoid administration may accelerate breakdown of lean tissue and enhance glucose intolerance owing to stimulation of gluconeogenesis. Patients with inflammatory bowel disease who require elective surgery should be evaluated for malnutrition preoperatively.

Patients with gastrointestinal fistulas can develop electrolyte, protein, fat, vitamin, and trace metal deficiencies; dehydration; and acid-base imbalance. Aggressive fluid replacement is often needed. Patients with fistulas often require nutritional support. The choice of feeding route or formula will depend on the level and length of dysfunctional bowel. Patients with proximal enterocutaneous fistulas (from the stomach to the mid-ileum) should receive TPN with no oral intake. Patients with low fistulas should receive TPN initially, but after infection is brought under control, they can often be switched to an enteral formula or even a low-residue diet.

Pancreatitis

The concept of pancreatic rest has evolved over the recent years. Ranson criteria can serve as a rough estimate of the need for nutritional support. Patients with acute pancreatitis who present with three or fewer Ranson criteria should be treated with fluid replacement, pain control, and brief bowel rest. Most of these patients can rapidly resume an oral diet and do not benefit from TPN. Those with more than three Ranson criteria should receive nutritional support. Recent data documents the successful use of enteral diets, particularly elemental products via jejunal access, avoiding TPN if feasible.

Short Bowel Syndrome

Inadequate intestinal absorptive surface leads to malabsorption, excessive water loss, electrolyte derangements, and malnutrition. The absorptive capacity of the small intestine is highly redundant, and resection of up to half its functional length is reasonably well tolerated. Short bowel syndrome typically occurs when less than 200 cm of anatomic small bowel remain, although the presence of the ileocecal valve may reduce this length to 150 cm. However, short bowel syndrome also may occur from functional abnormalities of the small bowel resulting from severe inflammation or motility disorder. The optimal nutritional therapy for a patient with short bowel syndrome must be tailored individually and depends upon the underlying disease process and the remaining anatomy. Following resection, the remaining bowel undergoes long-term adaptation, with observed increases in villous height, luminal diameter, and mucosal thickness. The estimated minimum length of small bowel required for adult patients to become independent of TPN is 120 cm.

Adaptation to short gut occurs over time, and initial management should be directed at avoiding electrolyte imbalance and dehydration while providing daily caloric requirements through TPN. Some patients may eventually supplement TPN with oral intake. In these patients, dietary management includes consuming frequent small meals, avoiding hyperosmolar foods, restricting fat intake, and limiting consumption of foods high in oxalate (precipitates nephrolithiasis).

▶ AIDS

Patients with AIDS frequently develop protein-calorie malnutrition and weight loss. Many factors contribute to deficiencies of electrolytes (sodium and potassium), trace metals (copper, zinc, and selenium), and vitamins (A, C, E, pyridoxine, and folate). Enteropathy may impair fluid and nutrient absorption and produce a voluminous, life-threatening diarrhea. Dehydration and further immune dysfunction occur as a consequence of refractory diarrhea.

Malnourished AIDS patients require a daily intake of 35-40 kcal and 2.0-2.5 g protein. Those with normal gut function should be given a high-protein, high-calorie, low-fat, lactose-free oral diet. Patients with compromised gut function require an enteral (amino acid or polypeptide) or parenteral nutrition.

▶ Solid Organ Transplant Recipients

Patients who have undergone organ transplantation present unique issues in relation to nutritional management due to both the preexisting disease state and the medications taken to prevent graft rejection. During the acute posttransplant phase, adequate nutrition is required to help prevent infection, promote wound healing, support metabolic demands, replenish lost stores, and mediate the immune response. Organ transplantation complications, including rejection, infection, wound healing, renal insufficiency, hyperglycemia, and surgical complications, require specific nutritional requirements and therapies.

Obesity is associated with both decreased patient survival and decreased graft survival, in part due to a greater incidence of surgical, metabolic, and cardiovascular complications. Patients with BMI greater than 30 kg/m^2 show a higher incidence of steroid-induced posttransplant diabetes mellitus. The first 6 weeks following transplantation is characterized by increased nutritional demands due to a combination of surgical metabolic stress and high doses of immunosuppressive medications. Daily protein intake recommendation in the immediate posttransplant phase, as well as during acute rejection episodes, is 1.5 g/kg actual body weight.

Long-term immunosuppression is associated with protein hypercatabolism, obesity, dyslipidemia, glucose intolerance, hypertension, hyperkalemia, and alteration of vitamin D metabolism. Approximately 60% of renal recipients develop dyslipidemia posttransplant. Alterations in lipid metabolism may be associated with corticosteroids, cyclosporine, thiazide diuretics, or beta-blockers, as well as with renal insufficiency, nephrotic syndrome, insulin resistance, or obesity. There is evidence that abnormal lipoprotein levels lead to glomerulosclerosis, renal disease progression, and even potential graft failure.

Dietary salt restriction is recommended in transplant patients, as salt intake may play a role in cyclosporine-induced hypertension caused by sodium retention. Sodium intake is recommended not to exceed 3 g/d. Cyclosporine is associated with hypomagnesemia and hyperkalemia, especially during the immediate posttransplant phase when the dosage is high. Additionally, antihypertensive treatment with beta-blocker agents or with angiotensin-converting enzyme (ACE) inhibitors may exacerbate hyperkalemia. Calcium, phosphorus, and vitamin D metabolism are influenced by prolonged therapy with steroids leading to osteopenia and osteonecrosis. The daily recommendation for dietary calcium is 800-1500 mg, and the recommended intake of phosphorus is 1200-1500 mg/d. Some patients may also require supplementation of active vitamin D. Patients on a low-protein diet often need multivitamin supplements. During the first year, the major nutritional goal is to treat preexisting malnutrition and prevent excessive weight gain.

▶ Major Trauma

In severely injured patients, metabolic changes must be acknowledged early and monitored during the posttraumatic phase. Severe trauma induces alteration of metabolic pathways and activation of the immune system. Depending on the severity of the initial injury, catabolic changes in posttraumatic metabolism can last from several days to weeks. The posttraumatic metabolic changes include hypermetabolism with increased energy expenditure, enhanced protein catabolism, insulin resistance associated with hyperglycemia, failure to tolerate glucose load, and high plasma insulin levels ("traumatic diabetes"). As a general rule, the metabolic demands of the patient can increase by 1.3-1.5 times the normal requirements.

After the state of traumatic-hemorrhagic shock has been compensated for, metabolic changes are characterized by an increased metabolic turnover, activation of the immune system, and induction of the hepatic acute-phase response. This results in increased consumption of energy and oxygen. In addition to the acute hypermetabolic state, the systemic inflammatory cascade is initiated, with the release of proinflammatory cytokines and activation of the complement system. Bacterial translocation from the gut may further aggravate these metabolic sequelae and inflammatory response.

Many severely injured patients require inotropic support, and vasoactive drugs promote catabolism by reducing serum levels of anabolic hormones. In contrast, endogenous catecholamines, cortisol, and glucagon levels are elevated after trauma, leading to increased energy substrate mobilization. Proteinolysis of skeletal muscle and glycolysis are increased to provide the substrates for hepatic gluconeogenesis and biosynthesis of acute-phase proteins. The equilibrium is shifted toward supporting the immune response and wound healing at the cost of enhanced proteinolysis of skeletal muscle. In addition, stimulation of the neuroendocrine axis through stress, pain, inflammation, and shock increases the caloric turnover significantly above baseline. This leads to increased serum levels of catabolic hormones, such as cortisol, glucagon, and catecholamines, and decreased levels of insulin.

Appropriate immunonutrition should be started in the ICU, preferably by enteral route, in order to counteract the effects of the hypermetabolic state after major trauma. Without absolute contraindications, guidelines clearly favor the concept of early enteral nutrition within 24-48 hours after admission in the ICU. It is important not to overfeed critically injured patients with calories, since this may contribute to adverse outcomes. Early overfeeding of severely injured patients leads to an increase in oxygen consumption, carbon dioxide production, lipogenesis, and hyperglycemia and contributes to secondary immune suppression.

Obese patients are particularly susceptible to the adverse effects of overfeeding. Current feeding recommendations for morbidly obese ICU patients are a high protein, hypocaloric diet. Caloric provision should approximate 60%-70% of caloric requirements determined by indirect calorimetry or other predictive equation. A simplistic weight-based approach approximates 22-25 kcal and 2-2.5 g of protein per kg ideal body weight per day.

▶ References

Almeida AI et al: Nutritional risk screening in surgery: valid, feasible, easy! *Clin Nutr.* 2012;31(2):206-211.

Anthony PS et al: Nutrition screening tools for hospitalized patients. *Nutr Clin Pract.* 2008;23(4):373-382.

Barlow R et al: Prospective multicenter randomized controlled trial of early enteral nutrition for patients undergoing major upper gastrointestinal surgical resection. *Clin Nutr.* 2011;30(5): 560-566.

Biesalski HK et al: Water, electrolytes, vitamins and trace elements: guidelines on parenteral nutrition, Chapter 7. *Ger Med Sci.* 2009;7:Doc21.

Bines JE. Intestinal failure: a new era in clinical management. *J Gastroenterol Hepatol.* 2009;24(Suppl 3):S86-92.

Braga M et al: ESPEN guidelines on parenteral nutrition: surgery. *Clin Nutr.* 2009;28(4):378-386.

Chen YY et al: Nutrition support in surgical patients with colorectal cancer. *World J Gastroenterol.* 2011;17(13):1779-1786.

Dhaliwal R et al: Guidelines, guidelines, guidelines: what are we to do with all of these North American guidelines? *JPEN J Parenter Enteral Nutr.* 2010;34(6):625-643.

Duggal S et al: HIV and malnutrition: effects on immune system. *Clin Dev Immunol.* 2012;2012:784740.

Elke G et al: Current practice in nutritional support and its association with mortality in septic patients: results from a national, prospective, multicenter study. *Crit Care Med.* 2008;36: 1762-1767.

Felekis D et al: Effect of perioperative immuno-enhanced enteral nutrition on inflammatory response, nutritional status, and outcomes in head and neck cancer patients undergoing major surgery. *Nutr Cancer.* 2010;62(8):1105-1112.

Fukatsu K et al: Nutrition and gut immunity. *Surg Clin North Am.* 2011;91(4):755-770, vii.

Hermsen JL et al: Food fight! parenteral nutrition, enteral stimulation and gut-derived mucosal immunity. *Langenbecks Arch Surg.* 2009; 394(1):17-30.

Ikezawa F et al: Reversal of parenteral nutrition-induced gut mucosal immunity impairment with small amounts of a complex enteral diet. *Trauma.* 2008;65(2):360-366.

Ioannidis O: Nutrition support in acute pancreatitis. *JOP.* 2008;9(4):375-390.

Metheny NA et al: Monitoring for intolerance to gastric tube feedings: a national survey. *Am J Crit Care.* 2012;21(2):e33-e40.

Kavanagh BP et al: Glycemic control in the ICU. *N Engl J Med.* 2010;363:2540-2546.

Klek S et al: Perioperative nutrition in malnourished surgical cancer patients: a prospective, randomized, controlled clinical trial. *Clin Nutr.* 2011;30(6):708-713.

Langer G et al: Nutritional interventions for liver-transplanted patients. *Cochrane Database Syst Rev.* 2012;8:CD007605.

Leyba OC et al: Guidelines for specialized nutritional and metabolic support in the critically-ill patient: update. Consensus SEMICYUC-SENPE: septic patient. *Nutr Hosp.* 2011;26 (Suppl 2):67-71.

Lomer MC et al: Review article: lactose intolerance in clinical practice: myths and realities. *Aliment Pharmacol Ther.* 2008;27(2):93-103.

Manzanares W et al: Antioxidant micronutrients in the critically ill: a systematic review and meta-analysis. *Crit Care.* 2012;16:R66.

McClave SA et al: Guidelines for the provision and assessment of nutrition support therapy in the adult critically ill patient: Society of Critical Care Medicine (SCCM) and American Society for Parenteral and Enteral Nutrition (A.S.P.E.N.). *JPEN J Parenter Enteral Nutr.* 2009;33:277-316.

McClave SA et al: Nutrition therapy of the severely obese, critically ill patient: summation of conclusions and recommendations. *JPEN J Parenter Enteral Nutr.* 2011;35(5 Suppl): S88-S96.

Mirtallo JM et al: International consensus guidelines for nutrition therapy in pancreatitis. *JPEN J Parenter Enteral Nutr.* 2012;36(3):284-291.

Okamoto Y et al: Attenuation of the systemic inflammatory response and infectious complications after gastrectomy with preoperative oral arginine and omega-3 fatty acids supplemented immunonutrition. *World J Surg.* 2009;33(9):1815-1821.

Owers CE et al: Perioperative optimization of patients undergoing bariatric surgery. *J Obes.* 2012;2012:781546.

Phillips MS et al: Overview of enteral and parenteral feeding access techniques: principles and practice. *Surg Clin North Am.* 2011;91(4):897-911, ix.

Plauth M et al: ESPEN guidelines on parenteral nutrition: hepatology. *Clin Nutr.* 2009;28:436-444.

Ryu SW et al: Comparison of different nutritional assessments in detecting malnutrition among gastric cancer patients. *World J Gastroenterol*. 2010;16(26):3310-3317.

Singer P et al: ESPEN guidelines on parenteral nutrition: intensive care. *Clin Nutr*. 2009;28:387-400.

Wernerman J: Clinical use of glutamine supplementation. *J Nutr*. 2008;138(10):S2040-S2044.

Wiesen P et al: Nutrition disorders during acute renal failure and renal replacement therapy. *JPEN J Parenter Enteral Nutr*. 2011;35(2):217-222.

Williams FN et al: What, how, and how much should patients with burns be fed? *Surg Clin North Am*. 2011;91(3):609-629.

Wischmeyer PE: Glutamine: role in critical illness and ongoing clinical trials. *Curr Opin Gastroenterol*. 2008;24(2):190-197.

Worthington PH et al: Parenteral nutrition: risks, complications, and management. *J Infus Nurs*. 2012;35(1):52-64.

Yang H et al: Enteral versus parenteral nutrition: effect on intestinal barrier function. *Ann N Y Acad Sci*. 2009;1165:338-346.

Zhang Y et al: Perioperative immunonutrition for gastrointestinal cancer: a systematic review of randomized controlled trials. *Surg Oncol*. 2012;21(2):e87-e95.

Zhang Y et al: Perioperative immunonutrition for gastrointestinal cancer: a systematic review of randomized controlled trials. *Surg Oncol*. 2012;21(2):e87-e95.

Ziegler TR: Parenteral nutrition in the critically ill patient. *N Engl J Med*. 2009;361(11):1088-1097.

MULTIPLE CHOICE QUESTIONS

1. Which of the following is not a proposed mechanism by which enteral feeding decreases bacterial intestinal wall translocation when compared to IV nutrition?

   A. Preserved local cytokine expression pattern
   B. Increased villous height and over all mucosal mass
   C. Bactericidal activity of enteral nutrition components
   D. Stimulation of intraluminal IgA transportation

2. Which of the following stressors results in the greatest increase in energy expenditure above basal metabolic needs?

   A. Sepsis
   B. Trauma
   C. Elective operations
   D. Burns

3. Regarding centrally administered parenteral nutrition in the critically ill patient, which of the following is not true?

   A. An initial formulation for nonamino acid calories is generally advised to consist of 70% dextrose and 30% fat emulsion.
   B. TPN should be avoided if anticipated use is less than 6-7 days.
   C. The recommended amino acid dose ranges from 0.8 to 1 g/kg.
   D. The line-related complication rate from CVCs is greater than 15%.

4. Which of the following is true?

   A. Lactose intolerance is most prevalent in European Caucasians when compared to other populations.
   B. Gastric residuals of 100 cc should prompt holding of tube feeds.
   C. Gastric bypass patients are prone to deficiencies of the fat-soluble vitamins, calcium, iron, vitamin B_{12}, and folate.
   D. Enteral nutrition carries a technical complication rate of 10%.

5. Regarding nutritional indices, which of the following is false?

   A. PNI has been validated in patients undergoing either major cancer or gastrointestinal surgery and found to accurately identify a subset of patients at increased risk for complications.
   B. The NRI is an excellent tool for tracking the adequacy of nutritional support.
   C. The MNA is a rapid and reliable tool for evaluating the nutritional status of the elderly.
   D. SGA is a reproducible clinical method that has been validated and encompasses the patient's history and physical examination.

Anesthesia

Theodore J. Sanford Jr, MD

Anesthesiology is a "team sport." Providing the best and safest care for patients depends on all members of the team—surgeons, nurses, and anesthesia providers—communicating in a timely, efficient, and patient-focused manner. Anesthesiologists today not only provide patient care in the operating room but also have patient responsibilities in other areas, including preoperative anesthesia clinics (PACs), postanesthesia care units (PACUs), obstetrics, ambulatory surgery centers, endoscopy suites, postoperative pain management, critical care units, and chronic pain management.

Anesthesia is a term derived from the Greek meaning "without sensation" and is commonly used to indicate the condition that allows patients to undergo a variety of surgical or nonsurgical procedures without the pain or distress they would otherwise experience. More importantly, this blocking of pain and/or awareness is reversible. Anesthesiology is the medical practice of providing anesthesia to patients and is most commonly provided by a medical doctor, an anesthesiologist, either alone or in conjunction with a certified registered nurse anesthetist (CRNA), anesthesia assistant, or resident physician-in-training. Anesthesia is most often described as being a general anesthetic, that is, a drug-induced loss of consciousness during which patients are not arousable even by noxious stimulus and often require a controlled airway. Anesthesia can also be provided without inducing unconsciousness by utilizing regional blockade, local anesthesia with monitored anesthesia care (MAC), or conscious sedation.

HISTORY OF ANESTHESIA

One of modern medicine's most important discoveries was that the application of diethyl ether (ether) could provide the classic requirements of anesthesia: analgesia, amnesia, and muscle relaxation in a reversible and safe manner. Crawford Long was the first to use ether in 1842, and William Morton's successful 1846 public demonstration of ether as

an anesthetic in the "Ether Dome" of Massachusetts General Hospital ushered in the modern day of anesthesia and surgery. Chloroform was used by Sir James Y. Simpson to provide analgesia to Queen Victoria in 1853 during the birth of Prince Leopold. This royal approval of inhalation agents led to the wide acceptance of their use as surgical anesthesia. Ether (flammability, solubility) and chloroform (liver toxicity) each had significant drawbacks, and over time, inhalation agents were developed with similar anesthetic effects but much safer physiologic and metabolic properties.

Cocaine's ability to produce topical anesthesia for ophthalmic surgery was discovered in the late 1800s. The hypodermic needle was introduced in 1890 and facilitated the injection of cocaine to produce reversible nerve blockade and later the injection of cocaine via a lumbar puncture to produce a spinal anesthetic and the first spinal headache. The chemical properties of cocaine were soon determined and manipulated to synthesize numerous other local anesthetic agents used to achieve what became known as regional anesthesia, which lacks the unconsciousness and amnesia of the general anesthetics but does produce analgesia and lack of motor movement in the "blocked" region.

Underwood EA: Before and after Morton. A historical survey of anaesthesia. *Br Med J.* 1946;2:525.

OVERALL RISK OF ANESTHESIA

Anesthesia is performed over 70 million times per year in the United States and is remarkably safe. The number of anesthesia-related deaths has decreased dramatically in the last 30 years because of intense scrutiny by the American Society of Anesthesiologists. The realization that most problems are related to airway compromise has led to advanced respiratory monitoring utilizing pulse oximetry and capnography for every patient undergoing anesthesia. The Institute of Medicine's *To Err Is Human* complimented the anesthesiology community for its marked decrease in morbidity and mortality from anesthesia. Overall, the risk of anesthesia-related death in the healthy patient is estimated to be as low as 1:100,000-200,000 anesthetics.

The combination of amnesia, with or without unconsciousness, analgesia, and muscle relaxation is purposely induced by an anesthetic caregiver and is achieved either by administering inhalation agents in appropriate doses to affect the central nervous system (CNS) or by using specific intravenous pharmacologic agents to produce the same effects as inhaled vapors. These agents include amnestics, for example, benzodiazepines (midazolam or diazepam); analgesics, for example, the opioids morphine and fentanyl derivatives; the neuromuscular blocking drugs succinylcholine, pancuronium, or vecuronium; and sedative hypnotics, for example, sodium pentothal and propofol. All of the agents have adverse physiologic consequences: respiratory depression, cardiovascular depression, and loss of consciousness. Furthermore, some of these agents may induce allergic reactions. Some have also been known to trigger malignant hyperpyrexia.

The most common problems associated with adverse outcomes today still relate to airway compromise, medication errors, and central venous cannulation. Other concerns are postoperative neurologic complications (eg, nerve injury), ischemic optic neuropathy, coronary ischemia, anesthesia in remote locations (eg, interventional radiology sites), and probably most importantly, inadequate preoperative evaluation and preparation.

The anesthesia provider must be able to (1) achieve a state of anesthesia quickly and safely by choosing the appropriate techniques and agents, taking into consideration the patient's medical condition; (2) maintain and monitor a state of anesthesia throughout the surgical procedure while compensating for the effects of varying degrees of surgical stimulation and blood and fluid losses; (3) reverse the muscle relaxation and amnesia as necessary; and (4) return the patient to physiologic homeostasis while maintaining sufficient analgesia to minimize postprocedure pain.

Kohn LT, Corrigan JM, Donaldson MS (editors): *To Err Is Human: Building a Safer Health System*. Washington, DC: National Academy Press, 2000.

PREOPERATIVE EVALUATION

A preoperative evaluation is a responsibility of the anesthesiologist and is a basic element of anesthesia care (Table 11–1). This evaluation consists of information gathered from multiple sources, including the patient's medical record, history and physical examinations, and findings from medical tests and consults or other evaluations performed prior to the patient being seen by the anesthesiologist. Improved patient outcome and satisfaction is the result of an adequate,

Table 11–1. Preoperative evaluation.

Goals
    Optimize patient condition
    Understand and control comorbidities and drug therapy
    Ensure patient's questions are answered
Timing
    High surgical invasiveness: at least 1 day prior
    Medium invasiveness: day before or day of surgery
    Low invasiveness: day of surgery
Content
    Review medical records
    Directed history and physical examination: airway, heart, and lungs
    Indicated laboratory or additional consultations

structured, formal presurgical, or preprocedure evaluation and preparation performed on all patients.

▶ Timing

The timing of the preoperative evaluation depends primarily on the degree of planned surgical invasiveness. For high surgical invasiveness, the initial assessment should be done at a minimum the day before the planned procedure by the anesthesia staff. Patients undergoing medium surgical invasive procedures can be evaluated the day before or even on the day of surgery, and for low surgical invasiveness, the initial assessment may be done the day of surgery. Time must be allotted to follow up on conditions discovered during the preoperative visit and to answer patient questions. Perioperative complications and deaths are most often a combination of patient comorbidities, surgical complexity, and anesthesia effects. The Physical Status Classification of the American Society of Anesthesiologists is the best known of many perioperative classification schemes (Table 11–2). This classification system does not assign risk but is a common language used to describe patients' preoperative physical status. The system is an alert to the anesthesia practitioner and all members of the patient care team.

Table 11–2. American Society of Anesthesiologists physical status classification.

ASA 1 (PS1): A normal healthy patient
ASA 2 (PS2): A patient with mild systemic disease
ASA 3 (PS3): A patient with severe systemic disease
ASA 4 (PS4): A patient with severe systemic disease that is a constant threat to life
ASA 5 (PS5): A moribund patient who is not expected to survive without the operation
ASA 6 (PS6): A declared brain-dead patient whose organs are being removed for donor purposes
E: Emergency

Patients should ideally be seen in a PAC staffed by anesthesia personnel who evaluate patients from the anesthetic perspective and who look for physical conditions (airway) and controlled, uncontrolled, or unrecognized medical conditions that can lead to perioperative morbidity and mortality. There must be adequate communication between anesthesiologist and surgeon such that any conditions that may result in patient compromise are optimally addressed. Optimally, a patient's medical status has been adequately addressed by the patient's primary care physician prior to being referred to the PAC. However, in some instances, only a cursory "cleared for anesthesia and surgery" may result in a necessary delay. Any patients other than healthy ASA 1 or 2 patients should be seen in a PAC. Prior to referring patients to the PAC, the surgeon should have already ordered the necessary preoperative labs and in many instances will have already detected uncontrolled medical conditions that require consultations from other specialties in order to recommend and in some instances improve a patient's status.

The optimal preoperative evaluation has the following two elements: (1) content—readily accessible medical records, patient interview, a directed preanesthesia examination, indicated preoperative laboratory tests, and additional consultations when indicated; the minimum acceptable examination includes an assessment of the airway, heart, and lungs well in advance of the planned date of surgery; and (2) preoperative tests—only as indicated by comorbidities and never as a screen, these tests should be specifically aimed at helping the anesthesiologist formulate an anesthetic plan.

Practice advisory for preanesthesia evaluation: a report by the American Society of Anesthesiologists Task Force on Preanesthesia Evaluation. *Anesthesiology*. 2012;116:1-17.

History & Physical Examination

The anesthesiologist should specifically ask the patient about previous operations, anesthetic type, and any complications, for example, allergic reactions, abnormal bleeding, delayed emergence, prolonged paralysis, difficult airway management, awareness, or jaundice. Each of these describes a possible specific anesthetic morbidity that must be further investigated either by history or specific testing. Medical conditions detected as decreased exercise tolerance, shortness of breath, orthopnea, kidney or liver disease, and metabolic abnormalities, for example, diabetes or thyroid disease, should be ascertained. A comprehensive history seeks to identify serious cardiac conditions, for example, unstable coronary syndromes, angina, myocardial infarctions either recent or past, decompensated congestive heart failure, significant arrhythmias, or severe valvular disease. Any recent changes in cardiac symptoms or other associated diseases, for example, diabetes, renal disease, or cerebrovascular disease symptoms, should be identified.

Any family history of adverse responses to anesthetics (malignant hyperthermia) and social history of smoking, drug use, and alcohol consumption is important. Finally, a comprehensive review of concurrent medications including antihypertensives, insulin, bronchodilators, or any other medications that can interact with anesthetic agents should be documented. Certain medications may result in increased or decreased anesthetic requirements, prolongation of muscle relaxants, abnormal responses to sympathomimetics, delayed or enhanced metabolism of anesthetics, and/or augmentation of the depressant effects of anesthetics. The patient's use of herbal medicines can have an adverse reaction with some anesthetics (Table 11–3) and all should be discontinued 2-3 weeks before surgery.

Wong A, Townley SA: Herbal medicines and anaesthesia. *Br J Anaesth*. 2011;11:15-17.

▶ Airway Examination & Classification

After the vital signs are obtained, the physical examination begins with the upper airway. Ability to control the airway is mandatory. The focus of the examination is to assess those factors that would make airway control (eg, endotracheal intubation) difficult or impossible. Seven keys to the upper airway examination should be documented:

1. Range of motion of the cervical spine: Patients should be asked to extend and flex their neck to the full range of possible motion so the anesthesiologist may look for any limitations.

2. Thyroid cartilage to mentum distance: ideal is greater than 6 cm.

3. Mouth opening: ideal is greater than 3 cm.

4. Dentition: dentures, loose teeth, poor conservation.

5. Jaw protrusion: ability to protrude the lower incisors past the upper incisors.

6. Presence of a beard.

7. Examination and classification of the upper airway based on the size of patient's tongue and the pharyngeal structures visible on mouth opening with the patient sitting looking forward. This visual description of the airway structures is known as the Mallampati score (Figure 11–1).

Grade I The soft palate, anterior and posterior tonsillar pillars, and uvula are visible—suggests easy airway intubation.

Grade II Tonsillar pillars and part of the uvula obscured by the tongue.

Grade III Only soft palate and hard palate visible.

Grade IV Only the hard palate is visible—suggests challenging airway.

Table 11–3. Perioperative effects of common herbal medicine.[1]

Name (Other Names)	Alleged Benefits	Perioperative Effects	Recommendations
Echinacea	Stimulates immune system	Allergic reactions; hepatotoxicity; interference with immune suppressive therapy (eg, organ transplants)	Discontinue as far in advance of surgery as possible
Ephedra (ma huang)	Promotes weight loss; increases energy	Ephedrine-like sympathetic stimulation with increased heart rate and blood pressure, arrhythmias, myocardial infarction, stroke	Discontinue at least 24 h prior to surgery; avoid monoamine oxidase inhibitors
Garlic (ajo)	Reduces blood pressure and cholesterol levels	Inhibition of platelet aggregation (irreversible)	Discontinue at least 7 days prior to surgery
Ginkgo (duck foot, maidenhair, silver apricot)	Improves cognitive performance (eg, dementia), increases peripheral perfusion (eg, impotence, macular degeneration)	Inhibition of platelet-activating factor	Discontinue at least 36 h prior to surgery
Ginseng	Protects against "stress" and maintains "homeostasis"	Hypoglycemia; inhibition of platelet aggregation and coagulation cascade	Discontinue at least 7 days prior to surgery
Kava (kawa, awa, intoxicating pepper)	Decreases anxiety	GABA-mediated hypnotic effects my decrease MAC (see Chapter 7); possible risk of acute withdrawal	Discontinue at least 24 h prior to surgery
St. John's wort (amber, goat-weed, *Hypericum perforatum*, klamathe-weed)	Reverses mild to moderate depression	Inhibits serotonin, norepinephrine, and dopamine reuptake by neurons; increases drug metabolism by induction of cytochrome P-450	Discontinue at least 5 days prior to surgery
Valerian	Decreases anxiety	GABA-mediated hypnotic effects may decrease MAC; benzodiazepinelike withdrawal syndrome	Taper dose weeks before surgery if possible; treat withdrawal symptoms with benzodiazepines

[1]For more details, see Ang-Lee MK, Moss J, Yuan C: Herbal medicine and perioperative care. *JAMA.* 2001;286:208.
GABA, γ-aminobutyric acid; MAC, minimum alveolar concentration.
Reproduced, with permission, from Mallampati SR: Clinical sign to predict difficult tracheal intubation (hypothesis), *Can Anaesth Soc J.* 1983 May;30(3 Pt 1):316–317.

The physical examination then focuses on heart and lungs, potential intravenous catheter sites, and potential sites for regional anesthesia. Range of motion of limbs must also be noted as this may affect positioning in the operating room. Finally, any neurologic abnormalities must be noted.

When a metabolic or physical finding or symptom is discovered during this visit, the anesthesiologist may believe that a specialty consultation is necessary to suggest ways to optimize the patient for surgery and anesthesia. If this is the case, the anesthesiologist should communicate with the surgeon in order to prevent unnecessary or unexpected delays in the surgical schedule. It is imperative that any consults ordered be completed and the results be available by the day of surgery.

The anesthesiologist can then advise the patient on appropriate options for general anesthesia versus regional techniques based on the patient's history, physical examination, and type of surgery. Although some surgical procedures must always be performed under general anesthesia, the anesthesiologist may discuss other options with the patient. If the referring surgeon has a particular preference for a type of anesthetic, such preferences should be communicated to the anesthesiologist directly rather than through the patient. It is also best if the referring surgeon does not promise any specific agent or technique without first consulting with the anesthesia care givers.

> Mallampati SR et al: A clinical sign to predict difficult tracheal intubation: a prospective study. *Can Anaesth Soc J.* 1985;32:429.

Preoperative Fasting

The anesthesiologist must discuss with the patient the requirements for preprocedure fasting and the management of medications up to the time of surgery or procedure.

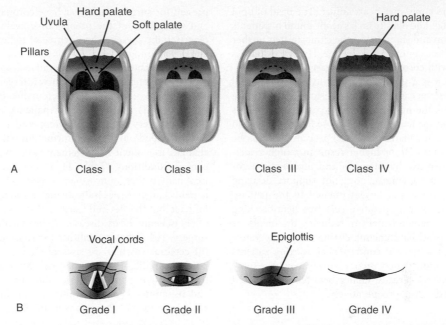

▲ **Figure 11–1.** Mallampati airway classification of oral opening. (Reproduced with permission from Morgan GE, Mikhail MS, Murray MJ: *Clinical Anesthesiology*, 4th ed. McGraw-Hill.)

Current guidelines for preoperative fasting are as follows: (1) No solid food should be eaten after the evening meal. At the minimum, most anesthesiologists delay an anesthetic so that the last solid food was 6-8 hours prior to nonemergent surgery or procedures involving anesthesia. (2) NPO after midnight except for sips of water to take oral medications. Water may be ingested up to 2 hours before checking in for surgery. Some institutions allow other clear liquids, for example, coffee, a few hours prior to surgery or procedure. However, because surgery schedules can change abruptly and procedure time may be moved forward, NPO after midnight is the best policy. (3) Pediatric fasting guidelines vary among institutions, so practitioners should consult with their particular pediatric anesthesia group.

> American Society of Anesthesiologists: Practice guidelines for preoperative fasting and the use of pharmacologic agents to reduce the risk of pulmonary aspiration: application to healthy patients undergoing elective procedures. *Anesthesiology.* 2011;114:495-511.

▶ Drugs to Continue Preoperatively

In the perioperative period patients should continue taking beta-blocking agents, statin medications, antihypertensives except the angiotensin II receptor blockers (ARBs) and angiotensin-converting enzyme inhibitors (ACE) antihypertensive medications. Patients taking ARBs or ACE inhibitors can experience marked hypotension with the induction of general anesthesia and respond poorly to common vasopressors. Patients taking anticoagulants such as Coumadin, clopidogrel, and the newer anticoagulants such as dabigatran (Pradaxa) should stop these medications prior to most surgeries. The timing and bridging of cessation of these anticoagulants is the responsibility of the surgical service. Continuation of low-dose aspirin for patients with coronary stents or atrial fibrillation is recommended. Oral antihyperglycemic agents need should not be taken the day of surgery. Insulin-dependent patients should receive instructions from the anesthesiologist during the preanesthesia visit as to the management of their insulin. Other medications should be discussed with the patient and surgery team at the time of the preoperative anesthesia visit.

▶ Comorbidities

Comorbidities should be well controlled in the preoperative period to avoid postprocedure morbidity, and even mortality.

▶ Cardiovascular Disease (Hypertension, Coronary Artery Disease, Congestive Heart Failure)

A. Hypertension

Hypertension is the most common preexisting medical disease identified preoperatively and is a major risk factor for renal, cerebrovascular, peripheral vascular, cardiac ischemia or infarction, and congestive heart failure. The triad of lipid disorders, diabetes, and obesity is classically found in patients with hypertension and should alert the clinician that further evaluation for these conditions is needed. Hypertension has an association with coronary artery disease, and the preoperative evaluation is a unique opportunity to identify and treat the nonessential causes of hypertension. The literature strongly supports the notion that all hypertensive patients should be treated medically to be as close to normotension as possible before any planned surgical procedure. Diastolic pressures of 110 mm Hg or higher result in a higher incidence of intraoperative hypotension and myocardial ischemia. However, the literature does not support delaying surgery if the delay would be detrimental to the patient. The introduction of perioperative selective beta-blocking drugs provides a marked benefit in reducing the incidence of significant myocardial ischemia during the perioperative period. Although somewhat controversial, starting patients on beta-blockers immediately preoperatively may have some risk, but any patient already taking beta-blockers should continue taking the drug preoperatively.

Sear JW, Giles JW, Howard G, Foex P: Perioperative beta-blockade, 2008: what does POISE tell us, and was our earlier caution justified? *Br J Anaesth.* 2008;101:135-138.

Wax DB et al: Association of preanesthesia hypertension with adverse outcomes. *J Cardiothorac Vasc Anesth.* 2010:24(6): 927-930.

B. Coronary Artery Disease

Ischemic heart disease is a leading cause of death in the United States and is the leading cause of morbidity and mortality in the perioperative period. About 25% of patients who present for surgery each year have coronary artery disease, and thus much of the preoperative evaluation focuses on detecting the presence and degree of ischemic heart disease and determining whether it is likely to impact anesthesia and surgery. A major goal of preoperative assessment of cardiac status is to determine what, if any, interventions—coronary artery bypass graft (CABG), percutaneous coronary intervention (PCI)—would benefit patients undergoing noncardiac surgery. In general, preoperative cardiac tests are recommended only if the information obtained will lead to changes in patient management. However, certain active clinical conditions (Table 11–4) demand evaluation and treatment before noncardiac surgery. Determining which patient characteristics indicate high perioperative risk is very difficult, but the Revised Cardiac Risk Index (RCRI) factors of (1) ischemic heart disease, (2) heart failure, (3) high-risk surgery, (4) diabetes mellitus, (5) renal insufficiency, and (6) cerebral vascular diseases are a validated set of independent predictors of cardiac risk for patients. The anesthesiologist in a pre-op clinic will screen for these factors and recommend further studies based on the presence or absence of RCRIs. Patients with no RCRIs have a very low (0.4%) cardiac risk while patients with three or more risk factors have a 5.4% risk of an adverse cardiac event and warrant further testing. Because of the high incidence of silent ischemia, some institutions will require patients older than 50 to have an electrocardiogram (EKG). A simple exercise tolerance description of the functional capacity of the patient (eg, ability to climb two flights of stairs without stopping) is also a practical screening. This initial history by the surgeon or anesthesiologist may be the first cardiac assessment the patient has ever had. The assessment of functional capacity may be the first indication of the need for further evaluation of potential cardiac pathology.

Table 11–4. Active cardiac conditions for which the patient should undergo evaluation and treatment before noncardiac surgery.

Condition	Examples
Unstable coronary syndromes	Unstable or severe angina Recent myocardial infarction (> 7 but < 30 days ago)
Decompensated heart failure (New York Heart Association class IV): worsening or new onset Significant arrhythmias	High-grade atrioventricular block Mobitz II atrioventricular block Third-degree atrioventricular block Symptomatic ventricular arrhythmias Supraventricular arrhythmias (including atrial fibrillation with uncontrolled ventricular rate [> 100] at rest) Symptomatic bradycardia Newly recognized ventricular tachycardia
Severe valvular disease	Severe aortic stenosis (mean pressure gradient > 40 mm Hg or aortic valve area < 1.0 cm^2 or symptomatic) Symptomatic mitral stenosis (progressive dyspnea on exertion, exertional syncope, or heart failure)

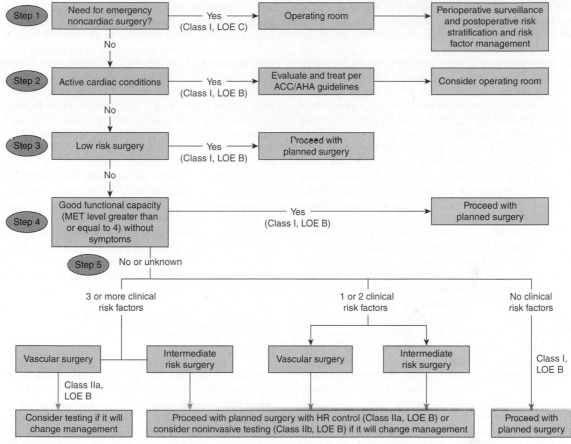

▲ **Figure 11–2.** Cardiac evaluation and care algorithm for noncardiac surgery based on active clinical conditions, known cardiovascular disease or cardiac risk factors for patients 50 years of age or greater. Summary of ACC/AHA 2007 perioperative guideline algorithm on cardiovascular evaluation and care for noncardiac surgery. HR = heart rate, LOE = loss of evidence, MET = metabolic equivalent.

The American Heart Association (AHA) developed a useful algorithm for all providers (Figure 11–2). This algorithm, updated in 2007, no longer focuses on stress testing but recommends testing only if the results could have an impact on surgery or anesthesia and lead to changes in patient management. The AHA guidelines state that most patients who have asymptomatic heart disease can safely undergo elective noncardiac surgery without performing invasive or even noninvasive cardiac testing.

Fleisher LA et al: 2009 ACCF/AHA Focused Update on Perioperative Beta Blockade Incorporated Into the ACC/AHA 2007 Guidelines on Perioperative Cardiovascular Evaluation and Care for Noncardiac Surgery A Report of the American College of Cardiology Foundation/American Heart Association Task Force on Practice Guidelines. *Circulation.* 2009;120: c169–c276.

Ford MK et al: Systematic review: prediction of perioperative cardiac complications and mortality by the revised cardiac risk index. *Ann Intern Med.* 2010:152:26.

C. Patients With Prior Percutaneous Coronary Intervention (Angioplasty and Stents)

There is much controversy about the best treatment for patients who have had a PCI procedure, angioplasty without stents, or angioplasty with either a bare metal or drug-eluting stent. Because of the risk for thrombosis at the site of intervention, patients are usually placed on a dual antiplatelet therapy of aspirin and clopidogrel for 2-4 weeks following angioplasty, 4-6 weeks for the bare metal stents, and up to 1 year for the drug-eluting stents. Stopping these antiplatelet drugs for a surgical intervention that falls in the therapy period presents a risk for perioperative cardiac events if the stent thromboses. The AHA guidelines recommend that if the procedure is elective, then the operation should be postponed until the case can be done with aspirin as the only antiplatelet drug. If the operation is urgent, then consideration must be given to the timing of the surgery and the risk of surgical bleeding. If the risk of bleeding is low, then a PCI with a stent should be considered and the patient placed on dual antiplatelet therapy. If the bleeding risk is high, the AHA recommends the following based on the timing of surgery: angioplasty for surgery within 14-29 days, bare metal stent for planned surgery within 30-365 days, and drug-eluting stent for surgery that can be delayed 1 year. Truly urgent and/or emergent surgery necessitates angioplasty for a procedure with a high risk of surgical bleeding and stenting for a case with a low risk for bleeding.

The AHA guidelines recommend several other measures: (1) Perioperative beta-blockade is indicated for patients previously on beta-blockers, patients undergoing major vascular surgery, and patients undergoing intermediate-risk surgery with one or more RCRIs. Beta-blockade may be started several days to weeks before planned surgery in order to produce a consistent targeted heart rate between 65 and 70 beats/min. The addition of statin class agents, alpha-2 agonists, and calcium channel blockers may also be effective. (2) Left ventricular function should be assessed preoperatively for patients with unexplained dyspnea or who have active or a history of compensated heart failure with changing symptoms. (3) Coronary revascularization is suggested for patients with left main disease, symptomatic three-vessel disease and poor ejection fraction (EF), two-vessel disease with left anterior descending coronary artery stenosis, poor EF and a positive stress test, or an acute ST segment elevation myocardial infarction. AHA does not recommend prophylactic CABG surgery in patients with stable coronary artery disease. (4) Blood glucose should be tightly controlled. (5) Patients with pacemakers or implanted defibrillator devices should have them checked 3-6 months before major surgery. (6) Patients with drug-eluting cardiac stents should continue aspirin therapy and discontinue other antiplatelet agents for as short a time as possible. (7) Beta-blockers and statin drugs should be continued in the perioperative period. (8) Cardiology consultants should be asked for specific recommendations that would reduce immediate perioperative cardiac risk.

Practice alert for perioperative management of patients with coronary artery stents. *Anesthesiology.* 2009:110:1-2.

D. Pulmonary Disease

The presence of significant pulmonary disease is suspected or confirmed by the history and physical examination. Poor functional capacity may be the first indication that further workup may be necessary. The presence of either obstructive or restrictive lung disease always puts the patient at risk for perioperative complications, for example, pneumonia and prolonged difficulty weaning from the ventilator. In some instances, arterial blood gas analysis or pulmonary function tests are necessary to determine responsiveness to bronchodilators. Asthmatic patients should be asked about the severity of their disease, hospitalizations, responsiveness to inhalers, and steroid usage. There is no value for routine preoperative chest x-rays. Surgical history and physical examination may be the first indication of significant pulmonary disease, and workup may be initiated before sending the patient to the PAC. Optimally, patients who smoke should stop smoking at least 8 weeks before scheduled surgery. Warner demonstrated that the highest rate of pulmonary complications in 200 patients undergoing CABG was in those who had stopped smoking 1-8 weeks preoperatively. Recent cessation of cigarette smoking may pose a greater risk of pulmonary complication because of the commonly observed increase in cough and sputum production. Patients should abstain from smoking for as long as possible both before and after surgery.

Warner DO: Helping surgical patients quit smoking: why, when, and how. *Anesth Analg.* 2005;101:481.

E. Obesity

The national epidemic of obesity poses particular problems for surgery and anesthesia. The body mass index (BMI), the ratio of weight (kg)/height (m^2), gives an idea of the degree of obesity. Normal BMI is about 21.6 kg/m^2, overweight is 25-30 kg/m^2, obese is 30-35 kg/m^2, and extreme obesity is more than 35 kg/m^2. Extreme obesity patients have a variety of perioperative issues and should be evaluated in a PAC. Particular attention should include the upper airway and evaluation of cardiovascular, respiratory, metabolic, and gastrointestinal systems. Abnormal BMI patients have cardiovascular issues with venous access, hypertension, cardiomegaly, decreased left ventricular function, and cor pulmonale, and they have twice the incidence of ischemic heart disease than patients at normal weight. Extreme obesity is associated with significant pulmonary problems, including restrictive lung volumes, obstructive sleep apnea, hypoxemia, increased Paco$_2$, increased hematocrit, and right heart failure. The extremely obese patient's airway is often difficult to maintain with mask ventilation secondary to decreased neck mobility and adiposity and requires careful preoperative evaluation. Almost all the major endocrine problems with extreme obesity involve the effects of diabetes mellitus and require preoperative assessment of glycemic control. Obesity also leads to abnormal fatty deposits in the liver that cause increased metabolism of inhalation anesthetics. Morbidly obese patients may have a higher risk of gastric aspiration and development of aspiration pneumonia. Finally, postoperative pain management must be considered.

F. Diabetes Mellitus

The most common metabolic abnormality is diabetes mellitus, and its presence should cause a high index of suspicion for cardiac problems. Patients on insulin therapy are at higher risk for cardiac morbidity and mortality, including myocardial infarction and heart failure. Glucose control may be very difficult to maintain in the perioperative period, and preoperative assessment of control should always be ascertained through history or laboratory testing. Tight glucose control may reduce infections postoperatively but it is controversial whether intensive insulin therapy decrease mortality, perioperative hypoglycemia, or cardiac events. Anesthesia providers are responsible for glucose control during the procedure, and the surgical service is typically responsible for this care in the postoperative period.

Hua J et al: Intensive intraoperative insulin therapy versus conventional insulin therapy during cardiac surgery: a meta-analysis. *J Cardiothoracic Vasc Anesth.* 2012;26(5):829-834. Epub Feb 14, 2012.

G. Patients on Low-Molecular-Weight Heparin

Patients taking low-molecular-weight heparin (LMWH) for deep venous thrombosis prophylaxis present an unusual problem for both surgeon and anesthesiologist. The current guidelines dictate that unless absolutely indicated, neuraxial anesthesia (spinal, epidural) should not be performed unless LMWH has been stopped for at least 12 hours and preferably 24 hours. That means that a substitute anticoagulant should be initiated if neuraxial anesthesia is to be done, or this approach is avoided.

H. Renal Impairment

Acute renal failure (ARF) occurs in approximately 1%-5% of all hospitalized patients and is responsible for increased length of stay and mortality. The preoperative visit can help to identify patient risk factors for ARF in those with previously normal renal function undergoing noncardiac surgery. The perioperative onset of ARF in patients with previously normal renal function is associated with increased postoperative mortality, especially significant within 1 year postsurgery. BMI higher than 32 kg/m^2, age, emergency surgery, liver disease, high-risk surgery (intrathoracic, intraperitoneal, suprainguinal vascular, large blood loss), peripheral vascular occlusive disease, and chronic obstructive pulmonary disease necessitating chronic bronchodilator therapy place patients at increased risk for perioperative renal impairment.

Kheterpal S et al: Predictors of postoperative acute renal failure after noncardiac surgery in patients with previously normal renal function. *Anesthesiology.* 2007;107:892.

Preoperative Medications

The use of preoperative medications is hampered by the fact that most patients are not in the medical facility until the day of surgery. Most premedications now consist of an anxiolytic agent (eg, midazolam) and an opiate (eg, fentanyl) given in the immediate preanesthesia period. These premedications are often given because patients have a preconceived notion that they need something to relax. Alternatively, a thorough explanation of what the patient can expect in terms of surgery and anesthesia has a significant calming effect comparable to that of medications given to relieve anxiety. Administration of premedication to prevent pulmonary aspiration syndrome is often considered with the use of agents that increase gastric pH (H$_2$ blockers, proton pump inhibitors, antacids) or agents that lower gastric volume.

Informed Consent

Many institutions and practices obtain a signed informed consent from patients for anesthesia, while other institutions include the anesthesia consent in the surgical consent. Regardless of the particular facility requirements, the anesthesiologist should write a note in the patient chart indicating that the patient has been informed of the issues surrounding anesthesia and understands the risks and complications as described. The informed consent for anesthesia should include a discussion of what to expect from the administration of anesthesia and possible adverse effects and risks. A number of issues should be discussed routinely, including timing of surgery, premedication, risks of dental injury, cardiac risks, sequence of events prior to anesthesia induction, awakening from anesthesia, presence of catheters, duration of time in the PACU, anticipated return to a hospital bed or discharge, postoperative pain management, and the likelihood of nausea and vomiting. Patients may have questions concerning perioperative awareness. Rather than cause undue worry, clinical judgment should dictate how detailed a description of each of these issues should be for each patient.

Choice of Anesthesia

Considerations in choosing an anesthetic technique include the planned surgical procedure, positioning requirements, patient preferences, surgeon preferences, the urgency of the operation, postoperative pain management, and potential for admission to a critical care unit. Some procedures (eg, thoracotomy) cannot be performed under a regional anesthetic or neuraxial blockade and necessitate a general anesthetic. Other procedures (eg, extremity surgery) can be performed under regional, neuraxial, or general anesthesia. Sometimes a combination of an epidural and a general anesthetic may be chosen with continuation of the epidural for postoperative pain management. Emergency surgery for patients with a full stomach may necessitate a rapid-sequence general anesthetic to protect from pulmonary aspiration. Regional anesthesia may provide anesthesia for hip surgery but may not provide much in the way of patient comfort because of the position requirements of a fracture table. Patient age and preference must also be included in the decision of choice of anesthetic technique. However, some regional anesthesia may be contraindicated for patients with the peripheral neuropathy of diabetes. Notation of the proposed type of anesthesia must be entered into record of the preanesthesia evaluation.

Holding Room & Operating Room

The nurse, surgeon, and anesthesiologist have many tasks to perform, starting in the holding area before the surgery can begin. The nurse checks the patient in and records vital signs, checks for a signed consent, and starts an intravenous line if needed. The surgeon should confirm and mark the site of surgery. The anesthesiologist should confirm the preoperative evaluation and type of anesthetic selected.

Wrong Site Surgery

In July 2004, the Joint Commission on the Accreditation of Healthcare Organizations (JCAHO) instituted a patient safety mandate known as the Universal Protocol for preventing wrong site, wrong procedure, wrong person surgery. All members of the care team must be familiar with and always participate in and perform the following three steps of this Universal Protocol.

Step 1: Initial verification of the intended patient, procedure, and site of the procedure. This step begins at the time the procedure is scheduled and again at the time of admission into the medical facility, anytime care responsibility is transferred to another caregiver, and before the patient leaves the preoperative area for the operating room.

Step 2: Marking the operative site. An unambiguous mark must be made using a marker that is sufficiently permanent to be visible after surgical prep and draping on or near the intended surgical incision site. This mark should not be an X, as in "X marks the spot," but rather a word or line representing the proposed incision. This mark must be made by the surgeon performing the procedure. If possible, the patient should participate when the site is marked.

Step 3: The time out immediately before starting the procedure. A time out must be conducted in the location where the surgical procedure will be done, and all members of the care team—surgeon, nurses, anesthesiologists—must actively participate in verification of correct patient identity, correct side and site of surgery, agreement on the scheduled procedure, and assurance that all of the necessary implants and special equipment are immediately available. This time out must take place before incision. JCAHO requires that the time out be documented in the medical record.

Joint Commission on the Accreditation of Healthcare Organizations: Universal protocol for preventing wrong site, wrong procedure, wrong person surgery. Available at: www.jointcommission.org/patientsafety/universalprotocol. Accessed November 28, 2008.

The Operating Room

The anesthesiologist must check the equipment in the operating room before helping to transport the patient. Once in the operating room, the patient is transferred to the operating table with the assistance of the nurses and anesthesiologist. It is standard anesthesia practice to apply monitors to measure arterial blood pressure (a-line, blood pressure cuff), heart rate, oxygenation (pulse oximeter), and ventilation (capnography) before induction of anesthesia (Table 11–5).

The anesthesiologist must be certain that a surgeon is present in the room before beginning induction. The final time out should then be performed, confirming site, patient, procedure, and surgical personnel.

General Anesthesia Management

Patients will be preoxygenated before induction of a general anesthetic. General anesthesia is commonly induced by administration of intravenous drugs (eg, propofol or thiopental) and, in cases when cardiovascular status is compromised, etomidate or ketamine. Patients receiving propofol may complain of discomfort at the IV sites, and patients receiving etomidate may have some athetoid movements that appear seizurelike. Almost all anesthetics are preceded by the

Table 11–5. Standards for basic anesthesia monitoring.

Parameter	Equipment
Oxygenation: Ensure patient concentration in inspired gas and blood during all anesthetics	*Oxygen analyzer:* Part of anesthesia machine *Pulse oximeter:* Continuously audible variable pitch pulse tone
Ventilation: Ensure adequate patient ventilation	*Capnography:* Continuous monitoring for the presence of end-tidal CO_2
Circulation: Ensure adequacy of patient circulatory function	*EKG:* Continuously displayed from the beginning until leaving the room *Arterial blood pressure monitor:* Measured at least every 5 minutes *Measurement of patient heart rate:* Usually from EKG or pulse oximeter
Temperature: Aid in maintenance of appropriate patient temperature	Oral, skin, nasal, or bladder temperature probe

administration of an opiate (eg, fentanyl) in a dose that is not intended to induce an anesthetic but that helps reduce the amount of induction agent. Most general anesthetics then include a muscle relaxant to facilitate endotracheal intubation. Tracheal intubation is almost always performed during general anesthesia and is especially important for patients presenting for emergent surgery with presumed full stomach or when positive pressure ventilation is required. The laryngeal mask airway (LMA) can also be used to maintain a patent airway. To minimize the time that the trachea is unprotected, a rapid-sequence induction of anesthesia using rapid administration of induction agent and rapid-acting muscle relaxant (eg, succinylcholine) can be utilized. The "crash induction" is a modification of this rapid sequence technique with the application of cricoid pressure by a caregiver other than the inducing anesthesia personnel.

General anesthesia may also be induced by mask using an inhalation anesthetic (eg, isoflurane or sevoflurane). This method is commonly used for children. Once adequate depth of anesthesia is assured, a muscle relaxant may be administered to help facilitate endotracheal intubation. Inhalation induction takes longer than rapid-sequence induction, and the airway may be unprotected for a longer time. A combination of inhalation agent and intravenous agent can also be used to induce general anesthesia.

Once an adequate depth of anesthesia and adequate muscle relaxation is attained, the trachea is intubated. Ease of endotracheal intubation can usually be predicted from the careful preoperative airway evaluation.

However, the anesthesiologist occasionally encounters an unexpected difficult intubation and additional maneuvers may be necessary: These can include cricoid manipulation, adjustment of the patient's head position, or use of a long, stiff catheter (eg, a bougie) or a fiberoptic bronchoscope. The American Society of Anesthesiologists provides an algorithm for the management of the difficult airway. If another provider is placing cricoid pressure, the anesthesiologist must directly state what maneuver would be the most helpful. If the airway cannot be secured after multiple attempts, patients can be awakened and a decision made to proceed with an awake fiberoptic intubation or to cancel the anesthetic until further workup can be performed. The most serious complication of endotracheal intubation, and the most common cause of serious anesthesia morbidity and mortality, is the failure to secure the airway. Other common complications are dental injuries, soft tissue injury to the lips, hypertension and tachycardia, and laryngospasm on extubation.

Following anesthetic induction, the patient must be properly positioned for the procedure. It is the responsibility of both surgeon and anesthesiologist to assure that the patient is positioned to avoid physical or physiologic complications. The American Society of Anesthesiologists' closed claims study notes that nerve damage from malpositioning during surgery is the second most common anesthetic complication.

Careful attention must be paid to adequately protect all potential pressure and vulnerable areas such as elbows, knees, heels, and eyes. The ulnar nerve is particularly susceptible to injury, as is the brachial plexus when patient's arms are abducted too far. Hemodynamics may also be compromised by position changes that may result in decreased venous return and resultant hypotension.

American Society of Anesthesiologists: Practice guidelines for management of the difficult airway: an updated report by the American Society of Anesthesiologists Task Force on Management of the Difficult Airway. *Anesthesiology*. 2003; 98:1269.
Cheney FW et al: Nerve injury associated with anesthesia: a closed claims study. *Anesthesiology*. 1999;90:1062.

► Maintenance of General Anesthesia

Once the airway is safely secured, anesthesiologists commonly maintain the anesthetic with a combination of an inhalation agent, nitrous oxide, opiate, and muscle relaxant. This "balanced anesthetic" allows for titration of agents to maintain the requirements of anesthesia: analgesia, amnesia (unconsciousness), skeletal muscle relaxation, and control of the hemodynamic responses to surgical stimulation. Drugs with specific pharmacologic profiles are chosen to help satisfy the anesthetic requirements. Analgesia is provided by opiates and inhalational agents; amnesia is provided by benzodiazepines, nitrous oxide, and inhalation agents; and muscle relaxation is provided by neuromuscular blocking drugs, inhaled agents, or local anesthetics. The provision of the right amount of muscle relaxation to facilitate the procedure but not too much to obscure a clinical sign of anesthetic depth or to result in prolonged relaxation postoperatively presents a challenge to the anesthesiologist. A peripheral nerve stimulator can monitor muscle relaxation such that the relaxant is reversible at the end of the case to allow for safe extubation.

► Regional Anesthesia for Surgery

Many operations require no general anesthetic. These include almost any procedure done below the waist, on lower abdomen, and on the upper extremities. Spinal or epidural anesthesia provide excellent muscle relaxation, profound analgesia, and avoidance of airway manipulation, and allows the patient to be conscious. Spinal or epidural anesthesia have additional advantages: decreased blood loss during orthopedic procedures, fewer thrombotic complications, less pulmonary compromise, maintenance of vasodilatation for postoperative vascular surgeries, earlier hospital discharge, and avoidance of immune response compromise.

A. Spinal Anesthesia

Most spinal anesthetics are performed in either the lateral position or with the patient sitting on the operating table.

Following sterile prep and local skin anesthetic, a small 25-27 gauge spinal needle is introduced in the lower lumbar spine, and the subdural space is identified by the presence of cerebrospinal fluid (CSF). Depending on the planned length of surgery, either lidocaine or bupivacaine (with or without epinephrine or an opiate) is injected. Lidocaine spinal anesthesia provides at most 2 hours of anesthesia, while bupivacaine provides up to 5 hours of anesthesia. However, due to patient discomfort from tourniquet break-through pain, the use of orthopedic tourniquets limits the usefulness of spinals no matter which local anesthetic is used to no more than 2 hours. Once the local agent is injected, patients are placed in the supine position for 5-10 minutes to allow for proper spread of the local anesthetic. During this time, blood pressure and heart rate are monitored; both hypotension and bradycardia can be induced by a sympathectomy due to the cephalad spread of the local. During this 5-10 minute period, patient movement should be limited. Once the block has stabilized, the surgical preparation and positioning can proceed. The anesthesiologist monitors the patient in the same manner as for general anesthesia and administers sedation as needed.

Other than expected hemodynamic changes, the most common complication of spinal anesthesia is postspinal headaches. The incidence is very low when smaller-gauge spinal needles are used and are more common in young women. The spinal headache is almost always positional and abates when the patient is recumbent. Severe headaches can result in diplopia because of stretching of the sixth cranial nerve as the brain sinks from loss of CSF. Patients usually complain of the headache a day or two following the operation. Conservative treatment is the maintenance of adequate hydration, remaining recumbent, and an analgesic such as acetaminophen. Severe headache may require a "blood patch" to plug the leak of CSF and is performed by an anesthesiologist.

B. Epidural Anesthesia

Epidural anesthesia has several distinct differences from spinal anesthesia. The epidural space is between the ligamentum flavum and the dural structures; in placing an epidural, the subdural space is not entered, so no CSF leak is created with the potential for a spinal headache. The epidural anesthetic may be continued by insertion of a small catheter into the epidural space. Additional local anesthetic can be added to move the block to higher spinal levels or to maintain the selected level of anesthesia. This continuous epidural technique can be used for postoperative pain control. The catheter can be placed at spinal levels in the midthoracic region for thoracotomy or lower thoracic or lumbar region for abdominal operations or lower extremity procedures. Epidural anesthesia requires the administration of high volumes of local anesthetics. There is the potential for intravascular injection with resultant cardiovascular compromise

or high block. There is also the potential for misplacement of the catheter or epidural needle in the subarachnoid space. Instillation of the larger volumes of local in the subarachnoid space can result in a total spinal or high block with resultant cardiovascular collapse. Therefore, small test doses of local anesthetic are administered to evaluate for signs of intravenous injection or high block. Another potential disadvantage of epidural anesthesia is that the onset is much slower than spinal anesthesia. The same hemodynamic changes observed with epidural can occur with spinals.

A common complication of both spinal and epidural anesthesia is prolonged blockade of parasympathetic fibers that innervate the bladder with resultant urinary retention and the need for a urinary bladder catheter.

C. Peripheral Nerve Block

True regional anesthesia is useful for procedures on the extremities. Useful anesthesia of the upper extremity can be obtained by blockade of the brachial plexus using an interscalene approach, a supraclavicular approach, or an axillary approach. Lower extremity surgery may be performed utilizing blockade of the lumbar plexus and its major branches: femoral nerve, sciatic nerve, lateral femoral cutaneous nerve, obturator nerve, and popliteal nerve. In some instances, a catheter can be placed near the nerve or plexus to allow for continuous blockade and postoperative pain control. The usefulness of these blocks for extremity surgery is limited in time by the use of tourniquets if the patient is to remain awake during the procedure. These blocks are very useful if avoidance of a general anesthetic is desired. Additional advantages of peripheral nerve blocks include earlier discharge from recovery areas and return to home, lack of administration of large doses of opiates, less nausea and vomiting, no instrumentation of patient airway, and earlier ambulation. Intraoperative sedation may be provided, and the anesthesiologist monitors the patient in the standard manner.

▶ Monitored Anesthesia Care

Monitored anesthesia care (MAC) was previously termed local anesthesia with standby. The "standby" is an anesthesia caregiver who monitors the patient's status while the surgeon performs a procedure under local anesthesia. The anesthesiologist can also provide sedation and analgesia as needed for the patient. This type of anesthesia is usually requested by the surgeon for patients who may be especially frail in health; it provides the option to convert to a general anesthetic if necessary.

▶ Completion of Surgery

At the end of the procedure, most often patients who have been intubated for the surgery have their muscle relaxation reversed and the anesthetic depth decreased to allow them to return to consciousness. Once the return of muscle function has been assured and the patient is able to respond to commands, the endotracheal tube can be removed and the patient closely observed to ensure adequate ventilation. Patients are then transferred to a stretcher and transported to the PACU, accompanied by a member of the anesthesia care team who monitors the patient's condition during transport. Many institutions require that a member of the surgical team also accompany the patient to the PACU along with the anesthesiologist. Some critically ill patients are transported directly to the intensive care unit (ICU), still intubated, sedated, and ventilated.

Postanesthesia Recovery Room

The PACU, most commonly known as the recovery room, is where most patients are transferred after surgery. The PACU is the designated area in which patients receive postanesthesia monitoring of vital signs as well as the beginning of the nursing care for their surgical recovery. It is the standard of the American Society of Anesthesiologists that all patients, regardless of the type of anesthesia, receive appropriate postanesthesia care, either in a PACU or an equivalent area such as a critical care unit. An exception to this standard can only be made by the anesthesiologist responsible for the patient's care. Once in the PACU, a verbal report is provided to the responsible PACU nurse by a member of the anesthesia care team who is familiar with and who accompanied the patient during transport. The surgeon can also give a report as to the surgical issues that may impact on the patient's recovery.

The PACU is equipped with essentially the same monitors as the operating room and with the drugs and equipment needed for emergency resuscitation. The PACU is a specialized, short-stay ICU. PACUs are staffed with specially trained nurses to monitor patients who are recovering from the anesthetic. Patients are continually monitored in the PACU for approximately 1 hour or until they fulfill specific objective criteria. Discharge from the PACU requires the clinical judgment of the PACU team. Particular attention is focused on the monitoring of oxygenation, ventilation, circulation, level of consciousness, and temperature.

Most PACUs use a discharge scoring system (egg, the Aldrete score) describing objective criteria that must be fulfilled before the patient can be discharged from the PACU. These criteria include quantitative analysis of patient's ability to move extremities in response to verbal commands, adequacy of ventilation (pulse oximetry) circulation (stable vital signs) level of consciousness, and pain control. After outpatient surgery, patients must have an adult to escort them home. Most institutions have policies requiring that anesthesiologists, in conjunction with the PACU nursing team, discharge patients from PACU.

Aldrete JA, Kroulik D: A postanesthetic recovery score. *Anesth Analg.* 1970;49:924.

Awad JT, Chung F: Factors affecting recovery and discharge following ambulatory surgery. *Can J Anaesth.* 2006;53:858.

COMMON POSTOPERATIVE PROBLEMS

There are many reasons why patients have other than a routine stay in the PACU. The three most common PACU problems are hypothermia, nausea and vomiting, and pain control. Hypotension/hypertension, hypoxemia, hypercapnia/hypoventilation, and agitation can also occur.

▶ Hypothermia

A very common complication of anesthesia and surgery is hypothermia. Every effort should be made in the operating room to avoid patients becoming hypothermic, even if this requires that the operating room temperature is maintained at a warmer-than-comfortable level. Patients who are admitted to the PACU and are hypothermic must be rewarmed to avoid the adverse consequence of shivering (ie, increased oxygen consumption). Hypothermia may also have an adverse effect on coagulation parameters and may delay recovery from anesthesia due to decreased drug metabolism. The most effective methods of rewarming are forced-air warming devices or water-jacket devices. Shivering can be actively treated with small doses of meperidine.

Rajagopalan S et al: The effects of mild perioperative hypothermia on blood loss and transfusion requirement. *Anesthesiology.* 2008;108:71.

▶ Postoperative Nausea & Vomiting

According to the Society of Ambulatory Anesthesia (SAMBA), untreated, postoperative nausea and vomiting (PONV) occurs in 20%-30% of the general surgical population and up to 70%-80% in the high-risk surgical population. The increased PACU stays and sometimes hospital admission to control PONV adds to patient discomfort and morbidity and adds a financial burden to the health care system. SAMBA's seven guidelines have been adopted by many health care facilities for the prevention and treatment of PONV.

1. Identify patients at high risk for PONV. The most consistent independent predictors for PONV are female gender, nonsmoking, and a history of PONV or motion sickness, coupled with the anesthesia-related factors of general anesthesia with volatile anesthetics, nitrous oxide, and postoperative opioids.

2. Reduce baseline risk factors for PONV. The most reliable strategy is to use regional anesthesia when possible. Otherwise, propofol used for induction; minimization of intraoperative volatile agents, opioids, and nitrous oxide; and epidurals for postoperative pain management may be the best strategy to reduce PONV.

3. Administer PONV prophylaxis using one or two interventions in adults at moderate risk for PONV. The 5-HT$_3$ receptor antagonists (ondansetron, dolasetron, granisetron), dexamethasone, and low-dose droperidol are among the most effective first-line antiemetics for PONV prophylaxis: Each independently reduces PONV by 25%. It is recommended that adults who present with moderate risk for PONV receive a combination therapy for prophylaxis with drugs from different classes and different mechanisms. A new drug, aprepitant, a neurokinin-1 (NK-1) receptor antagonist has been shown to significantly reduce PONV given alone or in combination with the 5-HT$_3$s.

4. For patients at high risk for PONV, SAMBA recommends a multimodal approach to prophylaxis that includes using two or more interventions and trying to reduce the baseline factors (eg, anxiolysis), minimizing the anesthetic agents chosen, and using the pharmacologic interventions mentioned above.

5. Administer prophylactic antiemetics to children at high risk for PONV. Use the same combination therapy as in adults.

6. Some patients have no risk factors for PONV and therefore receive no prophylaxis but develop PONV postoperatively. Recommended treatment is to begin with low-dose 5-HT$_3$ antagonist, which is the only class of drugs that has been adequately studied to be effective for the treatment of existing PONV.

7. If rescue therapy for patients who have received prophylaxis is required, it is recommended that the antiemetic(s) chosen should be from a different therapeutic class than the drugs used for prophylaxis.

Gan TJ et al: Society for Ambulatory Anesthesia guidelines for the management of postoperative nausea and vomiting. *Anesth Analg.* 2007;1051:615.

▶ Postoperative Acute Pain Management

The management of postoperative surgical pain is the responsibility of both the anesthesiology and surgery services. Other than PONV, inadequate postoperative pain control is a primary cause of unanticipated hospital admission for outpatient surgery. The severity of the pain is usually site dependent (upper abdominal procedures tend to be more painful than lower abdominal procedures; ie, appendectomy is more painful than inguinal hernia, which is more painful than minor chest wall surgery), but the individual patient's response to the pain and efforts to treat it vary widely. What may appear to be a minor incision to some may be very painful to others. The clinical challenge of providing adequate postoperative pain management is also a major mandate by JCAHO and the national media. Thus, almost every anesthesia department has an acute pain management team that can help with the management of patients in PACU and later in the surgical intensive care or general care unit.

Morphine has been the historical postoperative analgesic, administered either intramuscularly or intravenously. Patient response to a standardized administration protocol is variable, however, and can fail to control pain or cause symptoms of overdosage. Every patient is different in the required serum concentration of drug that results in adequate pain control.

There are four common modalities or approaches to postoperative pain management:

Oral medications. For minor procedures, for example, excision of skin lesions, nonsteroidal analgesics may be sufficient. For more intense levels of pain, oral narcotics in combination with acetaminophen are often effective.

Intravenous opioids. Occasionally, one or two intravenous doses of morphine, hydromorphone, or fentanyl may be sufficient to control postoperative pain. However, a more reliable method is the administration of small doses of narcotic given on demand by the patient. Patient-controlled analgesia (PCA) uses the same or even less total narcotic to control pain and is as safe as intramuscular medications. Patients are instructed on how to use the PCA device to administer narcotic on demand. PCA has widespread acceptance by patients, physicians, and nurses because it provides pain control in a timely manner that more closely matches the patient's requirements. Caution must be used when pain control appears to be inadequate and house staff covering the patient are tempted to give an intravenous "boost" of narcotic.

Epidural opiate analgesia. The application of opioids or narcotics at the neuraxial receptor sites via an epidural catheter is probably the modality of choice for severe acute postoperative pain control. An epidural catheter is preferably placed preoperatively at a spinal dermatome level close to the site of incision: midthoracic level for thoracic surgeries, lower thoracic for upper abdominal surgeries, or lumbar for lower abdominal incisions or lower extremity surgeries. This technique utilizes a continuous infusion of a combined solution of a low concentration of local anesthetic (bupivacaine 0.125 mg/cc) and an opioid (morphine, hydromorphone, or fentanyl). This modality does not require patient cooperation but can be used in a PCA mode. Epidural analgesia can be continued for multiple days; it has beneficial effects for maintaining peripheral vasodilatation after vascular procedures and improving respiratory mechanics due to reduced pain when patients are breathing on their own. Patients must be monitored for respiratory depression while receiving epidural analgesia, as respiratory depression is the major complication from this pain control therapy.

Specific nerve or plexus block. Local anesthesia block of single nerves or continuous catheter infusion of local anesthetic around major nerve plexuses is becoming more popular. Examples include single injection or placement of a continuous catheter around the femoral nerve for controlling pain from knee surgery and continuous catheters around the brachial plexus (usually supraclavicular) for controlling pain from upper extremity surgery.

► Complications of Anesthesia

No matter how well patients are prepared for anesthesia and surgery, there is always the possibility of a complication from the delivery of anesthesia. These complications can be minor in nature (eg, intravenous infiltration, hypothermia, or minor ocular injury) or major issues (eg, an unanticipated difficult airway that may result in significant morbidity or death). Many complications are preventable with good preoperative preparation, but some are not preventable (unexpected drug reactions or metabolic crisis, eg, malignant hyperthermia). Four common complications are anesthesia awareness, peripheral nerve injury, malignant hyperthermia, and visual loss.

► Awareness

Many patients are concerned about being aware during the surgical procedure. Intraoperative awareness under general anesthesia is rare with a reported incidence of 0.1%-0.2%. Intraoperative awareness does occur and can lead to significant psychological sequelae and extended disability for the patient. Certain types of surgery have a higher incidence of intraoperative awareness, including cardiac surgery, major trauma, and obstetrics. All are associated with critical or life-threatening situations of hemodynamic compromise that make awareness unavoidable if the caregiver is to achieve other critical anesthetic goals of maintaining cardiac, respiratory, and vascular homeostasis. The Practice Advisory from the American Board of Anesthesiologists defines intraoperative awareness: "When a patient becomes conscious when a surgical procedure is performed under a general anesthetic and subsequently has (explicit) recall of these events." The Advisory notes that the recall does not include the time before the general anesthetic is induced or the time of intentional emergence and return to consciousness.

Strategies suggested to lessen or eliminate the risk of intraoperative awareness include the following:

1. Preoperative evaluation. Patients with a history of previous intraoperative awareness, substance abuse, chronic use of opioids for pain control, and limited hemodynamic reserve have increased risk for intraoperative awareness. Such patients undergoing high-risk operations should be informed of the potential for awareness. There is no consensus that informing all patients about the possibility of intraoperative awareness leads to higher incidence of awareness.

2. Preanesthesia preparation. A strict preoperative equipment checklist involving the anesthesia machine and its components, for example, the volatile anesthesia vaporizer agent levels, is mandatory. Although this strategy does not prevent human errors, it does provide the anesthesiologist a constant reminder that there are preventable components to the complication of awareness.

3a. Intraoperative monitoring. The currently accepted strategy is to utilize all the standard anesthesia patient monitors (EKG, blood pressure measurements, heart rate monitors, continuous agent analyzers, and capnography) and to intermittently assess for purposeful or reflex movement to detect intraoperative consciousness. There are instances in which there were no reported changes in vital signs in patients who have reported recall.

3b. Monitoring brain electrical activity. Several monitoring devices are claimed to be able to interpret data from the processed, raw electroencephalogram of patients and correlate it to the depth of anesthesia and thus help prevent recall under general anesthesia. The commonest device currently available is known as the bispectral index monitor (BIS; Aspect Medical Systems, Natick, MA). Currently, the use of BIS for patients undergoing general anesthesia has not been shown to offer any advantage over a protocol that uses end-tidal anesthetic agent concentrations in decreasing the incidence of intraoperative awareness.

In conclusion, when awareness occurs, either reported spontaneously by the patient in the postoperative period or elicited during the postoperative visit by the anesthesiologist, the patient's report must be taken seriously. Some patients will require significant counseling and treatment postoperatively, and caregivers should be sensitive to the potential issue and offer any help requested.

American Board of Anesthesiologists: Practice advisory for intraoperative awareness and brain function monitoring. *Anesthesiology.* 2006;104:847.

Avidan MS et al: Prevention of intraoperative awareness in a high-risk surgical population. *N Engl J Med.* 2011;591-600.

► Peripheral Nerve Injury

Peripheral nerve injury is a known complication of anesthesia and can occur under general anesthesia or a regional technique. These injuries are almost always due to patient positioning and the patient's inability to report and respond to abnormal pressure points or awkward position of an extremity. The ulnar nerve at the elbow is the most common injury and occurs even if the patient has had what was felt to be adequate padding provided for protection. Other peripheral nerves that are less commonly injured include the peroneal nerve at the knee and the radial nerve as it passes through the spiral grove of the humerus. The peroneal nerve is typically injured by abnormal position against a lithotomy stirrup, and the radial nerve is injured by a blood pressure cuff or abnormal pressure from surgical towels. Patients usually report numbness along the course of the nerve, but some motor weakness may also occur. These injuries usually resolve in a short time period. Abnormal stretching of the brachial plexus from extreme abduction of the arms, improperly placed shoulder braces, or chest wall retractors during cardiac surgery may result in more serious injuries, including not only sensory but motor loss that may not recover as rapidly or completely as the ulnar, radial, or peroneal nerves. More severe injuries that involve motor loss need to have a baseline examination established and therapy started. Since most of these peripheral nerve injuries are due to malpositioning during surgery, it is the responsibility of surgeons, nurses, and anesthesiologists to adequately position patients and provide sufficient padding or other protection.

Welch MB, Brummett CM, Welch TD, et al: Perioperative peripheral nerve injuries: a retrospective study of 380,680 cases during a 10-year period at a single institution. *Anesthesiology.* 2009;111:490-497.

Malignant Hyperthermia

Malignant hyperthermia is a rare, genetically inherited disease characterized by intense muscle contraction. It results from an uncontrolled release of calcium from the sarcoplasmic reticulum and massive increase of intracellular calcium in skeletal muscle due to the inability of the calcium to be reabsorbed. This intense muscle contraction leads to a hypermetabolic state manifest by hyperthermia, hypercapnia, tachycardia, and metabolic acidosis. It is fatal if untreated. Malignant hyperthermia is commonly triggered by the administration of anesthetic agents; the depolarizing muscle relaxant succinylcholine alone or in conjunction with a volatile agent. The more modern anesthetic vapors sevoflurane and desflurane are less frequently implicated as triggers. Early clinical manifestations of malignant hyperthermia include unexplained tachycardia and metabolic acidosis, but temperature elevation may be a late finding. Although not always reliable, the earliest sign of malignant hyperthermia is sometimes masseter spasm following the administration of succinylcholine during induction. Careful monitoring must always ensue. Relying on temperature elevation alone is dangerous, and arterial blood gases must be monitored for unexplained metabolic acidosis. In some patients, malignant hyperthermia develops insidiously during the surgery, and temperature elevation can be the first manifestation.

Malignant hyperthermia is treatable and preventable. The treatment of choice is intravenous dantrolene. Every operating room must have a malignant hyperthermia protocol and a kit that includes multiple doses of dantrolene. Dantrolene is supplied as a powder and requires several minutes to mix it into a useable intravenous solution. Malignant hyperther-

mia is a true anesthesia emergency, and the anesthesiologist will require assistance from the operative team. The surgical procedure may have to be postponed. Successful treatment of malignant hyperthermia is the usual outcome. Patients should be monitored in a critical care unit for 24 hours or until stable and referred for confirmatory testing.

Malignant hyperthermic reactions can be prevented. Any patient with a personal or family history of malignant hyperthermia should be administered a completely nontriggering anesthetic without relying on succinylcholine or volatile agents.

Hopkins PH: Malignant hyperthermia. *Trends Anaesthes Crit Care.* 2008;19(1):22-33.

Perioperative Visual Loss

A recently described complication of prolonged (> 6.5 hours) spinal surgical procedures performed in the prone position, associated with large blood losses, is partial or complete visual loss. Vision loss seems to be associated with an ischemic optic neuropathy without any known etiology. There does not seem to be any identifiable pre-op patient characteristic. Intraoperative management for patients undergoing prolonged procedures involving substantial blood loss include continuous blood pressure monitoring and CVP monitoring. There is no consensus on lower limits of hematocrit, limits of vasopressors, or prone positioning. There is no known treatment. The risk of visual loss should be discussed with patients in the preoperative phase of surgery and anesthesia for those operations that require prone positioning.

Apfelbaum JL et al: Practice Advisory for Perioperative Visual Loss Associated with Spine Surgery. An Updated Report by the American Society of Anesthesiologists Task Force on Perioperative Visual Loss. *Anesthesiology.* 2012;116:274-285.

MULTIPLE CHOICE QUESTIONS

1. Many patients take over-the-counter herbal remedies. In the perioperative period patients should be advised

   A. To continue taking their usual herbal remedies
   B. Stop only those remedies that have been approved by their physician
   C. Continue taking only those remedies that have been approved by the FDA
   D. Stop all over-the-counter herbal remedies

2. Regarding the timing of the preoperative anesthesia workup for patients scheduled for a surgical procedure

   A. The initial assessment can be done the day of surgery for healthy patients undergoing procedures of high surgical invasiveness.

B. The initial assessment should be done at a minimum the day before surgery for patients undergoing procedures of high surgical invasiveness.

C. The preoperative assessment for healthy patients by an anesthesiologist is not required.

D. A note from the patient's primary care physician stating that the patient is "cleared for anesthesia and surgery" will suffice as the preoperative assessment.

3. Regarding patients who have had a recent drug-eluting stent placed and scheduled for an elective surgical procedure with a high risk of bleeding

A. Surgery may be performed within 4 weeks of stent placement as long as the patient continues taking aspirin and clopidogrel.

B. Surgery may be performed within 4 weeks of stent placement with the patient stopping the clopidogrel and continuing on low-dose aspirin.

C. Should have the surgical procedure delayed until the procedure can be performed with the patient only taking low-dose aspirin.

D. Surgery should be delayed for up to 1 year.

4. Strategies to prevent intraoperative awareness include

A. Strict monitoring of intraoperative vital signs by the anesthesiologist will always detect intraoperative awareness

B. Informing patients during the preoperative workup of the possibility of awareness

C. Monitoring brain electrical activity with the BIS monitor

D. None of the above

5. The preoperative assessment by an anesthesiologist includes an assessment of a patient's risk for an intraoperative cardiac event. The RCRI factors include all of the following except

A. A history of ischemic heart disease

B. Diabetes mellitus

C. Obesity

D. Renal insufficiency

E. High-risk surgery

F. Heart failure

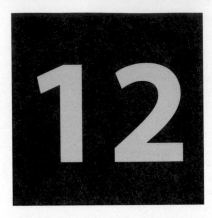

Shock & Acute Pulmonary Failure in Surgical Patients

James W. Holcroft, MD

John T. Anderson, MD

Matthew J. Sena, MD

INITIAL TREATMENT OF SHOCK

Cardiovascular failure, or shock, can be caused by (1) depletion of the vascular volume; (2) compression of the heart or great veins; (3) intrinsic failure of the heart itself or failure arising from excessive hindrance to ventricular ejection; (4) loss of autonomic control of the vasculature; (5) severe untreated systemic inflammation; and (6) severe but partially compensated systemic inflammation. If the shock is decompensated, the mean blood pressure or the cardiac output (more precisely, the product of the pressure and output) will be inadequate for peripheral perfusion. In compensated shock, the perfusion will be adequate but only at the expense of excessive demands on the heart. Depending on the type and severity of cardiovascular failure and on response to treatment, shock can go on to compromise other organ systems. This chapter discusses the cardiovascular and pulmonary disorders associated with shock.

HYPOVOLEMIC SHOCK

► Diagnosis

Hypovolemic shock (shock caused by inadequate circulating blood volume) is most often caused by bleeding but may also be a consequence of protracted vomiting or diarrhea, sequestration of fluid in the gut lumen (eg, bowel obstruction), or loss of plasma into injured or burned tissues. Regardless of the etiology, the compensatory responses, mediated primarily by the adrenergic nervous system, are the same: (1) constriction of the venules and small veins in the skin, fat, skeletal muscle, and viscera with displacement of blood from the peripheral capacitance vessels to the heart; (2) constriction of arterioles in the skin, skeletal muscle, gut, pancreas, spleen, and liver (but not the brain or heart); (3) improved cardiac performance through an increase in heart rate and contractility; and (4) increased sodium and

water reabsorption through renin-angiotensin-aldosterone as well as vasopressin release. The result is improved cardiac filling, increased cardiac output (both directly by the increase in contractility and indirectly through increased end-diastolic volumes), and increased blood flow to organs with no or limited tolerance for ischemia (brain and heart).

The symptoms and signs of hypovolemic shock are many and can be caused either by the inadequate blood volume or by the compensatory responses. Some signs manifest themselves early, in mild forms of shock. Some present late and only in severe forms of shock. The goal is to pick up on the early signs. Doing so can save a life.

As early signs of shock, the physician might find it difficult to gain intravenous access. The skin might be cold (a nonspecific sign, but an early sign). But, by far and away, the most important, that is, most sensitive, of all the early signs of hypovolemic shock is diminished blood flow to the skin and subcutaneous tissues. It is a sign that needs to be elicited with care. It can be missed. It is best detected in the skin on the plantar surface of the foot, an area without pigmentation, with the color determined solely by the blood contained in the tissues. One begins by compressing the skin over the plantar surface of a toe with intense pressure, just short of being painful, followed by milking of the blood contained in the compressed area proximally, to the skin over the metatarsal phalangeal joint. The compression is then suddenly released. The previously compressed area will be profoundly pale, but will fill quickly, within a few seconds, if the patient is not in shock (and does not have peripheral vascular disease). In a hypovolemic patient, the refill takes longer. The test is usually done with the foot at the level of the heart, but if the patient is reasonably stable and if the lower extremities are not injured, it is more sensitive if it can be done with the foot raised above the level of the heart, to a height of perhaps 30 cm. Although the toe is usually used, one can also use the skin over the heel. The heel affords a larger surface for observation. One has to use different criteria, however. If the toe is used, color should begin to return within 4 seconds; if the heel is used, color should return in 2 seconds.

Postural hypotension—a fall in the systolic blood pressure of more than 10 mm Hg that persists for more than 1 minute when the patient sits up—can be a sign of early or mild shock. It is very useful in patients who are suspected of being hypovolemic from either dehydration or occult internal blood loss (eg, in a patient who might have gastrointestinal bleeding). It cannot be used, however, in very ill patients and in injured patients, who might not tolerate changes in position.

Low filling pressures in the right atrium are always present in hypovolemic shock, even in cases of mild shock, assuming there is no accompanying cardiac compression. Filling pressures high enough to distend the neck veins when the patient's head, neck, and torso are elevated 30 degrees, in the absence of cardiac compression, rule out hypovolemic shock. Failure to see the veins suggests, but is not diagnostic of, hypovolemia.

Oliguria is a consistent finding in early shock, in the absence of a hyperosmolar-induced diuresis. A bladder catheter should be inserted in any patient suspected of being hypovolemic. Urine output is considered to be potentially inadequate if it is less than 0.5 mL/kg/h in an adult, less than 1 mL/kg/h in a child, or less than 2 mL/kg/h in an infant. The sign, if present, is both sensitive and specific. One must wait, however, for 30 minutes or so, before one knows that the sign is present.

The hematocrit will fall within minutes in the bleeding patient, or in the patient who has bled, even when the blood loss is mild, if the patient has been given asanguineous fluids. In the absence of fluid administration, however, the fall can take hours—restitution of the intravascular volume from interstitial albumin and water and electrolytes, takes time. One can make an estimate of the blood loss, if the patient has been given asanguineous fluids, by the magnitude of the fall in the hematocrit. A hematocrit fall of 3%-4% indicates that the blood volume was depleted by about 10%; a fall of 6%-8% indicates a depletion of about 20% (or 1 L in an average adult). These calculations assume that the patient has been given enough fluid to correct the hypovolemia. They also assume that the patient was not dehydrated, prior to the hemorrhage, and that the patient did not have large loses of plasma into the extravascular spaces, as in a patient with large burns, prior to a possible hemorrhage. The hematocrit in these patients can be normal in the face of even substantial bleeding.

Hypovolemic shock is easier to recognize when it becomes more severe. In moderate cases (a deficit of 20%-30% of the blood volume), the patient can be thirsty. Hypotension can be present, even in the supine position. A metabolic acidemia, usually with a compensatory rapid respiratory rate, can develop after initial resuscitation. (The acidemia is usually not present before resuscitation. The products of anaerobic metabolism in the ischemic tissues are only flushed into the circulating blood volume once some degree of reperfusion has been achieved.)

In profound hypovolemic shock (a deficit of more than 30% of blood volume), the blood pressure will always be low, even in the supine position. Cerebral and cardiac perfusion can become inadequate. Signs of the former include changes in mental status, restlessness, agitation, confusion, lethargy, or the appearance of inebriation; signs of the latter include an irregular heartbeat or electrocardiographic evidence of myocardial ischemia, such as ST–T segment depression and, over time, the appearance of Q waves. A metabolic acidemia will always be present, after initial resuscitation.

There are many pitfalls in making the diagnosis of hypovolemic shock, and every clinician will miss the diagnosis on occasion. In some patients, especially children and young adults, strong compensatory mechanisms can maintain the blood pressure at normal levels in the setting of mild to moderate shock. In other patients, one might not know if the observed pressure is abnormally low—a young patient might normally have systolic pressures in the low 100s; the same pressure in a chronically hypertensive patient might precede catastrophe. Pain-producing injuries in the absence of blood loss should produce hypertension; a normal pressure in a patient with a pain-producing injury suggests hypovolemia. Administration of a sedative or narcotic in the face of hypovolemia can produce hypotension but usually has no effect on the pressure in a normovolemic subject—one should not ascribe hypotension to sedatives or narcotics until the possibility of hypovolemia has been ruled out.

The heart rate is notoriously unreliable as a sign of hypovolemic shock. Although it increases in response to graded hemorrhage in anesthetized animals, the correlation between hypovolemia and heart rate in unanesthetized human beings is poor. Unanesthetized hypovolemic human beings often have normal heart rates. Severe hypovolemia can even produce bradycardia, as the cardiovascular system makes a last attempt to allow filling of the ventricles during diastole. A normal heart rate provides no assurance that the patient is not in shock. (A rapid heart rate, however, has to be taken seriously. It might be the only indication of shock. The pitfall is in the assumption that a normal heart rate rules out shock.)

There are at least three other pitfalls that can lead to missing the diagnosis of shock: (1) the cutaneous vasoconstriction of hypovolemic shock can be ablated by the vasodilation induced by alcohol or other pharmacologic agents, both therapeutic and recreational; the patient might have well-perfused skin even when hypovolemic; (2) the oliguria of shock can be overcome by an osmotic diuresis induced by high blood alcohol or glucose levels; and (3) shock can cause alterations in mental status that resemble intoxication with drug use or inebriation. If so, the patient might be in a preterminal state, in which the shock is so severe that cerebral blood flow becomes inadequate. The diagnosis of drug or alcohol use, as the cause of the mental abnormalities, should only be made after shock has been ruled out.

▶ Treatment

A. Airway and Ventilation

Resuscitation of patients in hypovolemic shock, either hemorrhagic or nonhemorrhagic, begins with ensuring adequacy of the airway. In many patients in shock, especially severe shock, this means preemptive intubation and mechanical ventilation. The physician cannot let uncertainty about the airway interfere with evaluation and resuscitation of other problems in the often confusing picture of shock. A patient who later turns out to need no support for the airway or ventilation can easily be extubated; failure to intubate a patient who later loses control of an airway or who can no longer ventilate means, at the least, an emergency intubation under difficult conditions and, at the worse, anoxic brain damage or death. This approach is different from the approach for medical patients with decompensated chronic obstructive lung disease, in whom intubation can mean prolonged mechanical ventilation and perhaps even failure to ever extubate. Those patients have such severe underlying pulmonary disease that even under baseline conditions they have trouble breathing. The baseline condition in surgical patients is usually perfectly adequate pulmonary function. Once the possible surgical problems are ruled out or dealt with, there is usually no problem with extubation.

If the patient requires mechanical ventilation, and almost all patients intubated for shock do, volume control ventilation, or some variant thereof, is preferable, in the initial phases of resuscitation (in the latter phases, after the dust has settled, we usually use pressure modulated ventilation—see the section in this chapter on Treatment of Acute Pulmonary Failure). The tidal volume is set at 7 mL/kg ideal body weight (IBW); the inspiratory time, at 1 second; the respiratory rate, at 15 breaths/min; and the end expiratory pressure, at 0 cm H_2O, with all of these settings designed to minimize the mean airway pressure. To maintain adequate arterial oxygen saturation, the inspired oxygen concentration is set at 1.00. (The oxygen concentrations can be decreased later, after blood gases come back and the patient is more stable.)

The quick-to-intubate-and-ventilate approach described above pertains to all patients in shock with one exception—patients who present immediately after injury with life-threatening torso hemorrhage. The bleeding can be into the abdomen or **into** the chest or **into** the pericardium. The diagnosis is usually made on the basis of the clinical setting or on sonographic imaging. Some of these patients have to be intubated in the emergency room. If possible, however, one should delay intubation until the patient is in the operating room (which is the immediate destination for all of

these patients, once the problem of exsanguinating cavitary hemorrhage is recognized).

A patient in profound shock from bleeding **into** the torso can suddenly deteriorate, to the point of losing his vital signs, with intubation and initiation of positive pressure ventilation. Positive pressure ventilation has effects on the cardiovascular system. All of them are bad, and all are worsened in the face of hypovolemia. The positive pressure compresses the superior and inferior venae cavae, increasing the time needed to fill the right atrium and right ventricle during diastole. (Normal negative pressure ventilation, spontaneous ventilation, decreases the time needed.) Positive pressure squeezes the thin-walled chambers of the heart (the atria and the right ventricle), making it harder for the chambers to fill during diastole. (Negative pressure ventilation makes it easier for the chambers to fill.) Positive pressure squeezes the pulmonary artery, pulmonary microvasculature, and pulmonary veins, making it hard for the right ventricle to transmit its generated energy into the pulmonary artery. (Negative pressure makes it easier to transmit the energy.) Positive pressure ventilation also compresses the pulmonary veins, mandating longer times for the left atrium to fill during diastole. (Negative pressure allows for quicker filling.)

If the patient loses his vital signs in the operating room, with intubation, the surgeon and anesthesiologist will be ideally situated to deal definitively with the underlying problems of hemorrhage and airway management. In contrast, if the patient is intubated in the emergency department and loses his vital signs, the team will be at a major disadvantage in dealing with the underlying problems. An example is in the patient with a gunshot wound to the abdomen who losses vital signs shortly after intubation in the emergency department. Opening the chest will be done hastily, under suboptimal conditions and it is unlikely to be of help. The maneuver does not deal with the underlying problem-bleeding **into** the abdomen. The patient needs a celiotomy, which cannot be done in the emergency department.

B. Bleeding

Direct pressure should be the first maneuver in controlling external bleeding from any part of the body. Commercially available tourniquets or improvised pneumatic tourniquets can be used for bleeding from extremities. They are easy to apply and are usually safe for up to 2 hours, with the caveat that bleeding should be controlled quickly so as to minimize tourniquet time. Several commercially available, FDA-approved hemostatic agents are available for temporary control of external bleeding. They have been proven to be effective in prehospital and combat environments and can be effective in the hospital setting as well. Blood in the pleural cavities should be drained with a chest tube. Expansion of the lung will decrease further bleeding from the pulmonary parenchyma through apposition of the visceral and parietal pleurae and will reestablish ventilation through the compressed lung. The tube will also allow monitoring for ongoing bleeding, providing key information that can prompt early operative intervention. Bleeding from pelvic fractures may require temporary binder placement. More definitive control can come later, with angiographic embolization or surgical control. Major long bone fractures should be immobilized. Although it might not be necessary to say, patients with intra-abdominal or intractable intrathoracic bleeding should be prepared for the operating room.

Blind clamping, without direct visualization, in the emergency room, should not be attempted, in the initial control of external bleeding. It can result in target vessel injury or, worse, adjacent venous laceration with increased bleeding.

C. Initial Fluid Resuscitation

Vascular access is best obtained with percutaneously placed, large-bore (ideally 14-gauge or larger) venous catheters. The catheters can be placed in superficial veins in the upper extremities, in central veins at the thoracic outlet, or in the femoral veins; catheters can also be placed in the saphenous veins, by cutdown, or directly into interosseous sites (sternum, tibia, or humerus) using specially designed needle introducer systems (FAST-1, EZ IO), the major advantage of the latter devices being the minimal training required to achieve successful access. Choice of access depends on severity of the shock, pattern of injury, provider experience, and consequences of a complication with the access, should one occur. If veins in the lower extremities are to be used, they must be decannulated within 24 hours to minimize the risk of thrombosis and infection. Gaining central venous access can be dangerous as patients in hypovolemic shock will frequently have collapsed central veins. Urgency of placement predisposes to errors in technique. A pneumothorax or an unintentional arterial puncture in the unstable patient might prove fatal.

Initial fluid resuscitation begins with a warmed crystalloid solution. Either normal saline or lactated Ringer solution can be used. Use of lactate in the resuscitative fluid is reasonable if the shock seems to be severe and if the arterial pH is likely to be less than 7.20. The lactate will buffer the hydrogen ions that are released into the central circulation with the initiation of resuscitation. The resultant lactic acid is then oxidized in the liver to carbon dioxide and water, which are excreted by the lungs and kidneys.

If the arterial pH is not likely to be excessively low, normal saline can be used as the initial resuscitative fluid. A modest hyperchloremic acidemia in the immediate postresuscitative state might favorably change the conformation of albumin molecules, decreasing movement of plasma **into** the interstitium. The acidemia might also increase myocardial contractility.

Blood flow to the liver is not a factor in deciding on lactated Ringer versus normal saline. Even minimal flow, as in severe shock, will be enough to deliver the buffered hydrogen ion to the liver parenchyma. Lactated Ringer should not be used, however, if the patient has preexisting liver disease. Adequate oxidation requires functioning liver cells.

The rate at which the initial crystalloid resuscitation should be given depends on two factors: (1) the severity of the shock and the presence of uncontrolled bleeding. When bleeding has been controlled, resuscitation to normovolemia is the goal. (2) Two L is given as fast as possible, followed by a third liter infused over 10 minutes if necessary. This amount of fluid will resuscitate most patients in whom hemorrhage has been arrested.

If the patient is not resuscitated with this amount of fluid, one should renew the search for bleeding, which might be **into** the chest, abdomen, or retroperitoneum. In addition, one should begin to use blood products, while cutting back on asanguineous fluids.

D. Blood Products

Transfusion therapy can be life saving, but it is not without risk. Transfusion reactions, transmission of blood-borne pathogens, acute lung injury (ALI), and immunomodulation can all arise from the administration of blood products. In the acutely bleeding patient, allogeneic packed red cells should be used when the estimated blood loss exceeds 1.5 L (30% of the blood volume), and possibly earlier if there is the potential for ongoing bleeding or if the patient is at risk for having coronary artery disease (Table 12–1).

In urgent settings, type-O blood should be given to restore circulating blood volume. Rh-positive blood can be given to men and women who are beyond childbearing age; Rh-negative blood has to be used in women of childbearing age. The patient's blood type can be determined within 10 minutes, in most hospitals, and type-specific, uncrossed matched red cells should be used when they become available (except in the case of massive casualties, when type O, Rh-negative universal donor cells should be used, to minimize the chance of giving the wrong type of blood to a misidentified patient). Type specific cells should also be used in the setting of massive transfusion, when crossmatching becomes impossible because of the heterogeneous origin of the circulating cells following rapid blood volume replacement.

If resuscitation is ongoing and if it appears as though the total blood loss is likely to exceed one blood volume in 12 hours, plasma and platelets should be given in amounts sufficient to approximate a 1:1:1 ratio. This should be determined as early as possible to avoid dilutional coagulopathy. "Massive transfusion protocols" can maximize efficient use of blood products through the utilization of predetermined component ratios, bedside refrigeration, and in some cases,

Table 12–1. Hematocrit triggers for transfusion: influence of coronary artery disease (CAD), environment in which the patient is being treated (emergency department vs. intensive care unit), and likelihood of bleeding.

Coronary Artery Disease (CAD)	Environment	Likelihood of Bleeding	Desired Hematocrit (%)
No	ICU	Unlikely	21
No	ICU	Possible	21
No	ED	Unlikely	24
No	ED	Possible	27
Yes	ICU	Unlikely	27[1]
Yes	ICU	Possible	30[2]
Yes	ED	Unlikely	33[2]
Yes	ED	Possible	36[2]

[1]Hematocrit values less than 27 may be sufficient in some patients with treated CAD when there is no risk of bleeding.
[2]Hematocrit values greater than 30 generally serve as a buffer for unanticipated or unmeasurable bleeding. They are not necessary in all patients with CAD.

protocol-driven laboratory monitoring. Crystalloid infusion can be restricted in the case of massive transfusions—adequate amounts of crystalloids will be infused in conjunction with the blood products.

E. Goals of Fluid Resuscitation

Giving excessive amounts of fluids in an effort to restore the blood pressure to normal or supranormal levels will create edema. Edema in the gut can create an abdominal compartment syndrome, with compression of the inferior vena cava, displacement of the diaphragm **into** the chest, and compression of the heart and lungs; edema in the liver can lead to compression of biliary ductules and inability to excrete bilirubin into the gut; edema in the lungs can hinder ventilation and oxygenation; and edema in wounded tissues can impede healing and the ability to fight off infection. Unnecessarily high blood pressures can also potentially exacerbate bleeding. On the other hand, inadequate resuscitation can leave the patient exposed to the many adverse late effects of prolonged shock, such as multiorgan failure.

The primary goal in fluid resuscitation for all forms of shock is the same: restoration of adequate end organ perfusion, the product of the mean pressure perfusing the organ and the blood flow to the organ. Resuscitating to a brachial systolic pressure of 80 mm Hg or a radial pulse

in the bleeding patient is reasonable until hemorrhage has been controlled. (The treating physician will not know the cardiac output or organ blood flow in the early phases of resuscitation, but he or she can use clinical criteria, such as skin perfusion, urine output, and mental status, in managing the patient, along with the blood pressure.) After the bleeding is controlled, a systolic pressure of 90 mm Hg might be reasonable. In the very old, the blood pressure goal should be higher to ensure a cushion of perfusion for the brain, heart, and other viscera that might be supplied by arteries obstructed by atherosclerosis.

One must keep in mind during the resuscitation, however, that using the blood pressure to define severity of shock or to assess the adequacy of resuscitation can be hazardous. Most patients in hypovolemic shock will be able to constrict the arterioles in their skin, muscle, and visceral organs in response to the hypovolemia (the exception being inebriated patients). They can often maintain a normal pressure even in the face of continued shock. One must consider many variables in assessing adequacy of resuscitation, including peripheral perfusion, urine output, mental status, acid-base balance, and resolution of any signs of myocardial ischemia.

F. Correction of Coagulation Abnormalities

After severe trauma or major sepsis, many patients will demonstrate signs of intravascular coagulation, with prolonged clotting times, low platelet counts, decreased fibrinogen levels, and production of fibrin degradation products or fibrin monomers. Correction requires administration of plasma and platelets, especially to patients who continue to bleed and to those with severe head injuries, in whom intracranial bleeding could be devastating.

Traditional replacement of coagulation factors has been done with thawed frozen plasma. The advantages of frozen plasma are logistical; the disadvantage is that it has to be thawed prior to use, which may take from 30 to 60 minutes. Increasingly, trauma centers are using either prethawed plasma or "liquid" plasma that has never been frozen. The advantage of the former is that the product does not have to be thawed; the major disadvantage is the potential for waste. "Liquid" plasma has the potential advantage of increased factor activity with the disadvantage of waste. Finally, there has been interest in developing freeze dried plasma, particularly by the military. Although the Europeans have extensive experience with the product (it is approved for use in Europe), there is currently no FDA approved formulation in the United States.

Over the last decade, pharmacologic therapy for hemorrhage-related coagulopathy has become a standard adjunct in the setting of hemorrhagic shock. In the recent past, recombinant activated factor VII has been used routinely for severely injured patients with ongoing traumatic coagulopathy. Administration of doses between 80 and

100 mcg/kg is generally recommended for coagulopathy in trauma patients. Smaller doses may be useful for warfarin reversal in the setting of intracranial hemorrhage. Due to the mechanism of action, platelet and fibrinogen levels need to be adequate at the time of administration.

Tranexamic acid (TXA) is an antifibrinolytic agent that has recently been adopted for routine use by the military as a pharmacologic adjunct for hemorrhage control (REF). It is being used with increasing frequency in civilian settings. The impetus for use in trauma originated from a large prospective international trial (CRASH-2) as well as a large retrospective cohort of combat casualties. Although there is no universally recommended monitoring when using the product, it seems reasonable to think that it should be particularly useful in the presence of excessive fibrinolysis, which can be assessed with the use of the thromboelastogram (TEG), a test that is being used more and more often in diagnosing fibrinolysis in the bleeding patient.

Using pharmacologic agents to improve hemostasis can lead to procoagulant side effects. These have been well documented with activated factor VII but are less well known with antifibrinolytic agents such as TXA. If the patient is not bleeding and is not at risk for a devastating consequence of rebleeding, one should not give procoagulant factors—they will only fuel the fire of systemic inflammation and coagulation. As with any intervention, the benefit to risk ratio should be individualized.

G. Hypothermia: Prevention and Treatment

Maintenance of normothermia is critical in the setting of hemorrhagic shock. Patients who have significant blood loss may lose the ability to increase metabolic heat production. In addition, initial fluid replacement is often done using room temperature or cold solutions such as crystalloid administered in the field by paramedics or unwarmed blood products in the hospital. The added stress of environmental or surgical exposure can make it difficult to maintain normothermia. The impact cannot be overstated. The adverse effects of hypothermia on coagulopathy can be profound.

For these reasons, hypothermia prevention and treatment should be an immediate and ongoing management priority during resuscitation from hemorrhagic shock. At the very least, one should keep the environment warm, infuse fluids through warmers, and keep the patient covered, as much as possible. These efforts should commence as soon as possible after the injury or after the onset of illness.

H. Modalities to Be Avoided

There is no role for using colloid solutions in the setting of hypovolemic shock except when size and weight of the crystalloid solutions limit their availability, as in treating mass casualties or under wartime conditions. Under these circumstances, solutions containing hetastarch or hypertonic

saline and dextran can be used. Otherwise, colloids provide no benefit over crystalloid solutions, and they add to cost. Vasopressors should not be used in resuscitating neurologically intact hypovolemic patients, except in desperate situations for short periods while the vascular volume is reexpanded. The idea that vasopressors divert flow from nonessential organs to essential organs is ill-conceived. Although some organs can withstand ischemia for longer periods of time than others, there are very few parts of the body that are not essential. Patients given vasopressors in shock are at risk for ischemic gangrene of the limbs, gut necrosis, liver failure, and acute tubular necrosis. Vasopressors, however, are often indicated in patients in neurogenic shock, because those patients may have lost critical physiological compensatory responses (see section on Neurogenic Shock).

Elevation of the lower extremities above the level of the heart (Trendelenburg position) in a normovolemic subject shifts blood to the heart and increases ventricular end-diastolic volumes. In the hypovolemic patient, however, adrenergically mediated venoconstriction has likely already achieved this shift. Thus the position is of little value in treating hypovolemic shock, and its awkwardness can make evaluation and treatment of other problems more complicated. The position, however, is useful for the treatment of neurogenic shock.

In trauma patients, the pneumatic antishock garment can be useful for temporary compression of bleeding sites that cannot be controlled by other means, for temporary stabilization of pelvic fractures, and as a temporary expedient to increase the blood pressure during transport in patients in neurogenic shock. It has no other uses. It limits the physical examination. It precludes use of the veins in the lower part of the body as sites for venous access. It can hinder filling of the ventricles by compressing the inferior vena cava and the renal and hepatic veins. It can hinder left ventricular ejection by compressing the arterioles in the lower body. It can push the diaphragm into the chest and interfere with ventilation. It is of no use in displacing blood from the periphery to the heart in neurologically intact patients—discharge of the adrenergic system will already have achieved that goal.

CARDIAC COMPRESSIVE SHOCK

▶ Diagnosis

Cardiac compressive shock can arise from any condition that compresses the heart or great veins, including pericardial tamponade, tension pneumothorax, massive hemothorax, rupture of the diaphragm with encroachment of abdominal viscera into the chest, and distention of the abdomen with compression of the intra-abdominal great veins and elevation of the diaphragm into the chest. All of these conditions are worsened if the patient has to be mechanically ventilated.

The signs of compressive shock are similar to those of hypovolemic shock—postural hypotension, poor cutaneous perfusion, oliguria, hypotension in the supine position, mental status changes, electrocardiographic signs of myocardial ischemia, metabolic acidemia, and hyperventilation—combined with distended neck veins. The only other type of shock that can produce the combination of poor perfusion associated with distended neck veins is cardiogenic shock, which rarely poses a problem in differential diagnosis. Cardiogenic shock usually develops against a background of evident disease that predisposes to primary myocardial dysfunction. Cardiac compression usually follows trauma or occurs in a setting where mechanical compromise of the heart or great veins can arise from imposition of external pressure (as in a possible pericardial tamponade).

The so-called paradoxic pulse is occasionally helpful in diagnosis. A spontaneous breath in a normovolemic subject without cardiac compression produces little effect on systemic blood pressure. If the heart is compressed, the systolic pressure can fall by more than 10 mm Hg. (In contrast, a fall in the blood pressure with positive pressure ventilation is common and nonspecific, especially in hypovolemic patients; the concept of a paradoxic pulse applies only to patients who are breathing on their own.)

The diagnosis of cardiac compression is facilitated if the patient can be monitored in an intensive care unit (ICU) with a pulmonary artery catheter, when small stroke volumes in the face of high filling pressures can be documented by direct measurement. In addition, the catheter can be used to compare pressures in the left and right atria. Under normal circumstances, the pressure in the left atrium is about 5 mm Hg higher than in the right. In tamponade, the pressures are the same.

▶ Treatment

Infusion of fluid can transiently overcome some of the ill effects of cardiac compression, but the cause of shock in these patients is mechanical, and definitive treatment must correct the mechanical abnormality. Treatment of compressive shock caused by large-volume, high-pressure mechanical ventilation is discussed later in this chapter in the section on mechanical ventilation.

CARDIOGENIC SHOCK

▶ Diagnosis

Cardiogenic shock can arise from several causes, including arrhythmias, ischemia-induced myocardial failure, valvular or septal defects, systemic or pulmonary hypertension, myocarditis, and myocardiopathies. Of all the forms of shock, it can be the most resistant to treatment. If the heart cannot pump, there may be nothing that can be done. On the other hand, in less severe cases, it is possible to improve the efficiency of the pumping capability that remains.

The diagnosis of cardiogenic shock usually depends on recognizing an underlying medical condition predisposing the heart to dysfunction in conjunction with an abnormal electrocardiogram. Given the relative oxygen demands of the left and right ventricles, shock caused by left ventricular failure is much more common in patients with ischemic heart disease and typically presents with chest pain, a third heart sound, rales, ST segment elevation on a 12-lead electrocardiogram, and, on chest film, an enlarged heart or pulmonary edema. Cardiogenic shock may be associated with distended neck veins if the right ventricle has failed, unless the patient is also hypovolemic, as in a bleeding patient with a recent myocardial infarction. In many cases, patients with recent shock or trauma may have mild to moderate forms of right ventricular dysfunction related primarily to the heart's response to systemic inflammation or elevated ventilator pressures. Right-sided dysfunction can be associated with peripheral edema, an enlarged and tender liver, and, on chest film, an enlarged heart. The diagnosis is usually easy, but two common situations may pose a problem.

The first is a ruptured abdominal aortic aneurysm in a patient with coronary artery disease. The patient might have abdominal pain consistent with a myocardial infarction and electrocardiographic signs of ischemia—the ischemia being caused by hypovolemia and shock. The key is to observe the neck veins.

The second is to ascribe shock to myocardial contusion in a patient who has just suffered a blunt injury to the chest. Although blunt chest trauma can damage the heart, the damage is usually either fatal, with death at the scene of the injury, or, more often, of no clinical significance. A contusion that produces failure but not death is rare. Shock after blunt trauma in a patient who survives to reach the hospital is almost never caused by contusion—it is far more likely to be caused by hypovolemia or by a mechanical problem.

▶ Treatment

A. Initial Management of Dysrhythmias

In the initial treatment of acute dysrhythmias, we use the approach described by Ursic and Harken (ref in the ACS textbook). A bradydysrhythmia in a hypotensive patient with a heart rate less than 50 beats/min deserves treatment, even if the ventricular contractions are well coordinated. One should begin with the intravenous administration of atropine, at a dose of 0.5 mg, repeated at 2-minute intervals for a maximum dose of 2 mg. If the rate remains slow and if the patient is still unstable, the heart should be paced by transvenous or external means.

A tachydysrhythmia can put a patient at risk for myocardial ischemia regardless of origin (sinus vs nonsinus) or etiology (hypovolemic or cardiogenic shock). Thus one has to decide if the rate is so rapid that it threatens the patient's myocardium. As a first approximation, the goal for most patients should be a ventricular rate between 50 and 100. But the goal can be different for different patients. The maximal ventricular rate, the rate that can be sustained for perhaps 5 minutes, but not longer, declines with age (220—age in years). The maximal aerobic rate, a rate that can be maintained indefinitely, but with strain, is 60%-90% of this value depending on the physical condition of the patient and the presence or absence of ischemic heart disease. For example, a healthy 20-year-old man in good condition should be able to tolerate and sustain a heart rate of 160 (80% of 200) without difficulty (although one should search for the cause of the tachycardia). On the other hand, a 65-year-old man with known coronary stenosis may have a myocardial aerobic threshold of 93 beats/min:

$$(220 - 65) \times 0.6$$

Rates exceeding these limits should be treated.

A moribund patient with a tachydysrhythmia should undergo electrical cardioversion, an intervention that result in full cardiac function with normal blood supply to the brain in a matter of seconds. No other treatment has this potential. Electrical cardioversion is the treatment of choice for coarse ventricular fibrillation, ventricular tachycardia, and for supraventricular dysrhythmias with unsustainably rapid ventricular responses. It is not the treatment of choice for asystole or fine ventricular fibrillation, but no treatment for these dysrhythmias has a chance of achieving resuscitation with full neurological function. Nothing will be gained with cardioversion in the patient in asystole or fine fibrillation, but nothing will be lost.

One hundred joules (J) should be used initially, with rapid escalation to 360 J, as needed. The cardioversion takes precedence over securing the airway, and it takes precedence over obtaining vascular access; it even takes precedence over making a diagnosis of the arrhythmia. Once converted, the patient should be given a single 100-mg dose of lidocaine. Serum electrolytes should be measured and corrected, if needed. One to two grams of magnesium sulfate should be given intravenously over 15 minutes, regardless of initial plasma concentrations. More should be given later if the values are low.

Treatment of any non-moribund patient with a tachydysrhythmia begins with ensuring euvolemia and treating other possible extracardiac causes of a tachycardia (such as fever, stress, pain, and anxiety). Dangerously rapid tachydysrhythmias associated with abnormal ventricular conduction should be electrically cardioverted, followed with lidocaine, electrolyte correction, and administration of a single dose of magnesium. In the non-moribund patient with a dangerously rapid tachydysrhythmia and normal ventricular conduction, the initial goal is to slow the rate. Give up to 10 mg of verapamil intravenously over 10 minutes. This will slow the rate in the large majority of the patients. If the initial dose fails to slow the rate, an additional dose can be given 30 minutes after the initiation of the first dose. If the ventricular response is still too rapid, give digoxin. The digoxin is administered as a loading dose of 0.5 g intravenously, followed by 0.25 g every 6 hours for two additional doses (total of 1.0 g). More might be needed—the goal is to block the AV node enough so that the ventricular response is acceptable. Daily maintenance doses are usually needed, for long-term control, and the serum levels should be measured. Electrolytes should be corrected; magnesium should be supplemented.

For continued control of the rate, we favor digoxin. But one can also continue to use verapamil or add a beta-blocker, for long-term control. All three classes of drugs–calcium channel blockers, digoxin, and beta-blockers-slow AV nodal conduction, but, of the three, only digoxin increases myocardial contractility. Surgical patients need contractility to perfuse wounded or infected tissues.

If more than one drug has to be used, the patient will need to be in a monitored setting. Complete heart block is a potentially disastrous side effect with all of these drugs, especially when used in combination.

If ventricular conduction is normal and the patient is in atrial fibrillation, and if it is thought that the fibrillation is going to be of long duration, and if the physician is sure that the patient needs an "atrial kick," the patient can be converted to a sinus rhythm with amiodarone. This set of conditions is rarely the case, however, in the noncardiac surgical patient. The "atrial kick" provides close to no added energy production from the heart in all but the most extreme cases of myocardial dysfunction. The atria in any reasonably functional heart serve only as reservoirs of energy, as capacitors, like other capacitance elements in the circulation, like the venules and small veins. The atria allow the ventricles to fill evenly under conditions of varying heart rates, but that goal is achieved with or without active contraction of the chambers.

Amiodarone frequently results in conversion of atrial fibrillation to a sinus rhythm, but the disadvantages of the drug, in the noncardiac patient, almost always outweigh the potential benefit. Conversion can lead to embolization of clot from the atrial appendage to the brain. The drug depresses myocardial contractility (potentially impeding wound healing and the ability to fight off infection). It has a long half-life. Its effects can last for weeks.

B. Opioids

Opioids can be especially effective in treating cardiac failure after myocardial infarction. They relieve pain, provide sedation, block adrenergic discharge to the arterioles, block discharge to the venules and small veins, redistribute the blood from the atria and ventricles to the venous capacitance vessels in the periphery, and decrease myocardial oxygen requirements.

C. Diuretics

Diuretics are the keystone of therapy in congestive heart failure with large ventricular end-diastolic volumes. By decreasing vascular volume, diuretics decrease atrial pressures and mobilize peripheral and pulmonary edema. Pulmonary vascular pressures and volumes decrease; effectiveness of right ventricular contraction increases. Coronary blood flow increases as coronary sinus pressure drops. Decreasing pressures in the ventricles during diastole, when the ventricular muscle receives its nutrient blood flow, alleviates compression of the coronary vasculature in the endocardium. Decreasing pressures in the right atrium decreases the stiffness of the coronary vasculature, which decreases the stiffness of the ventricles during diastole (the garden hose effect). The ventricular end-diastolic volumes potentially can increase without much of an associated increase in the end-diastolic pressures.

D. Beta-Blockers

Almost all patients in cardiac failure with ischemia and a rapid heart rate will benefit from a beta-adrenergic blocking agent (eg, esmolol or metoprolol). Decreasing the rate and reducing ventricular stiffness during systole decreases myocardial oxygen requirements. Increasing time in diastole and decreasing ventricular stiffness during diastole augments ventricular filling and increases efficiency of ventricular contraction. All of these effects reduce myocardial oxygen consumption and potentially salvage marginal myocardium. In many patients, the reduced oxygen requirements can be achieved with only minimal loss of energy output from the ventricles. The only contraindication to the use of beta-blockers, beyond the rare development of bronchospasm with administration of the drugs, is hypotension. This latter problem is easily monitored.

E. Vasodilators

Hypertension is unusual but not unheard of in patients with cardiogenic shock. The hypertension is usually associated with inefficient delivery of energy into the aortic root. Treatment should begin with opioids, if the patient is in pain, and then diuresis, if the ventricular end-diastolic volumes are large. Nitroprusside and nitroglycerin are the most useful short-term vasodilators in surgical patients in heart failure (besides opioids). Both drugs act quickly and are easy to monitor; both dilate the systemic arterioles; nitroglycerin also dilates the systemic venules and small veins. For long-term control of pressure, angiotensin-converting enzyme (ACE) inhibitors and calcium channel blockers should be used in place of the nitrates. If the patient has a tachycardia or, as may well be the case, if the patient is at risk for having coronary artery disease or myocardial ischemia, beta-blockade can be used.

Beneficial consequences of controlling the pressure include mobilization of edema, both pulmonary and systemic; enhanced perfusion of the myocardium; reduction of ventricular work and oxygen requirements and, consequently, relief of myocardial ischemia. On the other hand, excessive venous dilation can decrease cardiac filling enough so that stroke volumes and blood pressures fall; excessive arteriolar dilation can make the pressures fall further.

F. Inotropic Agents

Inotropic agents, such as dobutamine or milrinone, can increase cardiac output in some, but not all, patients in cardiogenic shock. Inotropic agents almost always result in increased myocardial oxygen requirements, but this is not usually a problem. Patients receiving the agents should be monitored in an ICU. Development of chest pain or ischemic electrocardiogram changes suggest that oxygen demand is exceeding supply. If it is necessary to use inotropic agents for more than 1 hour, a pulmonary artery catheter should be inserted. Systemic arterial pressures, atrial filling pressures, and cardiac output should be determined at different infusion rates. If any question remains about the adequacy of volume resuscitation, cardiovascular parameters should be measured before and after a fluid bolus is given.

Digitalis compounds should not be used in acute cardiac failure except to control ventricular rates in patients with supraventricular tachydysrhythmias. Toxicity may develop, especially when pH and electrolyte changes are unpredictable. The inotropic actions of digitalis are no different from those of dopamine and milrinone.

G. Chronotropic Agents

Although uncommon in the surgical setting, patients with cardiac failure and a low heart rate (< 70 beats/min) may temporarily benefit from the administration of a chronotropic agent, such as dopamine. (Isoproterenol is almost never used nowadays.) When using dopamine, the heart rate should be increased only to levels that can be tolerated comfortably. A 60-year-old patient with normal coronary arteries gains little with a heart rate that exceeds 120 beats/min; the limit is about 90 beats/min in the presence of coronary artery disease. In most cases, however, the price to be paid for using a chronotropic agent exceeds the potential benefit. Chronotropic agents increase myocardial work and oxygen requirements and shorten the time during diastole for coronary blood flow and ventricular filling. They should be used only as a temporary expedient. If they are used for more than 30 minutes, a pulmonary arterial catheter should be inserted. The goal of therapy is a normal or slightly supranormal cardiac output that provides adequate end-organ perfusion and reverses shock. Trying to achieve more than that only increases the risk of myocardial ischemia.

H. Vasoconstrictors

A vasoconstrictor is occasionally useful to increase coronary perfusion pressure in the setting of coronary stenoses. To be effective, the agent must increase aortic pressure enough so that the increased myocardial perfusion compensates for the increase in the myocardial oxygen requirements.

The major untoward effect of these agents is ischemic necrosis of noncardiac organs, such as the extremities or intestine. They will not increase perfusion to the brain in the setting of cardiogenic shock, assuming that the carotid arteries are open and that the patient has a functioning adrenergic nervous system. The endogenous adrenergic nervous system is ideally suited for ensuring adequate blood flow to the brain. Constrictors should be used only when absolutely necessary and for no more than 60 minutes unless a pulmonary arterial catheter is in place.

I. Transaortic Balloon Pump

The transaortic balloon pump decreases the hindrance that the left ventricle faces when it ejects its blood into the aortic root and can be very effective in resuscitating selected patients with severe reversible left ventricular dysfunction (eg, after cardiopulmonary bypass or acute myocardial infarction). It should be used only if a pulmonary arterial catheter is in place.

J. Extracorporeal Membrane Oxygenation

Extracorporeal membrane oxygenation is most often used in conditions in which one can expect cardiac function to recover within a matter of a few days. Bleeding complications make it impractical for periods exceeding that time.

K. Operative Correction

Although listed last, surgically correctable cardiac conditions should be identified and corrected early, prior to the development of irreversible organ dysfunction. Ruptured valves, occluded arteries, aneurysmal ventricular walls, and certain arrhythmias are examples of potentially correctable lesions. In these cases, early cardiac surgical consultation should be the rule.

NEUROGENIC SHOCK

▶ Diagnosis

Shock caused by failure of the autonomic nervous system can arise from regional or general anesthetics, injuries to the spinal cord, or administration of autonomic blocking agents. The venules and small veins lose tone, worsened by paralysis of surrounding skeletal muscles. Blood pools in the periphery, ventricular end-diastolic volumes decrease, and stroke volumes and blood pressure fall. Loss of arteriolar

tone in the denervated areas makes the pressure fall further. If the lesion is below the midthoracic sympathetic outflow (approximately T3), activation of the cardiac adrenergic nerves will increase the heart rate and augment ventricular systolic function; if the lesion is more cephalad, the heart will not be able to compensate. Cardiovascular decompensation in neurogenic shock can be profound.

The diagnosis rests on knowledge of the circumstances preceding the onset of shock and on the physical examination. The patient will always be hypotensive, and the skin will be warm and flushed in the denervated areas. The cause is usually obvious.

Nonfatal head injury—in contrast to spinal cord injury—does not produce neurogenic shock or any other kind of shock. In fact, increased intracranial pressure typically increases blood pressure and slows the heart rate (Cushing reflex). Hypotension and tachycardia should never be attributed to head injury—even severe head injury with cerebral dysfunction—until hypovolemia has been ruled out. It is a tragedy to ascribe shock to a head injury when the problem is bleeding from a ruptured spleen.

▶ Treatment

Trendelenburg position, if it does not complicate other aspects of care, is useful. Intravenous fluids to fill the dilated venules and small veins should be given. Vasoconstrictors should be used if fluids and Trendelenburg position are not enough. Norepinephrine and phenylephrine are good choices if the heart rate is rapid. Dopamine is a good choice if the heart rate is slow.

The primary purpose of vasoconstricting agents in this setting is to restore tone in the venules and small veins; a secondary goal is to constrict dilated arterioles. The blood pressure should be increased to the point that coronary perfusion is sustained—as judged by normal ST–T segments on electrocardiography and absence of chest pain—and to the point that perfusion to the brain and spinal cord is supported. The pressure also has to be high enough to perfuse organs with preexisting obstructing proximal arterial lesions. These patients should be placed in the ICU for both neurologic and hemodynamic monitoring. If vasoconstrictors are used for more than several hours, or if the patient is at high risk for bleeding from multisystem trauma, central venous pressure monitoring or a pulmonary arterial catheter should be used to ensure adequate cardiac filling and function.

LOW-OUTPUT INFLAMMATORY SHOCK

▶ Diagnosis

Bowel perforation, intestinal necrosis, abscesses, gangrene, and soft tissue infections can produce low-output inflammatory shock, as can ischemia-reperfusion and inadequate resuscitation of massive injuries or large burns.

The cytokinemia arising from the systemic inflammation can disrupt the microvascular endothelium and prompt the loss of plasma into the interstitium. The shock mimics the clinical picture of severe hypovolemic shock, with signs of adrenergic discharge, oliguria, obtundation, and metabolic acidemia. The EKG may show signs of ischemia. Hyperthermia or hypothermia may be present. The diagnosis is usually clear from the clinical circumstances.

▶ Treatment

Treatment consists of administration of intravenous fluids and antibiotics, correction of gastrointestinal leaks, debridement of dead tissue, and drainage of pus. The patient should be transferred to an ICU. Vasoconstrictors can be given for very short periods of time if the hypotension is so profound that it threatens the brain, the heart, or an organ with an obstructed arterial supply. Inotropes can be used more liberally, while the vascular volume is being replenished, but even then they should be used judiciously until additional physiologic data confirms a euvolemic state. This is easily obtained through the use of a central venous or pulmonary artery catheter. Alternatively, newer, noninvasive measurements of ventricular filling may prove useful. Successful volume expansion will convert the low-output inflammatory shock into a high-output state.

HIGH-OUTPUT INFLAMMATORY SHOCK

▶ Diagnosis

High-output inflammatory shock can precede low-output inflammatory shock or can be the result of successful treatment of low-output shock. The shock usually, but not always, is associated with a fever. The patient is hypotensive with warm, well-perfused extremities, as the body attempts to control its core temperature by off-loading heat to the environment. If a pulmonary arterial catheter is placed, the cardiac output is found to be high, assuming that the ventricular end-diastolic volumes have been brought back to normal levels. The outputs will remain high, occasionally as high as twice normal, as long as the inflammatory state persists. The oxygen consumption may be increased by a factor of 1.5.

▶ Treatment

Treatment consists of control of the underlying cause and fluid administration. Inotropes may be useful. If large amounts of fluids are necessary for the resuscitation and if inotropes are being considered, an assessment of ventricular end-diastolic volume should be made to ensure the heart is adequately filling and to assess the impact of the intervention. The most accurate means to accomplish this is through the use of a pulmonary artery catheter. As this

is not always possible, other, less invasive monitoring techniques include the measurement of central venous pressure and serial echocardiography. All have advantages, disadvantages, and in some cases, complications. Regardless, the goal is to perfuse the inflamed tissues with adequate power so that the product of the cardiac output and the mean arterial pressure is normal. In many patients, the result will be a cardiac output that is increased by a factor of 1.5 with a blood pressure that is decreased to a value that is two-thirds of normal. As in other forms of shock, the pressure has to be high enough to perfuse the heart and brain and organs with potentially obstructed arteries, but it does not have to be normal. Vasoconstrictors can be dangerous, potentially leading to necrosis of the limbs, the gut, and the kidneys, especially if there is any degree of hypovolemia. They should not be used unless the clinician is positive that both the right and left ventricular end-diastolic volumes are normally expanded.

American College of Surgeons: *ATLS: Advanced Trauma Life Support Student Manual.* 9th ed. American College of Surgeons; 2012.

Chan PS et al, American Heart Association National Registry of Cardiopulmonary Resuscitation Investigators: Delayed time to defibrillation after in-hospital cardiac arrest. *N Engl J Med.* 2008;358:9.

CRASH-2 trial collaborators, Shakur H, Roberts I, et al: Effects of tranexamic acid on death, vascular occlusive events, and blood transfusion in trauma patients with significant haemorrhage (CRASH-2): a randomized, placebo-controlled trial. *Lancet.* 2010;376:23-32.

Doyle, GS, Taillac PP: Tourniquets: a review of current use with proposals for expanded prehospital use. *Prehosp Emerg Care.* 2008;12:241.

Hess JR, Brohi K, Dutton RP, et al: The coagulopathy of trauma: a review of mechanisms. *J Trauma.* 2008;65:748-754.

Holcomb JB, de Junco DJ, Fox EE, et al: The prospective, observational, multicenter, major trauma transfusion (PROMMTT) study. *JAMA Surg.* 2013;148:127-136.

Holcomb JB, Minei KM, Scerbo ML, et al: Admission rapid thrombelastography can replace conventional coagulation tests in the emergency department. *Ann Surg.* 2012;256:476-486.

Holcomb JB, Wade CE, Michalek JE, et al: Increased plasma and platelet to red blood cell ratios improves outcome in 466 massively transfused civilian trauma patients. *Ann Surg.* 2008;248:447-458.

Martinaud C, Ausset S, Deshayes AV, et al: Use of freeze-dried plasma in French intensive care unit in Afghanistan. *J Trauma.* 2011;71:1761-1765.

Matijevic N, Wang Y, Cotton B, et al: Better hemostatic profiles of nevert-frozen liquid plasma compared with thawed fresh frozen plasma. *J Trauma Acute Care Surg.* 2013;74:84-91.

Nunez TC, Young PP, Holcomb JB, et al: Creation, implementation, and maturation of a massive transfusion protocol for the exsanguinating trauma patient. *J Trauma.* 2010;68:1498-1505.

Radwan ZA, Matijevic N, del Junco DJ, et al: An emergency department thawed plasma protocol for severely injury patients. *JAMA Surg.* 2013;148:170-175.

Shenkin HA et al: On the diagnosis of hemorrhage in man: a study of volunteers bled large amounts. *Amer J Med.* 1944;208:421.

Sperry JL, Ochao JB, Gunn SR, et al: An FFP:PRBC transfusion ratio >= 1:1.5 is associated with a lower risk of mortality after massive transfusion. *J Trauma.* 2008;65:986-993.

Spinella PC et al: The effect of recombinant activated factor VII on mortality in combat-related casualties with severe trauma and massive transfusion. *J Trauma.* 2008;64:286.

Tapia NM, Chang A, Norman M, et al: TEG-guided resuscitation is superior to standardized MTP resuscitation in massively transfused penetrating trauma patients. *J Trauma Acute Care Surg.* 2013;74:378-386.

INITIAL TREATMENT OF ACUTE PULMONARY FAILURE

DIAGNOSIS OF PULMONARY FAILURE IN SURGICAL PATIENTS

Most causes of pulmonary failure in the surgical patient can be ascribed to one or more of nine causes: the pulmonary failure of shock, trauma, and sepsis; mechanical failure caused by deranged respiratory system mechanics; atelectasis; aspiration; pulmonary contusion; pneumonia; pulmonary embolism; cardiogenic pulmonary edema; and, rarely, neurogenic pulmonary edema.

The pulmonary failure of shock, trauma, and sepsis arises from extrapulmonary trauma, infection, or ischemia-reperfusion in the setting of shock. Products of coagulation and inflammation are washed out from the damaged tissues and carried to the lungs (or to the liver, in the case of the splanchnic circulation, and from there to the lungs), where they set up an acute inflammatory reaction. The extrapulmonary causes are many and range from necrotizing infections to noninfective inflammatory responses (such as pancreatitis) to reperfusion of ischemic limbs to soft tissue injury to broken bones (and embolism of fat and clot from the bone marrow—the so-called fat embolism syndrome, now an outdated term).

The concept of pulmonary failure secondary to extrapulmonary ischemia-reperfusion, coagulation, and inflammation, which is common in surgical patients, can be subsumed into a broader category of pulmonary failure, known as the acute respiratory distress syndrome (ARDS). ARDS is defined by the sudden onset of hypoxemia with bilateral infiltrates, a Pao_2:Fio_2 less than 200 and the absence of left atrial hypertension (a pulmonary arterial wedge pressure < 18 if measured). A less severe form, ALI requires a Pao_2: Fio_2 less than 300 with the other criteria.

The causes of ARDS include those that are responsible for the pulmonary failure of shock, trauma, and sepsis and also include severe pneumonia and aspiration. The end result in all of these conditions is activation of macrophages and other inflammatory cells in the lungs. The mediators disrupt the microvascular endothelium, increasing its permeability. Plasma extravasates into the interstitium and, in the case of the lungs, into the alveoli. The resultant pulmonary edema impairs both ventilation and oxygenation; the microembolization to the lungs impairs perfusion. Arterial oxygen saturation decreases and carbon dioxide content increases—assuming that no compensatory mechanisms come into play. Lastly, to make things worse, the inflammatory process in the lungs releases mediators into the systemic circulation that can lead to inflammation and dysfunction in the liver, gut, and kidneys.

A number of different mediators of coagulation and inflammation have been implicated as causes of the increased permeability. Proteases, kinins, complement, oxygen radicals, prostaglandins, thromboxanes, leukotrienes, lysosomal enzymes, and other mediators are released from aggregates of platelets and white cells or from the endothelium or plasma as a consequence of the interaction between the aggregates and the vessel wall. Some of these substances are chemoattractants of more platelets and white blood cells, and a vicious cycle of inflammation develops that worsens the disruption of the vascular endothelium.

Pathologically, ARDS (and the pulmonary failure of shock, trauma, and sepsis) is characterized by diffuse alveolar damage and a nonspecific inflammatory reaction, with the loss of alveolar epithelium and hyaline membrane formation. Monocytes and neutrophils invade the interstitium. Edema appears within a few hours, alveolar flooding is florid within 1 day, and fibrosis begins in 1-2 weeks. If the process is unchecked, the lungs become sodden and resemble liver tissue on gross inspection; scar tissue appears within a week, and function-limiting fibrosis begins to develop within 2 weeks. If early treatment is effective, the lungs return to normal, both grossly and microscopically.

Mechanical failure can arise from chest wall trauma, pain and weakness after surgery and anesthesia, debility caused by the catabolic metabolism of long-term illness, or bronchopleural fistula. Massive trauma to the chest with multiple fractures of multiple ribs or bilateral disruption of the costochondral junctions can result in a free-floating segment of chest wall known as a *flail chest*. Expansion and relaxation of the chest wall during spontaneous breathing results in paradoxic motion of the free segment in response to changes in intrathoracic pressure; ventilation becomes compromised; and the partial pressure of arterial carbon dioxide ($Paco_2$) increases. In addition, hypoventilation leads to progressive atelectasis and hypoxemia. Lesser degrees of chest wall injury can lead to hypoventilation secondary to pain with similar results. Prolonged mechanical ventilation with loss of muscle mass and power in the diaphragm and the accessory muscles of respiration can require ventilatory support until muscle function returns to normal. A bronchopleural fistula—a communication from the airway to the pleural cavity to the atmosphere, either through a chest tube or through a hole in the chest wall—can develop after pulmonary surgery, trauma, or infection. Large air leaks can compromise ventilation to the uninvolved lung as well as to the diseased side because insufflated air preferentially goes to the side with the fistula.

Atelectasis—localized collapse of alveoli—can develop with prolonged immobilization, as during anesthesia or in association with bed rest. The problem is usually full-blown within a few hours after the initiating event. Only mechanical failure (to which it is related), aspiration, cardiogenic pulmonary edema, and pulmonary embolism can produce equivalent levels of hypoxemia so soon, and no other cause of hypoxemia can respond so quickly to therapy. The diagnosis is supported by auscultation of bronchial breath sounds at dependent portions of the lung and occasionally, if severe enough, by x-ray confirmation of plate-like collapse of pulmonary parenchyma. The most reliable confirmation of the diagnosis, however, comes with response to therapy, which can include pain control when necessary and encouragement of deep breathing, coughing, and ambulation when practical. When the hypoxia is severe and refractory to conservative measures, intubation and mechanical ventilation may be necessary, particularly if the underlying etiology (pain and immobility) cannot be reversed easily (eg, high spinal cord injury). Rarely, flexible bronchoscopy may be useful if the lung parenchymal volume loss is due to proximal bronchial obstruction. In general, most forms of atelectasis respond within a few hours to conservative therapy.

Aspiration of gastric contents or blood can occur in any patient who cannot protect the airway. Shock, severe brain injury, or pharmacologic depression (anesthesia, narcotics, or benzodiazepines) can result in a depressed level of consciousness and loss of airway protective reflexes. Gastric acid or particulate matter in the airways leads to disruption of the alveolar and microvascular membranes, causing interstitial and alveolar edema. The resultant hypoxemia is usually evident within a few hours and is associated with a localized infiltrate on x-ray. Recovery of gastric contents by suctioning from the endotracheal tree confirms the diagnosis.

Pulmonary contusion arises from direct trauma to the chest wall and the underlying lung parenchyma. Hypoxemia associated with a localized infiltrate on x-ray develops over 24 hours as the injured lung becomes edematous.

Pneumonia can arise primarily or may be superimposed on aspiration, pulmonary contusion, or the pulmonary failure of shock, trauma, and sepsis. The diagnosis is made by recovery of bacteria and purulent material from the endotracheal tree, hypoxemia, signs of systemic inflammation, and a localized infiltrate on x-ray. The Clinical Pulmonary Infection Score (CPIS), which is derived from these parameters, can be used to quantify the clinical, radiographic, and laboratory findings of pneumonia. It is useful both for diagnosis and for determining the length of treatment. Bronchoalveolar lavage and quantitative culture may occasionally be used to assist in distinguishing pneumonia from ARDS and other causes of pulmonary inflammation.

Pulmonary embolism typically presents with sudden deterioration of pulmonary function after an event—such as an operation, injury, or the beginning of immobilization—that can stimulate deposition of clot in a large systemic vein. Patients with cancer are at particularly high risk, and in any patient the greater the magnitude of operation or injury, the greater the chance of venous thrombosis and embolization. Clot emboli must be organized to be clinically significant; embolism to the lung of fresh soft clot rarely causes any difficulty. The pulmonary endothelium contains potent fibrinolysins that can break up any poorly organized embolus. Although uncommon in the initial 72 hours following an acquired risk factor (injury, surgery), early postinjury and postsurgical pulmonary embolism is well documented and has to be considered in the differential diagnosis of abrupt-onset hypoxemia.

The chest film is usually nonspecific. A definite diagnosis can be made by high-definition contrast enhanced computed tomograms of the pulmonary vasculature. Modern imaging is extremely sensitive. A negative study rules out an embolism. The CT can also identify atelectasis, infiltrates, and effusions that may not be readily apparent using a standard anterior-posterior radiograph done in the ICU. The major risk involves the physical movement of the patient to the radiology suite. The risk of contrast nephropathy is very low in a euvolemic patient, even in the setting of mild baseline renal disease.

Pulmonary arteriography, with right heart catheterization, can also be used to make the diagnosis of embolism but is seldom used nowadays, with one exception. The study can be very useful in hemodynamically unstable patients in whom a large "saddle embolus" is suspected. The catheter can be left in place, if an embolus is found, and used for catheter-directed thrombolysis.

Cardiogenic pulmonary edema arises from high left atrial and pulmonary microvascular hydrostatic pressures. Patients who have suffered an acute myocardial infarction can present this way, as can patients with underlying myocardial or coronary artery disease when faced with fluid shifts and surgical stress. Occasionally, the rapid administration of intravenous fluid—especially in elderly patients with poor myocardial performance—will outstrip the heart's ability to pump, and pulmonary edema will result. Acute valvular disease, though rare after injury or cardiac surgery, is another possible cause of inability of the left heart to pump effectively.

The diagnosis is made on the basis of hypoxemia, rales, a third heart sound, perihilar infiltrates, Kerley lines, and cephalization of blood flow on x-ray along with elevated pulmonary arterial wedge pressures on pulmonary arterial catheterization. A wedge (or left atrial) pressure of 24 mm Hg can produce cardiogenic pulmonary edema even in the presence of an intact endothelium in the pulmonary micro-vasculature. Pulmonary arterial wedge pressures less than 24 mm Hg will generally not produce edema if the pulmonary vascular endothelium is intact; pressures exceeding 16 mm Hg can worsen the edema associated with increased permeability (such as ARDS). The goal for the wedge pressure in a patient with uncomplicated cardiogenic pulmonary edema in the absence of an inflammatory process in the lungs should be 20 mm Hg or less; the goal in a patient with an inflammatory process should be 12-16 mm Hg.

Neurogenic pulmonary edema is associated both experimentally and clinically with head injury and increased intracranial pressure. The exact mechanism by which this occurs is unknown, but it is probably related to sympathetic discharge with postmicrovascular vasoconstriction in the lungs and a resultant increase in pulmonary microvascular hydrostatic pressure. This form of pulmonary edema and oxygenation defect is rare. In the great majority of patients with a head injury and pulmonary edema, the edema will be caused by some other mechanism, such as ARDS.

INDICATIONS FOR INTUBATION & USE OF MECHANICAL VENTILATION

The indications for intubation and mechanical ventilation are related but often assessed separately. Patients who have primary airway compromise—caused by stridor, maxillofacial trauma, facial and airway burns with edema, or a depressed mental status—may need intubation to protect the airway. In these cases, early intervention is the rule as rapid clinical deterioration can convert a semiurgent procedure into an emergency. In some cases, intubation should be performed before the patient shows evidence of airway compromise. In severe cases, such as massive facial edema, early cricothyroidotomy should be performed.

Intubation of the airway is also indicated if mechanical ventilation is needed for the treatment of established pulmonary failure or for prophylaxis against potential failure or for pulmonary toilet in the face of aspiration. The decision to intubate and initiate mechanical ventilation should be made on the basis of clinical criteria. A respiratory rate exceeding 36 breaths/min, labored ventilation, use of accessory muscles of ventilation, and tachycardia are all indications for intervention. Finally, intubation and mechanical ventilation should be considered in anticipation of treatment that can compromise the airway or worsen the pulmonary status. These include the need for excessive sedation or narcotics, massive fluid resuscitation, and the manipulation of fractures.

Arterial blood gas (ABG) measurements are of no value in making decisions about intubation and mechanical ventilation in patients in extremis. These patients should be intubated regardless of the blood gas results. ABG measurements, however, can assist in the decision to intubate

less severely stressed patients. In the setting of hypoxemia, intubation should be considered if the Pao_2 is less than 60 mm Hg and the patient's supplemental oxygen exceeds an O_2 concentration of 50%. For hypercapneic patients, a $Paco_2$ greater than 45 mm Hg in the setting of acidemia should prompt intubation, especially if serial measurements demonstrate a worsening respiratory acidosis. Regardless of the laboratory values, these guidelines should always be put in the clinical context. A $Paco_2$ of 40 mm Hg in a patient breathing 40 breaths/min is as alarming as a $Paco_2$ of 60 mm Hg in a patient with a respiratory rate of 10 breaths/min. A Pao_2 of 60 mm Hg on room air in a patient with chronic lung disease may be acceptable; the same value in a patient who is tensing the sternocleidomastoid and intercostal muscles with each breath, making excessive or discoordinated use of the abdominal musculature, and who seems to be struggling to draw in enough air, mandates immediate intubation.

The indications for intubation should be more liberal for a surgical patient than for a medical patient. The medical patient with an exacerbation of chronic obstructive lung disease can be poorly served by placement of a foreign body in the trachea. Airway resistance increases, coughing becomes less effective, and opportunistic organisms obtain a foothold on and near the tube. The benefit from intubation may be minimal and noninvasive ventilation techniques, such as bilevel positive airway pressure (BiPAP), may be all that is needed. This support can be given simultaneously with other treatments—such as administration of bronchodilators, antibiotics, and diuretics—in order to avoid intubation and its potential complications.

Circumstances for the seriously ill surgical patient are usually different. The patient who has multiple injuries, for example, can temporarily tolerate the increased airway resistance, loss of cough, and increased likelihood of tracheobronchial infection. What cannot be tolerated is respiratory arrest during trauma resuscitation or during preparation for an operation.

The indications for intubation in the patient with a suspected or known injury to the cervical spine are the same as those in patients with no likelihood of injury. Under no circumstances should concern about the cervical spine lead to procrastination about securing the airway. The consequences of respiratory arrest and anoxic brain damage are as tragic as those of exacerbating a cervical spine injury.

▶ Types of Intubation

The trachea can be intubated via the mouth, the nose, the cricothyroid membrane (cricothyroidotomy), or directly (tracheostomy). The tubes used for intubation used to come with either high pressure cuffs or low pressure cuffs. Because of problems with compromise of tracheal blood supply, and the subsequent problems of tracheomalacia, erosion into the innominate artery or the esophagus, and tracheal stenosis, the high pressure cuffs are no longer used. All modern tubes come with low pressure cuffs.

Of the four methods available for intubation, the orotracheal route is usually the easiest. Nasotracheal intubation requires the presence of spontaneous ventilation in order to guide tube placement; cricothyroidotomy and tracheotomy require surgical exposure. Orotracheal intubation allows for passage of a larger tube than the nasotracheal route and avoids the problems of sinusitis and necrosis of the nares, which can occur with nasotracheal intubation. On the other hand, nasotracheal intubation can be accomplished in the awake patient with minimal sedation, and some patients seem to find long-term presence of a nasotracheal tube more comfortable than that of an orotracheal tube. Neither nasotracheal nor orotracheal intubation requires neck flexion or axial rotation. Either approach can be used in patients with suspected injuries to the cervical spine, assuming that axial traction is maintained during the intubation.

Cricothyroidotomy is indicated when an urgent surgical airway is needed. Extensive maxillofacial trauma can make intubation by the orotracheal or nasotracheal route impossible. Translaryngeal intubation can also be difficult because of poor patient cooperation, altered anatomy, or airway or laryngeal swelling. If the patient is in extremis and respiratory collapse is imminent, attempts at orotracheal or nasotracheal intubation should not be prolonged. As a rule, if translaryngeal intubation is not successful after one or two attempts, cricothyroidotomy should be done. The cricothyroid membrane in the midline is bounded superiorly by the lower border of the thyroid cartilage. It is located by palpation and is incised by a stab incision. After the hole has been enlarged with the knife handle, a size 6 or 6.5 endotracheal tube should be inserted. After the airway is secured, the tube can be trimmed (without cutting the balloon tubing) to prevent accidental dislodgement. Alternatively a no. 4 or no. 6 tracheostomy tube can be used if available.

There are several advantages to using the endotracheal tube during an urgent cricothyroidotomy. These include increased tube compliance which facilitates insertion and, perhaps most importantly, universal availability. They are typically found in every airway kit or crash cart. A 6.5 tube will usually accommodate a bougie introducer which may facilitate insertion, particularly when the anatomy is difficult (obese or short neck) and the field is bloody. Larger endotracheal or tracheostomy tubes should not be used as they may not always pass easily through the cricothyroid space. In the short term, these smaller tubes are more than adequate as a rescue treatment and can easily be changed under more controlled circumstances.

Once the airway is secured and the patient stable, a more definitive airway can be planned as needed. The need to convert to a tracheotomy is not absolute. In some cases, the patient may no longer require airway protection. In others, endotracheal intubation may be a reasonable option. In the past, concerns over subglottic stenosis necessitated conversion of the cricothyroidotomy within several days. This has not been uniformly supported by the literature and should be individualized based on anticipated continued need for airway protection and mechanical ventilation.

Conversion of either an endotracheal airway or cricothyroidotomy to a tracheostomy should be done under controlled conditions. A transverse incision overlying the upper trachea is developed by separating the strap muscles of the neck in the midline. Often the thyroid isthmus must be either displaced or divided to allow for adequate exposure of the anterior surface of the trachea. The tracheostomy tube is placed through the second or third tracheal ring.

Tracheostomy placement is frequently performed for patients who require long-term mechanical ventilation. There are advantages and disadvantages to both the endotracheal tube and the tracheostomy. As a result, there are few absolute diagnostic or time standards for conversion beyond airway control.

One of the theoretical advantages of continued endotracheal intubation is the ease of tube repositioning, which allows distributing pressure on the tracheal mucosa over a larger area, compared with the balloon on the end of a tracheostomy tube, which is fixed in place. The result is a much lower incidence of late tracheal stenosis and tracheoinnominate artery and tracheoesophageal fistulas, compared with a tracheostomy. In addition, because the opening of a translaryngeal tube is well away from the neck and chest, intravenous catheters in these areas can be kept sterile. Finally, the cuffs on translaryngeal tubes usually lie in a more axial position in the trachea than those on a tracheostomy tube and are better able to maintain a seal in patients with poor pulmonary compliance and high inspiratory pressures.

On the other hand, for long-term care, airway resistance with a tracheostomy is lower, nursing care is simpler, suctioning is more direct, and the tubes do not damage the vocal cords or larynx. In addition and perhaps most importantly, accidental extubation is less serious. A well-established tracheostomy tract can be easily reintubated while the patient continues to breathe through the stoma. Tracheostomy is also of benefit when weaning from mechanical ventilation is slow and the patient has failed extubation on multiple occasions. The presence of a tracheostomy allows for prolonged periods off the ventilator without the need for reintubation. If the patient develops respiratory distress off the ventilator and a tracheostomy is present, the ventilator can simply be reconnected to the tracheostomy tube.

The timing of conversion from a translaryngeal intubation to a tracheostomy is controversial. Recommendations as short as 3 days have been made, but large numbers of patients have been intubated for months by the orotracheal or nasotracheal route without serious sequelae. Patients should be converted when airway protection, pulmonary toilet, or any of the other indications outlined above are present. If, in addition, the need for more than 2-3 weeks of intubation is obvious, the threshold for performing tracheostomy should be lowered.

▶ Modes of Mechanical Ventilation

Once the airway is controlled, the ventilator should be set up beginning with the mode of ventilation. There are three primary variables used to describe the mode of mechanical ventilation: trigger, limit, and cycle (Table 12–2). The trigger can be patient or time triggered with the latter often referred to as "machine triggered." This is the variable that determines when a patient receives a breath (starts inspiration). The second is the limit variable and refers to the setting that, when reached, is maintained constant throughout the inspiratory cycle (ie, the "upper limit"). Limit variables are either pressure or flow. When flow is the limit variable, the ventilator is said to be in volume control or volume limited because of the relationship *flow × time = volume*. Finally, the cycle variable is that which, once reached, terminates the inspiratory cycle and allows passive expiration. Using these three variables, different modes of ventilation have been created. Some are mostly of historical interest, and others are newer, combination modes designed to maximize patient physiology, safety, and comfort.

Machine triggers are time functions based on the set rate, inspiratory time, and inspiratory to expiratory ratio (I:E ratio). Two of the three can be set, and the third is determined. A rate of 20 breaths/min and an inspiratory time of 1 second results in an I:E ratio of 1:2 (1 s inspiration + 2 s expiration = 3 s for a complete cycle; 20 cycles/min).

Patient triggers for delivery of an assisted breath can be either pressure-based or "flow by" depending on the ventilator model. A pressure trigger requires the patient to generate negative pressure at the onset of inspiration—the pressure in the ventilator tubing falls below a preset value and the ventilator detects this fall in pressure and responds by delivering a breath. The time involved in generating and delivering the breath to the patient, however, can make this form of breathing uncomfortable for the patient. Modern ventilators avoid this problem of triggering by using a flow-by circuit. The ventilator delivers a constant flow of air through the ventilator tubing during expiration, usually at a low level of approximately 5 L/min. The ventilator compares the expiratory and inspiratory flow rates. If the patient is making no inspiratory effort, the flow rates will be the same. If the patient begins to take a breath, the expiratory rate will fall below the inspiratory rate. The ventilator is programmed to trigger a breath when the difference in the flow rates reaches a preset value, usually around 2 L/min, or when the expiratory flow rate falls to 3 L/min. The patient is rewarded with the free flow of at least some air as soon as the effort is initiated. The great majority of patients prefer flow-by over pressure triggering.

A. Volume Control Ventilation

Volume control ventilation is most often used today in situations in which the ventilation needs to be kept simple and the efforts made by the patient need to be minimized, as in the acutely injured or ill patient. The assist-control mode is the most commonly used mode of volume ventilation. It is designed to assist any ventilatory effort made by the patient by delivering a machine breath. Whenever the patient begins to inspire, the ventilator is triggered and the preset machine tidal volume is given. A machine backup rate is also set to ensure a minimal number of machine breaths in the absence of spontaneous ventilatory efforts.

Table 12–2. Characteristics of five commonly used modes of mechanical ventilation.

Mode	Trigger	Limit	Cycle	Notes
Intermittent mandatory ventilation (IMV)	Time (machine)	Flow (volume) or pressure	Time	Volume control IMV or pressure control IMV Can be synchronized to patients effort (SIMV) and/or used in conjunction with pressure support
Assist control (AC)	Patient and/or time	Flow (volume) or pressure	Time	Assist control volume control (AC VC) or Assist control pressure control (AC PC)
Pressure support (PS)	Patient	Pressure	Flow	Purely spontaneous mode and often referred to as a form of continuous positive airway pressure (CPAP) on the ventilator controls
Inverse ratio	Time	Pressure	Time	PC IMV mode with prolonged inspiratory phase to increase mean airway pressure and functional residual capacity
Pressure-regulated volume control	Patient and/or time	Pressure	Time	Variation of pressure control that limits pressure but adjusts between breaths to ensure preset tidal volume

B. Pressure Control Ventilation and Pressure Support Ventilation

In pressure control ventilation, the inspiratory pressure, inspiratory time, and I:E ratio are selected, and the ventilator automatically adjusts the gas flow rate to maintain a constant pressure during inspiration. The main advantage of this over volume control is that gas flow more closely matches the change in lung compliance that occurs during inspiration. This has the theoretical benefit of a more even distribution of inspired gas and possibly a lower risk of regional alveolar overdistention. It is also more comfortable for the awake patient. Although this can be achieved through manipulating the flow pattern in more advanced volume control ventilators, it is automatic in pressure control ventilation. Physiologic inspiratory times and I:E ratios are usually chosen to improve patient comfort. An inspiratory time of 1 second with an expiratory time of 2-3 seconds is typical. Longer inspiratory times with shorter expiratory times (inverse ratio ventilation) can be used if the physiologic times prove inadequate to provide enough support. The long inspiratory times, along with the short expiratory times, result in air trapping and increase the mean airway pressure. The net result is an increase in functional residual capacity (FRC), similar to that accomplished with high positive end-expiratory pressure (PEEP) levels.

Pressure support ventilation is also a pressure-limited form of ventilation and in most cases, can be considered a distinct mode of ventilation (Table 12–2). It differs from pressure control in that it is always patient triggered and the inspiratory time is determined by the patient and not set by the ventilator. As in pressure control ventilation, the ventilator adjusts the flow to maintain a constant pressure during inspiration. The inspiratory time, however, is determined by the interaction of the gas flow with the patient's inspiratory effort. To do this, the ventilator measures the peak inspiratory flow rate during inspiration. The flow rate usually reaches a maximum value early in the inspiration and then tapers off as the patient's inspiratory effort decreases. When the flow rate decreases to a predetermined fraction of the maximal flow (generally 25% of maximum), gas flow is terminated, and the patient is allowed to exhale. Pressure support can also be used in conjunction with the intermittent mandatory ventilation (IMV) mode (see next section).

The level of the pressure support is set so that the patient breathes comfortably at a reasonable rate, usually less than 24 breaths/min. The goal of the support is to ensure adequate oxygenation and a pH greater than 7.30. The tidal volume generated under these circumstances is generally unimportant.

The mode has many advantages. It is usually comfortable for the patient. It overcomes resistance to inspiratory flow in the endotracheal tube and in the ventilatory apparatus and decreases the work of breathing. It makes it impossible for the ventilator to deliver excessively high pressures. The flow is maintained for as long as the patient continues to make an inspiratory effort, so the patient can sigh at will. This minimizes the development of atelectasis. It is also ideally suited for preparing the patient for weaning and extubation.

C. Intermittent Mandatory Ventilation & Assist Control Ventilation

With IMV, all aspects of breathing are controlled including the rate, inspiratory time, and expiratory time (and as a result, I:E ratio). The limit variable can be either pressure (PC IMV) or volume (VC IMV). The breaths are generally synchronized (SIMV) if the patient has spontaneous respiratory effort. In this mode, any attempt to breathe at a greater frequency than the set rate is unsupported unless additional pressure support is added. In this case, the patient receives two different modes during mechanical ventilation. The first is the mandatory, machine-triggered breath at the set rate and inspiratory time. The second is a spontaneous, patient-triggered breath at a rate equal to the total minus the set rate with an inspiratory time determined by the patient (see previous discussion of pressure support ventilation). These two breaths will have different waveform characteristics on the ventilator display.

Assist control mode was originally set up to "assist" the patient's spontaneous effort with a completely supported mechanical breath. It can be used with a volume or pressure limit (VC or PC) and set up with a backup rate when spontaneous effort is minimal or absent. The main distinction from SIMV is that all of the patient's inspiratory efforts are completely supported (not just those at the set rate). This has the small disadvantage of air trapping when the patient's respiratory rate is excessively high (> 30-35 breaths per minute) and should be used with caution in patients at risk for hyperinflation (severe emphysema). There is no role for pressure support ventilation in this mode as all breaths are completely assisted.

D. Hybrid Modes

Over the past 15 years, it has become possible to ventilate patients with even more sophisticated hybrid modes. Some ventilators can be set up to deliver constant pressure during the inspiration in such a way that the tidal volume delivered falls in a preset range (pressure-limited volume control, PRVC). Some ventilators can be set up to deliver a preset tidal volume but without exceeding a preset pressure. Some ventilators can be set up with gradually decreasing ventilatory support with algorithms built into the system to minimize the need for physician adjustment of the ventilator during weaning.

▶ Setting Up the Ventilator

After choosing the mode (AC, SIMV, or PS; PC or VC), five parameters remain to be determined: the backup ventilatory rate, the goal tidal volume of the machine-delivered breaths, the inspiratory time, the inspired oxygen concentration (FIO_2), and the PEEP level. The first two of these parameters determine ventilation; the latter three are important in determining oxygenation.

Ventilation has three components: minute ventilation (V_E), alveolar ventilation (V_A), and dead space ventilation (V_D). Although V_A is most closely related to $PacO_2$, at steady state, the relationship with V_E and V_D is roughly constant, and therefore, V_E, which is easily quantified, can be used as a surrogate. In patients with uncomplicated pulmonary failure, the respiratory rate can be set at 12-15 breaths/min and the tidal volume set to 7 mL/kg IBW. This produces a V_E of 6-7.5 L/min and a V_A of 4-5 L/min (assuming V_D of 33% in a 70 kg patient). In the absence of significant pulmonary dysfunction, this will result in a $PacO_2$ of approximately 40 mm Hg and is a good starting point from which adjustments can be made.

If the $PacO_2$ is elevated, increases in the respiratory rate will often correct the problem. Although this is less efficient than increasing the tidal volume (due to the increased dead space ventilation that occurs with higher respiratory rates), it is a reasonable first step when the respiratory rate is less than 25 breaths/min. Excessively high respiratory rates (> 30 breaths/min) can result in air trapping, especially in patients with expiratory air flow obstruction (chronic obstructive pulmonary disease or severe asthma). On the other hand, excessively high volumes may be associated with elevated airway pressures and can result in barotrauma (pneumothorax), volutrauma (alveolar overdistention), or both. Except in certain circumstances (intracranial hypertension), it is better to accept a mild respiratory acidosis than to ventilate the patient using excessively large tidal volumes (> 10 mL/kg IBW) or excessively high airway pressures (plateau pressure > 30 cm H_2O). When the pH is less than 7.20, very high rates or volumes may be necessary until the pH can be brought into the normal range either through renal compensatory mechanisms or administered bicarbonate. Very high rates or volumes may also be necessary when a bronchopleural fistula is present, to compensate for the volume lost through the fistula.

The inspired oxygen concentration should be kept high enough so that, in most cases, the oxygen saturation of arterial blood exceeds 92%. Patients with chronic obstructive pulmonary disease and long-standing CO_2 retention are an exception. Such patients have lost the ability to increase their respiratory drive in response to increases in $PacO_2$ and rely instead on their response to hypoxemia. Increasing the arterial oxygen saturation by adding exogenous oxygen takes away this hypoxic ventilatory stimulus and makes weaning from ventilatory support more difficult.

All of the nonoxygen volume of ventilator gas is made up of nitrogen, which, unlike oxygen, is not absorbed from alveoli. Nitrogen can be of great value in stenting open the alveoli. When it is replaced by increasing concentrations of oxygen, increased atelectasis caused by oxygen absorption can occur. In addition, high concentrations of oxygen can cause chronic pulmonary fibrosis. Ideally, the inspired oxygen concentration should be kept at 0.50 or less.

Keeping the inspired oxygen levels at acceptably low levels is frequently facilitated by the use of PEEP. The pressure is generated by closure of a valve in the expiratory circuit of the ventilator to keep the airway pressure above a preset level during expiration and to minimize alveolar collapse. Placement of an endotracheal tube bypasses the normal physiologic PEEP present during spontaneous ventilation from closure of the glottis at the end of expiration. In addition, supine patients may have a lower FRC due to increased intra-abdominal pressure and cephalad displacement of the diaphragm into the chest. This can be overcome through the use of low levels of "physiologic" PEEP (5 cm H_2O). Increasing the PEEP should be considered when the respiratory system compliance is low or when adequate oxygenation requires an FIO_2 that exceeds 0.50.

Low levels of PEEP (< 10 cm H_2O) are well tolerated by most patients. The consequences of excessive PEEP are barotrauma and decreased cardiac output. First, the high pressure can compress the superior and inferior vena cava and the pulmonary veins, compromising diastolic filling of the ventricles (in contrast with a spontaneous inspiration, which augments filling). Second, the high pressures can compress the thin-walled atria and right ventricle, further compromising end-diastolic volumes (also in contrast with a spontaneous inspiration). Finally, the high pressures can compress the pulmonary microvasculature, making it difficult for the right ventricle to push blood through the pulmonary vasculature. The remedy for the decreased cardiac output is usually fluid infusion. The potential problem with this remedy is worsening of the pulmonary failure that prompted the use of the PEEP in the first place. Accounting for all of these factors, PEEP levels greater than 10-12 cm H_2O should generally be used with a pulmonary arterial catheter in place. Titrating to the optimal oxygen delivery, and not arterial PaO_2, will ensure a balance between the risks and benefits of high PEEP levels. Monitoring the mixed venous oxygen saturation serves as a reasonable method to achieve this goal. Even with invasive monitoring, PEEP levels greater than 15-20 cm H_2O are rarely of benefit.

▶ Ventilator Safety & Alarms

As can be inferred, modern ventilators are complex, and they should, in general, be used only in the setting of continuous cardiopulmonary monitoring to include electrocardiography and pulse oximetry. In addition, the ventilators themselves have alarms for early warning of apnea, changes in tidal volume or minute ventilation, and excessive inspiratory pressures. These should be individualized to each patient so that nurses, respiratory therapists, and physicians are notified early in the course of the physiologic derangement. In many cases, the ventilator alarm will precede changes in the pulse oximeter or electrocardiogram. All personnel taking care of the patient should be knowledgeable with both the equipment and the mode of ventilation.

Discontinuing Mechanical Ventilation

Patients who seem to be doing well and who have required mechanical ventilation for less than 24 hours can frequently be extubated quickly after undergoing a trial of spontaneous ventilation. Patients must be able to maintain their own airway, and their acute illness should be resolving. They should be able to maintain adequate oxygenation with an inspired oxygen concentration of 0.40 or less and with a PEEP of 8 cm water or less.

The majority of ventilated patients are most effectively weaned with daily spontaneous breathing trials. The breathing trial can be given with T-piece ventilation in which the endotracheal tube is attached to a length of tubing connected to a blow-by oxygen source. Alternatively, the trial can be accomplished with a low level (typically 5 cm of water) of pressure support with PEEP or with PEEP alone. In either case, the patient is asked to support his or her own breathing for 30 minutes. If the patient is breathing comfortably at the end of the trial, the patient can be extubated. If a question arises as to the degree of comfort, arterial blood should be drawn for gases, and the patient should be put back on the ventilator while waiting for the results of the blood gas analysis. If the patient was reasonably comfortable at the end of the 30-minute trial and if the pH comes back at a normal value, the patient can be extubated. Note that at the conclusion of the 30-minute trial, full ventilator support should be resumed pending the laboratory results. The patient needs to be well rested when the endotracheal tube is removed. If the patient fails the 30 minute trial, full support is resumed for the remainder of the day, and the trial is repeated the following day. In some cases, the duration of the breathing trial can be extended to up to 2 hours. Although the ability to predict successful extubation is not significantly different, the increased duration may be appropriate for patients who have already required reintubation following completion of a 30 minute SBT. There is generally no role for breathing trials of longer duration when the patient is endotracheally intubated. In fact, this may serve to unnecessarily fatigue the patient making successful extubation, less likely.

Weaning from mechanical ventilation can also be achieved with IMV. Although generally inferior to the once-daily spontaneous breathing trial, patients who are severely debilitated and have required mechanical ventilation for prolonged periods (> 2-3 weeks) can be successfully weaned using this technique when combined with a gradual reduction in pressure support. The IMV rate is gradually decreased, requiring the patient to contribute increasingly to the maintenance of adequate minute ventilation. The patient's overall clinical status, respiratory rate, and arterial P_{CO_2} are used as guidelines to determine the rate of weaning. When an IMV of 4/min or less is well tolerated for long periods, the patient is placed on pressure support, which is weaned daily until mechanical support is no longer needed. As noted above, patients with an endotracheal tube in place (vs tracheostomy) should only undergo brief periods where the pressure support is less than 5-8 cm H_2O (30-120 minutes). This amount of PS is required to mitigate the increased resistance of the endotracheal tube. Patients who repeatedly fail extubation or are severely deconditioned benefit from a more deliberate and gradual weaning of the ventilator. Frequently, these patients benefit from tracheostomy and optimization of nutritional status as adjuncts to weaning. Factors that increase the work of breathing such as reactive airway disease, large pleural effusions, and chest wall or visceral edema should be treated and minimized.

Extubation

The decision to extubate the patient depends both on the assessment for the need for airway protection as well as the need for mechanical ventilation. As mentioned previously, the latter can be determined based on the result of a 30-minute trial of spontaneous breathing. The former should be based on several factors, including the patient's level of consciousness, the presence of airway injury or edema, the need for ongoing endotracheal suctioning, and the possible need for further operative procedures within the next 24 hours. Finally, a subjective determination of a patient's ability to tolerate extubation and spontaneous ventilation should be made. An alert and communicative patient who can lift her head off the pillow is a good candidate for extubation; a lethargic, diaphoretic patient is not. For patients who require continued airway protection but no longer require mechanical ventilatory support, a tracheostomy should be considered.

ADJUVANT DIAGNOSTIC & THERAPEUTIC MEASURES

Chest Radiographs

Chest x-rays should be obtained daily in patients being treated with mechanical ventilation. A review of the film should confirm the placement of all lines and tubes, including the endotracheal tube, central venous catheters, pleural tubes (thoracostomies), and nas/orogastric or nas/oroenteric tubes. A search for specific pulmonary and pleural processes should be performed. Local infiltrates such as pneumonia or patchy/diffuse processes such as the ARDS should be identified.

In addition to a daily chest radiograph, a stat chest x-ray should be obtained whenever a patient's cardiopulmonary status rapidly deteriorates. Tubes or lines might be displaced; new problems with a reversible etiology such a pneumothorax, a lobar collapse, or a new infiltrate suggesting aspiration might be identified.

Sedation & Muscle Relaxants

Mechanically ventilated patients frequently require sedatives and/or analgesia to ameliorate the agitation and pain associated with their disease and treatment. Narcotic analgesia in the form of intermittent or continuous opiate infusion may be sufficient. Narcotics, however, should not be used to treat agitation and anxiety that is thought to be caused by the ventilator. Sedating agents, including propofol and benzodiazepines, should be used instead. In addition, haloperidol and risperidone may be useful adjuncts, either alone or in combination with benzodiazepines. As a general rule, intermittent dosing is preferred to continuous infusions. When the latter is used, the agent should be stopped at least once daily—giving the patient a so-called sedation holiday—to assess neurologic status and determine the need for continuing sedation.

Neuromuscular blocking agents add an additional level of patient control and can greatly simplify ventilatory management in patients with severe pulmonary insufficiency. These agents should be reserved for severe patient-ventilator dyssynchrony, a situation in which the patient's spontaneous respiratory efforts result in discoordinated and inadequate ventilation by the mechanical ventilator. This may have the untoward effect of life-threatening hypoxemia in a patient with little physiologic reserve.

Nonphysiologic ventilatory methods, such as inverse ratio or high-frequency oscillatory ventilation, may also require the use of neuromuscular blocking agents. Major side effects include a potential increased risk of ventilator-associated pneumonia (VAP), through loss of cough mechanism, and an association with late polyneuromyopathy of critical illness. As a result, they should be used only when absolutely necessary and for the shortest possible time.

Antibiotics

Ventilator-associated pneumonia is the most common nosocomial infection in the ICU. The risk of acquiring VAP is directly related to the duration of mechanical ventilation. There is no gold standard for VAP diagnosis. Possible criteria include a new or progressive infiltrate on chest radiograph, worsening hypoxemia, increased sputum quantity, new onset of purulent sputum associated with abundant white cells and organisms on Gram-stained smears, or positive sputum cultures with known pathogenic organisms. Signs of systemic sepsis with increased temperature, leukocytosis, increasing fluid requirements, and glucose intolerance are also common findings in VAP.

If all of these are present, antibiotics should be started. If only one or two are present, antibiotics are probably best withheld to avoid overgrowth of resistant organisms that could later cause fatal pneumonia. Exceptions to this approach include older, severely debilitated patients, immunocompromised patients, and those who are critically ill in whom delayed antibiotic therapy might result in irretrievable deterioration. Thus, an 80-year-old patient with flail chest and a new infiltrate should probably be given antibiotics early; a 20-year-old patient who was hospitalized for a gunshot wound involving the colon and who develops questionable pneumonia 2 weeks later is more likely to tolerate a delay in the initiation of antibiotics until the diagnosis is more definite. In addition, the latter patient may have an alternative explanation for his fever and leukocytosis, such as an intra-abdominal abscess. In this case, the wrong diagnosis might delay appropriate source control (abscess drainage). The CPIS can be useful to guide the diagnosis. The goal is to avoid overtreatment with the risk of antimicrobial resistance and superinfection. Antibiotics can safely be discontinued in patients empirically started on antibiotics for suspected pneumonia who have a CPIS value of 6 or less at 72 hours.

King DR: Emergent cricothyroidotomy in the morbidly obese: a safe, no-visualization technique. *J Trauma.* 2011;71:1873-1874.

Graham DB, Eastman AL, Aldy KN, et al: Outcomes and long-term follow up after emergent cricothyroidotomy: is routine conversion to tracheostomy necessary? *Am Surg.* 2011;77: 1707-1711.

Barr J, Fraser GL, Puntillo K, et al: Clinical practice guidelines for the management of pain, agitation, and delirium in adult patients in the intensive care unit. *Crit Care Med.* 2013;41: 263-306.

Schweickert WD, Pohlman MC, Pohlman AS, et al: Early physical and occupational therapy in mechanically ventilated, critically ill patients: a randomized controlled trial. *Lancet.* 2009;373:1874-1882.

▼ TREATMENT OF THE MORE CHALLENGING PATIENT

This discussion of shock and pulmonary failure in the surgical patient has concentrated on making a clinical diagnosis and directing treatment on the basis of that diagnosis. This approach works well in many patients, but in some it is not sufficient. Effective treatment in the more seriously ill patient frequently has to take into account the underlying physiological abnormalities if the treatment is to work. With this approach, the clinical diagnosis becomes less important. Dealing with the underlying physiological problem becomes paramount.

COMMON PHYSIOLOGICAL RESPONSES TO SEVERE SHOCK

The body responds to the shock state with compensatory responses. These responses help the patient deal with the initial abnormalities of the shock but can contribute to the later consequences of cardiac and pulmonary failure. Understanding these responses can help the physician in managing the consequences.

Neurohumoral Responses

The neurohumoral responses to shock include discharge of the cardiovascular nerves and release of vasoactive, metabolically active, and volume-conserving hormones. The responses can be lifesaving before therapy begins and serve to maintain homeostasis once therapy has started.

Adrenergic discharge constricts the arterioles, venules, and small veins in all parts of the body except the brain and heart and augments myocardial systolic function. The result is increased cardiac output and blood pressure and diversion of flow to the brain and heart.

The vasoactive hormones angiotensin II and vasopressin act in concert with discharge of the cardiovascular adrenergic nerves. Angiotensin II constricts the vasculature in the skin, kidneys, and splanchnic organs and diverts blood flow to the heart and brain. It also stimulates the adrenal medulla to release aldosterone, resulting in reabsorption of sodium ions from the glomerular filtrate. Vasopressin, like adrenergic discharge and angiotensin II, constricts the vascular sphincters in the skin and splanchnic organs (it does not constrict the renal vasculature) and diverts blood flow to the heart and brain. It also stimulates reabsorption of water from the distal tubules.

Metabolic Responses

In all severe shock states, intracellular hydrogen ion concentrations increase. To compensate, extracellular sodium flows down its electrochemical gradient into the cells, along with chloride and water, in exchange for intracellular hydrogen ion. Intracellular pH increases back toward normal, but the cells swell, with perhaps an increase of 3 L in the intracellular volume.

Hypovolemia, hypotension, pain, and other stresses of critical illness stimulate the release of cortisol, glucagon, and epinephrine—all of which increase extracellular glucose concentrations. Thus, glucose should not be used in the initial fluid resuscitation of the patient in shock—it is not necessary and can even induce an osmotic diuresis, worsening hypovolemia and confusing the clinical picture. Glucose-containing solutions should be reserved for those patients who might be in insulin shock.

On the other hand, the endogenously produced glucose generated by the physiological release of the counter-regulatory hormones provides fuel for nervous system function, metabolism of blood cells, and wound healing. The modest increase in extracellular osmolality also helps replenish vascular volume by drawing water out of the cells and by increasing the interstitial hydrostatic pressure. The increased pressure drives interstitial protein into the lymphatics and

from there into the vascular space. Interstitial oncotic pressure falls, and plasma oncotic pressure rises. The augmented oncotic gradient between the vascular and interstitial spaces draws water, sodium, and chloride into the vascular space from the interstitial space. This replenishment of vascular volume will continue as long as interstitial hydrostatic pressures are maintained and as long as interstitial protein stores, which constitute more than half of the total extracellular protein content, can be recruited. A certain degree of hyperglycemia might be beneficial in the postresuscitative phase. Once the patient has recovered, however, it appears that it is best to aggressively keep the blood glucose levels low, at 120 mg/dL or less.

Other hormones with potential metabolic actions, including insulin and growth hormone, are also released during critical illnesses. They have little effect, however, compared with cortisol, glucagon, and epinephrine. Indeed, infusion of cortisol, glucagon, and epinephrine in normal subjects can produce most of the metabolic changes of critical illness.

Microvascular Responses

In severely ill patients, three responses—dilation of systemic arterioles, failure of cell membrane function, and disruption of the vascular endothelium—serve to worsen the patient's condition. In decompensated shock, the systemic arterioles lose their ability to constrict, while the postcapillary sphincters remain constricted. Microvascular hydrostatic pressure rises. Water, sodium, and chloride are driven out of the vascular space and into the interstitium. The process is limited, however, because the oncotic gradient, which increases as fluid is lost from plasma, prevents further fluid losses.

Trauma and sepsis activate coagulation and inflammation, which can disrupt microvascular endothelial integrity in severely ill patients. Platelet and white cell microaggregates that form in injured or infected tissues embolize to the lungs or liver, where they lodge in the microvasculature. The microaggregates, endothelium, and plasma in the regions of embolization release kinins, platelet-activating factors, fibrin degradation products, thromboxanes, prostacyclin, prostaglandins, complement, leukotrienes, lysosomal enzymes, oxygen radicals, and other toxic factors, which damage the endothelium and dilate the vasculature in the region of the emboli and distally. Protein, water, sodium, and chloride extravasate into the interstitium. The amount of extravasation is limited by the increases in interstitial hydrostatic pressure that arise from interstitial flooding and by dilution of interstitial protein concentrations. The edema that results can be massive and can involve any tissue in the body.

PULMONARY ARTERY CATHETER (SWAN-GANZ CATHETER)

The pulmonary arterial catheter can be useful in evaluating the cardiovascular consequences associated with the physiological responses described above, and it can be invaluable in directing treatment in selected, seriously ill patients. The modern pulmonary arterial catheter is equipped with a thermistor and an oximeter on its tip. It permits measurement of the cardiac output; right atrial, pulmonary arterial, and pulmonary arterial wedge pressures; and mixed venous oxygen contents. Knowledge of the cardiac output and filling pressures can be used to assess ventricular function as fluid is administered or withheld. The mixed venous oxygen saturation reflects the adequacy of oxygen delivery to the periphery; a value less than 60% indicates inadequate peripheral oxygenation and can be used to evaluate adequacy of the cardiac output and of systemic arterial oxygen content. It can also be used to determine oxygen consumption, which is calculated as the cardiac output multiplied by the difference of the oxygen contents of blood in the systemic and pulmonary arteries. Oxygen consumption can fall in severely ill patients, and measurements of consumption can help assess the patient's response to resuscitation. All of this information can help in dealing with the physiological abnormalities of the shock state and the pulmonary failure that can arise from the shock.

The catheter is particularly useful when treatment of one organ system might harm another. For example, fluid administration might be needed to treat septic shock, but excess fluid might contribute to pulmonary failure; a diuretic might be indicated in an oliguric patient in congestive heart failure, but excessive diuresis might decrease the cardiac output to the point that the kidneys fail; and fluid might be needed for cardiovascular resuscitation in a patient with multiple injuries, but too much fluid might exacerbate cerebral edema. The pulmonary arterial catheter can be extremely helpful in these situations.

Data obtained from the Swan-Ganz catheter can be misleading, however, if mistakes are made in performing the measurements. The cardiac output, as measured by thermodilution, is obtained by creating a temperature differential in the blood in the right atrium and analyzing the change in temperature in the blood over time as it flows past a thermistor on the end of the pulmonary arterial catheter. The greater the area under the temperature curve, the smaller the flow through the right heart. If injections of cold saline are used to create the temperature differential, they should be made at random times during the respiratory cycle to give the best indication of the output available to the patient, but some prefer to make the injections at a consistent time in the cycle to minimize variability in the cardiac output–associated heart-lung interactions. If a heater coil in the catheter is used to create the temperature differential, the changes are made randomly by a program in the equipment used with the catheter. All calculations are made by a computer in the equipment.

When one is obtaining pulmonary arterial or mixed venous blood, the balloon on the end of the catheter should be deflated, and the blood should be withdrawn slowly. If the

blood is withdrawn too quickly, the walls of the pulmonary artery will collapse around the end of the catheter, and the specimen will be contaminated by blood that is pulled back, in a retrograde manner, past ventilated and nonperfused alveoli. The oximeter on the tip of the catheter has to be calibrated frequently by comparing the oxygen saturations of blood obtained from the pulmonary artery with the saturations readout by the oximeter. One must be certain that the blood that is to be used for calibration is truly representative.

The pressures measured with the pulmonary arterial catheter are displayed on an oscilloscope and include a mean pressure that is calculated by computer circuitry in the monitoring equipment. These mean pressures can be used in patient management. They have the advantage that they represent the pressures throughout the respiratory cycle and thus average in the variability associated with heart-lung interactions. Some clinicians prefer to read the end-expiratory pressures from the oscilloscope screen and use those values in patient management. Those pressures are relatively independent of heart-lung interactions, but they can be difficult to interpret, even by the most experienced ICU nurse or physician.

Of the five pressures obtained from the catheter, only two—the right atrial and the mean pulmonary arterial pressures—can be taken at face value; the other three—the pulmonary arterial systolic, diastolic, and wedge pressures—are subject to errors of measurement and interpretation. The pulmonary arterial wedge pressure usually is the same as the left atrial pressure. The wedge pressure will not reflect left atrial pressure; however, if the catheter is in a portion of the vasculature occluded by inflated alveoli. If the wedge pressure varies by more than 10 mm Hg with cycles of mechanical ventilation, one should assume that the tip of the catheter is facing the pressure in the alveoli rather than the pressure in the left atrium.

To account for variations in size of the patient, the cardiac output can be indexed to the calculated body surface area. Alternatively, however, one can use the patient's desirable body weight, calculated on the assumption that a desirable weight is one that is associated with longevity and freedom from diabetes. A body mass index (BMI) of 21 is convenient to use for both men and women. Making a rough approximation of the patient's height, to the nearest half-foot, the desirable weights associated with that height, assuming a BMI of 21, are indicated in Table 12–3. The cardiac outputs associated with that weight are also indicated, assuming that the subjects are supine, nonstressed, resting, fasting, and in a thermoneutral environment. The resting oxygen consumptions under these conditions are

$$3.5 \text{ mL} \times \text{weight} (-1) \times \text{min} (-1)$$

The outputs and the consumptions for patients older than 50 years are adjusted with the assumption that metabolic activity decreases by 10% per decade after age 50.

Table 12–3. Approximate desirable weight, cardiac output, and oxygen consumption in young resting, supine, fasting individuals of varying heights, in a thermoneutral environment.

Height (ft, in)	Desirable Weight[1] (kg)	Cardiac Output[2] (L/min)	Oxygen Consumption[3] (mL/min)
5'0"	49	5	170
5'6"	59	6	205
6'0"	70	7	245
6'6"	83	8	290

[1]Calculated with assumption that the desirable weight is that which gives a BMI of 21.
[2]Calculated as 100 mL · kg^{-1} · min^{-1}.
[3]Calculated as 3.5 mL · kg^{-1} · min^{-1}.

Thus, for a 70-year-old person who is 6 feet tall, a normal cardiac output is 7 L/min multiplied by 0.8, or 5.6 L/min. The oxygen consumption is 245 mL/min multiplied by 0.8 or 195 mL/min.

OXYHEMOGLOBIN DISSOCIATION

The amount of oxygen contained in the blood and the amount of oxygen available to be delivered to the tissues can be expressed as a concentration, a saturation, or a partial pressure. All three have their value. Understanding their relationships can help in understanding the cardiac and pulmonary pathophysiology of the critically ill surgical patient.

The concentration of oxygen in the blood, or oxygen content, is expressed as milliliters of O_2/dL of blood, or vol%. The oxygen content can be measured directly, but the measurement is time consuming, and the content is usually calculated on the basis of the other two measures of blood oxygenation, the oxygen saturation (So_2) and the Po_2. The oxygen content is related to these other quantities by the following formula:

$$Co_2 = 1.34 \times [Hb] \times So_2 + 0.0031 \times Po_2 \quad (1)$$

where [Hb] is expressed as g/dL and the Po_2 as mm Hg.

Thus, for example, the oxygen content of a blood specimen with a [Hb] of 12 g/dL, an So_2 of 90%, and a Po_2 of 60 mm Hg is 14.7 vol%.

The first term in the equation represents the O_2 carried by the hemoglobin molecule; the second, the O_2 dissolved in the blood water. This second term is small compared with the first as long as the [Hb] is greater than, say, 7 g/dL and the Po_2 is less than, say, 100 mm Hg. Omitting the second term then simplifies the formula to read as follows:

$$Co_2 = 1.34 \times [Hb] \times So_2 \quad (2)$$

For the previous set of blood gases, this would give a Co_2 of 14.5 vol%.

The formula can be made even simpler by substituting the fraction 4/3 for the decimal 1.34:

$$Co_2 = 4/3 \times [Hb] \times So_2 \quad (3)$$

Because [Hb] and the So_2 can usually be approximated by integers with little loss of accuracy, the calculation frequently allows cancellation of the three and can be done mentally. For the previous example, the oxygen content would be 14.4 vol%.

Calculation of the oxygen content requires knowledge of the So_2. Many pulmonary arterial catheters are now equipped with sensors mounted on their tips that directly measure the saturation of the blood in the pulmonary artery. Alternatively, blood can be withdrawn from the tip of the catheter and sent to the laboratory, where the So_2 can be easily measured by an instrument known as a co-oximeter. Most laboratories will make this measurement by specific request, but some will calculate the So_2 from the Po_2. This calculation is frequently inaccurate for mixed venous specimens but is usually accurate for arterial blood. The calculation is made from equations that are based on the oxyhemoglobin dissociation curve (Figure 12–1), an empirically derived relationship between the So_2 of nonfetal human blood and its Po_2. The saturation for a given Po_2 depends on blood temperature, [H$^+$], and Pco_2 and on the red cell concentration of 2,3-diphosphoglycerate (2,3-DPG). The laboratory should be told the temperature, and it will measure the [H$^+$] and Pco_2. It will then calculate the So_2

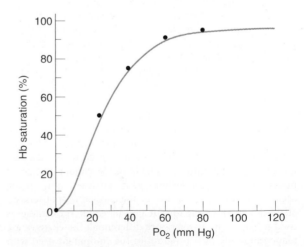

▲ **Figure 12–1.** Oxyhemoglobin dissociation curve for human blood at 37°C with a Pco_2 of 40 mm Hg, a pH of 7.40, and a normal 2,3-DPG red cell concentration. Approximate values from Table 12–4 fall close to the idealized curve.

Table 12–4. Approximate correlations for partial pressures of oxygen and oxygen saturation in blood at 37°C with a pH of 7.4, a P_{CO_2} of 40 mm Hg, and a normal 2,3-DPG red cell concentration.

P_{O_2} (mm Hg)	S_{O_2} (%)
0	0
25	50
40	75
60	90
80	95

from the P_{O_2} with the assumption that the 2,3-DPG concentration is normal.

It is helpful, however, to have some guidelines for converting back and forth between S_{O_2} and P_{O_2}. Five approximations for points on the dissociation curve for a patient with normal temperature, [H+], P_{CO_2}, and 2,3-DPG levels are given in Table 12–4. The P_{50} of human hemoglobin—the P_{O_2} at which the molecule is half-saturated—is 27 mm Hg (approximated as 25 mm Hg in the table). The P_{O_2} and S_{O_2} for mixed venous blood in a person with a [Hb] of 15 g/dL and a normal O_2 consumption and cardiac output are 40 mm Hg and 75%, respectively. A P_{O_2} of 60 mm Hg—a value that should be exceeded by most patients in an ICU—corresponds to a S_{O_2} of 90%. A P_{O_2} of 80 mm Hg corresponds to a S_{O_2} of 95%. Remembering the values in the table allows construction of a dissociation curve and facilitates conversion from one measure of oxygenation to the other. For example, in a patient with a normal temperature, [H+], P_{CO_2}, and 2,3-DPG, and a [Hb] of 10 g/dL, a P_{O_2} of 60 mm Hg in the systemic arterial blood would create an oxygen content of 12 vol% (from Equation 1), a value that would be adequate if the patient had normal coronary arteries and a good heart. Such a value would be inadequate, however, in the face of underlying heart disease.

CAUSES OF ELEVATED Pa_{CO_2}

The patient in pulmonary failure will frequently have an elevated arterial carbon dioxide tension. The arterial P_{CO_2} is proportionate to CO_2 production divided by alveolar ventilation—defined as the volume of air exchanged per unit time in functioning alveoli. Since CO_2 production is usually fairly constant in adequately perfused patients, the Pa_{CO_2} comes to be inversely proportionate to alveolar ventilation. An elevated Pa_{CO_2} in the presence of normal CO_2 production means inadequate alveolar ventilation. Ventilation should be assessed with respect to how much work is required to generate the Pa_{CO_2}. In the case of spontaneous ventilation,

this assessment involves the frequency and depth of breathing; in the case of mechanical ventilation, the frequency of the machine-generated breaths and the tidal volume of those breaths.

The Pa_{CO_2} also gives an indication of dead space ventilation—the ventilation of nonperfused airways. Since minute or total ventilation is dead space ventilation plus alveolar ventilation, a normal Pa_{CO_2} combined with a normal minute ventilation implies a normal dead space ventilation. A normal Pa_{CO_2} that must be generated by a supranormal minute ventilation implies increased dead space ventilation. Normal dead space ventilation is one-third of total ventilation, but many critically ill surgical patients will have dead space ventilation that is up to two-thirds of total ventilation. Increased dead space ventilation can be caused by hypovolemia with poor perfusion of nondependent alveoli, ARDS, pulmonary emboli, pulmonary vasoconstriction, and mechanical ventilation-induced compression of the pulmonary vasculature. Hypovolemia should be treated by expansion of the vascular volume. Emboli should be treated by anticoagulation or by elimination of their source. Dead space generated by mechanical ventilation should be minimized by adjustment of the ventilator, usually by decreasing tidal volumes or end-expiratory pressures, while at the same time maintaining enough mechanical support to generate a normal P_{CO_2} and alveolar ventilation.

CAUSES OF LOW Pa_{O_2}

Almost all surgical patients with pulmonary failure will have systemic arterial hypoxemia. There are five physiological causes: low inspired O_2 concentration, diffusion block between alveolar gas and capillary blood, subnormal alveolar ventilation, shunting of blood through completely nonventilated portions of the lung or bypassing of blood past the lung, and perfusion of parts of the lung that have low ventilation/perfusion ratios. In addition, any process that decreases the mixed venous oxygen content in the presence of any of the above can lower the arterial P_{O_2} even further. Low mixed venous oxygen content can be caused by a low arterial oxygen content, low cardiac output, or high O_2 consumption.

Arterial hypoxemia in the surgical patient is usually caused by shunting, low ventilation/perfusion ratios, low mixed venous oxygen content, or a combination of these factors. Low inspired O_2 concentrations at sea level are impossible so long as the ventilator is functioning properly. (This must be checked, however, as the first step in diagnosing and correcting the cause of a low Pa_{O_2}.) Diffusion block is exceedingly rare in surgical patients. Subnormal alveolar ventilation can be ruled out with a normal arterial P_{CO_2} assuming CO_2 production is not depressed. Thus, shunting and areas of low ventilation/perfusion ratios, along with low mixed venous oxygen content, remain as causes for almost all cases of hypoxemia in the surgical patient. Shunting and low ventilation/perfusion ratios do not need to be distinguished from each other very often, but the distinction can be made by increasing the inspired O_2 concentration to 100%: Hypoxemia caused by areas of low ventilation/perfusion ratios will be at least partially corrected by 100% O_2; hypoxemia caused by shunting will not. The mixed venous oxygen content can be measured with the pulmonary arterial catheter.

ACID-BASE BALANCE

Acid-base abnormalities can arise from the hypoventilation of pulmonary insufficiency or from the metabolic abnormalities of shock. The former has already been discussed. The latter can become more involved.

The hydrogen ion, carbon dioxide gas, and bicarbonate equilibrate with one another in the plasma water, and if two of the quantities are known, the third can be calculated. In practice, the P_{CO_2} and $[H^+]$, which are measured directly with the blood gas apparatus, will be known. The $[HCO_3^-]$ can then be calculated by the Henderson-Hasselbalch equation, which can be written in the following form:

$$[HCO_3^-] = \frac{24 \times P_{CO_2}}{[H^+]} \quad \textbf{(4)}$$

where $[HCO_3^-]$ is expressed as mmol/L, P_{CO_2} as mm Hg, and $[H^+]$ as nmol/L. This form of the equation requires conversion of pH, the more common expression of $[H^+]$, into nmol/L, the more logical expression, but the conversion is not difficult (Table 12–5). The values in the table are easy to remember if one notes that each value in the column under $[H^+]$ is 80% of the value immediately above, with the exception of 80 and 63, which are off by 1. Thus, by Equation 4, if the P_{CO_2} is 60 mm Hg and the pH is 7.30, the $[HCO_3^-]$ is 29 mmol/L.

The $[HCO_3^-]$ calculated by this equation is the amount of bicarbonate ion dissolved in the plasma water and can be obtained only from a specimen of blood that is obtained and processed without exposure to the atmosphere. The "CO_2 combining power" that is typically measured along with electrolyte concentrations in blood that is not processed anaerobically includes not only the $[HCO_3^-]$ but any CO_2 gas and carbonic acid that is dissolved in the plasma as well. The CO_2 combining power is usually about 2 mmol/L greater than the calculated (and actual) $[HCO_3^-]$.

The base deficit or excess is determined by comparing the calculated $[HCO_3^-]$ with the $[HCO_3^-]$ that might be expected in a patient with a given P_{CO_2} and $[H^+]$. These expected values have been determined by analyzing blood obtained from patients with a wide variety of pulmonary disorders. For example, the kidneys in a patient with chronic respiratory acidemia can usually compensate to the extent that a chronic elevation in P_{CO_2} of 10 mm Hg will generate an increase in $[HCO_3^-]$ of 3 mmol/L. A patient with

Table 12–5. Conversion of pH to hydrogen ion concentration.

pH	Hydrogen Ion Concentration (mol/L)
7.0	100
7.1	$100 \times 0.8 = 80$
7.2	$80 \times 0.8 = 63$
7.3	$63 \times 0.8 = 50$
7.4	$50 \times 0.8 = 40$
7.5	$40 \times 0.8 = 32$
7.6	$32 \times 0.8 = 25$

Values not indicated in the table can be derived by interpolation. For example, a pH of 7.35 corresponds to a hydrogen ion concentration of approximately 45.

chronic obstructive lung disease and a chronically elevated P_{CO_2} of 60 mm Hg would be expected to have a $[HCO_3^-]$ of 30 mmol/L—6 mmol/L more than a normal value of 24. If such a patient had a pH of 7.30, the actual $[HCO_3^-]$ would be 29 mmol/L (from Equation 4; see the example in the preceding paragraph). That is, the observed value would be 1 mmol/L less than predicted, and the patient would be said to have a base deficit of 1 mmol/L.

The difficulty with the concept of base deficit and excess is that it rests on historically determined values, which may not be applicable to the patient at hand. For example, if a surgical patient with previously normal lungs lost his or her airway after an operation and began to hypoventilate, one would expect the $[HCO_3^-]$ to be normal—24 mmol/L—because the kidneys would not have had time to compensate for the hypercapnia. If the P_{CO_2} was 60 mm Hg and the pH 7.30, the physician should be concerned because the $[HCO_3^-]$ is 29 mmol/L (these values are the same as in the preceding paragraphs). A value of 29 mmol/L should alert the physician to the fact that the $[HCO_3^-]$ is too high, perhaps because $NaHCO_3$ had been given unnecessarily. The base deficit, however, would be 1 mmol/L, suggesting that the patient's $[HCO_3^-]$ was appropriate. The base deficit would be misleading.

The use of base deficit and excess is ensconced in the literature, and the terms are used in this chapter. However, the concept of $[HCO_3^-]$ may be preferable. Errors in patient evaluation are more likely to be minimized if the physician interprets that value in the light of a particular patient's situation. If a chronically ill patient in the ICU has severe ARDS and a P_{CO_2} of 60 mm Hg with a pH of 7.30, no attempt should be made to change the accompanying $[HCO_3^-]$ of 29 mmol/L—that value represents the expected renal compensation for such a chronic hypercapnia (though the impaired alveolar ventilation should be of concern). Alternatively, if the patient's Pco_2 is 60 mm Hg and the pH is 7.45, the patient has an inappropriately high $[HCO_3^-]$ of approximately 40 mmol/L (calculated from Equation 4), perhaps because of unreplaced losses of hydrogen ion from the stomach, chronic use of a loop diuretic, or administration of excessive amounts of acetate in the patient's parenteral nutrition. In this situation, the $[HCO_3^-]$ should be brought down into the low 30s. The excessively high $[HCO_3^-]$ and its resultant alkalemia may be blunting the patient's ventilatory drive.

Thus, in dealing with acid-base disorders, the calculation of the bicarbonate concentration in arterial plasma can be taken from the blood gas laboratory or calculated by the clinician. In the case of a metabolic acidemia, the underlying abnormality should be corrected and then, if the pH remains less than 7.20, sodium bicarbonate can be used, but only after resuscitation has been initiated and only with the intent of bringing the pH up to a modestly higher level, such as a pH of 7.30. The bicarbonate produces carbon dioxide and water locally, in the interstitial fluid at the sites where the hydrogen ions are being produced. In the absence of resuscitation, the locally generated carbon dioxide can cross back into the cell, worsening intracellular acidosis. There is no problem with bicarbonate if it is given after some local flow has been achieved. The generated carbon dioxide will be washed centrally into the pulmonary vasculature, where it will be eliminated by the lungs.

Metabolic alkalemia in the surgical patient is usually easy to recognize and treat. Contraction alkalemia is treated with fluid expansion. Hypokalemic, hypochloremic metabolic alkalemia caused by unreplaced loss of gastric fluid (continuous nasogastric suction or protracted vomiting), is treated with normal saline supplemented with potassium chloride. Hypokalemic hypochloremic alkalemia caused by use of loop diuretics is treated by withholding diuresis. In situations where continued diuresis is warranted, the addition of acetazolamide to the diuretic regimen is helpful. Although the administration of 0.1 N hydrochloric acid can reverse severe alkalemia, it is rarely necessary and should only be given as a slow central intravenous drip over a period of 48 hours. The amount of acid to be given is calculated on the basis of the presumed extracellular chloride deficit, with the assumption that the interstitial chloride concentration is the same as the plasma concentration, that is, with the assumption that the Donnan factor for chloride is 1.

RISK ASSESSMENT

Predicting the likelihood of survival in critically ill surgical patients is best accomplished by evaluating clinical and laboratory findings. Computation of a severity of illness score is usually unnecessary. Nonetheless, several scoring systems have been developed with the intention of increasing the precision of the estimate. All such systems assign a mathematical probability for survival in groups of patients, and many are useful for research purposes because they allow comparisons of patients among different institutions. None of them, however, are accurate enough to predict survival for an individual patient, though some are still clinically useful for assessing the effects of therapy.

The APACHE II score, in which clinical data and 14 measured variables are entered into a formula to assess the probability of survival, takes about 30 minutes to calculate by hand—less by computer. The score can predict survival in critically ill medical patients; it has not been found to be of value in the usual surgical patient, and in any case, it is too cumbersome unless one has a particular interest in this kind of methodology.

Methods for predicting survival in trauma patients are well established, though most trauma systems are designed to evaluate all trauma patients and not the specific subset of critically ill trauma patients. The Injury Severity Score, the Revised Trauma Score, and the ASCOT score have proved to be most reliable. The Glasgow Coma Score is quite accurate for predicting survival in patients with head injuries. Combining the Glasgow Coma Score with a simple measurement of fluid requirement has also proved to be accurate in critically injured trauma patients.

MULTIPLE CHOICE QUESTIONS

1. Shock can be caused by

   A. Depletion of intravascular volume
   B. Loss of autonomic control of the vasculature
   C. Severe untreated systemic inflammation
   D. Both A and C
   E. All of A, B, and C

2. Hypothermia in hemorrhagic shock

   A. Is of limited risk in the initial 24 hours after injury
   B. Can contribute to coagulopathy
   C. Is unusual in the trauma population outside of cold-weather or water-immersion injuries
   D. Is best treated by warming the ambient room temperature
   E. Is a secondary concern that can be addressed after the care of injuries

3. Cardiac or great vessel compressive shock

   A. Can be caused by pericardial tamponade
   B. May accompany tension pneumothorax
   C. Is worsened by the need for positive pressure ventilation
   D. Cannot be caused by intra-abdominal injury
   E. All of A, B, and C

4. The pulmonary failure of shock, trauma, and sepsis

    A. Can be related to products of coagulation and inflammation that are washed out from the damaged tissues

    B. Can be effectively treated with a combination of antibiotics and corticosteroids

    C. Is always related to systemic infection

    D. Is caused by a decrease in pulmonary vascular permeability

    E. Both A and C

5. All of the following are true about pressure support ventilation, except

    A. PSV is a pressure-limited ventilator mode

    B. PSV includes a set inspiratory time

    C. PSV breaths are patient-triggered

    D. Inspiratory flow is adjusted to maintain airway pressure

    E. PSV can be combined with IMV

Management of the Injured Patient

Mark R. Hemmila, MD
Wendy L. Wahl, MD

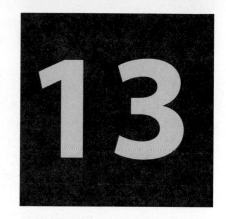

EPIDEMIOLOGY OF TRAUMA

As a "disease," trauma is a major public health problem. In the United States, it is the leading cause of death among people aged 1-45. For persons under age 30, trauma is responsible for more deaths than all other diseases combined. Because trauma adversely affects a young population, it results in the loss of more working years than all other causes of death. Presence of alcohol is a significant contributor to trauma fatalities, and one-third of all traffic deaths are alcohol related. The financial costs of injury are astounding and exceed $400 billion annually. Regrettably, nearly 40% of all trauma deaths could be avoided by injury prevention measures (50% of passenger vehicle occupants killed were unrestrained), alcohol cessation, and by the establishment of regional trauma systems that would expedite the evaluation and treatment of seriously injured patients.

Trauma deaths have been described as having a trimodal distribution (Figure 13–1), with peaks that correspond to the types of intervention that would be most effective in reducing mortality. The first peak, the **immediate deaths,** represents patients who die of their injuries before reaching the hospital. The injuries accounting for these deaths include major brain or spinal cord trauma and those resulting in rapid exsanguination. Few of these patients would have any chance of survival even with access to immediate care because almost 60% of these deaths occur at the same time as the injury. Prevention remains the major strategy to reduce these deaths.

The second peak, the **early deaths** are those that occur within the first few hours after injury. Half are caused by internal hemorrhage, and the other half, by central nervous system injuries. Almost all of these injuries are potentially treatable. However, in most cases, salvage requires prompt and definitive care of the sort available at a trauma center, which is a specialized institution that can provide immediate resuscitation, identification of injuries, and access to a ready operating room 24 hours a day. Development of well-organized trauma systems with rapid transport and protocol-driven care can reduce the mortality in this time period by 30%.

The third peak, the **late deaths,** consists of patients who die days or weeks after injury. Ten percent to 20% of all trauma deaths occur during this period. Mortality for this period has traditionally been attributed to infection and multiple organ failure. However, development of trauma systems has changed the epidemiology of these deaths. During the first week, refractory intracranial hypertension following severe head injury is now responsible for a significant number of these deaths. Improvements in critical care management continue to be essential in reducing deaths during this phase. It is paramount that surgeons caring for trauma patients have genuine expertise in surgical critical care.

TRAUMA SYSTEMS

The terrorist attacks of September 11, 2001, highlighted the need for national and state trauma systems that can handle both routine events and mass casualty situations. The purpose of a trauma system is to provide timely, organized care in order to minimize preventable morbidity and mortality following injury. The system includes prehospital care designed to identify, triage, treat, and transport victims with serious injuries. Criteria for staging patients with major trauma consist of standardized scoring systems based on readily discernible anatomic and physiologic variables. These criteria are designed to identify not only the more severe and complex single injuries but also combinations of injuries that require tertiary care. Trauma centers that are part of a larger trauma system are already organized to respond to unexpected multiple casualty events. Regional trauma centers have established links with emergency medical service

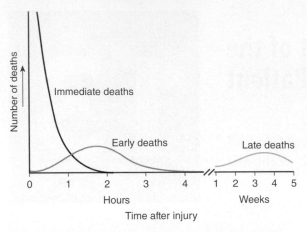

▲ **Figure 13–1.** Periods of peak mortality after injury. (Modified from Hoyt DB, Coimbra R: Trauma: introduction. In: Greenfield LJ, Mulholland MW, Oldham KT, et al. *Surgery, Scientific Principles and Practice,* 3rd ed. Lippincott Williams & Wilkins, 2001; p. 271.)

providers and participate in systemwide patient triage and quality improvement. Gaps remain, however, in areas of the country not served by trauma systems, and a wide range in the degree of disaster preparedness exists at all levels of trauma care.

The American College of Surgeons (ACS) defines four levels of institutional trauma care. Level I is the highest designation a trauma center can receive. It indicates that the hospital has committed itself to the care of trauma patients and offers the highest level of skill available in trauma care. A level I trauma center is directed by a board-certified surgeon specializing in trauma care and is staffed by a team of board-certified trauma care specialists available 24 hours a day—including emergency room physicians, trauma surgeons, neurosurgeons and neurologists, orthopedic surgeons, plastic surgeons, anesthesiologists, and radiologists. Level II trauma centers provide 24-hour care by in-hospital and on-call physicians. They can deliver the same quality of care as a level I center but without the same teaching and research obligations. The level III trauma center provides prompt assessment, resuscitation, and stabilization followed by surgical treatment or interhospital transfer as appropriate. Level III centers serve a valuable function in less populated areas where resuscitation and stabilization before transport may be lifesaving. Level IV centers are designed to provide advanced trauma life support (ATLS) prior to patient transfer in remote areas in which no higher level of care is available.

Determining if a victim of a vehicle crash requires care at a trauma center is a decision for emergency medical responders. The Centers for Disease Control (CDC) has sponsored research and policy making aimed at providing guidance to answer this question. It is established that care at a level 1 trauma center reduces the risk of death by 25% for severely injured patients, when compared to treatment at a hospital which does not have verified trauma center resources. The CDC has undertaken two initiatives based on research and expert panel findings: (1) guidelines for the field triage of injured patient and (2) advanced automatic collision notification and triage of the injured patient (AACN). The published guidelines for the field triage of injured patients provides a rapid easily understood algorithm which allows for determination of where to triage trauma patients based upon findings at the scene taking into account assessment of vital signs/level of consciousness, anatomic evidence of injury, and mechanism of injury with regard to the level of energy involved (Figure 13–2). Partnering with the automotive industry has allowed for development of sophisticated sensors and vehicle telematics that allow early notification of a crash, prediction of the likelihood of serious injury among the occupants, and assistance with the field triage decision making. In combination, the AACN system and the field triage algorithm are expected to decrease the time that it takes for a seriously injured patient to receive appropriate and definitive trauma care.

PREHOSPITAL CARE & IMMEDIATE MEASURES AT A CRASH SITE

At first glance, the trauma victim may not appear to be badly injured. Sometimes there may be little external evidence of injury; however, when the mechanism of trauma is sufficient to produce severe injury, the victim must be handled as if a severe injury has occurred. It is critical at the scene that the injured person be protected from further trauma; likewise, rescue personnel need to take precautions to avoid injury to themselves. First aid at the scene of an accident should be administered by trained personnel whenever possible.

Whether the patient is first seen on the battlefield, beside a road, in the emergency ward, or in the hospital, the basic principles of initial management are the same:

1. Is the victim breathing? If not, provide an airway and establish bag-mask ventilation.

2. Is there a pulse or heartbeat? If not, begin closed-chest compression.

3. Is there gross external bleeding? If so, elevate the part if possible and apply enough external pressure to stop the bleeding. A tourniquet when utilized by trained providers is acceptable in circumstances of extreme bleeding.

4. Is there any question of injury to the spine? If so, protect the neck and spine before moving the patient.

5. Splint obvious fractures.

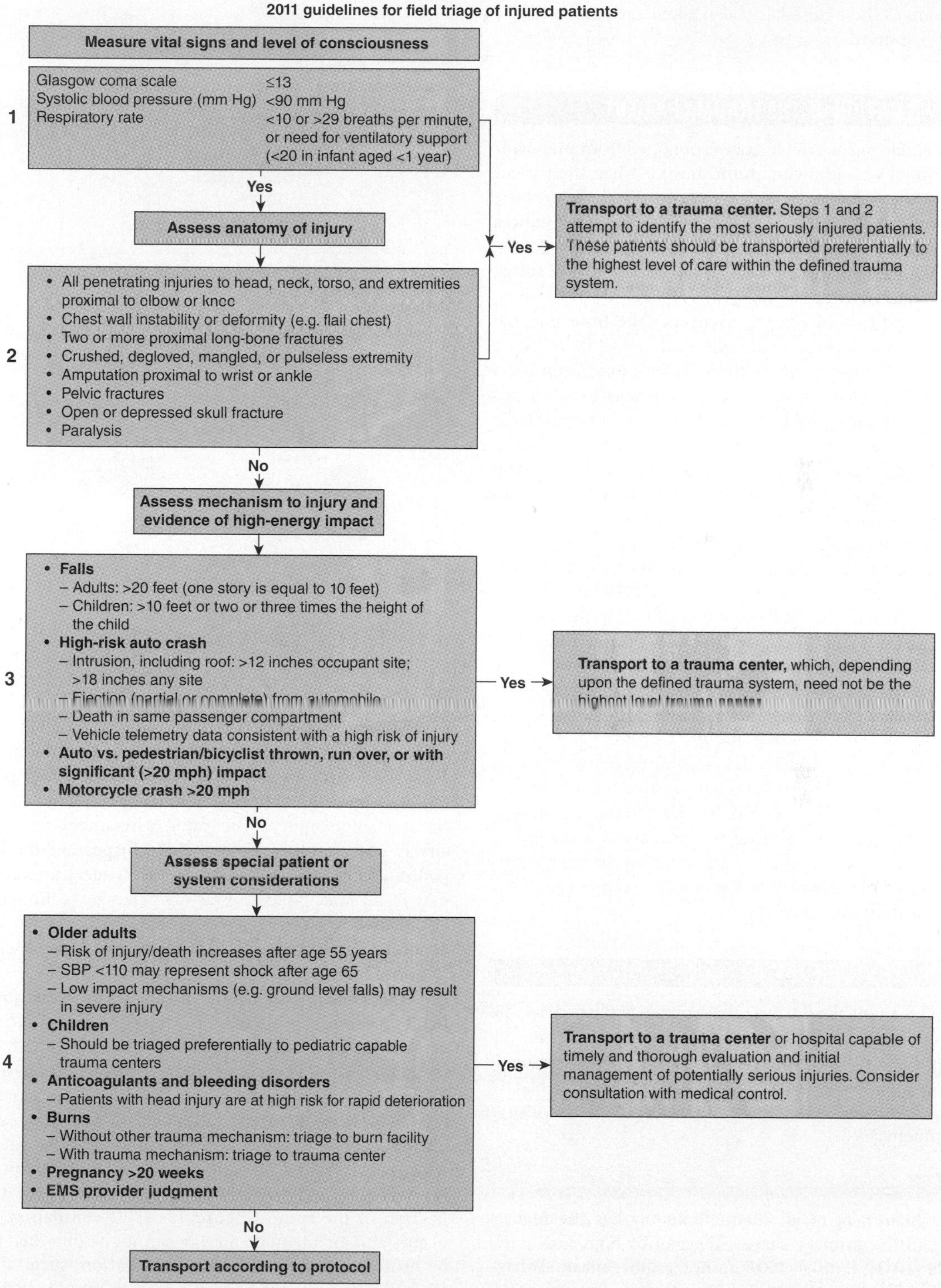

2011 guidelines for field triage of injured patients

▲ **Figure 13–2.** CDC 2011 guidelines for field triage of injured patients.

As soon as these steps have been taken, the patient can be safely transported.

EVALUATION OF THE TRAUMA PATIENT

In most situations, a brief history is obtained from prehospital personnel via radio communication or when the patient arrives at the hospital. In the case of motor vehicle crashes, for example, it is important to determine the circumstances of the injury, including the speed of impact, the condition of the vehicle, the position of the patient at the scene, type of restraint systems present, evidence of blood loss, and the condition of other passengers. The time that the injury occurred and the treatment rendered while en route is recorded. Knowing the mechanism of injury often gives a clue to concealed trauma. Information regarding serious underlying medical problems should be sought from Medic Alert bracelets or wallet cards. If the patient is conscious and stable, the examiner should obtain a complete history and use this information to direct the examination in order to avoid unnecessary tests.

Trauma victims require a precise, rapid, systematic approach to initial evaluation in order to ensure their survival. The ATLS system developed by the ACS Committee on Trauma represents the best current approach to the severely injured patient. The sequence of evaluation includes primary survey, resuscitation, secondary survey, and definitive management. The primary survey attempts to identify and treat immediate life-threatening conditions. Resuscitation is performed, and the response to therapy is evaluated. The secondary survey includes a comprehensive physical examination designed to detect all injuries and establish a treatment priority for potentially life-threatening and/or limb-threatening ones. During the primary and secondary surveys, appropriate laboratory and imaging studies are performed to aid in the identification of injuries and prepare the patient for definitive care.

1. PRIMARY SURVEY

The ATLS manual and provider course published by the ACS Committee on Trauma is the accepted guideline for the primary survey. The primary survey is a rapid assessment to detect life-threatening injuries following the ABCDE: airway, breathing, circulation, disability, and exposure/environment.

AIRWAY

The establishment of an adequate airway has the highest priority in the primary survey. Oxygen by high-flow nasal cannula (10-12 L/min), 100% nonrebreather mask, or bag-mask ventilation with pulse oximetry should be started if not already in place. Maneuvers used in the trauma patient

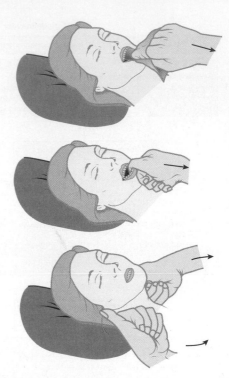

▲ **Figure 13–3.** Relief of airway obstruction.

to establish an airway must consider a possible cervical spine injury. Any patient with multisystem trauma, especially those with an altered level of consciousness or blunt trauma above the clavicles, should be assumed to have a cervical spine injury. The rapid assessment for signs of airway obstruction should include inspection for foreign bodies and facial, jaw, or tracheal/laryngeal fractures that may result in acute loss of airway patency. Techniques that can be used to establish a patent airway while protecting the cervical spine include the chin lift or jaw thrust maneuvers (Figure 13–3).

Patients who can communicate verbally without difficulty are unlikely to have an impaired airway. Repeated assessment of airway patency is always prudent. Those patients with severe head injury, altered level of consciousness, or Glasgow Coma Scale (GCS) score 8 or less usually require placement of a definitive airway. Orotracheal or nasotracheal intubation can be attempted with cervical spine precautions if a second person maintains axial immobilization of the head to prevent destabilization of the spine (Figure 13–4). If ventilatory failure occurs and an adequate airway cannot be obtained readily by orotracheal or nasotracheal intubation, surgical cricothyroidotomy should be performed as rapidly as possible (Figure 13–5).

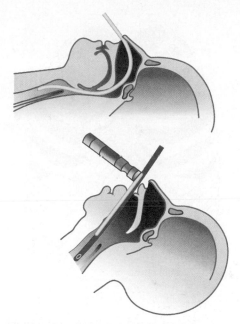

▲ **Figure 13–4.** A. Nasotracheal intubation.
B. Orotracheal intubation.

BREATHING

Once the airway has been established, it is necessary to ensure that oxygenation and ventilation is adequate. Examine the patient to determine the degree of chest expansion, breath sounds, tachypnea, crepitus from rib fractures, subcutaneous emphysema, and the presence of penetrating or open wounds. Immediately life-threatening

pulmonary injuries that must be detected and treated promptly include tension pneumothorax, open pneumothorax, flail chest, and massive hemothorax. Chest injury has the second highest case fatality rate in the trauma patient. The following are examples of life-threatening pulmonary injuries and their treatment:

1. Tension pneumothorax—This condition occurs when air becomes trapped in the pleural space under pressure. The harmful effects result primarily from shift of the mediastinum, impairment of venous return, and potential occlusion of the airway. Tension pneumothorax is difficult to diagnose even when the patient reaches the hospital. The clinical findings consist of hypotension in the presence of distended neck veins, decreased or absent breath sounds on the affected side, hyperresonance to percussion, and tracheal shift away from the affected side. These signs may be difficult to detect in a hypovolemic patient with a cervical collar in place. Cyanosis may be a late manifestation. Emergency treatment consists of insertion of a large-bore needle or plastic intravenous cannula (angiocath) through the chest wall into the pleural space in the second intercostal space along the midclavicular line to relieve the pressure and convert the tension pneumothorax to a simple pneumothorax. The needle or cannula should be left in place until a thoracostomy tube is inserted for definitive management (Figure 13–6).

2. Open pneumothorax—This condition results from an open wound of the chest wall with free communication between the pleural space and the atmosphere. The resulting impairment of the thoracic bellows, and its ability to expand the lung results in inadequate ventilation. With chest expansion during a breath, air moves in and out of the chest wall opening instead of through the trachea, producing

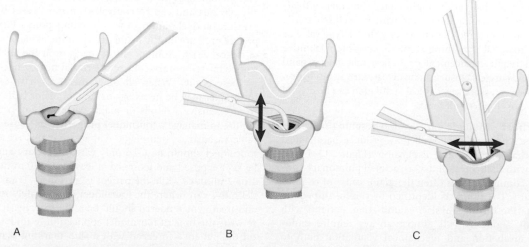

A   B   C

▲ **Figure 13–5.** Surgical cricothyroidotomy.

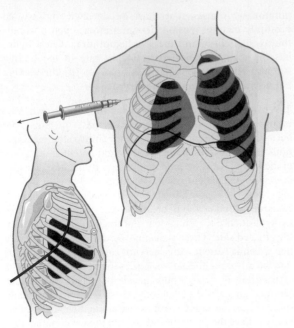

▲ Figure 13–6. Relief of pneumothorax. Tension pneumothorax must be immediately decompressed by a needle introduced through the second anterior intercostal space. A chest tube is usually inserted in the midaxillary line at the level of the nipple and is directed posteriorly and superiorly toward the apex of the thorax. The tube is attached to a "three-bottle" suction device, and the rate of escape of air is indicated by the appearance of bubbles in the second of the three bottles. Cessation of bubbling suggests that the air leak has become sealed.

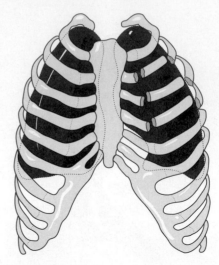

▲ Figure 13–7. Flail chest.

hypoventilation that can be rapidly fatal. Emergency treatment consists of sealing the wound with an occlusive sterile dressing taped on three sides to act as a flutter-type valve or with any material if nothing sterile is available. Definitive treatment requires placement of a chest tube to reexpand the lung and surgical closure of the defect. Airway intubation with positive-pressure mechanical ventilation can be helpful in massive open pneumothorax.

3. Flail chest—Multiple rib fractures resulting in a free-floating segment of chest wall may produce paradoxical motion that impairs lung expansion (Figure 13–7). In patients with flail chest, injury-associated pulmonary contusion is common and is often the major cause of respiratory failure. The injury is identified by careful inspection and palpation during physical examination. Patients with large flail segments will almost always require endotracheal intubation and mechanical ventilation both to stabilize the flail segment and to optimize gas exchange.

Smaller flail segments may be well tolerated if supplemental oxygen and adequate analgesia are provided. The work of breathing is increased considerably, and many patients who initially appear to be compensating well may suddenly deteriorate a few hours later. Therefore, most patients with flail chest require monitoring in an intensive care unit (ICU).

CIRCULATION

▶ Hemorrhage

Free hemorrhage from accessible surface wounds is usually obvious and can be controlled in most cases by local pressure and elevation of the bleeding point. Firm and precise pressure on the major artery in the axilla, antecubital space, wrist, groin, popliteal space, or at the ankle may suffice for temporary control of arterial hemorrhage distal to these points. When all other measures have failed, a tourniquet may be necessary to control major hemorrhage from extensive wounds or major vessels in an extremity. Failure to manage a tourniquet properly may cause irreparable vascular or neurologic damage. For this reason, the tourniquet should be used only when necessary and must be kept exposed and loosened at least every 20 minutes for 1 or 2 minutes while the patient is in transit. Transport to definitive care where the tourniquet can be safely removed and treatment rendered should be a top priority. It is wise to write the time of tourniquet application in military time on the patient's forehead with a skin-marking pen or on adhesive tape.

► Vascular Access & Resuscitation

All patients with significant trauma should have large-caliber peripheral intravenous catheters inserted immediately for administration of crystalloid fluids as needed. If any degree of shock is present, at least two 14-16 gauge peripheral intravenous lines should be established usually in the antecubital fossa. If venous access cannot be obtained by percutaneous peripheral or central venous cannulation, an intraosseous line in the tibia or other uninjured site should be placed. A venous cutdown of the saphenous vein at the ankle using an angiocath or intravenous extension tubing with the tip cut off can be performed, but is a difficult procedure in the field. A blood sample for type and cross-match should be sent from the venous line, if not already drawn.

As soon as the first intravenous line is inserted, rapid crystalloid infusion should begin. Adult patients should be given 2 L of Ringer lactate or normal saline. For children, the initial administered crystalloid volume should be 20 mL/kg. Patients who experience a transient response should receive an additional infusion of 2 L of crystalloid. Patients in hemorrhagic shock for whom there is no improvement in blood pressure from initial crystalloid infusion or who transiently respond but fail a second crystalloid bolus should be switched to resuscitation with blood products. Beyond the administration of the first two units of packed red blood cells (PRBC), it is important to also administer fresh plasma or thawed fresh frozen plasma (FFP) to avoid coagulopathy in the massively transfused patient. Massive transfusion is defined as at least 10 units of PRBC. The exact ratio of FFP to PRBC is still under active investigation, but a target range of 1:1 or 2:3 is considered acceptable. Military data has shown that the early use of plasma can reduce mortality by up to 50% in the massively transfused trauma patient. Giving platelets as part of the massive transfusion protocol is also supported by military data demonstrating a 20% reduction in mortality for patients who received platelets as fresh whole blood or apheresis platelets in conjunction with PRBC. The exact platelet-to-PRBC ratio for optimal treatment of the hemorrhaging trauma patient is not known, but giving a unit of platelets for every five units of PRBC is a reasonable ratio. Type O, Rh-negative PRBC should be immediately available in the emergency department for any patient with impending cardiac arrest or massive hemorrhage. Some high-volume trauma centers now also stock fresh or "prethawed" AB plasma as well. Type-specific blood should be available within 15-20 minutes of patient arrival to the hospital.

Tranexamic acid is an antifibrinolytic agent which inhibits the breakdown of clotted blood. It does not promote new blood clot formation. Two large clinical trials, one in the military setting and another in civilian population, have demonstrated the efficacy of tranexamic acid when utilized as part of a blood product resuscitation strategy in patients with traumatic hemorrhage. The survival benefit is greatest in patients who received massive transfusion and those in whom early treatment was accomplished ($\leq$ 1 hour after injury). Tranexamic acid started greater than 3 hours after injury increased the risk of death due to bleeding and is likely ineffective. Dosing is typically 1 g intravenously over 10 minutes, followed by a drip infusion of an additional 1 g over 8 hours.

Transfusion of blood products is not without risk. Despite rigorous screening programs, transmission of viral blood-borne diseases can occur. The current incidence of blood-borne pathogen transmission following red blood cell transfusion are hepatitis B, 1:350,000; hepatitis C 1:400,000; and HIV, 1:2 million. Transfusion of blood products is also associated with transfusion-related immunomodulation and transfusion-related acute lung injury. Both of these problems can increase morbidity and mortality. The storage age of blood transfused can also contribute to problems. Transfusion of a patient with older units of PRBC has been shown to cause generation of systemic proinflammatory mediators and increase the risk of wound infection.

► Monitoring

As intravenous access is obtained, electrocardiogram leads for continuous cardiac monitoring should be placed. Noninvasive blood pressure measurements should be acquired with a time-cycled blood pressure cuff. Pulse oximetry is valuable in ensuring that adequate hemoglobin oxygen saturation is present in the injured patient. Temperature is a crucial vital sign, and it should be measured and recorded along with the first pulse and blood pressure in the emergency department.

NEUROLOGIC DISABILITY

A brief neurologic examination should be documented to assess patients' degree of neurologic impairment. Many factors may contribute to altered levels of consciousness and should be considered in addition to central nervous system injury in all trauma patients. Other than the direct trauma, the most common contributing causes of altered mental status for trauma patients are alcohol intoxication, other central nervous system stimulants or depressants, diabetic ketoacidosis, cerebrovascular accident, and hypovolemic shock. Less common causes are epilepsy, eclampsia, electrolyte imbalances associated with metabolic and systemic diseases, anaphylaxis, heavy metal poisoning, electric shock, tumors, severe systemic infections, hypercalcemia, asphyxia, heat stroke, severe heart failure, and hysteria. These uncommon causes of coma or diminished mental status should be considered if routine testing such as blood alcohol and glucose level, urine toxicology, and head computerized tomography (CT) scanning are unrevealing as to the etiology of mental

Table 13–1. Glasgow Coma Scale score.

Parameter	Score
Best motor response	
Normal	6
Localizes	5
Withdraws	4
Flexion	3
Extension	2
None	1
Best verbal response	
Oriented	5
Confused	4
Verbalizes	3
Vocalizes	2
None	1
Eye opening	
Spontaneous	4
To command	3
To pain	2
None	1

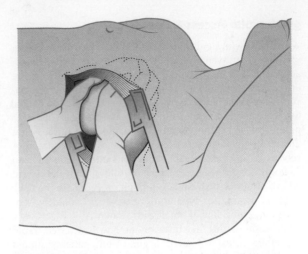

▲ **Figure 13–8.** Emergency thoracotomy and open cardiac massage.

impairment. In such cases, further laboratory and diagnostic testing may be warranted.

The differential diagnosis depends upon a careful history and complete physical examination, with particular attention to the neurologic examination with documentation of the patient's GCS score (Table 13–1), and an urgent head CT scan. The GCS score is useful in monitoring acute changes in neurologic function and is used for prognosticating outcomes after severe head injury. The motor component of the GCS score is the most accurate for predicting outcome and has a linear relationship with mortality. Lateralizing signs may also suggest evidence of an intracranial mass effect or carotid or vertebral artery injury, while loss of distal motor and/or sensory function may help localize potential spinal cord injuries.

EXPOSURE/ENVIRONMENT

All clothing should be removed (cut off with trauma shears, usually) from the seriously injured patient, with care taken to avoid unnecessary movement. The removal of helmets or other protective clothing may require additional personnel to stabilize the patient and prevent further injury. All skin surfaces should be examined to identify occult injuries that may not be readily apparent, such as posterior penetrating trauma or open fractures. After inspecting all surfaces, warm blankets or warming devices should be placed to avoid hypothermia in the seriously injured patient.

EMERGENCY ROOM THORACOTOMY

Certain injuries are so critical that operative treatment must be undertaken as soon as the diagnosis is made. In these cases, resuscitation is continued as the patient is being operated on. For cardiopulmonary arrest that occurs in the emergency room as a direct result of trauma, external cardiac compression is rarely successful in maintaining effective perfusion of vital organs. An emergency left anterolateral thoracotomy should be performed in the fourth or fifth intercostal space, and the pericardium should be opened anterior to the phrenic nerve (Figure 13–8). Open cardiac massage, cross-clamping of the descending thoracic aorta, repair of cardiac injuries, and internal defibrillation can be performed as appropriate. Wounds of the lung producing severe hemorrhage or systemic air embolus may require pulmonary hilar cross-clamping.

Emergency room thoracotomy is most useful for cardiac arrest due to penetrating thoracic trauma, particularly in patients with pericardial tamponade from stab wounds. This extreme procedure is ineffective for most patients with cardiac arrest due to blunt trauma and for all patients who have no detectable vital signs in the field (< 1% survival). If vital signs are present in the emergency room but arrest appears imminent, the patient should be transferred rapidly to the operating room if at all possible, since conditions in the operating room are optimal for surgical intervention.

RESUSCITATION PHASE

▶ Shock

Shock is defined as inadequate end-organ tissue perfusion. Some degree of shock accompanies most severe injuries and

Table 13–2. Classification of hypovolemic shock.

	Class I	Class II	Class III	Class IV
Blood loss (mL)	Up to 750	750–1500	1500–2000	> 2000
Blood loss (% BV)	Up to 15%	15–30%	30–40%	> 40%
Pulse rate (beats/min)	< 100	> 100	> 120	> 140
Blood pressure	Normal	Minimal decrease	Decreased	Significantly decreased
Pulse pressure	Normal	Narrowed	Narrowed	Unobtainable or very narrow
Hourly urine output	≥ 0.5 mL/kg	≥ 0.5 mL/kg	< 0.5 cc/kg	Minimal
CNS/mental status	Slightly anxious	Mildly anxious	Anxious & confused	Confused or lethargic

is manifested initially by pallor, cold sweat, weakness, light-headedness, tachycardia, hypotension, thirst, air hunger, and, eventually, loss of consciousness. Patients with any of these signs should be presumed to be in shock and evaluated thoroughly. All patients determined to be in any degree of shock should be reexamined at regular intervals. The degree of shock has been categorized to guide resuscitation and help caregivers recognize the severity of symptoms (Table 13–2).

A. Hypovolemic Shock

Hypovolemic shock is due to loss of whole blood or plasma. Blood pressure may be maintained initially by vasoconstriction. Tissue hypoxia increases when hypotension ensues, and shock may become irreversible if irreparable damage occurs to the vital organs. Massive or prolonged hemorrhage, severe crush injuries, major fractures, and extensive burns are the most common causes. The presence of any of these conditions is an indication for prompt intravenous fluid infusion.

In mild or class 1 shock (< 15% blood volume loss), compensatory mechanisms may preserve adequate perfusion, and no skin or physiologic changes may be apparent. In moderate or class 2 shock (15%-30% blood loss), the skin on the extremities becomes pale, cool, and moist as a result of vasoconstriction and release of epinephrine. Systolic blood pressure is often maintained at near-normal levels, but urine output will usually decrease. With severe or class 3 shock (30%-40% blood volume loss), these changes—particularly diaphoresis—become more marked, and urine output declines significantly. Hypotension ensues. In addition, changes in cerebral function become evident consisting chiefly of agitation, disorientation, and memory loss. A common error is to attribute uncooperative behavior to intoxication, drug use, or brain injury when in fact it may be due to cerebral ischemia from blood loss. With class 4 shock (> 40% blood volume loss), profound hypotension is typically accompanied by loss of consciousness and anuria.

In this situation, rapid resuscitation with crystalloid and blood products is necessary to prevent imminent death.

With any degree of shock, intravenous balanced salt solution (eg, lactated Ringer solution) should be given rapidly until the signs of shock abate and urine output returns to normal. If shock appears to be due to blood loss, blood transfusion should be given, starting with two units of uncross-matched O-negative blood if cross-matched blood is unavailable. Additional resuscitation with crystalloid and/or blood products is guided by the cause of volume loss and response to fluid administration. Successful resuscitation is indicated by warm, dry, well-perfused skin, a urine output of 30-60 mL/h, and an alert sensorium. Improvement in pH toward normal, correction of lactic acidosis, and minimization of base deficit as measured on an arterial blood gas sample are also indicators of successful resuscitation.

As a general principle, measurements of blood pressure and pulse are less reliable than changes in urine output in assessing the severity of shock. Young and athletic older patients may have compensatory mechanisms which maintain adequate blood pressure even with moderate volume loss. Older patients and those taking cardiac or blood pressure medications often do not exhibit tachycardia even with extreme volume loss. Therefore, a Foley catheter should be inserted into the bladder to monitor urine output in any patient with major injuries or shock. Oliguria is the most reliable sign of moderate shock, and successful resuscitation is indicated by a return of urine output to 0.5-1 mL/kg/h. Absence of oliguria is an unreliable index of the absence of shock if the patient has an osmotic diuresis due to alcohol, glucose, mannitol, or intravenous contrast material.

A patient who is receiving intravenous fluids at a high rate may not exhibit signs of shock even in the setting of ongoing hemorrhage. If a patient continues to require high volumes of fluid after initial resuscitation in order to maintain urine output, mental status, and blood pressure, further investigation must be performed to rule out occult hemorrhage. The patient must be kept recumbent and given reassurance and analgesics as necessary. If opioids are necessary for pain relief, they are best administered intravenously in small doses.

B. Neurogenic Shock

Neurogenic shock is due to the pooling of blood in autonomically denervated venules and small veins and is usually due to spinal cord injury. Neurogenic shock is not caused by an isolated head injury, and in those patients, other causes of shock should be sought. A patient exhibiting signs of neurogenic shock (warm and well-perfused distal extremities in the presence of hypotension) should be given a 2 L crystalloid fluid bolus—followed by an additional bolus if the response is suboptimal. If neurogenic shock persists with fluid resuscitation, phenylephrine or another vasopressor should be given as a drip with the dosage adjusted until the blood pressure is maintained at a satisfactory level. If the patient does not improve quickly, other kinds of shock must be considered. Patients with neurogenic shock may require central venous pressure monitoring to ensure an optimal volume status.

C. Cardiac Compressive Shock

Cardiac compressive shock is caused by compression of the thin-walled chambers of the heart—the atria and the right ventricle—or by compression or distortion of the great veins entering the heart. The usual causes of this type of shock in the trauma patient are pericardial tamponade, tension pneumothorax, massive hemothorax, diaphragmatic rupture with herniation of abdominal contents into the chest, and an elevated diaphragm from massive abdominal hemorrhage. Treatment consists of urgent decompression depending on the specific cause. In severe cases, emergency thoracotomy may be necessary to restore adequate cardiac function.

D. Cardiogenic Shock

Cardiogenic shock is caused by decreased myocardial contractility and is most commonly caused by myocardial infarction or arrhythmia. Older trauma patients may develop a myocardial infarction as a complication of their injuries. On occasion an acute myocardial infarction may precede a traumatic event and be a cause of injury or loss of consciousness. Rarely, a severe myocardial contusion may lead to cardiogenic shock. Treatment is supportive, with volume replacement guided by hemodynamic monitoring and administration of inotropic agents to augment cardiac output as necessary to maintain adequate end-organ perfusion. Unfortunately, patients with traumatic injuries are not usually candidates for anticoagulant or lytic therapy, and treatment of their acute myocardial ischemia is sometimes hindered by concerns about bleeding. Echocardiography is helpful for assessment of wall motion abnormalities from severe cardiac contusion.

▶ Laboratory Studies

Immediately after intravenous catheters are placed, a blood sample should be drawn for blood typing and cross-matching. If the patient has a history of renal, hepatic, or cardiac disease or is taking diuretics or anticoagulants, serum electrolytes and coagulation parameters should be measured. In most patients with serious injuries, an arterial blood gas provides rapid data about acidosis and base deficit, both of which are markers of under-resuscitation in addition to oxygenation (Pao_2) and ventilation ($Paco_2$). Gross blood in the urine indicates the need for further diagnostic testing with abdominal CT scan or, in selected cases, a cystogram and urethrogram. Patients with obvious severe head injury, where intracranial pressure monitoring may be indicated, should have coagulation studies and a platelet count performed. Measurement of blood alcohol level and urine toxicology screen may be useful in patients with altered mental status.

▶ Imaging Studies

Radiographic plain films of the chest and pelvis are required in all major injuries. Lateral C-spine films have been supplanted by formal CT scanning of the neck in patients with suspicion of or mechanism for cervical spine injury. Bedside focused assessment with sonography for trauma (FAST) is the preferred triage method for determining the presence of hemoperitoneum in blunt trauma patients or cardiac tamponade in blunt and penetrating trauma patients. The presence of hemoperitoneum in an unstable patient on FAST may be an indication for exploratory laparotomy. Presence of hemoperitoneum in a stable patient or a negative FAST in a patient with abdominal pain is indication for further evaluation with abdominal CT scan.

Patients who have an abnormal chest radiograph with a mechanism for blunt aortic injury should undergo further screening with either helical chest CT done at the time of abdominal imaging or with aortography, if necessary. Cervical spine CT scans should be obtained for patients who are unconscious, have pain in the cervical region, have neurologic deficits, or have painful or distracting injuries. CT scanning of the head should be performed in all patients with loss of consciousness or more serious neurologic impairment. Radiographs of the long bones and noncervical spine can usually be deferred until the more critical injuries of the thorax and abdomen have been delineated and stabilized.

2. SECONDARY SURVEY & PATTERNS OF INJURY

A rapid and complete history and physical examination are essential for patients with serious or multiple injuries. Progressive changes in clinical findings are often the key to correct diagnosis, and negative findings that change to positive may be of great importance in revising an initial clinical evaluation. This is particularly true in the case of abdominal, thoracic, and intracranial injuries, which frequently do not become manifest until hours after the trauma.

Recognition of injury patterns is also important in identifying all injuries. For example, fractures of the calcaneus resulting from a fall from a great height are often associated with central dislocation of the hip and fractures of the spine and of the skull base. A crushed pelvis is often combined with laceration of the posterior urethra or bladder, vagina, or rectum. Crush injuries of the chest are often associated with lacerations or rupture of the spleen, liver, or diaphragm. Penetrating wounds of the chest may involve not only the thoracic contents but also the abdominal viscera. These combinations occur frequently and should always be suspected.

TREATMENT PRIORITIES

In all cases of patients with multiple injuries, there must be a "captain of the team" who directs the resuscitation, decides which x-rays or special diagnostic tests should be obtained, and establishes priority for care by continuous consultation with other surgical specialists and anesthesiologists. A trauma surgeon or a general surgeon experienced in the care of injured patients usually has this role.

After controlling the airway if necessary, resuscitation and blood volume replacement have first priority. Deepening stupor in patients under observation should arouse suspicion of an expanding intracranial lesion requiring serial neurologic examinations and head CT. Too often, obvious signs of acute alcohol intoxication have been assumed to be the cause of unconsciousness, and intracranial hemorrhage has been overlooked.

Cerebral injuries take precedence in care when there is rapidly deepening coma. Extradural bleeding is a critical emergency, requiring operation for control of bleeding and cerebral decompression. Subdural bleeding may produce a similar emergency. If the patient's condition permits, CT scanning should be performed for localization of the bleeding within the cranium prior to other operative interventions being initiated. In many cases of combined cerebral and abdominal injury with massive bleeding, laparotomy and craniotomy should be performed simultaneously.

Most urologic injuries are managed at the same time as associated intra-abdominal injuries. Pelvic fractures present special problems and are discussed in Chapter 40. Unless there is associated vascular injury with threatened ischemia of the limb, fractures of the long bones can be splinted and treated on an urgent basis. Open contaminated fractures should be cleansed and debrided as soon as possible. Injuries of the hand run the risk of infection that may result in a lifelong handicap without early effective treatment.

Early treatment of the hand at the same time as treatment of any life-threatening injuries avoids infection and preserves the means of livelihood. Tetanus prophylaxis should be given in all instances of open contaminated wounds, puncture wounds, and burns.

Patients with a severe burden of trauma and shock may not be candidates for definitive treatment of all injuries in the immediate setting. Three physiological derangements comprise the "lethal triad" in the trauma literature: hypothermia, acidosis, and coagulopathy. These are boundaries of a patient's physiologic envelope beyond which the patient will develop irreversible shock and eventual death. Bailing out of the abdomen with damage control maneuvers in a patient headed for the lethal triad is not a sign of defeat; instead it is usually the intelligent option. Early warning signs of physiologic compromise that could lead to the lethal triad are edema of the small bowel, midgut distension, dusky serosal surfaces, tissue that is cool to the touch, noncompliant swollen abdominal wall, diffuse oozing from surgical or raw surfaces, and lack of obvious clot formation. Successful packing relies on clot formation, so employing a strategy of early packing is recommended rather than turning to it as a last resort.

Details of definitive management of injuries are discussed in the sections on trauma that follow and in the various organ system chapters of this book.

American College of Surgeons Committee on Trauma: *Advanced Trauma Life Support for Doctors Student Manual*, 8th ed. Chicago, IL: American College of Surgeons, 2008.

Centers for Disease Control and Prevention: Advances in motor vehicle crash response. Available at http://www.cdc.gov/injuryresponse/aacn.html. Accessed July 18, 2012.

Centers for Disease Control and Prevention: Injury Prevention and Control. Field triage. Available at http://www.cdc.gov/fieldtriage/. Accessed August 18, 2012.

CRASH-2 collaborators et al: Effects of tranexamic acid on death, vascular occlusive events, and blood transfusion in trauma patients with significant haemorrhage (CRASH-2): a randomized, placebo-controlled trial. *Lancet*. 2010;376:23.

CRASH-2 collaborators et al: The importance of early treatment with tranexamic acid in bleeding trauma patients: an exploratory analysis of the CRASH-2 randomised controlled trial. *Lancet*. 2011;377:1096.

Haas B et al: The mortality benefit of direct trauma center transport in a regional trauma system: a population-based analysis. *J Trauma Acute Care Surg*. 2012;72:1510.

Morrison JJ et al: Military application of tranexamic acid in trauma emergency resuscitation (MATTERs) study. *Arch Surg*. 2012;147:113.

NECK INJURIES

All injuries to the neck are potentially life threatening because of the many vital structures in this area. Injuries to the neck are classified as blunt or penetrating, and the treatment is different for each. The patient must be examined closely for associated head and chest injuries. The initial level of consciousness is of paramount importance; progressive depression of the sensorium may signify intracranial bleeding or cerebral ischemia and requires neurosurgical evaluation. Trauma to the base of the neck may lacerate major blood vessels or have associated pneumothorax. Hemorrhage into the pleural cavity may occur suddenly as contained hematomas rupture.

▶ Clinical Findings

Injuries to the larynx and trachea can be asymptomatic or may cause hoarseness, laryngeal stridor, or dyspnea secondary to airway compression or aspiration of blood. Subcutaneous emphysema in the neck can be present if the wall of the larynx or trachea has been disrupted.

Esophageal injuries are rarely isolated and by themselves may not cause immediate symptoms. Severe chest pain and dysphagia are characteristic of esophageal perforation. Hours later, as mediastinitis develops, progressive sepsis may occur. Mediastinitis results because the deep cervical space is in direct continuity with the mediastinum. Esophageal injuries can be recognized promptly if the surgeon is alert to the possibility and seeks out early diagnosis. Exploration of the neck, radiographic examination of the esophagus with contrast medium, and in selected cases flexible esophagoscopy confirms the diagnosis.

Cervical spine fractures and spinal cord injuries should always be suspected in deceleration injuries or following direct trauma to the neck. If the patient complains of cervical pain or tenderness or if the level of consciousness is depressed, the head and neck should be immobilized (eg, with a rigid cervical collar or sandbags) until cervical radiologic imaging can be performed to rule out a cervical fracture or ligamentous injury.

Injury to the great vessels (subclavian, common carotid, internal carotid, and external carotid arteries; subclavian, internal jugular, and external jugular veins) may follow blunt or penetrating trauma. Fractures of the clavicle or first rib may lacerate the subclavian artery and vein. With vascular injuries, the patient typically presents with visible external blood loss, neck hematoma formation, and in varying degrees of shock. Occasionally, bleeding may be contained and the injury may go undetected for a short time. Auscultation may reveal bruits that suggest arterial injury.

▶ Types of Injuries

A. Penetrating Neck Injuries

Penetrating injuries of the neck are divided into three anatomic zones (Figure 13–9). Zone I injuries occur at the thoracic outlet, which extends from the level of the cricoid cartilage to the clavicles. Included in this area are the proximal carotid arteries, the subclavian vessels, and the major

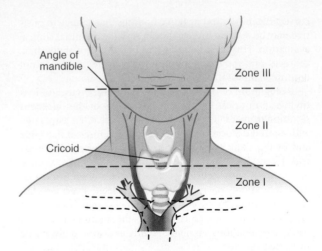

▲ **Figure 13–9.** Zones of the neck.

vessels of the chest. Proximal control of injuries to vascular structures in this zone often requires a thoracotomy or sternotomy. Zone II injuries occur in the area between the cricoid and the angle of the mandible. Injuries here are the easiest to expose and evaluate. Zone III injuries are between the angle of the mandible and the base of the skull. Exposure is much more difficult in this zone and in some cases may require disarticulation of the mandible. High injuries can be inaccessible, and control of hemorrhage may require ligation of major proximal vessels or angiographic embolization.

Penetrating trauma to the posterior neck may injure the vertebral column, the cervical spinal cord, the interosseous portion of the vertebral artery, and the neck musculature. Penetrating trauma to the anterior and lateral neck may injure the larynx, trachea, esophagus, thyroid, carotid arteries, subclavian arteries, jugular veins, subclavian veins, phrenic and vagus nerves, and thoracic duct.

With any penetrating cervical trauma, the likelihood of significant injury is high because there are so many vital structures in such a small space. Any patient with shock, expanding hematoma, or uncontrolled hemorrhage should be taken to the operating room for emergency exploration. The location of the injury suggests which structures may be involved. Vascular injuries at the base of the neck require thoracotomy or sternotomy to obtain proximal control of injured blood vessels before the site of probable injury is exposed. If the patient is stable after resuscitation, additional diagnostic testing may be considered.

Conventional angiography or computed tomography angiography is usually recommended for patients with stable injuries in zones I and III because precise identification of the location and extent of injury may alter the operative approach. If possible, angiography should be performed before exploration of any injury in which blood vessels may be damaged below the level of the cricoid cartilage or above a line connecting the mastoid process with the angle of the jaw. Arterial injuries above this line are practically inaccessible. If injury to the carotid artery at the base of the skull is confirmed by angiography, repair may not be possible and ligation may be required to control bleeding, or angiographic intervention may be required. Injured carotid arteries that have produced a neurologic deficit should be repaired if possible. The morbidity and mortality of patients undergoing carotid artery repair are significantly lower than those who have ligation of the carotid artery (15% vs 50%). Carotid artery ligation is indicated in the patient who presents with uncontrollable hemorrhage or coma with no prograde flow in the carotid artery.

Since exposure of injuries in zone II is relatively easy to obtain, a policy of mandatory exploration was the traditional recommendation for all injuries penetrating the platysma muscle. Although this approach is safe, reliable, and time-tested, studies have demonstrated that a selective approach is as safe provided that diagnostic testing does not detect a major injury and the patient is stable. High-resolution helical CT scanning of the neck can also be used to guide surgical decision making in zone II penetrating injuries. Invasive studies such as endoscopy and conventional angiography can often be eliminated if CT demonstrates a trajectory remote from vital structures such as blood vessels or the aerodigestive tract.

In the absence of an obvious vascular injury on clinical examination, ultrasound with color-flow Doppler has been demonstrated to be reliable in ruling out carotid artery injuries. Computed tomography angiography can also be used in this setting and may offer the advantage of identifying an unsuspected vertebral artery injury. Vertebral artery injuries should also be suspected when bleeding from a posterior or lateral neck wound cannot be controlled by pressure on the carotid artery or when there is bleeding from a posterolateral wound associated with fracture of a cervical transverse process. Flexible or rigid endoscopy can be used to evaluate the trachea and esophagus. A contrast study of the upper esophagus should be performed to identify esophageal injuries that might not be readily apparent on endoscopy. These injuries can be difficult to detect and are occasionally missed on surgical exploration. In either case, repeated, careful examinations should be performed.

B. Blunt Neck Injuries

The most important injuries resulting from blunt cervical trauma are: (1) cervical fracture, (2) cervical spinal cord injury, (3) vascular injury, and (4) laryngeal and tracheal injury. Radiographic examination of the cervical spine and soft tissues is essential. Careful neurologic examination can differentiate between injuries to the spinal cord, brachial plexus, and brain.

The diagnosis of a cervical spine fracture is reliant on the history, physical examination, and confirmatory studies. The use of plain radiographs has been supplanted by non-contrast computed tomography of the cervical spine. Awake, unimpaired patients with a negative physical examination are unlikely to have a clinically significant cervical spine injury. Obtunded patients with a negative CT scan and no clinical signs of cervical spine injury are also unlikely to have an injury. Following a negative CT scan, the cervical collar is typically removed once the patient is no longer obtunded and the examination can be repeated, or immediately if the patient is likely to remain obtunded/intubated in the ICU. The pediatric patient with an unreliable physical examination often requires additional imaging to clear the spine. Adult patients with a negative CT scan and pain often require flexion and extension views or a MRI to rule out ligamentous injury. Cervical fractures are often managed with external immobilization using rigid collars or a halo/vest apparatus. In some cases, unstable cervical spine fractures require reduction and internal fixation.

Vascular injuries may occur in cases of severe or localized blunt neck trauma. The common or internal carotid arteries can be torn or sustain intimal disruption and require intervention. Imaging of the cervical vessels is recommended in blunt trauma patients with lateralizing neurologic symptoms or GCS less than 8 with head CT findings that do not explain the neurologic symptoms. Screening should also be considered in patients with mandible or facial fractures, complex skull fractures, traumatic brain injury with thoracic injuries, scalp degloving, and thoracic vascular injuries. While four-vessel arteriography of bilateral carotid and vertebral arteries was the previous gold standard, newer imaging techniques such as a dedicated cervical CT-angiogram or MR-angiogram are the preferred screening tools. Formal arteriograms are reserved for patients who may have injuries amenable to angiographic intervention or if the diagnosis cannot be made by other means and would alter treatment. Most blunt carotid injuries are not amenable to operative intervention due to the location or extent of injury. The use of endovascular stent techniques to repair or control blunt carotid artery injuries is also an option. Patients with blunt carotid or vertebral artery injuries should be considered for anticoagulation or antiplatelet therapy. The value of anticoagulation continues to be debated due to associated bleeding complications, and antiplatelet therapy is a reasonable alternative to full systemic anticoagulation.

▶ Complications

The complications of untreated neck trauma are related to the individual structures injured. Injuries to the larynx and trachea can result in acute airway obstruction, late tracheal stenosis, and sepsis. Cervicomediastinal sepsis can result from esophageal injuries. Carotid artery injuries can produce death from hemorrhage, stroke or cerebral ischemia, and arteriovenous fistula with cardiac decompensation. Major venous injury can result in exsanguination, air embolism, and arteriovenous fistula formation if there is concomitant arterial injury. Cervical fracture can result in paraplegia, quadriplegia, or death.

Prevention of these complications depends upon immediate resuscitation by intubation of the airway, prompt control of external hemorrhage and blood replacement, protection of the head and neck when cervical fracture is possible, accurate and rapid diagnosis, and prompt operative treatment when indicated.

▶ Treatment

Control of the airway with early intubation is the first key maneuver to successful management of severe neck injuries. Any wound of the neck that penetrates the platysma requires prompt surgical exploration or diagnostic workup to rule out major vascular injury. In patients with zone II injuries, color-flow Doppler imaging may provide a reliable way to assess for vascular injury and can be a safe alternative to contrast angiography. Arteries damaged by high-velocity missiles require debridement. End-to-end anastomosis of the mobilized vessels is preferred, but if a significant segment is lost, an autogenous vein graft can be used. Vertebral artery injury presents a formidable technical problem because of the interosseous course of the artery shortly after it arises from the subclavian artery. Although unilateral vertebral artery ligation has been followed by fatal midbrain or cerebellar necrosis, because of inadequate communication to the basilar artery, only 3% of patients with left vertebral ligation and 2% of patients with right vertebral ligation develop these complications. Therefore, in the face of massive hemorrhage from a partially severed vertebral artery, ligation with surgical clips applied to the vessel between the transverse processes above and below the laceration is accepted.

Subclavian artery injuries are best approached through a combined cervicothoracic incision. Proper exposure is the key to success in the management of these difficult and too-often fatal injuries. Ligation of the subclavian artery is relatively safe, but primary repair is preferable. Care should be taken to avoid phrenic nerve and thoracic duct injury when operating in this region of the neck. If the patient is stable and a subclavian injury is identified at arteriography, an endovascular stent is another therapeutic option.

Venous injuries are best managed by ligation. The possibility of air embolism must be kept constantly in mind. A simple means of preventing this complication is to lower the patient's head using the Trendelenburg position until bleeding is controlled.

Esophageal injuries should be sutured closed primarily and drained. Use of muscle flaps using omohyoid or sternocleidomastoid muscles to cover the repair can be helpful.

Drainage is the mainstay of treatment. Extensive injury to the esophagus is often immediately fatal because of associated injuries to the spinal cord. Systemic antibiotics should be administered routinely to patients with esophageal injuries.

Minor laryngeal and tracheal injuries do not require treatment, but immediate tracheostomy should be performed when airway obstruction exists. If there has been significant injury to the thyroid cartilage, a temporary laryngeal stent (Silastic) should be employed to provide support. Mucosal lacerations should be approximated before insertion of the stent. Conveniently located small perforations of the trachea can be utilized for tracheostomy. Otherwise, the wounds can be closed after they are debrided and a distal tracheostomy performed. Extensive circumferential tracheal injuries may require resection and anastomosis or reconstruction using synthetic materials.

Cervical spinal cord injury should be managed in such a way as to prevent further damage. When there is cervical cord compression from hematoma, vertebral fractures, or foreign bodies, decompression laminectomy is necessary.

▶ Prognosis

Severe laceration of the cervical spinal cord often results in paralysis. Injuries to the soft tissues of the neck, trachea, and esophagus have a good to excellent prognosis if promptly treated. Major vascular injuries have a good prognosis if promptly treated before the onset of irreversible shock or neurologic deficit. The overall death rate for major cervical injuries is about 10%.

Bromberg WJ et al: Blunt cerebrovascular injury practice management guidelines: Eastern Association for the Surgery of Trauma. *J Trauma*. 2010;68:471.

Burlew CC et al: Blunt cerebrovascular injuries: redefining screening criteria in the era of noninvasive diagnosis. *J Trauma Acute Care Surg*. 2012;72:330.

Chung S et al: Trauma association of Canada pediatric subcommittee national pediatric cervical spine evaluation pathway: consensus guidelines. *J Trauma*. 2011;70:873.

Como JJ et al: Computed tomography alone may clear the cervical spine in obtunded blunt trauma patients: a prospective evaluation of a revised protocol. *J Trauma*. 2011;70:345.

DiCocco JM et al: Optimal outcomes for patients with blunt cerebrovascular injury (BCVI): tailoring treatment to the lesion. *J Am Coll Surg*. 2011;212:549.

Emmett KP et al: Improving the screening criteria for blunt cerebrovascular injury: the appropriate role for computed tomography angiography. *J Trauma*. 2011;70:1058.

Hennessy D et al: Cervical spine clearance in obtunded blunt trauma patients: a prospective study. *J Trauma*. 2010;68:576.

Inaba K et al: Evaluation of multidetector computed tomography for penetrating neck injury: a prospective multicenter study. *J Trauma Acute Care Surg*. 2012;72:576.

Wang AC et al: Evaluating the use and utility of noninvasive angiography in diagnosing traumatic blunt cerebrovascular injury. *J Trauma Acute Care Surg*. 2012;72:1601.

THORACIC INJURIES

Thoracic trauma accounts directly for or is a contributing factor in 50% of deaths from trauma. Early deaths are commonly due to: (1) airway obstruction, (2) flail chest, (3) open pneumothorax, (4) massive hemothorax, (5) tension pneumothorax, and (6) cardiac tamponade. Later deaths are due to respiratory failure, sepsis, and unrecognized injuries/complications. The majority of blunt thoracic injuries are the result of automobile accidents. Even what appears to be a minor blunt thoracic injury leading to rib fractures and pulmonary contusions can have a profound effect on patients. Near-side collisions are responsible for a higher incidence of blunt aortic injury among older adults and are associated with lower delta V forces compared to those in younger patients. Penetrating chest injuries from knives, bullets, etc, are deadly and can result in complex patterns of injury. The mortality rate in hospitalized patients with isolated chest injury is 4%-8%; it is 10%-15% when one other organ system is involved and rises to 35% if multiple additional organs are injured.

Combined injuries of multiple intrathoracic structures are typical. There are often other injuries to the abdomen, head, or skeletal system. When performing an operation on the chest for trauma, it is often necessary to operate on the abdomen as well. Therefore, when trauma patients are brought to the operating room for a laparotomy or thoracotomy, both body regions should be prepped into the operative field. Eighty-five percent of chest injuries do not require open thoracotomy, but immediate use of lifesaving measures is often necessary and should be within the competence of all surgeons.

A rapid estimate of cardiorespiratory status and possible associated injuries from the physical examination gives the physician a valuable overview of a patient who has sustained thoracic injuries. For example, patients with upper airway obstruction appear cyanotic, ashen, or gray; examination reveals stridor or gurgling sounds, ineffective respiratory excursion, constriction of cervical muscles, and retraction of the suprasternal, supraclavicular, intercostal, or epigastric regions. The character of chest wall excursions and the presence or absence of penetrating wounds should be observed. If respiratory excursions are not visible, ventilation is probably inadequate. Severe paradoxic chest wall movement in flail chest is usually located anteriorly and can be seen immediately. Sucking wounds of the chest wall should be obvious. A large hemothorax may be detected by percussion, and subcutaneous emphysema is easily detected on palpation as crepitus. Both massive hemothorax and tension pneumothorax may produce absent or diminished breath sounds and a shift of the trachea to the opposite side, but in massive hemothorax the neck veins are usually collapsed. If the patient has a thready or absent pulse and distended neck veins, the main differential diagnosis is between cardiac tamponade and tension pneumothorax.

In moribund patients, diagnosis must be immediate, and treatment may require chest tube placement, pericardiocentesis, or thoracotomy in the emergency room. The first priority of management should be to provide an airway and restore circulation. One can then reassess the patient and outline definitive measures. A cuffed endotracheal tube and assisted ventilation are required for apnea, ineffectual breathing, severe shock, deep coma, airway obstruction, flail chest, or open sucking chest wounds. Persistent shock or hypoxia due to thoracic trauma may be caused by any of the following: massive hemopneumothorax, cardiac tamponade, tension pneumothorax or massive air leak, or air embolism. If hemorrhagic shock is not explained readily by findings on chest x-ray or external losses, it is almost certainly due to intra-abdominal bleeding.

▶ Tube Thoracostomy

If time permits, the chest is prepared and draped in a sterile fashion. In awake patients, local anesthetic (1% lidocaine) is injected in the skin and surrounding tissues at the planned site of tube insertion. In an unconscious patient, this step is usually unnecessary. The location of the chest tube insertion site is the interspace between the fourth and fifth ribs in the **midaxillary** line. A 2- to 3-cm skin incision is created with a #10 scalpel and carried down into the subcutaneous tissue. Using a large hemostat, a soft tissue tunnel is created just superior to the cephalad edge of the fifth rib. A finger or blunt clamp is used to penetrate the parietal pleura and enter the pleural space. The wound is explored with an index finger to confirm entry into the pleural cavity and check for pulmonary adhesions. A 36F straight thoracostomy tube is inserted and directed posteriorly toward the apex of the lung. The tube is anchored to the skin with stitches and connected to a Pleur-Evac device set at 20 cm H_2O suction with a water seal.

▶ Types of Injuries

A. Chest Wall

Rib fracture, the most common chest injury, varies across a spectrum from simple fracture to fracture with hemopneumothorax to severe multiple fractures with flail chest, pulmonary contusion, and internal injuries. With simple fractures, pain on inspiration is the principal symptom; treatment consists of providing adequate analgesia. In cases of multiple fractures, intercostal nerve blocks or epidural analgesia may be required to ensure adequate ventilation. Multiple fractures can be associated with decreased ventilation and subsequent pneumonia, particularly in the elderly patient.

Flail chest occurs when a portion of the chest wall becomes isolated by multiple fractures and paradoxically moves in and out with inspiration and expiration with a potentially severe reduction in ventilatory efficiency. The magnitude of the effect is determined by the size of the flail segment and the amount of pain with breathing. The rib fractures are usually anterior, and there are at least two fractures of the same rib. Bilateral costochondral separation and sternal fractures can also cause a flail segment. An associated lung contusion may produce a decrease in lung compliance not fully manifest until 12-48 hours after injury. Increased negative intrapleural pressure is then required for ventilation, and chest wall instability becomes apparent. If ventilation becomes inadequate, atelectasis, hypercapnia, hypoxia, accumulation of secretions, and ineffective cough occur. Arterial Pao_2 is often low before clinical findings appear. Serial blood gas analysis is the best way to determine if a treatment regimen is adequate. For less severe cases, intercostal nerve block or continuous epidural analgesia may be adequate treatment. However, more severe cases require ventilatory assistance for variable periods of time with a cuffed endotracheal tube and a mechanical ventilator.

Most rib or sternal fractures will heal without treatment. In selected patients, internal fixation may be useful; however, determining the patient population who would most benefit is still under investigation. Commercially produced, implantable rib and sternal fracture plating systems are now available. A system with bioabsorbable plates has been described which allows fixation of fragments during the healing process and metabolism by the body within 24 months. Patients who would potentially benefit from an open reduction internal fixation procedure are those with nonunion, severely displaced rib fractures with overriding fragments, severe pain with respiratory compromise (eg, difficulty in being weaned off the mechanical ventilator), multiple unstable rib fractures, and those undergoing thoracotomy for other intrathoracic indication. Because of the peristomal bacterial burden associated with a tracheostomy, this procedure should be used with caution in patients with a prior tracheostomy and need for a surgical incision high on the chest wall.

B. Trachea and Bronchus

Blunt tracheobronchial injuries are often due to compression of the airway between the sternum and the vertebral column in decelerating or high-velocity crush accidents. The distal trachea or main stem bronchi are usually involved, and 80% of all injuries are located within 2.5 cm from the carina. Penetrating tracheobronchial injuries may occur at any location. Most patients have pneumothorax, subcutaneous emphysema, pneumomediastinum, and hemoptysis. Cervicofacial emphysema may be dramatic. Tracheobronchial injury should be suspected when there is a massive air leak or when the lung does not readily reexpand after chest tube placement. In penetrating injuries of the trachea or main stem bronchi, there is usually massive

hemorrhage and hemoptysis. Systemic air embolism resulting in cardiopulmonary arrest may occur if a bronchovenous fistula is present. If air embolism is suspected, emergency thoracotomy should be performed with cross-clamping of the pulmonary hilum on the affected side. The diagnosis is confirmed by aspiration of air from the heart. In blunt injuries, the tracheobronchial injury may not be obvious and may be suspected only after major atelectasis develops several days later. Diagnosis may require flexible or rigid bronchoscopy. Immediate primary repair with absorbable sutures is indicated for all tracheobronchial lacerations.

C. Pleural Space

Hemothorax (blood within the pleural cavity) is classified according to the amount of blood: minimal, 350 mL; moderate, 350-1500 mL; or massive, 1500 mL or more. The rate of bleeding after evacuation of the hemothorax is clinically even more important. If air is also present, the condition is called *hemopneumothorax.*

Hemothorax should be suspected with penetrating or severe blunt thoracic injury. There may be decreased breath sounds and dullness to percussion, and a chest x-ray should be promptly obtained. In experienced hands, ultrasound can diagnose pneumothorax and hemothorax, but this technique is not widely employed at this time. Tube thoracostomy should be performed expeditiously for all hemothoraces. In 85% of cases, tube thoracostomy is the only treatment required. If bleeding is persistent, as noted by continued output from the chest tubes, it is more likely to be from the chest wall and an intercostal artery rather than a pulmonary artery. The use of positive end-expiratory pressure can help tamponade pulmonary parenchymal bleeding in trauma patients who are intubated. When the rate of bleeding shows a steady trend of greater than 200 mL/h or the total hemorrhagic output exceeds 1500 mL, thoracoscopy or thoracotomy should usually be performed. The trend and rate of thoracic bleeding is probably more important than the absolute numbers in deciding to perform surgical intervention. Thoracoscopy has been shown to be effective in controlling chest tube bleeding in 82% of cases. This technique has also been shown to be 90% effective in evacuating retained hemothoraces. In most of these cases, the chest wall is the source of hemorrhage. Thoracotomy is required for management of injuries to the lungs, heart, pericardium, and great vessels.

Pneumothorax occurs in lacerations of the lung or chest wall following penetrating or blunt chest trauma. Hyperinflation (eg, blast injuries and diving accidents) can also rupture the lungs. After penetrating injury, 80% of patients with pneumothorax also have blood in the pleural cavity. Most cases of pneumothorax are readily diagnosed on chest x-ray. In some cases, an occult pneumothorax will be identified on a chest or abdominal CT scan. Pneumothorax or hemothorax may be identified on the lateral scans performed as part of the FAST examination of the abdomen for trauma (see section on abdominal trauma). Most cases of traumatic pneumothorax should be treated with immediate tube thoracostomy; however, small occult pneumothoraces in stable patients can be observed.

Tension pneumothorax develops when a flap-valve leak allows air to enter the pleural space but prevents its escape; intrapleural pressure rises, causing total collapse of the lung and a shift of the mediastinal viscera to the opposite side, interfering with venous return to the heart. It must be relieved immediately to avoid impairment of cardiac function. Immediate treatment involves placement of a large-bore needle or plastic angiocath in the pleural space with care being taken to avoid injury to the intercostal vessels. After this emergency measure has been instituted, tension pneumothorax should be treated definitively by tube thoracostomy.

Sucking chest wounds, which allow air to pass in and out of the pleural cavity, should be promptly treated by a three-sided occlusive dressing and tube thoracostomy. The pathologic physiology resembles flail chest except that the extent of associated lung injury is usually less. Definitive management includes surgical closure of the defect in the chest wall.

D. Lung Injury

Pulmonary contusion due to sudden parenchymal concussion occurs after blunt trauma or wounding with a high-velocity missile. Pulmonary contusion happens in 75% of patients with flail chest but can also occur following blunt trauma without rib fracture. Alveolar rupture with fluid transudation and extravasation of blood are early findings. Fluid and blood from ruptured alveoli enter alveolar spaces and bronchi, and produce localized airway obstruction and atelectasis. Increased mucous secretions and overzealous intravenous fluid therapy may combine to produce copious secretions and further atelectasis. The patient's ability to cough and clear secretions effectively is weakened because of chest wall pain or mechanical inefficiency from fractures. Elasticity of the lungs is decreased, resistance to air flow increases, and as the work of breathing increases, blood oxygenation and pH drop and $PaCO_2$ rises. The cardiac compensatory response may be compromised, because as many as 35% of these patients have an associated myocardial contusion.

Treatment is often delayed because clinical and x-ray findings may not appear until 12-48 hours after injury. The clinical findings are copious, thin, blood-tinged secretions; chest pain; restlessness; apprehensiveness; and labored respirations. Eventually, dyspnea, cyanosis, tachypnea, and tachycardia develop. X-ray changes consist of patchy parenchymal opacification or diffuse linear peribronchial densities that may progress to diffuse opacification ("white-out") characteristic for acute respiratory distress syndrome.

Mechanical ventilatory support permits adequate alveolar ventilation and reduces the work of breathing. Blood gases should be monitored and arterial saturation adequately maintained. There is some controversy over the best regimen for fluid management, but excessive hydration or blood transfusion should be avoided. Serial measurement of central venous pressure, mixed venous oxygen saturation, and cardiac output help avoid over- or underresuscitation. Despite optimal therapy, about 15% of patients with pulmonary contusion die. Use of protective mechanical ventilator strategies is essential in these patients to avoid progressive ventilator induced lung injury. Use of low-tidal volumes (6 mL/kg) and avoidance of plateau pressures greater than 35 cm H_2O are recommended.

Most lung lacerations are caused by penetrating injuries, and hemopneumothorax is usually present. Tube thoracostomy is indicated to evacuate pleural air or blood and to monitor continuing leaks. Since expansion of the lung tamponades the laceration, most lung lacerations do not produce massive hemorrhage or persistent air leaks. Should a pulmonary laceration require operative intervention, lung-sparing techniques rather than formal anatomic lung resection should be employed when feasible to reduce morbidity and mortality.

Lung hematomas are the result of local parenchymal destruction and hemorrhage. The x-ray appearance is initially a poorly defined density that becomes more circumscribed a few days to 2 weeks after injury. Cystic cavities occasionally develop if damage is extensive. Most hematomas resolve adequately with expectant treatment.

E. Heart and Pericardium

Blunt injury to the heart occurs most often from compression against the steering wheel in automobile accidents. This injury is in decline with the increasing prevalence of airbag technology in motor vehicles. The injury varies from localized contusion to cardiac rupture. Autopsy studies of victims of immediately fatal accidents show that as many as 65% have rupture of one or more cardiac chambers, and 45% have pericardial lacerations. The incidence of blunt myocardial injury in patients who reach the hospital is unknown but is probably higher than generally suspected. The clinical relevance of this diagnosis is widely debated. Most trauma surgeons advocate the diagnosis and treatment of the actual clinical problem such as acute heart failure, valvular injury, cardiac rupture, or dysrhythmia.

Early clinical findings include friction rubs, chest pain, tachycardia, murmurs, dysrhythmias, or signs of low cardiac output. Patients with risk factors for blunt myocardial injury should undergo evaluation with a 12-lead electrocardiogram (EKG). If the EKG is normal and the patient is asymptomatic, the work up is complete. An abnormal EKG should prompt further evaluation with an echocardiogram.

Patients with proven injury on echocardiogram and/or hemodynamic instability should be admitted to the ICU and managed appropriately for the diagnosed injury. An abnormal EKG with a normal echocardiogram merits at least 24 hours of monitoring in a telemetry unit and daily repeat EKGs until stable or the dysrhythmia resolves. Standard measurement of cardiac enzymes is not useful and has no role in the diagnosis of blunt myocardial injury. If the patient is suspected of having a myocardial infarction or acute myocardial ischemia, then cardiac enzymes should be obtained and a cardiology consultation arranged.

Management of symptomatic blunt myocardial injury should be the same as for acute myocardial infarction. Hemopericardium may occur without tamponade and can be treated by pericardiocentesis. Tamponade in blunt cardiac trauma is often due to myocardial rupture or coronary artery laceration. Tamponade produces distended neck veins, shock, and cyanosis. Immediate thoracotomy and control of the injury are indicated. If cardiopulmonary arrest occurs before the patient can be transported to the operating room, emergency room thoracotomy with relief of tamponade should be performed. Treatment of injuries to the valves, papillary muscles, and septum must be individualized; and when tolerated, delayed repair is usually recommended.

Pericardial lacerations from stab wounds tend to seal and cause tamponade, whereas gunshot wounds frequently leave a sufficient pericardial opening for drainage. Gunshot wounds produce more extensive myocardial damage, multiple perforations, and massive bleeding into the pleural space. Hemothorax, shock, and exsanguination occur in nearly all cases of cardiac gunshot wounds. The clinical findings are those of tamponade or acute blood loss. Use of ultrasound and the FAST examination technique can reveal the presence of clinically significant blood in the pericardial space.

Treatment of penetrating cardiac injuries requires prompt thoracotomy, pericardial decompression, and control of hemorrhage. Most patients do not require cardiopulmonary bypass. The standard approach has been to repair the laceration using mattress sutures with pledgets while controlling hemorrhage with a finger on the heart. Suture control of cardiac lacerations may be technically difficult when working with a beating heart or in patients with large or multiple lacerations. Several studies have demonstrated that in most cases, emergency temporary control of hemorrhage from cardiac lacerations can be achieved with the use of a skin stapler (Figure 13–10). Following stabilization of the patient, the staples can be removed after definitive suture repair is performed in the operating room. Hemostatic sealants such as FloSeal offer significant promise as additional tools in the surgical armamentarium when dealing with lacerations to the heart or great vessels. Regardless of the approach utilized, care must be taken to avoid injury to the coronary arteries.

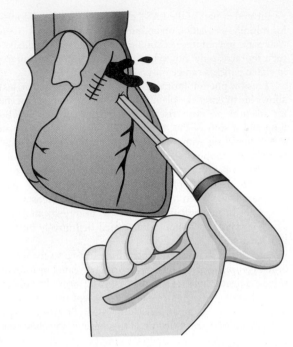

▲ **Figure 13–10.** Technique of cardiac stapling. Finger pressure (not shown) is used to maintain hemostasis during stapling. (Reproduced, with permission, from Macho JR, Markison RE, Schecter WP: Cardiac stapling in the management of penetrating injuries of the heart: rapid control of hemorrhage and decreased risk of personal contamination. *J Trauma.* 1993;34:711.)

Pericardiocentesis or creation of a pericardial window is reserved for selected cases when the diagnosis is uncertain or in preparation for thoracotomy. In approximately 75% of cases of stab wounds and 35% of cases of gunshot cardiac wounds, the patient survives the operation. However, it is estimated that 80%-90% of patients with gunshot wounds of the heart do not reach the hospital.

F. Esophagus

Anatomically, the esophagus is well protected, and perforation from external penetrating trauma is relatively infrequent. Blunt injuries are exceedingly rare. The most common symptom of esophageal perforation is pain; fever develops within hours in most patients. Hematemesis, hoarseness, dysphagia, or respiratory distress may also be present. Physical findings include shock, local tenderness, subcutaneous emphysema, or Hamman sign (pericardial or mediastinal "crunch" synchronous with cardiac sounds). Leukocytosis occurs soon after injury. X-ray findings on plain chest films include evidence of a foreign body or missile and mediastinal air or widening. Pleural effusion or hydropneumothorax is frequently seen, usually on the left side. Contrast x-rays of the esophagus should be performed but are positive in only about 70% of proven perforations.

A nasogastric tube should be passed to evacuate gastric contents. If recognized within 24-48 hours after injury, the esophageal perforation should be closed and pleural drainage instituted with large-bore catheters. Repair of these perforations requires special techniques that include buttressing of the esophageal closure with pleural or pericardial flaps; pedicles of intercostal, diaphragmatic, or cervical strap muscles; and serosal patches from stomach or jejunum. Illness and death are due to mediastinal and pleural infection.

G. Thoracic Duct

Chylothorax and chylopericardium are rare complications of trauma but are difficult to manage when they occur. Penetrating injuries of the neck, thorax, or upper abdomen can injure the thoracic duct or its major tributaries.

Symptoms are due to mechanical effects of the accumulations (eg, shortness of breath from lung collapse or low cardiac output from tamponade). The diagnosis is established when the fluid is shown to have characteristics of chyle.

The patient should be maintained on a fat-free, high-carbohydrate, high-protein diet and the effusion aspirated. Chest tube drainage should be instituted if the effusion recurs. Lipid-free total parenteral nutrition with no oral intake may be effective in treating persistent leaks. Three or 4 weeks of conservative treatment usually are curative. If daily chyle loss exceeds 1500 mL for 5 successive days or persists after 2-3 weeks of conservative treatment, the thoracic duct should be ligated via a right thoracotomy. Intraoperative identification of the leak may be facilitated by preoperative administration of fat-containing a lipophilic dye.

H. Diaphragm

Penetrating injuries of the diaphragm outnumber blunt diaphragmatic injuries by a ratio of at least 6:1. Diaphragmatic lacerations occur in 10%-15% of cases of penetrating wounds to the chest and in as many as 40% of cases of penetrating trauma to the left chest. Injuries to the right diaphragm are more common than previously thought. The injury is rarely obvious. Wounds of the diaphragm must not be overlooked because they rarely heal spontaneously and because herniation of abdominal viscera into the chest can occur with catastrophic complications either immediately or years after the injuries.

Associated injuries are usually present, and as many as 25% of patients are in shock when first seen. There may be abdominal tenderness, dyspnea, shoulder pain, or unilateral breath sounds. The diagnosis is often missed. Although chest radiography is a sensitive diagnostic tool, it may be entirely normal in 40% of cases. The most common finding is ipsilateral hemothorax, which is present in about

50% of patients. Occasionally, a distended, herniated stomach is confused with a pneumothorax. Passage of a nasogastric tube before x-rays will help to identify an intrathoracic stomach. CT scan or contrast x-rays may be necessary to establish the diagnosis in some cases. Newer generation helical CT scanners that allow sagittal reformatting can be helpful in definitively diagnosing diaphragmatic injury. Laparoscopy is a useful but invasive technique for detecting occult diaphragmatic injuries in patients who have no other indications for formal laparotomy.

Once the diagnosis is made, a transabdominal surgical approach should be used in cases of acute rupture. Laparoscopic suturing for repair of the injury may be possible in selected cases. The diaphragm should be reapproximated and closed with interrupted or running nonabsorbable sutures. Chronic herniation is associated with adhesions of the affected viscera to the thoracic structures and should be approached via thoracotomy, with the addition of a separate laparotomy when indicated. These cases can be quite challenging and appropriate preoperative planning is recommended.

Bhatnagar A et al: Rib fracture fixation for flail chest: what is the benefit? *J Am Coll Surg.* 2012;215:201-205.

Cook CC et al: Great vessel and cardiac trauma. *Surg Clin North Am.* 2009;89:797.

DuBose JJ et al: Isolated severe traumatic brain injuries sustained during combat operations: demographics, mortality outcomes, and lessons to be learned from contrasts to civilian counterparts. *J Trauma.* 2011;70:11.

Kaiser M et al: The clinical significance of occult thoracic injury in blunt trauma patients. *Am Surg.* 2010;76:1063.

Nagarsheth K et al: Ultrasound detection of pneumothorax compared with chest x-ray and computed tomography scan. *Am Surg.* 2011;77:480.

Neschis DG et al: Blunt aortic injury. *N Engl J Med.* 2008;359:1708.

Nirula R et al: Rib fracture fixation: controversies and technical challenges. *Am Surg.* 2010;76:793.

O'Connor J et al: Penetrating cardiac injury. *J R Army Med Corps.* 2009;155:185.

ABDOMINAL INJURIES

The specific type of abdominal injury varies according to whether the trauma is penetrating or blunt. Blunt injuries predominate in rural areas, while penetrating injuries are more common in urban areas. The mechanism of injury in blunt trauma is rapid deceleration, and noncompliant organs such as the liver, spleen, pancreas, and kidneys are at greater risk of injury due to parenchymal fracture. Occasionally, hollow viscous organs may be injured, with the duodenum and urinary bladder being particularly susceptible. The small bowel occupies a large portion of the total abdominal volume and is more likely to be injured by penetrating trauma. Most blunt abdominal injuries are related to motor vehicle accidents. Although the use of restraints has been associated with a decrease in the incidence of head, chest, and solid organ injuries, their use may be associated with pancreatic, mesenteric, and intestinal injuries due to organ compression against the spinal column. These injuries should be considered in patients who have signs of seat belt-related contusions of the abdominal wall. Internal abdominal injury may be present in as many as 30% of these cases. In any abdominal trauma, hemoperitoneum may not manifest clinical signs of peritoneal irritation, particularly in patients with other distracting injuries or depressed mental status. Retroperitoneal injury may be more subtle and difficult to diagnose during the initial evaluation.

Deaths from abdominal trauma result largely from early severe hemorrhage and coagulopathy or from later sepsis. Most deaths from abdominal trauma are preventable. Patients at risk of abdominal injury should undergo prompt and thorough evaluation. In most trauma centers, after physical examination, the initial diagnostic evaluation includes bedside FAST and portable radiographs of the pelvis and chest to assess for other potential sites of bleeding. In unstable patients who cannot be adequately evaluated with FAST due to size, technical problems, or subcutaneous air, diagnostic peritoneal lavage is warranted. After the initial FAST examination, patients who are stable or who respond to initial fluid resuscitation should have a CT scan of the abdomen and pelvis to evaluate for intra-abdominal and retroperitoneal injuries. Patients with persistent hypotension requiring fluid and blood resuscitation in the face of a positive FAST or diagnostic peritoneal lavage should be transported to the operating room emergently for exploratory laparotomy.

In some cases, dramatic physical findings may be due to abdominal wall injury in the absence of intraperitoneal injury. If the results of diagnostic studies are equivocal, diagnostic laparoscopy or exploratory laparotomy should be considered, since they may be lifesaving if serious injuries are identified early. Evaluation always includes a comprehensive physical examination with pelvic and rectal examinations included and may require specific laboratory and radiologic tests (eg, retrograde urethrogram or cystogram, rigid sigmoidoscopy, abdominal CT). Serial physical examinations may be necessary to detect subtle findings.

▶ Types of Injuries

A. Penetrating Trauma

Penetrating injuries to the abdomen that present with shock or ongoing resuscitation require prompt exploration. Lacerations of major blood vessels or the liver can cause severe and early shock. Penetrating injuries of the spleen, pancreas, or kidneys usually do not bleed massively unless a major vessel to the organ (eg, the renal artery) is damaged. Bleeding must be controlled promptly with packing and appropriate clamping for vascular control. A patient in shock with a penetrating injury of the abdomen who does not respond to 2 L of crystalloid fluid resuscitation should be operated on immediately following chest x-ray and switched blood product resuscitation.

Patients with hollow visceral injuries may have very few physical signs initially but will progress to sepsis if the injuries are not recognized. Increasing abdominal tenderness demands surgical exploration. White blood cell count elevations and fever appearing several hours following injury are keys to early diagnosis.

The treatment of hemodynamically stable patients with penetrating injuries to the lower chest or abdomen varies. All surgeons agree that patients with signs of peritonitis or hypovolemia should undergo surgical exploration, but operative treatment is less certain for patients with no signs of peritonitis or sepsis who are cardiovascularly stable.

Most stab wounds of the lower chest or abdomen should be explored, since a delay in treatment of a hollow viscous perforation can result in severe sepsis. Some surgeons recommend a selective policy in the management of these patients. When the depth of injury is in doubt, local wound exploration may rule out peritoneal penetration. Laparoscopy has a role in the evaluation of penetrating injuries in experienced hands, but requires considerable diligence to avoid missed injuries. All gunshot wounds of the lower chest and abdomen should be explored, unless there is a likely superficial scything wound, because the incidence of injury to major intra-abdominal structures exceeds 90% in such cases.

B. Blunt Trauma

A major advance in management of blunt trauma has been the FAST examination. Ultrasound has proven to be an ideal modality in the immediate evaluation of the trauma patient because it is rapid and accurate for the detection of intra-abdominal fluid or blood and is readily repeatable. It provides valuable information that augments the surgeon's diagnostic capabilities. Since its introduction in North America in 1989, ultrasonography has become commonplace, and a recent survey reports that 78% of United States trauma centers routinely use the FAST examination in the evaluation of patients.

The goal of the FAST examination is the identification of abnormal collections of blood or fluid. In this regard, it obviates the need for diagnostic peritoneal lavage. The primary focus is on the peritoneal cavity, but attention is also directed to the pericardium and to the pleural space. Unclotted blood or fluid allows transmission of ultrasound waves without echoes and thus appears black (Figure 13–11). In the standard FAST examination, four areas are scanned: the right upper quadrant, the subxiphoid area, the left upper quadrant, and the pelvis (Figure 13–12). Most surgeons recommend scanning initially in the right upper quadrant because

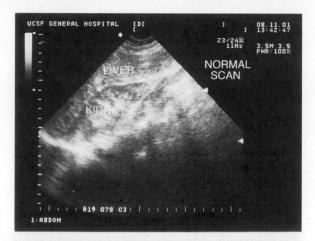

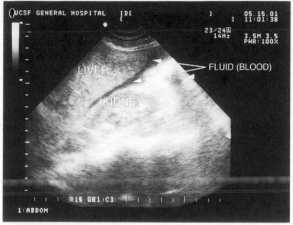

▲ **Figure 13–11.** A. Normal ultrasound of the right upper quadrant. B. Right upper quadrant ultrasound revealing blood between the liver and the kidney and between the liver and the diaphragm. (Courtesy of San Francisco General Hospital.)

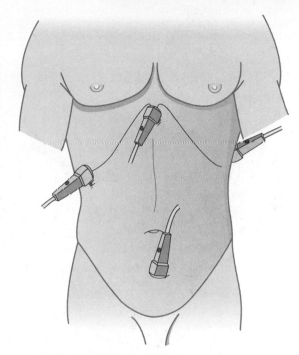

▲ **Figure 13–12.** Transducer positions for FAST. Pericardial area, right and left upper quadrants, and pelvis. (Reproduced, with permission, from Rozycki GS et al. Surgeon-performed ultrasound for the assessment of truncal injuries: lessons learned from 1540 patients. *Ann Surg.* 1998;228:557.)

more than half of the positive tests will reveal blood or fluid in this area. Unstable patients with a positive FAST examination should undergo urgent exploratory laparotomy.

The other diagnostic procedures most commonly used in patients without obvious indications for immediate laparotomy include diagnostic peritoneal lavage, CT scanning, and diagnostic laparoscopy.

▶ Diagnostic Peritoneal Lavage

Diagnostic peritoneal lavage is designed to detect the presence of intraperitoneal blood. Although its use has decreased to virtually nil at many centers with the use of the FAST examination, it is still an important test in certain circumstances because of its high sensitivity for the presence

of blood. Additional determinations of leukocytes, Gram stain, particulate matter, or amylase in the lavage fluid may indicate the presence of a bowel injury. Drainage of lavage fluid from a chest tube or urinary catheter may indicate a lacerated diaphragm or bladder. Lavage can be performed easily and rapidly, with minimal cost and morbidity. It is an invasive procedure that will affect the findings on physical examination and should be performed by a surgeon.

The procedure is neither qualitative nor quantitative. It cannot identify the source of hemorrhage, and relatively small amounts of intraperitoneal bleeding may result in a positive study. It may not detect small and large injuries to the diaphragm and cannot rule out injury to the bowel or retroperitoneal organs. The overall indications for diagnostic peritoneal lavage include abdominal pain or tenderness, low abdominal rib fractures, unexplained hypotension, spinal or pelvic fractures, paraplegia or quadriplegia, and assessment hampered by altered mental status due to neurologic injury or intoxication. Despite the many potential indications, FAST followed by abdominal pelvic CT scanning has replaced the need for most diagnostic

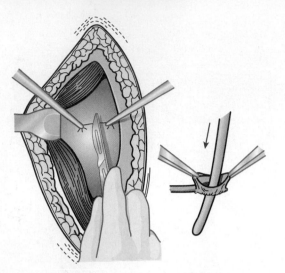

▲ **Figure 13–13.** Diagnostic peritoneal lavage.

Table 13–3. Criteria for evaluation of peritoneal lavage fluid.

Positive
= 100,000 red cells/μL
= 500 white cells/μL
= 175 units amylase/dL
Bacteria on Gram-stained smear
Bile
Food particles
Intermediate
Pink fluid on free aspiration
50,000–100,000 red cells/μL in blunt trauma
100–500 white cells/μL
75–175 units amylase/dL
Negative
Clear aspirate
< 100 white cells/μL
< 75 units amylase/dL

peritoneal lavages. The only contraindication is a need for emergency laparotomy.

The procedure may be performed with careful technique on patients with prior abdominal surgery and in pregnant patients. It should usually be performed through a small infraumbilical incision with placement of the catheter under direct vision (Figure 13–13). In pregnant patients and those with pelvic fractures, a supraumbilical approach is indicated. Closed techniques of catheter placement utilizing trocars or guidewires have been shown to be almost as safe as the open technique, but the rate of failure with the closed technique is higher, thus eliminating most of the potential advantage. After placement of the catheter, 1 L of normal saline solution is instilled into the peritoneal cavity and then allowed to drain by gravity. At least 200 mL of lavage fluid should be recovered to allow for accurate interpretation. A portion of the recovered fluid is sent for laboratory analysis of cell counts, the presence of particulate matter, and amylase. Criteria for evaluation of results are summarized in Table 13–3.

▶ Computed Tomography

Computed tomography (CT) is noninvasive, qualitative, sensitive, and accurate for the diagnosis of intra-abdominal and retroperitoneal injuries. Modern multi-slice spiral scanners have greatly decreased the time required for obtaining high-quality images. However, CT scanning remains expensive, involves the use of intravenous contrast administration, exposes the patient to radiation, and requires an experienced radiologist for proper interpretation of the scans. CT scanning also involves transport from the acute care area and should not be attempted in the unstable patient.

Computed tomography scanning has a primary role in defining the location and magnitude of intra-abdominal injuries related to blunt trauma. It has the advantage of detecting most retroperitoneal injuries, but it may not identify all gastrointestinal injuries. The information provided on the magnitude of injury allows for potential nonoperative management of patients with solid organ injuries. Nonsurgical therapy is now used in more than 80% of blunt liver and spleen injuries. Detection of high-grade solid organ injuries or bleeding pelvic fractures by CT in relatively stable patients can also lead to other minimally invasive interventions, such as angiographic embolization, which increases the success of nonoperative management. Table 13–4 compares the time, costs, advantages, and disadvantages of nonoperative methods used for evaluation of the injured abdomen.

▶ Diagnostic Laparoscopy

Laparoscopy has an important diagnostic role in stable patients with penetrating abdominal trauma. It can quickly establish whether peritoneal penetration has occurred and thus reduce the number of negative and nontherapeutic trauma laparotomies performed. In selected patients, therapeutic laparoscopy has been used to repair injuries to the bowel and diaphragm. This approach offers all the advantages and disadvantages of minimally invasive surgery. Laparoscopy has also been applied safely and effectively as a screening tool in stable patients with blunt abdominal trauma. However, its use in this context requires further study. Concerns regarding the use of laparoscopy in trauma include the possibility of missed injuries, air embolism, hemodynamic instability related to the pneumoperitoneum, and complications related to trocar placement.

Table 13–4. Comparison of diagnostic methods for abdominal trauma.

Methods	Time/Cost	Advantages/Disadvantages
Physical examination	Quick/no cost	Useful for serial examinations, very limited by other injuries, coma, drug intoxication, poor sensitivity and specificity.
Diagnostic peritoneal lavage (DPL)	Quick/ inexpensive	Rapid results in unstable patient but invasive and may be overly sensitive for blood and not specific for site of injury; requires experience and may be limited if previous surgery.
Focused assessment with sonography for trauma (FAST)	Quick/ inexpensive	Rapid detection of intra-abdominal fluid and pericardial tamponade; may be limited by operator experience, large body habitus, subcutaneous air; poor for detection of bowel injury. Fairly sensitive but not highly specific.
Helical computerized abdominal tomography (CT)	Slower/ expensive	Most specific for site of injury and can evaluate retroperitoneum; very good sensitivity but may miss bowel injury; risk of reaction to contrast dye.

Exploratory Laparotomy

The three main indications for exploration of the abdomen following blunt trauma are peritonitis, ongoing intra-abdominal hemorrhage, and the presence of other injuries known to be frequently associated with intra-abdominal injuries. Peritonitis after blunt abdominal trauma is rare and can arise from rupture of a hollow organ, such as the duodenum, bladder, intestine, or gallbladder; from pancreatic injury; or occasionally from the presence of retroperitoneal blood.

Emergency abdominal exploration should be considered for patients with profound hypovolemic shock and a normal chest x-ray unless extra-abdominal blood loss is sufficient to account for the hypovolemia. In most cases, a rapidly performed FAST examination or peritoneal lavage will confirm the diagnosis of intraperitoneal hemorrhage. Patients with blunt trauma and hypovolemia should be examined first for intra-abdominal bleeding even if there is no overt

evidence of abdominal trauma. For example, hypovolemia may be due to loss of blood from a large scalp laceration, but it may also be due to unsuspected rupture of the spleen. Hemoperitoneum may present with no signs except hypovolemia. The abdomen may be flat and nontender. Patients whose extra-abdominal bleeding has been controlled should respond to initial fluid resuscitation with an adequate urine output and stabilization of vital signs. If signs of hypovolemia (tachycardia, hypotension, low urine output, metabolic acidosis) recur, intra-abdominal bleeding must be considered to be the cause.

Other injuries frequently associated with abdominal trauma are rib fractures, pelvic fractures, abdominal wall injuries, and fractures of the thoracolumbar spine (eg, 20% of patients with fractures of the left lower ribs have a splenic laceration).

▶ Treatment

A. Splenic Injuries

The spleen is the most commonly injured organ in cases of blunt abdominal trauma. Splenic injuries in children are typically managed without surgery. Currently, 50%-88% of adults with blunt splenic injuries are also treated nonoperatively. Patients must be monitored closely and immediate availability of an operating room is essential. Patients should be evaluated frequently for the possibility of other missed injuries or recurrent bleeding. Stable patients who have high-grade splenic injuries on CT scan or have evidence of ongoing bleeding on CT scan may be candidates for angiographic embolization. Unstable patients with splenic injuries should undergo splenectomy or attempts at splenic repair if appropriate.

Associated injuries are uncommon for patients in whom nonoperative management is attempted. In unstable patients, emergent celiotomy should be performed. Splenic salvage procedures such as splenorrhaphy, partial resection, wrapping with Vicryl mesh, or topical therapy with hemostatic agents should be attempted if the patient's condition permits and there are a limited number of concomitant abdominal injuries. In the face of multiple injuries, ongoing cardiovascular compromise, or vascular avulsion of the spleen, total splenectomy is indicated. Following splenectomy, immunizations against *Pneumococcus* species, *Meningococcus* species, and *Haemophilus influenzae* are recommended postoperatively to reduce the risk of overwhelming postsplenectomy sepsis.

B. Liver Injuries

Approximately 85% of all patients with blunt hepatic trauma are stable following resuscitation. In this group, nonoperative management has been proven to be superior to open operation in avoiding complications and decreasing mortality. The primary requirement for nonoperative therapy is continued hemodynamic stability. Patients are monitored in the ICU with frequent assessment of vital signs and serial hematocrits. If transfusion with more than two units of PRBC is required, arteriography with possible embolization of bleeding vessels should be considered.

Nonoperative management of blunt hepatic trauma is successful in more than 90% of cases. With more severe injuries, repeat CT scanning may be necessary to evaluate for possible complications such as parenchymal infarction, hematoma, or biloma. Extrahepatic bile collections should generally be drained percutaneously. Intrahepatic collections of blood and bile usually resolve spontaneously over the course of several months. Patients with high-grade liver injuries have up to a 40% chance of developing bile leaks from the injured liver bed. Nuclear medicine scanning to delineate biliary flow with derivatives of iminodiacetic acid is useful in detection of bile leaks and should be done in the first few days after injury to reduce complications. Laparoscopic washout and placement of drains is an option for patients found to have evidence of extrahepatic bile leakage on HIDA scan. In addition, 1%-4% of patients with blunt liver injury will have injuries to other abdominal organs, which should prompt the clinician to consider the possibility of missed injury in patients who develop abdominal sepsis after injury.

Severe liver injury may result in exsanguinating hemorrhage with hypotension that does not respond to fluid resuscitation. For these patients, operative exploration is warranted. At laparotomy, immediate efforts should be directed to control of hemorrhage and stabilization of the patient by restoration of circulating blood volume. The initial techniques for the control of hepatic hemorrhage include manual compression, perihepatic packing, and the Pringle maneuver. Manual compression or perihepatic packing with laparotomy pads will control hemorrhage in most cases. The Pringle maneuver—clamping of the hepatic pedicle—should be performed when life-threatening hemorrhage is unresponsive to packing; it will control all hepatic bleeding except that from the hepatic veins or the intrahepatic vena cava. In most cases, the Pringle maneuver should not be maintained for more than 1 hour in order to prevent ischemic damage to the liver. Hepatic bleeding can be controlled by suture ligation or application of surgical clips directly to the bleeding vessels. Electrocautery or the argon beam coagulator can be used to control bleeding from raw surfaces of the liver. Microfibrillar collagen or hemostatic gelatin foam sponges soaked in thrombin can be applied to bleeding areas with pressure to control diffuse capillary bleeding. Fibrin glue has been used in treating both superficial and deep lacerations and appears to be the most effective topical agent but reports of fatal anaphylactic reactions have limited its use. When injury has already resulted in massive blood loss, packing of the abdomen with laparotomy pads and planned reexploration should be considered. Avoidance of the lethal triad of hypothermia, acidosis, and coagulopathy are paramount to successful surgical treatment of a major liver injury and may require further resuscitation in the ICU prior to return to the operating room. At the time of reexploration in 24-48 hours, hemorrhage is usually well controlled and can be managed with individual vessel ligation and debridement. Evidence of persistent hemorrhage should prompt earlier reexploration. Angiographic embolization may be a useful adjunct to surgical packing if arterial hemorrhage is still present or not well controlled. Rarely, selective hepatic artery ligation, resectional debridement, or hepatic lobectomy may be required to control hemorrhage. The raw surface of the liver may then be covered with omentum. Drains should always be used. Decompression of the biliary system is contraindicated, though sutures or clips should be used to control intraparenchymal bile ducts.

Hepatic vein injuries frequently bleed massively. Hepatic venous or intrahepatic vena caval injury should be suspected immediately when the Pringle maneuver fails to control bleeding. Several techniques have been described for isolation of the intrahepatic cava prior to attempted repair of these injuries. Unfortunately, even with the use of these techniques, mortality remains very high.

C. Biliary Tract Injuries

Biliary tract injuries are relatively uncommon, particularly for blunt trauma. Injury to the gallbladder should be treated in most cases by cholecystectomy. Minor injuries to the common bile duct can be treated by suture closure and insertion of a T-tube. Avulsion of the common bile duct or in combination with duodenal or ampullary trauma may require choledochojejunostomy in conjunction with total or partial pancreatectomy, duodenectomy, or other diversion procedures. Segmental loss of the common bile duct is best treated by choledochojejunostomy and drainage.

D. Pancreatic Injuries

Pancreatic injuries may present with few clinical manifestations. Injury should be suspected whenever the upper abdomen has been traumatized, especially when serum amylase and lipase levels remain persistently elevated. The best diagnostic study for pancreatic injury (other than exploratory celiotomy) is CT scan of the abdomen. Peritoneal lavage is usually not helpful. Upper gastrointestinal studies with water-soluble contrast material may suggest pancreatic injury by demonstrating widening of the duodenal C-loop. Endoscopic retrograde cholangiopancreatography may be used in selected cases to evaluate for injuries to the major ducts.

The treatment of pancreatic injury depends on its grade and extent. Minor injuries not involving a major duct may be treated nonoperatively. Moderate injuries usually require operative exploration, debridement, and the placement of external drains. More severe injuries, including those with major duct injury or transection of the gland, may require distal resection or external drainage. Traumatic injuries to the head of the pancreas often include associated vascular injuries and carry a high mortality rate. Efforts should be directed at controlling hemorrhage, and drains can be placed in the area of the pancreatic injury. In most cases, pancreaticoduodenectomy should not be attempted in the setting of an unstable patient with multiple injuries.

The late complications of pancreatic injuries include pseudocyst, pancreatic fistula, and pancreatic abscess. Patients treated without resection may require reoperation for resection or Roux-en-Y internal gastrointestinal drainage.

E. Gastrointestinal Tract Injuries

Most injuries of the stomach can be repaired. Large injuries, such as those from shotgun blasts, may require subtotal or total resection. Failure to identify posterior stomach wall injuries by opening the lesser space is a pitfall to guard against.

Duodenal injuries may not be evident from the initial physical examination or x-ray studies. Abdominal films will reveal retroperitoneal gas within 6 hours after injury in most patients. CT performed with a contrast agent will frequently identify the site of perforation. Most duodenal injuries can be treated with lateral repair. Some may require resection with end-to-end anastomosis. Occasionally, pancreaticoduodenectomy or duodenal diversion with gastrojejunostomy and pyloric closure is required to manage a severe injury. A duodenostomy tube is useful in decompressing the duodenum and can be used to control a fistula caused by an injury. Jejunal or omental patches may also aid in preventing a suture line leak. A distal jejunostomy feeding tube is helpful in the long-term recovery from these injuries.

Duodenal hematomas causing high-grade obstruction usually resolve with nonoperative management. Patients may require total parenteral nutrition. In some cases, a small-bore enteral feeding tube can be passed beyond the area of obstruction utilizing interventional radiology techniques. Large hematomas may require operative evacuation, particularly when the obstruction lasts for more than 10-14 days and a persistent hematoma is seen on CT scan.

Most small bowel injuries can be treated with a two-layer sutured closure, though mesenteric injuries leading to devascularized segments of small bowel will require resection. The underlying principle is to preserve as much small bowel as possible.

For injuries to the colon, the past approach has been to divert the fecal stream or exteriorize the injury. However,

more recent studies have shown a higher complication rate with colostomy formation than with primary repair. Wounds should be considered for primary repair if the blood supply is not compromised. Primary repair is more likely to be associated with complications in patients with ongoing shock, in those requiring multiple transfusions, if more than 6 hours elapse between injury and operation, or if there is gross contamination or peritonitis. Small, clean rectal injuries may be closed primarily if conditions are favorable. The treatment of larger rectal wounds involving pelvic fracture should include proximal diversion. Insertion of presacral drains is optional. In this latter case, direct repair of the rectal injury is not mandatory but should be performed if it can be readily exposed. Irrigation of the distal stump should be performed in most cases unless it would further contaminate the pelvic space.

F. Abdominal Wall Injuries

Abdominal wall injuries from blunt trauma are most often due to shear forces, such as being run over by the wheels of a tractor or bus. The shearing often devitalizes the subcutaneous tissue and skin, and if debridement is delayed, a serious necrotizing anaerobic infection may develop. The management of penetrating abdominal wall injuries is usually straightforward. Debridement and irrigation are appropriate surgical treatments. Every effort must be made to remove foreign material, shreds of clothing, necrotic muscle, and soft tissue. Abdominal wall defects may require insertion of absorbable mesh or coverage with a myocutaneous flap.

G. Genitourinary Tract Injuries

The most commonly injured genitourinary tract organs are the male genitalia, the uterus, the urethra, the bladder, the ureters, and the kidneys. The workup for these injuries consists primarily of radiologic examinations, which may include abdominal CT scan, cystogram, or retrograde urethrogram. In unstable patients with associated injuries, it may not be possible to obtain these studies prior to emergency laparotomy. In these patients, an intraoperative single-shot intravenous urogram is safe and of high quality in most cases. This study often provides important information that facilitates rapid and accurate decision making. It can confirm function in the noninjured kidney and help in identifying blunt renal injuries that may be safely observed.

1. Bladder injuries—Rupture of the bladder, like urethral disruption, is frequently associated with pelvic fractures. Seventy-five percent of ruptures are extraperitoneal and 25% intraperitoneal. Intraperitoneal bladder ruptures should be repaired through a mid-line abdominal incision. Rupture of the anterior wall of the bladder can be repaired by direct suture; rupture of the posterior wall can be repaired from inside the bladder after an opening has been made in the anterior wall. Care should be taken to avoid entering a pelvic hematoma. Retroperitoneal injuries can often be treated with urinary drainage, depending on the size of injury. Postoperatively, urine should be diverted for at least 7 days.

2. Urethral injuries—Membranous prostatic urethral disruption is often associated with pelvic fractures or deceleration injuries. Blood at the urethral meatus associated with scrotal hematoma and high-riding prostate on digital rectal examination are the classic signs of injury to the male urethra. The prostate may be elevated superiorly by the pelvic hematoma and will be free-riding and high on rectal examination. If these signs are present, a retrograde urethrogram should be performed before attempts at catheter placement, which may convert an incomplete injury to a complete disruption. If an injury is present, urethrography will demonstrate free extravasation of contrast from the urethra into the preperitoneal space.

Penetrating injuries are best treated with primary repair. Suprapubic bladder drainage and delayed reconstruction of blunt urethral disruption injuries are safe and effective in most cases. Immediate realignment with cystourethroscopy and placement of a urethral catheter is an attractive, minimally invasive alternative. In cases of partial disruption, it has been shown to result in stricture-free outcomes.

Major injuries to the bulbous or penile urethra should be managed by suprapubic urinary diversion. A voiding cystourethrogram may later reveal a stricture, but operative correction or dilation is usually not necessary.

3. Renal injuries—Advances in the imaging and staging of renal trauma as well as in treatment strategies have decreased the need for operation and increased renal preservation. More than half of renal injuries can be treated nonoperatively. Management criteria are based on radiographic, laboratory, and clinical findings. Nonoperative treatment of penetrating renal lacerations is appropriate in hemodynamically stable patients without other injuries. Small to moderate injuries can be treated nonoperatively, but severe injuries are associated with a significant risk of delayed bleeding if treated expectantly. Stable patients may be candidates for angiographic procedures to control bleeding, revascularize a dissection or injuries leading to vessel thrombosis. Renal exploration should be considered if laparotomy is indicated for associated injuries. A mid-line transabdominal approach is preferred. The renal artery and vein are secured before the Gerota fascia is opened. The injury should be managed by suture repair, partial nephrectomy, or, rarely, total nephrectomy. Pedicle grafts of omentum or free peritoneal patch grafts can be used to cover defects. Renal vascular injuries require immediate operation to save the kidney. Meticulous attention to reconstructive techniques in renal exploration can ensure an excellent renal salvage rate. Adherence to the principles of early proximal vascular control, debridement of devitalized tissue, hemostasis, closure of the collecting

system, and coverage of the defect will maximize the salvage of renal function while minimizing potential complications.

Perirenal hematomas found incidentally at celiotomy should be explored if they are expanding, pulsatile, or not contained by retroperitoneal tissues or if a preexploration urogram shows extensive urinary extravasation.

4. Injuries to the male genitalia—Injuries to the male genitalia usually result in skin loss only; the penis, penile urethra, and testes are usually spared. Skin loss from the penis should be treated with a primary skin graft. Scrotal skin loss should be treated by delayed reconstruction; an exposed testis can be temporarily protected by placing it in a subcutaneous tissue pocket in the thigh.

5. Uterine injuries—Injuries of the female reproductive organs are infrequent except in combination with genitourinary or rectal trauma. Injuries to the uterine fundus usually can be repaired with absorbable sutures; drainage is not necessary. In more extensive injuries, hysterectomy may be preferable. The vaginal cuff may be left open for drainage, particularly if there is an associated urinary tract or rectal injury. Injuries involving the uterus in a pregnant woman usually result in death of the fetus. Bleeding may be massive in such patients, particularly in women approaching parturition. Cesarean section plus hysterectomy may be the only alternative.

6. Ureteral injuries—Ureteral injuries are easily missed because urinalysis and imaging studies can be unreliable. Most such injuries can be successfully reconstructed by primary repair over stents, ureteral reimplantations, or ureteroureterostomy depending on the level of injury.

Bhullar IS et al: Age does not affect outcomes of nonoperative management of blunt splenic trauma. *J Am Coll Surg.* 2012;214:958.

Bhullar IS et al: Selective angiographic embolization of blunt splenic traumatic injuries in adults decreases failure rate of nonoperative management. *J Trauma Acute Care Surg.* 2012;72:1127.

Bjurlin MA et al: Comparison of nonoperative management with renorrhaphy and nephrectomy in penetrating renal injuries. *J Trauma.* 2011;71:554.

Burlew CC et al: Sew it up! A Western Trauma Association multi-institutional study of enteric injury management in the postinjury open abdomen. *J Trauma.* 2011;70:273.

Dabbs DN et al: Treatment of major hepatic necrosis: lobectomy versus serial debridement. *J Trauma.* 2012;69:562.

Natarajan B et al: FAST scan: is it worth doing in hemodynamically stable blunt trauma patients? *Surgery.* 2010;148:695.

Peitzman AB et al: Surgical treatment of injuries to the solid abdominal organs: a 50-year perspective from the Journal of Trauma. *J Trauma.* 2010;69:1011.

Piper GL, Peitzman AB: Current management of hepatic trauma. *Surg Clin North Am.* 2010;90:775.

Sharp JP et al: Adherence to a simplified management algorithm reduces morbidity and mortality after penetrating colon injuries: a 15-year experience. *J Am Coll Surg.* 2012;214:591.

Sharp JP et al: Impact of a defined management algorithm on out-come after traumatic pancreatic injury. *J Trauma Acute Care Surg.* 2012;72;100.

Wei B et al: Angioembolization reduces operative intervention for blunt splenic injury. *J Trauma.* 2008;64:1472.

VASCULAR INJURIES

▶ Historical Perspective

Much of our knowledge of blood vessel injuries was developed during the course of military conflicts in the 20th century. Although techniques for the management of vascular injuries were in use prior to World War I, arterial ligation to save a life rather than arterial repair to salvage a limb was generally employed, and amputation frequently resulted after vascular injury.

The current mortality rate for lower extremity arterial injury is low in both civilian and recent military series: 2%-6%. Limb salvage rates in civilian series are 85%-90%, with best results obtained for interposition vein grafts. Ligation, need for reoperation, and failed revascularization are associated with worse outcomes and higher amputation rates. Low mortality and improved limb salvage is a result of more rapid transport of injured people, improved blood volume replacement, selective use of arteriography and shunts, and better operative techniques.

▶ The Epidemiology of Vascular Trauma

The epidemiology of vascular trauma has been studied in three different settings: military conflicts, large urban locations, and, to a lesser extent, rural areas. The types of injuries seen in civilian vascular trauma, once much different from military settings, are now more similar to military wounds. The incidence is increasing as a result of the rise in urban violence, motor vehicle crashes, and iatrogenic injuries owing to more frequent use of minimally invasive diagnostic and therapeutic procedures.

Peripheral vascular trauma typically occurs in young men between the ages of 20 and 40 years. In both urban and rural environments, penetrating mechanisms dominate, accounting for 50%-90% of vascular injuries. Because many vascular injuries of the head, neck, and torso are immediately fatal, most patients with vascular injuries surviving transport have extremity trauma. This is especially true in the military experience where extremity vascular injuries account for approximately 90% of all arterial trauma. In the urban civilian experience, extremity vascular injuries comprise about 50% of arterial injuries. In rural vascular trauma, blunt injuries occur more frequently than in urban populations.

Mortality and utilization of medical resources is higher among patients with vascular injuries than among patients who do not have blood vessel injuries. Vascular injuries from automobile accidents or falls from heights and crush injuries account for up to half of all noniatrogenic vascular injuries in US hospitals. The likelihood of vascular injury after blunt trauma correlates with the overall severity of the injury and the presence of specific orthopedic injuries; for example, up to 45% of patients with posterior knee dislocations or severe instability from high-velocity blunt trauma sustain popliteal artery injury.

The number of iatrogenic vascular injuries has risen dramatically in recent decades. Most involve diagnostic and therapeutic procedures utilizing the femoral (less frequently the brachial or axillary) vessels, which serve as percutaneous access routes. In order of decreasing frequency, injuries include hemorrhage and hematoma, pseudoaneurysm, arteriovenous fistula formation, vessel thrombosis, and embolization. Rates of injury range from 0.5% for diagnostic procedures to as high as 10% for therapeutic procedures involving large catheters. Increasing age, female gender, use of anticoagulation, and the presence of atherosclerosis increase the risk of these complications. Complications remote from the puncture site include vessel rupture and dissection. Operative procedures (especially hepatic and pancreaticobiliary surgery) are associated with iatrogenic vascular trauma. In addition, anterior and retroperitoneal approaches to the lumbar spine and other orthopedic procedures such as total joint replacement and arthroscopy can produce vascular injuries.

▶ Types of Injuries

A. Penetrating Trauma

The local and regional effects of penetrating wounds are determined by the mechanism of vessel injury. Stab wounds, low-velocity (< 2000 ft/s) bullet wounds, iatrogenic injuries from percutaneous catheterization, and inadvertent intra-arterial injection of drugs produce less soft tissue injury and disrupt collateral circulation less than injuries from sources with greater kinetic energy. The high-velocity missiles responsible for war wounds produce more extensive vascular injuries, which involve massive destruction and contamination of surrounding tissues. The temporary cavitational effect of high-velocity missiles causes additional trauma to the ends of severed arteries and may produce arterial thrombosis due to disrupted intima even when the artery has not been directly hit. This blast effect can also draw material such as clothing, dirt, or pieces of skin along the wound tract, which contributes to the risk of infection. Associated injuries are often major determinants of the eventual outcome.

Shotgun blasts present special problems. Although muzzle velocity is low (about 1200 ft/s), the multiple pellets produce widespread damage, and shotgun wadding entering the wound enhances the likelihood of infection. Similar to high-velocity injuries, the damage is often much greater than might be anticipated from inspection of the entry wound. Moreover, the multiplicity of potential sites of arterial damage often mandates diagnostic arteriography even in the presence of obvious arterial insufficiency.

B. Blunt Trauma

Motor vehicle accidents are a major cause of blunt vascular trauma. Multiple injuries include fractures and dislocations; and while direct vascular injury may occur, in most instances the damage is indirect due to fractures. This is especially likely to occur with fractures near joints, where vessels are relatively fixed and vulnerable to shear forces. For example, the popliteal artery and vein are frequently injured in association with posterior dislocation of the knee. Fractures of large heavy bones such as the femur or tibia transmit forces that have cavitation effects similar to those caused by high-velocity bullets. There is extensive damage to soft tissues and neurovascular structures, and edema formation interferes with evaluation of pulses. Delay in diagnosis and the presence of associated injuries decrease the chances of limb salvage. Contusions or crush injuries may result in complete or partial disruption of arteries, producing intimal flaps or intramural hematomas that impede blood flow.

Blunt thoracic aortic injury (BTAI) is a serious traumatic injury that continues to have a high initial mortality and is associated with modern high-speed methods of transportation or significant falls. Autopsy data from cases of fatal BTAI demonstrated that 57% of patients were dead at the scene or on arrival to the hospital, 37% died during the first 4 hours at the hospital, and only 6% died after 4 hours in the hospital. The disruption generally occurs at the aortic isthmus (between the left subclavian artery and the ligamentum arteriosum) due to a deceleration injury in which the heart, the ascending aorta, and the transverse arch continue to move forward while movement of the isthmus and the descending aorta is limited by their posterior attachments. Clinical findings associated with traumatic rupture of the thoracic aorta are listed in Table 13–5 and radiographic

Table 13–5. Clinical features of traumatic aortic rupture.

History of high-speed deceleration injury
Flail chest
Fractured sternum
Superior vena cava syndrome
Multiple or first or second rib fractures
Upper extremity hypertension or pulse deficits
Hematoma in the carotid sheaths
Interscapular bruits
Hoarseness with normal larynx

Table 13–6. Radiographic features of traumatic aortic rupture.

Widening of mediastinum
Fractured sternum
Multiple or first rib or second rib fractures
Esophageal deviation to the right
Tracheal deviation to the right
Apical cap
Depression of left main stem bronchus
Obliteration of the aortic knob
Obliteration of the descending aorta
Obliteration of the aortopulmonary window
Obliteration of the medial left upper lobe
Widened paravertebral stripe

findings in Table 13–6. Blunt traumatic injury to the abdominal aorta is uncommon, but it has been reported from lap seat belt trauma.

Almost any vessel can be injured by blunt trauma, including the extracranial cerebral and visceral arteries. Blunt carotid arterial injuries are associated with mortality rates of 20%-30%, with over 50% of survivors having permanent, severe neurologic deficits. Whereas in the past vertebral artery injuries were considered innocuous, recent studies have reported devastating complications related to these injuries, including a 70% incidence of coexistent cervical spine injuries. Traumatic injury to the superior mesenteric artery is associated with a 50% mortality rate. The brachial and popliteal arteries, which cross joints and are exposed to direct trauma, are particularly susceptible to injury as a result of fractures and dislocations.

▶ Clinical Findings

A. Hemorrhage

When pulsatile external hemorrhage is present, the diagnosis of arterial injury is obvious, but when blood accumulates in deep tissues of the extremity, the thorax, abdomen, or retroperitoneum, the only manifestation may be shock. Peripheral vasoconstriction may make evaluation of peripheral pulses difficult until blood volume is restored. If the artery is completely severed, thrombus may form at the contracted vessel ends and a major vascular injury may not be suspected. The presence of arterial pulses distal to a penetrating wound does not preclude arterial injury; as many as 20% of patients with injuries of major arteries in an extremity have palpable pulses distal to the injury, either because the vessel has not thrombosed or because pulse waves are transmitted through soft clot. Conversely, the absence of a palpable pulse in an adequately resuscitated patient is a sensitive indicator of arterial injury.

B. Ischemia

Acute arterial insufficiency must be diagnosed promptly to prevent tissue loss. Ischemia should be suspected when the patient has one or more of the "five Ps": pain, pallor, paralysis, paresthesia, or pulselessness. The susceptibility of different cells to hypoxia varies (eg, sudden occlusion of the carotid artery results in brain damage within minutes unless collateral circulation can maintain adequate perfusion, but a kidney can survive severe ischemia for up to an hour). Peripheral nerves are quite vulnerable to ischemia because they have a high basal energy requirement to maintain ion gradients over large membrane surfaces and because they have few glycogen stores. Hence, interruption of arterial flow for relatively short periods can result in nerve damage due to interrupted substrate delivery. In contrast, skeletal muscle is more tolerant of decreased arterial flow. Muscle can be ischemic for up to 4 hours without developing histologic changes. In general, complete interruption of all arterial inflow (including collateral blood supply) results in neuromuscular ischemic damage after 4-6 hours. Restoration of flow can actually worsen this damage as part of the reperfusion syndrome and can increase the severity of the original ischemic insult.

Prolonged ischemia can produce muscle necrosis and rhabdomyolysis, which releases potassium and myoglobin into the circulation. Myoglobin is an oxygen-transporting protein similar in structure to hemoglobin; it is innocuous unless it dissociates into hematin, which is nephrotoxic in an acidic milieu. Precipitation of hematin pigment also occurs when urine flow is reduced by hypotension or hypovolemia, obstructing renal tubules and worsening nephrotoxicity. Myoglobinemia can lead to acute tubular necrosis and renal failure, hyperkalemia, and a risk of life-threatening arrhythmias. Thus, in addition to limb loss, acute arterial ischemia can produce organ failure and death.

C. False Aneurysm

Disruption of an arterial wall as a result of trauma may lead to formation of a false aneurysm. The wall of a false aneurysm is composed primarily of fibrous tissue derived from nearby tissues, not arterial tissue. Because blood continues to flow past the fistulous opening, the extremity is seldom ischemic. False aneurysms may rupture at any time. They continue to expand because they lack vascular wall integrity. Spontaneous resolution of pseudoaneurysms larger than 3 cm is unlikely, and operative repair becomes increasingly difficult as the aneurysms increase in size and complexity with time. Symptoms gradually appear as a result of compression of adjacent nerves or collateral vessels or from rupture of the aneurysm—or as a result of thrombosis with ischemic symptoms. Iatrogenic false aneurysms after arterial puncture thrombose spontaneously within 4 weeks when they are less than 3 cm in diameter.

Simple ultrasound follow-up rather than operative therapy is indicated. Color-flow duplex-guided compression of iatrogenic pseudoaneurysms is successful in 70%-90% of attempts, but the procedure is uncomfortable and may take hours of probe pressure. Ultrasound-guided thrombin injection has been effective for thrombosis of large false aneurysms in a matter of seconds, but distal arterial thrombosis has also been described using this technique.

D. Arteriovenous Fistula

With simultaneous injury of an adjacent artery and vein, a fistula may form that allows blood from the artery to enter the vein. Because venous pressure is lower than arterial pressure, flow through an arteriovenous fistula is continuous; accentuation of the bruit and thrill can be detected over the fistula during systole. Traumatic arteriovenous fistulas may occur as operative complications (eg, aortocaval fistula following removal of a herniated intervertebral disk). Iatrogenic femoral arteriovenous fistulas after arteriograms and cardiac catheterization are seen with increasing frequency. Long-standing large arteriovenous fistulas may result in high-output cardiac failure. Similar to iatrogenic pseudoaneurysms occurring after arteriography, spontaneous resolution of acute arteriovenous fistulas usually occurs.

▶ Diagnosis

Arterial injury must be considered in any injured patient. Patients who present in shock following penetrating injury or blunt trauma should be assumed to have vascular injury until proven otherwise. Any injury near a major artery should arouse suspicion. A plain film may be helpful in demonstrating a fracture whose fragments could jeopardize an adjacent vessel or a bullet fragment that could have passed near to a major vessel. Before the x-ray is taken, entrance and exit wounds should be marked with radiopaque objects such as a paper clip.

Diagnosis is usually established on the basis of physical examination looking for signs of injury (Table 13–7).

Table 13–7. Signs of extremity vascular injury.

Hard signs
Expanding or pulsatile hematoma
Limb ischemia
Bruit or thrill
Absence of distal pulse
Soft signs
History of hemorrhage at scene, now stopped
Deficit of nerve associated with vessel
Stable, nonexpanding hematoma
Proximity of wound to major extremity blood vessel
Ankle brachial index < 0.9

In addition to checking for obvious hemorrhage and the five Ps, the physician should listen for a bruit, palpate for a thrill (eg, of an arteriovenous fistula), and look for an expanding hematoma (eg, of a false aneurysm). Secondary hemorrhage from a wound is an ominous sign that may herald massive hemorrhage. The finding of these "hard" signs reliably reflects the presence of a vascular injury; hard signs mandate immediate exploration in most instances. The presence of "soft" signs (history of bleeding, diminished but palpable pulse, injury in proximity to a major artery, neurapraxia) requires further tests or serial observation.

Doppler flow studies have gained importance in the diagnosis of arterial trauma. An ankle brachial index (ABI), determined by dividing the systolic pressure in the injured limb by the systolic pressure in an uninjured arm, is highly reliable for excluding arterial injury after both blunt and penetrating trauma. An ABI less than 0.9 has sensitivity of 95%, specificity of 97%, and negative predictive value of 99% for determining the presence of clinically significant arterial injury. Thus, only patients with soft signs and an ABI less than 0.9 require arteriography.

Color-flow duplex ultrasonography combines real-time B mode (brightness modulation) ultrasound imaging with a steerable pulsed Doppler flow detector. This technology can provide images of vessels and velocity spectral analysis. Color-flow duplex scanning of an area of injury is noninvasive, painless, portable, and easily repeated for follow-up examinations. When compared with arteriography and performed by experienced examiners, duplex ultrasound identifies nearly all major injuries that require treatment, potentially at considerable cost savings. In addition to screening for arterial trauma, duplex scanning has been used to detect pseudoaneurysms, arteriovenous fistulas, and intimal flaps. However, potential logistical and resource problems exist. The technology is sophisticated and requires skill in operation and interpretation, which is not always immediately available.

Arteriography is the most accurate diagnostic procedure for identifying vascular injuries (Figure 13–14). Arteriography to exclude vascular injury for soft signs results in a negative exploration rate of 20%-35% and an arteriography-related complication rate of 2%-4%. Proximity as the sole indication for arteriography has an extremely low yield, ranging from 0% to 10%. Patients with unequivocal signs of arterial injury on physical examination or plain films should have urgent operation. The false-negative rate of arteriography is low, and a normal arteriogram precludes the need for surgical exploration. Virtually all arteriographic errors are due to false-positives, which occur in 2%-8% of patients. Technical considerations in performing arteriography include the following: (1) entrance and exit wounds should be marked with a radiopaque marker; (2) the injection site should not be near the suspected injury; (3) an area 10-15 cm proximal and distal to the suspected injury should

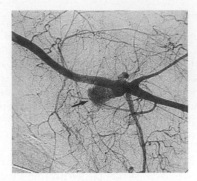

▲ **Figure 13–14.** Arteriogram showing traumatic pseudoaneurysm of subclavian/axillary artery from penetrating injury.

be included in the arteriographic field; (4) sequential films should be obtained to detect early venous filling; (5) any abnormality should be considered an indication of arterial injury unless it is obviously the result of preexisting disease; and (6) two different projections should be obtained.

Emergency center arteriography using micropuncture Seldinger technique or cannulating the artery to be studied with an 18-gauge catheter (antegrade in the lower extremity and prograde in the upper extremity arteries) is quick and accurate. The use of fluoroscopy, especially if equipped with subtraction capability, simplifies the timing of contrast injection and x-ray exposure. Fluoroscopy is particularly helpful to visualize distal arteries and minimize the amount of contrast media needed. Arteriography may be particularly useful in differentiating arterial injury from spasm. In general, it is risky to attribute abnormal physical findings in an injured patient to arterial spasm; an arteriogram is indicated in such patients.

Arteriography is also valuable when arterial injuries may have occurred at multiple sites or to localize an injury when a long parallel penetration makes this determination difficult. Complications of arteriography include groin hematomas, iatrogenic pseudoaneurysms, arteriovenous fistulas, embolic occlusions, and delays in diagnosis that may lead to irreversible ischemia in marginally perfused limbs. The availability of CT angiograms with latest generation multidetector contrast-enhanced spiral scanners is a viable alternative to traditional angiography. CT angiograms can diagnose intimal dissections, pseudoaneurysms, arteriovenous fistulas, thrombosis or occlusion, and active bleeding. Metallic foreign bodies can create artifacts that interfere with generation of optimal CT angiogram studies.

For patients suspected of having BTAI based on mechanism of injury, the chest x-ray is a good screening tool to determine the need for further investigation. The most significant radiographic findings for possible BTAI include widened mediastinum, obscured aortic knob, deviation

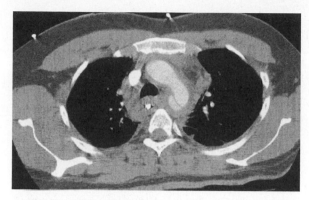

▲ **Figure 13–15.** Computed tomography scan of the chest showing traumatic disruption of the aorta from blunt injury.

of the left mainstem bronchus or nasogastric tube, and opacification of the aortopulmonary window. Helical chest CT scanning is a useful diagnostic tool for screening and diagnosis of BTAI (Figure 13–15). A negative chest CT scan can obviate the need for further evaluation with a contrast aortogram. Patients with indeterminate CT scans or positive scans should have confirmation and delineation of the extent of BTAI with arteriography or a CT angiogram. In selected instances, cardiothoracic and/or trauma surgeons may consider helical CT scanning alone to be an adequate and complete work-up for BTAI. In addition, a helical CT angiogram with 3D reconstruction guides potential endovascular approach for treatment of BTAI. The use of either transesophageal echocardiography or intraluminal ultrasound in the diagnosis of BTAI continues to evolve, but they are not considered standard diagnostic modalities.

► Management

A. Initial Treatment

A rapid but thorough examination should be performed to determine the complete extent of injury. The physician must establish the priority of arterial injury in the overall management of the patient and should remember that delay in arterial repair decreases chances of a favorable outcome. When repair is performed within 12 hours after injury, amputation is rarely necessary; if repair is performed later, the incidence of amputation is about 50%. Depending on the degree of ischemia, delay in arterial repair will lead to lasting neuromuscular damage after as short a period as 4-6 hours.

Restoration of blood volume and control of hemorrhage are done simultaneously. If exsanguinating hemorrhage precludes resuscitation in the emergency room, the patient should be moved directly to the operating room. External bleeding is best controlled by firm direct pressure or packing. Probes or fingers should not be inserted into the wound because a clot may be dislodged, causing profuse bleeding. Tourniquets occlude venous return, disturb collateral flow, and further compromise circulation and should not be employed unless exsanguinating hemorrhage cannot be controlled by other means. Atraumatic vascular clamps may be applied to accessible vessels by trained surgeons, but blind clamping can increase damage and injure adjacent nerves and veins.

After hemorrhage has been controlled and general resuscitation accomplished, further assessment is possible. The extent of associated injuries is determined and a plan of management made. Large-bore intravenous catheters should be placed in extremities with no potential venous injuries. It is prudent to preserve the saphenous or cephalic vein in an uninjured extremity for use as a venous autograft for vascular repair.

B. Nonoperative Treatment

Some arterial injuries remain asymptomatic and heal. Data supporting the practice of observation of small or asymptomatic arterial injuries have emerged from experimental animal studies and clinical reports showing resolution, improvement, or stabilization of arterial injuries. In well-defined settings, this strategy has proved safe in follow-up reports covering periods of up to 10 years. Thus, a nonoperative approach may be appropriate for compliant patients willing to return for follow-up who have: (1) no active hemorrhage; (2) low-velocity injuries (particularly stab wounds or iatrogenic punctures); (3) minimal arterial wall disruptions (< 5 mm); (4) small (< 5 mm) intimal defects; and (5) intact distal circulation.

Follow-up must include frequent physical examinations and carefully performed noninvasive studies, and patients should be asymptomatic and the strategy must be reconsidered if symptoms develop. Adjuvant therapy with antiplatelet agents is usually recommended to improve patency in patients with intimal flaps.

Endovascular management has assumed a greater role in the treatment of arterial trauma in recent years. Transcatheter embolization with coils or balloons has been successful in managing selected arterial injuries such as pseudoaneurysms, arteriovenous fistulas, and active bleeding from nonessential arteries. Coils are made of stainless steel with wool or polyester tufts. They are extruded at the site of vessel injury through 5F or 7F catheters. After deployment, the coils expand and lodge at the extrusion site and the tufts promote thrombosis. Catheter-based intra-arterial infusion of vasodilators has also been used to treat vasospasm in small distal arteries.

The recent popularity of endovascular grafting in elective vascular surgery (Chapter 34) has been applied to the treatment of arterial trauma. A fixation device such as a stent is attached to a graft, and the Stent graft is inserted endoluminally from a remote site and deployed at the site of injury to repair false aneurysms or arteriovenous fistulas. The indications for endovascular grafting are likely to change as technology advances, but the most frequent application currently is in stable patients with delayed presentations who have complex false aneurysms or arteriovenous fistulas. Use of Stent grafts in the acute setting requires the availability of a wide variety of sizes and lengths of grafts and advanced catheter skills.

Endovascular repair of BTAI can be performed either electively or even emergently (Figure 13–16). In a recent American Association for the Surgery of Trauma (AAST) multicenter study, two-thirds of patients underwent endovascular Stent graph repair as compared to one-third who underwent traditional open repair. When adjusted for confounding variables, the endovascular approach was associated with reduced mortality (odds ratio 8.42, 95% confidence interval 2.76-25.69) and fewer blood transfusions. Further study is needed to determine the long-term outcome using endovascular techniques to repair BTAI. Commercial grafts have yielded better results than the noncommercial "homemade" grafts. Thoracic aorta lacerations of more than 1.5 cm resulting in graft apposition length less than 2 cm or those near or in the curvature of the aortic arch are associated with an increased risk of endoleak. Endoleak occurred in 14% of the AAST BTAI trial patients, with half being successfully managed with the deployment of additional stent grafts.

In selected cases of BTAI repair, whether it is operative or endovascular, treatment is delayed because treatment and recovery from other more life-threatening injuries has priority (eg, severe pulmonary contusion, brain injury). This is acceptable, and the incidence of aortic rupture after 4 hours in the hospital is low. Systemic blood pressure and heart rate should be controlled with a beta-blocker and other pharmacologic agents as necessary to minimize the risk of rupture while waiting for definitive repair of the injured aorta.

C. Operative Treatment

General anesthesia is preferable to spinal or regional anesthesia. When vascular injuries involve the neck or thoracic outlet, endotracheal intubation must be performed carefully to avoid dislodging a clot and to protect the airway. Moreover, care is necessary to avoid neurologic damage in patients with associated cervical spine injuries. At least one uninjured extremity should also be prepared for surgery so that saphenous or cephalic vein conduit may be obtained if a vein graft is required. Provision should also be made for operative arteriography.

Incisions should be generous and parallel to the injured vessel. Meticulous care in handling incisions is essential to avoid secondary infections; all undamaged tissue should be conserved for use in covering repaired vessels. Preservation of all arterial branches is important in order to maintain collateral circulation. Atraumatic control of the vessel should be achieved proximal and distal to the injury so that the injured area may be dissected free of other tissues and inspected without risk of further bleeding. When large hematomas and multiple wounds make exposure and clamping of vessels difficult, it is wise to place a sterile orthopedic tourniquet proximal to the injury that can be inflated temporarily if needed.

The extent of arterial injury must be accurately determined. Arterial spasm generally responds to gentle hydraulic or mechanical dilation. Local application of warm saline or drugs such as papaverine, tolazoline, lidocaine, or nitroglycerin is occasionally effective in relieving spasm. Intra-arterial injection of nitroglycerin or papaverine is also very effective in alleviating spasm. If spasm persists, however, it is best to assume that it is caused by an intramural injury, and the

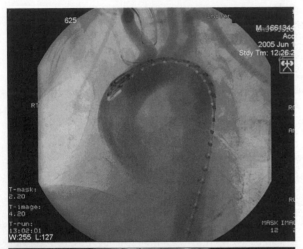

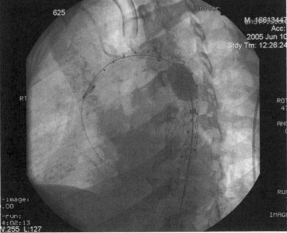

▲ **Figure 13–16.** Aortogram and placement of aortic stent graft to repair a blunt aortic disruption.

vessel should be opened for direct inspection. An old adage is that spasm is spelled "c-l-o-t."

All devitalized tissue, including damaged portions of the artery, must be debrided. One should resect only the grossly injured portion of the vessel. The method of reconstruction depends on the degree of arterial damage. In selected instances, the ends of injured vessels can be approximated and an end-to-end anastomosis created. If the vessels cannot be mobilized well enough to provide a tension-free anastomosis, an interposition graft should be used. Early experience with prosthetic interposition grafts was disappointing since postoperative infection, thrombosis, and anastomotic disruption were common. These problems have decreased considerably with the use of grafts made of expanded polytetrafluoroethylene (PTFE). Proponents of synthetic graphs focus on the fact that they fail well (cg, infected pseudoaneurysm), whereas a vein graft will disintegrate and result in a sudden blow-out type hemorrhage. Nevertheless, most surgeons still prefer to use an autogenous graft (ie, vein or artery) in severely contaminated wounds. Saphenous vein grafts should be obtained from the noninjured leg to avoid impairment of venous return on the side of the injury. Patch angioplasty using saphenous vein is performed when closure of a partially transected vessel would result in narrowing. Suturing should be done with fine 5-0 or 6-0 monofilament material.

In the unusual circumstance of isolated vascular injury, 5000-10,000 units of intravenous heparin can be given to prevent thrombosis. Otherwise, a small amount of dilute heparin solution (100 units/mL) may be gently injected into the proximal and distal lumen of the injured vessel before clamps are applied. Proximal and distal thrombi are removed with a Fogarty embolectomy catheter. Backbleeding from the distal artery is not a sure indication that thrombus is absent. A completion operative arteriogram is indicated to determine distal patency and to check on the adequacy of the reconstruction—even when distal pulses are palpable.

It was formerly taught that fractures should be stabilized before vascular injuries were repaired so that manipulation of bones would not jeopardize vascular repair. The disadvantages of this dictum were delay in restoration of flow to ischemic tissue and interference with vascular reconstruction and subsequent arteriographic study of the completed repair by the fixation device. It is currently recommended that vascular repair be performed first, followed by careful application of external traction devices that allow easy access to the wound for observation and dressing changes. Another alternative is to place an intraluminal shunt temporarily across the vascular injury to decrease ischemia while fractures or other injuries are treated. Once the fracture is stabilized, the temporary shunt can be removed and definitive vascular repair completed. Improved outcomes similar to civilian lower extremity vascular trauma have been

attributed to the use of temporary vascular shunts and damage control techniques in the current Iraq War.

Repaired vessels must be covered with healthy tissue. If left exposed, they invariably desiccate and rupture. Skin alone is inadequate, because subsequent necrosis of the skin would leave the vessels exposed, greatly endangering the reconstruction. Generally, an adjacent muscle (eg, sartorius muscle for coverage of the common femoral artery) can be mobilized and placed over the repair. Musculocutaneous flaps can be constructed by plastic surgeons to cover almost any site. In an extensive or severely contaminated wound, a remote bypass may be routed through clean tissue planes to circumvent difficult soft tissue coverage problems.

D. Venous Injuries

Venous injuries commonly accompany arterial injuries. In order of decreasing frequency, the most common extremity venous injuries are the superficial femoral vein, the popliteal vein, and the common femoral vein. The relative importance and timing of venous repair in an injured extremity is controversial. Advocates of routine venous repair contend that ligation is associated with significant postoperative morbidity, including more frequent failure of arterial repairs due to compromised outflow, venous insufficiency, compartment syndrome, and limb loss. Proponents of venous ligation argue that venous repairs are difficult (requiring interposition, compilation, and spiral grafting), time consuming (dangerous in the multiply-injured patient), and likely to cause occlusion (patency rates are only about 50%). The presence of postoperative edema after combined arterial and venous injuries is not reliably reduced by attempted venous repair. It seems reasonable to recommend repair of venous injuries when the repair is not too technically difficult (lateral venorrhaphy) and the patient is hemodynamically stable. Complex repair with autologous vein or ringed PTFE can yield good short term patency in experienced hands (77% primary repair, 67% vein graft, 74% PTFE). Thus, the decision to repair the vein depends on the condition of the patient and the condition of the vein. When venous ligation is necessary, postoperative edema can be controlled by elevation of the extremity and use of compression stockings or wraps. In patients undergoing venous repair, patency should be monitored using duplex scanning. If thrombosis of the repair is detected and there are no contraindications, anticoagulation should be instituted and maintained for at least 3 months postoperatively.

E. Fasciotomy

Fasciotomy is an important adjunctive treatment in many cases of arterial trauma. Indications include the following: (1) combined arterial and venous injury; (2) massive soft tissue damage; (3) delay between injury and repair (4-6 hours); (4) prolonged hypotension; and (5) excessive swelling or high tissue pressure measured by one of several techniques. Whenever compartment pressures (measured with a needle and manometer) approach 25-30 mm Hg, fasciotomy should be considered. Fasciotomies must be performed through adequate skin incisions because when edema is massive, the skin envelope itself can compromise neurovascular function.

Fasciotomies are not benign procedures. They create large open wounds, and chronic venous insufficiency is a recognized late complication even in the absence of venous reflux or obstruction. The chronic swelling is thought to be related to loss of integrity of the ensheathing fascia of the calf muscles, reducing the efficiency of the calf muscle pump. Thus, some authorities recommend against routine use of fasciotomies at the initial operation. This approach is dependent on the ability to conduct frequent serial physical examinations and the ready availability of an operating room should problems arise. In the postoperative period, compartmental pressures can be measured using a handheld solid-state transducer as often as clinically indicated. Normal intracompartment pressure is less than 10 mm Hg. In general, a pressure of 25-30 mm Hg requires either fasciotomy or continuous monitoring. When the pressure exceeds 30 mm Hg, fasciotomy is mandatory. In patients who are obtunded or who cannot cooperate with serial physical examination, earlier fasciotomy should be considered.

F. Immediate Amputation

High-energy or crush injuries of the extremities are associated with high morbidity and a poor prognosis for useful limb function—there is a high late amputation rate despite initial limb salvage. Vascular injuries are now repaired with a high rate of success, but associated orthopedic, soft tissue, and nerve injuries are the critical factors that determine long-term function. A number of scoring systems or indices have been proposed to help determine when to amputate immediately and thus reduce the number of protracted reconstructive procedures that ultimately fail. Management of the mangled extremity is particularly difficult, and none of the scoring systems are universally accepted. Evaluation and management of these patients should be multidisciplinary, and the decision to amputate emergently should be made by two independent surgeons whenever possible.

Avery LE et al: Evolving role of endovascular techniques for traumatic vascular injury: a changing landscape? *J Trauma Acute Care Surg.* 2012;72:41.

Demetriades D et al, the American Association for the Surgery of Trauma Thoracic Aortic Injury Study Group: Operative repair or endovascular stent graft in blunt traumatic thoracic aortic injuries: results of an American Association for the Surgery of Trauma Multicenter Study. *J Trauma.* 2008;64:561.

Feliciano DV, Shackford SR: Vascular injury: 50th anniversary year review article of the journal of trauma. *J Trauma.* 2010;68:1009.

Fox CJ et al: Damage control resuscitation for vascular surgery in a combat support hospital. *J Trauma.* 2008;65:1.

Karmy-Jones R et al: Endovascular repair compared with operative repair of traumatic rupture of the thoracic aorta: a nonsystemic review and a plea for trauma-specific reporting guidelines. *J Trauma.* 2011;71:1059.

Paul JS et al: Minimal aortic injury after blunt trauma: selective nonoperative management is safe. *J Trauma.* 2011;71:1519.

Patterson BO et al: Imaging vascular trauma. *Br J Surg.* 2012;99: 494-505.

Rasmussen TE et al: Tourniquets, vascular shunts, and endovascular technologies: esoteric or essential? A report from the 2011 AAST military liaison panel. *J Trauma Acute Care Surg.* 2012;73:282.

Sepehripour AH et al: Management of the left subclavian artery during endovascular stent grafting for traumatic aortic injury—a systematic review. *Eur J Vasc Endovasc Surg.* 2011;41:758.

Sohn VY et al: Demographics, treatment, and early outcomes in penetrating vascular combat trauma. *Arch Surg.* 2008;143:783.

Subramanian A et al: A decade's experience with temporary intravascular shunts at a civilian level I trauma center. *J Trauma.* 2008;65:316.

Woodward EB et al: Penetrating femoropopliteal injury during modern warfare: experience of the Balad Vascular Registry. *J Vasc Surg.* 2008;47:1259.

BLAST INJURY

Blast injuries in civilian populations occur as a result of fireworks, household explosions, or industrial accidents. Urban guerrilla warfare or terrorist tactics may take the form of letter bombs, suitcase bombs, vehicle bombs, and suicide bombers. Injuries occur from the effects of the blast itself, propelled foreign bodies, or, in large blasts, from falling objects. Military blast injuries may also involve personnel submerged in water. Water increases energy transmission and the possibility of injury to the viscera of the thorax or abdomen. The pathophysiology of blast injuries involves two mechanisms. Crush injury results from rapid displacement of the body wall and may result in laceration and contusion of underlying structures. Minor displacements may produce serious injury if the body wall velocity is high. In addition, the motion of the body wall generates waves that propagate within the body and transfer energy to internal sites.

▶ Clinical Findings

A. Symptoms and Signs

The injury is dependent upon proximity to the blast, space confinement, and detonation size. Large explosions cause multiple foreign body impregnations, bruises, abrasions, and lacerations. Gross soilage of wounds from clothing, flying debris, or explosive powder is common. About 10% of all casualties have deep injuries to the chest or abdomen. Blast-induced circulatory shock may be caused by immediate myocardial depression without a compensatory vasoconstriction.

Lung damage usually involves rupture of the alveolus with hemorrhage. Air embolism from bronchovenous fistula may cause sudden death. The mechanisms of lung injury are thought to be due to spalling effects (splintering forces produced when a pressure wave hits a fluid-air interface), implosion effects, and pressure differentials. Hypoxia may result from a ventilation-perfusion mismatch caused by the pulmonary hemorrhage. Patients with pulmonary blast injury may die despite intensive respiratory support.

Blast injury causing pneumatic disruption of the esophagus or bowel has been reported. Tension pneumoperitoneum is a known although rare complication of barotrauma. Letter bombs cause predominantly hand, face, eye, and ear injuries. Energy transmission within the fluid media of the eye can cause globe rupture, dialysis of the iris, hyphema of the anterior chamber, lens capsule tears, retinal rupture, or macular pucker. Ear injuries may consist of drum rupture or cochlear damage. There may be nerve or conduction hearing deficit or deafness. Tinnitus, vertigo, and anosmia are also seen in letter bomb casualties.

B. Imaging Studies

Chest x-ray may initially be normal or may show pneumothorax, pneumomediastinum, or parenchymal infiltrates. In mass casualty situations it may be necessary to reserve the use of CT scans for those patients with acute changing neurologic examinations during the immediate intake period. Patients with multiple penetrating injuries from shrapnel may benefit from full-body CT scanning following initial stabilization and evaluation. Correlation of radiologic imaging studies with clinical examination is useful in guiding which injuries may need operative intervention when the number of skin surface wounds is high and it is impractical to explore all of these wounds.

▶ Treatment

Severe injuries with shock from blood loss or hypoxia require resuscitative measures to restore perfusion and oxygenation. Penetrating injuries of the brain may require neurosurgical intervention along with intracranial pressure monitoring. The usual criteria for exploring penetrating wounds of the thorax or abdomen are employed. Perforation of hollow organs should be suspected in patients with appropriate histories, particularly those who were submerged at the time of injury. Respiratory insufficiency may result from pulmonary injury or may be secondary to shock, fat embolism, or other causes. Tracheal intubation and prolonged respiratory care with mechanical ventilation may be necessary. In cases of tension pneumoperitoneum, surgical decompression may dramatically improve respiratory and hemodynamic functions. Shrapnel is the main cause of abdominal injury following terrorist bombings. Surgical treatment of extremity injuries requires wide debridement of devitalized muscle,

thorough cleansing of wounds, and removal of foreign materials. The possibility of gas gangrene in contaminated muscle injuries may warrant open treatment. Eye injuries may require immediate repair. Ear injuries are usually treated expectantly.

Bala M et al: Abdominal trauma after terrorist bombing attacks exhibits a unique pattern of injury. *Ann Surg.* 2008;248:303.
Bala M et al: The pattern of thoracic trauma after suicide terrorist bombing attacks. *J Trauma.* 2010;69:1022.
Champion H et al: Improved characterization of combat injury. *J Trauma.* 2010;68:1139.
DuBose J et al: Management of post-traumatic retained hemothorax: a prospective, observational, multicenter AAST study. *J Trauma Acute Care Surg.* 2012;72:11.

MULTIPLE CHOICE QUESTIONS

1. A 31-year old man with a stab wound to the left neck over the sternocleidomastoid at the level of the lower pole of the thyroid gland

   A. Has a wound in an area that is easily explored in the operating room as most injuries here can be identified and controlled directly
   B. Has a penetrating injury in zone 3
   C. Should have an initial assessment including airway, breathing, and circulation
   D. Should be taken to angiography if unstable
   E. Has little risk of vascular injury

2. All of the following are correct about a patient with a systolic blood pressure of 75 torr after a roll-over automobile accident that resulted in the death of another passenger except

   A. Should be transported to a trauma center as expediently as possible
   B. Can have shock due to hypovolemia, cardiac failure, or neurogenic causes
   C. Should have an algorithmic approach to his care in the prehospital and trauma resuscitation phases of care
   D. Should bypass the trauma room and go directly to the operating room
   E. Has a mechanism of injury that places him at substantial risk of being severely injured

3. Thoracic injuries

   A. Are unusually contributors to the death of a trauma patient
   B. Can cause late deaths due to respiratory failure or sepsis
   C. Can include acceleration/deceleration as common mechanism of a severe aortic injury

D. Carry a similar mortality in older and younger patients

E. A, B, and C are all correct

4. Abdominal injuries

A. Can only be reliably assessed by CT scan or laparotomy

B. Require laparotomy and repair for all identified liver parenchyma injuries

C. Can routinely be evaluated by laparoscopy

D. Can be evaluated by diagnostic peritoneal lavage primarily to identify intraperitoneal bile

E. From gunshot wounds below the nipple line typically require laparotomy for evaluation and management

5. Peripheral vascular injuries

A. Are common in young men

B. Are more likely from penetrating than blunt injury

C. Are not often evaluated by CT scan

D. Can commonly be iatrogenic from medical procedures

E. All are correct

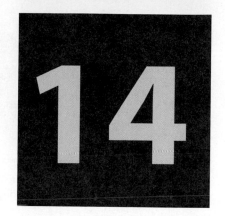

Burns & Other Thermal Injuries

14

Robert H. Demling, MD

▼ BURNS

A severe thermal injury is one of the most devastating physical and psychological injuries a person can suffer. Over 2 million injuries due to burns require medical attention each year in the United States, with 14,000 deaths resulting. Fires in the home are responsible for only 5% of burn injuries but for 50% of burn deaths—most due to smoke inhalation. About 75,000 patients require hospitalization every year, and 25,000 of those remain hospitalized for over 2 months—evidence of the severity of illness associated with this injury.

ANATOMY & PHYSIOLOGY OF THE SKIN

The skin is the largest organ of the body, ranging in area from 0.25 m² in the newborn to 1.8 m² in the adult. It consists of two layers: the epidermis and the dermis (corium). The outermost cells of the epidermis are dead cornified cells that act as a tough protective barrier against the environment, including bacterial invasion and chemical exposure. The inner cells of the epidermis are metabolically active, producing compounds like growth factor, which help the ongoing replication process every 2 weeks. The second, thicker layer, the dermis (0.06-0.12 mm), is composed chiefly of fibrous connective tissue. The dermis contains the blood vessels and nerves to the skin and the epithelial appendages of specialized function like sweat glands. The nerve endings that mediate pain are found in the dermis.

The dermis is a barrier that prevents loss of body fluids by evaporation and loss of excess body heat. Sweat glands help maintain body temperature by controlling the amount of water that evaporates. The dermis is also interlaced with sensory nerve endings that mediate the sensations of touch, pressure, pain, heat, and cold. This is a protective mechanism that allows an individual to adapt to changes in the physical environment.

The skin produces vitamin D, which is synthesized by the action of sunlight on certain intradermal cholesterol compounds.

DEPTH OF BURNS

The depth of the burn (Figure 14–1) significantly affects all subsequent clinical events. The depth may be difficult to determine and in some cases is not known until after spontaneous healing has occurred or when the eschar is surgically removed or separates, exposing the wound bed.

Traditionally, burns have been classified as first-, second-, and third-degree, but the current emphasis on burn healing has led to classification as partial-thickness burns, which can heal spontaneously, and full-thickness burns, which require skin grafting, although deep partial-thickness burns are usually excised and grafted as well.

A first-degree burn involves only the epidermis and is characterized by erythema and minor microscopic changes; tissue damage is minimal, protective functions of the skin are intact, skin edema is minimal, and systemic effects are rare. Pain, the chief symptom, usually resolves in 48-72 hours, and healing takes place uneventfully. In 5-10 days, the damaged epithelium peels off in small scales, leaving no residual scarring. The most common causes of first-degree burns are overexposure to sunlight and brief scalding.

Second-degree or partial-thickness burns are deeper, involving all of the epidermis and some of the corium or dermis. The systemic severity of the burn and the quality of subsequent healing are directly related to the amount of undamaged dermis. Superficial burns are often characterized by blister formation, while deeper partial-thickness burns have a reddish appearance or a layer of whitish, nonviable dermis firmly adherent to the remaining viable tissue. Blisters, when present, continue to increase in size in the postburn period as the osmotically active particles in the blister fluid attract water. Complications from superficial

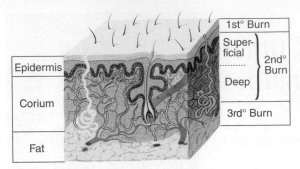

▲ **Figure 14–1.** Layers of the skin showing depth of first-degree, second-degree, and third-degree burns.

second-degree burns are mainly severe pain related. These burns usually heal with minimal scarring in 10-14 days unless they become infected.

Deep dermal burns heal over a period of 4-8 weeks with only a fragile epithelial covering developing that arises from the residual uninjured epithelium of the deep dermal sweat glands and hair follicles. Severe hypertrophic scarring occurs when such an injury heals; the resulting epithelial covering is prone to blistering and breakdown. Evaporative losses after healing remain high compared with losses in normal skin. Conversion of a partial thickness injury to a full-thickness burn by the actions of wound bacteria is common. Skin grafting of deep dermal burns, when feasible, improves the biologic quality and appearance of the skin cover.

Full-thickness (third-degree) burns have a characteristic white, dry, waxy appearance and may appear to the untrained eye as unburned skin. Burns caused by prolonged exposure to heat, with involvement of fat and underlying tissue, may be brown, dark red, or black. The diagnostic findings of full-thickness burns are lack of sensation in the burned skin, lack of capillary refill, and a leathery texture that is unlike normal skin. All dermal epithelial elements are destroyed, leaving no potential for reepithelialization.

DETERMINATION OF SEVERITY OF INJURY

Illness and death are related to the size (surface area) and depth of the burn, the age and prior state of health of the victim, the location of the burn wound, and the severity of associated injuries, particularly lung injuries caused by smoke inhalation.

The total body surface area involved in the burn is most accurately determined by using the age-related charts designed by Lund and Browder (Figure 14–2). A set of these charts should be filled out for every burn patient on admission and when resuscitation is begun.

A careful calculation of the percentage of total body burn is useful for several reasons. First, there is a general clinical tendency to both underestimate and overestimate the

size of the burn and thus its severity. The American Burn Association has adopted a severity index for burn injury (Table 14–1). Second, prognosis is directly related to the extent of injury both size and depth. Third, the decision about who should be treated in a specialized burn facility or managed as an outpatient is based on the estimate of burn size and depth.

Patients under age 2 years and over age 60 years have a significantly higher death rate for any given extent of burn. The higher death rate in infants results from a number of factors. First, the body surface area in children relative to body weight is much greater than in adults. Therefore, a burn of comparable surface area has a greater physiologic impact on a child. Second, immature kidneys and liver do not allow for removal of a high solute load from injured tissue or the rapid restoration of adequate nutritional support. Third, the incompletely developed immune system increases susceptibility to infection. Associated conditions such as cardiac disease, diabetes, or chronic obstructive pulmonary disease significantly worsen the prognosis in elderly patients.

Burns involving the hands, face, feet, or perineum are at risk for severe complications if not properly treated. Patients with such burns should always be admitted to the hospital, preferably to a burn center. Chemical and electrical burns or those involving the respiratory tract are invariably far more extensive than is evident on initial inspection. Therefore, hospital admission is also necessary in these cases.

PATHOLOGY & PATHOPHYSIOLOGY OF THERMAL INJURIES

The microscopic pathologic feature of the burn wound is principally surface coagulation necrosis. Burned tissue has three distinct zones. The first is the zone of "coagulation," or necrosis with irreversible cell death and no capillary blood flow. Surrounding this is a zone of injury or stasis, characterized by sluggish capillary blood flow and injured cells. Although damaged, the tissue is still viable. Further tissue injury can be caused by products of inflammation such as oxidants and vasoconstrictor mediators. Environmental insults such as hypoperfusion, desiccation, or infection can also cause the injured tissue to become necrotic. This process is called **wound conversion.** The third zone is that of "hyperemia," which is the usual inflammatory response of healthy tissue to nonlethal injury. Vasodilatation and increased capillary permeability is typically present.

A rapid loss of intravascular fluid and protein occurs through the heat-injured capillaries. The volume loss is greatest in the first 6-8 hours, with capillary integrity returning toward normal by 36-48 hours. A transient increase in vascular permeability also occurs in nonburned tissues, probably as a result of the initial release of vasoactive mediators. However, the edema that develops in nonburned tissues during resuscitation appears to be due in large part to

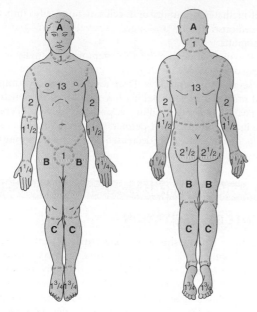

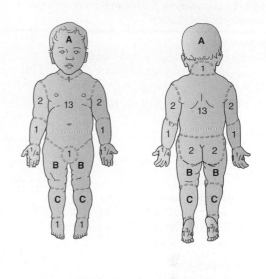

Relative percentages of areas affected by growth

	Age		
Area	10	15	Adult
A = half of head	5 1/2	4 1/2	3 1/2
B = half of one thigh	4 1/4	4 1/2	4 3/4
C = half of one leg	3	3 1/4	3 1/2

Relative percentages of areas affected by growth

	Age		
Area	0	1	5
A = half of head	9 1/2	8 1/2	6 1/2
B = half of one thigh	2 3/4	3 1/4	4
C = half of one leg	2 1/2	2 1/2	2 3/4

▲ **Figure 14–2.** Table for estimating extent of burns. In adults, a reasonable system for calculating the percentage of body surface burned is the "rule of nines": Each arm equals 9%, the head equals 9%, the anterior and posterior trunk each equal 18%, and each leg equals 18%; the sum of these percentages is 99%.

the marked hypoproteinemia caused by protein loss into the burn itself. A systemic inflammatory response occurs in response to a large body burn, resulting in the release of oxidants and other inflammatory mediators into unburned tissues. A generalized decrease in cell energy and membrane potential occurs as a result. This leads to a shift of extracellular sodium and water into the intracellular space. This process is also corrected as hemodynamic stability is restored but will return if the systemic inflammation is amplified. Smoke inhalation markedly increases the hemodynamic instability, fluid requirements, and mortality rates by adding another source of intense inflammation leading to local lung and systemic tissue damage.

METABOLIC RESPONSE TO BURNS & METABOLIC SUPPORT

The initial metabolic response appears to be activated by proinflammatory cytokines and in turn oxidants. The secretion of catecholamines, cortisol, glucagon, renin-angiotensin,

antidiuretic hormone, and aldosterone is also increased. Early in the response, energy is supplied by the breakdown of stored glycogen and by the process of anaerobic glycolysis.

Profound hypermetabolism and catabolism occur in the postburn period, characterized by an increase in metabolic rate that approaches doubling of the basal rate in severe burns and a rapid loss of the components of lean body mass with muscle loss exceeding a pound a day. The degree of response is proportionate to the degree of injury, with a plateau occurring when the burn involves about 70% of the total body surface. The initiating and perpetuating factors are the mediators of inflammation, especially the cytokines and endotoxin. Added environmental stresses such as pain, cooling, and sepsis syndrome increase the obligatory hypermetabolism and catabolism.

During the first postburn week, the metabolic rate (or heat production) and oxygen consumption rise progressively from the normal level present during resuscitation and remain elevated until the wound is covered and no other sources of inflammation remain. The specific pathophysiologic

Table 14–1. Summary of American Burn Association burn severity categorization.

Major Burn Injury

Second-degree burn of > 25% body surface area in adults

Second-degree burn of > 20% body surface area in children

Third-degree burn of > 10% body surface area

Most burns involving hands, face, eyes, ears, feet, or perineum

Most patients with the following:

    Inhalation injury

    Electrical injury

    Burn injury complicated by other major trauma

    Poor-risk patients with burns

Moderate Uncomplicated Burn Injury

Second-degree burn of 15%-25% body surface area in adults

Second-degree burn of 10%-20% body surface area in children

Third-degree burn of < 10% body surface area

Minor Burn Injury

Second-degree burn of < 15% body surface area in adults

Second-degree burn of < 10% body surface area in children

Third-degree burn of < 2% body surface area

mechanism remains undefined, but increased and persistent catecholamine and cortisol secretion are major factors, as is increased circulating endotoxin absorbed from wound or gut and proinflammatory cytokines.

The evaporative water loss from the wound may reach 300 mL/m^2/h (normal is about 15 mL/m^2/h). This produces a heat loss of about 580 kcal/L of water evaporated. Covering the burn with an impermeable membrane, such as skin substitute, reduces the heat loss. Similarly, placing the burn patient in a warm environment, where convection and radiant loss of heat are minimized, also modestly reduces the heat loss and the metabolic rate. The persistently elevated circulating levels of catecholamines and cortisol stimulate an exaggerated degree of gluconeogenesis and protein breakdown. Protein catabolism, glucose intolerance, and marked total body weight loss result.

Aggressive nutritional support along with rapid wound closure and control of pain, stress, and sepsis will help control the hypermetabolic catabolic state. Controlled use of a beta-blocker has been shown to decrease catabolism. In addition, insulin, growth hormones, and testosterone analogues have been shown to both decrease catabolism and increase anabolism.

IMMUNOLOGIC FACTORS IN BURNS

A number of immunologic abnormalities in burn patients predispose to infection. Serum IgA, IgM, and IgG are frequently depressed, reflecting depressed B-cell function.

Cell-mediated immunity or T-cell function is also impaired, as demonstrated by prolonged survival of homografts and xenografts.

Polymorphonuclear (PMN) chemotactic activity is suppressed. A decrease in chemotaxis predates evidence of clinical sepsis by several days. Decreased oxygen consumption and impaired bacterial killing have also been demonstrated in PMNs. Depressed killing is probably due to decreased production of hydrogen peroxide and superoxide; this has been demonstrated by decreased PMN chemiluminescent activity in burn patients.

▼ BURN MANAGEMENT

ACUTE RESUSCITATION

The burn patient should be assessed and treated like any patient with major trauma. The first priority is to ensure an adequate airway. If there is a possibility that smoke inhalation has occurred—as suggested by exposure to a fire in an enclosed space or burns of the face, nares, or upper torso—arterial blood gases and arterial oxygen saturation of hemoglobin and carboxyhemoglobin CoHgb levels should be measured, and 100% oxygen should be administered. If CoHgb is elevated, 100% oxygen should be administered until levels return to normal.

Endotracheal intubation is indicated if the patient is semicomatose, has deep burns to the face and neck, or is otherwise critically injured. Intubation should be done early in all doubtful cases, because delayed intubation will be difficult to achieve in cases associated with facial and pharyngeal edema or upper airway injury, and an emergency tracheostomy may become necessary later under difficult circumstances. Respiratory support is necessary for severe smoke damage to the lower airways. If the burn exceeds 20% of body surface area, a urinary catheter should be inserted to monitor urine output. A large-bore intravenous catheter should be inserted, preferably into a large peripheral vein. There is a significant complication rate with the use of central lines in burn patients owing to the increased risk of infection.

Severe burns are characterized by large losses of intravascular fluid, which are greatest during the first 8-12 hours. Fluid loss occurs as a result of the altered capillary permeability, severe hypoproteinemia, and the shift of sodium into the cells. Both fluid shifts diminish significantly by 24 hours postburn. The lung appears to be reasonably well protected from the early edema process, and pulmonary edema is uncommon during the resuscitation period unless there is a superimposed inhalation injury. Increasing perfusion rather than infusion of bicarbonates is the appropriate approach.

Initially, an isotonic crystalloid salt solution is infused to counterbalance the loss of plasma volume into the extravascular space and the further loss of extracellular fluid into the intracellular space. Lactated Ringer solution is commonly used, the rate being dictated by urine output, pulse (character and rate), state of consciousness, and, to a lesser extent, blood pressure. Urine output should be maintained at 0.5 mL/kg/h and the pulse at 120 beats/min or slower. Base deficit has been shown to be an excellent marker, with an increasing deficit indicating inadequate perfusion.

Swan-Ganz catheters and central venous pressure lines are seldom needed except in the case of severe smoke inhalation injury or unless the patient has sufficient cardiopulmonary disease that accurate monitoring of volume status would be difficult without measurement of filling pressures or unless a persistent base deficit is present, indicating continued impaired perfusion. The amount of lactated Ringer necessary in the first 24 hours for adequate resuscitation is approximately 3-4 mL/kg of body weight per percent of body burn, which is the amount of fluid needed to restore the estimated sodium deficit. At least half of the fluid is given in the first 8 hours because of the greater initial volume loss. Dextrose-containing solutions are not used initially because of early stress-induced glucose intolerance.

Although the importance of restoring colloid osmotic pressure and plasma proteins is well recognized, the timing of colloid infusion remains somewhat varied. Plasma proteins are ordinarily not infused until after the initial plasma leak begins to decrease. This usually occurs about 4-8 hours postburn. The addition of a protein infusion to the treatment regimen after this period will decrease the fluid requirements and—in very young or elderly patients and in patients with massive burns (in excess of 50% of body surface)—will improve hemodynamic stability.

After intravenous fluids are started and vital signs stabilized, the wound should be debrided of all loose skin and dirt. To avoid severe hypothermia, debridement is best done by completing one body area before exposing a second. An alternative is to use an overhead radiant heater, which will decrease net heat loss. Cool water is a very good analgesic on a small superficial burn; however, it should not be used for larger burns because of the risk of hypothermia. Pain is best controlled with the use of intravenous rather than intramuscular narcotics. Tetanus toxoid, 0.5 mL, should be administered to patients with any significant burn injury.

POSTRESUSCITATION PERIOD

Treatment should aim to decrease excessive catecholamine stimulation and provide enough calories to offset the effects of the hypermetabolism. Hypothermia, pain, and anxiety all need to be aggressively controlled. Hypovolemia should be prevented by giving enough fluid to make up for the body losses.

Ongoing management of any smoke inhalation injury will be necessary using vigorous pulmonary toilet to avoid airway plugging and hypoxia. Nutritional support should begin as early as possible in the postburn period to maximize wound healing and minimize immune deficiency. Patients with moderate body burns may be able to meet nutritional needs by voluntary oral intake. Patients with large burns invariably require calorie and protein supplementation to reach a goal of 30 cal/kg body weight for calories and 1.5 g/kg body weight for protein. This can usually be accomplished by administering a formula diet through a small feeding tube. Parenteral nutrition is also occasionally required, but the intestinal route is preferred if needs can be met this way. Early restoration of gut function will also decrease gut bacterial translocation and endotoxin leak.

Vitamins A, E, and C and zinc should be given until the burn wound is closed. Low-dose heparin therapy may be beneficial, as with other immobilized patients with soft tissue injury.

CARE OF THE BURN WOUND

In the management of superficial partial or second-degree burns, one must provide as aseptic an environment as possible to prevent infection. However, superficial burns generally do not require the use of topical antibiotics. Occlusive dressings are used to minimize exposure to air, increase the rate of reepithelialization, and decrease pain. The exception is the face, which can be treated open with an antibacterial ointment. If there is no infection, burns will heal spontaneously.

The goals in managing deep partial-thickness or full-thickness (third-degree) burns are to prevent invasive infection (ie, burn wound sepsis), to remove dead tissue, and to cover the wound with skin or skin substitutes as soon as possible.

All topical antibiotics retard wound healing to some degree and therefore should be used only on deep second- or third-degree burns or wounds, which have a high risk of infection.

▶ Topical Antibacterial Agents

Topical agents have definitely advanced the care of burn patients. Although burn wound sepsis is still a major problem, the incidence is lower and the death rate has been markedly reduced, particularly in burns of less than 50% of body surface area. A silver-containing product is the treatment of choice because silver has superior antimicrobial properties. Silver sulfadiazine is the most widely used preparation. Mafenide, silver nitrate, povidone-iodine, and gentamicin ointments are also used. Silver release dressings are now very popular. A secondary dressing is placed over the silver release dressing to retain heat and optimize the wound environment.

Silver sulfadiazine, a cream that is effective against a wide spectrum of gram-positive and gram-negative organisms, is only moderately effective in penetrating the burn eschar. A transient leukopenia secondary to bone marrow suppression often occurs with the use of silver sulfadiazine in large burns, but the process is usually self-limiting, and the agent does not have to be discontinued.

Silver release dressings are available in a slow-release form that release silver ions for several days, decreasing dressing changes and improving patient comfort.

Exposure Versus Closed Management

There are two methods of management of the burn wound with topical agents. In exposure therapy, no dressings are applied over the wound after application of the agent to the wound twice or three times daily. This approach is typically used on the face and head. Disadvantages are increased pain and heat loss as a result of the exposed wound and an increased risk of cross-contamination.

In the closed method, an occlusive dressing is applied over the agent and is usually changed twice daily. The disadvantage of this method is the potential increase in bacterial growth if the dressing is not changed twice daily, particularly when thick eschar is present. The advantages are less pain, less heat loss, and less cross-contamination. The closed method is generally preferred.

Temporary Skin Substitutes

Skin substitutes are another alternative to topical agents for the partial-thickness burn or the clean excised wound. A number of synthetic and biologically active temporary skin substitutes are in use. Reepithelialization is accelerated. Also, pain is better controlled. Homografts (human skin) work better for this purpose on large excised wounds but are difficult to obtain. Other alternatives include a number of tissue engineered skin substitutes, which contain bioactive matrix components.

Hydrotherapy

The use of immersion hydrotherapy for wound management has substantially decreased. A number of studies have shown that the infection rate is actually increased when patients are immersed in a tub because of the generalized inoculation of burn wounds with bacteria from what was previously a localized infection. Hydrotherapy, on a slant board, is a very useful approach once the wounds are in the process of being debrided and closed. Showering is also effective for wound cleansing in the more stable patient.

Debridement & Grafting

Burn wound inflammation, even in the absence of infection, can result in multiple organ dysfunction and perpetuation of the hypermetabolic catabolic state. Early wound closure would be expected to control this process more effectively. Surgical management of burn wounds has now become much more aggressive, with operative debridement

beginning within the first several days postburn rather than after eschar has sloughed. More rapid closure of burn wounds clearly decreases the rate of sepsis and significantly decreases the death rate. The approach to operative debridement varies from an extensive burn excision and grafting within several days of injury to a more moderate approach of limiting debridements to less than 15% of the burned area. Excision can be carried down to fascia or to viable remaining dermis or fat. Excision to fascia is more commonly used when the burn extends well into the fat. A meshed skin graft can be covered with a biologic dressing to avoid desiccation of the uncovered wound. Excision to viable tissue, referred to as tangential excision, is advantageous because it provides a vascular base for grafting while preserving remaining viable tissue, especially dermis. Tourniquets can be used to decrease blood loss. Blood loss is substantial in view of the vascularity of the dermis.

A number of permanent skin substitutes could further facilitate wound closure, particularly in large burns with insufficient donor sites. Autologous cultures of epithelium have been applied with some success. Permanent skin substitutes composed of both dermis and epidermis have been designed to maintain coverage and improve skin function.

Maintenance of Function

The maintenance of functional motion during the evolution of the burn wound is necessary to avoid loss of motion at joints. Wound contraction, a normal event during healing, may result in extremity contracture. Immobilization will produce joint stiffness. Contracture of the scar, muscles, and tendons across a joint causes loss of motion, which can be diminished by traction and early motion.

The scar is a metabolically active tissue, continually undergoing reorganization. The extensive scarring that frequently occurs after burns can lead to disfiguring and disabling contractures, but it may be avoided by the use of splints and elevation to maintain a functional position. Following application of the skin graft, maintenance of proper positioning with splints is indicated along with active motion exercises.

If reinjury does not occur, the amount of collagen in the scar tends to decrease with time (usually over a year). Stiff collagen becomes softer, and on flat surfaces of the body, where reinjury and inflammation are prevented, remodeling may totally eliminate contracture. However, around joints or the neck, contractures can persist, and surgical reconstruction is necessary. The sooner the burn wound can be covered with skin grafts, the less likely is contracture formation.

MANAGEMENT OF COMPLICATIONS

Infection remains a critical problem in burns, though the incidence has been reduced by modern therapy with the combination of early excision and grafting along with

Table 14–2. Diagnosis of burn wound infection.

Systemic Changes	Colonized or Clean	Wound Infection
Body temperature	Increased	Variable
White blood cell count	Increased Mild left shift	High or low Severe left shift
Wound appearance	Variable—may appear purulent or benign	Purulence may be present, or wound surface may appear dry and pale
Bacterial Content		
Surface	Scant to large amount	Variable
Quantitative	Usually $< 10^5/g$	Usually $> 10^5/g$
Biopsy	No invasion of normal tissue	Invasion of normal tissue by organisms

topical antibacterial agents. An infection is present when a quantitative culture of the burn indicates a concentration of 10^5 organisms; a semiquantitative swab culture is used more commonly. The cultures also show the sensitivity of the bacteria, and when the bacterial concentration passes 10^5 organisms per gram, systemic administration of specific antibiotics should be instituted (Tables 14–2 and 14–3).

Sepsis syndrome occurs in all major burns. Fever, hypermetabolism, catabolism, and often leukocytosis are typical characteristics, the result of local burn and total body inflammation. Infection is often not present as this process can be attributed to an autodestructive response to inflammation. This intense inflammatory response can lead to death from multisystem organ failure and hemodynamic parameters comparable to sepsis shock.

Any significant infection can further perpetuate this response. Continued deterioration of a wound is likely due to invasive infection. A more common cause of infection today is a pulmonary complication—either a chemical or bacterial insult leading to pneumonia. Catheter sepsis is the third most common cause of infection. If infection is found, an aggressive antibiotics regime is indicated. Early excision and wound closure is the best way to avoid later development of burn wound sepsis.

Circumferential burns of an extremity or of the trunk pose special problems. Swelling beneath the unyielding eschar may act as a tourniquet to blood and lymph flow, and the distal extremity may become swollen and tense. More extensive swelling may compromise the arterial supply. Escharotomy, or excision of the eschar, may be required. To avoid permanent damage, escharotomy must be performed before arterial ischemia develops. Constriction involving the chest or abdomen may severely restrict ventilation and may require longitudinal escharotomies. Anesthetics are rarely required, and the procedure can usually be performed in the patient's room.

Acute gastroduodenal (Curling) ulcers were at one time a frequent complication of severe burns, but the incidence is now extremely low, largely as a result of the early and routine institution of antacid and nutritional therapy and the decrease in the rate of sepsis.

A complication unique to children is seizures, which may result from electrolyte imbalance, hypoxemia, infection, or drugs; in one-third of cases, the cause is unknown. Hyponatremia is the most frequent cause. Systemic hypertension occurs in about 10% of cases in the postresuscitation period.

RESPIRATORY INJURY IN BURNS

Today the major cause of death after burns is respiratory failure or complications in the respiratory tract. The problems include inhalation injury, aspiration in unconscious

Table 14–3. Most common pathogens in burn infections.

	Staphylococcus aureus	Pseudomonas aeruginosa	Candida albicans
Wound appearance	Loss of wound granulation	Surface necrosis; patchy, black	Minimal exudate
Course	Slow onset over 2-5 days	Rapid onset over 12-36 hours	Slow (days)
CNS signs	Disorientation	Modest changes	Often no change
Temperature	Marked increase	High or low	Modest changes
White blood count	Marked increase	High or low	Modest changes
Hypotension	Modest	Often severe	Minimal change
Mortality rate	5%	20%-30%	30%-50%

Table 14–4. Carbon monoxide poisoning.

Carboxyhemoglobin Level	Severity	Symptoms
< 20%	Mild	Headache, mild dyspnea, visual changes, confusion
20%-40%	Moderate	Irritability, diminished judgment, dim vision, nausea, easy fatigability
40%-60%	Severe	Hallucinations, confusion, ataxia, collapse, coma
> 60%	Fatal	

patients, bacterial pneumonia, pulmonary edema, and post-traumatic pulmonary insufficiency. Smoke inhalation markedly increases mortality from burn injury.

Smoke inhalation injuries, caused by incomplete products of combustion and which predispose to other complications, are divided into three categories: carbon monoxide poisoning (Table 14–4), upper airways injury, and inhalation of noxious compounds in the lower airways (Table 14–5).

Carbon monoxide poisoning must be considered in every patient suspected of having inhalation injury on the basis of having been burned in a closed space and physical evidence of inhalation. Arterial blood gases and carboxyhemoglobin levels must be determined. Levels of carboxyhemoglobin above 5% in nonsmokers and above 10% in smokers indicate carbon monoxide poisoning. Carbon monoxide has an affinity for hemoglobin 200 times that of oxygen, displaces oxygen, and produces a leftward shift in the oxyhemoglobin dissociation curve (P_{50}, the oxygen tension at which half the hemoglobin is saturated with oxygen, is lowered). Calculations of oxyhemoglobin saturation may be

Table 14–5. Sources of toxic chemicals in smoke.

Wood, cotton	Aldehydes (acrolein), nitrogen dioxide, CO
Polyvinylchloride	Hydrochloric acid, phosgene, CO
Rubber	Sulfur dioxide, hydrogen sulfide, CO
Polystyrene	Copious black smoke and soot—CO_2, H_2O, and some CO
Acrylonitrile, polyurethane, nitrogenous compounds	Hydrogen cyanide
Fire retardants may produce toxic fumes	Halogens (F_2, Cl_2, Br_2), ammonia, hydrogen cyanide, CO

misleading because the hemoglobin combined with carbon monoxide is not detected and the percentage saturation of oxyhemoglobin may appear normal.

Mild carbon monoxide poisoning (< 20% carboxyhemoglobin) is manifested by headache, slight dyspnea, mild confusion, and diminished visual acuity. Moderate poisoning (20%-40% carboxyhemoglobin) leads to irritability, impairment of judgment, dim vision, nausea, and fatigability. Severe poisoning (40%-60% carboxyhemoglobin) produces hallucinations, confusion, ataxia, collapse, and coma. Levels in excess of 60% carboxyhemoglobin are usually fatal.

Various toxic chemicals in inspired smoke produce tracheobronchial respiratory injuries. Inhalation of kerosene smoke, for example, is relatively innocuous. Smoke from a wood fire is extremely irritating because it contains aldehyde gases, particularly acrolein. Direct inhalation of acrolein, even in low concentrations, irritates mucous membranes and causes severe airway damage. Smoke from some plastic compounds, such as polyurethane, is the most serious kind of toxic irritant, and some plastics give off poisonous gases such as chlorine, sulfuric acid, and cyanides. Cyanide absorption can be lethal. Oxidants are released after all smoke exposures, causing mucosal and alveolar injury.

Inhalation injury causes severe mucosal edema followed soon by sloughing of the mucosa. The destroyed mucosa in the larger airways is replaced by a mucopurulent membrane. The edema fluid enters the airway and, when mixed with the pus in the lumen, may form casts and plugs in the smaller bronchioles. Terminal bronchioles and alveoli contain carbonaceous material. Acute bronchiolitis and bronchopneumonia commonly develop within a few days. Sputum smears should be examined daily to detect early bacterial tracheobronchial infection.

When inhalation injury is suspected, early endoscopic examination of the airway with fiberoptic bronchoscopy is helpful in determining the area of injury (ie, the extent of upper and lower airway involvement). Unfortunately, the severity of the injury cannot be accurately quantified by bronchoscopy—it can only be shown that an injury is present. Direct laryngoscopy probably gives as much information.

After several days, small bronchi become obstructed by inflammation and mucin plugs, leading to severe atelectasis and resulting hypoxia. This process is typically confined to the airways; in severe cases, alveolar edema will be present.

The most common cause of respiratory failure is a chemical tracheobronchitis due to the inhalation injury. Airway clearance is impeded due to ciliary damage and denuded airways. Alteration of oropharyngeal normal flora with colonization by pathogens then leads to bronchopneumonia.

Pulmonary insufficiency is associated with systemic sepsis. Differentiating acute respiratory distress syndrome (ARDS) from bacterial pneumonia may be difficult in severe cases of inhalation of sepsis. There is damage to the pulmonary capillaries and leakage of fluid and protein into the interstitial spaces of the lung, resulting in loss of compliance and difficulty in oxygenation of the blood. Modern methods of ventilatory support and vigorous pulmonary toilet have significantly reduced the death rate from pulmonary insufficiency.

▶ Treatment

Management of a burn patient should include frequent evaluation of the lungs throughout the hospital course. All patients who initially have evidence of smoke inhalation should receive humidified oxygen in high concentrations. If carbon monoxide poisoning has occurred, 100% oxygen should be given until the carboxyhemoglobin content returns to normal levels and symptoms of carbon monoxide toxicity resolve. With severe exposures, carbon monoxide may still be bound to the cytochrome enzymes, leading to cell hypoxia even after carboxyhemoglobin levels have returned to near normal. Continued oxygen administration will also reverse this process. Hyperbaric oxygen is often used in these cases.

The use of corticosteroids for inhalation injuries is no longer controversial and is clearly contraindicated with the exception of chronic bronchiolitis obliterans. The exception is the patient with a relative steroid insufficiency.

Bronchodilators by aerosol or aminophylline given intravenously may help if wheezing is due to the reflex bronchospasm typically present. Chest physical therapy is also required.

When endotracheal intubation is used without mechanical ventilation (eg, for upper airway obstruction), mist and continuous positive pressure ventilatory assistance should be included. The humidity will help loosen the secretions and prevent drying of the airway; the continuous positive pressure will help prevent atelectasis and closure of lung units distal to the swollen airways. Tracheostomy is indicated in the first several days for patients who are expected to require ventilatory support for a few weeks or more. If the neck is burned, excision and grafting followed by tracheostomy is indicated in order to improve pulmonary toilet.

Mechanical ventilation should be instituted early if a significant pulmonary injury is anticipated. A large body burn with chest wall involvement will result in decreased chest wall compliance, increased work of breathing, and subsequent atelectasis. Tracheobronchial injury from inhaled chemicals is accentuated by the presence of a body burn, with a resultant increase in the potential for atelectasis and infection. Controlled ventilation along with sedation will diminish the degree of injury and also conserve energy expenditure. Early excision of the deep chest wall burn will help remove the constricting component. Wound closure in turn will decrease the excessive CO_2 production caused by the hypermetabolic state.

REHABILITATION OF THE BURNED PATIENT

Plastic surgical revisions of scars are often necessary after the initial grafting, particularly to release contractures over joints and for cosmetic reasons. The physician must be realistic in defining an acceptable result, and the patient should be told that it may take years to achieve. Burn scars are often unsightly, and—although hope should be extended that improvement can be made—total resolution is not possible in many cases.

Skin expansion techniques utilizing a subdermal Silastic bag that is gradually expanded have greatly improved scar revision management. The ability to enlarge the available skin to be used for replacement of scar improves both cosmetic appearance and function. Advances in microvascular flap surgery have also resulted in substantial improvements in outcome.

The patient must take special care of the skin of the burn scar. Prolonged exposure to sunlight should be avoided, and when the wound involves areas such as the face and hands, which are frequently exposed to the sun, ultraviolet screening agents should be used. Hypertrophic scars and keloids are particularly bothersome and can be diminished with the use of pressure garments, which must be worn until the scar matures—approximately 12 months. Since the skin appendages are often destroyed by full-thickness burns, creams and lotions are required to prevent drying and cracking and to reduce itching. Substances such as lanolin, vitamin A and D ointment, and Eucerin cream are all effective

Fraburg C: Effects of differences in percent total surface burn surface area estimation on fluid resuscitation of transferred burn patients. *J Burn Care Res.* 2007;28:42.

Hall JJ: Use of high frequency percussive ventilation in inhalation injury. *J Burn Care Res.* 2007;3:396.

Ipaktchi K: Attenuating burn wound inflammation improves pulmonary function and survival in a burn pneumonia model. *Crit Care Med.* 2007;35:2139.

Jeschke M: Effect of insulin on the inflammatory and acute phase response after burn injury. *Crit Care Med.* 2007;9:519.

Palmieri T: Inhalation injury research progress and needs. *J Burn Care.* 2007;4:594.

Rubino C: Total upper and low eyelid replacement following thermal injury using an ALT flap. *J Plast Reconstruct Aesthet Surg.* 2007;20:215.

Tenenhaus M: Burn surgery. *Clin Plast Surg.* 2007;34:697.

Wascak J: Early versus later internal nutritional support in adults with burn injury: a systemic review. *J Hum Nutr Diet.* 2007;20:25.

▼ ELECTRICAL INJURY

There are three kinds of electrical injuries: electrical current injury, electrothermal burns from arcing current, and flame burns caused by ignition of clothing. Occasionally, all three are present in the same victim.

Electrical current injury, or "hidden injury," results from the passage of electrical current through the body. Flash or arc burns are thermal injuries to the skin caused by a high-tension electrical current creating local heat and damaging skin. The thermal injury to the skin is intense and deep, because the electrical arc has a temperature of about 2500°C (high enough to melt bone). Flame burns from ignited clothing are often the most serious part of the injury. Treatment is the same as for any thermal injury.

Once current enters the body, its pathway depends on the resistances it encounters in the various organs. The following are listed in descending order of resistance: bone, fat, tendon, skin, muscle, blood, and nerve. The pathway of the current determines immediate survival; for example, if the current passes through the heart or the brain stem, death may be immediate from ventricular fibrillation or apnea. Current passing through muscles may cause spasms severe enough to produce long-bone fractures or dislocations.

The type of current is also related to the severity of injury with low-voltage (150 V) current. The usual 60-cycle alternating current that causes most injuries in the home is particularly severe. Alternating current causes tetanic contractions, and the victim may become "locked" to the contact. Cardiac arrest is common from contact with low-voltage house current.

High-voltage electrical current injuries are more than just burns. Focal deep burns occur at the points of entrance and exit through the skin. These burns often extend through local muscle, resulting in fourth-degree burn. Once inside the body, the current travels through muscles, causing an injury more like a crush than a thermal burn. This leads to blood and fluid extravasation, increasing interstitial pressure in the muscle compartments. A fasciotomy is often necessary, opening all the muscle compartments involved. Early action is necessary to avoid severe vascular insufficiency or nerve damage. Thrombosis frequently occurs in vessels deep in an extremity, causing a greater depth of tissue necrosis than is evident at the initial examination. The greatest muscle injury is usually closest to the bone, where the highest heat of resistance is generated. The treatment of electrical injuries depends on the extent of deep muscle and nerve destruction more than on any other factor.

Severe myoglobinuria may develop with the risk of acute tubular necrosis as the muscle pigment is released from muscle and precipitates in renal tubules. The urine output must be kept two to three times normal with intravenous fluids. Alkalinization of the urine and osmotic diuretics may be indicated if myoglobinuria is present to more rapidly clear the pigment.

A rapid drop in hematocrit sometimes follows as sudden destruction of red blood cells by the electrical energy occurs. Bleeding into deep tissues may occur as a result of disruption of blood vessels and tissue planes. In some cases, thrombosed vessels disintegrate later and cause massive interstitial hemorrhage. Increased fluid infusion is required for initial resuscitation compared to extent of external thermal burns alone.

The skin burn at the entrance and exit sites is usually a depressed gray or yellow area of full-thickness destruction surrounded by a sharply defined zone of hyperemia. Charring may be present. The lesion should be debrided to underlying healthy tissue. Frequently, there is deep destruction not initially evident, especially to muscles beneath the skin surface. This dead and devitalized tissue must also be excised as soon as possible. Amputation rate for extremity involved is still high but decreasing. A second debridement is usually indicated 24-48 hours after the injury, because the necrosis is found to be more extensive than originally thought. The strategy of obtaining skin covering for these burns can tax ingenuity because of the extent and depth of the wounds. Microvascular flaps are now used routinely to replace large tissue losses.

In general, the treatment of electrical injuries is complex at every step, and these patients are referred to specialized centers. There are no formulas for determining severity and outcome of high-voltage electrical injuries.

Edlich R: Modern concepts of treatment and prevention of electrical burns. *J Long Term Eff Med Implants*. 2005;15:511.

Moughsoudi H: Electrical and lightning injuries. *J Burn Care Res*. 2007;28:255.

▼ HEAT STROKE & RELATED INJURIES

Heat stroke occurs when core body temperature exceeds 40°C and produces severe central nervous system dysfunction. Two related syndromes induced by exposure to heat are heat cramps and heat exhaustion.

In humans, heat is dissipated from the skin by radiation, conduction, convection, and evaporation. When the ambient temperature rises, heat loss by the first three is impaired; loss by evaporation is hindered by a high relative humidity. Predisposing factors to heat accumulation are dermatitis; use of phenothiazines, beta-blockers, diuretics, or anticholinergics; intercurrent fever from other disease; obesity; alcoholism; and heavy clothing. Cocaine and amphetamines may increase metabolic heat production.

Heat cramps—muscle pain after exertion in a hot environment—are usually attributed to salt deficit. It is probable, however, that many cases are really examples of **exertional rhabdomyolysis.** This condition, which may also be a complicating factor in heat stroke, involves acute muscle injury due to severe exertional efforts beyond the limits for which the individual has trained. It often produces myoglobinuria, which rarely affects kidney function except when it occurs in patients also suffering from heat stroke. Complete recovery is the rule after uncomplicated heat cramps.

Heat exhaustion consists of fatigue, muscular weakness, tachycardia, postural syncope, nausea, vomiting, and an urge to defecate caused by dehydration and hypovolemia from heat stress. Temperature usually exceeds 39°C. Although body temperature is normal in heat exhaustion, there is a continuum between this syndrome and heat stroke.

Heat stroke, a result of imbalance between heat production and heat dissipation, kills about 4000 persons yearly in the United States. Exercise-induced heat stroke most often affects young people (eg, athletes, military recruits, laborers) who are exercising strenuously in a hot environment, usually without adequate training. Heat production exceeds the ability to dissipate the heat; core temperature then rises and hypovolemia is evident. Sedentary heat stroke is a disease of elderly or infirm people whose cardiovascular systems are unable to adapt to the stress of a hot environment and release sufficient heat such that body temperature rises. Epidemics of heat stroke in elderly people can be predicted when the ambient temperature surpasses 32.2°C and the relative humidity reaches 50%-76%.

The mechanism of injury is direct damage by heat to the parenchyma and vasculature of the organs. In addition, there is a marked cytokine-induced activation of inflammation similar to sepsis, leading to inflammation-induced organ damage. The central nervous system is particularly vulnerable, and cellular necrosis is found in the brains of those who die of heat stroke. Hepatocellular and renal tubular damage are apparent in severe cases. Subendocardial damage and occasionally transmural infarcts are discovered in fatal cases even in young persons without previous cardiac disease. Disseminated intravascular coagulation may develop, aggravating injury in all organ systems and predisposing to bleeding complications.

▶ Clinical Findings

A. Symptoms and Signs

Heat stroke should be suspected in anyone who develops sudden neurological changes in a hot environment. If the patient's temperature is above 40°C (range: 40-43°C), the diagnosis of heat stroke is definitive. Measurements of body temperature must be made rectally. A prodrome including dizziness, headache, nausea, chills, and goose-flesh of the chest and arms is seen occasionally but is not common. In most cases, the patient recalls having experienced no warning symptoms except weakness, tiredness, or dizziness. Confusion, belligerent behavior, or stupor may precede coma. Convulsions may occur.

The skin is pink or ashen and sometimes, paradoxically, dry and hot; dry skin in the presence of hyperpyrexia is virtually pathognomonic of heat stroke. Profuse sweating is usually present in runners and other athletes who have heat stroke. The heart rate ranges from 140 beats/min to 170 beats/min; central venous or pulmonary wedge pressure is high;

and in some cases the blood pressure is low. Hyperventilation may reach 60 breaths/min and may give rise to respiratory alkalosis. Pulmonary edema and bloody sputum may develop in severe cases. Jaundice is frequent within the first few days after onset of symptoms.

Dehydration, which may produce the same central nervous system symptoms as heat stroke, is an aggravating factor in about 50% of cases.

B. Laboratory Findings

There is no characteristic pattern to the electrolyte changes. The serum sodium concentration may be normal or high, and the potassium concentration is usually low on admission or at some point during resuscitation. In the first few days, the aspartate aminotransferase (AST), lactate dehydrogenase (LDH), and creatine kinase (CK) may be elevated, especially in exertional heat stroke. Proteinuria and granular and red cell casts are seen in urine specimens collected immediately after diagnosis. If the urine is dark red or brown, it probably contains myoglobin. The blood urea nitrogen and serum creatinine rise transiently in most patients and continue to climb if renal failure develops. Hematologic findings may be normal or may be typical of disseminated intravascular coagulation (ie, low fibrinogen, increased fibrin split products, slow prothrombin and partial thromboplastin times, and decreased platelet count).

C. Prevention

For the most part, heat stroke in military recruits and athletes in training is preventable by adhering to a graduated schedule of increasing performance requirements that allows acclimatization over 2-3 weeks and increasing fluid replacement using water and some electrolytes, especially sodium. Heat produced by exercise is dissipated by increased cardiac output, vasodilation in the skin, and increased sweating. With acclimatization, there is increased efficiency for muscular work, increased myocardial performance, expanded extracellular fluid volume if hydration is maintained, greater output of sweat for a given amount of work (releasing more heat), a lower salt content of sweat, and a lower central temperature for a given amount of work.

Access to drinking water should be unrestricted during vigorous physical activity in a hot environment. Free water is preferable to electrolyte-containing solutions. Clothing and protective gear should be lightened as heat production and air temperature rise, and heavy exercise should not be scheduled at the hottest times of day, especially at the beginning of a training schedule.

▶ Treatment

The patient should be cooled rapidly. The most efficient method is to induce evaporative heat loss by spraying the patient with water at 15°C and fanning with cool air. Immersion in an ice water bath or the use of ice packs is also effective but causes cutaneous vasoconstriction and shivering and makes patient monitoring more difficult. Monitor the rectal temperature frequently. To avoid overshooting the end point, vigorous cooling should be stopped when the temperature reaches 38.9°C. Shivering should be controlled with parenteral phenothiazines. Oxygen should be administered, and if the Pao_2 drops below 65 mm Hg, tracheal intubation should be performed to control ventilation. Fluid, electrolyte, and acid-base balance must be controlled by frequent monitoring. Intravenous fluid administration should be based on the central venous or pulmonary artery wedge pressure, blood pressure, and urine output; overhydration must be avoided. Intravenous mannitol (12.5 g) may be given early if myoglobinuria is present to avoid renal dysfunction. Disseminated intravascular coagulation may require treatment with heparin. Occasionally, inotropic agents (eg, isoproterenol, dopamine) may be indicated for cardiac insufficiency, which should be suspected if hypotension persists after hypovolemia has been corrected.

Prognosis

Bad prognostic signs are temperature of 42.2°C or more, coma lasting over 2 hours, shock, hyperkalemia, and an AST greater than 1000 units/L during the first 24 hours. The death rate is about 10% in patients who are correctly diagnosed and treated promptly. Deaths in the first few days are usually due to cerebral damage; later deaths may be from bleeding or may be due to cardiac, renal, or hepatic failure.

Jardine DS: Heat illness and heat stroke. *Pediatr Rev.* 2007;28:249.
Leon LR: Heat stroke and cytokines. *Prog Brain Res.* 2007;162:481.

▼ FROSTBITE

Frostbite involves freezing of tissues. Ice crystals form between and in the cells and grow at the expense of intracellular water. The resulting ischemia due to vasoconstriction and increased blood viscosity is the mechanism of tissue injury. Skin and muscle are considerably more susceptible than tendons and bones to freezing damage due to a lower oxygen requirement, which explains why the patient may still be able to move severely frostbitten digits.

Frostbite is caused by cold exposure, the effects of which can be magnified by moisture or wind; for example, the chilling effects on skin are the same with an air temperature of 6.7°C and a 40-mph wind as with an air temperature of −40°C and only a 2-mph wind. Contact with metal or gasoline in very cold weather can cause virtually instantaneous freezing; skin will often stick to metal and be lost. The risk of frostbite is increased by generalized hypothermia, which produces peripheral vasoconstriction as part of the mechanism for preservation of core body temperature.

Two related injuries, trench foot and immersion foot, involve prolonged exposure to wet cold above freezing (eg, 10°C). The resulting tissue damage is produced by tissue ischemia.

▶ Clinical Findings

Frostnip, a minor variant of this syndrome, is a transient blanching and numbness of exposed parts that may progress to frostbite if not immediately detected and treated. It often appears on the tips of fingers, ears, nose, chin, or cheeks and should be managed by rewarming through contact with warm parts of the body or warm air.

Frostbitten parts are numb, painless, and of a white or waxy appearance. With superficial frostbite, only the skin and subcutaneous tissues are frozen, so the tissues beneath are still compressible with pressure. Deep frostbite involves freezing of underlying tissues, which imparts a wooden consistency to the extremity.

After rewarming, the frostbitten area becomes mottled blue or purple and painful and tender. Blisters appear that may take several weeks to resolve. The part becomes edematous and to a varying degree painful.

▶ Treatment

The frostbitten part should be rewarmed (thawed) in a water bath at 40-42.2°C for 20-30 minutes. Thawing should not be attempted until the victim can be kept permanently warm and at rest. It is far better to continue walking on frostbitten feet even for many hours than to thaw them in a remote cold area where definitive care cannot be provided. If a thermometer is unavailable, the temperature of the water should be adjusted to be warm but not hot to a normal hand. Never use the frozen part to test the water temperature or expose it to a source of direct heat such as a fire. The risk of seriously compounding the injury is great with any method of thawing other than immersion in warm water.

After thawing has been completed, the patient should be kept recumbent and the injured part left open to the air, protected from direct contact with sheets, clothing, or other material. Blisters should be left intact and the skin gently debrided by immersing the part in a whirlpool bath for about 20 minutes twice daily. No scrubbing or massaging of the injured part should be allowed, and topical ointments, antiseptics, and so on, are of no value. Vasodilating agents and surgical sympathectomy do not appear to improve healing.

The tissue will heal gradually, and any dead tissue will become demarcated and usually slough spontaneously. Early in the course, it is nearly impossible, even for someone with considerable experience in the treatment of frostbite, to judge the depth of injury; most early assessments tend to overestimate the extent of permanent damage. Therefore, expectant treatment is the rule, and surgical debridement should be avoided even if evolution of the injury requires many months. Surgery may be indicated to release constricting circumferential eschars, but rarely should the process of spontaneous separation of gangrenous tissue be surgically facilitated. Even in severe injuries, amputation is rarely indicated before 2 months unless invasive infection supervenes. Nuclear scans may be useful to delineate tissue viability.

Concomitant fractures or dislocations create challenging and complex problems. Dislocations should be reduced immediately after thawing. Open fractures require operative reduction, but closed fractures should be managed with a posterior plastic splint. Anterior tibial compartment syndrome, which may develop in patients with associated fractures, may be diagnosed by arteriography and treated by fasciotomy.

After the eschar separates, the skin is noted to be thin, shiny, tender, and sensitive to cold; occasionally it exhibits a tendency to perspire more readily. Gradually, it returns toward normal, but pain on exposure to cold may persist indefinitely.

▶ Prognosis

The prognosis for normal function is excellent if appropriate treatment is provided. Individuals who have recovered from frostbite have increased susceptibility to another frostbite injury on exposure to cold.

Affleck DG et al: Assessment of tissue viability in complex extremity injuries: utility of the pyrophosphate nuclear scan. *J Trauma.* 2001;50:263.

Murphy JV et al: Frostbite: pathogenesis and treatment. *J Trauma.* 2000;48:171.

▼ ACCIDENTAL HYPOTHERMIA

Accidental hypothermia consists of the uncontrolled lowering of core body temperature below 35°C by exposure to cold. The syndrome may be seen, for example, in elderly people living alone in inadequately heated homes, in alcoholics exposed to the cold during a binge, in those engaged in winter sports, and in people who become lost in cold weather. Alcohol facilitates the induction of hypothermia by producing sedation (inhibiting shivering) and cutaneous dilation. Other sedatives, tranquilizers, and antidepressants are occasionally implicated. Diseases that predispose to hypothermia include myxedema, hypopituitarism, adrenal insufficiency, cerebral vascular insufficiency, mental impairment, and cardiovascular disorders.

The heart is the organ most sensitive to cooling and is subject to ventricular fibrillation or asystole when the temperature drops to 21-24°C. Hypothermia affects the oxyhemoglobin dissociation curve, so less oxygen is released to the tissues. Cardiac standstill may cause death in less than 1 hour in shipwreck victims immersed in cold water (6.7°C).

Increased capillary permeability, manifested by generalized edema and pulmonary, hepatic, and renal dysfunction, may develop as the patient is rewarmed. Coagulopathies and disseminated intravascular coagulation are seen occasionally. Pancreatitis and acute renal failure are common in patients whose temperature on admission is below 32°C.

▶ Clinical Findings

A. Symptoms and Signs

The patient is mentally depressed (somnolent, stuporous, or comatose), cold, and pale to cyanotic. The clinical findings are not always striking and may be mistaken for the effects of alcohol. The core temperature ranges from 21°C to 35°C. Shivering is absent when the temperature is below 32°C. Respirations are slow and shallow. The blood pressure is usually normal and the heart rate slow. When the core temperature drops below 32°C, the patient may appear to be dead. The extremities may be frostbitten or frozen.

B. Laboratory Findings

Dehydration may increase the concentration of various blood constituents. Severe hypoglycemia is common, and unless detected and treated immediately, it may become dangerously worse as rewarming produces shivering. The serum amylase is elevated in about half of cases, but autopsy studies show that it does not always reflect pancreatitis. Diabetic ketoacidosis becomes a management problem in some patients whose amylase values are elevated on entry. The AST, LDH, and CK enzymes are usually elevated but are of no predictive significance. The electrocardiogram shows lengthening of the PR interval, delay in interventricular conduction, and a pathognomonic J wave at the junction of the QRS complex and ST segment.

▶ Treatment

Hypothermic patients should never be considered dead until all measures for resuscitation have failed, because cardiopulmonary arrest in severe hypothermia is still compatible with some recovery.

Mild hypothermia (body temperature 32-35°C) can be treated in most cases by passive rewarming (heavy clothing and blankets in a warm environment) for a few hours—especially when the patient is shivering. The patient's temperature should be continuously monitored with a rectal or esophageal probe until body temperature reaches normal. Since the volume of intravenous fluids required for resuscitation is often substantial, their temperature can affect the outcome. Consequently, intravenous fluids should be warmed with a heat exchanger during administration.

Active rewarming is indicated for temperature below 32°C, cardiovascular instability, or failure of passive rewarming. The methods include immersion in a warm water bath, inhalation of heated air, pleural lavage, and blood warming with an extracorporeal bypass machine. Active external rewarming is most often performed by immersion in a warm (40-42°C) water bath, which will raise body temperature at a rate of 1-2 degrees per hour. A disadvantage of this method is that the core temperature may continue to decline after initiation of the rewarming efforts (known as afterdrop), which is associated with worsening cardiovascular function.

Closed pleural irrigation should be performed by flushing the right hemithorax with warm (40-42°C) saline solution through two large thoracostomy tubes, one anterior and the other posterior. Rewarming by peritoneal lavage involves giving warm (40-45°C) crystalloid solutions, 6 L/h, which raises core temperature by 2-4 degrees per hour.

Active core rewarming with partial cardiopulmonary bypass, the most efficient technique, is indicated for patients with ventricular fibrillation and severe hypothermia or those with frozen extremities. At a flow rate of 6-7 L/min, core temperature can be raised by 1-2°C every 3-5 minutes.

In severe cases, endotracheal intubation should be used for better management of ventilation and protection against aspiration, a common lethal complication. Arterial blood gases should be monitored frequently. Bretylium tosylate in an initial dose of 10 mg/kg is the best drug for ventricular fibrillation. Antibiotics are often indicated for coexisting pneumonitis. Serious infections are often unsuspected upon admission, and delay in appropriate therapy may contribute to the severity of the illness. Hypoglycemia calls for intravenous administration of 50% glucose solution. Fluid administration must be gauged by central venous or pulmonary artery wedge pressures, urine output, and other circulatory parameters. Increased capillary permeability following rewarming predisposes to the development of pulmonary edema and compartment syndromes in the extremities. To minimize these complications, the central venous or wedge pressure should be kept below 12-14 cm water. Drugs should not be injected into peripheral tissues, because absorption will not take place while the patient is cold and because drugs may accumulate to produce serious toxicity as rewarming occurs.

As rewarming proceeds, the patient should be continually reassessed for signs of concomitant disease that may have been masked by hypothermia, especially myxedema and hypoglycemia. Any inexplicable failure to respond should suggest adrenal insufficiency.

▶ **Prognosis**

Survival can be expected in only 50% of patients whose core temperature drops below 32.2°C. Coexisting diseases (eg, stroke, neoplasm, myocardial infarction) are common and increase the death rate to 75% or more. Survival does not correlate closely with the lowest absolute temperature

reached. Death may result from brain damage pneumonitis, heart failure, or renal insufficiency.

MULTIPLE CHOICE QUESTIONS

1. Burn severity can be informed by each of the following except

   A. Fraction of body surface area affected
   B. Patient's age
   C. Death of others in the same incident
   D. Accompanying other major trauma
   E. Concurrent inhalational injury

2. Hypermetabolism after burn injuries

   A. Can contribute to coagulopathy
   B. Causes a disproportionate loss of muscle mass
   C. Can approach a threefold increase in basal metabolic rate after severe burns
   D. Can be slowed with beta-adrenergic blockade
   E. Is not catabolic and can be limited by decreased caloric intake

3. Care of the burn wound may include each of the following except

   A. Closed method occlusive dressings with twice daily dressing changes
   B. May accompany tension pneumothorax
   C. Exposure therapy with topical agents applied to uncovered areas of the face
   D. Primary management with bismuth-containing antimicrobial topical agents
   E. Temporary coverage with a skin substitute

4. Maintenance of functional motion during burn wound healing

   A. Benefits from early consideration with functional position splinting and active motion
   B. Is benefitted, in general, by the tendency of the wounds to contract
   C. Suffers after early skin grafting due to promotion of wound contracture
   D. Is easier to maintain around joints due to increased natural motion
   E. A and C

5. Respiratory compromise after burn wounds is commonly due to

   A. Early pulmonary emboli (12-36 hours after injury)
   B. Inhalational injury
   C. Cardiogenic pulmonary edema
   D. Fungal bronchitis
   E. Viral pneumonitis

Otolaryngology: Head & Neck Surgery

Paul M. Weinberger, MD

David J. Terris, MD

INTRODUCTION

From hearing loss or nasal hemorrhage (epistaxis) to endocrine surgery and expert management of acute airway emergencies, otolaryngology/head and neck surgery is a surgical subspecialty which focuses on the management of a wide range of disorders of the head and neck. As a colleague once put it, "Otolaryngology pretty much covers everything above the clavicles except the eyes, the brain, and the spinal cord." The limits inherent to a single book chapter preclude covering such a broad field comprehensively. Therefore this chapter will present an overview of selected disease processes in otolaryngology that are of importance to the general surgeon in training. Other important parts of otolaryngology such as surgical endocrine disorders of the neck (eg, thyroid and parathyroid), facial plastic and reconstructive surgery, and facial skeletal trauma are covered in separate chapters.

DISORDERS OF THE EAR, AUDITORY, VESTIBULAR SYSTEMS, AND TEMPORAL BONE

▶ Anatomy and Physiology

The external ear consists of two parts, the auricle (projecting from the lateral aspect of the head) and the external auditory canal (EAC) projecting medially to the tympanic membrane. Functioning as resonant amplifiers of sound energy, the concha of the auricle (Figure 15–1) has a resonance frequency of approximately 5 KHz, and the EAC has a resonance frequency of approximately 3.5 KHz. Combined, the external ear amplifies sound by approximately 10-15 dB in the 2-5 KHz range.

The tympanic membrane is positioned in an oblique plane, separating the EAC from the middle ear. It functions in transforming acoustic energy from sound waves to mechanical energy, which is transmitted via the ossicles—malleus, incus, and stapes to the oval window of the cochlea. The mechanics of the middle ear further amplify sound

energy using two methods. First, the tympanic membrane is approximately 17 times larger than the footplate of the stapes; second, the ossicles act as a lever, providing a mechanical advantage of 1:1.3 from the tympanic membrane to the oval window. Combined, the result in a 25-30 dB gain in amplification.

The temporal bone houses the bony portion of the EAC, the middle, and the inner ear. The otic capsule of the inner ear is the hardest bone in the human body. Other important structures passing through or adjacent to the temporal bone include the carotid artery, the jugular vein, and the facial nerve (seventh cranial nerve). All of these structures are at risk for injury from temporal bone trauma.

The inner ear consists of the cochlea, which is both the auditory and vestibular sense organ. The vestibular system senses both linear acceleration (gravity) and angular acceleration (rotation). The hearing portion of the cochlea is a coiled tube that resembles a snail. Divided into three separate chambers, the scala vestibule and the scala tympani are filled with perilymph (similar in composition to extracellular fluid), while the scala media is filled with endolymph (similar in composition to intracellular fluid). The endolymph composition is maintained by Na+/K+ ATPase pumps within the stria vascularis found on the lateral walls of the scala media. These different chambers thus have different electrolyte composition, creating an electrical potential between the compartments. The sound energy, once transferred through the ossicles to the oval window of the cochlea, is coupled directly to the perilymph of the scala vestibule.

The resulting traveling wave is in the form of mechanical energy, which is then converted to electrical (neural) impulses within the scala media by the organ of Corti. The organ of Corti consists of inner hair cells (which are the sensory cells) and outer hair cells (which function as modulators of the inner hair cells), support cells and tectorial membrane. These nerve impulses produced by the inner hair cells are transmitted to the brainstem by the eighth cranial nerve,

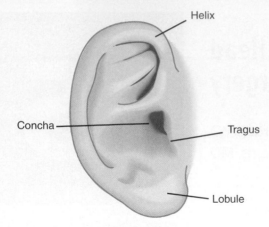

Helix

Concha

Tragus

Lobule

▲ **Figure 15–1.** Normal external ear anatomy.

which travels from the cochlea through the internal auditory canal (IAC).

The vestibular system consists of the utricle, saccule, and three semicircular canals. Enveloped within the endolymphatic membrane, which is filled with endolymph, they are surrounded by perilymph, and then the very hard bone of the otic capsule. The utricle detects horizontal acceleration while the saccule detects vertical acceleration. Three semicircular canals, situated at right angles to each other, and paired with a semicircular canal on the opposite side of the head, detect angular acceleration.

Simplified, linear or angular motion causes their respective sensory cells to deflect, and the sensory cell body to depolarize. Depending on the direction, each vestibular apparatus will either increase or decrease the discharge rate relative to the basal rate, providing both direction, and speed of acceleration. Vestibular information is transmitted to the brainstem by the vestibular branch of the eighth cranial nerve.

▶ Urgencies and Emergencies

A. Sudden Sensorineural Hearing Loss

The sudden onset of unilateral (or more uncommonly bilateral) hearing loss occurs at an annual incidence of 5-20 cases per 100,000 persons and can be an extremely unsettling experience for a patient. Most experts use a definition based on at least a 30 dB hearing loss occurring over 3 days or less. The causes of SSHL include viral infection (particularly herpes-family viruses), trauma, vascular compromise from thromboembolic phenomena or vasospasm, autoimmune disease, ototoxic (from chemotherapy, antibiotics, or salicylates), and congenital anatomic defects.

Prompt evaluation and initiation of treatment is critical, and may improve the prognosis for hearing improvement. Because of the multitude of potential mechanisms,

a careful history should be performed. Often, the cause remains unknown. Patients may report an antecedent loud noise exposure such as an explosion (suggesting traumatic perilymphatic fistula), or upper respiratory tract infection symptoms (suggesting possible viral mechanism). Recent heart surgery or thromboembolic phenomenon could suggest a vascular etiology. Patients should be questioned about coincident imbalance or vertiginous symptoms, and tinnitus (ringing in the ears), indicative of vestibular as well as auditory pathology.

Formal pure-tone audiometry testing should be obtained. If the patient reports vestibular or balance symptoms, investigation of the vestibular system should be performed. Dix–Hallpike and Baranay maneuvers test for vertigo in response to specific position changes with respect to gravity. Simple tests of the auditory system (Weber and Rinne tests) can also be performed at the bedside using a 512 KHz tuning fork (Table 15–1). Pneumatic otoscopy should be performed, to evaluate for fistula sign (vertigo on pneumotoscopy insufflation).

Workup should include evaluation for a vestibular schwannoma, as this represents approximately 1%-3% of the sudden sensorineural hearing loss (SSHL). This can be done by the auditory evoked brainstem response (ABR), or a magnetic resonance imaging (MRI) with contrast using IAC protocols. Some experts advocate a less expensive screening MRI without contrast as an acceptable first step, followed by more definitive evaluations if any abnormalities are present. Laboratory studies should include a CBC with differential, ESR, PT/PTT, and cochlear antibodies. Additional studies

Table 15–1. Weber and Rinne tuning fork tests.

Condition	Weber	Rinne
Left sensorineural hearing loss	Louder on *right*	A>B bilaterally
Left conductive hearing loss	Louder on *left*	A>B on right A=B or A<B on left
Normal hearing	Midline/no difference	A>B bilaterally

In the **Weber** test, the tuning fork is struck and applied in the midline to the skull or teeth. This stimulates both cochlea by direct bone conduction. The patient is asked whether they hear the sound the same on both sides or louder on one side.

In the **Rinne** test, a tuning fork is struck and held by the auricle (condition "A," air conduction). Sound is conducted through the ossicular chain and to the cochlea. The fork is then applied to the mastoid tip, and acoustic energy transmitted to the cochlea by direct bone conduction (condition "B," bone conduction). The patient is then asked which is louder, A or B. In a normal hearing ear, A (air) is greater than B (bone). In sensorineural hearing loss, A will still be greater than B. In conductive hearing loss, A=B or even B>A.

that may be helpful include syphilis testing (either MHA-TP or FTA-Abs), and thyroid function tests. If there is a family history of sudden hearing loss, a computed tomography (CT) scan looking for enlarged vestibular aqueduct can be obtained.

If the workup reveals a cause for the SSHL, this should be addressed. Unfortunately, the majority remain idiopathic. In this case, unless contraindicated due to comorbidities, initial treatment should be started empirically. Oral corticosteroids, such as a prednisone taper (60 mg daily for 9 days then tapering over 5 days), and antiviral medication (such as acyclovir) should be administered for a minimum of 2 weeks. Other treatments such as hyperbaric oxygen, carbogen inhalation, anticoagulation, and diuretics have been proposed for the treatment of SSHL but results of these therapies have been inconclusive.

The prognosis for spontaneous recovery of function is hopeful, and approximately 60% of patients will recover full or partial hearing. With corticosteroid treatment, this may increase to 80% according to some studies. The addition of acyclovir has not been shown to be effective, but some experts recommend it due to low side effects and a plausible mechanism of action.

B. Acute Facial Nerve Paralysis

The seventh cranial nerve (facial nerve) innervates the muscles of facial expression (as well as special motor afferents to the parotid and lacrimal glands). A careful history will help define the onset of paralysis (eg, acute deterioration over less than 2-3 days, or gradual decline). Antecedent events (temporal bone trauma, acute otitis media [AOM], hearing loss or imbalance, and recent viral illness) should be elicited and can help guide further workup and management.

Potential causes of acute facial nerve paralysis are numerous; however over 50% are idiopathic and termed "Bell Palsy." Note that Bell Palsy is a diagnosis of exclusion, and therefore a focused but complete workup must be performed. Fully 20% of facial nerve paralyses are caused by trauma. Other common causes (but by no means an inclusive list) include herpes zoster oticus (Ramsey Hunt syndrome), complications from otitis media and mastoiditis, Lyme disease, cholesteatoma, and neoplasm.

A complete physical examination with emphasis on the neurologic system and cranial nerves is critical. An important consideration in evaluating the patient with acute facial nerve paralysis is distinguishing between central and peripheral lesions. In central lesions, there is sparing of forehead elevation on the affected side due to decussating fibers from the contralateral side. In peripheral lesions the fibers have already crossed and there is no forehead sparing. The degree of facial nerve functional loss should be documented and has important bearing on prognosis. Several grading systems have been proposed; the House–Brackmann scale is the most

Table 15–2. House-Brackmann facial nerve paralysis scale.

Grade	Characteristics
I (Normal)	Normal function in all branches
II (Mild dysfunction)	Slight weakness to visual inspection Normal symmetry and tone at rest Forehead: moderate to good function Eye: complete closure, minimal effort Mouth: slight asymmetry
III (Moderate dysfunction)	Mild difference to gross inspection between sides Normal symmetry and tone at rest Forehead: slight to moderate movement Eye: compete closure, requires effort Mouth: slightly weak, requires effort
IV (Moderately severe dysfunction)	Obvious weakness to gross inspection between sides Normal symmetry and tone at rest Forehead: no motion even with effort Eye: incomplete closure even with effort Mouth: asymmetric with maximum effort
V (Severe dysfunction)	Only barely perceptible motion to gross inspection Asymmetry at rest Forehead: no motion even with effort Eye: incomplete closure even with effort Mouth: slight movement even with maximum effort
VI (Total paralysis)	No movement

widely used and is presented in Table 15–2. Facial nerve function is graded from I (normal) to VI (total paralysis) for each side.

Evaluation should include pure-tone audiometry and electrophysiologic testing. A high-resolution CT of the temporal bone is the imaging study of choice for evaluating bone changes (from mastoiditis, temporal bone trauma, cholesteatoma, or neoplasm) whereas MRI with contrast is helpful when inflammation (eg, herpes zoster oticus) or neoplasm affecting the nerve is suspected. Laboratory studies should include a CBC with differential and ESR or CRP. If these are clinically suspected, autoimmune serologies and Lyme titers can be obtained.

If the facial nerve paralysis is caused by traumatic injury, management depends on the onset of paralysis; immediate and complete paralysis will often benefit from surgical decompression. In delayed or partial dysfunction, spontaneous recovery is likely and surgical intervention may not be beneficial. For idiopathic paralysis (Bell Palsy), initial medical therapy is targeted to reducing inflammation and targeting a possible viral etiology. A corticosteroid course should be initiated, either prednisone or prednisolone. Previous recommendations for the use of acyclovir (or similar antiherpetic analog) have recently been questioned. A large-scale randomized double blind study by Sullivan et al demonstrated no benefit for acyclovir, but significant benefit for prednisolone in the treatment of Bell Palsy. If the paralysis progresses, surgical decompression may be beneficial. Most experts also argue a significant benefit to performing surgical decompression of the facial nerve if a patient progresses to severe paralysis, provided the decompression is performed within 14 days of the onset of paralysis. Severe paralysis is usually defined as developing greater than 90% degeneration on electroneurography (ENoG) and lacking voluntary motor potentials on EMG.

C. Foreign Body in the External Auditory Canal–Button Batteries

The vast majority of cases of foreign bodies in the EAC occur in children, or mentally impaired adults. Many otologic foreign bodies, if carefully selected, are actually amenable to removal under direct visualization in an emergency department or primary care office setting. In a large series of over 600 cases of ear foreign bodies, Shulze et al found an overall 77% success rate for the removal under direct visualization by emergency physicians. It is important to note that the majority of those foreign bodies successfully removed in this manner fit the category of "soft, irregular" material such as paper or cotton, and "pliable or rubber-like" such as silly putty or erasers. Success with hard objects, and especially spherical objects such as plastic beads was markedly lower. Thus, an argument can be made for a single attempt by the pediatrician or emergency physician under direct visualization, if the object meets the former criteria. This should be tempered, however, with the understanding that complication rates are much higher with removal under direct vision. Complications of foreign body removal most commonly include canal wall lacerations (47%), with tympanic membrane perforations less common (4%). More serious complications such as ossicular chain injury and oval window perforation are possible but rare. When initial foreign body removal is performed instead by the otolaryngologist using binocular otomicroscopy either in the office or operative setting, the complication rate is quite low (6.3%).

Foreign body removal using binocular otomicroscopy is the primary method used by most otolaryngologists. Specific techniques depend on the characteristics of the foreign body. Objects with sharp edges can often be grasped with alligator or duck-bill forceps. Soft objects are often amenable to removal with otologic suction. Removal of spherical and hard, irregular objects requires more finesse. In these cases a 90-degree probe is invaluable. The probe is carefully guided behind the object under binocular otomicroscopic visualization. Then the probe is rotated along its axis to bring the end behind the object. The object is then guided out of the EAC. Another special case is an insect within the EAC, most

commonly cockroaches. This can be quite alarming to the patient if the insect is still alive. The proximity of the insect to the tympanic membrane translates movement of the insect to distressingly loud perceived sound levels. In such cases the external ear canal can be gently irrigated with either mineral oil or lidocaine to suffocate the insect followed by prompt removal.

Some non-otolaryngologists advocate the use of gentle irrigation to attempt dislodgement of EAC foreign bodies. This technique can be used successfully, but requires caution. First, if there is any suspicion of tympanic membrane perforation, irrigation is contraindicated as it could flush debris into the middle ear space. Second, if the foreign body is composed of vegetable material (such as a popcorn kernel) irrigation should be avoided. If the object is not successfully flushed out, subsequent swelling of the vegetable foreign body can result in extreme pain as the EAC skin is compressed against the bony canal. Removal, once this occurs can be problematic, and may require general anesthesia and the use of an operating microscope. For this reason, otologic medications are also contraindicated in vegetable material otologic foreign bodies. The third condition where irrigation (and otologic medications) is specifically contraindicated is in the case of EAC button-batteries.

While the previously described foreign bodies can be managed on an outpatient basis, the finding of a button battery in the EAC is considered an emergent situation, requiring urgent removal by an otolaryngologist. If left in place for any length of time, batteries in the EAC can result in severe complications. In an early description of this problem by Kavanagh et al, 100% of patients experienced multiple, serious sequelae. These included tympanic membrane perforation or total destruction (75%), marked dermal destruction with bone exposure (88%), impairment of hearing (38%), ossicular chain erosion (25%), and even facial nerve paralysis (13%). Both leakage of corrosive battery acid and electrical current discharge resulting in chlorine gas and sodium hydroxide by electrolysis have been hypothesized to contribute to the destructive effects of button batteries. Removal is accomplished under binocular otomicroscopy in the operating room, and sometimes requires piecemeal removal of the battery. Following removal of the battery, the EAC should be flushed with copious amounts of saline, and careful inspection of the external canal and tympanic membrane should be performed.

▶ Disorders and Diseases

A. Otitis Externa

Otitis externa is an infection of the EAC, usually from bacterial species such as *Pseudomonas, Proteus, Klebsiella, Streptococcus,* and *Enterobacter.* Evaluation and management of a patient with suspected otitis externa includes a complete history and physical examination with emphasis on the otologic examination. Patients will often give a history of recent water exposure to the external ear, such as from swimming, or other predisposing factors such as chronic hearing aid use. The external pinna should be manipulated gently. In otitis media this should not elicit pain, whereas for patients with otitis externa movement of the pinna is extremely painful. On handheld otoscopy the canal wall will appear edematous and erythematous. Sometimes the edema is severe enough the tympanic membrane cannot be visualized. In this case, insertion of a Pope otowick is indicated to carry ototopical medications the length of the external ear canal past the obstructed site. Severe cases may require frequent suction debridement under microscopic visualization. Patients should be placed on ototopical antibiotic drops containing a topical corticosteroid, such as ciprofloxacin 0.3%/dexamethasone 0.1% suspension (Ciprodex). Some (largely nonotolaryngologist) physicians allow the use of hydrocortisone 1%/polymyxin/neomycin (Cortisporin) as an alternative. This is not recommended for several reasons. First, several authors have demonstrated up to 10% risk of contact dermatitis with polymyxin/neomycin ototopical drops. Second, if a possibility of tympanic membrane perforation exists, these drops carry the possibility of ototoxicity, according to laboratory studies in animals; they are not approved for the middle ear use (unlike fluoroquinolones). Additionally, some studies have demonstrated faster pain relief with Ciprodex compared to Cortisporin. It is essential to note that failure to respond to appropriate therapy within 48-72 hours should prompt the clinician to reassess the patient to confirm a diagnosis of otitis externa.

Of note, patients with a history of diabetes (or any immunocompromising condition) should demand more aggressive therapy targeted toward *Pseudomonas*. This will usually involve an ototopical fluoroquinolone, ototopical corticosteroid, and oral or IV fluoroquinolone therapy. In the past, this subset of otitis externa carried the misnomer "malignant otitis externa" due to the high mortality rate even with surgical debridement and antibiotics. Modern antibiotic therapy and earlier diagnoses and intervention have dramatically improved outcomes, and mortality from this disease is now relatively rare.

Otomycosis is otitis externa due to a fungal infection, usually due to *Aspergillus* or *Candida* species. On otoscopy, there is usually far less edema and erythema than with bacterial infection. The use of ototopical antibiotic solutions will not improve these patients, and usually worsens their condition. Otomycosis can be notoriously difficult to treat, but many cases do respond to suction debridement followed by acidic eardrops and a topical corticosteroid. A commonly used topical preparation is acetic acid 2% with hydrocortisone 1% (Vosol HC). Topical antifungals such as nystatin or amphotericin B are also available but use of these should be reserved for difficult cases under the care of an otolaryngologist.

B. Otitis Media

Classification of common middle ear pathology is often poorly understood by nonotolaryngologists. There are multiple disease processes of the middle ear which include the root term "otitis media." Additionally, the acronyms used to represent diseases of abnormal middle ear fluid are quite similar.

The first condition, AOM, represents what is commonly referred to as "a middle ear infection." The typical patient is a young child, with history of upper respiratory tract symptoms, fever, and pulling at one ear. Handheld otoscopy will reveal a bulging, erythematous tympanic membrane. Unlike otitis externa (above) there is no pain with manipulation of the auricle. Several studies from Europe have demonstrated that the majority of AOM cases resolve spontaneously without intervention. Nevertheless, in the United States most parents would be unhappy with a decision not to treat, and antibiotic therapy for AOM is routine. Usual pathogens include bacteria such as *Streptococcus*, *Haemophilus*, and *Moraxella*. The latter two are often resistant to penicillins and thus treatment with amoxicillin may not clear the infection; thus many practitioners recommend a second-generation cephalosporin. Failure to respond to these agents often necessitates a second-line antibiotic such as amoxicillin-clavulanic acid (Augmentin).

Otitis media with effusion (OME) is defined as fluid in the middle ear but no active signs of an infection. OME often results from eustachian tube dysfunction, which predisposes to accumulation of a sterile serous fluid in the middle ear cleft that does not clear. OME is common in young children, with a prevalence approaching 30% according to some reports. Patients with OME present with complaints of muffled or decreased hearing. Examination reveals fluid in the middle ear cleft. Chronic serous otitis media (CSOM) results when middle ear fluid after an episode of AOM fails to clear after a reasonable time span (4-6 weeks).

The most common surgical intervention to treat these problems is myringotomy and tympanostomy (M&T), so-called "ventilation tube" placement. Basic indications for M&T include multiple episodes of AOM (four episodes in 6 months, or six episodes in 12 months), CSOM with hearing impairment present for 3 months or longer, or presence of complications of AOM. Some authors have advocated for a more stratified approach to indications, where patients presenting with problems at an early age warrant surgical intervention with less stringent criteria.

C. Vestibular Schwannoma

Vestibular schwannomas (also sometimes referred to by the misnomer "acoustic neuromas") represent a nonmalignant but neoplastic proliferation of Schwann cells ensheathing the eighth cranial nerve. These tumors represent nearly 10% of all intracranial tumors, and usually present with a unilateral high-frequency sensorineural hearing loss, followed later by development of imbalance symptoms. Even a mild degree of hearing loss may be misleading, as sensory processing (as evidenced by speech discrimination scores) are often more impaired than pure-tone averages would predict. Tinnitus and true vertigo are less common symptoms. Interestingly, these tumors arise more often from the vestibular division than the auditory division of cranial nerve eight. The symptoms associated with vestibular schwannomas are associated with compressive effects from the neoplastic growth. In the case of larger tumors, patients can sometimes present with facial nerve weakness. One important syndrome associated with vestibular schwannomas is neurofibromatosis-2 (NF2). Patients with NF2 can present with bilateral vestibular schwannomas, and consideration of hearing preservation strategies thus is extremely important for these patients.

Presumptive diagnosis of vestibular schwannoma is usually made by MRI with gadolinium. Schwannomas enhance brightly on T1 or T2 weighted images with gadolinium. Other diagnostic tests can include auditory brainstem response (ABR), electronystagmography (ENG). All patients with suspected vestibular schwannomas should have audiometric testing (pure-tone averages and speech discrimination scores) performed.

Management of vestibular schwannomas remains controversial. Many authors advocate that small schwannomas confined to the IAC can be successfully watched via serial imaging. Tumors demonstrating no growth (<2 mm) can continue to be watched, while most authors would argue for intervention if more than 2 mm growth occurs. If intervention is elected, treatment can be microsurgical (often involving combined neurosurgical and otologist collaboration) or by stereotactic radiosurgery (gamma knife) for small tumors. The goal of treatment is eradication of the tumor while preserving hearing and facial nerve function when possible. Preservation of facial nerve function (House-Brackman grade 2 or better) is generally successful in up to 70% of patients, regardless of surgical approach used.

D. Benign Paroxysmal Positional Vertigo

Dizziness is an extremely common phenomenon, and has been estimated to affect as many as 30% of patients. An important distinction should be made at this point between various sensations commonly described by patients as "dizziness." For patients describing dizziness symptoms, an attempt to elicit a more accurate description should always be sought. Vertigo is defined as the illusion of rotation. This should be distinguished from sensations of imbalance or unsteadiness, or of almost losing consciousness (presyncope).

Benign paroxysmal positional vertigo (BPPV) is the most common cause of acute-onset vertigo. Patients will describe sudden onset of intense vertigo lasting seconds rather than minutes, usually brought on by changes in head or body position relative to gravity. There is sometimes an associated history of head trauma. The etiology is thought to be due to dislocation of micro-crystals of calcium hydroxyapatite (otoconia) from the vestibule into the posterior semicircular canal. Certain head movements cause the otoconia to abnormally trigger copular deflection and thus elicit imbalanced vestibular input to the brainstem triggering intense vertigo. Diagnosis of BPPV can be made by positional testing, such as the Dix–Hallpike maneuver. In this test, the patient's head is turned to one side and the patient is laid into a recumbent position with the head maintained in the rotated position. Elicitation of vertigo, often accompanied by the expected rotatory nystagmus, essentially confirms the diagnosis. Treatment consists of directed repositioning techniques such as the Epley maneuver. These maneuvers are designed to rotate the otoconia through the semicircular canal, depositing them back in a more physiologic location within the vestibule. Often several treatments are required, and patients can be instructed in the self-application of these maneuvers.

E. Méniére Disease

Méniére disease is characterized by waxing and waning sensorineural hearing loss (typically low frequency more than high), episodes of vertigo, sensation of aural fullness, and tinnitus. Hearing loss typically follows an episodic but slowly progressive course, with times of worse hearing followed by partial recovery. The hearing loss (and vestibular dysfunction) is most commonly unilateral, although bilateral disease can develop. The vertigo attacks associated with Méniére disease can be debilitating, and are often accompanied by nausea, vomiting, and inability to perform normal activities.

Diagnosis of Méniére disease is made based on clinical presence of the tetrad of symptoms, combined with evidence of hearing loss and vestibular dysfunction. The episodic nature of the disease is an important characteristic; a single episode of hearing loss and vertigo should not prompt a diagnosis of Méniére disease. In this case, viral labyrinthitis is a more likely culprit.

First described in 1861 by Prosper Méniére, the pathogenesis of Méniére disease remains essentially unknown. It is thought to relate to dilation of the membranous labyrinth, possibly from dysfunction within the endolymphatic sac. Anatomic cadaver studies have demonstrated endolymphatic hydrops (swelling of the scala media and endolymphatic sac) in patients with Méniére disease. Unfortunately, these anatomic changes have also been demonstrated in presumably normal (or at least asymptomatic) patients.

The mainstay of treatment for Méniére disease remains medical therapy. Patients are typically begun on a low-salt diet initially. Patients are also instructed to avoid caffeine, nicotine, and alcohol. Diuretics can be added, along with vestibular suppressants such as diazepam. Antihistamines (meclizine, dimenhydrinate, etc) have also demonstrated benefit in ameliorating vertigo symptoms associated with Méniére disease.

Patients suffering from severe, incapacitating vertigo and failing medical therapy can be offered several surgical interventions. Many authors advocate unilateral chemical ablation of the vestibular system. This is most often accomplished by transtympanic injection of gentamycin, and while efficacious for vertigo resolution is associated with sensorineural hearing loss in up to 25% of patients. For patients with intact hearing, many experts feel endolymphatic sac decompression and shunting can offer significant relief with preservation of hearing, although this remains unproven in randomized controlled trials. Similarly unproven, vestibular neurectomy (selective sectioning of the vestibular branch of the eighth cranial nerve) may conserve hearing and provide vertigo relief. For patients with severe hearing loss and vertigo, a total transmastoid labyrinthectomy relieves vertigo in over 90% of patients, at the cost of complete hearing loss on the affected side.

F. Cholesteatoma

A cholesteatoma is a cyst-like, expansile lesion of the temporal bone consisting of stratified squamous epithelium and trapped desquamated keratin. It occurs in the pneumatized temporal bone, most commonly the middle ear and mastoid (Figure 15–2). There are two types of cholesteatoma (acquired and congenital) with the former being the most common. Acquired cholesteatomas arise from either retraction pockets within the tympanic membrane, or secondarily from a tympanic membrane perforation. Congenital cholesteatomas are thought to arise from epithelial cell rests that fail to undergo apoptosis during development. Whatever the origin, once formed cholesteatomas behave in a locally destructive manner. Bone erosion is common, especially of the ossicular chain but also potentially the bone surrounding the inner ear (the otic capsule). If left untreated cholesteatomas can even invade intracranially.

Early cholesteatomas have few if any symptoms, and usually start with a slowly progressive hearing loss. If an infection develops in a cholesteatoma, a foul otorrhea will develop, and this sometimes is the presenting symptom. If a cholesteatoma is suspected, careful inspection under binocular otomicroscopy is essential. All debris must be removed to allow a full visualization of the entire visible portion of the tympanic membrane. Cholesteatomas will appear as a whitish keratin mass. A pneumatic otoscopy test is essential; if vertigo is elicited the surgeon must suspect erosion into the inner ear structures.

The treatment for cholesteatoma is surgery, usually involving removal of the mastoid air cell septations by otologic drill, exposing the middle ear space. This accomplishes two

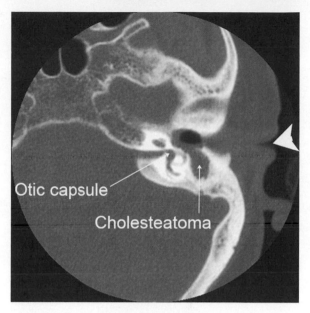

▲ **Figure 15–2.** Cholesteatoma of the left middle ear. Large arrowhead indicates the external ear canal. Note the soft tissue density (cholesteatoma) in the middle ear space and the absence of any visible ossicular chain. Part of the bony covering of the inner ear semicircular canal (the otic capsule) has also been eroded.

goals providing safe visualization and access and removal of all cholesteatoma tissue. This procedure is performed under careful microscopic visualization as many important structures (such as the facial nerve and the inner ear) should be preserved. The primary goal of surgery is creation of a safe, dry ear. All other considerations, including preservation of hearing, take second place.

DISORDERS OF THE NOSE AND PARANASAL SINUSES

▶ Anatomy and Physiology

The nose and paranasal sinuses serve to warm, filter, and humidify inspired air, to modulate vocalizations and speech, and provide for the sense of smell. The external nose consists of soft tissue and skin resting on a largely cartilaginous framework. The internal nose (nasal cavity) begins at the nasal vestibule anteriorly and extends posteriorly to the choana (which forms the boundary between the nasal cavity and the nasopharynx).

The nasal cavity (Figure 15–3) is divided in the sagittal plane in largely symmetric halves by the nasal septum. These cavities are partially filled by the three turbinates (superior, middle, and inferior, and occasionally a fourth supreme

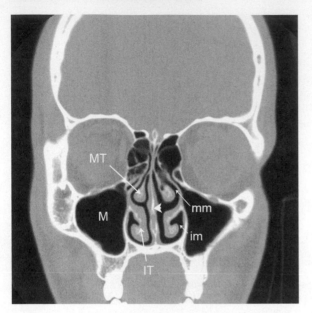

▲ **Figure 15–3.** Sinonasal anatomy. In this coronal plane CT scan, several key sinonasal landmarks can be seen. M, maxillary sinus; IT, inferior turbinate; MT, middle turbinate; im, inferior meatus; mm, middle meatus; arrowhead indicates nasal septum.

turbinate), which arise from the lateral nasal wall. The spaces below each turbinate are called meati (eg, superior meatus, middle meatus, and inferior meatus). These meati are important for localizing the outflow tracts of the various paranasal sinuses, which drain in a characteristic pattern. The nasolacrimal duct drains into the inferior meatus. The maxillary, frontal, and anterior ethmoid sinuses all drain into the middle meatus. The sphenoid sinus and posterior ethmoids drain into the superior meatus. Additionally, the olfactory nerve endings (the end organ for the sense of smell) are located on the superior nasal septum and superior turbinate mucosa.

The paranasal sinuses consist of hollow cavities that derive from pneumatization into the frontal, ethmoid, sphenoid, and maxillary bones of the craniofacial skeleton. They are lined with respiratory epithelium (pseudostratified ciliated columnar epithelium), which serves to circulate and drain mucous along with entrapped particulate matter. They are normally air-filled but can become fluid-filled if the ostia become obstructed by inflammation, anatomic problems, or disease process.

▶ **Urgencies and Emergencies**

A. Nasal Foreign Body

As is the case for foreign bodies of the external ear, nasal foreign bodies are typically encountered in children.

Typical presentation is a young child with several day history of *unilateral* foul rhinorrhea. Oftentimes, the offending foreign body was inserted days to weeks before symptom onset, and the patient or parents may not recall a specific event precipitating the symptoms.

Offending foreign bodies can include vegetative, inert (plastic/metal) material and button batteries. Unlike external ear foreign bodies, nasal foreign bodies should always be treated as relative urgencies regardless of the type of object present. This is because of the anatomic relationship of the nose to the upper airway—if the object becomes dislodged, it could easily become an airway foreign body (a true emergency).

For this reason, many otolaryngologists advocate recommend removal of all but the most anteriorly placed nasal foreign bodies under general anesthesia using endoscopic visualization. The threshold for performing retrieval under sedation should likewise be low. In our practice, nasal foreign bodies confined to the nasal vestibule, or easily visible by anterior rhinoscopy can be safely removed without sedation *in a cooperative patient*. Young children, superior or posterior location or difficult visualization all result in removal in the operating room with endoscopic visualization. Another advantage to removing nasal foreign bodies in this manner is that postremoval inspection of the nasal cavity is easily performed. Oftentimes the nasal mucosa can be significantly inflamed and placement of absorbable material can prevent unwanted adhesions between opposing mucosal surfaces.

Nasal button batteries present a similar situation to external ear button batteries (see External Ear Foreign Body, above). The potential for extensive tissue damage from leakage of acid and electrical current discharge usually necessitates removal under general anesthesia. Following removal, extensive flushing with normal saline and careful inspection of the nasal cavity should be performed.

B. Invasive Fungal Sinusitis

Invasive fungal sinusitis is almost always encountered in immunocompromised patients, most often patients undergoing chemotherapy for malignancy, or poorly controlled diabetics. It is caused by uncontrolled infiltrative growth of usually non-pathogenic fungal organisms. Offending agents are ubiquitous in the environment, and are commonly found in the nasal secretions of healthy normal patients. The two most common fungi are *Aspergillus* and *Rhizopus* species. The latter is more aggressive and is termed Mucormycosis. *Rhizopus* tends to preferentially grow in acidic environments, and is thus found more often in the setting of diabetic ketoacidosis. Even with early diagnosis and maximal surgical therapy, and modern antifungal agents, the disease still carries a significant mortality rate. This varies depending on causative agent, from approximately 10% (*Aspergillus*) to 30% (*Rhizopus*).

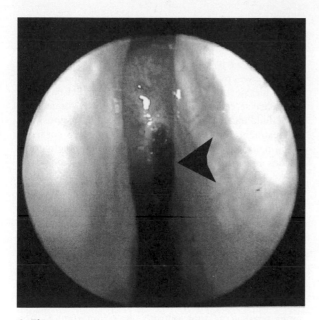

▲ **Figure 15–4.** Invasive fungal sinusitis. In this patient with invasive fungal sinusitis, the initial finding was a dark area (arrowhead) on the inferior face of the middle turbinate found on bedside nasal endoscopy.

The index of suspicion for invasive fungal sinusitis must be high for any immunocompromised patient, as the symptoms can be subtle and the disease rapidly progressive. Patients are usually ill appearing and complain of facial pain, headache, nasal discharge, and may have mental status changes. Careful inspection of the face, oral cavity, and nasal cavity is mandatory. Dark ulcers (Figure 15–4) may be noted on the anterior face of the middle turbinate, inferior turbinate, lateral nasal wall, septum, or palate. Cranial nerve deficits may be noted in later stages of the disease.

If invasive fungal sinusitis is suspected, biopsies should be taken of the suspicious areas and sent for immediate pathologic examination. The pathologist should be alerted that invasive fungal sinusitis is suspected, so that special fungal stains can be performed. A worrisome finding is lack of bleeding at the biopsy site, as this may signify retrograde tissue infarction secondary to angioinvasive fungus.

Once invasive fungal sinusitis is confirmed, therapy consists of rapid reversal of immunosupression followed by aggressive surgical debridement of all necrotic tissue (down to healthy, bleeding tissue) and systemic antifungal therapy. Two commonly used agents are voriconazole and amphotericin B. Usually multiple surgical debridements are required. Typically, patients do not recover unless the underlying immunosuppression is resolved; for example absolute neutrophil counts greater than 500 or diabetic ketoacidosis

rapidly reversed. Adjuvant therapy with donor neutrophil transfusion is an emerging treatment addition especially in cases failing to respond to conventional treatment. A multidisciplinary team including otolaryngology, hematology/oncology, and infectious disease specialists should closely follow these patients. Many patients develop metastatic fungal infections and can develop necrotic cavitation at distant sites. This often occurs as the patient's immune system recovers, and can result in lethal pulmonary hemorrhage, strokes, and other serious systemic sequelae.

Invasive fungal sinusitis should not be confused with other forms of fungal disease of the paranasal sinuses. In allergic fungal sinusitis, chronic host immunologic/inflammatory response to noninvasive fungal elements results in tissue eosinophilia, nasal polyps (hyperplastic growth that obstructs normal drainage and airflow), and bony remodeling.

C. Epistaxis

Epistaxis most commonly arises from the anterior portion of the nasal septum, referred to as Little's area. In this region, blood vessels derived from both the internal and external carotid anastomose to form Kiesselbach plexus. This rich blood supply can result in quite dramatic amounts of bleeding which can be distressing for the patient. Fortunately, many of these episodes respond to simple external pressure (pinching the anterior external nose) for 10 minutes.

The etiology of epistaxis is primarily related to disruption of nasal mucosa, thus exposing small blood vessels that can rupture. In children this often relates to nose picking. In adults, the etiology often relates to turbulent nasal airflow, such as from a deviated nasal septum. Other predisposing factors include drying of the nasal mucosa, and hypertension. The latter is particularly important in the acute management of epistaxis; often the bleeding will not be controllable until the accompanying hypertension is dealt with.

Epistaxis not responding to conservative management may require intranasal tamponade. Several different packing devices, including petrolatum gauze, thrombin containing collagen products, sponges, and inflatable balloons can be used to perform anterior packing. Anterior bleeding from Little's area can also sometimes be controlled with topical silver nitrate chemical cauterization, usually under endoscopic visualization.

Another common source of epistaxis is bleeding from branches of the anterior ethmoid or sphenopalatine artery. Epistaxis from these often requires posterior packing (such as with Foley catheter occlusion of the choanae and complete obliteration of the nasal airspace with gauze packing). Patients requiring posterior packing should be hospitalized and placed on pulse oximetry. Of note, nasal packing materials should be covered with topical antibiotics before placement, and all patients with intranasal packing should be placed on antistaphylococcal antibiotics to prevent possible toxic shock syndrome. Epistaxis recalcitrant to anterior and posterior packing can be managed by surgical ligation of the offending arterial supply (internal maxillary, sphenopalatine, and anterior ethmoid) or by arterial embolization by an interventional radiologist.

Chronic medical management of patients predisposed to epistaxis includes management of hypertension, and promoting moist nasal mucosa. Patients are commonly placed on two to three times daily application of nasal saline spray, and topical petroleum jelly or antibiotic ointment to the anterior septum. Patients with severe, recurrent epistaxis should be evaluated for possible systemic disease (such as hereditary hemorrhagic telangiectasia, Wegener granulomatosis, etc).

▶ Disorders and Diseases

A. Acute Rhinosinusitis

Rhinosinusitis refers to inflammation of the mucosal lining of the nose and paranasal sinuses. Acute rhinosinusitis is present for less than 3 weeks, and is usually precipitated by a viral upper respiratory tract infection. It is important to emphasize that only a minority of cases of acute rhinosinusitis become complicated by bacterial superinfection (0.5%-2%). Similarly, change in color of nasal discharge is not a specific sign of bacterial rhinosinusitis.

Symptoms initially reflect the precipitating upper respiratory viral infection (cough, sneezing, fever, nasal congestion, facial pain/pressure, rhinorrhea, and sore throat) followed by development of rhinosinusitis symptoms. A set of diagnostic symptoms for rhinosinusitis (both acute and chronic) have been established. Patients must have two major, or one major and two minor criteria. These criteria are outlined in Table 15–3.

Table 15–3. Major and minor criteria for diagnoses of rhinosinusitis.

Major Criteria	Minor Criteria
Facial pain or pressure	Headache
Nasal obstruction	Fever (for chronic rhinosinusitis)
Nasal discharge or purulence	Halitosis
Purulence in nasal cavity	Fatigue
Anosmia or hyposmia	Dental pain
Fever (for acute rhinosinusitis)	Cough
	Ear pain/pressure/fullness

Adapted from Lanza DC, Kennedy DW. *Otolaryngol Head Neck Surg.* 1997; 117(3 Pt 2): S1-S7.

Acute bacterial rhinosinusitis should be suspected if symptoms persist after 10 days, or worsen within 10 days after an initial improvement. Physical examination may reveal purulent nasal secretions, nasal mucosal erythema, and tenderness overlying the sinuses. Nasal endoscopy (with middle meatal cultures) can be very useful, and visualization of purulent secretions emanating from the osteomeatal complex should increase suspicion for bacterial rhinosinusitis.

Treatment of acute rhinosinusitis is largely conservative in nature. Nasal saline lavage helps to eliminate excess mucous and inflammatory mediators, and restore mucocilliary clearance. Topical decongestants (such as oxymetazoline) can help reduce mucosal edema and restore sinus ostia drainage. Use should be restricted to 3 days, as tachyphylaxis and dependence can result from overuse of topical decongestants. Mucolytics such as guaifenesin can help thin mucous secretions, allowing easier mucocilliary transport. The only therapy tested and confirmed by placebo-controlled trials is intranasal topical steroids (such as mometasone or flunisolide). Topical steroids have been demonstrated to reduce time to symptom resolution, both for bacterial and nonbacterial acute rhinosinusitis. It is important to note that antihistamines have no proven benefit in acute rhinosinusitis, and may actually cause symptom exacerbation by drying mucous secretions. Antibiotics should be reserved for patients suspected of having acute bacterial rhinosinusitis. Current recommendations specify first-line antibiotic therapy should consist of amoxicillin. After 7 days, if a patient fails to improve clinically a broader-spectrum antibiotic such as a fluoroquinolone, trimethoprim/sulfamethoxazole, azithromycin, or amoxicillin/clavulanic acid can be tried. All of these have greater than 80% efficacy in clearing acute bacterial rhinosinusitis.

Patients experiencing multiple episodes of acute rhinosinusitis should be evaluated carefully for predisposing conditions. These may include anatomic obstruction (which may be relieved by septoplasty and/or functional endoscopic sinus surgery), underlying impairment of mucociliary clearance (such as from immotile cilia/Kartagener syndrome, or cystic fibrosis), or immune system dysfunction. Complications of acute bacterial rhinosinusitis can include orbital cellulitis and subperiosteal abscess formation, meningitis, and cavernous sinus thrombosis.

B. Chronic Rhinosinusitis

Chronic rhinosinusitis is extremely common, and affects between 2% and 15% of people in the United States. It is defined as the presence of rhinosinusitis symptoms for greater than 12 weeks (major criteria from Table 15–3) combined with evidence of inflammation. The latter can include findings of purulent mucous in the middle meatus or ethmoid region, nasal polyps or polypoid degeneration of the nasal mucosa. Radiographic findings (Figure 15–5)

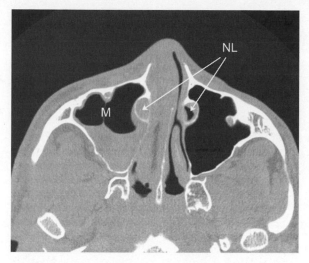

▲ **Figure 15–5.** Chronic sinusitis. In this axial plane CT of a patient with chronic sinusitis, radiographic evidence of inflammation can be seen. The right nasolacrimal duct (NL) mucosa is edematous. There is an air-fluid level and opacification of the right maxillary sinus (M).

can also document inflammation, most commonly by CT. Findings can include diffuse mucosal thickening, chronic bony remodeling, and sinus opacification.

Management of chronic rhinosinusitis is primarily by topical and systemic medication. Most otolaryngologists place chronic rhinosinusitis patients on topical nasal steroids for at least 1 month. At this time if symptoms persist, a CT scan may be useful in demonstrating any anatomic abnormalities that may be amenable to surgical correction. Surgery is aimed at removing the obstruction to natural mucous flow from the paranasal sinuses, and most patients will continue to require medication after surgery to prevent return of symptoms.

The etiology of chronic rhinosinusitis is not fully elucidated. Most otolaryngologists feel that there are several disease processes currently described together under the generic heading chronic rhinosinusitis. Tissue eosinophilia may play an important role in differentiating these groups; current molecular evidence supports this distinction. Future research will undoubtedly change our understanding of these disease processes and how they are managed.

C. Rhinitis Medicamentosa

As mentioned above, extended use of topical nasal decongestants (such as oxymetazoline) or other vasoconstrictors (such as intranasal cocaine) can lead to tachyphylaxis and mucosal dependence. The resulting severe mucosal edema, hyperemia, and nasal obstruction are termed *rhinitis*

medicamentosa. Patients will report daily topical vasoconstrictor/decongestant use, and absolute dependence on these medications for any appreciable nasal airflow. It is not unusual for patients suffering from rhinitis medicamentosa to carry their topical vasoconstrictor medication with them due to their frequent use. This is often a telltale sign of dependence. On physical examination the nasal mucosa will be thickened, erythematous and edematous, and lack appreciable decongestion on topical decongestant application.

Treatment requires complete cessation of the offending agent. Patients should be started on nasal saline lavage and nasal topical steroids. Oral decongestants and a course of oral corticosteroids may help hasten symptom resolution and increase patient compliance. Resolution usually takes 3-4 weeks, and may require much more time in the case of long-term vasoconstrictor use, or intranasal cocaine abuse.

Complications of untreated rhinitis medicamentosa include poor healing after nasal surgery, septal perforation, and formation of synechiae. For this reason, it is important to recognize and treat rhinitis medicamentosa preoperatively, before embarking on any nasal surgical treatment.

DISORDERS OF THE ORAL CAVITY AND PHARYNX

▶ Anatomy and Physiology

The oral cavity is bounded anteriorly by the vermilion border of the lips, and posteriorly by the anterior pillars of the palatine tonsils. The superior aspect of the oral cavity includes the hard and soft palate, and inferiorly includes the lingual mucosa and the anterior two-thirds of the tongue. This region of the tongue is bounded by the circumvallate papilla, which lie along the sulcus terminalis and separate the oral tongue from the base of tongue (part of the oropharynx).

The pharynx connects the nasal and oral cavities to the esophagus and larynx. It consists of three segments— the nasopharynx, the oropharynx, and the hypopharynx (Figure 15–6). The nasopharynx begins as an extension from the posterior aspect of the nasal cavity and extends from the nasal choana to the soft palate. The oropharynx extends from the soft palate to the level of the hyoid bone, and is bounded laterally by the tonsillar pillars (the palatoglossal and palatopharyngeal arches). It includes the base of tongue, lateral/posterior pharyngeal wall, and tonsillar fossae. The hypopharynx extends from the level of the hyoid bone to the inferior aspect of the cricoid cartilage, and includes the pyriform sinuses, postcricoid region, and posterior hypopharyngeal wall.

The primary functions of the oral cavity are related to chewing and swallowing (mastication and deglutition) and shaping of phonatory vibrations to produce intelligible speech. Taste buds on the dorsum of the tongue are

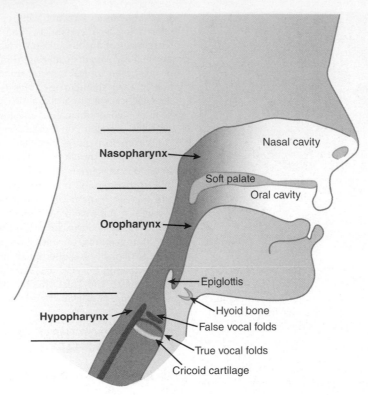

Nasal cavity

Nasopharynx

Soft palate

Oral cavity

Oropharynx

Epiglottis

Hyoid bone

Hypopharynx

False vocal folds

True vocal folds

Cricoid cartilage

▲ **Figure 15–6.** Relationship of the three sections of the pharynx. The nasopharynx extends from the nasal choanae to the soft palate. The oropharynx then extends from the soft palate to the level of the hyoid bone. The hypopharynx extends from the level of the hyoid bone to the level of the cricoid cartilage.

responsible for basic taste perception—sweet, salty, bitter, and sour. This sensory information is transmitted to the facial nerve via the chorda tympani nerve for the anterior two-thirds of the tongue. General sensation of the tongue is carried by the lingual nerve. All sensory information from the posterior one-third of the tongue is carried by the glosso-pharyngeal nerve. Complex nuances of taste are mediated by olfactory receptors in the superior-most aspect of the nasal cavity and are not directly related to the tongue or oral cavity.

The tongue has four pairs of intrinsic muscles, which interdigitate throughout the tongue. These muscles act to lengthen or shorten the tongue, curl the apex and edges, and flatten or round the dorsal surface. The intrinsic tongue muscles originate and insert within the tongue itself. Extrinsic tongue muscles (genioglossus, hyoglossus, stylo-glossus, and palatoglossus) also act to protrude, depress, elevate, and retract the tongue. All motor function of the tongue is mediated by cranial nerve XII (the hypoglossal nerve).

The act of swallowing, or deglutition, is complex and consists of three main phases—oral, pharyngeal, and esoph-ageal. The oral phase is under voluntary control, while the remaining phases proceed under reflex control. The oral phase of swallowing consists of preparation of the food bolus by mastication to soften and shape the bolus. Following this, oral transport ensues and the food bolus is transported to the posterior tongue. The anterior tongue then elevates against the hard palate, contracts and propels the bolus to the oropharynx. Simultaneously, the naso-pharynx is sealed off preventing nasal regurgitation. In the pharyngeal phase, several complex actions occur which elevate the larynx, temporarily halt respirations and protect the airway from aspiration, and relax the cricopharyngeus muscle to allow passage of the food bolus. The esophageal phase then propels the food bolus distally by means of sequential peristaltic contractions. Alteration of the timing or execution of any of these phases can result in dysphagia, or difficulty swallowing.

▶ **Urgencies and Emergencies**

A. Acute Angioedema and Ludwig Angina

Acute angioedema is characterized by localized swelling of subcutaneous and submucosal tissue of the head and neck.

The swelling may begin with mild facial involvement but may progress to involve the oral cavity, tongue, pharynx, and larynx. It is often self-limited but may present as a medical emergency. Tongue or laryngeal involvement may rapidly lead to airway obstruction and asphyxiation. Angioedema has a rapid onset and with proper medical treatment usually resolves within 24-48 hours. The underlying pathophysiology of angioedema involves vasoactive mediators such as bradykinin and histamine, causing interstitial edema through endothelial-mediated vasodilation of arterioles with subsequent capillary and venule leakage. The three major etiologies are drug-induced, hereditary, and allergic angioedema. Drug-induced and hereditary angioedema appear to be mediated by the kallikrein-kinin system while allergic angioedema appears to be mast cell-mediated.

Initial management of acute angioedema is focused on airway maintenance. Depending on clinical presentation, this may include nebulized epinephrine inhalation, intubation (either oral or transnasal fiberoptic), or tracheotomy. Due to the potentially rapid progression of this disease process, there should be a low threshold for securing an airway by the latter two methods. Many authors advocate the use of glucocorticoids (10 mg dexamethasone IV every 8 hours) combined with histamine receptor antagonists (both an H1 antagonist such as benadryl 25 mg IV every 6 hours, and an H2 antagonist such as ranitidine 50 mg IV every 6 hours) for 24 hours. Recent evidence has shown that the latter therapies may not be beneficial in drug-induced or hereditary angioedema. This should be balanced with the understanding that in clinical practice, rapid differentiation of the exact subtype of angioedema may not be as practical as empiric therapy given the relatively benign nature of these medications compared to the potentially life-threatening threat of airway obstruction.

Drug-induced angioedema has classically been associated with the use of angiotensin-converting enzyme inhibitors (ACE inhibitors), although many other medications can also (less commonly) cause this phenomenon. The incidence of angioedema secondary to ACE inhibitor use has been noted to be 0.4%-0.7%. The pathophysiology of ACE inhibitor-induced angioedema appears to be secondary to a localized increase in bradykinin levels related to the inhibition of ACE. Studies have shown that one-half of all cases of ACE inhibitor-induced angioedema occur within the first week of initiating treatment. However, some patients undergo years of ACE inhibitors therapy without incident before their first attack of acute angioedema. Treatment should begin with emergent airway maintenance with discontinuation of any possible drugs that may be inducing the edema. Other drugs with known complications of angioedema include rituximab, alteplase, fluoxetine, laronidase, lepirudin, and tacrolimus. Studies involving angiotensin II receptor antagonists (ARBs) have revealed a decreased incidence of angioedema in comparison to ACE inhibitors therapy. However, clinicians should still use caution when initiating an ARB in a patient with known ACE inhibitor-induced angioedema.

Hereditary angioedema involves a deficiency or dysfunction of C1-esterase inhibitor, which leads to increased levels of vasoactive bradykinin. It is autosomally dominant in inheritance and the defect has been mapped to chromosome 11q. Clinically, hereditary angioedema often presents with recurrent episodes of facial and oral swelling, as well as abdominal pain secondary to intestinal wall edema. Studies have revealed that certain drugs (estrogen, ACE inhibitors, ARBs), surgery, and infections may elicit acute angioedema attacks in hereditary angioedema patients. After airway maintenance has been ensured, intravenous C1-esterase inhibitor is the treatment modality of choice. The synthetic steroid danazol has also been used prophylactically to help prevent future acute episodes by increasing the functional levels of C1-esterase inhibitor.

Allergic angioedema is mast cell-mediated and histamine plays the major role in its pathophysiology. In contrast to drug-induced and hereditary angioedema, skin changes including urticaria and pruritis are commonly seen in allergic angioedema. Clinically, the pruritic wheals are spread by scratching and lesions are usually limited to the lips and periorbital areas and less commonly the extremities and genitalia. This form of angioedema is frequently seen in patients who also suffer from atopic dermatitis, allergic rhinitis, and asthma. Triggers of acute attacks of allergic angioedema include certain drugs, infections, food, and plant products.

Ludwig angina is an uncommon life threatening condition characterized by cellulitis involving the submental, sublingual, and submandibular spaces. The source of the infection is odontogenic and spreads rapidly. The infection is usually polymicrobial with aerobic and anaerobic gram-positive cocci and gram-negative rods. Prior to antibiotics the mortality rate exceeded 50%. Clinically, patients present with painful neck swelling and edema of the floor of mouth often leading to elevation and displacement of the tongue. Patients will have a prominent "hot potato" voice and palpation of the floor of mouth reveals woody edema. The most common cause of death in these patients is airway compromise, and therefore, primary treatment should be centered on airway maintenance with early involvement of anesthesiology and otolaryngology physicians. Intubation is often anatomically difficult and tracheotomy under local anesthesia is often the preferred method of ensuring a patent airway. Recent case studies have shown the benefit of intravenous dexamethasone and nebulized epinephrine to aid with temporizing the airway and transnasal intubation. Airway observation in the intensive care unit may be an option for less severe cases. After the airway has been secured, proper systemic antibiotic therapy should be initiated immediately followed by incision and drainage for most cases. Major complications include extension of the infection posteriorly to involve the parapharyngeal and retropharyngeal spaces as well as the superior mediastinum. The diagnosis is clinical, but CT may be used to assess the retropharyngeal extension of the infection.

B. Peritonsillar Abscess

Peritonsillar abscess (PTA) is a common infection of the peritonsillar space between the palatine tonsil, tonsillar pillars, and the superior pharyngeal constrictor muscle. Its prevalence in the United Stated has been estimated at 30 per 100,000 people annually. The infection is suppurative in nature and thought to be secondary to either extension of adjacent acute tonsillitis or obstruction of Weber glands (minor salivary glands) at the tonsillar pole. PTA is seen in both children and adults. The typical patient presents complaining of a 4- to 5-day history of sore throat and fever, with worsening trismus, odynophagia, dysphagia, and inability to tolerate secretions. PTA should be managed acutely, as the infection may progress and spread to the deep neck tissue and compromise the airway.

The gold standard in diagnosis of PTA is physical examination, which reveals bulging soft tissue, tonsillar erythema and exudate, and possible uvular deviation. Needle aspiration or incision and drainage confirms the diagnosis. Recent studies have revealed the benefit of intraoral ultrasound in the diagnosis of PTA. CT may be necessary in patients with severe trismus or young uncooperative patients and can aid in differentiating PTA from retropharyngeal abscess.

The management of PTA is dependent on the patient characteristics. Needle aspiration can be performed quickly, is relatively safe, and can be both diagnostic and therapeutic. Incision and drainage should only be performed by physicians with an understanding of the relevant pharyngeal anatomy, as multiple vital structures including cranial nerves and the carotid artery potentially lie within the surgical field. In cooperative adults, it can usually be performed using local anesthesia but patients with severe trismus may require general anesthesia. In our practice (for adult patients), pre-procedure administration of 900 mg clindamycin, 10 mg dexamethasone, IV fluid hydration, and IV morphine for analgesia can greatly facilitate the procedure by reducing trismus and promoting patient comfort and cooperation. After instillation of local anesthetic, a needle aspiration can be used to confirm the site of incision. A limited mucosal incision is made with a scalpel, taking care not to penetrate the underlying muscular layer. Blunt dissection is then used to penetrate the abscess cavity. Oral suction should be in place before penetration of the abscess cavity to prevent possible aspiration of purulence. Studies have shown both needle aspiration and incision and drainage to be greater than 90% effective but both carry a 10%-15% risk of recurrent PTA. The pediatric patient usually will not tolerate either needle aspiration or incision and drainage under local anesthesia and general anesthesia is often necessary.

Antibiotic therapy against *Streptococcus pyogenes* and oral anaerobes with either penicillin or clindamycin should follow abscess drainage. Most patients with PTA can be treated as outpatients.

Emergent tonsillectomy in the setting of acute infection ("Quincy tonsillectomy") is usually reserved for cases of PTA that are not successfully drained by simple incision and drainage. While some authors advocate this as a first-line therapeutic option, the increased operative difficulty secondary to acute inflammation, and increased incidence of postoperative hemorrhage make this a less attractive option. It requires general anesthesia and most otolaryngologists would advocate overnight hospitalization postoperatively for observation.

If needle aspiration or incision and drainage of a PTA is performed, it is important to counsel the patient that future risk of PTA is increased. Many otolaryngologists therefore recommend an elective tonsillectomy be performed 2-3 months following a PTA.

C. Deep Neck Space Infections

Although greatly decreased in incidence since the advent of modern antibiotics, deep neck space infections remain a potentially life-threatening condition and require acute recognition and treatment. The source of deep neck space infection is most commonly odontogenic. Other sources of infection include adjacent tonsillar, upper respiratory and salivary infections as well as instrumentation and foreign bodies. These infections are usually polymicrobial, composed predominantly of anaerobes mixed with various streptococcal and staphylococcal species. Drug-resistant bacteria are commonly seen in intravenous drug users who present with deep neck space infections secondary to needle injection disruption of the cervical fascia. Presenting symptoms depend on the exact location of the abscess, but patients commonly present with fever, painful sore throat, decreased neck range of motion, dysphagia, and odynophagia. Physical examination can reveal trismus, a toxic appearance with facial and neck edema, cervical lymphadenopathy, and purulent oral secretions. It is not uncommon for patients to present several days after being discharged on antibiotics for a less severe, local infection. It is important to note that patients on antibiotic or immunosuppression therapy may have more subtle signs of infection and systemic toxicity may be masked.

A thorough understanding of the anatomy of the cervical fascia and deep spaces of neck is paramount in diagnosing and managing these rapidly spreading infections. The cervical fascia is divided into two layers, the superficial cervical fascia and the deep cervical fascia. The deep cervical fascia is further divided into three separate layers—superficial layer of deep cervical fascia, middle layer of deep cervical fascia, and deep layer of deep cervical fascia.

Furthermore, the middle layer of deep cervical fascia is subdivided into muscular and visceral divisions and the deep layer of deep cervical fascia is subdivided into alar and prevertebral layers.

These divisions of the deep cervical fascia separate the neck into numerous potential spaces, which may harbor these life-threatening infections. One easy way of categorizing these spaces is by their relationship to the hyoid bone. Potential spaces that exist entirely above the hyoid bone include the submandibular space and the parapharyngeal space. The pretracheal space exists entirely below the hyoid bone. The prevertebral space, danger space, and retropharyngeal space extend along the entire length of the neck.

Parapharyngeal abscess must be differentiated from PTA, as the former requires external drainage via the submaxillary fossa while the latter is best drained intraorally. Retropharyngeal abscesses are most commonly seen in children and are located between the visceral layer of the middle layer of deep cervical fascia and the alar division of the deep layer of deep cervical fascia. Because of the smaller caliber airway in children, retropharyngeal abscess represents a potential source of airway obstruction and should be managed accordingly. The danger space is the region between the alar and prevertebral layers of the deep cervical fascia, which extends from the base of the skull to the diaphragm. Infection of the danger space usually arises from contiguous spread from retropharyngeal, prevertebral, or pharyngo-maxillary infections. The lack of definitive anatomic barriers in the danger space offers very little resistance to spread of infection. The prevertebral space is directly posterior to the danger space between the prevertebral division of deep cervical fascia and the paravertebral fascia. Infection of prevertebral space is usually secondary to penetrating trauma or tuberculosis.

Lateral and anteroposterior neck films have traditionally been used to help localize an abscess, although this has now largely been replaced by CT. Recent studies have shown a potential benefit of MRI in delineating soft tissue and vascular spread of infection, although the time required to obtain MRI imaging makes its use of questionable value. Deep neck space infections can progress rapidly and patients usually require hospitalization under close supervision.

Initial treatment should focuses on an evaluation of need for securing an airway with either endotracheal intubation or tracheotomy. Once airway patency has been verified or secured, needle aspiration can sometimes be performed (in the case of easily accessible abscesses) to obtain culture and gram stain. Intravenous antibiotics are started immediately and should cover both aerobic and anaerobic organisms. Ampicillin-sulbactum or clindamycin are commonly used. If methicillin-resistant *Staphylococcus aureus* is suspected, vancomycin should also be initiated. If the patient does not improve clinically on antibiotic therapy after 48 hours, open surgical drainage of the abscess may be necessary.

Major complications of deep neck space infections include mediastinitis, osteomyelitis, Horner syndrome, and cranial nerve deficits. Involvement of the carotid sheath may also lead to suppurative jugular thrombophlebitis (Lemierre syndrome). Early diagnosis and proper treatment may help limit these serious complications.

▶ Disorders and Diseases

A. Oral Cavity Lesions

Inspection and palpation of the oral cavity is an essential part of the head and neck examination. There are numerous lesions that may affect the oral cavity and this review focuses on those which may predispose patients to oral cavity neoplasms. Approximately half of all head and neck cancers occur in the oral cavity.

Leukoplakia is actually a descriptive term rather than a true pathologic term. It represents an asymptomatic white plaque that cannot be scraped off. It is frequently found on the oral and buccal mucosa as well as the tongue. Its prevalence has been estimated from 1% to 5% of the population. Some studies have linked leukoplakia to tobacco use although the true etiology is still uncertain. Leukoplakia represents the clinically evident result of hyperplastic epithelial growth. Many authors recommend a short 1-2 week trial of oral topical steroid preparation (kenalog in orobase) for initial management. Leukoplakia is associated with a malignant transformation rate of approximately 5%, and persistent lesions should be biopsied to assess for premalignant dysplasia or malignancy. The rates of dysplasia are highest for lesions found on the floor of the mouth, tongue, and lower lip. Treatment is aimed at preventing malignant transformation to oral cavity squamous cell carcinoma (OCSCC). Surgical excision, KTP laser, and CO_2 laser excision have all been shown to be effective. Recent studies have also revealed potential efficacy of medical treatment with both topical bleomycin in dimethyl sulfoxide and retinoid compounds.

Erythroplakia is categorized as a nonhomogenous leukoplakia and is described as a velvety red plaque that cannot be removed. It is found in similar regions of the oral cavity as leukoplakia and is also usually asymptomatic at presentation. It is less common than traditional homogenous white leukoplakia with prevalence estimated at 0.2%-0.8%. However, it boasts a higher degree of premalignant dysplasia than leukoplakia, with over half of cases having *in situ* or overtly invasive squamous cell carcinoma on histologic examination.

Lichen planus is a common dermatologic lesion that may present in the oral cavity. The skin lesions are classically described as pruritic, planar, purple, polygonal papules, while the oral lesions have several different phenotypic subtypes. Reticular, plaque-like, atrophic, erosive, and bullous forms have all been described in the literature. The oral lesions have a questionable capacity for malignant transformation. The data is controversial but one study has estimated the rate of malignant transformation to OCSCC between 1% and 5%. The lesions require biopsy to confirm the diagnosis. Treatment includes vigorous oral hygiene, topical steroids, and immunosuppressive agents.

B. Sialadenitis and Sialothithiasis

There are several nonneoplastic and inflammatory conditions that may affect the major and minor salivary glands. Infection of the salivary glands may be either viral or bacterial in etiology. Viral sialadenitis is most commonly secondary to mumps, which presents with a flu-like prodrome followed by parotid gland swelling. Mumps normally affects children and may be complicated by orchitis, oophoritis, aseptic meningitis, and encephalitis. The incidence of mumps has declined significantly since routine vaccination has been instituted. Other viruses known to cause sialadenitis include cytomegalovirus, coxsackievirus A and B, echovirus, Epstein-Barr virus, and influenza A.

Bacterial sialadenitis may be acute or chronic. Acute suppurative sialadenitis occurs most commonly in dehydrated patients who are postoperative, elderly, or those on diuretic therapy. The parotid gland is affected in the majority of cases secondary to the diminished bacteriostatic activity of its serous saliva. Salivary stasis, ductal obstruction, and decreased saliva production appear to be predisposing conditions to acute sialadenitis. Patients usually present with fever, systemic toxicity, and tender swelling and enlargement of the affected glands. The most common organism isolated is *S aureus*, though culture may reveal a polymicrobial infection with both aerobic and anaerobic organisms. Treatment involves ample hydration, warm facial compresses, sialogogues (such as lemon wedges) to stimulate saliva secretion in the affected gland. Antibiotics targeted against *S aureus* should be started immediately and continued for 7-10 days. CT may be necessary to rule out abscess formation or stone (sialolithiasis) in patients who do not improve clinically after several days of appropriate therapy.

Sialolithiasis may occur in the setting of acute or chronic sialadenitis or it may be an incidental finding on routine imaging studies. Salivary calculi affect males more than females and are seen most frequently between ages 30 and 60. In contrast to sialadenitis, sialolithiasis preferentially affects the submandibular glands because of their alkaline, high calcium, mucus-rich environment. Large, solitary, radio-opaque stones are usually found in the submandibular glands, while the parotid glands are more likely to have multiple smaller, radiolucent stones. Calculus formation is believed to be secondary to partial obstruction of the salivary duct combined with calcium-rich stagnant saliva. Salts composed of calcium phosphate, magnesium, ammonium, and carbonate precipitate in this environment. Contributing factors to the development of salivary calculi include underlying acute or chronic sialadenitis, dehydration, and

anticholinergic medications. Uric acid salivary calculi may also be seen in the setting of gout.

Patients with sialolithiasis frequently present with pain and swelling of the affected gland, although many patients have asymptomatic calculi discovered incidentally. Eating usually exacerbates the pain. Physical examination may reveal the location of the calculi by simple palpation. Obstruction of the flow of saliva can be analyzed by massaging the gland. It is important to note that stones are more commonly found in the salivary ductal structures rather than their associated glands. CT is the preferred method of imaging if sialolithiasis is suspected but a calculus is unable to be palpated on physical examination. CT has a 10-fold greater sensitivity than plain films in detecting salivary calculi. Ultrasound may also have benefit in locating calculi when CT is unavailable. Sialography is no longer routinely used and is contraindicated in patients with acute sialadenitis.

Treatment of sialolithiasis should begin conservatively with hydration, salivary gland massage, heating pads applied to the affected gland, and sialogogues. Anticholinergic medications should be discontinued and antibiotics should be initiated if there is concern for acute suppurative sialadenitis. There are several options for more invasive therapy for patients who do not respond to conservative management. Transoral removal of submandibular stones, sialadenectomy, lithotripsy, wire-basket removal, and sialoendoscopy have all been shown to be effective in the appropriate patient.

C. Acute and Chronic (Recurrent) Tonsillitis

Tonsillitis is one of the most common problems encountered by the otolaryngologist. In general, tonsillitis refers to inflammation of the palatine tonsils located on the lateral walls of the oropharynx between the palatoglossal and palatopharyngeal folds. The pharyngeal tonsils or adenoids, while part of Waldeyer's ring of lymphatic tissue are anatomically separate from the palatine tonsils. The adenoids are located on the posterior wall of the nasopharynx in close proximity to the eustachian tube opening.

Acute tonsillitis is primarily a pediatric disease that tends to affect children aged 5-15. It is most commonly caused by group A beta-hemolytic streptococcal species, although anaerobes, *Haemophilus influenzae*, and viruses can also be causative agents. Patients usually present with fever, painful sore throat, halitosis, and dysphagia. It is important to note the distinction in clinical presentation between acute tonsillitis, viral pharyngitis, and infectious mononucleosis (caused by the Epstein-Barr virus). Viral pharyngitis commonly presents with a triad of cough, coryza, and conjunctivitis, while patients with mononucleosis typically present with anterior and posterior cervical lymphadenopathy, odynophagia, and a grayish tonsillar exudate. On physical examination, the acute tonsillitis patient has erythematous tonsils, purulent tonsillar exudate, and anterior cervical lymphade-nopathy.

Tonsillar hyperplasia is measured in the medial-to-lateral plane of the oropharynx and helps in the assessment of upper airway obstruction. They are traditionally rated on a 1–4 scale, with 1+ being confined below the level of the tonsillar pillars, 2+ at the pillars, 3+ extending past the pillars, and 4+ meeting in the midline. Tonsillar hyper-trophy in the pediatric population may predispose to the development of sleep-disordered breathing. Patients typi-cally present with heroic snoring, voice changes, observed episodes of sleep apnea, and daytime somnolence. In these cases, elective tonsillectomy (usually combined with adenoidectomy) can often provide resolution of obstruc-tive symptoms.

The diagnosis of acute tonsillitis is clinical although many practitioners rely on a positive streptococcal test or culture. The mainstay in treatment of acute tonsillitis continues to be a 7-10 day course of penicillin or a comparable cephalospo-rin. However, it is now estimated that failure with penicillin therapy occurs in up to 30% of cases. Following up culture results and adjusting the antibiotic therapy has therefore become an important step in management. Complications from acute tonsillitis include the formation of PTA and neck abscess formation. Antibiotic use has greatly decreased the incidence of rare systemic complications like poststrepto-coccal glomerulonephritis and rheumatic fever.

Many patients have a solitary episode of acute tonsillitis, which responds favorably to antibiotic treatment, while some patients have recurrent acute tonsillitis with mul-tiple infections over the course of years. Chronic tonsillitis is a state of persistent tonsillar inflammation for greater than 3 months following an episode of acute infection. It is characterized by chronic sore throat and odynophagia with tonsillar enlargement, tonsillolithic debris, and cervi-cal lymphadenitis present on physical examination. Recent studies have suggested that polymicrobial infections, drug-resistant organisms, *H influenzae*, *S aureus*, anaerobes, and actinomycetes may all play a role in chronic tonsillar disease. Treatment of chronic tonsillitis, therefore, should begin with the use of broader spectrum antibiotics like amoxicillin-clavulanate or clindamycin, which may target these offending organisms.

The critical question in the treatment of both acute and chronic tonsillitis is whether or not to perform a tonsillec-tomy. Medical management with antibiotics is always the first-line therapy for acute tonsillitis. Tonsillectomy for acute episodes (also known as "Quincy tonsillectomy") is usually considered only when complications such as deep neck-space abscess or acute airway obstruction are concurrently present. Tonsillectomy is generally performed for patients with recurrent acute tonsillitis, defined as seven episodes within 1 year, five episodes each year for the past 2 years, or three episodes per year for 3 successive years.

D. Obstructive Sleep Apnea

Obstructive sleep apnea is an intrinsic dyssomnia that affects roughly 15-20 million people in the United States. It is classi-cally described as the presence of hypopneic episodes, apneic episodes, and respiratory effort related arousals that occur during sleep. An apneic event requires 10 or more seconds of cessation of airflow, followed by arousal with restoration of normal ventilation. The definition of hypopnea varies between sleep laboratories, but generally refers to an epi-sode of decreased airflow (>50% reduction) for greater than 10 seconds, associated with decreased oxygen saturation or arousal. Patients usually present with nighttime snoring, daytime hypersomnolence, irritability, morning headaches, cognitive impairment, and often witnessed apneic events with cessation of airflow followed by choking or gasping. When taking a history, it is important to confer with the patient's bed partner, as the patient may be unaware of his/her nighttime symptoms. Cardiovascular disease, hyper-tension, metabolic dysfunction, respiratory failure, and cor pulmonale are among the serious long-term effects of obstructive sleep apnea.

The pathophysiology of obstructive sleep apnea appears to be a combination of upper airway collapse and decreased neural output from the respiratory center in the brainstem. During normal inspiration, the pharyngeal muscles are stim-ulated via a central nervous system reflex pathway to help maintain pharyngeal airway patency. During sleep, however, these neural reflexes are attenuated and the airway becomes more susceptible to collapse. Patients who are predisposed to airway obstruction due to anatomic reasons are at high risk for developing obstructive sleep apnea. Documented anatomic risk factors for obstructive sleep apnea include macroglossia, adenotonsillar hypertrophy, elongation of the soft palate, and retrognathia.

Obstructive sleep apnea is more common in men and the overall incidence appears to increase with age. The most significant risk factor is obesity and the recent increase in prevalence is thought to relate to the current obesity epidemic. Other known risk factors include nasal obstruc-tion, smoking, diabetes mellitus, alcohol consumption, and the previously mentioned anatomic abnormalities. Physical examination may reveal obesity with an increased neck cir-cumference. A thorough head and neck examination should be performed to fully assess airway patency. Oral cavity examination may reveal tonsillar hyperplasia. The nasal cavity and nasopharynx should be examined using a flexible fiberoptic endoscope to rule out nasal obstruction secondary to deviated septum, nasal polyps, or turbinate hyperplasia. The modified Müller maneuver should be performed to assess for site of upper airway collapse during inspiration. Patients are asked to inspire against a closed mouth while their nose is pinched shut, thus creating a column of nega-tive pressure within the upper airway. The airway at the level of the soft palate, lateral pharyngeal wall, and base of tongue are then observed for luminal collapse and graded on a 1-3 scale.

Polysomnography remains the gold standard in diagnosing obstructive sleep apnea, which can be defined by either the apnea-hypopnea index (AHI) or the respiratory disturbance index (RDI). The AHI includes the number of hypopneas and apneas which occur per hour of sleep, while the RDI is the number of hypopneas, apneas, and respiratory effort related arousals per hour of sleep. The generally accepted guidelines for diagnosis of obstructive sleep apnea are an AHI of 15 or greater in an asymptomatic patient or an AHI of greater than 5 in a symptomatic patient. Imaging studies are usually not required to diagnose obstructive sleep apnea, although they may help assess for upper airway anatomic abnormalities.

Treatment of obstructive sleep apnea should begin with the identification and prevention of risk factors. Behavior modifications such as weight loss, smoking and alcohol cessation, and discontinuation of any CNS depressants may help improve the patient's apneic index. Safety precautions related to daytime hypersomnolence need to be discussed for high-risk patients like pilots and commercial truck drivers.

Continuous positive airway pressure (CPAP) is considered first-line therapy after behavioral modifications. The positive pressure helps keep the airway patent and has been shown to be highly effective in reducing obstructive sleep apnea symptoms. Some patients experience difficulty tolerating CPAP therapy. Breathing against the positive pressure airflow can be difficult to adjust to, and this must be considered when treating the obstructive sleep apnea patient. Bi-level positive airway pressure (BiPAP) is another system that employs a higher inspiratory pressure with a lower expiratory pressure to allow for easier expiration. There are numerous oral appliances, which may help adjust the airway during sleep to improve patency, although studies have shown these appliances to be less effective than CPAP in improving the apneic index.

Several surgical options are available for patients who do not respond well to initial treatment. Routine adenoidectomy and tonsillectomy has been shown to be effective in pediatric patients with isolated adenotonsillar hypertrophy contributing to their obstructive sleep apnea symptoms. For adult patients, more extensive surgery is usually required. Uvulopalatopharyngoplasty (UP3) is the first-line surgical therapy in which the uvula, a small amount of soft palate, and the palatine tonsils are removed. The concept of "multi-level sleep surgery" is important, as UP3 alone is associated with a significant (>50%) failure rate. Most commonly UP3 is combined with additional procedures to address other areas of obstruction. Septoplasty and inferior turbinate reduction can improve nasal airflow. The tongue base can be advanced by suture suspension, hyoid suspension, or genioglossus advancement. Other more invasive surgical interventions include maxillomandibular advancement. Some authors have advocated less-invasive therapy including palatal stiffening implants and radiofrequency ablation, but the long-term data are lacking. Life-threatening obstructive sleep apnea that does not respond to CPAP/BiPAP or surgical intervention may require permanent tracheostomy. A repeat polysomnogram should be performed in surgical patients 1-3 months postoperatively to monitor for improvements.

DISORDERS OF THE LARYNX AND TRACHEA

▶ Anatomy and Physiology

The anatomy of the larynx (Figures 15–7 and 15–8) is best understood in the context of its function. The primary function of the larynx is to protect the airway from aspiration during swallowing. The epiglottis and aryepiglottic folds help direct food and liquids laterally into the pyriform sinuses and away from the midline laryngeal inlet. The paired arytenoid cartilages act as attachment points for most of the intrinsic muscles of the larynx, serving to move the vocal folds together (adduction) and apart (abduction). The false vocal folds and true vocal folds adduct to prevent entry of food or liquids into the airway.

The larynx also functions in respiration. Owing to reflex pathways in the brainstem, the glottis opens just prior to inspiration. Other laryngeal reflexes respond to subglottic

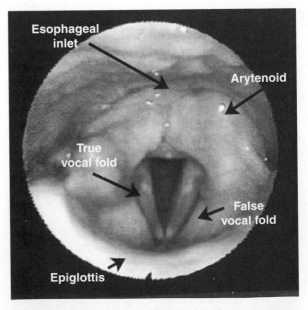

▲ **Figure 15–7.** Internal anatomy of the larynx as seen on endoscopy.

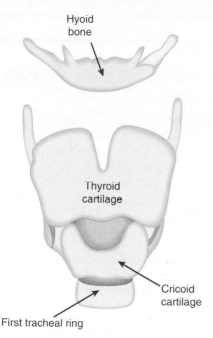

Hyoid
bone

Thyroid
cartilage

Cricoid
cartilage

First tracheal ring

▲ **Figure 15–8.** Cartilaginous and bony laryngeal framework.

pressure and hypercapnea. Additionally, initiation of swallowing causes a reflex period of involuntary apnea.

Phonation is the most uniquely human of the three functions of the larynx. At its most basic description, the glottic larynx produces a fundamental tone by the vibration of the free edge of the true vocal folds. This vibration is due to passive vibration of the vocal folds from air moving past the opposed free edges. Changing the tension within the vocal fold changes the pitch at which the vocal fold vibrates.

Several cartilages comprise the framework of the larynx (Figure 15–8). The thyroid cartilage is the largest laryngeal cartilage. This shield-shaped cartilage is responsible for the anterior neck prominence, sometimes called the "Adam's apple" in lay terminology, and it provides protection to the internal components of the larynx. The cricoid cartilage lies inferior to the thyroid cartilage and serves as the major support for the larynx. It is the only complete cartilaginous ring within the upper airway. Internally, the paired arytenoid cartilages articulate with the cricoid cartilage, and attach to the vocal folds. Movement of the arytenoids results in abduction or adduction of the vocal folds. The epiglottis is a flexible cartilage located above the larynx. It is not involved in structural support of the larynx, but serves to assist in protecting the airway during deglutition (swallowing).

Innervation to the larynx is provided by the vagus nerve (cranial nerve X). The vagus nerve originates from three nuclei located within the medulla—the nucleus ambiguous,

the dorsal nucleus, and the solitary tract nucleus. All motor fibers (and thus laryngeal motor innervation) originate from the nucleus ambiguous. The dorsal (parasympathetic) nucleus is the origination for efferents to involuntary muscles of the bronchi, esophagus, heart, stomach, and intestine. Sensory innervation from the pharynx, larynx, and esophagus terminates in the solitary tract nucleus. The vagus nerve exits the skull base through the jugular foramen. It descends in the neck behind the jugular vein and carotid artery and sends pharyngeal branches to the muscles of the pharynx and soft palate. The superior laryngeal nerve arises directly from the vagus, and has an internal and external branch. The internal superior laryngeal nerve enters the larynx through the thyrohyoid membrane and supplies sensation to the larynx above the true vocal cords. The external superior laryngeal nerve innervates the cricothyroid muscle, the only muscle of the larynx not innervated by the recurrent laryngeal nerve. The right recurrent laryngeal nerve arises from the vagus and loops around the subclavian artery. The left recurrent laryngeal nerve arises more distally in the thorax, and loops around the aortic arch. Both recurrent laryngeal nerves then ascend in the tracheo-esophageal grooves, and enter the larynx near the cricothyroid joint. The recurrent laryngeal nerves provide motor innervation to all of the intrinsic muscles of the larynx except the cricothyroid. A summary of the laryngeal muscles is provided in Table 15–4.

▶ Urgencies and Emergencies

A. Pediatric Airway Obstruction

The rapid and accurate evaluation of a child in respiratory distress is one of the most critical skills an otolaryngologist must master. Noisy breathing and respiratory distress have multiple etiologies, and differentiation between acute emergencies and chronic conditions is essential. An important point to learn early on is that not all noisy breathing is stridor.

True stridor may represent an impending airway failure, and thus must be distinguished from other upper airway noises that are sometimes mistakenly referred to as "stridor." Airway obstruction at the level of the nasopharynx produces snoring sounds, or stertor. Tracheobronchitis can produce a wheezy, barking cough characteristic of croup. Asthma, tracheobronchial foreign bodies, and bronchomalacia can produce wheezing. "Stridor" specifically refers to the noise that is produced by air movement through a partially obstructed airway. Inspiratory stridor usually signifies an obstruction above the level of the vocal cords, while expiratory stridor most often occurs with subglottic obstruction. Biphasic stridor usually signifies an obstruction at the level of the vocal cords or subglottis.

The immediate concern in evaluating a child with stridor is verifying or establishing a stable airway. The initial evaluation should consist of non-invasive examination to

Table 15–4. Major muscles of the larynx.

Muscle	Function	Innervation	Key Point
Posterior cricoarytenoid	Abducts vocal folds, tenses vocal folds	Recurrent laryngeal nerve	ONLY abductor of vocal folds
Lateral cricoarytenoid	Adducts true vocal folds	Recurrent laryngeal nerve	
Interarytenoid	Adducts posterior glottis	Recurrent laryngeal nerve	ONLY laryngeal muscle receiving bilateral innervation
Oblique arytenoids	Closes laryngeal inlet during swallowing	Recurrent laryngeal nerve	
Thyroarytenoid	Adducts, tenses vocal fold	Recurrent laryngeal nerve	
Cricothyroid	Increase vocal fold tension, especially at higher pitches	External branch of superior laryngeal nerve	ONLY muscle not innervated by recurrent laryngeal nerve

avoid exacerbating a potentially unstable airway. If the child is in acute respiratory distress, evaluations such as flexible fiberoptic laryngoscopy should not routinely be performed.

A careful history should be obtained, including the duration of the stridor and relationship to feedings. Parents should be questioned about any change in symptoms with position changes. Presence of any birth or intrauterine complications, history of intubation, as well as congenital anomalies should be determined.

If the child is not in acute distress, flexible fiberoptic laryngoscopy may provide valuable diagnostic information. This can be done with the child awake and restrained, or under general anesthesia with spontaneous ventilations. This allows determination of nasopharyngeal and supraglottic anatomy, as well as vocal cord motion. If available, the examination should be recorded to allow playback and review, as real-time examination can be problematic in an often-uncooperative child.

Other investigations should be based on the presence of suggestive symptoms. Swallowing function is often impaired in children with stridor, and should be evaluated. Vascular rings may produce extrinsic compression of the esophagus and trachea leading to stridor, feeding difficulties and failure to thrive. An altered, weak, or absent cry from birth can suggest neurologic impairment. Recurrent pneumonia or excessive cough with feeding may be present with vocal cord impairment, severe reflux, or tracheoesophageal fistula.

One of the most common causes of pediatric stridor is laryngotracheobronchitis, or croup. This is an acute viral illness, most commonly caused by the parainfluenza virus. The typical patient is an infant or young child with low-grade fever, seal-like barking cough, and occasionally biphasic stridor. The classic radiographic finding is a "steeple" sign visible on AP views, indicative of the characteristic narrowed subglottic airway from edema. The typical course for most patients is resolution over several days and few patients require hospitalization. Signs of respiratory distress including tachypnea, retractions, and cyanosis may necessitate closer observation such as hospitalization. For these more severe cases, treatment with humidified air, nebulized racemic epinephrine, and systemic steroids may be indicated. Manipulation of the airway may exacerbate the clinical situation, and should be avoided unless clearly indicated.

Epiglottitis is fortunately becoming vanishingly rare in most industrialized countries, owing to nearly universal vaccination of children against *H influenzae* type B. If recognized and managed appropriately (with aggressive airway control) outcomes are usually excellent. If managed conservatively, epiglottitis is associated with up to 6%-10% mortality. Patients present with high fever, drooling, and odynophagia and are usually toxic in appearance. Of note, epiglottitis tends to progress quite rapidly; patients can decompensate clinically in a matter of hours. The characteristic position naturally assumed by patients with epiglottitis is the leaning forward position, to maximize their marginal airway opening. Even oral cavity examination with a tongue blade can precipitate an airway crisis; therefore evaluation and treatment ideally consists of immediate control of the airway in the operating room under general inhalational anesthesia. A cherry-red epiglottis will be visible on endoscopic examination. Pharyngeal and blood cultures should be obtained, and the child started on broad spectrum IV antibiotics such as ceftriaxone. Once definitive identification of the culprit organism is made antibiotic selection can be narrowed appropriately. Children are left intubated until air leak around the endotracheal tube is evident.

Chronic pediatric stridor is most often due to laryngomalacia. Parents will usually report onset of symptoms shortly after birth. It often worsens initially, but in the vast majority of cases resolves without the need for intervention, usually by 12-18 months. A variety of factors have been hypothesized to contribute to laryngomalacia including neurologic, muscular, and reflux-induced inflammation. The stridor is worsened while crying or in an excited state, and is usually

Table 15–5. Summary of the Cotton grading system for subglottic stenosis.

Grades	Degree of Subglottic Obstruction
Grade 1	Less than 50% obstruction
Grade 2	50%-70% obstruction
Grade 3	71%-99% obstruction
Grade 4	100% obstruction

relieved by placement in the prone position. Flexible fiber-optic laryngoscopy reveals collapse of floppy supraglottic structures such as the epiglottis and aryepiglottic folds. There is a strong association of laryngomalacia with reflux, and presumptive treatment with an acid blocking medication (such as ranitidine) may be beneficial. Surgical treatment of the supraglottis is reserved for severe cases such as patients with cyanosis or failure to thrive. The most common procedure is aryepiglottiplasty, where cold knife or carbon dioxide laser is used to excise redundant mucosa over the arytenoid cartilages. Rarely, tracheostomy may be necessary.

Subglottic stenosis is the second most common cause of chronic pediatric stridor. Causes include both congenital stenosis, and acquired (most often from prolonged intubation). Typically, patients have recurrent "croup" and biphasic stridor. If present in older children, the patient may only become symptomatic periodically, in association with upper respiratory tract infections. Diagnosis requires endoscopic evaluation, and can be defined as a subglottic airway diameter of less than 4 mm in full-term infants and less than 3 mm in premature infants. Pediatric subglottic stenosis is traditionally graded according to the Cotton scale (Table 15–5). Tracheotomy may be required in moderate to severe cases. Treatment of subglottic stenosis can consist of tracheal dilatation (either by rigid serial dilation or controlled radial expansion balloon), debridement by microdebrider or carbon dioxide laser, cricoid split, or laryngotracheoplasty.

B. Foreign Body Aspiration

Airway foreign body typically involves children between 1 and 4 years of age, but can occur in any age group. Children in this age range tend to place objects in their mouths and lack molars for grinding of food. Objects can range from peanuts (most common) to coins, marbles, and toy products. Adult foreign body aspiration is usually associated with food, typically meat. Foreign body aspiration is potentially life threatening and it is recognized as the fifth most common cause of unintentional-injury related mortality in the United States. Pharyngeal foreign body (most

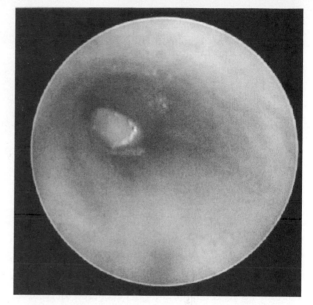

▲ **Figure 15–9.** Airway foreign body in a 4 year old. The patient in question had a history of brief choking while eating dinner three nights earlier, followed by intermittent nonproductive cough. He had a normal chest x-ray and slight wheezing heard on one side only. On rigid bronchoscopy, a soft green bean was found in a right distal bronchus.

commonly in the vallecula) represents a potential impending airway foreign body, and should be treated as such.

The clinical presentation of patients with airway foreign body depends on the anatomic location. Patients with pharyngeal or hypopharyngeal foreign bodies typically present with dysphagia, odynophagia, and occasionally drooling from inability to tolerate secretions. If large objects become lodged in the larynx, patients may present with pain, dysphonia, inspiratory stridor, and dyspnea. Tracheal foreign bodies produce both inspiratory and expiratory stridor. Distally located foreign bodies (Figure 15–9) often lodge in the right bronchus (especially in adults). This is due to the angles at which the left and right mainstem bronchi branch off the trachea, with the right being a less acute angle. Distal foreign bodies typically produce unilateral wheezing and decreased breath sounds. A history of acute choking episode is very common and is 76%-92% sensitive in diagnosing foreign body aspiration.

Acute management of airway foreign body is dictated by patient condition. In a conscious patient who is able to exchange air and cough, an attempt at foreign body removal should not be made immediately. Unconscious patients, or victims unable to cough or move air require immediate intervention. If the means for performing a cricothyrotomy or tracheotomy are not available, the Heimlich maneuver can be performed as three manual abdominal thrusts to compress the lungs and potentially produce enough airway pressure to dislodge the foreign body. For patients without impending loss of airway, anteroposterior and lateral radiographs of the airway including larynx and chest can be helpful. While only radio-opaque foreign bodies can be visualized, radiographs may demonstrate obstructive emphysema, atelectasis, or consolidation. Additionally, they can provide a baseline study for future comparison.

Definitive removal of an airway foreign body requires general anesthesia, and direct laryngoscopy. Distally located foreign bodies are best addressed with rigid bronchoscopy for removal. A clear history consistent with aspiration often should prompt operative evaluation, even if specific symptoms (stridor, unilateral wheezing, decreased breath sounds) are lacking, as these may be absent in up to 40% of cases. Suspected nut aspiration (common in children) should be treated aggressively. Local tissue reactions to the nut oils and proteins are common, and can be robust. Post removal, patients with peanut aspiration may require intensive care unit observation and ventilatory support while the inflammatory reaction resolves.

C. Laryngeal Trauma

Laryngeal trauma is rare, representing 1 out of every 14,000-42,000 emergency room visits. Quick recognition of laryngeal trauma is essential as it can rapidly lead to death. Up to one-third of laryngeal trauma victims die prior to arrival to a hospital setting.

Laryngeal trauma can be classified as blunt or penetrating. Blunt laryngeal trauma results from crushing of the laryngeal framework against the cervical spine, and usually results from motor vehicle accidents. Other common etiologies include strangulation type injuries, and clothesline injuries. Penetrating laryngeal trauma usually results from projectile injury, such as a gunshot, or knife wounds to the neck.

Every patient with trauma to the neck should be evaluated for potential laryngeal trauma. Patients may report dyspnea, hoarseness, or aphonia. Other less common symptoms include dysphagia, anterior neck pain, and odynophagia. Evaluation should begin with the ABCs of trauma–airway, breathing, circulation. Severe laryngeal trauma (particularly clothesline-type injuries) can result in loss of airway and necessitate the need for immediate tracheotomy. Physical findings common in patients with laryngeal trauma include stridor, subcutaneous crepitance (emphysema), bruising or edema to the anterior neck, loss of palpable landmarks, and hemoptysis. As outlined above (stridor and airway obstruction) the type of stridor can often give an indication of the site of airflow obstruction.

Further evaluation of laryngeal trauma is dictated by the patient's condition. If an adult patient's airway is unstable, most experts would advocate awake tracheostomy or cricothyrotomy under local anesthesia, as endotracheal intubation in the setting of laryngeal trauma can be problematic. For unstable pediatric laryngeal trauma, inhalational anesthetic followed by rigid endoscopic intubation is recommended by many experts. Once a stable airway has been determined or secured, evaluation can proceed.

Flexible fiberoptic laryngoscopy is advocated for awake, stable patients. The airway should be evaluated for vocal cord mobility, edema, laryngeal lacerations, and hematomas. Because the underlying mechanism of injury often results in damage to other adjacent structures, laryngeal trauma patients should undergo complete cervical spine radiography, and evaluation for esophageal or vascular injury should be considered. Some authors recommend fine-cut CT imaging of the larynx to help guide treatment planning. It should be emphasized that CT scanning rarely provides useful information regarding the immediate airway management for patients suspected of having laryngeal trauma, but often provide helpful information regarding surgical planning for repair.

Management of the patient with laryngeal trauma depends on the severity of injury. Patients with small laryngeal hematomas, small lacerations not involving the vocal fold edge or anterior commissure, and nondisplaced stable thyroid cartilage fractures can often be managed without tracheostomy. Most such patients should be hospitalized for 24 hours of airway observation and placed on systemic steroids, humidified air, and proton pump inhibitor (PPI) therapy. If mucosal disruption is present antibiotics should be initiated.

More severe laryngeal traumas often require tracheotomy and direct laryngoscopy or even open laryngeal exploration and repair. This should ideally be performed within 24 hours of the initial injury. Open laryngeal exploration is performed via a midline thyrotomy approach. A horizontal skin incision is made at the level of the cricothyroid membrane. Subplatysmal flaps are elevated, and the strap muscles divided at the midline. The airway is then entered in the midline of the cricothyroid membrane, and a vertical incision through the midline thyroid cartilage extended superiorly. Care must be taken to avoid injury to the underlying endolaryngeal mucosa. Following this, the mucosa is incised allowing inspection of the endolarynx. Once the endolarynx is exposed, all mucosal lacerations should be repaired to cover all exposed cartilage. If the anterior commissure is disrupted, a laryngeal stent may need to be placed, although placement of a stent itself leads to some degree of laryngeal injury. If placed, stents should be removed as soon as possible, usually around 2 weeks.

Outcomes for laryngeal trauma patients are fairly good once initial control of the airway is obtained. Most patients usually achieve a stable airway and undergo decannulation, which may take from 1 to 6 months or longer depending on the extent of injury. Overall, up to 90% of patients can recover a satisfactory vocal quality if managed appropriately.

▶ Disorders and Diseases

A. Hoarseness

Hoarseness or *dysphonia* is defined as an alteration in the quality or character of phonation. Patients may describe their voice as breathy, harsh, or rough. Common etiologies of hoarseness include viral illness, vocal fold paralysis, laryngopharyngeal reflux (LPR), laryngeal polyps, allergy, vocal abuse, dysplasia, and cancer.

Patients should be questioned about onset, frequency, and nature of the hoarseness. As previously discussed, the larynx is an essential part of swallowing, and any history of coughing or choking after eating should be elicited. Likewise the patient should be questioned about recurrent episodes of pneumonia. Any history of intubation, head and neck trauma, or previous head and neck surgery should be sought. Patients should be questioned about smoking and alcohol use.

Physical examination begins with a full head and neck examination. It is important to visualize the larynx. Methods of visualization include indirect mirror examination, rigid endoscopy, or transnasal flexible fiberoptic laryngoscopy. Videostroboscopy offers invaluable information about vocal fold motion and can identify adynamic segments and altered areas of mucosal wave propagation.

One common benign cause of hoarseness is vocal polyps. These are due to local tissue inflammation. Vocal nodules are distinct from polyps, and always occur bilaterally. They are most often a result of vocal abuse/misuse and usually respond dramatically to voice therapy. Vocal fold granulomas are usually due to extra-esophageal acid reflux damage.

Hoarseness can also be the presenting symptom for cancer, most often for cancer of the true vocal folds. The vast majority of laryngeal cancer is squamous cell cancer, and smoking is the biggest risk factor for its development. Laryngeal cancer is discussed further in the section Head and Neck Cancer. While early stage laryngeal cancer is highly curable, advanced stage carries a dramatically reduced prognosis. Thus, any patient with hoarseness lasting longer than 2 weeks should be evaluated and undergo visualization of their larynx.

B. Laryngopharyngeal Reflux

LPR impacts hundreds of thousands of patients annually, with some studies estimating as many as 30% of Americans may suffer from some degree of LPR. It is increasingly clear that LPR is a disease separate and distinct from classic gastroesophageal reflux disease (GERD). Patients with LPR typically present with frequent throat clearing, globus sensation, cough and hoarseness (as opposed to postprandial heartburn with GERD).

Physical examination of patients suspected of LPR should include an examination of the larynx, most commonly by flexible transnasal fiberoptic laryngoscopy. Hoarseness is not pathognomonic for LPR, and can also be present in more serious disorders. Several laryngeal findings are common in patients with LPR. Presence of vocal cord granuloma or pseudosulcus vocalis, although uncommon, is highly suggestive of LPR. Other common laryngoscopic findings consistent with LPR include posterior laryngeal hypertrophy, laryngeal edema and erythema, cobblestoning, or posterior commissure bar.

The diagnosis of LPR relies on a combination of symptoms and physical findings rather than one isolated factor being pathognomonic. Several studies have demonstrated the presence of many of the above symptoms and laryngeal findings in healthy, normal control patients. Many clinicians advocate the use of a metric scale that combines multiple common symptoms or physical findings. Two such instruments are the reflux finding score (RFS) and the reflux symptom index (RSI). In general, an RFS of greater than 8 is suggestive for LPR, and a score of greater than 13 on the RSI is likewise indicative of LPR.

Treatment for LPR currently consists of PPIs as a first-line therapy with surgery (eg, Nissen fundoplication) for selected treatment failures. It should be pointed out that although multiple uncontrolled studies have demonstrated benefit of PPIs for the treatment of LPR, the majority of randomized controlled trials have failed to confirm this. Possible confounding factors include lack of clear "gold standard" for the diagnosis of LPR, and differing treatment regimens. Our current practice is to place patients with LPR on once-daily PPI therapy for a 3- to 6-month period, after which response to treatment is assessed. The extended length of time is critical, as studies have shown that resolution of laryngeal findings can take up to 6 months to resolve once PPI therapy is initiated. If there is no response to once-daily PPI therapy, the patient can be advanced to twice-daily PPI therapy. Disease severity can prompt initiation of PPI therapy at twice-daily dosing; severe laryngeal edema or presence of subglottic stenosis would be two such indications.

It should also be mentioned that if a patient is diagnosed with LPR, some form of evaluation of the esophagus should be undertaken. There is up to a 20% incidence of unsuspected esophageal abnormalities in patients with LPR. This evaluation can take the form of imaging modalities such as barium swallow, or endoscopic examination such as esophagoscopy.

C. Vocal Cord Immobility/Paralysis

Vocal cord mobility problems represent a wide range of etiologies characterized by diverse patient presentation and prognostic outcomes. The distinction between unilateral and bilateral, and between paretic (hypomobile) versus paralyzed cords is imperative.

Patients with unilateral vocal cord paralysis may be asymptomatic, but often present with a hoarse, breathy voice. Their voice often starts out stronger in the morning and worsens throughout the day as they develop vocal fatigue. Accompanying symptoms can include frequent throat clearing, cough, vague globus sensation, and aspiration. Often patients will report subjective shortness of breath or a feeling of "running out of air" despite normal pulmonary function. This is secondary to glottal incompetence (lack of apposition of the vocal folds) resulting in escaped air during phonation. Thus a patient with unilateral vocal fold paralysis may be able to climb a flight of stairs without difficulty, yet feel short of breath when attempting to carry on a telephone conversation. Patients should be questioned specifically about swallowing, weight loss, recent illnesses or intubations, and surgeries (especially cardiac, cervical spine, and thyroid procedures).

The etiologies of vocal cord paralysis reflect the diverse nature of illnesses and injuries that can result in the final common pathway of vocal cord immobility or paralysis. The vocal cords derive their innervation from the vagus nerve, and any injury along the course of this nerve may result in vocal cord paralysis. Unilateral vocal cord paresis is by far the most common, with bilateral representing less than 20% of all paralysis. Historically, the most common cause of unilateral vocal cord paralysis was malignancy (such as lung cancer or skull base tumors). More recent studies show that iatrogenic surgical injury is now the most common cause. Nonthyroid surgical procedures (including anterior approaches to the cervical spine and carotid endarterectomy) now account for the majority of these iatrogenic injuries. Thyroid surgery remains the most common cause of bilateral vocal cord paralysis. Table 15–6 summarizes the most common causes of vocal fold paralysis. It should be noted that laryngeal manifestations of rheumatoid arthritis can rarely mimic vocal cord paralysis, although the underlying problem in this case is vocal cord immobility secondary to fixation of the arytenoid cartilages.

It is important to note that vocal cord immobility or paralysis is a *sign of pathology* and not a diagnosis. Thus the first concern when evaluating a patient with vocal cord paralysis should be investigation of the etiology. Often the cause is not identifiable, and the vocal cord paralysis is deemed idiopathic. A thorough head and neck examination should be performed, including endoscopic evaluation of the larynx. This most often is by flexible fiberoptic laryngoscopy, with most laryngologists recommending videostroboscopy as well. For unilateral recurrent laryngeal nerve injury, the affected immobile cord will usually lie in a paramedian position. This is due to lack of abduction, with some retained adduction (due to the cricothyroid muscle, which

Table 15–6. Most common causes of vocal cord paralysis.

Unilateral Vocal Cord Paralysis (%)	
Surgical injury	37
Cardiovascular, anterior cervical spine procedures	(51)
Thyroid surgery	(33)
Idiopathic (viral, inflammatory)	19
Malignancy	18
Intubation-related injury	6
Trauma	6
Bilateral Vocal Cord Paralysis (%)	
Surgical injury	37
Cardiovascular, anterior cervical spine procedures	(10)
Thyroid/parathyroid surgery	(90)
Malignancy	14
Intubation	13
Idiopathic (viral, inflammatory)	11
Neurologic (Wallenberg syndrome, Parkinson, multiple sclerosis, Guillain-Barre, others)	11
Trauma	7

is innervated by the superior laryngeal nerve). For more proximal vagal lesions, the affected cord will usually rest in intermediate position, due to loss of both abduction and adduction innervation. There is also loss of sensation to the affected hemilarynx, and aspiration is common.

Diagnostic testing should include a chest radiograph and CT scan following the entire vagus nerve course (ie, neck and chest, from skull base to the mid-chest). More esoteric tests are likely to be low yield and poorly cost-effective, and should be reserved for more selective use. Many laryngologists advocate the use of laryngeal electromyography (EMG). This test is performed percutaneously, and tests the superior laryngeal nerve and recurrent laryngeal nerve by evaluating motor unit electrical activity in the cricothyroid and thyroarytenoid muscles, respectively. Laryngeal EMG can provide useful information regarding the degree and likely site of injury (central vs peripheral), as well as the potential for spontaneous recovery. It is most predictive if performed 6 weeks to 6 months after initial injury.

Initial therapy for unilateral vocal cord paralysis consists of observation and speech therapy. Often the opposing vocal cord can compensate by crossing the midline and closing the glottal gap. This can produce an acceptable vocal quality, usually occurring within a 3-6 months time span.

Patients not obtaining a good result using these conservative measures can be treated by a variety of surgical interventions. The goal of surgical treatment for unilateral vocal cord paralysis is medialization of the affected cord. This reduces the glottic gap and allows the opposing, innervated cord to contact the other vocal fold with less effort. Treatment selection for unilateral vocal cord paralysis depends on the potential for recovery. In cases such as iatrogenic surgical injury with little chance of spontaneous recovery, definitive therapy can be initiated early. For idiopathic causes, a more conservative approach is usually advocated. Overall, up to 60% of patients with idiopathic unilateral vocal cord paralysis will recover to a near normal voice within 8-12 months. Thus, most experts would recommend waiting at least 1 year before proceeding with definitive therapy. Clear indications for earlier intervention include significant dysphagia and aspiration from glottic incompetence.

Definitive surgical procedures for unilateral vocal fold paralysis include laryngeal framework surgery, injection of longer lasting material, and reinnervation techniques. The thyroplasty technique (a laryngeal framework surgical procedure) is performed through an external skin incision. After exposing the thyroid cartilage, a window is cut in the thyroid ala overlying the position of the vocal fold on the affected side. An implant is then placed in a subperichondrial window, thus pushing the vocal fold toward the midline. Implants can include Silastic, autologous cartilage, and Gore-Tex. Most laryngologists perform this procedure with the patient lightly sedated. A flexible fiberoptic laryngoscope can be suspended in position, and the patient is asked to phonate periodically so that the surgical effects can be evaluated in real time and adjusted accordingly.

Another common surgical intervention is injection medialization. This can be performed as an office-based procedure using only local anesthesia, or in the operating room under general anesthesia. In either case, a variety of injectable materials are placed within the vocal fold lateral to the vocal process, to medialize the cord. In the past, Teflon was commonly used for this purpose, but has now largely fallen out of favor secondary to a high rate of complications. An alternative, long lasting (but not permanent) injectable is calcium hydroxyapetite microspheres in methylcarboxycellulose carrier gel (Radiesse Voice). Temporary injectables include gelfoam paste, hyaluronic acid, micronized cadaveric dermis (Cymetra), cross-linked collagen (Zyderm), and methylcarboxycellulose gel (Radiesse Voice Gel).

Surgical reinnervation for unilateral vocal cord paralysis is gaining popularity. Approaches can include nerve-muscle pedicle (using the omohyoid and ansa hypoglossi nerve) and direct nerve-nerve reinnervation (ansa cervicalis to recurrent laryngeal nerve). Results from these techniques are generally good, but can take 6 months or longer to be realized. For this reason, many surgeons combine reinnervation with injection medialization using a temporary substance.

For bilateral vocal cord paralysis, treatment approaches have a different perspective. Whereas restoration of voice is the primary goal for unilateral paralysis, resolution of potential or actual airway compromise is of tantamount importance in cases of bilateral paralysis. Most patients are initially treated with a tracheotomy to bypass the glottic obstruction. One common surgical procedure is lateralization of the vocal folds by arytenoidectomy. While this usually provides a patent airway and allows decannulation (reversal of the tracheotomy) the patient's vocal quality usually suffers significantly.

Another surgical approach, partial posterior cordectomy) can often preserve vocal quality to some degree, while providing improved airway. This approach uses a laser through a surgical laryngoscope to remove a c-shaped wedge from the posterior portion of one vocal cord. This preserves a bilateral vibratory margin anteriorly while providing an airway posteriorly. The technique is often best performed as multiple less aggressive procedures to fine-tune vocal quality versus airway, rather than a single definitive procedure.

D. Recurrent Respiratory Papillomatosis

Recurrent respiratory papillomatosis is caused by the human papilloma virus, specifically types 6 and 11. Human papilloma virus is a small nonenveloped virus that infects the nuclei of host cells for replication. Papillomaviruses show a preference for infection of epithelial tissues and are very common in humans. Human papillomavirus (HPV) is responsible for a variety of disease including skin warts, recurrent respiratory papillomatosis, and invasive cancers such as cervical or oropharyngeal carcinoma. Transmission is hypothesized to involve vertical transmission during childbirth; maternal presence of condylomata during the perinatal period confers a 200-fold increase in relative risk for developing respiratory papillomatosis.

Benign, recurrent hyperplastic tissue growth of the upper airway characterizes this disease. It has a bimodal age distribution, with incidence peaks in children (infants to 12 years old), and in adults (30-40 years of age). Patients typically present with dysphonia or aphonia, although advanced disease can cause stridor from impending airway obstruction.

The primary site affected is the larynx, with the glottis being the most common area followed by the supraglottic larynx (Figure 15–10). Respiratory papillomatosis generally remains confined to the larynx but can spread distally to affect the trachea, bronchi, and lungs. Disease recurrence is frequent, and reports of children requiring more than 100 surgical procedures are not uncommon.

The primary therapy for respiratory papillomatosis remains surgical debulking, primarily by microdebrider or carbon dioxide laser ablation. Adjuvant medical treatments include cidofovir, indole-3-carbinol, ribavirin, mumps vaccine, and photodynamic therapy. The role for these adjuvant

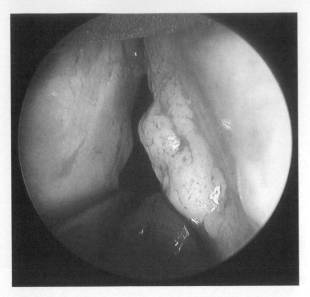

▲ **Figure 15–10.** Adult recurrent respiratory papillomatosis. The right true vocal fold is involved with respiratory papillomatosis. In this patient, the disease was confined mostly to the single true vocal fold, although some disease was also present in the anterior portion of the contralateral vocal fold.

therapies in the treatment of respiratory papillomatosis is still being elucidated. Many otolaryngologists advocate avoidance of tracheotomy if possible, because this has been epidemiologically associated with increased risk of spread of papillomas to the lower respiratory tract. It is possible because patients with inherently more aggressive disease are also those who are more likely to require tracheostomy.

HEAD AND NECK CANCER

▶ Pathophysiology of Head and Neck Squamous Cell Carcinoma

Excluding skin cancer, the vast majority of head and neck cancers are squamous cell cancers. This is the sixth most common malignancy; over 500,000 patients worldwide are diagnosed with head and neck squamous cell carcinoma each year. Head and neck squamous cell carcinoma is a potentially curable malignancy when diagnosed at an early stage. Unfortunately, patients often present with locally advanced disease. Overall, the prognosis is poor in this latter group of patients. For patients with advanced disease, between 60% and 70% develop loco-regional recurrences within 2 years.

Despite numerous advances in our understanding of this disease and in development of improved medical and

surgical therapies, mortality rates have not changed significantly over the last two decades. Additionally, current therapies (both surgical and nonsurgical) carry a high level of treatment-related morbidity; patients with advanced-stage disease often suffer significant speech and swallowing impairment following treatment.

Development of head and neck squamous cell carcinoma is traditionally attributed to the synergistic carcinogenic effects of tobacco and alcohol. Other factors, such as poor oral dentition, gastroesophageal reflux, betel nut chewing, and viral infection may also be important contributors to the development of head and neck squamous cell carcinoma. It is now accepted that high-risk types (eg, 16, 18, and 31) of HPV are a causal agent in the development of some head and neck squamous cell carcinomas, particularly cancers of the oropharynx. While as many as 50% of oropharyngeal cancers have detectable HPV-16 DNA, only 25%-30% of all oropharyngeal cancers are thought to have a viral etiology (as opposed to the usual insults of tobacco and alcohol). In HPV-mediated transformation, oncoproteins (primarily E6 and E7) encoded by the HPV genome are transcribed by infected human epithelial cells, resulting in the degradation and inactivation of host tumor suppressor genes p53 and Rb. This is thought to allow unchecked cell cycle progression and development of genetic instability. Head and neck squamous cell carcinomas with active (eg, transcribed) HPV share a common molecular phenotype, similar to that of HPV-caused cervical cancer. Head and neck squamous cell carcinomas with inactive HPV appear to share a molecular phenotype in common with HPV-negative head and neck squamous cell carcinomas. The role, if any, of HPV in these latter cancers is under investigation.

Head and neck cancers are thought to progress through characteristic stages of premalignancy (dysplasia, carcinoma *in situ*, until finally reaching invasive carcinoma). This progression reflects the accumulation of multiple genetic changes from mutation, gene silencing (via methylation), chromosomal rearrangements, deletions and duplications. Common changes include mutational inactivation of p53 and Rb tumor suppressors, abrogation of the tumor suppressor p16 axis, amplification of the CCND1 locus (the gene encoding the cell cycle mediator cyclin D1), and various changes resulting in overexpression of epidermal growth factor receptor (EGFR), c-Met and transforming growth factor alpha (TGF-α).

Another important concept in head and neck cancer biology is that of *field cancerization*. According to this theory, first described in 1953, the entire mucosa of the upper aerodigestive tract is exposed to the same carcinogenic insults. Thus, premalignant changes are likely in a wide field, not just at the site of the original cancer. Even if that cancer is successfully treated, the patient remains at high risk for developing subsequent malignancies throughout the upper aerodigestive tract. Recent molecular-based investigations have provided strong support for this concept, and multiple studies have demonstrated genetic alterations in histologically normal tissue from high-risk individuals. For this reason, patients with a history of head and neck squamous cell carcinoma should be closely followed with yearly screening examinations for life.

► Evaluation of the Patient With Head and Neck Cancer

A. History and Physical Examination

Any patient with a significant history of alcohol and tobacco use who presents with complaints related to the upper aerodigestive system should be evaluated with an index of suspicion for head and neck squamous cell carcinoma. Common symptoms of head and neck cancer can be quite subtle. Mechanical obstruction and dysfunction from tumor mass can produce dysphagia. Head and neck cancers are often associated with significant pain, and odynophagia is common for cancers of the oral cavity and oropharynx. Referred pain from neck metastases can result in otalgia, as can cancers arising in the nasopharynx or those affecting the EAC. Cancers of the true vocal cords often produce significant hoarseness early in the course of disease progression. Other symptoms can include hemoptysis, globus sensation, trismus, and weight loss. Sometimes the presenting symptom is a neck mass representing nodal metastases from an asymptomatic primary source.

Patients should be asked about family history of cancers and personal risk factors such as alcohol use and all forms of tobacco–cigarettes, cigars, chewing tobacco, etc. Certain ethnic populations (specifically emigrants from the country of India) may give a history of betel nut chewing. This nut has been found, like tobacco, to have synergistic carcinogenic risk when present in combination with alcohol consumption.

Physical examination should include a comprehensive evaluation of all sites of the head and neck. Inspection of the face and scalp for skin lesions, masses, and asymmetry should be performed. Otoscopy and anterior rhinoscopy allow evaluation of the EAC, tympanic membrane, and nasal cavity. Unilateral serous fluid in the middle ear space in an adult should raise suspicion for a nasopharyngeal lesion. The entire oral cavity should be evaluated, including each gingivo-buccal sulcus. The floor of mouth and base of tongue should be manually palpated for induration, pain on palpation, and asymmetry. Evaluation of the larynx and base of tongue can be performed by headlamp and mirror examination (indirect laryngoscopy). Flexible fiberoptic evaluation often provides additional detail and visualization not possible with the former method. Additionally, the nasal cavity and nasopharynx can easily be evaluated during the same procedure. A complete evaluation of the cranial nerves should be performed. This can often give insight into nerves affected by tumor mass effect (compression) or direct nerve invasion (perineural spread).

The neck should be carefully palpated for cervical lymphadenopathy. This is most easily accomplished by standing behind the patient and palpating each area of the neck symmetrically using both hands. This allows tactile comparison between sides. The pads of the fingers and thumbs are the most sensitive parts of the hands and should be used instead of the tips of the digits.

B. Imaging

Imaging is an important part of the diagnostic evaluation of a patient with head and neck cancer. Goals of imaging include preoperative identification of site and extent of tumor infiltration, presence of suspicious lymph nodes, and presence of anatomic variations. The imaging modality of choice for most suspected head and neck tumors is CT scan with intravenous contrast. This allows adequate soft tissue and bony detail. Most head and neck cancers will demonstrate enhancement on IV contrast administration, and the contrast additionally makes delineation of soft tissue structures much easier. In some cases contrasted MRI may offer additional information. These cases include evaluation of the skull base, parapharyngeal space and orbit, and evaluation of cranial nerves for signs of perineural spread.

Increasingly, evaluation of head and neck squamous cell carcinoma patients for distant metastases and monitoring for posttreatment disease recurrence or persistence involves the use of tumor imaging by 18F-fluorodeoxyglucose positron emission tomography (FDG-PET) (Figure 15–11). The use of FDG-PET and combined PET/CT modalities is extremely important as early identification of persistent/recurrent disease has the potential to impact survival, especially for patients with advanced nodal disease. While CT and MRI rely on contrast enhancement patterns and differences in tissue attenuation, FDG-PET works somewhat independently of these criteria. FDG follows a cellular uptake pathway similar to glucose and becomes concentrated in cells with elevated glucose utilization. Because changes in tumor metabolism often precede changes discernable on clinical examination this makes FDG-PET potentially valuable in discovering clinically nondetectable tumor spread or recurrence. PET-CT results are generally reported as standardized uptake values (SUV). This is a ratio of tissue FDG uptake normalized to injected dose of FDG, patient body weight, and serum glucose levels. Higher SUV values indicate increased FDG uptake. Multiple tissue metabolic changes can lead to increased FDG uptake, including inflammation, infection, radiation response, and malignancy. While still a matter of debate, general consensus is that SUV greater than 2.5-3.5 should be considered suspicious for malignancy.

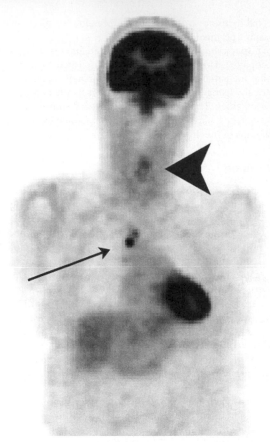

▲ Figure 15–11. Positron emission tomography (PET scan). PET scan showing uptake in the original primary site (palate, indicated by large arrowhead) as well as new mediastinal uptake indicative of nodal metastases (thin arrow). Note the normal physiologic uptake in the liver (moderate intensity) and heart and brain (high intensity) demonstrating the relatively high glucose utilization of these organs.

C. Staging and Treatment of Head and Neck Squamous Cell Carcinoma: TNM Staging

Staging for head and neck squamous cell carcinoma in the United States uses a TNM system. Staging is important because it allows estimation of prognosis, treatment planning, and expected response to treatment. The TNM system classifies cancers by **T**–primary tumor size, **N**–locoregional nodal metastases, and **M**–distant metastatic spread. The rules for classification vary by subsite within the head and neck. In general cancers of subsites that can be seen directly (ie, oral cavity, oropharynx, etc) are T-staged by size. By comparison, cancers of subsites not visible directly (ie, larynx, hypopharynx, sinonasal, etc) are T-staged by anatomic spread of disease.

Initial evaluation of the primary site and T-staging is best accomplished by operative direct laryngoscopy and esophagoscopy. This allows examination of the primary site and evaluation of the entire upper aerodigestive tract for simultaneous second primary tumors and biopsy of suspicious areas. Some authors propose trans-nasal esophagoscopy as an acceptable alternative to operative endoscopy. This method allows evaluation (and biopsy) of the most common areas for malignancy with the exception of the postcricoid region and subglottis. Transnasal esophagoscopy has the advantage of being able to be performed as an office-based procedure without the need for sedation.

It should be mentioned that cancers of Waldeyer's ring which includes the palatine tonsil and base of tongue (lingual tonsil), while usually squamous cell cancer, can also be lymphoid in origin (such as lymphoma). If there is a suspicion for lymphoma, biopsy specimens should be sent as fresh material and not placed into formaldehyde. Often, flow cytometry and other pathologic tests useful for evaluation of lymphomas cannot be performed on formaldehyde-fixed specimens.

N-stage is determined by the presence of clinically evident regional lymph node metastases. It is important to point out that for head and neck cancer suspicious lymphadenopathy identified only on CT or MRI scan is included in the clinical staging. Radiologic findings suspicious for malignant lymph node metastases include lymph nodes that are round, heterogeneously enhancing, and larger than 1 cm. The current criteria for N-staging (for subsites other than nasopharynx) is summarized in Table 15–7.

M-stage is determined by the presence of distant metastatic disease. The most common sites of metastases for head and neck squamous cell carcinoma are the liver and the lungs. Therefore part of the initial staging workup for a patient with head and neck cancer includes some method of

Table 15–7. Determination of N-stage for cancers of the oral cavity, oropharynx, hypopharynx, and larynx.

Nx	Regional lymph nodes cannot be assessed
N0	No regional lymph node metastases
N1	Metastases in a single ipsilateral lymph node, 3 cm or less
N2 N2a	Metastases in a single ipsilateral lymph node, > 3 cm but not more than 6 cm
N2b	Metastases in multiple ipsilateral lymph nodes < 6 cm
N2c	Metastases in bilateral or contralateral lymph nodes < 6 cm
N3	Metastases in lymph node(s) greater than 6 cm

Table 15–8. Summary of TNM staging for cancers of the oral cavity, oropharynx, hypopharynx, and larynx.

Stage	T-Stage	N-Stage	M-Stage
Stage 0	T-is (*in situ*)	N0	M0
Stage I	T1	N0	M0
Stage II	T2	N0	M0
Stage III	T3 T1-T3	N0 N1	M0
Stage IVa	T4a T1-T4a	N0-N1 N2	M0
Stage IVb	T4b Any T	N0-N2 N3	M0
Stage IVc	Any T	Any N	M1

evaluating these structures. This most commonly consists of liver function blood tests and a chest roentgenogram, although at some institutions whole-body CT-PET scan is becoming more prevalent. M-stage is reported as Mx (cannot be determined), M0 (no distant metastases) or M1 (distant metastatic disease).

Overall staging is achieved by combining the T, N, and M stages to yield four broad stages (stage I-IV, with I carrying the best prognosis and IV the worst). Stage IV is further split into IV-a (simplified, denoting a surgically treatable cancer) and IV-b and -c (surgically unresectable). The overall staging system (based on the *AJCC Cancer Staging Manual*, sixth edition) for sites other than nasopharynx is summarized in Table 15–8 and Figure 15–12.

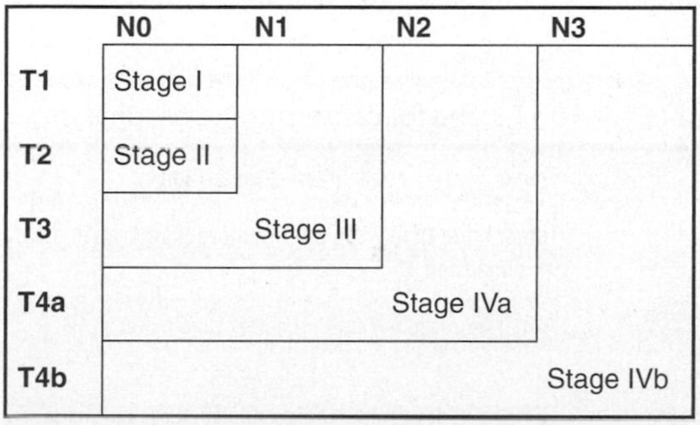

▲ **Figure 15–12.** Summary of staging criteria for cancers of the oral cavity, oropharynx, hypopharynx, and larynx. Carcinoma in situ is stage 0, and presence of distant metastases (M1) is staged as stage IVc regardless of T or N stage.

Therapy

Traditional therapy for head and neck squamous cell carcinoma depends on the stage of the cancer and varies by subsite. Simplified, early stage cancers are usually treated with single modality therapy, either surgical excision or radiation therapy. Advanced stage (stages III and IV) cancers are best treated by combined modality therapy, either surgery and postoperative radiotherapy, or chemotherapy/radiation therapy. Current research has shown that the latter is best delivered as concurrent chemotherapy-radiation therapy.

One new modality being investigated for head and neck squamous cell carcinoma includes molecularly targeted therapy. These therapies are designed to be specific for cancer cells, and include monoclonal antibodies and small molecule protein inhibitors. The most studied targeted therapy in head and neck squamous cell carcinoma is cetuximab, which targets the EGFR. In the initial randomized controlled clinical trial, researchers found that concurrent cetuximab and radiotherapy improved survival and locoregional disease control compared to radiotherapy alone. Studies have also demonstrated improvement in survival when cetuximab is combined with traditional chemotherapy. The EXTREME (Erbitux in First Line Treatment of Recurrent or Metastatic Head and Neck Cancer) trial randomized 442 patients from 17 countries to either chemotherapy (5-fluorouracil plus either cisplatin or carboplatin) or the same chemotherapy plus cetuximab. Patients in the cetuximab arm had 20% reduction in risk of death, and overall survival was increased from a median 7.4 months to 10.1 months. Other targeted therapies currently being studied include bevacizumab (an inhibitor of VEGF receptor, involved in angiogenesis) and various orally administered EGFR small-molecule tyrosine kinase inhibitors. Particularly promising are combination targeted therapies which include agents addressing both the EGF and VEGF pathways.

SPECIFIC HEAD AND NECK SQUAMOUS CELL CANCER SITES

Cancers of the Oral Cavity

Patients with oral cavity cancer typically present with a painful mass of the tongue, buccal mucosa, floor of mouth, or alveolar ridge. Appearance to visual examination alone can be misleading. While most cancers have either an ulcerative or an exophytic appearance, many can have only subtle visually detectable changes. On palpation, the involved area is usually firm and indurated. A bimanual examination of the floor of mouth is mandatory for a complete examination. The mass should be manipulated to discern mobility. Oral cavity cancers can invade the mandible quite readily, and immobility should raise concern for bone invasion.

As with other head and neck subsites where the primary tumor can be directly visualized, T-staging is assessed by

Table 15–9. T Stage for cancers of the oral cavity.

T1	Tumor 2 cm or less in greatest dimension
T2	Tumor more than 2 cm, but not more than 4 cm in greatest dimension
T3	Tumor more than 4 cm in greatest dimension
T4	
T4a	Tumor invades through adjacent structures
	Lip: cortical bone, floor of mouth, facial skin of chin or nose
	Oral cavity proper: cortical bone, deep muscles of tongue (genioglossus, palatoglossus, hyoglossus, styloglossus), skin.
T4b	Tumor invades masticator space, pterygoid plates, skull base, and/or encases carotid artery

tumor size (summarized in Table 15–9). Cancers which invade adjacent structures are, in general, up-staged to T4 regardless of size. Note that superficial erosion of the bony tooth socket by a gingival primary tumor is not sufficient to upstage to T4.

The nodal drainage patterns of oral cavity cancers are of particular concern, because the incidence of occult metastases can approach 30% depending on T-stage and depth of invasion. Cancers of the upper lip can drain to the parotid bed in addition to level I. When planning treatment of occult metastases, it is important to remember that midline cancers of the oral cavity often drain bilaterally.

Treatment for oral cavity cancer is primarily surgical. Cancers of the lip can often be addressed with simple wedge excision, with 5-mm borders of surrounding normal tissue. If less than one-third of the lip is excised, a reasonable result can be obtained with simple closure. Larger excisions require a reconstructive procedure, often involving transfer of lip tissue from the contralateral lip. Cancers of the tongue, floor of mouth, and buccal mucosa are excised with a margin of 1 cm normal appearing tissue. Often primary closure, with or without a split thickness skin graft, will provide acceptable functional outcomes. Large resections usually require a flap reconstruction, especially if bone is involved, and a segmental mandibulectomy needs to be performed. The flap reconstruction can be either a pedicled flap (such as pectoralis major flap), or a free flap (radial forearm and fibular being common flap harvest sites).

Assuming appropriate treatment, outcomes for patients with oral cavity cancer are generally good. The prognosis for squamous cell carcinoma of the lip is excellent, with 5-year survival of 91% for stage I-II, 83% for stage III-IVb, and 52% for stage IVc. Squamous cell carcinoma of the oral cavity proper carries a reduced, yet still relatively good prognosis. Five-year survival rates are 72% for stage I-II, 44% for stage III-IVb, and 35% for stage IVc.

▶ Cancers of the Oropharynx

The oropharynx consists of the soft palate, base of tongue, palatine tonsils, and posterior/lateral oropharyngeal walls. Patients with cancer of the soft palate usually present with relatively early stage lesions, which typically remain fairly superficial. They usually arise on the anterior aspect of the palate and patients may report noticing a lump in the palate while swallowing. This contrasts with cancers of the tongue base, tonsillar region and pharyngeal walls, which typically present at advanced stage. These anatomic regions lack the rich supply of pain nerve fibers typical of the oral cavity and soft palate, and cancers can spread significantly before being noticed. Typical presenting symptoms usually are attributable to sequelae from invasion of adjacent structures, and can include dysphagia, cranial nerve defects, referred otalgia, trismus (from pterygoid muscle invasion), or neck mass (from nodal metastases). Because early-stage oropharyngeal cancers often are asymptomatic, any erythroplastic or suspicious lesion in these areas should be biopsied even if no associated symptoms are present.

As is the case for oral cavity cancer, T-staging for squamous cell cancer of the oropharynx is generally determined by tumor size (summarized in Table 15–10). Again, invasion of adjacent structures results in classification as T4 regardless of size. Oropharyngeal cancer N-staging is the same as other head and neck squamous cell carcinoma subsites (except nasopharynx). Nodal metastases from oropharyngeal cancers are common, with 70% of patients with oropharyngeal cancer having ipsilateral cervical nodal metastases at the time of presentation. Bilateral cervical nodal metastases are also relatively common, up to 30%-50%, depending on size and subsite of the primary tumor.

Treatment for oropharyngeal cancer, especially the tongue base and soft palate, is often weighted toward non-surgical therapy. This is because surgical resection can result in extensive morbidity in terms of velopharyngeal insufficiency (for palate) and dysphagia (for tongue base).

Table 15–10. T stage for cancers of the oropharynx.

T1	Tumor 2 cm or less in greatest dimension
T2	Tumor more than 2 cm, but not more than 4 cm in greatest dimension
T3	Tumor more than 4 cm in greatest dimension
T4	
T4a	Tumor invades through adjacent structures (larynx; deep muscles of tongue such as genioglossus, palatoglossus, hyoglossus, styloglossus; medial pterygoid, hard palate, mandible)
T4b	Tumor invades masticator space, pterygoid plates, lateral nasopharynx, skull base, and/or encases carotid artery

Because of interruption of the blood supply to the remainder of the tongue, large base of tongue cancers usually require total glossectomy even if the anterior tongue is spared. Surgical resections of all but the smallest oropharyngeal cancers usually require flap reconstruction; in the modern era this is most often in the form of a free flap with microvascular anastomoses. A tracheotomy is usually performed during the initial surgical resection for maintenance of adequate airway. As collective experience with robot-assisted oropharyngeal surgery advances, surgical treatment is likely to become more common as this approach appears to have decreased morbidity compared to open techniques.

As with other head and neck squamous cell carcinomas, early stage (I-II) cancers are treated with single modality therapy, and advanced stage (III-IV) cancers require multiple modalities. It should be noted that nonsurgical modalities have their own set of consequences, and there is some evidence demonstrating worse swallowing outcomes following chemotherapy-radiation compared to surgery and postoperative radiotherapy for advanced stage oropharyngeal lesions.

The association between HPV and oropharyngeal cancers deserves special mention. HPV is the accepted etiologic cause of greater than 95% of cervical cancer. Since the first demonstration of HPV in a head and neck squamous cell carcinoma tumor in 1985, numerous studies have found HPV DNA in head and neck squamous cell carcinomas from various subsites, most commonly the oropharynx. It now appears that of oropharyngeal squamous cell carcinomas, approximately 50% have no association with HPV, 25% are likely to be caused by HPV (similar to cervical cancer), and 25% have HPV DNA but an unclear relationship between the virus and the cancer. Future studies assessing the role of HPV in this latter group are currently being developed.

Survival for oropharyngeal cancer is generally worse than that of oral cavity cancer. Five-year survival for stage I-II oropharyngeal cancer is 58%, stage III-IVb is 41%, and stage IVc only 20%.

▶ Cancers of the Larynx

Interestingly, laryngeal cancer was an extremely rare disease until the 20th century. Mass-produced cigarettes came into vogue in the 1900s; soon after this a dramatic rise in the incidence of laryngeal cancer began to be noted. Tobacco exposure is now accepted as the primary etiologic agent responsible for laryngeal cancer. Other possible additive factors include laryngo-pharyngeal reflux and possibly certain viruses such as herpes simplex or HPV.

Laryngeal cancers can arise from above the true vocal folds (supraglottic region), below the true vocal folds (subglottic region) or from the true vocal folds (glottic region). The latter represents greater than 75% of all laryngeal cancers.

For patients with glottic laryngeal cancer, dysphonia (hoarseness) is the most common presenting symptom. Any hoarseness that persists longer than 2 weeks, especially in a patient with associated risk factors of tobacco or alcohol use, should undergo laryngeal examination. Patients with hoarseness, however, are more likely to have a non-malignant cause for their symptoms than to have laryngeal cancer.

Laryngeal cancers arising from the subglottis or supraglottis usually present at a later stage than do glottic cancers, as hoarseness does not develop until late in the disease process. Oftentimes, the presenting symptom can be life-threatening stridor from an obstructive mass. Emergent awake tracheotomy is sometimes required to secure a stable patent airway in these cases. Other symptoms can include globus sensation ("lump in throat") and dysphagia. Evaluation for preexisting swallowing dysfunction is emerging as an essential part of the diagnostic workup for laryngeal cancers. Because of the emphasis on organ-preservation strategies, identification of patients likely to end up with a nonfunctioning larynx may alter treatment planning. Currently this is an area of active investigation.

Unlike oral cavity and oropharyngeal cancer (T-staged by tumor size), cancers of the larynx are T-staged by anatomic spread of disease (Table 15–11). One important factor is determination of vocal cord fixation. This can be reliably determined with greater than 90% accuracy based on in-office flexible fiberoptic evaluation combined with high-resolution CT imaging of the larynx. Laryngeal cancer N staging follows the convention for other head and neck subsites (except nasopharynx).

Therapy for early (T1-T2) glottic cancer has traditionally been radiation therapy, especially for early, diffuse disease involving both true vocal folds and the anterior commissure. In these cases, surgical resection would result in significant disruption of the normal vocal fold architecture and function. This should be balanced with the knowledge that radiation therapy is essentially a one-time treatment modality, which carries its own spectrum of side effects and sequelae.

The goal of organ preservation (ie, preserving a functional ability to phonate and protect the airway during deglutition) should be kept in mind when planning treatment options. In the now famous "fireman's study," McNeil et al found that many people would accept a 20% decrease in survival, rather than lose their larynx. Surgical organ preservation strategies include endoscopic microsurgical excision, supracricoid laryngectomy, and vertical partial laryngectomy. Endoscopic microsurgical excision can allow maximal preservation of vocal function in selected T1 glottic cancers, while maintaining a sound oncologic outcome. In this approach, dissection is meticulously performed just deep to the most involved layer of the true vocal fold (epithelium, superficial lamina propria, deep lamina propria or vocal ligament, vocalis muscle). Partial laryngectomies

Table 15–11. T stage for cancers of the larynx.

Supraglottis	
T1	Tumor limited to one subsite of the supraglottis. Normal vocal cord mobility.
T2	Tumor invades mucosa of more than one subsite of the supraglottis, glottis, or adjacent structure (tongue base, vallecula, medial wall of pyriform). Normal vocal cord mobility.
T3	Tumor limited to the larynx but presence of vocal cord fixation, and/or invades postcricoid, preepiglottic tissues, paraglottic space, *inner cortex only* invasion of thyroid cartilage.
T4	
T4a	Tumor invades through thyroid cartilage and/or extends to other tissues beyond the larynx (eg, trachea, deep extrinsic tongue muscles, strap muscles, thyroid, esophagus).
T4b	Tumor invades prevertebral space, encases carotid artery, or invades mediastinal structures.
Glottis	
T1	
T1a	Tumor limited to unilateral true vocal cord with normal mobility (may involve anterior or posterior commisure).
T1b	Tumor limited to bilateral true vocal cords with normal mobility (may involve anterior or posterior commisure).
T2	Tumor extends to supraglottis and/or subglottis and/or impaired vocal cord mobility.
T3	Tumor limited to larynx with vocal cord fixation and/or invades paraglottic space, and/or minor thyroid cartilage invasion (*inner cortex only*).
T4	
T4a	Tumor invades through the thyroid cartilage and/or invades tissues beyond the larynx (trachea, soft tissues of the neck including deep extrinsic tongue muscles, strap muscles, thyroid, esophagus).
T4b	Tumor invades prevertebral space, encases carotid artery or invades mediastinal structures.
Subglottis	
T1	Tumor limited to subglottis.
T2	Tumor extends to true vocal cord(s) with normal or impaired mobility (but no fixation).
T3	Tumor limited to larynx, with vocal cord fixation.
T4	
T4a	Tumor invades cricoid or thyroid cartilage and/or invades tissues beyond larynx (trachea, soft tissues of the neck including deep extrinsic tongue muscles, strap muscles, thyroid, esophagus).
T4b	Tumor invades prevertebral space, encases carotid artery, or invades mediastinal structures.

(vertical partial and supracricoid) can yield satisfactory voice and swallowing function, but require extensive patient cooperation in the postoperative period. Supracricoid laryngectomy involves removal of the supraglottis, false and true vocal cords, and thyroid cartilage. The hyoid bone, cricoid cartilage, and at least one arytenoid are preserved. The movement of the remaining arytenoid against the tongue base allows phonation and (eventual) preservation of swallowing function. Postoperatively, aspiration is to be expected and patients with poor preoperative pulmonary function should not be offered this option. Total laryngectomy is the treatment of choice for salvage of organ-preservation failures, as well as the primary treatment for most advanced glottic (T3 and T4) cancers.

Outcomes for patients with laryngeal cancer can be excellent. For early stage I glottic carcinoma (tumor limited to the true vocal folds), 5-year overall survival rates of 90% can be expected. Overall, laryngeal cancer carries a 5-year survival for stage I-II disease of 79%. With invasion of adjacent structures characteristic of stage III-IVb disease, 5-year survival decreases to 55%, and with distant metastases (stage IVc) the 5-year survival is 35%.

▶ Cancers of the Hypopharynx

The hypopharynx is a continuation of the oropharynx, and extends superiorly from the level of the hyoid bone to the level of the inferior aspect of the cricoid cartilage. It consists of the pyriform sinuses (the most common subsite for hypopharyngeal cancer), the posterior pharyngeal wall and postcricoid regions. The hypopharynx is lined with stratified squamous epithelium and is invested with an abundant lymphatic drainage network. Patients with hypopharyngeal cancer typically present with advanced stage disease, stage III or worse. There are several contributing factors, including lack of specific symptoms for small lesions in this region, and a lack of anatomic boundaries to prevent spread of disease. Typical presenting symptoms can include referred otalgia, odynophagia, and dysphagia. Other symptoms can include a neck mass (from nodal metastases), hoarseness (due to laryngeal involvement), and weight loss. Like laryngeal cancer, hypopharyngeal cancer is chiefly related to excessive alcohol and tobacco exposure. There is also some evidence for a possible contribution of GERD to hypopharyngeal cancer. This may explain the increased likelihood for patients with Plummer–Vinson syndrome to develop hypopharyngeal cancer, regardless of tobacco or alcohol exposure. In Plummer–Vinson syndrome, patients develop esophageal webs, and chronic acid exposure above the site of webbing is thought to possibly result in chronic inflammation predisposing to malignancy.

Hypopharyngeal cancer T-staging is somewhat unique, as it is a combination of tumor size (as for oral cavity and oropharyngeal tumors) and anatomic spread (as for laryngeal cancer). The T-staging criteria for hypopharyngeal

Table 15–12. T stage for cancers of the hypopharynx.

T1	Tumor limited to 1 subsite and 2 cm or less in greatest dimension
T2	No fixation of hemilarynx, and tumor – invades more than subsite or an adjacent area (larynx, oropharynx) and/or – more than 2 cm, but not more than 4 cm in greatest dimension
T3	Tumor more than 4 cm in greatest dimension or fixation of hemilarynx
T4 T4a	Tumor invades through adjacent structures (thyroid/cricoid cartilage, hyoid bone, thyroid gland, esophagus, central compartment)
T4b	Tumor involves prevertebral fascia, mediastinal structures, and/or encases carotid artery

cancer are summarized in Table 15–12. N-staging and M-staging are the same as for the majority of head and neck sites (except nasopharynx).

Early stage (T1-T2 tumors) hypopharyngeal cancer is often treated with primary radiotherapy. Surgical resection is more likely in these instances to lead to dysphagia and aspiration. Alternatively, laryngeal conservation surgery may be a reasonable option for some of these early-stage cancers. More advanced (T3-T4) tumors can be treated by surgical resection with postoperative radiotherapy, or chemotherapy/radiation therapy. The standard surgical procedure is total laryngectomy with partial pharyngectomy. Tumor extension into the esophagus requires a cervical esophagectomy. The resulting alimentary tract defects require repair by various methods, including microvascular jejunal free flap, gastric pull up, or microvascular myocutaneous flap (most often tubed radial forearm or anterolateral thigh). Organ preservation surgical strategies can achieve laryngeal preservation rates of up to 40% for highly selected cases, but these remain somewhat controversial. As previously described for laryngeal cancer, preoperative evaluation of a patient's pulmonary function status is critical, as significant postoperative aspiration can be expected. Because of the high incidence of occult nodal metastases, treatment of the neck lymphatics should be included in any therapeutic plan. For clinically evident neck disease, neck dissection is indicated. For patients with a clinically negative neck, optimal management is still being elucidated. Elective neck dissection represents one option for the clinically negative neck. Alternatively, if radiation therapy is planned for treatment of the primary site, the radiation fields can be adjusted to include treatment doses to the neck lymphatics.

Hypopharyngeal cancer carries the worst prognosis of any head and neck subsite. The underlying reasons for this are still unclear, and several hypotheses have been suggested. A distinctive pathologic feature of hypopharyngeal cancer is the propensity for submucosal spread of disease, often resulting in clinically understaging disease extent. The abundant lymphatic drainage of the hypopharynx may also predispose the patient to early nodal metastases. It has also been suggested that the lack of definitive anatomic boundaries may allow early spread of disease. Given all of these factors, it should not be surprising that 5-year survival for stage I-II hypopharyngeal cancer is 47%, stage III-IVb is 30%, and stage IVc only 16%.

▶ Salivary Gland Neoplasms

Neoplasms (both benign and malignant) of the salivary glands are relatively uncommon, representing approximately 2% of all head and neck neoplasms. In general, the larger the salivary gland, the higher the overall incidence of neoplasms—but these neoplasms are also less likely to be malignant. Major salivary glands include the parotid, submandibular, and sublingual glands. The minor salivary glands are scattered mainly throughout the mucosa of the lips and oral cavity, and to a lesser extent the entire upper aerodigestive tract. For these smaller glands, the incidence of neoplasms is lower, but if one does occur it is more likely to be malignant. The parotid gland accounts for 80% of all neoplasms, while 15% arise from the submandibular glands and 5% from the sublingual and minor salivary glands. For any given tumor, the incidence of malignancy is 20% for parotid tumors, 60% for submandibular tumors, and 80% for sublingual and minor salivary gland tumors. Unlike squamous cell carcinoma, tobacco and alcohol exposure do not appear to play an etiologic role in salivary gland malignancy. It should be noted that the parotid gland contains lymph nodes that drain the preauricular and temporal skin; any parotid mass should raise suspicion for a skin cancer with intraparotid nodal metastases and a complete examination of the scalp and preauricular skin is indicated.

The most common benign salivary gland tumor is pleomorphic adenoma (also called benign mixed tumor), representing 60% of all salivary gland neoplasms. Patients typically present with a slowly enlarging, painless firm mass (most often in the parotid gland). Facial nerve paralysis is exceedingly rare, even with very large tumors, due to the slow-growing nature of these neoplasms. Malignant transformation of pleomorphic adenoma is rare but does occur; the resultant malignancy is highly aggressive. Treatment for pleomorphic adenoma is complete surgical excision including a surrounding margin of normal tissue. Due to microscopic transcapsular tumor infiltration, simple enucleation is insufficient for these benign neoplasms.

The second most common benign salivary neoplasm is papillary cystadenoma lymphomatosum (also known as Warthin tumor). This benign tumor is responsible for

10% of parotid neoplasms, but is rare outside of the parotid gland. Bilateral tumors are present in up to 10% of patients so careful palpation and/or imaging of both parotid beds is important if this tumor is suspected. Patients typically present with a slowly enlarging parotid mass, which is painless and rubbery upon palpation. Standard treatment is complete surgical excision (such as superficial parotidectomy with facial nerve preservation) although some authors advocate that enucleation of these tumors may be adequate therapy.

The most common salivary gland malignancy is mucoepidermoid carcinoma. Despite the propensity of the smaller salivary gland neoplasms to be malignant, the most common site for mucoepidermoid carcinoma is still the parotid gland. Approximately 45%-70% of mucoepidermoid carcinomas arise from the parotid gland, while 20% occur in minor salivary glands of the palate. Typical symptoms at presentation can be quite similar to those of benign salivary neoplasms, with a painless enlarging mass. Symptoms such as pain or facial paralysis are uncommon, but when present should raise suspicion for a high-grade aggressive lesion. Mucoepidermoid cancers are graded as low grade (mostly mucus cells), intermediate grade, and high grade (characterized by a hypercellular solid tumor). The latter can be difficult to distinguish from squamous cell carcinoma without immunohistochemical staining. Treatment is tailored to both the extent of disease, tumor grade, and location. Localized disease is usually amenable to surgical excision (parotidectomy with facial nerve preservation, submandibular gland excision, or wide local excision for minor salivary gland origin). Advanced disease requires extensive resection, often combined with neck dissection and/or postoperative radiotherapy.

The second most common salivary gland malignancy is adenoid cystic carcinoma. It is most common in the submandibular, sublingual, and minor salivary glands. Of all parotid neoplasms, adenoid cystic carcinoma is more likely to present with pain or paresthesias, although an asymptomatic mass is still the more common presentation. Adenoid cystic carcinoma is characterized by a propensity for perineural spread. Thus, preoperative imaging with gadolinium-enhanced MRI is often helpful in therapeutic planning. Treatment consists of complete surgical resection (sometimes requiring facial nerve sacrifice) and postoperative radiation therapy. There is some evidence that postoperative proton-beam therapy offers improved outcomes compared to traditional radiation therapy, although the former is available at only a few centers in the United States. Adenoid cystic carcinoma rarely spreads to cervical lymphatics, so neck dissection is not routinely advocated. It does, however, have a propensity for distant metastases—especially the lung. The disease is also characterized by frequent local recurrence, up to 40% even after adequate local excision. Because of the relatively slow growing nature of this disease, survival for adenoid cystic carcinoma at 5 years is favorable, approximately 65% for all stages. Due to the propensities for local

Table 15–13. T stage for major salivary gland cancer.

T1	Tumor 2 cm or less in greatest dimension, no extraparenchymal extension
T2	Tumor more than 2 cm, but not more than 4 cm in greatest dimension, no extraparenchymal extension
T3	Tumor more than 4 cm in greatest dimension and/or extraparenchymal extension
T4	
T4a	Tumor invades through adjacent structures (skin, mandible, external auditory canal, and/or facial nerve involvement)
T4b	Tumor invades skull base, pterygoid plates, and/or encases carotid artery

recurrence and distant metastases, however, this statistic decreases to 12%-15% at 15 years.

As mentioned above, malignant degeneration of pleomorphic adenomas can occur although it is uncommon. Some authors have estimated the risk of malignant degeneration at 1.5% for the first 5 years, increasing to 9.5% by 15 years or longer. The resulting malignant tumor is termed "carcinoma ex-pleomorphic adenoma" and is characterized by an aggressive natural history and poor clinical outcome. The most common presentation is sudden rapid growth of a previously stable parotid mass. Histologically, the malignant cells can take the form of any epithelial malignancy except acinic cell. Carcinoma ex-pleomorphic adenoma is characterized by frequent lymph node metastases, and up to 25% of patients will have clinically evident cervical lymphadenopathy on presentation. Treatment includes radical surgical resection, often combined with neck dissection and/or postoperative radiotherapy.

The prognosis of salivary gland malignancies varies according to histologic type, location, extent of disease, and grade. The criteria for T-staging are similar to other head and neck sites with directly measurable tumor size, and are summarized in Table 15–13. Overall, early stage (stage I-II) salivary gland cancers carry an excellent prognosis, greater than 80% at 5 years. Advanced (stage III-IV) salivary gland cancers on the other hand, have overall 5-year survival rates ranging from 23% to 56% depending on type and grade.

References

Baugh RF, Archer SM, Mitchell RB, et al: Clinical practice guideline: tonsillectomy in children. *Otolaryngol Head Neck Surg.* Jan 2011;144(suppl 1):S1-S30.

Carter KB, Jr., Loehrl TA, Poetker DM: Granulocyte transfusions in fulminant invasive fungal sinusitis. *Am J Otolaryngol.* 2012;33(6):663-666.

Chandana SR, Conley BA: Salivary gland cancers: current treatments, molecular characteristics and new therapies. *Expert Rev Anticancer Ther.* Apr 2008;8(4):645-652.

Chau JK, Lin JR, Atashband S, Irvine RA, Westerberg BD: Systematic review of the evidence for the etiology of adult sudden sensorineural hearing loss. *Laryngoscope.* May 2010;120(5):1011-1021.

Coelho DH, Lalwani AK: Medical management of Meniere's disease. *Laryngoscope.* 2008;118(6):1099-1108.

Danner CJ: Facial nerve paralysis. *Otolaryngol Clin North Am.* Jun 2008;41(3):619-632.

DelGaudio JM, Clemson LA: An early detection protocol for invasive fungal sinusitis in neutropenic patients successfully reduces extent of disease at presentation and long term morbidity. *Laryngoscope.* Jan 2009;119(1):180-183.

Edge SB, Byrd DR, Compton CC, et al: *AJCC Cancer Staging Manual,* 7th ed. New York: Springer-Verlag; 2009.

Ferri GG, Modugno GC, Pirodda A, et al: Conservative management of vestibular Schwannomas: an effective strategy. *Laryngoscope.* 2008;118(6):951-957.

Gallagher TQ, Derkay CS: Recurrent respiratory papillomatosis: update 2008. *Curr Opin Otolaryngol Head Neck Surg.* Dec 2008;16(6):536-542.

Gifford TO, Orlandi RR: Epistaxis. *Otolaryngol Clin North Am.* Jun 2008;41(3):525-536.

Gupta R, Sataloff RT: Laryngopharyngeal reflux: current concepts and questions. *Curr Opin Otolaryngol. Head Neck Surg.* Jun 2009;17(3):143-148.

Hamilos DL. Chronic rhinosinusitis: epidemiology and medical management. *J Allergy Clin Immunol.* Oct 2011;128(4):693-707; quiz 708-699.

Higgins TS, McCabe SJ, Bumpous JM, Martinez S: Medical decision analysis: indications for tympanostomy tubes in RAOM by age at first episode. *Otolaryngol Head Neck Surg.* Jan 2008;138(1):50-56.

Higgins KM, Wang JR: State of head and neck surgical oncology research-a review and critical appraisal of landmark studies. *Head Neck.* Dec 2008;30(12):1636-1642.

Joe SA, Thambi R, Huang J: A systematic review of the use of intranasal steroids in the treatment of chronic rhinosinusitis. *Otolaryngol Head Neck Surg.* Sep 2008;139(3):340-347.

Kim S, Grandis JR, Rinaldo A, Takes RP, Ferlito A: Emerging perspectives in epidermal growth factor receptor targeting in head and neck cancer. *Head Neck.* May 2008;30(5):667-674.

Leibowitz MS, Nayak JV, Ferris RL: Head and neck cancer immunotherapy: clinical evaluation. *Curr Oncol Rep.* Mar 2008;10(2):162-169.

Lin HC, Friedman M, Chang HW, Gurpinar B: The efficacy of multilevel surgery of the upper airway in adults with obstructive sleep apnea/hypopnea syndrome. *Laryngoscope.* May 2008;118(5):902-908.

Oosthuizen JC: Paediatric blunt laryngeal trauma: a review. *Int J Otolaryngol.* 2011;2011:183047.

Pearlman AN, Conley DB: Review of current guidelines related to the diagnosis and treatment of rhinosinusitis. *Curr Opin Otolaryngol Head Neck Surg.* Jun 2008;16(3):226-230.

Psyrri A, DiMaio D: Human papillomavirus in cervical and head-and-neck cancer. *Nat Clin Pract Oncol.* Jan 2008;5(1):24-31.

Pullens B, Giard JL, Verschuur HP, van Benthem PP: Surgery for Meniere's disease. *Cochrane Database Sys Rev.* 2010(1): CD005395.

Pullens B, van Benthem PP: Intratympanic gentamicin for Meniere's disease or syndrome. *Cochrane Database Sys Rev.* 2011(3):CD008234.

Schreiber BE, Agrup C, Haskard DO, Luxon LM: Sudden sensorineural hearing loss. *Lancet.* Apr 3 2010;375(9721):1203-1211.

Weinberger PM, Yu Z, Kountourakis P, et al: Defining molecular phenotypes of human papillomavirus-associated oropharyngeal squamous cell carcinoma: validation of three-class hypothesis. *Otolaryngol Head Neck Surg.* Sep 2009;141(3):382-389 e381.

Zalmanovici A, Yaphe J: Intranasal steroids for acute sinusitis. *Cochrane Database Sys Rev.* 2009(4):CD005149

MULTIPLE CHOICE QUESTIONS

1. You are asked to evaluate a 6-year-old child with nasal pain. She is on the pediatric hematology-oncology service, and is undergoing chemotherapy for acute lymphoblastic leukemia. She has no other pertinent medical history. The pain has been present for 12 hours. On examination, you note no abnormalities in the oral cavity, oropharynx, or external head and neck examination. Her pulse is regular and her respirations are nonlabored. On nasal examination you note a slight duskiness to the anterior face of the left middle turbinate. An appropriate response would be

   A. Reassure the child and her parents that she is most likely fine, and schedule a follow-up visit for the following day

   B. Take her to the operating room immediately for an emergent biopsy

   C. Order a contrasted MRI of the nose/face/orbits and a complete blood count (CBC) with differential

   D. Start her on nasal decongestant spray (oxymetazoline) twice daily, nasal saline irrigations, and an oral antihistamine once daily

2. You are asked to evaluate a patient in the emergency room with rapid onset of lip and tongue swelling. He develops shortness of breath and stridor during your examination. Following an emergent tracheotomy to establish his airway you do a thorough review of his medication history. Which of the following drug class(es) is/are known to be associated with acute angioedema?

   A. Angiotensin converting enzyme inhibitors (ACE inhibitors, such as lisinopril)

   B. Angiotensin II receptor blockers (ARBs, such as losartan)

   C. Recombinant tissue plasminogen activators (r-tPAs, such as alteplase)

   D. Anticoagulant direct thrombin inhibitors (such as lepirudin)

   E. All of the above

3. A 34-year-old woman is seen in the emergency department with submandibular swelling, fever, and pain. She is unable to open her mouth more than a few millimeters. One hour later she collapses, and she has only minimal air movement with bag-mask ventilation. Attempts at oral intubation are unsuccessful. Fortunately, you are standing nearby and offer to perform an emergency cricothyrotomy. Where is the best place to rapidly create an airway inferior to the vocal cords with a minimum danger of hemorrhage?

A. Immediately superior to the cricoid cartilage
B. Immediately superior to the hyoid bone
C. Immediately superior to the jugular notch
D. Immediately superior to the third tracheal ring
E. Immediately superior to the thyroid cartilage

4. A 25-year-old man sees his surgeon for follow up care 1 month after undergoing a parathyroidectomy. The patient has vocal hoarseness, so a transnasal endoscopy is performed. The left vocal fold is found to be immobile and paramedian. Denervation of which of the following muscles is most likely responsible for the vocal fold position noted?

A. Left cricothyroid muscle
B. Left lateral cricoarytenoid muscle
C. Left posterior cricoarytenoid muscle
D. Left thyroarytenoid muscle
E. Left vocalis muscle

5. Which of the following patients with squamous cell carcinoma of the head and neck most likely has the worse prognosis?

A. 46-year old woman, nonsmoker and occasional drinker with oral tongue cancer measuring 2.5 cm × 1.0 cm. No neck nodes or distant metastases are noted on examination.
B. 84-year old woman, 48 pack-year smoking history and drinks 2-3 liquor drinks per day. Has a hoarse voice for 3 months and is found to have a T2N0M0 laryngeal cancer.
C. 45-year old man, nonsmoker who drinks 1 glass of red wine daily. Has a prominent right level III neck mass. On oral examination has a 2.5 cm right tonsil mass consistent with an oropharyngeal primary.
D. 25-year old man with 12 pack-year tobacco history and chronic severe gastroesophageal reflux. Presents with throat pain and dysphagia (trouble swallowing). On fiberoptic endoscopy is found to have a 3 cm ulcerated hypopharyngeal mass. No palpable neck adenopathy is present.

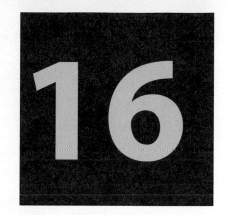

Thyroid & Parathyroid

Gerard M. Doherty, MD

▼ THE THYROID GLAND

EMBRYOLOGY & ANATOMY

The main anlage of the thyroid gland develops as a median endodermal downgrowth from the first and second pharyngeal pouches (Figure 16–1). During its migration caudally, it contacts the ultimobranchial bodies developing from the fourth pharyngeal pouches. When it reaches the position it occupies in the adult, with the isthmus situated just below the cricoid cartilage, the thyroid divides into two lobes. The site from which it originated persists as the foramen cecum at the base of the tongue. The path the gland follows may result in thyroglossal remnants (cysts) or ectopic thyroid tissue (lingual thyroid). A pyramidal lobe is frequently present. Agenesis of one thyroid lobe, almost always the left, may occur.

The normal thyroid weighs 15-25 g and is attached to the trachea by loose connective tissue. It is a highly vascularized organ that derives its blood supply principally from the superior and inferior thyroid arteries. A thyroid ima artery may also be present.

PHYSIOLOGY

The function of the thyroid gland is to synthesize, store, and secrete the hormones thyroxine (T_4) and triiodothyronine (T_3). Iodide is absorbed from the gastrointestinal tract and actively trapped by the acinar cells of the thyroid gland. It is then oxidized and combined with tyrosine in thyroglobulin to form monoiodotyrosine (MIT) and diiodotyrosine (DIT). These are coupled to form the active hormones T_4 and T_3, which initially are stored in the colloid of the gland. Following hydrolysis of the thyroglobulin, T_4 and T_3 are secreted into the plasma, becoming almost instantaneously bound to plasma proteins. Most T_3 in euthyroid individuals, however, is produced by extrathyroidal conversion of T_4 to T_3.

The function of the thyroid gland is regulated by a feedback mechanism that involves the hypothalamus and pituitary. Thyrotropin-releasing factor (TRF), a tripeptide amide, is formed in the hypothalamus and stimulates the release of the thyroid-stimulating hormone (TSH) thyrotropin, a glycoprotein, from the pituitary. Thyrotropin binds to TSH receptors on the thyroid plasma membrane, stimulating increased adenylyl cyclase activity; this increases cyclic adenosine monophosphate (cAMP) production and thyroid cellular function. Thyrotropin also stimulates the phosphoinositide pathway and—along with cAMP—stimulates thyroid growth.

EVALUATION OF THE THYROID

In a patient with enlargement of the thyroid (goiter), the history (including local and systemic systems and family history) and examination of the gland are most important and are complemented by the selective use of thyroid function tests. The surgeon must develop a systematic method of palpating the gland to determine its size, contour, consistency, nodularity, and fixation and to examine for displacement of the trachea and the presence of palpable cervical lymph nodes. Normal or abnormal structures that are attached to the larynx, such as the thyroid gland, move cephalad with deglutition, whereas adjacent lymph nodes typically do not. The isthmus of the thyroid gland crosses the front of the trachea immediately caudal to the cricoid cartilage.

Thyroid function is assessed by highly sensitive TSH assays that can differentiate among patients with hypothyroidism (increased TSH levels), euthyroidism, and hyperthyroidism (decreased TSH levels). In most cases, therefore, serum T_3, T_4, and other variables need not be measured. A free T_4 level is helpful in monitoring patients during treatment for Graves disease because the TSH level may remain suppressed despite the patient's status

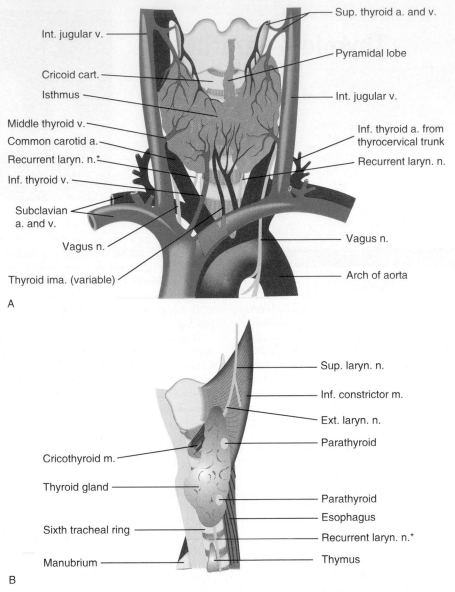

Int. jugular v. —

Cricoid cart. —

Isthmus —

Middle thyroid v. —
Common carotid a. —
Recurrent laryn. n.* —
Inf. thyroid v. —

Subclavian
a. and v. —

Vagus n. —

Thyroid ima. (variable) —

— Sup. thyroid a. and v.

— Pyramidal lobe

— Int. jugular v.

— Inf. thyroid a. from
thyrocervical trunk

— Recurrent laryn. n.

— Vagus n.

— Arch of aorta

A

— Sup. laryn. n.

— Inf. constrictor m.

— Ext. laryn. n.

— Parathyroid

Cricothyroid m. —

Thyroid gland —

Sixth tracheal ring —

Manubrium —

— Parathyroid

— Esophagus

— Recurrent laryn. n.*

— Thymus

B

▲ **Figure 16–1.** Thyroid anatomy. *The recurrent laryngeal nerve runs in the tracheoesophageal groove on the left and has a slightly more oblique course on the right before it enters the larynx just posterior to the cricothyroid muscle at the level of the cricoid cartilage.

improving. A serum T_3 level is useful for diagnosing T_3 toxicosis (high T_3 and low TSH), or the euthyroid sick, low T_3 syndrome (low T_3 and normal or slightly increased TSH).

Radioactive iodine (RAI) uptake is useful for differentiating between hyperthyroidism and increased secretion of thyroid hormone (low TSH and increased RAI uptake) on the one hand and subacute thyroiditis (low TSH and low RAI uptake) on the other. Patients with the latter "leak" thyroid hormone from the gland, which suppresses serum TSH levels and, consequently, iodine uptake by the thyroid. Patients with Graves disease have increased levels of thyroid-stimulating immunoglobulins that increase iodine uptake despite low TSH levels.

DISEASES OF THE THYROID

HYPERTHYROIDISM (THYROTOXICOSIS)

 ESSENTIALS OF DIAGNOSIS

▶ Nervousness, weight loss with increased appetite, heat intolerance, increased sweating, muscular weakness and fatigue, increased bowel frequency, polyuria, menstrual irregularities, infertility

▶ Goiter, tachycardia, atrial fibrillation, warm moist skin, thyroid thrill and bruit, cardiac flow murmur; gynecomastia

▶ Eye signs: stare, lid lag, exophthalmos

▶ TSH low or absent; TSI, iodine uptake, T_3 and T_4 increased; T_3 suppression test abnormal (failure to suppress radioiodine uptake)

▶ General Considerations

Hyperthyroidism is caused by the increased secretion of thyroid hormone (Graves disease, Plummer disease, iodine-induced [jodbasedow effect], amiodarone toxicity, TSH-secreting pituitary tumors, human chorionic gonadotropin [hCG]-secreting tumors), or by other disorders that increase thyroid hormone levels without increasing thyroid gland secretion (excess exogenous thyroid hormone intake, subacute thyroiditis, struma ovarii, and, rarely, metastatic thyroid cancers that secrete excess thyroid hormone). The most common causes of hyperthyroidism are diffusely hypersecretory goiter (Graves disease) and nodular toxic goiter (Plummer disease).

In all forms, the symptoms of hyperthyroidism are due to increased levels of thyroid hormone in the blood stream. The clinical manifestations of thyrotoxicosis may be subtle or marked and tend to go through periods of exacerbation and remission. Some patients ultimately develop hypothyroidism spontaneously (~ 15%) or as a result of treatment. Graves disease is an autoimmune disease—often with a familial predisposition—whereas the etiology of Plummer disease is unknown. Most cases of hyperthyroidism are easily diagnosed on the basis of the signs and symptoms; others (eg, mild or apathetic hyperthyroidism—which occurs most commonly in the elderly) may be recognized only with laboratory testing for a suppressed TSH level.

Thyrotoxicosis has been described with a normal T_4 concentration, normal or elevated radioiodine uptake, and normal protein binding but with increased serum T_3 by RIA (T_3 toxicosis). T_4 pseudothyrotoxicosis is occasionally seen in critically ill patients and is characterized by increased

levels of T_4 and decreased levels of T_3 due to failure to convert T_4 to T_3. Thyrotoxicosis associated with toxic nodular goiter is usually less severe than that associated with Graves disease and is only rarely if ever associated with the extrathyroidal manifestations of Graves disease such as exophthalmos, pretibial myxedema, thyroid acropathy, or periodic hypocalcemic paralysis.

If left untreated, thyrotoxicosis causes progressive and profound catabolic disturbances and cardiac damage. Death may occur in thyroid storm or because of heart failure or severe cachexia.

▶ Clinical Findings

A. Symptoms and Signs

The clinical findings are those of hyperthyroidism as well as those related to the underlying cause (Table 16–1). Nervousness, increased diaphoresis, heat intolerance, tachycardia, palpitations, fatigue, and weight loss in association with a nodular, multinodular, or diffuse goiter are the classic findings in hyperthyroidism. The patient may have a flushed and staring appearance. The skin is warm, thin, and moist, and the hair is fine.

In Graves disease, there may be exophthalmos, pretibial myxedema, or vitiligo, virtually never seen in single or multinodular toxic goiter. The Achilles reflex time is shortened in hyperthyroidism and prolonged in hypothyroidism. The patient on the verge of thyroid storm has accentuated symptoms and signs of thyrotoxicosis, with hyperpyrexia, tachycardia, cardiac failure, neuromuscular excitation, delirium, or jaundice.

B. Laboratory Findings

Laboratory tests reveal a suppressed TSH and an elevation of T_3, free T_4, and radioactive iodine. A history of medications is important, since certain drugs and organic iodinated compounds affect some thyroid function tests, and iodide excess may result in either iodide-induced hypothyroidism or iodine-induced hyperthyroidism (jodbasedow effect). In mild forms of hyperthyroidism, the usual diagnostic laboratory tests are likely to be only slightly abnormal. In these difficult-to-diagnose cases, two additional tests are helpful: the T_3 suppression test and the thyrotropin-releasing hormone (TRH) test. In the T_3 suppression test, hyperthyroid patients fail to suppress the thyroidal uptake of radioiodine when given exogenous T_3. In the TRH test, serum TSH levels fail to rise in response to administration of TRH in hyperthyroid patients.

Other findings include a high thyroid-stimulating immunoglobulin (TSI) level, low serum cholesterol, lymphocytosis, and occasionally hypercalcemia, hypercalciuria, or glycosuria.

Table 16–1. Clinical findings in thyrotoxicosis.

Clinical Manifestations	Frequency
Tachycardia	Nearly all
Nervousness	Nearly all
Goiter	Nearly all
Skin changes	Nearly all
Tremor	Nearly all
Increased sweating	Majority
Hypersensitivity to heat	Majority
Palpitations	Majority
Fatigue	Majority
Weight loss	Majority
Bruit over thyroid	Majority
Dyspnea	Majority
Eye signs	Majority
Weakness	Majority
Increased appetite	Majority
Eye complaints	Majority
Leg swelling	Some
Hyperdefecation (without diarrhea)	Some
Diarrhea	Some
Atrial fibrillation	Some
Splenomegaly	Few
Gynecomastia	Few
Anorexia	Few
Liver palms	Few
Constipation	Few
Weight gain	Few

▶ Differential Diagnosis

Anxiety neurosis, heart disease, anemia, gastrointestinal disease, cirrhosis, tuberculosis, myasthenia and other muscular disorders, menopausal syndrome, pheochromocytoma, primary ophthalmopathy, and thyrotoxicosis factitia may be clinically difficult to differentiate from hyperthyroidism.

Differentiation is especially difficult when the thyrotoxic patient presents with minimal or no thyroid enlargement. Patients may also have painless or spontaneously resolving thyroiditis and are hyperthyroid because of increased release of thyroid hormone from the thyroid gland. This condition, however, is self-limited, and treatment with antithyroid drugs, radioactive iodine, or surgery is rarely necessary.

Anxiety neurosis is perhaps the condition most frequently confused with hyperthyroidism. Anxiety is characterized by persistent fatigue usually unrelieved by rest, clammy palms, a normal sleeping pulse rate, and normal laboratory tests of thyroid function. The fatigue of hyperthyroidism is often relieved by rest, the palms are warm and moist, tachycardia persists during sleep, and thyroid function tests are abnormal.

Organic disease of nonthyroidal origin that may be confused with hyperthyroidism must be differentiated largely on the basis of evidence of specific organ system involvement and normal thyroid function tests.

Other causes of exophthalmos (eg, orbital tumors) or ophthalmoplegia (eg, myasthenia) must be ruled out by ophthalmologic, ultrasonographic, computed tomography (CT) or magnetic resonance imaging (MRI) scans, and neurologic examinations.

▶ Treatment

Hyperthyroidism may be effectively treated by antithyroid drugs, radioactive iodine, or thyroidectomy. Treatment must be individualized and depends on the patient's age and general state of health, the size of the goiter, the underlying pathologic process, and the patient's ability to obtain follow-up care.

A. Antithyroid Drugs

The principal antithyroid drug used in the United States is methimazole, 30-100 mg orally daily; propylthiouracil (PTU), 300-1000 mg orally daily has become an infrequent choice due to side effects. These agents interfere with organic binding of iodine and prevent coupling of iodotyrosines in the thyroid gland. One advantage over thyroidectomy and radioiodine in the treatment of Graves disease is that drugs inhibit the function of the gland without destroying tissue; therefore, there is a lower incidence of subsequent hypothyroidism. This form of treatment is usually used in preparation for surgery or RAI treatment but may be used as definitive treatment. Reliable patients with small goiters are good candidates for this regimen. A prolonged remission after 18 months of treatment occurs in 30% of patients, some of whom eventually become hypothyroid. Side effects of PTU include rashes and fever (3%-4%), agranulocytosis (0.1%-0.4%), and, rarely, liver failure. Patients must be warned to immediately stop the drug, see a physician, and have a white blood cell count if sore throat or fever develops.

B. Radioiodine

Radioiodine (^{131}I) may be given safely after the patient has been treated with antithyroid medications and has become euthyroid. Radioiodine is indicated for patients who are over 40 years or are poor risks for surgery and for patients with recurrent hyperthyroidism. It is less expensive than operative treatment and is effective. Radioiodine treatment at doses necessary to treat hyperthyroidism does not appear to increase the risk of leukemia or of congenital anomalies. However, an increased incidence of benign thyroid tumors and, rarely, thyroid cancer has been noted to follow treatment of hyperthyroidism with radioiodine. In young patients, the radiation hazard is certainly increased, and the chance of developing hypothyroidism is virtually 100%. After the first year of treatment with radioiodine, the incidence of hypothyroidism increases about 3% per year.

Hyperthyroid children and pregnant women should not be treated with radioiodine.

C. Surgery

1. Indications for Thyroidectomy—The main advantages of thyroidectomy is a more rapid and certain control of the disease than can be achieved with radioiodine treatment. Surgery is often the preferred treatment: (1) in the presence of a very large goiter or a multinodular goiter with relatively low RAI uptake, (2) if there is a suspicious or malignant thyroid nodule, (3) for patients with ophthalmopathy, (4) for the treatment of pregnant patients or children, (5) for the treatment of women who wish to become pregnant within 1 year after treatment, and (6) for patients with amiodarone-induced hyperthyroidism.

2. Preparation for Surgery—The risk of thyroidectomy for toxic goiter is small since the introduction of the combined preoperative use of iodides and antithyroid drugs. Methimazole or another antithyroid drug is administered until the patient becomes euthyroid and is continued until the time of operation. Three drops of potassium iodide solution or Lugol iodine solution are then given for about 10 days before surgery in conjunction with the propylthiouracil as this may decrease the friability and vascularity of the thyroid, thereby technically facilitating thyroidectomy.

An occasional untreated or inadequately treated hyperthyroid patient may require an emergency operation for some unrelated problem such as acute appendicitis and thus require immediate control of the hyperthyroidism. Such a patient should be treated in a manner similar to one in thyroid storm, since thyroid storm or hyperthyroid crises may be precipitated by surgical stress or trauma. Treatment of hyperthyroid patients requiring an emergency operation or those in thyroid storm is as follows: prevent release of preformed thyroid hormone by administration of Lugol iodine solution or with ipodate sodium; give β-adrenergic blocking agents to antagonize the peripheral manifestations of thyrotoxicosis; and decrease thyroid hormone production and extrathyroidal conversion of T_4 to T_3 by giving propylthiouracil.

The combined use of β-blocking agents and iodide lowers serum thyroid hormone levels. Other important considerations are to treat precipitating causes (eg, infection, drug reactions); to support vital functions by giving oxygen, sedatives, intravenous fluids, and corticosteroids; and to reduce fever. Benzodiazepines may be useful in the patient in whom nervousness is a prominent symptom, and a cooling blanket should be used in patients if needed fir temperature control.

3. Subtotal Thyroidectomy—The treatment of hyperthyroidism by subtotal, near-total, or total thyroidectomy eliminates both the hyperthyroidism and the goiter. As a rule, nearly all of the thyroid gland is removed, sparing the parathyroid glands and the recurrent laryngeal nerves. A very complete total thyroidectomy is generally indicated for patients with Graves ophthalmopathy.

The death rate associated with these procedures is extremely low—less than 0.1%. Thyroidectomy thus provides safe and rapid correction of the thyrotoxic state. The frequency of recurrent hyperthyroidism and hypothyroidism depends on the amount of thyroid remaining and on the natural history of the hyperthyroidism. Given an accomplished surgeon and good preoperative preparation, injuries to the recurrent laryngeal nerves and parathyroid glands occur in less than 2% of cases. Adequate exposure and avoidance of injury to the recurrent laryngeal nerves and parathyroid glands are essential.

▶ Ocular Manifestations of Graves Disease

The pathogenesis of the ocular problems in Graves disease remains unclear. Evidence originally supporting the role of either long-acting thyroid stimulator (LATS) or exophthalmos-producing substance (EPS) has not been authenticated.

The eye complications of Graves disease may begin before there is any evidence of thyroid dysfunction or after the hyperthyroidism has been appropriately treated. Usually, however, the ocular manifestations develop concomitantly with the hyperthyroidism. Relief of the eye problems is often difficult to accomplish until coexisting hyperthyroidism or hypothyroidism is controlled.

The eye changes of Graves disease vary from no signs or symptoms to loss of sight. Mild cases are characterized by upper lid retraction and stare with or without lid lag or proptosis. These cases present only minor cosmetic problems and usually require no treatment unless the eyes are dry. When moderate to severe eye changes occur, there is retro-orbital soft tissue involvement with proptosis, extraocular muscle involvement, and finally optic nerve involvement. Some cases may have marked chemosis, periorbital edema, conjunctivitis, keratitis, diplopia, ophthalmoplegia, and impaired vision. Ophthalmologic consultation is required.

Treatment of the ocular problems of Graves disease includes maintaining the patient in a euthyroid state without increase in TSH secretion, protecting the eyes from light and dust with dark glasses and eye shields, elevating the head of the bed, using diuretics to decrease periorbital and retrobulbar edema, and giving methylcellulose or guanethidine eye drops. High doses of glucocorticoids are beneficial in certain patients, but their effectiveness is variable and unpredictable. If exophthalmos progresses despite medical treatment, lateral tarsorrhaphy, retrobulbar irradiation, or surgical decompression of the orbit may be necessary. Total thyroidectomy is the treatment of choice when it can be done with a low risk of complications. Graves disease is more likely to worsen after radioiodine treatment than after thyroidectomy. It is important that patients with ophthalmopathy be made aware of the natural history of the disease and also that they be kept euthyroid, since hyperthyroidism and hypothyroidism may produce visual deterioration. Operations to correct diplopia should be deferred until after the ophthalmopathy has stabilized.

EVALUATION OF THYROID NODULES & GOITERS

▶ Thyroid Nodules

The clinician should determine whether a nodular goiter or thyroid nodule is causing localized or systemic symptoms and whether it is benign or malignant. The differential diagnosis includes benign goiter, intrathyroidal cysts, thyroiditis, benign and malignant tumors, and, rarely, metastatic tumors to the thyroid. The history should specifically emphasize the duration of swelling, recent growth, local symptoms (dysphagia, pain, or voice changes), and systemic symptoms (hyperthyroidism, hypothyroidism, or those from possible tumors metastatic to the thyroid). The patient's age, gender, place of birth, family history, and history of radiation to the neck are most important. Low-dose therapeutic radiation (6.5-2000 cGy) in infancy or childhood is associated with an increased incidence of benign goiter (~ 35%) or thyroid cancer (~ 13%) in later life. A thyroid nodule is more likely to be a cancer in a man than in a woman, and in younger (under 20 years) and older (over 60 years) patients rather than in others. In certain geographic areas, endemic goiter and benign nodules are common. Thyroid cancer is familial in about 25% of patients with medullary thyroid cancer (familial medullary thyroid cancer, multiple endocrine neoplasia [MEN] types 2A and 2B) and in about 7% of patients with papillary or Hürthle cell cancer. Papillary thyroid cancer occurs more often in patients with Cowden syndrome, Gardner syndrome, or Carney syndrome.

The clinician must systematically palpate the thyroid to determine whether there is a solitary thyroid nodule or if it is a multinodular gland and whether there are palpable lymph nodes. A solitary hard thyroid nodule is likely to be malignant, whereas most multinodular goiters are benign. Ultrasound evaluation helps document the number of nodules, whether a nodule is suspicious for cancer, and whether there are coexistent suspicious lymph nodes.

In many patients, the possibility of cancer is difficult to exclude without microscopic examination of the gland itself. Percutaneous needle biopsy is the most cost-effective diagnostic test and, along with ultrasound, has replaced radioiodine scanning for the evaluation of nodules. Cytologic results are classified by the Bethesda criteria (Table 16–2). False-positive diagnoses of cancer are rare, but about 20% of biopsy specimens reported as one of the indeterminate categories (follicular lesion of unknown significance or neoplasms) and there are more rare falsely benign results. If the specimen is reported as inadequate, biopsy should be repeated. Needle biopsy is not as helpful in patients with a history of irradiation to the neck because radiation-induced tumors are often multifocal, and a negative biopsy may therefore be unreliable. About 40% of these patients will have thyroid cancer. Radioiodine scanning can be used selectively to determine whether a follicular neoplasm by cytologic examination is functioning (warm or hot) or nonfunctioning (cold). Hot solitary thyroid nodules may cause hyperthyroidism but are rarely malignant, whereas cold solitary thyroid nodules have an incidence of cancer of 15%-20%. Thyroid carcinoma is uncommon (~ 3%) in

Table 16–2. Bethesda classification for thyroid cytology.

Cytology Result	Likelihood of Malignancy	Usual Management
Nondiagnostic	Unknown	Reaspiration
Benign	< 1%	Follow
Follicular lesion of undetermined significance	5%-10%	Consider follow, reaspiration or molecular testing of aspirate
Follicular or Hürthle cell neoplasm	20%-30%	Consider follow, reaspiration or molecular testing of aspirate
Suspicious for malignancy	50%-75%	Generally treat as for malignancy
Malignant	100%	Treat for malignancy

multinodular goiters, but if there is a dominant nodule or one that enlarges, it should be biopsied or removed. Thyroid cancer occurs in nearly 40% of the children with solitary thyroid nodules; therefore, fine-needle biopsy or thyroidectomy is indicated. Ultrasound differentiates solid and cystic lesions and, as mentioned, may detect enlarged lymph nodes. About 15% of cold solitary lesions are cystic. CT or MRI scans are usually not necessary but are helpful when the limits of the tumor cannot be defined, such as in patients with large, invasive, or substernal goiters or tumors.

The principal indications for surgical removal of a nodular goiter are: (1) suspicion of or documented cancer, (2) symptoms of pressure, (3) hyperthyroidism, (4) substernal extension, and (5) cosmetic deformity. Incidentally discovered thyroid nodules by ultrasonography, CT, MRI, or positron emission tomography (PET) scans should be evaluated by ultrasound, then, if indicated, fine-needle aspiration biopsy. Nonoperative treatment is indicated in patients with small or moderately sized multinodular goiters and Hashimoto thyroiditis unless there is a clinically suspicious area, a nodule that is growing, a personal history of radiation exposure or a family history of thyroid carcinoma.

▶ Simple or Nontoxic Goiter (Diffuse & Multinodular Goiter)

Simple goiter may be physiologic, occurring during puberty or pregnancy, or it may occur in patients from endemic (iodine-poor) regions or as a result of prolonged exposure to goitrogenic foods or drugs. As the goiter persists, there is a tendency to form nodules. Goiter may also occur early in life as a consequence of a congenital defect in thyroid hormone production or in patients with Hashimoto thyroiditis. It is generally assumed that nontoxic goiter represents a compensatory response to inadequate thyroid hormone production, although thyroid growth immunoglobulins may also be important. Nontoxic diffuse goiter usually responds favorably to thyroid hormone administration.

Symptoms are usually awareness of a neck mass and dyspnea, dysphagia, or symptoms caused by interference with venous obstruction. In diffuse goiter, the thyroid is symmetrically enlarged and has a smooth surface; however, most patients have multinodular glands by the time they seek medical care. Thyroid function is usually normal, though the sensitive TSH may be suppressed and the radioiodine uptake increased. Surgery is indicated to relieve the pressure symptoms of a large goiter for substernal goiter or to rule out cancer when there are localized areas of hardness or rapid growth. Aspiration biopsy cytology is helpful in these patients.

Baloch ZW et al: Diagnostic terminology and morphologic criteria for cytologic diagnosis of thyroid lesions: a synopsis of the National Cancer Institute Thyroid Fine-Needle Aspiration State of the Science Conference. *Diagn Cytopathol*. 2008;36:425.

Cibas ES et al: Indications for thyroid FNA and pre-FNA requirements: a synopsis of the National Cancer Institute Thyroid Fine-Needle Aspiration State of the Science Conference. *Diagn Cytopathol*. 2008;36:390-399.

INFLAMMATORY THYROID DISEASE

The inflammatory diseases of the thyroid are termed acute, subacute, or chronic thyroiditis, which can be either suppurative or nonsuppurative.

Acute suppurative thyroiditis is uncommon and is characterized by the sudden onset of severe neck pain accompanied by dysphagia, fever, and chills. It usually follows an acute upper respiratory tract infection; can be diagnosed by percutaneous aspiration, smear, and culture; and is treated by surgical drainage. The organisms are most often streptococci, staphylococci, pneumococci, or coliforms. It may also be associated with a piriform sinus fistula. A barium swallow is therefore recommended in persistent or recurrent cases.

Subacute thyroiditis, a noninfectious disorder, is characterized by thyroid swelling, head and chest pain, fever, weakness, malaise, palpitations, and weight loss. Some patients with subacute thyroiditis have no pain (silent thyroiditis), in which case the condition must be distinguished from Graves disease. In subacute thyroiditis, the erythrocyte sedimentation rate and serum gamma globulin are almost always elevated, and radioiodine uptake is very low or absent with increased or normal thyroid hormone levels. The illness is usually self-limited, and aspirin and corticosteroids relieve symptoms. Most of these patients eventually become euthyroid.

Hashimoto thyroiditis, the most common form of thyroiditis, is usually characterized by enlargement of the thyroid with or without pain and tenderness. It is much more common in women (~ 15% of US women) and occasionally causes dysphagia or hypothyroidism.

Hashimoto thyroiditis is an autoimmune disease. Serum titers of antimicrosomal and antithyroglobulin antibodies are elevated. Appropriate treatment for most patients consists of giving small doses of thyroid hormone. Operation is indicated for marked pressure symptoms, for suspected malignant tumor, and for cosmetic reasons. If the thyroid is large or asymmetric, or if it contains a discrete nodule, or grows rapidly, percutaneous needle biopsy or thyroidectomy is recommended. Thyroid lymphoma can rarely occur in patients with Hashimoto thyroiditis.

Riedel thyroiditis is a rare condition that presents as a hard woody mass in the thyroid region with marked fibrosis and chronic inflammation in and around the gland. The inflammatory process infiltrates muscles and causes symptoms of tracheal compression. Hypothyroidism is usually present, and hypoparathyroid may develop. Surgical treatment is required to relieve tracheal or esophageal obstruction.

BENIGN TUMORS OF THE THYROID

Benign thyroid tumors are adenomas, involutionary nodules, cysts, or localized thyroiditis. Most adenomas are of the follicular type. Adenomas are usually solitary and encapsulated and compress the adjacent thyroid. The major reasons for removal are a suspicion of cancer, functional overactivity producing hyperthyroidism, and cosmetic disfigurement.

MALIGNANT TUMORS OF THE THYROID

ESSENTIALS OF DIAGNOSIS

▶ History of irradiation to the neck in some patients

▶ Painless or enlarging nodule, dysphagia, or hoarseness

▶ Firm or hard, fixed thyroid nodule; ipsilateral cervical lymphadenopathy

▶ Normal thyroid function; nodule stippled with microcalcifications and solid (ultrasound), cold (radioiodine scan); positive or suspicious cytology

▶ Family history of thyroid cancer

▶ General Considerations

An appreciation of the classification of malignant tumors of the thyroid is important, because thyroid tumors demonstrate a wide range of growth and malignant behavior. At one end of the spectrum is papillary carcinoma, which usually occurs in young adults, grows very slowly, metastasizes through lymphatics, and is compatible with long life even in the presence of metastases (Figure 16–2). At the other extreme is undifferentiated carcinoma, which appears late in life and is nonencapsulated and invasive, forming large infiltrating tumors composed of small or large anaplastic cells. Most patients with anaplastic thyroid carcinoma succumb as a consequence of local recurrence, pulmonary metastasis, or both within 9 months. Between these two extremes are follicular, Hürthle cell, and medullary carcinomas, sarcomas, lymphomas, and metastatic tumors. The prognosis depends on the histologic pattern, the age and gender of the patient, the extent of tumor spread at the time of diagnosis, whether the tumor takes up radioiodine, and other factors. On average, 5% of patients with papillary, 10% of those with follicular, 15% of those with Hürthle cell, and 20% of those with medullary thyroid cancer will die within 10 years from these tumors.

The cause of most cases of thyroid carcinoma is unknown, although persons who received low-dose (6.5-2000 cGy) therapeutic radiation to the thymus, tonsils, scalp, and skin in infancy, childhood, and adolescence have an increased risk of developing thyroid tumors. Children are most susceptible to radiation exposure such as occurred with the

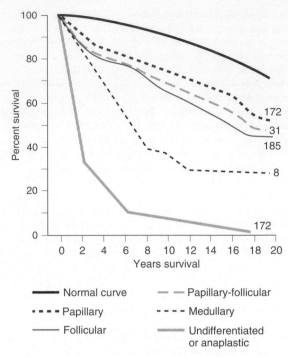

▲ **Figure 16–2.** Survival rates after thyroidectomy for papillary, mixed papillary-follicular, follicular, medullary, and undifferentiated thyroid cancer.

Chernobyl nuclear accident, but adults up to 50 years of age who were exposed to the atomic blast at Hiroshima had an increased incidence of benign and malignant thyroid tumors. The incidence of thyroid cancer increases for at least 30 years after irradiation. *RET/PTC* rearrangements occur in about 80% of radiation associated papillary thyroid cancers.

▶ Types of Thyroid Cancer

A. Papillary Carcinoma

Papillary adenocarcinoma accounts for 85% of cancers of the thyroid gland. The tumor usually appears in early adult life and presents as a solitary nodule. It then spreads via intraglandular lymphatics within the thyroid gland and then to the subcapsular and pericapsular lymph nodes. Fifty percent of children and 20% of adults present with palpable lymph nodes. The tumor may metastasize to lungs or bone. Microscopically, it is composed of papillary projections of columnar epithelium. Psammoma bodies are present in about 60% of cases. Mixed papillary-follicular, follicular variants of papillary carcinoma, and poorly differentiated cancers including tall cell and columnar cell papillary thyroid cancers are sometimes found. The rate of growth may be stimulated by TSH. A *BRAF* mutation is the most common mutation in papillary thyroid cancer and is associated with lymph node metastases and a higher recurrence rate.

B. Follicular Adenocarcinoma

Follicular adenocarcinoma accounts for approximately 10% of malignant thyroid tumors. It appears later in life than the papillary form and may be rubbery or even soft on palpation. Follicular tumors are encapsulated. Microscopically, follicular carcinoma may be difficult to distinguish from normal thyroid tissue. Capsular (invasion through the capsule) and vascular invasion distinguish follicular carcinoma from follicular adenoma. Follicular thyroid cancers only occasionally (~5%) metastasize to the regional lymph nodes, but they have a greater tendency to spread by the hematogenous route to the lungs, the skeleton, and, rarely, the liver. Metastases from this tumor often demonstrate avidity for RAI after total thyroidectomy. Skeletal metastases may appear years after resection of the primary lesion. Hürthle cell carcinoma is considered a clinical variant of follicular carcinoma. It is more likely to be multifocal and involve lymph nodes than follicular carcinoma. Like follicular carcinoma, it makes thyroglobulin, however it does not usually take up radioiodine. The prognosis is not as good for either follicular or Hürthle cell cancers as with the papillary type (Figure 16–3).

C. Medullary Carcinoma

Medullary carcinoma accounts for approximately 7% of malignant tumors of the thyroid and 15% of thyroid cancer deaths. It contains amyloid and is a solid, hard, nodular

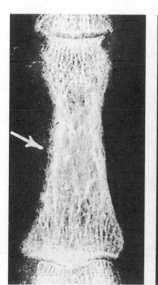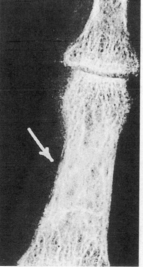

▲ **Figure 16–3.** Subperiosteal resorption of radial side of second phalanges.

tumor that does not take up radioiodine and secretes calcitonin. Medullary carcinomas arise from parafollicular cells of the ultimobranchial bodies or C cells. Familial medullary carcinoma occurs in about 25% of patients. It may be isolated or occur with pheochromocytomas (often bilateral), lichen planus amyloidosis, and hyperparathyroidism (MEN2A, Table 16–3). It may also occur with or without pheochromocytomas (usually bilateral), marfanoid habitus, multiple neuromas, and ganglioneuromatosis (MEN2B). Hirschsprung disease occurs more frequently in patients with familial medullary cancer. All patients with medullary thyroid cancer should be screened for an *RET* point mutation on chromosome 10 because 10% of patients without a positive family history have de novo mutations. For patients detected by family genetic screening, most experts recommend prophylactic total thyroidectomy at an age determine by the risk associated with the specific mutation. Isolated familial medullary thyroid cancer is the least aggressive form, whereas this cancer is most aggressive in MEN2B patients.

D. Undifferentiated Carcinoma

This rapidly growing tumor, also known as anaplastic carcinoma, occurs principally beyond middle life and accounts for 1% of all thyroid cancers. This tumor usually evolves from a papillary or follicular neoplasm. It is a solid, quickly enlarging, hard, irregular mass diffusely involving the gland and often invades the trachea, muscles, and neurovascular structures. The tumor may be painful and somewhat tender, may be fixed on swallowing, and may cause laryngeal or esophageal obstructive symptoms. Microscopically, there are three major types: giant cell, spindle cell, and small cell. Mitoses are frequent. Cervical lymphadenopathy and pulmonary metastases are common. Local recurrence after surgical treatment is the rule. Combination treatment with external radiation therapy, chemotherapy, and surgery offers palliation to some patients but is rarely curative (Figure 16–2).

▶ Treatment

The treatment of differentiated thyroid carcinoma (which does not include anaplastic carcinoma or medullary thyroid cancer) is operative removal. For papillary carcinoma over 1 cm, acceptable operations are near-total or total thyroidectomy. For solitary papillary carcinomas less than 1 cm, thyroid lobectomy is adequate treatment. Subtotal or partial lobectomy is contraindicated because the incidence of tumor recurrence is greater and survival is shorter. Total thyroidectomy is recommended for papillary (> 1.0 cm), follicular, Hürthle cell, and medullary carcinomas if the operation can be done without producing permanent hypoparathyroidism or injury to the recurrent laryngeal nerves. Total thyroidectomy is preferred over other operations because of the high incidence of multifocal tumor within the gland, a clinical recurrence rate of

Table 16–3. Multiple endocrine neoplasia syndromes.

Syndrome	Major Clinical Components	Associated Clinical Components	Site of Genetic Abnormality
MEN1	• Hyperparathyroidism • Duodenopancreatic neuroendocrine tumors • Pituitary adenomas	• Thyroid adenoma • Adrenal adenoma • Thymic carcinoid tumor • Subcutaneous lipoma • Cutaneous collagenomas and angiofibromas	• *Menin*-tumor suppressor gene • Mutation eliminates function from one allele
MEN2A	• Medullary thyroid cancer • Hyperparathyroidism • Pheochromocytoma	• Lichen planus	• *RET* protooncogene • Mutation causes constitutive receptor activation
MEN2B	• Medullary thyroid cancer • Pheochromocytoma • Neurofibromas of lips and tongue • Marfanoid habitus	• Colonic dysfunction similar to Hirschsprung disease	
Familial medullary thyroid cancer	• Medullary thyroid cancer		

about 7% in the contralateral lobe if it is spared, and the ease of assessment for recurrence by serum thyroglobulin assay and neck ultrasound examinations during follow-up examinations. This also allows one to use adjuvant or therapeutic radioiodine treatment. Preoperative ultrasound is essential in patients with papillary cancer, and all abnormal central and lateral neck lymph nodes should be removed. Whether an ipsilated prophylactic central neck dissection should be done is controversial.

A functional modified radical neck dissection preserving the jugular vein, sternocleidomastoid muscle, spinal accessory nerve, and sensory nerves is performed if lymph nodes in the lateral neck are clinically involved.

Medullary carcinoma is associated with such a high incidence of nodal involvement that a bilateral central neck node compartment dissection should be done in all patients. Concomitant ipsilateral and contralateral modified radical neck dissection may be indicated selectively for primary tumors more than 1.5 cm in diameter and when the central neck nodes are involved. When serum calcitonin or carcinoembryonic antigen (CEA) levels remain elevated after thyroidectomy, ultrasound or MRI examination of the neck and MRI of the mediastinum should be done. Laparoscopic evaluation of the liver for the common miliary metastases is recommended for patients with markedly elevated calcitonin levels. If there is no metastatic in the liver, then central neck dissection and bilateral functional neck dissections should be done, if not already done, including removal of nodes from the superior mediastinum.

Isolated distant metastatic deposits of differentiated thyroid carcinoma should be removed surgically if possible and treated with ^{131}I after total thyroidectomy or thyroid ablation with radioactive iodine. All patients with thyroid cancer should be maintained indefinitely on suppressive doses of thyroid hormone (mild suppression for low-risk patients). For follow-up, it is helpful to measure basal and TSH-stimulated serum levels of thyroglobulin (a tumor marker for differentiated thyroid cancer), which are usually increased (> 2 ng/mL) in patients with residual tumor after total thyroidectomy.

For **undifferentiated carcinoma, malignant lymphoma,** or **sarcoma,** the tumor should be excised as completely as possible and then treated by radiation and chemotherapy. It is common that no operation beyond a diagnostic biopsy is useful for these patients, as they may be locally inoperable with a course dictated by the systemic disease.

Bilimoria KY et al: Extent of surgery affects survival for papillary thyroid cancer. *Ann Surg.* 2007;246:375.
Cooper DS et al: Revised American Thyroid Association management guidelines for patients with thyroid nodules and differentiated thyroid cancer. *Thyroid.* 2009;19:1167.
Kloos RT et al: Medullary thyroid cancer: management guidelines of the American Thyroid Association. *Thyroid.* 2009;19:565.
Smallridge RC et al: American Thyroid Association guidelines for management of patients with anaplastic thyroid cancer. *Thyroid.* 2012;2:1104.

THE PARATHYROID GLANDS

EMBRYOLOGY & ANATOMY

Phylogenetically, the parathyroids appear rather late, being first seen in amphibia. They arise from pharyngeal pouches

III and IV and may be arrested as high as the level of the hyoid bone during their descent to the posterior capsule of the thyroid gland. Four parathyroid glands are present in 85% of the population, and 85% are situated on the posterior lateral surface of the thyroid gland. About 15% of people have more than four glands. Occasionally, one or more may be incorporated into the thyroid gland or thymus and hence are intrathyroidal or intrathymic in location. Parathyroid III, which normally assumes the inferior position, may be found in the anterior mediastinum, usually in the thymus. The upper parathyroids (parathyroid IV) usually remain in close association with the upper portion of the lateral thyroid lobes at the level of the cricoid cartilage but may be loosely attached by a long vascular pedicle and migrate caudally in the tracheoesophageal groove into the posterior mediastinum. About 85% of parathyroid glands lie within 1 cm of where the inferior thyroid artery and recurrent laryngeal nerve cross.

The normal parathyroid gland has a distinct yellowish-brown color, is ovoid, tongue-shaped, polypoid, or spherical, and averages $2 \times 3 \times 7$ mm. The total mean weight of four normal parathyroid glands is about 150 mg. These encapsulated glands are usually supplied by a branch of the inferior thyroid artery but may be supplied by the superior thyroid artery. The vessels can be seen entering a hilum-like structure, a feature that differentiates parathyroid glands from fat.

PHYSIOLOGY

Parathyroid hormone (PTH), vitamin D, and calcitonin play vital roles in calcium and phosphorus metabolism in bone, kidney, and gut. Specific radioimmunoassays are available to measure PTH, vitamin D, and calcitonin. Ionized calcium, the physiologically important fraction, can now be accurately measured. Total serum calcium concentration is composed of approximately 48% ionized calcium, 46% protein-bound calcium, and 6% calcium complexed to organic anions. Total serum calcium varies directly with plasma protein concentrations, but calcium ion concentrations are unaffected.

PTH and calcitonin work in concert to modulate fluctuations in plasma levels of ionized calcium. When the ionized calcium level falls, the parathyroid glands secrete more PTH, and the parafollicular cells within the thyroid secrete less calcitonin. The rise in PTH and fall in calcitonin produce increased bone resorption and increased resorption of calcium in the renal tubules. More calcium enters the blood, and ionized calcium levels return to normal.

In the circulation, immunoreactive PTH is heterogeneous, consisting of the intact hormone and several hormonal fragments. The amino terminal (N-terminal) fragment is biologically active, whereas the carboxyl terminal (C-terminal) fragment is biologically inert. Measurement of intact PTH by immunoassay is best for screening for hyperparathyroidism and for selective venous catheterization to localize the source of PTH production. PTH-related peptide (PTHrP) that is secreted by nonparathyroid malignant tumors does not cross-react with intact PTH assays.

Because PTH levels rise in normal subjects if ionized calcium levels are low, calcium and PTH must be determined from samples drawn simultaneously to diagnose hyperparathyroidism. The combination of increased PTH levels and hypercalcemia without hypocalciuria is almost always diagnostic of hyperparathyroidism.

▼ DISEASES OF THE PARATHYROIDS

PRIMARY HYPERPARATHYROIDISM

ESSENTIALS OF DIAGNOSIS

▶ Increased fatigue, weakness, arthralgias, nausea, vomiting, dyspepsia, constipation, polydipsia, polyuria, nocturia, psychiatric disturbances, renal colic, bone pain, and joint pain ("stones, bones, abdominal groans, psychic moans, and fatigue overtones"). Some patients are asymptomatic

▶ Nephrolithiasis and nephrocalcinosis, osteopenia, osteoporosis, osteitis fibrosa cystica, peptic ulcer disease, renal dysfunction, gout, pseudogout, chondrocalcinosis, pancreatitis

▶ Hypertension, band keratopathy, neck masses

▶ Serum calcium, PTH, chloride, usually increased; serum phosphate low or normal; uric acid and alkaline phosphatase sometimes increased; urine calcium increased, normal, or, rarely, decreased; urine phosphate increased; tubular reabsorption of phosphate decreased, osteocalcin and deoxypyridinoline cross-links increased

▶ X-rays: subperiosteal resorption of phalanges, demineralization of the skeleton (osteopenia or osteoporosis), bone cysts, and nephrocalcinosis or nephrolithiasis

▶ General Considerations

Primary hyperparathyroidism is due to excess or nonsuppressed PTH secretion from a single parathyroid adenoma (83%), multiple adenomas (6%), hyperplasia (10%), or carcinoma (1%). Once thought to be rare, primary hyperparathyroidism is now found in 0.1%-0.3% of the general population and is the most common cause of hypercalcemia in unselected patients. It is uncommon before puberty; its peak incidence is between the third and fifth decades, and it is two to three times more common in women than in men.

Overproduction of PTH in spite of upper normal or elevated serum levels of calcium results in mobilization of calcium from bone and inhibition of the renal reabsorption of phosphate, thereby producing hypercalcemia and hypophosphatemia. This causes a wasting of calcium and phosphorus, with osseous mineral loss and osteopenia or osteoporosis. Other associated or related conditions that offer clues to the diagnosis of hyperparathyroidism are nephrolithiasis, nephrocalcinosis, osteitis fibrosa cystica, peptic ulcer, pancreatitis, hypertension, and gout or pseudogout. Hyperparathyroidism also occurs in both MEN1, known as **Wermer syndrome**, and MEN2, known as Sipple syndrome (Table 16–3). The former is characterized by tumors of the parathyroid, pituitary, and pancreas (hyperparathyroidism, pituitary tumors, and functioning or nonfunctioning islet cell pancreatic tumors) that may cause Zollinger-Ellison syndrome (gastrinoma), hypoglycemia (insulinoma), glucagonoma, somatostatinoma, and pancreatic polypeptide tumors (PPomas). Other tumors in MEN1 syndrome include adrenocortical tumors, carcinoid tumors, multiple lipomas, and cutaneous angiomas. MEN2A consists of hyperparathyroidism (20%) in association with medullary carcinoma of the thyroid (98%), pheochromocytoma (50%), and lichen planus amyloidosis. MEN2B patients have a marfanoid habitus, multiple neuromas, and pheochromocytomas but rarely have hyperparathyroidism. Familial hyperparathyroidism can also occur alone or in the presence of jaw tumor syndrome.

Parathyroid adenomas range in weight from 65 mg to over 35 g, and the size usually parallels the degree of hypercalcemia. Microscopically, these tumors may be of chief cell, water cell, or, rarely, oxyphil cell type.

Primary parathyroid hyperplasia involves all of the parathyroid glands. Microscopically, there are two types: chief cell hyperplasia and water-clear cell (wasserhelle) hyperplasia. Hyperplastic glands vary considerably in size but are usually larger than normal (65 mg).

Parathyroid carcinoma is rare but is more common in patients with profound hypercalcemia and in patients with familial hyperparathyroidism and jaw tumor syndrome. Parathyroid cancers are palpable in half the patients and should be suspected in patients at operation when the parathyroid gland is hard, has a whitish or irregular capsule, or is invasive. Parathyromatosis is a rare condition causing hypercalcemia due to multiple embryologic rests or, more commonly, due to seeding when a parathyroid tumor has ruptured or the tumor capsule has been disrupted.

▶ Clinical Findings

A. Symptoms and Signs

Historically, the clinical manifestations of hyperparathyroidism have changed. Forty years ago, the diagnosis was based on bone pain and deformity (osteitis fibrosa cystica), and in later years on the renal complications (nephrolithiasis and nephrocalcinosis). At present, over two-thirds of patients are detected by routine screening, or because of osteopenia or osteoporosis, and some are asymptomatic. Patients with even mild primary hyperparathyroidism are predisposed to cardiovascular events and fractures. After successful surgical treatment, many patients thought to be asymptomatic become aware of improvement in unrecognized preoperative symptoms such as fatigue, mild depression, weakness, constipation, polydipsia and polyuria, and bone and joint pain. Hyperparathyroidism should be suspected in all patients with hypercalcemia and the above symptoms, especially if associated with nephrolithiasis, nephrocalcinosis, hypertension, left ventricular hypertrophy, peptic ulcer, pancreatitis, or gout. Patients with primary hyperparathyroidism appear to have a shortened life expectancy that improves after successful parathyroidectomy. Younger patients and those with less severe hypercalcemia after parathyroidectomy have the best prognosis.

B. Laboratory Findings, Imaging Studies, and Differential Diagnosis (Approach to the Hypercalcemic Patient)

1. Laboratory Findings—Together, hyperparathyroidism and humoral hypercalcemia of malignancy (nonparathyroid cancer) are responsible for about 90% of all cases of hypercalcemia. Hyperparathyroidism is the most common cause of hypercalcemia detected by undirected methods such as routine screening, whereas cancer is the most common cause of hypercalcemia in hospitalized patients. Other causes of hypercalcemia are listed in Table 16–4. In many patients the diagnosis is obvious, while in others it may be difficult. At times, more than one reason for hypercalcemia may exist in the same patient, such as cancer or sarcoidosis plus hyperparathyroidism. A careful history must be obtained documenting: (1) the duration of any symptoms possibly related to hypercalcemia; (2) symptoms related to malignant disease; (3) conditions associated with hyperparathyroidism, such as renal colic, peptic ulcer disease, pancreatitis, hypertension, or gout; and (4) possible excess use of milk products, antacids, baking soda, or vitamins. In patients with a recent cough, wheeze, or hemoptysis, epidermoid carcinoma of the lung should be considered. Hematuria might suggest hypernephroma, bladder tumor, or renal lithiasis. A long history of renal stones or peptic ulcer disease suggests that hyperparathyroidism is likely.

The most important tests for the evaluation of hypercalcemia are, in order of importance, serum calcium, PTH, phosphate, chloride, alkaline phosphatase, creatinine; uric acid and urea nitrogen; urinary calcium; blood hematocrit and pH; serum magnesium; and erythrocyte sedimentation rate (Table 16–5). Measurement of 25-hydroxy and 1,25-hydroxy vitamin D levels, and serum protein electrophoresis are helpful in selected patients when other tests are equivocal.

Table 16–4. Causes of hypercalcemia.

	Approximate Frequency
Cancer	Common
Metastatic breast cancer	
PTH-related peptide secreting (lung, kidney)	
Multiple myeloma	
Leukemia	
Other metastatic cancer	
Endocrine Disorders	Common
Hyperparathyroidism	
Hyperthyroidism	
Addison disease, pheochromocytoma	
Hypothyroidism, VIPoma	
Increased Calcium or Vitamin Intake and Drugs	Uncommon
Milk-alkali syndrome	
Vitamin D and A overdosage	
Thiazide diuretics, lithium	
Granulomatous Diseases	Uncommon
Sarcoidosis	
Tuberculosis	
Benign Familial Hypocalciuric Hypercalcemia and Other Disorders	Rare
Paget disease	
Immobilization	
Idiopathic hypercalcemia of infancy	
Aluminum intoxication	
Dysproteinemias	
Rhabdomyolysis	

Table 16–5. Laboratory evaluation of hypercalcemia.

Essential	Selective
Blood Tests	
Calcium	Creatine and BUN
Phosphate	Chloride
PTH (intact or two-site assay)	Uric acid
Alkaline phosphatase	pH
	Protein electrophoresis or albumin: globulin ratio
	25-dihydroxyvitamin D and 1,25-dihydroxyvitamin D
Radiographic or Nuclear Medicine Procedures	
Chest x-ray	Sestamibi scan of neck and ultrasound of neck
Abdominal plain films	
Ultrasound of kidneys	
Bone density (hip, lumbar spine, wrist)	
Urine Tests	
24-hour urinary calcium[1]	Urinalysis
	Deoxypyridinoline cross-links
	Osteocalcin

[1]When urine calcium is < 100 mg/24 h, a diagnosis of benign familial hypocalciuric hypercalcemia must be considered.

A high serum calcium and a low serum phosphate suggest hyperparathyroidism, but about half of patients with hyperparathyroidism have normal serum phosphate concentrations. Patients with vitamin D intoxication, sarcoidosis, malignant disease without metastasis, and hyperthyroidism may also be hypophosphatemic, but patients with breast cancer and hypercalcemia are only rarely so. In fact, if hypophosphatemia and hypercalcemia are present in association with breast cancer, concomitant hyperparathyroidism is probable. Measurement of serum PTH has its greatest value in this situation, since the PTH level is low or nil in patients with hypercalcemia due to all causes other than primary hyperparathyroidism or familial hypocalciuric hypercalcemia. In general, serum PTH levels should be measured in all patients with persistent hypercalcemia without an obvious cause and in normocalcemic patients who are suspected of having hyperparathyroidism. Determination of intact serum PTH levels is sensitive and is not influenced by tumors that secrete parathyroid-related peptide. Nonparathyroid tumors that secrete pure PTH are extremely rare.

An elevated serum chloride concentration is a useful diagnostic clue found in about 40% of hyperparathyroid patients. PTH acts directly on the proximal renal tubule to decrease the resorption of bicarbonate, which leads to increased resorption of chloride and mild hyperchloremic renal tubular acidosis. An increased serum chloride is not found in other causes of hypercalcemia. Calculation of the serum chloride to phosphate ratio takes advantage of slight increases in serum chloride and slight decreases in serum phosphate concentrations. A ratio above 33 suggests hyperparathyroidism; this was a more clinically useful observation before the availability of rapid and accurate PTH measurement.

A 24-hour urine calcium level is helpful for diagnosing hypercalcemic patients who have low urinary calcium levels resulting from benign familial hypocalciuric hypercalcemia (BFHH) and for patients with marked hypercalciuria (> 400 mg/24 h). Patients with BFHH do not benefit from parathyroidectomy.

Serum protein electrophoretic patterns are helpful for diagnosis of multiple myeloma and sarcoidosis. Hypergammaglobulinemia is rare in hyperparathyroidism but is not uncommon in patients with multiple myeloma and sarcoidosis. Roentgenograms of the skull or site of bone pain in patients with elevated alkaline phosphatase levels will often reveal typical "punched-out" bony lesions, and the diagnosis of myeloma can be firmly established by bone marrow examination. Sarcoidosis can be difficult to diagnose, because it may exist for years with limited clinical findings. A chest x-ray revealing a diffuse fibronodular infiltrate and prominent hilar adenopathy is suggestive, and the demonstration of noncaseating granuloma in lymph nodes is diagnostic.

Serum alkaline phosphate levels are elevated in about 10% of patients with primary hyperparathyroidism and may also be increased in patients with Paget disease and cancer. When the serum alkaline phosphatase level is elevated, serum 5′-nucleotidase, which parallels liver alkaline phosphatase, should be measured to determine if the increase is from bone, which suggests parathyroid disease, or liver.

2. Bone Studies—Bone densitometry and radiographic examination of bone frequently reveals osteopenia (1 standard deviation below normal density) or osteoporosis (2.5 standard deviations below normal), but overt skeletal changes such as subperiosteal resorption or brown tumor are found in less than 10% of patients with hyperparathyroidism. Dual photon bone density studies of the femur, lumbar spine, and radius help document osteopenia that occurs in about 70% of women with hyperparathyroidism. Bone changes of osteitis fibrosa cystica are rare on x-ray unless the serum alkaline phosphatase concentration is increased. Primary and secondary hyperparathyroidism can produce subperiosteal resorption of the phalanges and bone cysts (Figure 16–3). A ground-glass appearance of the skull with loss of definition of the tables and demineralization of the outer aspects of the clavicles are less frequently seen. In patients with markedly elevated serum alkaline phosphatase levels without subperiosteal resorption on x-ray, Paget disease or cancer must be suspected. A 24-hour urine test for deoxypyridinoline cross-link assay or osteocalcin detects increased bone loss.

3. Differential Diagnosis—The differentiation between hyperparathyroidism because of primary parathyroid disease and that due to humoral hypercalcemia of malignancy can now almost always be determined by measuring intact PTH, which is increased in primary hyperparathyroidism but suppressed in humoral hypercalcemia of malignancy.

The most common tumors causing humoral hypercalcemia of malignancy are squamous cell carcinoma of the lung, renal cell carcinoma, and bladder cancer. Less commonly it is due to hepatoma or to cancer of the ovary, stomach, pancreas, parotid gland, or colon. Recent onset of symptoms, increased sedimentation rate, anemia, serum calcium greater than 14 mg/dL, and increased alkaline phosphatase activity without osteitis fibrosa cystica suggest humoral hypercalcemia of malignancy; mild hypercalcemia with a long history of nephrolithiasis or peptic ulcer suggests primary hyperthyroidism. Documented hypercalcemia of 6 months or longer essentially rules out malignancy-associated hypercalcemia.

In milk-alkali syndrome, a history of excessive ingestion of milk products, calcium-containing antacids, and baking soda is often obtained. These patients become normocalcemic after discontinuing these habits. Patients with milk-alkali syndrome usually have renal insufficiency and low urinary calcium concentrations and are usually alkalotic rather than acidotic. Because of the high incidence of ulcer disease in hyperparathyroidism, milk-alkali syndrome may occasionally coexist with that disorder. This is very infrequent now that acid-suppressing medications, such as proton pump inhibitors, are available to manage peptic ulcer disease.

Hyperthyroidism, another cause of hypercalcemia and hypercalciuria, can usually be differentiated because manifestations of thyrotoxicosis rather than hypercalcemia bring the patient to the physician. Occasionally, an elderly patient with apathetic hyperthyroidism may be hypercalcemic. A sensitive TSH test should be evaluated in hypercalcemic patients whose PTH levels are not increased. Treatment of hyperthyroidism with antithyroid medications causes serum calcium to return to normal levels within 8 weeks.

Normal subjects taking **thiazide diuretics** may develop a transient increase in serum calcium levels, usually less than 1 mg/dL. Larger rises in serum calcium induced by thiazides have been reported in patients with primary hyperparathyroidism and idiopathic juvenile osteoporosis. Most patients who have hypercalcemia while taking thiazides have another reason for the increase. The best way to evaluate these patients is to switch them to a nonthiazide antihypertensive agent or diuretic and to measure the PTH level. Thiazide-induced hypercalcemia is not associated with increased serum PTH in patients without hyperparathyroidism.

Benign familial hypocalciuric hypercalcemia is one of the few conditions that causes chronic hypercalcemia and mildly elevated PTH levels. It can be difficult to distinguish from mild primary hyperparathyroidism. The best way to diagnose this disorder is to document a low urinary calcium and a family history of hypercalcemia, especially in children.

Other miscellaneous causes of hypercalcemia are Paget disease, immobilization (especially in Paget disease or in young patients), dysproteinemias, idiopathic hypercalcemia of infancy, aluminum intoxication, and rhabdomyolysis (Table 16–4).

C. Approach to the Normocalcemic Patient With Possible Hyperparathyroidism

Renal failure, hypoalbuminemia, pancreatitis, deficiency of vitamin D or magnesium, and excess phosphate intake may cause serum calcium levels to be normal in hyperparathyroidism. Correction of these disorders results in hypercalcemia if hyperparathyroidism is present. The incidence of normocalcemic hyperparathyroidism in patients with hypercalciuria and recurrent nephrolithiasis (idiopathic hypercalciuria) is not known. Because the serum calcium concentration may fluctuate, it should be measured on more than three separate occasions. Determination of serum ionized calcium is also sometimes revealing, since it may be increased in patients with normal total serum calcium levels.

If a patient has elevated serum levels of ionized calcium and PTH, the diagnosis of normocalcemic hyperparathyroidism has been confirmed. There are three major causes of hypercalciuria and nephrolithiasis: (1) increased absorption of calcium from the gastrointestinal tract (absorptive hypercalciuria), (2) increased renal leakage of calcium (renal hypercalciuria) and (3) primary hyperparathyroidism. Patients with absorptive hypercalcemia absorb too much calcium from the gastrointestinal tract and therefore have low serum PTH levels. Patients with renal hypercalciuria lose calcium from leaky renal tubules and have increased PTH levels. They can be distinguished from patients with normocalcemic hyperparathyroidism by their response to treatment with thiazides. In renal leak hypercalcemia, serum PTH levels become normal because thiazides correct the excessive loss of calcium, whereas in primary hyperparathyroidism increased serum PTH levels persist and the patient often becomes hypercalcemic.

▶ Natural History of Untreated & Treated Hyperparathyroidism

Patients with untreated hyperparathyroidism have an increased risk of dying prematurely, mainly from cardiovascular and malignant disease. There is decreased respiratory muscular capacity and increased frequency of hypertrophic cardiomyopathy with left ventricular hypertrophy and decreased vascular compliance even in hyperparathyroid patients without hypertension. Hyperparathyroid patients have more hypertension, nephrolithiasis, osteopenia, peptic ulcer disease, gout, renal dysfunction, and pancreatitis. After successful parathyroidectomy, previously hyperpara-

thyroid patients still have an increased risk of premature death, however, younger patients and those with less severe disease return to a normal survival curve sooner than do older patients or those with more severe hyperparathyroidism. Most patients with hyperparathyroidism—even those with normocalcemic hyperparathyroidism—have symptoms and associated conditions. In 80% of patients, these clinical manifestations improve or disappear after parathyroidectomy.

▶ Treatment

The only curative treatment of primary hyperparathyroidism is parathyroidectomy. There are no convincing data to support a plan of medical observation, and considerable data support a surgical approach. Once associated conditions such as hypertension and renal dysfunction become well established, they seem to progress despite correction of the primary hyperparathyroidism. Thus, it appears to be better to intervene early while it is still possible to correct these problems. In all patients, however, the diagnosis should be established, and short delays to clarify the diagnosis are justified. The criteria for intervention in asymptomatic patients have been revised several times over two decades (Table 16–6), but have always also included the option for correction of the abnormality based on individual patient and physician judgments.

A. Marked Hypercalcemia (Hypercalcemic Crisis)

The initial treatment in patients with marked hypercalcemia and acute symptoms is hydration and correction of hypokalemia and hyponatremia. While the patient is being hydrated, assessment of the underlying problem is essential so that more specific therapy may be started. Milk and alkaline products, estrogens, thiazides, and vitamins A and D should be immediately discontinued. Furosemide is useful to increase calcium excretion in the rehydrated patient. Etidronate, plicamycin, and calcitonin are usually effective for short periods in treating hypercalcemia regardless of cause. Glucocorticoids are very effective in vitamin D intoxication, hyperthyroidism, and sarcoidosis and in many patients with cancer, including those with peptide-secreting tumors, but are less effective when there is extensive bone disease. As mentioned previously, hyperparathyroid patients only occasionally respond to glucocorticoid administration.

In patients with marked hypercalcemia, once the diagnosis of hyperparathyroidism is established, localization studies, cervical exploration, and parathyroidectomy should be performed in a vigorously hydrated patient, since this is the most rapid and effective method of normalizing the serum calcium.

Table 16–6. Indications for parathyroidectomy in asymptomatic primary hyperparathyroidism.

Criterion	1990	2002	2008
Hypercalcemia	Serum calcium > 1.5 mg/dL above normal	Serum calcium > 1 mg/dL above normal	Serum calcium > 1 mg/dL above normal
Hypercalciuria	24 h urine calcium > 400 mg	24 h urine calcium > 400 mg	Not included
Renal insufficiency	Reduced by 30%	Reduced by 30%	GFR < 60 mL/min
Osteoporosis	Z-score < 2	T-score < 2.5	T-score < 2.5 or h/o fragility fracture
Age	< 50 y	< 50 y	< 50 y

B. Localization

Preoperative localization of parathyroid tumors can now be accomplished in about 80%-90% of patients with ultrasonography and sestamibi scans. These studies, however, are helpful in fewer patients with parathyroid hyperplasia (Figure 16–4). Localization studies are essential in patients with persistent or recurrent hyperparathyroidism and can direct a focused exploration in patients with primary hyperparathyroidism. An experienced surgeon can find the tumors in about 95% of patients who have not had previous parathyroid or thyroid surgery without preoperative tests, however preoperative knowledge of the location of the abnormal glands can simplify the operation.

For patients who have had prior neck operations, including thyroid and parathyroid procedures, preoperative localization is especially important. CT scan with specially timed contrast enhancement and selective venous catheterization with PTH immunoassay are often helpful. The surgeon must carefully evaluate these cases prior to exploration to optimize the opportunity for a successful operation. A frequently employed preference is that two concordant studies identify the site of the parathyroid abnormality prior to operating.

C. Operation

Three approaches are now acceptable for patients with sporadic primary hyperparathyroidism. A bilateral neck exploration (exposing all four parathyroid glands) is safe and does not depend upon preoperative tests or intraoperative PTH testing for success. A unilateral approach can be elected when one or more localization tests lateralize a solitary parathyroid tumor. At operation, a normal and abnormal parathyroid should be identified on the side of the localized tumor. A focal operation can be done in similar patients and the operation completed when the intraoperative PTH level decreases according to some planned criteria. When the sestamibi and ultrasound scans both independently identify the same tumor, a successful operation occurs in approximately 96% of patients. Videoscopic parathyroidectomy is recommended by a minority of surgeons.

In over 80% of cases, the parathyroid tumor is found attached to the posterior capsule of the thyroid gland. The parathyroid glands are usually symmetrically placed, and lower parathyroid glands are situated anterior to the recurrent laryngeal nerve, whereas the upper parathyroid glands lie posterior to the recurrent laryngeal nerve, where it enters the cricothyroid muscle. Parathyroid tumors may also lie cephalad to the superior pole of the thyroid gland, along the great vessels of the neck in the tracheoesophageal area, in thymic tissue, in the substance of the thyroid gland itself, or in the mediastinum. Care must be taken to avoid bleeding and not to traumatize the parathyroid gland or tumors, since color is useful in distinguishing them from surrounding thyroid, thymus, lymph node, and fat. Furthermore, rupture of the parathyroid gland may result in parathyromatosis (seeding of parathyroid tissue) and possible recurrent hyperparathyroidism. Two helpful maneuvers for localizing parathyroid tumors at operation are following the course of a branch of the inferior thyroid artery and looking for the fat that is usually associated with the parathyroid glands. One should attempt to identify four parathyroid glands when a bilateral approach is elected, though there may be more than four or fewer than four.

In a focused parathyroidectomy, if a probable parathyroid adenoma is found, it is removed and the diagnosis of adenoma confirmed by a decrease in PTH of greater than 50% from baseline and into the normal range. If the intraoperative PTH does not fall appropriately, then further exploration to identify additional abnormal parathyroid tissue should be undertaken during the same anesthetic. If normal glands are identified, they should be carefully documented. If two adenomas are found, both are removed, and both normal glands can be biopsied for confirmation but should not be removed.

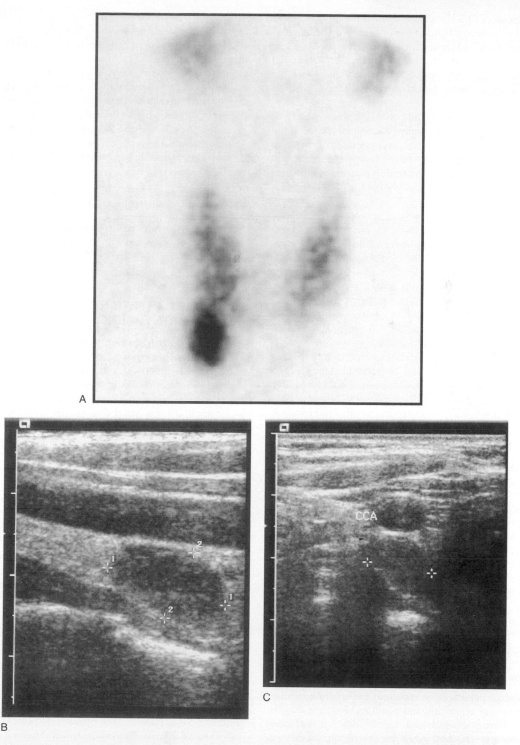

▲ **Figure 16–4.** Parathyroid adenomas. **A:** Sestamibi scan of right lower parathyroid adenoma. **B:** Longitudinal ultrasound scan of left lower parathyroid adenoma. **C:** Transverse ultrasound scan of left lower parathyroid adenoma.

The presence of a completely normal parathyroid gland at operation indicates that the tumor removed is adenomatous rather than hyperplastic, since in hyperplasia all the parathyroid glands are involved. However, the variation in the appearance of normal parathyroid glands, and the subtlety of hyperplastic glands can make this distinction complex.

When all parathyroid glands are hyperplastic, the most normal gland should be partially resected, leaving a 50 mg remnant, and confirmed to be well-vascularized prior to removal of the remaining glands. The upper thymus and perithymic tract should be removed in patients with hyperplasia, because a fifth parathyroid gland is present in 15% of cases.

If exploration fails to reveal a parathyroid tumor, a missing lower gland is often in the thymus (anterior mediastinum), whereas a missing upper gland is usually paraesophageal (or in the posterior mediastinum). One should therefore perform a careful and thorough exploration of the areas in which parathyroid tissue is likely to reside.

The recurrence rate of hyperparathyroidism after the removal of a single adenoma in patients with sporadic hyperparathyroidism is 2% or less. In patients with multiple endocrine neoplasia and familial hyperparathyroidism, recurrent hyperparathyroidism is expected as long as they have residual parathyroid tissue. Thus, the plan for management of these patients over their lifetime should be to limit both the complications from hyperparathyroidism, and the number and complexity of operations required to manage it.

D. Postoperative Care

Following removal of a parathyroid adenoma or hyperplastic glands, the serum calcium concentration falls to normal or below normal in 24-48 hours. Patients with severe skeletal depletion ("hungry bones"), long-standing hyperparathyroidism, vitamin D deficiency, or high preoperative serum calcium levels may develop profound hypocalcemia with paresthesias, carpopedal spasm, or even seizures. If the symptoms are mild and serum calcium falls slowly, oral supplementation with calcium is all that is required. When marked symptoms develop, it can be necessary to administer intravenous calcium gluconate. If the response is not rapid, the serum magnesium concentration should be determined and replenished. Treatment with calcitriol, 0.5 micrograms twice daily is sometimes required. (See section on Hypoparathyroidism.)

E. Reoperation

Treatment of persistent or recurrent hyperparathyroidism requires careful evaluation and planning. First the diagnosis must be reestablished, and the rationale for correcting the hyperparathyroidism must be specifically confirmed. If operation is planned, then preoperative localization is mandatory. Most surgeons perform noninvasive localization tests (ultrasound, sestamibi scan, CT scan) initially. If the localization is not clear, then invasive testing follows (selective venous catheterization with PTH measurement, rarely angiography). Most patients have a parathyroid tumor that can be removed through a cervical incision, making mediastinal exploration unnecessary. The success rate for patients requiring reoperation is about 90%, and the complication rate is higher depending upon the nature of the prior operation(s) and the location of the abnormal gland. The success rate is lower in patients with negative or equivocal localization tests and in patients with parathyromatosis and parathyroid cancer.

Bilezikian JP: Primary hyperparathyroidism. *Endocr Prac.* 2012;18:781.

Bilezikian JP et al: Guidelines for the management of asymptomatic primary hyperparathyroidism: summary statement from the third international workshop. *J Clin Endocrinol Metab.* 2009;94:335.

SECONDARY & TERTIARY HYPERPARATHYROIDISM

In secondary hyperparathyroidism, there is an increase in PTH secretion in response to low plasma concentrations of ionized calcium, usually due to renal disease or vitamin D deficiency, and malabsorption,. This results in chief cell hyperplasia. When secondary hyperparathyroidism occurs as a complication of renal disease, the serum phosphorus level is usually high, whereas in malabsorption, osteomalacia, or rickets it is frequently low or normal. Secondary hyperparathyroidism with renal osteodystrophy is a frequent complication of hemodialysis and peritoneal dialysis. Factors that play a role in renal osteodystrophy are: (1) phosphate retention secondary to a decrease in the number of nephrons; (2) failure of the diseased or absent kidneys to hydroxylate 25-dihydroxyvitamin D to the biologically active metabolite 1,25-dihydroxyvitamin D, with decreased intestinal absorption of calcium; (3) resistance of the bone to the action of PTH; and (4) increased serum calcitonin concentrations. The resulting skeletal changes are identical with those of primary hyperparathyroidism but are often more severe.

Most patients with secondary hyperparathyroidism are treated medically. Maintaining relatively normal serum concentrations of calcium and phosphorus during hemodialysis and treatment with calcitriol (orally or intravenously) have decreased the incidence of bone disease.

Indications for operation in patients with secondary hyperparathyroidism include: (1) a calcium × phosphate product > 70, (2) severe bone disease and pain, (3) pruritus, (4) extensive soft tissue calcification with tumoral calcinosis, and (5) calciphylaxis. Most patients with secondary hyperparathyroidism requiring parathyroidectomy have very high serum PTH levels. In the patient with secondary hyperparathyroidism in whom subtotal parathyroidectomy or total parathyroidectomy with autotransplantation is indicated, all but about 50 mg of the most normal parathyroid gland should be removed, or 15 (1-mm) slices of parathyroid tissue should be transplanted into individual muscle pockets in the forearm.

Following parathyroidectomy patients usually respond with dramatic relief of bone and joint pain and pruritus. Profound hypocalcemia frequently results following subtotal or total parathyroidectomy with autotransplantation for renal osteodystrophy, both because of "hungry bones" and because of decreased PTH secretion. Hypocalcemia due to hungry bones can be anticipated in patients with markedly elevated alkaline phosphatase levels and hand films documenting subperiosteal resorption.

Occasionally, a patient with secondary hyperparathyroidism develops relatively autonomous hyperplastic parathyroid glands. In most patients after successful renal transplantation, the serum calcium concentration returns to normal, and the hyperplastic parathyroid glands regress. In some patients, however, profound hypercalcemia develops (tertiary hyperparathyroidism). In general, surgical therapy for so-called tertiary hyperparathyroidism should be delayed until all medical approaches, including treatment with vitamin D, calcium supplementation, and phosphate binders, have been exhausted; if the condition persists beyond 1 year posttransplant, or if the hypercalcemia is severe, then operation for tertiary disease should be considered.

Kasiske BL et al: KDIGO clinical practice guideline for the care of kidney transplant recipients: a summary. *Kidney Int.* 2010 Feb;77(4):299-311.

Kidney disease: improving global outcomes (KDIGO) CKD-MBD work group: KDIGO clinical practice guideline for the diagnosis, evaluation, prevention, and treatment of chronic kidney disease-mineral and bone disorder (CKD-MBD). *Kidney Int Suppl.* 2009 Aug;(113):S1-S130.

Kovacevic B et al: Parathyroidectomy for the attainment of NKF-K/DOQI™ and KDIGO recommended values for bone and mineral metabolism in dialysis patients with uncontrollable secondary hyperparathyroidism. *Langenbeck Arch Surg.* 2012;397:413.

HYPOPARATHYROIDISM

 ESSENTIALS OF DIAGNOSIS

▶ Paresthesias, muscle cramps, carpopedal spasm, laryngeal stridor, convulsions, malaise, muscle and abdominal cramps, tetany, urinary frequency, lethargy, anxiety, psychoneurosis, depression, and psychosis

▶ Surgical neck scar. Positive Chvostek and Trousseau signs

▶ Brittle and atrophied nails, defective teeth, cataracts

▶ Hypocalcemia and hyperphosphatemia, low or absent urinary calcium, low or absent circulating parathyroid hormone

▶ Calcification of basal ganglia, cartilage, and arteries as seen on x-ray

▶ General Considerations

Hypoparathyroidism, although uncommon, occurs most often as a complication of thyroidectomy, especially when performed for carcinoma or recurrent goiter. Idiopathic hypoparathyroidism, an autoimmune process associated with autoimmune adrenocortical insufficiency, is also unusual, and hypoparathyroidism after ^{131}I therapy for Graves disease is rare. Neonatal tetany may be associated with maternal hyperparathyroidism. Hypothyroidism as well as hypoparathyroidism may occur in patients with Riedel struma.

▶ Clinical Findings

A. Symptoms and Signs

The manifestations of acute hypoparathyroidism are due to hypocalcemia. Low serum calcium levels precipitate tetany. Latent tetany may be indicated by mild or moderate paresthesias with a positive Chvostek or Trousseau sign. The initial manifestations are paresthesias, circumoral numbness, muscle cramps, irritability, carpopedal spasm, convulsions, opisthotonos, and marked anxiety. Chronically, dry skin, brittleness of the nails, and spotty alopecia including loss of the eyebrows are common. Since primary hypoparathyroidism is rare, a history of thyroidectomy is almost always present. Generally speaking, the sooner the clinical manifestations appear postoperatively, the more serious the prognosis. After many years, some patients become adapted to a low serum calcium concentration, so that tetany is no longer evident.

B. Laboratory Findings

Hypocalcemia and hyperphosphatemia are demonstrable. The urine phosphate is low or absent, tubular resorption of phosphate is high, and the urine calcium is low.

C. Imaging Studies

In chronic hypoparathyroidism, x-rays may show calcification of the basal ganglia, arteries, and external ear.

Differential Diagnosis

A good history is most important in the differential diagnosis of hypocalcemic tetany. Occasionally, tetany occurs with alkalosis and hyperventilation. Symptomatic hypocalcemia occurring after thyroid or parathyroid surgery is due to parathyroid removal or injury, or is secondary to hungry bones. Other major causes of hypocalcemic tetany are intestinal malabsorption and renal insufficiency. These conditions may also be suggested by a history of diarrhea, pancreatitis, steatorrhea, or renal disease. Laboratory abnormalities include decreased concentrations of serum proteins, cholesterol, and carotene and increased concentrations of stool fat in malabsorption and an increased blood urea nitrogen and creatinine in renal failure.

Serum PTH concentrations are low in hypocalcemia secondary to idiopathic or iatrogenic hypoparathyroidism. In hypocalcemia secondary to malabsorption and renal failure, serum PTH concentrations are elevated and the serum alkaline phosphatase concentration is normal or increased.

Treatment

The aim of treatment is to raise the serum calcium concentration, to bring the patient out of tetany, and to lower the serum phosphate level so as to prevent metastatic calcification. Most postoperative hypocalcemia is transient; if it persists longer than 2-3 weeks or if treatment with calcitriol (1,25-dihydroxyvitamin D) is required, the hypoparathyroidism may be permanent.

A. Acute Hypoparathyroid Tetany

Acute hypoparathyroid tetany requires emergency treatment. Make certain an adequate airway exists. Reassure the anxious patient to avoid hyperventilation and resulting alkalosis, which exacerbates the hypocalcemia. Calcium gluconate IV, 10-20 mL of 10% solution administered slowly resolves the tetany. Fifty milliliters of 10% calcium gluconate may then be added to 500 mL of 5% dextrose solution and administered by intravenous drip at a rate of 1 mL/kg/h. Adjust the rate of infusion so that hourly determinations of serum calcium are normal.

To make the transition to oral supplements to support the serum calcium level, calcitriol (1,25-dihydroxyvitamin D), 0.25-0.5 μg twice daily, is very helpful and takes effect within 48-72 hours. This enables the GI tract to absorb increased amounts of calcium. Calcitriol has a rapid onset of action compared to other vitamin D preparations. Oral calcium supplements of up to 6 g/d can then generally resolve the hypocalcemia even in patients with permanent, severe hypoparathyroidism. Hypomagnesemia is present in some cases of tetany not responding to calcium treatment. In such cases, magnesium (as magnesium sulfate) should

be given in a dosage of 4-8 g/d intramuscularly or 2-4 g/d intravenously.

B. Chronic Hypoparathyroidism

Once tetany has responded to intravenous calcium, change to oral calcium (citrate, gluconate, lactate, or carbonate) three times daily or as necessary. The management of the hypoparathyroid patient is difficult, because the difference between the controlling and intoxicating dose of vitamin D may be quite small. Episodes of hypercalcemia in treated patients are often unpredictable and may occur in the absence of symptoms. Vitamin D intoxication may develop after months or years of good control on a given therapeutic regimen. Dihydrotachysterol is useful in the exceptional case to supplement treatment with calcium and 1,25-dihydroxyvitamin D, when the usual measures fail to control the hypocalcemia. Frequent serum calcium determinations are necessary to regulate the proper dosage of vitamin D and to avoid vitamin D intoxication. The dose of vitamin D required to correct hypocalcemia may vary from 25,000 to 200,000 IU/d. Phosphorus should also be limited in the diet; in most patients, simple elimination of dairy products is sufficient. In some patients, aluminum hydroxide gel may be necessary to bind phosphorus in the gut to increase fecal losses.

Exogenous PTH analogs may be helpful in the long-term management of bone disease in patients with hypoparathyroidism. The optimal strategies are under development.

Cusano NE et al: The effect of PTH(1-84) on quality of life in hypoparathyroidism. *J Clin Endocrinol Metab.* 2013 Jun;98(6): 2356-2361.
Sikjaer T et al: PTH (1-84) replacement therapy in hypoparathyroidism: a randomized controlled trial on pharmacokinetic and dynamic effects following 6 months of treatment. *J Bone Miner Res.* 2013 Oct;28(10):2232-2243.

MULTIPLE CHOICE QUESTIONS

1. The best test to assess the thyroid function status of a patient who does not have known pituitary disease is

   A. Free T_4
   B. T_3
   C. T_4
   D. TSH
   E. T_4/T_3 ratio

2. Indications for surgery to correct hyperthyroidism include

   A. Pregnancy
   B. Age over 50 years
   C. Large goiter with low radioiodine uptake
   D. Both A and C
   E. None of the above

3. Follicular thyroid cancer

   A. Is separated from papillary thyroid cancer because it develops from the follicular cells of the thyroid
   B. Is less likely to spread to lymph nodes than is papillary thyroid cancer
   C. Is commonly inoperable because of local invasion and encompassment of surrounding structures
   D. Commonly makes thyroid hormone producing hyperthyroidism
   E. Is best treated with radioiodine therapy, followed by thyroidectomy

4. The differential diagnosis of hypercalcemia includes

   A. Vitamin A toxicity
   B. Vigorous exercise
   C. Hypothyroidism
   D. Myasthenia gravis
   E. None of the above

5. Patient characteristics that would meet current indications for surgery to correct asymptomatic hyperparathyroidism include

   A. Renal insufficiency with a glomerular filtration rate of 72 mL/min
   B. Age of 57 years
   C. Positive localization tests with concordant ultrasound and sestamibi scans
   D. Osteoporosis with a T-score of −2.8
   E. A serum calcium level of 10.8 mg/dL with an upper limit of normal of 10.3 mg/dL

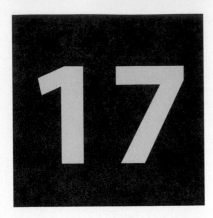

Breast Disorders

Armando E. Giuliano, MD

Sara A. Hurvitz, MD

▼ BENIGN BREAST DISORDERS

FIBROCYSTIC CONDITION

ESSENTIALS OF DIAGNOSIS

- ▶ Painful, often multiple, usually bilateral masses in the breast
- ▶ Rapid fluctuation in the size of the masses is common
- ▶ Frequently, pain occurs or worsens and size increases during premenstrual phase of cycle
- ▶ Most common age is 30-50 years. Rare in postmenopausal women not receiving hormonal replacement

▶ General Considerations

Fibrocystic condition is the most frequent lesion of the breast. Although commonly referred to as "fibrocystic disease," it does not, in fact, represent a pathologic or anatomic disorder. It is common in women 30-50 years of age but rare in postmenopausal women who are not taking hormonal replacement. Estrogen is considered a causative factor. There may be an increased risk in women who drink alcohol, especially women between 18 and 22 years of age. Fibrocystic condition encompasses a wide variety of benign histologic changes in the breast epithelium, some of which are found so commonly in normal breasts that they are probably variants of normal but have nonetheless been termed a "condition" or "disease."

The microscopic findings of fibrocystic condition include cysts (gross and microscopic), papillomatosis, adenosis, fibrosis, and ductal epithelial hyperplasia. Although fibrocystic condition has generally been considered to increase the risk of subsequent breast cancer, only the variants with a component of epithelial proliferation (especially with atypia) or increased breast density on mammogram represent true risk factors.

▶ Clinical Findings

A. Symptoms and Signs

Fibrocystic condition may produce an asymptomatic mass in the breast that is discovered by accident, but pain or tenderness often calls attention to it. Discomfort often occurs or worsens during the premenstrual phase of the cycle, at which time the cysts tend to enlarge. Fluctuations in size and rapid appearance or disappearance of a breast mass are common with this condition as are multiple or bilateral masses and serous nipple discharge. Patients will give a history of a transient lump in the breast or cyclic breast pain.

B. Diagnostic Tests

Mammography and ultrasonography should be used to evaluate a mass in a patient with fibrocystic condition. Ultrasonography alone may be used in women under 30 years of age. Because a mass due to fibrocystic condition is difficult to distinguish from carcinoma on the basis of clinical findings, suspicious lesions should be biopsied. Fine-needle aspiration (FNA) cytology may be used, but if a suspicious mass that is nonmalignant on cytologic examination does not resolve over several months, it should be excised or biopsied by core needle. Surgery should be conservative, since the primary objective is to exclude cancer. Occasionally, FNA cytology will suffice. Simple mastectomy or extensive removal of breast tissue is rarely, if ever, indicated for fibrocystic condition.

▶ Differential Diagnosis

Pain, fluctuation in size, and multiplicity of lesions are the features most helpful in differentiating fibrocystic condition from carcinoma. If a dominant mass is present, the diagnosis of cancer should be assumed until disproven by biopsy. Mammography may be helpful, but the breast tissue in these young women is usually too radiodense to permit a worthwhile study. Sonography is useful in differentiating a cystic mass from a solid mass, especially in women with dense breasts. Final diagnosis, however, depends on analysis of the excisional biopsy specimen or needle biopsy.

Treatment

When the diagnosis of fibrocystic condition has been established by previous biopsy or is likely because the history is classic, aspiration of a discrete mass suggestive of a cyst is indicated to alleviate pain and, more importantly, to confirm the cystic nature of the mass. The patient is reexamined at intervals thereafter. If no fluid is obtained by aspiration, if fluid is bloody, if a mass persists after aspiration, or if at any time during follow-up a persistent or recurrent mass is noted, biopsy should be performed.

Breast pain associated with generalized fibrocystic condition is best treated by avoiding trauma and by wearing a good supportive brassiere during the night and day. Hormone therapy is not advisable, because it does not cure the condition and has undesirable side effects. Danazol (100-200 mg orally twice daily), a synthetic androgen, is the only treatment approved by the US Food and Drug Administration (FDA) for patients with severe pain. This treatment suppresses pituitary gonadotropins, but androgenic effects (acne, edema, hirsutism) usually make this treatment intolerable; in practice, it is rarely used. Similarly, tamoxifen reduces some symptoms of fibrocystic condition, but because of its side effects, it is not useful for young women unless it is given to reduce the risk of cancer. Postmenopausal women receiving hormone replacement therapy may stop or change doses of hormones to reduce pain. Oil of evening primrose (OEP), a natural form of gamolenic acid, has been shown to decrease pain in 44%-58% of users. The dosage of gamolenic acid is six capsules of 500 mg orally twice daily. Studies have also demonstrated a low-fat diet or decreasing dietary fat intake may reduce the painful symptoms associated with fibrocystic condition. Further research is being done to determine the effects of topical treatments such as topical nonsteroidal anti-inflammatory drugs as well as topical hormonal drugs such as topical tamoxifen.

The role of caffeine consumption in the development and treatment of fibrocystic condition is controversial. Some studies suggest that eliminating caffeine from the diet is associated with improvement while other studies refute the benefit entirely. Many patients are aware of these studies and report relief of symptoms after giving up coffee, tea, and chocolate. Similarly, many women find vitamin E (400 international units daily) helpful; however, these observations remain anecdotal.

Prognosis

Exacerbations of pain, tenderness, and cyst formation may occur at any time until menopause, when symptoms usually subside, except in patients receiving hormonal replacement. The patient should be advised to examine her own breasts regularly just after menstruation and to inform her practitioner if a mass appears. The risk of breast cancer developing in women with fibrocystic condition with a proliferative or atypical component in the epithelium or papillomatosis is higher than that of the general population. These women should be monitored carefully with physical examinations and imaging studies.

Kabat GC et al: A multi-center prospective cohort study of benign breast disease and risk of subsequent breast cancer. *Cancer Causes Control.* 2010 Jun;21(6):821-828. [PMID: 20084540]

Pruthi S et al: Vitamin E and evening primrose oil for management of cyclical mastalgia: a randomized pilot study. *Altern Med Rev.* 2010 Apr;15(1):59-67. [PMID: 20359269]

Salzman B et al: Common breast problems. *Am Fam Physician.* 2012 Aug 15;86(4):343-349. [PMID:22963023]

FIBROADENOMA OF THE BREAST

This common benign neoplasm occurs most frequently in young women, usually within 20 years after puberty. It is somewhat more frequent and tends to occur at an earlier age in black women. Multiple tumors are found in 10%-15% of patients.

The typical **fibroadenoma** is a round or ovoid, rubbery, discrete, relatively movable, nontender mass 1-5 cm in diameter. It is usually discovered accidentally. Clinical diagnosis in young patients is generally not difficult. In women over 30 years, fibrocystic condition of the breast and carcinoma of the breast must be considered. Cysts can be identified by aspiration or ultrasonography. Fibroadenoma does not normally occur after menopause but may occasionally develop after administration of hormones.

No treatment is usually necessary if the diagnosis can be made by needle biopsy or cytologic examination. Excision with pathologic examination of the specimen is performed if the diagnosis is uncertain. Cryoablation, or freezing of the fibroadenoma, appears to be a safe procedure if the lesion is consistent with fibroadenoma on histology prior to ablation. Cryoablation is not appropriate for all fibroadenomas because some are too large to freeze or the diagnosis may not be certain. There is no obvious advantage to cryoablation of a histologically proven fibroadenoma except that some patients may feel relief that a mass is gone. However, at times a mass of scar or fat necrosis replaces the mass of the fibroadenoma. Reassurance seems preferable. It is usually not possible to distinguish a large fibroadenoma from a phyllodes tumor on the basis of needle biopsy results or imaging alone.

Phyllodes tumor is a fibroadenoma-like tumor with cellular stroma that grows rapidly. It may reach a large size and, if inadequately excised, will recur locally. The lesion can be benign or malignant. If benign, phyllodes tumor is treated by local excision with a margin of surrounding breast tissue. The treatment of malignant phyllodes tumor is more controversial, but complete removal of the tumor with a rim of normal tissue avoids recurrence. Because these tumors may be large, simple mastectomy is sometimes necessary. Lymph node dissection is not performed, since the sarcomatous portion of the tumor metastasizes to the lungs and not the lymph nodes.

Abe M et al: Malignant transformation of breast fibroadenoma to malignant phyllodes tumor: long-term outcome of 36 malignant phyllodes tumors. *Breast Cancer.* 2011 Oct;18(4):268-272. [PMID: 22121516]

El Hag IA et al: Cytological clues in the distinction between phyllodes tumor and fibroadenoma. *Cancer Cytopathol.* 2010 Feb 25;118(1):33-40. [PMID: 20094997]

Tse GM et al: Phyllodes tumor of the breast: an update. *Breast Cancer.* 2010;17(1):29-34. [PMID: 19434472]

NIPPLE DISCHARGE

In order of decreasing frequency, the following are the most common causes of nipple discharge in the nonlactating breast: duct ectasia, intraductal papilloma, and carcinoma. The important characteristics of the discharge and some other factors to be evaluated by history and physical examination are listed in Table 17–1.

Spontaneous, unilateral, serous or serosanguineous discharge from a single duct is usually caused by an intraductal papilloma or, rarely, by an intraductal cancer. A mass may not be palpable. The involved duct may be identified by pressure at different sites around the nipple at the margin of the areola. Bloody discharge is suggestive of cancer but is more often caused by a benign papilloma in the duct. Cytologic examination may identify malignant cells, but negative findings do not rule out cancer, which is more likely in women over age 50 years. In any case, the involved bloody duct—and a mass if present—should be excised. A ductogram (a mammogram of a duct after radiopaque dye has been injected) is of limited value since excision of the suspicious ductal system is indicated regardless of findings. Ductoscopy, evaluation of the ductal system with a small scope inserted through the nipple, has been attempted but is not effective management.

In premenopausal women, spontaneous multiple duct discharge, unilateral or bilateral, most noticeable just before menstruation, is often due to fibrocystic condition. Discharge may be green or brownish. Papillomatosis and ductal ectasia are usually detected only by biopsy. If a mass is present, it should be removed.

Table 17–1. Characteristics of nipple discharge in the nonpregnant, nonlactating woman.

Finding	Significance
Serous	Most likely benign FCC, ie, duct ectasia
Bloody	More likely neoplastic–papilloma, carcinoma
Associated mass	More likely neoplastic
Unilateral	Either neoplastic or non-neoplastic
Bilateral	Most likely non-neoplastic
Single duct	More likely neoplastic
Multiple ducts	More likely FCC
Milky	Endocrine disorders, medications
Spontaneous	Either neoplastic or non-neoplastic
Produced by pressure at single site	Either neoplastic or non-neoplastic
Persistent	Either neoplastic or non-neoplastic
Intermittent	Either neoplastic or non-neoplastic
Related to menses	More likely FCC
Premenopausal	More likely FCC
Taking hormones	More likely FCC

FCC, fibrocystic condition.

A milky discharge from multiple ducts in the nonlactating breast may occur from hyperprolactinemia. Serum prolactin levels should be obtained to search for a pituitary tumor. Thyroid-stimulating hormone (TSH) helps exclude causative hypothyroidism. Numerous antipsychotic drugs and other drugs may also cause a milky discharge that ceases on discontinuance of the medication.

Oral contraceptive agents or estrogen replacement therapy may cause clear, serous, or milky discharge from a single duct, but multiple duct discharge is more common. In the premenopausal woman, the discharge is more evident just before menstruation and disappears on stopping the medication. If it does not stop, is from a single duct, and is copious, exploration should be performed since this may be a sign of cancer.

A purulent discharge may originate in a subareolar abscess and require removal of the abscess and the related lactiferous sinus.

When localization is not possible, no mass is palpable, and the discharge is nonbloody, the patient should be reexamined every 3 or 4 months for a year, and a mammogram and an ultrasound should be performed. Although most discharge is from a benign process, patients may find it annoying or disconcerting. To eliminate the discharge, proximal duct excision can be performed both for treatment and diagnosis.

Chen L et al: Bloody nipple discharge is a predictor of breast cancer risk: a meta-analysis. *Breast Cancer Res Treat*. 2012 Feb;132(1):9-14. [PMID: 21947751]

Kamali S et al: Ductoscopy in the evaluation and management of nipple discharge. *Ann Surg Oncol*. 2010 Mar;17(3):778-783. [PMID: 20012502]

Montroni I et al: Nipple discharge: is its significance as a risk factor for breast cancer fully understood? Observational study including 915 consecutive patients who underwent selective duct excision. *Breast Cancer Res Treat*. 2010 Oct;123(3):895-900. [PMID: 20354781]

Morrogh M et al: Lessons learned from 416 cases of nipple discharge of the breast. *Am J Surg*. 2010 Jul;200(1):73-80. [PMID: 20079481]

Zervoudis S et al: Nipple discharge screening. *Womens Health (Lond Engl)*. 2010 Jan;6(1):135-151. [PMID: 20050819]

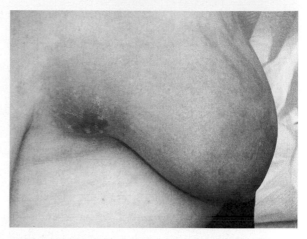

▲ **Figure 17–1.** Breast abscess and cellulitis. (Copyright Richard P. Usatine, MD; from Usatine RP, Smith MA, Mayeaux EJ Jr, Chumley H. *The Color Atlas of Family Medicine*. 2nd ed. New York, NY: McGraw-Hill; 2013.)

FAT NECROSIS

Fat necrosis is a rare lesion of the breast but is of clinical importance because it produces a mass (often accompanied by skin or nipple retraction) that is usually indistinguishable from carcinoma even with imaging studies. Trauma is presumed to be the cause, though only about 50% of patients give a history of injury. Ecchymosis is occasionally present. If untreated, the mass effect gradually disappears. The safest course is to obtain a biopsy. Needle biopsy is often adequate, but frequently the entire mass must be excised, primarily to exclude carcinoma. Fat necrosis is common after segmental resection, radiation therapy, or flap reconstruction after mastectomy.

BREAST ABSCESS

During nursing, an area of redness, tenderness, and induration may develop in the breast. The organism most commonly found in these abscesses is *Staphylococcus aureus*.

Infection in the nonlactating breast is rare. A subareolar abscess may develop in young or middle-aged women who are not lactating (Figure 17–1). These infections tend to recur after incision and drainage unless the area is explored during a quiescent interval, with excision of the involved lactiferous duct or ducts at the base of the nipple. In the nonlactating breast, inflammatory carcinoma must always be considered. Thus, incision and biopsy of any indurated tissue with a small piece of erythematous skin is indicated when suspected abscess or cellulitis in the nonlactating breast does not resolve promptly with antibiotics. Often needle or catheter drainage is adequate to treat an abscess, but surgical incision and drainage may be necessary.

Trop I et al: Breast abscesses: evidence-based algorithms for diagnosis, management, and follow-up. *Radiographics*. 2011 Oct;31(6):1683-1699. [PMID: 21997989]

Rizzo M et al: Management of breast abscesses in nonlactating women. *Am Surg*. 2010 Mar;76(3):292-295. [PMID: 20349659]

DISORDERS OF THE AUGMENTED BREAST

At least 4 million American women have had breast implants. Breast augmentation is performed by placing implants under the pectoralis muscle or, less desirably, in the subcutaneous tissue of the breast. Most implants are made of an outer silicone shell filled with a silicone gel, saline, or some combination of the two. Capsule contraction or scarring around the implant develops in about 15%-25% of patients, leading to a firmness and distortion of the breast that can be painful. Some require removal of the implant and surrounding capsule.

Implant rupture may occur in as many as 5%-10% of women, and bleeding of gel through the capsule is noted even more commonly. Although silicone gel may be an immunologic stimulant, there is no increase in autoimmune disorders in patients with such implants. The FDA has advised symptomatic women with ruptured silicone implants to discuss possible surgical removal with their clinicians. However, women who are asymptomatic and have no evidence of rupture of a silicone gel prosthesis should probably not undergo removal of the implant. Women with symptoms of autoimmune illnesses often undergo removal, but no benefit has been shown.

Studies have failed to show any association between implants and an increased incidence of breast cancer.

However, breast cancer may develop in a patient with an augmentation prosthesis, as it does in women without them. Detection in patients with implants is more difficult because mammography is less able to detect early lesions. Mammography is better if the implant is subpectoral rather than subcutaneous. The prosthesis should be placed retropectorally after mastectomy to facilitate detection of a local recurrence of cancer, which is usually cutaneous or subcutaneous and is easily detected by palpation. Recently there has been an association of lymphoma of the breast with silicone implants.

If a cancer develops in a patient with implants, it should be treated in the same manner as in women without implants. Such women should be offered the option of mastectomy or breast-conserving therapy, which may require removal or replacement of the implant. Radiotherapy of the augmented breast often results in marked capsular contracture. Adjuvant treatments should be given for the same indications as for women who have no implants.

De Jong D et al: *JAMA.* 2008 Nov 5;300(17):2030-5. [PMID 18984890]

Jewell ML: *Aesthet Surg J.* 2012 Nov;32(8):1031-1034. [PMID: 23012658]

Taylor CR et al: *Appl Immunohistochem Mol Morphol.* 2012 Dec 11. [Epub ahead of print] [PMID: 23235342]

Yang N et al: The augmented breast: a pictorial review of the abnormal and unusual. *AJR Am J Roentgenol.* 2011 Apr; 196(4):W451-460. [PMID: 21427311]

Zakhireh J et al: Application of screening principles to the reconstructed breast. *J Clin Oncol.* 2010 Jan 1;28(1):173-180. [PMID: 19884555]

CARCINOMA OF THE FEMALE BREAST

ESSENTIALS OF DIAGNOSIS

▶ Risk factors include delayed childbearing, positive family history of breast cancer or genetic mutations (*BRCA1*, *BRCA2*), and personal history of breast cancer or some types of proliferative conditions.

▶ *Early findings:* Single, nontender, firm to hard mass with ill-defined margins; mammographic abnormalities and no palpable mass.

▶ *Later findings:* Skin or nipple retraction; axillary lymphadenopathy; breast enlargement, erythema, edema, pain; fixation of mass to skin or chest wall.

▶ Incidence & Risk Factors

Breast cancer will develop in one of eight American women. Next to skin cancer, breast cancer is the most common cancer in women; it is second only to lung cancer as a cause of death. In 2012, there were approximately 229,060 new cases and 39,920 deaths from breast cancer in women in the United States. An additional 63,300 cases of breast carcinoma in situ were detected, principally by screening mammography. Worldwide, breast cancer is diagnosed in approximately 1.38 million women, and about 458,000 die of breast cancer each year, with the highest rates of diagnosis in Western and Northern Europe, Australia, New Zealand, and North America and lowest rates in Sub-Saharan Africa and Asia. These regional differences in incidence are likely due to the variable availability of screening mammography as well as differences in reproductive and hormonal factors. In Western countries, incidence rates decreased with a reduced use of postmenopausal hormone therapy and mortality declined with increased use of screening and improved treatments. In contrast, incidence and mortality from breast cancer in many African and Asian countries has increased as reproductive factors have changed (such as delayed childbearing) and as the incidence of obesity has risen.

The most significant risk factor for the development of breast cancer is age. A woman's risk of breast cancer rises rapidly until her early 60s, peaks in her 70s, and then declines. A significant family history of breast or ovarian cancer may also indicate a high risk of developing breast cancer. Germline mutations in the *BRCA* family of tumor suppressor genes accounts for approximately 5%-10% of breast cancer diagnoses and tend to cluster in certain ethnic groups, including women of Ashkenazi Jewish descent. Women with a mutation in the *BRCA1* gene, located on chromosome 17, have an estimated 85% chance of developing breast cancer in their lifetime. Other genes associated with an increased risk of breast and other cancers include *BRCA2* (associated with a gene on chromosome 13); ataxia-telangiectasia mutation; and mutation of the tumor suppressor gene *p53*. If a woman has a compelling family history (such as breast cancer diagnosed in two first-degree relatives, especially if diagnosed younger than age 50; ovarian cancer; male breast cancer; or a first-degree relative with bilateral breast cancer), genetic testing may be appropriate. In general, it is best for a woman who has a strong family history to meet with a genetics counselor to undergo a risk assessment and decide whether genetic testing is indicated.

Even when genetic testing fails to reveal a predisposing genetic mutation, women with a strong family history of breast cancer are at higher risk for development of breast cancer. Compared with a woman with no affected family members, a woman who has one first-degree relative (mother, daughter, or sister) with breast cancer has double the risk of developing breast cancer and a woman with two first-degree relatives with breast cancer has triple the risk of developing breast cancer. The risk is further increased for a woman whose affected family member was premenopausal at the time of diagnosis or had bilateral breast cancer. Lifestyle and reproductive factors also contribute to risk of breast cancer. Nulliparous women and women whose first full-term pregnancy occurred after the age of 30 have an elevated risk. Late menarche and artificial menopause are associated with a lower incidence, whereas early menarche (under the age of 12) and late natural menopause (after the age of 55) are associated with an increase in risk. Combined oral contraceptive pills may increase the risk of breast cancer. Several studies show that concomitant administration of progesterone and estrogen to postmenopausal women may markedly increase the incidence of breast cancer, compared with the use of estrogen alone or with no hormone replacement treatment. The Women's Health Initiative prospective randomized study of hormone replacement therapy stopped treatment with estrogen and progesterone early because of an increased risk of breast cancer compared with untreated women or women treated with estrogen alone. Alcohol consumption, high dietary intake of fat, and lack of exercise may also increase the risk of breast cancer. Fibrocystic breast condition, when accompanied by proliferative changes, papillomatosis, or atypical epithelial hyperplasia, and increased breast density on mammogram are also associated with an increased incidence. A woman who had cancer in one breast is at increased risk for cancer developing in the other breast. In these women, a contralateral cancer develops at the rate of 1% or 2% per year. Women with cancer of the uterine corpus have a risk of breast cancer significantly higher than that of the general population, and women with breast cancer have a comparably increased risk of endometrial cancer. Socioeconomic and racial factors have also been associated with breast cancer risk. Breast cancer tends to be diagnosed more frequently in women of higher socioeconomic status and is more frequent in white women than in black women.

Women at greater than average risk for developing breast cancer (Table 17–2) should be identified by their practitioners and monitored carefully. Risk assessment models have been developed and several have been validated (most extensively the Gail 2 model) to evaluate a woman's risk of developing cancer. Those with an exceptional family history should be counseled about the option of genetic testing. Some of these high-risk women may consider prophylactic mastectomy, oophorectomy, or tamoxifen, an FDA-approved preventive agent. The Prevention and Observation of Surgical Endpoints (PROSE) consortium monitored women with deleterious *BRCA1/2* mutations from 1974 to 2008 and reported that 15% of women with a known *BRCA* mutation underwent bilateral prophylactic mastectomy, and none of them developed breast cancer during the 3 years of follow-up. In contrast, subsequent breast cancer developed in 98 (7%) of the 1372 women who did not have surgery. Moreover, women who underwent prophylactic salpingo-oophorectomy had a lower risk of ovarian cancer, all-cause mortality, as well as breast cancer- and ovarian cancer-specific mortality.

Table 17–2. Factors associated with increased risk of breast cancer.

Race	White
Age	Older
Family history	Breast cancer in parent, sibling, or child especially bilateral or premenopausal)
Genetics	*BRCA1* or *BRCA2* mutation
Previous medical history	Endometrial cancer Proliferative forms of fibrocystic disease Cancer in other breast
Menstrual history	Early menarche (under age 12) Late menopause (after age 50)
Reproductive history	Nulliparous or late first pregnancy

Women with genetic mutations in whom breast cancer develops may be treated in the same way as women who do not have mutations (ie, lumpectomy), though there is an increased risk of ipsilateral and contralateral recurrence after lumpectomy for these women. One study showed that of patients with a diagnosis of breast cancer who were found to be carriers of a *BRCA* mutation, approximately 50% chose to undergo bilateral mastectomy.

▶ Prevention

The National Surgical Adjuvant Breast Project (NSABP) conducted the first Breast Cancer Prevention Trial (BCPT) P-1, which evaluated tamoxifen, a selective estrogen receptor modulator (SERM), as a preventive agent in women with no personal history of breast cancer but at high risk for developing the disease. Women who received tamoxifen for 5 years had about a 50% reduction in noninvasive and invasive cancers compared with women taking placebo. However, women over age 50 who received the drug had an increased incidence of endometrial cancer and deep venous thrombosis.

The SERM raloxifene, effective in preventing osteoporosis, is also effective in preventing breast cancer. The NSABP Study of Tamoxifen and Raloxifene (STAR) P-2 trial compared raloxifene with tamoxifen for the prevention of breast cancer in a high-risk population. With a median follow-up of 81 months, raloxifene was associated with a higher risk of invasive breast cancer but had an equivalent risk for noninvasive disease compared with tamoxifen. Uterine cancer, cataracts, and thromboembolic events were significantly lower in the raloxifene-treated patients than in tamoxifen-treated patients. While SERMs have been shown to be effective at reducing the risk of breast cancer, the uptake of this intervention by women has been relatively low, possibly due to the perceived risks and side effects of therapy.

A cost-effectiveness study based on a meta-analysis of four randomized prevention trials showed that tamoxifen saves costs and improves life expectancy when higher risk (Gail 5-year risk at least 1.66%) women under the age of 55 years were treated.

Similar to SERMs, aromatase inhibitors (AI) such as exemestane have shown great success in preventing breast cancer with a lower risk of uterine cancer and thromboembolic events, although bone loss is a significant side effect of this treatment. In an international phase III clinical trial, 4560 postmenopausal women at high risk for breast cancer were randomly assigned to receive exemestane or placebo for 5 years. "High risk" was defined as at least one of the following: at least 60 years of age, Gail 5-year risk score > 1.66%; prior atypical ductal or lobular hyperplasia or lobular carcinoma in situ (LCIS); or ductal carcinoma in situ (DCIS) with mastectomy. With a median follow up of 35 months, there was a 65% relative risk reduction in the annual risk of invasive breast cancer (0.19% vs 0.55%; hazard ratio, 0.35; 95% CI, 0.18, 0.70; $P = 0.002$) for patients who received exemestane. While exemestane use was associated with a higher rate of adverse events (88% vs 85%; $P = 0.003$), there were no significant differences between the groups in terms of skeletal fractures or cardiovascular events, though longer follow up is needed to accurately assess these outcomes. Based on these data, exemestane is a reasonable risk-reducing option for postmenopausal women at higher risk for breast cancer.

Collaborative Group on Hormonal Factors in Breast Cancer: Menarche, menopause, and breast cancer risk: individual breast cancer risk: individual participant meta-analysis, including 118 964 women with breast cancer from 117 epidemiological studies. *Lancel Oncol.* 2012;13(11):1141-1151.

Ehemen C et al: Annual report to the nation on the status of cancer, 1975-2008, featuring cancers associated with excess weight and lack of sufficient physical activity. *Cancer.* 2012;118(9): 2338-2366. [PMID: 22460733]

Goss PE et al: CTG MAP.3 Study Investigators. Exemestane for breast-cancer prevention in postmenopausal women. *N Engl J Med.* 2011 Jun 23;364(25):2381-2391. [PMID: 21639806]

Jemal A et al: Global cancer statistics. *CA Cancer J Clin.* 2011 Mar-Apr;61(2):69-90. [PMID: 21296855]

Meads C et al: A systematic review of breast cancer incidence risk prediction models with meta-analysis of their performance. *Breast Cancer Res Treat.* 2012 Apr;132(2):365-377. [PMID: 22037780]

Schwartz MD et al: Long-term outcomes of BRCA1/BRCA2 testing: risk reduction and surveillance. *Cancer.* 2012;118(2):510-517. [PMID: 21717445]

Siegel R et al: Cancer statistics, 2012. *CA Cancer J Clin.* 2012;62(1):10-29. [PMID: 22237781]

Vogel VG et al: National Surgical Adjuvant Breast and Bowel Project. Update of the National Surgical Adjuvant Breast and Bowel Project Study of Tamoxifen and Raloxifene (STAR) P-2 Trial: preventing breast cancer. *Cancer Prev Res (Phila).* 2010 Jun;3(6):696-706. [PMID: 20404000]

▶ Early Detection of Breast Cancer

A. Screening Programs

A number of large screening programs, consisting of physical and mammographic examination of asymptomatic women, have been conducted over the years. On average, these programs identify 10 cancers per 1000 women over the age of 50 and 2 cancers per 1000 women under the age of 50. Screening detects cancer before it has spread to the lymph nodes in about 80% of the women evaluated. This increases the chance of survival to about 85% at 5 years.

About one-third of the abnormalities detected on screening mammograms will be found to be malignant when biopsy is performed. The probability of cancer on a screening mammogram is directly related to the Breast Imaging Reporting and Data System (BIRADS) assessment, and workup should be performed based on this classification. Women 20-40 years of age should have a breast examination as part of routine medical care every 2-3 years. Women over age 40 years should have annual breast examinations. The sensitivity of mammography varies from approximately 60%-90%. This sensitivity depends on several factors, including patient's age (breast density) and tumor size, location, and mammographic appearance. In young women with dense breasts, mammography is less sensitive than in older women with fatty breasts, in whom mammography can detect at least 90% of malignancies. Smaller tumors, particularly those without calcifications, are more difficult to detect, especially in dense breasts. The lack of sensitivity and the low incidence of breast cancer in young women have led to questions concerning the value of mammography for screening in women 40-50 years of age. The specificity of mammography in women under 50 years varies from about 30%-40% for nonpalpable mammographic abnormalities to 85%-90% for clinically evident malignancies. In 2009, the US Preventive Services Task Force recommended against routine screening mammography in this age range, and also recommended mammography be performed every 2 years for women between the ages of 50 and 74. The change in recommendation for screening women age 40-50 were particularly controversial in light of several meta-analyses that included women in this age group and showed a 15%-20% reduction in the relative risk of death from breast cancer with screening mammography. To add to the controversy, an analysis of the Surveillance, Epidemiology and End Results (SEER) database from 1976 to 2008 suggests that screening mammography has led to substantial increases in the number of breast cancer cases diagnosed but has only had a minor impact on the rate of women presenting with advanced disease. These data should all be taken into consideration when advising a patient regarding the utility of screening mammography. The American Cancer Society continues to recommend yearly mammography for women beginning at the age of 40, continuing as long as good health lasts.

B. Clinical Breast Examination and Self-Examination

Breast self-examination (BSE) has not been shown to improve survival. Because of the lack of strong evidence demonstrating value, the American Cancer Society no longer recommends monthly BSE. The recommendation is that patients be made aware of the potential benefits, limitations, and harms (increased biopsies or false-positive results) associated with BSE. Women who choose to perform BSE should be advised regarding the proper technique. Premenopausal women should perform the examination 7-8 days after the start of the menstrual period. First, breasts should be inspected before a mirror with the hands at the sides, overhead, and pressed firmly on the hips to contract the pectoralis muscles causing masses, asymmetry of breasts, and slight dimpling of the skin to become apparent. Next, in a supine position, each breast should be carefully palpated with the fingers of the opposite hand. Some women discover small breast lumps more readily when their skin is moist while bathing or showering. While BSE is not a recommended practice, patients should recognize and report any breast changes to their clinicians as it remains an important facet of proactive care. A small number of studies have reported a reduction in breast cancer mortality with screening clinical breast examination (CBE). While the evidence is only fair, in contrast to BSE, the ACS recommends CBE every 3 years in women ages 20-39 and annually starting at the age of 40.

C. Imaging

Mammography is the most reliable means of detecting breast cancer before a mass can be palpated. Most slowly growing cancers can be identified by mammography at least 2 years before reaching a size detectable by palpation. Film screen mammography delivers < 0.4 cGy to the mid-breast per view. Although full-field digital mammography provides an easier method to maintain and review mammograms, it has not been proven that it provides better images or increases detection rates more than film mammography. In subset analysis of a large study, digital mammography seemed slightly superior in women with dense breasts. Computer-assisted detection has not shown any increase in detection of cancers.

Calcifications are the most easily recognized mammographic abnormality. The most common findings associated with carcinoma of the breast are clustered pleomorphic microcalcifications. Such calcifications are usually at least five to eight in number, aggregated in one part of the breast and differing from each other in size and shape, often including branched or V- or Y-shaped configurations. There may be an associated mammographic mass density or, at times, only a mass density with no calcifications. Such a density usually has irregular or ill-defined borders and may lead to architectural distortion within the breast but may be subtle and difficult to detect.

Indications for mammography are as follows: (1) to screen at regular intervals asymptomatic women at high risk for developing breast cancer (see above); (2) to evaluate each breast when a diagnosis of potentially curable breast cancer has been made, and at regular intervals thereafter; (3) to evaluate a questionable or ill-defined breast mass or other suspicious change in the breast; (4) to search for an occult breast cancer in a woman with metastatic disease in axillary nodes or elsewhere from an unknown primary; (5) to screen women prior to cosmetic operations or prior to biopsy of a mass, to examine for an unsuspected cancer; (6) to monitor those women with breast cancer who have been treated with breast-conserving surgery and radiation; and (7) to monitor the contralateral breast in those women with breast cancer treated with mastectomy.

Patients with a dominant or suspicious mass must undergo biopsy despite mammographic findings. The mammogram should be obtained prior to biopsy so that other suspicious areas can be noted and the contralateral breast can be evaluated. Mammography is never a substitute for biopsy because it may not reveal clinical cancer, especially in a very dense breast, as may be seen in young women with fibrocystic changes, and may not reveal medullary cancers.

Communication and documentation among the patient, the referring practitioner, and the interpreting physician are critical for high-quality screening and diagnostic mammography. The patient should be told about *how* she will receive timely results of her mammogram; that mammography does not "rule out" cancer; and that she may receive a correlative examination such as ultrasound at the mammography facility if referred for a suspicious lesion. She should also be aware of the technique and need for breast compression and that this may be uncomfortable. The mammography facility should be informed in writing by the clinician of abnormal physical examination findings. The Agency for Health Care Policy and Research (AHCPR) Clinical Practice Guidelines strongly recommend that all mammography reports be communicated in writing to the patient and referring practitioner.

Magnetic resonance imaging (MRI) and ultrasound may be useful screening modalities in women who are at high risk for breast cancer but not for the general population. The sensitivity of MRI is much higher than mammography; however, the specificity is significantly lower and this results in multiple unnecessary biopsies. The increased sensitivity despite decreased specificity may be considered a reasonable trade-off for those at increased risk for developing breast cancer but not for normal-risk population. In 2009, the National Comprehensive Cancer Network (NCCN) guidelines recommended MRI in addition to screening mammography for high-risk women, including those with *BRCA1/2* mutations, those who have a lifetime risk of breast cancer of > 20%, and those with a personal history of LCIS. Women who received radiation therapy to the chest in their teens or twenties are also known to be at high risk for developing breast cancer and screening MRI may be considered in addition to mammography. MRI is useful in women with breast implants to determine the character of a lesion present in the breast and to search for implant rupture and at times is helpful in patients with prior lumpectomy and radiation.

Allen SS et al: The mammography controversy: when should you screen? *J Fam Pract.* 2011 Sep;60(9):524-531. [PMID: 21901178]

Bleyer A et al: Effect of three decades of screening mammography on breast-cancer incidence. *N Engl J Med.* 2012;367(21): 1998-2005. [PMID: 23171096]

Hendrick RE et al: United States Preventive Services Task Force screening mammography recommendations: science ignored. *AJR Am J Roentgenol.* 2011 Feb;196(2):W112-116. [PMID: 21257850]

James JJ et al: Mammographic features of breast cancers at single reading with computer-aided detection and at double reading in a large multicenter prospective trial of computer-aided detection: CADET II. *Radiology.* 2010 Aug;256(2):379-386. [PMID: 20656831]

Kalager M et al: Effect of screening mammography on breast-cancer mortality in Norway. *N Engl J Med.* 2010 Sep 23;363(13): 1203-1210. [PMID: 20860502]

Meissner HI et al: Breast cancer screening beliefs, recommendations and practices: primary care physicians in the United States. *Cancer.* 2011 Jul 15;117(14):3101-3111. [PMID: 21246531]

Morrow M et al: MRI for breast cancer screening, diagnosis, and treatment. *Lancet.* 2011;378(9805):1804-1811. [PMID 22098853]

Warner E: Clinical practice. Breast-cancer screening. *N Engl J Med.* 2011 Sep 15;365(11):1025-1032. [PMID: 21916640]

Clinical Findings Associated With Early Detection of Breast Cancer

A. Symptoms and Signs

The presenting complaint in about 70% of patients with breast cancer is a lump (usually painless) in the breast. About 90% of these breast masses are discovered by the patient. Less frequent symptoms are breast pain; nipple discharge; erosion, retraction, enlargement, or itching of the nipple; and redness, generalized hardness, enlargement, or shrinking of the breast. Rarely, an axillary mass or swelling of the arm may be the first symptom. Back or bone pain, jaundice, or weight loss may be the result of systemic metastases, but these symptoms are rarely seen on initial presentation.

The relative frequency of carcinoma in various anatomic sites in the breast is shown in Figure 17–2.

Inspection of the breast is the first step in physical examination and should be carried out with the patient sitting, arms at her sides, and then overhead. Abnormal variations in breast size and contour, minimal nipple retraction, and slight edema, redness or retraction of the skin can be identified (Figure 17–3). Asymmetry of the breasts and retraction or dimpling of the skin can often be accentuated by having

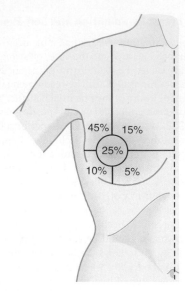

▲ **FIGURE 17–2.** Frequency of breast carcinoma at various anatomic sites.

the patient raise her arms overhead or press her hands on her hips to contract the pectoralis muscles. Axillary and supraclavicular areas should be thoroughly palpated for enlarged nodes with the patient sitting (Figure 17–4). Palpation of the breast for masses or other changes should be performed with the patient both seated and supine with the arm abducted

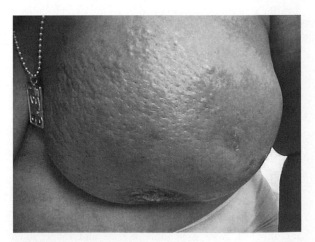

▲ **Figure 17–3.** Peau d'orange sign (resemblance to the skin of an orange due to lymphedema) in advanced breast cancer. (Copyright Richard P. Usatine, MD; from Usatine RP, Smith MA, Mayeaux EJ Jr, Chumley H. *The Color Atlas of Family Medicine.* 2nd ed. New York, NY: McGraw-Hill; 2013)

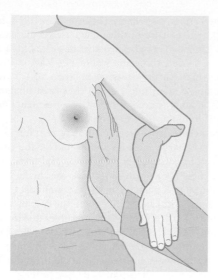

▲ **Figure 17–4.** Palpation of axillary region for enlarged lymph nodes.

(Figure 17–5). Palpation with a rotary motion of the examiner's fingers as well as a horizontal stripping motion has been recommended.

Breast cancer usually consists of a nontender, firm or hard mass with poorly delineated margins (caused by local infiltration). Very small (1-2 mm) erosions of the nipple epithelium may be the only manifestation of Paget disease of the breast. Watery, serous, or bloody discharge from the nipple is an occasional early sign but is more often associated with benign disease.

A small lesion, less than 1 cm in diameter, may be difficult or impossible for the examiner to feel but may be discovered by the patient. She should always be asked to demonstrate the location of the mass; if the practitioner fails

to confirm the patient's suspicions and imaging studies are normal, the examination should be repeated in 2-3 months, preferably 1-2 weeks after the onset of menses. During the premenstrual phase of the cycle, increased innocuous nodularity may suggest neoplasm or may obscure an underlying lesion. If there is any question regarding the nature of an abnormality under these circumstances, the patient should be asked to return after her menses. Ultrasound is often valuable and mammography essential when an area is felt by the patient to be abnormal but the physician feels no mass. MRI may be considered, but the lack of specificity should be discussed by the clinician and the patient. MRI should not be used to rule out cancer because MRI has a false-negative rate of about 3%-5%. Although lower than mammography, this false-negative rate cannot permit safe elimination of the possibility of cancer. False negatives are more likely seen in infiltrating lobular carcinomas and DCIS.

Metastases tend to involve regional lymph nodes, which may be palpable. One or two movable, nontender, not particularly firm axillary lymph nodes 5 mm or less in diameter are frequently present and are generally of no significance. Firm or hard nodes larger than 1 cm are typical of metastases. Axillary nodes that are matted or fixed to skin or deep structures indicate advanced disease (at least stage III). On the other hand, if the examiner thinks that the axillary nodes are involved, that impression will be borne out by histologic section in about 85% of cases. The incidence of positive axillary nodes increases with the size of the primary tumor. Noninvasive cancers (*in situ*) do not metastasize. Metastases are present in about 30% of patients with clinically negative nodes.

In most cases, no nodes are palpable in the supraclavicular fossa. Firm or hard nodes of any size in this location or just beneath the clavicle should be biopsied. Ipsilateral supraclavicular or infraclavicular nodes containing cancer indicate that the tumor is in an advanced stage (stage III or IV). Edema of the ipsilateral arm, commonly caused by metastatic infiltration of regional lymphatics, is also a sign of advanced cancer.

B. Laboratory Findings

Liver or bone metastases may be associated with elevation of serum alkaline phosphatase. Hypercalcemia is an occasional important finding in advanced cancer of the breast. Carcinoembryonic antigen (CEA) and CA 15-3 or CA 27-29 may be used as markers for recurrent breast cancer but are not helpful in diagnosing early lesions. Investigational breast cancer markers through proteomics and hormone assays may prove to be helpful in early detection or evaluation of prognosis.

C. Imaging for Metastases

For patients with suspicious symptoms or signs (bone pain, abdominal symptoms, elevated liver enzymes) or

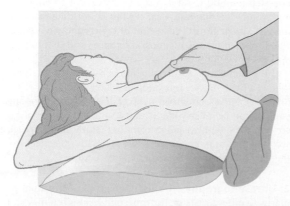

▲ **Figure 17–5.** Palpation of breasts. Palpation is performed with the patient supine and arm abducted.

locally advanced disease (clinically abnormal lymph nodes or large primary tumors), staging scans are indicated prior to surgery or systemic therapy. Chest imaging with CT or radiographs may be done to evaluate for pulmonary metastases. Abdominal imaging with CT or ultrasound may be obtained to evaluate for liver metastases. Bone scans using ^{99m}Tc-labeled phosphates or phosphonates are more sensitive than skeletal radiographs in detecting metastatic breast cancer. Bone scanning has not proved to be of clinical value as a routine preoperative test in the absence of symptoms, physical findings, or abnormal alkaline phosphatase or calcium levels. The frequency of abnormal findings on bone scan parallels the status of the axillary lymph nodes on pathologic examination. Positron emission tomography (PET) scanning alone or combined with CT (PET-CT) is effective for detecting soft tissue or visceral metastases in patients with symptoms or signs of metastatic disease.

D. Diagnostic Tests

1. Biopsy—The diagnosis of breast cancer depends ultimately on examination of tissue or cells removed by biopsy. Treatment should never be undertaken without an unequivocal histologic or cytologic diagnosis of cancer. The safest course is biopsy examination of all suspicious lesions found on physical examination or mammography, or both. About 60% of lesions clinically thought to be cancer prove on biopsy to be benign, while about 30% of clinically benign lesions are found to be malignant. These findings demonstrate the fallibility of clinical judgment and the necessity for biopsy.

All breast masses require a histologic diagnosis with one probable exception, a nonsuspicious, presumably fibrocystic mass, in a premenopausal woman. Rather, these masses can be observed through one or two menstrual cycles. However, if the mass is not cystic and does not completely resolve during this time, it must be biopsied. Figures 17–6 and 17–7 present algorithms for management of breast masses in premenopausal and postmenopausal patients.

The simplest biopsy method is needle biopsy, either by aspiration of tumor cells (FNA cytology) or by obtaining a small core of tissue with a hollow needle (core biopsy).

FNA cytology is a useful technique whereby cells are aspirated with a small needle and examined cytologically. This technique can be performed easily with virtually no morbidity and is much less expensive than excisional or open biopsy. The main disadvantages are that it requires a pathologist skilled in the cytologic diagnosis of breast cancer and it is subject to sampling problems, particularly because deep lesions may be missed. Furthermore, noninvasive cancers usually cannot be distinguished from invasive cancers and immunohistochemical tests to determine expression of hormone receptors and the amplification of the HER2

oncogene cannot be reliably performed on FNA biopsies. The incidence of false-positive diagnoses is extremely low, perhaps 1%-2%. The false-negative rate is as high as 10%. Most experienced clinicians would not leave a suspicious dominant mass in the breast even when FNA cytology is negative unless the clinical diagnosis, breast imaging studies, and cytologic studies were all in agreement, such as a fibrocystic lesion or fibroadenoma.

Large-needle (core needle) biopsy removes a core of tissue with a large cutting needle and is the diagnostic procedure of choice for both palpable and image-detected abnormalities. Hand-held biopsy devices make large-core needle biopsy of a palpable mass easy and cost effective in the office with local anesthesia. As in the case of any needle biopsy, the main problem is sampling error due to improper positioning of the needle, giving rise to a false-negative test result. This is extremely unusual with image-guided biopsies. Core biopsy has the advantage that tumor markers, such as estrogen receptor (ER), progesterone receptor (PR), and HER2 overexpression can be performed on cores of tissue.

Open biopsy under local anesthesia as a separate procedure prior to deciding upon definitive treatment is becoming less common with the increasing use of core needle biopsy. Needle biopsy, when positive, offers a more rapid approach with less expense and morbidity, but when nondiagnostic it must be followed by open biopsy. It generally consists of an excisional biopsy, which is done through an incision with the intent to remove the entire abnormality, not simply a sample. Additional evaluation for metastatic disease and therapeutic options can be discussed with the patient after the histologic or cytologic diagnosis of cancer has been established. As an alternative in highly suspicious circumstances, the diagnosis may be made on frozen section of tissue obtained by open biopsy under general anesthesia. If the frozen section is positive, the surgeon can proceed immediately with the definitive operation. This one-step method is rarely used today except when a cytologic study has suggested cancer but is not diagnostic and there is a high clinical suspicion of malignancy in a patient well prepared for the diagnosis of cancer and its treatment options.

In general, the two-step approach—outpatient biopsy followed by definitive operation at a later date—is preferred in the diagnosis and treatment of breast cancer, because patients can be given time to adjust to the diagnosis of cancer, can consider alternative forms of therapy, and can seek a second opinion if they wish. There is no adverse effect from the few week delay of the two-step procedure.

2. Ultrasonography—Ultrasonography is performed primarily to differentiate cystic from solid lesions but may show signs suggestive of carcinoma. Ultrasonography may show

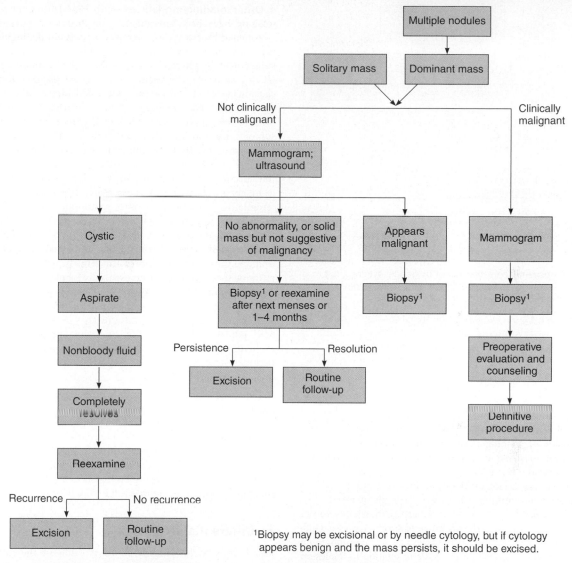

▲ **Figure 17–6.** Evaluation of breast masses in premenopausal women. (Adapted, with permission, from Chang S, Haigh PI, Giuliano AE. Breast disease. In: Berek JS, Hacker NF, eds. *Practical Gynecologic Oncology*, 4th ed. LWW, 2004.)

an irregular mass within a cyst in the rare case of intracystic carcinoma. If a tumor is palpable and feels like a cyst, an 18-gauge needle can be used to aspirate the fluid and make the diagnosis of cyst. If a cyst is aspirated and the fluid is nonbloody, it does not have to be examined cytologically. If the mass does not recur, no further diagnostic test is necessary. Nonpalpable mammographic densities that appear benign should be investigated with ultrasound to determine

whether the lesion is cystic or solid. These may even be needle biopsied with ultrasound guidance.

3. Mammography—When a suspicious abnormality is identified by mammography alone and cannot be palpated by the clinician, the lesion should be biopsied under mammographic guidance. In the **computerized stereotactic guided core needle** technique, a biopsy needle is inserted

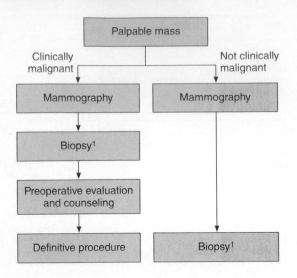

¹Biopsy may be excisional or by needle cytology, but if cytology appears benign and the mass persists, it should be excised.

▲ **Figure 17–7.** Evaluation of breast masses in post-menopausal women. (Adapted, with permission, from Chang S, Haigh PI, Giuliano AE. Breast disease. In: Berek JS, Hacker NF, eds. *Practical Gynecologic Oncology,* 4th ed. LWW, 2004.)

into the lesion with mammographic guidance, and a core of tissue for histologic examination can then be examined. Vacuum assistance increases the amount of tissue obtained and improves diagnosis.

Mammographic localization biopsy is performed by obtaining a mammogram in two perpendicular views and placing a needle or hook-wire near the abnormality so that the surgeon can use the metal needle or wire as a guide during operation to locate the lesion. After mammography confirms the position of the needle in relation to the lesion, an incision is made and the subcutaneous tissue is dissected until the needle is identified. Often, the abnormality cannot even be palpated through the incision—as is the case with microcalcifications—and thus it is essential to obtain a mammogram of the specimen to document that the lesion was excised. At that time, a second marker needle can further localize the lesion for the pathologist. Stereotactic core needle biopsies have proved equivalent to mammographic localization biopsies. Core biopsy is preferable to mammographic localization for accessible lesions since an operation can be avoided. A metal clip should be placed after any image-guided core biopsy to facilitate finding the site of the lesion if subsequent treatment is necessary.

4. Other imaging modalities—Other modalities of breast imaging have been investigated for diagnostic purposes. Automated breast ultrasonography is useful in distinguishing cystic from solid lesions but should be used only as a supplement to physical examination and mammography. Ductography may be useful to define the site of a lesion causing a bloody discharge, but since biopsy is almost always indicated, ductography may be omitted and the blood-filled nipple system excised. Ductoscopy has shown some promise in identifying intraductal lesions, especially in the case of pathologic nipple discharge, but in practice, this technique is rarely used. MRI is highly sensitive but not specific and should not be used for screening except in highly selective cases. For example, MRI is useful in differentiating scar from recurrence postlumpectomy and may be valuable to screen high-risk women (eg, women with *BRCA* mutations). It may also be of value to examine for multicentricity when there is a known primary cancer; to examine the contralateral breast in women with cancer; to examine the extent of cancer, especially lobular carcinomas; or to determine the response to neoadjuvant chemotherapy. Moreover, MRI-detected suspicious findings that are not seen on mammogram or ultrasound may be biopsied under MRI guidance. PET scanning does not appear useful in evaluating the breast itself but is useful to examine for distant metastases.

5. Cytology—Cytologic examination of nipple discharge or cyst fluid may be helpful on rare occasions. As a rule, mammography (or ductography) and breast biopsy are required when nipple discharge or cyst fluid is bloody or cytologically questionable. Ductal lavage, a technique that washes individual duct systems with saline and loosens epithelial cells for cytologic evaluation, is being evaluated as a risk assessment tool but appears to be of little value.

▶ Differential Diagnosis

The lesions to be considered most often in the differential diagnosis of breast cancer are the following, in descending order of frequency: fibrocystic condition of the breast, fibroadenoma, intraductal papilloma, lipoma, and fat necrosis.

▶ Staging

The American Joint Committee on Cancer and the International Union Against Cancer have agreed on a TNM (tumor, regional lymph nodes, distant metastases) staging system for breast cancer. Using the TNM staging system enhances communication between researchers and clinicians. Table 17–3 outlines the TNM classification.

Table 17–3. TNM staging for breast cancer.

Primary Tumor (T)

Definitions for classifying the primary tumor (T) are the same for clinical and for pathologic classification. If the measurement is made by physical examination, the examiner will use the major headings (T1, T2, or T3). If other measurements, such as mammographic or pathologic measurements, are used, the subsets of T1 can be used. Tumors should be measured to the nearest 0.1 cm increment.

TX	Primary tumor cannot be assessed
T0	No evidence of primary tumor
Tis	Carcinoma in situ
Tis (DCIS)	Ductal carcinoma in situ
Tis (LCIS)	Lobular carcinoma in situ
Tis (Paget)	Paget disease of the nipple with no tumor

Note: Paget disease associated with a tumor is classified according to the size of the tumor.

T1	Tumor 2 cm or less in greatest dimension
T1mic	Microinvasion 0.1 cm or less in greatest dimension
T1a	Tumor more than 0.1 cm but not more than 0.5 cm in greatest dimension
T1b	Tumor more than 0.5 cm but not more than 1 cm in greatest dimension
T1c	Tumor more than 1 cm but not more than 2 cm in greatest dimension
T2	Tumor more than 2 cm but not more than 5 cm in greatest dimension
T3	Tumor more than 5 cm in greatest dimension
T4	Tumor of any size with direct extension to: (a) chest wall; or (b) skin, only as described below
T4a	Extension to chest wall, not including pectoralis muscle
T4b	Edema (including peau d'orange [Figure 17–3]) or ulceration of the skin of the breast, or satellite skin nodules confined to the same breast
T4c	Both T4a and T4b
T4d	Inflammatory carcinoma

Regional Lymph Nodes (N)

Clinical

NX	Regional lymph nodes cannot be assessed (eg, previously removed)
N0	No regional lymph node metastasis
N1	Metastasis in movable ipsilateral axillary lymph node(s)
N2	Metastases in ipsilateral axillary lymph nodes fixed or matted, or in clinically apparent[1] ipsilateral internal mammary nodes in the *absence* of clinically evident axillary lymph node metastasis
N2a	Metastasis in ipsilateral axillary lymph nodes fixed to one another (matted) or to other structures
N2b	Metastasis only in clinically apparent[1] ipsilateral internal mammary nodes and in the *absence* of clinically evident axillary lymph node metastasis
N3	Metastasis in ipsilateral infraclavicular lymph node(s) with or without axillary lymph node involvement, or in clinically apparent[1] ipsilateral internal mammary lymph node(s) and in the *presence* of clinically evident axillary lymph node metastasis; or metastasis in ipsilateral supraclavicular lymph node(s) with or without axillary or internal mammary lymph node involvement
N3a	Metastasis in ipsilateral infraclavicular lymph node(s)
N3b	Metastasis in ipsilateral internal mammary lymph node(s) and axillary lymph node(s)
N3c	Metastasis in ipsilateral supraclavicular lymph node(s)

Regional Lymph Nodes (pN)[2]

Pnx	Regional lymph nodes cannot be assessed (eg, previously removed, or not removed for pathologic study)
pN0	No regional lymph node metastasis histologically, no additional examination for isolated tumor cells

(continued)

Table 17–3. TNM staging for breast cancer. (*Continued*)

Note: Isolated tumor cells (ITC) are defined as single tumor cells or small cell clusters not > 0.2 mm, usually detected only by immunohistochemical (IHC) or molecular methods but which may be verified on hematoxylin and eosin stains. ITCs do not usually show evidence of malignant activity, eg, proliferation or stromal reaction.

pN0(i⁻)	No regional lymph node metastasis histologically, negative IHC
pN0(i⁺)	No regional lymph node metastasis histologically, positive IHC, no IHC cluster > 0.2 mm
pN0(mol⁻)	No regional lymph node metastasis histologically, negative molecular findings (RT-PCR)[3]
pN0(mol⁺)	No regional lymph node metastasis histologically, positive molecular findings (RT-PCR)[3]
pN1	Metastasis in one to three axillary lymph nodes, and/or in internal mammary nodes with microscopic disease detected by sentinel lymph node dissection but not clinically apparent[4]
pN1mi	Micrometastasis (> 0.2 mm, none > 2.0 mm)
pN1a	Metastasis in one to three axillary lymph nodes
pN1b	Metastasis in internal mammary nodes with microscopic disease detected by sentinel lymph node dissection but not clinically apparent[4]
pN1c	Metastasis in one to three axillary lymph nodes and in internal mammary lymph nodes with microscopic disease detected by sentinel lymph node dissection but not clinically apparent.[4] (If associated with greater than three positive axillary lymph nodes, the internal mammary nodes are classified as pN3b to reflect increased tumor burden)
pN2	Metastasis in four to nine axillary lymph nodes, or in clinically apparent[1] internal mammary lymph nodes in the *absence* of axillary lymph node metastasis
pN2a	Metastasis in four to nine axillary lymph nodes (at least one tumor deposit > 2.0 mm)
pN2b	Metastasis in clinically apparent[1] internal mammary lymph nodes in the *absence* of axillary lymph node metastasis
pN3	Metastasis in 10 or more axillary lymph nodes, or in infraclavicular lymph nodes, or in clinically apparent[1] ipsilateral internal mammary lymph nodes in the *presence* of one or more positive axillary lymph nodes; or in more than three axillary lymph nodes with clinically negative microscopic metastasis in internal mammary lymph nodes; or in ipsilateral supraclavicular lymph nodes
pN3a	Metastasis in 10 or more axillary lymph nodes (at least one tumor deposit > 2.0 mm), or metastasis to the infraclavicular lymph nodes
pN3b	Metastasis in clinically apparent[1] ipsilateral internal mammary lymph nodes in the *presence* of one or more positive axillary lymph nodes; or in more than three axillary lymph nodes and in internal mammary lymph nodes with microscopic disease detected by sentinel lymph node dissection but not clinically apparent[4]
pN3c	Metastasis in ipsilateral supraclavicular lymph nodes

Distant Metastasis (M)

MX	Distant metastasis cannot be assessed
M0	No distant metastasis
M1	Distant metastasis

Stage Grouping

Stage 0	Tis	N0	M0
Stage 1	T1[5]	N0	M0
Stage IIA	T0	N1	M0
	T1[5]	N1	M0
	T2	N0	M0
Stage IIB	T2	N1	M0
	T3	N0	M0
Stage IIIA	T0	N2	M0
	T1[5]T2	N2	M0
	T3	N2	M0
	T3	N1	M0
		N2	M0

(continued)

Table 17–3. TNM staging for breast cancer. (*Continued*)

Stage IIIB	T4	N0	M0
	T4	N1	M0
	T4	N2	M0
Stage IIIC	Any T	N3	M0
Stage IV	Any T	Any N	M1

Note: Stage designation may be changed if postsurgical imaging studies reveal the presence of distant metastases, provided that the studies are carried out within 4 months of diagnosis in the absence of disease progression and provided that the patient has not received neoadjuvant therapy.
[1]*Clinically apparent* is defined as detected by imaging studies (excluding lymphoscintigraphy) or by clinical examination or grossly visible pathologically.
[2]Classification is based on axillary lymph node dissection with or without sentinel lymph node dissection. Classification based solely on sentinel lymph node dissection without subsequent axillary lymph node dissection is designated (sn) for "sentinel node," eg, pN0(i+)(sn).
[3]RT-PCR, reverse transcriptase/polymerase chain reaction.
[4]*Not clinically apparent* is defined as not detected by imaging studies (excluding lymphoscintigraphy) or by clinical examination.
[5]T1 includes T1mic.
Reproduced, with permission, of the American Joint Committee on Cancer (AJCC), Chicago, Illinois, *AJCC Cancer Staging Manual*, 7th ed. New York: Springer-Science and Business Media LLC, 2010. Available at www.springer.com.

► Pathologic Types

Numerous pathologic subtypes of breast cancer can be identified histologically (Table 17–4).

Except for the *in situ* cancers, the histologic subtypes have only a slight bearing on prognosis when outcomes are compared after accurate staging. The noninvasive cancers by definition are confined by the basement membrane of the ducts and lack the ability to spread. Histologic parameters for invasive cancers, including lymphovascular invasion and tumor grade, have been shown to be of prognostic value. Immunohistochemical analysis for expression of hormone receptors and for overexpression of HER2 in the primary tumor offers prognostic and therapeutic information.

SPECIAL CLINICAL FORMS OF BREAST CANCER

► Paget Carcinoma

Paget carcinoma is not common (about 1% of all breast cancers). Over 85% of cases are associated with an underlying invasive or noninvasive cancer, usually a well-differentiated infiltrating ductal carcinoma or a DCIS. The ducts of the nipple epithelium are infiltrated, but gross nipple changes are often minimal, and a tumor mass may not be palpable.

Because the nipple changes appear innocuous, the diagnosis is frequently missed. The first symptom is often itching or burning of the nipple, with superficial erosion or ulceration. These are often diagnosed and treated as dermatitis or bacterial infection, leading to delay or failure in detection. The diagnosis is established by biopsy of the area of erosion. When the lesion consists of nipple changes only, the incidence of axillary metastases is less than 5%, and the prognosis is excellent. When a breast mass is also present, the incidence of axillary metastases rises, with an associated marked decrease in prospects for cure by surgical or other treatment.

Table 17–4. Histologic types of breast cancer.

Type	Frequency of Occurrence (%)
Infiltrating ductal (not otherwise specified)	80-90
Medullary	5-8
Colloid (mucinous)	2-4
Tubular	1-2
Papillary	1-2
Invasive lobular	6-8
Noninvasive	4-6
Intraductal	2-3
Lobular in situ	2-3
Rare cancers	< 1
Juvenile (secretory)	
Adenoid cystic	
Epidermoid	
Sudoriferous	

▶ Inflammatory Carcinoma

This is the most malignant form of breast cancer and constitutes less than 3% of all cases. The clinical findings consist of a rapidly growing, sometimes painful mass that enlarges the breast. The overlying skin becomes erythematous, edematous, and warm. Often there is no distinct mass, since the tumor infiltrates the involved breast diffusely. The inflammatory changes, often mistaken for an infection, are caused by carcinomatous invasion of the subdermal lymphatics, with resulting edema and hyperemia. If the clinician suspects infection but the lesion does not respond rapidly (1-2 weeks) to antibiotics, biopsy should be performed. The diagnosis should be made when the redness involves more than one-third of the skin over the breast and biopsy shows infiltrating carcinoma with invasion of the subdermal lymphatics. Metastases tend to occur early and widely, and for this reason inflammatory carcinoma is rarely curable. Radiation, hormone therapy, and chemotherapy are the measures most likely to be of value rather than operation. Mastectomy is indicated when chemotherapy and radiation have resulted in clinical remission with no evidence of distant metastases. In these cases, residual disease in the breast may be eradicated.

▶ Breast Cancer Occurring During Pregnancy or Lactation

Breast cancer complicates approximately 1 in 3000 pregnancies. The diagnosis is frequently delayed, because physiologic changes in the breast may obscure the lesion and screening mammography is not done in young or pregnant women. When the cancer is confined to the breast, the 5-year survival rate is about 70%. In 60%-70% of patients, axillary metastases are already present, conferring a 5-year survival rate of 30%-40%. A retrospective analysis of women who were younger than 36 years when breast cancer was diagnosed showed that while women with pregnancy-associated breast cancer were more frequently diagnosed with later stage breast cancer, they had similar rates of locoregional recurrence, distant metastases, and overall survival as women with nonpregnancy-associated breast cancer. It is thus important for primary care and reproductive specialists to aggressively workup any breast abnormality discovered in a pregnant woman. Pregnancy (or lactation) is not a contraindication to operation or treatment, and therapy should be based on the stage of the disease as in the nonpregnant (or nonlactating) woman. Overall survival rates have improved, since cancers are now diagnosed in pregnant women earlier than in the past and treatment has improved. Breast-conserving surgery may be performed and chemotherapy given even during the pregnancy.

▶ Bilateral Breast Cancer

Bilateral breast cancer occurs in less than 5% of cases, but there is as high as a 20%-25% incidence of later occurrence of cancer in the second breast. Bilaterality occurs more often in familial breast cancer, in women under age 50 years, and when the tumor in the primary breast is lobular. The incidence of second breast cancers increases directly with the length of time the patient is alive after her first cancer—about 1%-2% per year.

In patients with breast cancer, mammography should be performed before primary treatment and at regular intervals thereafter, to search for occult cancer in the opposite breast or conserved ipsilateral breast. MRI may be useful in this high-risk group.

▶ Noninvasive Cancer

Noninvasive cancer can occur within the ducts (DCIS) or lobules (LCIS). DCIS tends to be unilateral and most often progresses to invasive cancer if untreated. In approximately 40%-60% of women who have DCIS treated with biopsy alone, invasive cancer develops within the same breast. LCIS, although thought to be a premalignant lesion or a risk factor for breast cancer, in fact may behave like DCIS. In a 2004 analysis of multiple NSABP studies, invasive lobular breast cancer not only developed in patients with LCIS but it developed in the same breast and indexed location as the original LCIS. Although more research needs to be done in this area, the invasive potential of LCIS is being reconsidered. Higher grade and pleomorphic LCIS may behave more like DCIS, and may be associated with invasive carcinoma. For this reason, some surgeons are now recommending that pleomorphic LCIS be surgically removed with clear margins.

The treatment of intraductal lesions is controversial. DCIS can be treated by wide excision with or without radiation therapy or with total mastectomy. Conservative management is advised in patients with small lesions amenable to lumpectomy. Although research is defining the malignant potential of LCIS, it can be managed with observation. Patients unwilling to accept the increased risk of breast cancer may be offered surgical excision of the area in question or bilateral total mastectomy. Currently, the accepted standard of care offers the alternative of chemoprevention, which is effective in preventing invasive breast cancer in both LCIS and DCIS that has been completely excised. Axillary metastases from *in situ* cancers should not occur unless there is an occult invasive cancer. Sentinel node biopsy may be indicated in large DCIS treated with mastectomy.

Amant F et al: Breast cancer in pregnancy. *Lancet.* 2012;379(9815):570-579. [PMID 22325662]

Bruening W et al: Systematic review: comparative effectiveness of core-needle and open surgical biopsy to diagnose breast lesions. *Ann Intern Med.* 2010 Feb 16;152(4):238-246. [PMID: 20008742]

Rakha EA et al: The prognostic significance of lymphovascular invasion in invasive breast carcinoma. *Cancer.* 2012 Aug 1;118(15):3670-3680. [PMID: 22180017]

Robertson FM et al: Inflammatory breast cancer: the disease, the biology, the treatment. *CA Cancer J Clin.* 2010 Nov-Dec; 60(6):351-375. [PMID: 20959401]

Sinclair S et al: Primary systemic chemotherapy for inflammatory breast cancer. *Cancer.* 2010 Jun 1;116(Suppl 11):2821-2828. [PMID: 20503414]

Veronesi U et al: Sentinel lymph node biopsy in breast cancer: ten-year results of a randomized controlled study. *Ann Surg.* 2010 Apr;251(4):595-600. [PMID: 20195151]

BIOMARKERS & GENE EXPRESSION PROFILING

Determining the ER, PR, and HER2 status of the tumor at the time of diagnosis of early breast cancer and, if possible, at the time of recurrence is critical, both to gauge a patient's prognosis and to determine the best treatment regimen. In addition to ER status and PR status, the rate at which tumor divides (assessed by an immunohistochemical stain for Ki-67) and the grade and differentiation of the cells are also important prognostic factors. These markers may be obtained on core biopsy or surgical specimens. Patients whose tumors are hormone receptor-positive tend to have a more indolent disease course than those whose tumors are receptor-negative. Moreover, treatment with an antihormonal agent is an essential component of therapy for hormone-receptor positive breast cancer at any stage. While up to 60% of patients with metastatic breast cancer will respond to hormonal manipulation if their tumors are ER-positive, less than 5% of patients with metastatic, ER-negative tumors will respond.

Another key element in determining treatment and prognosis is the amount of the HER2 oncogene present in the cancer. HER2 overexpression is measured by an immunohistochemical assay that is scored using a numerical system: 0 and 1+ are considered negative for overexpression, 2+ is borderline/indeterminate, and 3+ is overexpression. In the case of 2+ expression, fluorescence in situ hybridization (FISH) is recommended to more accurately assess HER2 amplification. According to the College of American Pathologists, a FISH score of less than 1.8 is negative for amplification, 1.8-2.2 is indeterminant, and greater than 2.2 is amplified. The presence of HER2 amplification and overexpression is of prognostic significance and predicts the response to trastuzumab.

Individually these biomarkers are predictive and thus provide insight to guide appropriate therapy. Moreover, when combined they provide useful information regarding risk of recurrence and prognosis. In general, tumors that lack expression of HER2, ER, and PR ("triple negative") have a higher risk of recurrence and metastases and are associated with a worse survival compared with other types. Neither endocrine therapy nor HER2-targeted agents are useful for this type of breast cancer, leaving chemotherapy as the only treatment option. In contrast, patients with early stage, hormone receptor-positive breast cancer may not benefit from the addition of chemotherapy to hormonal treatments. Several molecular tests have been developed to assess risk of recurrence and to predict which patients are most likely to benefit from chemotherapy. Oncotype DX (Genomic Health) evaluates the expression of 21 genes relating to ER, PR, HER2, and proliferation in a tumor specimen and categorizes a patient's risk of recurrence (recurrence score) as high, intermediate, or low risk. In addition to providing prognostic information, the test also has predictive value since studies have shown that patients in the high-risk category are most likely to respond to chemotherapy. This test is primarily indicated for ER-positive, node-negative tumors but at least one study has shown that it may also have value in node-positive tumors. Centralized testing for ER, PR, HER2, and Ki67 by standard immunohistochemical techniques is able to provide as much prognostic information as Oncotype DX. Mammaprint (Agendia) is another assay that is available for evaluating prognosis. This 70-gene signature is FDA-approved and may be performed on fresh frozen tumor tissue taken at the time of a patient's surgery. This test classifies patients into good and poor prognostic groups to predict clinical outcome and may be used on patients with hormone receptor positive or negative breast cancer. Several other assays are in development to better stratify patients based on risk assessment.

Albain KS et al: For The Breast Cancer Intergroup of North America. Prognostic and predictive value of the 21-gene recurrence score assay in postmenopausal women with node-positive, oestrogen-receptor-positive breast cancer on chemotherapy: a retrospective analysis of a randomised trial. *Lancet Oncol.* 2010 Jan;11(1):55-65. [PMID: 20005174]

Capala J et al: Molecular imaging of HER2-positive breast cancer: a step toward an individualized "image and treat" strategy. *Curr Opin Oncol.* 2010 Nov;22(6):559-566. [PMID: 20842031]

Cuzick J et al: Prognostic value of a combined estrogen receptor, progesterone receptor, Ki-67, and human epidermal growth factor receptor 2 immunohistochemical score and comparison with the Genomic Health recurrence score in early breast cancer. *J Clin Oncol.* 2011 Nov 10;29(32):4273-4278. [PMID: 21990413]

Foulkes WD et al: Triple-negative breast cancer. *N Engl J Med.* 2010 Nov 11;363(20):1938-1948. [PMID: 21067385]

Galanina N et al: Molecular predictors of response to therapy for breast cancer. *Cancer J.* 2011 Mar-Apr;17(2):96-103. [PMID: 21427553]

Macrinici V et al: Clinical updates on EGFR/HER targeted agents in early-stage breast cancer. *Clin Breast Cancer.* 2010;10(Suppl 1): E38-E46. [PMID: 20587406]

Sparano JA et al: Clinical application of gene expression profiling in breast cancer. *Surg Oncol Clin N Am.* 2010 Jul;19(3):581-606. [PMID: 20620929]

▶ **Treatment: Curative**

Clearly, not all breast cancer is systemic at the time of diagnosis. For this reason, a pessimistic attitude concerning the management of breast cancer is unwarranted. Most patients with early breast cancer can be cured. Treatment with a curative intent is advised for clinical stage I, II, and III disease (see Tables 17–3 and 39–4). Patients with locally advanced (T3, T4) and even inflammatory tumors may be cured with multimodality therapy, but in most, palliation is all that can be expected. Treatment with palliative intent is appropriate for all patients with stage IV disease and for patients with unresectable local cancers.

A. Choice and Timing of Primary Therapy

The extent of disease and its biologic aggressiveness are the principal determinants of the outcome of primary therapy. Clinical and pathologic staging help in assessing extent of disease (Table 17–3), but each is to some extent imprecise. Other factors such as tumor grade, hormone receptor assays, and HER2 oncogene amplification are of prognostic value and are key to determining systemic therapy, but are not important in determining the type of local therapy.

Controversy has surrounded the choice of primary therapy of stages I, II, and III breast carcinoma. Currently, the standard of care for stage I, stage II, and most stage III cancer is surgical resection followed by adjuvant radiation or systemic therapy, or both, when indicated. Neoadjuvant therapy is becoming more popular since large tumors may be shrunk by chemotherapy prior to surgery, making some patients who require mastectomy candidates for lumpectomy. It is important for patients to understand all of the surgical options, including reconstructive options, prior to having surgery. Patients with large primary tumors, inflammatory cancer, or palpably enlarged lymph nodes should have staging scans performed to rule out distant metastatic disease prior to definitive surgery. In general, adjuvant systemic therapy is started when the breast has adequately healed, usually within 4-8 weeks after surgery. While no prospective studies have defined the appropriate timing of adjuvant chemotherapy, one retrospective population-based study has suggested that chemotherapy should be initiated within 12 weeks of surgery to avoid a compromise in relapse-free and overall survival.

B. Surgical Resection

1. Breast-conserving therapy—Multiple, large, randomized studies including the Milan and NSABP trials show that disease-free and overall survival rates are similar for patients with stage I and stage II breast cancer treated with partial mastectomy (breast-conserving lumpectomy) plus axillary dissection followed by radiation therapy and for those treated by modified radical mastectomy (total mastectomy plus axillary dissection).

Tumor size is a major consideration in determining the feasibility of breast conservation. The lumpectomy trial of the NSABP randomized patients with tumors as large as 4 cm. To achieve an acceptable cosmetic result, the patient must have a breast of sufficient size to enable excision of a 4-cm tumor without considerable deformity. Therefore, large tumor size is only a relative contraindication. Subareolar tumors, also difficult to excise without deformity, are not contraindications to breast conservation. Clinically detectable multifocality is a relative contraindication to breast-conserving surgery, as is fixation to the chest wall or skin or involvement of the nipple or overlying skin. The patient—not the surgeon—should be the judge of what is cosmetically acceptable. Given the relatively high risk of poor outcome after radiation, concomitant scleroderma is a contraindication to breast-conserving surgery. A history of prior therapeutic radiation to the ipsilateral breast or chest wall (or both) is also a contraindication for breast conservation.

Axillary dissection is primarily used to properly stage cancer and plan radiation and systemic therapy. Intraoperative lymphatic mapping and sentinel node biopsy identify lymph nodes most likely to harbor metastases if present (Figure 17–8). Sentinel node biopsy is a reasonable alternative to axillary dissection in selected patients with invasive cancer. If sentinel node biopsy reveals no evidence of axillary metastases, it is highly likely that the remaining lymph nodes are free of disease and axillary dissection may be omitted. An important study from the American College of Surgeons Oncology group randomized women with sentinel node metastases to undergo completion of axillary dissection or to receive no further axillary treatment after lumpectomy; no difference in survival was found, showing that axillary dissection for selected node-positive women is not necessary. These results challenge standard treatment regimens.

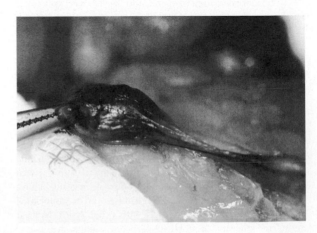

▲ **Figure 17–8.** Sentinel node. (Used with permission from Giuliano AE.)

Breast-conserving surgery with radiation is the preferred form of treatment for patients with **early-stage breast cancer**. Despite the numerous randomized trials showing no survival benefit of mastectomy over breast-conserving partial mastectomy and irradiation, breast-conserving surgery still appears to be underutilized.

2. Mastectomy—Modified radical mastectomy is the standard therapy for most patients with early-stage breast cancer. This operation removes the entire breast, overlying skin, nipple, and areolar complex as well as the underlying pectoralis fascia with the axillary lymph nodes in continuity. The major advantage of modified radical mastectomy is that radiation therapy may not be necessary, although radiation may be used when lymph nodes are involved with cancer or when the primary tumor is large (≥ 5 cm). The disadvantage of mastectomy is the cosmetic and psychological impact associated with breast loss. Radical mastectomy, which removes the underlying pectoralis muscle, should be performed rarely, if at all. Axillary node dissection is not indicated for noninfiltrating cancers because nodal metastases are rarely present. Skin-sparing and nipple-sparing mastectomy is currently gaining favor but is not appropriate for all patients. Breast-conserving surgery and radiation should be offered whenever possible, since most patients would prefer to save the breast. Breast reconstruction, immediate or delayed, should be discussed with patients who choose or require mastectomy. Patients should have an interview with a reconstructive plastic surgeon to discuss options prior to making a decision regarding reconstruction. Time is well spent preoperatively in educating the patient and family about these matters.

C. Radiotherapy

Radiotherapy after partial mastectomy consists of 5-7 weeks of five daily fractions to a total dose of 5000-6000 cGy. Most radiation oncologists use a boost dose to the cancer location. Early results of studies examining the utility and recurrence rates after intraoperative radiation or dose dense radiation in which the time course of radiation is shortened show promising results similar to standard techniques. Accelerated partial breast irradiation, in which only the portion of the breast from which the tumor was resected is irradiated for 1-2 weeks, appears effective in achieving local control. The American Society of Breast Surgeons Registry Trial reported that in 1440 patients treated with brachytherapy, the 3-year actuarial rate of ipsilateral breast cancer recurrence was 2.15% and no unexpected adverse events were seen. Long-term follow-up will be necessary as will results from ongoing randomized clinical trials comparing brachytherapy to standard external beam radiation.

Current studies suggest that radiotherapy after mastectomy may improve recurrence rates and survival in patients with tumors 5 cm or more or positive lymph nodes. Researchers are also examining the utility of axillary irradiation as an alternative to axillary dissection in the clinically node-negative patient with sentinel node micrometastases. A Canadian trial (MA20) of postoperative nodal irradiation after lumpectomy and axillary dissection shows improved survival with nodal irradiation.

D. Adjuvant Systemic Therapy

The goal of systemic therapy, including hormone modulating drugs (endocrine therapy), cytotoxic chemotherapy, and the HER2-targeted agent trastuzumab, is to kill cancer cells that have escaped the breast and axillary lymph nodes as micrometastases before they become macrometastases (ie, stage IV cancer). Systemic therapy improves survival and is advocated for most patients with curable breast cancer. In practice, most medical oncologists are currently using adjuvant chemotherapy for patients with either node-positive or higher-risk (eg, hormone receptor-negative or HER2-positive) node-negative breast cancer and using endocrine therapy for all hormone receptor–positive invasive breast cancer unless contraindicated. Prognostic factors other than nodal status that are used to determine the patient's risks of recurrence are tumor size, ER and PR status, nuclear grade, histologic type, proliferative rate, oncogene expression (Table 17–5), and patient's age and menopausal status. In general, systemic chemotherapy decreases the chance of recurrence by about 30% and hormonal modulation

Table 17-5. Prognostic factors in node-negative breast cancer.

Prognostic Factors	Increased Recurrence	Decreased Recurrence
Size	T3, T2	T1, T0
Hormone receptors	Negative	Positive
DNA flow cytometry	Aneuploid	Diploid
Histologic grade	High	Low
Tumor labeling index	< 3%	> 3%
S phase fraction	> 5%	< 5%
Lymphatic or vascular invasion	Present	Absent
Cathepsin D	High	Low
HER-2/neu oncogene	High	Low
Epidermal growth factor receptor	High	Low

decreases the risk of recurrence by 40%-50% (for hormone receptor–positive cancer). Systemic chemotherapy is usually given sequentially, rather than concurrently with radiation. In terms of sequencing, typically chemotherapy is given before radiation and endocrine therapy is started concurrent with or after radiation therapy.

The long-term advantage of systemic therapy has been well established. All patients with invasive hormone receptor–positive tumors should consider the use of hormone-modulating therapy. Most patients with HER2-positive tumors should receive trastuzumab-containing chemotherapy regimens. In general, adjuvant systemic chemotherapy should not be given to women who have small node-negative breast cancers with favorable histologic findings and tumor markers. The ability to predict more accurately which patients with HER2-negative, hormone receptor-positive, lymph node-negative tumors should receive chemotherapy is improving with the advent of prognostic tools, such as Oncotype DX and mammaprint. These tests are undergoing prospective evaluation in two clinical trials (TAILORx and MINDACT).

1. Chemotherapy—The Early Breast Cancer Trialists' Collaborative Group (EBCTCG) meta-analysis involving over 28,000 women enrolled in 60 trials of adjuvant polychemotherapy versus no chemotherapy demonstrated a significant beneficial impact of chemotherapy on clinical outcome in early breast cancer. This study showed that adjuvant chemotherapy reduces the risk of recurrence and breast cancer–specific mortality in all women but also showed that women under the age of 50 derive the greatest benefit. On the basis of the superiority of anthracycline-containing regimens in metastatic breast cancer, both doxorubicin and epirubicin have been studied extensively in the adjuvant setting. Studies comparing Adriamycin (doxorubicin) and cyclophosphamide (AC) or epirubicin and cyclophosphamide (EC) to cyclophosphamide-methotrexate-5-fluorouracil (CMF) have shown that treatments with anthracycline-containing regimens are at least as effective, and perhaps more effective, than treatment with CMF. The EBCTCG analysis including over 14,000 patients enrolled in trials comparing anthracycline-based regimens to CMF, showed a small but statistically significant improved disease-free and overall survival with the use of anthracycline-based regimens. It should be noted, however, that most of these studies included a mixed population of HER2-positive and HER2-negative breast cancer patients and were performed before the development of trastuzumab. Retrospective analyses of a number of these studies suggest that anthracyclines may be primarily effective in tumors with HER2 overexpression or alteration in the expression of topoisomerase IIa (the target of anthracyclines and close to the HER2 gene). Given this, for HER2-negative,

node-negative breast cancer, four cycles of AC or six cycles of CMF are probably equally effective.

When taxanes (T = paclitaxel and docetaxel) emerged in the 1990s, multiple trials were conducted to evaluate their use in combination with anthracycline-based regimens. The majority of these trials showed an improvement in disease-free survival and at least one showed an improvement in overall survival with the taxane-based regimen. A meta-analysis of taxane versus nontaxane anthracycline-based regimen trials showed an improvement in disease-free and overall survival for the taxane-based regimens.

Several regimens have been reported including AC followed by paclitaxel or docetaxel (AC-T), TAC (docetaxel concurrent with AC), 5-fluorouracil (F)EC-docetaxel, and FEC-paclitaxel. Results from CALGB 9741 showed that compared with a standard dose regimen, administration of "dose-dense" AC-P chemotherapy (that is, in an accelerated fashion, in which the frequency of administration is increased without changing total dose or duration) with granulocyte colony stimulating factor (G-CSF) support led to improved both disease-free (82% vs 75% at 4 years) and overall survival (92% vs 90%). Exploratory subset analysis suggested that patients with hormone receptor–negative tumors derived the most benefit from the dose-dense approach.

The US Oncology trial 9735 compared four cycles of AC with four cycles of taxotere (docetaxel) and cyclophosphamide (TC). With a median of 7 years follow-up, this study showed a statistically significantly improved disease-free survival and overall survival in the patients who received TC. Until this, no trial had compared a non-anthracycline taxane-based regimen to an anthracycline-based regimen.

An important ongoing study (US Oncology 06090) is prospectively evaluating whether anthracyclines add any incremental benefit to a taxane-based regimen by comparing six cycles of TAC to six cycles of TC in HER2-negative breast cancer patients. A third arm was added to evaluate the benefit of adding bevacizumab, a monoclonal antibody directed against vascular endothelial growth factor (VEGF), to TC. While awaiting the results of this trial, oncologists are faced with choosing from among the above treatment regimens for HER2-negative breast cancer. It is interesting to note a sharp decline in the use of anthracyclines has been observed since 2006. Given the benefits described above, taxanes are now used for most patients receiving chemotherapy for early breast cancer.

The overall duration of adjuvant chemotherapy still remains uncertain. However, based on the meta-analysis performed in the Oxford Overview (EBCTCG), the current recommendation is for 3-6 months of the commonly used regimens. Although it is clear that dose intensity to a specific threshold is essential, there is little, if any, evidence to support the long-term survival benefit of high-dose chemotherapy with stem cell support.

Chemotherapy side effects are now generally well controlled. Nausea and vomiting are abated with drugs that directly affect the central nervous system, such as ondansetron and granisetron. Infertility and premature ovarian failure are common side effects of chemotherapy, especially in women over the age of 40, and should be discussed with patients prior to starting treatment. The risk of life-threatening neutropenia associated with chemotherapy can be reduced by use of growth factors such as pegfilgrastim and filgrastim (G-CSF), which stimulate proliferation and differentiation of hematopoietic cells. Long-term toxicities from chemotherapy, including cardiomyopathy (anthracyclines), peripheral neuropathy (taxanes), and leukemia/myelodysplasia (anthracyclines and alkylating agents), remain a small but significant risk.

2. Targeted Therapy—

A. HER2 overexpression Approximately 20% of breast cancers are characterized by amplification of the HER2 oncogene leading to overexpression of the HER2 oncoprotein. The poor prognosis associated with HER2 overexpression has been drastically improved with the development of HER2-targeted therapy. Trastuzumab (Herceptin [H]), a monoclonal antibody that binds to HER2, has proved effective in combination with chemotherapy in patients with HER2 overexpressing metastatic and early breast cancer. In the adjuvant setting, the first and most commonly studied chemotherapy backbone used with trastuzumab is AC-T. Subsequently, the BCIRG006 study showed similar efficacy for AC-TH and a nonanthracycline-containing regimen, TCH (docetaxel, carboplatin, trastuzumab). Both were significantly better than AC-T in terms of disease-free and overall survival and TCH had a lower risk of cardiac toxicity. Both AC-TH and TCH are FDA-approved for nonmetastatic, HER2-positive breast cancer. In these regimens, trastuzumab is given with chemotherapy and then continues beyond the course of chemotherapy to complete a full year. The reporting of two trials in 2012 (the Herceptin Adjuvant [HERA] evaluating 1 vs 2 years of trastuzumab and the Protocol for Herceptin as Adjuvant therapy with Reduced Exposure [PHARE] study evaluating 6 vs 12 months of trastuzumab) have thus far confirmed that 1 year of trastuzumab should remain the standard of care. At least one study (N9831) suggests that concurrent, rather than sequential, delivery of trastuzumab with chemotherapy may be more beneficial. Another question being addressed in trials is whether to treat small (> 1 cm), node-negative tumors with trastuzumab plus chemotherapy. Retrospective studies have shown that even small (stage T1a,b) HER2-positive tumors have a worse prognosis compared with same-sized HER2-negative tumors. The NSABP B43 study is also ongoing to evaluate whether the addition of trastuzumab to radiation therapy is warranted for DCIS.

Cardiomyopathy develops in a small but significant percent (1%-4%) of patients who receive trastuzumab-based regimens. For this reason, anthracyclines and trastuzumab are rarely given concurrently and cardiac function is monitored periodically throughout therapy.

B. Endocrine Therapy Adjuvant hormone modulation therapy is highly effective in decreasing recurrence and mortality by 25% in women with hormone receptor–positive tumors regardless of menopausal status. The traditional regimen has been 5 years of the estrogen-receptor antagonist/agonist tamoxifen until the 2012 reporting of the Adjuvant Tamoxifen Longer Against Shorter (ATLAS) trial in which 5 versus 10 years of adjuvant tamoxifen were compared. In this study, women who received 10 years of tamoxifen had a significantly improved disease free as well as overall survival, particularly after year 10. Though these results are impressive and potentially practice changing, the clinical application of long-term tamoxifen use must be discussed with patients individually, taking into consideration risks of tamoxifen such as secondary uterine cancers, venous thromboembolic events as well as side effects that impact quality of life. Ovarian ablation in premenopausal patients with ER-positive tumors may produce a benefit similar to that of adjuvant systemic chemotherapy. Whether the use of ovarian ablation plus tamoxifen (or an AI) is more effective than either measure alone is still unclear. In the Stockholm subset of the Zoladex in Premenopausal Patients (ZIPP) study, 927 premenopausal women were randomly assigned to goserelin, tamoxifen, the combination of both, or to no endocrine therapy for 2 years. With a median follow-up of 12.3 years, this substudy showed that goserelin and tamoxifen each significantly reduce the risk of recurrence of hormone receptor–positive breast cancer compared to control (goserelin 32%, [$P = 0.005$] and tamoxifen 27% [$P = 0.018$]), yet the combination of goserelin and tamoxifen was not superior to either treatment alone. This issue is still not settled and is being addressed in ongoing clinical trials (Suppression of Ovarian Function Trial [SOFT] and Tamoxifen and Exemestane Trial [TEXT]) that have not yet reported. AIs, including anastrozole, letrozole, and exemestane, reduce estrogen production and are also effective in the adjuvant setting for postmenopausal women. Approximately seven large randomized trials enrolling more than 24,000 patients have compared the use of AIs with tamoxifen or placebo as adjuvant therapy. All of these studies have shown small but statistically significant improvements in disease-free survival (absolute benefits of 2%-6%) with the use of AIs. In addition, AIs have been shown to reduce the risk of contralateral breast cancers and to have fewer associated serious side effects (such as endometrial cancers and thromboembolic events) than tamoxifen. However, they are associated with accelerated bone loss and an increased risk of fractures as well as a musculoskeletal syndrome characterized by arthralgias or myalgias (or both) in up to 50% of patients. The American Society of Clinical Oncology and the NCCN have recommended that postmenopausal women with hormone receptor–positive breast cancer be offered an AI either initially or after tamoxifen therapy. HER2 status should not affect the use or choice of hormone therapy.

3. Bisphosphonates—Two randomized studies (ZO-FAST and ABCSG-12) have evaluated the use of an adjuvant intravenous bisphosphonate (zoledronic acid) in addition to standard local and systemic therapy. The results showed a 32%-40% relative reduction in the risk of cancer recurrence for hormone receptor–positive nonmetastatic breast cancer. In fact, at the San Antonio Breast Cancer Symposium in 2011, with a median follow-up of 76 months, the ABCSG-12 study reported improved overall survival for patients treated with zoledronic acid. Conflicting results have been reported from the AZURE study. In this randomized study that enrolled premenopausal and postmenopausal patients, there was no disease-free or overall survival benefits associated with the addition of zoledronic acid to endocrine therapy for the overall study population. However, a prespecified subset analysis in patients who were postmenopausal for at least 5 years did demonstrate a significant disease-free and overall survival benefit with the addition of the bisphosphonate. Side effects associated with intravenous bisphosphonate therapy include bone pain, fever, osteonecrosis of the jaw (rare), and renal failure. Currently, the adjuvant use of bisphosphonates and other bone stabilizing drugs, such as inhibitors of receptor activator of nuclear factor kappa B ligand (RANK-B), remains investigational.

4. Adjuvant therapy in older women—Data relating to the optimal use of adjuvant systemic treatment for women over the age of 65 are limited. Results from the EBCTCG overview indicates that while adjuvant chemotherapy yields a smaller benefit for older women compared with younger women, it still improves clinical outcomes. Moreover, individual studies do show that older women with higher risk disease derive benefits from chemotherapy. One study compared the use of oral chemotherapy (capecitabine) to standard chemotherapy in older women and concluded that standard chemotherapy is preferred. Another study (USO TC vs AC) showed that women over the age of 65 derive similar benefits from the taxane-based regimen as women who are younger. The benefits of endocrine therapy for hormone receptor-positive disease appear to be independent of age. In general, decisions relating to the use of systemic therapy should take into account a patient's comorbidities and physiological age, more so than chronologic age.

E. Neoadjuvant Therapy

The use of chemotherapy or endocrine therapy prior to resection of the primary tumor (neoadjuvant) is gaining popularity. This enables the assessment of in vivo chemosensitivity. Patients with hormone receptor–negative or HER2 positive breast cancer (or both) are more likely to have a pathologic complete response to neoadjuvant chemotherapy than those with hormone receptor–positive breast cancer. A complete pathologic response at the time of surgery is associated with improvement in survival. Neoadjuvant chemotherapy also increases the chance of breast conservation by shrinking the primary tumor in women who would otherwise need mastectomy for local control. Survival after neoadjuvant chemotherapy is similar to that seen with postoperative adjuvant chemotherapy. Neoadjuvant AI therapy has been evaluated in a phase II study involving 115 postmenopausal patients with hormone receptor-positive breast cancer. The overall response rate was 62% in this study, and 38% of patients initially ineligible for breast conservation were able to have lumpectomy. There is considerable concern as to the timing of sentinel lymph node biopsy (SLNB), since the chemotherapy may affect any cancer present in the lymph nodes. Several studies have shown that sentinel node biopsy can be done after neoadjuvant therapy. However, a large multicenter study, ACOSOG 1071, demonstrated a false-negative rate of 10.7%, well above the false-negative rate outside the neoadjuvant setting (< 1%-5%). Many physicians recommend performing SLNB before administering the chemotherapy in order to avoid a false-negative result and to aid in planning subsequent radiation therapy. Others prefer to perform SLNB after neoadjuvant therapy to avoid a second operation and assess postchemotherapy nodal status. If a complete dissection is necessary, this can be performed at the time of the definitive breast surgery.

Important questions remaining to be answered are the timing and duration of adjuvant and neoadjuvant chemotherapy, which chemotherapeutic agents should be applied for which subgroups of patients, the use of combinations of hormonal therapy and chemotherapy as well as possibly targeted therapy, and the value of prognostic factors other than hormone receptors in predicting response to therapy.

▶ Treatment: Palliative

Palliative treatments are those to manage symptoms, improve quality of life, and even prolong survival, without the expectation of achieving cure. Only 10% of patients have *de novo* metastatic breast cancer at the time of diagnosis. However, in most patients who have a breast cancer recurrence after initial local and adjuvant therapy, the recurrence presents as metastatic rather than local (in breast) disease. Breast cancer most commonly metastasizes to the liver, lungs, and bone, causing symptoms such as fatigue, change in appetite, abdominal pain, respiratory symptoms, or bone pain. Triple negative (ER-, PR-, HER2-negative) and HER2-positive tumors have a higher rate of brain metastases than hormone-receptor positive, HER2-negative tumors. Headaches, imbalance, vision changes, vertigo, and other neurologic symptoms may be signs of brain metastases.

A. Radiotherapy and Bisphosphonates

Palliative radiotherapy may be advised for primary treatment of locally advanced cancers with distant metastases to control ulceration, pain, and other manifestations in the breast and regional nodes. Irradiation of the breast and chest wall and the axillary, internal mammary, and supraclavicular nodes should be undertaken in an attempt to cure locally advanced and inoperable lesions when there is no evidence of distant metastases. A small number of patients in this group are cured in spite of extensive breast and regional node involvement.

Palliative irradiation is of value also in the treatment of certain bone or soft-tissue metastases to control pain or avoid fracture. Radiotherapy is especially useful in the treatment of isolated bony metastases, chest wall recurrences, brain metastases, and acute spinal cord compression.

In addition to radiotherapy, bisphosphonate therapy has shown excellent results in delaying and reducing skeletal events in women with bony metastases. Zoledronic acid is an FDA-approved intravenous bisphosphonate given monthly for bone metastases from breast cancer. Denosumab, a fully human monoclonal antibody that targets RANK-ligand, was approved by the FDA in 2010 for the treatment of advanced breast cancer causing bone metastases, based on data showing that it reduced the time to first skeletal-related event (eg, pathologic fracture) compared to zoledronic acid.

Caution should be exercised when combining radiation therapy with chemotherapy because toxicity of either or both may be augmented by their concurrent administration. In general, only one type of therapy should be given at a time unless it is necessary to irradiate a destructive lesion of weight-bearing bone while the patient is receiving another regimen. The regimen should be changed only if the disease is clearly progressing. This is especially difficult to determine for patients with destructive bone metastases, since changes in the status of these lesions are difficult to determine radiographically.

B. Targeted Therapy

1. Endocrine Therapy for Metastatic Disease—Targeted therapy refers to agents that are directed specifically against a protein or molecule expressed uniquely on tumor cells or in the tumor microenvironment. The first targeted therapy was the use of antiestrogen therapy in hormone receptor–positive breast cancer. The administration of hormones (eg, estrogens, androgens, progestins; Table 17–6); ablation of the ovaries, adrenals, or pituitary; administration of drugs that block hormone receptors (such as tamoxifen) or drugs that block the synthesis of hormones (such as AIs) have all been shown to be effective in hormone receptor–positive metastatic breast cancer. Palliative treatment of metastatic cancer should be based on the ER status of the primary tumor or the metastases. Because only 5%-10% of women with ER-negative tumors respond, they should not receive endocrine therapy except in unusual circumstances, for example, in an older patient who cannot tolerate chemotherapy. The rate of response is nearly equal in premenopausal and postmenopausal women with ER-positive tumors. A favorable response to hormonal manipulation occurs in about one-third of patients with metastatic breast cancer. Of those whose tumors contain ER, the response is about 60% and perhaps as high as 80% for patients whose tumors contain PR as well. The choice of endocrine therapy depends on the menopausal status of the patient. Women within 1 year of their last menstrual period are arbitrarily considered to be premenopausal and should receive tamoxifen therapy or rarely ovarian ablation, whereas women whose menses ceased more than a year before are postmenopausal and may receive tamoxifen or an AI. Women with ER-positive tumors who do not respond to first-line endocrine therapy or experience progression should be given a different form of hormonal manipulation. Because the quality of life during endocrine manipulation is usually superior to that during cytotoxic chemotherapy, it is best to try endocrine manipulation whenever possible. However, when receptor status is unknown, disease is progressing rapidly or involves visceral organs, chemotherapy should be used as first-line treatment.

Table 17–6. Agents commonly used for hormonal management of metastatic breast cancer.

Drug	Action	Dose, Route, Frequency	Major Side Effects
Tamoxifen citrate (Nolvadex)	SERM	20 mg orally daily	Hot flushes, uterine bleeding, thrombophlebitis, rash
Fulvestrant (Faslodex)	Steroidal estrogen receptor antagonist	500 mg intramuscularly day 1, 15, 29 and then monthly	Gastrointestinal upset, headache, back pain, hot flushes, pharyngitis
Toremifene citrate (Fareston)	SERM	40 mg orally daily	Hot flushes, sweating, nausea, vaginal discharge, dry eyes, dizziness
Diethylstilbestrol (DES)	Estrogen	5 mg orally three times daily	Fluid retention, uterine bleeding, thrombophlebitis, nausea
Goserelin (Zoladex)	Synthetic luteinizing hormone releasing analogue	3.6 mg subcutaneously monthly	Arthralgias, blood pressure changes, hot flushes, headaches, vaginal dryness
Megestrol acetate (Megace)	Progestin	40 mg orally four times daily	Fluid retention
Letrozole (Femara)	AI	2.5 mg orally daily	Hot flushes, arthralgia/arthritis, myalgia, bone loss
Anastrozole (Arimidex)	AI	1 mg orally daily	Hot flushes, skin rashes, nausea and vomiting, bone loss
Exemestane (Aromasin)	AI	25 mg orally daily	Hot flushes, increased arthralgia/arthritis, myalgia, bone loss

AI, aromatase inhibitor; SERM, selective estrogen receptor modulator.

A. The Premenopausal Patient

(i). *Primary Hormonal Therapy* The potent SERM tamoxifen is by far the most common and preferred method of hormonal manipulation in the premenopausal patient, in large part because it can be given with less morbidity and fewer side effects than cytotoxic chemotherapy and does not require oophorectomy. Tamoxifen is given orally in a dose of 20 mg daily. The average remission associated with tamoxifen lasts about 12 months.

There is no significant difference in survival or response between tamoxifen therapy and bilateral oophorectomy. Bilateral oophorectomy is less desirable than tamoxifen in premenopausal women because tamoxifen is so well tolerated. However, oophorectomy can be achieved rapidly and safely either by surgery, by irradiation of the ovaries if the patient is a poor surgical candidate, or by chemical ovarian ablation using a gonadotropin-releasing hormone (GnRH) analog. Oophorectomy presumably works by eliminating estrogens, progestins, and androgens, which stimulate growth of the tumor. AIs should not be used in a patient with functioning ovaries since they do not block ovarian production of estrogen.

(ii). *Secondary or Tertiary Hormonal Therapy* Patients who do not respond to tamoxifen or ovarian ablation may be treated with chemotherapy or may try a second endocrine regimen, such as GnRH analog plus AI. Whether to opt for chemotherapy or another endocrine measure depends largely on the sites of metastatic disease (visceral being more serious than bone-only, thus sometimes warranting the use of chemotherapy), the disease burden, the rate of growth of disease, and patient preference. Patients who take chemotherapy and then later have progressive disease may subsequently respond to another form of endocrine treatment (Table 17–6). The optimal choice for secondary endocrine manipulation has not been clearly defined for the premenopausal patient.

Patients who improve after oophorectomy but subsequently relapse should receive tamoxifen or an AI; if one fails, the other may be tried. Megestrol acetate, a progesterone agent, may also be considered. Adrenalectomy or hypophysectomy, procedures rarely done today, induced regression in 30%-50% of patients who previously responded to oophorectomy. Pharmacologic hormonal manipulation has replaced these invasive procedures.

B. The Postmenopausal Patient

(i). *Primary Hormonal Therapy* For postmenopausal women with metastatic breast cancer amenable to endocrine manipulation, tamoxifen or an AI is the initial therapy of choice. The side effect profile of AIs differs from tamoxifen and may be more effective. The main side effects of tamoxifen are nausea, skin rash, and hot flushes. Rarely, tamoxifen induces hypercalcemia in patients with bony metastases. Tamoxifen also increases the risk of venous thromboembolic events and uterine hyperplasia and cancer. The main side effects of AIs include hot flushes, vaginal dryness, and joint stiffness; however, osteoporosis and bone fractures are significantly higher than with tamoxifen. Phase II data from the randomized Fulvestrant fIRst-line Study comparing endocrine Treatments (FIRST) suggest that the pure estrogen antagonist, fulvestrant may be even more effective than front-line anastrozole in terms of time to progression. The combination of fulvestrant plus anastrozole may also be more effective than anastrozole alone, though two studies evaluating this question have yielded conflicting results.

(ii). *Secondary or Tertiary Hormonal Therapy* AIs are also used for the treatment of advanced breast cancer in postmenopausal women after tamoxifen treatment. In the event that the patient responds to AI but then has progression of disease, fulvestrant, has shown efficacy with about 20%-30% of women benefiting from use. Postmenopausal women who respond initially to a SERM or AI but later manifest progressive disease may be crossed over to another hormonal therapy. Until recently, patients who experienced disease progression on or after treatment with a SERM or AI were routinely offered chemotherapy. This standard practice changed in 2012 with the approval of everolimus (Afinitor), an oral inhibitor of the mammalian target of rapamycin (MTOR)—a protein whose activation has been associated with the development of endocrine resistance. A phase III, placebo-controlled trial (BOLERO-2) evaluated exemestane with or without everolimus in 724 patients with AI-resistant, hormone receptor–positive metastatic breast cancer, and at interim analysis found that patients treated with everolimus had a significantly improved progression free survival (10.6 months vs 4.1 months; HR, 0.36; 95% CI, 0.27-0.47; $P <$

0.001). Androgens (such as testosterone) have many toxicities and should be used infrequently. As in premenopausal patients, neither hypophysectomy nor adrenalectomy should be performed. High-dose estrogen therapy has also paradoxically been shown to induce responses in advanced breast cancer. A study that evaluated the use of low-dose (6 mg) versus high-dose (30 mg) estradiol daily orally for postmenopausal women with metastatic AI-resistant breast cancer showed that the two doses yielded similar clinical benefit rates (29% and 28%, respectively) and, as expected, the higher dose was associated with more adverse events than the low dose.

(iii). *Newer Agents in Development* Although endocrine therapy can lead to disease control for months to years in some patients, *de novo* and acquired resistance to hormonal manipulation remains an enormous barrier to the effective treatment of these patients. Thus, molecularly targeted agents are still needed to circumvent signaling pathways that lead to drug resistance. A randomized phase II study evaluating letrozole with or without an oral cyclin-D kinase (cdk) 4/6 inhibitor for the first-line treatment of postmenopausal women with hormone receptor-positive advanced breast cancer was reported at the San Antonio Breast Cancer Symposium in December 2012. A striking and highly significant 18.6 months improvement in progression free survival was observed with the cdk4/6-inhibitor (26.1 months with cdk 4/6 inhibitor vs 7.5 months in control arm). Phase III evaluation of this promising molecule is being planned.

2. HER2 targeted agents—For patients with HER2 overexpressing or amplified tumors, trastuzumab plus chemotherapy has been shown to significantly improve clinical outcomes including survival compared to chemotherapy alone. Trastuzumab plus chemotherapy was therefore the standard first-line treatment for HER2-positive metastatic breast cancer until 2012 when pertuzumab was granted FDA approval. Pertuzumab is a monoclonal antibody that targets the extracellular domain of HER2 at a different epitope than targeted by trastuzumab and inhibits receptor dimerization. A phase III placebo-controlled randomized study (CLEOPATRA) showed that patients treated with the combination of pertuzumab, trastuzumab, and docetaxel had a significantly longer progression free survival (18.5 months vs 12.4 months; HR, 0.62; 95% CI, 0.51-0.75; $P < 0.001$) compared with those treated with docetaxel and trastuzumab. Longer follow up revealed a significant overall survival benefit associated with pertuzumab as well.

A. Trastuzumab-Pretreated Disease

Lapatinib is an oral targeted drug that works by inhibiting the intracellular tyrosine kinases of the epidermal growth factor and HER2 receptors. This drug is FDA-approved for the treatment of trastuzumab-resistant HER2-positive metastatic breast cancer in combination with capecitabine, thus, a completely oral regimen. The combination of trastuzumab plus lapatinib has been shown to be more effective than lapatinib alone for trastuzumab-resistant metastatic breast cancer. Moreover, several trials have shown a significant clinical benefit for continuing HER2-targeted agents beyond progression. T-DM1 (trastuzumab emtansine) is a novel antibody drug conjugate in which trastuzumab is stably linked to a derivative of maytansine, enabling targeted delivery of the cytotoxic chemotherapy to HER2-overexpressing cells. The phase III trial (EMILIA) that evaluated T-DM1 in patients with HER2-positive, trastuzumab-pretreated advanced disease showed that T-DM1 is associated with improved progression free and overall survival compared to lapatinib plus capecitabine (EMILIA). Regulatory approval of T-DM1 is expected in 2013. Evaluation of T-DM1 in combination with pertuzumab for the first-line treatment of advanced breast cancer is ongoing in the phase III MARIANNE study and trials evaluating the use of these agents in early breast cancer are being planned. Several other drugs targeting the HER2 pathway are in development including everolimus, afatinib, neratinib, and HER2-targeted vaccines.

3. Targeting angiogenesis—Bevacizumab is a monoclonal antibody directed against VEGF. This growth factor stimulates endothelial proliferation and neoangiogenesis in cancer. A phase III randomized trial (E2100) in women with metastatic breast cancer showed increased response rate and progression-free survival rate with the combination of bevacizumab and paclitaxel as first-line treatment compared with paclitaxel alone; however, there was no significant overall survival benefit. This led to the accelerated FDA approval of bevacizumab in early 2008. Since that time, two additional prospective randomized clinical trials (AVADO and RIBBON-1) have reported that the addition of bevacizumab to standard chemotherapy improves disease-free survival and objective response rates compared with single-agent chemotherapy alone. A benefit in overall survival has not been demonstrated. Side effects from bevacizumab include hypertension, bleeding, and thromboembolic events.

While initial results were promising, the lack of both survival benefit and data to identify those tumor types most likely to benefit from bevacizumab resulted in the FDA revoking its approval of bevacizumab for metastatic breast cancer in 2011.

4. Targeting "triple-negative" breast cancer—Until very recently, breast cancers lacking expression of the hormone receptors ER and PR, and HER2 have only been amenable to therapy with cytotoxic chemotherapy. This type of "triple-negative" breast cancer, while heterogeneous, generally behaves aggressively and is associated with a poor prognosis. Newer classes of targeted agents are being evaluated specifically for triple-negative breast cancer. Some triple-negative breast cancers may be characterized by an inability to repair double-strand DNA breaks (due to mutation or epigenetic silencing of the BRCA gene). **Poly-ADP ribose-polymerase (PARP) inhibitors** are a class of agents that prevent the repair of single strand DNA breaks and are showing promise in BRCA-mutated and triple-negative breast cancer. One relatively small randomized phase II clinical trial evaluating gemcitabine plus carboplatin with or without an agent that inhibits PARP (BSI-201) for triple-negative metastatic breast cancer showed improved clinical outcomes, including improved overall survival for PARP inhibitor–treated patients. However, the phase III randomized study of this agent failed to meet its endpoints, possibly relating to its relative weak inhibition of PARP. Research in this area is rapidly expanding with multiple clinical trials of other PARP inhibitors and other molecularly targeted agents ongoing.

▶ Palliative Chemotherapy

Cytotoxic drugs should be considered for the treatment of metastatic breast cancer: (1) if visceral metastases are present (especially brain, liver, or lymphangitic pulmonary); (2) if hormonal treatment is unsuccessful or the disease has progressed after an initial response to hormonal manipulation; or (3) if the tumor is ER-negative or HER2-positive. Prior adjuvant chemotherapy does not seem to alter response rates in patients who relapse. A number of chemotherapy drugs (including vinorelbine, paclitaxel, docetaxel, gemcitabine, ixabepilone, carboplatin, cisplatin, capecitabine, albumin-bound paclitaxel, eribulin, and liposomal doxorubicin) may be used as single agents with first-line objective response rates ranging from 30% to 50%.

Combination chemotherapy yields statistically significantly higher response rates and progression-free survival rates, but has not been conclusively shown to improve overall survival rates compared with sequential single-agent therapy. Combinations that have been tested in phase III studies and have proven efficacy compared with single-agent therapy include capecitabine/docetaxel, gemcitabine/paclitaxel, and capecitabine/ixabepilone. Various other combinations of drugs have been tested in phase II studies, and a number of clinical trials are ongoing to identify effective combinations. For patients whose tumors have progressed after several lines of therapy and who are considering additional therapy, clinical trial participation with experimental drugs in phase I, II, or III testing should be encouraged.

In the past, high-dose chemotherapy and autologous bone marrow or stem cell transplantation aroused widespread interest for the treatment of metastatic breast cancer. However, multiple clinical trials failed to show any improvement in survival with high dose chemotherapy with stem cell transplant over conventional chemotherapy and the procedure is now rarely, if ever, performed for stage IV breast cancer.

Baselga J et al: CLEOPATRA Study Group. Pertuzumab plus trastuzumab plus docetaxel for metastatic breast cancer. *N Engl J Med.* 2012 Jan 12;366(2):109-19. [PMID: 22149875]

Baselga J et al: Everolimus in postmenopausal hormone-receptor-positive advanced breast cancer. *N Engl J Med.* 2012 Feb 9;366(6);520-529. [PMID: 22149876]

Berger AM et al: Cancer-related fatigue: implications for breast cancer survivors. *Cancer.* 2012;118(8 Suppl):2261-2269. [PMID 22488700]

Cortazar P et al: Meta-analysis results from the collaborative trials in neoadjuvant breast cancer (CTNeoBC). *Cancer Res.* 2012;72(24 Suppl):93s, Abstract S1-S11.

Davies C et al: Long-term effects of continuing adjuvant tamoxifen to 10 years versus stopping at 5 years after diagnosis of oestrogen receptor-positive breast cancer: ATLAS, a randomized trial. *Lancet.* 2013 Mar 9;381(9869):805-816 [PMID: 23219286]

Finn RS et al: Results of a randomized phase 2 study of PD 0332991, a cyclin-dependent kinase (cdk) 4/6 inhibitor, in combination with letrozole vs. letrozole alone for first-line treatment of ER+/HER2- advanced breast cancer. *Cancer Res.* 2012;72(24 Suppl):91s, Abstract S1-S6.

Giordano S et al: Decline in the use of anthracyclines for breast cancer. *J Clin Oncol.* 2012;30(18):2232-2239. [PMID: 22614988]

Giuliano AE et al: Axillary dissection vs no axillary dissection in women with invasive breast cancer and sentinel node metastasis: a randomized clinical trial. *JAMA.* 2011 Feb 9;305(6): 569-575. [PMID: 21304082]

Goldhirsch A et al: HERA trial: 2 years versus 1 year of trastuzumab after adjuvant chemotherapy in women with HER2-positive early breast cancer at 8 years of median follow up. *Cancer Res.* 2012;72(24 Suppl):103s, Abstract S5-S2.

Huang WW et al: Zoledronic acid as an adjuvant therapy in patients with breast cancer: a systematic review and meta-analysis. *PLoS One.* 2012;7(7):e40783. [PMID:22844410]

Khan SA et al: Optimal surgical treatment of breast cancer: implications for local control and survival. *J Surg Oncol.* 2010 Jun 15;101(8):677-686. [PMID: 20512943]

Martin M et al: GEICAM 9805 investigators. Adjuvant docetaxel for high-risk, node-negative breast cancer. *N Engl J Med.* 2010 Dec 2;363(23):2200-2210. [PMID: 21121833]

Mehta R et al: Combination anastrozole and fulvestrant in metastatic breast cancer. *N Engl J Med.* 2012;367:435-444. [PMID: 22853014]

National Comprehensive Cancer Network. NCCN Guidelines: Breast Cancer. Available at http://www.nccn.org/professionals/physician_gls/f_guidelines.asp.

Perez EA et al: Sequential versus concurrent trastuzumab in adjuvant chemotherapy for breast cancer. *Clin Oncol.* 2011 Dec 1;29(34):4491-4497. [PMID: 22042958]

Pivot X et al: PHARE trial results comparing 6 to 12 months of trastuzumab in adjuvant early breast cancer. *Cancer Res.* 2012;72(24 Suppl):104s, Abstract S5-S3.

Roberston J et al: Fulvestrant 500 mg versus anastrozole 1 mg for the first-line treatment of advanced breast cancer: follow-up analysis from the randomized 'FIRST' study. *Breast Cancer Res Treat.* 2012;136(2):503-511. [PMID: 23065000]

Rossari JR et al: Bevacizumab and breast cancer: a meta-analysis of first-line phase III studies and a critical reappraisal of available evidence. *J Oncol.* 2012;2012:417673. [PMID: 23008712]

Serletti JM et al: Breast reconstruction after breast cancer. *Plast Reconstr Surg.* 2011 Jun;127(6):124e-35e. [PMID: 21617423]

Slamon D et al: Breast Cancer International Research Group. Adjuvant trastuzumab in HER2-positive breast cancer. *N Engl J Med.* 2011 Oct 6;365(14):1273-1283. [PMID: 21991949]

Stopeck AT et al: Denosumab compared with zoledronic acid for the treatment of bone metastases in patients with advanced breast cancer: a randomized, double-blind study. *J Clin Oncol.* 2010 Dec 10;28(35):5132-5139. [PMID: 21060033]

Sverrisdottir A et al: Interaction between goserelin and tamoxifen in a prospective randomised clinical trial of adjuvant endocrine therapy in premenopausal breast cancer. *Breast Cancer Res Treat.* 2011 Aug;128(3):755-763. [PMID: 21625929]

Ovana MM et al: Tamoxifen therapy: Tamoxifen use in patients with survival in early breast cancer. *N Engl J Med.* 2010 Jun 3;362(22):2053-2065. [PMID: 20519679]

Verma S et al: Trastuzumab emtansine for HER2-positive advanced breast cancer. *N Engl J Med.* 2012;367(19):1783-1791. [PMID: 23020162]

▶ Prognosis

Stage of breast cancer is the most reliable indicator of prognosis (Table 17–7). Axillary lymph node status is the best-analyzed prognostic factor and correlates with survival at all tumor sizes. When cancer is localized to the breast with no evidence of regional spread after pathologic examination, the clinical cure rate with most accepted methods of therapy ranges from 75% to greater than 90%. In fact, patients with small mammographically detected biologically favorable tumors and no evidence of axillary spread have a 5-year survival rate greater than 95%. When the axillary lymph nodes are involved with tumor, the survival rate drops to 50%-70% at 5 years and probably around 25%-40% at 10 years. Increasingly, the use of biologic markers, such as ER, PR, grade, and HER2, is helping to identify high-risk tumor types as well as direct treatment used (see Biomarkers & Gene Expression Profiling). Tumors with marked aneuploidy have a poor prognosis (Table 17–5). Gene analysis

Table 17–7. Approximate survival (%) of patients with breast cancer by TNM stage.

TNM Stage	5 Years	10 Years
0	95	90
I	85	70
IIA	70	50
IIB	60	40
IIIA	55	30
IIIB	30	20
IV	5-10	2
All	65	30

studies, such as Oncotype Dx, can predict disease-free survival for some subsets of patients.

The mortality rate of breast cancer patients exceeds that of age-matched normal controls for nearly 20 years. Thereafter, the mortality rates are equal, though deaths that occur among breast cancer patients are often directly the result of tumor. Five-year statistics do not accurately reflect the final outcome of therapy.

In general, breast cancer appears to be somewhat more malignant in younger than in older women, and this may be related to the fact that fewer younger women have ER-positive tumors. Adjuvant systemic chemotherapy, in general, improves survival by about 30% and adjuvant hormonal therapy by about 25%.

For those patients whose disease progresses despite treatment, studies suggest supportive group therapy may improve survival. As they approach the end of life, such patients will require meticulous palliative care (see Chapter 5).

Kim C et al: Gene-expression-based prognostic assays for breast cancer. *Nat Rev Clin Oncol.* 2010 Jun;7(6):340-347. [PMID: 20440284]

Wishart GC et al: PREDICT: a new UK prognostic model that predicts survival following surgery for invasive breast cancer. *Breast Cancer Res.* 2010;12(1):R1. [PMID: 20053270]

▶ Follow-up Care

After primary therapy, patients with breast cancer should be monitored long-term in order to detect recurrences and to observe the opposite breast for a second primary carcinoma. Local and distant recurrences occur most frequently within the first 2-5 years. During the first 2 years, most patients should be examined every 6 months (with mammogram every 6 months on the affected breast), then annually there-

after. Since these women are at an increased risk for local or contralateral breast tumor, MRI is being used by many breast surgeons to monitor patients with prior malignancies. Most insurance companies will reimburse for this. Special attention is paid to the contralateral breast because a new primary breast malignancy will develop in 20%-25% of patients. In some cases, metastases are dormant for long periods and may appear 10-15 years or longer after removal of the primary tumor. Although studies have failed to show an adverse effect of hormonal replacement in disease-free patients, it is rarely used after breast cancer treatment, particularly if the tumor was hormone receptor positive. Even pregnancy has not been associated with shortened survival of patients rendered disease free—yet many oncologists are reluctant to advise a young patient with breast cancer that it is safe to become pregnant, and most will not support prescribing hormone replacement for the postmenopausal breast cancer patient. The use of estrogen replacement for conditions such as osteoporosis, vaginal dryness, and hot flushes may be considered for a woman with a history of breast cancer after discussion of the benefits and risks; however, it is not routinely recommended, especially given the availability of nonhormonal agents for these conditions (such as bisphosphonates and denosumab for osteoporosis). Vaginal estrogen is frequently used to treat vaginal atrophy with no obvious ill effects.

A. Local Recurrence

The incidence of local recurrence correlates with tumor size, the presence and number of involved axillary nodes, the histologic type of tumor, the presence of skin edema or skin and fascia fixation with the primary tumor, and the type of definitive surgery and local irradiation. Local recurrence on the chest wall after total mastectomy and axillary dissection develops in as many as 8% of patients. When the axillary nodes are not involved, the local recurrence rate is less than 5%, but the rate is as high as 25% when they are heavily involved. A similar difference in local recurrence rate was noted between small and large tumors. Factors such as multifocal cancer, in situ tumors, positive resection margins, chemotherapy, and radiotherapy have an effect on local recurrence in patients treated with breast-conserving surgery. Adjuvant systemic therapy greatly decreases the rate of local recurrence.

Chest wall recurrences usually appear within the first several years but may occur as late as 15 or more years after mastectomy. All suspicious nodules and skin lesions should be biopsied. Local excision or localized radiotherapy may be feasible if an isolated nodule is present. If lesions are multiple or accompanied by evidence of regional involvement in the internal mammary or supraclavicular nodes, the disease is best managed by radiation treatment of the entire chest wall including the parasternal, supraclavicular, and axillary areas and usually by systemic therapy.

Local recurrence after mastectomy usually signals the presence of widespread disease and is an indication for studies to search for evidence of metastases. Distant metastases will develop within a few years in most patients with locally recurrent tumor after mastectomy. When there is no evidence of metastases beyond the chest wall and regional nodes, irradiation for cure after complete local excision should be attempted. After partial mastectomy, local recurrence does not have as serious a prognostic significance as after mastectomy. However, those patients in whom a recurrence develops have a worse prognosis than those who do not. It is speculated that the ability of a cancer to recur locally after radiotherapy is a sign of aggressiveness and resistance to therapy. Completion of the mastectomy should be done for local recurrence after partial mastectomy; some of these patients will survive for prolonged periods, especially if the breast recurrence is DCIS or occurs more than 5 years after initial treatment. Systemic chemotherapy or hormonal treatment should be used for women in whom disseminated disease develops or those in whom local recurrence occurs.

B. Breast Cancer Survivorship Issues

Given that most women with nonmetastatic breast cancer will be cured, a significant number of women face survivorship issues stemming from either the diagnosis or the treatment of the breast cancer. These challenges include psychological struggles, upper extremity lymphedema, cognitive decline (also called "chemo brain"), weight management problems, cardiovascular issues, bone loss, postmenopausal side effects, and fatigue. One randomized study reported that survivors who received psychological intervention from the time of diagnosis had a lower risk of recurrence and breast cancer–related mortality. A randomized study in older, overweight cancer survivors showed that diet and exercise reduced the rate of self-reported functional decline compared with no intervention. Cognitive dysfunction is a commonly reported symptom experienced by women who have undergone systemic treatment for early breast cancer. Studies are ongoing to understand the pathophysiology leading to this syndrome. An interesting study reported that 200 mg of modafinil daily improved speed and quality of memory as well as attention for breast cancer survivors dealing with cognitive dysfunction. This promising study requires validation in a larger clinical trial.

1. Edema of the arm—Significant edema of the arm occurs in about 10%-30% of patients after axillary dissection with or without mastectomy. It occurs more commonly if radiotherapy has been given or if there was postoperative infection. Partial mastectomy with radiation to the axillary lymph nodes is followed by chronic edema of the arm in 10%-20%

of patients. Sentinel lymph node dissection has proved to be a more accurate form of axillary staging without the side effects of edema or infection. Judicious use of radiotherapy, with treatment fields carefully planned to spare the axilla as much as possible, can greatly diminish the incidence of edema, which will occur in only 5% of patients if no radiotherapy is given to the axilla after a partial mastectomy and lymph node dissection.

Late or secondary edema of the arm may develop years after treatment, as a result of axillary recurrence or infection in the hand or arm, with obliteration of lymphatic channels. When edema develops, a careful examination of the axilla for recurrence or infection is performed. Infection in the arm or hand on the dissected side should be treated with antibiotics, rest, and elevation. If there is no sign of recurrence or infection, the swollen extremity should be treated with rest and elevation. A mild diuretic may be helpful. If there is no improvement, a compressor pump or manual compression decreases the swelling, and the patient is then fitted with an elastic glove or sleeve. Most patients are not bothered enough by mild edema to wear an uncomfortable glove or sleeve and will treat themselves with elevation or manual compression alone. Benzopyrones have been reported to decrease lymphedema but are not approved for this use in the United States. Rarely, edema may be severe enough to interfere with use of the limb. Traditionally, patients were advised to avoid weight lifting with the ipsilateral arm to prevent a worsening in lymphedema. However, a prospective randomized study has shown that twice weekly progressive weight lifting improves lymphedema symptoms and exacerbations and improves extremity strength.

2. Breast reconstruction—Breast reconstruction is usually feasible after total or modified radical mastectomy. Reconstruction should be discussed with patients prior to mastectomy, because it offers an important psychological focal point for recovery. Reconstruction is not an obstacle to the diagnosis of recurrent cancer. The most common breast reconstruction has been implantation of a silicone gel or saline prosthesis in the subpectoral plane between the pectoralis minor and pectoralis major muscles. Alternatively, autologous tissue can be used for reconstruction.

Autologous tissue flaps are aesthetically superior to implant reconstruction in most patients. They also have the advantage of not feeling like a foreign body to the patient. The most popular autologous technique currently is the transrectus abdominis muscle flap (TRAM flap), which is done by rotating the rectus abdominis muscle with attached fat and skin cephalad to make a breast mound. The free TRAM flap is done by completely removing a small portion of the rectus with overlying fat and skin and using microvascular surgical techniques to reconstruct the vascular supply on the chest wall. A latissimus dorsi flap can be swung from the back but offers less fullness than the TRAM flap and is therefore less acceptable cosmetically. An implant often is used to increase the fullness with a latissimus dorsi flap. Reconstruction may be performed immediately (at the time of initial mastectomy) or may be delayed until later, usually when the patient has completed adjuvant therapy. When considering reconstructive options, concomitant illnesses should be considered, since the ability of an autologous flap to survive depends on medical comorbidities. In addition, the need for radiotherapy may affect the choice of reconstruction as radiation may increase fibrosis around an implant or decrease the volume of a flap.

3. Risks of pregnancy—Data are insufficient to determine whether interruption of pregnancy improves the prognosis of patients who are identified to have potentially curable breast cancer and who receive definitive treatment during pregnancy. Theoretically, the high levels of estrogen produced by the placenta as the pregnancy progresses could be detrimental to the patient with occult metastases of hormone-sensitive breast cancer. However, retrospective studies have not shown a worse prognosis for women with gestational breast cancer. The decision whether or not to terminate the pregnancy must be made on an individual basis, taking into account the clinical stage of the cancer, the overall prognosis for the patient, the gestational age of the fetus, the potential for premature ovarian failure in the future with systemic therapy, and the patient's wishes. Women with early-stage gestational breast cancer who choose to continue their pregnancy should undergo surgery to remove the tumor and systemic therapy if indicated. Retrospective reviews of patients treated with anthracycline-containing regimens for gestational cancers (including leukemia and lymphomas) have established the relative safety of these regimens during pregnancy for both the patient and the fetus. Taxane-based and trastuzumab-based regimens have not been evaluated extensively, however. Radiation therapy should be delayed until the pregnant patient has delivered.

Equally important is the advice regarding future pregnancy (or abortion in case of pregnancy) to be given to women of child-bearing age who have had definitive treatment for breast cancer. To date, no adverse effect of pregnancy on survival of women who have had breast cancer has been demonstrated. When counseling patients, oncologists must take into consideration the patients' overall prognosis, age, comorbidities, and life goals.

In patients with inoperable or metastatic cancer (stage IV disease), induced abortion is usually advisable because of the possible adverse effects of hormonal treatment, radio-therapy, or chemotherapy upon the fetus in addition to the expectant mother's poor prognosis.

Bergh J et al: FACT: an open-label randomized phase III study of fulvestrant and anastrozole in combination compared with anastrozole alone as first-line therapy for patients with receptor positive postmenopausal breast cancer. *J Clin Oncol.* 2012;30(16):1919-1925. [PMID: 22370325]

Chalasani P et al: Caring for the breast cancer survivor: a guide for primary care physicians. *Am J Med.* 2010 Jun;123(6): 489-495. [PMID: 20569749]

Del Mastro L et al: Effect of the gonadotropin-releasing hormone analogue triptorelin on the occurrence of chemotherapy-induced early menopause in premenopausal women with breast cancer: a randomized trial. *JAMA.* 2011 Jul 20;306(3):269-276. [PMID: 21771987]

Fong DY et al: Physical activity for cancer survivors: meta-analysis of randomized controlled trials. *BMJ.* 2012;344:e70. [PMID: 22294757]

Hermelink K: Acute and late onset cognitive dysfunction associated with chemotherapy in women with breast cancer. *Cancer.* 2011 Mar 1;117(5):1103. [PMID: 20960507]

Rourke LL et al: Breast cancer and lymphedema: a current overview for the healthcare provider. *Womens Health (Lond Engl).* 2010 May;6(3):399-406. [PMID: 20426606]

Schmitz KH et al: Weight lifting for women at risk for breast cancer-related lymphedema: a randomized trial. *JAMA.* 2010 Dec 22;304(24):2699-2705. [PMID: 21148134]

Siegel R et al: Cancer treatment and survivorship statistics, 2012. *CA Cancer J Clin.* 2012;62(4):220-2241. [PMID: 22700443]

▼ CARCINOMA OF THE MALE BREAST

 ESSENTIALS OF DIAGNOSIS

► A painless lump beneath the areola in a man usually over 50 years of age

► Nipple discharge, retraction, or ulceration may be present

► Generally poorer prognosis than in women

► General Considerations

Breast cancer in men is a rare disease; the incidence is only about 1% of that in women. The average age at occurrence is about 70 years and there may be an increased incidence of breast cancer in men with prostate cancer. As in women, hormonal influences are probably related to the development of male breast cancer. There is a high incidence of both breast cancer and gynecomastia in Bantu men, theoretically owing to failure of estrogen inactivation by a liver damaged by associated liver disease. It is important to note that first-degree relatives of men with breast cancer are considered to be at high risk. This risk should be taken into account when discussing options with the patient and family. In addition, *BRCA2* mutations are common in men with breast cancer. Men with breast cancer, especially with a history of prostate cancer, should receive genetic counseling. The prognosis, even in stage I cases, is worse in men than in women. Blood-borne metastases are commonly present when the male patient appears for initial treatment. These metastases may be latent and may not become manifest for many years.

▶ Clinical Findings

A painless lump, occasionally associated with nipple discharge, retraction, erosion, or ulceration, is the primary complaint. Examination usually shows a hard, ill-defined, nontender mass beneath the nipple or areola. Gynecomastia not uncommonly precedes or accompanies breast cancer in men. Nipple discharge is an uncommon presentation for breast cancer in men but is an ominous finding associated with carcinoma in nearly 75% of cases.

Breast cancer staging is the same in men as in women. Gynecomastia and metastatic cancer from another site (eg, prostate) must be considered in the differential diagnosis. Benign tumors are rare, and biopsy should be performed on all males with a defined breast mass.

▶ Treatment

Treatment consists of modified radical mastectomy in operable patients, who should be chosen by the same criteria as women with the disease. Breast conserving therapy is rarely performed. Irradiation is the first step in treating localized metastases in the skin, lymph nodes, or skeleton that are causing symptoms. Examination of the cancer for hormone receptor proteins and HER2 overexpression is of value in determining adjuvant therapy. Men commonly have ER-positive tumors and rarely have overexpression of HER2. Adjuvant systemic therapy and radiation is used for the same indications as in breast cancer in women.

Because breast cancer in men is frequently a disseminated disease, endocrine therapy is of considerable importance in its management. Tamoxifen is the main drug for management of advanced breast cancer in men. Tamoxifen (20 mg orally daily) should be the initial treatment. There is little experience with AIs though they should be effective. Castration in advanced breast cancer is a successful measure and more beneficial than the same procedure in women but is rarely used. Objective evidence of regression may be seen in 60%-70% of men with hormonal therapy for metastatic disease—approximately twice the proportion in women. The average duration of tumor growth remission is about 30 months, and life is prolonged. Bone is the most frequent site of metastases from breast cancer in men (as in women), and hormonal therapy relieves bone pain in most patients so treated. The longer the interval between mastectomy and recurrence, the longer the remission following treatment is likely. As in women, there is correlation between ERs of the tumor and the likelihood of remission following hormonal therapy.

AIs should replace adrenalectomy in men as they have in women. Corticosteroid therapy alone has been considered to be efficacious but probably has no value when compared with major endocrine ablation. Either tamoxifen or AIs may be primary or secondary hormonal manipulation.

Estrogen therapy—5 mg of diethylstilbestrol three times daily orally   may be effective hormonal manipulation after others have been successful and failed, just as in women. Androgen therapy may exacerbate bone pain. Chemotherapy should be administered for the same indications and using the same dosage schedules as for women with metastatic disease or for adjuvant treatment.

▶ Prognosis

Men with breast cancer seem to have a worse prognosis than women with breast cancer because breast cancer is diagnosed in men at a later stage. However, a large population based, international study reported that after adjustment for prognostic features (age, stage, treatment), men had a significantly improved relative survival from breast cancer compared to women. For node-positive disease, 5-year survival is approximately 69%, and for node-negative disease, it is 88%. A practice-patterns database study reported that based on NCCN guidelines, only 59% of patients received the recommended chemotherapy, 82% received the recommended hormonal therapy, and 71% received the recommended postmastectomy radiation, indicating a relatively low adherence to NCCN guidelines for men.

For those patients whose disease progresses despite treatment, meticulous efforts at palliative care are essential (see Chapter 5).

Kiluk JV et al: Male breast cancer: management and follow-up recommendations. *Breast J.* 2011 Sep-Oct;17(5):503-509. [PMID: 21883641]

Miao H et al: Incidence and outcome of male breast cancer: an international population-based study. *J Clin Oncol.* 2011 Nov 20;29(33):4381-4386. [PMID: 21969512]

Ravi A et al: Breast cancer in men: prognostic factors, treatment patterns, and outcome. *Am J Mens Health.* 2012 Jan;6(1):51-58. [PMID: 21831929]

Wauters CA et al: Is cytology useful in the diagnostic workup of male breast lesions? A retrospective study over a 16-year period and review of the recent literature. *Acta Cytol.* 2010 May-Jun;54(3):259-264. [PMID: 20518408]

Zurrida S et al: Male breast cancer. *Future Oncol.* 2010 Jun;6(6):985-991. [PMID: 20528235]

MULTIPLE CHOICE QUESTIONS

1. Fibrocystic condition of the breast is

   A. Communicable disease
   B. Common in postmenopausal women
   C. Caused at least in part by estrogen stimulation of breast tissue
   D. Carries a threefold increased risk of breast cancer
   E. Does not actually include any cysts on histology

2. Risk factors for breast cancer include

   A. Early childbearing
   B. Iodine deficiency
   C. *BRCA1* mutation only in families of Ashkenazi Jewish descent
   D. A personal history of breast cancer
   E. None of the above

3. Breast cancer screening in asymptomatic women

   A. Identifies about 2 cancers per 1000 women over age 50 years
   B. Identifies cancer without node involvement in about 80% of detected cases
   C. Includes a history, physical examination, bilateral mammogram, and ultrasound for women between ages 40 and 50 years
   D. Is followed by a 5-year survival of 95% for women diagnosed through screening
   E. Should include all women yearly after the age of 30 years

4. The clinical findings at breast cancer presentation most commonly include

   A. A painless mass identified by the patient
   B. A new mass discovered during a clinician physical examination (60% of cases)
   C. Nipple discharge (60% of cases)
   D. An axillary mass due to metastatic lymph nodes (40% of cases)
   E. None of the above

5. Axillary lymph node metastases from breast cancer

   A. Are not important for predicting patient survival in women with breast cancer
   B. Are generally palpable if present
   C. Can be reliably detected by sestamibi scintigraphy
   D. Can be reliably detected by sentinel lymph node biopsy in women with clinically uninvolved axillary lymph nodes
   E. Are frequently present in residual lymph nodes when sentinel lymph node biopsy shows no evidence of disease

Thoracic Wall, Pleura, Mediastinum, & Lung

K. Barrett Deatrick, MD

Jason Long, MD

Andrew C. Chang, MD

ANATOMY & PHYSIOLOGY

ANATOMY OF THE CHEST WALL & PLEURA

The physiology of respiration and the anatomy of the chest wall are tightly linked. The chest wall is an airtight, expandable, cone-shaped cage. Normal ventilation occurs when expansion of the rib cage and simultaneous diaphragmatic excursion create negative intrathoracic pressure, allowing inward flow of air.

The function of the chest wall is made possible by its segmentally arranged anatomy. The ventral wall of the bony thorax extends from the suprasternal notch to the xiphoid, approximately 18 cm in the adult. It is formed by the manubrium, sternum, and xiphoid process. The remainder of the anterior wall and the lateral walls are formed by 12 ribs. The first seven pairs of ribs articulate directly with the sternum, the next three pairs connect to the lower border of the preceding rib, and the last two terminate in the wall of the abdomen. The sides of the chest wall consist of the upper 10 ribs, which slope obliquely downward from their posterior attachments. The posterior chest wall is formed by the twelve thoracic vertebrae, their transverse processes, and the 12 ribs (Figure 18–1). The upper ventral portion of the thoracic cage is covered by the clavicle and the subclavian vessels. Laterally, it is covered by the shoulder girdle and axillary nerves and vessels; dorsally, it is covered in part by the scapula.

The superior aperture of the thorax (also called either the thoracic inlet or the thoracic outlet) is a downwardly slanted 5- to 10-cm kidney-shaped opening bounded by the first costal cartilages and ribs laterally, the manubrium anteriorly, and the body of the first thoracic vertebra posteriorly. The inferior aperture of the thorax is bounded by the twelfth vertebra and ribs posteriorly and the cartilages of the seventh to tenth ribs and the xiphisternal joint anteriorly. It is much wider than the superior aperture and is occupied by the diaphragm.

The blood supply and innervation of the chest wall are via the intercostal vessels and nerves (Figures 18–2 and 18–3). The upper thorax also receives vessels and nerves from the cervical and axillary regions. The underside of the sternum's blood supply derives from the internal thoracic artery branches, which anastomose with the intercostal vessels along the lateral aspect of the chest wall.

The entirety of the thoracic cavity is lined by a pleural membrane. The parietal pleura is the innermost lining of the chest wall and is divided into four parts: the cervical pleura (cupola or cupula), costal pleura, mediastinal pleura, and diaphragmatic pleura. The visceral pleura is a mesodermal layer investing the lungs and is continuous with the parietal pleura, joining it at the hilum of the lung. The potential pleural space is a capillary gap that normally contains only a few drops of serous fluid. However, this space may be enlarged when fluid (hydrothorax), blood (hemothorax), pus (pyothorax or empyema), lymphatic fluid (chylothorax), or air (pneumothorax) fills this potential cavity.

PHYSIOLOGY OF THE CHEST WALL & PLEURA

▶ Mechanics of Respiration

Ventilation is the process of moving gas through the conducting airways, to and from the alveoli, and occurs when elevation of the rib cage and descent of the diaphragm cause an increase in thoracic volume and generate negative intrathoracic pressure. In infants, the ribs have not yet assumed their oblique contour and ventilation depends on diaphragmatic breathing. Furthermore, accessory muscles of respiration contribute to the conformational change in the thoracic cage during periods of intense exercise or respiratory distress (Figure 18–4).

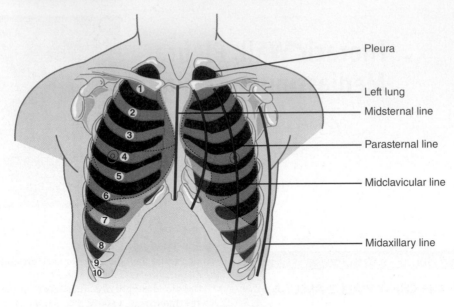

▲ **Figure 18–1.** The thorax, showing rib cage, pleura, and lung fields.

Expiration is mainly passive, resulting from elastic recoil of the lungs. An exception to this is deep breathing, when the abdominal musculature contracts, pulling the rib cage downward and simultaneously elevating the diaphragm by compressing the abdominal viscera against it.

▶ Physiology of the Pleural Space

A. Pressure

The pleural cavity pressure is normally negative, owing to the opposing forces of elastic recoil of the lung and active

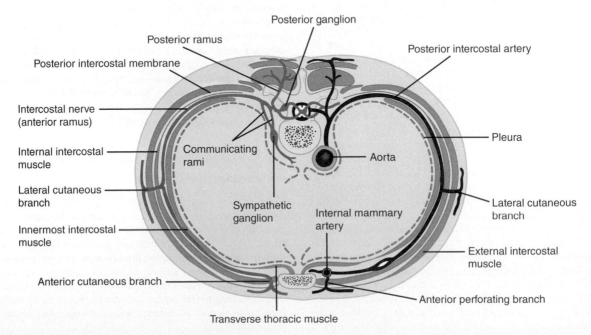

▲ **Figure 18–2.** Transverse section of thorax.

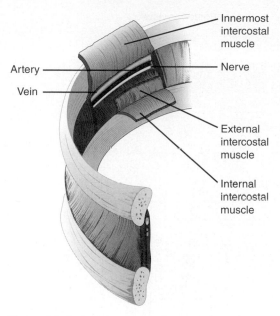

▲ Figure 18–3. Intercostal muscles, vessels, and nerves.

expansion of the space by the chest wall. During quiet respiration, it varies from -15 cm H_2O with inspiration to 2 cm H_2O during expiration. Larger pressure changes (eg, -60 cm H_2O during forced inspiration to $+30$ cm H_2O during vigorous expiration) may occur with deep breathing. Because of gravity, pleural pressure at the apex is more negative when the body is upright and changes about 0.2 cm H_2O per centimeter of vertical height.

B. Fluid Formation and Reabsorption

The formation (transudation) and reabsorption of fluid within the pleural space depends on hydrostatic, colloid, and tissue pressures (the Starling equation) in addition to permeability of the pleural membrane. In health, fluid is formed by the parietal pleura and absorbed by the visceral pleura (Figure 18–5). Since systemic capillary hydrostatic pressure is 30 cm H_2O, and intrapleural negative pressure averages -5 cm H_2O there is a net *hydrostatic* pressure of 35 cm H_2O. Additionally, the colloid osmotic pressure of the systemic capillaries is 34 cm H_2O and an opposing 8 cm H_2O of pleural space osmotic pressure. Thus, a net 26 cm H_2O osmotic pressure draws fluid back into systemic capillaries. Since systemic hydrostatic pressure (35 cm H_2O) exceeds osmotic capillary pressure (26 cm H_2O) by 9 cm H_2O, there is a 9 cm H_2O net drive of fluid into the pleural space by systemic capillaries in the chest wall. Similar calculations for the visceral pleura involving the low-pressure pulmonary circulation will show that there is a resulting net drive of 10 cm H_2O that attracts pleural fluid into pulmonary

capillaries. Thus, there is normally a balance favoring neither loss nor gain of fluid in this space.

In health, pleural fluid is low in protein (<100 mg/dL). When it increases in disease to about 1 g/dL, the net colloid osmotic pressure of the visceral pleural capillaries is equaled and pleural fluid reabsorption becomes dependent on lymphatic drainage. Thus, abnormal amounts of pleural fluid may accumulate: (1) when hydrostatic pressure is increased, such as in heart failure; (2) when capillary permeability is increased, as in inflammatory or neoplastic disease; or (3) when colloid osmotic pressure is decreased.

ANATOMY OF THE MEDIASTINUM

The mediastinum is the compartment between the pleural cavities. It extends anteriorly from the suprasternal notch to the xiphoid process and posteriorly from the first to the eleventh thoracic vertebrae. Superiorly, fascial planes in the neck are in direct communication; inferiorly, the mediastinum is limited by the diaphragm. Apertures through the inferior extent of the mediastinum are traversed by the aorta, inferior vena cava, esophagus, and vagus nerve.

The mediastinum may be divided into a number of compartments in several ways. Classically, it may be divided into the superior, anterior, middle, and posterior compartments. The superior compartment extends above a line drawn from the fourth thoracic vertebrae to the sternomanubrial junction (Angle of Louis.) In the three-compartment Darliell alaosification (Figure 18–9), the anterior mediastinum contains the thymus gland, the lymph nodes, the ascending aorta and transverse aorta, the great vessels, and areolar tissue. The middle mediastinum contains the heart, the pericardium, the trachea, the hila of the lungs, the phrenic nerves, lymph nodes, and areolar tissue. The posterior mediastinum contains the sympathetic chains, the vagus nerves, the esophagus, the thoracic duct, lymph nodes, and the descending aorta.

Congenital abnormalities within the mediastinum are numerous. A defect in the anterior mediastinal pleura with communication of the right and left hemithorax is rare. This retrosternal part of the anterior mediastinum is normally thin, and overexpansion of one pleural space may cause "mediastinal herniation" or a bulge of mediastinal pleura toward the opposite side.

Displacements of the mediastinum occur from masses or from accumulations of air, fluid, blood, or chyle interfering with vital functions. Tracheal compression, vena caval obstruction, and esophageal obstructions cause clinical symptoms. The mediastinum can also be displaced laterally when pathologic processes of one hemithorax cause mediastinal shift. Fibrosis and lung volume loss can shift the mediastinum toward the affected side. Open pneumothorax and massive hemothorax shift the mediastinum away from the affected side. Open pneumothorax produces

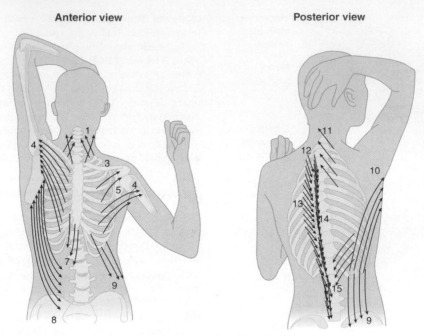

Anterior view　　　**Posterior view**

Secondary muscles of inspiration
(1) sternocleidomastoideus　(3) scalenes　(4) pectoralis major　(5) pectoralis minor
(10) serratus anterior　(11) serratus posterior superior　(12) upper iliocostalis

Secondary muscles of expiration
(8) external oblique　(9) internal oblique　(7) rectus abdominus　(13) lower iliocostalis
(14) lower longissimus　(15) serratus posterior inferior

▲ **Figure 18–4.** Accessory muscles of respiration. (From Kapandji IA. The respiratory muscle. In: Kapandji IA, ed. *The Physiology of the Joints.* vol. 3. *The Trunk and the Vertebral Column.* Churchill Livingstone, 1974.)

alternating paradoxic mediastinal shifts with respiration and will adversely affect ventilation. Acute mediastinal displacement may produce hypoxia or reduced venous return and cause dysrhythmias, hypotension, or cardiac arrest.

ANATOMY OF THE LUNG

The fundamental unit of lung anatomy is a bronchopulmonary segment (Figure 18–7). The right lung has three lobes: upper, middle, and lower. The left lung consists of two lobes: upper and lower. On the left, the lingular segments of the upper lobe are the homolog of the right middle lobe. Two fissures of varying completeness separate the lobes on the right side. The major, or oblique, fissure divides the upper and middle lobes from the lower lobe. The minor, or horizontal, fissure separates the middle from the upper lobe. On the left side, the single oblique fissure separates the upper and lower lobes. The parenchymal anatomy can be seen by studying the sequential division of the bronchopulmonary tree. The trachea and main stem bronchi and

their branches contain a posterior membranous area and are prevented from collapsing by horseshoe-shaped anterior segments of cartilage in their walls. The cartilaginous reinforcement of the airway gradually becomes less complete as the branches become smaller, and reinforcement ceases with bronchi of 1-2 mm. The bronchopulmonary segmental anatomy is designated by numbers (Boyden) or by name (Jackson and Huber). There are typically 18 bronchopulmonary segments (right upper 3, right middle 2, right lower 5, left upper 4, left lower 4) as shown in Figure 18–7. The segmental bronchial anatomy is most constant with the pulmonary vascular structures showing more variability.

The lungs have a dual blood supply: the pulmonary and the bronchial arterial systems. The pulmonary arteries transmit deoxygenated blood from the right ventricle for oxygenation. They closely accompany the bronchi. The bronchial arteries usually arise directly from the aorta or nearby intercostal arteries and are variable in number. They transmit oxygenated blood to the bronchial wall up to the level of the terminal bronchioles. The pulmonary veins

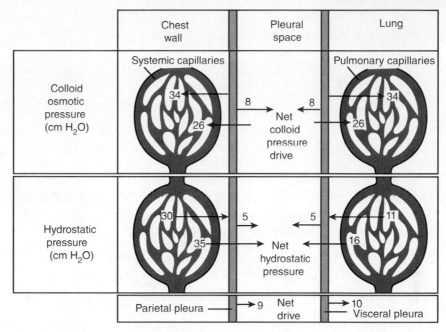

▲ **Figure 18–5.** Movement of fluid across the pleural space, showing production and absorption of pleural fluid.

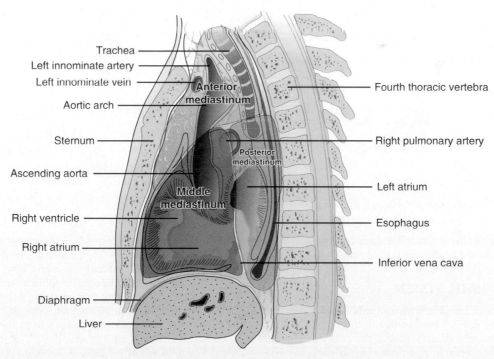

▲ **Figure 18–6.** Divisions of the mediastinum (Burkell classification). Light screening: anterior mediastinum; lower dark screening: middle mediastinum; dotted area at right: posterior mediastinum.

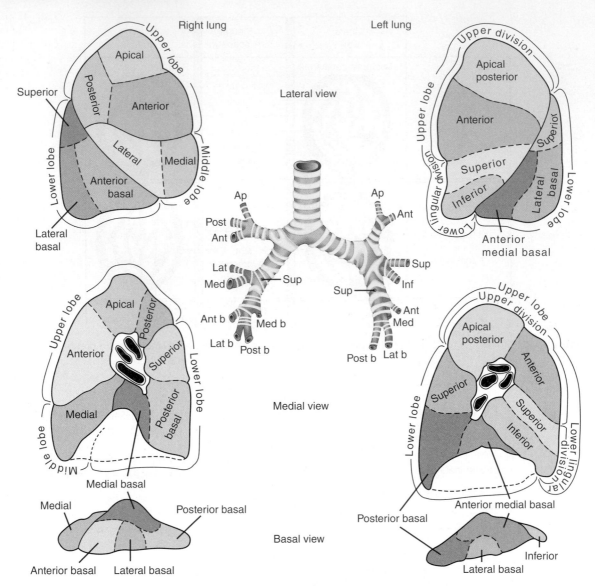

▲ **Figure 18–7.** Segmental anatomy of the lungs.

travel in the interlobar septa and do not correspond to the distribution of the bronchi or the pulmonary arteries.

THE LYMPHATIC SYSTEM

The lymphatics travel in intersegmental septa centrally as well as to the parenchymal surface to form subpleural networks. Drainage continues toward the hilum in channels that follow the bronchi and pulmonary arteries. The lymphatics eventually enter lymph nodes in the major fissures of the lungs, the hilum, and the paratracheal regions.

The direction of lymphatic drainage—irrespective of the primary site—is cephalad and ipsilateral, but contralateral flow may occur from any lobe. The usual sequence of lymphatic spread of pulmonary cancer is first to the regional parabronchial nodes and then to the ipsilateral paratracheal, subcarinal, scalene, or inferior deep cervical nodes. The lymphatics from the left lower lobe may be almost equally distributed to the left and right. From the left upper lobe, distribution is often to the anterior mediastinal group (A-P window and para-aortic lymph nodes).

▶ Skin Tests

Skin tests are used in the diagnosis of tuberculosis, histoplasmosis, and coccidioidomycosis. Tuberculin testing is usually done with purified protein derivative (PPD) injected intradermally. Intermediate-strength PPD should be used in patients who seem likely to have active disease. Induration of 10 mm or more at the injection site after 48-72 hours is positive and indicates either active or arrested disease. Because false-negative reactions are rare, a negative test fairly reliably rules out tuberculosis. Mumps antigen is usually placed on the opposite forearm to test for anergy. Skin tests for histoplasmosis and coccidioidomycosis are performed in a similar way, but skin tests for fungal infections are unreliable and serologic tests should be performed instead.

▶ Endoscopy

A. Laryngoscopy

Indirect laryngoscopy is used to assess vocal cord mobility in patients suspected of having lung carcinoma when there has been a voice change. It should also be performed to search for an otherwise occult source for malignant cells in sputum or metastases in cervical lymph nodes.

B. Bronchoscopy

Roentgenographic evidence of bronchial obstruction, unresolved pneumonia, foreign body, suspected carcinoma, hemoptysis, aspiration pneumonia, and lung abscess are only a few of the indications for bronchoscopy. Depending on the indication, either flexible or rigid bronchoscopy may be performed. Rigid bronchoscopy must be done under general anesthesia and is most often used for clearing major airways of bulky obstructing lesions such as tumors, foreign bodies, or blood clots. Tumor ablation may be done via multiple techniques, including the use of Nd:YAG laser.

Flexible bronchoscopy is a highly effective diagnostic and therapeutic tool. It can be performed under local and intravenous sedation. Washings are usually obtained for bacterial or fungal culture and cytologic examination. Visible lesions are biopsied directly and brush biopsies are obtained from specific bronchopulmonary segments. Occasionally, transcarinal needle biopsy of a subcarinal node is obtained.

Bronchoscopically, 30%-50% of lung tumors are visible. Brushing, random biopsies, and sputum cytology may still yield a positive diagnosis of cancer or tuberculosis in the absence of a visible lesion. The yield is influenced by size, location, and histologic cell type of the lesion.

Additional techniques available during bronchoscopy include the use of endo-bronchial ultrasound (EBUS) and electromagnetic navigational bronchoscopy. EBUS enables visualization of masses and lymph nodes from the central airways, and facilitates fine needle aspiration of these lesions. Navigational bronchoscopy integrates use of a virtual bronchoscopy obtained from cross-sectional imaging (usually CT scan) and a tracking system based on three dimensional feedback from electromagnetic signals to allow access to lesions deep within the lung parenchyma.

▶ Mediastinoscopy

Cervical mediastinoscopy remains a mainstay of evaluation of the mediastinum despite advances in imaging. Properly performed mediastinoscopy samples nodes from at least three stations, including ipsilateral and contralateral paratracheal levels 2 and 4 and subcarinal level 7. Cervical mediastinoscopy is performed through a 3- to 4-cm incision one fingerbreadth above the sternal notch. Dissection proceeds beneath the pretracheal fascia, allowing safe access to mediastinal nodes and avoiding major vascular structures. After palpation, the mediastinoscope can be inserted and nodes biopsied under direct vision. Unclear structures care aspirated prior to attempted biopsy.

Enlarged lymph nodes in the aorticopulmonary window are technically inaccessible by means of standard cervical mediastinoscopy. Extended cervical mediastinoscopy provides access to these aorticopulmonary window nodes. It is performed through the same neck incision as standard mediastinoscopy except the dissection is carried laterally beside the left carotid artery toward and then over the aorta into the aorticopulmonary space. Because of the surrounding structures, this procedure carries significant risks and in patients with dilated or calcific aortas or previous cardiac operations, is contraindicated.

In experienced hands, the complications of mediastinoscopy are minimal (< 1%-2%). Major bleeding complications requiring sternotomy or thoracotomy for repair are infrequent (1%-2%). Other possible complications include pneumothorax, recurrent nerve injury, infection, and esophageal injury.

Mediastinoscopy is almost invariably accurate in the diagnosis of sarcoidosis. It is also useful to diagnose tuberculosis, histoplasmosis, Castleman silicosis, metastatic carcinoma, lymphoma, and carcinoma of the esophagus. It should not be used in the investigation of primary mediastinal tumors, which should be approached by an incision permitting definitive excision.

▶ Chamberlain Procedure

Anterior mediastinotomy (the Chamberlain procedure) is used to sample nodes and biopsy tissue in the anterior mediastinum, most commonly in the aortopulmonary window. A small (3-4 cm) incision is made over the second or third interspace on the appropriate side of the lesion. Alternatively, the procedure can be performed with videoscopic guidance (video-assisted thoracoscopic surgery [VATS]). The mediastinum is approached through the interspace directly or after excising the costochondral cartilage using either the mediastinoscope or an open technique. Careful attention is paid to preserving the mammary vessels encountered in the dissection. The mediastinum is approached extrapleurally unless lesions specifically within the thorax—effusions, tumors invading the hilum or chest wall—need to be investigated. Furthermore, if additional access is required to facilitate the dissection or to treat a complication, the incision can be converted to a larger anterior thoracotomy.

Complications resulting from anterior mediastinotomy include bleeding, recurrent nerve injury, and infection. Major morbidity is less than 1%-2%.

Scalene lymph node biopsy has been largely replaced by mediastinoscopy although remains important particularly for evaluation of suspicious supracervical lymphadenopathy.

▶ Video-Assisted Thoracoscopic Surgery

VATS plays an important role in the diagnosis and staging of thoracic malignancies as well as in the resection of isolated peripheral pulmonary nodules and bullous lung disease. Furthermore, it has been an advance in lung biopsy and pleurodesis procedures. Although some oncologic concerns persist, thoracoscopic procedures are the standard of care for many resections, although they have not entirely supplanted open resection. As instruments and techniques have evolved, complications from VATS procedures (persistent air leaks, hemorrhage, tumor seeding, etc) have decreased. Overall, major complication rates of 1%-2% are reported. Faster patient recovery, shorter hospital stays, decreased pain are major advantages of VATS, although long-term differences between videoscopic and formal thoracotomy using muscle-sparing incisions are yet to be demonstrated.

▶ Pleural Biopsy

Biopsies of the pleura can be performed either using percutaneous needle techniques, VATS, or open surgical approaches. It is indicated when the cause of a pleural effusion cannot be determined by analysis of the fluid or when tuberculosis is suspected. A definitive diagnosis can be obtained in 60%-80% of cases of tuberculosis or cancer. The principal complication is pneumothorax. Five percent to 10% of biopsy specimens are inadequate for diagnosis. Biopsy of the pleura can be performed via videoscopic or open technique with minimal morbidity, providing the pathologist with a specimen superior to that of needle biopsy.

Kuździał J et al: Current evidence on transcervical mediastinal lymph nodes dissection. *Eur J Cardiothorac Surg* 2011;40(6):1470.

Yasufuku K et al: A prospective controlled trial of endobronchial ultrasound-guided transbronchial needle aspiration compared with mediastinoscopy for mediastinal lymph node staging of lung cancer. *J Thorac Cardiovasc Surg* 2011;142(6):1393.

▶ Lung Biopsy

A. Needle Biopsy

The most common indication for the use of transthoracic needle biopsy of the lung is the evaluation of a solitary pulmonary nodule. It may also be used to confirm the presence of metastatic disease. Lung biopsy may also be indicated in diffuse parenchymal disease and in some patients with localized lesions. Most commonly, lung biopsies are now performed under CT guidance. Complications following percutaneous needle biopsy include pneumothorax (5%-30%), hemothorax, hemoptysis, and air embolism. Pulmonary hypertension or cysts and bullae are contraindications. Several deaths have been reported. There is about a 60% chance of obtaining useful information. Additionally, there is controversy concerning the risks of spreading the tumor by needle biopsy in localized disease.

B. Surgical Biopsy

Thoracoscopy is the standard approach for open lung biopsy in patients who can tolerate single lung ventilation. Techniques for port placement vary, but all allow introduction of a stapler and operating thoracoscope. In addition to allowing smaller incisions, thoracoscopy allows for the visualization of multiple segments and taking multiple biopsies in diffuse diseases. For open biopsies a limited intercostal or anterior parasternal incision is used to remove a 3- to 4-cm wedge of lung tissue in diffuse parenchymal lung disease. The site of incision is selected for accessibility and potential diagnostic value. The incision is generally made at the fifth interspace on the right at the anterior axillary line to allow for access to all three lobes for biopsy. The middle lobe and lingula are selected in specific cases when pathology exists only in these areas, as they generally yield results of the poorest quality. Open lung biopsy is associated with a lower death rate, fewer complications, and greater diagnostic yield than needle biopsy. It is especially useful in critically ill, immunosuppressed patients for differentiation of infectious infiltrative lesions from neoplastic infiltrative lesions. Peripheral lesions are totally excised by wedge or segmental resection, and deeply placed lesions are removed by lobectomy in suitable candidates.

▶ Sputum Analysis

Sputum cytology can be valuable for detecting lung cancer. Specimens are obtained by deep coughing or by abrasion with a brush, or bronchial washings are obtained by either bronchoscopic or percutaneous transtracheal washing techniques. Specimens should be collected in the morning and delivered to the laboratory promptly. Centrifugation or filtration can be used to concentrate the cellular elements.

In primary lung cancer, sputum cytology is positive in 30%-60% of cases. Repeated sputum examination improves the diagnostic return. Examination of the first broncho-scopic washing material yields a diagnosis in 60% of cases. Postbronchoscopy sputum analysis should always be made at 6-12 and 24 hours, as findings may be positive at these times when previous tests were negative. Cytologic analysis using immunohistochemistry to molecular markers (cyto-keratins, hnRNP, etc) has improved accuracy and sensitivity and the ability to detect premalignant lesions.

Computed Tomography Scan

Computed tomography (CT) is a cornerstone of evaluation of chest pathology. CT scanning is critical in the staging of carcinoma, and has value in defining the extent of metastatic disease.

Magnetic Resonance Imaging

Although the major value of magnetic resonance imaging (MRI) in the thorax has been in cardiovascular imaging, it can also show invasion of lung cancer into the chest wall, vertebrae, and spinal cord as well as mediastinal structures. MRI has a particular niche in the evaluation of superior sulcus (Pancoast) tumors to establish involvement of the brachial plexus, subclavian vessel, or bony chest wall.

Positron Emission Tomography

Positron emission tomography (PET) is an important tool in staging and workup of the cancer patient. PET scanners are widely available. PET scanning may identify unsuspected regional or distant disease in up to 20%-30% of patients with lung cancer or esophageal cancer compared with conventional imaging methods (CT, bone scan). PET scanning is more accurate than CT scan in detection of cancer spread to mediastinal lymph nodes. Because of the high negative predictive value of PET scanning, a negative PET scan in the mediastinum permits direct progression to thoracotomy. The presence of a positive PET scan in the mediastinum mandates either mediastinoscopy or, more recently, endo-scopic evaluation of mediastinal lymph nodes because of false-positive PET scan results.

The combined PET/CT is highly accurate (> 90%), but by itself it has a 10%-20% false-positive rate in the medi-astinum. Therefore, interpretations of PET results must be accepted with caution and must be confirmed by surgical staging when inconsistent with the overall clinical picture.

DISEASES OF THE CHEST WALL

LUNG HERNIA

A lung hernia results from a defect in the chest wall may be congenital or acquired as the result of trauma or a surgical operation. Most lung hernias are thoracic in location, but cervical (defects of Sibson fascia) or diaphragmatic hernia-tion may occur occasionally. Lung hernias may present as a tender subcutaneous mass that enlarges with cough or Valsalva. Other than this mass, they are usually asymptom-atic. Once diagnosed, these hernias should be repaired, with repair of the skeletal defect and prosthetic mesh reinforce-ment. This may be done open or with VATS techniques.

CHEST WALL INFECTIONS

Infections of the chest wall or pleural spaces may pose complex challenges in medical management. Infections that appear to involve only the skin and soft tissues may actu-ally represent outward extensions of deeper infection of the ribs, cartilage, sternum, or even the pleural space (empyema necessitatis). Inadequate drainage of superficial infection can lead to inward extension into the pleural space, causing empyema.

Subpectoral abscess is caused by suppurative adenitis of the axillary lymph nodes, rib or pleural infection, or poste-rior extension of a breast abscess. It may also occur as a com-plication of chest wall surgery (eg, mastectomy, pacemaker placement). Symptoms include erythema, induration of the pectoral region, and obliteration of the normal infraclavicu-lar depression and may progress to systemic sepsis. Shoulder movement is painful. Organisms most commonly involved include hemolytic streptococci and *Staphylococcus aureus*. Treatment involves incisional drainage along the lateral border of the pectoralis major muscle and administration of systemic antibiotics.

Subscapular abscess may arise from osteomyelitis of the scapula but most commonly follows thoracic opera-tions such as thoracotomy or thoracoplasty. Winging of the scapula or paravertebral induration of the trapezius muscle is usually present. A pleural communication is suggested if a cough impulse is present or if the size of the mass varies with position or direct pressure. The diagnosis is established by needle aspiration. Open drainage is indicated for pyogenic infections not involving the pleural space. Tubercular lesions should be treated by chemotherapy and needle aspiration, if possible.

Osteomyelitis of the Ribs

In the past, osteomyelitis of the ribs was often caused by typhoid fever and tuberculosis. Except in children, hematog-enous osteomyelitis is a rare problem today. Thoracotomy incisions may result in osteomyelitis.

Sternal Osteomyelitis

Infection of the sternum most commonly follows median sternotomy incisions, particularly in diabetics. It presents as a postoperative wound infection or mediastinitis with drain-age, fever, leukocytosis, and instability of the sternal closure.

Treatment consists of control of systemic sepsis with appropriate antibiotics, open drainage, resection of the involved sternum, and reconstruction of the defect with pectoralis muscle, serratus muscle, or omental coverage. Occasionally, sternal osteomyelitis will be due to tuberculosis.

▶ Infection of the Costal Cartilages & Xiphoid

Costal cartilage infections are relatively unresponsive to antibiotic therapy. Once devascularized, perichondral tissue necroses and acts as a foreign body to perpetuate the infection and favor sinus tract formation. The most common cause is direct extension of other surgical infections (eg, wound infection, subphrenic abscess). Surgical division of costal cartilages, as in a thoracoabdominal incision, may predispose to cartilage infection postoperatively if local sepsis develops. A wide variety of organisms have been implicated.

Erythema and induration with fluctuance and often spontaneous drainage can occur. The course can be fulminant or may be indolent over months or years, with periodic exacerbations. Associated osteomyelitis of the sternum, ribs, or clavicle may occur.

The treatment of choice includes resection of the involved cartilage and adjacent involved bony structures. Recurrence is due to underestimation of the extent of disease and inadequate resection.

▶ Reconstruction of the Chest Wall

Chest wall reconstruction may be necessary following trauma, surgical resection, or infection resulting in destruction of chest wall structures. Rigid reconstruction of the chest wall is generally recommended for defects greater than 5 cm, although posterior resections covered by the scapula will not necessarily need rigid mesh reconstruction. Advances in the use of musculocutaneous flaps and the supportive use of methyl methacrylate and Marlex mesh to produce solidity below these muscular flaps have facilitated repairs. In massive chest wall defects, vascularization of the area is essential and can be accomplished by use of omental flaps as well as pectoralis, latissimus dorsi, and rectus flaps. Microsurgical techniques for repair of such defects have greatly expanded the ability of plastic surgeons to deal with extensive resectional and infective processes.

Mahabir RC, Butler CE: Stabilization of the chest wall: autologous and alloplastic reconstructions. *Semin Plast Surg* 2011; 25: 34-42.

TIETZE SYNDROME (COSTOCHONDRITIS)

Tietze syndrome is a painful, nonsuppurative inflammation of the costochondral cartilages and is of unknown cause. Recent evidence suggests that costochondritis may represent a manifestation of seronegative rheumatic disease. Local swelling and tenderness are the only symptoms; they usually disappear without therapy. The syndrome may recur.

Several reports have suggested the use of bone scintigraphy and chest CT for diagnosis of infected costochondritis. Bone scanning was effective in localizing and identifying inflamed costochondral junctions. Treatment is symptomatic and may include analgesics (NSAIDs) and local or systemic corticosteroids. When symptoms persist longer than 3 weeks and tumefaction suggests neoplasm, excision of the involved cartilage may be indicated and is usually curative.

Stochendahl MJ, Christe.nsen HW: Chest pain in focal musculoskeletal disorders. *Medical Clin North Am* 2010;94(2):259-273.

MONDOR DISEASE (THROMBOPHLEBITIS OF THE THORACOEPIGASTRIC VEIN)

Mondor disease consists of localized thrombophlebitis of the anterolateral chest wall. It is more prominent in women than in men and occasionally follows mastectomy. There are few symptoms other than the presence of a localized tender, cordlike structure in the subcutaneous tissues of the abdomen, thorax, or axilla. The disease is self-limited and does not pose a risk of thromboembolism. The possibility of an infective origin or stasis of the interrupted venous return due to neoplasm must be ruled out.

CHEST WALL TUMORS

Chest wall tumors may be simulated by enlarged costal cartilages, chest wall infection, fractures, rickets, scurvy, hyperparathyroidism, and other conditions. Most commonly, chest wall lesions present as a mass with localized or referred pain; less than 25% are asymptomatic. Approximately 60% of all chest wall masses prove to be malignant. Lesions arise from one of the three components of the chest wall, including soft tissues (eg, muscle, nerve ,fascia), bone, and cartilage.

The majority of tumors arise from either bone or cartilage. Rib involvement is more common than sternal presentation. Chest CT offers the most information for diagnosis and staging. Chest wall sarcomas are associated with pulmonary metastasis. Simple chest x-rays may initially identify a mass, especially if it is calcified. Bone scans should be obtained in all cases.

Initial diagnosis is obtained by limited incisional biopsy (transverse) if the mass is large (> 4 cm). Smaller lesions are excised en bloc, ensuring negative margins, with full knowledge that a malignancy is present in many cases. Classic teaching has been to perform en bloc wide local excisions with immediate reconstruction for all lesions at initial presentations. Progress with adjuvant multimodality therapy, however, for tumors such as rhabdomyosarcomas and Ewing sarcoma supports the use of initial limited biopsy for tissue diagnosis to guide treatment planning.

▶ Specific Neoplasms

A. Benign Soft Tissue Tumors

1. Lipomas—Lipomas are the most common benign tumors of the chest wall. Occasionally, they are very large and lobulated, and they may have dumbbell-shaped extensions that indent the endothoracic fascia beneath the sternum through an intercostal space. They may communicate with a large mediastinal or supraclavicular component.

2. Neurogenic tumors—These may arise from intercostal or superficial nerves. Solitary neurofibromas are most common, followed by neurolemmomas.

3. Cavernous hemangiomas—Hemangiomas of the thoracic wall are usually painful and occur in children. Tumors may be isolated or may involve other tissues (eg, lung), as in Rendu-Osler-Weber syndrome.

4. Lymphangiomas—This rare lesion is seen most often in children. It may have poorly defined borders that make complete excision difficult.

B. Malignant Soft Tissue Tumors

Roughly 50% of all chest wall masses are sarcomas, yet overall they represent only a small percentage (5%) of all malignant soft tissue sarcomas. Survival is determined by the histologic grade, the completeness of resection, and the presence and development of metastases (synchronous or metachronous). Low-grade tumors have 5-year and 10-year survivals approaching 90% and 82%, respectively. With high-grade lesions, however, 5-year survival rates are only 30%-50%. The development of metastasis greatly reduces the chances of survival.

Treatment is directed at a complete resection with emphasis on achieving negative margins (1-2 cm). En bloc resection techniques include raising skin flaps and reconstruction with soft tissue flaps, Marlex mesh, and methyl methacrylate to correct chest wall deformity and prevent paradoxic chest movement.

There are many histologic subtypes of soft tissue sarcoma. Typically, low-grade sarcomas include desmoids or liposarcomas with low-grade features. Next most frequently seen are malignant fibrosarcoma, rhabdomyosarcoma, and malignant fibrous histiocytoma, which are usually high-grade lesions.

Individual histologic subtype is *not* by itself a significant prognostic variable, but histologic grade *is* significant. Metastases—either synchronous or metachronous—are most commonly to the lungs (75%) and should be resected if negative margins can be achieved and adequate lung function preserved. Therapy for low-grade lesions should consist of a complete resection. Incompletely resected lesions should be treated with external beam radiation therapy. High-grade lesions should be resected and patients enrolled in clinical trials evaluating the efficacy of systemic adjuvant chemotherapy. Postoperative radiotherapy is often helpful in the setting of close margins or tumor spillage.

1. Fibrosarcomas—Fibrosarcoma is the most common primary soft tissue cancer of the chest wall. It occurs most frequently in young adults. Treatment is neoadjuvant chemotherapy followed by resection. A subtype of these tumors includes neurofibrosarcomas, which involve the thoracic wall almost twice as often as other parts of the body. Also referred to as malignant peripheral nerve sheath tumors or malignant schwannomas, they often occur in patients with neurofibromatosis and usually originate from intercostal nerves.

2. Malignant fibrous histiocytoma/high-grade pleomorphic sarcoma—Malignant fibrous histiocytoma has a bimodal distribution, with peaks between 20 and 30 years of age and between 50 and 60. Although they are the most common soft tissue sarcoma of adults, they rarely rise from the chest wall. Treatment is neoadjuvant chemotherapy followed by resection, followed by additional adjuvant chemotherapy.

3. Rhabdomyosarcoma—Rhabdomyosarcoma is an uncommon tumor in adults but is the second most common chest wall tumor in children. Treatment is neoadjuvant chemoradiation, surgical resection, then ongoing chemotherapy and radiation. These tumors are aggressive and often unresectable.

4. Liposarcomas—These tumors account for approximately one-third of all primary cancers of the chest wall. They occur more often in men.

C. Benign Skeletal Tumors

1. Chondromas, osteochondromas, and myxochondromas—The combined frequency of these three cartilaginous tumors is about 30%-45% of all benign skeletal tumors. Cartilaginous tumors are usually single and occur with equal frequency in males and females between childhood and the fourth decade. The tumors are usually painless and tend to occur anteriorly along the costal margin or in the parasternal area. Wide local excision is curative.

2. Fibrous dysplasia—Fibrous dysplasia (bone cyst, osteofibroma, fibrous osteoma, and fibrosis ossificans) accounts for a third or more of benign skeletal tumors of the chest wall. This cystic bone tumor can occur in any portion of the skeletal system, but approximately half involve the ribs. The differential diagnosis includes cystic bone lesions associated with hyperparathyroidism. The tumor is usually single and may be related to previous trauma. Some patients experience swelling, tenderness, or vague discomfort, but the lesion is usually silent and is detected on routine chest x-ray. Treatment consists of local excision.

3. Eosinophilic granuloma—Eosinophilic granuloma may occur in the clavicle, the scapula, or (rarely) the sternum. Coexisting infiltrates of the lung are often present. This condition often represents a more benign form of Langerhans cell histiocytosis or Hand–Schüller–Christian disease. Fever, malaise, leukocytosis, eosinophilia, or bone pain may be present. Rib involvement presents as a swelling with cortical bone destruction and periosteal new growth. The clinical picture can resemble osteomyelitis or Ewing sarcoma. When the disease is localized, excision will result in cure.

4. Hemangioma—Cavernous hemangioma of the ribs presents as a painful mass in infancy or childhood. The tumor appears on chest x-ray either as multiple radiolucent areas or as a single trabeculated cyst.

4. Miscellaneous—Fibromas, lipomas, osteomas, and aneurysmal bone cysts are all relatively rare lesions of the chest wall. The diagnosis is established after excisional biopsy.

D. Malignant Skeletal Tumors

1. Chondrosarcomas—Chondrosarcomas are the most common primary malignant tumor of the chest wall (20%-40%). They most commonly develop from the costochondral junctions of the first four ribs but can involve the sternum. About 15%-20% of all skeletal chondrosarcomas occur in the ribs or sternum. Most appear in patients 20-40 years of age. Local involvement of pleura, adjacent ribs, muscle, diaphragm, or other soft tissue may develop. Pain is uncommon and most patients complain only of the mass. Chest x-ray shows destroyed cortical bone, usually with diffuse mottled calcification, and the border of the tumor is indistinct. Successful treatment necessitates wide local excision and en bloc resection to achieve negative margins. Incomplete excision carries a significantly worse prognosis. Overall survival, as in all soft tissue sarcomas, is heavily dependent on the histologic grade. Completely resected low-grade chondrosarcoma has a 60%-80% 5-year survival rate. Patients with high-grade lesions who subsequently develop distant metastasis have only 20%-30% 5-year survival.

Although a complete resection can often be curative, local recurrence portends future metastatic disease and poor survival. Therefore, even in the setting of large tumors (> 15–20 cm), resection should be considered even if it necessitates removal of more than eight ribs. With epidural pain control and immediate reconstruction techniques, most patients will do well. Despite large chest wall resections, most patients can be immediately extubated and will not suffer drastic changes in pulmonary function or chest wall dynamics.

2. Ewing sarcoma (hemangioendothelioma, endothelioma)—Ewing sarcoma is a small, round cell-type tumor which most commonly occurs in a single rib. It accounts for 10%-15% of all primary chest wall tumors. Presentation as a primary chest lesion is not common (< 15%). Typically, Ewing sarcoma presents as a large, warm, painful soft tissue mass usually associated with pleural effusion. Systemic symptoms such as fever, malaise, and weight loss are common. Radiologic studies demonstrate the classic "onion skin" appearance caused by widening and sclerosis of the cortex as multiple layers of new bone are produced.

Diagnosis can usually be made by fine-needle aspirate or incisional biopsy. Histologically, these tumors are unique and consist of broad sheets of small polyhedral cells with pale cytoplasm and small hyperchromatic nuclei. They stain periodic acid-Schiff-positive.

Ewing sarcoma is commonly a disease of childhood and adolescence. The most important prognostic indicator for survival is development of distant metastases. Current therapy consists of neoadjuvant chemotherapy (including cyclophosphamide, dactinomycin, doxorubicin, and vincristine) surgical resection if the tumor is well demarcated and can be completely resected. Radiotherapy may be indicated as postoperative adjuvant treatment, or in the case of tumors that are not completely resectable. Overall, 5-year survivals range from 15% to 60%. Long-term survivals (10 years) are achievable in patients who do not develop metastases.

3. Osteogenic sarcoma (osteosarcoma)—Osteosarcoma occurs in the second and third decades, and 60% of cases occur in men. It is more aggressive than chondrosarcoma. X-ray findings consist of bone destruction and recalcification at right angles to the bony cortex, which gives the characteristic "sunburst" appearance. Osteogenic sarcoma most commonly presents as an extremity lesion, with only a small percentage of cases being chest wall primaries. Overall, less than 5% of all osteogenic sarcomas arise in the chest wall. Osteogenic sarcoma occurs in the second to fourth decades of life, half-again more commonly in men than in women. It is associated with environmental triggers, as well as with mutations in the retinoblastoma gene (RB1, 500-1000x risk) and Li-Fraumeni syndrome (p53, 15x risk). Typically, they are more aggressive tumors with a propensity for early metastasis to lung and bone.

Osteogenic sarcoma differs from chondrosarcoma in that it is usually sensitive to chemotherapy. They are treated with neoadjuvant chemotherapy followed by surgical resection. Even with neoadjuvant treatment, however overall 5-year survival after complete resection and postoperative chemotherapy may only be 15%.

4. Myeloma (solitary plasmacytoma)—Solitary plasmacytomas of the chest wall are comparatively rare lesions. They constitute 5%-20% of all chest wall tumors. Radiologically, they present as classic "punched-out" lytic lesions without evidence of new bone formation. They are more common in men than in women and typically present in the fifth to seventh decades of life. Over 75% of the time, solitary chest wall plasmacytomas are associated with diffuse multiple myeloma. Survival is based on the development of systemic disease. Local control and relief of pain are achieved with radiation therapy (usually 3000-4600 cGy). Once systemic disease is diagnosed, treatment consists of chemotherapy. Overall, 5-year and 10-year survivals for solitary plasmacytomas of the chest wall are 35%-40% and 15%-20%, respectively. Typical median survivals after treatment with radiation therapy and chemotherapy average 56 months.

E. Metastatic Chest Wall Tumors

Metastases to bones of the thorax are often multiple and are usually from tumors of the kidney, thyroid, lung, breast, prostate, stomach, uterus, or colon. Renal cell and thyroid malignancies have a high propensity for metastasizing to the sternum. Occasionally, they present as a pulsatile mass due to the excessive vascularity of the metastasis. An aneurysm of the ascending thoracic aorta, while rare, must be considered in the differential diagnosis and ruled out prior to attempts at excisional biopsy. Involvement by direct extension occurs in carcinoma of the breast and lung. Primary lung cancer with direct extension to chest wall without nodal involvement (T3 N0) carries a reasonable 5-year survival (10%-50%) when treated with radical en bloc resection. Lung metastasis with direct chest wall extension should be treated with radical en bloc resection of the chest wall and underlying lung.

Ferraro P et al: Principles of chest wall resection and reconstruction. *Thorac Surg Clin* 2010;20(4):465.
Hemmati SH et al: The prognostic factors of chest wall metastasis resection. *Eur J Cardiothorac Surg*. 2011;40(2):328.
Smith SE, Keshavjee S: Primary chest wall tumors. *Thoracic Surg Clin* 2010;20(4):495.

▼ DISEASES OF THE PLEURA

Diseases of the pleura may be benign or malignant and may represent primary pleural processes, localized extrapleural diseases, or systemic illnesses. The most common pleural problem is the presence of air (pneumothorax) within the pleural space. Pleural effusions—accumulations of fluid—result from benign sterile fluid, malignant fluid, pus, chyle, or blood. Primary pleural tumors are uncommon, but involvement of the pleura with metastatic cancer is common.

The most common symptoms of pleural disease are pain and dyspnea. The pain is sharp, and it is characteristically worsened by respiratory movements, often inhibiting inspiration. Pleural pain is mediated through somatic intercostal

nerves of the chest wall (cervical and costal pleura) and through the phrenic nerve (diaphragmatic and mediastinal pleura), causing chest wall or back pain and pain referred to the shoulder, respectively. The visceral pleura contains only sympathetic and parasympathetic nerve fibers and therefore is insensate; however, extension of visceral processes to involve the parietal pleura can produce typical pleuritic chest pain.

PLEURAL EFFUSION

Pleural effusion is the presence of fluid within the pleural space. More specific terminology may be used when the nature of the fluid is known. Hydrothorax is a collection of serous (most often transudative but also exudative) fluid, while pus in the pleural cavity is referred to as a pyothorax or empyema. Additional terms are used for blood (hemothorax) and chyle (chylothorax). Abnormal pleural fluid accumulates as a result of one or more of the following mechanisms: (1) increase in the pulmonary vascular hydrostatic pressure (congestive heart failure, mitral stenosis); (2) decrease in the vascular colloid oncotic pressure (hypoproteinemia); (3) increase in the capillary permeability due to inflammation (eg, pneumonia, pancreatitis, sepsis); (4) decrease in the intrapleural pressure (atelectasis); (5) decrease in the lymphatic drainage (carcinomatosis); (6) transdiaphragmatic movement of abdominal fluid through lymphatics or physical defects (ascites, pancreatic pseudocyst rupture); and (7) rupture of a vascular or lymphatic structure (traumatic injury).

Decreased respiratory excursion, diminished breath sounds, dullness to percussion, a pleural friction rub, and local tenderness are signs that indicate the presence of pleural effusion. With long-standing and advanced disease, contraction of the hemithorax with narrowed intercostal spaces and localized bulging, swelling, or redness may occur. Chest radiographs demonstrate varying degrees of opacification of the ipsilateral hemithorax. Accumulation of 300-500 mL fluid causes blunting of the costophrenic angle on x-ray. If the entire hemithorax is opacified, 2000-2500 mL may be present. The mediastinum may be shifted to the contralateral side in the presence of a large effusion, or it may remain in the midline—particularly if proximal bronchial obstruction results in lobar or total lung atelectasis, if the mediastinum is fixed from fibrosis or tumor infiltration, if the ipsilateral lung is infiltrated with tumor, or if malignant mesothelioma is present. CT scanning may be required to evaluate complex, loculated, or recurrent pleural fluid collections. Interventional radiology services are useful for loculated pleural effusions that may be managed by percutaneous drain placement under CT guidance.

Generally, serous effusions are separated into two broad categories—transudates and exudates—based on the physical and cellular characteristics of the pleural fluid. Identification of the specific type of effusion aids in determination of the cause and most often depends on examination of at least

20 mL of fluid obtained by thoracentesis. Basic tests should include total protein, lactate dehydrogenase (LDH), total and differential cell counts, glucose, pH, cytology, and Gram stain with culture. Furthermore, simultaneous serum total protein, LDH, and glucose should be measured. Effusions with total protein content less than 3 g/dL (or a fluid-serum ratio lower than 0.5), an LDH level less than 200 units/dL (or a fluid-serum ratio < 0.6), and a specific gravity below 1.016 represent transudates, while all other effusions are classified as exudates. The results of these basic tests frequently allow the underlying pathologic process to be elucidated (Table 18–1).

Table 18–1. Differential diagnosis of pleural effusions.[1]

	Tuberculosis	Cancer	Congestive Heart Failure	Pneumonia and Other Nontuberculous Infections	Rheumatoid Arthritis and Collagen Disease	Pulmonary Embolism
Clinical context	Younger patient with history of exposure to tuberculosis.	Older patient in poor general health.	Presence of congestive heart failure.	Presence of respiratory infection.	History of joint involvement; subcutaneous nodules.	Postoperative immobilized, or venous disease.
Gross appearance	Usually serous; often sanguineous.	Often sanguineous.	Serous.	Serous.	Turbid or yellow-green.	Often sanguineous.
Microscopic examination	May be positive for acid-fast bacilli; cholesterol crystals.	Cytology positive in 50%.	—	May be positive for bacilli.	—	—
Cell count	Few have > 10,000 erythrocytes; most have > 1000 leukocytes, mostly lymphocytes.	Two-thirds bloody; 40% >1000 leukocytes, mostly lymphocytes.	Few have > 10,000 erythrocytes or > 1000 leukocytes.	Polymorphonuclears predominate.	Lymphocytes predominate.	Erythrocytes predominate.
Culture	May have positive pleural effusion; few have positive sputum or gastric washings.	—	—	May be positive.	—	—
Specific gravity	Most > 1.016.	Most > 1.016.	Most > 1.016.	> 1.016.	> 1.016.	> 1.016.
Protein	90% 3 g/dL or more.	90% 3 g/dL or more.	75% > 3 g/dL.	3 g/dL or more.	3 g/dL or more.	3 g/dL or more.
Sugar	60% < 60 mg/dL.	Rarely < 60 mg/dL.	—	Occasionally < 60 mg/dL.	5–17 g/dL (rheumatoid arthritis).	—
Other	No mesothelial cells on cytology. Tuberculin test usually positive. Pleural biopsy positive.	If hemorrhagic fluid, 65% will be due to tumor; tends to recur after removal.	Right-sided in 55%–70%.	Associated with infiltrate on x-ray.	Rapid clotting time; LE cell or rheumatoid factor may be present.	Source of emboli may be noted.

Other exudates: spgr > 1.016
Fungal infection: Exposure in endemic area. Source fluid. Microscopy and culture may be positive for fungi. Protein 3 g/dL or more. Skin and serologic tests may be helpful.
Trauma: Serosanguineous fluid. Protein 3 g/dL or more.
Chylothorax: History of injury or cancer. Chylous fluid with no protein but with fat droplets.

[1]Modified from: Therapy of pleural effusion: A statement by the Committee on Therapy of the American Thoracic Society. *Am Rev Respir Dis.* 1968;97:479.

1. Hydrothorax

▶ Malignancy

More than 25% of all pleural effusions are secondary to cancer, and 35% of patients with lung cancer, 23% of patients with breast cancer, and 10% of patients with lymphoma develop malignant pleural effusions during the course of their disease. Approximately 10% of malignant effusions are secondary to primary pleural tumors, mostly mesothelioma. The mechanism is primarily through lymphatic obstruction in either the peripheral lung or central lymph node channels of the mediastinum. Malignant pleural effusions can be serous, serosanguineous, or bloody and are diagnosed primarily by demonstrating malignant cells in the fluid. Cytologic confirmation is successful 50%, 65%, and 70% of the time after one, two, or three thoracenteses, respectively. Closed pleural biopsy alone is successful in only 50% of cases, but coupled with thoracentesis it can increase the diagnostic yield to 80%. Thoracoscopy with direct pleural biopsy, however, is successful in 97% of patients and should be considered in any patient with a suspicious effusion after two negative thoracenteses.

Treatment of malignant effusions is strictly palliative: Most patients die within 3-6 months of developing a malignant pleural effusion, so prompt diagnosis and therapy are essential. The goals of treatment are lung reexpansion and pleural symphysis. This is most readily accomplished with placement of a chest tube (2028F) and closed-tube drainage for 24-48 hours. Generally, no more than 1 L is allowed to drain initially. Subsequently, 200-500 mL is allowed to drain every 1-2 hours until the effusion is fully drained. This controlled draining avoids the rare complication of reexpansion pulmonary edema. Once full lung expansion is obtained pleurodesis should be performed with an appropriate agent before loculations have formed. Different chemical, radioactive, and infectious agents have been used in the past with varying success rates, but most commonly used are talc (87%-100% insufflation; 83%-100% slurry), or doxycycline. Finally, mechanical pleurectomy without chemical instillation can control pleural effusions in over 99% of patients, but this requires an operative procedure. Talc is inexpensive, highly effective, and easily administered either as a powder insufflated into the open chest or as a slurry instilled through a chest tube.

Complications following pleurodesis include pneumothorax, loculated hydrothorax, fever, infection (empyema), acute respiratory distress syndrome (particularly following bilateral simultaneous pleurodesis, which for this reason alone are contraindicated), and recurrence. Problems are uncommon, and most patients can have their chest tubes removed within 48-72 hours following talc pleurodesis.

▶ Cardiovascular Disease

Pleural effusions are common findings in patients with moderate to severe congestive heart failure. Heart failure may be secondary to ischemia, valvular heart disease, viral myocarditis, congenital heart disease, and other less common lesions. The effusion may be bilateral or unilateral. When unilateral, the right hemithorax is most often affected. Fluid frequently involves the interlobar fissures (most commonly the minor fissure on the right) and can form localized collections simulating mass lesions known as "pseudotumors." Other cardiovascular causes of pleural effusions include constrictive pericarditis and pulmonary venous obstruction.

▶ Renal Disease

Hydronephrosis, nephrotic syndrome, and acute glomerulonephritis are on occasion associated with pleural effusions. Rupture of the collecting system into the pleural space can also produce a hydrothorax. In this latter case, the pleural fluid creatinine will be elevated (fluid-serum creatinine ratio significantly > 1.0).

▶ Pancreatitis

Moderate to severe pancreatitis is associated with a pleural effusion that characteristically occurs on the left and contains fluid with an amylase concentration substantially higher than that in the serum. Rarely pseudocysts of the capsule of the pancreas may communicate with the pleural space, resulting in high-volume pleural effusions.

▶ Cirrhosis

Approximately 5% of patients with cirrhosis and ascites will develop a pleural effusion. In contrast to pancreatitis, nearly all of these effusions occur on the right side.

▶ Thromboembolism

Pulmonary thromboemboli are sometimes accompanied by a pleural effusion. These effusions are typically serosanguineous and small, but they may be frankly bloody and massive. Characteristic x-ray findings are almost always present in the lung. Since the fluid is usually reabsorbed in a short period of time, drainage is seldom necessary.

2. Thoracic Empyema

Pyothorax (empyema thoracis) is the accumulation of pus within the pleural cavity. The pus is usually thick, creamy, and malodorous. If empyema occurs in the setting of underlying suppurative lung disease (ie, pneumonia, lung abscess, or bronchiectasis), it is referred to as a parapneumonic empyema (60% of cases). Other causes of thoracic empyema are surgery (20%), trauma (10%), esophageal rupture, other chest wall or mediastinal infections, bronchopleural fistula, extension of a subphrenic or hepatic abscess, instrumentation of the pleural space (thoracentesis, chest tube placement, etc), and, rarely, hematogenous seeding from a distant site of infection.

Empyemas are divided into three phases based on their natural history: acute exudative, fibrinopurulent, and chronic organizing. The *acute exudative phase* is characterized by the outpouring of sterile pleural fluid (incited by pleural inflammation), with a low viscosity, white blood cell count, and LDH concentration as well as normal glucose level and normal pH. The pleura remains mobile during this phase. The *fibrinopurulent phase* develops at approximately 2-7 days, marked by an increase in the turbidity, white blood cell count, and LDH levels in the fluid. Glucose levels and pH of the fluid decrease and fibrin is deposited on pleural surfaces, limiting the empyema but also fixing (trapping) the lung. The chronic organizing phase begins 7-28 days after the onset of the disease and is characterized by a pleural fluid glucose level less than 40 mg/dL and a pH less than 7.0. The pleural exudate becomes thick, and the pleural fibrin deposits thicken and begin to organize, further immobilizing the lung. In patients with inadequately treated chronic empyema, erosion through the chest wall (empyema necessitatis), chondritis, osteomyelitis of the ribs or vertebral bodies, pericarditis, and mediastinal abscesses may occur.

The bacteriology of thoracic empyema has evolved over the years. Prior to the discovery of penicillin in the 1940s, most empyemas were caused by pneumococci and streptococci. With modern antibiotics and improved anaerobic culture techniques, however, the most common isolates from adult empyemas are now anaerobic bacteria, particularly bacteroides species as well as fusobacterium and *Peptococcus* species.

Staphylococcus is the most common organism causing empyema (92% in children under 2 years), and staphylococcal empyema is one of the most common complications of staphylococcal pneumonias in both adults and children (Table 18–2). Gram-negative bacteria also continue to be significant pathogens, particularly in parapneumonic empyemas. *Escherichia coli* and pseudomonas species account for 66% of aerobic gram-negative empyemas, and

other organisms include *Klebsiella pneumoniae, Proteus* species, *Enterobacter aerogenes,* and *Salmonella.* Rarely, fungi (*Aspergillus, Coccidioides immitis, Blastomyces,* and *Histoplasma capsulatum*) and parasites such as *Entamoeba histolytica* can cause empyemas. In a review, empyemas were found to contain anaerobic bacteria in only 35% of cases, aerobic bacteria in only 24%, and a combination in 41%. In addition, the average number of bacterial species isolated was 3.2 per patient.

Aspiration of oropharyngeal flora may represent a source of polymicrobial infection. Although patients may rarely be completely asymptomatic, most patients with thoracic empyemas present with varying symptoms depending on the underlying disease process, the extent of the pleural involvement, and the immunologic state of the patient. Patients typically complain of fever, pleuritic chest pain or a sense of chest heaviness, dyspnea, hemoptysis, and a cough usually productive of purulent sputum. Signs of thoracic empyema include anemia, tachycardia, tachypnea, diminished breath sounds with dullness to percussion on the involved side, clubbing of fingertips, and occasionally pulmonary osteoarthropathy.

Although the medical history and physical examination often suggest the presence of thoracic empyema, the plain chest radiograph is the most important noninvasive diagnostic test. Empyemas may be associated with an underlying pneumonia, lung abscess, or pleural effusion and appear as posterolateral D-shaped densities on x-ray. In large empyemas, the mediastinum may be shifted away from the affected side. Bronchoscopy should be performed on all patients to exclude the presence of endobronchial obstruction. CT scanning provides critical anatomic detail regarding loculations and can assist in differentiation of empyema from lung abscess.

Thoracentesis is the procedure of choice for the diagnosis of thoracic empyema. Aspiration of pus establishes the diagnosis, permitting identification of the offending organisms. In early empyemas—particularly those partially treated with antibiotics—the pleural fluid may not be frankly purulent. In these cases, a pleural fluid pH less than 7.0, glucose less than 40 mg/dL, and an LDH level greater than 1000 units/L strongly suggest an evolving empyema even if Gram stain and cultures fail to identify organisms.

Goals for the treatment of thoracic empyemas include: (1) control of the infection; (2) removal of the purulent material with obliteration and sterilization of the pleural space and reexpansion of the lung; and (3) elimination of the underlying disease process.

Options for treatment include repeated thoracentesis, closed tube thoracostomy, rib resection and open drainage, decortication and empyemectomy, thoracoplasty, and muscle flap closure. Adjunctive maneuvers reported to aid in the disruption and drainage of loculated empyemas include instillation of fibrinolytic enzymes (such as tPA) and video-

Table 18–2. Incidence of various complications of staphylococcal pneumonia in adults and children (in %).

	Adults	Children
Abscess	25	50
Empyema	15	15
Pneumatocele	1	35
Effusion	30	55
Bronchopleural fistula	2	5

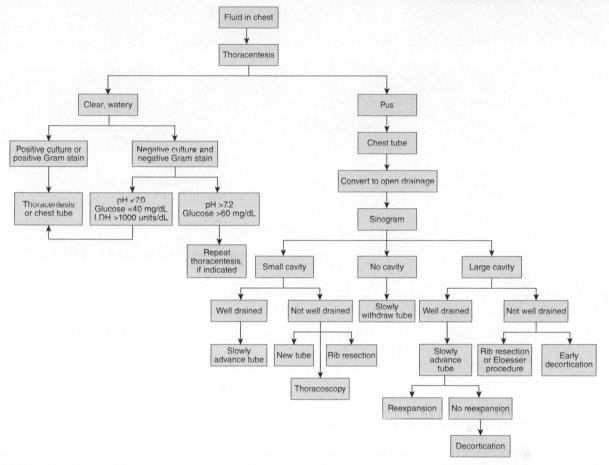

▲ **Figure 18–8.** Management of empyema. (Modified and reproduced with permission from Shields TW. *General Thoracic Surgery,* 3rd ed. Williams & Wilkins, Baltimore, 1989.)

assisted thoracoscopic debridement. A rational approach to empyema management is outlined in Figure 18–8. Initially, an intercostal catheter of adequate size is carefully inserted into the most dependent portion of the empyema cavity. If after 24–72 hours sepsis persists—or if there is any question as to the adequacy of drainage—a CT scan should be obtained. If, on the other hand, complete drainage and reexpansion of the lung are achieved, no further drainage procedures are necessary.

Patients with residual spaces that are inadequately drained, patients with continued sepsis, and patients thought to require prolonged tube drainage are candidates for open drainage procedures. These can usually be safely performed 10–14 days after closed-tube drainage, since the pleurae fuse by that time and the risk of pneumothorax and lung collapse is eliminated. Options for an open drainage include simple rib resection and open flap drainage

(Eloesser procedure). Simple rib resection involves the removal of short segments (3-6 cm) of one, two, or three ribs at the most dependent portion of the empyema cavity (at or anterior to the posterior axillary line). A tube can be placed through this opening and effective drainage established. A second approach involves the creation of a U-shaped flap of chest wall that is sewn to the parietal pleura after resection of short segments (3-6 cm) of one, two, or three ribs. This creates an epithelialized tract for long-term tubeless drainage of empyema cavities. This type of an open drainage allows the empyema cavity to drain reliably and to be easily debrided, irrigated, and cleaned. Ultimately, through lung reexpansion, wound contraction, and granulation, the cavity often completely disappears.

Another option is early decortication and empyemectomy. This is especially useful for good-risk patients with early loculated empyemas and inadequate tube drainage

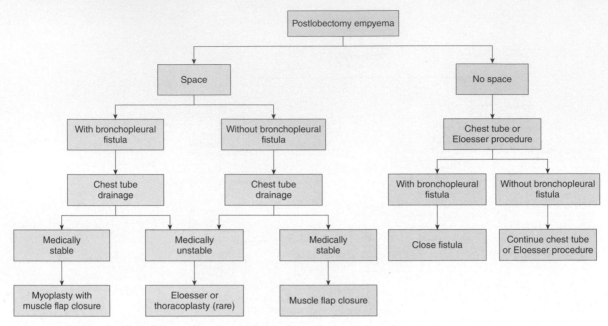

▲ **Figure 18–9.** Postlobectomy empyema. (Modified and reproduced with permission from Shields TW. *General Thoracic Surgery,* 3rd ed. Williams & Wilkins, Baltimore, 1989.)

or lung expansion. Furthermore, if performed early in the course of the process, resection of both parietal and visceral pleural peels (decortication) can be performed as a thoracoscopic procedure. More advanced or chronic disease involves a thoracotomy with decortication with resection of the intact empyema itself (empyemectomy), if possible. The best results with this approach are obtained when the underlying lung is entirely normal and reexpands fully. Posttraumatic empyema, in particular, has been amenable to this treatment.

Empyemas that occur following pulmonary resection may be difficult to manage. If residual lung is present (resections less than pneumonectomy), the general principles outlined above still apply, although a complicating bronchopleural fistula is often present (Figure 18–9). Simple tube drainage is instituted initially followed by open drainage if necessary. Empyemas following pneumonectomy, however, pose a special problem because there is no longer any lung to obliterate the infected space. In addition, postpneumonectomy empyemas frequently are associated with bronchopleural fistulas. In these patients, specific surgical procedures designed to obliterate residual intrathoracic spaces and in many cases close remaining bronchopleural fistulas may be required (Figure 18–10). In the absence of a bronchopleural fistula, sterilization and closure of a postpneumonectomy space (without obliteration) may be attempted using an irrigation catheter inserted into the apex of the chest cavity.

An antibiotic solution specific for the organisms present is then infused into the chest. The solution is allowed to drain through a dependent tube or opening created by simple rib resection. After 2-8 weeks, the catheters are removed and the cavity is closed. The success rate with this technique is quite variable and is reported to be 20%-88%. For patients who fail this approach and for those patients with bronchopleural fistulas, the main goal of therapy is to obliterate the residual space and close any bronchopleural fistulas. This is most readily accomplished by the transposition of muscle with or without omentum into the empyema cavity. Multiple muscles may be required, including pectoralis major, latissimus dorsi, serratus anterior, intercostal muscle, and rectus abdominis (Figure 18–11). Use of these muscles is highly successful in closing any remaining bronchopleural fistulas and in completely obliterating the remaining intrathoracic space. The success of muscle flap closure of empyema spaces has made thoracoplasty (once a common procedure for reducing empyema spaces) a rare operation.

Antibiotics are an important adjunct in the treatment of empyemas, but it must be emphasized that drainage is the primary treatment modality. Although antibiotic therapy is always instituted early in the course of therapy when signs of systemic infection generally are present, they need not be continued once effective drainage is established. In fact, overuse of antibiotics may lead to the generation of resistant bacteria and therefore compromise the success of

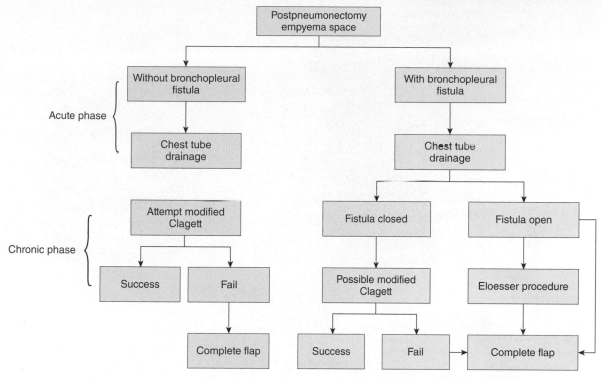

▲ **Figure 18–10.** Postpneumonectomy empyema. (Modified and reproduced with permission from Shields TW. *General Thoracic Surgery,* 3rd ed. Williams & Wilkins, Baltimore, 1989.)

any subsequent procedures designed to obliterate residual intrathoracic space.

Krassas A et al: Current indications and results for thoracoplasty and intrathoracic muscle transposition. *Eur J Cardiothorac Surg* 2010;37(5):1215.

3. Hemothorax

Blood in the pleural space usually occurs secondary to trauma, surgery, diagnostic or therapeutic procedures, neoplasms, pulmonary infarction, and infections (tuberculosis). Most hemothoraces can be treated effectively with large-bore (32-36F) closed chest tube drainage, particularly since small amounts of blood (occupying less than one-third of the hemithorax) are readily reabsorbed by the body. However, if significant blood clot has formed (occupying more than one-third of the hemithorax) or if secondary infection occurs, further measures must be taken to avoid the development of an empyema or fibrothorax with pulmonary compromise. Many hemothoraces requiring more than simple tube drainage can be managed with VATS procedures. Rarely, open thoracotomy may be required for complete decortication and evacuation.

4. Chylothorax

Accumulation of chyle within the pleural space is most often due to surgical procedures, particularly cardiothoracic and esophageal operations. Trauma, malignancy, central venous catheterization, congenital lymphatic malformations, thoracic aortic aneurysms, filariasis, and cirrhosis may also rarely cause chylothorax. Penetrating thoracic trauma can lacerate the thoracic duct at any level, but blunt thoracic trauma usually causes a shearing of the duct at the right crus of the diaphragm. This may also occur with violent coughing or hyperextension of the spine. The initial treatment of chylothorax is similar to that of a malignant pleural effusion. Closed chest tube drainage is instituted; the lung is fully reexpanded; and a low-fat diet is started. In some cases, intravenous hyperalimentation (either peripheral or central) may greatly improve the patient's condition. Some evidence supports the use of somatostatin to decrease the output from chylous effusions. The irritating nature of chyle promotes pleurodesis, and in half of patients the leak will stop spontaneously. The instillation of sclerosing agents (see section on pleural effusion, above) has also been advocated to increase the chances of success. If chyle continues to drain for more than 7 days or if significant drainage

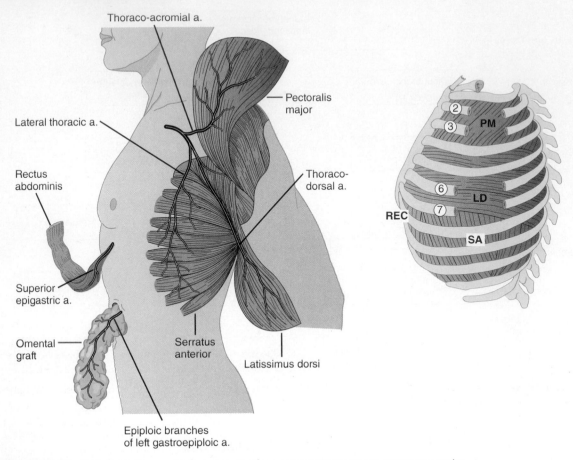

Thoraco-acromial a.

Pectoralis major

Lateral thoracic a.

Thoraco-dorsal a.

Rectus abdominis

Superior epigastric a.

Omental graft

Serratus anterior

Latissimus dorsi

Epiploic branches of left gastroepiploic a.

PM

LD

REC

SA

▲ **Figure 18–11.** Extrathoracic muscle flap closure of a postpneumonectomy empyema cavity.

continues for even a shorter period of time, serious consideration should be given to operation since patients quickly become malnourished from the large associated protein losses. Video-assisted thoracoscopic techniques are usually ideal, making open thoracotomy rarely necessary. The standard approach is via the right chest, where the thoracic duct may be identified as it emerges from beneath the diaphragm between the aorta and the azygos vein. Ligation of the tissues in this area is usually all that is needed.

PNEUMOTHORAX

Air in the pleural space (pneumothorax) can occur as a result of a breach in either the parietal (trauma, esophageal perforation, surgery, etc) or visceral pleura (bulla, fine-needle aspirations, etc). Rarely, infections of the pleural space with gas-forming organisms may produce a pneumothorax. Since a chest radiograph is only a two-dimensional representation of a three-dimensional space, a relatively small separation of

the pleural surfaces (eg, 1 cm) on a chest x-ray can translate into a relatively large pneumothorax. A large amount of intrapleural air that causes a shift of the mediastinum toward the contralateral lung is referred to as a tension pneumothorax. A pneumothorax associated with an open chest wound may be termed an open pneumothorax or sometimes a "sucking chest wound." *Tension and open pneumothoraces are surgical emergencies because both ventilation and venous return of blood to the heart are compromised.* Intrapleural air may mix with blood, as frequently occurs after trauma (hemopneumothorax) or esophageal perforation (pyopneumothorax).

Pneumothoraces usually are classified as either spontaneous or acquired (those caused by a specific event such as trauma, invasive procedures, etc). Spontaneous pneumothoraces sometimes are divided into "primary" and "secondary" categories; however, all spontaneous pneumothoraces are secondary to some underlying pathologic process, and such a division is therefore strictly artificial. Most commonly, spontaneous pneumothoraces are caused by rupture of small subpleural blebs due to increased transpulmonary pressure most pronounced at the apex of the lung (apex of the upper lobe and superior segment of the lower lobe). Coughing, rapid falls in atmospheric pressure (> 10 millibars/24 h), rapid decompression (scuba divers), and high altitudes (jet pilots) all are associated with increased transpulmonary pressures and spontaneous pneumothorax. In addition, normal transpulmonary pressures can cause rupture of blebs in patients with connective tissue disorders such as Marfan syndrome. Other causes of spontaneous pneumothorax include apical bullae (patients with chronic obstructive pulmonary disease [COPD]), *Pneumocystis* pneumonia (patients with AIDS), metastatic cancer (particularly sarcomas), lymphangioleiomyomatosis, eosinophilic granuloma, rupture of the esophagus or of a lung abscess, cystic fibrosis, and menstruation (catamenial pneumothorax). Classically, however, spontaneous pneumothoraces occur in asthenic males (male-to-female ratio 6:1) between the ages of 16 and 24, often with a history of smoking. The true incidence is unknown, since up to 20% of patients remain asymptomatic and do not seek medical attention.

Patients with pneumothoraces complain of pleuritic chest pain and dyspnea. If severe underlying cardiopulmonary disease exists or if a tension pneumothorax develops, symptoms become much more dramatic and include diaphoresis, cyanosis, weakness, and symptoms of hypotension and cardiovascular collapse. Physical examination reveals tachypnea, tachycardia, deviation of the trachea away from the involved side (tension pneumothorax), decreased breath sounds, hyperresonance, and diminished vocal fremitus on the involved side. Arterial blood gases may demonstrate hypoxia and occasionally hypocapnia from hyperventilation, and the EKG may show axis deviations, nonspecific ST segment changes, and T wave inversion. The standard test for the diagnosis of pneumothoraces is the posteroanterior (PA) and lateral chest radiograph. Exhalation accentuates the contrast between the collapsed lung and the intrapleural air as well as the magnitude of the collapse. Rarely, a CT scan may be necessary to differentiate a pneumothorax from a large bulla in patients with severe emphysema. In 5%-10% of patients, a small pleural effusion may be present and can be hemorrhagic.

The treatment of spontaneous pneumothoraces varies depending on the patient's symptoms and condition, the degree of collapse, the cause, and the estimate of the chance of recurrence. Small (< 20%-25%), stable, asymptomatic pneumothoraces in otherwise healthy patients can be followed (often on an outpatient basis) with the expectation of complete resolution within several weeks, since air is normally reabsorbed at a rate of 1%-1.25% per day. Larger asymptomatic pneumothoraces taking longer than 2-3 weeks to resolve place the patient at risk for developing trapped lung as a result of deposition of fibrin on the visceral pleura. These patients—as well as patients with symptoms, increas-

ing pneumothoraces, or pneumothoraces associated with pleural effusions—should have them evacuated. In highly selected patients, this can be accomplished with simple aspiration as long as the immediate and 2-hour delayed chest radiographs document reexpansion. It should be emphasized, however, that some small breaks in the visceral pleural seal once the lung collapses and can reopen with reexpansion. The chance of recurrence is 20%-50% with this method, and follow-up x-ray is therefore mandatory after 24 hours.

Most patients with significant pneumothoraces (> 30%) require placement of a closed-chest catheter (8-20F) for acceptable reexpansion. This catheter then can be placed either to underwater suction drainage or to a Heimlich (one-way) valve. If a Heimlich valve maintains full expansion, the patient may be treated as an outpatient; however, if a Heimlich valve fails to reexpand the lung fully or if the patient's condition is not optimal, admission to hospital and underwater chest tube suction drainage is required. Unless some contraindication exists, chest tubes should be placed in the midaxillary line at the level of the fifth intercostal space (nipple line). In women, the breast tissue should be retracted medially and avoided in the dissection to the chest wall. Placement with the use of blunt clamp dissection avoids the dangers of trocar insertion and should almost always be used. Following resolution of any air leakage, the tube may be taken off suction (water seal) and removed if the lung remains fully inflated. In patients with classic spontaneous pneumothoraces, the chance of recurrence increases with each episode. Following a single episode, the risk of a recurrent pneumothorax is 40%-50%. After two episodes, the risk increases to 50%-75%, and with three previous episodes, the risk is in excess of 80%. Currently, most first-time patients are treated initially with simple chest tube drainage; however, with subsequent recurrences, additional therapy generally is indicated. Furthermore, with the development of VATS, some feel that a more aggressive approach should be taken even for first-time pneumothoraces.

Patients with air leaks lasting longer than 7 days, patients who do not fully reexpand their lungs, patients in high-risk occupations (scuba divers, airline pilots, etc), patients with large bullae or poor pulmonary function, and patients with bilateral or recurrent pneumothoraces are candidates for additional medical (pleurodesis) or surgical intervention. Furthermore, patients who frequently travel to places distant from medical care are offered early surgical intervention. Previously, tetracycline pleurodesis was used to decrease the incidence of recurrent pneumothoraces. The use of this substance, however, was associated with significant pain and controversy. It is currently no longer available. The use of talc slurry or powder in this setting is also controversial due to the potential for long-term fibrothorax and restrictive lung disease but has been shown to reduce the recurrence rate to as low as 2%. Many other chemical agents have been used in the past, including mechlorethamine, doxycycline, iodoform, guaiacol, urea, and hypertonic glucose, with varying success rates. Since pleurodesis can make subsequent surgical procedures more difficult, the use of this treatment option continues to generate controversy.

Medically fit patients who are candidates for pleurodesis are also candidates for operation. The procedures used to prevent recurrent pneumothoraces include: (1) axillary thoracotomy with apical bullectomy, mechanical pleurodesis, and partial pleurectomy; and (2) complete parietal pleurectomy. Both procedures can be performed with either open or VATS techniques. Complete parietal pleurectomy generally is avoided, since some patients may require future thoracic surgical procedures that are extremely difficult in the face of total parietal pleurectomy. Apical bullectomy, mechanical pleurodesis, and partial apical pleurectomy have been shown to reduce the recurrence rate to near zero. In addition, this procedure is easily accomplished either with VATS techniques or through a small transaxillary thoracotomy, both of which are well tolerated.

Several special situations exist that require particular expertise in treatment decisions. Patients with cystic fibrosis and severe COPD may be candidates for lung transplantation, and both pleurodesis and operation may make subsequent transplantation more dangerous. Therefore, consultation with a transplant surgeon is advisable prior to considering these therapies. AIDS patients with *Pneumocystis* pneumonia and pneumothorax are extremely difficult to manage, having a high rate of persistent bronchopleural fistula, treatment failure, and death. For optimal management, the pulmonary surgeon should have extensive experience in the management of chest catheters.

PRIMARY PLEURAL TUMORS

Primary pleural tumors are uncommon neoplasms of two main types: diffuse malignant pleural mesotheliomas and localized fibrous tumors of the pleura (previously referred to as localized mesotheliomas). Although diffuse malignant pleural mesothelioma is the most common primary pleural tumor, involvement of the pleura with metastatic disease is more frequent and represents the most likely cause of any newly diagnosed pleural malignancy.

1. Localized Fibrous Tumors of the Pleura

Localized fibrous tumors of the pleura arise from subpleural fibroblasts than produce an array of lesions varying from peripheral pulmonary nodules to sessile subpleural masses to the more typical large pedunculated neoplasms. The visceral pleura is involved more often than the parietal pleural, and both benign (70%) and malignant (30%) variations exist. Histologically, benign tumors can exhibit three patterns—fibrous, cellular, and mixed—while malignant ones also have three distinct appearances: tubulopapillary, fibrous, and dimorphic. These tumors behave more like sarcomas

of the pleura than diffuse malignant mesotheliomas. Most localized fibrous tumors of the pleura are asymptomatic, discovered only incidentally on chest radiography. Extremely large tumors, however, may produce symptoms of bronchial compression with dyspnea, cough, and chest heaviness—and, rarely, symptoms of hypoglycemia from the production of an insulin-like peptide (4% of patients). On physical examination, signs of clubbing and hypertrophic pulmonary osteoarthropathy (20%-35%) may be present. Chest radiography most often demonstrates a well-circumscribed mass that may move with changes in position if the tumor is pedunculated. A pleural effusion is present in 15% of cases and can be bloody, though this does not indicate unresectability. Fine-needle aspiration cytology may be suggestive; however, the diagnosis generally can be established with certainty only at surgery.

The treatment of these lesions is a complete resection. Although lobectomy is usually not required for lesions involving the visceral pleura, wedge resection of the pulmonary parenchyma in the area of the tumor is recommended. For neoplasms arising from the parietal pleura, chest wall resection is prudent. Following complete surgical excision, no further therapy is indicated and the prognosis is good, with some patients surviving for over 10 years without recurrence; however, if the resection is incomplete, radiation therapy should be contemplated because the prognosis is poor, with a median survival of only 7 months.

2. Diffuse Malignant Pleural Mesothelioma

Diffuse malignant pleural mesothelioma is the most common primary tumor of the pleura. Since 1960, the disorder has been strongly linked to the use of asbestos. Thick serpentine asbestos fibers (chrysotile) generally are deposited in the proximal airways and are easily cleared with less risk of the development of tumors; however, thin needle-like amphibole fibers (crocidolite, amosite, actinolite, anthophyllite, and tremolite) and the soil silicate zeolite, found in the Anatolia region of Turkey, usually lodge in the terminal airways and migrate to the pleura, thereby increasing the risk of diffuse malignant pleural mesothelioma to more than 300 times that of the general population. The increased incidence of mesothelioma in shipbuilders exposed to asbestos-laden insulation from World War II-era ships further implicates asbestosis in the pathophysiology of the disease. The latency period after exposure ranges from 15 to 50 years. Recent research suggests that the generation of free radicals (including nitric oxide), depression of the immune system (both cellular and humoral), induction of cytokines (tumor necrosis factor [TNF]-α, interleukin [IL]-1α, IL-1β, and IL-6), and the production of genetic defects, such as abnormalities of chromosomes 1, 3, 4, 6, 7, 9, 11, 17 (p53), and 22 (involves *c-sis,* which encodes for one chain of platelet-derived growth factor) all may play a role in the mechanism of asbestos-related disease.

Histologically, diffuse malignant pleural mesotheliomas are divided into four categories: (1) epithelial or tubopapillary (35%-40%), which are associated with pleural effusions and a slightly better prognosis; (2) fibrosarcomatous or mesenchymal (20%), which are often "dry" mesotheliomas; (3) mixed (35%-40%); and (4) undifferentiated (5%-10%). The right hemithorax (60%) is affected more often than the left (35%) and 5% are bilateral.

Most patients with diffuse malignant pleural mesotheliomas complain of dyspnea on exertion and chest wall discomfort, but other symptoms, such as cough, fever (paraneoplastic), malaise, weight loss, and dysphagia, also occur. Complaints of severe chest wall pain, abdominal distention, pericardial tamponade, and superior vena cava syndrome suggest advanced disease. Although most patients develop distant metastases at some time during the course of their disease, these lesions rarely become symptomatic. Chest radiographs are distinctly abnormal, showing pleural thickening, effusion (75%), and narrowing of intercostal spaces. CT often suggests the diagnosis because of diffuse irregular pleural thickening. The diagnosis generally requires substantial tissue samples and is not generally obtainable from fine-needle aspiration cytology. Tissue can be easily acquired with VATS techniques.

Immunohistochemical stains for carcinoembryonic antigen, LeuM1, B72.3, and BerEP4 are usually negative, while those for vimentin and keratin are generally positive. Calretinin stain, which is specific for cells of mesothelial origin, has recently become available. This immunohistochemical marker can with near certainty determine whether an epithelial malignant tumor is either metastatic to pleura, for example, an adenocarcinoma (calretinin-negative) or a primary malignant mesothelioma (calretinin-positive). This stain has become an important clinical tool and should be performed on all suspected cases of diffuse malignant pleural mesothelioma. Electron microscopy may also be helpful in distinguishing this disorder from metastatic adenocarcinoma, with which it is often confused. Pathologic staging of diffuse malignant pleural mesothelioma, like its treatment (see below), has been controversial. The original Butchart staging system and a more recently promulgated tumor, node, metastases (TNM) staging system are set forth in the Table 18–3; however, neither is widely accepted or utilized.

The treatment of diffuse malignant pleural mesothelioma also remains variable. Owing to the low incidence of this disease, its natural history has not been carefully defined with regard to various prognostic factors, and few randomized trials have been conducted to compare treatment strategies. The reported median survival for all patients ranges from 7 months to 16 months. Recent randomized prospective trials have demonstrated benefit of platinum-based chemotherapy in combination with the antifolates pemetrexed or raltitrexed. Vogelzang and co-workers randomized 448 patients with unresectable pleural mesothelioma to receive cisplatin

Table 18–3. Staging systems for malignant mesothelioma.

BUTCHART STAGING SYSTEM

Stage I: Tumor is confined within the "capsule" of the parietal to pleura, ie, involving the ipsilateral pleura, lung, diaphragm, and external surface of the pericardium within the pleural reflection only.

Stage II: Tumor invades the chest wall or mediastinum (esophagus, trachea, or great vessels). Alternatively, lymph nodes within the chest are involved with metastatic disease.

Stage III: Tumor penetrates the diaphragmatic muscle to involve the peritoneum or retroperitoneum, the pericardium to involve the internal surface of heart, and the mediastinum to involve the contralateral pleura. Alternatively, lymph nodes outside the chest are involved with metastatic disease.

Stage IV: Distant hematogenous metastatic.

TNM STAGING SYSTEM

Tumor stage

TX: The primary tumor cannot be assessed.

T0: No evidence of primary tumor exists.

T1: The primary tumor is limited to the ipsilateral parietal or visceral pleura.

T2: Tumor invades any of the following: ipsilateral lung, endothoracic fascia, diaphragm, pericardium.

T3: Tumor invades any of the following: ipsilateral chest wall muscles, ribs, mediastinal organs or tissues.

T4: Tumor extends to any of the following: contralateral pleura or lung by direct extension, peritoneum or intra-abdominal organs by direct extension, cervical tissues.

Lymph node stage

NX: Regional lymph nodes cannot be assessed.

N0: No regional lymph node metastases are present.

N1: Metastases are present in ipsilateral bronchopulmonary or hilar lymph nodes.

N2: Metastases are present in ipsilateral mediastinal lymph nodes.

N3: Metastases are present in contralateral mediastinal, internal mammary, supraclavicular, or scalene lymph nodes.

Metastatic stage

MX: The presence of distant metastases cannot be assessed.

M0: No distant metastases exist.

M1: Distant metastases are present.

STAGE GROUPINGS

Stage I: T1–2, N0, M0

Stage II: T1–2, N1, M0

Stage III: T3, N0–1, M0; T1–3, N2, M0

Stage IV: T4, any N, M0; any T, N3, M0; any T, any N, M1

versus cisplatin in combination with pemetrexed. Patients treated with pemetrexed in addition to cisplatin demonstrated improved median survival (12.1 vs 9.3 months) and progression-free survival. The improved survival came at a cost of increased bone marrow–related toxicity (neutropenia and leukopenia). van Meerbeeck and co-workers demonstrated similar findings in a randomized sample of patients comparing cisplatin and combination cisplatin and raltitrexed. Mean survival in the cohort receiving combination cisplatinum and raltitrexed was 11.2 months versus 8.8 months in patients receiving cisplatin alone. Newer chemotherapeutic agents under active investigation include ranpirnase, intrapleural IL-2, and vascular endothelial-derived growth factor antagonists (bevacizumab).

Surgery alone has also been used in attempts to improve survival, and two major approaches have been utilized: radical pleuropneumonectomy or parietal pleurectomy with decortication. The initial experience with radical pleuropneumonectomy demonstrated only a higher associated morbidity but not better long-term survival when compared to less radical pleurectomy and decortication. When combined with postoperative chest wall irradiation, the latter procedure results in a median survival of up to 25 months. Other approaches have combined preoperative chemotherapy (MD Anderson), intraoperative and postoperative chemotherapy (Lung Cancer Study Group, Cleveland Clinic), photodynamic therapy (NCI), and immunotherapy with TNF-α as well as interferon (IFN)-α and IFN-Γ (NCI, SWOG) with limited success. Currently, the use of intraoperative radiation therapy (UCSF, MSKCC) and gene therapy are also being investigated. Although the general impression is that multimodality therapy is superior to any one therapy alone, the exact combination of treatment options for this disease is yet to be defined. It is clear, however, that new therapies are needed.

Chapman A et al: Population based epidemiology and prognosis of mesothelioma in Leeds, UK. *Thorax* 2008;63(5):435.

Kadota K et al: Pleomorphic epithelioid diffuse malignant pleural mesothelioma: a clinicopathological review and conceptual proposal to reclassify as biphasic or sarcomatoid mesothelioma. *J Thorac Oncol* 2011;6(5):896.

Rusch V et al: The role of surgical cytoreduction in the treatment of malignant pleural mesothelioma: meeting summary of the International Mesothelioma Interest Group Congress, September 11-14, 2012, Boston, Mass. *J Thorac Cardiovasc Surg* 2013;145(4):909.

▼ DISEASES OF THE MEDIASTINUM

MEDIASTINITIS

Mediastinitis may be acute or chronic. There are four sources of mediastinal infection: direct contamination, hematogenous or lymphatic spread, extension of infection from the neck or retroperitoneum, and extension from the lung or pleura. The most common direct contamination is esophageal perforation. Acute mediastinitis may follow esophageal, cardiac, and other mediastinal operations. Rarely, the mediastinum is directly infected by suppurative conditions involving the ribs or vertebrae. Most direct mediastinal infections are caused by pyogenic organisms. Most mediastinal infections that invade via the hematogenous and lymphatic routes are granulomatous. Contiguous involvement of the mediastinum along fascial planes from cervical infection is frequent; this

occurs less commonly from the retroperitoneum because of the influence of the diaphragm. Empyema often loculates to form a paramediastinal abscess, but extension to form a true mediastinal abscess is uncommon. Extension of mediastinal infections to involve the pleura is common.

1. Acute Mediastinitis

Esophageal perforation, the source of 90% of acute mediastinal infections, can be caused by vomiting (Boerhaave syndrome), iatrogenic trauma (endoscopy, dilation, operation), external trauma (penetrating or blunt), cuffed endotracheal tubes, ingestion of corrosives, carcinoma, or other esophageal disease. Mediastinal infection secondary to cervical disease may follow oral surgery; cellulitis; external trauma involving the pharynx, esophagus, or trachea; and cervical operative procedures such as tracheostomy, mediastinoscopy, and thyroidectomy.

▶ Clinical Findings

Emetogenic esophageal perforation (Boerhaave syndrome) is usually associated with a history of vomiting but in some cases is insidious in onset. Severe boring pain located in the substernal, left or right chest, or epigastric regions is the chief complaint in over 90% of cases. One-third of patients have radiation to the back, and in some cases pain in the back may predominate. Low thoracic mediastinitis can sometimes be confused with acute abdominal diseases or pericarditis. Acute mediastinitis is often associated with chills, fever, or shock. If pleural extension develops, breathing may aggravate the pain or cause radiation to the shoulder. Swallowing increases the pain, and dysphagia may be present. The patient is febrile, and tachycardia is noted. About 60% of patients have subcutaneous emphysema or pneumomediastinum. A pericardial crunching sound with systole (Hamman sign) is often a late sign. Fifty percent of patients with esophageal perforation have pleural effusion or hydropneumothorax. Pneumomediastinum or pneumothorax following esophageal endoscopy is sine qua non of esophageal perforation. Neck tenderness and crepitation are more often found in cervical perforations.

The diagnosis may be confirmed by contrast x-ray examination of the esophagus, preferably using thin barium. If no esophageal leak is evident then the study is completed using standard concentration barium. The use of water-soluble media is to be avoided to prevent consequences of water-soluble contrast aspiration in this population that is at increased risk for repiratory complication. Endoscopic visualization of the perforation is not recommended as an initial diagnostic maneuver as this may inadvertently extend the perforation. Chest CT scan with oral and intravenous contrast is helpful in determining the level of the perforation and the degree of mediastinal soilage as well as possible underlying esophageal or pulmonary pathology. The patient, however, must be clinically stable to be subjected to the rigors of these tests. For more critically ill patients, simple oral administration (or administration through a proximally placed nasogastric tube) of contrast and a simultaneous portable chest x-ray in an intensive care setting can often confirm the diagnosis. Myocardial infarction is sometimes mistakenly diagnosed in patients with esophageal perforation when a predisposing cause of pneumomediastinum is not apparent.

▶ Treatment

Surgical management of intrathoracic esophageal perforation depends on the underlying cause (iatrogenic, tumor, stricture, etc) and the amount of elapsed time from leak to diagnosis. All intrathoracic leaks should be surgically explored. Initial management includes immediate drainage of associated pleural contamination by large-bore chest tubes and decompression of the occasional pneumothorax. Broad-spectrum antibiotics, including antifungal therapy, are initiated and vigorous fluid hydration administered.

Typically, a right thoracotomy offers the most access to the intrathoracic esophagus and should be used through the sixth interspace. Even distal left-sided perforations can be managed from the right side. A left thoracotomy, however, is useful when a perforated esophagus from a distal esophageal stricture is encountered.

Treatment of an immediately recognized (< 24 h) iatrogenic esophageal perforation in an otherwise normal esophagus includes primary two-layer closure with careful attention to complete mucosal closure by interrupted absorbable sutures or surgical staplers. Esophageal muscle is then closed over the mucosal injury and buttressed with either a flap of parietal pleura, diaphragm, or intercostal muscle. Copious irrigation and wide drainage is performed. Occasionally, closure over a T-tube drain has been successful.

Esophageal perforations more than 48 hours old are widely drained and the esophagus either defunctionalized or resected. This depends on the degree of mediastinal soilage discovered upon exploration, the extent of sepsis, and the patient's performance status. When perforation occurs secondary to esophageal cancer or manipulation for severe reflux stricture, achalasia, or an otherwise abnormal esophagus, different surgical options exist. If the perforation is recognized immediately and the patient is not floridly septic, esophageal resection is preferred. Reconstruction (usually using a gastric conduit) can be done at the same setting but only if the patient is stable and the degree of contamination minimal. Otherwise, reconstruction is performed at a later date when the patient has fully recovered from the septic event. Esophageal stent placement and adequate drainage of the mediastinal and pleural spaces also can be considered.

The mortality associated with esophageal perforation remains high (30%-60%) despite advances in critical care, nutritional support, and operative management. The specific surgical approach—repair, resection, or endoscopic—must be tailored to the individual circumstances (mechanism of perforation, underlying pathology, time to diagnosis, and patient performance status) in order to achieve optimal results.

2. Chronic Mediastinitis

Chronic mediastinitis usually involves specific granulomatous processes with associated mediastinal fibrosis and chronic abscesses. Histoplasmosis, tuberculosis, actinomycosis, nocardiosis, blastomycosis, and syphilis have been incriminated. Amebic abscesses and parasitic disease such as echinococcal cysts are rare causes. The infectious process is usually due to histoplasmosis or tuberculosis and involves the mediastinal lymph nodes. Esophageal obstructions may occur. Adjacent mediastinal structures may become secondarily infected. Granulomatous mediastinitis and fibrosing mediastinitis are different manifestations of the same disease. Mediastinal fibrosis is a term used synonymously with idiopathic, fibrous, collagenous, or sclerosing mediastinitis. Eighty or more cases of mediastinal fibrosis have been reported, but the cause has been determined in only 16%, and of these over 90% were due to histoplasmosis. In only 25% of 103 cases of granulomatous mediastinitis has the cause been identified. Histoplasmosis was the most common known cause (60%) and tuberculosis the second-most common (25%).

About 85% of patients with mediastinal fibrosis have symptoms from entrapment of mediastinal structures as follows: superior vena caval obstruction in 82%; tracheobronchial obstruction, 9%; pulmonary vein obstruction, 6%; pulmonary artery occlusion, 6%; and esophageal obstruction, 3%. Rarely, inferior vena caval obstruction or involvement of the thoracic duct, atrium, recurrent laryngeal nerve, or stellate ganglion is found. Multiple structures may be simultaneously involved.

Seventy-five percent of patients with granulomatous mediastinitis have no symptoms, and disease is discovered by chest x-ray, which shows a mediastinal mass. The mass is in the right paratracheal region in 75% of cases. In the 25% of patients with symptoms, about half have superior vena caval obstruction and one-third have esophageal obstruction. Occasional patients have bronchial obstruction, bronchoesophageal fistula, or pulmonary venous obstruction.

A mediastinal tuberculous or fungal abscess occasionally dissects long distances to present on the chest wall paravertebrally or parasternally. Secondary rib or costal cartilage infections with multiple draining sinus tracts occur.

▶ Clinical Findings

A. Symptoms and Signs

Granulomatous and fibrosing mediastinitis affects women two to three times more commonly than men. Women aged 20-30 years are most typically affected, though the disorder may present in the fourth to fifth decades. Esophageal involvement results in dysphagia or hematemesis. Tracheobronchial involvement may cause severe cough, hemoptysis, dyspnea, wheezing, and episodes of obstructive pneumonitis. Pulmonary vein obstruction—the most common serious manifestation—produces congestive heart failure resembling advanced mitral stenosis and is usually fatal. Although not diagnostic, the respective skin tests in cases due to histoplasmosis or tuberculosis are strongly positive.

B. Imaging Studies

X-ray findings demonstrate a right paratracheal or anterior mediastinal mass. There may be spotty or subcapsular calcifications. Classically, histoplasmosis presents with hilar node calcification or so-called popcorn granuloma appearance. Calcification can also occur in thymoma or teratoma located in the anterior mediastinum. Chest CT (with intravenous and oral contrast) is most effective in defining the extent of mediastinal fibrosis and impingement on vital structures.

▶ Treatment

Specific antimicrobial therapy is indicated when an infecting organism is identified. Patients with symptomatic mediastinal masses and fibrosis can require resection for relief of obstruction.

▶ Prognosis

The prognosis following surgical excision of granulomatous mediastinal masses is good. Operative procedures do not appear to activate fibrosing mediastinitis, but success in treatment has been unpredictable. Most patients with fibrosing mediastinitis—whether treated or not—survive but have persistent symptoms.

Athanassiadi KA: Infections of the mediastinum. *Thorac Surg Clin* 2009;19(1):37.

Baillot R et al: Impact of deep sternal wound infection management with vacuum-assisted closure therapy followed by sternal osteosynthesis: a 15-year review of 23,499 sternotomies. *Eur J Cardiothorac Surg* 2010;37(4):880.

Kaye AE et al: Sternal wound reconstruction: management in different cardiac populations. *Ann Plast Surg* 2010;64(5):658.

SUPERIOR VENA CAVAL SYNDROME

Superior vena caval obstruction produces a distinctive clinical syndrome. Malignant tumors are the cause in 80%-90% of cases; lung cancer accounts for about 90%. The incidence of superior vena caval syndrome in lung cancer patients is 3%-5%. The male-to-female ratio is about 5:1. Other primary mediastinal tumors that may cause superior vena caval obstruction include thymoma, Hodgkin disease, and lymphosarcoma. Metastatic tumors from the breast or thyroid or from melanoma also occasionally cause superior vena caval obstruction. Benign tumors are an unusual cause, but substernal goiter, any large benign mediastinal masses, and atrial myxoma have been implicated. Thrombotic conditions, either idiopathic or associated with polycythemia, mediastinal infection, or indwelling catheters, are unusual causes. The association of superior vena caval obstruction with chronic mediastinitis is discussed in the preceding section. Trauma may produce acute venous obstruction (eg, traumatic asphyxia, mediastinal hematoma).

The clinical manifestations depend on the abruptness of onset, the location of the obstruction, the completeness of occlusion, and the availability of collateral pathways.

Venous pressure measured in the arms or head varies from 200 to 500 mm H_2O, and severity of symptoms is correlated with the pressure. Fatal cerebral edema can occur within minutes of an acute complete obstruction, whereas a slowly evolving one permits development of collaterals and may be only mildly symptomatic. Symptoms are milder when the azygos vein is patent. Azygous blood flow—normally about 11% of the total venous return—can increase to 35% of the venous return from the head, neck, and upper extremities. Thus, the most severe cases occur when occlusion is complete and the azygos vein is involved. The thrombus may propagate proximally to occlude the innominate and axillary veins.

▶ Clinical Findings

Symptoms include puffiness of the face, arms, and shoulders and a blue or purple discoloration of the skin. Central nervous system symptoms include headache, nausea, dizziness, vomiting, distortion of vision, drowsiness, stupor, and convulsions. Respiratory symptoms include cough, hoarseness, and dyspnea, often due to edema of the vocal cords or trachea. Nasal congestion is often an early presenting symptom. These symptoms are made worse when the patient lies flat or bends over. In long-standing cases, esophageal varices may develop and produce gastrointestinal bleeding. The veins of the neck and upper extremities are visibly distended, and in long-standing cases there are marked collateral venous channels over the anterior chest and abdomen. Chronic pleural effusions may develop as a result of impaired lymphatic drainage. Onset of symptoms in fibrosing mediastinitis may be insidious, consisting initially of early morning edema of the face and hands. Occasionally, symptoms and findings are localized to one side when the level of obstruction is above the vena cava and only the innominate vein is blocked. In this situation, symptoms are mild because communicating veins in the neck usually decompress the affected side.

The diagnosis can be confirmed by measuring upper extremity venous pressure; in patients with severe symptoms, a pressure of 350 mm H_2O or more is usual. Of patients with malignant vena caval obstruction studied by venography, 35% have thrombosis involving the innominate or axillary veins, 15% have complete caval obstruction without thrombosis, and 50% have partial superior vena caval obstruction. If patency of the azygos vein is in question, interosseous azygography may be useful. Chest x-ray may show a right upper lobe lung lesion or right paratracheal mass. Aortography is occasionally required to exclude aortic aneurysm. CT or MRI scan with contrast enhancement provides sufficient anatomic detail, supplanting the need for arteriography or venography as a diagnostic modality for this syndrome. The differential diagnosis may include angioneurotic edema, congestive heart failure, constrictive pericarditis, and fibrosing mediastinitis. Effort thrombosis of the axillary vein and innominate vein obstruction from elongation and buckling of the innominate artery can be considered in unilateral cases.

▶ Complications

In patients with partial superior vena caval obstruction, thrombosis may suddenly change mild symptoms to marked venous distention, cyanotic swelling, vocal cord edema, and impaired cerebration. Bleeding from esophageal varices is rare except in severe long-standing cases.

▶ Treatment

Superior vena caval obstruction caused by cancer should be treated with diuretics, restriction, avoidance of upper extremity intravenous lines, head elevation, and prompt radiation therapy. Cases of superior vena cava obstruction due to tumor begin to subside by 7-10 days of treatment. Because of the possibility of thrombosis in malignant cases, the use of fibrinolytic agents has been suggested. Caution must be advised in using anticoagulants, however, because many patients have advanced disease and may harbor occult cerebral metastases. Therefore, before starting therapy, patients should undergo CT or MRI brain scanning to prevent the occurrence of intracerebral hemorrhage. Recently, the use of intravascular expansile stents has been pioneered. Limited early experience suggests that the lumen can be reopened and that good venous drainage and decompression can be achieved by minimally invasive interventional radiologic techniques. Long-term results have not been reported, and disadvantages include the need for anticoagulation to prevent recurrent thrombosis. Chemotherapy is sometimes used alone or with radiotherapy. Most cases of malignant superior vena caval obstruction are not remediable by operation. Tissue diagnosis is important for diagnosis and for guiding therapy. Invasive procedures, however, must be tailored to the individual patient and the severity of the caval obstruction. Patients with new, severe, or rapidly progressive symptoms should receive immediate palliative radiation therapy. Patients with subacute presentations can better tolerate the time required to make the diagnosis.

Fine-needle aspiration, bronchoscopy, cervical mediastinoscopy, and anterior mediastinotomy—and even, occasionally, thoracotomy—offer possible approaches for obtaining tissue. Caution must be advised, however, in the setting of acute fulminant superior vena caval obstruction because any invasive procedure will carry a significantly higher morbidity due to bleeding from venous obstruction. In this case, attempts at invasive techniques for tissue diagnosis should be avoided. Most frequently, the disease process has been previously histologically confirmed because superior vena caval obstruction presents typically as a complication of locally advanced disease. In benign incomplete superior vena caval obstruction, surgical excision of the compressing mass can provide an excellent result. In total obstruction, such as occurs in fibrosing mediastinitis, most patients will gradually improve without treatment. There are numerous surgical procedures designed to bypass caval obstruction, replace the superior vena cava, or recanalize the vena caval lumen. These procedures have been dramatically effective in some cases, but only recently have they been sufficiently successful to warrant consideration.

▶ Prognosis

Radiotherapy is most effective when superior vena caval obstruction is incomplete. Mean survival of patients with malignant caval obstruction from lung cancer is 6-8 months. The death rate from causes related to vena caval obstruction itself is only 1%-2%.

MEDIASTINAL MASS LESIONS

Lesions within the mediastinum include a variety of masses, both malignant and benign, that arise from the diverse organs and tissues which occupy the central thorax. Overall, the incidence of all mediastinal masses is low, especially compared with the frequency of lesions arising within the lung (bronchogenic cancer, etc). Mediastinal malignancies constitute less than 20% of all thoracic tumors.

Mediastinal masses arise from specific structures that reside in relatively constant anatomic arrangement. The mediastinum itself is defined laterally by the mediastinal pleura of each lung; superiorly and inferiorly by the thoracic inlet and diaphragm, respectively; anteriorly by the sternum; and posteriorly by the vertebral bodies. For purposes of definition, the mediastinum is divided loosely into three main compartments: anterior (or anterosuperior), middle, and posterior. The anterior mediastinum contains the thymus, fat, and lymph nodes while the middle mediastinum contains the heart, pericardium, ascending and transverse aorta, brachiocephalic veins, trachea, bronchi, and lymph nodes. The posterior mediastinum consists of the descending thoracic aorta, esophagus, azygous vein, autonomic ganglia and nerves, lymph nodes, and fat. This has important implications for diagnosing suspected masses. The likelihood of malignancy is influenced primarily by three main factors: anatomic location, age, and the presence or absence of symptoms. Although two-thirds of mediastinal tumors are benign, masses in the anterior compartment are more likely to be malignant. Age is an important predictor as well with many lymphomas and germ cell tumors presenting between the second and fourth decade of life. Symptomatic patients are more likely to have a malignancy. Although classically in adults the majority of mediastinal masses tend to be benign (cysts, neurogenic tumors, etc), recent series have demonstrated a shift toward malignant processes being more prevalent.

An anterior mediastinal mass can indicate the following: thymoma (the most common), thymic hyperplasia, thymolipoma, thymic cyst, thymic carcinoid, thymic carcinoma, germ cell tumor (teratoma, seminoma, and non-seminomatous germ cell tumor), lymphoma, parathyroid adenoma, substernal thyroid, and lymphangioma. A middle mediastinal mass can include lymphoma, pericardial cyst, bronchogenic cyst, aneurysm, and lymphadenopathy. A posterior mediastinal mass can include neurogenic tumor, enteric cyst, bronchogenic cyst, meningocele, diaphragmatic or hiatus hernia, and paravertebral abscess. The most common mediastinal masses in children are neurogenic tumors (50%-60%). In young children (< 4 years of age), they are invariably malignant (neuroblastomas). In the adults, a neurogenic tumor is the most common mediastinal mass. This arises in the posterior compartment (typically from a peripheral nerve sheath) and is usually benign, occasionally calcified, and well circumscribed.

An extensive workup of a mediastinal lesion is usually not required for diagnosis since surgery is usually required both to establish the diagnosis and provide effective treatment. Standard PA and especially lateral chest films will often provide much useful information; however, contrast CT scanning has become the diagnostic test of choice. MRI, while helpful for assessing vascular or spinal cord extension, has not proved to be more effective than dynamic CT scanning.

Fluoroscopy may show pulsation or variation of shape or location with change of position and respiration. Tomography may reveal calcification or air-fluid levels. Barium swallow is used to evaluate intrinsic esophageal lesions or esophageal displacement by extrinsic masses. Contrast studies of the intestinal tract may reveal the stomach, colon, or small bowel in a hernia. Myelography can be of crucial importance in neurogenic tumors to explain symptoms or to plan operative management. CT angiography can identify aneurysms or displacement. Pulmonary arteriography may be useful to distinguish mediastinal and pulmonary tumors.

Scintigraphy scanning is important in evaluating possible substernal goiter in anterior mediastinal lesions, since goiters can generally be removed by the standard cervical approach. Skin tests and serologic studies may be used in suspected granulomatous disease. Bone marrow examination, hormone assays, and serum tumor markers (α-fetoprotein [AFP], β-human chorionic gonadotropin [β-HCG], and LDH) are important adjuncts to evaluate a suspected germ cell tumor.

Bronchoscopy and esophagoscopy are occasionally useful to identify primary lung lesions or lesions of the esophagus. Mediastinoscopy and mediastinal biopsy must be used cautiously in mediastinal tumors that are potentially curable. Excisional biopsy is imperative in lesions (eg, thymomas) that are histologically difficult to evaluate since a curable but locally invasive malignancy might be dispersed. Mediastinoscopy is useful for the diagnosis of sarcoidosis, Castleman disease, or disseminated lymphoma.

▶ Clinical Findings

Symptoms are more frequent among patients with malignant rather than benign lesions. About one-third of patients have no symptoms. Those patients who become symptomatic can present with cough (60%), chest pain (30%), fevers/chills (20%), or dyspnea (16%). Hemoptysis and, rarely, expectoration of cyst contents may occur. Weight loss and dysphagia are found each in about 10% of patients. Myasthenia gravis (MG) (15%-20% with thymoma), fever, and superior vena caval obstruction are each found in about 5% of patients.

Symptoms can be categorized into two groups: localizing symptoms and systemic symptoms. Localizing symptoms are secondary to tumor invasion and include respiratory compromise, dysphagia, paralysis of the limbs, diaphragm, and vocal cords, Horner syndrome, and superior vena cava syndrome. These findings are concerning for a malignant process. Malignant tumors, especially lymphomas, may produce chylothorax. Systemic symptoms are typically due to the release of excess hormones, antibodies, or cytokines. Thymoma has been associated with myasthenia, hypogammaglobulinemia, Whipple disease, red blood cell aplasia, and Cushing disease. Hypoglycemia is a rare complication of mesothelioma, teratoma, and fibroma. Hypertension and diarrhea occur with pheochromocytoma and ganglioneuroma. Neurogenic tumors may produce specific neurologic findings from cord pressure or may be associated with hypertrophic osteoarthropathy and peptic ulcer disease.

A. Neurogenic Tumors

Neurogenic tumors are derived from tissue of the neural crest, including cells of the peripheral, autonomic, and paraganglionic nervous systems. Neurogenic tumors almost always occur in the posterior mediastinum—often the superior portion—arising from intercostal or sympathetic nerves. Rarely, the vagus or phrenic nerve is involved. Seventy to eighty percent of all neurogenic tumors are benign. The most common tumor (40%-65%) arises from the nerve sheath (schwannoma and neurofibroma) and is usually benign. Malignant tumors occur more frequently in children. Most malignant tumors (neuroblastoma, etc) arise from the nerve cells. Neurogenic tumors may be multiple or dumbbell in type, with widening of the intervertebral foramen. In these cases, MRI is necessary to determine if the mass extends within the spinal canal. Dumbbell tumors have been removed in the past by a two-stage approach, though a single-stage approach is now more widespread. [123]I metaiodobenzylguanidine scintigraphy can be applicable particularly for patients with middle metastinal tumor suspected to be a pheochromocytoma.

B. Mediastinal Cystic Lesions

Cysts of the mediastinum may arise from the pericardium, bronchi, esophagus, or thymus. Pericardial cysts are also called "springwater" or mesothelial cysts. Seventy-five percent are located near the cardiophrenic angles and 75% of these are on the right side. Ten percent are actually diverticula of the pericardial sac that communicate with the pericardial space. Bronchogenic cysts arise close to the main stem bronchus or trachea, often just below the carina. Histologically, these contain elements found in bronchi, such as cartilage, and are lined by respiratory epithelium. Enterogenous cysts are known by several names, including esophageal cyst, enteric cyst, or duplication of the alimentary tract. They arise along the surface of the esophagus and may be embedded within its wall. They may be lined by squamous epithelium similar to the esophagus or gastric mucosa. Enterogenous cysts are occasionally associated with congenital abnormalities of the vertebrae. About 10% of cysts in the mediastinum are nonspecific, without a recognizable lining.

C. Germ Cell Tumors

Germ cell tumors are common mass lesions found in young adults and represent 15% of anterior mediastinal mass lesions. Malignant germ cell tumors are more common in men (>90%). Historically, they are both solid and cystic, and the more differentiated tumors can contain hair or teeth. Microscopically, ectodermal, endodermal, and mesodermal elements are present. These tumors occasionally rupture into the pleural space, lung, pericardium, or vascular structures. Most germ cell tumors of the mediastinum are metastatic and present with concomitant retroperitoneal disease.

Primary mediastinal extragonadal germ cell malignancies are rare, representing less than 5% of all mediastinal germ cell cancers and less than 5% of all primary mediastinal tumors. As pluripotent cells, germ cell tumors (GCTs) can give rise to several histologically distinct malignancies, including seminoma (40%), embryonal carcinomas and nongestational choriocarcinomas (20%), and yolk sac tumors (20%). Teratomas (20%) can have both benign and malignant components. Almost all such tumors (> 90%) produce

tumor markers, including β-HCG and AFP. LDH—a nonspecific tumor marker—is produced by most bulky mediastinal germ cell tumors and is often an effective indicator of tumor burden.

Much progress in treating these tumors has been made with multi-modality therapy (surgery, radiation therapy, and chemotherapy). Currently, over 50% 5-year survival is achievable for nonseminomatous GCT, and over 90% 5-year survival is typical for seminomatous mediastinal GCT. Patients should be screened and followed with AFP, β-HCG, and LDH markers. Resection should be offered after combination chemotherapy has been administered and only after all elevated tumor markers have normalized.

Residual mediastinal masses following chemotherapy and normalization of tumor markers should be resected. At surgery, approximately 40% will be mature teratomas (with the potential for malignant degeneration), 40% necrotic tumors, and 20% residual tumors (requiring postoperative salvage chemotherapy). Rarely is palliative debulking surgery indicated if tumor markers remain elevated after several cycles of chemotherapy. Instead, alternative chemotherapy or investigational therapy should be offered.

D. Lymphoma

Lymphoma is usually associated with disseminated disease metastatic to the mediastinum. It is typically identified in the anterior compartment but can present anywhere through the mediastinum. This is the second-most common mass in the anterior mediastinum. Occasionally, lymphosarcoma, Hodgkin disease, or reticulum cell sarcoma arises as a primary mediastinal lesion.

▶ Treatment

Treatment is tailored to the specific disease process causing the mediastinal mass. In almost all cases, tissue diagnosis is imperative for guiding appropriate therapy. Minimally invasive techniques (fine-needle aspiration or core-needle biopsy) or mediastinoscopy and mediastinotomy are appropriate for diagnosis of a mediastinal mass that is secondary to metastatic disease (eg, lymphomas and germ cell tumors). Mediastinal masses that represent primary malignancies (thymoma, neurogenic tumors, etc) are treated usually with initial resection. Percutaneous biopsy of primary malignancies should be reserved for patients with locally advanced disease, considered either unresectable or suitable for preoperative systemic therapy and/or radiation therapy prior to attempted resection.

Surgical approaches include median sternotomy (anterior masses), posterolateral thoracotomy (posterior and middle mediastinal masses) as well as VATS or bilateral anterior thoracotomy (all mediastinal compartments). Adjuvant chemotherapy is important for malignant germ cell lesions, malignant neurogenic tumors, and bulky or advanced thymomas. Postoperative radiation therapy decreases local recurrence in higher stage thymoma and in other incompletely resected lesions. Radiation and chemotherapy constitutes the principal therapy for primary mediastinal lymphoma.

Complete resection is the treatment of choice for all neurogenic tumors. A standard posterolateral thoracotomy offers optimal exposure; however, more limited incisions, including thoracoscopy, can be effective for resection of clinically benign small (< 6 cm) lesions. Dumbbell lesions involving the spinal canal warrant a neurosurgical consultation. For lesions that cannot be completely excised, postoperative radiation may decrease local recurrence and symptoms. Incompletely excised or especially large or infiltrative neuroblastomas should receive combination radiation and chemotherapy in conjunction with surgery.

▶ **Prognosis**

Overall, the outlook for patients with mediastinal masses has improved, with advances in combined chemotherapy and multimodality therapy. Surgical morbidity and mortality remain low (1%-4%). Patients with benign mediastinal lesions do significantly better (> 95% cure rates) than those who have malignant mediastinal masses (< 50% overall survival).

Albany C et al: Extragonadal germ cell tumors: clinical presentation and management. *Curr Opin Oncol* 2013;225(3):261-265.
Boateng et al: Vascular lesions of the mediastinum. *Thorac Surg Clin* 2009;19:91-105.

TUMORS OF THE THYMUS & MYASTHENIA GRAVIS

The thymic gland is the site of a variety of neoplasms that include thymoma, lymphoma, (eg, Hodgkin disease), granuloma, and other less common tumors. Cell types of the thymus include epithelial cells, myoid cells, thymic lymphocytes, and B lymphocytes. Tumors of the thymus can arise from any of these cell types with thymic epithelial tumors (thymoma, thymic carcinoma, and neuroendocrine tumor) being the most common. Lymphoid or hematopoietic neoplasms and mesenchymal tumors occur less frequently. Thymoma is a primary neoplasm of the thymus gland arising from thymic epithelial cells without cytologic or histologic signs of malignancy. A well-differentiated thymic carcinoma has some cytologic features of atypia, and thymic cancer cells are cytologically malignant. Thymoma is the most common tumor of the anterior mediastinum composing approximately 50% of all tumors of the anterior mediastinum and 15%-20% of all mediastinal tumors.

Thymoma may be classified according to predominant cell type into lymphocytic (25%), epithelial (25%), and lymphoepithelial (50%) varieties. Spindle cell tumor, which is sometimes associated with red cell aplasia, is considered among the epithelial tumors. The histologic subtypes have not been associated with prognostic significance. The World Health Organization (WHO) consensus guidelines provide a histologic classification system for thymoma and thymic carcinoma based on both morphology and lymphocyte-to-epithelial cell ratio. The WHO classification system classifies thymoma and thymic carcinoma in categories ranging from type A (bland spindle cells and limited lymphocytes) to type C (grossly atypical cells that are indicative of thymic carcinoma). The identification of a single pathologic subtype is difficult however, since there is considerable histologic heterogeneity. The Masaoka staging system, originally described in 1981 and revised in 1994, is the most frequently used staging method of thymoma and thymic carcinoma. This staging system classifies thymoma into four stages based on the presence of invasion and anatomic extent of involvement observed both clinically and histopathologically. The Masaoka staging system has been shown to be a significant independent factor for survival, with 5-year survival rates by stage approaching 98%-100% for stage I and II diseases, 88% in stage III disease, and 70% for patients with stage IVa and 52% for IVb, respectively. The WHO classification system as well as the Masaoka staging system is set forth in Table 18–4.

MG is a neuromuscular disorder characterized by weakness and fatigability of voluntary muscles owing to decreased numbers of acetylcholine receptors at neuromuscular junctions. Because of the high incidence of thymic abnormalities, improvement after thymectomy, association with other autoimmune disorders, and presence in the serum of 90% of patients of an antibody against acetylcholine receptors, MG is thought to be of autoimmune etiology. About 30% of patients with thymoma have MG, and about 15% of patients with myasthenia develop a thymoma. Thymic carcinoma, which carries a worse prognosis than other thymomas, is

Table 18–4. Staging system for malignant thymoma.

STAGE	DESCRIPTION
I	Macroscopically, completely encapsulated; microscopically, no capsular invasion.
IIa	Macroscopic invasion into surrounding fatty tissues or mediastinal pleura (without microscopic invasion).
IIb	Microscopic evidence of capsular invasion or microscopic invasion of surrounding fatty tissues or mediastinal pleura.
III	Macroscopic invasion into a neighboring organ (pericardium, great vessels, or lung).
IVa	Pleural or pericardial dissemination.
IVb	Lymphatic or hematogenous distant metastases.

rarely associated with MG. About 85% of patients with MG have thymic abnormalities consisting of germinal center formation in 70% and thymoma in 15%. MG can occur in association with tumors of any cell type but is more common with the lymphocytic variety. The mean age of patients with thymoma-associated MG is between 44 and 49 years of age without significant differences between males and females. Patients with thymoma-associated MG tend to be younger than those with non-MG thymoma.

▶ Clinical Findings

Fifty percent of thymomas are first identified in an asymptomatic patient on a chest x-ray obtained for another purpose. Symptomatic patients may present with chest pain, dysphagia, myesthenic symptoms, dyspnea, or superior vena caval syndrome. Paraneoplastic symptoms are fairly common in the setting of thymoma and account for approximately 60% of all presentations of thymoma.

CT with intravenous contrast of the chest provides information on the size, density, and relationship of the tumor to the surrounding intrathoracic organs and vessels. It may also reveal any pleural metastases. MRI is occasionally helpful to assess vascular invasion.

The diagnosis of MG can be made from the patient's history of easy fatigability and associated decremental response in muscular contraction to repeated stimulation of the motor nerve or from improvement in these abnormalities in response to edrophonium (Tensilon), a short-acting anticholinesterase drug.

Level of clinical suspicion for thymoma may dictate the need for biopsy prior to resection. In patients with a high likelihood of thymoma, excision without biopsy may be both diagnostic and therapeutic. CT-guided core needle biopsy is a useful and less invasive technique for determining histology of an anterior mediastinal mass, but should be considered only if there is evidence for local invasion such that a greater extent of resection might be necessary. Definitive diagnosis of thymoma is based on histologic study of a tissue sample usually after excisional biopsy or a complete resection has been performed. Small, well-encapsulated anterior mediastinal masses should not be biopsied, as the procedure penetrates the tumor capsule and can lead to tumor seeding and recurrence, thus jeopardizing the opportunity for cure of an early-stage thymoma.

▶ Treatment

The surgical approaches to thymectomy are varied and reflect the balance between complete, curative resection and the magnitude and morbidity of a procedure. All approaches enable a complete resection of the capsular thymus with the extent of peri-thymic mediastinal and cervical tissue resection distinguishing each of the procedures. The goal of the operation is total thymectomy. Transsternal thymectomy with en bloc resection of the anterior mediastinal fat tissue from phrenic to phrenic laterally and the diaphragm to the thyroid gland is considered the standard, classical operative approach. Alternative approaches include transcervical thymectomy and minimally invasive approaches such as VATS thymectomy and robotic-assisted thymectomy. The latter approaches, while useful for thymectomy for benign conditions (myasthenia, etc), arguably have a limited role in the surgical treatment of malignant thymoma.

Despite a paucity of randomized controlled trials, summary treatment guidelines for each stage of the disease have been established by consensus in the literature. Multidisciplinary discussion is encouraged to assure appropriate therapy is recommended and provided. For disease stages I and II (see Table 18-4), complete resection alone is the standard of care. Radiotherapy may be considered for patients at risk for recurrence. Risk factors for recurrence include invasion through the capsule, close surgical margins, WHO grade B type, and a tumor adherent to the pericardium. Patients presenting with resectable or potentially resectable stage III disease should be evaluated for multimodality therapy. Surgical resection can be considered either initially or following neoadjuvant therapy if complete resection is not initially feasible. Neoadjuvant or induction chemotherapy may decrease the volume of the tumor, thereby facilitating complete resection. If resection is not appropriate then chemotherapy, either concurrent or sequential, with radiotherapy can be considered. For patients with stage IVA disease, operation can be considered only if pleural or pericardial metastases are resectable.

Anticholinesterase drugs (eg, neostigmine bromide) are given as initial treatment to patients with MG. Corticosteroids may be given in selected cases, but a high incidence of side effects makes them unsuitable for more liberal use. Early thymectomy is now recommended for all patients with symptomatic MG whether or not a thymoma is suspected. The course of the disease is usually improved, and subsequent development of a malignant thymoma is eliminated. Thymectomy can be postponed in the occasional patient with mild disease well controlled by anticholinesterase therapy.

Following thymectomy, about 75% of patients with MG are improved and 30% achieve complete remission. Younger patients benefit more from thymectomy than do those over the age of 40 years, but a positive effect also accrues to the latter group. Recently, minimally invasive approaches to thymectomy for myasthenia patients has resulted in reduced length of stay, decreased blood loss, and decreased pain in comparison with more traditional partial sternal splitting procedures.

▶ Prognosis

The rates of complication and death with thymectomy are low except in the setting of locally advanced disease.

Respiratory care of patients with MG in the immediate postoperative period now presents little difficulty because of the availability of anticholinesterase drugs. Recent evidence including a retrospective review by Okereke et al suggests that neither MG nor paraneoplastic syndromes are associated with a poor prognosis and there are no differences in survival between those with and without MG.

The Masaoka staging system has been widely accepted as the best predictor of survival in thymoma patients. Although in general the WHO histologic classification of thymoma has been considered reproducible, issues have been raised regarding interobserver variability which may impact its prognostic ability. Completeness of resection has been shown to be an important independent predictor of survival.

Overall survival rates are extremely good for early-stage thymomas, and 10-year survival rates are excellent. Stage I lesions approach 100% 10-year survival rates. Stage II tumors with resection and postoperative radiation therapy have approximately 75% 10-year survival rates. Patients with locally advanced stage III thymoma, however, have long-term survival rates of less than 25%. Outcomes with multimodality therapy (neoadjuvant chemotherapy, surgery followed by chemotherapy and radiation therapy) are improving, as marked by significant tumor responses and enhanced resectability rates. Long-term disease specific survival can be expected not only after surgery for early-stage thymoma but also after surgery for advanced disease, including select patients with pleural metastases. However, patients who undergo surgery for stage IVa disease have reduced disease-free survival.

THYMIC CARCINOMA

This tumor is a rare variant (< 15%) of thymic lesions and is histologically and biologically quite different from invasive or malignant thymoma. A large number of histologic types of thymic carcinoma have been described and range from low-grade, well-differentiated neoplasms to high-grade, poorly differentiated malignancies. The most common type of thymic carcinoma in Western patients is poorly differentiated, nonkeratinizing squamous cell carcinoma. Thymic carcinomas tend to be very invasive and difficult to resect completely. Unfortunately, even in the setting of a complete resection, recurrence is common both locally and at distant sites. Still, when at all possible, an aggressive combined-modality approach (induction chemotherapy, resection, and postoperative chemoradiotherapy) should be employed. Typically, these are young men (< age 50 years) with an otherwise excellent performance status. While a good response to induction therapy and a complete resection will provide a significant disease-free interval, long-term survival is still unlikely. Better systemic agents and a molecular understanding of this cancer holds hope for significant improvements in cure rates.

Casey EM et al: Clinical management of thymoma patients. *Hematol Oncol Clin N Am* 2008;22(3):457.

Falkson CB et al: The management of thymoma: a systematic review and practice guidelines. *J Thorac Oncol* 2009;4(7):911.

Moran CA, Suster S: Thymic carcinoma: current concepts and histologic features. *Hematol Oncol Clin N Am* 2008:22(3):393.

Okereke IC et al: Prognostic indicators after surgery for thymoma. *Ann Thorac Surg* 2010;89(4):1071.

▼ DISEASES OF THE LUNGS

CONGENITAL CYSTIC ANOMALIES OF THE LUNG

Congenital lesions of the lung include primarily tracheobronchial atresia, bronchogenic cysts, pulmonary dysplasia, pulmonary sequestration, congenital cystic adenomatoid malformations (CCAM), and congenital lobar emphysema (CLE). Although many of these lesions present early in life with dramatic symptoms and physical findings, most remain occult until late childhood and even into adult life. These uncommon lesions arise from aberrations in normal aerodigestive tract development, which begins during the fourth week of fetal life when the lung bud forms at the caudal end of a groove in the primordial pharynx. An initial phase of sequential airway branching occurs until as many as 20-25 generations are reached by the sixteenth week of fetal life. These branches are divided into three zones: a proximal conductive zone (branches 1-16), an intermediate transitional zone (branches 17-19), and a distal respiratory zone (branches 20-25). A second canalicular phase is then entered as capillaries develop in the distal air passages. Finally, the alveolar phase begins at approximately 26 weeks of fetal life as prototype alveolar air sacs appear complete with both type I and type II pneumocytes. The number and size of alveoli continue to increase until the total alveolar surface reaches the adult size of nearly 100 m^2.

A. Tracheobronchial Atresia

Atresia of the tracheobronchial tree can occur at any level and may involve an isolated segment or multiple diffuse areas of the airway. Tracheal atresia is associated with polyhydramnios, prematurity, esophageal atresia, and tracheoesophageal fistula. Typically, neonates present with intractable cyanosis and despite a normal-appearing larynx are unable to be intubated. Emergency tracheostomy can be life-sustaining in babies with isolated subglottic atresia; in other infants with more diffuse disease, mask ventilation can achieve some palliation through anomalous esophagobronchial connections. Diffuse airway involvement, however, is invariably fatal.

Isolated bronchial atresia results in a bronchus that ends in a blind pouch. A mucocele develops distal to the obstruction and, as a result of compression of neighboring normal bronchial structures, causes emphysematous changes in the surrounding lung. Since children frequently develop wheezing, stridor, and pulmonary infections in the involved segments, resection is almost always indicated. Like bronchial atresia, true congenital bronchial stenosis is rare, although right main stem bronchial stenosis occurs not infrequently from iatrogenic airway trauma in chronically ventilated patients.

Related anomalies of the tracheobronchial tree include anomalous tracheal or esophageal bronchi and tracheal diverticula. These rare lesions often present with symptoms of bronchial obstruction and in many cases require resection of involved lung tissue due to chronic infection and the development of bronchiectasis (see section on Bronchiectasis). Similar to pulmonary sequestration, these lesions can have a dominant systemic arterial blood supply that must be kept in mind if operation is contemplated.

B. Bronchogenic Cysts

Bronchogenic cysts are the most common cystic lesions of the mediastinum and arise from abnormal budding of the foregut during development. The cyst wall consists of fibroelastic tissue, smooth muscle, and cartilage, whereas the cyst itself is lined with respiratory tract epithelia. It may also contain mucus-producing cuboidal cells, which contribute to enlargement of the cyst with mucus. They may occur anywhere along the tracheobronchial tree but occur most commonly in the vicinity of the right pulmonary hilum and subcarinal region. Less frequently, they present in the neck, lower lobes of the lung, pleura, pericardium, or below the diaphragm. When large, cysts can compress surrounding vital structures, including the aerodigestive tract causing dysphagia, pneumothorax, cough, or hemoptysis or become infected. The diagnosis is confirmed by CT as a spherical fluid- or mucus-filled nonenhancing mass. An air-fluid level may be present thus suggesting communication with the airway. Cysts within the pulmonary parenchyma more commonly communicate with a bronchus, as opposed to those in the mediastinum. In general, mediastinal bronchogenic cysts present with airway compression and parenchymal cysts are manifested by pulmonary infection. Some cysts have been noted to enlarge rapidly and rupture into the pleural space, causing tension pneumothorax. Rare cases of malignant transformation have been reported. All bronchogenic cysts—regardless of location—are best treated with either simple or segmental resection by VATS or thoracotomy. Rarely, lobectomy is required.

Correia-Pinto J, et al. Congenital lung lesions underlying molecular mechanisms. *Semin Pediatr Surg* 2010;19(3):171.
Masters IB: Congenital airway lesions and lung disease. *Pediatr Clin North Am* 2009;56(1):227.

C. Bronchopulmonary Dysplasia

Bronchopulmonary dysplasia (BPD) is a form of chronic lung disease that occurs in infants, usually in preterm infants receiving respiratory support with mechanical ventilation or prolonged oxygen supplementation. With the introduction of positive pressure ventilation in newborn infants Northway et al originally described a pattern of lung injury characterized by airway injury, inflammation, and parenchymal fibrosis in preterm infants who had received mechanical ventilation. Since the introduction and implementation of antenatal corticosteroids and postnatal surfactant replacement BPD now more commonly affects those of extremely low birth weight and born less than 26 weeks of gestation. BPD nowadays is fundamentally viewed as the result of abnormal reparative processes in response to injury and inflammation occurring in an immature lung of a genetically susceptible infant. The pathogenesis of BPD begins with a very immature lung complicated by iatrogenic damage from therapy with oxygen and volume ventilation with superimposed infection and inflammation as well as pulmonary edema complicated by poor nutrition. Treatment is supportive combining new approaches to ventilation (nasal CPAP and inhaled nitric oxide) with vitamin A. The American Thoracic Society has recently published a position paper on the care of the child with chronic lung disease of infancy and childhood that addresses many of these issues.

D. Pulmonary Aplasia and Agenesis

Pulmonary hypoplasia is a relatively common abnormality of lung development and is defined pathologically as an abnormally low radial alveolus count and low ratio of lung weight to body weight. Pulmonary hypoplasia is termed primary pulmonary hypoplasia when no inciting cause is identified and is likely caused by abnormalities of the transcription factors that regulate early lung morphogenesis. These neonates present with tachypnea and hypoxemia resistant to administration of supplemental oxygen due to abnormal thickening of the pulmonary arteriolar wall. Persistent fetal circulation, hypoxemia, hypercapnia, and acidosis lead to early death in over 75% of patients. Secondary pulmonary hypoplasia is associated with a restriction of lung growth or the absence of fetal breathing. Any reduction of the chest cavity by a mass, effusion, or external compression can impact lung growth. The most common of these abnormalities is congenital diaphragmatic hernia (see Chapter 43). Other conditions associated with secondary pulmonary hypoplasia include those that produce oligohydramnios and direct chest compression (eg, bilateral renal agenesis [Potter syndrome], renal dysplasia, and amniotic fluid leaks); those with abnormal bone development and small rigid chest walls (eg, achondroplasia, chondrodystrophia fetalis calcificans, osteogenesis imperfecta, and spondyloepiphyseal dysplasia); those with decreased fetal respiratory movements (eg, phrenic nerve agenesis, abdominal masses or ascites with elevation of the diaphragm, arthrogryposis multiplex congenita, camptodactyly, and congenial myotonic dystrophy); those with intrathoracic mass lesions (eg, CCAM, cystic hygroma, esophageal duplication cysts); and those with pulmonary vascular abnormalities (eg, scimitar syndrome, pulmonary artery agenesis).

Unilateral pulmonary agenesis occurs when one lung and the associated vascular structures fail to develop. Neonates with pulmonary agenesis may present with tachypnea and cyanosis, particularly if associated cardiac anomalies exist (50% of cases). Some patients, however, remain asymptomatic until childhood, when they complain of dyspnea and wheezing suggestive of asthma. Physical examination in these patients reveals marked tracheal deviation toward the side of the agenesis, and chest x-ray, barium esophagography, and chest CT may be required to exclude other diagnostic possibilities such as total lung atelectasis from foreign body aspiration, total lung sequestration, and esophageal bronchus.

E. Pulmonary Sequestration

Pulmonary sequestration describes a mass of lung parenchyma that arises through abnormal budding of the caudal embryonic foregut and consequently has *no bronchial communication* with the otherwise normal tracheobronchial tree. Sequestration may occur either within normal lung tissue, termed intralobar sequestration, or as separate masses with their own visceral pleura, referred to as extralobar sequestration. The majority (85%) of sequestrations are of the intralobar type. Intralobar sequestrations receive their blood supply from the thoracic or abdominal aorta and splenic artery and their venous drainage from the pulmonary veins. In some cases this may be associated with anomalous venous drainage of the normal lung. Intralobar sequestrations are most commonly found on the left side in the lower lobe. Extralobar sequestrations are less common and receive their blood supply from the thoracic or abdominal aorta and the venous drainage via the systemic veins such as the hemiazygos or azygous veins or inferior vena cava. Both are associated with foregut communications but more commonly in extralobar sequestrations.

Intralobar sequestrations are usually diagnosed later in childhood or adolescence with multiple episodes of pneumonia. Common symptoms include a chronic or recurrent cough. Extralobar sequestrations usually present in infancy with respiratory distress and chronic cough or manifest as gastrointestinal symptoms if a communication with the gastrointestinal tract exists. In rare instances, patients may present with hemoptysis or congestive heart failure from large left-to-right shunts through the sequestration. The diagnosis is usually suspected on chest x-ray and confirmed with a CT scan of the chest delineating the arterial and venous

drainage. Angiography can be used to confirm the diagnosis and elucidate aberrant vascular anatomy. Treatment consists of segmental resection or, if necessary, lobectomy via thoracotomy or video-assisted procedure. Great care must be taken to identify the nature of both the arterial blood supply and the venous drainage to avoid exsanguinating hemorrhage from division of an unrecognized systemic artery or venous infarction of the normal lung from ligation of the common draining vein. Following successful resection, the prognosis is favorable.

F. Congenital Cystic Adenomatoid Malformation

CCAM is the second most common cause of newborn respiratory distress, secondary to structural problems. CCAM is a discrete, space-occupying intrapulmonary mass that contain variable-sized cysts. These lesions do not function in normal gas exchange yet airspaces within these masses communicate with the tracheobronchial tree. Histologically, CCAM is distinguished from other lesions and normal lung by polypoid projections of the mucosa, an increase in smooth muscle and elastic tissue within cyst walls, an absence of cartilage, the presence of mucus-secreting cells, and the absence of inflammation. The classification system described by Stocker organizes these lesions on pathologic appearance and clinical outcome. Class I consists of large cysts greater than 2 cm; class II consists of small cysts less than 2 cm; class III consists of solid lesions without cysts. Children will present either at birth or in early childhood with recurrent respiratory infections. The growth of CCAMs usually plateaus between 25 and 28 weeks, at which time the fetus appears to grow around the lesion. The vast majority of small- to moderate-sized CCAMs remain asymptomatic during fetal life. Approximately 15% of CCAMs will shrink significantly before birth. However, large lesions represent 5%-10% of CCAMs and may produce significant mass effect, which can lead to pulmonary hypoplasia, impaired fetal swallowing and polyhydramnios, and impaired venous return and heart failure. Fetal hydrops can result and appears to depend on the size and rate of growth of the mass, and result from compression of the superior vena cava and impaired venous return. As therapeutic fetal interventions have become feasible, the ability to predict which infants will progress to hydrops has become critical. High-resolution fetal MRI can calculate a cyst volume ratio which is useful in predicting progression to hydrops. Fetal interventions including a short course of maternal betamethasone for microcystic CCAM and minimally invasive *in utero* thoracoamniotic shunting for macrocystic CCAM have been shown to be successful. If fetal development is uncomplicated, early delivery is not encouraged. At birth, the infants are stratified based on symptoms. Critically ill infants require immediate resection of the involved lobe. An asymptomatic neonate should be initially evaluated with chest radiography. While surgery can be delayed in those patients with small lesions, any patient with known CCAM should undergo elective resection due to possible future complications including pneumonia and malignant transformation.

G. Congenital Lobar Emphysema

CLE is the cause of half of the episodes of newborn respiratory distress due to structural abnormalities and is defined as an overdistended lobe resulting from the obstruction of a lobar bronchus. Obstruction can arise from abnormal cartilage development or an ischemic event during bronchial development. CLE also can develop as the result of meconium aspiration, lobar torsion, or an extrinsic cause such as obstructing lymph nodes. The left upper lobe is most commonly involved, and with the right middle lobe next in prevalence. In addition, neonates who require prolonged mechanical ventilation (eg, those with hyaline membrane disease) can develop lobar emphysema from a combination of suction catheter trauma and barotrauma. The right lower lobe is most frequently affected in such patients. Most infants present within the first 6 months of life with respiratory distress. In some patients, severe respiratory distress may occur in the neonatal period, requiring emergency evaluation and treatment. Almost all infants present with tracheal and mediastinal deviation away from the affected side, hyperresonance and decreased breath sounds on the affected side, and a chest radiograph demonstrating hyperlucency in the area of the affected lobe with compression of adjacent lung. A chest radiograph often is sufficient before proceeding with operation. Occasional patients, particularly older children, may require chest CT scans to exclude other pathology (eg, bronchogenic cysts, anomalous pulmonary vessels, and hilar lymphadenopathy). Bronchoscopy also may be necessary to rule out the presence of a foreign body causing ball-valve airway obstruction. Successful therapy in all patients requires pulmonary resection, which almost uniformly consists of lobectomy. Great care is necessary with airway management at the time of induction of general anesthesia in these patients as positive-pressure ventilation can result in further shifting of the mediastinum resulting in impaired venous return and cardiovascular collapse. If such a situation arises, an emergent thoracotomy should be preformed to allow for the affected lobe to "herniate out" of the incision decompressing mediastinal pressure. Even after lung resection, patients may have bronchomalacia and a tendency toward bronchospasm.

CONGENITAL VASCULAR LESIONS OF THE LUNG

Vascular diseases of the lung include two main processes: arteriovenous malformations and vascular rings. Arteriovenous malformations are uncommon congenital lesions that develop as a result of abnormal capillary formation during the canalicular phase of development. Most arise from the pulmonary artery, but occasionally a systemic arterial source can be involved similar to that in pulmonary sequestration. Rarely, an arteriovenous malformation can arise from a coronary artery, with the right coronary artery involved 55% of the time. Coronary arteriovenous fistulas drain into the right ventricle (40%), right atrium (25%), pulmonary artery (20%), coronary sinus (7%), superior vena cava (1%), or left-sided heart chambers (7%). Patients are either asymptomatic or develop signs of congestive heart failure. Myocardial infarction is rare. A continuous murmur and signs of reduced left ventricular afterload may be present. Although the diagnosis often can be established with echocardiography and color Doppler imaging, the definitive diagnosis, shunt fraction, and complete preoperative planning require catheterization and angiography. Operation is indicated for symptomatic patients and for those asymptomatic patients with large shunts.

Vascular rings occur from abnormal development of the aortic arches and major branches, with resulting compression of the trachea and esophagus. In normal fetal development, a dual system of six aortic arches regresses in such a way that the left fourth arch becomes the main left-sided aorta, the left sixth arch develops as the ductus arteriosus, and the right fourth arch persists as the right innominate artery and subclavian artery. Most vascular rings, however, are associated with a right-sided aortic arch and are classified as complete vascular rings or incomplete rings (arterial slings). Complete vascular rings include a double aortic arch (67%, the most common complete ring), a right aortic arch with a left subclavian and left ductus arteriosus (30%), a right aortic arch with mirror-image branching and a left ductus arteriosus (rare), and a left aortic arch with an aberrant right subclavian and right ductus arteriosus (very rare). Incomplete rings consist of an aberrant right subclavian artery that originates on the left side and passes posterior to the esophagus (most common incomplete ring) and an anomalous left pulmonary artery arising from the right pulmonary artery and passing between the trachea and the esophagus (pulmonary artery sling).

Most patients present with symptoms of tracheal or esophageal compression. Patients with an anomalous right subclavian artery may present later in life with obstructive symptoms (dysphagia lusoria), while those with complete vascular rings and pulmonary artery slings typically present early in life (within 6 months) with symptoms of respiratory distress (often frank stridor), particularly with neck flexion and poor feeding. The diagnosis is often suggested by characteristic findings on barium esophagogram. Bilateral indentations imply double aortic arch. A posterior indentation suggests an aberrant right subclavian artery, large right-sided indentations suggest complete rings associated with a right aortic arch, and an anterior impression is typical of a pulmonary artery sling. Often, the diagnosis can be confirmed by echocardiography. MRI/MRA often provides useful anatomic details. Surgical repair of these lesions is indicated once the diagnosis is established and is accomplished by dividing the vascular ring usually through a left thoracotomy. With double aortic arches, the smaller of the two arches is divided distal to the subclavian artery, while other complete rings generally are treated by division of the ligamentum arteriosum. Aberrant right subclavian arteries may be simply divided or, if necessary, divided and transposed to the right side. Pulmonary artery slings require reimplantation of the left pulmonary artery and often resection of the compressed trachea, which often has severe tracheomalacia and stenosis. Rarely, tracheomalacia secondary to vascular ring compression necessitates suspension of the aortic arch from the sternum.

SUPPURATIVE DISEASES OF THE LUNG

1. Lung Abscess

A lung abscess usually begins as a necrotizing pneumonia progessing to liquefactive necrosis of the lung parenchyma. The liquefied necrotic material eventually empties into a draining bronchus, forming a necrotic cavity of pus containing an air-fluid level. With rupture, the infection can extend into the pleural space, producing an empyema. Arbitrarily, abscesses are termed acute if the duration is less than 6 weeks and chronic if more than 6 weeks. Although the incidence of lung abscesses fell dramatically following the introduction of effective antibiotics in the 1940s and 1950s, a recent increase in the number of immunocompromised individuals secondary to organ transplantation, chemotherapy, and AIDS has resulted in a resurgence in the numbers of lung abscesses requiring treatment.

Lung abscesses can be divided into two major categories based on etiology: primary and secondary. Lung abscesses are termed primary when they arise in a previously healthy individual or secondary to an underlying cause. Most commonly a primary abscess occurs as a result of aspiration owing to impaired consciousness or swallowing dysfunction due to neuromuscular or esophageal diseases. Sixty to seventy percent of lung abscesses present in the right lung in the dependent posterior segment of the right-upper lobe and superior segment of the lower lobe. They are most commonly polymicrobial with a predominance of anaerobic organisms including *Peptostreptococcus, Bacteroides fragilis*, and *Fusobacterium*. Conditions that predispose to aspiration include anesthesia (both general and monitored), neurologic disorders (cerebrovascular accidents, seizures, diabetic coma, head trauma, etc), drug ingestion (alcohol, narcotics, etc), normal sleep, poor oral hygiene (increases bacterial load), and esophageal disease (gastroesophageal reflux, achalasia, cancer, tracheoesophageal fistula). Secondary causes include bronchial obstruction (tumor, foreign body, hilar lymphadenopathy), necrotizing pneumonia (*S auerus, K pneumoniae*),

chronic pneumonia (due to fungi, tubercle bacilli), and opportunistic infection in an immunodeficient host. Over the years the incidence of secondary lung abscess arising in the setting of an immunocompromised state has increased. As a result, virulent aerobic species such as *Klebsiella, Pseudomonas, Proteus, Enterobacter*, and *S aureus* now comprise the majority of these infections as opposed to anaerobic species. Gram-negative lung abscess occurs in elderly and immunocompromised patients with nosocomial pneumonia. Cavitating lesions may arise in the setting of a malignancy or pulmonary infarct. Direct extension of a localized infection such as amebiasis or subphrenic abscess may also progress to a secondary lung abscess. Blood-borne infections can give rise to multiple lung abscesses in the periphery of the lung and are the result of septic emboli from bacteria, endocarditis, septic thrombophlebitis, or subphrenic infection. It should be noted that secondary infections of congenital or acquired cystic lesions, such as bronchogenic cysts, bullae, tuberculous cavities, and hydatid cysts, are not true pulmonary abscesses because they occur in a preformed space.

▶ Clinical Findings & Diagnosis

Patients with lung abscesses typically reports symptoms of cough, fever, putrid sputum, hemoptysis, dyspnea, pleuritic chest pain, and weight loss. Symptoms are often insidious in onset and associated with malaise and weight loss if chronic. Complications include rupture into a bronchus, with initial hemoptysis followed by the production of foul-smelling, purulent sputum (and the potential for life-threatening pneumonia from aspiration of pus into normal lung); rupture into the pleural space with resulting pyopneumothorax, sepsis, and possibly empyema necessitatis; and, rarely, massive hemoptysis requiring emergent pulmonary resection. On physical examination, signs of lobar consolidation predominate; but clubbing, signs of pleural effusion, cachexia, and rarely a draining chest wound (empyema necessitatis) can be present. Laboratory studies should include a differential white blood cell count and sputum culture. Chest radiography and CT scan of the thorax are usually sufficient to aid diagnosis and differentiate between empyema and abscess. Cavitation is generally apparent on chest radiographs 2 weeks after the onset of symptoms. Radiological resolution lags behind clinical and biochemical improvement, taking up to 3 months to resolve in up to 70%. In cases of suspected bronchial obstruction or in all patients with unexplained lung abscesses, bronchoscopy is indicated. Fine-needle aspiration of the abscess cavity for diagnostic culture has been shown to isolate the offending pathogens in 94% of patients compared with only 11% and 3% from sputum culture and bronchoalveolar lavage, respectively. Early fine-needle aspiration can prompt a change of the antibiotic regimen in 43% of cases and can be life-saving in immunocompromised patients with unusual organisms.

Treatment

Antibiotic administration has been the mainstay of therapy following general resuscitation measures. First-line treatment should include aerobic and anaerobic coverage for a period of 4-6 weeks. Once the acute sepsis subsides (after up to 2 weeks), therapy can frequently be changed to an oral outpatient regimen and continued until complete resolution of the abscess occurs (3-5 months). Important adjuncts to antibiotic administration include chest physiotherapy, postural drainage, bronchoscopy (may require repeated examinations to maintain bronchial drainage), and health maintenance measures (general nutrition, dental hygiene, etc).

In patients who do not respond to this initial regimen and who do not have surgical indications (see below), early percutaneous drainage has been shown to be a safe and effective procedure (mortality rate, 1.5%; morbidity rate, 10%). Specific proposed indications for percutaneous drainage include: (1) an abscess under tension as evidenced by mediastinal shift, displacement of fissures, or downward displacement of the diaphragm; (2) radiographic verification of contralateral lung contamination; (3) unremitting signs of sepsis after 72 hours of adequate antibiotic therapy; (4) abscess size larger than 4 cm or increasing abscess size; (5) rising fluid level; and (6) persistent ventilatory dependency.

In addition to drainage, intervention permits microbiological analysis of the aspirate. In up to 47% of patients, initial antibiotic regimens require adjustment based on microbial speciation and sensitivity analyses. Tube thoracostomy carries risk of parenchymal injury with resulting chronic air leak and/or bronchopleural fistula (BPF). Operative intervention is rarely indicated in the management of lung abscess but should be considered in patients with failure of clinical or radiological improvement after 4-6 weeks of antibiotic therapy, abscesses larger than 6 cm, massive or life-threatening hemoptysis (4%), empyema or BPF (4%), and bronchial obstruction (particularly if secondary to resectable cancer). Furthermore, acute rupture into the pleural space (pyopneumothorax) is still a surgical emergency. When surgery is indicated, either thoracoscopic or open lobectomy generally is the preferred procedure and can be accomplished with low morality (0%-2%) and morbidity. A double-lumen tube is mandatory to protect the airway due to the high risk of spillage of abscess into the contralateral lung. Routine buttressing of the bronchial stump with a vascularized pedicle (intercostal muscle or pericardial fat) is recommended to prevent BPF.

Prognosis

Antibiotics given over 4-6 weeks with percutaneous drainage is effective in 85%-95% of patients. Mortality for lung abscess has decreased from 30% to 40% in the preantibiotic era to 10% in the present era, but remains greater for elderly individuals, immunocompromised patients, or those who have abscess larger than 6 cm, bronchial obstruction, multiple abscesses, necrotizing pneumonia, or gram-negative pneumonia.

Agasthian T. Results of surgery for bronchiectasis and pulmonary abscesses. *Thorac Surg Clin* 2012;22:333.

2. Bronchiectasis

Bronchiectasis is defined as irreversible dilation of the peripheral airways secondary to damage of the structural components of the bronchial wall (elastin, muscles, and cartilage). Mechanisms of damage include bronchial wall injury, bronchial lumen obstruction, and traction from adjacent fibrosis seen in end-stage lung fibrosis. Cole's "vicious cycle" hypothesizes that initial infection, in a background of genetic susceptibility or impaired mucosal clearance, results in retention of microorganisms in the bronchial tree. Overproduction of thick inflammatory mucus in the setting of persistent microbial colonization of dilated airways, together with impairment of mucociliary clearance mechanisms causes a vicious cycle of repeated and prolonged episodes of chronic inflammation resulting in progressive airway and lung damage.

The clinical syndrome manifests as chronic dilation of bronchi, a paroxysmal cough that produces variable amounts of fetid, mucopurulent sputum, and recurrent pulmonary infections. Aspirated foreign bodies, endobronchial neoplasms, and hilar lymphadenopathy (see section on Middle Lobe Syndrome, later) also can cause retention of secretions, infections, and progressive bronchiectasis. The presence of true established bronchiectasis, however, must be distinguished from pseudobronchiectasis, which is a cylindric bronchial dilation that is associated with acute bronchopneumonia. When left untreated, true bronchiectasis progresses, while pseudobronchiectasis reverses completely after weeks to months.

Most cases are related to acquired disorders and are caused by two factors: infection and bronchial obstruction. Acquired viral and bacterial infections in infancy and childhood (eg, pertussis, measles, influenza, tuberculosis, bronchopneumonia) were common predisposing conditions that led to bronchiectasis in the past and are still common in developing countries. With the reemergence of tuberculosis postinfectious bronchiectasis is also becoming more prevalent, and is seen 11% of patients. In developed countries, immune deficiency syndromes (hypogammaglobulinemia and leukocyte dysfunction), metabolic defects (cystic fibrosis, alspha-1 antitrypsin deficiency), ultrastructural defects (primary ciliary dyskinesia, Young syndrome, Kartagener syndrome, congenital defects of cartilage), and pulmonary sequestration are more common causes.

Reid categorized bronchiectasis into three main types based on pathologic appearance: (1) tubular or cylindrical, characterized by smooth dilation of the bronchi; (2) varicose, in which the bronchi are dilated with multiple indentations; and (3) cystic or saccular, in which dilated bronchi terminate in blind ending sacs of pus with no communication with the rest of the lung. Saccular bronchiectasis follows severe infections and cases of bronchial obstruction, while the cylindrical variant is associated with tuberculosis and immune disorders. Varicose consists of alternating areas of cylindrical and saccular types.

Bronchiectasis can be classified also as perfused or nonperfused types according to functional hemodynamic perfusion studies as described by Ashour. The perfused type has cylindrical bronchiectatic changes with intact pulmonary artery flow, whereas the nonperfused type involves cystic bronchiectasis with absent pulmonary artery flow and retrograde filling of the pulmonary artery through the systemic circulation.

Taken together, tubular or cylindric bronchiectasis tends to have better prognosis than cystic/varicose varieties, as the lung areas affected by the former tend to have good function and perfusion. Cystic bronchiectasis tends to indicate a completely destroyed, nonfunctional, and nonperfused lung. Additionally, all parameters of respiratory function are worse in the saccular type as compared with the tubular type. Saccular type bronchiectasis also is associated with higher bacterial loads with virulent strains, such as *Pseudomonas.*

In general, bronchiectasis involves the second-order to fourth-order branches of the segmental bronchi, and its distribution is largely characteristic of the underlying pathology. The left lung tends to be more involved than the right lung in 55%-80% of cases. This may be because the left mainstem bronchus is narrower and longer than the right and subject to greater compression pressures, especially by the aortic arch. The lower lobes are commonly affected owing to gravity-dependent retention of infected secretions. Congenital disorders, for example, are associated with diffuse bilateral bronchiectasis, while tuberculosis and granulomatous diseases are characterized by unilateral or bilateral disease, most commonly limited to the upper lobes and superior segments of the lower lobes. Furthermore, bronchiectasis following pyogenic and viral pneumonias usually involves only the lower lobes, middle lobe, and lingula, and postobstructive bronchiectasis is generally limited to the obstructed segments (see also Middle Lobe Syndrome, later). Common pathogens in patients with bronchiectasis include *H influenzae, S aureus, K pneumoniae, E coli,* and, in the chronic setting, *Pseudomonas* species. Mycobacteria, fungi, and *Legionella* should also be cultured.

▶ Clinical Findings & Diagnosis

Patients with a history of recurrent febrile episodes often complain of a chronic or intermittent cough that produces variable amounts of foul-smelling sputum (up to 500 mL/d).

Hemoptysis occurs in 41%-66%, but rarely is it massive. Bronchiectasis associated with granulomatous disease may not be associated with a productive cough (so-called dry bronchiectasis). Exacerbations and advanced disease are manifested by increased sputum production, fever, dyspnea, anorexia, fatigue, and weight loss. A history of sinus problems, infertility, or a family history of similar problems suggests the presence of an inherited disorder associated with bronchiectasis. Physical examination may reveal cyanosis, clubbing, pulmonary osteoarthropathy, evidence of malnutrition, and, in advanced disease, signs of cor pulmonale. Although bronchiectasis is suspected, an imaging study is usually required for confirmation. Bronchograms were at one time required, but high-resolution chest CT scans are now the imaging procedure of choice to document bronchial dilation, particularly with saccular disease. Even with the diagnosis of bronchiectasis, however, endobronchial neoplasm or foreign body must be excluded by flexible fiberoptic bronchoscopy.

▶ Treatment

In nearly all patients, conservative medical therapy is indicated and generally is sufficient. This includes broad-spectrum antibiotics, bronchodilators, humidification, expectorants, mucolytics, and effective routine postural drainage. In patients with continued infection, bronchoscopy with bronchoalveolar lavage should be considered to obtain more accurate culture results. Other adjunctive therapies include influenza and pneumococcal vaccines and, in some patients, chronic "prophylactic" antibiotic administration with trimethoprim-sulfamethoxazole, erythromycin, or ciprofloxacin. A recent advance in controlling underlying bacterial (especially pseudomonas) infection and symptoms associated with bronchiectasis has been the use of inhaled antibiotics. In the cystic fibrosis and chronic bronchiectasis population, nebulized tobramycin or gentamicin has proven effective in controlling infection, sputum production, and symptoms in a significant proportion of patients.

Patients who fail intensive medical therapy may be candidates for surgical resection if the following criteria are met: (1) the disease must be localized and completely resectable; (2) pulmonary reserve must be adequate; (3) the process must be irreversible (ie, not pseudobronchiectasis, bronchial stricture, foreign body, etc); and (4) significant symptoms must persist. Preoperative assessment requires a high-resolution chest CT scan, although some surgeons still prefer a bronchogram as a "road map." Pulmonary function studies generally are not necessary, since the involved segments do not function.

The goals of surgery are to remove all active disease and to preserve as much functioning lung parenchyma as possible. The surgical approach includes complete segmental resection of the involved areas. Partial resection almost always ends in recurrence. Resection most commonly involves all basal segments (unilaterally or bilaterally) along with the middle lobe or lingula. With tuberculosis, however, removal of the upper lobe or lobes with or without the superior segment of the lower lobes is more likely. During operation, meticulous maintenance of a clear airway devoid of mucopurulent secretions and blood is essential. Careful dissection of the bronchovascular structures is difficult in patients with chronic inflammation and scarring but is essential to avoid complications.

▶ Prognosis

Although most patients are successfully treated with medical therapy, some require operation. The results of pulmonary resection depend on the cause and type of parenchymal involvement. Success with elimination of symptoms occurs in up to 80% of patients with limited localized disease but only 36% of those with diffuse disease. Prognostic factors include: (1) unilateral disease restricted to the basal segments; (2) young age; (3) absence of sinusitis and rhinitis; (4) history of pneumonia; and (5) no major airway obstruction. Overall morbidity and mortality rates are surprisingly low at 3%-5% and less than 1%, respectively.

3. Middle Lobe Syndrome

Middle lobe syndrome (MLS) is characterized by recurrent or chronic collapse of the middle lobe of the right lung but can also involve the lingula of the left lung. There are two forms of MLS: obstructive and nonobstructive. Obstructive MLS occurs as a result of an endobronchial lesion or extrinsic compression of the middle lobe bronchus from hilar lymphadenopathy or tumor causing postobstructive atelectasis and pneumonitis. The most common cause of extrinsic compression of the right-middle lobe bronchus is enlargement of peribronchial lymph nodes due to fungal infections such as histoplasmosis or atypical mycobacterial infections. Adenopathy due to sarcoidosis or lymph node metastases has also been described in obstructive MLS. Less common causes include aspirated foreign objects, broncholiths, inspissated mucus (associated with cystic fibrosis), and endoluminal granulomas associated with sarcoidosis.

Nonobstructive MLS is characterized by the absence of a mechanical obstruction of the middle lobe bronchus on bronchoscopy and/or CT of the chest. Though poorly understood the narrow diameter and long length of the middle lobe bronchus, combined with an acute angle at its origin, create poor conditions for adequate drainage. This form of MLS is the most common cause and commonly occurs in adults and children with recurrent pneumonia. It is often related to asthma, bronchitis, and cystic fibrosis.

The diagnosis of MLS should be entertained in a patient with repeated episodes of right-sided pneumonia, only after other causes of obstruction (bronchogenic cancer, foreign body, etc), have been ruled out. Evaluation includes chest radiography, bronchoscopy and CT of the chest. Most patients respond to intensive medical therapy including bronchodilators, mucolytics, and broad spectrum antibiotics in addition to therapeutic bronchoscopy. Those who do not respond should be offered resection of the right-middle lobe and/or debulking lymphadenopathy, which is associated with a low mortality rate and favorable outcome. Other indications for surgery include bronchiectasis, fibrosis (bronchial stenosis), abscess, unresolved or intractable recurrent pneumonia, hemoptysis, and suspicion of neoplasm.

Gudbjartsson T et al: Middle lobe syndrome: a review of clinicopathological features, diagnosis and treatment. *Respiration* 2012;84:80.

4. Broncholithiasis

Broncholithiasis is defined as the presence of calculi (broncholiths) within the tracheobronchial tree. In most cases, a broncholith is formed by erosion and extrusion of a calcified adjacent lymph node into the bronchial lumen and is usually associated with long-standing foci of necrotizing granulomatous lymphadenitis. Calcified lymph nodes can remain attached to the bronchial wall, lodge in a bronchus, or be expectorated (lithoptysis). The most common cause of broncholithiasis in the United States is histoplasmosis. Tuberculosis is another frequent cause in some parts of the world.

Patients with broncholithiasis often complain of hemoptysis, lithoptysis (30%), cough, sputum production, fever, chills, and pleuritic chest pain. The hemoptysis is characteristically sudden and self-limited, though rarely it may be massive. Symptoms of pneumonia may indicate bronchial obstruction from an impacted broncholith. Signs suggesting broncholithiasis include localized wheezing on physical examination, evidence of hilar calcifications or segmental atelectasis and pneumonia on chest x-ray, and bronchoscopic evidence of peribronchial disease. The diagnosis is confirmed by documentation of lithoptysis or the presence of an endobronchial "lung stone."

The complications of broncholithiasis include hemoptysis, which on occasion can be massive and life threatening; suppurative lung diseases (eg, pneumonia and bronchiectasis); midesophageal traction diverticula; and, rarely, tracheobronchoesophageal fistula.

In addition to instituting appropriate therapy for underlying pulmonary diseases, treatment is primarily directed at removal of endobronchial stones. This can be accomplished at the time of bronchoscopy if the broncholith is freely floating within the tracheobronchial tree or if it extends well into the bronchial lumen and can be removed without excessive force or traction (20% of cases). The main danger of transbronchoscopic removal of broncholiths is the risk for massive hemorrhage. This results during inappropriate removal of broncholiths that remain substantially attached to the parabronchial tissues. Because of intense peribronchial fibrosis in this situation, the broncholith not infrequently becomes adherent to vascular structures such as the pulmonary artery, which may be torn with vigorous attempts at broncholith removal.

Nearly 80% of patients with broncholiths that remain *in situ* require surgical removal. The goal of surgery in this disease is preservation of lung function. The broncholith may be removed safely with bronchotomy; however, most patients require segmentectomy or lobectomy, particularly if destruction of lung parenchyma has occurred from postobstruction suppurative lung disease. Fistulas between the airway and the esophagus should be repaired with interposition of normal tissue (intercostal muscle flap, etc) between the two structures to prevent recurrence. Following surgery, the prognosis is excellent.

Cerfolio R et al: Rigid bronchoscopy and surgical resection for broncholithiasis and calcified mediastinal lymph nodes. *J Thorac Cardiovasc Surg* 2008;136:186.

5. Cystic Fibrosis and Mucoid Impaction of the Bronchi

Cystic fibrosis is an autosomal recessive multisystem congenital disorder that is characterized by chronic airway obstruction and infection and by exocrine pancreatic insufficiency and gastrointestinal tract dysfunction with consequent effects on nutrition, growth, and maturation. The disorder is the result of several characterized mutations in the cystic fibrosis transmembrane regulator (CFTR) gene, most commonly the ΔF508 mutation. Such mutations cause abnormalities of chloride and likely sodium transport leading to abnormal regulation and reduction of airway surface liquid volume. The result is a viscous and tenacious mucus that adheres to the airway surface epithelium resulting in airflow obstruction and bacterial infection (*S auerus, P aeruginosa,* and *Burkholderia cepacia*). Once established, infection of the CF lung is rarely eradicated. Pulmonary manifestations of the disorder include mucoid impaction, bronchitis, bronchiectasis, pulmonary fibrosis, emphysema, and lung abscess. Mucoid plugs are rubbery, semisolid, gray to greenish-yellow in color, and round, oval, or elongated in shape. There is often a history of recurrent upper respiratory infection, fever, and chest pain. Expectoration of hard mucus plugs or hemoptysis may occur.

The earliest manifestation of CF lung disease is a cough that progressively worsens to becoming a daily event and productive. It often becomes paroxymal and associated with gagging and emesis. Sputum is usually tenacious, purulent, and often green, reflecting bacterial infection. Hyperinflation of the lungs due to airway obstruction is noted early in the progression of lung disease. Asthmatic or bronchiolitic-type

wheezing is common. CF patients typically have mild bronchitis symptoms for long periods of time punctuated by increasingly frequent acute exacerbations of symptoms that include increased intensity of cough, tachypnea, shortness of breath, decreased activity and appetite, and weight loss. Intense antibiotic therapy and assistance with clearance of mucus are usually required to reduce lung symptoms and improve lung function. End-stage lung disease is characterized by substantial hypoxemia, pulmonary hypertension, cor pulmonale, and death.

The primary objectives of CF treatment are to control infection, promote mucus clearance, and improve nutrition. Therapy includes postural drainage with chest percussion, expectorants, detergents, bronchodilators, antibiotics, and aerosol inhalation. More novel therapies include inhaled hypertonic saline which osmotically draws water onto the airway surface thereby "rehydrating" the airway mucus allowing for easier expectoration, aerosolized rhDNase which lyses the viscous DNA contained within airway mucus and ibuprofen which has been shown to slow the decline in lung function. Surgery including partial lung resection is indicated for apparently localized disease (lung abscess and bronchiectasis) and recurrent severe exacerbations. Lobectomy is occasionally indicated for massive hemoptysis that is refractory to bronchial artery embolization.

Double lung transplantation has become an accepted therapy for respiratory failure secondary to CF. Patients should be referred when their prognosis is about equal to the waiting time for donor lungs, currently about 2 years after acceptance as a lung transplant candidate. Relative contraindications to transplant include severe malnutrition (ideal body weight < 70%), chronic steroid use greater than 20 mg of prednisone daily and mechanical ventilation (center dependent). Multiresistant *P aeruginosa* infection is not a contraindication for transplantation although panresistant *P aeruginosa* is considered, at some centers, to be a contraindication. *Burkholderia cepacia* is viewed by some to be a contraindication to lung transplantation. The transplanted lungs remain free of CF, but are subject to secondary infection, acute rejection, and chronic rejection (bronchiolitis obliterans syndrome). The 5-year survival following lung transplantation is 48%. The median survival in all CF patients now exceeds 31 years.

O'Sullivan BP et al: Cystic fibrosis. *Lancet* 2009;373:1891.

6. Tuberculosis

Tuberculosis markedly declined as a cause of death between 1953 and 1984, but since 1985, this disease has experienced resurgence due to increased immigration of infected individuals and HIV infection. A reservoir of about 5000-8000 clinical cases exists, and an additional 25,000 new cases occur annually. Multidrug-resistant tuberculosis (MDR-TB) and, most recently, extensively drug-resistant tuberculosis (XDR-TB) have emerged over the last 20 years. MDR-TB is defined as those strains resistant to at least isoniazid and rifampicin. XDR-TB strains are defined as those resistant to rifampicin, isoniazid, flurooquinolones, and any of capreomycin, kanamycin, or amikacin. Resistance to these antituberclar drugs is the result of spontaneous mutations in the genome and is due to a myriad of factors most commonly inadequate treatment of active pulmonary tuberculosis. Less than 20% of the United States population is tuberculin-positive, but tuberculosis remains a common infectious cause of death worldwide. It is estimated that there are 440,000 new MDR-TB cases identified each year worldwide, many of these arising in previously treated patients. Nearly 50% of cases occur in India and China. The prognosis of treatment of MDR-TB or XDR-TB is significantly worse than for drug-susceptible disease.

Several species of the genus mycobacterium may cause lung disease, but 95% of cases of lung disease are due to *Mycobacterium tuberculosis*. Several "atypical" species of *Mycobacterium*, such as *Mycobacterium bovis* and *Mycobacterium avium,* that are chiefly soil-dwellers, have become clinically more important in recent years because they are less responsive to preventive and therapeutic measures. Mycobacteria are nonmotile, nonsporulating, weakly gram-positive rods classified in the order Actinomycetales. Dormant organisms remain alive for the life of the host.

The initial infection often involves pulmonary parenchyma in the midzone of the lungs. When hypersensitivity develops after several weeks, the typical caseation appears. Regional hilar lymph nodes become enlarged. Most cases arrest spontaneously at this stage. Should the infection progress, caseation necrosis develops and giant cells produce a typical tubercle. A cause of latent disease in the elderly or debilitated patient is dormant reactivation tubercles. Sites in the apical and posterior segments of the upper lobes and superior segments of the lower lobes are the usual areas of infection.

▶ Clinical Findings

A. Symptoms and Signs

Patients may present with minimal symptoms, including fever, cough, anorexia, weight loss, night sweats, excessive perspiration, chest pain, lethargy, and dyspnea. Extrapulmonary disease may be associated with more severe symptoms, such as involvement of the pericardium, bones, joints, urinary tract, meninges, lymph nodes, or pleural space. Erythema nodosum is seen occasionally in patients with active disease.

B. Laboratory Findings

False-negative tests with intermediate-strength PPD are usually due to anergy, improper testing, or outdated tuberculin. Anergy is sometimes associated with disseminated tuberculosis, measles, sarcoidosis, lymphomas, or recent vac-

cination with live viruses (eg, poliomyelitis, measles, rubella, mumps, influenza, or yellow fever). Immunosuppressive drugs (eg, corticosteroids, azathioprine) and disease states (eg, AIDS, organ transplantation) may also cause false-negative responses. Mumps skin tests are negative in patients taking immunosuppressive drugs. Culture of sputum, gastric aspirates, and tracheal washings as well as pleural fluid and pleural and lung biopsies may establish the diagnosis.

C. Imaging Studies

Radiographic findings include involvement of the apical and posterior segments of the upper lobes (85%) or the superior segments of the lower lobes (10%). Seldom is the anterior segment of the upper lobe solely involved, as in other granulomatous diseases such as histoplasmosis. Involvement of the basal segments of the lower lobes is uncommon except in women, blacks, and diabetics, but endobronchial disease usually involves the lower lobes, producing atelectasis or consolidation. Differing x-ray patterns correspond to the pathologic variations of the disease: the local exudative lesion, the local productive lesion, cavitation, acute tuberculous pneumonia, miliary tuberculosis, Rasmussen aneurysm, bronchiectasis, bronchostenosis, and tuberculoma.

▶ Differential Diagnosis

It is critical to distinguish the x-ray findings from bronchogenic carcinoma, particularly when there is tuberculoma without calcification.

▶ Treatment

A. Medical Treatment

Active disease should be treated with one of the chemotherapeutic regimens that have recently been shown to shorten the period of treatment while maintaining their potency. Such drugs include isoniazid, streptomycin, rifampin, and ethambutol.

Treatment of MDR-TB and XDR-TB is less well defined. The World Health Organization (WHO) recently updated and put forth recommendations for treating MDR-TB. This includes:

- Rapid drug-susceptibility testing of isonizaid and rifampicin should be performed at the initial diagnosis of tuberculosis.

- The use of sputum microscopy and culture should be used instead of microscopy alone.

- Later generation flurooquinolones, as well as ethionamide, should be used in patients with MDR-TB.

- The treatment of MDR-TB should include at least pyrazinamide, a flouroquinolone, a parenteral agent (kanamycin, amikacin, or capreomycin), ethionamide, and either cycloserine or p-aminosalicyclic acid.

- An intensive treatment of at least 8-months duration is recommended.

The success of MDR-TB therapy ranges from 36% to 79% with a mortality rate of 11%. It is estimated that less than 10% of people with MDR-TB are receiving appropriate treatment according to international guidelines.

B. Surgical Treatment

The role of surgery in treatment of tuberculosis has diminished dramatically since chemotherapy became available. It is now confined to the following indications: (1) failure of chemotherapy; (2) performance of diagnostic procedures; (3) destroyed lung; (4) postsurgical complications; (5) persistent bronchopleural fistula; and (6) intractable hemorrhage. The most common parenchymal resections include lobectomy, followed by pneumonectomy. Muscle flap coverage is strongly recommended. The infectious process often involves the pleural space and it is useful to perform an extrapleural dissection to minimize contamination or bacterial superinfection of the resection cavity.

Pulmonary resection is adjunctive to chemotherapy. The rationale for lung resection of parenchyma affected by MDR-TB is to remove a large focal burden of organisms present in destroyed nonviable lung tissue. The destroyed lung parenchyma and associated cavities are an ideal environment for the bacillus to grow due to its isolation from the circulation and therefore the host's defenses. Surgery is recommended in MDR-TB patients with extensive drug resistance—those with localized disease amenable to resection and those with high drug activity. Pretreatment with chemotherapeutic regimens for at least 2 months is required before operation to reduce the bacterial burden, followed by 12-24 months of treatment after surgery.

Diagnostic lung resection may be necessary to rule out other diseases, such as cancer, or to obtain material for cultures. Patients with destroyed lobes or cavitary tuberculosis of the right-upper lobe containing large infected foci may sometimes be candidates for resection.

The disease can become reactivated in some patients who have had thoracoplasty, plombage, or resection, and a few will require reoperation. The most common indications for surgery after plombage therapy are pleural infection (pyogenic or tuberculous) and migration of the plombage material, causing pain or compression of other organs. Following pulmonary resection, tuberculous empyema may develop in the postpneumonectomy space, sometimes associated with a bronchopleural fistula or bony sequestration. Persistent bronchopleural fistula after chemotherapy and closed tube drainage may require direct operative closure. Use of muscle flaps (intercostal, etc) is highly recommended to cover any bronchial stumps, especially in the setting of pneumonectomy.

Tuberculous empyema poses unique problems of management. Treatment depends on whether the empyema is:

(1) associated with parenchymal disease; (2) mixed tuberculous and pyogenic or purely tuberculous; and (3) associated with bronchopleural fistula. The ultimate objective is complete expansion of the lung and obliteration of the empyema space. Pulmonary decortication or resection may be used for tuberculosis, but open or closed drainage is necessary when the process is complicated by pyogenic infection or bronchopleural fistula.

▶ Prognosis

The prognosis is excellent in most cases treated medically; the death rate decreased from 25% in 1945 to less than 10% currently. Perioperative mortality for pulmonary resections for tuberculosis ranges from 10% for pneumonectomy to 3% for lobectomy and 1% for segmentectomy and subsegmental resections.

The morbidity of surgical resection ranges from 12% to 39% with the most common complications being bleeding, empyema, wound complications, and bronchopleural fistula. The rate of sputum sterilization ranges from 78% to 96% in MDR-TB patients. Factors leading to poorer outcomes include retreatment cases, XDR-TB, bilateral disease, and low body mass index.

Falzon D et al: WHO guidelines for the programmatic management of drug-resistant tuberculosis: 2011 update. *Eur Respir J* 2011;38:516-528.

Kang MW et al: Surgical treatment for multidrug-resistant and extensive drug-resistant tuberculosis. *Ann Thorac Surg* 2010;89:1597-1602.

Kempker RR et al: Surgical treatment of drug-resistant tuberculosis. *Lancet Infect Dis* 2012;12(2):157-166.

Massard G et al: Surgery for the sequelae of postprimary tuberculosis. *Thorac Surg Clin* 2012;22(3):287-300.

FUNGAL INFECTIONS OF THE LUNG

Pulmonary fungal infections are increasing due to the widespread use of broad-spectrum antibiotics, the use of corticosteroids and other immunosuppressive drugs, and the spread of HIV infection. However, infection can occur in immunocompetent hosts. Fungal infections frequently involve the respiratory tract and include histoplasmosis, coccidioidomycosis, blastomycosis, cryptococcosis, aspergillosis, mucormycosis, and candidiasis. Fungal infections, though ubiquitous, are notable for several characteristic endemic areas. Candidiasis rarely if ever requires operative treatment and thus will not be discussed here.

1. Histoplasmosis

Histoplasma capsulatum is a dimorphic soil fungus found in soil enriched by the nitrogen contained in bird and bat guano. Abandoned buildings, attics, lofts, and areas under trees that serve as bird and bat roosts and caves are especially likely to contain high concentrations. In endemic areas, exposure is common, and most infections are sporadic. Outbreaks have been traced to spelunking, demolition of buildings, and activities that disrupt contaminated soil. This organism is found primarily in the Ohio and Mississippi River valleys and in Central America. Mammals, including humans, inhale the organism and macrophages engulf the fungus. It then transforms into the budding yeast form, causing activation of inflammatory cytokines. Over several months the ongoing inflammation causes granuloma formation in lymph nodes with resulting caseation, necrosis, fibrosis, and calcification. The diagnosis of histoplasmosis is made definitively by growth of the organism from either sputum, BAL fluid, lung tissue, or mediastinal lymph nodes—though incubation periods of 4-6 weeks are required. Serology also plays an important role in the diagnosis. Both complement fixation and immunodiffusion tests should be ordered. Serology is not useful in immunosuppressed patients who are unable to mount an antibody response. The *Histoplasma* EIA has been under development as a diagnostic aid and detects the galactomannan component of the cell wall of *H capsulatum*. The original assay was marked by poor sensitivity; however, with modifications its sensitivity has increased to 65% in patients with acute pulmonary histoplasmosis.

Most infections in immunocompetent individuals are asymptomatic. Infections are classified as acute, chronic, or disseminated. Acute infections are manifested: (1) as a flu-like syndrome with fever, chills, dry cough, headache, retrosternal discomfort, arthralgias, and a rash suggesting erythema nodosum; (2) with symptoms similar to a flu-like syndrome but limited to the lungs and occasionally accompanied by a productive cough; or (3) as an acute diffuse nodular disease with mild symptoms. Radiographic findings in these three acute syndromes typically demonstrate ill-defined upper lobe nonsegmental opacities; nonsegmental areas of consolidation that tend to change; and diffuse, discrete 3- to 4-mm nodules, respectively. Hilar adenopathy on chest x-ray is common. Physical examination can be normal or may reveal signs of pneumonia.

In contrast, chronic infections include: (1) an asymptomatic solitary, discrete nodule less than 3 cm in diameter known as a histoplasmoma (most common), often with central and concentric calcifications ("target lesion") and frequently located in the lower lobes; (2) chronic cavitary histoplasmosis, which typically occurs in patients with underlying obstructive disease, characteristically mild symptoms, fibronodular upper lobe infiltrates, and centrilobular emphysematous spaces; (3) mediastinal granulomas that may result in broncholithiasis, esophageal traction diverticula, superior vena cava compression, and tracheobronchoesophageal fistulas; and (4) fibrosing mediastinitis, which can produce compression of the superior vena cava, tracheobronchial tree, or esophagus.

Disseminated disease includes an acute, subacute, and chronic form. These infections occur in children (acute and subacute) as well as adults (subacute and chronic). Fever and abdominal pain are common. Other findings include hepatosplenomegaly, pancytopenia, meningitis, endocarditis, adrenocortical insufficiency, and oropharyngeal ulceration (chronic form).

Radiographic imaging in disseminated disease may demonstrate diffuse interstitial pneumonitis (25%) or minimal findings. The symptoms and roentgenographic findings of histoplasmosis resemble those of tuberculosis, although the disease appears to progress more slowly. There may be cough, malaise, hemoptysis, low-grade fever, and weight loss. As many as 30% of cases coexist with tuberculosis. Pulmonary fibrosis, bulla formation, and pulmonary insufficiency occur in advanced cases of histoplasmosis. Mediastinal involvement is quite frequent and may take the form of granuloma formation, or dysphagia. Furthermore, mediastinal fibrosis is among the most common benign causes of superior vena caval syndrome (discussed earlier in the chapter). Erosion of inflammatory lymph nodes into bronchi may cause expectoration of broncholiths, hemoptysis, wheezing, or bronchiectasis. Traction diverticula of the esophagus may lead to development of tracheoesophageal fistula. Pericardial involvement may lead to constrictive pericarditis.

In lesions that present as solitary pulmonary nodules, histoplasmosis is diagnosed in about 15%-20% of cases. Radiologically, early infections appear as diffuse mottled parenchymal infiltrations surrounding the hila, with enlargement of hilar lymph nodes. Cavitation indicates advanced infection and is the complication about which the surgeon is most often consulted. The diagnosis rests on finding a positive skin test or complement fixation test and culturing the fungus from sputum or a bronchial aspirate.

Medical therapy of histoplasmosis is indicated only in cavitary and severe disease and for most infections in immunocompromised hosts. Azoles are recommended as first-line treatment for patients who have mild to moderate pulmonary histoplasmosis. Itraconazole (200-400 mg/d for 6 months) is the drug of choice for cavitary disease, while amphotericin B (1-2 g total dose) is reserved for patients with more serious infections and infections in immunocompromised patients. Reflecting increasing use of corticosteroids for ARDS in the last decade, the current American Thoracic Society Guidelines recommend the use of intravenous methylprednisilone as adjunctive therapy for severe acute pulmonary histoplasmosis. Operative intervention is reserved for treatment of complications and to rule out neoplastic disease in the case of suspicious pulmonary nodules. Broncholithectomy via rigid bronchoscopy with or without pulmonary resection, repair of tracheobronchoesophageal fistulas, decompression of mediastinal granulomas, and spiral saphenous vein bypass of severe symptomatic superior vena cava obstruction are typical examples. The Infectious Diseases Society of America recommends pericardiectomy for recurrent pericardial effusions. In cases of vascular fibrosis of the superior vena cava and pulmonary vessels percutaneous intravascular dilation and stenting is recommended as first-line treatment.

2. Coccidioidomycosis

Coccidioides immitis is a dimorphic soil fungus endemic to the Sonoran life zone (Utah, Arizona, California, Nevada, and New Mexico) and is associated with creosote brush. Dry heat with brief intense rain is essential for this fungus, which is spread by strong winds. Infection occurs through inhalation of as few as 1-10 arthrospores, which then germinate as parasitic spherules. Spherules have a double refractile cell wall and produce endospores that cause the spherule to rupture, spreading the infection to the surrounding tissues. Caseation, suppuration, abscess formation, and fibrosis follow. The diagnosis of coccidioidomycosis relies on the detection of acutely elevated titers of immunoglobulin M (IgM) antibodies (by latex agglutination and confirmed by immunodiffusion tube precipitin tests) or rising serum immunoglobulin G (IgG) antibody complement fixation titers (seroconversion or fourfold rise) in the appropriate clinical context. The coccidioidin and Spherulin skin tests, which become positive 3-21 days following infection, are generally useful only for epidemiologic studies and not for the diagnosis of acute disease. *C immitis* grows well in culture, but it is extremely hazardous to handle and requires a laminar flow hood due to the highly infectious nature of the arthrospores. Identification of the spherules in tissue, lavage samples, and fine-needle aspirates is helpful in making the diagnosis in some patients. Although many stains can be used, including routine fungal (potassium hydroxide, KOH) preparations, Pap staining is most sensitive. Gram stains, however, fail to demonstrate spherules.

Primary infection is asymptomatic in 60% of patients, while most others develop desert fever, with fever, productive cough, pleuritic chest pain, pneumonitis, and a rash typical of erythema nodosum or erythema multiforme. Disease that includes arthralgias is known as desert rheumatism. Radiographic findings demonstrate segmental or nonsegmental, homogeneous or mottled infiltrates with a predilection for the lower lobes. Physical examination is often unrevealing, but rales and rhonchi may be present. Other findings include eosinophilia (66%), hilar adenopathy (20%), and small exudative pleural effusions (2%-20%). Symptomatic persistent infection associated with chest x-ray findings 6-8 weeks after primary infection is classified as one of five types: persistent pneumonia, chronic progressive pneumonia, miliary coccidioidomycosis, coccidioidal nodules, or pulmonary cavities. Persistent pneumonia manifests with symptoms of fever, productive cough, and pleuritic

chest pain in association with protracted infiltrates and consolidation on chest x-ray generally resolving within 8 months. Patients with chronic progressive pneumonia complain of fever, cough, dyspnea, hemoptysis, and weight loss, with bilateral apical nodular densities and multiple cavities lasting years. This presentation closely resembles tuberculosis and chronic histoplasmosis. Miliary coccidioidomycosis occurs early and rapidly, associated with bilateral diffuse infiltrates. This form of disease implies the presence of impaired immunity and has an associated mortality rate of 50%. Nearly half of patients with coccidioidal nodules are asymptomatic. These nodular densities (coccidiomas) appear in the middle and upper lung fields, often within 5 cm of the hilum; range from 1 to 4 cm in size; and do not calcify, making it hard to distinguish them from malignancy. In endemic areas, 30%-50% of all nodules are coccidiomas. Patients develop pulmonary cavities in 10%-15% of cases of coccidioidomycosis. Typically, these are solitary (90%), thin-walled, located in the upper lobes (70%), less than 6 cm in size (90%), and close spontaneously within 2 years (50%). Some cavities, however, cross fissures; cause hemoptysis (25%-50%), usually mild; rupture, producing a pyopneumothorax with a bronchopleural fistula; or become infected with *Aspergillus*. Uncommonly, dissemination can occur, particularly in immunocompromised individuals, in pregnancy (third trimester), and in non-Caucasian individuals. Although pulmonary symptoms in disseminated disease are mild, meningeal involvement is common and the mortality rate is high (50%).

Medical therapy is not indicated in asymptomatic, immunocompetent individuals. Patients with persistent or chronic pneumonia, miliary disease, and those at risk for dissemination should be treated with antifungal therapy. Amphotericin B (0.5-2.5 g intravenously as total dose) is the standard treatment, though the newer azole compounds (fluconazole, ketoconazole, and itraconazole) may be used for long-term maintenance therapy, since the relapse rate may be as high as 25%-50%. Surgery is reserved for patients with coccidiomas when cancer is a concern and in patients with cavities that have an associated radiographic abnormality suggesting carcinoma (ie, thick wall) or that develop a complication (eg, hemoptysis and pyopneumothorax from rupture). Resection should include all diseased tissue and most often requires lobectomy.

3. Blastomycosis

Blastomyces dermatitidis is a dimorphic soil fungus found in warm, wet, nitrogen-rich soil in an endemic area that extends east of a line from the Texas Gulf coast to the border between Minnesota and North Dakota (except Florida and New England). Infection occurs characteristically in males (male-to-female ratio 6:1-15:1) from 30-60 years of age through inhalation of conidia (asexual spores). At 37°C, the conidia germinate as yeasts, producing caseation in a manner similar to tuberculosis. Rarely, infection may develop through direct skin inoculation. Risk factors include poor hygiene, exposure to dust and wood, manual labor, and poor housing conditions. Since no accurate skin or serologic tests exist, the diagnosis depends on culture or histologic identification of the yeast form. Culture of the mycelial form can be hazardous. *B dermatitidis* grows as white to tan colonies of septate hyphae at room temperature but changes to budding yeast at 37°C. This temperature-dependent change reflects the uncoupling of oxidative phosphorylation. The yeast form can be found in sputum (33%), bronchoalveolar lavage specimens (38%), lung biopsies (21%), and fine-needle aspirates (7%) and can be demonstrated with standard KOH preparations or many other histologic stains (but not Gram stain). The yeast, however, does not have a large capsule (distinguishes it from *Cryptococcus neoformans*) and does not grow intracellularly (differentiates it from *H capsulatum*).

Manifestations of blastomycosis can occur in many organ systems, including the lungs, skin, bone, genitourinary tract (prostatitis and epididymo-orchitis), and central nervous system. Pulmonary infection can be asymptomatic or may present with flu-like symptoms, evidence of pneumonia, or pleurisy. Cough (36%), weight loss (20%), pleuritic pain (26%), fever (23%), hemoptysis (21%), erythema nodosum, and ulcerative bronchitis are common. Radiographic findings include homogeneous or patchy consolidation in a nonsegmental distribution with pleural effusions or thickening or cavitation (15%-25%). In some patients, the appearance of pulmonary masses may mimic carcinoma. A predilection for the upper lobes has been noted; however, unlike histoplasmosis and coccidioidomycosis, in blastomycosis, hilar and mediastinal adenopathy is unusual.

Limited disease in asymptomatic immunocompetent patients requires no specific therapy. Itraconazole, 100-200 mg/d orally for at least 2-3 months, is now the therapy of choice for nonmeningeal disease, with a response rate of over 80%. Amphotericin B (0.5-2 g), however, is indicated in patients with meningeal disease or failed therapy. Surgical resection is rarely necessary except when the possibility of malignancy cannot be excluded.

4. Cryptococcosis

Cryptococcus neoformans is an encapsulated yeast-like budding fungus. It is a saprophyte existing on the skin, nasopharynx, gastrointestinal tract, and vagina of humans as well as in pigeon excreta, grasses, trees, plants, fruits, bees, wasps, insects (cockroaches), birds, milk products, pickle brine, and soil. Cryptococcal infection generally indicates the presence of an underlying debilitating disease in an immunocompromised host. Infection occurs from inhalation of the yeast form. The diagnosis can be established by the detection of serum antigen (via complement fixation tests) in patients with appropriate clinical and radiographic findings. More commonly, however, histologic identification with India ink stains is used; routine cultures are not performed because they are extremely time-consuming and require multiple biochemical tests for differentiation of cryptococcus from other fungi. No accurate skin test exists for cryptococcosis.

The most common sites of infection are the lungs and central nervous system. Pulmonary infection may remain asymptomatic, or patients may complain of cough, pleuritic chest pain, and fever. Radiographically, cryptococcus can appear as a localized, well-defined 3-10-cm pleural-based mass without smooth borders; as single or multiple areas of consolidation, usually within one lobe but in nonsegmental distribution; or as a disseminated miliary nodular infiltrate. A predilection for the lower lobes has been noted. Central nervous system infection usually follows an asymptomatic pulmonary infection. Central nervous system symptoms are highly variable, since many patients are severely immunocompromised and do not manifest the usual signs and symptoms of meningitis or cerebritis.

Medical therapy is indicated in most cases of pulmonary infection except for rare cases of limited localized disease. Amphotericin B (0.5-2 g) remains the treatment of choice and is often combined with flucytosine (150/mg/kg/d) for synergy. New azole compounds (eg, fluconazole, itraconazole, and voriconazole) have been used with increasing frequency as first-line therapy both as single agents and in combination. Surgery is rarely indicated and is useful only to exclude the possibility of malignancy or to determine the etiology of an undiagnosed diffuse pulmonary infiltrate by open lung biopsy.

5. Aspergillosis

Aspergillus species are ubiquitous dimorphic soil fungi found in soil and decaying organic matter. The most common pathogenic species include *Aspergillus fumigatus* (most common), *Aspergillus niger*, *Aspergillus flavus*, and *Aspergillus glaucus*. In culture, these fungi resemble an aspergillum, which is a brush used to sprinkle holy water. Aspergillosis represents the second-most common (after candidiasis) opportunistic fungal infection in immunocompromised hosts and the third-most common systemic fungal infection requiring hospital care. Infection occurs almost exclusively through inhalation of conidia into areas of lung with impaired mucociliary function (eg, tuberculous cavities). Although the diagnosis is supported by demonstrating immediate and delayed-type hypersensitivity skin reactions, by culturing uniform septate hyphae with dichotomous branching at 45 degrees, and by detecting specific IgG and IgE antibodies, a definitive diagnosis requires demonstration of hyphal tissue invasion or documentation of hyphae on methenamine silver stain in a suspected aspergilloma. Galactomannan enzyme-linked immunosorbent assays have recently become available and serve as a sensitive serum measure of invasive infection.

Infection with *Aspergillus* species usually takes one of three forms: allergic bronchopulmonary aspergillosis, invasive aspergillosis, and aspergilloma. Allergic bronchopulmonary aspergillosis occurs in patients who are atopic (asthmatics) and in patients with cystic fibrosis. Endobronchial fungal growth leads to dilated airways filled with mucus and fungus. Continuous exposure to fungal antigens results in precipitating antibodies, increased IgE levels (which correlate with disease activity), and both immediate and delayed-type hypersensitivity. Patients complain of cough, fever, wheezing, dyspnea, pleuritic pain, and hemoptysis. Chest x-ray shows homogeneous densities in a "gloved-finger," inverted Y, or "cluster of grapes" pattern. Five stages have been defined depending on disease activity and steroid dependency: Stage 1 includes acute infection with characteristic x-ray and laboratory evidence of disease; stage 2 occurs with steroid-induced remission; stage 3 is characterized by asymptomatic exacerbations of laboratory and x-ray findings; steroid-dependent asthma with worsening laboratory tests (total IgE, precipitins, etc) is indicative of stage 4 disease; and end-stage fibrosis, bronchiectasis, and obstruction define stage 5.

Invasive aspergillosis is found exclusively in immunocompromised patients, particularly in patients with leukemia (50%-70% of cases). Dissemination occurs frequently, and three types of pulmonary disease have been described: tracheobronchitis (uncommon), necrotizing bronchopneumonia, and hemorrhagic infarction (most common). In tracheobronchitis, disease is usually limited to the larger airways (bronchus more so than trachea) with little parenchymal involvement. Focal or diffuse mucosal ulceration, pseudomembranes, and intraluminal fungal plugs are common. Patients often present with cough, dyspnea, wheezing, and hemoptysis. Occasionally, patchy areas of atelectasis secondary to bronchial obstruction can be seen on chest x-ray. Necrotizing bronchopneumonia should be suspected in patients with unremitting fever, dyspnea, tachypnea, radiologic evidence of bronchopneumonia, and a poor response to standard antibiotic therapy. Finally, hemorrhagic infarction due to vascular permeation with nonthrombotic occlusion of small- to medium-sized arteries and necrosis typically results in either a well-defined nodule or a wedge-shaped, pleura-based density. Symptoms are nonspecific and include fever, dyspnea, dry cough, pleuritic chest pain, and hemoptysis. Cavitation is common, and radiologic examination may reveal "round" pneumonia or "air crescents" of a mycotic lung sequestrum.

Aspergillomas ("fungus balls" or mycetomas) are divided into two types: simple, thin-walled cysts lined with ciliated epithelium and surrounded by normal parenchyma; and complex cavities associated with markedly abnormal surrounding lung tissue. Aspergillomas most often occur in the upper lobes and in the superior segments of the lower lobes. Although they may be multiple (22%), calcification and air-fluid levels are rare. Most aspergillomas—particularly complex ones—are associated with cavitary lung disease, that is, tuberculosis (most common), histoplasmosis, sarcoidosis, bronchiectasis, and others. Hemoptysis occurs in 50%-80% and can present with frequent minor episodes (30% subsequently have massive bleeding), repeated moderate episodes, or a single episode of massive hemoptysis. Chest x-ray may reveal a 3- to 6-cm round, mobile density with a crescent of air.

Corticosteroids are indicated in patients with allergic bronchopulmonary aspergillosis in addition to measures to relieve bronchospasm (inhaled β-agonists or anticholinergics). In invasive aspergillosis, amphotericin B (0.5-2 g intravenously as total dose) has been standard therapy despite a mortality of 90%. In addition, some patients with complex aspergillomas and severe pulmonary disease are not candidates for surgical resection, and intracavitary amphotericin has been used with modest success. Surgery is indicated for complications of *Aspergillus* infection. Hemoptysis due to aspergillomas is usually best treated by surgical resection. Furthermore, hemoptysis associated with localized invasive aspergillosis (particularly once cavitation has occurred) can be treated by resection and amphotericin B. Generally, wide excision (lobectomy) is required; however, in some high-risk patients with aspergillomas, cavernostomy, and muscle flap closure is an alternative.

6. Mucormycosis

Infection with *Rhizopus arrhizus*, *Absidia* species, and *Rhizomucor* species of the class *Zygomycetes* and the order Mucorales occurs in certain distinct immunosuppressed patient populations: people with poorly controlled diabetes and leukemia patients. These fungi are ubiquitous organisms that are found in decaying fruit, vegetable matter, soil, and manure. Infection occurs following inhalation of sporangiospores, which germinate in a hyphal form. The diagnosis is made by demonstrating the organism in symptomatic patients. No accurate skin or serologic tests exist. Although the fungi do grow in culture as broad, irregular nonseptate hyphae that branch at angles up to 90 degrees (occasionally being confused with *Aspergillus* species), most commonly the diagnosis is made on histologic examination. The sine qua non for mucormycosis is hyphal vascular invasion between the internal elastic membrane and the media of blood vessels, causing thrombosis, infarction, and necrosis.

In addition to pulmonary infections, mucormycosis manifests as distinct clinical syndromes such as rhinocerebral infection (direct extension into the central nervous system from paranasal sinus infection), cutaneous infection (burn patients), gastrointestinal infection (children with protein-calorie malnutrition), and disseminated infection (uremic patients receiving deferoxamine therapy). Patients with pulmonary infection complain of fever, cough, pleuritic chest pain, and hemoptysis. Frequently, this type of infection occurs in immunocompromised hosts and follows a fulminant course. Three patterns of infection are noted on chest x-ray: limited disease with involvement of a single lobe or segment, diffuse or disseminated disease with involvement of both lungs and the mediastinum, and endobronchial disease with bronchial obstruction and secondary bacterial infection. Characteristic CT findings include a halo sign (area of low attenuation around a dense infiltrate), ring enhancement, and an air-crescent sign (area of contrast between normal lung and a radiodense cavitating lesion). Amphotericin B is the standard treatment. In nonneutropenic patients, the newer azole compounds may be useful; however, infection with these fungi remains highly lethal, with a mortality of 90%. The cause of death in these patients is often fungal sepsis, progressive pulmonary dysfunction, and hemoptysis. In the small group of patients with limited disease, aggressive surgical resection in combination with amphotericin B has lowered the mortality to only 50%. In contrast, the endobronchial form can be effectively treated with transbronchoscopic resection (using the Nd:YAG laser) in a large proportion of patients.

7. Pneumocystosis

Pneumocystis carinii is a fungal organism that has been found in the lungs of a variety of domesticated and wild mammals and is distributed worldwide in humans. Pulmonary involvement leads to progressive pneumonia and respiratory insufficiency. Disease has been seen with increasing frequency in recipients of organ transplants who are undergoing immunosuppressive therapy. Diagnosis is made by open lung biopsy. Without treatment with trimethoprim-sulfamethoxazole, pentamidine, or inhaled antimicrobial therapy, the course is one of relentless progression. With improved antiviral therapy for HIV infections, the incidence of pneumocystosis has been declining.

LoCicero J et al: Surgery for other pulmonary fungal infections, *Actinomyces*, and *Nocardia. Thorac Surg Clin* 2012;22:363-374.
Smith JA et al: Pulmonary fungal infections. *Respirology* 2012;17:913-926.

SARCOIDOSIS (BOECK SARCOID, BENIGN LYMPHOGRANULOMATOSIS)

Sarcoidosis is a noncaseating granulomatous disease of unknown cause involving the lungs, liver, spleen, lymph nodes, skin, and bones. The highest incidence is reported in Scandinavia, England, and the United States. The incidence in blacks is 10-17 times that in whites. Half of patients are

between ages 20 and 40 years, with women more frequently affected than men.

▶ Clinical Findings

A. Symptoms and Signs

Sarcoidosis may present with symptoms of pulmonary infection, but usually these are insidious and nonspecific. Erythema nodosum may herald the onset, and weight loss, fatigue, weakness, and malaise may appear later. Fever occurs in approximately 15% of cases. Pulmonary symptoms occur in 20%-30% and include dry cough and dyspnea. Hemoptysis is rare. One-fifth of patients with sarcoidosis have myocardial involvement, and heart block or failure may occur. Peripheral lymph nodes are enlarged in 75%, scalene lymph nodes are microscopically involved in 80% and mediastinal nodes in 90%, and cutaneous involvement is present in 30%. Hepatic and splenic involvement can be shown by biopsy in 70% of cases. There may be migratory or persistent polyarthritis, and central nervous involvement occurs in a few patients.

B. Imaging Studies

The x-ray findings in sarcoidosis are classified into five descriptive categories or stages (Table 18–5). Pulmonary disease can manifest as a reticulonodular infiltrate, an acinar pattern of opacities, or large nodules with or without mediastinal adenopathy. Mediastinal lymph node involvement characteristically includes bilateral symmetric hilar and paratracheal lymphadenopathy. Anterior or posterior mediastinal adenopathy or asymmetric hilar involvement should prompt a suspicion of other diseases, particularly Hodgkin disease and non-Hodgkin lymphomas. Pleural effusions and cavitation are rare and, if present, necessitate an evaluation for tuberculosis, congestive heart failure, and coincidental pneumonia.

C. Diagnosis

Although no single test exists to confirm absolutely the diagnosis of sarcoidosis (the diagnosis remains one of exclusion), it may be suggested by the characteristic radiographic appearance of bilateral hilar and mediastinal lymphadenopathy, by

Table 18–5. Radiographic stages of sarcoidosis.

Stage 0: No x-ray abnormality
Stage 1: Hilar and mediastinal lymph node enlargement without pulmonary abnormalities
Stage 2: Hilar and mediastinal lymph node enlargement with pulmonary abnormalities
Stage 3: Diffuse pulmonary disease without adenopathy
Stage 4: Pulmonary fibrosis

gallium 67 scanning, and by elevated serum and bronchoalveolar fluid levels of angiotensin-converting enzyme and lysozyme. Pathologic documentation of noncaseating granulomas should normally be obtained either via transbronchial biopsy or mediastinoscopy (more reliable, with > 95% success rate). Culture for mycobacteria, fungi, and other atypical infections must also be negative.

D. Treatment

Asymptomatic patients and those with minimal clinical disease may require no therapy. Corticosteroids have been used in patients with pulmonary impairment and symptomatic disease with good success. Despite the indolent nature of the disease and steroid therapy, long-term mortality is reported as high as 10%. Lung transplantation has been utilized with success in patients refractory to medical management.

▼ NEOPLASMS OF THE LUNG

PRIMARY LUNG CANCER

Lung cancer is the most common cause of cancer-related death in both men and women in the United States. In 2013, it is estimated that 228,190 new cases and 159,480 deaths will occur due to pulmonary malignancies. This represents 14% of all new cancer cases and 27% of all cancer-related deaths. Tobacco smoking accounts for 85% of all lung cancer cases. The effect is greatest for cigarettes and least for pipe smoking and is directly related to the amount of tobacco smoked. Following 5-6 years of smoking cessation, the risk exponentially declines, and after 15 years approaches, but never reaches, that of nonsmokers. "Passive" exposure to cigarette smoke, on the other hand, increases the risk in nonsmokers by two to three times. Exposure to all forms of asbestos (amosite, chrysotile, and crocidolite) has been implicated in as many as 23% of lung cancers, accounting for the high incidence among shipyard workers, insulators, cement makers, truck drivers, and plumbers. The effect is particularly pronounced in smokers and is most commonly associated with squamous cell and small cell carcinoma. Exposure to radon and its alpha-emitting daughter isotopes have been implicated in the increased incidence of lung cancer in both uranium miners and populations living in geographic areas naturally contaminated with high levels of radon gas. Although it has been known for some time that people with high activity of 4-debrisoquine hydroxylase, the so-called debrisoquine metabolic phenotype, have a 10-fold increased risk of lung cancer, only recently has the role of genetic factors been appreciated.

Chromosome deletions (particularly 11p, 13q, 17p, and 3p), tumor suppressor gene mutations (p53, Hap-1, ErbAb, etc), and constitutive, high-level expression of both growth factor genes (insulin-like and transferrin-like growth factors), epidermal growth factor receptors (HER2/neu, EGFR1,

etc), and protooncogenes (c-, N-, and L-myc; H-, N-, and K-ras; and c-myb) have all been implicated in the pathogenesis of lung cancer. Other factors such as vitamin A deficiency, air pollution; exposure to arsenic, cadmium, chromium, ether, and formaldehyde; and employment as bakers, cooks, construction workers, cosmetologists, leather workers, pitchblende miners, printers, rubber workers, and pottery workers have also been incriminated. Finally, certain diseases (eg, progressive systemic sclerosis [scleroderma]) have a defined predisposition for the development of lung cancer. Silencing of genes by aberrant promoter hypermethylation is viewed as a crucial component in lung cancer pathobiology. High throughput genomic analysis has identified scores of genes and metabolic pathways that appear to be associated with the progression of lung cancer.

▶ Pathology

Lung cancer occurs more commonly in the right lung than the left, and the upper lobes are involved more commonly than the lower lobes or the right-middle lobe. Synchronous primary lung cancers occur in up to 7% of patients, and 10% of patients will develop a metachronous new tumor (2% per year risk postresection of early stage disease). Furthermore, patients with lung cancer are at higher risk of developing cancers of the upper respiratory tract, oral cavity, esophagus, bladder, and kidney presumably related to the "field effect" of smoking. Lung cancers typically spread by local extension to involve the visceral and parietal pleura, chest wall, great vessels, pericardium, diaphragm, esophagus, and vertebral column. Common sites of metastatic involvement include the ipsilateral pulmonary and hilar lymph nodes, the mediastinal lymph nodes, the lung, liver, bone, brain, adrenal glands, pancreas, kidney, soft tissues, and myocardium. The exact pathologic classification of lung cancer has not been uniform despite attempts at standardization by the World Health Organization. Functionally, however, squamous cell carcinoma, large cell carcinoma, and adenocarcinoma are grouped together under the designation of non-small cell carcinomas and constitute 80% of all lung tumors. Small cell carcinoma represents 15%-20%, while bronchial gland adenomas, including carcinoids, comprise the remaining 5%. The differential locations of some of these neoplasms are summarized in Table 18–6.

A. Squamous Cell Carcinoma

The major pathologic features of squamous cell carcinoma are keratinization, cellular stratification, and intercellular bridges. Squamous cell carcinomas account for about 20% of all cases of lung cancer and 70% of non–small cell tumors. Two-thirds are located centrally near the hilum and one-third peripherally. The growth rate and the rate of metastasis tend to be slower than those of other lung tumors.

Table 18–6. Location of lung cancer by histologic type.

Histology	Central (%)	Peripheral (%)
Squamous cell carcinoma	64–81	19–36
Adenocarcinoma	5–29	71–95
Large cell carcinoma	42–49	51–58
Small cell carcinoma	74–83	17–26
Overall	63	37

Reproduced, with permission, from Cameron RB: Malignancies of the lung. In Cameron RB, ed: *Practical Oncology*. New York, NY: McGraw-Hill; 1994.

B. Adenocarcinoma

Adenocarcinomas, which constitute 30% of lung cancers and 60% of non–small cell tumors, are characterized as acinar, papillary, lepidic (formerly nonmucinous bronchioloalveolar [BAC] with > 5 mm invasion), micropapillary and solid, as well as preinvasive lesions including atypical adenomatous hyperplasia and adenocarcinoma *in situ* (≤ 3 cm formerly BAC) and minimally-invasive (≤ 3 cm lepidic predominant tumor with a 5 mm invasion). Acinar adenocarcinoma is composed of glands lined by columnar cells that secrete mucin. Lepidic carcinoma is characterized by intraluminal papillary fragments that appear in alveoli or small bronchioles. The incidence of adenocarcinoma of the lung is increasing relative to squamous cell carcinoma, perhaps as a consequence of the rise in lung cancer among women, although the exact cause remains unclear.

C. Small Cell Carcinoma

Small cell (oat cell) carcinomas have small, round nuclei with nuclear chromatin and cytoplasm. They are biologically and clinically distinct from all other cell types such that the term non–small cell lung cancer (NSCLC) often is applied to all other cell types. Small cell carcinomas comprise 15%-20% of all lung cancers. They occur centrally, metastasize early but also can exhibit significant partial response to combined-modality treatment, albeit with limited 5-year survival.

D. Large Cell Carcinoma

Large cell carcinomas are composed of large polygonal spindle or oval cells arranged in sheets, nests, or clusters. Multinucleated giant cells, intracellular hyalin droplets, glycogen, and acidophilic nuclear inclusions may be present. These tumors are seen peripherally and are less common.

E. Adenosquamous Tumors

Adenosquamous tumors show both cellular features and are more biologically aggressive than other NSCLC. Survival percentages of patients with adenosquamous tumors are significantly lower than what is reported for adenocarcinoma or squamous cell cancer.

F. Bronchial Gland Adenomas

Bronchial gland adenoma is a misnomer, since the vast majority of these tumors are malignant. Included in this group are carcinoid tumors, adenoid cystic carcinomas, mucoepidermoid carcinoma, mixed tumors of the salivary gland type, and mucous gland adenoma. Carcinoid tumors are derived from Kulchitsky cells, have a vascular stroma, and tend to be located centrally in proximal airways. Although they are slow-growing, they can metastasize widely. Carcinoid syndrome is rarely associated with bronchial carcinoids, as opposed to intestinal carcinoids that metastasize to the liver. Adenoid cystic carcinomas—also referred to as cylindromas—feature groups of epithelial cells that form duct-like structures interspersed with cystic spaces. These neoplasms are locally aggressive and often extend beyond apparent gross pathologic margins. Metastases from adenoid cystic carcinomas often involve the lung, are slow growing, and are amenable to surgical excision. Mucoepidermoid carcinomas are rare tumors characterized by the presence of squamous cells, mucus-secreting cells, and an intermediate cell type. The cells are bland and less aggressive than those of adenosquamous carcinomas. Mixed tumors of the salivary type are extremely rare infiltrating tumors that are curable with wide local excision. Finally, mucus gland adenomas (papillary or bronchial cyst adenomas) are the only true benign "adenomas" of this group with no metastatic potential. These neoplasms are rare tumors of the major bronchi and consist of numerous mucus-filled cysts lined by a well-differentiated epithelium. Generally, bronchoscopic removal can be accomplished and results in long-term cure.

▶ Clinical Presentation

Nearly 94% of patients present with symptoms from the effects of the primary tumor, regional spread, or metastatic disease. Local effects of the primary tumor account for 27% of presenting symptoms and vary depending on the location of the tumor. Central tumors are associated with cough, hemoptysis, respiratory difficulty (wheezing, stridor, or dyspnea), pain, and pneumonia. Peripheral tumors can cause cough, chest wall pain, pleural effusions, pulmonary abscess, Horner syndrome (ipsilateral miosis, ptosis, and anhidrosis), and Pancoast syndrome (ipsilateral shoulder and arm pain in the C8-T1 nerve root distribution, Horner syndrome, and a superior sulcus—usually squamous—lung cancer). Symptoms due to the effect of regional spread include hoarseness from recurrent nerve paralysis, dyspnea due to phrenic nerve paralysis, dysphagia from compression of the esophagus, superior vena cava syndrome from compression or invasion of the superior vena cava, and pericardial tamponade from invasion of the pericardium. Metastatic disease may present with symptoms of systemic illness (anorexia, weight loss, weakness, and malaise), local manifestations of distant metastases (jaundice, abdominal mass, bony pain or fracture, neurologic deficits, mental status changes, seizures, and soft tissue masses). A number of paraneoplastic syndromes associated with lung cancer have been identified (Table 18–7).

▶ Diagnosis & Evaluation

Lung cancer is usually suspected from abnormal findings on a chest x-ray obtained in the course of a routine physical examination or, more commonly, after a complaint of pul-

Table 18–7. Paraneoplastic syndromes associated with lung cancer.

Cardiovascular
  Thrombophlebitis
  Nonbacterial thrombotic endocarditis
  Neuromuscular
  Subacute cerebellar degeneration
  Dementia
  Limbic encephalitis
  Optic neuritis, retinopathy
  Subacute necrotic myelopathy
  Autonomic neuropathy (small cell)
  Myasthenic (Eaton-Lambert) syndrome (small cell)
  Polymyositis
Gastrointestinal
  Carcinoid syndrome (carcinoid and small cell)
  Anorexia, cachexia
Hematologic
  Erythrocytosis
  Leukocytosis
Metabolic
  Inappropriate adrenocorticotropic hormone (ACTH) (small cell)
  Inappropriate antidiuretic hormone (ADH) (small cell)
  Hypercalcemia (squamous cell carcinoma)
  Inappropriate gonadotropins
Dermatologic
  Acanthosis nigricans (adenocarcinoma)
  Dermatomyositis
  Erythema gyratum
  Ichthyosis
Other
  Hypertrophic pulmonary osteoarthropathy (squamous cell, large cell, and adenocarcinoma)
  Nephrotic syndrome
  Fever

monary symptoms (see previous discussion). Findings vary from a small peripheral nodule to an unresolving infiltrate or even total lung atelectasis. Occasionally, the location of the abnormality may suggest certain cell types (see Table 18–7). Once the diagnosis of lung cancer is suspected, a definitive diagnosis can be obtained in over 90% of patients with either bronchoscopy for proximal lesions or fine-needle aspiration cytology for peripheral lesions.

CT scanning is an integral part of the assessment of patients with lung cancer. Chest CT scans should also include the upper abdomen to assess two of the most common sites of metastases (liver and adrenal glands). Injection of intravenous contrast while the scan is obtained facilitates evaluation of the mediastinum. Additional radiographic evaluation includes tests to evaluate other common sites of metastases, such as bone and brain. A serum alkaline phosphatase is essential, and a bone scan and brain CT scan (or preferably MRI) should be obtained if indicated by elevated alkaline phosphatase levels, neurologic symptoms, or bone pain or if advanced-stage disease (stage III or beyond) is present. Fluorodeoxyglucose (FDG) PET has evolved into a critical staging test. It is most effective as a tool for assessing for distant occult disease. It can be helpful for predicting mediastinal node involvement, but it is not definitive. False-positive rates as high as 15%-20% have been reported. Furthermore, nodules less than 1 cm in diameter generally are not imaged reliably by PET scanning. Combination high-resolution CT scan and PET scan assessment permits improved correlation of abnormal CT findings with FDG uptake suggestive of tumor.

Thoracentesis or thoracoscopy (or both) should be performed in any patient with evidence of a pleural effusion to exclude diffuse involvement of the pleura (M1 or stage IV disease) which indicates metastatic disease. Despite increasing reliance on PET scan to stage the mediastinum, patients with NSCLC but without metastatic disease should be evaluated with endobronchial ultrasound guided FNA, cervical mediastinoscopy or parasternal mediastinotomy (Chamberlain) if necessary to document the status of the mediastinal nodes in equivocal cases. PET scanning is informative but tissue confirmation typically is necessary. For small cell lung cancer staging should be directed at assessing the presence of extrathoracic disease, to confirm limited-stage tumor extent. The use of CT scans alone is inaccurate in 40%-60% of patients with enlarged lymph nodes over 1 cm (false positive) and 15% of patients without "significant" lymphadenopathy (false negative).

Once all the information from these staging procedures is in hand, the patient with NSCLC can be classified into one of three categories: (1) early lung cancer without mediastinal involvement, that is, stage I/II (see next section); (2) locally advanced lung cancer, that is stage IIIA/B; and (3) metastatic lung cancer, or stage IV. Therapy is determined by disease stage. Patients with small cell lung cancer usually are grouped into two categories: disease limited to the ipsilateral hemithorax, including supraclavicular nodes (limited disease), or disease extending beyond the thorax (extensive disease, eg, below the diaphragm or brain metastases).

Several recent analyses indicate that lung cancer screening by either regular routine chest radiography or sputum cytology is not recommended. Low-dose screening chest CT can be considered, but only among select individuals in the context of multidisciplinary comprehensive care that includes not only screening but also image interpretation, evaluation, management and appropriate treatment of findings.

▶ Staging

By 1987, the American Joint Committee on Cancer (AJCC) and the Union Internationale Contre le Cancer (UICC) had developed a joint staging system for lung carcinoma based on data gathered primarily by Clifford Mountain of the MD Anderson Cancer Center. The most recent iteration (7th edition) of the lung cancer staging system, published in 2007, is based on the tumor (T), the status of regional lymph nodes (N), and the presence or absence of distant metastases (M), as outlined in Table 18–8.

▶ Treatment

Treatment for small cell carcinoma consists primarily of chemotherapy and radiation, although recent data indicate that for early disease (T1-T2 lesions without hilar adenopathy) resection may improve local control and result in increased long-term survival (as high as 50%), particularly when combined with postoperative chemotherapy.

Treatment for NSCLC varies with stage. Early-stage disease (stage I/II) has historically been treated with surgery alone. Notably, several randomized prospective trials have demonstrated a statistically significant improvement in lung cancer survival among patients treated with adjuvant chemotherapy for early stage (stages II and III) NSCLC. Combined-modality therapy utilizing induction chemotherapy or chemoradiotherapy appears to confer a survival advantage for patients with potentially resectable stage IIIA disease, although overall survival was not improved compared with patients receiving chemotherapy with definitive-dose radiation therapy. Locally advanced and surgically unresectable disease (stage IIIB) is best managed with concurrent platinum-based chemotherapy and fractionated radiation therapy. Among patients with metastatic disease (stage IV), chemotherapy is best for palliation of symptoms. Radiotherapy in this case also is reserved primarily for symptomatic lesions. Combined-agent chemotherapy offers 2-3 months (20%) survival extension to advanced-stage patients. It has been shown to be cost-effective and improve quality of life and is generally well tolerated by patients with reasonable performance status. New biologic agents—so-called targeted therapies—are showing activity in clinical trials and

Table 18–8. TNM stage groupings.

Primary tumor	
TX	Primary tumor cannot be assessed, or cytologic evidence of malignant cells in sputum or bronchial washings but not visualized by imaging or bronchoscopy
T0	No evidence of primary tumor
Tis	Carcinoma in situ
T1	Tumor ≤ 3 cm in greatest diameter, completely surrounded by lung or visceral pleura, and without bronchoscopic evidence of involvement of more proximal than a lobar bronchus
T2	Tumor > 3 cm in greatest diameter, invading the visceral pleura, involving the main stem bronchus but > 2 cm distal to the carina, or tumor associated with atelectasis or obstructive pneumonitis extending to the hilum but not involving the entire lung
T3	Tumor of any size invading the chest wall, diaphragm, mediastinal pleura, parietal pericardium; tumor involving the main stem bronchus within 2 cm of but not involving the carina; or tumor associated with atelectasis or obstructive pneumonitis of the entire lung
T4	Tumor of any size invading the mediastinum, heart, great vessels, trachea, esophagus, vertebral body, or carina or tumor associated with a malignant pleural effusion

Regional lymph nodes (N stage)	
NX	Regional lymph nodes cannot be assessed
N0	No evidence of regional lymph node metastases
N1	Metastases in ipsilateral peribronchial or hilar lymph nodes, including by direct extension
N2	Metastases in ipsilateral mediastinal or subcarinal lymph nodes
N3	Metastases in contralateral mediastinal or hilar lymph nodes or ipsilateral or contralateral scalene or supraclavicular nodes

Distant metastases (M stage)	
MX	Presence of distant metastases cannot be assessed
M0	No evidence of distant metastases
M1	Distant metastases are present

Stage grouping	
Occult disease	TX, N0, M0
Stage 0	Tis, N0, M0
Stage IA	T1, N0, M0
Stage IB	T2 N0 M0
Stage IIA	T1 N1 M0
Stage IIB	T2 N1 M0
	T3 N0 M0
Stage IIIA	T1–2, N2, M0, or T3, N0–2, M0
Stage IIIB	T4, any N, M0, or any T, N3, M0
Stage IV	Any T, Any N, M1

should improve overall survival statistics. It is hoped that with advances in targeted and conventional therapies, the current overall survival (< 15% at 5 years) of patients with lung cancer can be improved.

▶ Induction Chemotherapy

Recently completed clinical trials and several ongoing studies suggest survival benefit of treatment with platinum-based chemotherapy prior to resection. Induction chemotherapy has been standard for locally advanced surgically resectable disease, but evidence is accumulating to support induction therapy in early stage NSCLC.

A. Surgical Treatment

1. Surgical Staging—As noted earlier, almost all patients with NSCLC limited to the thorax should undergo cervical mediastinoscopy or EBUS-FNA to exclude involvement of N2 mediastinal lymph nodes (N2 or N3 disease). A possible exception is a small peripheral (T1) nodule, especially of squamous cell histology without any evidence for mediastinal adenopathy on chest CT scan. PET scan is used with increasing frequency to stage the mediastinum. Surgical staging with cervical mediastinoscopy remains the most accurate staging maneuver. Adenocarcinomas with negative mediastinal nodes by CT have an 18%-25% false-negative rate. For left-sided lesions, left parasternal mediastinotomy (Chamberlain) may be required to assess the status of the aorticopulmonary lymph nodes. Without pathologic confirmation of the status of mediastinal lymph nodes, CT scans have been associated with high false-positive and false-negative rates. A surgical assessment of the proximal airways is also required even if this means repeating this invasive procedure, often previously performed by the pulmonologist. Because treatment decisions are based on accurate staging, and treatment of early-stage disease (stage I/II) differs significantly from locally advanced disease (stage IIIA/B); this approach is essential. The importance of accurate staging for patients with NSCLC cannot be overstated.

2. Indications and Preoperative Assessment—Pulmonary resection is indicated for early-stage lung cancer (stage I/II) and in combination with chemotherapy and radiation in locally advanced resectable disease (stage IIIA or resectable T4, IIIb). In addition, resection may be indicated for patients with a single site of metastatic disease, such as a solitary brain or adrenal gland metastasis. Both relative and absolute contraindications to surgical resection are listed in Table 18–9.

Preoperative assessment is directed toward evaluating both cardiopulmonary reserve and overall patient fitness. The patient's general performance status or functional classification is probably the most accurate factor

Table 18–9. Medical and surgical contraindications to pulmonary resection.

Absolute	Relative
Myocardial infarction within previous 3 months	Myocardial infarction within previous 6 months
SVC syndrome (due to metastatic tumor)	SVC syndrome (due to primary tumor)
Bilateral endobronchial tumor	Recurrent laryngeal nerve paralysis (due to primary tumor in aortico-pulmonary window)
Contralateral lymph node metastases (N3)	Horner syndrome
Malignant pleural effusion	Small cell histology
Distant metastases (except solitary brain and adrenal metastases)	Metastases higher than the midtracheal lymph nodes
	Pericardial involvement
	$FEV_1 < 0.8$ L (< 50%)
	FEV_1 0.9–2.4 and insufficient pulmonary reserve for planned resection
	Main pulmonary artery involvement

in predicting a successful outcome following operation. Advanced age alone is not a contraindication to resection. A thorough cardiac evaluation is also necessary since lung cancer and cardiovascular disease share common risk factors (eg, smoking). Patients with cardiac symptoms, an abnormal EKG, or other findings suggestive of ischemic heart disease should be screened by a stress test (eg, exercise treadmill, dipyridamole- or adenosine-thallium study, dobutamine echocardiogram). Significant coronary artery disease should be treated with coronary artery bypass or catheter-based intervention as indicated, prior to any contemplated pulmonary resection. Furthermore, significant pulmonary hypertension and myocardial infarction within 3 months has been associated with up to 20% perioperative mortality and constitute absolute contraindications to standard resection. Other high-risk findings include myocardial infarction within 6 months, ventricular arrhythmias and heart block, particularly left posterior fascicular hemiblock. Finally, the patient's pulmonary function and predicted ability to tolerate the required pulmonary resection should be assessed. This is accomplished with pulmonary function tests (spirometry, diffusing capacity, exercise oximetry) and with differential (quantitative) ventilation-perfusion scanning when appropriate. In a 70-kg patient, the following preoperative studies suggest high risk for perioperative morbidity and are relative contraindications to resection: forced expiratory volume in 1 second (FEV_1) below 0.8 L, a predicted postoperative FEV_1 below 0.8, a predicted maximum voluntary ventilation under 50%, a $Paco_2$ higher than 45 mm Hg, and a Pao_2 less than 50 mm Hg. A diffusion limitation capacity of carbon monoxide (DLCO) less than 60% predicted is correlated with an increase in perioperative mortality. Generally, for patients whose predicted postoperative values for FVC, FEV_1, or DLCO are projected to be less than 40% predicted, further assessment of functional status and operability are recommended.

3. Pulmonary Resection

A. EARLY AND LOCALLY ADVANCED NON-SMALL CELL LUNG CANCER—The extent of pulmonary resection is dictated by the location of the primary tumor and the presence or absence of involved hilar (interlobar) lymph nodes. Limited segmental resection for stage I/II NSCLC has been evaluated by the Lung Cancer Study Group and found to result in an increased local recurrence rate (15% vs 3%) and lower overall survival, although more recent cohort studies suggest that sublobar resection, particularly segmentectomy rather than non-anatomic wedge excision, may be considered for smaller lung nodules without evidence for local (N1) lymph node involvement. Lobectomy remains the standard of care for resection of early stage NSCLC. Recent case series have suggested that sublobar resection actually might be adequate in terms of local recurrence and disease-free survival particularly for stage I carcinoma; this is the focus of an ongoing multicenter clinical trial. Samples of interlobar (hilar) lymph nodes are submitted for immediate pathologic examination to exclude involvement that would require pneumonectomy. A "sleeve" resection of main stem bronchus can also be included in the resection, particularly with the right-upper lobe. Pneumonectomy may be necessary for proximal lesions involving the main stem bronchus or the interlobar (hilar) lymph nodes, although bronchial and/or vascular sleeve resections should be considered. In addition, techniques are available for more extensive resection such as intrapericardial pneumonectomy and tracheal sleeve pneumonectomy.

The overall mortality rates following segmental resection, lobectomy, and pneumonectomy are 1.4%, 2.9%, and 6.2%, respectively, in centers with large experience. Complications following pulmonary resection include cardiac arrhythmias, hemorrhage, infection (empyema), bronchopleural fistula, respiratory insufficiency, and pulmonary embolism.

B. ADVANCED (METASTATIC) NON-SMALL CELL LUNG CANCER—Patients with solitary brain and adrenal metastases, especially if metachronous, are still candidates for resection and have benefited by prolonged survival in a few small retrospective studies in comparison with historical controls. Systemic preoperative (induction) chemotherapy and radiotherapy, however, should be administered initially. In addition, transbronchial Nd:YAG laser resection of tumors obstructing the proximal airways can provide satisfactory palliation for selected patients. Improvements in the design and deployment techniques of expansile stents have been a significant advance for palliation of proximal airway obstruction. Finally, photodynamic laser therapy with photosensitizers can alleviate airway obstruction from tumors, albeit not as quickly as Nd:YAG laser ablation.

C. SMALL CELL LUNG CANCER—Resection for small peripheral tumors followed by aggressive postoperative chemotherapy may increase the local control rate and potentially the overall survival rate in the early small cell lung cancer. Survival rates as high as 50% with this approach have been reported.

B. Radiation Therapy

1. Non–Small Cell Lung Cancer— Radiation therapy can be administered with curative intent in stage I/II disease in patients who refuse or are not medically suitable candidates for surgery. The 5-year survival rate with this approach, however, is only 22%-33%. With locally advanced disease (stage IIIA/B), radiation therapy (5500-6000 cGy) until recently has been the treatment of choice. Although local or nodal recurrence rates are less than 30%, long-term survival is less than 10% in these patients, and the type of fractionation scheme has not altered the outcome. Stereotactic radiation techniques appear to have early efficacy in terms of tumor control and overall survival, particularly for medically inoperable patients.

Adjuvant radiation therapy following resection has been extensively studied by the Lung Cancer Study Group and has been found to decrease local or nodal recurrence but not to prolong overall survival. A much-disputed meta-analysis (the PORT study) showed a decrease in survival for stage II patients treated with postoperative radiation. Differences in radiotherapy techniques within the analysis may account for the worse outcomes. Preoperative radiation has been used with T3 lesions, particularly Pancoast tumors, with improved survival; however, there is no objective evidence that radiation must be given preoperatively. A multicenter intergroup trial (SWOG) has shown a significant survival advantage for combined chemoradiotherapy (etoposide, platinum, and 4500 cGy) prior to resection for Pancoast (superior sulcus) tumors that were N1 or less. Complete resection rates were improved, 20%-25% complete pathologic responses were achieved, and survival was significantly improved (45%-50% at 3 years) over surgery alone or preoperative radiotherapy and surgery. Intraoperative radiation has been investigated but to date has been associated with unacceptably high morbidity. Among patients with metastatic disease, therapeutic radiation is indicated in patients with symptoms of pain, neurologic symptoms, and symptoms of superior vena cava compression.

2. Small Cell Lung Cancer—Multiple randomized trials comparing the combination of radiation and chemotherapy to chemotherapy alone in limited-stage small cell lung cancer have been conducted. The majority show improved local control and modest (3-4 months) prolonged survival with the combination. This was at the cost of increased morbidity, however. In extensive disease, no benefit has been demonstrated for radiation therapy other than for palliative radiation of symptomatic metastases. Prophylactic cranial irradiation may be beneficial but can cause significant cognitive deficits.

C. Chemotherapy

1. Non–Small Cell Lung Cancer—Although chemotherapy alone has not generally been used in the treatment of early or locally advanced NSCLC, combinations of chemotherapy and radiotherapy have been evaluated in locally advanced unresectable disease. In some instances, no benefit to the combination was demonstrated, particularly when only single agents were used; however, improved results with both radiation and combined-agent chemotherapy have recently been documented. In the presence of metastatic disease, multiple trials of combination chemotherapy have demonstrated a modest improvement in overall survival (14 weeks or 25% improved survival) but not without some toxicity. Even so, quality of life assessments and cost analyses support the use of outpatient combined-agent chemotherapy over palliative care alone.

A. Postoperative adjuvant therapy—A progressive trend in lung cancer therapy has evolved in favor of far more widespread use of adjuvant chemotherapy. Three large multicenter randomized trials in Europe and North America have served as a basis for the increased application of postoperative platinum-based chemotherapy (Italian Stage IB, the International Adjuvant Lung Cancer Trial [IALT], Cancer and Leukemia Group B [CALGB] 9633, and National Cancer Institute of Canada [NCIC] BR10). The benefit of chemotherapy appears to vary based on patient selection but is estimated to be an increase of 5%-15% survival measured at 5 years from diagnosis (Table 18–10).

2. Small Cell Lung Cancer— Combination chemotherapy currently produces 85%-95% and 75%-85% response rates in limited-stage and extensive-stage disease, respectively. Furthermore, median survival is 12-16 months and 7-11 months in each group. Regimens of doublet therapy consisting of cisplatin and etoposide, irinotecan, or paclitaxel have had good efficacy with less toxicity than prior alkylator-based treatment regimens. The optimal duration of therapy has not been defined, but the majority of the effect appears to occur within the first four cycles.

D. Immunotherapy

Immunotherapy using bacillus Calmette-Guérin (BCG), levamisole, IL-2, TNF-α, lymphokine-activated killer (LAK) cells, and tumor-infiltrating lymphocytes has not proved beneficial in any clinical studies to date.

E. Targeted Therapies

Molecular-based therapies targeting overexpressed growth receptors (*EGFR1*, HER-2/*neu*) by monoclonal antibody or small molecules have demonstrated clinical effectiveness among select patient populations. Additional agents targeting signal transduction pathways (eg, farnesyl transferase inhibitors) for the *ras* pathway as well as antisense oligonucleotide and gene therapies are all in advanced clinical testing stages and in combination with standard cytotoxic chemotherapy appear to enhance response rates. Prospective randomized trials evaluating the efficacy of

Table 18–10. Adjuvant trials favoring use of chemotherapy in completely resected non–small cell lung cancer.[1]

Study	CT Regimen	Radiation Therapy	5-Year Survival CT vs Control
Italian Stage IB Study	Cis/Etoposide × 6	No	63% vs 45%
IALT LeChevalier	Various platinum	Yes ±	44.5% vs 40.4%
CALGB 9633 Strauss	Carbo/Taxol × 4	No	69% vs 54%
JBR.10 Alam	Vin/P × 4	No	71% vs 59%[2]

[1]CT, Carbo/Taxol, carboplatin paclitaxel; Vin/P, vinorelbine cisplatin; Cis, cisplatin.
[2]4-year survival statistics.

EGFR tyrosine kinase inhibitor therapy have not been able to validate the findings of earlier non-randomized (phase I/II) trials.

▶ Prognosis

A. Non–Small Cell Lung Cancer

The survival of patients with NSCLC is highly dependent on the pathologic stage. Overall, the 5-year survival of patients with stages I, II, IIIA, IIIB, and IV is 43%-64%, 20%-40%, 15%-25%, 5%-7%, and less than 2%, respectively. A breakdown of survival by TNM classification is set forth in Table 18–11. Improved survival will likely depend on earlier diagnosis and further coordinated efforts among surgeons, medical oncologists, and radiation oncologists.

B. Small Cell Lung Cancer

Patients with limited-stage disease achieve a median survival of 12-16 months with 5%-25% 2-year survival, while those with extensive-stage disease have a median survival of only 7-11 months, with only 1%-3% surviving 2 years.

Albain KS et al: Radiotherapy plus chemotherapy with or without surgical resection for stage III non-small-cell lung cancer: a phase III randomised controlled trial. *Lancet* 2009;374:379.

Beroukhim R et al: The landscape of somatic copy-number alteration across human cancers. *Nature* 2010;463:899.

Detterbeck FC et al: Screening for lung cancer: diagnosis and management of lung cancer, 3rd ed. American College of Chest Physicians Evidence-Based Clinical Practice Guidelines. *Chest* 2013;143(5 suppl):e78S-e92S. doi:10.1378/chest.12-2350.

Howlader N et al: (eds). *SEER Cancer Statistics Review, 1975-2010.* Bethesda, MD: National Cancer Institute. Available at http://seer.cancer.gov/csr/1975_2010/, based on November 2012 SEER data submission, posted to the SEER web site, April 2013.

Jett JR et al: Treatment of small cell lung cancer: diagnosis and management of lung cancer, 3rd ed. American College of Chest Physicians Evidence-Based Clinical Practice Guidelines. *Chest* 2013;143(5 suppl):e400S-e419S. doi:10.1378/chest.12-2363.

Pignon JP et al: Lung adjuvant cisplatin evaluation: a pooled analysis by the LACE Collaborative Group. *J Clin Oncol* 2008;26:3552.

Shah A et al: Cost-effectiveness of stereotactic body radiation therapy versus surgical resection for stage I non-small cell lung cancer. *Cancer* Online publication May 29, 2013.

Timmerman R et al: Stereotactic body radiation therapy for inoperable early stage lung cancer. *JAMA* 2010;303:1070.

Travis WD et al: IASLC/ATS/ERS international multidisciplinary classification of lung adenocarcinoma. *J Thorac Oncol* 2011;6:244.

UNUSUAL PULMONARY NEOPLASMS

▶ Malignant Neoplasms

Bronchial adenomas are a group of low-grade malignancies arising from the bronchial tree. Carcinoid tumors constitute 85%-90% of these neoplasms, with adenoid cystic carcinoma (10%) and mucoepidermoid carcinoma (< 5%) accounting for most of the remainder. Carcinoid tumors are classified as either typical or atypical, with markedly different histologic characteristics (Table 18–12). Adenoid cystic carcinomas occur in the lower trachea; infiltrate locally along submucosal and perineural tissue planes, often far beyond the boundaries of gross tumor; and metastasize late. Mucoepidermoid carcinomas resemble salivary tumors, with varying numbers of three distinct cell types: mucous, squamous, and intermediate. Patients with bronchial adenomas complain of cough, recurrent pulmonary infections, hemoptysis, pain, and wheezing. Only 15% of patients are completely asymptomatic. Carcinoid syndrome is rare with pulmonary carcinoid tumors. Most bronchial adenomas are diagnosed with a combination of plain chest radiography, CT, and bronchoscopy. Biopsy at the time of bronchoscopy

Table 18–11. Survival in non–small cell lung cancer.

Stage	TNM Description	Five-Year Survival
I		70–76%
a	T1, N0	80–83%
b	T2, N0	60–65%
II		30–40%
a	T1, N1	32–40%
b	T2, N1	28–35%
	T3, N0	
IIIA		10–30%
	T3, N1	30–45%
	T1–2, N2	7–30%
	T3, N2	0–5%
IIIB		<10%
	T4, any N	<10%
	Any T, N3	<10%
IV	M1	<5%
Overall		14.5%

Table 18–12. Characteristics of typical and atypical carcinoid tumors.

	Typical %	Atypical %
Incidence	90	10
Central location	80	50
Peripheral location	20	50
Metastases	10–15	50–70

can be associated with significant bleeding, and measures to control this must be readily available.

Lung resection is indicated for these tumors, with lobectomy being the most common procedure. Sleeve and bronchoplastic resections are particularly useful to preserve pulmonary function in these patients and make standard pneumonectomy rare. Removal of adenoid cystic carcinomas requires generous margins and frozen section examination of the margins at the time of surgery. Up to 8 cm of trachea can be removed with primary anastomosis. In addition, postoperative radiation may be indicated for close margins. With the possible exception of atypical carcinoid, chemotherapy is generally not indicated in the treatment of these neoplasms.

The long-term outlook is good for patients with metastatic disease. Even patients with adenoid cystic carcinoma and distant metastases may do well for extended periods due to the slow-growing nature of this malignancy; however, lymph node and distant metastases in patients with carcinoid tumors generally carry a poor prognosis.

▶ **Benign Neoplasms**

Benign neoplasms of the lung are uncommon, accounting for less than 1% of all pulmonary tumors. Most are hamartomas, but fibromas, leiomyomas, neurofibromas, myoblastomas, and benign metastasizing leiomyomas also occur. Most lesions are peripheral and asymptomatic; however, central lesions can produce symptoms of cough, wheezing, hemoptysis, and recurrent pneumonia. Typically, the lesions are discovered on routine chest radiographs and appear as a 1- to 2-cm well-circumscribed, bosselated lower lung nodule with calcifications in 10%–30%. Central lesions may require bronchoscopy for diagnosis, but a pathologic diagnosis is most often obtained by fine-needle aspiration biopsy or surgery. Surgical resection should be conservative and limited to wedge excision unless the lesion occupies the proximal bronchial airway and is associated with recurrent distal infections or bronchiectasis. In such cases, lobectomy is indicated. Following resection, the prognosis is excellent.

SPECIAL PROBLEM: THE SOLITARY PULMONARY NODULE

With the frequent use of chest radiography, solitary pulmonary nodules ("coin lesions") are frequently found in patients without pulmonary symptoms. These lesions pose a diagnostic problem for clinicians because they may represent something as benign as a nipple shadow or as malignant as lung cancer. The overall incidence of cancer in coin lesions is as low as 10%. Other diagnostic possibilities include: (1) infections due to mycobacteria (tuberculosis), fungi (histoplasmosis, coccidioidomycosis), and helminths (echinococcosis); (2) inflammatory nodules from rheumatoid arthritis, focal pneumonitis, and Wegener granulomatosis; (3) congenital anomalies, such as bronchogenic cysts and arteriovenous malformations; (4) benign neoplasms such as hamartomas, hemangiomas, papillary tumors, fibrous tumors of the pleura; (5) malignant neoplasms of the lung; and (6) miscellaneous processes such as hematomas, pulmonary infarcts, pleural plaques, loculated effusions, chest wall masses, and mucoid impaction. Although certain radiographic findings may suggest malignancy or benignity, solid pathologic proof that the nodule does not represent a malignancy rests with the clinician. In general, malignant neoplasms are larger and grow rapidly, appear spiculated, often with surface umbilication or notching and eccentric excavation. In addition, cancers often occur in smokers (or former smokers) over the age of 40 with negative skin tests for tuberculosis, histoplasmosis, or coccidioidomycosis (although positive tests do not exclude cancer), and in nodules that lack calcium (CT Hounsfield units < 175). In contrast, benign lesions are small (< 1 cm), stable (> 2 years), and calcified ("target" or "popcorn" distribution; CT Hounsfield units > 175) and are associated with positive skin tests in 70%-90% of patients.

Evaluation of these patients usually includes chest CT scan, but sputum cytology, cultures, bronchoscopy, and mediastinoscopy are sometimes helpful. FDG-PET scanning plays an important role in the evaluation of tumors that are suspicious for malignancy. PET scan can often differentiate among lesions suspicious for malignancy.

With the advent of spiral CT scanning, the incidence of asymptomatic pulmonary nodules can vary from 25% to 70%. The vast majority of these lesions now identified are less than 1 cm and often as small as 2-3 mm. In one series, the incidence of lung cancer in the asymptomatic 10 pack-year smoking history population over the age of 50 years was 27% of all lesions identified, followed, and treated. Ongoing trials are assessing the efficacy and cost-effectiveness of CT screening for lung cancer. In the properly selected high-risk patient population (eg, over 60 years of age, moderate COPD, FEV_1 < 70%), and an over 20 pack-year smoking history), spiral CT may prove to be cost-effective and will save lives.

Ultimately, a pathologic diagnosis must be made. In some instances, fine-needle aspiration cytology may be helpful, particularly if a tissue diagnosis of hamartoma can be made or if cultures demonstrating infectious organisms are obtained. The vast majority of solitary pulmonary nodules require excisional biopsy to exclude the possibility of malignancy. Currently, this is accomplished with video-assisted techniques in most patients, particularly if the lesion is in the periphery of the lung. If a benign lesion is encountered, nothing further is warranted, but if a lung cancer is diagnosed, immediate lobectomy is indicated. The prognosis following resection of a coin lesion that turns out to be a bronchogenic carcinoma is good, with a 5-year survival of as high as 80%-90% for lesions smaller than 1 cm.

SECONDARY LUNG CANCER

Autopsy studies have demonstrated that 30% of all patients with malignancies develop pulmonary metastases, and 12% have been shown to have isolated lung disease that is totally resectable. In addition, 10% of these latter patients (1.2% of all patients) have solitary lung metastases. Most pulmonary metastases occur through hematogenous spread from the primary site—lymphatic or transbronchial spread is extremely rare. Secondary metastatic spread to the pulmonary and mediastinal lymph nodes, however, can also occur.

In patients with known extrathoracic primary cancers, multiple pulmonary lesions almost always represent metastatic disease. Solitary lesions, however, may be due to benign disease (18%) or new primary lung cancer (18%) as well as metastatic disease (64%). Most patients with pulmonary metastases are asymptomatic even with extensive disease. If symptoms do develop, cough, hemoptysis, fever, dyspnea, and pain are common. The diagnosis is generally initially suggested by routine chest radiography, and CT of the chest should always be ordered to assess the lungs for other nodules. Although CT scans are more sensitive, detecting nodules as small as 3 mm, they are also less specific (false-positive rate of 55%) than plain x-rays. Pathologic confirmation of the diagnosis is essential and usually is obtained at the time of resection. For patients who are not surgical candidates, fine-needle aspiration cytology is useful for peripheral lesions, while central lesions may require bronchoscopy for tissue diagnosis.

Medically fit patients with resectable disease are surgical candidates as long as the following criteria are fulfilled: (1) the primary tumor must be controlled or imminently controllable; (2) no other sites of disease may exist; (3) no other therapy can offer comparable results; and (4) the operative risk must be low. Since adenocarcinomas (especially breast cancer) commonly involve multiple organs, it is imperative that with this histology a full evaluation be performed, including bone scan and head CT or MRI. Solitary squamous cell nodules, even in the presence of a previous squamous cell carcinoma (eg, head and neck tumors), should be addressed as a new primary (lung) cancer.

Pulmonary resection can be accomplished through a standard posterolateral thoracotomy, median sternotomy, or bilateral anterior thoracotomies. The latter approach is particularly beneficial for bilateral disease involving the lower lobes. Video-assisted thoracoscopy is increasingly applied to metastatic disease in an attempt to reduce the morbidity of multiple resections. On occasion, during open operations for metastatic disease, several unsuspected nodules are found by direct palpation that might be missed with thoracoscopy. Wedge resection is the treatment of choice unless the lesion is a solitary squamous cell carcinoma or adenocarcinoma. These latter lesions cannot be distinguished from primary lung cancer on frozen section pathologic examination, and they must therefore be treated as primary lung cancers with lobectomy and mediastinal lymph node dissection. Occasionally, other malignant tumors identified by histologic examination may require lobectomy or, rarely, even pneumonectomy because of involvement of the proximal pulmonary artery or bronchus.

The success rate with surgical removal of pulmonary metastases has been greatest with testicular (51% 5-year survival) and head-neck cancers (47% 5-year survival). Other types of tumors, such as osteogenic and soft tissue sarcomas, renal cell carcinoma, and colon carcinoma, are all associated with prolonged survival in 20%-35% of patients. Results of resection for melanoma are less favorable (10%-15% survival benefit). Isolated, resectable pulmonary metastases from rectal cancer can have as high as a 55% 5-year survival with metastasectomy alone.

Furthermore, multiple thoracotomies over periods in excess of 10 years are not unusual with the sarcomas. Numerous studies have been conducted in attempts to identify prognostic factors that could aid in the selection of patients for resection. Adverse prognostic factors have included: (1) multiple or bilateral lesions; (2) more than four lesions seen on CT scan; (3) tumor doubling time less than 40 days; (4) a short disease-free interval; and (5) advanced age.

Although no consensus has developed regarding the selection of candidates for surgical exploration, it is generally agreed that no single criterion should be used to exclude patients from surgical resection. In all series, long-term benefit and survival hinges on complete resection. If a complete resection is not deemed possible, resection should not be offered.

Blackmon SH, Shah N, Roth JA, et al: Resection of pulmonary and extrapulmonary sarcomatous metastases is associated with long-term survival. *Ann Thorac Surg* 2009;88(3):877.

Gossot D, Radu C, Girard P, et al: Resection of pulmonary metastases from sarcoma: can some patients benefit from a less invasive approach? *Ann Thorac Surg* 2009;87(1):238.

Internullo E, Cassivi SD, Van Raemdonck D, Friedel G, Treasure T: Pulmonary metastasectomy: a survey of current practice amongst members of the European Society of Thoracic Surgeons. *J Thorac Oncol* Nov 2008;3(11):1257.

Lou F, Huang J, Sima CS, et al: Patterns of recurrence and second primary lung cancer in early-stage lung cancer survivors followed with routine computed tomography surveillance. *J Thorac Cardiovasc Surg* 2013;145(1):75.

von Meyenfeldt EM, Wouters MW, Fat NL, et al: Local treatment of pulmonary metastases: from open resection to minimally invasive approach? Less morbidity, comparable local control. *Surg Endosc* 2012;26(8):2312.

MULTIPLE CHOICE QUESTIONS

1. Chest wall masses

   A. Are nearly always benign
   B. Are common in postmenopausal women
   C. Mostly arise from bone or cartilage
   D. Most commonly arise from muscle, nerve, or fascia
   E. Are rarely resectable

2. Risk factors for lung cancer include all of the following except

   A. Exposure to asbestos
   B. Tobacco smoking
   C. Vitamin A deficiency
   D. Iodine deficiency
   E. Exposure to arsenic

3. Pleural effusion, the presence of fluid within the pleural space, can collect through all of the following mechanisms except

   A. Increase in the pulmonary vascular hydrostatic pressure (congestive heart failure and mitral stenosis)
   B. Ureteral obstruction with transdiaphragmatic urine leak
   C. Decrease in the vascular colloid oncotic pressure (hypoproteinemia)
   D. Increase in the capillary permeability due to inflammation (pneumonia, pancreatitis, and sepsis)
   E. Pancreatic pseudocyst rupture with transdiaphragmatic movement of abdominal fluid

4. The four sources of mediastinal infection include the following, except

   A. Spontaneous bacterial mediastinitis of sarcoidosis
   B. Direct contamination
   C. Hematogenous or lymphatic spread
   D. Extension of infection from the neck or retroperitoneum
   E. Extension from the lung or pleura

5. Cystic fibrosis is all of the following except

   A. An autosomal recessive multisystem congenital disorder
   B. Characterized by chronic airway obstruction and infection
   C. The result of mutation in the cystic fibrosis transmembrane regulator gene
   D. Effectively cured by double lung transplantation with a 10-year graft survival exceeding 85%
   E. A predisposing factor for chronic lung infection

The Heart: I. Surgical Treatment of Acquired Cardiac Disease

Jonathan W. Haft, MD

CORONARY ARTERY DISEASE

▶ Pathophysiology

The heart has the highest metabolic demands when compared to other organs. The vast majority of the energy substrate utilization is expended during unrelenting periodic contraction of the myocardium. Blood flow is delivered at a rate of 1 mL/g of cardiac tissue per minute at rest. Increases in myocardial oxygen consumption, via adenosine diphosphate and adenosine mediated arteriolar vasodilation, can result in a reciprocal increase in blood flow, up to five times normal. This increased blood flow is accommodated by recruitment of an extensive capillary bed within the myocardium, with nearly 1 capillary per myocyte. Between 70% and 80% of available oxygen is extracted from coronary blood flow at rest. Thus, the metabolic needs of the heart are tightly coupled to the availability of coronary blood flow, since additional extraction is limited. In addition, blood flow through the left ventricular epicardial arteries is phasic. During myocardial contraction, extravascular compression of intramyocardial capillaries prevents forward flow during systole, limiting flow to the diastolic phase of the cardiac cycle. This is even more pronounced in the subendocardial region where myocardial oxygen demands are greatest as a result of increased wall tension and greater sarcomere shortening. Because of the elevated and insistent myocardial oxygen consumption, the restriction of blood flow to diastole, and the high basal level of oxygen consumption, the heart is particularly susceptible to ischemic injury related to stenosis of the epicardial coronary arteries.

The heart receives its blood supply from the left and right coronary arteries (Figure 19–1). These epicardial vessels originate as the first branches off of the aortic root, in their respective sinuses of Valsalva. The coronary circulation is traditionally divided into three territories or regions: the left anterior descending (LAD), the circumflex (arising from the left coronary artery), and the right (from the right coronary artery). The dominance of the heart refers to which major artery terminates as the posterior descending branch. Ninety percent of individuals are right dominant, as the right coronary artery supplies the posterior descending artery. The remaining 10% are left dominant, as the terminal branch of the circumflex artery supplies the posterior descending artery.

The left coronary artery is referred to as the left main coronary artery. After its origin in the left sinus of Valsalva, it courses between the left atrial appendage and the pulmonary artery. The left main coronary artery varies in length but is typically less than 2 cm long. It terminates in two branches: the LAD and the circumflex coronary arteries. In less than 1% of patients, the left main artery is absent, with the LAD and circumflex originating as separate ostia from the left sinus of Valsalva.

The LAD, or anterior interventricular artery, courses anteriorly and inferiorly in the interventricular groove toward the apex of the heart. Several branches of the LAD travel along the anterolateral surface of the left ventricle and are known as diagonal arteries. Their number and size are highly variable. Branches to the interventricular septum take off perpendicularly, the first of which is often sizable. The LAD is the most prominent of the three coronary territories and carries approximately 50% of myocardial blood flow.

After arising from the left main, the circumflex coronary artery dives posteriorly along the atrioventricular groove. Several obtuse marginal branches supply the lateral wall of the left ventricle; these branches vary in both size and number. In 10% of patients, the circumflex continues posteriorly and gives rise in its terminal branch to the posterior descending coronary artery, running from the posterior atrioventricular groove toward the posterior apex in the interventricular groove. Some patients have a third branch of the left main referred to as the ramus intermedius. If present, this branch is often large and supplies the anterolateral wall of the left ventricle.

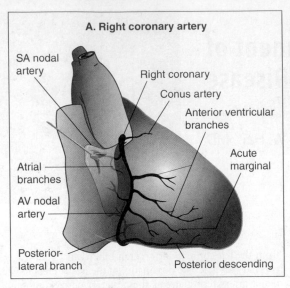

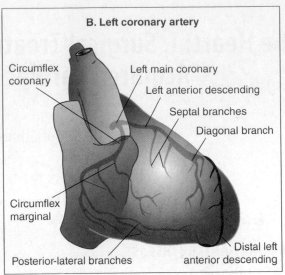

A. Right coronary artery

SA nodal artery

Right coronary

Conus artery

Anterior ventricular branches

Acute marginal

Atrial branches

AV nodal artery

Posterior-lateral branch

Posterior descending

B. Left coronary artery

Circumflex coronary

Left main coronary

Left anterior descending

Septal branches

Diagonal branch

Circumflex marginal

Posterior-lateral branches

Distal left anterior descending

▲ **Figure 19–1.** Anatomy of the coronary circulation.

The right coronary artery originates from the right sinus of Valsalva in the aortic root. It courses anteriorly and rightward until reaching the right atrioventricular groove. The vessel then descends around the acute margin of the heart, giving rise to one or more branches supplying the right ventricle. In 90% of patients, the right coronary artery continues posteriorly, terminating as the posterior descending coronary artery and the posterolateral artery.

Atherosclerosis, a progressive multifocal disease of medium and large muscular arteries of the systemic circulation, tends to occur predominantly at vessel bifurcations, sharp curvatures, and other regions creating pressure wave reflections and recirculation. Because of these flow-related considerations, atherosclerotic stenotic lesions are generally restricted to the proximal regions of the large epicardial coronary arteries. In particular, stenosis found in the LAD and circumflex vessels are frequently isolated, short, and in the proximal segments. The right coronary artery, however, develops diffuse obstructions, although rarely extending into the posterior descending or intramural branches.

The pathologic mechanism of coronary atheroma formation is identical to the lesions found elsewhere in the vascular tree. Endothelial injury from cigarette smoke, hypercholesterolemia, hyperglycemia, hypertension, or other causes of inflammation initiate a cascade of events. These include endothelial dysfunction with reduced nitric oxide production, monocyte adhesion and migration, lipid accumulation, and smooth muscle cell proliferation. The end result is an enlarging plaque encroaching on the arterial lumen, separated from the blood stream by a collagen-rich fibrous plaque. The lesion can cause flow limitations, particularly

when the luminal cross-sectional area is reduced by at least 75%. With this degree of obstruction, the vasodilatory reserve required during increased myocardial demand is restricted, resulting in transient myocardial ischemia until demand returns to baseline. The atherosclerotic plaque also causes coronary ischemia when the lesion becomes unstable. The fibrous plaque can fracture, causing rupture of the plaque contents and complete epicardial thrombosis, the presumed mechanism of ST-segment elevation myocardial infarction (STEMI). Additionally, subtotal plaque disruption can cause vasoconstriction, platelet activation, and embolization, resulting in ischemia without total occlusion of the epicardial vessel. This is the presumed mechanism of unstable angina and non-ST-segment elevation myocardial infarction (NSTEMI).

▶ Patient Presentation

Patients with coronary atherosclerosis can present with a variety of symptoms depending on the severity and nature of their occlusive lesions as well as on their other medical comorbidities. Chronic stable angina is the most frequent complaint of the patient with coronary artery disease. At rest, coronary blood flow is adequate to meet myocardial demand, and patients are without symptoms. However, during exercise or stress, as myocardial oxygen demand increases, autoregulatory mechanisms vasodilate to increase myocardial blood flow fivefold to sixfold. Stable coronary obstructions become flow limiting, resulting in an imbalance of oxygen demand and supply. Chest pain develops rapidly and is typically described as tightness, squeezing, constricting, or aching. It is usually midsternal and radiates to the left shoulder, arm, or neck. The classically described Levine sign with a clenched fist over the sternum is a common finding. Some patients, however, describe symptoms that are collectively referred to as "anginal equivalents." These include dyspnea, diaphoresis, nausea, heartburn, and dizziness or presyncope. Although the clinical manifestations of angina are variable, the pathognomonic feature of chronic stable angina is that the symptoms occur predictably with exertion and are always relieved with rest.

Acute coronary syndrome (ACS) encompasses a spectrum of conditions related to coronary occlusive disease, including unstable angina, NSTEMI, and STEMI. Patients with unstable angina experience chest pain or an anginal equivalent that is new, occurs at rest, or occurs with increasing severity from their baseline chronic stable symptoms, also called crescendo angina. Patients who develop NSTEMI have evidence of myocardial injury with elevated blood levels of myocardial enzymes (troponin and the myoglobin [Mb] fraction of creatine kinase). Unstable angina and NSTEMI are important prognostic indicators, as 10% of patients will die of cardiovascular causes within 6 months.

STEMI represents the consequences of large epicardial vessel occlusion typically associated with plaque rupture. Patients usually describe severe retrosternal chest pain that persists for more than 30 minutes. Patients with previous chronic stable angina will report that the current pain does not resolve with rest or nitroglycerine and is more intense in quality. Patients often describe additional symptoms such as diaphoresis, nausea, and dizziness. Although improvements in health systems have drastically increased survival from myocardial infarction, mortality for STEMI remains near 10%.

Diagnostic Evaluation

Patients with suspected coronary artery disease should undergo a resting electrocardiogram. Although most patients with chronic stable angina have a normal electrocardiogram pattern, evidence of previous myocardial infarctions may be identified with the presence of either Q waves or conduction abnormalities. The most widely used diagnostic test to evaluate for coronary artery disease is exercise electrocardiography. Using standardized protocols, patients are exercised on a treadmill or bicycle ergometer while a 12-lead electrocardiogram is continuously recorded. The test is continued until the patient's symptoms are noted or until the development of significant ST segment shifts suggesting myocardial ischemia. The diagnostic accuracy of exercise stress electrocardiogram testing can be enhanced with myocardial perfusion imaging. Several radioactive tracers are used clinically, the most frequent of which is thallium-201. Because of its similarities to potassium ions, it is taken up preferentially by the viable cardiac myocytes. Its distribution within the myocardium is proportional to the rate of perfusion. In some cases, patients are unable to exercise because of additional physical or psychological limitations. Pharmacologic agents can substitute for exercise by increasing myocardial oxygen demand (dobutamine) or by directly vasodilating coronary arteries (adenosine), thus demonstrating regions with fixed restrictions in myocardial blood flow. Echocardiography can be used as an alternative to nuclear perfusion imaging to increase the accuracy of exercise electrocardiogram testing. Echocardiography demonstrates regional changes in wall motion that can be observed during myocardial ischemia. It can also identify valvular abnormalities or other conditions that may influence treatment choices.

Coronary angiography, also known as cardiac catheterization, is indicated in symptomatic patients with suspected coronary occlusive lesions. After percutaneous access is obtained in the arterial system, preformed catheters of varying sizes are advanced fluoroscopically to selectively engage the ostia of the left and right coronary arteries. Radiopaque contrast is injected with imaging of the opacified coronary artery. Standardized views are obtained of both the right and left coronary systems to provide different projections to clearly define the vascular anatomy and to quantify the severity of occlusive lesions (Figure 19–2). Additionally, catheters can be inserted across the aortic valve into the left ventricular cavity. Contrast injection for ventriculography can provide information about ventricular systolic function, cavity size, and the presence of left-sided valvular abnormalities. During cardiac catheterization, stenotic lesions in the epicardial vessels can be treated using percutaneous techniques, described in the section on Percutaneous Intervention. Newer imaging techniques using high-resolution multislice CT scanning with 3D reconstruction and magnetic resonance imaging (MRI) are increasingly utilized. These noninvasive approaches have the potential to improve the safety and convenience of coronary imaging; however, resolution remains inferior to standard coronary angiography.

Medical Treatment

Medical therapy of coronary artery disease begins with controlling risk factors that contribute to formation and destabilization of the atherosclerotic plaque. The most important intervention is cessation of cigarette smoking. Other interventions include control of hypertension, diabetes, and hypercholesterolemia. Dietary modifications and exercise can improve all of these conditions, but pharmacologic treatment is often necessary.

Statins can improve cholesterol levels and improve the ratio of low-density to high-density lipoproteins, and they have been demonstrated to reduce rates of myocardial infarction and death. Angiotensin-converting inhibitors have been shown to reduce mortality and myocardial

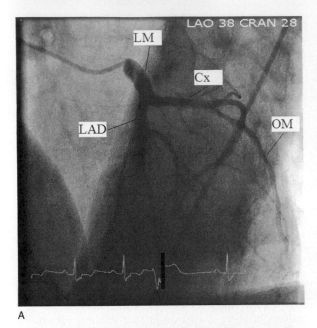

A

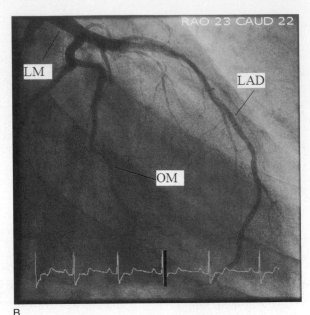

B

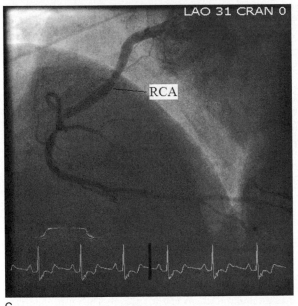

C

▲ **Figure 19–2. A:** Left anterior oblique (LAO) view of the left coronary artery. **B:** Right anterior oblique (RAO) view of the left coronary artery. **C:** LAO view of the right coronary artery. LM, left main; LAD, left anterior descending; Cx, circumflex; RCA, right coronary artery; OM, obtuse marginal.

infarction in patients with coronary artery disease coupled with hypertension, diabetes, or left ventricular dysfunction. Aspirin, by inhibiting platelet activity, reduces death and myocardial infarctions in patients with coronary artery disease and should be prescribed to all patients unless significant contraindications exist. Beta-blocking agents reduce myocardial oxygen consumption by reducing heart rate and wall tension, and they increase oxygen delivery by increasing the diastolic phase and thus subendocardial perfusion. Despite these perceived benefits, beta-blockers have not been shown to reduce cardiovascular mortality or morbidity in patients without left ventricular dysfunction or hypertension. Nitrates also decrease myocardial oxygen consumption via venodilation, reducing cardiac preload and waltension, and vasodilation, reducing afterload. Some epicardial vasodilation will occur, improving coronary blood flow. Nitrates can control symptoms, either immediately when given sublingually or prophylactically when used as an oral long-acting agent. Headaches are notable side effects, and the vasodilatory properties of nitrates can be exaggerated by phosphodiesterase inhibitors frequently used for the treatment of erectile dysfunction. Medical treatment alone is appropriate for patients with coronary artery disease affecting one or two epicardial vessel territories and satisfactory symptom control.

► Percutaneous Intervention

In 1977, Dr. Andreas Gruentzig performed the first percutaneous intervention with balloon angioplasty on a stenotic lesion in the LAD. This pioneer laid the foundation for a revolution in the treatment of coronary artery disease worldwide. Percutaneous coronary intervention is among the most frequently performed medical procedures in the world, and its use continues to expand. These interventions include balloon angioplasty, intracoronary stent implantation, as well as rotational and laser atherectomies. Using the same techniques described for cardiac catheterization, small, highly flexible and steerable guidewires can be advanced percutaneously down the lumen of stenotic epicardial coronary arteries. Over this guidewire, balloon tipped-catheters can be advanced across the stenosis and inflated to supraatmospheric pressures. This stretches and dilates the affected vessel, restoring the lumen to its predisease dimensions. Restenosis with balloon angioplasty was common, occurring in nearly 40% of patients. The use of nitinol scaffolding stents has greatly reduced restenosis rates to nearly 15% and they are now used in nearly 90% of percutaneous procedures in the United States. The latest addition in the armamentarium of percutaneous coronary interventions is the drug-eluting stent. The drugs impregnated into the walls of the stent are antiproliferative, similar to agents used to prevent replication of immune cells in transplant recipients. The sirolimus eluting and paclitaxel eluting stents have further reduced the rate of target vessel restenosis and the need for repeat interventions. However, reports of late stent thrombosis have raised concerns, and indefinite use of antiplatelet regimens has been recommended.

► Surgical Treatment

Although alternative surgical approaches to myocardial ischemia had been attempted previously, René Favaloro is credited with creation of the coronary bypass procedure from his work at the Cleveland Clinic. Since its inception in 1967, coronary artery bypass grafting (CABG) has increased in volume until the last decade, with minimal growth, presumably from improved percutaneous and medical treatments (Figure 19–3). Despite the recent trends, CABG

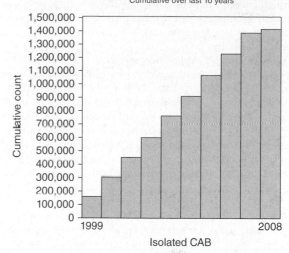

Number of isolated CAB procedures
Cumulative over last 10 years

▲ **Figure 19–3.** Trend in reduction of coronary bypass graft procedures in the United States.

continues to be among the most frequent, successful, and well-studied procedures performed in medicine.

A. Indications

Three large prospective multicenter randomized clinical trials evaluating CABG versus medical therapy are widely quoted and should be understood when considering the indications for coronary bypass grafting. Despite the historical nature of these studies and the evolution in both surgical technique and medical treatment, these trials continue to provide important information about the benefits of surgical revascularization in patients with advanced coronary atherosclerosis.

The Veterans Administration Cooperative Study enrolled 1000 patients between 1970 and 1974. Patients had chronic anginal complaints and were free of myocardial infarction within 6 months. Medical treatment consisted largely of nitrates and aspirin, and surgical mortality was extremely high when compared to contemporary results. A statistically significant survival advantage was seen in the surgical group versus the medical group at 7 years (77% vs 72%), despite 38% of medical patients crossing over to surgical treatment. Subgroup analysis demonstrated more pronounced survival advantages for patients with three-vessel disease, patients with left ventricular dysfunction, and patients with significant stenosis of the left main coronary artery.

The European Coronary Surgery Study recruited 767 men with chronic angina from 1973 to 1976. Only patients with preserved left ventricular function were included. A survival advantage for the surgical group was seen in the overall cohort, but particularly in patients with three-vessel disease and those with proximal LAD stenosis. There were also advantages demonstrated in reduction of angina and exercise capacity.

The Coronary Artery Surgery Study enrolled patients from a nonrandomized registry of patients who underwent coronary angiography from 1974 to 1979 at 15 centers. Patients with mild angina were randomized to medical treatment and CABG. There was no survival advantage in the 790 randomized patients; however, the cohort with left ventricular dysfunction had better survival with surgery, particularly those with left ventricular dysfunction and three-vessel disease. Evaluation of the nonrandomized patients in the registry also found survival advantages for surgically treated patients with left main stenosis or left main equivalent stenosis.

Although these three landmark studies are nearly 30 years old, some important principles continue to apply: patients with more advanced coronary atherosclerosis, particularly those with left ventricular dysfunction, stand to achieve the most benefit from surgical revascularization.

Numerous clinical trials have more recently compared CABG with percutaneous interventions. The Randomized Intervention Treatment of Angina (RITA) trial compared balloon angioplasty with CABG for patients with single and multivessel disease. There was no difference in survival, but repeat intervention was required five times more frequently in the angioplasty group. The Bypass Angioplasty Revascularization Investigation (BARI) enrolled 1829 patients with chronic or unstable angina from 1988 to 1991. There was no survival advantage at 5 years; however, 31% of the patients in the percutaneous group crossed over for CABG. The need for repeat revascularization was again five times higher in the percutaneous group, and the subgroup of patients with diabetes had improved survival at 5 years (81% vs 66%).

A recent comparison between patients with multivessel coronary disease treated with PCI versus CABG was performed using Medicare claims data as well as the Society of Thoracic Surgeons Database and the American College of Cardiology Foundation PCI Data Registry. Adjusted and unadjusted survival rates were superior for those undergoing CABG at 4 years. As technology and pharmacology continue to evolve, additional studies will be required. However, CABG offers survival and quality-of-life advantages in selected patients with coronary artery disease. The most recent recommendations from the American Heart Association and the American College of Cardiology regarding the indications for coronary bypass surgery are presented in Table 19–1.

B. Techniques

The principles of coronary bypass surgery are to restore normal myocardial perfusion by creating alternative routes

Table 19–1. American heart association guidelines for coronary bypass graft surgery[*]

Asymptomatic
- Left main coronary artery disease or left main equivalent (proximal LAD, proximal circumflex) (class I)
- Three-vessel coronary artery disease (class I)
- Proximal LAD disease and one- or two-vessel disease (class IIa, particularly if there is decreased LV function or extensive ischemia on noninvasive study

Symptomatic
　Stable angina
- Left main coronary artery disease or left main equivalent (class I)
- Three-vessel coronary artery disease (class I)
- Two-vessel coronary artery disease and proximal LAD with decreased LV function or significant ischemia on noninvasive study (class I)
- One- or two-vessel disease not involving the proximal LAD but with high-risk findings on noninvasive study (class I)
　One-vessel disease involving the proximal LAD (class IIa)

Unstable angina/NSTEMI
- Left main coronary artery disease or left main equivalent (class I)
- Three-vessel coronary artery disease (class I)
- One- or two-vessel disease with ongoing ischemia; vessels are not amenable to percutaneous therapy (class I)
- One- or two-vessel disease not involving the proximal LAD (class IIa)

STEMI
- Ongoing chest pain or hemodynamic instability with lesions not amenable to percutaneous treatment (class I)
- Surgical complications of myocardial infarction, such as ruptured papillary muscle or postinfarct ventricular septal defect (class I)
- Cardiogenic shock (class I)
- Recurrent malignant arrhythmias (class I)

Decreased LV function
- Left main, left main equivalent, or three-vessel coronary artery disease (class I)
- Two-vessel coronary artery disease (class I)
- Proximal LAD disease (class IIa)

Failed PTCA
- Ongoing ischemia with adequate distal target (class I)
- Hemodynamic instability (class I)

[*]Evidence class I: Evidence of or general agreement that the treatment is effective. Class IIa: Conflicting evidence or diverging opinion, but evidence favors treatment. Class IIb: Conflicting evidence or diverging opinion, but efficacy is less well established. Class III: Evidence suggests the treatment is *not* helpful.
LAD, left anterior descending; LV, left ventricular; NSTEMI, non-ST-segment elevation myocardial infarction; STEMI, ST-segment elevation myocardial infarction.

for blood to reach the jeopardized territories. This strategy has several advantages, including the large-caliber conduits, their extramyocardial location in avoiding the compressive forces during systole, and their attachment at strategic locations to maximize return of normal blood flow. The most important aspect of the procedure is construction of a technically sound and strategically well-created bypass graft.

A variety of conduits may be chosen; the most traditional and still most frequently utilized is the saphenous vein. The vessel is easily harvested with minimal morbidity, and it is technically easy to create the precise anastomosis. Minimally invasive approaches using endoscopic techniques now reduce the impact on the patient. Limitations of the saphenous vein are primarily based on its tendency to develop accelerated atherosclerotic lesions. The vein graft plaque is more frequently circumferential and diffuse, with a weaker fibrous cap and a higher predilection for distal embolization. Patency of saphenous vein grafts is approximately 50% at 10 years. In addition, suitable vein conduit may not be available, either harvested for previous coronary or peripheral bypass procedures or unusable from varicosities or sclerosis.

The left internal mammary artery can be mobilized from its pedicle on the left subclavian artery and anastomosed to the anterior or lateral epicardial vessels of the heart, most frequently to the LAD. This strategy has several well-described advantages owing to the improved patency rate of the internal mammary graft when compared to saphenous vein grafts. The right internal mammary artery can also serve as a bypass conduit; however, harvesting of both internal mammary vessels increases the risk of sternal ischemia and surgical wound-healing complications. Because of the improved patency of arterial grafts as compared to saphenous vein grafts, the radial and gastroepiploic artery have been explored as alternatives to vein grafts. However, improved long term patency has not been reliably established, and morbidity from harvesting has slowed widespread adoption of this approach.

The standard approach for coronary bypass grafting is via the median sternotomy, where the sternum is divided longitudinally, exposing the heart and great vessels. The left thoracotomy could be alternatively used, particularly after previous heart surgery where sternal reentry could hazard injury to adhesed cardiac structures or patent grafts. Preparation is then made to institute cardiopulmonary bypass (CPB). Anticoagulation with 300 IU heparin per kilogram is infused to achieve an activated clotting time of greater than 400 seconds. Typically, the ascending aorta is used for arterial inflow, and venous return is accomplished via a cannula in the right atrial appendage (Figure 19–4). CPB is commenced, evacuating venous blood into the cardiotomy reservoir. Mechanical ventilation can be discontinued. Using a heat exchanger, the blood is actively cooled to 28-32°C to reduce tissue oxygen requirements and organ injury. Shed mediastinal blood can be scavenged and returned to the CPB system, reducing blood loss during the anticoagulation period. Cardioplegic arrest is then initiated by cross-clamping the ascending aorta and infusing cold blood cardioplegia solution into the aortic root. The makeup of cardioplegia solutions differs among centers and even among surgeons; however, most centers combine autologous blood obtained from the CPB system with crystalloid solution cooled to 12°C containing citrate to bind ionic calcium, dextrose, pH buffers, and potassium (~ 30 mM/L) to arrest all cardiac activity. Cardioplegia is administered intermittently to maintain myocardial temperature and diastolic arrest during the cross-clamp period.

With the arrested heart, a dry and motionless surgical field is created, allowing creation of precise surgical anastomoses on even the smallest of epicardial coronary

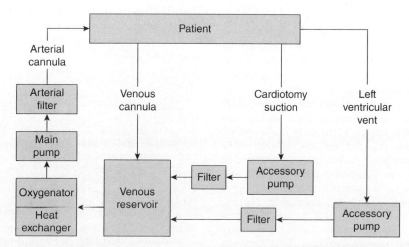

▲ **Figure 19–4.** Schematic of cardiopulmonary bypass (CPB). (From Morgan GE, Mikhail MS, Murray MJ: *Clinical Anesthesiology*, 4th ed. McGraw-Hill, 2006.)

arteries. The targets are identified on the epicardial surface, and the sites for anastomotic reconstruction are determined on the basis of information from the preoperative cardiac catheterization and suitability of the native vessel. An arteriotomy is created on the exposed vessel, and it is extended for approximately 5 mm. The conduit is fashioned with an appropriately sized bevel or spatulation, and the anastomosis is created, typically in running fashion with fine polypropylene suture. The conduits are tested for patency and hemostasis, and they are cut to the appropriate size, avoiding tension or kinking. Saphenous vein or free arterial conduits are typically connected to the ascending aorta. A 4-5 mm punch device is used to create a circular aortotomy. The anastomoses are constructed in running fashion with polypropylene suture. If conduit length is limited, the proximal anastomoses can be created as Y grafts off of other vein grafts or off of the pedicled internal mammary artery graft.

After completion of all anastomoses, weaning from CPB is prepared. The patient is warmed to normothermia. As the heart begins to warm, ventricular fibrillation often occurs, requiring electrical defibrillation. Temporary conduction abnormalities may require epicardial pacing, but it is often transient. Mechanical ventilation is resumed, and the patient is gradually weaned from CPB. Pharmacologic inotropic support may be required but is often unnecessary if ventricular function was preserved preoperatively. An appropriate dose of protamine is infused to reverse the effects of heparin, and cannulae for bypass are removed. Once hemostasis is adequate, chest closure is performed with stainless steel wires. The pericardium is typically left open to avoid constriction of the atria or kinking of the bypass grafts. The pedicled left internal mammary artery graft is positioned posterior to the anterior surface of the left lung to protect it from injury should sternal reentry be required in the future.

Recently, attempts to reduce the invasive nature of coronary bypass grafting and the potential complications of CPB have been introduced. Techniques to perform bypass grafting without CPB have improved and are promoted by its advocates. Off-pump coronary bypass grafting (OPCAB) have potential advantages in reducing neurologic complications associated with air and atheroemboli, as well as reducing blood transfusion requirements and cost. The procedure involves manipulation and stabilization of the beating heart to expose the epicardial targets. Particularly for vessels on the posterior and posterolateral surfaces, hemodynamic instability can result while the heart is elevated and rotated for optimal exposure. The anesthesiologist must be capable of responding to these rapid changes, and the surgeon must have the judgment and ability to immediately abandon off-pump attempts and institute CPB before significant organ injury occurs. The anastomoses are more challenging, with blood in the moving operative field. Although several single-center reports have demonstrated satisfactory short-term results and mid-term graft patency rates, multi-center randomized and observation studies have suggested that OPCAB techniques may offer some benefits but at the expense of reduced graft patency rates and increased incomplete revascularization. As a result, OPCAB penetrance has not markedly increased over the last several years.

C. Results

Since the creation of the Society of Thoracic Surgeons voluntary reporting database in 1989, short-term outcomes of coronary bypass grafting are widely available to the public, providing information for patients, referring physicians, and practicing surgeons to compare their results to national averages. The Society also provides a validated risk assessment scoring system, creating mortality estimates based on an individual patient's clinical data. Overall, risk of perioperative death is 1%-3%. Multivariate predictors of death include advanced age, recent myocardial infarction, decreased ventricular function, renal insufficiency, and female gender. Conduit patency is determined from clinical trials that included angiographic assessments at varying time intervals in the absence of symptoms. Data are largely historical and are subject to biases of patient selection but are largely considered to be reliable. Saphenous vein grafts occlude 20%-30% by 1 year. Early graft loss is felt to be attributable to anastomotic imperfections or graft kinking, endothelial injury during harvest, limited native coronary runoff, or progression of native occlusive disease. Late failures appear to occur at a rate of 5% per year, with 10-year patency approximately 40%-50%. Late failures are primarily attributed to accelerated atherosclerosis of the vein conduit. The pedicled internal mammary artery has far superior patency, particularly when anastomosed to the LAD. With adequate target vessel runoff, 10-year patency rates of 90%-95% have been reported in multiple independent studies. Radial arteries and free mammary artery conduits appear to have patency rates intermediate to saphenous vein and pedicled mammary arteries and are more frequently utilized in younger patients.

Afilalo J et al: Off-pump vs. on-pump coronary artery bypass surgery: an updated meta-analysis and meta-regression of randomized trials. *Eur Heart J* 2012;33:1257.

Kelbaek H et al: Drug-eluting versus bare metal stents in patients with st-segment-elevation myocardial infarction: eight-month follow-up in the Drug Elution and Distal Protection in Acute Myocardial Infarction (DEDICATION) trial. DEDICATION Investigators. *Circulation* 2008;118:1155.

Lamy A et al: Off-pump or on-pump coronary-artery bypass grafting at 30 days. *N Engl J Med* 2012;366:1489.

Reddy GP et al: MR imaging of ischemic heart disease. *Magn Reson Imaging Clin N Am* 2008;16:201.

Schroeder S et al: Cardiac computed tomography: indications, applications, limitations, and training requirements. Working Group Nuclear Cardiology and Cardiac CT. *Eur Heart J* 2008;29:531.

Weintraub WS et al: Comparative effectiveness of revascularization strategies. *N Engl J Med* 2012;366:1467.

Wenaweser P et al: Incidence and correlates of drug-eluting stent thrombosis in routine clinical practice. 4-year results from a large 2-institutional cohort study. *J Am Col Cardiol* 2008;52:1134.

▼ VALVULAR HEART DISEASE

MITRAL REGURGITATION

▶ Pathophysiology

A. Anatomy

The mitral valve separates the left atrium from the left ventricle. It should be considered as the sum of its three components: the leaflets, the annulus to which the leaflets attach, and the subvalvar apparatus, consisting of the cords and papillary muscles. The mitral valve has two leaflets, anterior and posterior (Figure 19–5). The anterior leaflet is larger in surface area, but its attachment to the annulus represents only one-third of the circumference. The anterior portion of the mitral valve annulus is in direct continuity with the annulus of the left and noncoronary cusps of the aortic valve, also known as the aortomitral continuity. The posterior leaflet is shorter, but its annular attachments cover two-thirds of the circumference. The posterior leaflet often can be separated into three distinct scallops, although the prominence of these separations varies among individuals. The anterior

and posterior leaflets are separated from each other by the anterolateral and posteromedial commissures, which mark the location of the right and left fibrous trigones respectively. The trigones are dense collagenous structures within the annulus representing a portion of the fibrous skeleton of the heart. The mitral annulus is elliptical in shape, and its dimensions change dynamically during cardiac contraction, reducing its cross-sectional area by as much as 40%. The anterolateral and posteromedial papillary muscles are vertically oriented bundles of cardiac myocytes. Chordae tendineae originate from the heads of the papillary muscles and span the distance to both the anterior and posterior mitral valve leaflets. Chords are designated as primary if they attach to the leading edge of the leaflet, secondary if they attach to the ventricular surface of the leaflets, or tertiary if they attach to the ventricular surface of the mitral annulus. The chords play an important role in preventing leaflet prolapse. The posteromedial papillary muscle is prone to ischemic injury, since it relies on a single right coronary artery for circulation. In contrast, the anterolateral papillary muscle gains its blood supply from the LAD and circumflex branches and tends to be more resistant to ischemic injury.

B. Classification of Mitral Regurgitation

Regurgitation through the mitral valve can result from a variety of pathologic conditions. Alain Carpentier developed a simplified classification scheme based on leaflet motion (Table 19–2) to organize the different disease processes that can cause mitral regurgitation. In Carpentier type I mitral regurgitation, the leaflet motion is normal. The regurgitation is a result of either dilation of the annulus, as can be seen in cardiomyopathy with progressive ventricular enlargement, or of leaflet perforation, as can be seen with destructive endocarditis. Type II is associated with excessive leaflet motion. Patients with type II mitral regurgitation have ruptured chordae or papillary muscles from ischemia or endocarditis, or they have with pathologically redundant mitral leaflet tissue. Redundant, prolapsing, or myxomatous mitral leaflets can be either acquired from fibroelastic deficiency or hereditary from weak connective tissue. In either case, the

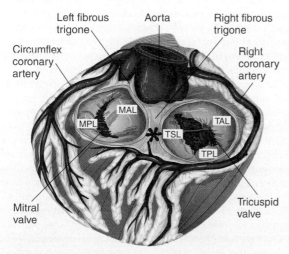

▲ **Figure 19–5.** Anatomy of the mitral and tricuspid valves (MAL, mitral anterior leaflet; MPL, mitral posterior leaflet; TAL, tricuspid anterior leaflet; TSL, tricuspid septal leaflet; TPL, tricuspid posterior leaflet).

Table 19–2. Carpentier classification of mitral regurgitation.

I	Normal leaflet motion
	Annular dilation, leaflet perforation
II	Excessive leaflet motion
	Prolapsed or myxomatous leaflet, ruptured chord
III	Restricted leaflet motion
	Rheumatic disease, ischemic mitral regurgitation

excessive leaflet motion prevents proper coaptation of the anterior and posterior leaflets. Patients with type III have restricted leaflet motion. Type III is often associated with rheumatic heart disease, where leaflets can become calcified, and the chords are thickened and foreshortened. The leaflets do not adequately rise in systole, and coaptation is impaired. Alternatively, some patients develop severe mitral regurgitation owing to ischemic injury. Typically, a previous myocardial infarction has resulted in ventricular remodeling, resulting in dilation and retraction of the papillary muscles. As a result, the leaflets are tethered into the ventricle, limiting mobility and preventing proper coaptation.

Mitral regurgitation is always pathologic but can be tolerated surprisingly well when the onset is gradual, allowing for a series of physiologic adaptations. On the other hand, acute mitral regurgitation, as can be associated with infective endocarditis or ischemic papillary muscle rupture, results in immediate pulmonary congestion because the unprepared left atrium is incapable of handling the additional volume load. Several compensatory mechanisms occur as mitral regurgitation develops and progressively worsens. The left atrium and pulmonary venous system gradually dilates, thus increasing compliance to better accommodate the excess volume. The backwards flow of mitral regurgitation reduces ventricular afterload, reducing myocardial wall tension. The reduction in forward flow is accounted for by increased diastolic filling, increasing preload. This maintains cardiac output and can delay onset of symptoms for significant time. Gradually, left ventricular end diastolic volume continues to rise, resulting in pathologic remodeling, creating a dilated and more spherical ventricular cavity. Systolic function is progressively and inexorably impaired as a result of both mechanical considerations owing to the altered shape and molecular mechanisms both intracellular and extracellular. A vicious cycle ensues, with deteriorating systolic function and rising end diastolic volume promoting further ventricular remodeling and dilation and worsening mitral regurgitation. Longstanding mitral regurgitation will result in sustained elevation in left atrial pressure and volume, resulting in pulmonary vascular changes, pulmonary hypertension, and eventually, right ventricular dysfunction.

C. Symptoms

Acute mitral regurgitation is poorly tolerated and is typically associated with pulmonary congestion and low cardiac output. Patients describe dyspnea, poor exercise tolerance, and fatigue. Often, the etiology of the mitral regurgitation is more dominant in the clinical presentation. Patients with acute endocarditis may have fever, shaking chills, and manifestations of septic embolization such as stroke and intestinal or extremity ischemia. Patients suffering from acute myocardial infarction with a ruptured papillary muscle complain of chest pain and diaphoresis.

Chronic mitral regurgitation can be asymptomatic for many years as a result of progressive atrial and ventricular adaptation. Eventually, patients develop symptoms of heart failure, including dyspnea, fatigue, and lower extremity edema. When left atrial dilation results in atrial fibrillation, patients may describe heart palpitations. Often, the onset of atrial fibrillation is the initial presentation of symptoms, as rapid ventricular response decreases diastolic filling time and creates a sudden reduction in cardiac output. As ventricular function deteriorates and pulmonary vascular changes occur, signs of right-sided heart failure develop, such as lower extremity edema and ascites.

▶ Diagnostic Testing

The physical findings of mitral regurgitation vary depending on the duration and the degree of compensation. For patients with longstanding mitral regurgitation, ventricular dilation displaces the point of maximal impulse (PMI) laterally. On auscultation, an S3 gallop is often heard, resulting from increased diastolic flow. The systolic murmur is characteristically described as blowing, best heard over the cardiac apex and radiating to the axilla. In acute mitral regurgitation, the murmur tends to be limited to early in systole. With more chronicity, the murmur is progressively holosystolic.

The chest radiograph often demonstrates cardiomegaly from ventricular dilation. With severe uncompensated heart failure, pulmonary edema may be evident; however, this is more commonly seen with acute mitral regurgitation. The electrocardiogram is often nonspecific but may demonstrate evidence of previous myocardial infarction and will confirm the presence of atrial fibrillation.

Echocardiography is the mainstay in the diagnosis of mitral regurgitation; it provides information about the mechanism of the disease, which is essential in planning surgical intervention. Images of the leaflets can determine if the leaflet motion is normal, restricted, or excessive. Information about annular size and mobility can be obtained. Using color Doppler, the size and direction of the regurgitant jet can quantify the severity and give clues as to the mechanism (Figure 19–6). The severity of the regurgitation is determined by the width and length of the regurgitant jet or the presence of reversed flow within the pulmonary veins. Echocardiography also provides information about the chronicity of the disease and can document progressive adaptation such as left atrial and ventricular dilation. This information is often used in determining timing of surgical intervention, particularly in asymptomatic patients. Echocardiography is usually performed transthoracic. However, in some patients, the views are obscured by body habitus or emphysema, limiting the image quality. Transesophageal echocardiography (TEE) can improve the resolution of images and better clarify the severity and mechanism of the mitral valve pathology.

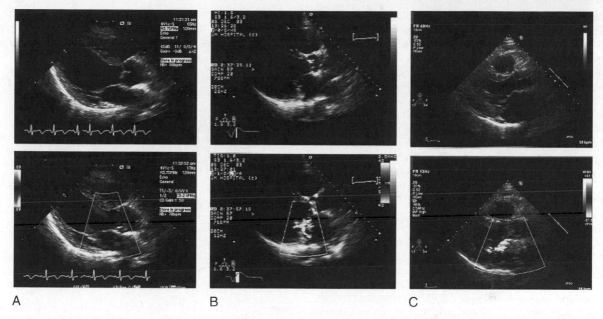

▲ **Figure 19–6.** Echocardiographic view of the mitral valve. **A:** Normal valve. **B:** Dilated annulus with central regurgitation. **C:** Prolapsing posterior leaflet with eccentric regurgitation.

Cardiac catheterization is an important adjunctive tool, helping to identify additional cardiac pathology, and can determine the adequacy of preoperative medical optimization. Coronary angiography is performed preoperatively to identify coronary arterial occlusive lesions that may require bypass grafting at the time of mitral valve repair or replacement. Although contrast ventriculography can demonstrate the regurgitant jet, it is no longer necessarily used to quantify the regurgitant volume, since echocardiography has become the standard technique. Right heart catheterization will demonstrate intravascular volume overload and low cardiac output. It may also be helpful in diagnosing pulmonary vascular changes in patients who deny symptoms.

▶ Surgical Treatment

A. Indications

The indications for operation on the mitral valve depend on the specific pathology as well as clinical symptoms. In addition, the indications have evolved in recent years owing to improved outcomes related to better surgical techniques, anesthetic considerations, myocardial protection, and postoperative care. Furthermore, intervention on the mitral valve may be performed for less severe disease if operation is indicated for coronary artery disease or aortic valve pathology.

Certainly, among patients who represent reasonable operative risks, those with severe mitral regurgitation and heart failure symptoms should be offered an operation. In addition, those with severe mitral regurgitation and signs of left ventricular dysfunction should undergo operation because myocardial decompensation can progress rapidly without corrective action. There is insufficient evidence that operative intervention for asymptomatic severe mitral regurgitation and normal ventricular function improves survival. Historically, these patients were observed with close clinical follow-up and serial echocardiography. Signs of left ventricular dilation, dysfunction, or new-onset symptoms prompted surgical referral. Some have argued that the presence of pulmonary hypertension or atrial fibrillation represent maladaptive changes and suggest surgical correction.

Surgical techniques of addressing the mitral valve have changed dramatically in recent years. Increasingly, operations have focused on repair rather than prosthetic replacement of the mitral valve. Valve preservation has several advantages. The interaction of the mitral valve and the left ventricle goes beyond just competence and the handling of blood volume. A complex interdependence exists between ventricle and valve, and long-term ventricular function depends on its relationship with the mitral annulus, papillary muscles, and chordae tendineae. Surgical techniques to correct mitral regurgitation that preserve these relationships are more likely to maintain normal ventricular function. In addition to the effects on ventricular function, prosthetic mitral valves carry limitations. Bioprosthetic devices (porcine or bovine) have limited durability because of structural valvular degeneration. The rate of bioprosthetic valve failure is proportional to age, with faster deterioration in younger patients. Mechanical valves are more durable but require lifelong systemic anticoagulation with warfarin. Because of the limitations imposed by prosthetic valves (durability and anticoagulation), surgical referral for mitral regurgitation is often delayed if there is a high likelihood of valve replacement. If valve repair is expected because of mitral pathology and surgeon experience, earlier operation for mitral regurgitation is often considered, particularly in the absence of symptoms or ventricular dilation.

Surgical indications for operation in endocarditis of the mitral valve are different than for other pathologies. Certainly, valvular destruction with severe mitral regurgitation, heart failure, and ventricular dilation requires operative intervention. However, there are other specific indications for valve replacement. A history of systemic embolization or the presence of large, highly mobile vegetations at risk of embolization necessitates urgent surgical intervention. In addition, ongoing bacteremia despite appropriate antibiotic treatment coverage mandates early operation. The presence of certain organisms, such as highly resistant bacteria or fungal endocarditis warrants surgical treatment. Surgery is required for the presence of mitral annular abscess with incipient cardiac conduction abnormalities or creation of an intracardiac fistula. Prior to surgery, attempts at controlling the original source of infection should be made, including dental extractions and drainage of abscesses.

B. Techniques

Approach to the mitral valve is best accomplished via a median sternotomy. Although the mitral valve can be exposed via a right or left thoracotomy, the median sternotomy offers the best access for initiation of CPB as well as the ability to perform other cardiac procedures if necessary, such as coronary bypass grafting or aortic valve replacement. CPB is initiated, typically draining the superior and inferior vena cavae separately, and infusing into the ascending aorta. The heart is arrested using cold cardioplegia delivered into the aortic root. The left ventricle is vented, typically using the right superior pulmonary vein.

A variety of incisions can be used to expose the mitral valve, and the quality of exposure is essential in obtaining a good surgical result. The most frequent approach is by an incision directly into the left atrium. The interatrial groove of Sondergaard can be developed using sharp technique, lifting the right atrium anteriorly off of the left atrium (Figure 19–7). A vertical incision is made in the left atrium, just medial to the confluence of the right-sided pulmonary veins. Self-retaining retractors are available to elevate the atriotomy and provide visualization. Often, rotation of the table to the left away from the surgeon improves the

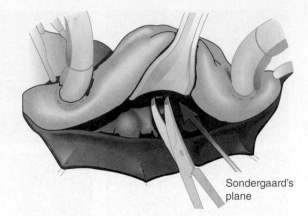

▲ **Figure 19–7.** Exposure of the mitral valve via the interatrial groove. (From Cohn LH: *Cardiac Surgery in the Adult,* 3rd ed. McGraw-Hill, 2007.)

exposure. Alternatively, an approach across the interatrial septum can be chosen. The superior and inferior vena cavae are controlled with snares, and the right atrium is opened. The fossa ovalis is identified and incised vertically. This incision is extended superiorly toward the superior vena cava through the muscular portion of the interatrial septum. The septal incision can also be extended medially along the dome of the left atrium, the so-called superior septal approach. While exposure of the mitral valve is excellent, there is a risk of injury to the sinus node, requiring implantation of a permanent pacemaker.

Once the valve has been exposed, assessment of the mitral valve is performed to determine the mechanism of mitral regurgitation and the technique for repair or replacement. Injection of cold saline into the left ventricle will identify the location of regurgitation and the presence of flail or significantly prolapsed leaflets. The leaflets are inspected for their mobility and the presence of calcifications or perforations. The annulus is inspected for dilation and calcium. Once the mechanism of regurgitation is clear, a plan is made for repair or replacement. The strategy used depends on the pathologic mechanism (Figure 19–8).

When the mitral regurgitation is purely a result of annular dilation or posterior leaflet restriction from a previous myocardial infarction, mitral annuloplasty alone often adequately alleviates the leak. Horizontal sutures are placed along the mitral annulus, including the fibrous trigones. Care must be taken to avoid injury to underlying structures, such as the circumflex coronary artery, the coronary sinus, and the atrioventricular node. Annuloplasty is typically performed with the assistance of prosthetic rings or bands of varying degrees of rigidity. Some of the rings completely encircle the entire annulus, and some are incomplete,

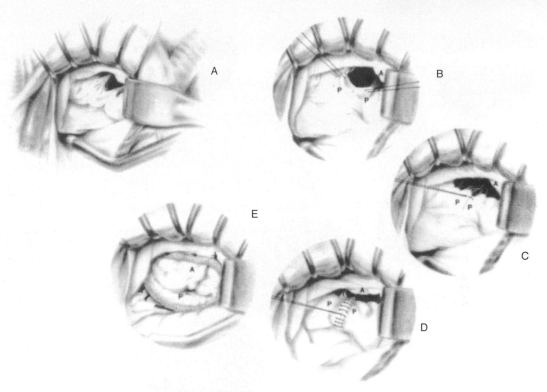

▲ **Figure 19–8.** Panels **A–E** represent atrial views of posterior leaflet reconstruction for isolated posterior leaflet prolapse and insertion of an annuloplasty ring.

designed to extend posteriorly from trigone to trigone (Figure 19–9). The annular mattress sutures are brought up through the sewing cuff of the ring and tied down. The size of the ring is selected to match the area of the anterior leaflet and the distance between the trigones. Competence is tested with saline injection, and the cardiac chambers are closed. After weaning from CPB, the valve is inspected using transesophageal echocardiography. An adequate repair must demonstrate both competence and low resistance, as evidenced by low pressure gradients across the valve.

Myxomatous degeneration of the mitral valve typically involves the posterior leaflet, particularly the P2 scallop. This lesion can be reproducibly repaired using techniques with the potential for indefinite durability. After exposure of the mitral valve, the point of prolapse is identified. A quadrangular portion of the prolapsing section is excised to the annulus. The gap is bridged by undercutting the annular attachments of the adjacent portion of the posterior leaflet. The mobilized edge of the posterior leaflet is sewn back to the annulus with running suture (Figure 19–10), reducing its effective height. An annuloplasty can be performed to address any annular dilation as well as to provide reinforcement to the posterior annular reconstruction.

When prolapse or chordal rupture involve the anterior leaflet, repair is more difficult. A variety of approaches have been described, but the likelihood of durable repair is far

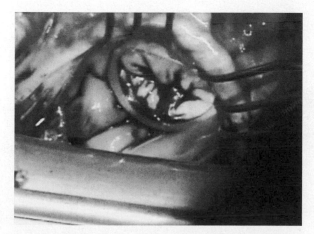

▲ **Figure 19–9.** Operative photograph of a mitral ring annuloplasty for ischemic mitral regurgitation. The ring plicates the posterior annulus to restore leaflet coaptation.

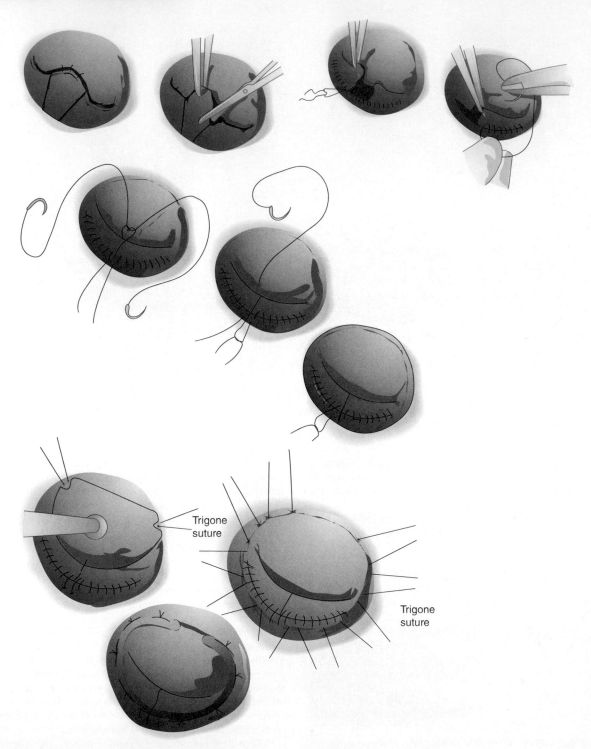

▲ Figure 19–10. Quadrangular resection and sliding annuloplasty for prolapse of the posterior mitral valve leaflet. (From Cohn LH: *Cardiac Surgery in the Adult,* 3rd ed. McGraw-Hill, 2007.)

less when compared to the more common posterior leaflet prolapse. One approach involves the creation of artificial cords. Typically, polytetrafluoroethylene is used to create neochords from the papillary muscle to the edge of the leaflet. The challenge is to create the precise length to allow coaptation without prolapse. Alternatively, the flail anterior segment can be removed and is replaced with a resected portion of the posterior leaflet, including its attached chords. A simpler approach is the edge-to-edge technique, in which the opposing edges of the anterior and posterior leaflets are sewn together with a single suture, creating a double-orifice mitral valve. Popularized by Alfieri and colleagues, this approach has been applied using catheter-based techniques, obviating the need for open surgery.

Often, the regurgitant mitral valve cannot be repaired, such as when there is severe valvular destruction from infective endocarditis or extensive calcifications as can be seen with rheumatic mitral valve disease. The mitral valve is exposed, and the leaflets are excised. Attempts are made to preserve chordal attachments to the annulus, and portions of the posterior leaflet can be plicated to the annulus to preserve secondary chords. This is typically not possible with rheumatic disease because the calcified annulus will require extensive debridement. Annular mattress sutures with felt or Teflon pledgets are placed circumferentially. For mechanical prostheses, the pledgets are oriented on the atrial side to avoid interference with the actuation of the disk. For bioprosthetic implants, the pledgets can be placed on the ventricular side, which allows for a slightly larger prosthetic (Figure 19–11). After sutures are placed, the annulus is sized and an appropriate prosthetic is chosen. The sutures are driven through the sewing ring of the valve and tied down. After weaning from CPB, the valve is carefully inspected using transesophageal echocardiography for signs of paravalvular leak, normal motion of the leaflets or disks, and a low pressure gradient across the valve.

C. Results

Repair or replacement of the mitral valve for regurgitation preserves ventricular function and allows some remodeling by eliminating the volume overload and its associated incipient changes. However, loss of myocardial contractility, as a result of longstanding mitral regurgitation or otherwise, typically does not recover. Only its progressive decline can be halted. This reinforces the need to intervene before severe ventricular dilation has occurred, even in asymptomatic patients.

Mitral regurgitation associated with prolapsing myxomatous leaflets carries low perioperative mortality, and the freedom from degeneration of a repaired valve is greater than 90% at 10 years. Some of the low periprocedural mortality is related to the young age and low incidence of comorbidities in this patient population. Mitral valve repair associated with

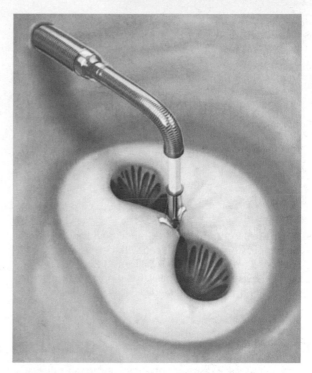

▲ **Figure 19–11.** Percutaneous device for mitral valve repair, currently in clinical trials. (Reproduced with permission from Abbott Laboratories, Abbott Park, Illinois.)

coronary bypass grafting carries a perioperative mortality of approximately 5%, with ejection fraction, renal function, and age being independent predictors of death. Although mortality after coronary bypass grafting is associated with the severity of preoperative mitral regurgitation, there is no evidence that mitral repair reduces this mortality. Repairing the mitral valve, however, is associated with improved long-term survival, as compared to replacing the valve.

MITRAL VALVE STENOSIS

▶ Pathophysiology

Rheumatic heart disease is the most common cause of mitral valve stenosis. Although nearly 20 million people are affected with rheumatic fever in underdeveloped countries, the incidence in the United States and Western Europe has declined markedly, largely a result of advanced medical care and use of antibiotics to treat infections caused by group A streptococci. Untreated infection results in an immunologic response to bacterial antigens that resemble cardiac tissue. The degree of the immunologic response and the severity of ongoing valvular destruction appear to be related to genetic factors. Although the damage can affect the entire

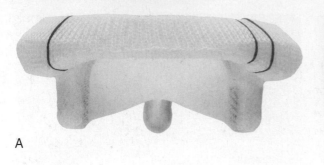

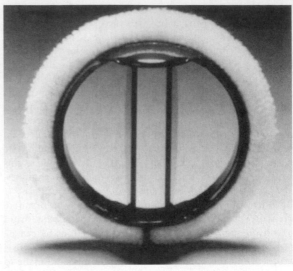

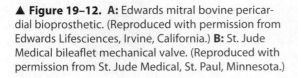

▲ **Figure 19–12. A:** Edwards mitral bovine pericardial bioprosthetic. (Reproduced with permission from Edwards Lifesciences, Irvine, California.) **B:** St. Jude Medical bileaflet mechanical valve. (Reproduced with permission from St. Jude Medical, St. Paul, Minnesota.)

endocardium and even the pericardium, the mitral valve is the most commonly involved, with 40% of patients having only mitral valve disease. Mitral and aortic valve disease is also frequently seen, and rarely patients will have isolated aortic valve involvement. It remains unclear why right-sided valves are rarely affected.

The characteristic features of rheumatic mitral valve disease include leaflet and chordal thickening and retraction (Figure 19–12). Commissural fusion is also apparent, and a late feature is dense calcification of the annulus and leaflets. Turbulence created by impaired leaflet mobility exacerbates the valve destruction, accelerating further fibrosis and calcification.

Mitral valve stenosis can also be caused by mitral annular calcification, which can become quite bulky, protruding into the valve orifice. The posterior leaflet can become contracted and fixed, while the anterior leaflet thickens and becomes less mobile. Structural valvular degeneration of bioprosthetic mitral valves can cause mitral valve stenosis as well as thrombosis or pannus formation in mechanical prostheses. Advanced endocarditis can result in effective mitral valve stenosis, as bulky vegetations obstruct the inflow path. Congenital abnormalities, such as the parachute mitral valve with a single papillary muscle, can become stenotic, requiring intervention.

The stenotic mitral valve results in a pressure gradient between the left atrium and ventricle. This fixed resistance increases the left atrial pressure even further during exercise, as cardiac output increases, but resistance across the valve is unchanged. Severe mitral valve stenosis is associated with a mean transvalvular gradient of 10-15 mm Hg at rest. Cardiac

output is dependent on ventricular filling, and left ventricular end diastolic pressure and volume are typically low. Exercise-induced tachycardia decreases diastolic filling time, producing a paradoxical reduction in cardiac output. Left ventricular function is typically normal or hyperdynamic, but some patients have combined mitral valve stenosis and mitral regurgitation, as well as significant aortic valve insufficiency, and will develop chronic left ventricular volume overload and dysfunction. Thus, the hemodynamic consequences of mitral valve stenosis depend to a certain degree on the presence of mitral regurgitation and other associated valvular pathology.

As the mitral transvalvular gradient worsens, the left atrial wall hypertrophies. The a-wave on the atrial pressure tracing is accentuated during atrial contraction. Progressively, the left atrium dilates, creating disorganized electrical conduction pathways. Reentry pathways lead to frequent premature atrial contractions and eventually to atrial fibrillation. The onset of atrial fibrillation often is the inciting clinical event, with the reduced diastolic filling time from rapid ventricular response and the loss of atrial contraction both resulting in reduced left ventricular filling and a drop in cardiac output. The sustained elevation in left atrial pressure results in pulmonary vascular changes producing pulmonary hypertension. These changes can lead to right ventricular pressure overload with tricuspid valve insufficiency and to right ventricular volume overload.

Symptoms of mitral valve stenosis often do not develop until the disease is advanced, owing to ventricular and atrial adaptive responses. Patients describe dyspnea from pulmonary congestion or reduced cardiac output, initially limited to exertion. Onset of atrial fibrillation often prompts urgent evaluation, as the loss of atrial contraction and tachycardia cause a precipitous drop in cardiac output and pulmonary congestion. Late findings include signs of right-sided heart failure such as ascites and lower extremity edema. Cerebrovascular events or other thromboembolic complications from an intracardiac thrombus are not uncommon with longstanding mitral valve stenosis, as the dilated left atrium and left atrial appendage have regions of stagnation and thrombus formation, particularly in the setting of atrial fibrillation. Since two-thirds of the patients with mitral valve stenosis are women, symptoms often present during later stages of pregnancy as the increased cardiac output results in higher left atrial pressures and pulmonary congestion.

▶ Diagnostic Evaluation

Because presentation tends to be late, many patients present with signs of longstanding heart failure, including cachexia, ascites, and lower extremity edema. On auscultation, the low diastolic rumble is best heard over the cardiac apex. An opening snap can be heard in the early stages of the disease, and the systolic murmur of tricuspid regurgitation is a late finding, as is a parasternal heave from right ventricular hypertrophy.

The electrocardiogram will diagnose atrial fibrillation, and right axis deviation may be present, suggesting advanced pulmonary hypertension. The chest radiograph is often normal but may demonstrate straightening of the left heart border caused by dilation of the pulmonary arteries. Pulmonary edema may be present on initial evaluation when atrial fibrillation is the inciting event. Cardiac catheterization is important in identifying associated coronary arterial pathology and can confirm the severity of the mitral stenosis using simultaneous left and right heart catheterization with pressure measurements. The degree of pulmonary hypertension and its reversibility with provocative agents may be assistive in determining surgical candidacy in advanced cases.

Echocardiography is the mainstay in diagnosis of mitral valve stenosis. Surface or transthoracic echocardiography is preferred because it is noninvasive, and can usually provide images demonstrating the characteristic thickening and restricted mobility of the mitral leaflets. If images are obscured by patient body habitus or obstructive lung disease, a transesophageal echocardiogram can be performed. The proximity of the esophagus with the left atrium provides excellent visualization and can easily demonstrate the thickened mitral subvalvar apparatus typical of rheumatic disease. Color Doppler can be used to show turbulent flow across the valve orifice, and the pressure gradients can be estimated by measuring the peak and mean velocity of blood through the valve.

▶ Treatment

Medical treatment is limited to control of symptoms. Recurrent episodes of infection must be prevented, as accel-erated progression of the disease can be seen. Prompt initiation of antibiotics for suspected infections is prudent. Complications of mitral valve stenosis should be addressed and controlled. Rapid ventricular response to atrial fibrillation can be treated with a number of pharmacologic agents, and attempts at cardioversion should be made once the presence of intracardiac thrombus has been excluded. It is often difficult to maintain sinus rhythm in the mitral valve stenosis patient with a significantly dilated left atrium in whom rate control alone may be acceptable. Systemic anticoagulation with warfarin should be initiated if there has been a history of atrial fibrillation. Once the patient describes symptoms of heart failure, intervention on the mitral valve should be considered. For symptomatic patients not candidates for catheter-based or surgical intervention, diuretics and oral sodium restriction to control heart failure symptoms is all that is available.

Catheter-based balloon mitral valvotomy can reduce the obstructing pressure gradient and improve symptoms in selected patients. Patients with severe mitral valve stenosis and symptoms and asymptomatic patients with severe mitral valve stenosis and pulmonary hypertension are eligible if there is no mitral regurgitation, no left atrial thrombus, and favorable valve morphology, such as absence of extensive subvalvular fibrosis and calcification. The procedure is performed by femoral venous puncture and transeptal access to the mitral valve across the interatrial septum. A 25-mm hourglass Inoue balloon is advanced across the valve orifice and inflated. Significant improvement in hemodynamics is seen immediately, with reduction in transvalvular pressure gradients by as much as 15 mm Hg. The incidence of restenosis in selected patients is approximately 25% at 4 years.

Indications for surgical treatment are the same as for balloon valvuloplasty, including symptomatic patients with moderate or severe mitral valve stenosis and asymptomatic patients with pulmonary hypertension. Valve repair can be performed in carefully selected patients with reasonable long-term results. CPB is initiated in the same manner as for mitral repair for mitral regurgitation. After cardioplegic arrest, the mitral valve is exposed. Any thrombus within the atrium or atrial appendage is removed. The left atrial appendage can be transected and oversewn at its base to remove its future embolic potential. The areas of commissural fusion are cut, and the leaflets are decalcified. Occasionally, fused chords are divided to increase leaflet mobility. In carefully selected patients, recurrent mitral valve stenosis is less than 20% in up to 15 years.

In most cases, however, severe leaflet and subvalvular calcification has made the valve unreconstructable, requiring valve replacement. Overaggressive debridement of the posterior mitral annulus can result in perforation and atrioventricular separation and should be avoided. The selection of valve prosthetic depends on the unique clinical circumstances. Bioprosthetic valves are minimally thrombogenic

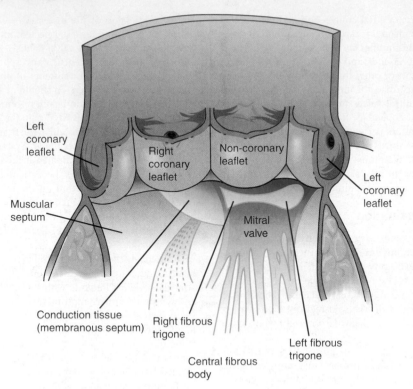

▲ Figure 19–13. Anatomic relationships of the aortic root. (From Cohn LH: *Cardiac Surgery in the Adult,* 3rd ed. McGraw-Hill, 2007.)

and do not require lifelong anticoagulation with warfarin. However, they are prone to structural valvular degeneration resulting in recurrent mitral valve stenosis or mitral regurgitation. Valve prosthetics are improving, and freedom from structural valvular degeneration is as high as 85% at 10 years. Mechanical valves are thrombogenic and require lifelong anticoagulation, such as warfarin, which is associated with a 1%-2% annual incidence of major bleeding complications. They are more durable and reduce the need for reoperation. In general, patients younger than 60 years of age or those already requiring warfarin for atrial fibrillation should be considered for a mechanical valve.

AORTIC VALVE DISEASE

The aortic valve separates the outflow tract of the left ventricle with the ascending aorta. It is a trileaflet structure, with three semilunar cusps named for the coronary arteries that arise within the underlying sinuses. The left and right coronary arteries originate within these respective sinuses, with no coronary artery arising within the *noncoronary* sinus. The free edges of the cusps are thickened at regions called the nodules of Arantius. The valve leaflets attach to

the wall of the aorta at the annulus, and the locations where two adjacent cusps meet are the commissures. Important structures can be identified under these triangular-shaped zones (Figure 19–13). The commissure between the right and noncoronary cusp serves as the superior border to the membranous interventricular septum and the atrioventricular conduction center. The non-left commissure guards the aortomitral curtain and the center of the anterior leaflet of the mitral valve. The left-right commissure overlies the muscular interventricular septum and the medial border of the right ventricular outflow tract. These intimate intracardiac relationships are no more apparent than within the left ventricular outflow tract.

The thin-walled aortic valve leaflets easily open and close during the cardiac cycle, purely following the pressure changes and blood flow path. Under normal circumstances, opening offers very little resistance to flow. The aortic sinuses have an important role during valve closure, as the volume of blood within the space between the opened valve cusp and the aortic wall develop vortices as blood velocity falls. These vortices exert central pressure and initiates valve closure. The sudden reversal of flow from deceleration completes the diastolic closure.

AORTIC STENOSIS

▶ Pathophysiology

The most common cause of aortic stenosis is senile calcific aortic stenosis. It is believed to represent degenerative changes at the cellular level, including lipid accumulation and inflammatory infiltrates, similar to atherosclerotic changes seen in the medium-sized arterial tree. Not surprisingly, it is associated with elevated cholesterol, hypertension, cigarette smoking, diabetes, and other risk factors for atherosclerosis. It is most common in the seventh and eighth decades of life and occurs in patients whose valves previously appeared normal. The cusps become progressively immobilized and calcified, starting at the flexion points and extending both along the leaflets and into the wall of the aortic root.

Congenital bicuspid aortic valve represents the most common congenital cardiac lesion, occurring in 2% of the general population. Turbulent flow across the valve causes trauma, leading to fibrosis and calcium deposition, further increasing turbulence, and accelerating the process. Significant stenosis typically occurs in the fifth and sixth decades of life, although they can present earlier. Patients with congenital bicuspid aortic valves often have dilation or aneurysmal degeneration of the ascending aorta. Some evidence suggests a genetic etiology, with the presence of abnormal microfibrils causing premature cystic medial necrosis.

Rheumatic heart disease can affect the aortic valve, although it is unusual for the disease to be limited to the aorta, with mitral involvement far more common. As with rheumatic mitral stenosis, fusion of the commissures tends to be the initial feature, followed by progressive thickening and retraction of the leaflets. The reduced leaflet mobility results in a clinical picture of combined aortic valve stenosis and insufficiency.

Aortic stenosis develops gradually, allowing adaptive changes to maintain cardiac output. The left ventricle gradually hypertrophies in response to the severity of the outflow tract obstruction, often resulting in pressure gradients exceeding 100 mm Hg. As a result, patients can remain asymptomatic until severely advanced disease is present. While concentric left ventricular hypertrophy maintains systolic function in the face of severe outflow obstruction, diastolic function of the thickened and noncompliant ventricle is progressively impaired. Diastolic dysfunction can be overcome to a certain degree with atrial hypertrophy and enhanced atrial kick. In addition, as left ventricular end diastolic pressure rises, intravascular volume status and peripheral vascular resistance adjust to maintain the required preload. Certain triggers can disrupt this delicate balance, including loss of atrial contribution from atrial fibrillation or reduced diastolic filling time from increased heart rate, as might be seen during exercise. These triggers can create sudden clinical decompensation, producing markedly reduced cardiac output and pulmonary edema, even in a previously asymptomatic patient.

The most common clinical presentation in a patient with aortic stenosis is gradual decrease in exercise tolerance. The fixed outflow obstruction prevents an increase in stroke volume typically seen in exercise with elevated circulating catecholamines. Any change in cardiac output is limited to an increase in heart rate, decreasing diastolic filling time for the stiff and noncompliant ventricle. As a result, there is limited boost in cardiac output during exercise, producing premature exertional fatigue and dyspnea. Some patients describe angina, as myocardial oxygen demand exceeds supply. The hypertrophied heart consumes more oxygen without reciprocal increase in epicardial delivery. In addition, the outflow obstruction prolongs systole, further increasing oxygen demand. Symptoms are typically exertional, as the increased heart rate reduces diastolic coronary perfusion time. Syncope or presyncope is occasionally described in patients with aortic stenosis, presumable related to systemic vasodilation during exercise without a reciprocal increase in cardiac output. Advanced heart failure with symptoms at rest or with minimal activity suggest a decrease in systolic function, likely a result of longstanding disease with alterations within the myocardium at the cellular level.

▶ Diagnostic Evaluation

Physical examination of the patient reveals several findings specific for aortic stenosis. There is a characteristic systolic crescendo/decrescendo murmur heard best over the base of the heart and radiating up the carotid arteries. The murmur becomes harsher and peaks later in systole as the severity worsens. Palpation of the carotid pulses reveals parvus and tardus, or a late peaking and low-amplitude pulse. A palpable thrill may be felt over the right second intercostal space.

The electrocardiogram demonstrates left ventricular hypertrophy in the majority of patients. Conduction or rhythm abnormalities are identified in some patients. The chest radiograph typically is normal but may demonstrate dilation of the ascending aorta in patients with congenital bicuspid valve. Cardiac catheterization provides important information about associated cardiac pathology, particularly coronary occlusive disease. In addition, hemodynamic assessment can confirm the severity of the aortic valve stenosis and quantify the degree of pulmonary hypertension.

The standard evaluation of patients with suspected aortic stenosis is echocardiography. Images of the valve reveal the severity of the stiffness and calcifications. Images also differentiate bicuspid from tricuspid anatomy and identify associated dilation of the ascending aorta. Ventricular function and additional valvular pathology, particularly in patients with rheumatic heart disease, is essential. Doppler echocardiography can measure the velocity of the aortic jet, allowing reliable estimates of the pressure gradients using the modified Bernoulli equation.

▶ Treatment

A. Medical Therapy

Because aortic stenosis can progress over 10-15 years, patients with mild to moderate disease and without symptoms can be followed without intervention. Serial echocardiography should be performed annually or every other year to assess for disease progression. The most important aspect of medical therapy is education of the patient about potential symptoms. Since symptoms can develop gradually, many patients will unconsciously alter their lifestyles and activity levels without recognizing the presence of limitations. Although there is some suggestion that cholesterol reduction with statins can reduce the calcifications, there is little evidence that medications can adequately palliate the symptomatic patient or can alter the timing of surgical intervention in asymptomatic patients.

B. Indications for Surgery

The indications for surgery on the stenotic aortic valve have been largely determined by the presence of symptoms. Numerous studies have demonstrated reasonably good prognosis in asymptomatic patients managed without surgery. However, symptoms may be equivocal, particularly in the elderly population. Exercise stress testing under the observation of a physician can help elucidate significant limitations that may not be apparent by merely questioning the patient. Surgery is also indicated for patients with moderate to severe aortic stenosis who are undergoing cardiac surgery for other indications, such as coronary bypass grafting or mitral valve replacement.

Handling of the asymptomatic patient with severe aortic stenosis is under some controversy. The severity of aortic stenosis can be quantified using Doppler echocardiography to estimate the pressure gradient across the aortic valve using the velocity of the outflow jet and the modified Bernoulli equation. Severe aortic stenosis is present when the mean gradient exceeds 40 mm Hg in the normal ventricle. Although some have described an increase in the rate of sudden death in patients with severe aortic stenosis, there remains no evidence to justify aortic valve replacement in the absence of symptoms.

AORTIC INSUFFICIENCY

▶ Pathophysiology

Several conditions can cause incompetence of the aortic valve. Any of the disease processes that cause aortic stenosis can also cause some degree of aortic valve insufficiency, including senile calcific aortic stenosis, degenerated bicus-

pid aortic valve, and rheumatic aortic valve disease. Aortic valve endocarditis is another common cause of aortic valve insufficiency. The most common cause of incompetence of the aortic valve is related to pathology within the aortic root and ascending aorta. Aneurysmal dilation of the ascending aorta, either from congenital conditions such as Marfan disease, from degenerative age-related changes, or from changes associated with a bicuspid aortic valve, can cause aortic valve insufficiency. As the wall of the aorta enlarges, the aortic valve annulus dilates and the leaflets separate, causing incompetence.

As with mitral valve regurgitation, aortic valve insufficiency is best tolerated when it occurs gradually. As the volume of regurgitation worsens, the ventricle adapts by dilating to accommodate the increased preload, and it hypertrophies to maintain the same level of systolic pressure at larger volumes. Despite progressive dilation, ventricular output and systolic function are maintained for long periods of time, leaving many patients asymptomatic for years. While end diastolic volume is elevated, end systolic volume is normal. With severe degrees of chronic aortic insufficiency, the heart can require ejecting as much as two to three times the circulating cardiac output, resulting in longstanding volume overload. Eventually, systolic function declines, resulting in a rapid and progressive rise in end diastolic volume, and heart failure symptoms ensue.

Most patients with chronic aortic insufficiency do not develop symptoms of heart failure until there is severe left ventricular dilation. Some patients describe palpitations or the sensation of ventricular heave, particularly when lying down. Acute aortic valve insufficiency, as can occur with aortic valve endocarditis, can present with cardiogenic shock because the relatively noncompliant ventricle is unprepared for the excess volume during both systole and diastole. There is a combination of high intracardiac filling pressures and low cardiac output. Patients are tachycardic and hypotensive as well as acutely dyspneic at rest. The patient with endocarditis may also be febrile with signs of embolization of vegetations, causing stroke, or extremity or intestinal ischemia.

▶ Diagnostic Testing

Certain characteristic physical examination findings are pathognomonic for chronic aortic valve insufficiency. The water-hammer pulse can be appreciated, with accentuated systole and abrupt collapse. Patients may have a head bob with each heart beat, or a pulse may be seen in the uvula. A systolic thrill is also described over the femoral artery from the augmented forward flow. The apical impulse is displaced laterally and inferiorly from cardiomegaly, and diastolic blood pressure is low. Auscultation will reveal a high-pitched diastolic murmur heard immediately after the second heart sound. The severity of the valvular lesion usually correlates with the duration of the murmur, not the intensity. The murmur is best heard with the patient leaning forward during a breath hold.

Echocardiography will establish the etiology of the aortic valve insufficiency, visualizing the motion of the leaflets and dilation of the aorta or the presence of vegetations or leaflet perforations. In addition, the ventricular size can be followed, as elevated end systolic volumes or reduced ejection fraction are indications for surgery. Reversal of flow seen in the descending aorta is a sign of severe aortic valve insufficiency. More sophisticated techniques can quantify the regurgitant volume, such as evaluating the regurgitant jet velocity/time integral.

▶ Treatment

For asymptomatic patients with moderate aortic insufficiency and normal ventricular dimensions, no treatment is necessary. Patients with severe aortic valve insufficiency and normal ventricular size should be followed every 6 months with assessment of symptoms and echocardiography. Some advocate the use of afterload reduction agents to reduce the volume of regurgitant blood, but no evidence demonstrates reduced need for surgery. Symptomatic patients who are not candidates for surgery should be treated with afterload reduction agents, such as calcium channel blockers or inhibitors of angiotensin-converting enzyme. Diuretics and salt restrictions may help in alleviating heart failure symptoms.

For operative candidates, development of heart failure symptoms is an indication for surgery. Asymptomatic patients with decreased left ventricular systolic function or elevated left ventricular end systolic volumes should also undergo operative treatment. Because ventricular dilation is associated with irreversible changes at the cellular level, intervention is best performed before these permanent changes occur.

▶ Surgical Techniques

As with most other cardiac surgical procedures, median sternotomy is the standard incision utilized for access to the aortic valve. The pericardium is opened longitudinally, and the reflection is mobilized off of the great vessels. The pulmonary artery and aorta are separated as they emanate from the heart, taking care to avoid injury to the takeoff of the right pulmonary artery or the left main coronary artery. The patient is anticoagulated with 300 IU heparin, and an activated clotting time of at least 400 seconds is confirmed. Cannulation for CPB is performed, using the distal ascending aorta or the transverse aortic arch to maximize the distance between the aortic cross-clamp and the aortotomy. Venous return is via the right atrial appendage. CPB is initiated, and the left ventricle is vented via a catheter advanced from the right superior pulmonary vein. The patient is cooled systemically to 32°C. An aortic cross-clamp is applied to the distal ascending aorta just proximal to the CPB cannula. The heart is arrested with cold blood cardioplegia

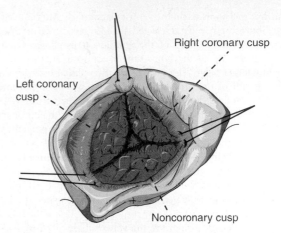

▲ Figure 19–14. Surgeon's view of the stenotic trileaflet aortic valve. (From Cohn LH: *Cardiac Surgery in the Adult,* 3rd ed. McGraw-Hill, 2007.)

solution with dextrose, phosphate, and potassium at 8°C. The cardioplegia is delivered antegrade down the coronary arteries using a catheter in the aortic root. Cardioplegia solution is also delivered retrograde via a balloon-tipped catheter in the coronary sinus. If severe aortic valve insufficiency is present, only retrograde cardioplegia can be delivered. Once diastolic cardiac arrest is achieved, the ascending aorta is opened transversely approximately 1-2 cm above the takeoff of the right coronary artery. The aortotomy is extended two-thirds of the circumference of the aorta, providing excellent visualization of the valve, the coronary ostia, and the ventricular outflow tract (Figure 19–14).

Excision of the stenotic aortic valve can be time consuming and requires meticulous attention to detail. The extensive calcifications can extend deep into the annulus and up the wall of the aortic root or down along the anterior leaflet of the mitral valve. The calcium buildup must be debrided aggressively enough to allow proper seating of the valve prosthesis without a paravalvular leak while avoiding residual outflow tract obstruction. However, overaggressive debridement can result in perforations of the aortic wall, ventricular septal defect, or unhinging of the mitral leaflet with resultant severe mitral regurgitation. In cases of endocarditis, any granulation tissue or residual vegetations must be removed and debrided to avoid recurrent infection of the implanted prosthetic. The outflow tract and aortic root is thoroughly irrigated to ensure removal of loose deposits and debris.

Once the native valve has been removed and the annulus satisfactorily debrided, the outflow tract is sized using tools provided by each manufacturer of valve prostheses. The appropriately sized valve is selected and secured in place. Mechanical valve prosthetics are implanted using a pledgeted mattress technique, leaving the pledgets on the aortic side. This eliminates the likelihood of the bulky pledgets interfering with the disk mechanisms on the ventricular surface. Alternatively, if a bioprosthetic valve is selected, the pledgets can be oriented on the ventricular side of the annulus. This allows supra-annular seating of the bioprosthetic and implantation of a slightly larger valve. The sutures are then placed through the sewing cuff of the prosthetic, and the valve is lowered into the surgical field. The sutures are tied, ensuring that the valve has seated properly to the annulus. The ostia of the coronary arteries should be inspected and clearly free of impingement by the prosthetic valve. The aortotomy is then closed with running polypropylene suture, occasionally reinforced with Teflon felt in the older patient with a thin aortic wall.

The patient is then gradually weaned from CPB, thoroughly deairing with gentle suction applied using the left ventricular vent and the aortic root catheter. Using the transesophageal echocardiogram, the valve is carefully inspected for competency and adequacy of the size. There should be no paravalvular leak, and the gradients across the valve should be low. Elevated pulmonary artery pressures or reduced cardiac output should alert the surgeon of the possibility of an unrecognized paravalvular leak.

Aortic valve endocarditis also poses unique surgical challenges. The infective process often results in abscess formation and occasionally intracardiac fistulas. The most important first step in addressing these problems is aggressive debridement of infected and devitalized tissue. Not only will residual infection colonize the implanted prosthetic but inadequate debridement with securing of the prosthetic to infected and devitalized tissue will lead to dehiscence with

need for early reoperation. Abscesses are common within the intervalvular fibrous body. The annular defect should be covered with a pericardial patch. Often, the entire root requires excision, requiring replacement with a valved conduit and reimplantation of the coronary ostia. Results for endocarditis are dependent on the clinical status of the patient at the time of surgery as well as the etiology of the infection. Intravenous drug users carry the worst prognosis, in large part related to recurrence of their addiction with subsequent reinfection.

TRANSCATHETER AORTIC VALVE REPLACEMENT

Recently, aortic valve replacement has been approached without sternotomy using endovascular techniques. Bioprosthetic valves of bovine or porcine pericardium are crimped and loaded onto a metallic frame (Figure 19–15). A 18-24 French delivery system can be inserted via the femoral vessels and expanded at the level of the left ventricular outflow tract either by balloon or using self-expanding titanium alloys. The native aortic valve is displaced by the prosthetic rather than removed as is done in surgical aortic valve replacement. The procedure can often be performed under local anesthesia, dramatically reducing perioperative morbidity. Current indications for this approach are patients with severe aortic stenosis and either prohibitive surgical risk or as an alternative to surgery in higher risk patients (estimated perioperative mortality of 15%). While the femoral access route is most frequently utilized, some

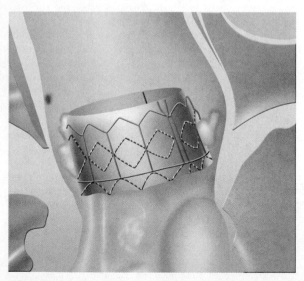

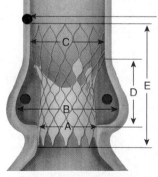

Note the position of any SVGs

A Annulus diameter
B Sinus of Valsalva diameter
C Ascending aorta diameter
D Sinus of Valsalva height
E Frame height (≈ 5 cm)

▲ **Figure 19–15. A:** Edwards Sapien percutaneous aortic valve (Reproduced with permission from Edwards Lifesciences, Irvine, California.) **B:** Medtronic CoreValve, currently in clinical trials. (Reproduced with permission from Medtronic CV Luxembourg SARL. The CoreValve System is an investigational device and is limited by US law to investigational use. CoreValve is a registered trademark of Medtronic CV Luxembourg SARL.)

patients with small peripheral vessels or extensive atherosclerotic disease may not accommodate the large size delivery systems. Alternative approaches include the iliac artery, axillary artery, ascending aorta, and the left ventricular apex. The latter two require mini-thoracotomies for exposure. Paravalvular leaks are common, with moderate to severe regurgitation occurring in 10%-15% of patients. Long-term survival is diminished in patients with significant aortic insufficiency. Stroke represents a concern as the large catheters traverse the aortic arch and the calcified aortic valve is dilated, hazarding cerebral embolization. When directly compared to surgery in high risk patients, the risk of neurologic event was twice as high with transcatheter aortic valve replacement (TAVR) (5.5% vs 2.4%). This risk may be justified in the context of an overall reduction in perioperative mortality for TAVR as compared to surgical aortic valve replacement in these high risk patients (3.4% vs 6.5%). While TAVR appears to be efficacious for high risk patients with severe aortic stenosis, it remains unclear if this approach will expand to a lower risk population.

Kodali SK et al: Two-year outcomes after transcatheter or surgical aortic valve replacement. *New Engl J Med* 2012;366:1686.

Webb JG, Wood DA: Current status of transcatheter aortic valve replacement. *J Am Coll Cardiol* 2012;60:483.

Whitlow PL et al: Acute and 12-month results with catheter-based mitral valve leaflet repair. *J Am Col Cardiol* 2012;59:130.

THORACIC AORTA

The ascending aorta represents a continuation of the aortic root at the sinotubular junction. The aortic arch extends from the ascending aorta, traveling posteriorly and to the left as it gives off the three "head vessels" superiorly: the innominate, left carotid, and left subclavian arteries. The thoracic aorta continues from the aortic arch into the descending thoracic aorta beyond the left subclavian artery. The descending thoracic aorta continues until the level of the diaphragm, where it becomes the abdominal aorta. The only branches originating from the descending thoracic aorta are the bronchial and esophageal arteries and multiple intercostal vessels that contribute important sources of blood flow to the spinal cord.

Some common variants are seen in the branch pattern of the thoracic aorta. The most common is the "bovine arch" in which the left carotid originates from the innominate artery. An aberrant right subclavian artery originates from the distal aortic arch on the lesser curvature and travels posterior to the esophagus from left to right. It has been associated with unusual causes of dysphagia from mechanical compression of the esophagus. Other abnormal variants of the aortic arch include a right-sided arch and double ligamentum arteriosum, which can cause tracheal or esophageal compression early in life and are discussed in the second part of this chapter, Congenital Heart Disease.

THORACIC AORTIC ANEURYSMS

▶ Pathophysiology

During systole, kinetic energy imparted by ventricular ejection is absorbed in the compliance of the aorta, resulting in transient expansion and recoil. The amount of energy absorption is proportional to the proximity to the left ventricle. As such, the ascending, descending, and abdominal aorta have different cellular features to accommodate their unique fluid-mechanical environments. Elastin fiber content is typically higher in the ascending aorta. These fibers are synthesized and degraded continuously by the smooth muscle cells, and a progressive fragmentation of these fibers is associated with aging, which is the reason for gradual dilation of the ascending aorta in the elderly. However, certain acquired conditions can accelerate the process, producing the pathologically enlarged aorta resulting in aneurysms. Aortic atherosclerosis is associated with aneurysm formation, predominantly in the descending thoracic aorta. The inflammatory process extends from the intima to the media, causing elastin fiber breakdown. Cystic medial degeneration is the end result of any of the acquired degenerative processes, resulting in elastin fiber fragmentation and loss of smooth muscle cells. The weakened aortic media progressively dilates and can become prone to rupture or dissection. Infection, inflammatory conditions, and trauma can also cause localized medial degeneration and aneurysm formation.

Certain heritable conditions are also associated with aneurysmal disease of the thoracic aorta. Most notable is Marfan syndrome, an autosomal dominant abnormality of fibrillin, an important component in elastin. Patients with Marfan syndrome present with aneurysmal degeneration of the thoracic aorta at any level, most notably in the ascending aorta, in the second and third decades of life. Patients with bicuspid aortic valves are prone to develop aneurysms of the ascending aorta, likely related to abnormalities of their aortic smooth muscle.

The natural history of unresected thoracic aortic aneurysms is dependent on the size and the etiology. The larger the aneurysm, the greater the wall tension and thus the risk of rupture or dissection. Beyond 5.5 cm in maximal diameter, there is a significant increase in the risk of rupture, dissection, or death. Although it varies with age and etiology, there is a reasonably predictable growth rate, estimated at approximately 0.1-0.2 cm per year. Marfan syndrome and other genetic causes of thoracic aortic pathology tend to have a higher likelihood of rupture at smaller aneurysm sizes, and the growth rate is faster than in acquired thoracic aneurysms.

Most patients with thoracic aortic aneurysms are asymptomatic. The diagnosis is often established on screening chest radiograph, CT, or echocardiography performed for other indications. Occasionally, patients with unrup-

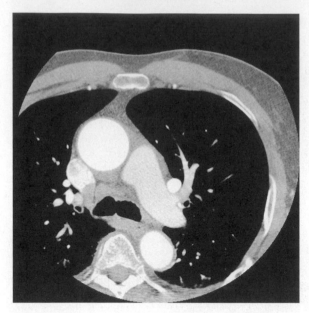

▲ **Figure 19–16.** CT scan of a dilated ascending aorta.

tured aneurysms describe chest pain presumably related to rapid enlargement or encroachment on adjacent structures. Unfortunately, many patients are not diagnosed with a thoracic aortic aneurysm until the time of rupture or dissection. Rupture of ascending aneurysms typically presents with crushing chest pain, whereas descending aneurysms cause tearing back or flank pain.

▶ **Diagnostic Testing**

In a patient presenting with a thoracic aneurysm without rupture, the physical examination is typically unremarkable. Chest radiograph may demonstrate a widened mediastinum. The electrocardiogram is helpful only for associated cardiac pathology. An echocardiogram demonstrates enlargement of the ascending aorta or descending aorta. The aortic arch is typically obscured from view by the trachea and the lungs.

Contrast-enhanced CT scanning is the most widely used test for aneurysms of the thoracic aorta (Figure 19–16). The CT scan can diagnose the aneurysm and accurately describe its size and extent, can be used for direct comparison for patients managed expectantly, and can differentiate isolated aneurysmal disease from an aortic dissection. Three-dimensional reconstruction is helpful in accurately assessing size and location of branch vessels. The limitation of CT scanning is the need for intravenous iodinated contrast, with its inherent nephrotoxic properties.

MRI provides quality resolution similar to CT scanning but can provide dynamic imaging for cardiac assessment and does not require iodinated contrast material. MRI, however,

is more time consuming and less available in many centers. Cardiac catheterization and aortography are performed only in planning operative intervention to exclude coronary artery disease or pulmonary hypertension.

▶ **Surgical Therapy**

The most frequent indication for operation on the aneurysmal ascending aorta is incidental to other cardiac pathology. It is generally agreed that an asymptomatic ascending aorta greater than 4.5-5 cm in size should be replaced at the time of aortic valve replacement or coronary bypass surgery, assuming the risk of the procedure would not be significantly altered. Any patient with a symptomatic ascending aneurysm should receive urgent surgery, although it is unusual for patients with ruptured ascending aortas to survive long enough to be given this opportunity. For asymptomatic patients without associated cardiac pathology, the indication for surgery is when the maximal diameter of the ascending aorta is greater than 5.5 cm. For patients with Marfan syndrome, surgery is indicated for lesser degrees of dilation. Additionally, for patients followed with serial CT scans, interval enlargement of the ascending aorta by a least 1 cm warrants consideration for surgical resection.

Sudden rupture or dissection is less frequent in the descending aorta, and thus the indications for operation are less stringent. In general, operation should be considered when the aneurysm reaches 6 cm in maximal diameter or if there is interval enlargement by at least 1 cm over 1 year. Patients with Marfan syndrome require surgery at smaller aortic sizes to prevent catastrophic complications. Increasingly, the descending thoracic aorta is treated using endovascular techniques. Balloon or self expanding stents are covered with vascular grafts and inserted via peripheral vessels and deployed creating a seal at the proximal and distal extent of the descending thoracic aneurysm, the so called "landing zones." Although the aneurysm is not removed, pressurized blood is excluded from the sac, eliminating the risk of rupture (Figure 19–17). Because the procedure does not require thoracotomy and aortic clamping, morbidity is substantially lower. However, endoleaks are frequent, in which there is failure to completely exclude blood flow into the aneurysm sac. These endoleaks may result in late aneurysm related complications. Endovascular treatment of descending thoracic aneurysm continues to evolve with experience and refinement of technology.

Medical treatment of small ascending or descending aneurysms involves aggressive blood pressure control using beta-blocking agents to reduce the forceful contraction against the weakened aortic wall, activity restriction to avoid straining, cessation of cigarette smoking, and weight loss. Patients followed with ascending or descending aortic aneurysms should receive repeat imaging for signs of interval growth prompting surgical intervention.

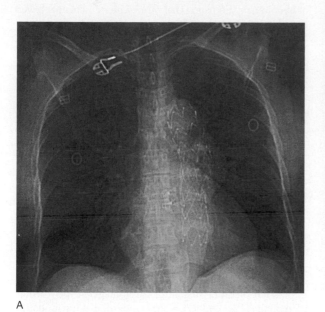

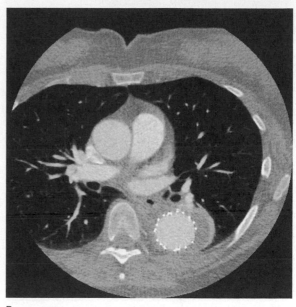

A

B

▲ **Figure 19–17.** Endovascular repair of a descending thoracic aneurysm. **A:** Chest radiograph. **B:** CT image. Note exclusion of contrast into the old aneurysm sac.

AORTIC DISSECTION

▶ **Pathophysiology**

Dissection of the thoracic aorta is among the most feared entities in all of medicine because of the exceedingly high mortality and the speed with which its injuries become irreversible. An intimal tear of the aorta allows blood flow to exit the lumen and travel a variable distance within the media. Depending on the location of the intimal tear and the direction in which blood travels, aortic dissections can be categorized using two prominent classification schemes. The DeBakey classification describes the location and the extent, whereas the more simplified Stanford classification looks at location alone. A Stanford type A dissection involves the ascending aorta; a Stanford type B involves the arch or descending aorta (Figure 19–18).

The precise etiology of aortic dissections is unclear, but there is an unambiguous association with a variety of conditions, including aortic aneurysms, hypertension, smoking, pregnancy, and recent intravascular trauma. Once blood enters the medial plane, the intima "floats" within the aortic lumen and has a characteristic appearance on CT scans (Figure 19–19). The blood within the false lumen reenters the true lumen through any number of naturally created fenestrations or holes, either from disruption of the side branches or from reentry at the termination of the false lumen. Blood flow to any of the side branches off of the aorta can be com-

promised by the intimal flap, causing ischemia, a condition referred to as malperfusion. Malperfusion can involve the coronary arteries, branches of the aortic arch to the brain, the renal arteries, the mesenteric arteries, or branches to the

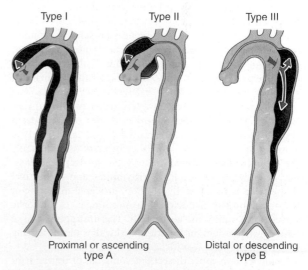

Type I   Type II   Type III

Proximal or ascending type A   Distal or descending type B

▲ **Figure 19–18.** DeBakey and Stanford Classifications of aortic dissection. DeBakey types I and II represent Stanford type A, whereas DeBakey type III is the same as a Stanford type B.

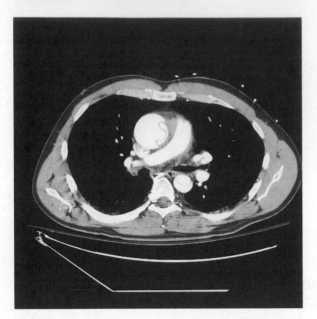

▲ **Figure 19–19.** CT scan of an acute aortic dissection. This Stanford type A dissection involves both the ascending and descending aortae. The large false lumen is nearly obstructing the true lumen.

lower extremities or the spinal cord. Blood can also exit the false lumen pathway into the adventitial space, causing free rupture. Rupture is more likely in Stanford type A dissections because of the intrapericardial location of the ascending aorta and the increased mechanical forces related to the proximity to the left ventricular outflow tract. Type B dissections in the descending aorta do not experience the same mechanical forces, because the more proximal aorta absorbs a significant amount of the kinetic energy. In addition, the extrapleural tissue helps reinforce the weakened adventitia, containing potential ruptures.

In addition to the free intrapericardial rupture of type A dissections, there are two other modes of early death responsible for the nearly 50% mortality associated with type A dissections. Malperfusion of the coronary ostia, typically the right coronary artery, causes acute myocardial infarction resulting in ventricular arrhythmias and myocardial dysfunction with shock. In addition, proximal migration of the dissection flap can disrupt the attachments of the aortic valve to the wall of the aortic root. The unsupported valve tissue prolapses into the ventricle during diastole, producing massive aortic valve insufficiency.

Patients with aortic dissections complain of tearing back pain or crushing chest pain. They are often hypertensive and tachycardic. The diagnosis can often be confused with acute myocardial infarction, ureterolithiasis, cholelithiasis, or pancreatitis. Patients with malperfusion can present with flank

or abdominal pain from renal or mesenteric ischemia, lower extremity pain or paresthesias from iliac occlusion, stroke from carotid occlusion, or acute paralysis from occlusion of the multiple branches to the spinal cord. These symptoms of malperfusion can often overwhelm the chest or back pain from the dissection, clouding the diagnostic evaluation. Delay in diagnosis is exceedingly common in acute aortic dissection.

▶ **Diagnostic Testing**

On physical examination, patients appear acutely ill and are tachycardic and hypertensive. Hypotension should warrant suspicion of pericardial tamponade, myocardial infarction, aortic valve insufficiency, or free rupture. Blood pressure should be assessed in all four extremities to document perfusion abnormalities from the dissection flap. Abdominal pain should prompt evaluation of possible mesenteric or renal malperfusion. Neurologic deficits suggest either cerebral embolization or spinal ischemia.

Chest radiographs are often performed as the initial diagnostic test. They may reveal widening of the mediastinum, a left pleural effusion, or cardiomegaly if pericardial tamponade is present. CT is the standard imaging modality used to diagnose aortic dissection and should be obtained promptly in a patient with new-onset tearing back or chest pain. The CT scan diagnoses the dissection and identifies associated aneurysmal disease as well as organs at risk for malperfusion. Transesophageal echocardiography has a critical role in patients with aortic dissection. TEE excludes involvement of the ascending aorta in cases that are equivocal on CT scan. In addition, TEE identifies cardiac dysfunction and, most importantly, aortic valve insufficiency from extension of the dissection into the aortic root.

▶ **Treatment**

A. Medical Therapy

Initial management of the patient with an acute aortic dissection is immediate control of elevated blood pressure. Narcotic agents can be given initially to control pain and reduce the catecholamine surge. Beta-blocking agents are particularly critical not only to reduce blood pressure but also to lower the force of contraction and the sheer stress directly impacting the weakened aortic tissue. Esmolol is a short-acting agent that can be administered as a continuous infusion to obtain fine control of blood pressure, avoiding excessive bradycardia or hypotension. If high blood pressure persists, an arterial vasodilator can be given, such as nitroprusside, with a goal of maintaining systolic blood pressure of 100-120 mm Hg.

Patients with type B aortic dissections are frequently treated with medical therapy only, consisting of pain and blood pressure control, as well as observation for signs of malperfusion or rupture. Most patients with type B dissections can be safely discharged from the hospital once blood pressure control is adequate and the pain has resolved. They are carefully followed for good antihypertensive control as well as surveillance CT scanning to assess for interval growth in the size of the descending aorta. The indications for operative intervention in an acute type B aortic dissection is ongoing chest pain despite adequate blood pressure control, aneurysmal enlargement of the descending aorta greater than 6 cm, or evidence of impending rupture on CT scanning.

B. Surgical Therapy

1. Indications—Patients with type A aortic dissections should undergo emergency surgery to avoid one of the three fatal complications associated with 95% of patients with untreated dissections. These complications include intrapericardial rupture with tamponade, aortic valve insufficiency, or acute myocardial infarction. Once the diagnosis of a type A dissection has been established, either by CT scan or TEE, the patient should be taken emergently to the operating room in preparation for emergency surgery. The only exception to immediate emergency surgery is when signs of malperfusion of the abdominal viscera exist. Although this strategy remains controversial, some advocate angiographic investigation for signs of malperfusion. Using a combination of contrast fluoroscopy, intravascular ultrasound, and selective cannulation of all branches from the aorta with pressure measurements, the extent of the dissection can be evaluated and areas of definite malperfusion can be identified. If the intimal flap is obstructing blood flow to any of the aortic branches, fenestration using balloon catheters can restore flow from the false to the true lumen, reperfusing ischemic organs. While patients with severe visceral malperfusion can have mortality rates of nearly 80%, more recent series adopting a strategy of initial catheter-based fenestration followed by surgical repair show estimated mortality rates in selected patients of less than 20%. Since catheter-based techniques are becoming more universally available, this strategy of delayed surgical repair may become more widespread.

2. Techniques—Once a patient with a type A dissection has been diagnosed, emergency surgery is usually indicated. The femoral or axillary artery is exposed for arterial cannulation for CPB. A median sternotomy is performed, exposing the dilated and dissected ascending aorta. After administration of 300 IU/kg of heparin, the patient is cannulated for CPB, using the right atrium for venous drainage. The patient is cooled aggressively to 18°C in preparation for hypothermic circulatory arrest. A catheter is placed in the coronary sinus to deliver retrograde cardioplegia for myocardial protection. A left ventricular vent is placed in the right superior pulmonary vein. Once the core body temperature has reached 18°C, CPB is discontinued, and the ascending aorta can be opened. The dissected aorta is

removed, typically extending along the lesser curvature of the aortic arch. The remaining arch is carefully inspected for additional intimal tears. An appropriately sized and spatulated Dacron graft is anastomosed to the aortic arch using running polypropylene suture buttressed with Teflon felt. CPB can be reinstituted, flushing air and debris out of the open anastomosis. The aortic cross-clamp can then be applied to the graft material. The proximal ascending aorta is resected to the sinotubular junction, and the Dacron graft is trimmed to size. The proximal anastomosis is performed in a similar fashion using running polypropylene suture buttressed with felt. A deairing needle is placed in the graft, and the aortic cross-clamp is removed. The patient is rewarmed and weaned from CPB.

Occasionally, the pathology extends proximally into the aortic root, requiring reconstruction or resection. If the root is not significantly enlarged, the dissection flap can be obliterated by inserting Teflon felt into the false lumen and reapproximating the intima to the adventitia using polypropylene suture. The aortic valve commissures can be resuspended to the aortic wall with pledgeted sutures from intima to adventitia. If the aortic root is dilated, the sinuses and valve tissue can be excised and replaced with a mechanical valve conduit, reattaching the coronary ostia using the Bentall technique (Figure 19–20). Under certain scenarios, the entire aortic arch must be removed and replaced with Dacron graft material. When the aortic arch is significantly aneurysmal, if the intimal tear is within the aortic arch, or in a patient with Marfan syndrome, the entire arch should be replaced. Each branch of the arch can be individually reimplanted to the graft, the three vessels can be attached as an island, or a multibranch graft of Dacron with side branches preattached can be anastomosed to the individual arch branches. When the arch is reconstructed, a longer duration of hypothermic circulatory arrest will be required. Cerebral perfusion can be initiated using balloon-tipped catheters inserted directly into the innominate and left carotid arteries. Blood flow at a rate of 600 cc/min at 18°C is generally considered adequate to prevent neurologic compromise.

3. Results—As previously described, the mortality of acute aortic dissection may be as high as 50%, since many patients will rupture before arrival at a qualified hospital. Operative mortality is in the range of 10%-20%, which includes consideration of the selection bias of choosing operative candidates. Cause of death is primarily related to malperfusion syndrome, resulting in neurologic, intestinal, or extremity ischemia. Cerebral injury related to hypothermic circulatory arrest is limited and should result in clinically significant stroke in less than 5% of patients. Long-term survival following repair of acute aortic dissection is good, approximately 50%-60% at 10 years.

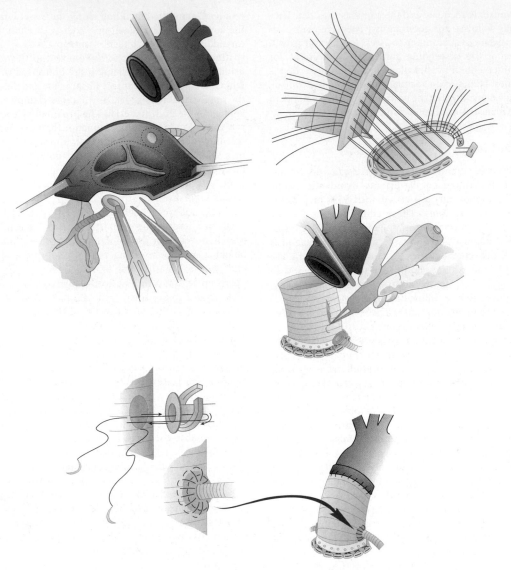

▲ **Figure 19–20.** Aortic root replacement with a mechanical valve conduit using the Bentall technique. The aortic valve and root are replaced and the coronary arteries are directly reimplanted. (From Cohn LH. *Cardiac Surgery in the Adult,* 3rd ed. McGraw-Hill, 2007.)

El-Sayed H, Ramlawi B: The current status of endovascular repair of thoracic aortic aneurysms. *Methodist Debakey Cardiovasc J* 2011;7:15.

Goddney PP et al: Survival after open versus endovascular thoracic aortic aneurysm repair in an observational study of the Medicare population. *Circulation* 2011;124:2661.

Patel HJ et al: Operative delay for peripheral malperfusion syndrome in acute type A aortic dissection: a long-term analysis. *J Thorac Cardiovasc Surg* 2008;135:1288.

▼ SURGICAL TREATMENT OF HEART FAILURE

HEART TRANSPLANTATION

▶ Indications

The incidence of congestive heart failure (CHF) is steadily rising, owing to the increase in the aging population and the reduced mortality of myocardial infarction. Nearly 5 million

Americans live with heart failure, and 500,000 new cases are diagnosed annually. Causes are multifactorial, but by far the most frequent etiology is related to coronary occlusive disease, with repeated ischemic insults and loss of viable myocardial contractility. Chronic ventricular volume overload from conditions such as undiagnosed valvular pathology or intracardiac septal defects can result in cardiomyopathy and advanced heart failure. Other causes of heart failure include viral myocarditis, peripartum cardiomyopathy, and idiopathic dilated cardiomyopathy.

All of these processes lead to the same result: loss of myocardial contractility with decreased cardiac output, elevated diastolic cardiac filling pressures, and pathologic neurohormonal adaptive responses. This leads to increased sympathetic tone, elevated peripheral vascular resistance, and salt and water retention, creating a vicious cycle with further reduction in cardiac output, edema, and pulmonary congestion.

Medical therapy includes reduction in salt intake and modest exercise to reduce sympathetic activation. Diuretics and aldosterone inhibitors counteract the inappropriately activated renin-angiotensin system. Angiotensin-converting enzyme inhibitors decrease peripheral vascular resistance and alter the myocardial intercellular matrix, allowing opportunities for reverse cardiac remodeling. The inotropic properties of digitalis glycosides have been demonstrated to reduce hospital admission for heart failure exacerbations, although at higher levels can increase mortality because of its proarrhythmic properties. Beta-blocking agents reduce sympathetic tone, allow upregulation of beta-receptors, and significantly reduce mortality in advanced heart failure patients. As the left ventricle dilates, electrical reentry pathways are generated, predisposing to malignant ventricular arrhythmias and sudden cardiac death. Strong evidence now demonstrates that implantation of automated internal cardiac defibrillators reduces mortality, and their use has become standard practice in heart failure management. In addition, selected patients with conduction system disturbances may benefit from cardiac resynchronization therapy by insertion of biventricular pacemakers that stimulate both the left and right ventricles simultaneously.

The effectiveness of medical therapy is often described by the New York Heart Association (NYHA) classification (Table 19–3). As a patient's NYHA functional class deteriorates despite adequate medical therapy, consideration for transplantation should be made. Because heart transplantation remains a scarce resource, selection of patients is crucial to maximize outcomes. Exclusion criteria have been established on the basis of solid evidence of increased perioperative or reduced long-term survival; criteria are listed in Table 19–4. The most frequently applied exclusion criteria include advanced age, end-organ injury from diabetes mellitus, chronic renal insufficiency (serum creatinine > 2.5), poor medical compliance or psychosocial instability, and morbid obesity (body mass index > 35).

Table 19–3. New York Heart Association classification of heart failure symptoms.

I	No limitations
II	Dyspnea with ordinary activity
III	Dyspnea with less than ordinary activity
IV	Dyspnea

Creation of concrete inclusion criteria has been more elusive because it is often difficult to predict mortality in this population. Historically, patient selection has relied on exercise stress evaluation and determination of maximal oxygen consumption (VO_2 max). Patients with a VO_2 max of less than 10 mL/kg/min have a definite survival advantage with transplantation, and those with a peak VO_2 of less than 14 mL/kg/min with NYHA class III or IV limitations appear to have a survival advantage. Recently, several scoring models have allowed more accurate risk stratification of mortality for ambulatory patients with advanced heart failure. These models have proven helpful for those patients in whom exercise testing appears intermediate in risk assessment, such as those with peak VO_2 between 10 and 14 mL/kg/min. The Heart Failure Survival Score (HFSS) uses seven independent predictors of mortality and creates high-, medium-, and low-risk groups for 1-year mortality. These variables include peak VO_2, QRS interval, ejection fraction, serum sodium, resting heart rate, ischemic versus nonischemic etiology, and mean blood pressure. Patients with intermediate peak VO_2 scores should be considered for transplantation if scoring models such as the HFSS predict high or medium risk for mortality.

Heart transplants are allocated according to a protocol prioritizing based on need and geographic distribution. Patients are assigned within a classification system as listed in Table 19–5. Status 1A patients receive the highest priority, as they require mechanical circulatory support with a device that will not allow discharge from the hospital, are supported by a device that is failing, or require infusion of inotropic agents at high doses and require pulmonary artery

Table 19–4. Heart transplant exclusion criteria.

Severe renal insufficiency
Recent malignancy
Advanced age
Obesity
Elevated pulmonary vascular resistance
Medication noncompliance

catheters to continuously monitor intracardiac filling pressures. Patients are assigned status 1B if they are supported with implantable circulatory support devices that allow ambulatory support or if they require continuous inotropic infusions at modest doses and do not require pulmonary artery catheters. Patients are considered status 2 if they do not require inotropes or mechanical circulatory support. Patients are designated status 7 if they are temporarily unsuited for a transplant. Organs are allocated with a complex algorithm that considers patient status, size, blood type compatibility, and geography.

▶ Technique

Patients are briefly evaluated to ensure that there have been no interval changes in their health status since their transplant evaluation. In particular, anticoagulation status is assessed and reversed if necessary, renal function should be reasonably stable, and a pulmonary artery catheter should be inserted to ensure that pulmonary vascular resistance has not changed appreciably since the most recent evaluation. Potential concerns should be discussed between the transplant surgeon and heart failure cardiologist.

Upon confirmation by the procuring team that the donor heart is visibly suitable, the recipient is anesthetized and prepared. A median sternotomy is performed. In the current era, the majority of recipients have undergone previous cardiac surgery, often including insertion of ventricular assist devices. As such, significant time may be required for dissection and identification of cardiac structures, and appropriate time should be allowed. The patient is heparinized to achieve an activated clotting time of at least 450 seconds. Arterial cannulation is preferred high on the lesser curvature of the aortic arch to allow for significant aortic removal, particu-

Table 19–5. United network for organ sharing listing status for heart transplantation.

Listing Status	Clinical Criteria
1A	Dependent on extracorporeal membrane oxygenation, intra-aortic balloon pump, total artificial heart, mechanical ventilation, or ventricular assist device with evidence of device malfunction or device-related complications
	Dependent on 2 inotropic infusions or 1 high-dose inotrope (7.5 mcg/kg/min dobutamine, dopamine, or 0.5 mcg/kg/min milrinone) with pulmonary artery catheter in place
1B	Dependent on ventricular assist device or inotropic infusion
2	Eligible for transplant but not dependent on inotropes or mechanical circulatory support
7	Hold; temporarily medically unsuitable for transplant

larly if the recipient has a ventricular assist device. Venous cannulation is in the superior and inferior vena cavae, and CPB is initiated. The cavae are controlled with snares, and an aortic cross-clamp is applied when the donor heart is within 20-30 minutes of arrival. Recipient cardiectomy is performed initially along the right atrioventricular groove and extending down into the coronary sinus. The aorta is transected just above the coronary arteries, avoiding entry into the dome of the left atrium or injury to the right pulmonary artery. The pulmonary artery is transected at the level of the pulmonary valve. The interatrial septum is opened, and the left atrium is divided along the mitral valve annulus. Once the recipient heart is removed, the left atrium is trimmed, removing the appendage and a portion of the interatrial septum.

The donor heart is carefully inspected for abnormalities, including a patent foramen ovale. The atrial cuff is trimmed to size-match the recipient. The left atrial anastomosis is performed with polypropylene in running fashion, everting the edges to minimize incorporation of epicardial tissue within the atria. Before completion of the anastomosis, the left ventricular vent is inserted via the right superior pulmonary vein through the mitral valve. This facilitates deairing and prevents premature rewarming from pulmonary effluent. The donor and recipient ascending aortas are trimmed appropriately, and the anastomosis is performed with running polypropylene suture. At the completion of this suture line, the aortic cross-clamp can be removed, thus terminating the period of cold ischemia. The ascending aorta and left ventricle are vented of residual air. Spontaneous resumption of cardiac activity typically occurs. The inferior vena cava anastomosis is completed with running polypropylene suture. A flexible cardiotomy suction catheter is placed through the donor superior vena cava and advanced into the coronary sinus to improve visualization. The superior vena cava is anastomosed with running polypropylene suture, and the caval snares can be removed. The pulmonary artery anastomosis is performed with running polypropylene, typically imbricating the posterior wall for greater strength. Care must be taken to avoid excess length and potential kinking of the pulmonary artery. The technique just described is for a *bicaval* implant. With a *biatrial* technique, the recipient cardiectomy preserves the superior and inferior vena caval attachments, instead creating an atriotomy along the lateral wall of the right atrium. The donor superior vena cava is ligated, and an incision in the inferior vena cava is extended several centimeters along the posterolateral atrial wall. This older approach is technically easier but is associated with more tricuspid valve regurgitation and atrial arrhythmias, and thus less desirable.

The patient is rewarmed, ventilated, and then weaned off of CPB. If sinus rhythm is less than 100-110 beats/min, atrial pacing is initiated. Inotropic support is typically required in light of the cold ischemic time, even for young and vigorous donor hearts. Right ventricular dysfunction is the most frequently seen complication, attributed to recipient pulmonary hypertension in the "untrained" heart and the inherent sensitivity of the right ventricle to preservation injury. This can be exacerbated by postoperative bleeding necessitating blood product transfusions with volume overload and worsening of pulmonary vascular resistance. Judicious volume administration, rapid pacing, and catecholamine infusions can overcome right ventricular dysfunction. Inhaled nitric oxide or prostacycline can selectively reduce pulmonary vascular resistance and improve hemodynamic stability.

Immunosuppression after heart transplantation is similar to that for other solid organs and includes antimetabolite agents such as mycophenolate, calcineurin inhibitors such as cyclosporine or tacrolimus, and corticosteroids. Because of their nephrotoxicity, initiation of calcineurin inhibitors is often delayed during the immediate postoperative period. As an alternative, induction therapy with either monoclonal or polyclonal antibodies against specific immune cells can be administered. Although routine use of induction therapy has not been demonstrated to improve outcomes, selected use for patients with perioperative renal insufficiency may be beneficial.

Outcomes

Despite the absence of any prospective randomized evidence, heart transplantation offers long-term survival advantages over medical therapy for appropriately selected patients with advanced heart failure. Survival rates have improved since the introduction of the procedure in 1967, with 1-year survival now approximately 85%. Most early deaths are attributable to perioperative complications or severe rejection. After this early period of attrition, there continues to be a linear decrement in survival, at a rate of approximately 3%-4% per year, and this rate has not decreased over the last 20 years. Causes of late mortality include transplant vasculopathy, opportunistic infections, immunosuppressive related malignancies, and rejection. Transplant vasculopathy is an accelerated coronary artery disease unique to the heart transplant recipient and is a result of repetitive vascular injury and sustained inflammatory response. Statins and vitamin supplements appear to slow the progression of vasculopathy, but the diffuse nature makes the disease less amenable to percutaneous or surgical revascularization. Median survival after heart transplant is estimated to be between 10 and 11 years (Figure 19–21).

MECHANICAL CIRCULATORY SUPPORT

Indications

Although heart transplantation has long been considered the gold standard treatment for advanced heart failure, the limited availability of suitable donors affords support for only a small percentage of those in need. Mechanical circulatory support to assist or replace the failing heart has made enormous progress over the last 40 years. Since the introduction

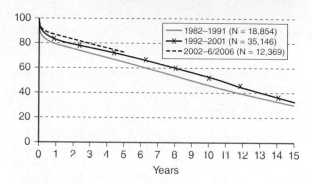

▲ **Figure 19–21.** Kaplan-Meier survival for adult heart transplants performed between January 1982 and June 2006 by era. All comparisons are significant at $p < 0.0001$. (Reproduced with permission from Taylor DO et al: Registry of the International Society for Heart and Lung Transplantation: twenty-fifth official adult heart transplant report—2008. *J Heart Lung Transplant* 2008;27:943.)

of CPB by Gibbon in 1953, the engineering of mechanical blood pumps has become more sophisticated, allowing treatment of an increasing population of patients on an ambulatory basis with reduced size, better blood biocompatibility and improved pump durability. As this rapid evolution continues, the indications, techniques, and expected results will change dramatically. More than any other aspect of cardiac surgery, the treatment of today will likely be remarkably different only a few years in the future.

The indications for implantable circulatory support are severe cardiac dysfunction despite maximal medical therapy. However, there are three distinct goals of support that represent vastly different patient populations and clinical scenarios: bridge to recovery, bridge to transplant, and destination therapy. Cardiogenic shock may have reversible causes, such as viral or peripartum cardiomyopathy, acute myocardial infarction, and postcardiotomy shock. Initiation of mechanical circulatory support can restore hemodynamics, unload the ventricle, and allow time for myocardial recovery. Chronic heart failure patients felt to be suitable candidates for heart transplantation can rapidly deteriorate, causing end-organ dysfunction and closing their window of opportunity. Implantable circulatory support can reverse acute organ injury and allow functional rehabilitation, improving their candidacy for and potentially their outcomes after heart transplantation. Patients with advanced heart failure and contraindications for transplantation, such as older age, chronic renal insufficiency, obesity, or fixed pulmonary hypertension, may benefit from implantable circulatory support as destination therapy.

Pumps

A variety of devices are available for mechanical circulatory support to satisfy each of the goals, and many more are currently in clinical trials or preclinical testing. Device selection depends on the clinical circumstances, with considerations including ease of implantation, adequacy and flexibility of support, patient quality of life, durability, and cost. The available devices are discussed in the context of their most frequently used application.

A. Short-term Devices

Intra-aortic balloon pumps provide counterpulsation during diastole, increasing coronary perfusion and reducing afterload and myocardial oxygen consumption. They are typically inserted percutaneously via the femoral artery and advanced into the descending thoracic aorta. Balloon timing automatically coincides with the electrocardiogram tracing or the arterial pressure waveform. They can be easily removed and have few complications. Intra-aortic balloon pump support is limited, improving cardiac output only by as much as 20%. The Abiomed BVS 5000 and AB 5000 are pneumatically driven extracorporeal blood pumps capable of up to 6 L/min of blood flow (Figure 19–22). The devices can be connected to any of the cardiac chambers to provide support for the failing left or right ventricle in a variety of configurations. A pneumatic compressor phasically actuates a diaphragm within the pump, producing pulsatile flow. The rate of actuation varies with the pump chamber filling, thus automatically adjusting output according to the patient's volume status. The Thoratec CentriMag is a centrifugal blood pump with a magnetically levitated rotor to improve

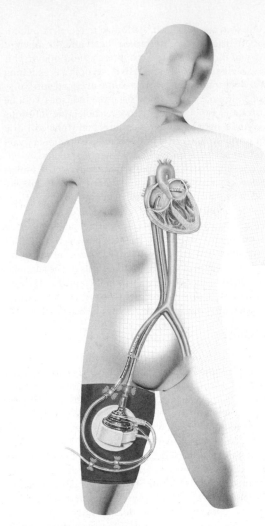

▲ **Figure 19–23.** TandemHeart percutaneous ventricular assist device. (Reproduced with permission from CardiacAssist, Inc, Pittsburgh, PA.)

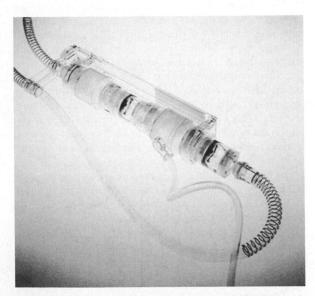

▲ **Figure 19–22.** Abiomed AB 5000 ventricular assist device. (Reproduced with permission from Abiomed, Inc., Danvers, MA.)

biocompatibility. There are no valve sinuses or other zones of stagnation, improving thrombogenicity. It produces continuous flow and requires manual pump speed adjustment under conditions of changing preload. The TandemHeart percutaneous ventricular assist device (VAD) uses a venous drainage cannula inserted from the femoral vein and advanced across the inter-atrial septum. Blood is drained from the left atrium using a centrifugal pump and infused into a cannula inserted into the femoral artery (Figure 19–23). Because of its femoral access, it requires a supine and immobilized patient. The Impella catheters are microaxial blood pumps placed across the aortic valve, draining blood from the left ventricular

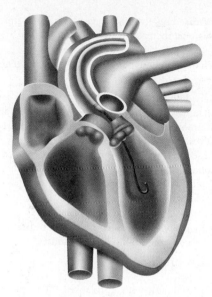

▲ **Figure 19–24.** Impella percutaneous microaxial blood pump. (Reproduced with permission from Abiomed, Inc, Danvers, MA.)

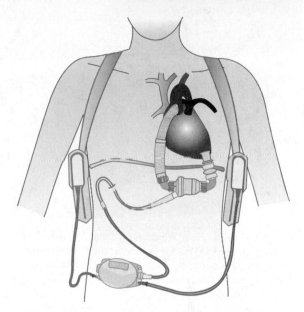

▲ **Figure 19–25.** HeartMate II left ventricular assist device. (Reproduced with permission from Thoratec, Inc., Pleasanton, CA.)

cavity and infusing into the aortic root (Figure 19–24). The catheters can be inserted peripherally, such as via the femoral artery, or directly into the ascending aorta. The largest of the Impella catheters can produce up to 5 L/min of flow.

B. Long-term Devices

Implantable mechanical circulatory support, such as left ventricular assist devices (LVADs) are increasingly used for patients with end stage irreversible heart failure, either as bridge to heart transplantation or for lifelong support (destination therapy). There have been substantial technologic advances in this field and the use of implantable circulatory support pumps is increasing at rapid pace.

Early LVADs were large, pulsatile pumps which used either electric or pneumatic force to actuate a diaphragm producing pulsatile ejection. These devices were limited by their large size and the tendency for the motor bearings to fail after prolonged support.

The current generation of circulatory support devices are valveless continuous-flow pumps which use continuously spinning impellers to generate blood flow. Since there is no displacement chamber to generate the flow pulse, the devices are smaller and silent, allowing support to smaller patients and improved patient satisfaction. In addition, the continuous nature of the mechanical load on a single bearing has the important advantage of improved durability.

The first of these pumps to gain Food and Drug Administration (FDA) approval is the HeartMate II

(Figure 19–25). After median sternotomy and creation of a small preperitoneal pocket, the diaphragm is divided allowing access to the left ventricular apex. On CPB, the inlet cannula of the HeartMate II is inserted into the left ventricular apex. The outflow graft is sutured to the ascending aorta. A percutaneous lead exits the right upper quadrant and is connected to a controller allowing interface with the pump. The controller is connected to a power source, either a power base unit plugged into standard wall outlets, or connected to wearable batteries which can provide untethered support for up to 10 hours. Early experience demonstrates improved success when compared to predicate devices. While median survival of VAD patients continues to improve, complications continue to limit the potential success of VAD therapy. Gastrointestinal bleeding occurs in approximately 30% of patients with continuous flow VADs, likely related to the combination of the required warfarin anticoagulation and acquired platelet dysfunction from device sheer forces. The incidence of stroke is approximately 8%-10% per year from both primary intracerebral hemorrhage and embolic events. Infections at the driveline insertion site can require debridement, prolonged intravenous antibiotics, and when severe, require complete pump exchange.

The next generation of LVADs is continuous-flow pumps with centrifugal design, utilizing magnetically levitated rotors. These LVADs eliminate entirely the need for contacting bearings, creating the potential for indefinite support without mechanical failure. In addition, these devices

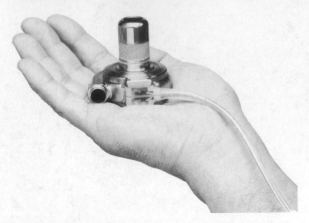

▲ **Figure 19–26.** HeartWare® Ventricular Assist System featuring the HVAD® Pump. The HeartWare® Ventricular Assist System is currently in clinical trial. (Reproduced with permission from HeartWare International, Inc., Framingham, MA.)

may have improved blood handling characteristics and could reduce some of the complications seen in prolonged mechanical assistance. The HeartWare Ventricular Assist System is currently in US clinical trials. Its miniature design allows implantation within the pericardial space, obviating the need for a preperitoneal pocket or incision of the diaphragm. Approval by the FDA is imminently expected at the time of this (Figure 19–26). The significant technological progress in mechanical circulatory support will likely have an enormous impact on the nature of surgical treatment of heart failure in the near future.

Slaughter MS et al: Advanced heart failure treated with continuous-flow left ventricular assist device. *N Engl J Med* 2009;361:2241.

Stehlik J et al: The registry of the International Society of Heart and Lung Transplantation: twenty-eighth adult heart transplant report—2011. *J Heart Lung Transplant* 2011;30:1078.

MULTIPLE CHOICE QUESTIONS

1. Which of the following does NOT contribute to the susceptibility of coronary ischemia?

   A. High baseline oxygen extraction
   B. Coronary flow limited largely during diastole
   C. Atherosclerosis tends to occur diffusely in small coronary vessels
   D. Increased myocardial oxygen demand requires proportional increase in coronary blood flow

2. Which of the following is true about aortic stenosis?

   A. Senile calcific aortic stenosis is associated with ascending aortic aneurysms
   B. Rheumatic heart disease affects the aortic valve most commonly, followed by the mitral and tricuspid valves
   C. Presence of left ventricular hypertrophy is an indication for surgery in patients with aortic stenosis
   D. Typical symptoms are exertional dyspnea, angina or syncope

3. For patients with mitral regurgitation, indications for mitral reconstruction do NOT include:

   A. Left ventricular dilation
   B. Dyspnea
   C. Asymptomatic with a prolapsed anterior mitral leaflet
   D. Moderate mitral regurgitation at the time of coronary bypass surgery

4. Which of the following is true of the thoracic aorta?

   A. Fibrosis results in contraction of the ascending aorta with age
   B. The ascending aorta should only be replaced when its maximum diameter exceeds 5.5 cm in the absence of symptoms
   C. Stanford type B dissections cause early death from intrapericardial rupture, aortic valve insufficiency or coronary malperfusion
   D. Malperfusion of the abdominal viscera can occur with either Stanford type A or type B aortic dissections

5. Which of the following is true regarding advanced heart failure?

   A. Beta-blockers improve survival in heart failure in part by up-regulation of beta-receptors
   B. The incidence of heart failure is decreasing because of advances in medical treatment
   C. The use of mechanical circulatory support does not affect priority status for heart transplantation
   D. Left ventricular dysfunction is the most frequent early complication following heart transplantation

II. Congenital Heart Disease

19

Jennifer S. Nelson, MD

Jennifer C. Hirsch-Romano, MD, MS

Richard G. Ohye, MD

Edward L. Bove, MD

DIAGNOSIS

Congenital heart disease encompasses a wide range of anomalies that result from abnormal fetal development of the heart. Defects can range from simple to complex. The age of presentation of these defects depends primarily on the physiologic impact of the anomaly. After birth, patients can present within minutes to hours with profound hypoxemia or hemodynamic collapse. Others may present weeks to months later with evidence of a new murmur or signs of congestive heart failure. Relatively asymptomatic lesions can go undetected until children are school age or adolescents. With current ultrasound imaging, many cardiac anomalies are identified on prenatal examination.

Early and accurate diagnosis of congenital heart disease requires careful identification of signs and symptoms of heart disease. The initial workup begins with a focused history and physical examination. Classification of heart murmurs can be highly suggestive of underlying cardiac anomalies. Early signs of heart disease include cyanosis, tachypnea, unequal pulses, and failure to thrive. Key symptoms of congenital heart disease in the patient's history include feeding difficulties, irritability, and frequent respiratory infections.

Standard diagnostic studies include a chest radiograph (CXR) and electrocardiography (EKG). Some cardiac defects have pathognomonic findings on CXR. Other anomalies may be suspected based on heart size, increased or decreased pulmonary markings, aortic arch sidedness, or situs abnormalities (the heart located in the mid- or right chest rather than the typical location in the left chest). EKG can identify rhythm disturbances, axis deviation, atrial enlargement, and ventricular hypertrophy. Transthoracic echocardiography is often the only diagnostic test needed to provide the anatomic detail required for surgical planning. Cardiac catheterization, cardiac magnetic resonance imaging (cMRI), and computed tomography angiography (CTA) are used as adjunct diagnostic tests when additional information on flow, pressure, resistance, or anatomic detail is required.

PREOPERATIVE MANAGEMENT

The care of congenital heart disease patients requires a collaborative effort of a multidisciplinary team of cardiologists, surgeons, interventionalists, echocardiographers, and radiologists. For the majority of congenital heart defects, surgical correction or catheter-based intervention is necessary for definitive treatment. Careful timing and planning of operative and catheter-based interventions along with highly skilled preoperative and postoperative care are essential to a successful outcome.

Certain defects such as atrial septal defects (ASDs), ventricular septal defects (VSDs), and patent ductus arteriosus (PDA) may resolve spontaneously over the first several years of life. The remaining defects require intervention when the risk of surgery is reasonable, when symptoms can no longer be managed medically, and/or prior to the onset of irreversible complications.

Neonates presenting with ductal-dependent lesions require ductal blood flow to maintain systemic or pulmonary perfusion. Ductal patency is achieved with intravenous prostaglandin E_1 therapy. Supplemental oxygen is supplied only as necessary for cyanosis as newborns tolerate relative cyanosis (oxygen saturations > 70%) quite well. The remainder of therapy is directed toward managing congestive heart failure symptoms with diuretics, afterload reduction, and maximal caloric intake.

OPERATIVE MANAGEMENT

For most congenital heart defects, surgical correction is possible. For more complex defects, staged repair with early palliation as well as staged palliation remain options. The anticipated somatic growth of the child must be considered when determining the surgical approach. Invasive monitoring lines are essential for monitoring patients during surgery and postoperatively. All patients have arterial and central venous catheters placed along with peripheral intravenous catheters and a Foley catheter. For neonates, the umbilical vessels are the desired venous and arterial access. Avoidance of long-standing and repeated femoral lines is important because patency of these vessels is often essential for diagnostic and interventional catheter procedures later in life. Due to variable blood flow with perfusion techniques and underlying cardiac anomalies, it is possible to have differential cooling and rewarming. Therefore, temperature probes are placed in the nasopharynx, the rectum, and on the skin to allow for accurate monitoring.

Most surgical repairs require cardiopulmonary bypass. This involves drainage of venous blood from the patient via cannulae placed in the superior and inferior vena cava (for intracardiac repairs) or a single cannula in the right atrium. Blood passes through the bypass circuit, which warms or cools the blood to the desired temperature, adds oxygen and removes carbon dioxide, and pumps the blood back into the body via an arterial cannula, usually in the ascending aorta. Hypothermia may be employed to decrease the metabolic demands of the body and heart, which provides additional protection against ischemia. The degree of hypothermia, 18-34°C, depends on the complexity and time needed to complete the procedure. The heart can be arrested with high-potassium cardioplegic solution delivered through the coronary arteries antegrade (through a cannula proximal to an aortic cross-clamp in the aorta) or retrograde (through a cannula placed in the coronary sinus). Arresting the heart allows the surgeon to operate safely with a still and bloodless field. An additional vent can be placed via the right superior pulmonary vein to capture pulmonary venous return and to assist in deairing of the heart.

Hypothermic circulatory arrest is required for complex aortic arch reconstructions. This involves cooling the patient to 18°C for a minimum of 20 minutes to ensure even cooling of the brain and body. The head is packed in ice, the patient's blood is drained into the venous reservoir, and the pump is turned off. The cannulae can then be removed from the field to aid in visualization and repair of the arch. No absolute safe duration of hypothermic circulatory arrest has been determined, but it is generally felt that it should be limited to no more than 45 minutes. Alternative techniques, such as regional cerebral perfusion and intermittent low-flow perfusion, have been employed to minimize the need for hypothermic circulatory arrest. To date, however, there is no literature to support that these techniques have additional benefit without additional risk.

POSTOPERATIVE MANAGEMENT

Patients are brought to the intensive care unit intubated and mechanically ventilated. All patients have temporary pacing wires in place for management of bradyarrhythmias and tachyarrhythmias. Many patients have additional intracardiac lines in place for pulmonary artery and left atrial pressure monitoring. Drainage catheters are placed within the mediastinum to prevent accumulation of blood and fluid. These are usually removed 2-4 days following surgery. Prophylactic antibiotics are given preoperatively as well as postoperatively when drainage tubes are in place.

Cardiopulmonary bypass produces a significant inflammatory response due to activation of cytokines. Patients exhibit fluid retention and pulmonary dysfunction as a result, requiring aggressive use of diuretics and mechanical ventilation as needed. Bleeding is a common complication following cardiac surgery and infrequently requires surgical exploration (< 2%). Postoperative coagulopathy results from a multitude of factors, including hemodilution, platelet damage, factor consumption, immature hepatic production of clotting factors, and incomplete reversal of heparin with protamine sulfate. Approximately 30% of all patients will have some arrhythmia after surgery, ranging from simple premature ventricular contractions to malignant tachyarrhythmias. The risk for long-term arrhythmias requiring chronic medication or heart block requiring a permanent pacemaker is approximately 1%. Most patients require hemodynamic support with vasopressors along with afterload reduction as necessary for ventricular dysfunction. Dopamine, epinephrine, and vasopressin are the first-line vasopressors for pediatric patients. Milrinone is used primarily for afterload reduction. Critically ill neonates may have thyroid and adrenal hypofunction, which can further exacerbate postoperative hemodynamic instability. Profound hemodynamic compromise occasionally requires additional mechanical assistance. Extracorporeal membrane oxygenation (ECMO) is the most widely and acutely available mechanical support for the pediatric population. The survival for congenital heart disease patients requiring ECMO support is approximately 50%. For patients in low cardiac output state, it is essential to rule out residual defects or repair failures that could be readdressed surgically or in the catheterization laboratory.

The pediatric population has highly reactive pulmonary vasculature that is unique from the adult cardiac surgery population. Postoperative pulmonary hypertensive crises can occur in the newborn and infant population. Crises can be initiated with agitation such as endotracheal suctioning. Maneuvers to minimize and treat pulmonary hypertensive crises include high-dose opioid anesthesia with fentanyl, paralysis, respiratory alkalosis, high fraction of inspired oxygen, and inhaled nitric oxide. Chronic agents to treat persistent pulmonary hypertension include phosphodiesterase inhibitors (eg, sildenafil) and prostacyclin (eg, Flolan).

CYANOTIC HEART DEFECTS

Cyanotic heart defects result from shunting of deoxygenated blood from the right side of the heart to the oxygenated left side of the heart or inadequate pulmonary blood flow. The relative mixing of deoxygenated and oxygenated blood produces desaturation of the arterial blood. The majority of cyanotic heart defects are diagnosed within the first few days to months of life. Cyanotic heart defects represent approximately 25% of all congenital heart defects.

The classic 5 T's of cyanotic heart defects—(1) tetralogy of Fallot (TOF); (2) transposition of the great arteries (TGAs); (3) truncus arteriosus; (4) total anomalous pulmonary venous return; and (5) tricuspid atresia are presented in this chapter along with hypoplastic left heart syndrome (HLHS).

▶ Tetralogy of Fallot

A. General Considerations

TOF is the most common cyanotic congenital heart defect. It occurs in 0.6 per 1000 live births and has a prevalence of about 4% among all patients with congenital heart disease. The pathologic anatomy is frequently described as having four components: VSD, overriding aorta, pulmonary stenosis, and right ventricular (RV) hypertrophy (Figure 19–27). Embryologically, the anatomy of TOF is thought to result from a single defect: anterior malalignment of the infundibular septum. The infundibular septum normally separates

the primitive outflow tracts and fuses with the ventricular septum. Anterior malalignment of the infundibular septum creates a VSD due to failure of fusion with the ventricular septum and also displaces the aorta over the VSD and right ventricle. Infundibular malalignment also crowds the RV outflow tract, causing pulmonary stenosis and, secondarily, RV hypertrophy. Prominent muscle bands also extend from the septal insertion of the infundibular septum to the RV free wall and contribute to the obstruction of the RV outflow tract. The pulmonary valve is usually stenotic and is bicuspid in 58% of cases. Pulmonary atresia occurs in about 7% of cases. The branch pulmonary arteries in TOF may exhibit mild diffuse hypoplasia or discrete stenosis (most frequently of the left pulmonary artery at the site of ductal insertion). Coronary artery anomalies are frequently present. The origin of the left anterior descending artery from the right coronary artery, which occurs in 5% of cases, is clinically important because the vessel crosses the RV infundibulum and is vulnerable to injury at the time of surgery. A right aortic arch is present in 25% of patients. Associated defects include ASD, complete atrioventricular septal defect (AVSD), PDA, or multiple VSDs.

B. Clinical Findings

Patients with TOF develop cyanosis due to right-to-left shunting across the VSD. The degree of cyanosis depends on the severity of obstruction of the RV outflow tract. Frequently, cyanosis is mild at birth and may remain undetected for

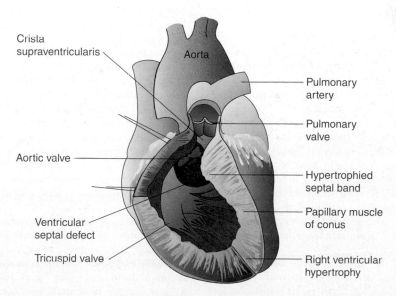

▲ **Figure 19–27.** Tetralogy of Fallot. The aorta overrides the ventricular septum. A large ventricular septal defect is present, and the hypoplastic infundibulum with hypertrophied muscle bands obstructs blood to the pulmonary arteries.

weeks or months. Neonates with severe infundibular obstruction or pulmonary atresia will develop symptoms shortly after birth and require a prostaglandin infusion to maintain ductal patency to ensure adequate pulmonary blood flow. In other patients, the RV outflow tract obstruction is minor, and the predominant physiology is that of a large VSD with left-to-right shunting and congestive heart failure.

The occurrence of intermittent cyanotic spells is a well-known feature of tetralogy. The etiology of "spelling" is still controversial but is clearly related to a transient imbalance between pulmonary and systemic blood flow. A spell may be triggered by hypovolemia or peripheral vasodilation (eg, after a bath or vigorous physical exertion). Spells may occur in neonates but are most frequently reported in infants between the ages of 3 and 18 months. Most spells resolve spontaneously within a few minutes, but some spells may be fatal. Older children have been observed to spontaneously squat to terminate spells. The squatting position is thought to increase systemic vascular resistance, which thereby favors pulmonary blood flow.

Cyanosis is the most frequent physical finding in TOF. Auscultation reveals a normal first heart sound and a single second heart sound. A systolic ejection murmur is present at the left upper sternal border. Older children may develop clubbing of the fingers and toes. Chest radiography typically demonstrates a boot-shaped heart due to elevation of the cardiac apex from RV hypertrophy. Pulmonary vascular markings are usually reduced. A right aortic arch may be present. An electrocardiogram shows RV hypertrophy. Echocardiography is definitive, and catheterization is not necessary in most cases.

C. Treatment

The medical management of TOF is directed toward the treatment and prevention of cyanotic spells. The immediate treatment of the spelling patient includes administration of oxygen, narcotics for sedation, and correction of acidosis. Transfusion is indicated for anemic infants. Alpha-agonists are useful for increasing systemic vascular resistance (which favors pulmonary blood flow). Some centers have used beta-blockers as a form of long-term therapy to suppress the incidence of spells. Long-term complications of untreated TOF include clubbing of the fingers and toes, severe dyspnea on exertion, brain abscesses (secondary to right-to-left shunting), paradoxical embolization, and polycythemia (which may lead to cerebral thrombosis). Long-term survival is unlikely for most patients with untreated TOF.

All patients with TOF should undergo surgical repair. Asymptomatic patients should be repaired electively between 4 and 6 months of age. Early repair is indicated for neonates with severe cyanosis and for infants who have had a documented spell or worsening cyanosis.

Classically, the repair of TOF was accomplished in two stages. During the first stage, pulmonary blood flow was augmented by creating a connection (or shunt) between a systemic artery and the pulmonary artery. At the second stage, the shunt was taken down, and a complete repair was performed. The first shunt procedure was the Blalock-Taussig shunt, in which the subclavian artery was mobilized and divided distally, and an end-to-side anastomosis was created between the inferiorly deflected subclavian and the ipsilateral pulmonary artery. The modified Blalock-Taussig shunt is the most common type of shunt used today and consists of an interposition graft (polytetrafluoroethylene) between the innominate or subclavian artery and the ipsilateral pulmonary artery. Creation of a shunt may be accomplished with or without the use of cardiopulmonary bypass.

Currently, one-stage repair of TOF is preferred by most centers. Initial palliation with a shunt is still indicated for some patients who present a high risk for complete repair, such as those with multiple congenital anomalies, significant prematurity, severe concurrent illness, or an anomalous coronary artery crossing a hypoplastic infundibulum.

Complete repair of TOF is performed using a median sternotomy and cardiopulmonary bypass with bicaval venous cannulation. By a transatrial approach, the RV outflow tract can be examined through the tricuspid valve. Muscle bundles obstructing the RV outflow tract are divided or resected. The VSD is closed with a patch. Pulmonary valvotomy is performed, when indicated, via a vertical incision in the main pulmonary artery. When the pulmonary valve annulus or infundibulum is severely hypoplastic, a transannular outflow tract patch may be necessary to relieve the obstruction. When an anomalous coronary artery crosses the infundibulum, a transannular incision may be contraindicated. In these cases, and in patients with pulmonary atresia, placement of a conduit (cryopreserved homograft or bioprosthetic heterograft) between the right ventricle (via a separate ventriculotomy) and main pulmonary artery will be necessary. Patients who undergo construction of a transannular patch develop pulmonary insufficiency as a consequence. This is surprisingly well tolerated in most infants, as long as the tricuspid valve is competent.

As these patients grow older, some will develop RV failure due to chronic pulmonary insufficiency, and pulmonary valve replacement may be necessary. Currently, pulmonary valve replacement is indicated for symptomatic patients or those at risk of life-threatening arrhythmias. For asymptomatic patients, it is generally agreed that pulmonary valve replacement should be undertaken before irreversible RV dysfunction occurs. cMRI has evolved as a valuable diagnostic tool for evaluating RV size, function, anatomic detail, and other hemodynamic parameters. An RV size "cutoff" is debated, but recent recommendations suggest considering valve replacement before RV end-diastolic volume index exceeds approximately 160 mL/m^2.

Catheter-based pulmonary valve replacement is an option for some patients depending on the RV outflow tract anatomy.

D. Prognosis and Complications

The early mortality following repair of TOF is 1%-5%. The results are worse for patients with TOF and pulmonary atresia. Long-term complications include recurrent obstruction of the RV outflow tract and development of RV dysfunction due to chronic pulmonary insufficiency. Actuarial survival at 20 years is 90% with excellent functional status.

Cheung EW, Wong WH, Cheung YF: Meta analysis of pulmonary valve replacement after operative repair of tetralogy of Fallot. *Am J Cardiol* 2010;106:552-557.

Kalfa DM, Serraf AE, Ly M, et al: Tetralogy of Fallot with an abnormal coronary artery: surgical options and prognostic factors. *Eur J Cardiothorac Surg* 2012;42:e34-e39.

Lee C, Kim YM, Lee CH, et al: Outcomes of pulmonary valve replacement in 170 patients with chronic pulmonary regurgitation after relief of right ventricular outflow tract obstruction: implications for optimal timing of pulmonary valve replacement. *JACC* 2012;60:1005-1014.

Valente AM, Gauvreau K, Assenza GE, et al: Rationale and design of an international multicenter registry of patients with repaired tetralolgy of Fallot to define risk factors for late adverse outomes: the INDICATOR cohort. *Pediatr Cardiol* 2012. PMID:22669402.

van de Woestijne PC, Mokhles MM, de Jong PL, et al: Right ventricular outflow tract reconstruction with an allograft conduit in patients after tetralogy of Fallot correction: long-term follow-up. *Ann Thorac Surg* 2011;92:161-166.

▶ Transposition of Great Arteries

A. General Considerations

TGA is a congenital cardiac anomaly in which the aorta arises from the right ventricle and the pulmonary artery originates from the left ventricle (Figure 19–28). TGA is divided into *dextro*-looped (d-TGA) and *levo*-looped (l-TGA). The looping refers to the right or left looping of the primitive heart tube during fetal development, which determines whether the atria and ventricles are concordant (right atrium attaches to the right ventricle and left atrium attaches to the left ventricle) or discordant. l-TGA is associated with atrioventricular (AV) discordance (right atrium attaches to the left ventricle and left atrium attaches to the right ventricle) and is also termed congenitally corrected TGA. l-TGA is a rare variant of TGA and is beyond the scope of this chapter, which focuses on d-TGA. The defect can be subdivided into d-TGA with intact ventricular septum (IVS) (55%-60%) and d-TGA with VSD (40%-45%), one-third of which are hemodynamically insignificant. Pulmonic stenosis, causing significant left ventricular outflow tract obstruction, occurs rarely with an IVS and in approximately 10% of d-TGA/VSD.

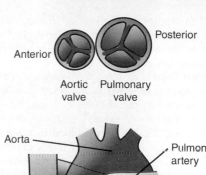

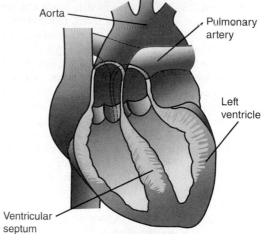

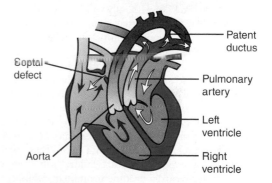

▲ **Figure 19–28.** Typical transposition of the great arteries. The aorta arises from the morphologic right ventricle and is anterior and slightly to the right of the pulmonary artery, which originates from the morphologic left ventricle. Inset at bottom illustrates the independent systemic and pulmonary circulations, which may be connected by a patent ductus arteriosus or atrial septal defect. Inset at top illustrates a common relationship of the two great arteries in typical transposition.

B. Clinical Findings

d-TGA is a relatively common cardiac anomaly and is the most common form of congenital heart disease presenting as cyanosis in the first week of life. The malformation accounts for approximately 10% of all congenital cardio-vascular malformations in infants. The degree of cyanosis depends on the amount of mixing between the pulmonary and systemic circulations. In d-TGA, oxygenated pulmonary venous blood is returned to the lungs, and desaturated systemic blood is returned to the body. Because the two circulations exist in parallel, some mixing between them must occur to allow oxygenated blood to reach the systemic circulation and the desaturated blood to reach the lungs. Mixing may occur at a number of levels, most commonly at the atrial level through an ASD or a patent foramen ovale (PFO). Generally, two levels of mixing are necessary to maintain adequate systemic oxygen delivery with a VSD or PDA serving as an additional site for cardiac mixing. In d-TGA, there can be no fixed shunt in one direction without an equal amount of blood passing in the other direction; otherwise, one circulation would eventually empty into the other. Therefore, the amount of desaturated blood reaching the lungs (effective pulmonary blood flow) must equal the amount of saturated blood reaching the aorta (effective systemic blood flow). Clinical characteristics are dependent on the degree of mixing and the amount of pulmonary blood flow. These factors relate to the specific anatomic subtype of d-TGA. Neonates with d-TGA/IVS (or small VSD) have mixing limited to the atrial level and PDA. The ASD may be restrictive, and the PDA generally will close over the first days to week of life. As the degree of mixing decreases, the patient becomes increasingly cyanotic and will eventually suffer cardiovascular collapse. Fortunately, the majority of these neonates will manifest cyanosis early in life, which is recognized by a nurse or physician within the first hour in 56% and in the first day in 92%. In d-TGA with a large VSD, there is additional opportunity for mixing and increased pulmonary blood flow. The neonate with d-TGA/VSD may manifest only mild cyanosis, which may be initially overlooked. However, generally within 2-6 weeks, signs and symptoms of congestive heart failure will emerge. Tachypnea and tachycardia become prominent, while cyanosis may remain mild. Auscultatory findings are consistent with congestive heart failure with increased pulmonary blood flow, including a pansystolic murmur, third heart sound, mid-diastolic rumble, gallop, and narrowly split second heart sound with an increased pulmonary component. Neonates with d-TGA and significant pulmonary stenosis present with severe cyanosis at birth. Lesser degrees of pulmonary stenosis will result in varying levels of cyanosis.

In cases of d-TGA, the electrocardiogram is normal at birth, demonstrating the typical pattern of RV dominance. Although the classic chest radiographic appearance of an egg-shaped heart with a narrow superior mediastinum may be seen, this finding is often obscured by an enlarged thymic shadow. The abnormal ventriculoarterial connection is clearly seen on echocardiography, which demonstrates that the posterior great vessel arising from the left ventricle is a pulmonary artery that bifurcates soon after its origin. The anterior great vessel is the aorta and arises from the RV. Associated lesions, including VSD, left ventricular outflow tract obstruction, and coarctation, may also be diagnosed. Although used less frequently for diagnosis, cardiac catheterization may be helpful to improve cardiac mixing by means of balloon atrial septostomy.

C. Treatment

The infant with d-TGA and severe cyanosis requires prompt diagnosis and treatment to improve mixing and increase the arterial oxygen saturation. The first intervention to improve mixing in a cyanotic newborn suspected of having TGA is to insure ductal patency by beginning an infusion of prostaglandin E_1. In the presence of a restrictive ASD, a balloon atrial septostomy, a technique developed by William Rashkind in 1966, is performed. The procedure involves inserting a balloon-tipped catheter across the foramen ovale into the left atrium. Inflation and forcible withdrawal of the catheter tears the septum primum and enlarges the ASD. Mixing generally increases immediately, with a substantial increase in arterial oxygen saturation. Without intervention, d-TGA is universally fatal. Untreated, 30% of neonates will die in the first week of life, 50% by the first month, 70% within 6 months, and 90% by 1 year. The definitive surgical treatment of patients with d-TGA has changed dramatically with the advent of the arterial switch operation (ASO). The ASO, first successfully performed by Jatene in 1975, has become the optimal surgical procedure for infants with this condition. Current techniques have reduced the operative mortality to 2%-4%. The operative technique involves transection of both great vessels and direct reanastomosis to reestablish ventriculoarterial concordance. Additionally, the coronary arteries are removed from the anterior aorta and relocated to the posterior great vessel (neoaorta). The extensive experience gained with this procedure has confirmed that any variant of coronary artery anatomy can be successfully repaired, although certain unusual forms impose a higher risk. Because many patients with d-TGA have an IVS, left ventricular pressure falls early in life as pulmonary vascular resistance decreases. In this situation, it is essential that the arterial repair be performed within the first 2-3 weeks of life, while the left ventricle is still able to meet systemic workloads. In patients presenting later, the left ventricle can be retrained with a preliminary pulmonary artery band and aortopulmonary shunt followed by the definitive arterial repair. Although patients with large VSDs do not require early repair because of their decreased left ventricular pressure, experience has indicated that even in this subgroup, the operation is best performed within the first month of life, before secondary complications such as pulmonary hypertension, congestive heart failure, or infection develop.

Patients with fixed left ventricular outflow tract obstruction are not candidates for the arterial repair because correction would result in systemic ventricular outflow tract obstruction. Most of these patients also have large VSDs. Palliation early in life with systemic-to-pulmonary artery shunting is an option, with definitive repair postponed until somatic growth results in cyanosis as the shunt is outgrown. At that time, the Rastelli procedure is performed, in which left ventricular blood is redirected through the VSD to the anterior aorta by placement of an intraventricular patch. The pulmonary artery is ligated, and right ventricle-to-distal pulmonary artery continuity is reestablished with a valve-bearing conduit. An increasing number of experienced centers currently recommend early complete repair in the neonatal period using a Rastelli procedure. Early repair eliminates the interim morbidity and mortality associated with a systemic-to-pulmonary artery shunt and chronic cyanosis.

D. Prognosis

Current hospital survival for the ASO is 96.6%-97.2%. Generally, dTGA/IVS has had a lower mortality than d-TGA/VSD or d-TGA/VSD/PS. Hospital mortality for d-TGA/IVS is 2.2%, compared to 4.3% for d-TGA/VSD. Long-term survivals at 5-10 years and 15-20 years are 92.2%-97.9% and 91.6%-96%, respectively. The most common cause for reintervention is supravalvar pulmonary stenosis, occurring in 19.7%-30.3%. A recent study of 40 patients undergoing a Rastelli operation over a 20-year period revealed a hospital mortality of 0%, with Kaplan–Meier survival of 93% at 5, 10, and 20 years. Freedom from conduit replacement was 86% at 5 years and 59% at 20 years.

Brown JW, Ruzmetov M, Huynh D, et al: Rastelli operation for transposition of the great arteries with ventricular septal defect and pulmonary stenosis. *Ann Thorac Surg* 2011:91:188-193.

Dodge-Khatami A, Mavroudis C, Mavroudis CD, et al: Past, present, and future of the arterial switch operation: historical review. *Cardiol Young* 2012:22:724-731.

Fricke TA, d'Udekem Y, Richardson M, et al: Outcomes of the arterial switch operation for transposition of the great arteries: 25 years of experience. *Ann Thorac Surg* 2012;94:139-145.

Kempny A, Wustmann K, Borgia F, et al: Outcome in adult patients after arterial switch operation for transposition of the great arteries. *Int J Cardiol* 2012. [epub ahead of print]

Lange R, Cleuziou J, Hörer J, et al: Risk factors for aortic insufficiency and aortic valve replacement after the arterial switch operation. *Eur J Cardiothorac Surg* 2008;34:711-717.

Oda S, Nakano T, Sugiura J, et al: Twenty-eight years' experience of arterial switch operation for transposition of the great arteries in a single institution. *Eur J Cardiothoracic Surg* 2012;42:674-679.

▶ Truncus Arteriosus

A. General Considerations

Truncus arteriosus is a rare anomaly that accounts for 0.4%-4% of all cases of congenital heart disease. A single arterial vessel arises from the heart, overriding the ventricular septum, and gives rise to the systemic, coronary, and pulmonary circulations. The Collett and Edwards classification of truncus arteriosus focuses on the origin of the pulmonary arteries from the common arterial trunk, as follows:

> *Type I:* Common arterial trunk gives rise to a main pulmonary artery and the aorta.
>
> *Type II:* Right and left pulmonary arteries arise directly from and in close proximity to the posterior wall of the truncus.
>
> *Type III:* Right and left pulmonary arteries arise from more widely separated orifices on the posterior truncal wall.
>
> *Type IV:* Branch pulmonary arteries are absent. Pulmonary blood flow is derived from aortopulmonary collaterals.

Persistent truncus arteriosus is the result of failed development of the aortopulmonary septum and subpulmonary infundibulum (conal septum). Normal septation leads to the development of both pulmonary and systemic outflow tracts, division of the semilunar valves, and formation of the aorta and pulmonary arteries. Failure of septation results in a VSD (absence of the infundibular septum), a single semilunar valve, and a single arterial trunk. Most cases are associated with a VSD with the superior margin of the defect formed by the truncal valve. The truncal valve leaflets are generally dysmorphic and their motion may be restricted. Leaflet number is highly variable, with about 65% tricuspid, 22% quadricuspid, 9% bicuspid, and rarely unicuspid or pentacuspid. As a result of these abnormally developed valve leaflets, a moderate or greater degree of truncal insufficiency is present in 20%-26% of patients. The pulmonary arteries are usually of normal size and most often arise from the left posterolateral aspect of the truncal artery, often in close proximity to the truncal valve and ostium of the left coronary artery.

Other cardiac anomalies are common and include an ASD (9%-20%), an interrupted aortic arch (10%-20%), and coronary ostial abnormalities (37%-49%) with the left coronary artery frequently noted to have a high origin, not uncommonly near the takeoff of the pulmonary arteries. Extracardiac anomalies are reported in approximately 28% of patients with truncus arteriosus. Described abnormalities include skeletal, genitourinary, gastrointestinal, and DiGeorge syndrome (11%).

B. Clinical Findings

The anatomy of truncus arteriosus results in obligatory mixing of systemic and pulmonary venous blood at the level of the VSD and truncal valve, which produces arterial saturations of 85%-90%. The systemic arterial saturation depends on the volume of pulmonary blood flow, which in turn is determined by the pulmonary vascular resistance (PVR). As the resistance begins to fall, excessive pulmonary circulation ensues and leads to pulmonary congestion and signs and symptoms of congestive heart failure. This nonrestrictive left-to-right shunt may cause early development of irreversible pulmonary vascular obstructive disease.

The presence of truncal valve abnormalities poses further hemodynamic burdens. Truncal valve regurgitation leads to ventricular dilation and low diastolic coronary perfusion pressures that can result in myocardial ischemia. Truncal valve stenosis promotes ventricular hypertrophy, increases the myocardial oxygen demand, and limits coronary and systemic perfusion, especially with the large volume of runoff into the pulmonary vascular bed.

Neonates with truncus arteriosus present with signs of congestive heart failure and collapsing peripheral pulses. Chest radiography shows marked cardiomegaly, pulmonary plethora, often with minimal thymus shadow, and a right aortic arch. The electrocardiogram most often depicts biventricular hypertrophy. Echocardiography is the diagnostic procedure of choice and can demonstrate the truncal vessel, the structure and function of the truncal valve, associated lesions such as interrupted aortic arch, and often the pulmonary arterial anatomy. Cardiac catheterization is not performed unless the anatomy is unclear, further information is needed about the status of the truncal valve, or the status of the pulmonary vasculature is unclear (ie, infants older than 3 months at diagnosis).

C. Treatment

The natural history of patients born with truncus arteriosus is early demise. Approximately 40% of infants are dead within 1 month, 70% by 3 months, and 90% by 1 year. Early death is caused by congestive heart failure. Survivors may do well for a period of time until the development of pulmonary vascular obstructive disease and Eisenmenger syndrome. The ultimate treatment of truncus arteriosus is surgical correction in the neonatal period. Medical treatment is palliative and directed toward controlling congestive heart failure with fluid restriction, diuretics, and afterload reduction. Complete repair entails separating the pulmonary arteries from the truncus, repairing the resulting defect in the aorta, closing the VSD, and restoring continuity of the RV outflow tract with an extracardiac conduit (Figure 19–29). Severe truncal valve regurgitation requires truncal valve repair or replacement. An associated interrupted aortic arch is repaired by constructing a primary end-to-end anastomosis of the distal ascending aorta with proximal augmentation if necessary.

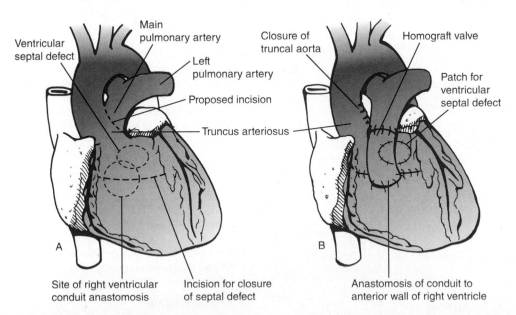

▲ **Figure 19–29.** Type 1 truncus arteriosus. **A:** The main pulmonary artery arises from the truncus arteriosus downstream to the truncal valve. A ventricular septal defect is present. **B:** The main pulmonary artery is incised from the truncus. The ventricular septal defect is closed with a patch. A valved conduit is sutured to the anterior wall of the right ventricle and the distal pulmonary artery.

D. Prognosis

The results of truncus arteriosus repair have improved greatly during the last two decades. Before the importance of early operation to avoid irreversible pulmonary vascular disease was appreciated, patients underwent repair at most institutions at an average age of 2-5 years with high mortality rates. Current hospital mortality for the neonatal repair of truncus arteriosus ranges between 4.3% and 17%, with the majority of deaths occurring in complex truncus arteriosus or in truncus arteriosus with associated severe truncal valve regurgitation. All patients will ultimately require reoperation for replacement of the right ventricle to pulmonary artery conduit with only 30%-42% being free from reoperation at 10 years. Thirty-year survival is approximately 75%-83%.

Chaker L, Marzouk BS, Hakim K, et al: Late reinterventions after repair of common arterial trunk. *Tunis Med* 2008;86:529-533.

de Siena P, Ghorbel M, Chen Q, et al: Common arterial trunk: review of surgical strategies and future research. *Expert Rev Cardiovasc Ther* 2011;12:1527-1538.

Henaine R et al: Fate of the truncal valve in truncus arteriosus. *Ann Thorac Surg* 2008;85:172.

Kaza AK, Lim HG, Dibardino DJ: Long-term results of right ventricular outflow tract reconstruction in neonatal cardiac surgery: options and outcomes. *J Thorac Cardiovasc Surg* 2009;138:911-916.

Raisky O, Ali WB, Bajolle F, et al: Common arterial trunk repair: with conduit or without? *Eur J Cardiothorac Surg* 2009;36:675.

▶ Total Anomalous Pulmonary Venous Connection

A. General Considerations

Total anomalous pulmonary venous connection (TAPVC) is a relatively uncommon congenital defect representing approximately 2% of all congenital heart anomalies. TAPVC encompasses a group of anomalies in which the pulmonary veins connect directly to the systemic venous circulation via persistent splanchnic connections. This abnormality results from failed transfer, in the normal developmental sequence, of pulmonary venous drainage from the splanchnic plexus to the left atrium. The most common classification system consists of four types: supracardiac (type 1), cardiac (type 2), infracardiac (type 3), and mixed (Figure 19-30). Partial anomalous pulmonary venous connection defines patients in whom some but not all venous drainage enters the left atrium, while the remaining veins connect to one or more persistent splanchnic veins.

TAPVC can also be classified by the presence of obstruction. Impingement from surrounding structures or inadequate caliber of the draining pulmonary vein(s) can result in varying degrees of obstruction. Obstruction in supracardiac TAPVC can occur by compression of the ascending vertical

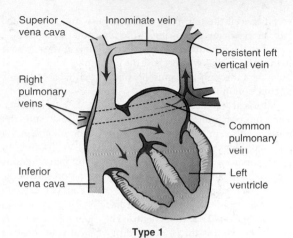

Type 1

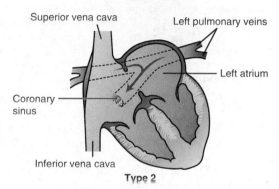

Type 2

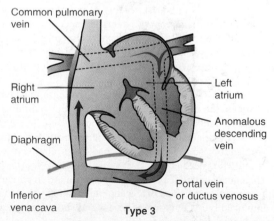

Type 3

▲ **Figure 19–30.** Common types of total anomalous pulmonary venous connection. Type 1: The pulmonary veins connect to a persistent left vertical vein, the innominate vein, and the right superior vena cava. Type 2: The pulmonary veins connect to the coronary sinus and the right atrium. Type 3: The pulmonary veins connect to an anomalous descending vein, a portal vein or persistent ductus venosus, and eventually enter the inferior vena cava.

vein between the left main stem bronchus and left pulmonary artery or by narrowing at the insertion of the vertical vein into the innominate vein. Obstruction is always present in the infracardiac type because the pulmonary venous blood must pass through the sinusoids of the liver. Obstruction is uncommon in the cardiac type.

Supracardiac occurs in approximately 45% of patients. The common pulmonary vein drains superiorly into the innominate vein, superior vena cava, or azygous vein via an ascending vertical vein. Cardiac TAPVC occurs in approximately 25% of patients. The pulmonary venous confluence drains into the coronary sinus or, on rare occasions, individual pulmonary veins will connect directly into the right atrium. Infracardiac TAPVC occurs in approximately 25% of patients. The pulmonary venous confluence drains into a descending vertical vein through the diaphragm into the portal vein or ductus venosus. Finally, a mixed type of TAPVC occurs in approximately 5% of patients and can involve any or all components of the previous three types.

B. Clinical Findings

TAPVC produces a mixing lesion because oxygenated blood from the pulmonary system drains back into the systemic venous circulation. The size of the ASD dictates the distribution of blood flow. Most patients with unobstructed TAPVC have few or no symptoms in infancy and present with signs and symptoms similar to an ASD. In the neonate with obstructed TAPVC, venous drainage from the pulmonary vasculature is impaired, leading to pulmonary venous hypertension and pulmonary edema. In severe cases, this increased pressure will lead to reflexive vasoconstriction of the pulmonary vasculature with pulmonary hypertension. Patients with obstruction present early in life with profound cyanosis from pulmonary edema.

The diagnosis can be made with echocardiographic identification of the anomalous connection of the pulmonary venous confluence to the systemic venous system. The ASD and other associated anomalies can be delineated. Cardiac catheterization is rarely necessary unless accurate measurement of PVR is needed.

The management of TAPVC is surgical repair. In patients with obstruction, medical management for stabilization may be employed but is often unsuccessful and should not delay surgical intervention.

C. Treatment

The principle of operative repair is to establish an unobstructed communication between the pulmonary venous confluence and the left atrium, interrupt the connections with the systemic venous circulation, and close the ASD. The specific repair is dependent on the type of anomalous connection.

1. **Supracardiac TAPVC** The repair of supracardiac TAPVC may be performed with moderate hypothermia (28-32°C) and bicaval cannulation or with a brief period of hypothermic (18°C) circulatory arrest. The optimal approach is to retract the ascending aorta to the left and the superior vena cava to the right to expose the pulmonary venous confluence. This approach provides excellent exposure without distortion of the heart or venous structures. The vertical vein can be identified and ligated (just prior to opening the confluence) outside the pericardium at the level of the innominate vein. A transverse incision is made in the pulmonary venous confluence, and a parallel incision is placed in the dome of the left atrium beginning at the base of the left atrial appendage. The common pulmonary vein is then anastomosed to the left atrium, taking care to construct an unrestrictive connection. A right atriotomy is made to close the ASD.

2. **Cardiac TAPVC** The repair of cardiac TAPVC can be performed with bicaval cannulation and moderate hypothermia with the use of a vent or a cardiotomy sucker to capture the pulmonary venous return. A right atriotomy is performed with identification of the ASD and the orifice of the coronary sinus. The roof of the coronary sinus is excised into the left atrium. A patch of pericardium or prosthetic material is then placed to close the enlarged ASD, effectively channeling the pulmonary venous and coronary sinus return into the left atrium. The conduction system travels in proximity to the coronary sinus, and care must be taken while suturing the patch in this area to avoid heart block.

3. **Infracardiac TAPVC** For infracardiac connections, a brief period of hypothermic circulatory arrest is often required. The heart is rotated superiorly. The descending vertical vein is identified by opening the posterior pericardium. The connection to the descending vertical vein is ligated at the level of the diaphragm. An incision is made along the length of the pulmonary venous confluence with a parallel incision on the posterior wall of the left atrium. The pulmonary venous confluence is then anastomosed to the left atrium, taking care not to narrow the connection. Tissue from the descending vertical vein can be used in the anastomosis. A right atriotomy is performed through which the ASD is closed.

4. **Recurrent pulmonary venous obstruction** The approach to recurrent pulmonary venous obstruction is dependent on the level of obstruction. Obstruction can develop at the anastomosis or within the individual pulmonary veins. The latter may initially present as an anastomotic constriction, as the true extent of obstruction is not always apparent at first. Isolated narrowing of the anastomosis between the common pulmonary

vein and left atrium often can be repaired with revision or patch augmentation of the anastomosis.

Obstruction of the individual pulmonary venous ostia is the greater challenge. Although the obstruction may initially appear to be limited to the ostium, progressive narrowing along the entire length of the vein into the hilum of the lung may occur with time. Repair of this lesion is technically challenging, and recurrent early obstruction is common. A new approach to recurrent pulmonary vein stenosis employs a "sutureless" technique utilizing in situ pericardium to create a neoatrium. The theory behind this repair is based on the concept that pulmonary venous obstruction results from inflammation induced locally by suture placement. Repair involves wide unroofing of the narrowed portion of each involved pulmonary vein from the left atrial anastomosis to the hilum. A wide flap of pericardium is then elevated with care taken to avoid disruption of posterior adhesions and injury to the phrenic nerve. This flap of pericardium is rotated over the unroofed pulmonary veins and sutured to the left atrial wall away from the venous ostia. A large neoatrium is then created into which pulmonary venous return can drain.

D. Prognosis

Early mortality in patients undergoing repair of TAPVC is associated with the initial degree of obstruction present. Early diagnosis and repair as well as optimal postoperative management, including aggressive treatment of pulmonary hypertension, have resulted in a dramatic reduction in operative risk. For patients surviving the perioperative period, the long-term survival and functional status are excellent.

Recurrent venous obstruction develops in 5%-17.5% of patients. Results following balloon angioplasty and/or stent insertion have been disappointing, and recurrent stenoses are the rule. Individual patch angioplasty of the ostia has also been utilized with poor long-term results. Lung transplantation has been considered in severe cases of extensive, bilateral disease. The mortality associated with reoperation for obstruction can be up to 59% when bilateral stenoses are present. The use of the sutureless technique for recurrent pulmonary vein obstruction has demonstrated improved survival and decreased recurrence.

Aquirre J, Mavroudis C, Jacobs M, et al: Direct operating room triage of neonates with total anomalous pulmonary venous connection. *Pediatr Cardiol* 2013;34(8):1874-1876. PMID: 22797519.

Hammel JM, Hunt PW, Abdullah I, et al: "Closed-vein" technique for primary sutureless repair of anomalous pulmonary venous connection. *Ann Thorac Surg* 2012;94:1021-1022.

Hickey EJ, Caldarone CA: Surgical management of post-repair pulmonary vein stenosis. *Semin Thorac Cardiovasc Surg Pediatr Card Surg Annu* 2011;14:101-108.

Seale AN, Uemura H, Webber SA, et al: Total anomalous pulmonary venous connection: outcome of postoperative pulmonary venous obstruction. *J Thorac Cardiovasc Surg* 2013;145(5):1255-1262. PMID: 22892140.

Yoshimura N, Fukahara K, Yamashita A, et al: Management of pulmonary venous obstruction. *Gen Thorac Cardiovasc Surg* 2012;60(12):785-791. PMID:23054615.

▶ Tricuspid Atresia

A. General Considerations

Tricuspid atresia refers to single-ventricle hearts that lack a communication between the right atrium and right ventricle. The only outlet for the right atrium is the ASD. If present, aneurysmal tissue of the septum primum may prolapse into the left atrium. The left atrium is normal in morphology but is often dilated. A normal communication with a mitral valve between the left atrium and left ventricle is present. The right ventricle is diminutive in size without an inlet portion. It is connected to the left ventricle by a VSD surrounded completely by muscle. The anatomic subtypes of tricuspid atresia are based on the relationship of the great arteries. Type I defects (70%) have normally related great vessels, type II (30%) have transposed great arteries, and type III (rare) have congenitally corrected TGAs. These types are further subclassified by the degree of obstruction to pulmonary blood flow, which is present in 45%-75% of patients. Aortic valve (10%) and aortic arch (25%) obstruction may also be present. Patients with tricuspid atresia are at increased risk for Wolff–Parkinson–White syndrome due to congenital and surgically acquired pathways.

B. Clinical Findings

The clinical presentation depends on the relationship of the great vessels and degree of restriction at the level of the atrial and ventricular septum. Most infants present with some degree of cyanosis. Systemic output is usually unobstructed. Prostaglandins may be necessary to maintain ductal patency in infants with severe obstruction to pulmonary blood flow.

C. Treatment

The initial palliation for most patients is the placement of a modified Blalock-Taussig shunt to maintain adequate pulmonary blood flow. A more complex initial palliation with a Norwood procedure may be necessary in the case of transposed great vessels. The remainder of the palliation involves a hemi-Fontan and Fontan procedure (discussed in the section on Hypoplastic Left Heart Syndrome).

D. Prognosis

The overall survival for tricuspid atresia is similar to that reported for other single-ventricle lesions palliated with a

Fontan procedure. The survival is 83% at 1 year, 70% at 10 years, and 60% at 20 years.

Abdul-Sater Z, Yehya A, Beresian J, et al: Two heterozygous mutations in NFATC1 in a patient with tricuspid atresia. *PLoS One* 2012;7:e49532.

Berg C, Lachmann R, Kaiser C, et al: Prenatal diagnosis of tricuspid atresia: intrauterine course and outcome. *Ultrasound Obstet Gynecol* 2010;35:183-190.

Ho PK, Lai CT, Wong SJ, et al: Three-dimensional mechanical dyssynchrony and myocardial deformation of the left ventricle in patients with tricuspid atresia after Fontan procedure. *J Am Soc Echocardiogr* 2012;25:393-400.

Wald RM et al: Outcome after prenatal diagnosis of tricuspid atresia: a multicenter experience. *Am Heart J* 2007;153:772.

▶ Hypoplastic Left Heart Syndrome

A. General Considerations

A variety of congenital cardiovascular malformations may result in a functional single-ventricle anatomy, most commonly tricuspid atresia, pulmonary atresia, unbalanced AVSD, and HLHS. The most common lesion is HLHS. Approximately 1000 infants with HLHS are born in the United States each year. It is the most common severe congenital heart defect, comprising 7%-9% of all anomalies diagnosed within the first year of life. All single-ventricle lesions share the common physiology of only a single ventricle capable of supporting cardiac output. HLHS refers to a constellation of congenital cardiac anomalies characterized by marked hypoplasia or absence of the left ventricle and severe hypoplasia of the ascending aorta. The systemic circulation is dependent on the right ventricle via a PDA, and there is obligatory mixing of pulmonary and systemic venous blood in the right atrium. There is associated aortic valve stenosis or atresia and mitral valve stenosis or atresia. The descending aorta is essentially a continuation of the ductus arteriosus, and the ascending aorta and aortic arch represents a diminutive branch of this vessel. Initial management includes a prostaglandin infusion to maintain ductal patency and correction of metabolic acidosis. The patient may require intubation and ventilator adjustment to reduce supplemental oxygen and maintain a Pco_2 of about 40 mm Hg to avoid excessive pulmonary flow.

B. Treatment

Surgical approaches to the treatment of this problem include cardiac transplantation and staged reconstruction. In the context of improving results for staged reconstruction, risks of immunosuppression, and limited donor availability, competing risk analysis favors staged repair, and most centers pursue this option as primary therapy for HLHS. Transplantation is generally reserved for very high-risk patients, such as those with depressed RV function, severe tricuspid regurgitation, or significant coronary sinusoids.

The first successful palliation of HLHS was reported by Norwood on a series of infants operated between 1979 and 1981. This procedure has been technically refined over the years, but three essential components remain: atrial septectomy, anastomosis of the proximal pulmonary artery to the aorta with homograft augmentation of the aortic arch, and aortopulmonary shunt. A "hybrid Norwood" procedure is an alternate form of stage I palliation. This procedure involves bilateral pulmonary artery bands and PDA stenting with or without concommittant balloon atrial septostomy. The ultimate goal of surgical palliation in patients with a univentricular heart is the total diversion of all vena caval blood directly into the pulmonary arteries. The Fontan procedure was first successfully performed in a patient with tricuspid atresia but has since evolved as an excellent way to establish physiologic repair for patients with more complex forms of univentricular heart. The superior vena caval blood returns directly via an end-to-side anastomosis with the pulmonary artery (bidirectional Glenn) or through a right atrial-pulmonary artery connection (hemi-Fontan) performed at 4-6 months of age. The inferior vena caval flow is directed to the pulmonary artery with an intra-atrial baffle (lateral tunnel technique) or an extracardiac conduit at 2-4 years of age. All oxygenated pulmonary venous flow empties into the ventricular chamber through the AV valves to be ejected to the systemic circulation, while superior and inferior vena caval blood flows directly to the lungs to acquire oxygen prior to returning to the heart. For the Fontan procedure to be performed with a low operative mortality and an acceptable functional result, certain criteria must be met. Normal pulmonary artery pressure (< 20 mm Hg) and PVR (< 2 Woods units·m²) are the most important prerequisites. Additionally, it is essential that ventricular function and AV valve function be normal. Although the Fontan procedure cannot be considered a truly corrective operation, it offers benefits that cannot be equaled by those of any of the other palliative procedures. The major advantages include restoration of normal systemic oxygen saturation and reduction of ventricular volume overload.

C. Prognosis

Universally fatal only three decades ago, tremendous strides have been made in improving the outcomes for patients with HLHS. Of the three stages, the highest-risk stage of the repair remains the Norwood operation. During the 1990s, the hospital survival for the Norwood procedure across the United States was approximately 40%. A recent Society of Thoracic Surgeons Congenital Heart Surgery Database study reported 81% hospital survival rate for more than 2000 Norwood operations performed in 2009. Currently, interstage (time between the Norwood and hemi-Fontan operation) mortality is about 12%. Reported survivals for the hemi-Fontan and Fontan procedures have also been excellent at 98% for both operations. Overall, 75% of patients diagnosed with HLHS will survive through the Fontan procedure.

The current results for the Fontan procedure are excellent with hospital mortality ranging from 2% to 9%. The condition of survivors is generally good, and most attain a functional status of New York Heart Association class I or II. The long-term results have been reported with a 93% 5-year survival and a 91% 10-year survival. Although long-term results are encouraging, late complications may be seen. Continued surveillance for arrhythmias, congenital heart failure, protein-losing enteropathy, and hepatic dysfunction remains important.

Ghanayem NS, Allen KR, Tabbutt S, et al: Interstage mortality after the Norwood procedure: results of the multicenter single ventricle reconstruction trial. *J Thorac Cardiovasc Surg* 2012;144:896-906.

Hornik CP, He X, Jacobs JP, et al: Complications after the Norwood operation: an analysis of The Society of Thoracic Surgeons Congenital Heart Surgery Database. *Ann Thorac Surg* 2011;92:1734-1740.

Lee TM, Aiyagari R, Hirsch JC, et al: Risk factor analysis for second-stage palliation of single ventricle anatomy. *Ann Thorac Surg* 2012;93:614-618.

Lowry AW: Resuscitation and perioperative management of the high-risk single ventricle patient: first-stage palliation. *Congenital Heart Disease* 2012;7:466-478.

Tabbutt S, Ghanayem N, Ravishankar C, et al: Risk factors for hospital morbidity and mortality after the Norwood procedure: a report from the Pediatric Heart Network Single Ventricle Reconstruction trial. *J Thorac Cardiovasc Surg* 2012;144:882-895.

ACYANOTIC HEART DEFECTS

1. Left-to-Right Shunting

▶ **Atrial Septal Defect**

A. General Considerations

Cardiac septation occurs between the third and sixth weeks of fetal development. The septum primum, which arises from the roof of the common atrium and descends inferiorly, initially divides the common atrium. The ostium primum is the opening below the inferior edge of the septum primum, which is obliterated as the septum primum fuses with the endocardial cushions. The ostium secundum forms in the midportion of the septum primum prior to closure of the ostium primum. The septum secundum also arises from the roof of the atrium and descends along the right side of the septum primum and covers the ostium secundum. This creates a flap valve whereby blood from the inferior vena cava may preferentially stream beneath the edge of the septum secundum and through the ostium secundum into the left atrium. After birth, the increase in left atrial pressure usually closes this pathway.

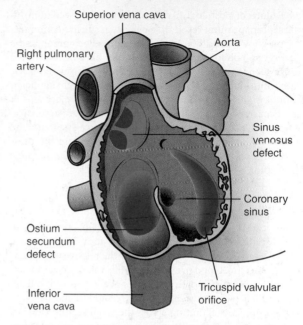

▲ **Figure 19–31.** Sinus venosus and ostium secundum defects in the atrial septum as viewed from the opened right atrium.

An ASD is a hole in the atrial septum (Figure 19–31). ASDs are the third-most common congenital heart defect, occurring in 1 out of 1000 live births and representing 10% of congenital heart defects. The most common ASD is the secundum defect, which occurs when the ostium secundum is too large for complete coverage by the septum secundum. Ostium secundum defects account for about 80% of ASDs. An ostium primum ASD, representing 10% of ASDs, occurs as a result of failure of fusion of the septum primum with the endocardial cushions (ostium primum defect is discussed later in the section on Atrioventricular Septal Defects [AVSD]). A third type of ASD is the sinus venosus defect, seen in about 10% of cases. Sinus venosus ASDs are caused by abnormal fusion of the venous pathways with the atrium and are characterized by defects high in the atrial septum near the orifice of the superior vena cava or, less commonly, low in the atrial septum near the inferior vena cava. Sinus venosus defects are frequently associated with partial anomalous pulmonary venous connection, usually with the right upper pulmonary vein draining into the superior vena cava near the cavoatrial junction. The rarest type of ASD is the unroofed coronary sinus septal defect. This occurs when there is loss of the common wall between the coronary sinus and the left atrium adjacent to the atrial septum. This unroofing of the coronary sinus leads to a communication between the right and left atria at the site of the coronary sinus.

Failure of postnatal fusion of the septum secundum to the septum primum results in a persistent slit-like communication known as a PFO. PFOs are extremely common in the general population, and autopsy studies have demonstrated a prevalence of 27%. PFOs are generally considered separate from other ASDs because of the absence of significant shunting, but they remain important clinically because of the occurrence of paradoxical embolization. A paradoxical embolus is usually a blood clot arising from a systemic vein, which would normally pass to the lungs, but in the presence of a septal defect may instead cross into the systemic circulation.

B. Clinical Findings

ASDs lead to increased pulmonary blood flow secondary to left-to-right shunting. Shunting at the atrial level is determined by the size of the defect and by the relative ventricular compliance (ie, blood preferentially fills the more compliant ventricle). At birth, both chambers are equally compliant, but as PVR falls, the right ventricle remodels and becomes more compliant. Shunting across the atrial septum causes a volume load on the right heart. A volume load is created by additional venous return to a chamber during diastole.

The volume overload from an ASD is usually well tolerated, and patients are frequently asymptomatic. Symptoms tend to develop when the ratio of pulmonary to systemic blood flow (Q_p/Q_s) exceeds two. The most common symptoms are fatigue, shortness of breath, exercise intolerance, and recurrent respiratory infections. Older patients with untreated ASDs tend to develop atrial dysrhythmias, and adults may develop congestive heart failure and RV dysfunction. Pulmonary vascular obstructive disease may develop rarely as a late complication of untreated ASD. Paradoxical embolization is also an important potential complication of ASD.

The classic physical findings in patients with ASDs include fixed splitting of the second heart sound and a systolic ejection murmur at the left upper sternal border due to increased flow across a normal pulmonary valve. A diastolic flow murmur across the tricuspid valve is occasionally audible. A prominent RV lift and increased intensity of the pulmonary component of the second heart sound may occur with pulmonary hypertension. Chest radiography shows cardiomegaly, with enlargement of the right atrium, right ventricle, and pulmonary artery. EKG frequently demonstrates right axis deviation and an incomplete right bundle branch block. When right bundle branch block occurs with a leftward or superior axis, the diagnosis of AVSD should be considered. Echocardiography confirms the diagnosis of ASD and defines the anatomy. Cardiac catheterization is important in selected cases to assess PVR in older patients, but it is used more frequently with therapeutic intent for device closure of ASDs.

C. Treatment

Because of the long-term complications associated with ASD, repair is recommended for all patients with symptomatic defects and in asymptomatic patients in whom the Q_p/Q_s is greater than 1.5. Repair is usually performed in children prior to school age. Closure of ASDs may be performed surgically or using a device deployed in the cardiac catheterization lab.

Surgical repair is usually recommended for large secundum defects and for most other types of ASDs. The heart is usually exposed by median sternotomy. Other surgical approaches have been proposed, including minimally invasive techniques, but there are technical drawbacks associated with each of the alternative approaches. In most cases, a limited midline incision with a partial lower sternal split provides adequate exposure and a cosmetically acceptable scar. The atrial septum is exposed through a right atriotomy. Small secundum defects or PFOs may sometimes be closed primarily by suturing the edge of the septum primum to the edge of the septum secundum. More commonly, larger defects are closed using a patch (polytetrafluoroethylene or autologous pericardium) and a running polypropylene suture. When anomalous pulmonary venous drainage is present, a baffle is created to redirect the flow across the ASD. In all cases, care is taken to deair the left atrium to avoid the complication of air embolization.

The first transcatheter device closure of an ASD was performed in 1976. A number of devices are currently available for percutaneous closure of a secundum ASD, and success rates for device deployment are greater than 90%. Device closure has the advantages of fewer complications and a shorter hospitalization. Device closure of small to moderate secundum ASDs and PFOs has now become the standard of care at most large centers.

Occasionally, adults will present with a newly diagnosed ASD. Many studies have confirmed that ASD closure in adults over the age of 40 increases survival and limits the development of heart failure. When the Q_p/Q_s is less than 1.5 and the ratio of pulmonary to systemic vascular resistance (R_p/R_s) is greater than 0.7, significant pulmonary vascular obstructive disease is usually present. A PVR in excess of 10-12 Woods units·m² represents a contraindication to ASD closure.

D. Prognosis

Operative mortality for ASD repair is close to 0%. Atrial arrhythmias (1.2%) and postpericardiotomy syndrome (4.7%) are the most common postoperative complications. The long-term survival for patients undergoing ASD repair in childhood is normal. The major long-term complication following surgical closure of ASD is the development of supraventricular arrhythmias, although the risk is lowered when the ASD is closed in childhood. The persistence of this risk despite relief of right-sided volume overload is thought to be related to incomplete atrial remodeling or due to the presence of the atriotomy scar. Longer follow-up is required to determine whether device closure alters the risk of atrial dysrhythmias.

Butera G, Biondi-Zoccai G, Sangiorgi G, et al: Percutaneous versus surgical closure of secundum atrial septal defects: a systematic review and meta-analysis of currently available clinical evidence. *EuroIntervention* 2011;7:377-385.

Butera G, Romagnoli E, Carminati M, et al: Treatment of isolated secundum atrial septal defects: impact of age and defect morphology in 1,013 consecutive patients. *Am Heart J* 2008;156:706-712.

Irwin B, Ray S: Patent foramen ovale—assessment and treatment. *Cardiovasc Ther* 2012;30:c128-e135.

Nyboe C, Fenger-Grøn M, Nielsen-Kudsk JE, et al: Closure of secundum atrial septal defects in the adult and elderly patients. *Eur J Cardiothorac Surg* 2012. [epub ahead of print]

Saito T, Ohta K, Nakayama Y, et al: Natural history of medium-sized atrial septal defect in pediatric cases. *J Cardiol* 2012;60:248-251.

Stewart RD, Bailliard F, Kelle AM, et al: Evolving surgical strategy for sinus venosus atrial septal defect: effect on sinus node function and late venous obstruction. *Ann Thorac Surg* 2007;84:1651-1655.

▶ Ventricular Septal Defect

A. General Considerations

Ventricular septation is a complex process that requires accurate development and alignment of a number of structures including the muscular interventricular septum, the AV septum (arising from the endocardial cushions), and the infundibular septum (which divides the outflow tracts of the right and left ventricles). The membranous septum is a fibrous portion of the ventricular septum, which is adjacent to the central fibrous body (where the mitral, tricuspid, and aortic valve annuli make contact).

VSDs are the most common congenital heart anomalies (with the exception of bicuspid aortic valve, which occurs in about 1.3% of the population). VSDs are present in about 4 of 1000 live births and represent about 40% of congenital heart defects. VSDs are classified based on their location in the ventricular septum (Figure 19–32). The most common defects are perimembranous (80%), which are located in the area of the membranous septum. Inlet defects (5%) are located beneath the septal leaflet of the tricuspid valve and are sometimes called atrioventricular (AV) canal-type defects. Defects located high in the ventricular septum are outlet defects (10%). Outlet VSDs are typically adjacent to both the pulmonary and aortic valves. Outlet defects are also known by several other names, including supracristal, infundibular, or doubly committed subarterial. Outlet defects are more common in the Asian population. Muscular (or trabecular) VSDs (5%) are completely bordered by muscle.

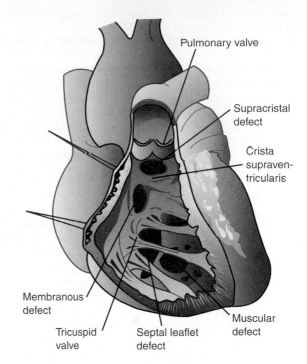

▲ **Figure 19–32.** Anatomic locations of various ventricular septal defects. The wall of the right ventricle has been excised to expose the ventricular septum.

Muscular VSDs are frequently multiple and may be associated with perimembranous or outlet defects. The size of VSDs varies. By definition, a VSD is nonrestrictive when its size (or the cumulative size of multiple defects) is greater than or equal to the size of the aortic annulus.

B. Clinical Findings

A VSD causes increased pulmonary blood flow due to left-to-right shunting primarily during systole. This creates a volume load on the left heart (the left atrium and ventricle receive the increased venous return during diastole). The right ventricle is not volume loaded (blood is ejected from the left ventricle through the VSD and directly into the pulmonary circulation), but it does experience a pressure load. The volume of shunt flow is determined by the size of the defect and by the ratio of R_p/R_s. After birth, the PVR is still high, and shunting across a VSD is sometimes minimal. Over the first several weeks of life, shunting tends to increase as the PVR normally falls. Therefore, a patient with a large VSD may be asymptomatic at birth but eventually develop severe congestive heart failure.

The natural history for patients with isolated VSDs is highly variable. Most VSDs are restrictive and tend to close spontaneously during the first year of life. Large VSDs are nonrestrictive, resulting in RV and pulmonary pressures that are systemic or nearly systemic, and high pulmonary blood flow with Q_p/Q_s ratios greater than 2.5-3. Moderate VSDs are restrictive, with pulmonary pressures that are one-half systemic (or less) and Q_p/Q_s ratios of 1.5-2.5. Small VSDs are highly restrictive; RV pressures remain normal, and the Q_p/Q_s is less than 1.5. Patients with large VSDs tend to develop symptoms of congestive heart failure by 2 months of age. Untreated, excessive pulmonary blood flow leads to pulmonary vascular obstructive disease by the second year of life. Patients with smaller VSDs may remain asymptomatic. In patients with outlet VSDs, prolapse of the aortic valve may occur, producing aortic insufficiency.

Signs of heart failure in infants with large VSDs include tachypnea, hepatomegaly, poor feeding, and failure to thrive. On physical examination, there is a pansystolic murmur at the left sternal border. Usually, the murmur is louder with smaller defects. The precordium is active. The pulmonary component of the second heart sound is accentuated in the presence of pulmonary hypertension. Chest radiography shows increased pulmonary vascular markings and cardiomegaly. EKG is significant for RV hypertrophy.

Patients with small VSDs have little shunting and are usually asymptomatic, having only a pansystolic murmur. Patients with moderate VSDs manifest symptoms and signs proportional to the degree of shunting.

In patients who have developed significant pulmonary vascular obstructive disease, the volume of left-to-right shunting is decreased, and the murmur may disappear. Eisenmenger physiology results when the shunt flow reverses to right-to-left, creating cyanosis.

The diagnosis of VSD is confirmed by echocardiography, which accurately defines the anatomy and excludes the presence of associated defects. Cardiac catheterization is used selectively in older children and adults in whom elevated PVR is suspected. Pulmonary vascular resistance is calculated by the following formula:

$$PVR = (PA_{mean} - LA)/Q_p$$

where PA_{mean} is the mean pulmonary artery pressure and LA is the left atrial pressure. The units of resistance by this formulation (using pressures in millimeters of mercury and pulmonary flow in liters per minute) are Woods units (which can be expressed in dynes·sec/cm^5 by multiplying by 80). PVR may be fixed or reactive, and at the time of cardiac catheterization, response to various pulmonary vasodilators may be assessed.

C. Treatment

The management of a patient with a VSD depends on the size of the defect, the type of the defect, the shunt volume, and the PVR. In general, patients with large defects who have intractable congestive heart failure or failure to thrive should undergo early surgical repair. If the congestive symptoms can be moderated by medical therapy, then surgery may be deferred until 6 months of age. Patients with moderate VSDs may be safely followed. If closure has not occurred by school age, then surgical closure is indicated. Small VSDs with Q_p/Q_s of less than 1.5 do not require closure. There is a small long-term risk of endocarditis for these patients, but this can be minimized with the appropriate use of prophylactic antibiotics. Patients with outlet VSDs have a significant risk of developing aortic insufficiency due to leaflet prolapse, and, therefore, all of these patients should undergo surgical closure. Older children and adults must undergo catheterization to assess the pulmonary circulation. When there is a fixed PVR greater than 8-10 Woods units·m^2, then surgery is contraindicated.

Exposure of the ventricular septum is most often achieved by making a right atriotomy and retracting the leaflets of the tricuspid valve. This provides access to perimembranous, inlet, and most trabecular VSDs. Outlet VSDs are frequently best exposed via a pulmonary arteriotomy because the defect lies just beneath the valve. Muscular VSDs located near the ventricular apex can be very difficult to expose, and an apical ventriculotomy may be necessary. Once the defect is exposed, it is closed using a polytetrafluoroethylene patch and a running polypropylene suture, although some centers may prefer other patch material or interrupted suture technique. It is important to understand the anatomy of the conduction tissue when closing VSDs. The AV node is an atrial structure that lies at the apex of an anatomic triangle (known as the triangle of Koch) formed by the coronary sinus, the tendon of Todaro (a prominent band leading from the inferior vena cava and inserting in the atrial septum), and the septal attachment of the tricuspid valve. The node then gives rise to the bundle of His, which penetrates the AV junction beneath the membranous septum. The bundle of His then bifurcates into right and left bundle branches, which pass along either side of the muscular ventricular septum. In the presence of a perimembranous VSD, the bundle of His passes along the posterior and inferior rim of the defect, generally on the left ventricular side. In this critical area, sutures must be placed superficially on the RV side a few millimeters from the edge of the defect. The bundle of His tends to run along the posterior and inferior margin of inlet VSDs as well. The conduction tissue is usually remote from outlet and trabecular VSDs.

Pulmonary artery banding is a palliative maneuver used to protect the pulmonary circulation from excessive blood flow. Pulmonary artery banding is currently performed only in patients who are felt to be poor candidates for VSD closure because of either associated illness or anatomic complexity, such as multiple muscular VSDs ("Swiss cheese" septum). A band is placed around the main pulmonary artery and tightened to achieve a distal pulmonary artery pressure of about one-half systemic. The band is secured to the adventitia of the pulmonary artery to prevent its migration. Distal migration may result in narrowing and poor growth of one or both branch pulmonary arteries, while proximal migration can cause deformity of the pulmonary valve. Later, when the patient is a candidate for VSD closure, the band must be removed. Repair of the main pulmonary artery at the band site is usually necessary and can typically be accomplished by scar resection and primary closure or patch repair.

Transcatheter devices allow closure of some VSDs in the cardiac catheterization lab. For specific VSDs, such as muscular, device closure may be preferable. Complications with device closure include complete heart block (3.8%), device embolization (0.01%), and aortic insufficiency (0.03%). For simple perimembranous VSDs, the risk of device closure is in excess of traditional surgical closure.

D. Prognosis

Surgical closure of a VSD is associated with a mortality of less than 1%. Potential complications include injury to the conduction tissue and injury to the tricuspid or aortic valves. Transient heart block may result from tissue swelling or injury from retraction, but permanent heart block occurs in less than 2% of cases. When heart block develops after surgery, patients are usually observed for a period of 7-10 days prior to permanent pacemaker implantation. Tricuspid insufficiency may be precipitated by annular distortion or chordal restriction by the VSD patch or sutures. The aortic valve may also be injured by inaccurate suturing (especially in perimembranous and outlet defects). A residual VSD is seen in about 5% of cases, and reoperation is indicated when significant shunting persists ($Q_p/Q_s > 1.5$) or the residual defect is larger than 2 mm in size. The Q_p/Q_s ratio can be calculated by measuring oxygen saturations and using the following formula derived from the Fick equation:

$$Q_p/Q_s = (Ao - SVC)/(PV - PA)$$

where Ao is the aortic (or systemic) saturation, SVC is the saturation in the superior vena cava, PV is the saturation in the pulmonary veins (which is usually estimated to be 95%-100%), and PA is the saturation in the pulmonary arteries. Intraoperative echocardiography is used routinely to identify residual defects, which can then be repaired before the patient leaves the operating room.

Anderson JB, Czosek RJ, Knilans TK, et al: Postoperative heart block in children with common forms of congenital heart disease: results from the KID database. *J Cardiovasc Electrophysiol* 2012. [Epub ahead of print].

Liu S, Chen F, Ding X, et al: Comparison of results and economic analysis of surgical and transcatheter closure of perimembranous ventricular septal defect. *Eur J Cardiothoracic Surg* 2012;42:e157-e162.

Oses P, Hugues N, Dahdah N: Treatment of isolated ventricular septal defects in children: Amplatzer versus surgical closure. *Ann Thorac Surg* 2010;90:1593-1598.

Spicer DE, Anderson RH, Backer CL: Clarifying the surgical morphology of inlet ventricular septal defects. *Ann Thorac Surg* 2013;95(1):236-241.

Zuo J, Xie J, Yi W, et al: Results of transcatheter closure of perimembranous ventricular septal defect. *Am J Cardiol* 2010;106:1034-1037.

▶ Atrioventricular Septal Defect

A. General Considerations

AVSDs represent a group of congenital abnormalities bound by a variable deficiency of the atrioventricular septum immediately above and below the AV valves. Other terms commonly applied to an AVSD include AV canal defects, endocardial cushion defects, and atrioventricular communis. Complete AVSDs have a single common AV valve orifice resulting in a single five-leaflet valve overlying both the right and left ventricles. Incomplete AVSDs have two separate AV valve orifices (tricuspid and mitral) with the mitral valve invariably having a cleft in the anterior leaflet. While most incomplete AVSDs have no ventricular level shunting, the classification of AVSDs as complete and incomplete depends only on the valve anatomy, not on the presence or absence of a VSD. Incomplete defects without associated ventricular level shunting have also been termed ostium primum ASDs, while those with a VSD have been described as intermediate or transitional AVSDs. AVSDs represent approximately 4% of congenital cardiac anomalies and are frequently associated with other cardiac malformations. AVSDs comprise 30%-40% of the cardiac abnormalities seen in patients with Down syndrome.

A complete AVSD is characterized by a common atrioventricular orifice, rather than separate mitral and tricuspid orifices, and a deficiency of endocardial cushion tissue, which results in an ASD and an inlet type of VSD (Figure 19–33). AVSDs were subclassified by Rastelli into the following three types according to the morphology of the anterior leaflet of the common AV valve:

Type A: The anterior bridging leaflet is divided and attached to the septum by multiple chordae.

Type B: The anterior bridging leaflet is attached to a papillary muscle in the right ventricle.

Type C: The anterior bridging leaflet is free-floating with no attachments except to the valve annulus.

When both left and right AV valves equally share the common AV valve orifice, the AVSD is termed balanced. Occasionally, the orifice may favor the right AV valve (right dominance) or the left AV valve (left dominance). In marked right dominance, the left AV valve and left ventricle are hypoplastic and frequently coexist with other left-sided abnormalities, including aortic stenosis, hypoplasia of the aorta, and coarctation. Conversely, marked left dominance results in a deficient right AV valve with associated hypoplasia of

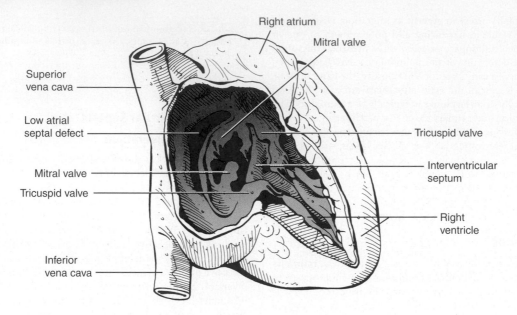

Right atrium

Mitral valve

Superior vena cava

Low atrial septal defect

Tricuspid valve

Interventricular septum

Mitral valve

Tricuspid valve

Right ventricle

Inferior vena cava

▲ **Figure 19–33.** Complete atrioventricular canal. The most common type has a divided anterior bridging leaflet. Both the left and right valvular components are attached to the interventricular septum with long, nonfused chordae. The left and right components of the posterior bridging leaflet are not separated.

the right ventricle, pulmonary stenosis or atresia, and TOF. Patients with severe imbalance require staged single-ventricle reconstruction.

The conduction tissue is displaced in an ASVD and is at risk during the surgical repair. The AV node is located posteriorly and inferiorly of its normal position toward the coronary sinus in the triangle of Koch. This triangle is bounded by the coronary sinus, the posterior attachment of the inferior bridging leaflet, and the rim of the ASD. The bundle of His courses posteriorly and inferiorly to run along the leftward aspect of the crest of the VSD, giving off the left bundle branch and continuing as the right bundle branch.

Cardiac anomalies associated with AVSDs include: PDA (10%) and TOF (10%). Important abnormalities of the left AV valve include single papillary muscle (parachute mitral valve) (2%-6%) and double orifice mitral valve (8%-14%). A persistent left superior vena cava with or without an unroofed coronary sinus is encountered in 3% of patients with an AVSD. Double-outlet right ventricle (2%) significantly complicates or may even preclude complete surgical correction. As mentioned previously, left ventricular outflow tract obstruction from subaortic stenosis or redundant AV valve tissue occurs in 4%-7%.

B. Clinical Findings

The predominant hemodynamic features of an AVSD are the result of left-to-right shunting at the atrial and ventricular

levels. In the absence of ventricular level shunting, the hemodynamics and clinical presentation of a patient with an incomplete AVSD resemble that of a typical secundum ASD with right atrial and RV volume overload. Patients with a complete AVSD with both atrial-level and ventricular-level shunting generally present early in infancy with signs and symptoms of congestive heart failure. In addition, moderate or severe left AV valve regurgitation occurs in approximately 10% of patients with an AVSD worsening the clinical picture. On physical examination, the precordium is hyperactive, often with a prominent thrill. Auscultatory findings include a systolic murmur along the left sternal border, a high-pitched murmur at the apex from the left AV valve regurgitation, and a middiastolic flow murmur across the common A-V valve. In the presence of elevated PVR, there may be a split first heart sound. Significant cardiomegaly and pulmonary overcirculation are found on the CXR. Electrocardiogram reveals biventricular hypertrophy, atrial enlargement, prolonged PR interval, leftward axis, and counterclockwise frontal plane loop. Echocardiography is diagnostic, defining the atrial and ventricular level shunting, valvular anatomy, and any associated anomalies. Up to 90% of untreated individuals with a complete AVSD develop pulmonary vascular disease by 1 year of age due to the large left-to-right shunt, potentially exacerbated by the associated AV valve regurgitation. Patients with trisomy 21 tend to develop pulmonary vascular obstructive disease earlier than chromosomally normal infants due to small airway disease, chronic hypoventilation, and elevated P_{CO_2}. Initial aggressive medical management is undertaken to relieve the symptoms of congestive heart failure. Elective surgical correction should be performed by age 3-6 months. Earlier intervention is indicated for failure of medical management.

Cardiac catheterization should be performed for patients over the age of 1 year, for patients with signs or symptoms of increased PVR, or in some cases to further evaluate other associated major cardiac anomalies. If the PVR is high, it is important to remeasure it while the child is breathing 100% oxygen with and without nitric oxide. If the pulmonary resistance falls, it implies that much of the elevated resistance is dynamic and can be managed in the perioperative period by ventilatory manipulation, supplemental oxygen, and nitric oxide. More recently, sildenafil has been shown to decrease elevation in PVR in children with congenital heart disease. Markedly elevated PVR (> 10 Woods units·m²) that does not respond to oxygen administration is generally considered a contraindication to repair.

C. Treatment

Operative treatment is almost always necessary as soon as symptoms are observed to prevent further clinical deterioration. Even in the absence of symptoms, operation is best performed before 6 months of age. Pulmonary artery banding, which permits delaying the repair until the child is larger, is no longer used today except in select complex or single-ventricle cases, extremely low birth weight or prematurity, and very poor clinical condition. This approach exposes the child to the risks of two operations, and the overall mortality exceeds that of primary repair in infancy. Patients with incomplete AVSDs usually require repair within the first few years of life.

Two techniques are widely employed for the repair of complete AVSDs: a 1-patch technique and a 2-patch technique. Incomplete AVSDs are repaired with the single-patch technique. Regardless of which approach is selected, the goals are to close the ASD and VSD and to separate the common AV valve into two nonstenotic, competent valves. The cleft in the anterior leaflet of the mitral valve is generally closed to lessen the risk of long-term mitral regurgitation. For the 2-patch technique, separate patches are used for the ASD and VSD. For the 1-patch technique, the superior and inferior bridging leaflets are divided along a line separating them into right and left components. A single patch is utilized to close both the ventricular and ASDs. The cut edges of the leaflets are then resuspended to the patch. For defects with a small VSD component, a modified single-patch technique may be employed. For this method, a single patch is sewn directly to the rim of the VSD, sandwiching the bridging leaflets between the patch and the crest of the VSD.

The short-term and long-term success of the operation is highly dependent on the status of the PVR and the surgeon's ability to maintain competence of the mitral valve. In developed countries, it is fortunately relatively uncommon for patients to present late in with an AVSD and refractory PVR elevations. Although earlier reports recommend that the cleft in the left AV valve should not be closed and the valve should be treated as a trileaflet structure, most authors now believe that closure of the cleft is an important mechanism in preventing postoperative left AV valve regurgitation. Significant AV valve regurgitation at the conclusion of surgery, severe dysplasia of the left AV valve, and failure to close the cleft of the left AV valve have been identified as important risk factors for reoperation. Significant postoperative left AV valve regurgitation is also a risk factor for operative and long-term mortality. The cleft should not be completely closed in the presence of a single papillary muscle to avoid causing the left AV valve stenosis. In the case of a double-orifice valve, the bridging tissue should not be divided to create a single opening in the valve.

D. Prognosis

Operative mortality is related largely to associated cardiac anomalies and left AV valve regurgitation. Mortality for repair of uncomplicated incomplete AVSDs is 0%-1.6%, while the addition of left AV valve regurgitation increases mortality to 4%-6%. For complete AVSDs, the mortality without left AV valve regurgitation is approximately 4%-5%, compared with 13% when significant degrees of regurgitation are present. The difference in operative mortality between patients with and without regurgitation underscores the importance of careful management of the left AV valve.

The majority of reoperations after repair of AVSD are due to left AV valve regurgitation or the development of subaortic stenosis. Significant postoperative AV valve regurgitation occurs in 6%-26% of patients, necessitating reoperation for valve repair or replacement in 3%-12%. The incidence of permanent complete heart block is approximately 1%-2%. Heart block encountered in the immediate postoperative period may be transient due to edema of or trauma to the AV node or bundle of His. However, right bundle branch block is common (22%).

Backer CL, Stewart RD, Mavroudis C: What is the best technique for repair of complete atrioventricular canal? *Semin Thorac Cardiovasc Surg* 2007;19:249.

Harmander B, Aydemir NA, Karaci AR, et al: Results for surgical correction of complete atrioventricular septal defect: associations with age, surgical era, and technique. *J Card Surg* 2012;27:745-753.

Kaza AK, Colan SD, Jaggers J, et al: Surgical interventions for atrioventricular septal defect subtypes: the pediatric heart network experience. *Ann Thorac Surg* 2011;92:1468-1475.

Shuhaiber JH, Ho Sy, Rigby M, et al: Current options and outcomes for the management of atrioventricular septal defect. *Eur J Cardiothorac Surg* 2009;35:891-900.

Stulak JM, Burkhart HM, Dearani JA, et al: Reoperations after repair of partial atrioventricular septal defect: a 45-year single-center experience. *Ann Thorac Surg* 2010;89:1352-1359.

Welke KF et al: Population-base perspective of long-term outcomes after surgical repair of partial atrioventricular septal defect. *Ann Thorac Surg* 2007;82:624.

▶ Patent Ductus Arteriosus

A. General Considerations

The ductus arteriosus is a normal fetal vascular structure that allows blood from the right ventricle to bypass the high-resistance pulmonary vascular bed and pass directly to the systemic circulation. The ductus communicates between the main pulmonary artery (or proximal left pulmonary artery) and the proximal descending thoracic aorta. Histologically, the media of the ductus contains a predominance of smooth muscle cells, while the media of the aorta and pulmonary artery contain well-developed elastic fibers. Vasocontrol of the ductus is mediated by two important mechanisms: oxygen tension and prostaglandin levels. During fetal development, low oxygen tension and high levels of circulating prostaglandin maintain ductal patency. During the final trimester, the ductus becomes less sensitive to prostaglandins and more sensitive to the effects of oxygen tension. Following birth, the rise in oxygen tension and fall in prostaglandins (which were previously supplied principally by the placenta) lead to ductal closure, which is usually complete by 12-24 hours. After closure, the ductus becomes a fibrous cord known as the ligamentum arteriosum. Failure of closure of the ductus leads to the condition called patent ductus arteriosus (PDA) which occurs in about 1 out of 1200 live births and accounts for 7% of congenital heart defect. The incidence is much higher in premature infants (> 20%). This elevated incidence is thought to be related to immaturity of the ductal wall resulting in impaired sensitivity to oxygen tension.

PDA may occur as an isolated defect, or it may occur in association with a number of other anomalies. Patency of the ductus arteriosus is desirable in a number of defects in which there is either inadequate pulmonary blood flow (such as pulmonary atresia) or inadequate systemic blood flow (as in severe coarctation of the aorta). The discovery that extrinsic delivery of prostaglandins can maintain ductal patency has played a critical role in improving the survival of these patients.

B. Clinical Findings

The physiologic manifestation of PDA is shunting of blood across the ductus. The shunt volume is determined by the size of the ductus and by the ratio of pulmonary to systemic vascular resistance. At birth, the PVR drops dramatically and continues to decline over the first several weeks of life. As a result, shunting across a PDA is from left-to-right. Excessive pulmonary blood flow can lead to congestive heart failure. In extreme cases, hypotension and systemic malperfusion may result. Patients with a large PDA who survive infancy tend to develop pulmonary vascular obstructive disease. Eisenmenger physiology results when the PVR exceeds the systemic vascular resistance, producing a reversal of shunting across the ductus to right-to-left. This leads to cyanosis and, eventually, RV failure. Small PDAs may persist to adulthood without producing any symptoms or physiologic derangement. Endocarditis and endarteritis have been reported as long-term complications of PDA.

In patients with PDA, symptoms are proportional to the shunt volume and the presence of associated defects. Left-to-right shunting produces volume overload of the left heart. Infants with congestive heart failure demonstrate symptoms of tachypnea, tachycardia, and poor feeding. Older children may present with recurrent respiratory infections, fatigue, and failure to thrive. Physical findings include a widened pulse pressure and a continuous "machinery" murmur heard best along the left upper sternal border. Chest radiography shows increased pulmonary vascular markings and left heart enlargement. Left ventricular hypertrophy and left atrial enlargement may be evident on the electrocardiogram. Echocardiography is the diagnostic method of choice. Diagnostic cardiac catheterization is performed only in older patients with suspected pulmonary hypertension to evaluate for pulmonary vascular obstructive disease. More frequently, catheterization is utilized for transcatheter occlusion of the ductus.

C. Treatment

PDA closure is performed for all symptomatic patients. Closure is also recommended for asymptomatic patients due to the risk of heart failure, pulmonary hypertension, and endocarditis. Closure of the ductus may be accomplished by one of three approaches: pharmacologic, surgical, and endovascular. Indomethacin, which is a prostaglandin inhibitor, stimulates PDA closure in premature infants. It is rarely effective in full-term infants. The dosing regimen is 0.1-0.2 mg/kg intravenously at 12- or 24-hour intervals for a total of three doses. This is effective in about 80% of premature babies. Due to its side effects, indomethacin is contraindicated in patients with sepsis, renal insufficiency, intracranial hemorrhage, or bleeding disorders. Failure of indomethacin after two complete courses results in referral for surgical closure.

The surgical approach to PDA is through a left posterolateral thoracotomy via the third or fourth intercostal space. The pleura is incised over the proximal descending thoracic aorta, which allows medial retraction of the vagus nerve. The recurrent laryngeal nerve curves behind the ductus and should be protected throughout the procedure. Dissection is then performed to demonstrate the pertinent anatomy. In many cases, the ductus is the largest vascular structure present, and it must not be confused with the aorta. Ductal tissue is extremely friable, so direct manipulation is minimized. In premature infants, the ductus is controlled with a single surgical clip; this procedure is commonly performed in the neonatal intensive care unit, thereby avoiding problems associated with patient transfer. In older patients, occlusion of the ductus is achieved with simple silk ligature or, preferably, by division between ligatures to minimize recurrence.

Recently, thoracoscopic techniques have been developed to perform PDA ligation. This approach has the potential benefits of decreased pain and quicker recovery. Disadvantages include a substantial learning curve and increased operating time.

A number of endovascular devices have been developed for the purpose of transcatheter occlusion of the PDA. This approach is very successful in older infants, children, and adults with small and moderate sized PDAs and has become the treatment of choice at many centers. Surgical therapy is reserved for PDAs having a large diameter or very short length.

Rarely, an adult will present with a significant PDA. These patients must be carefully evaluated for the presence of pulmonary vascular obstructive disease prior to ductal closure. If the patient is not a candidate for device closure, surgical closure can be problematic. Calcification of the ductal wall is common in adults, which makes ligation hazardous. In some cases, cardiopulmonary bypass may be required with patch closure of the ductus from within the pulmonary artery.

D. Prognosis

Closure of the ductus by surgical or transcatheter techniques is achieved with a mortality that approaches zero. Potential complications include pneumothorax, recurrent laryngeal nerve injury, and chylothorax (from injury to the thoracic duct). Long-term survival should be normal following PDA ligation in most patients. Survival in premature infants depends primarily on the extent of prematurity with its attendant complications.

Drighil A, Al Jufan M, Al Omrane K, et al: Safety of transcatheter patent ductus arteriosus closure in small weight infants. *J Interv Cardiol* 2012;4:391-394.

Giroud JM, Jacobs JP: Evolution of strategies for management of the patent arterial duct. *Cardiol Young* 2007;17:68.

Malviya M, Ohlsson A, Shah S: Surgical versus medical treatment with cyclooxygenase inhibitors for symptomatic patent ductus arteriosus in preterm infants. *Cochrane Database Syst Rev* 2013;3:CD003951.

Mosalli R, Alfaleh K: Prophylactic surgical ligation of patent ductus arteriosus for prevention of mortality and morbidity in extremely low birth weight infants. *Cochrane Database Syst Rev* 2008;(1):CD006181.

Van der Linde D, Konings EEM, Slager MA, et al: Birth prevalence of congenital heart disease world-wide: a systematic review and meta-analysis. *J Am Coll Cardiol* 2011;58:2241-2247.

2. Right-Sided Anomalies

▶ Pulmonary Stenosis

A. General Considerations

Isolated pulmonary stenosis occurs in 5%-8% of all congenital cardiac anomalies. The pulmonary valve is usually trileaflet with fusion of the commissures. The valve can appear thickened and domed on echocardiography. Most patients have an associated PFO or a secundum ASD. Pulmonary stenosis may be valvar or subvalvar due to muscular narrowing of the infundibulum (Figure 19-34).

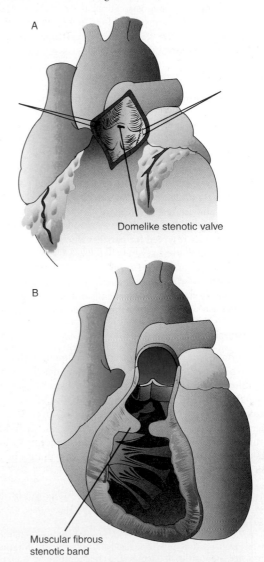

A

Domelike stenotic valve

B

Muscular fibrous
stenotic band

▲ **Figure 19-34.** Pulmonary stenosis. **A:** Valvular pulmonary stenosis. **B:** Infundibular pulmonary stenosis.

B. Clinical Findings

Young infants with severe pulmonary stenosis present with failure to thrive, right heart failure, and possibly hypoxic spells. Older children tend to have mild to moderate stenosis that is asymptomatic. They may, however, complain of shortness of breath with exertion or arrhythmias. The murmur of pulmonary stenosis tends to be prominent and therefore is not missed on routine examination. The presence of a systolic ejection murmur should prompt further workup, including an echocardiogram, which is diagnostic. Patients may be followed symptomatically with mild to moderate pulmonary stenosis. Surgical or catheter-based intervention should be considered for a gradient higher than 50 mm Hg, progressive ventricular hypertrophy, or new tricuspid regurgitation.

C. Treatment

Neonates presenting with profound cyanosis from severe pulmonary stenosis need to be placed on PGE_1 to maintain ductal patency. The ductus will maintain adequate pulmonary blood flow so that the patient can be stabilized. For isolated pulmonary stenosis, balloon valvuloplasty by an interventional cardiologist is highly successful and has replaced surgical intervention for the majority of patients. Asymptomatic infants with systemic RV pressures from pulmonary stenosis are also excellent candidates for balloon dilation. Surgical valvotomy or a transannular patch for pulmonary stenosis is reserved for patients who have failed balloon dilation, who have a severely hypoplastic valve annulus, or who have other associated anomalies including muscular infundibular narrowing. Older patients with progressive isolated pulmonary stenosis are excellent candidates for elective balloon dilation when they develop elevated RV pressures.

D. Prognosis

Early mortality for patients with critical pulmonary stenosis is 3%-10%. Restenosis occurs in 10%-25% of patients. Once the outflow obstruction is relieved, the RV hypertrophy and tricuspid insufficiency regress. Although overall survival is excellent for isolated pulmonary stenosis, over 50% of patients will require additional interventions, including repeat balloon dilation, pulmonary valve replacement, and ASD closure. Late atrial and ventricular arrhythmias occur in 38% of patients. Twenty-five year survival is 90%-96%.

Cuypers JA, Witsenburg M, van der Linde D, et al: Pulmonary stenosis: update on diagnosis and therapeutic options. *Heart* 2013. [epub ahead of print].

Harrild DM, Powell AJ, Tran TX, et al: Long-term pulmonary regurgitation following balloon valvuloplasty for pulmonary stenosis risk factors and relationship to exercise capacity and ventricular volume and function. *J Am Coll Cardiol* 2010;55:1041-1047.

Rigby ML: Severe aortic or pulmonary valve stenosis in premature infants. *Early Hum Dev* 2012;88:291-294.

Voet A, Rega F, de Bruaene AV, et al: Long-term outcome after treatment of isolated pulmonary valve stenosis. *Int J Cardiol* 2012;156:11-15.

▶ Ebstein's Anomaly

A. General Considerations

Ebstein's malformation was first described by Wilhelm Ebstein in 1866 as a constellation of clinical findings resulting from an abnormality of the tricuspid valve. It has become evident over time that the malformation is a disease of the entire right ventricle and the development of the tricuspid valve. It involves a spectrum of anatomical abnormalities of variable severity, which include apical displacement of the septal and mural leaflets of the tricuspid valve, which have failed to delaminate from the underlying myocardium; thinning or atrialization of the inlet component of the right ventricle, with variable dilation; and malformation of the anterosuperior leaflet, with anomalous attachments, redundancy, and fenestrations. Several other cardiac anomalies are often associated with the RV changes, such as atrial and VSDs, obstruction of the RV outlet, and Wolff–Parkinson–White syndrome. Ebstein's malformation can also afflict the left-sided systemic AV valve in the setting of congenitally corrected transposition.

B. Clinical Findings

The malformation is rare, accounting for no more than 1% of all congenital cardiac anomalies. Due to the significant anatomic variability in the abnormalities of the tricuspid valve and right ventricle, the age at presentation and severity of symptoms can also be highly variable. Patients who present in infancy have the poorest prognosis. There is a high rate of fetal death, hydrops, and pulmonary hypoplasia when the diagnosis is made during fetal life. Cyanosis is the most common presentation in infancy. These patients have severe tricuspid regurgitation with a poorly functioning right ventricle in the face of elevated pulmonary arterial resistance. The result is a state of low cardiac output dependent on right-to-left shunting across the fossa ovalis.

With less severe derangements of the tricuspid valve and preserved ventricular function, patients tend to present later in adolescence or early adulthood. Many patients are asymptomatic and present with a murmur noted on physical examination. In symptomatic patients, a common presentation involves the new onset of atrial arrhythmias or reentrant tachycardia. Exercise tolerance may be diminished, with cyanosis during extreme exertion if an ASD is present. Those patients with an intact atrial septum will often progress to congestive heart failure with increasing cardiomegaly.

Echocardiography is usually sufficient for accurate diagnosis and anatomic evaluation. The degree of displacement, tethering, and dysplasia of the valvar leaflets, as well as the amount of regurgitation, can be determined. Ventricular function and the extent of atrialization of the right ventricle can also be evaluated. Additional abnormalities, including the presence and direction of a shunt at the atrial level, can be assessed. Electrocardiographic findings include incomplete right bundle branch block, right axis deviation, ventricular preexcitation, and atrial arrhythmias. The CXR can vary from normal, in patients with mild anatomic abnormalities, to the classic "wall-to-wall" heart. Cardiac catheterization is rarely necessary.

C. Treatment

As noted previously, neonates often present with profound cyanosis and may require prostaglandins to maintain adequate flow of blood to the lungs during the early neonatal period when pulmonary resistance is high. It is important to distinguish functional from anatomic pulmonary atresia. In patients with functional atresia, it may be possible to wean them from the infusion of prostaglandins while maintaining adequate saturations of oxygen as pulmonary resistance falls. These patients can then be followed for development of further symptoms.

In neonates who cannot be weaned from prostaglandins due to unacceptable levels of hypoxemia, or in those with anatomic pulmonary atresia, it is necessary to construct a systemic-to-pulmonary shunt to maintain adequate pulmonary blood flow. For neonates who also develop significant symptoms of congestive heart failure while on prostaglandin, it is necessary to address the underlying valvar pathology. The options include closure of the tricuspid valve, with or without fenestration, along with construction of a modified Blalock-Taussig shunt, repair of the tricuspid valve if ventricular function is reasonable, or cardiac transplantation.

In the older patient with progressive symptoms, a variety of surgical options exist to address the malformed tricuspid valve. Most are based on techniques designed to mobilize the leading edge of the anterosuperior leaflet, aiming to create a competent monocusp valve with or without plication of the atrialized portion of the right ventricle. There is ongoing debate as to the necessity of obliterating the atrialized portion of the right ventricle. Historically, plication of this portion of the ventricle has been an integral part of most repairs, albeit that no clear physiologic benefit with regards to improved ventricular function has been demonstrated. In addition, the potential exists for injury to the right coronary artery as a result of the plication, which may adversely impact late outcomes and contribute to ventricular arrhythmias.

Replacement of the tricuspid valve is a final option. The late survival free from reoperation, however, has been equivalent to valvar repair. If replacement is required,

heterografts are preferred over mechanical valves due to risks of thrombosis. Other options using tissue valves include the insertion of pulmonary autografts, mitral valve homografts, and "top hat" mounted pulmonary or aortic homografts. When replacing the valve, the sutures should be brought around the coronary sinus, leaving it to drain into the right ventricle so as to minimize potential injury to the AV node. An open antiarrhythmia procedure is frequently performed concomitantly.

D. Prognosis

Ebstein's malformation is a rare but challenging congenital cardiac defect. The high degree of anatomic variability makes it difficult to have a standardized approach to these children. The symptomatic neonate carries a very grave prognosis. The presence of associated cardiac and other congenital anomalies often make survival impossible. Surgical options are limited at this age and often still result in a poor outcome. Medical management, if possible, is the best, as surgical success improves with age. If surgery is required, conversion to functional tricuspid atresia often offers the best survival, as the ventricle in the severely symptomatic neonate functions poorly. Transplantation remains an option, but the availability of organs limits its utility.

Patients who are not symptomatic in the neonatal period will often remain free from symptoms well into adolescence. Electrophysiologic symptoms usually precede symptoms of congestive heart failure. Indications for repair at these ages include symptoms, cyanosis, and progressive cardiomegaly.

Brown ML, Dearani JA, Danielson GK, et al: Functional status after operation for Ebstein anomaly: the Mayo Clinic experience. *J Am Cull Cardiol* 2008;52:460-466.

Dearani JA, Said SM, O'Leary PW, et al: Anatomic repair of Ebstein's malformation: lessons learned with cone reconstruction. *Ann Thorac Surg* 2013;95:220-228.

Malhotra SP, Petrossian E, Reddy VM, et al: Selective right ventricular unloading and novel technical concepts in Ebstein's anomaly. *Ann Thorac Surg* 2009;88:1975-1981.

Paranon S, Acar P: Ebstein's anomaly of the tricuspid valve: from fetus to adult: congenital heart disease. *Heart* 2008;94:237.

Shinkawa T, Polimenakos AC, Gomez-Fifer CA, et al: Management and long-term outcome of neonatal Ebstein anomaly. *J Thorac Cardiovasc Surg* 2010;139:354-358.

3. Left-Sided Anomalies

▶ Aortic Stenosis

A. General Considerations

Aortic stenosis is a form of left ventricular outflow tract obstruction that may occur at a valvar (70%), subvalvar (25%), or supravalvar (5%) level. Aortic stenosis occurs in about 4% of patients with congenital heart disease. The severity of aortic stenosis may be graded as mild (peak pressure gradient < 50 mm Hg), moderate (50 to 75 mm Hg), or severe (> 75 mm Hg).

Valvar aortic stenosis occurs secondary to maldevelopment of the aortic valve. Most commonly, a bicuspid valve is present, although tricuspid and unicuspid valves are also represented. In valvar aortic stenosis, the leaflets are thickened and frequently dysmorphic, and there is a variable degree of leaflet fusion along the commissures. The aortic annulus may be hypoplastic. In 20% of cases, valvar aortic stenosis is associated with other cardiac defects, most commonly coarctation of the aorta, PDA, VSD, or mitral stenosis. Men with valvar aortic stenosis outnumber women by a ratio of 4:1. There is a wide spectrum of clinical presentations of valvar aortic stenosis, but patients tend to present in one of two groups. Neonates and infants with severe aortic stenosis develop symptoms of rapidly progressive congestive heart failure, while older children generally have less severe obstruction and a more slowly progressive course.

Subvalvar aortic stenosis occurs below the level of the aortic valve and may be discrete (80%) or diffuse (20%). Discrete (or membranous) subaortic stenosis is rarely seen in infants and tends to progress over time. This lesion consists of a crescent or circumferential fibrous or fibromuscular membrane that protrudes into the left ventricular outflow tract. The pathogenesis of discrete subaortic stenosis is unknown, but it is thought to be an acquired lesion that develops secondary to a congenital abnormality of the left ventricular outflow tract in which abnormal flow patterns lead to endocardial injury with resultant fibrosis. Although the aortic valve leaflets are usually normal in discrete subaortic stenosis, the turbulent flow created by the obstruction can cause leaflet thickening and progressive aortic insufficiency. Diffuse subaortic stenosis is a more severe form of stenosis that creates a long, tunnel-like obstruction. Diffuse subaortic stenosis should be distinguished from hypertrophic cardiomyopathy. Both forms of subaortic stenosis are associated with a high risk of endocarditis.

Supravalvar aortic stenosis is characterized by thickening of the wall of the ascending aorta. The lesion may be localized (80%) to the region of the sinotubular ridge (at the level of the valve commissures), creating an hourglass deformity, or it may be more diffuse (20%), extending into the aortic arch and its branches. In both varieties, the aortic valve leaflets may be abnormal. The free edges of the aortic valve leaflets may adhere to the aortic wall in the region of intraluminal thickening, and this may lead to reduced coronary blood flow during diastole. Aortic wall thickening may also extend into the coronary ostia and further impair coronary blood flow. Associated cardiac lesions are common, particularly branch pulmonary artery stenoses. A genetic basis for supravalvar aortic stenosis has been established. About 50% of cases of supravalvar aortic stenosis are associated with Williams syndrome, in which a partial deletion of chromosome 7 (including the elastin gene) leads to the triad of supravalvar stenosis, mental retardation, and a characteristic "elfin" facies. Isolated mutations in the elastin gene have also been shown to produce familial supravalvar aortic stenosis with an autosomal dominant pattern of transmission. There is a significant incidence of endocarditis in patients with supravalvar aortic stenosis. Sudden death is frequently reported and is probably related to coronary obstruction.

B. Clinical Findings

Severe aortic stenosis is usually well-tolerated during fetal development. Although left ventricular output and antegrade flow across the aortic valve are decreased, the right ventricle compensates with increased output, and systemic perfusion is maintained by flow across the ductus. After birth, there is increased venous return to the left heart, and this exacerbates the pressure load created by the stenotic aortic valve, leading to left ventricular dysfunction. As the ductus closes during postnatal life, systemic malperfusion may develop with resulting hypotension, acidosis, and oliguria. Coronary perfusion is also impaired due to the combination of systemic hypotension and elevated left ventricular end-diastolic pressures. Patients with critical aortic stenosis typically exhibit severe left ventricular dysfunction. These patients usually show signs of distress soon after birth. On examination, there is impaired distal perfusion with poor capillary refill and diminished, thready pulses. A systolic ejection murmur may be absent if the cardiac output is severely diminished. Differential cyanosis may be observed due to perfusion of the lower body with desaturated blood shunting through the ductus. The electrocardiogram shows left ventricular hypertrophy, and the CXR displays cardiomegaly and pulmonary congestion. Echocardiography establishes the diagnosis.

In contrast to infants with critical aortic stenosis, older children with valvar aortic stenosis usually present with less severe stenosis (mild or moderate), and most are asymptomatic. Symptoms of angina, syncope, and congestive heart failure are not commonly reported. Congenital valvar aortic stenosis is a progressive lesion, however, and survival is dependent on the severity of stenosis and its rate of progression. Sudden cardiac death is the most common cause of mortality. Endocarditis occurs in less than 1% of patients. The diagnosis of valvar aortic stenosis in older children can frequently be made on physical examination. There is a classic systolic crescendo-decrescendo murmur at the upper sternal border, which radiates to the neck. An ejection click is often present. A visible apical impulse is suggestive of significant left ventricular hypertrophy. In severe cases, the pulse may be weak and delayed (pulsus tardus et parvus). The electrocardiogram shows left ventricular hypertrophy. The CXR is usually normal. Echocardiography accurately defines the level of stenosis and its severity. Using Doppler techniques, the pressure gradient across the stenotic valve may be estimated using a simplified form of the Bernoulli equation $P = 4V^2$, where P is the pressure gradient and V is the peak flow velocity. Cardiac catheterization is generally reserved for therapeutic intervention.

The clinical findings in subvalvar aortic stenosis are similar to those for valvar stenosis. The signs and symptoms of supravalvar aortic stenosis are similar to those in other forms of left ventricular outflow tract obstruction. The diagnosis is made by echocardiography, but cardiac catheterization or cardiac MRI is essential to define the aortic, coronary, and pulmonary arterial anatomy prior to surgical intervention.

C. Treatment

The neonate or infant with critical aortic stenosis represents a true emergency. Endotracheal intubation and inotropic support is routine. Ductal patency is maintained with prostaglandins, and acidosis is corrected. All patients with critical aortic stenosis require some form of urgent intervention. The approach is determined by the valve morphology and by the presence of associated defects. In its most extreme form, critical aortic stenosis may be associated with underdeveloped left-sided cardiac chambers and therefore may represent a form of HLHS. In these cases, single-ventricle palliation must be undertaken. For patients with adequate left-sided chambers, relief of aortic stenosis may be achieved by one of the following three approaches: percutaneous balloon valvuloplasty, surgical valvotomy, or aortic valve replacement. Balloon valvuloplasty is generally considered the procedure of choice when the aortic valve annulus is adequate and there are no associated cardiac defects. Alternatively, surgical valvotomy may be accomplished by closed or open techniques. The closed approach is performed using cardiopulmonary bypass without aortic cross-clamping. Dilators of increasing size are passed through a ventriculotomy in the left ventricular apex and advanced across the aortic valve. Some centers prefer open surgical valvotomy, which allows a precise valvotomy under direct vision, although aortic cross-clamping with cardioplegia is necessary. In all cases, the goal of therapy is to relieve stenosis without creating excessive aortic insufficiency. Dramatic clinical improvement is expected following balloon or surgical valve valvotomy, and early survivals of greater than 80% have been reported. The incidence of aortic insufficiency is slightly higher following balloon valvotomy. In most cases, however, stenosis will recur and repeat valvotomy or aortic valve replacement will eventually be required. Aortic valve replacement is problematic in the neonate due to small patient size. In these cases, many consider the best valve replacement to be a pulmonary autograft (Ross procedure) with enlargement of the aortic annulus (Konno aortoventriculoplasty). The Ross–Konno procedure has been used successfully for neonates with critical aortic stenosis in whom the aortic annulus is hypoplastic and for

selected patients in whom valvuloplasty was unsuccessful. Survival following the Ross-Konno procedure in infants has been shown to be excellent. Growth of the pulmonary autograft has been documented, thereby making it an ideal valve replacement for children. Unfortunately, as part of the Ross procedure, the pulmonary valve must be replaced using a cryopreserved homograft, which does not grow, and homograft replacement must be anticipated at intervals as the patient grows.

All patients with severe valvar aortic stenosis should undergo intervention, as should all symptomatic patients with moderate stenosis. Asymptomatic patients with mild or moderate stenosis are generally observed. As described for critical aortic stenosis, the techniques used to relieve aortic stenosis in older patients include percutaneous balloon valvuloplasty, surgical valvulotomy, and valve replacement. Balloon valvuloplasty is usually performed as the primary intervention and is associated with a success rate of nearly 90% and a mortality of less than 1%. Open surgical valvotomy is an alternative approach with similar results. For valves that are severely dysplastic, develop restenosis after intervention, or become insufficient as a result of prior intervention, valve replacement may be necessary. For older children, there are more options for valve replacement. The choices include mechanical prostheses, bioprosthetic valves, and tissue substitutes, such as porcine xenografts, cryopreserved human allografts, and pulmonary autografts (Ross procedure). The mechanical valves are the most durable but require chronic anticoagulation. The bioprosthetic and tissue valves do not require long-term anticoagulation but tend to deteriorate over time (with the exception of the pulmonary autograft). The pulmonary autograft has the potential advantage of growth but the homograft used to replace the pulmonary valve will require replacement. Selection of the appropriate replacement valve is a complex decision requiring input from all involved parties.

Intervention for discrete subvalvar stenosis is usually undertaken when the gradient exceeds 30-50 mm Hg or when aortic insufficiency is present. In these patients, resection of the membrane is readily performed by a transaortic approach. In order to reduce the incidence of restenosis, many centers advocate concurrent performance of a septal myomectomy to alter the geometry of the left ventricular outflow tract.

When diffuse subaortic stenosis is associated with hypoplasia of the aortic annulus, repair is best achieved with a Konno aortoventriculoplasty, whereby an incision is carried across the aortic annulus and subjacent ventricular septum, the opening patched, and an aortic valve implanted. Patients with an adequate aortic annulus may undergo a septoplasty (modified Konno), in which the septal incision is confined to the immediate subvalvar area and a patch is used to widen the left ventricular outflow tract without replacing the aortic valve.

Operative intervention is indicated for patients with supravalvar aortic stenosis in whom the gradient exceeds 50 mm Hg. A number of operations have been proposed for the treatment of localized supravalvar stenosis. The classical repair involves a longitudinal incision across the obstruction in the ascending aorta, which is extended into the noncoronary sinus. The thickened, hypertrophic ridge is resected by endarterectomy, and the aortotomy is augmented with an elliptical patch. A variation of this repair involves creation of an inverted-Y aortotomy with one limb of the Y extended into the noncoronary sinus and the other into the right coronary sinus. A Y-shaped patch is then used to augment the aortotomy. Finally, the Brom repair is performed by transection of the ascending aorta beyond the supravalvar ridge. Separate incisions are then made through the supravalvar ridge into each sinus of Valsalva. Triangular patches are placed to augment each of these incisions, thereby relieving the supravalvar obstruction. Reconnection of the aortic root to the ascending aorta completes the repair. The repair of the diffuse type of supravalvar stenosis is performed under circulatory arrest with extensive patching of the ascending aorta, transverse arch, and involved arch arteries. Branch pulmonary stenoses are best managed using transcatheter techniques.

D. Prognosis

Operative mortality approaches zero for resection of discrete subaortic stenosis. The recurrence rate of discrete stenosis following membrane resection and myomectomy has been reported to be as low as 4%. Despite the technical complexity of repair of diffuse subaortic stenosis, excellent results have been reported with high survival and freedom from reoperation. The results of surgery for localized supravalvar aortic stenosis are generally good with low operative mortality and excellent long-term survival. The diffuse form is more difficult to treat, and recurrence is more likely. Overall results are much worse when severe bilateral pulmonary artery stenoses are present. The mortality for aortic valve replacement regardless of valve choice is 2%-5%. The need for reoperation is dependent on valve choice and patient size. Early and late ventricular arrhythmias may occur commonly in patients with significant left ventricular hypertrophy.

Brown JW, Rodefeld MD, Ruzmetov M, et al: Surgical valvuloplasty versus balloon aortic dilation for congenital aortic stenosis: are evidence-based outcomes relevant? *Ann Thorac Surg* 2012;94:146-153.

Coskun KO, Popov AF, Tirilomis T, et al: Aortic valve surgery in congenital heart disease: a single-center experience. *Artif Organs* 2010;34:E85-E90.

Hickey EJ, Caldarone CA, Blackstone EH, et al: Biventricular strategies for neonatal critical aortic stenosis: high mortality associated with early reintervention. *J Thorac Cardiovasc Surg* 2012;144:409-417.

Maskatia SA, Ing FF, Justino H, et al: Twenty-five year experience with balloon aortic valvuloplasty for congenital aortic stenosis. *Am J Cardiol* 2011;108:1024-1028.

Piccardo A, Ghez O, Gariboldi V, et al: Ross and Ross-Konno procedures in infants, children, and adolescents: a 13-year experience. *J Heart Valve Dis* 2009;18(1):76-82.

▶ Aortic Coarctation

A. General Considerations

Coarctation of the aorta is a narrowing of the proximal descending thoracic aorta distal to the origin of the left subclavian artery, near the insertion of the ductus arteriosus (or ligamentum arteriosum). The severity of luminal narrowing and the length of the aorta affected are variable. Coarctation is thought to occur as a result of ectopic tissue from the ductus arteriosus that migrates into the wall of the adjacent aorta. After birth, as the ductus closes, the ectopic tissue in the aorta also constricts. Frequently, a posterior shelf of tissue is present at the point of most severe obstruction. The aortic obstruction caused by coarctation creates a pressure load on the left ventricle.

The incidence of coarctation is about 0.5 per 1000 live births, and its prevalence is about 7% of congenital heart defects. Coarctation is commonly associated with other heart defects, including bicuspid aortic valve (in more than 50% of cases), PDA, and VSD. Other left-sided obstructive lesions may also be present, such as aortic arch hypoplasia, aortic stenosis, mitral stenosis, and left ventricular hypoplasia. Coarctation is also recognized to occur in association with Turner syndrome.

B. Clinical Findings

Patients with severe coarctation present in the newborn period. Aortic obstruction is so significant that perfusion of the lower body is dependent upon flow from the ductus arteriosus. Spontaneous ductal closure typically worsens the aortic obstruction and may lead to malperfusion of tissues distal to the coarctation. The pressure load on the left ventricle may precipitate congestive heart failure. Patients may develop shock with severe acidosis, oliguria, and diminished distal pulses. Infants with severe coarctation will generally not survive without intervention.

Older children with coarctation are usually asymptomatic. The diagnosis is commonly made on the basis of hypertension in the upper extremities with decreased pulses in the lower extremities. Noninvasive blood pressure measurements in all four extremities help to quantify the severity of aortic obstruction. Older patients tend to develop extensive collateral arteries that bypass the obstruction. Life expectancy for these patients is 34 years without operation typically due to the development of heart failure. Other long-term complications of coarctation include aortic dissection (21%), endocarditis (18%) (frequently involving a bicuspid aortic valve), intracranial hemorrhage (12%) (from Berry aneurysms, which occur more commonly in patients with coarctation), endarteritis (in the poststenotic area of the aorta at the site of the jet of turbulent flow), and aortic aneurysm.

The diagnosis of coarctation can usually be made clinically. The infant with significant coarctation is frequently asymptomatic at birth but following closure of the ductus develops signs of heart failure such as irritability, tachypnea, and poor feeding. Lower extremity pulses are absent, and upper extremity pulses may be weak. Chest radiography shows cardiomegaly and pulmonary venous congestion. There is a left ventricular strain pattern on the electrocardiogram. Echocardiography is usually diagnostic, demonstrating narrowing of the aorta at the coarctation site with a loss of pulsatility in the descending aorta.

In older children and adults with coarctation, a pressure gradient between the arms and legs usually can be demonstrated by measuring cuff pressures in all four extremities. On chest radiography, rib notching may be evident, secondary to erosion of the inferior rib borders from the development of large intercostal collateral vessels. Echocardiography usually confirms the diagnosis. Anatomic details may also be clarified with CTA and cMRI. Cardiac catheterization is usually not necessary.

C. Treatment

Generally, all patients with coarctation should undergo surgical repair if the gradient is greater than 20 mm Hg. For neonates, the acute medical management includes initiation of PGE$_1$ for the purpose of reopening the ductus; this maneuver partially relieves the aortic obstruction and augments perfusion of the lower body due to improved antegrade flow across the arch as well as right-to-left flow across the ductus. Prostaglandins are usually effective for reopening the ductus when initiated within 3-7 days of life but are less successful thereafter.

Surgical repair of coarctation is usually performed through a left posterolateral thoracotomy via the third or fourth intercostal space. The descending thoracic aorta, ductus (or ligamentum), transverse aortic arch, and brachiocephalic vessels are mobilized. Care is taken to preserve the vagus nerve and its recurrent laryngeal branch.

The coarctation is usually evident externally by narrowing or posterior indentation; however, the degree of internal narrowing is usually much more severe. A dose of heparin (100 units/kg) may be given intravenously for patients younger than 2 years. Proximal and distal control of the aorta is achieved using clamps. Usually, the proximal clamp is positioned on the transverse arch between the innominate and left carotid vessels with concomitant occlusion of the left carotid and left subclavian. In infants and children, the preferred surgical approach to coarctation is resection

with extended end-to-end repair. A generous resection of the coarctation segment is performed. The proximal aorta is then spatulated along the lesser curvature and the distal aorta along the greater curvature. An extended end-to-end anastomosis is then performed.

In older children and adults, it may not be possible to perform a resection with primary repair without creating excessive tension on the anastomosis, which may lead to hemorrhage or scarring with recurrent coarctation. An alternative strategy is necessary in these cases. Patch aortoplasty may be performed in children in whom further growth is anticipated. The subclavian flap repair augments the narrowed aorta using native arterial tissue. Blood flow to the left arm is maintained by collateral vessels, although long-term studies have demonstrated a slight discrepancy in limb length in some patients. Prosthetic patch material may also be used. By avoiding circumferential prosthetic material, growth potential of the native aorta is preserved. The disadvantage of patch repair is a high risk of aneurysm formation. In adults, where growth is no longer an issue, resection of the coarctation may be performed with subsequent placement of a prosthetic interposition graft (either Dacron or polytetrafluoroethylene).

One of the principal concerns during coarctation repair is interruption of distal aortic blood flow, especially to the spinal cord. The anterior spinal artery is fed by major radicular branches from intercostal arteries. In patients without well-formed collaterals, ischemia of the spinal cord may be precipitated by aortic cross-clamping, and paraplegia may result. Protective measures include induction of mild hypothermia, maintenance of a high proximal aortic pressure, and minimization of cross-clamp time. In older patients, distal aortic perfusion may be maintained by the technique of left heart bypass, where oxygenated blood is taken from the left atrium and delivered to the femoral artery or distal aorta using a centrifugal pump. Overall, the incidence of paraplegia following coarctation repair is less than 1%.

Transcatheter therapy has been proposed for the primary therapy of coarctation, but this approach is controversial due to the incidence of recurrent coarctation, need for multiple interventions, injury to the femoral vasculature (for access), and aneurysm formation. Improved results have been achieved with balloon angioplasty with concurrent stent placement in older children and adults in whom further aortic growth is not anticipated. Balloon angioplasty is widely accepted for the treatment of recurrent coarctation following surgery, with 88%-94% achieving a gradient less than 20 mm Hg.

D. Prognosis

The early mortality following repair of coarctation in neonates is 1%-3%, while the risk in older children and adults is about 1%-2%. The incidence of recurrent coarctation following resection and end-to-end repair is about 10% whereas catheter-based interventions are associated with reintervention rates of 25% for balloon angioplasty and 5%-40% for stent placement. The long-term survival following repair of coarctation is determined by the presence of associated defects and the persistence of hypertension.

Following repair, patients may develop severe hypertension. This can be managed using intravenous beta-blockers (eg, esmolol) or vasodilators (eg, sodium nitroprusside). Uncontrolled hypertension can lead to the complication of mesenteric arteritis. Hypertension usually resolves within days to weeks after repair, although older children and adults may require lifelong antihypertensive therapy. Repair of coarctation during infancy is thought to minimize the risk of late hypertension.

Brown JW, Ruzmetov M, Hoyer MH, et al: Recurrent coarctation: is surgical repair of recurrent coarctation of the aorta safe and effective? *Ann Thorac Surg* 2009;88:1930-1931.

Burch PT, Cowley CG, Holubkov R, et al: Coarctation repair in neonates and young infants: is small size or low weight still a risk factor? *J Thorac Cardiovasc Surg* 2009;138:547-552.

Egan M, Holzer RJ: Comparing balloon angioplasty, stenting and surgery in the treatment of aortic coarctation. *Expert Rev Cardiovasc Ther* 2009;11:1401-1412.

Reich O, Tax P, Bartakova H, et al: Long-term (up to 20 years) results of percutaneous balloon angioplasty of recurrent aortic coarctation without use of stents. *Eur Heart J* 2008;29:2042-2048.

Thanopoulos BV, Eleftherakis N, Tzanos K, et al: Stent implantation for adult aortic coarctation. *J Am Coll Cardiol* 2008;52:1815-1816.

▶ Vascular Rings

A. General Considerations

Vascular rings comprise a spectrum of vascular anomalies of the aortic arch, pulmonary artery, and brachiocephalic vessels. The clinically significant manifestation of these lesions is a varying degree of tracheoesophageal compression. These vascular anomalies can be divided into complete vascular rings and partial vascular rings. Complete vascular rings can be divided into double aortic arch and right aortic arch with left ligamentum arteriosum. These two categories can be further subdivided on the basis of the specific anatomy. Incomplete vascular rings include aberrant right subclavian artery, innominate artery compression, and pulmonary artery sling. Other rare variations, which have been described, include left aortic arch with right descending aorta and right ligamentum, and left aortic arch with aberrant right subclavian artery and right ligamentum. The incidence of clinically significant vascular rings is 1%-2% of all congenital heart defects.

Vascular rings and pulmonary slings have been described in conjunction with other cardiac defects, including, TOF, ASD, branch pulmonary artery stenosis, coarctation, AVSD, VSD, interrupted aortic arch, and aortopulmonary window. Significant associated cardiac anomalies occur in 11%-20% of patients with a vascular ring. A right aortic arch is generally associated with a greater incidence of coexisting anomalies.

By the end of the fourth week of embryonic development, the six aortic or branchial arches have formed between the dorsal aortae and ventral roots. Subsequent involution and migration of the arches results in the anatomically normal or abnormal development of the aorta and its branches. The majority of the first, second, and fifth arches regress. The third arch forms the common carotid artery and proximal internal carotid artery. The right fourth arch forms the proximal right subclavian artery. The left fourth arch contributes to the portion of the aortic arch from left carotid to left subclavian arteries. The proximal portion of the right sixth arch becomes the proximal portion of the right pulmonary artery, while the distal segment involutes. Similarly, the proximal left sixth arch contributes to the proximal left pulmonary artery, and the distal sixth arch becomes the ductus arteriosus.

The pulmonary artery is formed from two vascular precursors as well as through a combination of angiogenesis, the de novo development of new blood vessels, and vasculogenesis, the budding and migration of existing vessels. As stated previously, the proximal pulmonary arteries are based on the sixth arches, whereas the primitive lung buds initially derive their blood supply from the splanchnic plexus. Ultimately, these two segments of the pulmonary artery join to form the vascular network of the lung parenchyma.

B. Clinical Findings

Children with a complete vascular ring generally present within the first weeks to months of life. Typically, children with a double aortic arch present earlier in life than those with a right arch and retroesophageal left ligamentum. In the younger age group, respiratory symptoms predominate, as liquids are generally well tolerated. Respiratory symptoms may include stridor, nonproductive cough, apnea, or frequent respiratory infections. The cough is classically described as "seal bark," or "brassy." These symptoms may mimic asthma, respiratory infection, or reflux, and children with vascular rings are often initially misdiagnosed. With the transition to solid food, dysphagia becomes more apparent.

The presentation of a patient with an incomplete vascular ring is variable. Children with innominate artery compression usually present within the first 1-2 years of life with respiratory symptoms. Although, aberrant right subclavian artery is the most common arch abnormality, occurring in approximately 0.5%-1% of the population, it rarely causes symptoms. Classically, when symptoms do occur, they present in the seventh and eighth decade, as the aberrant vessel becomes ectatic and calcified, causing dysphagia lusoria due to impingement of the artery on the posterior esophagus. An aberrant right subclavian rarely causes symptoms except when it is of an abnormally large caliber or associated with tracheomalacia.

Children with pulmonary artery slings generally present with respiratory symptoms within the first few weeks to months of life. As with complete rings, respiratory symptoms may include stridor, nonproductive cough, apnea, or frequent respiratory infections and may mimic other conditions leading to misdiagnosis. Pulmonary artery slings are associated with complete tracheal rings in 30%-40% of patients, leading to focal or diffuse tracheal stenosis.

The methods for diagnosing a vascular ring are multiple because of the variability in presentation and the spectrum of diagnostic tests available. A child with a presumptive diagnosis of asthma or tracheomalacia may be referred to a pulmonologist and a diagnosis of vascular ring made or suspected initially by CXR and bronchoscopy. In some situations, the diagnosis is made by echocardiography during evaluation for concurrent cardiac defects. Regardless, the diagnosis generally begins with a CXR. Complementary studies may include barium esophagogram, CTa, cMRI, and bronchoscopy. Important modalities to define the tracheal anatomy in a patient with a pulmonary artery sling include CTA, cMRI, or bronchoscopy. Echocardiography may be diagnostic and may be used to rule out other cardiac anomalies. Tracheograms and cardiac catheterizations, which have been used extensively in the past, are rarely currently indicated.

C. Treatment

A double aortic arch occurs when the distal portion of the right dorsal aorta fails to regress. The two arches form a complete ring, encircling the trachea and esophagus. The right arch is dominant in the majority of the cases, followed by left dominant, with codominant arches being the least common. The left and right carotid and subclavian arteries generally arise from their respective arches. The ligamentum arteriosum and descending aorta usually remain on the left.

The approach to repair of a double aortic arch is via a left posterolateral thoracotomy. The procedure can easily be accomplished through a limited, muscle-sparing incision through the third or fourth intercostal space. The pleura is incised, after identifying the vagus and phrenic nerves. The ligamentum or ductus arteriosum is divided while preserving the recurrent laryngeal nerve. The nondominant arch is then divided between two vascular clamps at the point where brachiocephalic flow is optimally preserved. If there is concern regarding the location for division, the arches can be temporarily occluded at various points while monitoring pulse and blood pressure in each limb. If there is an atretic segment, the division is done at the point of the atresia. Dissection around the esophagus and trachea in the region

of the ligamentum/ductus and nondominant arch allows for retraction of the vascular structures and lysis of any residual obstructing adhesions.

There are three anatomic variations for a right arch with a left ligamentum, which cause a complete vascular ring. If the left fourth arch regresses between the aorta and left subclavian, a right aortic arch with aberrant left subclavian artery results. The ligamentum arteriosum is retroesophageal, bridging the left pulmonary artery and aberrant left subclavian, forming a complete vascular ring. If the left fourth arch regresses after the origin of the left subclavian artery but before the arch reaches the dorsal aorta to communicate with the left sixth arch (which becomes the ductus arteriosus), there is mirror-image branching. The ligamentum arteriosum arises directly from the descending aorta, or from a Kommerell diverticulum off of the descending aorta, forming the complete ring. If communication is maintained between the left fourth and sixth arches, there is mirror-image branching with the ligamentum arising from the anterior, mirror-image left subclavian, and a ring is not formed.

The surgical approach for a right aortic arch with retroesophageal left ligamentum arteriosum is the same as for a double arch. The ligamentum is divided, and any adhesions around the esophagus and trachea are lysed. Rarely, the Kommerell diverticulum has been reported to cause compression even after division of the ligamentum. As such, it may be prudent to resect or suspend the diverticulum posteriorly.

In innominate artery compression syndrome, the aortic arch and ligamentum are in their normal leftward position. However, the innominate artery arises partially or totally to the left of midline. As the artery courses from left to right anterior to the trachea, it causes tracheal compression. The symptoms of innominate artery compression may be mild to severe. With mild symptoms and minimal tracheal compression on bronchoscopy, children can be observed expectantly because the symptoms may resolve with growth. Indications for surgery include apnea, severe respiratory distress, significant stridor, or recurrent respiratory tract infection. Several approaches for the correction of innominate artery compression syndrome have been described. These include simple division, division with reimplantation into the right side of the ascending aorta, and suspension to the overlying sternum.

An aberrant right subclavian artery occurs when there is regression of the right fourth arch between the right common carotid and right subclavian arteries. The right subclavian then arises from the leftward descending aorta, laying posterior to the esophagus as it crosses from left to right. Although the artery can compress the esophagus posteriorly, it is rarely the cause of symptoms in children. Surgical treatment involves simple division via a left posterolateral thoracotomy. Rarely, reimplantation or grafting from the right carotid or aortic arch may be necessary.

Normally, the right and left sixth aortic arches contribute to the proximal portions of their respective pulmonary arteries. If the proximal left sixth arch involutes and the bud from the left lung migrates rightward to meet the right pulmonary artery, a pulmonary artery sling is formed. Pulmonary artery slings are associated with complete tracheal rings and tracheal stenosis in 30%-40% of patients. Origin of the right upper lobe bronchus from the trachea ("pig bronchus" or "bronchus suis") has been reported in frequent association with pulmonary artery sling.

Initial attempts at the repair of a pulmonary artery sling involved reimplantation after division of the left pulmonary artery and translocation of the trachea without cardiopulmonary bypass. These early reports had a high incidence of left pulmonary artery thrombosis. This has led some authors to advocate division of the trachea and translocation of the left pulmonary artery. This approach would seem sensible if the trachea were being divided in the course of tracheal reconstruction. However, currently most authors advocate the reimplantation of the left pulmonary artery, which has resulted in excellent results. The procedure is done via a median sternotomy on cardiopulmonary bypass to insure optimal visualization of the repair. Aortic cross-clamping is not necessary. The left pulmonary artery is divided off of the right pulmonary artery, translocated anterior to the trachea, and reimplanted into the main pulmonary artery.

Any necessary reconstruction of the trachea for complete tracheal rings is done concurrently with bronchoscopic assistance. Many techniques for tracheal reconstruction have been described, with resection and primary reanastomosis and sliding tracheoplasty offering the most reliable results.

Over 95% of vascular rings without concurrent cardiac defects can be performed through a left thoracotomy. A right thoracotomy is indicated for the rare cases where there is a right ligamentum arteriosum. A right ligamentum occurs in the setting of a left aortic arch with right descending aorta, where the ligamentum bridges from the descending aorta to the right pulmonary artery forming a complete ring. Right ligamentum arteriosum has also been described with a left aortic arch with aberrant right subclavian artery. In this case, the ligamentum may arise from the aberrant subclavian artery, from a diverticulum off of the arch, or directly from the left arch to the right pulmonary artery. In addition, a double aortic arch with an atretic segment proximal to the right carotid artery is more easily divided through a right thoracotomy. The approach to these anomalies is the same as for a left-sided ring division, with the caveat that the right recurrent laryngeal nerve will loop around the right ligamentum.

Repair of vascular rings has been described using video-assisted thoracoscopic surgery (VATS) both with and without robotic assistance. Candidates for thoracoscopic division are limited to those patients requiring only the division of nonpatent vascular structures. In general, VATS is used for patients weighing more than15 kg due to current size limitations of the instruments.

D. Prognosis

Hospital mortality for the repair of a vascular ring was 1.6% in a recent series of 183 patients by Ruzmetov and colleagues. Overall survival was 96% at 35 years. Eight patients were repaired utilizing left pulmonary artery division and reimplantation for pulmonary artery sling, three of whom also required cardiopulmonary bypass for tracheal reconstruction. Of the 183 patients there were no operative mortalities and eight late deaths. All deaths were in patients with other complex cardiac anomalies. The major source of morbidity, as well as mortality, in this and other series is related to the tracheal reconstruction.

Dillman JR, Attili AK, Agarwal PP, et al: Common and uncommon vascular rings and slings: a multi-modality review. *Pediatr Radiol* 2011;41:1440-1454.

Kir M, Saylam GS, Karadas U, et al: Vascular rings: presentation, imaging strategies, treatment, and outcome. *Pediatr Cardiol* 2012;33:607-617.

Phelan E, Ryan S, Rowley H: Vascular rings and slings: interesting vascular anomalies. *J Laryngol Otol* 2011;125:1158-1163.

Russell HM, Backer CL: Pediatric thoracic problems: patent ductus arteriosus, vascular rings, congenital tracheal stenosis, and pectus deformities. *Surg Clin North Am* 2010;90:1091-1113.

Ruzmetov M, Vijay P, Rodefeld MD, et al: Follow-up of surgical correction of aortic arch anomalies causing tracheoesophageal compression: a 38-year single institution experience. *J Pediatr Surg* 2009;44:1328-1332.

▶ Coronary Anomalies

A. General Considerations

Coronary artery anomalies occur in between 0.2% and 1.2% of the population. They can be classified as minor, secondary, or major on the basis of their clinical significance. Minor defects have no functional significance and are usually detected as incidental findings at cardiac catheterization. Secondary defects have no intrinsic significance but alter surgical management when they are present. An example of a secondary defect is an anomalous origin of the left anterior descending from the right coronary artery, which crosses the hypoplastic infundibulum in a patient with TOF. The presence of this vessel may prevent the safe performance of a transannular incision and thereby mandate the use of a conduit. Major defects are the most important form of coronary anomaly because they exert an intrinsically adverse effect on the myocardium. Major anomalies can be subdivided based on anatomy: coronary arteriovenous fistula, anomalous pulmonary origin of a coronary artery, anomalous aortic origin of a coronary artery, myocardial bridging, or coronary artery aneurysm.

Coronary arteriovenous fistula is the most common major coronary anomaly. An abnormal connection exists between a coronary artery (usually the right) and another vascular structure (usually one of the right heart chambers). Most fistulas are isolated and solitary. The fistula leads to left-to-right shunting, which can produce congestive heart failure. Other symptoms include angina, endocarditis, myocardial infarction, arrhythmia, and sudden death. The diagnosis is suggested by echocardiography and confirmed by catheterization.

The second-most common major coronary anomaly is the origin of a coronary artery from the pulmonary artery. The most common manifestation is the anomalous left coronary artery arising from the pulmonary artery (ALCAPA). The right coronary (or both coronaries) may also arise anomalously from the pulmonary artery but only in very rare cases. ALCAPA is usually well tolerated during fetal development, but after birth, the pulmonary systolic pressure usually drops (following ductal closure and decline in PVR) and the anomalous coronary is perfused with desaturated blood at low pressure. Collateral vessels develop between the normal right coronary artery and the abnormal left coronary, but the benefit is negated due to the development of coronary steal, whereby the collateral blood shunts left to right by retrograde flow in the anomalous coronary into the low-pressure pulmonary artery. Most patients will present between 6 weeks and 3 months of life. Typical symptoms include irritability, difficulty in feeding, and other signs of congestive heart failure. Untreated, ALCAPA is nearly always fatal. Rarely, patients will survive to adulthood and present with symptoms of angina or sudden death. On examination, patients with ALCAPA frequently have a holosystolic murmur of ischemic mitral regurgitation. The pulmonary component of the second heart sound may be pronounced because of pulmonary hypertension. Chest radiography is significant for cardiomegaly and pulmonary edema. Electrocardiographic evidence of ischemia and infarction is usually present. Echocardiography is usually diagnostic and is useful for assessing the severity of left ventricular dysfunction and ischemic mitral regurgitation that are commonly present. Catheterization is occasionally necessary to clarify the anatomy, but this technique is used less frequently because of the risk of inducing life-threatening arrhythmias.

Anomalous aortic origins of the coronary arteries are usually minor defects, but a potentially dangerous abnormality exists when the left main coronary artery arises from the right coronary sinus and passes between the pulmonary artery and aorta. This defect has been associated with cardiac symptoms and sudden death, as has the origin of the right coronary artery from the left coronary sinus (usually when the right coronary is dominant). The etiology of ischemia in both defects is thought to be related to the acute angle of origin and slit-like orifice of the anomalous vessel and the extrinsic compression created by the apposing walls of the aorta and pulmonary artery. These defects usually present in older patients. Symptomatic patients are treated surgically by coronary artery bypass.

Myocardial bridging occurs when a segment of an epicardial coronary artery (usually the left anterior descending) takes an intramyocardial course over a short segment. Although this is a common incidental finding at cardiac catheterization, this defect has been associated in some cases with myocardial ischemia. Treatment involves dividing the muscle bridge to free the coronary, coronary bypass beyond the bridge, or transcatheter stenting.

Coronary aneurysms occur rarely, usually in conjunction with an inflammatory condition such as Kawasaki syndrome, polyarteritis nodosa, Takayasu arteritis, or syphilis. Coronary aneurysms may thrombose or lead to distal coronary stenosis or embolization. Rupture occurs uncommonly. Treatment ranges from antiplatelet therapy to coronary artery bypass grafting, and possible transplantation.

B. Treatment

All symptomatic fistulas should be occluded, either surgically or by transcatheter techniques. In some cases, coronary bypass grafting may be necessary when distal flow is compromised by fistula occlusion. Treatment of asymptomatic fistulas is controversial, but occlusion should probably be undertaken when significant left-to-right shunting is present.

Surgical repair is indicated for all patients with ALCAPA. Historically, the initial surgical approach involved ligation of the proximal left coronary artery. This served to eliminate coronary steal and allow perfusion of the left coronary system by collaterals from the right. Despite the ease of simple ligation, most centers have abandoned this approach in favor of establishment of a 2-coronary system, which offers better long-term freedom from ischemia. In older patients, this may be achieved by proximal ligation of the left coronary artery in conjunction with coronary artery bypass, ideally with a left internal mammary graft. Coronary bypass is technically difficult in neonates, and a number of alternative operations have been devised to create a direct connection between the aorta and the anomalous coronary artery. Most commonly, this can be achieved by removing the origin of the left coronary artery (along with a button of adjacent pulmonary artery) and reimplanting the vessel directly into the side of the aorta. Another approach involves creation of a side-to-side connection between the aorta and pulmonary artery with placement of an intrapulmonary baffle to direct flow from this connection to the anomalous left coronary ostium.

C. Prognosis

Survival following surgical repair of ALCAPA has improved over the years. Recent reports have suggested an operative mortality of 0%-6%. Ventricular function tends to normalize after surgery. In most patients, mitral valve function also improves, but for patients with severe mitral regurgitation, concurrent mitral valve repair may be indicated.

Attili A, Hensley AK, Jones FD, et al: Echocardiography and coronary CT angiography imaging of variations in coronary anatomy and coronary abnormalities in athletic children: detection of coronary abnormalities that create a risk for sudden death. *Echocardiography* 2013;30(2):225-233.

Bartoli CR, Wead WB, Giridharan GA: Mechanism of myocardial ischemia with an anomalous left coronary artery from the right sinus of valsalva. *J Thorac Cardiovasc Surg* 2012;144:402-408.

Camarda J, Berger S: Coronary artery abnormalities and sudden cardiac death. *Pediatr Cardiol* 2012;33:434-438.

Mavroudis C, Dodge-Khatami A, Steward RD, et al: An overview of surgery options for congenital coronary artery anomalies. *Future Cardiol* 2010;6:627-645.

Sundaram B, Kreml R, Patel S: Imaging of coronary anomalies. *Radiol Clin North Am* 2010;48:711-727.

MULTIPLE CHOICE QUESTIONS

1. Which of the following statements about ventricular septal defects (VSDs) is *false*?

   A. The most common type of VSD is perimembranous.
   B. Left-to-right shunting through a VSD causes a volume load on the right ventricle.
   C. A patient with a large VSD may be asymptomatic at birth, but eventually develop congestive heart failure due to a drop in pulmonary vascular resistance.
   D. In the presence of a perimembranous VSD, the bundle of His passes along the posterior and inferior rim of the defect, generally on the left ventricular side.

2. Which of the following infants would benefit most from the initiation of PGE$_1$?

   A. Neonate with prenatal diagnosis of aortic coarctation who develops acidosis, oliguria, and diminished pedal pulses 8 hours after birth.
   B. Two-day-old neonate with prenatal diagnosis of complete atrioventricular canal with O$_2$ saturation of 80% and poor systemic perfusion.
   C. Six-week-old infant presenting with irritability, poor feeding, and tachypnea who is diagnosed with ALCAPA and no PDA is seen on echocardiogram.
   D. One-week-old infant with double aortic arch presenting with increasing respiratory distress.

3. A newborn with d-transposition of the great arteries (d-TGA) remains severely cyanotic despite initiation of PGE$_1$ to maintain ductal patency. What is the recommended next step in management?

   A. Initiate inhaled nitric oxide therapy
   B. Diuresis with furosemide IV
   C. Balloon atrial septostomy
   D. Emergent arterial switch operation

4. What is the most common major coronary anomaly?

   A. Left coronary from the pulmonary artery (ALCAPA)
   B. Left anterior descending from the right coronary artery
   C. Coronary AV fistula
   D. Single coronary

5. In which of the following diagnoses is a *primary* catheter-based approach most likely to be recommended over surgery?

   A. Isolated aortic coarctation in a neonate
   B. Isolated pulmonary stenosis in a neonate
   C. PDA in a 1-kg premature infant with heart failure symptoms
   D. Symptomatic perimembranous VSD in a 6-month-old infant

Esophagus & Diaphragm

Marco E. Allaix, MD

Marco G. Patti, MD

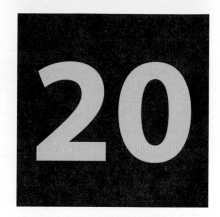

▼ THE ESOPHAGUS

ANATOMY

The esophagus (Figure 20–1) is a muscular tube that serves as a conduit for the passage of food and fluids from the pharynx to the stomach. It originates at the level of the sixth cervical vertebra, posterior to the cricoid cartilage. In the thorax, the esophagus passes behind the aortic arch and the left main stem bronchus, enters the abdomen through the esophageal hiatus of the diaphragm, and terminates in the fundus of the stomach. Its muscle fibers originate from the cricoid cartilage and pharynx above and interdigitate with those of the stomach below. About 2-4 cm of the esophagus is normally located below the diaphragm. The junction between the esophagus and stomach is maintained in its normal intra-abdominal position by the reflection of the peritoneum onto the stomach and of the phrenoesophageal ligament onto the esophagus. The latter is a fibroelastic membrane that lies beneath the peritoneum, on the inferior surface of the diaphragm. When it reaches the esophageal hiatus, the ligament is reflected in an orad direction onto the lower esophagus, where it inserts into the circular muscle layer above the gastroesophageal sphincter, 2-4 cm above the diaphragm.

Three anatomic areas of narrowing occur in the esophagus: (1) at the level of the cricoid cartilage (pharyngoesophageal or upper esophageal sphincter [UES]); (2) in the mid thorax, from compression by the aortic arch and the left main stem bronchus; and (3) at the level of the esophageal hiatus of the diaphragm (gastroesophageal or lower esophageal sphincter [LES]).

In the adult, the distance as measured from the upper incisor teeth to the cricopharyngeus muscle is 15-20 cm; to the aortic arch, 20-25 cm; to the inferior pulmonary vein, 30-35 cm; and to the gastroesophageal junction, approximately 40-45 cm.

The mucosal lining of the esophagus consists of stratified squamous epithelium that contains scattered mucous glands throughout. The musculature of the pharynx and upper third of the esophagus is skeletal in type (striated muscle); the remainder is smooth muscle. Physiologically, the entire organ behaves as a single functioning unit, so that no distinction can be made between the upper and lower esophagus from the standpoint of propulsive activity. As in the intestinal tract, the muscle fibers are arranged into inner circular and outer longitudinal layers. The esophagus has no serosal layer. The arterial supply to the esophagus is quite consistent. The upper end is supplied by branches from the inferior thyroid arteries. The thoracic portion receives blood from the bronchial arteries and from esophageal branches originating directly from the aorta. The intercostal arteries may also contribute. The diaphragmatic and abdominal segments are nourished by the left inferior phrenic artery and by the esophageal branches of the left gastric artery. The venous drainage is more complex and variable. The most important veins are those that drain the lower esophagus. Blood from this region passes into the esophageal branches of the coronary vein, a tributary of the portal vein. This connection constitutes a direct communication between the portal circulation and the venous drainage of the lower esophagus and upper stomach. When there is portal hypertension, as in cirrhosis of the liver, blood is shunted upward through the coronary vein and the esophageal venous plexus to eventually pass by way of the azygos vein into the superior vena cava. The esophageal veins may eventually form varices as they become distended when portal hypertension is present.

PHYSIOLOGY

The coordinated activity of the UES, the esophageal body and the LES is responsible for the motor function of the esophagus.

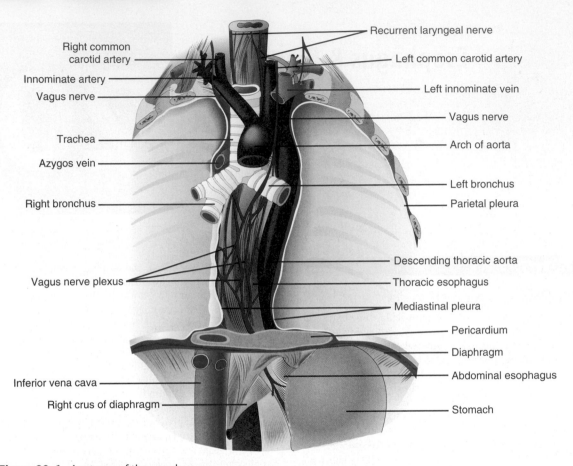

▲ **Figure 20–1.** Anatomy of the esophagus.

1. Upper Esophageal Sphincter

The UES receives motor innervation directly from the brain (nucleus ambiguous). The sphincter is continuously in a state of tonic contraction, with a resting pressure of about 100 mm Hg (anteroposterior axis). The sphincter prevents passage of air from the pharynx into the esophagus and reflux of esophageal contents into the pharynx. During swallowing, a food bolus is moved by the tongue into the pharynx, which contracts while the UES relaxes. After the food bolus has reached the esophagus, the UES regains its resting tone (Figure 20–2).

2. Esophageal Body

When food passes through the UES, a contraction is initiated in the upper esophagus, which progresses distally toward the stomach. The wave initiated by swallowing is referred as primary peristalsis (Figure 20–2). It travels at

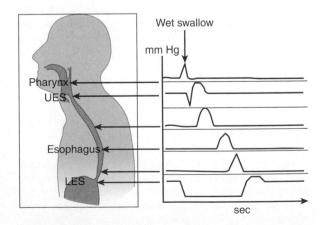

▲ **Figure 20–2.** Swallowing process. Upper esophageal sphincter, esophageal peristalsis, and lower esophageal sphincter in response to swallowing.

a speed of 3-4 cm/s and reaches amplitudes of 60-140 mm Hg in the distal esophagus. Local stimulation by distention at any point in the body of the esophagus will elicit a peristaltic wave from the point of stimulus. This is called secondary peristalsis and aids esophageal emptying when the primary wave has failed to clear the lumen of ingested food, or when gastric contents reflux from the stomach. Tertiary waves are considered abnormal, but they are frequently seen in elderly subjects who have no symptoms of esophageal disease.

3. Lower Esophageal Sphincter

The LES measures 3-4 cm in length and its resting pressure ranges between 15 and 24 mm Hg. At the time of swallowing, the LES relaxes for 5-10 seconds to allow the food bolus to enter the stomach and then regains its resting tone (Figure 20–2). The LES relaxation is mediated by vasoactive intestinal polypeptide and nitric oxide, both nonadrenergic, noncholinergic neurotransmitters. The resting tone depends mainly on intrinsic myogenic activity. The LES has a tendency to relax periodically at times independent from swallowing. These periodic relaxations are called transient

lower esophageal sphincter relaxations to distinguish them from relaxations triggered by swallows. The cause of these transient relaxations is not known, but gastric distention probably plays a role. Transient LES relaxations account for the small amount of physiologic gastroesophageal reflux present in any individual, and are also the most common cause of reflux in patients with gastroesophageal reflux disease (GERD). Decrease in length or pressure of the LES (or both) is responsible for abnormal reflux in the remaining patients. Overall, it is thought that while transient LES relaxation is the most common mechanism of reflux in volunteers and patients with either absent or mild esophagitis, the prevalence of a mechanically defective sphincter (hypotensive and short) increases in patients with severe esophagitis, particularly when Barrett metaplasia is present. The crus of the esophageal hiatus of the diaphragm contributes to the resting pressure of the LES. This *pinchcock* action of the diaphragm is particularly important because it protects against reflux caused by sudden increases of intra-abdominal pressure, such as with coughing or bending. This synergistic action of the diaphragm is lost when a sliding hiatal hernia is present, as the gastroesophageal junction is displaced above the diaphragm (Figure 20–3).

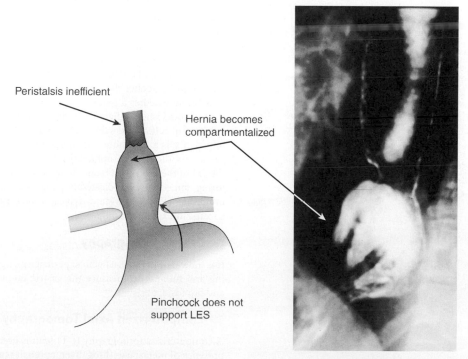

Peristalsis inefficient

Hernia becomes compartmentalized

Pinchcock does not support LES

▲ **Figure 20–3.** Pathophysiology of hiatal hernia.

DIAGNOSTIC APPROACH TO ESOPHAGEAL DISEASES

Symptomatic Evaluation

Esophageal symptoms can be divided into two groups: (1) typical, such as dysphagia, heartburn, and regurgitation and (2) atypical such as chest pain, cough, and hoarseness (Table 20–1). Dysphagia is a unique symptom as it points to an esophageal disorder, either functional (secondary to abnormalities of esophageal peristalsis or lack of coordination between different parts of the esophagus) or mechanical (secondary to a peptic or malignant stricture or an intraluminal mass). Heartburn can also be caused by non-esophageal disorders such as biliary disease, irritable bowel syndrome, coronary artery disease, and psychiatric diseases.

Upper Gastrointestinal Series

The upper gastrointestinal series test is performed by giving the patient barium to swallow. Subsequently, multiple images are taken, including the esophagus, the gastroesophageal junction, the stomach, and the duodenum (a barium swallow focuses just on the esophagus and the gastroesophageal junction). This test characterizes a hiatal hernia, an esophageal stricture, an esophageal diverticulum, or an intraluminal mass. A cine-esophagram is instead a dynamic evaluation of the swallowing process, and it

Table 20–1. Clinical presentation of GERD.

Esophageal	Heartburn
	Regurgitation
	Dysphagia
Gastric	Bloating
	Early satiety
	Belching
	Nausea
Pulmonary	Aspiration
	Asthma
	Wheezing
	Cough
	Dyspnea
	Fibrosis
Ears, nose, throat	Globus
	Water brash
	Hoarseness
Cardiac	Chest pain

is particularly useful in patients with functional dysphagia (secondary to a motility disorder, in the absence of a mechanical cause).

Upper Endoscopy

This test allows visualization of the mucosal surface of the esophagus, the stomach, and the duodenum. The presence and degree of esophagitis and the presence of an intraluminal mass can be determined, and biopsies taken.

Endoscopic Ultrasound

This test is used in patients with esophageal cancer to define the depth of penetration of the tumor through the esophageal wall (T) and the presence of enlarged periesophageal lymph nodes (N). Fine-needle aspiration of these nodes can be done, and cytologic analysis of the aspirate performed.

Esophageal Manometry

Esophageal manometry allows determination of: (1) LES location, length, pressure, and relaxation in response to swallowing; (2) pressure, duration, and velocity of propagation of the peristaltic waves; and (3) location, pressure, relaxation of the UES, and coordination with the pharyngeal contraction.

Ambulatory 24-Hour pH Monitoring

This test measures reflux of acid from the stomach into the esophagus, and it is considered the gold standard for the diagnosis of GERD. By convention, the catheter is placed 5 cm above the upper border of the manometrically determined LES and is kept in place for 24 hours, during which the patient does not alter the daily activities and diet. In addition to defining whether a pathologic amount of GER is present, the test establishes if there is a temporal correlation between episodes of reflux and symptoms (Figure 20–4). Esophageal impedance is a technique that measures flow of liquids and gas across the gastroesophageal junction, independently of the pH of the gastric refluxate. In association with pH monitoring, impedance is indicated in patients with proton pump inhibitors (PPIs)—resistant typical reflux symptoms and chronic unexplained cough.

Gastric Scintigraphy

It is indicated in patients who experience postprandial bloating and fullness to measure the gastric emptying of solids and liquids.

Computerized Axial Tomography

A computerized tomography (CT) scan is used to assess the presence of metastases (lung, liver, adrenals) in patients with esophageal cancer (M).

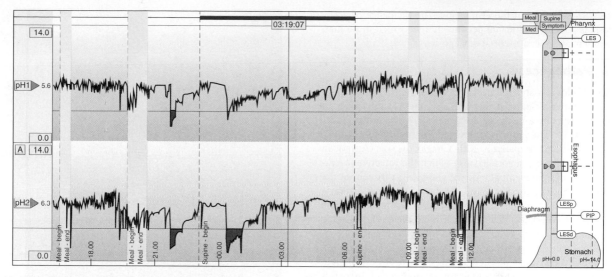

▲ **Figure 20–4.** Ambulatory pH monitoring. The superior plot reports the 24-hour pH recording in the proximal esophagus 20 cm above the upper border of the manometrically determined LES. The inferior plot reports the 24-hour pH recording in the distal esophagus 5 cm above the upper border of the manometrically determined LES. A reflux episode occurs when pH falls below pH = 4 and ends when pH returns above 4.

▶ Positron Emission Tomography

A positron emission tomography (PET) scan is used to assess the metastatic spread of esophageal cancer (M). In addition, it might help predict the response of esophageal cancer to neoadjuvant therapy.

▶ Laparoscopy/Thoracoscopy

Laparoscopy or thoracoscopy can be used to stage esophageal cancer, particularly when liver metastases or extensive lymphadenopathy are suspected.

Fisichella PM et al: The evolution of esophageal function testing and its clinical applications in the management of patients with esophageal disorders. *Dig Liver Dis* 2009;41:626-629.

Low DE: Update on staging and surgical treatment options for esophageal cancer. *J Gastrointest Surg* 2011;15:719-729.

Pech O et al: Accuracy of endoscopic ultrasound in preoperative staging of esophageal cancer: results from a referral center for early esophageal cancer. *Endoscopy* 2010;42:456-461.

van Heijl M et al: Accuracy and reproducibility of 3D-CT measurements for early response assessment of chemoradiotherapy in patients with oesophageal cancer. *Eur J Surg Oncol* 2011;37:1064-1071.

Weber C et al: Current applications of evolving methodologies in gastroesophageal reflux disease testing. *Dig Liver Dis* 2011;43:353-357.

Yoon HH et al: The role of FDG-PET and staging laparoscopy in the management of patients with cancer of the esophagus or gastroesophageal junction. *Gastroenterol Clin North Am* 2009;38:105-120.

ESOPHAGEAL MOTILITY DISORDERS

The named primary esophageal motility disorders are achalasia, diffuse esophageal spasm, nutcracker esophagus, and the hypertensive LES. They occur in the absence of any other esophageal disorder such as reflux, and their cause is unknown. These disorders present with a combination of dysphagia, regurgitation, chest pain, and heartburn. Esophageal manometry is the key test that differentiates these disorders.

ACHALASIA

 ESSENTIALS OF DIAGNOSIS

▶ Dysphagia

▶ Regurgitation

▶ Absence of esophageal peristalsis on esophageal manometry

▶ Radiologic evidence of distal esophageal narrowing

▶ General Considerations

Esophageal achalasia is characterized by the absence of esophageal peristalsis. In most patients, the LES is hypertensive and fails to relax appropriately in response to swallowing. These abnormalities lead to impaired emptying of food with consequent stasis in the esophagus. The incidence of achalasia is about 1 in 100,000 persons. It affects men more than women, and it can occur at any age.

▶ Pathogenesis

The etiology is still unknown, but two theories exist: (1) a degenerative disease of the neurons; and (2) infections of the neurons by a virus (eg, herpes zoster) or another infectious agent. The latter is supported by the fact that similar findings occur in patients with Chagas disease (American trypanosomiasis), a condition in which the infective organism destroys parasympathetic ganglion cells throughout the body, including the heart and the gastrointestinal, urinary, and respiratory tracts. The degeneration of the myenteric plexus of Auerbach determines loss of the postganglionic inhibitory neurons (which contain nitric oxide and vasoactive intestinal polypeptide), which mediate LES relaxation. Because the postganglionic cholinergic neurons are spared, there is unopposed cholinergic stimulation, which increases LES resting pressure and decreases LES relaxation. There is no propagation of peristaltic waves in response to swallowing, but rather the presence of simultaneous contractions.

▶ Clinical Findings

A. Symptoms and Signs

Dysphagia is the most common symptom, experienced by about 95% of patients. It is often for both solids and liquids. Most patients adapt with changes in their diet and are able to maintain a stable weight, while others eventually experience some weight loss. Regurgitation of undigested food is the second-most common symptom and it is present in about 60% of patients. It occurs more often in the supine position and may lead to aspiration. Heartburn is present in about 40% of patients. It is not due to GER, but rather to stasis and fermentation of undigested food in the distal esophagus. Chest pain also occurs in about 40% of patients, due to esophageal distension, and it is usually experienced at the time of a meal.

B. Imaging Studies

Endoscopy is usually the first test performed to rule out a mechanical obstruction such as a peptic stricture or cancer. A barium swallow usually shows narrowing at the level of the gastroesophageal junction, and slow emptying of contrast (Figure 20–5). A dilated, sigmoid esophagus may be present in patients with longstanding achalasia.

C. Special Tests

Esophageal manometry is the gold standard for establishing the diagnosis of esophageal achalasia. The classic manometric findings are: (1) absence of esophageal peristalsis and (2)

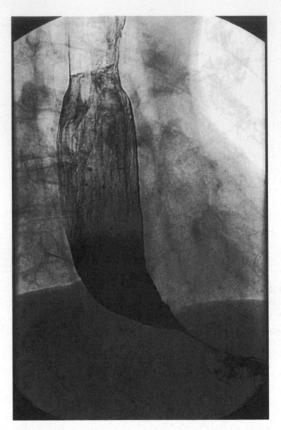

▲ **Figure 20–5.** Esophageal achalasia. Note dilation of the esophageal body, retained barium, and distal esophageal narrowing (bird's beak).

hypertensive LES (in about 50% of patients) that relaxes only partially in response to swallowing. When the esophagus is dilated and sigmoid in shape, it may be difficult to pass the catheter through the gastroesophageal junction into the stomach. In these cases, the catheter may be placed under fluoroscopic or endoscopic guidance. Recently, a new classification of esophageal achalasia has been proposed based on high-resolution manometry: type I, classic, with minimal esophageal pressurization; type II, achalasia with esophageal compression; and type III, achalasia with spasm.

▶ Differential Diagnosis

Benign strictures due to GER and esophageal carcinoma may mimic the clinical presentation of achalasia. Sometimes an infiltrating tumor of the gastroesophageal junction can mimic not only the clinical and radiological presentation of achalasia but also the manometric profile. This condition, called secondary or pseudo-achalasia, should be suspected in patients older than 60 years with recent onset of dysphagia (< 6 months) and excessive weight loss. An endoscopic ultrasound or a CT scan with fine cuts is recommended to rule out an underlying malignancy.

Complications

Aspiration of retained and undigested food can cause repeated episodes of pneumonia. Achalasia is also a risk factor for esophageal squamous cell carcinoma, probably due to the continuous irritation of the mucosa by the retained and fermenting food. Adenocarcinoma can occur in patients who develop GER after either pneumatic dilation or myotomy.

Treatment

Therapy is palliative, and it is directed toward relief of symptoms by decreasing the outflow resistance caused by the dysfunctional LES. Because peristalsis is absent and does not return after any form of treatment, gravity becomes the key factor that allows emptying of food from the esophagus into the stomach.

Medical Therapy

Calcium-channel blockers are used to decrease LES pressure. However, because only 10% of patients benefit from this treatment, it should be used primarily in patients who have contraindications to either pneumatic dilation or to surgery.

A. Endoscopic Treatment

Intrasphincteric injection of botulinum toxin is used to block the release of acetylcholine at the level of the LES, thereby restoring the balance between excitatory and inhibitory neurotransmitters. This treatment, however, is of limited value. Only 60% of treated patients still have relief of dysphagia 6 months after treatment, and this number further decreases to 30% (even after multiple injections) 2.5 years later. In addition, it often causes an inflammatory reaction at the level of the gastroesophageal junction, which makes a subsequent myotomy more difficult. It should be used primarily in patients who are poor candidates for dilatation or surgery.

Pneumatic dilation of the LES is considered the most effective nonsurgical treatment of achalasia and has been the main modality of treatment for many years until the advent of minimally invasive surgery in the early 1990s. A balloon is inflated at the level of the gastroesophageal junction to rupture the muscle fibers while trying to leave the mucosa intact. The initial success rate is around 90%, but it decreases in most patients to 50% at 10 years, even after multiple dilations. The perforation rate is about 2%-5%. If a free perforation occurs, patients are taken emergently to the operating room, where closure of the perforation and a myotomy on the contralateral side of the esophagus are performed. The

incidence of post-dilation GER is about 25%-35%. Patients who fail pneumatic dilation are usually treated by a laparoscopic Heller myotomy.

A recent novel approach to achalasia is the per-oral endoscopic esophageal myotomy (POEM). During this procedure the circular muscle fibers of the lower esophagus and the upper stomach are cut through a sub-mucosal tunnel. Long-term follow-up will be needed to assess the long-term results of this procedure.

B. Surgical Treatment

A laparoscopic Heller myotomy and partial fundoplication has progressively become the procedure of choice for esophageal achalasia during the last 20 years. The operation consists of a controlled section of the muscle fibers (myotomy) of the lower esophagus (6 cm) and proximal gastric wall (2-2.5 cm), followed by an anterior or a posterior partial fundoplication to prevent reflux. Patients spend 24-48 hours in the hospital, and return to regular activities in about 2 weeks. The operation effectively relieves symptoms in about 90% of patients, and it is effective even in patients who have a low LES pressure after previous dilation or when the esophagus is dilated. Therefore, it should be preferred to pneumatic dilation whenever surgical expertise is available. The incidence of postoperative reflux is around 25%-35%, and it is usually controlled by acid reducing medications. Persistent or recurrent dysphagia after myotomy can be treated with pneumatic dilation or another myotomy. Esophagectomy is reserved for patients with severe dysphagia who have failed both dilation and myotomy.

DIFFUSE ESOPHAGEAL SPASM

ESSENTIALS OF DIAGNOSIS

- ▶ Dysphagia
- ▶ Chest pain
- ▶ Intermittent symptoms
- ▶ Radiologic evidence of tertiary contractions (corkscrew esophagus)
- ▶ Intermittent normal and absent peristaltic waves on manometry (> 10%, < 100%)
- ▶ Normal 24-h ambulatory pH monitoring

General Considerations

The cause of diffuse esophageal spasm is not known. Stress might play a role. Progression of diffuse esophageal spasm to achalasia has been documented.

► Clinical Findings

A. Symptoms and Signs

The most common symptom is intermittent chest pain, which varies from slight discomfort to severe spasmodic pain that simulates the pain of coronary artery disease. Most patients complain of dysphagia, but weight loss is uncommon.

B. Imaging Studies

The barium swallow is abnormal in about 70% of patients. Fluoroscopic studies show segmental spasms, areas of narrowing, and irregular uncoordinated peristalsis (corkscrew esophagus) in about 30% of patients. An epiphrenic diverticulum is sometimes present.

C. Manometry

Esophageal manometry is the key test for establishing the diagnosis of diffuse esophageal spasm. The classic manometric findings are: (1) alternation of esophageal peristalsis and simultaneous contractions (> 10% and < 100%) and (2) normal LES function or abnormalities similar to those seen in achalasia.

D. Ambulatory 24-Hour pH Monitoring

This test is essential as the symptoms and the manometric picture of diffuse esophageal spasm can be caused by GERD. In such cases, treatment should be directed toward reflux because the dysmotility is secondary to the reflux. Therefore, it is crucial to be certain about the diagnosis, as treatment of GERD (acid-reducing medications or a fundoplication) is completely different from that of a primary esophageal motility disorder (pneumatic dilation or myotomy).

► Differential Diagnosis

When chest pain is the predominant symptom, a complete cardiac workup is necessary to exclude a cardiac reason for the pain. Once the heart disease has been excluded, ambulatory pH monitoring must be performed to rule out abnormal GER, which is the most common cause of noncardiac chest pain. Esophageal manometry is the only test that distinguishes diffuse esophageal spasm from other primary esophageal motor disorders. An endoscopy should be performed to confirm the absence of intraluminal lesions.

► Complications

Regurgitation and aspiration may occur, possibly leading to repeated episodes of pneumonia. An epiphrenic diverticulum may be present, secondary to the motor disorder.

► Treatment

The therapeutic approach to diffuse esophageal spasm is similar to that of achalasia. Both disorders can be conceptualized as different points in a spectrum of esophageal motility, where peristalsis is progressively lost. In patients with diffuse esophageal spasm, dysphagia is secondary to abnormalities of the peristalsis and the LES, while the chest pain probably results from esophageal distension from poor emptying. Medical therapy (long-acting nitrates, calcium-channel blocking agents) is relatively ineffective. Pneumatic dilation improves the dysphagia in about 25% of patients. Intrasphincteric injection of botulinum toxin has also given poor results. In contrast, a laparoscopic Heller myotomy and partial fundoplication (as for patients with achalasia) improves both dysphagia and chest pain in about 80% of patients.

The hypertensive lower esophageal sphincter is a rare disorder that manifests with dysphagia and is characterized manometrically by a hypertensive LES (resting pressure > 45 mm Hg), which relaxes in response to swallowing, and normal esophageal peristalsis. Treatment is similar to that of esophageal achalasia.

NUTCRACKER ESOPHAGUS

ESSENTIALS OF DIAGNOSIS

► Chest pain
► Dysphagia
► Intermittent symptoms
► Peristaltic waves propagate normally but have very high amplitude and long duration
► Normal 24-h ambulatory pH monitoring

► General Considerations

The cause of this disorder is not known.

► Clinical Findings

A. Symptoms and Signs

Chest pain is the most common symptom. Patients often come to the attention of gastroenterologists only after a thorough cardiac workup has been performed. About half of the patients complain of dysphagia in addition to chest pain.

B. Imaging Studies

The barium swallow is usually normal. An epiphrenic diverticulum is sometimes present.

C. Manometry

Esophageal manometry is the key test for establishing the diagnosis of nutcracker esophagus. The classic manometric findings are as follows: (1) normal propagation of the peristalsis waves (there are no simultaneous contractions)—the peristaltic waves in the distal esophagus, however, have very high amplitude (> 180 mm Hg) and duration (> 6 sec) and (2) normal LES function or abnormalities similar to those seen in achalasia and diffuse esophageal spasm.

D. Ambulatory 24-Hour pH Monitoring

This test is essential because the symptoms and the manometric picture of nutcracker esophagus can be caused by GERD. In such cases, treatment should be directed toward reflux because the dysmotility is secondary.

▶ Differential Diagnosis

When chest pain is the predominant symptom, a complete cardiac work up is necessary to exclude a cardiac reason for the pain. Once the heart has been excluded as a cause of the symptom, ambulatory pH monitoring must be performed to rule out abnormal GER, which is the most common cause of noncardiac chest pain. Esophageal manometry is the only test that distinguishes nutcracker esophagus from other primary esophageal motility disorders.

▶ Complications

Regurgitation and aspiration may occur, possibly leading to repeated pneumonic infections. An epiphrenic diverticulum may be present, secondary to the motor disorder.

▶ Treatment

The nutcracker esophagus is not as well defined as the other primary esophageal motility disorders for both pathophysiology and treatment. Initially, it was thought that the high pressure of the peristaltic contractions was the cause of the chest pain, so treatment was aimed at decreasing the high amplitude of the peristaltic waves. However, calcium-channel blockers are unable to improve the chest pain even though they decrease the strength of the contractions. Similarly, the results of surgery have been disappointing, as chest pain persists after myotomy in about 50% of patients. Dysphagia is improved in 80% of patients.

Bello B et al: Esophageal achalasia: a changing treatment algorithm. *World J Surg* 2011;35:1442-1446.

Boeckxstaens GE et al: Pneumatic dilation versus laparoscopic Heller's myotomy for idiopathic achalasia. *N Engl J Med* 2011;364:1807-1816.

Campos GM et al: Endoscopic and surgical treatments for achalasia: a systematic review and meta-analysis. *Ann Surg* 2009;249:45-57.

Inoue H et al: Peroral endoscopic myotomy (POEM) for esophageal achalasia. *Endoscopy* 2010;42:265-271.

Pandolfino JE et al: Achalasia: a new clinically relevant classification by high-resolution manometry. *Gastroenterology* 2008;135:1526-1533.

Patti MG et al: Achalasia and other esophageal motility disorders. *J Gastrointest Surg* 2011;15:703-707.

Patti MG et al: Esophageal achalasia 2011: pneumatic dilatation or laparoscopic myotomy? *J Gastrointest Surg* 2012 Apr;16:870-873.

Patti MG et al: Fundoplication after laparoscopic Heller myotomy for esophageal achalasia: what type? *J Gastrointest Surg* 2010;14:1453-1458.

Stefanidis D et al: SAGES guidelines for the surgical treatment of esophageal achalasia. *Surg Endosc* 2012;26:296-311.

ESOPHAGEAL DIVERTICULA

Esophageal diverticula are rare. They are located above the UES (pharyngoesophageal or Zenker diverticulum) or the LES (epiphrenic diverticulum). They are considered pulsion diverticula and are secondary to abnormalities of the sphincters in terms of resting pressure, relaxation in response to swallowing, and coordination with the segment above the sphincter. As a consequence, mucosa and submucosa protrude through the muscular layers, forming the outpouching.

1. Pharyngoesophageal Diverticulum (Zenker Diverticulum)

 ESSENTIALS OF DIAGNOSIS

▶ Dysphagia

▶ Regurgitation of undigested food (with risk of aspiration)

▶ Gurgling sounds in the neck

▶ Halitosis

▶ General Considerations

This is the most common of the esophageal diverticula and is three times more frequent in men than in women. Most patients are over age 60 years. The condition originates from the posterior wall of the esophagus, in a triangular area of weakness (Killian triangle), limited inferiorly by the upper border of the cricopharyngeal muscle and laterally by the oblique fibers of the inferior constrictor muscles of the pharynx. As the diverticulum enlarges, it tends to deviate from the midline, mostly to the left.

▶ Pathogenesis

A Zenker diverticulum is due either to lack of coordination between the pharyngeal contraction and the opening time of the UES or to a hypertensive UES. Because of the increased intraluminal pressure, there is progressive herniation of mucosa and submucosa through the Killian triangle. Occasionally, UES dysfunction can occur in the absence of a diverticulum (cricopharyngeal achalasia). A hereditary syndrome called oculopharyngeal muscular dystrophy, consisting of ptosis and dysphagia, has been described in patients of French-Canadian ancestry. The dysphagia is the result of weak pharyngeal musculature in the face of normal UES function; it is considerably improved by UES myotomy. This syndrome also manifests with cervical dysphagia. A chronic cough may develop in some patients from aspiration of saliva and ingested food.

▶ Clinical Findings

A. Symptoms

Dysphagia is the most common symptom and occurs in about 80%-90% of patients. Regurgitation of undigested food from the diverticulum often occurs, and can lead to aspiration into the tracheobronchial tree and pneumonia. Patients frequently have halitosis and can hear gurgling sounds in the neck. About 30% of patients have associated GERD.

B. Imaging Studies

A barium swallow clearly shows the position and size of the diverticulum or a prominent cricopharyngeal bar without diverticulum (Figure 20–6).

C. Special Tests

Esophageal manometry shows a lack of coordination between the pharynx and the cricopharyngeus muscle and often a hypertensive UES. In addition, it can show a hypotensive LES and abnormal esophageal peristalsis. Ambulatory pH monitoring determines if abnormal esophageal acid exposure is present. Endoscopy may be dangerous because the instrument can enter the diverticulum rather than the esophageal lumen and cause a perforation.

▶ Differential Diagnosis

Differential diagnosis includes esophageal stricture, achalasia, and esophageal cancer.

▶ Treatment

The standard treatment consists of eliminating the functional obstruction at the UES level (myotomy of the cricopharyngeus muscle and the upper 3 cm of the posterior esophageal wall) and excision or suspension of the diverticulum. For small diverticula (< 2 cm), the myotomy alone is sufficient. As an alternative to the conventional

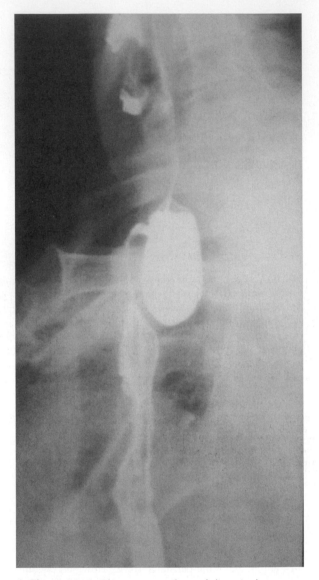

▲ **Figure 20–6.** Pharyngoesophageal diverticulum (Zenker diverticulum).

surgical treatment, a transoral endoscopic approach (using staplers, laser or coagulation through an endoscope that ablate the septum between the diverticulum and the cervical esophagus) can be used for diverticula between 3 and 6 cm in size. If present, GER should be corrected before dividing the UES in order to avoid aspiration. The prognosis is excellent in about 90% of cases. Complications are rare and the patients are usually able to eat the day after the procedure.

Al-Kadi AS et al: Endoscopic treatment of Zenker diverticulum: results of a 7-year experience. *J Am Coll Surg* 2010;211:239-243.

Herbella FA et al: Esophageal diverticula and cancer. *Dis Esophagus* 2012;25:153-158.

Herbella FAM et al: Modern pathophysiology and treatment of esophageal diverticula. *Langenbecks Arch Surg* 2012;397:29-35.

Koch M et al: Endoscopic laser-assisted diverticulotomy versus open surgical approach in the treatment of Zenker's diverticulum. *Laryngoscope* 2011;121:2090-2094.

2. Epiphrenic Diverticulum

ESSENTIALS OF DIAGNOSIS

▶ Dysphagia

▶ Regurgitation

▶ Diverticulum evident on barium swallow

▶ Esophageal motility disorder shown by esophageal manometry

General Considerations

Epiphrenic diverticulum is located in the distal 10 cm of the esophagus. It is not a primary anatomic abnormality but rather the consequence of an underlying motility disorder of the esophagus that causes an outflow obstruction at the level of the gastroesophageal junction, with consequent increase in intraluminal pressure and progressive herniation of mucosa and submucosa through the esophageal muscle layers.

Clinical Findings

A. Symptoms

The symptoms experienced by the patient are in part due to the underlying motility disorder (dysphagia, chest pain) and in part due to the diverticulum *per se* (regurgitation with the risk of aspiration). Some diverticula, however, can be asymptomatic.

B. Imaging Studies

A chest radiograph can show an air-fluid level in the posterior mediastinum. A barium swallow clearly shows the position and size of the diverticulum (Figure 20–7). Endoscopy is important to rule out an esophageal malignancy.

C. Special Tests

In the majority of cases, esophageal manometry shows the underlying motility disorder. Sometimes it is difficult to position the manometry catheter, and endoscopic or fluoroscopic guidance might be necessary.

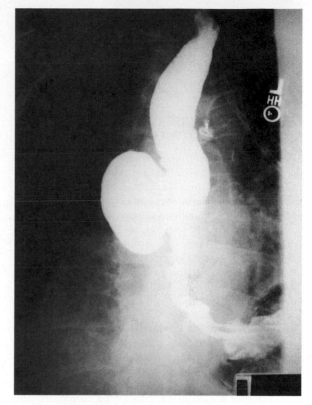

▲ **Figure 20–7.** Epiphrenic diverticulum.

Differential Diagnosis

A paraesophageal hernia can be confused with an epiphrenic diverticulum. The barium swallow and the endoscopy help in establishing the diagnosis.

Treatment

The treatment is surgical, and the laparoscopic approach is preferred. It consists of: (1) resection of the diverticulum; (2) long myotomy—it is performed in the side of the esophagus opposite to where the diverticulum is located, it extends proximally to the upper border of the neck of the diverticulum and distally for about 2 cm onto the gastric wall; and (3) a partial fundoplication to prevent GER. A laparoscopic diverticulectomy, with myotomy and fundoplication, is successful in 80%-90% of cases.

Soares R et al: Epiphrenic diverticulum: from pathophysiology to treatment. *J Gastrointest Surg* 2010;14:2009-2015.

Soares RV et al: Laparoscopy as the initial approach for epiphrenic diverticula. *Surg Endosc* 2011;25:3740-3746.

Vicentine FP et al: High resolution manometry findings in patients with esophageal epiphrenic diverticula. *Am Surg* 2011;77:1661-1664.

Zaninotto G et al: Therapeutic strategies for epiphrenic diverticula: systematic review. *World J Surg* 2011;35:1447-1453.

ESOPHAGEAL MANIFESTATIONS IN SCLERODERMA & OTHER SYSTEMIC DISEASES

Scleroderma and several other systemic diseases may involve the esophagus. In scleroderma or progressive systemic sclerosis, there is involvement of the gastrointestinal tract in up to 90% of patients. The most common site of gastrointestinal involvement is the smooth muscle portion of the esophagus, where atrophy and fibrosis occur. The upper esophagus (striated muscle) and the UES are not involved. As a consequence, LES pressure is low and the peristalsis is weak (low amplitude or abnormal propagation of the peristaltic waves). These changes can be followed by an increased amount of GER with delayed clearance of the refluxed gastric contents. Esophageal symptoms usually appear in patients with the characteristic skin changes and Raynaud syndrome. In addition to heartburn and regurgitation, patients may have respiratory symptoms due to the upward extent of the gastric refluxate and aspiration. Dysphagia may be due to the abnormal peristalsis or to the presence of a peptic stricture. The diagnostic approach is similar to that of patients with GERD:

- A barium swallow may show a hiatal hernia or a stricture.

- Endoscopy shows esophagitis in 50%-60% of patients. Barrett esophagus (BE) is present in about 10% of patients.

- Esophageal manometry usually shows a hypotensive LES. Dysmotility is frequent and can progress to complete loss of peristalsis.

- Ambulatory pH monitoring is essential to establish the diagnosis. It can also measure the presence of acid in the proximal esophagus and pharynx in patients with cough or vocal cord problems.

- Gastric scintigraphy is indicated in patients who experience postprandial bloating and fullness to measure the gastric emptying of solids and liquids.

Similar esophageal changes may also occur in rheumatoid arthritis, Sjögren syndrome, Raynaud disease, and systemic lupus erythematosus. Similar motor abnormalities are occasionally seen in alcoholism, diabetes mellitus, myxedema, multiple sclerosis, and amyloidosis.

Medical management should always be tried first. A PPI is the drug of choice. If gastroparesis is present, a prokinetic medication such as metoclopramide should be added. A fundoplication should be considered particularly in patients with regurgitation, cough, or vocal cord problems.

Ebert EC et al: Gastrointestinal and hepatic manifestations of systemic lupus erythematosus. *J Clin Gastroenterol* 2011;45:436-441.

Gregersen H et al: Mechanical characteristics of distension-evoked peristaltic contractions in the esophagus of systemic sclerosis patients. *Dig Dis Sci* 2011;56:3559-3568.

Lahcene M et al: Esophageal dysmotility in scleroderma: a prospective study of 183 cases. *Gastroenterol Clin Biol* 2009;33:466-469.

GASTROESOPHAGEAL REFLUX DISEASE

ESSENTIALS OF DIAGNOSIS

- ▶ Heartburn
- ▶ Regurgitation
- ▶ Sliding hiatal hernia on barium swallow
- ▶ Esophagitis on endoscopy
- ▶ Abnormal esophageal motility on manometry
- ▶ Abnormal esophageal exposure on ambulatory pH monitoring

▶ General Considerations

GERD is the most common upper gastrointestinal disorder of the Western world and accounts for about 75% of esophageal diseases. Heartburn, usually considered synonymous with the presence of abnormal gastroesophageal reflux, is experienced by 20%-40% of the adult population of Western countries. However, because many symptomatic patients treat themselves with over-the-counter medications without consulting a physician, the prevalence of the disease is probably higher than reported. The incidence of reflux symptoms increases with age, and both sexes seem to be equally affected. Symptoms are more common during pregnancy, probably due to hormonal effects on the LES and the increased intra-abdominal pressure due to the enlarging uterus. Recent studies have demonstrated a link between obesity and GERD whereby the body mass index has a direct effect on the severity of reflux.

▶ Pathogenesis

GERD is caused by the abnormal retrograde flow of gastric contents into the esophagus, resulting in symptoms and mucosal damage. A defective LES is the most common cause of GERD. Transient LES relaxations account for the majority of reflux episodes in patients without mucosal damage or with mild esophagitis, while a short and hypotensive LES is more frequently found in patients with more severe esophagitis. In 40%-60% of patients with GERD, abnormalities of esophageal peristalsis are also present. Because esophageal peristalsis is the main determinant of esophageal clearance (the ability of the esophagus to clear gastric contents refluxed through the LES), patients with abnormal esophageal peristalsis have more severe reflux and slower clearance. Therefore, these patients often have more severe mucosal injury and more frequent atypical symptoms such as cough or hoarseness. A hiatal hernia also contributes to the incompetence of the gastroesophageal junction by altering the anatomic relationship between the esophageal crus and the LES. As the gastroesophageal junction is displaced above the diaphragm, the pinchcock action of the esophageal crus is lost. In patients with large hiatal hernias, the LES is usually shorter and weaker, and the amount of reflux is greater.

▶ Clinical Findings

A. Symptoms

Heartburn, regurgitation, and dysphagia are considered typical symptoms of GERD; however, a clinical diagnosis of GERD based on these symptoms is correct in only 70% of patients (when compared with the results of pH monitoring). A good response to therapy with PPIs is a good predictor of the presence of abnormal reflux. GERD can also cause atypical symptoms such as cough, wheezing, chest pain, hoarseness, and dental erosions. Two mechanisms have been postulated for GERD-induced respiratory symptoms: (1) a vagal reflex arc resulting in bronchoconstriction and (2) microaspiration into the tracheobronchial tree. Ear, nose, and throat symptoms such as hoarseness or dental erosions are instead secondary to the upward extent of the acid with direct damage of the vocal cords or teeth.

B. Barium Swallow

A barium swallow provides information about the presence and size of a hiatal hernia, the presence and length of a stricture, and the length of the esophagus. This test, however, is not diagnostic of GERD, as a hiatal hernia or reflux of barium can be present in the absence of abnormal reflux.

C. Endoscopy

Fifty percent of patients with abnormal reflux do not have esophagitis on endoscopy. Therefore, endoscopy is useful for diagnosing complications of GERD such as esophagitis, BE, or a stricture. In addition, there is major interobserver variation among endoscopists for the low grades of esophagitis (Table 20–2).

D. Esophageal Manometry

This test provides information about the LES (resting pressure, length, and relaxation) and the quality of esophageal peristalsis. In addition, manometry is essential for proper placement of the pH probe for ambulatory pH monitoring (5 cm above the upper border of the LES).

Table 20–2. Endoscopic grading system for esophagitis.

Grade 1	Reddening of the mucosa without ulceration.
Grade 2	Linear ulcerations lined with granulation tissue that bleeds easily when touched.
Grade 3	Ulcerations have coalesced to leave islands of epithelium.
Grade 4	Stricture.

E. Ambulatory pH Monitoring

This test has a sensitivity and specificity of about 92% and is considered the gold standard for diagnosing GERD (Table 20–3). Medications that affect the production of acid by the parietal cells must be stopped 3 days (H_2-blocking agents) to 14 days (PPIs) prior to the study. Diet and exercise are unrestricted during the test in order to mimic a typical day of the patient's life. This test should be performed: (1) in patients who do not respond to medical therapy, (2) in patients who relapse after discontinuation of medical therapy, (3) before antireflux surgery, or (4) when evaluating atypical symptoms such as cough, hoarseness, and chest pain. Because fewer than 50% of these patients with atypical symptoms experience heartburn or have esophagitis on endoscopy, a pH monitoring study becomes the only way to determine whether abnormal reflux is present, establishing a temporal link between episodes of reflux and symptoms. A pH probe with two sensors, located 5 and 20 cm above the LES, allows determination of the upward extent of the reflux. Tracings are analyzed for a temporal correlation between symptoms and episodes of reflux.

Table 20–3. Normal values for ambulatory 24-hour pH monitoring.

Percentage of total time pH < 4.0	4.5
Percentage of upright time pH < 4.0	8.4
Percentage of supine time pH < 4.0	3.5
Number of episodes of reflux < 4.0	47
Number of episodes > 5 minutes	3.5
Longest episode (minutes)	20
Composite score[1]	14.7

[1]The composite score indicates the extent to which the patient's values deviate from the normal means of the six variables. It allows one to express in a single figure the degree of the patient's abnormality.

Differential Diagnosis

Heartburn can be the presenting symptom of irritable bowel syndrome, achalasia, cholelithiasis, coronary artery disease, or psychiatric disorders. Esophageal manometry and pH monitoring are essential to determine with certainty if GERD is present and if reflux is the cause of the symptoms.

Complications

Esophagitis is the most common complication. Peptic strictures are uncommon, particularly in the era of PPIs. BE is found in about 10%-15% of patients with reflux documented by pH monitoring. Some patients may eventually progress to high-grade dysplasia (HGD) and adenocarcinoma. Respiratory complications vary from chronic cough to asthma, aspiration pneumonia, and even pulmonary fibrosis. Vocal cord and dental damage can also occur.

Treatment

A. Lifestyle Modifications

Patients should eat frequent small meals during the day (to avoid gastric distention), avoiding fatty foods, spicy foods, and chocolate, as they lower LES pressure. The last meal should be no less than 2 hours before going to bed. In order to increase the effect of gravity, the head of the bed should be elevated over 4- to 6-inch blocks.

B. Medical Therapy

Antacids are useful for patients with mild intermittent heartburn. Acid-suppressing medications are the mainstay of medical therapy. H_2-blocking agents are usually prescribed for patients with mild symptoms or mild esophagitis. PPIs are superior to H_2-blocking agents because they determine a more profound control of the acid secretion, with healing of esophagitis in 80%-90% of patients. However, symptoms and esophagitis tend to recur in the majority of patients after discontinuation of therapy, so most patients need chronic maintenance therapy. In addition, about 50% of patients on maintenance PPIs require increasing doses to maintain healing of esophagitis. Acid-suppressing medications only alter the pH of the gastric refluxate, but reflux and aspiration can still occur because of an incompetent LES and ineffective esophageal peristalsis. Moreover, medical therapy is largely ineffective for the treatment of the extraesophageal manifestations of GERD due to the upward extension of the refluxate. PPIs can interfere with calcium absorption causing osteoporosis and fractures. In addition, PPIs can cause *Clostridium difficile* infection, delay in gastric emptying and abnormal cardiac activity due to decreased magnesium levels.

C. Surgical Therapy

The ideal patient for antireflux surgery is the one in whom ambulatory pH monitoring shows abnormal GER and whose heartburn is well controlled by PPIs. A careful selection of patients for surgery is mandatory. The operation is indicated in: (1) young patients who require chronic therapy with PPIs for control of symptoms, (2) patients in whom regurgitation persists during therapy, (3) patients with respiratory symptoms (cough, asthma, aspiration pneumonia, and pulmonary fibrosis), (4) patients with vocal cord damage, and (5) patients with BE. Recent evidence suggests that an effective antireflux operation may promote regression of the columnar epithelium in up to 50% of patients who have a short segment of BE (< 3 cm). In addition, it may arrest the progression from metaplasia to dysplasia. However, since the response to therapy is unpredictable, endoscopic surveillance after laparoscopic fundoplication in patients with BE is recommended.

The goal of surgical therapy is to restore the competence of the LES. A laparoscopic Nissen fundoplication (360°) is considered today the procedure of choice (Figure 20–8) because it increases the resting pressure and length of the LES, decreases the number of transient LES relaxations and improves quality of esophageal peristalsis. The operation is equally safe and effective in young and elderly patients.

The success of the operation is based on the following technical elements:

1. Dissection of the esophagus in the posterior mediastinum to allow 3-4 cm of esophagus to lie without tension below the diaphragm. By bringing the entire stomach and gastroesophageal junction below the diaphragm, a sliding hiatal hernia is reduced.

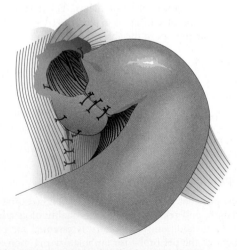

▲ **Figure 20–8.** Nissen fundoplication (360°).

2. Division of the short gastric vessels in order to create a "floppy" fundoplication.

3. Approximation of the esophageal crus to decrease the size of the esophageal hiatus, thereby avoiding herniation of the wrap.

4. Construction of a 360° fundoplication over a 56-60 French bougie.

The hospital stay is short (usually 1-2 days), and the postoperative discomfort is minimal. Most patients return to work within 2-3 weeks. Control of symptoms is obtained in about 80%-90% of patients at 10 years after a fundoplication. Failures are treated with either medications or a second operation.

Broeders JA et al: Laparoscopic anterior versus posterior fundoplication for gastroesophageal reflux disease: systematic review and meta-analysis of randomized clinical trials. *Ann Surg* 2011;254:39-34.

Davis CS et al: The evolution and long-term results of laparoscopic antireflux surgery for the treatment of gastroesophageal reflux disease. *JSLS* 2010;14:332-341.

Fisichella PM et al: Gastroesophageal reflux disease and morbid obesity: is there a relation? *World J Surg* 2009;33:2034-2038.

Galmiche JP et al: LOTUS Trial Collaborators. Laparoscopic antireflux surgery vs esomeprazole treatment for chronic GERD: the LOTUS randomized clinical trial. *JAMA* 2011;305:1969-1977.

Herbella FA et al: Gastroesophageal reflux disease: from pathophysiology to treatment. *World J Gastroenterol* 2010;16:3745-3749.

Soares RV et al: Interstitial lung disease and gastroesophageal reflux disease: key role of esophageal function tests in the diagnosis and treatment. *Arq Gastroenterol* 2011;48:91-97.

Sweet M et al: Gastroesophageal reflux disease and aspiration in patients with advanced lung disease. A review. *Thorax* 2009;64:167-173.

Tutuian R et al: Characteristics of symptomatic reflux episodes on acid suppressive therapy. *Am J Gastroenterol* 2008;103:1090-1096.

Symons NR et al: Laparoscopic revision of failed antireflux surgery: a systematic review. *Am J Surg* 2011;202:336-343.

Thijssen AS et al: Cost-effectiveness of PPIs versus laparoscopic Nissen fundoplication for patients with gastroesophageal reflux disease: a systematic review of the literature. *Surg Endosc* 2011;25:3127-3134.

BARRETT ESOPHAGUS

 ESSENTIALS OF DIAGNOSIS

▶ GERD symptoms (typical and atypical)

▶ Endoscopic evidence of "salmon pink" epithelium above gastroesophageal junction

▶ Specialized columnar epithelium on esophageal biopsy

General Considerations

BE is defined as a change in the esophageal mucosa with replacement of the squamous epithelium by columnar epithelium. About 10%-12% of patients undergoing endoscopy for symptoms of GERD are found to have BE, classified in short segment (< 3 cm in length) or long segment (3 cm or longer). Metaplasia may progress to high-grade dysplasia (HGD) and eventually adenocarcinoma. Thus, adenocarcinoma represents the final step of a sequence of events in which a benign disease (GERD) evolves into a preneoplastic disease and eventually into cancer.

Pathogenesis

BE is due to reflux of gastric contents (acid and duodenal juice) into the esophagus. When compared to patients with GERD with no mucosal injury or less severe esophagitis, patients with BE have a shorter and weaker LES and decreased amplitude of esophageal peristalsis. As a consequence, the amount of reflux is greater and esophageal clearance is slower. In addition, hiatal hernia is more common in patients with Barrett metaplasia.

Clinical Findings

A. Symptoms

Patients with BE typically have a long history of GERD. While most patients experience both typical and atypical symptoms of GERD, others may become asymptomatic over time due to the decreased sensitivity of the metaplastic epithelium.

B. Imaging Studies

Barium swallow may show ulcerations, a stricture, or a hiatal hernia. Endoscopy shows presence of "salmon pink" epithelium above the gastroesophageal junction, replacing the whitish squamous epithelium. The diagnosis is confirmed by pathologic examination of the esophageal mucosa and requires the identification of goblet cells, typical for intestinal epithelium.

C. Special Tests

Esophageal manometry often shows a short and hypotensive LES and abnormal esophageal peristalsis (decreased amplitude of peristaltic waves, simultaneous waves). Ambulatory pH monitoring usually shows a severe amount of acid reflux. Esophageal exposure to duodenal juice can be quantified by a fiberoptic probe that measures intraluminal bilirubin as a marker for duodenal reflux. In GERD patients, the prevalence of esophageal bilirubin exposure parallels the degree of mucosal injury, being higher in patients with BE. Nonacid reflux can be measured by impedance-pH monitoring.

▶ Treatment

A. Barrett Esophagus: Metaplasia

The treatment options are similar to those of patients with GERD without metaplasia and consist of either PPIs or a fundoplication. A surgical approach might offer an advantage over medical therapy for the following reasons:

1. Successful elimination of reflux symptoms with PPIs does not guarantee control of an acid reflux. When pH monitoring is performed in asymptomatic BE patients treated with these medications, up to 80% of them still have abnormal acid reflux.

2. PPIs do not eliminate the reflux of bile, a major contributor to the pathogenesis of BE. In contrast, an antireflux operation prevents any form of reflux by restoring the competence of the gastroesophageal junction.

3. A fundoplication may promote regression of the columnar epithelium. Many studies have shown that regression occurs in 15%-50% of patients when the length of the BE segment is less than 3 cm. Regardless of the effect of the fundoplication on symptoms, surveillance endoscopy should be performed every 12-24 months.

B. Barrett Esophagus: Low-Grade Dysplasia

Patients with low-grade dysplasia (LGD) should be treated for 1-2 months with high doses of PPIs (3-4 pills/d), and subsequently the endoscopy should be repeated with multiple biopsies. The rationale for this approach is to decrease the mucosal inflammation by blocking acid secretion, allowing the pathologist a more accurate reading. If the repeated biopsies show metaplasia or HGD, the patient will be treated accordingly. If LGD is confirmed, the patient can continue taking acid-reducing medications or have a laparoscopic fundoplication with ablation of the dysplastic epithelium. Although there is evidence that regression to metaplasia or even disappearance of the columnar epithelium can occur after a successful fundoplication, endoscopic surveillance should be performed every 6-12 months, because of the higher risk of developing esophageal cancer in these patients compared to patients with non-dysplastic BE.

C. Barrett Esophagus: High-Grade Dysplasia

When HGD is found and confirmed by two experienced pathologists, two treatment options are available:

1. Patients can enroll in a program of strict endoscopic surveillance, with endoscopy performed every 3 months and 4-quadrant biopsies obtained for every centimeter of BE. The goal is to detect cancer as soon as it develops but before it becomes invasive and spreads to lymph nodes: the risk of lymph node metastasis is about 20%-30% in patients with submucosal invasive carcinoma

(pT1b). Progression from HGD to cancer occurs in about 50% of patients 5 years after the initial diagnosis is established. This approach is reasonable if the patient is willing to undergo endoscopy every 3 months but unwilling to have an esophagectomy or if severe comorbidities are present.

2. For young and medically fit patients who are unwilling to undergo endoscopy every 3 months, an esophagectomy should be considered. The rationale for an operation is based on the following considerations: (a) cancer is already found in about 30% of patients thought to have HGD; (b) cancer develops in about 50% of patients during follow-up; (c) recent studies have shown that in specialized centers the operation can be performed with minimal morbidity and mortality, and postoperative quality of life similar to that of the general population; and (d) because the prognosis depends on the pathologic staging, waiting exposes patients to the risk of development of invasive cancer with lymph node metastases.

Esophagectomy remains the treatment of choice when: (1) endoscopic expertise is not available; (2) preoperative staging by endoscopic ultrasound is greater than T1aN0; (3) lymph node involvement is shown; (4) patients can not have a rigid follow-up; (5) multi focal dysplasia is present in a long segment; (6) complete eradication is not possible.

D. Endoscopic Treatment Modalities

Because either acid-reducing medications or a fundoplication determine regression in some patients with a short segment only, and because there is no evidence that they block progression to cancer, different modalities have been developed for the endoscopic treatment of the BE. Endoscopic resection is the basis of endoscopic therapy for BE and has been advocated not only as a therapeutic approach but also as a staging tool. The major advantage of the resection is the ability to provide samples of appropriate size and depth for an accurate histopathological diagnosis. Endoscopic Mucosal Resection (EMR) is curative in HGD and T1a lesions, with 5-year survival rates of 98%-100%.

Ablative therapies destroy the BE epithelium allowing replacement with neo-squamous epithelium. Photodynamic therapy is based on the administration of a photosensitizing drug, which is retained in the BE. Light of proper wavelength is then delivered endoscopically, producing an oxidative reaction with complete destruction of the abnormal mucosa in about 50% of patients. This technique, however, is associated with the development of esophageal strictures in about 30% of patients. In addition, islands of columnar epithelium can still be present under the regenerated squamous epithelium. The radio frequency ablation (RFA) seems to avoid these problems and is effective in about 70% of patients.

Feo C et al: Importance of a multidisciplinary approach in the treatment of Barrett's esophagus. *Updates Surg* 2011;63:5-9.

Konda VJ et al: Is the risk of concomitant invasive esophageal cancer in high-grade dysplasia in Barrett's esophagus overestimated? *Clin Gastroenterol Hepatol* 2008;6:159-164.

Patti MG et al: Role of minimally invasive surgery in the modern treatment of Barrett's esophagus. *Gastrointest Endosc Clin N Am* 2011;21:135-144.

Pech O et al: Comparison between endoscopic and surgical resection of mucosal esophageal adenocarcinoma in Barrett's esophagus at two high-volume centers. *Ann Surg* 2011;254:67-72.

Pech O et al: Endoscopic therapy of Barrett's esophagus. *Curr Opin Gastroenterol* 2009;25:405-411.

Pech O et al: Value of high-frequency miniprobes and conventional radial endoscopic ultrasound in the staging of early Barrett's carcinoma. *Endoscopy* 2010;42:98-103.

Rees JRE et al: Treatment for Barrett's oesophagus (Review). *Cochrane Database Syst Rev* Jan 20, 2010;(1):CD004060.

Shaheen NJ et al: Durability of radiofrequency ablation in Barrett's esophagus with dysplasia. *Gastroenterology* 2011;141:460-468.

HIATAL HERNIA

ESSENTIALS OF DIAGNOSIS

▶ May be asymptomatic

▶ Symptoms secondary to mechanical obstruction: dysphagia, epigastric discomfort, anemia

▶ Symptoms secondary to gastroesophageal reflux: heartburn, regurgitation

▶ General Considerations

Obesity, aging, and general weakening of the musculofascial structures set the stage for enlargement of the esophageal hiatus and herniation of the stomach into the posterior mediastinum. Hiatal hernias are divided into sliding hiatal hernias (type 1) (Figures 20–9 and 20–10) and paraesophageal hiatal hernias (types 2, 3, or 4) (Figures 20–11 and 20–12). The most common (95%) is the sliding hernia, where the gastroesophageal junction moves above the diaphragm together with some or the entire stomach. Type 2 hernias are characterized by herniation of the gastric fundus into the mediastinum alongside the esophagus, with the gastroesophageal junction remaining in an intra-abdominal position. Since the gastroesophageal sphincteric mechanism functions normally in most of these cases, reflux of gastric contents is uncommon. Type 3 hernias, also called mixed hernias, involve herniation of the stomach with the gastroesophageal junction into the mediastinum. In types 1 and 3, symptoms due to GER may occur along with symptoms secondary to the mechanical obstruction.

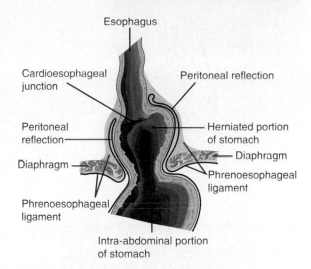

▲ **Figure 20–9.** Sliding esophageal hiatal hernia.

Finally, the rare type 4 hernias are characterized by an intrathoracic stomach along with associated viscera such as the spleen, colon, small bowel, or pancreas.

▶ Clinical Findings

Small hiatal hernias are in most cases asymptomatic, while large hiatal hernias may cause a wide variety of symptoms such as epigastric discomfort, chest pain, postprandial bloating, dysphagia, or respiratory problems (asthma, cough, or dyspnea caused by chronic aspiration). Anemia is secondary to gastric erosions, and it can be the only presenting symptom. In addition, patients may experience symptoms due to GER.

▶ Diagnosis

A barium swallow will delineate the anatomy and the type of hiatal hernia. Endoscopy is important to determine if gastric or esophageal inflammation is present and to rule out cancer. If reflux symptoms are present, manometry and pH monitoring should be performed.

▶ Complications

The most frequent complications of paraesophageal hernia are hemorrhage, incarceration, obstruction, and strangulation. The herniated portion of the stomach often becomes congested, and bleeding occurs from erosions of the mucosa. Obstruction may occur, most often at the esophagogastric junction as a result of torsion and angulation at this point—especially if a large portion (or all) of the stomach herniates into the chest. In paraesophageal hiatal hernia—in contrast to the sliding type—other viscera such as the small and large intestines and spleen may also enter the mediastinum along with the stomach.

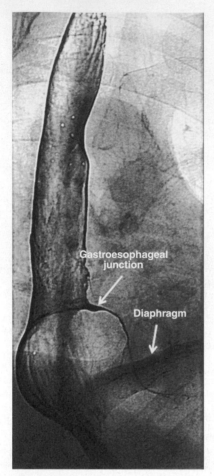

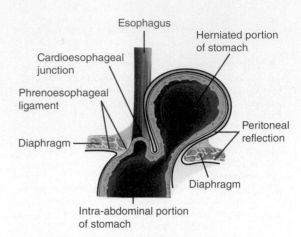

▲ **Figure 20–11.** Paraesophageal hernia.

▲ **Figure 20–10.** Large sliding hiatal hernia. Diaphragmatic hiatus is circled.

▶ Treatment

Operative repair is indicated in symptomatic patients. The usual method is to return the herniated stomach below the diaphragm into the abdomen, repair the enlarged esophageal hiatus, and then add a fundoplication. In most cases, the operation can be performed laparoscopically. The results of surgical management are excellent in about 90% of patients.

Dallemagne B et al: Laparoscopic repair of paraesophageal hernia. Long-term follow-up reveals good clinical outcome despite high radiological recurrence rate. *Ann Surg* 2011;253:291-296.

Herbella FAM, et al. Hiatal Mesh Repair—Current Status. *Surg Laparosc Endosc Percutan Tech* 2011;21:61-66.

Oelschlager BK et al: Biologic prosthesis to prevent recurrence after laparoscopic paraesophageal hernia repair: long-term follow-up from a multicenter, prospective, randomized trial. *J Am Coll Surg* 2011;213:461-468.

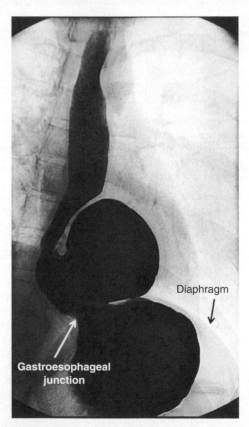

▲ **Figure 20–12.** Paraesophageal hernia. Note that the cardioesophageal junction remains in its normal anatomic position below the diaphragm.

TUMORS OF THE ESOPHAGUS

1. Benign Tumors of the Esophagus

ESSENTIALS OF DIAGNOSIS

▶ Dyesphagia, epigastric discomfort

▶ Radiographic demonstration of a smooth filling defect within the esophageal lumen

► General Considerations

Esophageal leiomyomas are the most common benign tumors of the esophagus. They represent 10% of all gastrointestinal leiomyomas. They originate in the smooth muscle layers, mostly in the lower two-thirds of the esophagus, and they narrow the esophageal lumen. These tumors consist of smooth muscle cells surrounded by a capsule of fibrous tissue. The mucosa overlying the tumor is generally intact, but occasionally it may become ulcerated as a result of pressure necrosis by an enlarging lesion. Leiomyomas are not associated with the development of cancer. Other tumors such as fibromas, lipomas, fibromyomas, and myxomas are rare. Congenital cysts or duplications of the esophagus (the second-most common benign lesion after leiomyomas) may occur at any level, although they are most common in the lower esophagus.

► Clinical Findings

Many benign lesions are asymptomatic and are discovered incidentally during the upper gastrointestinal fluoroscopic examination. Benign tumors or cysts grow slowly and become symptomatic only after reaching a size of 5 cm or more. On barium swallow, leiomyomas appear as a smooth filling defect within the esophageal lumen (Figure 20–13). An intraluminal mass covered by normal mucosa can be easily recognized during endoscopy, but biopsies should not be taken because they may make subsequent enucleation of the tumor more difficult. Endoscopic ultrasound and chest CT help in the characterization of the tumor and in the differential diagnosis.

► Differential Diagnosis

Leiomyomas, cysts, and duplications can be distinguished from cancer by their classic radiographic appearance. Intraluminal papillomas, polyps, or granulomas may be indistinguishable radiographically from early carcinoma, so their exact nature must be confirmed histologically.

► Treatment

Small polypoid intraluminal lesions may be removed endoscopically. The treatment of choice for symptomatic

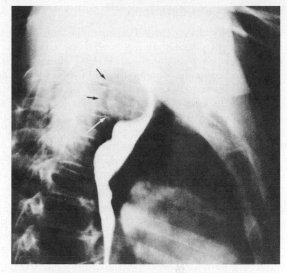

▲ **Figure 20–13.** Leiomyoma of esophagus. Note smooth, rounded density causing extrinsic compression of esophageal lumen.

leiomyomas is enucleation. While in the past a thoracotomy or a laparotomy was used, today enucleation can be accomplished by either a thoracoscopic or a laparoscopic approach.

Gullo R et al: Laparoscopic excision of esophageal leiomyoma. *Updates Surg* 2012;64(4):315-318.

Linde EM et al: Solitary esophageal leiomyoma with eosinophilic infiltrate: case report and review of the literature. *Dis Esophagus* 2011;24(1):E5-E7.

Watson TJ et al: Benign diseases of the esophagus. *Curr Probl Surg* 2009;46:195-259.

2. Carcinoma of the Esophagus

ESSENTIALS OF DIAGNOSIS

▶ Progressive dysphagia, initially for solids and later for liquids.

▶ Progressive weight loss.

▶ Diagnosis established by endoscopy and biopsies.

▶ Staging established by endoscopic ultrasound, computed tomography of chest and abdomen, and positron emission tomography. Bronchoscopy indicated for cancer of the midthoracic esophagus.

General Considerations

The epidemiology of esophageal cancer in the United States has changed considerably during the last 30 years. In the 1970s, squamous cell carcinoma was the most common type of esophageal cancer, accounting for about 90% of the total cases. It was located in the thoracic esophagus and affected mostly black men. Over the past three decades, there has been a progressive increase in the incidence of adenocarcinoma of the distal esophagus and gastroesophageal junction, so that today it accounts for more than 70% of all new cases of esophageal cancer. It is more frequent in white men with GERD and it is linked to BE.

Pathogenesis

The most common contributing factors for squamous cell carcinoma are cigarette smoking and chronic alcohol exposure. Chronic ingestion of hot liquids or foods, poor oral hygiene, and nutritional deficiencies may play a role. Certain medical conditions such as achalasia, caustic injuries of the esophagus, and Plummer–Vinson syndrome are associated with an increased incidence of squamous cell cancer. GERD is the most common predisposing factor for adenocarcinoma of the esophagus, where adenocarcinoma represents the last event of a sequence that starts with GERD and progresses to metaplasia, HGD, and cancer. Esophageal cancer arises in the mucosa and subsequently invades the submucosa and the muscle layers. Ultimately, structures located next to the esophagus may be infiltrated (tracheobronchial tree, aorta, recurrent laryngeal nerve). At the same time, the tumor tends to metastasize to the lymph nodes (mediastinal, celiac, cervical) and to the liver, lungs, peritoneum, adrenals, and bones.

Clinical Findings

A. Symptoms

Early esophageal cancer may be asymptomatic. As the cancer grows, dysphagia is the most common symptom. It is initially for solids but eventually it progresses to liquids. Weight loss occurs in more than 50% of patients. Patients can have pain when swallowing. Pain over bony structures may be due to metastases. Hoarseness is usually due to invasion of the right or left recurrent laryngeal nerves with paralysis of the ipsilateral vocal cord. Respiratory symptoms may be due to regurgitation and aspiration of undigested food or to invasion of the tracheobronchial tree, with development of a tracheoesophageal fistula.

B. Imaging Studies

Barium swallow shows the location and the extent of the tumor. Esophageal cancer usually presents as an irregular intraluminal mass or a stricture (Figure 20–14). Endoscopy allows direct visualization and biopsies of

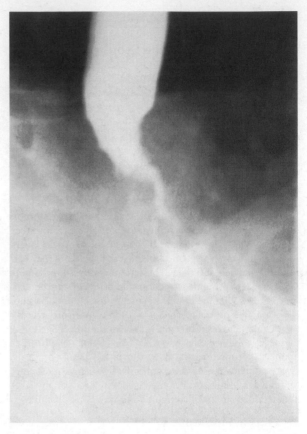

▲ **Figure 20–14.** Barium swallow demonstrating a distal esophageal carcinoma.

the tumor. For tumors of the upper and midesophagus, bronchoscopy is indicated to rule out invasion of the tracheobronchial tree.

C. Special Tests

After the diagnosis is established, it is important to determine the staging of the cancer (Table 20–4). Abdominal and chest CT scans and PET are useful to detect distant metastases and invasion of structures next to the esophagus. Endoscopic ultrasound is the most sensitive test to determine the depth of penetration by the tumor, the presence of enlarged periesophageal lymph nodes, and invasion of structures next to the esophagus. Furthermore, it allows a fine-needle aspiration of enlarged periesophageal lymph nodes. A bone scan is indicated in patients with new onset of bone pain.

Differential Diagnosis

The differential diagnosis includes peptic strictures due to reflux, achalasia, and benign esophageal tumors.

Table 20–4. AAJCC Staging System (ptnm) of Esophageal Cancer

Primary Tumor (T)	
Tx	Primary tumor cannot be assessed
T0	No evidence of primary tumor
Tis	Carcinoma in situ/high-grade dysplasia
T1	Tumor invades lamina propria, muscularis mucosae, or submucosa
T1a	Tumor invades lamina propria or muscularis mucosae
T1b	Tumor invades submucosa
T2	Tumor invades muscularis propria
T3	Tumor invades aventitia
T4	Tumor invades adjacent structures
T4a	Resectable tumor invading pleura, pericardium or diaphragm
T4b	Unresectable tumor invading other adjacent structures, eg, aorta, vertebral body, trachea
Regional Lymph Nodes (N)	
Nx	Regional lymph nodes cannot be assessed
N0	No regional lymph node metastasis
N1	1-2 regional lymph nodes involved
N2	3-6 regional lymph nodes involved
N3	7 or more regional lymph nodes involved
Distant Metastasis (M)	
M0	No distant metastasis
M1	Distant metastasis

Reproduced, with permission, from American Joint Committee on Cancer (AJCC) Cancer Staging Manual, 7th edition. Springer; 2011.

▶ Treatment

Treatment is based on the stage of the cancer. In patients with early esophageal cancer (pT1a), an esophagectomy can be avoided, because of the very low risk of lymph nodes metastasis (0%-3%), and EMR and RFA are very effective. However, patients need to undergo a very strict endoscopic follow-up to detect possible early recurrence.

Patients with invasive esophageal cancer (T1b and T2) are considered candidates for esophagectomy if the following criteria are met: (1) no evidence of spread of the tumor to structures next to the esophagus such as the tracheobronchial tree, the aorta, or the recurrent laryngeal nerve; (2) no evidence of distant metastases; (3) the patient is fit from a cardiac and respiratory point of view. An esophagectomy can be performed by using an abdominal and a cervical incision (with blunt dissection of the thoracic esophagus through the esophageal hiatus; *transhiatal esophagectomy*) or by using an abdominal and a right chest incision (*transthoracic esophagectomy*). After removal of the esophagus, continuity of the gastrointestinal tract is reestablished by using either the stomach or the colon. The transhiatal esophagectomy offers the advantage of avoiding the chest incision, with decreased compromise of lung function and decreased postoperative discomfort. The validity of the trans-hiatal esophagectomy as a cancer operation was initially questioned because part of the operation is not done under direct vision and because of the small number of resected lymph nodes. However, many retrospective studies and prospective randomized trials have shown no difference in survival between the two operations, suggesting that it is not the type of operation that influences survival but rather the stage of the disease at the time the operation is performed. The morbidity rate of the operation is around 30%, and it is mostly due to cardiac (arrhythmias), respiratory (atelectasis, pleural effusion), and septic complications (anastomotic leak, pneumonia). The mortality rate in specialized and "high volume" centers is less than 5%. These results are due to the presence of an experienced team composed of surgeons, anesthesiologists, intensivists, cardiologists, radiologists, and nurses.

The best treatment for patients with locally advanced cancer (T3-4N0-3, T2-N1-3) includes a combination of radiotherapy and chemotherapy used in order to improve local (radiotherapy) and distant control of the disease (chemotherapy), followed by surgery. Overall, it seems that the combination of neoadjuvant therapy followed by surgery offers the best survival benefit. This is particularly true in the subgroup of patients (about 20%) who have a "complete pathologic response" (no tumor found in the specimen).

Nonoperative therapy is reserved for patients who are not candidates for surgery because of local invasion of the tumor, metastases, or a poor functional status. The goal of therapy in these patients is palliation of the dysphagia. The following treatment modalities are available to achieve this goal:

1. Expandable, coated, metallic stents can be deployed by endoscopy under fluoroscopic guidance in order to keep the esophageal lumen open. They are particularly useful when a tracheoesophageal fistula is present.

2. Laser therapy (Nd:YAG laser) relieves dysphagia in up to 70% of patients. However, multiple sessions are usually required to keep the esophageal lumen open.

3. Radiation therapy is successful in relieving dysphagia in about 50% of patients.

The stage of the disease is the most important prognostic factor. Overall 5-year survival for esophageal cancer remains around 25%.

Boshier PR et al: Transthoracic versus transhiatal esophagectomy for the treatment of esophagogastric cancer: a meta-analysis. *Ann Surg* 2011;254:894-906.

Butler N et al: Minimally invasive oesophagectomy: current status and future direction. *Surg Endosc* 2011;25:2071-2083.

Gasper WJ et al: Has recognition of the relationship between mortality rates and hospital volume for major cancer surgery in California made a difference? A follow-up analysis of another decade. *Ann Surg* 2009;250:472-483.

Raz DJ et al: Side-to-side stapled intra-thoracic esophagogastric anastomosis reduces the incidence of leaks and stenosis. *Dis Esophagus* 2008;21:69-72.

Rice TW et al: 7th edition of the AJCC Cancer Staging Manual: esophagus and esophagogastric junction. *Ann Surg Oncol* 2010;17:1721-1724.

Scarpa M: Systematic review of health-related quality of life after esophagectomy for esophageal cancer. *World J Gastroenterol* 2011;17:4660-4674.

Wijnhoven BPL et al. Neoadjuvant chemoradiotherapy for esophageal cancer: a review of meta-analyses. *World J Surg* 2009;33:2606-2614.

Yoon HH et al: The role of FDG-PET and staging laparoscopy in the management of patients with cancer of the esophagus or gastroesophageal junction. *Gastroenterol Clin North Am* 2009;38:105-120.

OTHER SURGICAL DISORDERS OF THE ESOPHAGUS

PERFORATION OF THE ESOPHAGUS

ESSENTIALS OF DIAGNOSIS

▶ History of recent instrumentation of the esophagus or severe vomiting

▶ Pain in the neck, chest, or upper abdomen

▶ Signs of mediastinal or thoracic sepsis within 24 hours

▶ Radiographic evidence of an esophageal leak

▶ General Considerations

Esophageal perforations can result from iatrogenic instrumentation (eg, endoscopy, balloon dilation), severe vomiting, external trauma, and other rare causes. The subsequent clinical manifestations are influenced by the site of the perforation (ie, cervical or thoracic) and, in the case of thoracic perforations, whether or not the mediastinal pleura has been ruptured. Morbidity resulting from esophageal perforation is principally due to infection. Immediately after injury, the tissues are contaminated by esophageal contents, but infection has not become established; surgical closure of the defect will usually prevent the development of serious infection. If more than 24 hours have elapsed since the time of injury, severe contamination has occurred. At this time, the esophageal defect usually breaks down if it is surgically closed, and measures to treat mediastinitis and empyema may not be adequate to avoid a fatal outcome. Although serious infection usually occurs if surgical repair is delayed, a few cases of minor instrumental perforations can be managed by antibiotics without operation.

A. Instrumental Perforations

Medical instrumentation is the most common cause of esophageal perforation (diagnostic or therapeutic endoscopy). Instrumental perforations are most likely to occur in the cervical esophagus. The endoscope may press the posterior wall of the esophagus against osteoarthritic spurs of the cervical vertebrae, causing contusion or laceration. The cricopharyngeal area is the most common site of injury. Perforations of the thoracic esophagus may occur at any level but are most common at the natural sites of narrowing, at the level of the left main stem bronchus and at the diaphragmatic hiatus. Perforations during pneumatic dilatation for achalasia (2%-6%) occur proximal to the gastroesophageal junction.

B. Spontaneous (Postemetic) Perforation (Boerhaave Syndrome)

Spontaneous perforation usually occurs in the absence of preexisting esophageal disease, but 10% of patients have reflux esophagitis, esophageal diverticulum, or carcinoma. Most cases follow a bout of heavy eating and drinking. The perforation most frequently occurs in the left posterolateral wall, 3-5 cm above the gastroesophageal junction. The tear results from excessive intraluminal pressure, usually caused by violent retching and vomiting. Some cases have also been associated with childbirth, defecation, convulsions, heavy lifting, and forceful swallowing. The overlying pleura are also torn, so both the mediastinum and the pleural cavity are contaminated with esophageal contents. The second-most common site of perforation is at the midthoracic esophagus, on the right side at the level of the azygous vein.

▶ Clinical Findings

A. Signs and Symptoms

The principal early manifestation is pain, which is felt in the neck with cervical perforations and in the chest or upper abdomen with perforations of the thoracic esophagus. The pain may radiate to the back. With cervical perforations, pain is followed by crepitus in the neck, dysphagia, and signs of infection. Perforations of the thoracic esophagus, which communicate with the pleural cavity in about 75% of cases, are usually accompanied by tachycardia, tachypnea, dyspnea, and the early development of hypotension. With perforation into the chest, pneumothorax is produced, followed by hydrothorax and, if not promptly treated, empyema. The left chest is involved in 70% and the right chest in 20%; involvement is bilateral in 10%. Escape of air into the mediastinum may result in a "mediastinal crunch," which is produced by the heart beating against air-filled tissues (Hamman sign). If the pleura remain intact, mediastinal emphysema appears more rapidly, and pleural effusion is slow to develop.

B. Imaging Studies

X-ray studies are important to demonstrate that perforation has occurred and to locate the site of the injury. In perforations of the cervical esophagus, x-rays show air in the soft tissues, especially along the cervical spine. The trachea may be displaced anteriorly by air and fluid. Later, widening of the superior mediastinum may be seen. With thoracic perforations, mediastinal widening and pleural effusion with or without pneumothorax are the usual findings. An esophagogram using water-soluble contrast medium should be performed promptly in every patient suspected of having an esophageal perforation (Figure 20–15). If a leak is not seen, the examination should be repeated using barium. A CT scan of the chest is also useful to localize the perforation and eventually to drain mediastinal fluid collections.

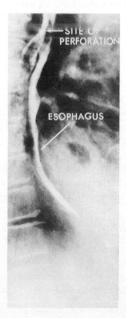

▲ **Figure 20–15.** Extravasation of contrast material through instrumental perforation of upper thoracic esophagus. Note loculi of air and fluid anterior to esophagus, indicating that mediastinitis has already developed.

C. Special Studies

Thoracentesis will reveal cloudy or purulent fluid, depending on how much time has passed since the time of perforation. The amylase content of the fluid is elevated, and serum amylase levels may also be high as a result of absorption of amylase from the pleural cavity.

▶ Treatment

Broad-spectrum antibiotics should be given immediately. The infection is usually polymicrobial with *Staphylococcus*, *Streptococcus*, *Pseudomonas*, and *Bacteroides*. Early operation is appropriate for all but a few cases, and every effort should be made to operate before the perforation is 24 hours old. For lesions treated within this time limit, the operation should consist of closure of the perforation and external drainage. External drainage alone may suffice for small cervical perforations, which may be difficult to find. Patients with achalasia in whom perforation has resulted from balloon dilation should have the tear in the esophagus repaired and a Heller myotomy performed on the opposite side of the esophagus. Definitive therapy (eg, resection) should also be performed in patients with other surgical conditions, such as esophageal carcinoma.

Primary repair has a high failure rate if the perforation is older than 24 hours. The classic recommendation in this situation has been to isolate the perforation (ie, to minimize further contamination) by performing a temporary cervical esophagostomy, ligating the esophagus just proximal to the gastroesophageal junction, and placing a feeding jejunostomy for enteral nutrition. Alternatively, the segment of esophagus where the perforation is located can be resected, bringing the proximal end of esophagus out through the neck and closing the distal end. The mediastinum is drained, and a feeding jejunostomy is created. Later, the esophagostomy is taken down, and stomach or colon interposed to bridge the gap. Blunt esophagectomy may be feasible as emergency treatment of instrumental perforation in a patient with lye stricture.

Nonoperative management consisting of antibiotics alone may be all that is necessary in a few selected cases of instrumental perforation. This approach should be confined to patients without thoracic involvement (eg, pneumothorax or hydrothorax) whose esophagogram demonstrates just a short extraluminal sinus tract without wide mediastinal spread (ie, the contamination is limited) and who have no systemic signs of sepsis (eg, hypotension and tachypnea). Recently, esophageal stents have been placed for the treatment of iatrogenic, intrathoracic esophageal perforations.

The survival rate is 90% when surgical treatment is accomplished within 24 hours. The rate drops to about 50% when treatment is delayed.

Carrott PW Jr et al: Advances in the management of esophageal perforation. *Thorac Surg Clin* 2011;21:541-545.

Dua KS: Expandable stents for benign esophageal disease. *Gastrointest Endosc Clin N Am* 2011;21:359-376.

Søreide JA et al: Esophageal perforation: diagnostic work-up and clinical decision-making in the first 24 hours. *Scand J Trauma Resusc Emerg Med* 2011;19:66.

INGESTED FOREIGN OBJECTS

Most cases of ingested foreign objects occur in children who swallow coins or other small objects. In adults, the problem most often consists of esophageal meat impaction or, less commonly, lodged bones or toothpicks. Dentures and esophageal disease, such as a benign stricture, are the principal predisposing factors in adults. Prisoners and mentally ill persons occasionally swallow foreign objects intentionally.

About 90% of swallowed foreign objects pass into the stomach and from there into the intestine and are eventually passed without problems. Ten percent hang up in the esophagus. If they traverse the esophagus, objects whose dimensions exceed 2-5 cm tend to remain in the stomach. Ten percent of ingested foreign objects require endoscopic removal, and 1% requires surgery. About 10% of ingested foreign objects enter the tracheobronchial tree.

The patient's history usually defines the problem adequately. The patient with a foreign object in the esophagus may or may not experience dysphagia or chest pain.

▶ Specific Kinds of Ingested Foreign Objects

A. Coins

Pennies and dimes usually pass into the stomach, but larger coins will lodge in the esophagus at or just beyond the cricopharyngeus. It is important to know if a swallowed coin has remained in the esophagus, and whether or not the patient has symptoms is an unreliable basis for making the determination. Therefore, anteroposterior and lateral chest x-rays should be obtained to determine whether the coin is in the esophagus or trachea. Small children should be x-rayed from the base of the skull to the anus in order to find any additional coins in the gut.

Coins in the esophagus should be removed promptly, since complications may occur if treatment delay exceeds 24 hours. The procedure is best accomplished with a grasping forceps passed through a flexible endoscope. Sedation is adequate for older children or adults, but general endotracheal anesthesia is required in order to protect the airway of infants and young children. A smooth foreign body too large to grasp with a forceps can be removed by passing a dilating balloon beyond it and then withdrawing the endoscope and balloon as a unit. If the object is small enough (< 20 mm), it may be pushed into the stomach.

Once a coin has passed into the stomach, it can be observed by periodic x-rays for as long as a month before the conclusion is reached that spontaneous elimination is unlikely and endoscopic removal is indicated.

B. Meat Impaction

Meat is the most common foreign object that lodges in the esophagus of adults, and many affected patients have underlying esophageal disease. The site of meat impaction is usually at the cricopharyngeus muscle or in the distal esophagus in patients with achalasia, diffuse esophageal spasm, or a stricture.

No x-rays (especially barium studies) are indicated, for they make the endoscopist's task more difficult. If obstruction is complete and the patient cannot handle saliva, endoscopy should be performed as an emergency to prevent aspiration. If the clinical findings are minor, however, endoscopy can be postponed for up to 12 hours to see whether the food will pass spontaneously.

Meat can usually be removed as a single piece using a polypectomy snare passed through a flexible endoscope. In some cases, a meat bolus can be pushed into the stomach, which is safe so long as it passes with minimal pressure. After the esophagus has been cleared, it should be checked endoscopically for underlying disease. An esophageal stricture should be dilated if the esophageal wall is not acutely inflamed as a result of the meat impaction.

C. Sharp and Pointed Objects

Bones, safety pins, hat pins, razor blades, toothpicks, nails, and many others constitute this group of foreign objects. The general principles of management are: (1) to remove these objects endoscopically by grasping and pulling a blunt side (eg, the hinge of an open safety pin) with forceps, (2) to remove a piece of glass or a razor blade by pulling it into the lumen of a rigid esophagoscope, or (3) to operate if neither of these methods appears to be safe. Sharp or pointed objects in the stomach should be removed surgically, since 25% of them will perforate the intestine, usually near the ileocecal valve, if they exit the pylorus.

D. Button Batteries

These small batteries are swallowed by children, just like coins, but unlike coins, they are highly corrosive and should be removed urgently before a serious complication such as an esophagotracheal or esophagoaortic fistula develops.

E. Cocaine Packets

Cocaine smugglers may swallow small packets of cocaine in balloons or condoms. Rupture of just one of these packets can be fatal, so attempts at endoscopic removal are unsafe.

If it appears that the packets will pass spontaneously, the patient may be watched; otherwise, surgical removal is indicated.

ASGE Standards of Practice Committee et al: Management of ingested foreign bodies and food impactions. *Gastrointest Endosc* 2011;73:1085-1091.

Sung SH et al: Factors predictive of risk for complications in patients with oesophageal foreign bodies. *Dig Liver Dis* 2011;43:632-635.

CAUSTIC INJURIES OF THE ESOPHAGUS

 ESSENTIALS OF DIAGNOSIS

► History of ingestion of caustic liquids or solids
► Burns of the lips, mouth, tongue, and oropharynx
► Chest pain and dysphagia

► General Considerations

Ingestion of strong solutions of acid or alkali or of solid substances of similar nature produces extensive chemical burns. The injury usually represents a suicide attempt in adults and accidental ingestion in children. Strong alkali produces "liquefaction necrosis," which involves dissolution of protein and collagen, saponification of fats, dehydration of tissues, thrombosis of blood vessels, and deep penetrating injuries. Acids produce a "coagulation necrosis" involving eschar formation, which tends to shield the deeper tissues from injury. Depending on the concentration and the length of time the irritant remains in contact with the mucosa, sloughing of the mucous membrane, edema and inflammation of the submucosa, infection, perforation, and mediastinitis may develop.

Ingested lye in solid form tends to adhere to the mucosa of the pharynx and proximal esophagus. Severe acute esophageal necrosis is rare, and the main clinical problems are early edema and late stricture formation, principally of the proximal esophagus. Liquid caustics commonly produce much more extensive esophageal necrosis, and occasionally even tracheoesophageal and esophagoaortic fistulas. If the patient survives the acute phase, a lengthy nondilatable stricture often develops.

Ingestion of strong acid characteristically produces greatest injury to the stomach, with the esophagus remaining intact in over 80% of cases. The result may be immediate gastric necrosis or late antral stenosis.

Nearly all severe injuries are caused by strong alkali. Weak alkali and acid are associated with less extensive lesions.

► Clinical Findings

A. Symptoms and Signs

Systemic symptoms roughly parallel the severity of the caustic burn. The most common finding is inflammatory edema of the lips, mouth, tongue, and oropharynx; in the absence of visible injury in this area, severe esophageal damage is rare. Patients with serious esophageal burns often experience chest pain and dysphagia and drooling of large amounts of saliva. Pain on swallowing may be intense. If the damage is severe, the patient often appears toxic, with high fever, prostration, and shock. The absence of toxicity does not rule out severe injury. Tracheobronchitis accompanied by coughing and increased bronchial secretions is frequently noted. Stridor may be present, and in a few patients respiratory obstruction progresses rapidly and requires tracheostomy for relief. Complete esophageal obstruction due to edema, inflammation, and mucosal sloughing may develop within the first few days.

B. Esophagoscopy

Endoscopy is the key test in the evaluation of caustic trauma to the esophagus. Determination of the extent of injury by esophagoscopy contributes substantially to therapeutic decisions. Endoscopy should be performed after the initial resuscitation, usually within 24 hours of admission. The scope is inserted far enough to gauge the most serious degree of burn, which is classified as first-, second-, or third-degree, as defined in Table 20–5.

Table 20–5. Endoscopic grading of corrosive burns of esophagus and stomach.

Grade	Definition	Endoscopic Findings
First-degree	Superficial mucosal injury	Mucosal hyperemia and edema; superficial mucosal desquamation
Second-degree	Full-thickness mucosal involvement. No or partial-thickness muscular injury	Sloughing of mucosa. Hemorrhage, exudate, ulceration, pseudomembrane formation, and granulation tissue when examined late
Third-degree	Full-thickness esophageal or gastric injury with extension into adjacent tissues	Sloughing of tissues with deep ulceration. Complete obliteration of esophageal lumen by edema; charring and eschar formation; full-thickness necrosis; perforation

Reproduced, with permission, from Estrera A et al: Corrosive burns of the esophagus and stomach: a recommendation for an aggressive surgical approach. *Ann Thorac Surg* 1986;41:276.

C. Radiology

A chest x-ray should be taken in all patients. It may show signs of esophageal perforation (subcutaneous emphysema, pneumomediastinum, pneumothorax) or aspiration (pulmonary infiltrates). An esophagogram is indicated in the initial evaluation if perforation is suspected and in later stages to detect the presence of a stricture.

▶ Treatment

Patients should be hospitalized and intravenous fluids antibiotics should be administered. The use of steroids is still controversial. A nasogastric tube placed under fluoroscopic or endoscopic guidance allows stenting of the esophagus, preventing complete obstruction of the lumen.

Patients with first-degree burns do not require aggressive therapy and may be discharged from the hospital after a short period of observation. Second-degree and minor spotty third-degree injuries are treated by inserting a nasogastric tube. Nutrition can be given through the nasogastric tube or parenterally. Periodic esophagograms are obtained in follow-up to look for stricture formation, which is treated early in its development by dilations and eventually resection.

Third-degree burns involving extensive esophagogastric necrosis require emergency esophagogastrectomy, esophagostomy, and feeding jejunostomy. Esophagectomy is best performed by the blunt technique using a laparotomy and cervical incision. It is sometimes necessary to resect adjacent organs (eg, transverse colon) that have also been damaged. Reconstruction by substernal colon interposition is performed 8-12 weeks later.

Early and proper management of caustic burns provides satisfactory results in most cases. The ingestion of strong acid or alkaline solutions with extensive immediate destruction of the mucosa produces profound pathologic changes that may result in fibrous strictures that require dilations and, in some cases, esophagectomy and colon interposition.

Cabral C et al: Caustic injuries of the upper digestive tract: a population observational study. *Surg Endosc* 2012;26:214-221.
Chirica M et al: Late morbidity after colon interposition for corrosive esophageal injury: risk factors, management, and outcome. A 20-years experience. *Ann Surg* 2010;252:271-280.

ESOPHAGEAL BANDS, WEBS, OR RINGS

A narrow mucosal ring (Schatzki ring) may develop at the lower end of the esophagus. Most patients are relatively free from symptoms. Dysphagia occurs when the ring is less than 12 mm in diameter. In most cases, the ring is located at the squamocolumnar junction and occurs in a patient with GERD. Being confined to the mucosa, it differs from an inflammatory (peptic) stricture, which involves all layers of the esophagus. A barium swallow clearly identifies the problem. Treatment consists of endoscopic dilation of the ring and treatment of the associated reflux (acid-reducing medications or fundoplication).

de Wijkerslooth LR et al: Endoscopic management of difficult or recurrent esophageal strictures. *Am J Gastroenterol* 2011;106:2080-2091; quiz 2092.
Müller M et al: Is the Schatzki ring a unique esophageal entity? *World J Gastroenterol* 2011;21(17):2838-2843.

▼ THE DIAPHRAGM

The diaphragm (Figure 20–16) is a musculotendinous, dome-shaped structure attached posteriorly to the first, second, and third lumbar vertebrae, anteriorly to the lower sternum and laterally to the costal arches. It separates the abdominal and the thoracic cavities. The diaphragm allows the passage of various normal structures through anatomic foramina. The aortic hiatus lies posteriorly at the level of the twelfth thoracic vertebra, and through it pass the aorta, the thoracic duct, and the azygos venous system. The esophageal hiatus lies immediately anteriorly and slightly to the left at the level of the tenth thoracic vertebra and is separated from the aortic hiatus by the decussation of the right crus of the diaphragm. Through this hiatus pass the esophagus and the vagus nerves. At the level of the ninth thoracic vertebra and slightly to the right of the esophageal hiatus is the vena caval foramen, which allows passage of the inferior vena cava and small branches of the phrenic nerve. The phrenic arteries arising directly from the aorta supply the diaphragm along with the lower intercostal arteries and the terminal branches of the internal mammary arteries.

PARASTERNAL OR RETROSTERNAL (FORAMEN OF MORGAGNI) HERNIA & PLEUROPERITONEAL (FORAMEN OF BOCHDALEK) HERNIA

Failure of fusion of the sternal and costal portions of the diaphragm anteriorly in the midline creates a defect (foramen of Morgagni) through which hernias can occur. Normally, the diaphragm becomes fused, allowing only the internal mammary arteries and their superior epigastric branches, along with lymphatics, to pass through this area. Posterolaterally, failure of fusion of the pleuroperitoneal canal creates a defect through which viscera may herniate to produce a foramen of Bochdalek hernia (Figure 20–17).

Although both types of hernia are congenital, symptoms in the Morgagni hernia usually do not develop until middle life or later. This type of hernia is more frequent in women. These hernias are mostly right-sided and have a hernia sac. The most common contents are the omentum, the colon, and the stomach. On the other hand, the Bochdalek hernia occurs more frequently on the left side and may cause severe respiratory distress at birth, requiring an emergent opera-

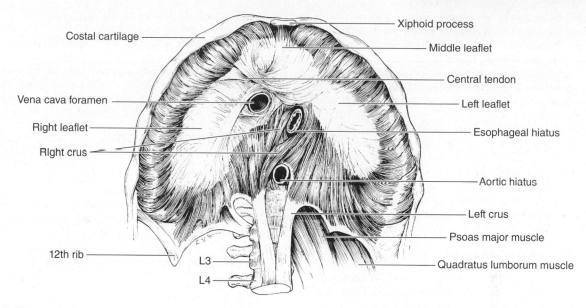

▲ **Figure 20–16.** Inferior surface of the diaphragm.

tion. Routine chest films show a retrosternal solid mass, a retrosternal air-filled viscus, or similar findings in the posterolateral thorax if a Bochdalek hernia is present. Chest CT confirms the diagnosis and identifies the contents of the hernia.

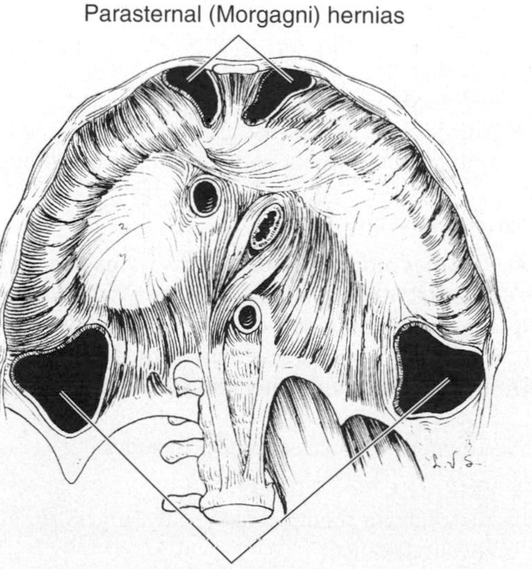

Elective surgical repair is indicated in most instances to prevent complications. An emergent operation may become necessary in the newborn infant who develops progressive cardiorespiratory insufficiency. Repair of the defect by a transabdominal approach is preferable, and the results are excellent. A minimally invasive approach (laparoscopic or thoracoscopic) has been recently used.

Laituri CA et al: Morgagni hernia repair in children: comparison of laparoscopic and open results. *J Laparoendosc Adv Surg Tech* 2011;21:89-91.

Nasr A et al: Foramen of Morgagni hernia: presentation and treatment. *Thorac Surg Clin* 2009;19:463-468.

TRAUMATIC DIAPHRAGMATIC HERNIA

Traumatic rupture of the diaphragm may occur as a result of penetrating wounds or severe blunt external trauma. Lacerations usually occur in the tendinous portion of the diaphragm, most often on the left side. The liver provides protection to diaphragmatic injury on the right side except from penetrating wounds. Abdominal viscera may immediately herniate through the defect in the diaphragm into the pleural cavity or may gradually insinuate themselves into the thorax over a period of months or years.

▶ **Clinical Findings**

Diaphragmatic ruptures present in two ways. In the acute form, the patient has recently experienced blunt trauma or a penetrating wound to the chest, abdomen, or back. The

Parasternal (Morgagni) hernias

Pleuroperitoneal (Bochdalek) hernias

▲ **Figure 20–17.** Sites of congenital diaphragmatic herniation.

clinical manifestations are essentially those of the associated injuries, but occasionally, massive herniation of abdominal viscera through the diaphragm causes respiratory insufficiency. In the chronic form, the diaphragmatic tear is unrecognized at the time of the original injury. Sometime later, symptoms (eg, pain, bowel obstruction) appear from herniation of viscera. Respiratory symptoms in such cases are less common.

Plain films of the chest may show a radiopaque area and occasionally an air-fluid level if hollow viscera have herniated. If the stomach has entered the chest, the abnormal path of a nasogastric tube may be diagnostic. Ultrasonography, CT scan, and MRI may demonstrate the diaphragmatic rent. Barium study of the colon may show irregular patches of barium in the colon above the diaphragm or a smooth colonic outline if the colon does not contain feces.

▶ **Differential Diagnosis**

Traumatic rupture of the diaphragm must be differentiated from atelectasis, space-consuming tumors of the lower pleural space, pleural effusion, and intestinal obstruction due to other causes.

▶ **Complications**

Hemorrhage and obstruction may occur. If herniation is massive, progressive cardiorespiratory insufficiency may threaten life. The most severe complication is strangulating obstruction of the herniated viscera.

▶ **Treatment**

For acute ruptures, a transabdominal (most commonly) or transthoracic route is used depending on the procedure required to treat ancillary injuries. When the diaphragmatic tear is the only injury, it is usually fixed by laparotomy. Chronic injuries can be repaired by either approach. Asymptomatic tears of the diaphragm with herniated viscera should be repaired, because the risk of strangulating obstruction is high. Laparoscopy is very useful for both diagnosis and treatment. Surgical repair of the rent in the diaphragm is curative, and the prognosis is excellent. The diaphragm supports sutures well, so recurrence is practically unknown.

Fiscon V et al: Laparoscopic repair of intrathoracic liver herniation after traumatic rupture of the diaphragm. *Surg Endosc* 2011;25:3423-3425.
Hanna WC et al: Acute traumatic diaphragmatic injury. *Thorac Surg Clin* 2009;19:485-489.

TUMORS OF THE DIAPHRAGM

Primary tumors of the diaphragm are not common. The majority are benign lipomas. Pericardial cysts develop in the space between the heart and the diaphragm and are usually unilocular and on the right side. Fibrosarcoma, the most common primary malignant diaphragmatic tumor, is extremely rare.

Benign tumors are usually asymptomatic. Since their benign nature cannot be established except by histology, all lesions of this type should be excised through an appropriate thoracotomy or thoracoabdominal approach.

MULTIPLE CHOICE QUESTIONS

1. Esophageal achalasia is characterized by

    A. Absence of esophageal peristalsis
    B. Heartburn in more than 50% of patients
    C. Low intraluminal pH due to GERD
    D. All of the above

2. Which of the following sentences about Zenker diverticulum is wrong?

    A. It is the most common diverticulum of the esophagus.
    B. It is a consequence of an underlying esophageal motility disorder.
    C. Aspiration of diverticular contents is frequent.
    D. The surgical treatment consists of LES myotomy, resection of the diverticulum or its suspension.

3. A 54-year-old patient has heartburn. The correct workup includes

    A. Esophageal manometry, 24-hour pH monitoring and upper endoscopy.
    B. Upper endoscopy and 24-hour pH monitoring.
    C. Nothing, the patient has gastro-esophageal reflux and needs surgery.
    D. Nothing; the patient has gastro-esophageal reflux and needs treatment with proton pump inhibitors.

4. Barrett esophagus

    A. Becomes more symptomatic over time due to the mucosal inflammation
    B. Is linked to duodeno-gastro-esophageal reflux
    C. Is classified short if less than 2 cm
    D. Is characterized by the presence of fundic type cells

5. Treatment of esophageal cancer includes

    A. EMR/RFA for a T1a lesion
    B. Neoadjuvant therapy followed by surgery for locally advanced cancer
    C. Intraesophageal stenting for patients with dysphagia and solid organ metastases
    D. All of the above

The Acute Abdomen

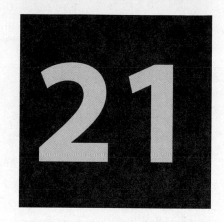

Elisha G. Brownson, MD
Katherine Mandell, MD

An "acute abdomen" denotes any sudden, spontaneous, nontraumatic, severe abdominal pain, typically of less than 24 hours duration. The acute abdomen requires rapid and specific diagnosis as several etiologies demand urgent operative intervention. Because there is frequently a progressive underlying intra-abdominal disorder, undue delay in diagnosis and treatment may adversely affect outcome.

The approach to a patient with an acute abdomen must be orderly and thorough. An acute abdomen should be suspected even in a patient with only mild or atypical presentations. Increasingly, certain patient populations present with atypical complaints, including the immunocompromised, elderly and gastric bypass patients. The history and physical examination often suggest the probable cause, allow formation of a differential diagnosis, and guide the choice of initial diagnostic studies. The clinician must then decide if in-hospital observation is warranted, if additional tests are needed, if early operation is indicated, or if nonoperative treatment would be more suitable.

All clinicians should be familiar with the presenting pattern of the most common causes of an acute abdomen (Table 21–1) and their atypical presentations in certain patient populations. Moreover, they should be familiar with regional specific disease patterns. While the most common cause of abdominal pain in patients presenting to the emergency department is nonspecific discomfort, missing treatable causes of abdominal pain can be disastrous for the patient.

HISTORY

▶ Abdominal Pain

History taking by an experienced physician is key to focusing the evaluation of a patient with an acute abdomen. Taking a patient history is an active process whereby a large number of diagnostic possibilities are considered in order to systematically eliminate less likely conditions.

Pain is the most common and predominant presenting feature of an acute abdomen. Careful consideration of the location, severity, mode of onset and progression, and the character of the pain will suggest a preliminary list of diagnoses.

A. Location of Pain

The location of pain serves only as a rough guide to the diagnosis; "typical" descriptions are reported in only two-thirds of cases. This variability is due to atypical pain patterns, a shift of maximum intensity away from the primary site, or advanced or severe disease. In patients presenting with diffuse peritonitis, generalized pain may completely obscure the precipitating event. Fortunately, some general patterns do emerge that provide clues to diagnosis and narrow the differential of the acute abdomen. Pain confined to either upper quadrant may be evaluated by anatomic consideration of acute conditions affecting underlying organs.

Because of the complex dual visceral and parietal sensory networks innervating the abdominal area, pain is not as precisely localized in the abdomen as in the extremities. Visceral sensation is mediated primarily by afferent C fibers located in the walls of hollow viscera and in the capsules of solid organs. Unlike cutaneous pain, visceral pain is elicited by distention, inflammation or ischemia stimulating the receptor neurons, or by direct involvement (eg, malignant infiltration) of sensory nerves. Visceral pain is a centrally perceived sensation, generally slow in onset, dull, poorly localized and protracted. The pain may be due to increased wall tension or luminal distention or forceful smooth muscle contraction (colic) producing diffuse, deep-seated pain. Visceral pain is most often felt in the midline because of the bilateral sensory supply to the spinal cord. Because different visceral structures are associated with different sensory levels in the spine

Table 21–1. Common causes of the acute abdomen.[1]

Gastrointestinal Tract Disorders
 Nonspecific abdominal pain
 Appendicitis
 Small and large bowel obstruction
 Perforated peptic ulcer
 Incarcerated hernia
 Bowel perforation
 Meckel's diverticulitis
 Boerhaave syndrome
 Diverticulitis
 Inflammatory bowel disorders
 Mallory–Weiss syndrome
 Gastroenteritis
 Acute gastritis
 Mesenteric adenitis
 Parasitic infections
Liver, Spleen, and Biliary Tract Disorders
 Acute cholecystitis
 Acute cholangitis
 Hepatic abscess
 Ruptured hepatic tumor
 Spontaneous rupture of the spleen
 Splenic infarct
 Biliary colic
 Acute hepatitis
Pancreatic Disorders
 Acute pancreatitis
Urinary Tract Disorders
 Ureteral or renal colic
 Acute pyelonephritis
 Acute cystitis
 Renal infarct
Gynecologic Disorders
 Ruptured ectopic pregnancy
 Twisted ovarian tumor
 Ruptured ovarian follicle cyst
 Acute salpingitis
 Dysmenorrhea
 Endometriosis
Vascular Disorders
 Ruptured aortic and visceral aneurysms
 Acute ischemic colitis
 Mesenteric thrombosis
Peritoneal Disorders
 Intra-abdominal abscesses
 Primary peritonitis
 Tuberculous peritonitis
Retroperitoneal Disorders
 Retroperitoneal hemorrhage

[1]The most common causes are marked with an asterisk (*). Conditions in italic type often require urgent operation. Please see specific chapters for management.

Table 21–2. Sensory levels associated with visceral structures.

Structures	Nervous System Pathways	Sensory Level
Liver, spleen and central part of diaphragm	Phrenic nerve	C3-5
Peripheral diaphragm, stomach, pancreas, gallbladder and small bowel	Celiac plexus and greater splanchnic nerve	T6-9
Appendix, colon and pelvic viscera	Mesenteric plexus and lesser splanchnic nerve	T10-11
Sigmoid colon, rectum, kidney, ureters and testes	Lowest splanchnic nerve	T11-L1
Bladder and rectosigmoid	Hypogastric plexus	S2-4

In contrast, parietal pain is mediated by both C and A delta nerve fibers, the latter being responsible for the transmission of more acute, sharper, better localized pain sensation. Direct irritation of the somatically innervated parietal peritoneum by pus, bile, urine, or gastrointestinal secretions leads to a more precisely localized pain. Parietal pain is more easily localized than visceral pain because the somatic afferent fibers are directed to only one side of the nervous system. The cutaneous distribution of parietal pain corresponds to the T6-L1 areas. Abdominal parietal pain is conventionally described as occurring in one of the four abdominal quadrants or in the epigastric or central abdominal area.

Abdominal pain may be referred or may shift to sites removed from the primarily affected organs (Figure 21–2). Referred pain denotes noxious (usually cutaneous) sensations perceived at a site distant from that of a strong primary stimulus. Distorted central perception of the site of pain is due to the confluence of afferent nerve fibers from disparate areas within the posterior horn of the spinal cord. For example, pain due to subdiaphragmatic irritation by air, peritoneal fluid, blood, or a mass lesion is referred to the shoulder via the C4-mediated (phrenic) nerve. Pain may also be referred to the shoulder from supradiaphragmatic lesions such as pleurisy or lower lobe pneumonia. Although more often perceived in the right scapular region, referred biliary pain may mimic angina pectoris if it is perceived in the anterior chest or left shoulder areas.

Spreading or shifting pain parallels the course of the underlying condition. The site of pain at onset should be distinguished from the site at presentation. The chronology of a patient's pain may be as important as the location itself. Beginning classically in the epigastric or periumbilical region, the initial visceral pain of acute appendicitis shifts

(Table 21–2), visceral pain may be felt in the midepigastrium, periumbilical area, lower abdomen, or flank areas (Figure 21–1) depending on the organ involved.

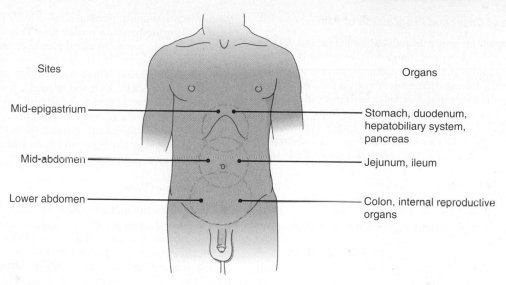

▲ **Figure 21–1.** Visceral pain sites.

to become sharper parietal pain localized in the right lower quadrant when the overlying peritoneum becomes directly inflamed (Figure 21–2). With a perforated peptic ulcer, pain almost always begins in the epigastrium, but as leaked gastric contents track down the right paracolic gutter, pain may descend to the right lower quadrant.

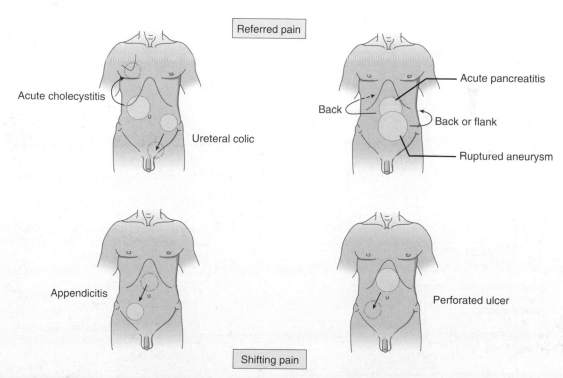

▲ **Figure 21–2.** Referred pain and shifting pain in the acute abdomen. Solid circles indicate the site of maximum pain; dashed circles indicate sites of lesser pain.

B. Mode of Onset and Progression of Pain

The mode of onset of pain reflects the nature and severity of the underlying process. Onset may be explosive (within seconds), rapidly progressive (within 1-2 hours), or gradual (over several hours). Unheralded, excruciating generalized pain suggests an intra-abdominal catastrophe such as a perforated viscus or rupture of an aneurysm, ectopic pregnancy, or abscess. Accompanying systemic signs (tachycardia, sweating, tachypnea, shock) soon supersede the abdominal disturbances and underscore the need for rapid resuscitation and laparotomy.

A less dramatic clinical picture is steady, mild pain becoming intensely centered in a well-defined area within 1-2 hours. Any of the above conditions may present in this manner, but this is more typical of acute cholecystitis, acute pancreatitis, strangulated bowel, mesenteric infarction, renal or ureteral colic and proximal small bowel obstruction.

Finally, some patients initially have slight—at times only vague—abdominal discomfort that is fleetingly present diffusely throughout the abdomen. It may be unclear whether these patients even have an acute abdomen or whether the illness is likely to be a matter for medical rather than surgical attention. Associated gastrointestinal symptoms are infrequent at first, and systemic symptoms are absent. Eventually, the pain and abdominal findings become more pronounced, steady and are localized to a smaller area. This gradual onset pattern leading to a more localized pain may reflect a slowly developing condition or the body's defensive efforts to cordon off an acute process. This broad category includes acute appendicitis (especially with the appendix in a retrocecal position), incarcerated hernias, distal small bowel and large bowel obstructions, uncomplicated peptic ulcer disease, walled-off (often malignant) visceral perforations, some genitourinary and gynecologic conditions, and milder forms of the rapid-onset group mentioned in the first paragraph.

C. Character of Pain

The nature, severity and periodicity of pain provide useful clues to the underlying pathology (Figure 21–3). Pain may be continual or intermittent. Steady pain is more common and often indicates a process that will lead to peritoneal inflammation. It may be constant in severity or fluctuate, but it is always present. Sharp superficial constant pain due to peritoneal irritation is typical of perforated ulcer or a ruptured appendix, ovarian cyst, or ectopic pregnancy. Intermittent, crampy pain (colic) may occur for short or long periods but is punctuated by pain free intervals and is most characteristic of obstruction of a hollow viscus. The gripping, mounting pain

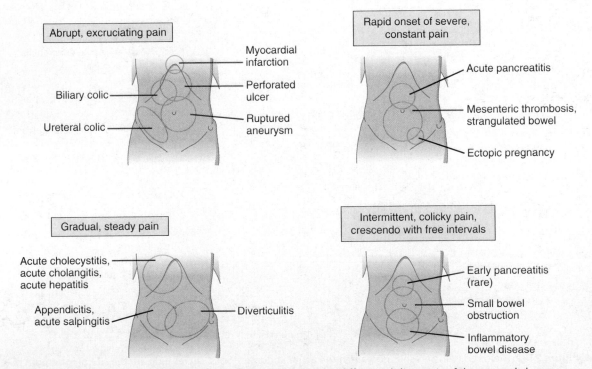

▲ **Figure 21–3.** The location and character of pain are helpful in the differential diagnosis of the acute abdomen.

of small bowel obstruction (and occasionally early pancreatitis) is usually intermittent, vague, deep-seated and crescendo at first but becomes sharper, unremitting and better localized. Unlike the disquieting but bearable pain associated with bowel obstruction, pain caused by lesions occluding smaller conduits (bile ducts, uterine tubes, ureters) rapidly becomes unbearably intense. The pain-free intervals reflect intermittent smooth muscle contractions. In the strict sense, the term "biliary colic" is a misnomer because biliary pain does not remit as bile ducts do not have peristaltic movements.

The quality of a patient's pain leads to the use of certain descriptors to describe different types of pain and may be typical of certain pathologies. The "aching discomfort" of ulcer pain, the "stabbing, breathtaking" pain of acute pancreatitis and mesenteric infarction, the "gripping" pain of a bowel obstruction and the "tearing" pain of ruptured aortic aneurysm remain apt descriptions. Despite the use of such descriptive terms, the quality of visceral pain is not a reliable clue to its cause.

The intensity of a patient's pain may relate to the severity of the insult. Agonizing pain denotes serious or advanced disease. Colicky pain is usually promptly alleviated by analgesics. Ischemic pain due to strangulated bowel or mesenteric thrombosis is only slightly assuaged even by narcotics. Nonspecific abdominal pain is usually mild, but mild pain may also be found with perforated ulcers that have become localized and in mild acute pancreatitis. An occasional patient will deny pain but complain of a vague feeling of abdominal fullness that feels as though it might be relieved by a bowel movement. This visceral sensation (gas stoppage sign) is due to reflex ileus induced by an inflammatory lesion walled off from the free peritoneal cavity, as in retrocecal appendicitis.

Past episodes of pain and factors that aggravate or relieve pain should be noted. Pain caused by localized peritonitis, especially when it affects upper abdominal organs, tends to be exacerbated by movement or deep breathing.

The location, character and severity of the pain in relation to its duration of onset and presence of systemic symptoms help to differentiate rapidly progressive surgical conditions (eg, intestinal ischemia) from more indolent or medical causes (eg, ruptured ovarian cyst) and allows formation of a differential diagnosis.

▶ Other Symptoms Associated with Abdominal Pain

Anorexia, fever, nausea and vomiting, constipation/obstipation, or diarrhea, often accompany abdominal pain, but are nonspecific symptoms and have limited diagnostic value.

A. Vomiting

When sufficiently stimulated by secondary visceral afferent fibers, the medullary vomiting centers activate efferent fibers to induce reflex vomiting. Hence, pain in the acute surgical abdomen usually precedes vomiting, whereas the reverse holds true in medical conditions. Vomiting is a prominent symptom in upper gastrointestinal diseases such as Boerhaave syndrome, Mallory–Weiss syndrome, acute gastritis and acute pancreatitis. Severe, uncontrollable retching provides temporary pain relief in moderate attacks of pancreatitis. The absence of bile in the vomitus is a feature of pyloric stenosis or gastric outlet obstruction. Where associated findings suggest bowel obstruction, the onset and character of vomiting may indicate the level of the lesion. Recurrent vomiting of bile-stained fluid is typical of proximal small bowel obstruction. In distal small or large bowel obstruction, prolonged nausea precedes vomiting, which may become feculent in late cases. Although vomiting may present in either acute appendicitis or nonspecific abdominal pain, coexisting nausea and anorexia are more suggestive of the former condition.

B. Constipation

Reflex ileus is often induced by visceral afferent fibers stimulating efferent fibers of the sympathetic autonomic nervous system (splanchnic nerves) to reduce intestinal peristalsis. Hence, paralytic ileus undermines the value of constipation in the differential diagnosis of an acute abdomen. Constipation itself is hardly an absolute indicator of intestinal obstruction. However, obstipation (the absence of passage of both stool and flatus) strongly suggests mechanical bowel obstruction if there is progressive painful abdominal distention or repeated vomiting.

C. Diarrhea

Copious watery diarrhea is characteristic of gastroenteritis and other medical causes of an acute abdomen. Blood-stained diarrhea suggests ulcerative colitis, Crohn disease, or bacillary or amebic dysentery. It is also found with ischemic colitis but often absent in intestinal infarction due to superior mesenteric artery occlusion.

D. Fever

Fever is a marker of inflammation and may be present in a variety of surgical conditions in the abdomen if they are allowed to progress. The sensitivity of this finding is low as the ability of many patient populations to mount a fever is compromised and for most diseases leading to acute abdomen fever is low grade or absent.

E. Other Specific Symptoms

These are extremely helpful if present. Significant weight loss may suggest cancer or more chronic mesenteric ischemia. Jaundice suggests hepatobiliary disorders. Hematochezia or hematemesis may suggest a gastroduodenal lesion or

Mallory–Weiss syndrome; melena a lower GI bleed or colonic ischemia and hematuria, ureteral colic, or cystitis. The passage of blood clots or necrotic mucosal debris may be the sole evidence of advanced intestinal ischemia.

▶ Other Relevant Aspects of the History

A. Past Medical History

A complete past medical history is crucial to identify both medical conditions related to the presentation of the acute abdomen as well as conditions of associated pulmonary, renal and cardiac systems that may mimic the acute abdomen in their presentation. Many chronic medical conditions complicate the patient's presentation and increase their surgical risk. An assessment of the patient's cardiovascular and pulmonary status should always be done before proceeding to the operating room. Liver disease should be noted as it increases risk for gastrointestinal bleeding, and in severe disease may be complicated by ascites and spontaneous bacterial peritonitis. In patients with vascular disease or atrial fibrillation mesenteric ischemia should be included in the differential. Inflammatory bowel disease can cause severe abdominal pain often treated medically but may be complicated by processes requiring more emergent intervention including intra-abdominal abscess, stricture, obstruction, or perforation.

A patient should also be asked about any history of recent trauma. Delayed splenic bleeding is one of the more common examples of traumatic injuries presenting in delayed fashion.

B. Operation History

Any history of a previous abdominal, groin, vascular, or thoracic operation may be relevant to the current illness. Particular attention to the mode of operation (laparoscopic, open, endovascular) and any anatomic reconstructions may clarify aspects of the current complaint. If possible within the time constraints imposed by the urgency of the current problem, operative notes and pathology reports should be obtained and reviewed.

C. Gynecologic History

The menstrual history is crucial to the diagnosis of ectopic pregnancy, mittelschmerz (due to a ruptured ovarian follicle) and endometriosis. A history of vaginal discharge or dysmenorrhea may denote pelvic inflammatory disease. A complete sexual history should be performed if indicated, and all women of childbearing age should be evaluated for possibility of pregnancy.

D. Medication History

The average patient is taking an increasing number of medications, which may have direct impact on their man-

agement. NSAIDs or aspirin may be a cause of a gastric or duodenal ulcer. Anticoagulants have been implicated in retroperitoneal and intramural duodenal and jejunal hematomas. Additionally, patients who are anticoagulated, or are on antiplatelet therapy may require correction or further consideration prior to operative management. Oral contraceptives have been implicated in the formation of benign hepatic adenomas and in mesenteric venous infarction. Corticosteroids or other chemotherapeutics and immunosuppressive medications, may mask the clinical signs of even advanced peritonitis.

Alcohol use should be interrogated as it can be associated with liver disease, ulcers, gastritis and pancreatitis.

E. Family History

Family history often provides the best information about medical or hereditary causes of an acute abdomen.

F. Travel History

Travel history may raise the possibility of amebic liver abscess or hydatid cyst, malarial spleen, tuberculosis, *Salmonella typhi* infection of the ileocecal area, or dysentery.

▼ FORMING A DIFFERENTIAL DIAGNOSIS LIST

Following a thorough history, the examiner should formulate an early differential diagnosis list using the subsequent physical examination findings to test the various diagnostic possibilities. The age and gender of the patient should assist in guiding the development of the differential diagnosis. Mesenteric adenitis mimics acute appendicitis in the young, gynecologic disorders complicate the evaluation of abdominal pain in women of childbearing age, and malignant and vascular diseases are more common in the elderly. Knowledge of the common causes of abdominal pain and their incidence in various populations is also helpful. Acute cholecystitis, appendicitis, bowel obstruction, cancer and vascular conditions are the common causes of a surgical acute abdomen in older patients. In children, appendicitis accounts for one-third of all abdominal pain and nonspecific abdominal pain for much of the remainder. Causes of an acute abdomen reflect disease patterns of the indigenous population, and awareness of common causes within the physician's locale improves diagnostic accuracy.

PHYSICAL EXAMINATION

The tendency to concentrate on the abdomen should be resisted in favor of a methodical and complete physical examination. Examination should begin with an initial assessment of the patient's vital signs. A patient with systemic signs of shock should be aggressively resuscitated concurrently with any ongoing evaluation. Auscultation of the heart and lungs should also be performed both to rule out sources of abdominal pain due to disorders within the chest (esophageal, cardiac, pulmonary) as well as being part of the preoperative evaluation.

The abdominal examination should be done with the patient in the supine position. A systematic approach to the abdominal examination (Table 21–3) is key to success. The physical examination allows the clinician to search for specific signs that confirm or rule out differential diagnostic possibilities (Table 21–4).

1. **General observation** General observation affords a fairly reliable indication of the severity of the clinical situation. Most patients, although uncomfortable, remain calm. The writhing of patients with visceral pain (eg, intestinal or ureteral colic) contrasts with the rigidly motionless bearing of those with parietal pain (eg, acute appendicitis, generalized peritonitis). Diminished responsiveness or an altered sensorium is suggestive of more advance or significant disease and may herald imminent cardiopulmonary collapse.

2. **Systemic signs** Systemic signs usually accompany rapidly progressive or advanced disorders of the acute abdomen. Extreme pallor, hypotension, hypothermia, tachycardia, tachypnea and diaphoresis suggest major intra-abdominal hemorrhage (eg, ruptured aortic aneurysm or tubal pregnancy). Given such findings, one must proceed rapidly with the examination and any tests to exclude extra-abdominal causes and institute treatment. If extra-abdominal pathology is excluded, these are markers of severe or rapidly progressive intra-abdominal pathology and are indication for emergent laparotomy.

3. **Fever** Constant low-grade fever is common in inflammatory conditions such as diverticulitis, acute cholecystitis and appendicitis. High fever with lower abdominal tenderness in a young woman without signs of systemic illness suggests acute salpingitis.

Table 21–3. Steps in physical examination of the acute abdomen.

1. Global assessment, vital signs	7. Special signs
2. Inspection	8. External hernias and male genitalia
3. Auscultation	9. Rectal examination
4. Cough tenderness	10. Pelvic examination
5. Percussion	
6. Palpation	
• Guarding or rigidity	
• Local palpation	
• Rebound tenderness	
• Deep tenderness	
• Bump tenderness	
• Masses	

Table 21–4. Physical findings in various causes of acute abdomen.

Condition	Helpful Signs
Perforated viscus	Scaphoid, tense abdomen; diminished bowel sounds (late); loss of liver dullness; guarding or rigidity.
Peritonitis	Motionless; absent bowel sounds (late); cough and rebound tenderness; guarding or rigidity.
Inflamed mass or abscess	Tender mass (abdominal, rectal, or pelvic); bump tenderness; special signs (Murphy, psoas, or obturator).
Intestinal obstruction	Distention; visible peristalsis (late); hyperperistalsis (early) or quiet abdomen (late); diffuse pain without rebound tenderness; hernia or rectal mass (some).
Paralytic ileus	Distention; minimal bowel sounds; no localized tenderness.
Ischemic or strangulated bowel	Not distended (until late); bowel sounds variable; severe pain but little tenderness; rectal bleeding (some).
Bleeding	Pallor, shock; distention; pulsatile (aneurysm) or tender (eg, ectopic pregnancy) mass; rectal bleeding (some).

Disorientation or extreme lethargy combined with a very high fever (> 39°C) or fever with chills and rigors signifies impending septic shock. This is most often due to advanced peritonitis, acute cholangitis, or pyelonephritis. However, fever is often mild or absent in elderly, chronically ill, or immunosuppressed patients despite a serious acute abdomen.

4. **Examination of the Acute Abdomen**

(a) **Inspection** The abdomen should be thoughtfully inspected before palpation. One should look for old surgical scars, hernias, evidence of trauma, stigmata of liver disease, obvious masses, distension and signs of peritonitis. A tensely distended abdomen with an old surgical scar suggests both the presence and the cause (adhesions) of small bowel obstruction. A scaphoid contracted abdomen is seen with perforated ulcer; visible peristalsis occurs in thin patients with advanced bowel obstruction; and soft doughy fullness is seen in early paralytic ileus or mesenteric thrombosis.

(b) **Auscultation** Auscultation of the abdomen should also precede palpation. Peristaltic rushes synchronous with colic are heard in mid-small bowel obstruction and in early acute pancreatitis. They differ from the high-pitched hyperperistaltic sounds unrelated to the crampy pain of gastroenteritis, dysentery and fulminant ulcerative colitis. An abdomen that is silent except for infrequent tinkly or squeaky sounds characterizes late bowel obstruction or diffuse peritonitis. Except for these more extreme patterns, the many auscultatory variants heard in abdominal conditions render them largely useless for specific diagnosis.

(c) **Coughing to elicit pain** The patient should be asked to cough and point to the area of maximal pain. Peritoneal irritation so demonstrated may be confirmed afterward without causing unnecessary pain by rigorous testing for rebound tenderness. This same localization may also be achieved with a foot tap or bed bump. Unlike the parietal pain of peritonitis, colic is visceral pain and is seldom aggravated by deep inspiration or coughing.

(d) **Percussion** Percussion serves several purposes. Tenderness on percussion is akin to eliciting rebound tenderness; both reflect peritoneal irritation and parietal pain. With a perforated viscus, free air accumulating under the diaphragm may efface normal liver dullness. Tympany near the midline in a distended abdomen denotes air trapped within distended bowel loops. Free peritoneal fluid may be detected by demonstrating shifting dullness.

(e) **Palpation** Palpation is performed with the patient resting in a comfortable supine position. Incisional and periumbilical hernias are noted. Tenderness that connotes localized peritoneal inflammation is the most important finding in patients with an acute abdomen. Its extent and severity are determined first by one- or two-finger palpation, beginning away from the area of cough tenderness and gradually advancing toward it. Tenderness is usually well demarcated in acute cholecystitis, appendicitis, diverticulitis and acute salpingitis. If there is poorly localized tenderness unaccompanied by guarding, one should suspect gastroenteritis or some other inflammatory intestinal process without peritonitis. Compared with the degree of pain, unexpectedly little or vaguely localized tenderness is elicited in uncomplicated hollow viscus obstruction, walled-off or deep-seated perforations (eg, retrocecal appendicitis or diverticular phlegmon) and in very obese patients. Severe pain out of proportion to examination is a hallmark for mesenteric ischemia.

Rebound tenderness is elicited by applying deep gentle pressure to the area of concern and then releasing the pressure rapidly. It is a marker of peritoneal inflammation but its usefulness may be confounded if the patient is startled by the abrupt release and interprets that as pain.

Guarding is assessed by placing both hands over the abdominal muscles and depressing the fingers gently. Properly performed, this maneuver is comforting to the patient. If there is voluntary spasm, the muscle will be felt to relax when the patient inhales deeply through the mouth. With true involuntary spasm, however, the muscle will remain taut and rigid (board like) throughout respiration. Except for rare neurologic disorders—and, for unknown reasons, renal colic—only peritoneal inflammation produces rectus muscle rigidity. Unlike peritonitis, renal colic induces spasm confined to the ipsilateral rectus muscle.

When the patient raises his or her head from the bed, the abdominal muscles will be tensed. Tenderness persists in abdominal wall conditions (eg, rectus hematoma), whereas deeper peritoneal pain due to intraperitoneal disease is lessened (Carnett test). Hyperesthesia may be demonstrable in abdominal wall disorders or localized peritonitis, but it is more prominent in herpes zoster, spinal root compression and other neuromuscular problems. Trigger point sensitivity, lateral costal rib tip tenderness and pain exacerbated by spinal motion reflect parietal abdominal wall conditions that subside dramatically after infiltration with local anesthetic agents.

Abdominal masses are usually detected by deep palpation. Superficial lesions such as a distended gallbladder or appendiceal abscess are often tender and have discrete borders. Deeper masses may be adherent to the posterior or lateral abdominal wall and are often partially walled off by overlying omentum and small bowel. As a result, their borders are ill-defined and only dull pain may be elicited by palpation. Examples include pancreatic phlegmon and ruptured aortic aneurysm.

(f) **Maneuvers** Even if a mass cannot be directly felt, its presence may be inferred by other maneuvers. A large psoas abscess may cause pain when the hip is passively extended or actively flexed against resistance (iliopsoas sign). Internal and external rotation of the flexed thigh may exert painful pressure (obturator sign) on a loop of the small bowel entrapped within the obturator canal (obturator hernia). Bump tenderness over the lower costal ribs indicates an inflammatory condition affecting the diaphragm, liver, spleen, or its adjacent structures. Referred pain to McBurney's point from the left lower quadrant (Rovsing's sign), is associated with acute appendicitis. If one suspects abdominal guarding is masking an acutely inflamed gallbladder, the right subcostal area should be palpated while the patient inhales deeply. Inspiration will be arrested abruptly by pain (Murphy's sign), or the gallbladder fundus may be felt as it strikes the examining fingers during descent of the diaphragm. Pain in the shoulder indicates irritation of the diaphragm by fluid such as blood, pus, gastric contents, or stool. Kehr sign is left shoulder pain associated with hemoperitoneum. Costovertebral angle tenderness is common in acute pyelonephritis.

Since they are not invariably present, these special signs are helpful in conjunction with a compatible history and related physical findings.

    (g) **Inguinal and femoral rings; male genitalia** The inguinal and femoral rings in both sexes and the genitalia in male patients should be examined.

    (h) **Rectal examination** A rectal examination should be performed in most patients with an acute abdomen. Diffuse tenderness is nonspecific, but right-sided rectal tenderness accompanied by lower abdominal rebound tenderness is indicative of peritoneal irritation due to pelvic appendicitis or abscess. Other useful findings include a rectal tumor, blood stained stool, or occult blood (detected by guaiac testing).

    (i) **Pelvic examination** An acute abdomen is incorrectly diagnosed more often in women than in men, particularly in younger age groups. A pelvic examination is vital in women with vaginal discharge, dysmenorrhea, menorrhagia, or left lower quadrant pain. A properly performed pelvic examination is invaluable in differentiating among acute pelvic inflammatory diseases that do not require operation and acute appendicitis, twisted ovarian cyst, or tubo-ovarian abscess.

INVESTIGATIVE STUDIES

The history and physical examination by themselves provide the diagnosis in two thirds of cases of an acute abdomen. Supplementary laboratory and radiologic examinations are indispensable for diagnosis of many surgical conditions, for exclusion of medical causes not treated by operation and for assistance in preoperative preparation. Even in the absence of a specific diagnosis, there may be enough information on which to base a rational decision about management. Additional studies are worthwhile if they are likely to significantly alter or improve therapeutic decisions. A more liberal use of diagnostic studies is justified in elderly or seriously ill patients, in whom the history and physical findings may be less reliable.

The availability and reliability of certain studies vary in different hospitals. When selecting a study the invasiveness, risk and cost-effectiveness should be considered. Test results must be interpreted within the clinical context of each case. Basic studies should be obtained in all but the most desperately ill patients, while other less vital tests may be requested later as indicated.

▶ Laboratory Investigations

A. Blood Studies

Hemoglobin, hematocrit, white blood cell and differential counts taken on admission are highly informative. Both a rising or marked leukocytosis ($> 13,000/\mu L$) as well as a leucopenia ($< 5000/\mu L$) are indicative of serious infection. The differential counts should be reviewed as the presence of increased neutrophils (left shift) may suggest the presence of infection, even when the white blood cell count is normal. Additionally, the presence of bands may indicate severe infection.

Serum electrolytes, urea nitrogen and creatinine are important, especially if hypovolemia is expected (ie, due to shock, copious vomiting or diarrhea, or delay in presentation). Creatinine is considered imperative prior to obtaining radiographic imaging with iodized contrast agents due to potential renal injury. Arterial blood gas with lactate should be obtained in patients with hypotension, generalized peritonitis, pancreatitis, possible ischemic bowel and septicemia. Elevated serum lactate may indicate bowel ischemia due to the correlation with anaerobic metabolism. However, this is nonspecific and may be elevated in other clinical scenarios, such as dehydration, cocaine use, or liver failure. Unsuspected metabolic acidosis may be the first clue to serious disease.

A raised serum amylase or more specifically lipase level corroborates a clinical diagnosis of acute pancreatitis. Moderately elevated amylase values must be interpreted with caution, since abnormal levels frequently accompany strangulated or ischemic bowel, twisted ovarian cyst, or perforated ulcer. Lipase is more specific to pancreatitis.

In patients with suspected hepatobiliary disease, liver function tests (serum bilirubin, alkaline phosphatase, aspartate aminotransferase, alanine aminotransferase, albumin and globulin) are useful to differentiate medical from surgical hepatic disorders and to gauge the severity of underlying parenchymal disease.

Clotting studies (platelet counts, prothrombin time and partial thromboplastin time) may be obtained in certain patients in anticipation of surgical intervention. They should be evaluated in patients on anticoagulants such as Coumadin, to ensure therapeutic levels or alert the clinician that correction is needed prior to surgical intervention. Prothrombin time is also a marker of the synthetic function of the liver in those with advanced liver disease. A peripheral blood smear should be considered if the history hints at a hematologic abnormality (cirrhosis, petechiae, etc). The erythrocyte sedimentation rate, often nonspecifically raised in the acute abdomen, is of dubious diagnostic value; a normal value does not exclude serious surgical illness.

A specimen of clotted blood for cross matching should be sent whenever urgent surgery is anticipated or there is suspicion of hemorrhage. **Beta** HCG serum testing is routinely performed at many institutions in lieu of urine testing. This should be performed on all women of childbearing age.

B. Urine Tests

Urinalysis is easily performed and may reveal useful information. Dark urine or a raised specific gravity reflects mild dehydration in patients with normal renal function. Hyperbilirubinemia may give rise to tea-colored urine that froths when shaken. Microscopic hematuria or pyuria can confirm ureteral colic or urinary tract infection and obviate a needless operation. Dipstick testing (for albumin, bilirubin, glucose and ketones) may reveal a medical cause of an acute abdomen. Pregnancy tests should be ordered on all women of childbearing age if serum testing was not performed.

C. Stool Tests

Gastrointestinal bleeding is not a common feature of the acute abdomen. Nonetheless, testing for occult fecal blood should be routinely performed. A positive test points to a mucosal lesion that may be responsible for large bowel obstruction or chronic anemia, or it may reflect an unsuspected carcinoma.

Stool samples for culture should be taken in patients with suspected gastroenteritis, dysentery, or cholera. *Clostridium difficile* should be on the differential of anyone with a recent course of antibiotic therapy.

▶ Imaging Studies

Radiographic imaging has become an invaluable aid in the evaluation, diagnosis and even treatment of the acute abdomen. It is of utmost importance that the surgeon, who is familiar with the clinical scenario of the patient, reviews all images. It should be remembered that patients in distress with concern for abdominal catastrophe may be moved to the operating room without any confirmatory imaging.

A. Plain Chest X-Ray Studies

An upright chest x-ray is essential in all cases of an acute abdomen. Not only is it vital for preoperative assessment, but it may also demonstrate supradiaphragmatic conditions that simulate an acute abdomen (eg, lower lobe pneumonia or ruptured esophagus). An elevated hemidiaphragm or pleural effusion may direct attention to subphrenic inflammatory lesions. Subdiaphragmatic air, if present, suggests perforated viscous and may forego the need for additional imaging. An upright chest radiograph is more sensitive than abdominal plain films for free intraperitoneal air.

B. Plain Abdominal X-Ray Studies

Plain supine films of the abdomen should be obtained only selectively. In general, erect (or lateral decubitus) views contribute little additional information except in suspected intestinal obstruction and rarely eliminate the need for further imaging. Plain films are indicated in patients with signs and symptoms of intestinal obstruction, or in patients with suspected foreign body ingestion. They are inappropriate in pregnant patients, unstable individuals in whom clear physical signs mandating laparotomy already exist,

or patients with only mild, resolving nonspecific pain. When looking at plain radiographs one should observe the gas pattern of the hollow viscera; an abnormal bowel gas pattern suggests paralytic ileus, mechanical bowel obstruction, or pseudo-obstruction. Bowel obstructions are usually accompanied with findings of gaseous distention, air-fluid levels, distended cecum and a paucity of air in the rectum. Colonic dilatation is seen in toxic megacolon or volvulus (Figure 30–15). "Thumbprint" impressions on the colonic wall are noted in about half of patients with ischemic colitis. Radiopaque densities may be seen with biliary, renal, or ureteral calculi; as well as in the case of foreign bodies. Although gallstones and renal calculi can be seen on plain films further imaging is almost always obtained obviating the need for a plain radiograph.

Free air under the hemidiaphragm suggests a perforated viscous, although it does not identify the source. Its presence in approximately 80% of perforated ulcers corroborates the clinical diagnosis. Massive pneumoperitoneum is observed in free colonic perforations. Biliary tree air designates a biliary-enteric communication, such as a gallstone ileus. Air delineating the portal venous system characterizes pylephlebitis.

C. Ultrasonography

Ultrasonography is becoming more common in the early evaluation of abdominal pain and may be used at the bedside by a trained physician. It is one of the first examinations for right upper quadrant pain that is biliary in nature. Ultrasonography has a diagnostic sensitivity of about 80% for acute appendicitis and is most useful in pregnant patients due to its safe modality and lower cost. It becomes technically difficult in the third trimester due to the large gravid uterus. Ultrasound also plays a role in evaluating a variety of gynecologic causes of abdominal pain. Color Doppler studies can distinguish avascular cysts and twisted masses from inflammatory and infectious processes. Ultrasound with Doppler may also be useful in evaluating for flow through the mesenteric vessels.

D. Computed Tomography Scan

Computed tomography (CT) scan of the abdomen is now generally routinely and rapidly available. This has proved extremely useful in the evaluation of abdominal complaints for patients who do not already have clear indications for laparotomy or laparoscopy. CT provides excellent diagnostic accuracy. Whether contrast is used should be carefully weighed on an individual basis. IV contrast administration may be limited by creatinine impairment. Oral contrast is useful to distinguish bowel from remaining abdominal contents. It can be administered orally or rectally; oral administration adds significant time to obtaining imaging and may not be appropriate in severely ill patients. With newer scanners the use of oral contrast is often unnecessary unless looking for bowel perforation or anastomotic leak. Newer low-dose CT scans are becoming available which reduce radiation exposure and provide advantages for pediatric imaging. CT scans should be used sparingly in pregnancy because of the risk radiation poses to the fetus, especially in the first trimester. Ultrasound or MRI are preferred imaging techniques in pregnancy.

CT can identify small amounts of free intraperitoneal gas and sites of inflammatory diseases that may prompt (appendicitis, tubo-ovarian abscess) or postpone (noncomplicated diverticulitis, pancreatitis, hepatic abscess) operation. It should not replace or delay operation in a patient for whom the findings will not change the decision to operate. CT has proven helpful in the diagnosis of appendicitis, especially where examination and laboratory data may not be clear, and is recommended in women, where other pelvic pathology may explain the presence of right lower quadrant pain.

E. Angiography

CT angiography (CTA), percutaneous invasive angiographic studies, or magnetic resonance angiography (MRA), are indicated if intestinal ischemia or ongoing hemorrhage are suspected. They should precede any gastrointestinal contrast study that might obscure film interpretation. Selective visceral angiography is a reliable method of diagnosing mesenteric infarction. Emergency angiography may confirm a ruptured liver adenoma or carcinoma or an aneurysm of the splenic artery or other visceral artery. Additionally it can be therapeutic for coiling or embolizing aneurysmal disease. In patients with massive lower gastrointestinal bleeding, angiography may identify the bleeding site, suggest the likely diagnosis (eg, vascular ectasia, polyarteritis nodosa), and be therapeutic if embolization can be performed. Angiography is of little value in ruptured aortic aneurysm or if frank peritoneal findings (peritonitis) are present. It is contraindicated in unstable patients with severe shock or sepsis and seldom warranted if other findings or tests already dictate the need for laparotomy or laparoscopy. A patient's renal function should be considered before contrast is administered. MRA is useful when a patient is unable to undergo IV contrast administration (due to either renal impairment or contrast dye allergy). It is additionally used as an alternative imaging modality in pregnancy.

F. Gastrointestinal Contrast X-Ray Studies

Gastrointestinal contrast studies should not be requested routinely or be regarded as screening studies. They are helpful only if a specific condition being considered can be verified or treated by a contrast x-ray examination. For suspected perforations of the esophagus or gastroduodenal area without pneumoperitoneum, a water-soluble contrast medium (eg, meglumine diatrizoate [Gastrografin]) is pre-ferred. If there is no clinical evidence of bowel perforation, a barium enema may identify the level of a large bowel obstruction or even reduce a sigmoid volvulus or intussusception. Upper GI contrast studies can also be helpful in the bariatric patient population to evaluate for leak or gastric pouch emptying.

G. Radionuclide Scans

The utility of radionuclide scans has been greatly decreased by the routine availability of urgent CT scans. Liver-spleen scans, HIDA scans and gallium scans may be useful for localizing intra-abdominal abscesses in rare cases. Radionuclide blood pool or Tc-sulfur colloid scans may identify sources of slow or intermittent intestinal bleeding. Technetium pertechnetate scans may reveal ectopic gastric mucosa in Meckel diverticulum.

▶ Endoscopy

Proctosigmoidoscopy is indicated in any patient with suspected large bowel obstruction, grossly bloody stools, or a rectal mass. Minimal air should be used for bowel insufflation to minimize iatrogenic bowel perforation. Besides reducing a sigmoid volvulus, colonoscopy may also locate the source of bleeding in cases of lower gastrointestinal hemorrhage that has subsided. Gastroduodenoscopy and endoscopic retrograde cholangiopancreatography (ERCP) are usually done electively to evaluate less urgent inflammatory conditions (eg, gastritis, peptic disease) in patients without alarming abdominal signs. However, urgent ERCP may be indicated in cases of suspected cholangitis.

▶ Paracentesis

Although performing paracentesis is becoming increasingly rare, it is important to understand that in patients with free peritoneal fluid, aspiration of blood, bile, or bowel contents is a strong indication for laparotomy. On the other hand, infected ascitic fluid may establish a diagnosis in spontaneous bacterial peritonitis, tuberculous peritonitis, or chylous ascites, which rarely require surgery.

▶ Laparoscopy

Laparoscopy is a therapeutic as well as diagnostic modality. The role of laparoscopy has broadened to be a useful modality in the treatment of abdominal emergencies. In certain cases it has been associated with decreased pain and faster recovery times. Its use is dependent on surgeon experience and hospital and OR equipment and staffing.

In cases of unclear diagnosis, laparoscopy helps guide surgical planning and avoid unneeded laparotomies. In young women, it may distinguish a nonsurgical problem (ruptured graafian follicle, pelvic inflammatory disease, tubo-ovarian disease) from appendicitis. In obese patients, it may allow for a smaller, less morbid incision. In obtunded, elderly, or critically ill patients, who often have deceptive manifestations of an acute abdomen, it may facilitate earlier treatment in those with positive findings while eliminating the added morbidity of a laparotomy in negative cases. Any patient undergoing laparoscopy must be suited to tolerate conversion to an open procedure when necessary.

Laparoscopy has become the standard of care for operative treatment of appendicitis and cholecystitis. For acute cholecystitis, laparoscopy performed within 48 hours of symptom onset significantly reduces the risk of conversion to an open procedure, reinforcing the importance of early diagnosis. Laparoscopy may also be used in treating small bowel obstructions, and can result in lower morbidity and a faster return to normal diet.

DIAGNOSTIC UNCERTAINTY

As the surgeon gathers data, the differential diagnosis is narrowed and associated with a clear direction of plan. The plan of action should focus on whether the patient will need to:

- go directly to the operating room,
- be admitted for surgical observation and expected operative intervention,
- be admitted for surgical observation or further diagnostics, or
- be admitted to medical service for nonoperative abdominal pain.

Several patient populations may fall out of the expected presentation of the patient with an acute abdomen. The clinical picture in early cases is often unclear. The following observations should be borne in mind:

1. Acute abdominal pain persisting for over 6 hours should be regarded as having a surgical problem requiring in-hospital evaluation. Well-localized pain and tenderness usually indicate a surgical condition. Systemic hypoperfusion with generalized abdominal pain is seldom nonsurgical.

2. Acute appendicitis and intestinal obstruction are the most frequent final diagnoses in cases erroneously believed at first to be nonsurgical. Appendicitis should remain a foremost concern if sepsis or an inflammatory lesion is suspected. It is the commonest cause of bizarre peritoneal findings producing ileus or intestinal obstruction. Pelvic appendicitis, with mild abdominal pain, vomiting and frequent loose stools, simulates gastroenteritis. Atypical presentations of appendicitis are encountered during pregnancy.

3. Salpingitis, dysmenorrhea, ovarian lesions and urinary tract infections complicate the evaluation of the acute abdomen in young women. Diagnostic errors can be avoided by taking a careful gynecologic history and performing a pelvic examination and urinalysis. Always consider a pregnancy test.

4. Unusual types or atypical manifestations of intestinal obstruction are easily missed. Emesis, abdominal distention and air-fluid levels on x-ray may be negligible in Richter hernia, proximal or closed-loop small bowel obstructions and early cecal volvulus. Intestinal obstruction in an elderly woman who has not had a previous operation suggests an incarcerated femoral hernia or, rarely, an obturator hernia or gallstone ileus.

5. Elderly or cardiac patients with severe unrelenting diffuse abdominal pain but no peritoneal signs may have intestinal ischemia. Arterial blood pH and lactate should be measured and visceral angiography or CTA performed expediently.

6. Medical causes of the acute abdomen should be considered and excluded if possible before exploratory laparotomy is planned (Table 21–5). Upper abdominal pain may be encountered in myocardial infarction, acute pulmonary conditions, pancreatitis and acute hepatitis. Generalized or migratory abdominal discomfort may be felt in acute rheumatic fever, polyarteritis nodosa and other vasculitides. Acute bursitis and hip joint disorders can produce pain radiating into the lower quadrants.

7. Beware of acute cholecystitis, acute appendicitis and perforated peptic ulcer in patients already hospitalized for an illness affecting another organ system.

Table 21–5. Medical causes of an acute abdomen for which surgery is not indicated.

Endocrine and Metabolic Disorders	Infections and Inflammatory Disorders
Uremia	Tabes dorsalis
Diabetic crisis	Herpes zoster
Addisonian crisis	Acute rheumatic fever
Acute intermittent porphyria	Henoch-Schönlein purpura
Acute hyperlipoproteinemia	Systemic lupus erythematosus
Hereditary Mediterranean fever	Polyarteritis nodosa
Hematologic Disorders	**Referred Pain**
Sickle cell crisis	Thoracic region
Acute leukemia	Myocardial infarction
Other dyscrasias	Acute pericarditis
	Pneumonia
Toxins and Drugs	Pleurisy
Lead and other heavy metal poisoning	Pulmonary embolus
Narcotic withdrawal	Pneumothorax
Black widow spider poisoning	Empyema
	Hip and back

SPECIAL POPULATIONS

Elderly

Due to the rising elderly population, physicians should expect to encounter more patients in this age group. Elderly patients presenting with an acute abdomen are more likely to require surgical intervention. These patients often have one or more medical comorbidities complicating their presentation. For example, patients with cardiovascular disease, whether known or unknown, will be more likely to present with acute mesenteric ischemia as a cause of abdominal pain. One of the most frequent causes of acute abdominal pain in the elderly is bowel obstruction. The etiology of these bowel obstructions will differ from younger populations with malignancy and hernias higher on the differential. Elderly patients tend to present later in their course of illness. Many will have past surgical history, which can make operative intervention technically challenging. Although surgical intervention for the acute abdomen in the elderly is safe and necessary, the perioperative morbidity and mortality rates are higher, largely due to medical comorbidities and more limited reserve.

Bariatrics

Obesity is increasingly prevalent in the United States and weight loss surgery has become relatively commonplace. This patient population presents both its own differential for the acute abdomen and its own anatomic challenge to the surgeon. Physical examination findings may be vague due to the patient's body habitus. Tachycardia is an ominous sign that should not be dismissed. Common causes of acute abdomen in the bariatric population include marginal ulcers, obstruction due to internal hernias or adhesions and gastric band complications. Due to the common formation of gallstones following rapid weight loss, cholecystitis is another frequent cause of the acute abdomen in post bypass patients.

Pregnancy

Pregnant women can present with confounding symptoms. Normal pregnancy may be associated with nausea and vomiting, or mild leukocytosis. Physical examination may also be misleading due to the shift in organs secondary to their enlarged uterus. The most common cause of the acute abdomen in pregnancy is appendicitis. Appendicitis in pregnancy may present with pain in atypical locations due to displacement by the uterus. Pain may be present in the right upper quadrant or if the appendix is pushed posteriorly, patients may not demonstrate peritoneal pain. Once diagnosed, early operative intervention is indicated as ruptured appendicitis leads to increased risk of fetal loss.

Table 21–6. Indications for urgent operation in patients with an acute abdomen.

Physical Findings
Involuntary guarding or rigidity, especially if spreading
Increasing or severe localized tenderness
Tense or progressive distention
Tender abdominal or rectal mass with high fever or hypotension
Rectal bleeding with shock or acidosis
Equivocal abdominal findings along with septicemia (high fever, marked or rising leukocytosis, mental changes, or increasing glucose intolerance in a diabetic patient)
    Bleeding (unexplained shock or acidosis, falling hematocrit)
    Suspected ischemia (acidosis, fever, tachycardia)
    Deterioration on conservative treatment
Radiologic Findings
Pneumoperitoneum
Gross or progressive bowel distention
Free extravasation of contrast material
Space-occupying lesion on scan, with fever
Mesenteric occlusion on angiography
Endoscopic Findings
Perforated or uncontrollably bleeding lesion

Immunocompromised

Immunosuppressed patients present a unique challenge, as their immune response will not mount the same presentation as an otherwise healthy patient. This population includes patients with HIV/AIDS, diabetics, patients on chemotherapy, transplant patients and patients on steroid therapy. Immunosuppressed patients have a wider differential including many obscure medical etiologies, such as various opportunistic infections. Due to the lack of inflammatory response, physical examination may present as not concerning. The examiner should be wary of a "benign examination" in light of an otherwise concerning clinical picture. These patients often do not mount an expected leukocytosis. Delayed diagnosis may be devastating as patients often present with advanced disease, shock, or peritonitis, with limited reserve.

INDICATIONS FOR SURGICAL EXPLORATION

The need for operation is apparent when the diagnosis is certain, but surgery sometimes must be undertaken before a precise diagnosis is reached. Table 21–6 lists some indications for urgent laparotomy or laparoscopy. Among patients with acute abdominal pain, those over age 65 years more often require operation (33%) than do younger patients (15%).

A liberal policy of exploration is advisable in patients with inconclusive but persistent right lower quadrant tenderness. Pain in the left upper quadrant infrequently requires urgent laparotomy and its cause can usually await elective confirmatory studies.

PREOPERATIVE MANAGEMENT

After initial assessment, parenteral analgesics for pain relief should not be withheld. In moderate doses, analgesics neither obscure useful physical findings nor mask their subsequent development. Indeed, abdominal masses may become obvious once rectus spasm is relieved. Pain that persists in spite of adequate doses of narcotics suggests a serious condition often requiring operative correction.

Resuscitation of acutely ill patients should proceed based on their intravascular fluid deficits and systemic diseases. Medications should be restricted to essential requirements. Particular care should be given to use of cardiac drugs and corticosteroids and to control of diabetes. Antibiotics are indicated for some infectious conditions or as prophylaxis in the perioperative period.

A nasogastric tube should be inserted in patients with hematemesis or copious vomiting, suspected bowel obstruction, or severe paralytic ileus. This precaution may prevent aspiration in patients suffering from drug overdose or alcohol intoxication, patients who are comatose or debilitated, or elderly patients with impaired cough reflexes. A urinary catheter should be placed in patients with systemic hypoperfusion. In some elderly patients, it eliminates the cause of pain (acute bladder distention) or unmasks relevant abdominal signs.

Informed consent for surgery may be difficult to obtain when the diagnosis is uncertain. It is prudent to discuss with the patient and family the possibility of multiple-staged operations, temporary or permanent stomal openings, impotence or sterility and postoperative mechanical ventilation. Whenever the exact diagnosis is uncertain—especially in young or frail or severely ill patients—a frank preoperative discussion of the diagnostic dilemma and reasons for laparotomy or laparoscopy will reduce postoperative anxieties and misunderstanding.

▶ References

Caruso C, La Torre M, Benini B, et al: Is laparoscopy safe and effective in nontraumatic acute abdomen? *J Laparoendosc Adv Surg Tech A* 2011;21(7):589-593. [Epub Jul 20, 2011].

Costamagna D, Pipitone Federico NS, Erra S et al: Acute abdomen in the elderly. A peripheral general hospital experience. *G Chir* 2009; 30(6/7):315-322.

Greenstein AJ, O'Rourke RW: Abdominal pain after gastric bypass: suspects and solutions. *Am J Surg* 2011;201:819-827.

Katz DS, Klein MA, Ganson G, Hines JJ: Imaging of abdominal pain in pregnancy. *Radiol Clin North Am* 2012;50(1):149-171.

Long SS, Long C, Lai H, Macura KJ: Imaging strategies for right lower quadrant pain in pregnancy. *Am J Roentgenol* 2011;196(1):4-12.

Van Randen A, Lameris W, van Es HW et al on behalf of the OPTIMA study group: The role of plain radiographs in patients with acute abdominal pain at the ED. *Am J of EM* 2011;29:582-589.e2.

MULITPLE CHOICE QUESTIONS

1. Of the following causes of abdominal pain, which occurs more frequently in patients less than 50 years old compared with older patients?

   A. Bowel obstruction
   B. Cholecystitis
   C. Appendicitis
   D. Diverticulitis
   E. Mesenteric Ischemia

2. Which of the following is correct regarding the role of the abdominal plain films in evaluation of the acute abdomen?

   A. They can exclude serious disease.
   B. They are most useful when intestinal obstruction is part of the differential diagnosis.
   C. They are an important part of the work up in patients presenting to the emergency department with abdominal pain.
   D. They are the most sensitive test for a perforated viscus.
   E. They have a high sensitivity in detecting disease including appendicitis, cholecystitis, renal stones and GI bleeding.

3. A 65-year-old man is brought to the ED with abrupt onset of acute abdominal pain. He appears uncomfortable and moaning. Initial vitals: BP 110/88 mm Hg, HR 125 beats/min and irregular, respiratory rate 24 breaths/min. His abdominal examination is remarkable for a non-distended abdomen with no tenderness elicited on examination. Which of the following would be the most helpful next step?

   A. Admit with observation
   B. PO challenge
   C. Basic labs including CBC, basic metabolic panel, amylase and lipase
   D. Upright plain abdominal x-ray
   E. ABG and Lactate

4. A 32-year old woman with 30 week pregnancy arrives to the emergency department complaining of nausea, one episode of emesis and right lower quadrant pain. Ultrasound performed does not visualize the appendix. WBC is 14. The next best step is

   A. Admit with observation
   B. CT scan abdomen/pelvis with PO/IV contrast
   C. MRI abdomen/pelvis
   D. Exploratory laparoscopy
   E. Exploratory laparotomy

5. All of the following are indications for urgent operative intervention EXCEPT

   A. A 49-year-old man with 12 hours of right lower quadrant pain, rebound tenderness and WBC 17.

   B. A 45-year-old diabetic woman with 18 hours of right upper quadrant pain, WBC 12 and ultrasound demonstrating pericholecystic fluid, thickened gallbladder wall and gallstones.

   C. A 52-year-old man with 2 days of bilateral lower quadrant pain and guarding on physical examination, WBC 18 and CT abdomen/pelvis which showing peri-sigmoidal fat stranding and extraluminal air.

   D. A 65-year-old man with 1 day of mild abdominal pain and reports of bright red blood per rectum. Normotensive, but hematocrit on admission 24% (baseline Hct 42%).

   E. A 78-year-old intubated woman, HR 110 beats/min, BP 95/60 mm Hg. Chest x-ray obtained to confirm endotrachial tube placement shows sub-diaphragmatic air.

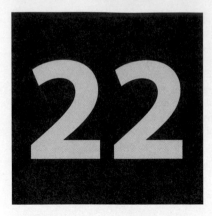

22

Peritoneal Cavity

Matthew Brady, MD

Eric Mahoney, MD

▼ THE PERITONEUM AND ITS FUNCTIONS

The peritoneum is the thin serous membrane that lines the peritoneal cavity. It is the largest serous surface layer in the human body and its surface area is similar to the skin. The structure is made up of a single, flat, layer of mesothelial cells, rich in microvilli. Beneath the mesothelium are a basement membrane and a loose collagen network containing vascularized connective tissue with scattered fibroblasts and macrophages. Normally there is between 5 and 20 mL of free peritoneal fluid, this can vary in women, peaking after ovulation. Normal peritoneal fluid has a specific gravity less than 1.016, protein concentration less than 3g/dL, pH between 7.5 and 8, and a white blood cell count less than 3000/μL. The peritoneum is divided anatomically into parietal and visceral components. The parietal peritoneum underlies the anterior, later, and posterior abdominal walls as well as the undersurface of the diaphragm and pelvic basin. The visceral peritoneum is reflected over the viscera within the abdominal cavity.

Once thought to be a passive barrier, the peritoneum is now understood to have numerous functions. The mesothelial cells secrete phosphatidylcholine, which provides a near frictionless environment within the peritoneum and allows intraperitoneal organs to glide over one another during peristalsis and movement. With its large surface area and semi permeable nature, it participates in fluid exchange with the extracellular fluid space at rates of over 500 mL/h. The circulation of peritoneal fluid is directed toward lymphatics on the undersurface of the diaphragm where particulate matter, up to 20 μm in size, is cleared via stomas in the diaphragmatic mesothelium and emptied into the right thoracic duct.

The peritoneum has a vigorous response to injury and inflammation. Normally sterile, the peritoneum participates in recognizing and eliminating bacteria. Mesothelial cells secrete opsonins that promote bacterial destruction, express CD40 and are aid in antigen presentation, and express intercellular adhesion molecule 1 (ICAM-1) and vascular cell adhesion molecule 1 (VCAM-1) which aid in attachment and activation of lymphocytes, granulocytes, and monocytes in response to infectious pathogens. The mesothelial cells secrete tPA under normal conditions which participates in intraperitoneal adhesiolysis. The peritoneum has significant wound healing functions as well, secreting multiple inflammatory mediators including vascular endothelial growth factor (VEGF), PAI, and nitrogen monoxide, TGF beta, and TNF alpha in response to trauma. In response to injury, the peritoneum produces a large proinflammatory response with fibrin deposition and activation of coagulation pathways as well. Imbalance between fibrin deposition and fibrinolysis following peritoneal traumatization can lead to the organization of fibrin deposits between adjacent structures and development of intraperitoneal adhesions which will be discussed further in later sections. Unlike with cutaneous wound healing, following injury to the mesothelium there is uniform recreation of the mesothelial monolayer within 5-10 days.

Brochhausen C et al: Current strategies and future perspectives for intraperitoneal adhesion prevention. *J Gastrointest Surg* 2012;16:1256.

Brochhausen C et al: Intraperitoneal adhesions–an ongoing challenge between biomedical engineering and the life sciences. *J Biomed Mater Res A* 2011;98:143.

Dinarvand P et al: Novel approach to reduce postsurgical adhesions to a minimum: administration of losartan plus atorvastatin intraperitoneally. *J Surg Res* 2012.

DiZerega GS et al: *Peritoneal Surgery*. New York: Springer-Verlag, 2000.

Hellebrekers BW et al: Pathogenesis of postoperative adhesion formation. *Br J Surg* 2011;98(11):1503-1516.

Maciver AH et al: Intra-abdominal adhesions: cellular mechanisms and strategies for prevention. *Int J Surg* 2011;9:589.

PRIMARY PERITONITIS

Primary (spontaneous) peritonitis occurring in the absence of gastrointestinal perforation is caused mainly by hematogenous spread but occasionally by transluminal or direct bacterial invasion of the peritoneal cavity. Impairment of the hepatic reticuloendothelial system and compromised peripheral destruction of bacteria by neutrophils promotes bacteremia, which readily infects ascitic fluid that has reduced bacterium-killing capacity. Primary peritonitis is most closely associated with cirrhosis and advanced liver disease with a low ascitic fluid protein concentration. It is also seen in patients with the nephrotic syndrome or systemic lupus erythematosus, or after splenectomy during childhood. Recurrence is common in cirrhosis and often proves fatal.

▶ Clinical Findings

The clinical presentation simulates secondary bacterial peritonitis, with abrupt onset of fever, abdominal pain, distention, and rebound tenderness. However, one-fourth of patients have minimal or no peritoneal symptoms. Most have clinical and biochemical manifestations of advanced cirrhosis or nephrosis. Leukocytosis, hypoalbuminemia, and a prolonged prothrombin time are characteristic findings. The diagnosis hinges upon examination of the ascitic fluid, which reveals a white blood cell count greater than $500/\mu L$ and more than 25% polymorphonuclear leukocytes. A blood-ascitic fluid albumin gradient greater than 1.1 g/dL, a raised serum lactic acid level, or a reduced ascitic fluid pH (< 7.31) supports the diagnosis. Bacteria are seen on Gram-stained smears in only 25% of cases. Culture of ascitic fluid inoculated immediately into blood culture media at the bedside usually reveals a single enteric organism, most commonly *Escherichia coli*, *Klebsiella*, or streptococci, but *Listeria monocytogenes* has been reported in immunocompromised hosts.

▶ Treatment

Antibiotic prophylaxis is of no proven value. Systemic antibiotics with third-generation cephalosporins (eg, cefotaxime) or a β-lactam-clavulanic acid combination along with supportive treatment are begun once the diagnosis has been established.

TUBERCULOUS PERITONITIS

▶ Pathophysiology

Tuberculosis peritonitis is encountered in 0.5% of new cases of tuberculosis. It presents as a primary infection without active pulmonary, intestinal, renal, or uterine tube involvement. Its cause is reactivation of a dormant peritoneal focus derived from hematogenous dissemination from a distant nidus or breakdown of mesenteric lymph nodes. Some cases occur as a systemic manifestation of extra-abdominal infection. Multiple small, hard, raised, whitish tubercles studding the peritoneum, omentum, and mesentery are the distinctive finding. A cecal tuberculoma, matted lymph nodes, or omental involvement may form a palpable mass.

The disease affects young persons, particularly women, and is more prevalent in countries where tuberculosis is still endemic. AIDS patients are especially susceptible to development of extrapulmonary tuberculosis such as this.

▶ Clinical Findings

Chronic symptoms (lasting more than a week) include abdominal pain and distention, fever, night sweats, weight loss, and altered bowel habits. Ascites is present in about half of cases, especially if the disease is of long standing, and may be the primary manifestation. A mass may be felt in a third of cases. The differential diagnosis includes Crohn disease, carcinoma, hepatic cirrhosis, and intestinal lymphoma. One-fourth of patients have acute symptoms suggestive of acute bowel obstruction or peritonitis that mimics appendicitis, cholecystitis, or a perforated ulcer.

Detection of an extra-abdominal site of tuberculosis, evident in half of cases, is the single most useful diagnostic clue. Pleural effusion is present in up to 50% of patients. Paracentesis, laparoscopy, or peritoneal biopsy is applicable only in patients with ascites. The peritoneal fluid is characterized by a protein concentration above 3 g/dL with less than 1.1 g/dL serum ascitic fluid albumin difference and lymphocyte predominance among white blood cells. Definitive diagnosis is possible in 80% of cases by culture (often taking several weeks) and direct smear. A purified protein derivative (PPD) skin test is useful only when positive (about 80% of cases). Hematologic and biochemical studies are seldom helpful, and leukocytosis is uncommon. The sedimentation rate is elevated in many cases. The presence of high-density ascites or soft tissue masses on ultrasonography or computed tomography (CT) scan supports the diagnosis. Young patients from endemic areas who present with classic symptoms or who have suggestive imaging findings should undergo diagnostic laparoscopy, which may obviate laparotomy.

▶ Treatment

In chronic cases, nonoperative therapy is preferable if the diagnosis can be established. Most patients presenting with acute symptoms are diagnosed only by laparotomy. In the absence of intestinal obstruction or perforation, only a biopsy of a peritoneal or omental nodule should be taken. Obstruction due to constriction by a tuberculous lesion usually develops in the distal ileum and cecum, although multiple skip areas along the small bowel may exist. Localized short segments of diseased bowel are best treated by resection with primary anastomosis. Multiple strictured areas may be managed either by side-to-side bypass or a stricturoplasty of partially narrowed segments.

Combination antituberculosis chemotherapy should be started once the diagnosis is confirmed or considered likely. A favorable response is the rule, but isoniazid and rifampin must be continued for 18 months postoperatively.

GRANULOMATOUS PERITONITIS

▶ Pathophysiology

Talc (magnesium silicate), cornstarch glove lubricants, gauze fluffs, and cellulose fibers from disposable surgical fabrics may elicit a vigorous granulomatous (a delayed hypersensitivity) response in some patients 2-6 weeks after laparotomy. The condition is uncommon now that surgeons wipe clean their gloves before handling abdominal viscera. Less rarely, granulomatous peritonitis may develop as a hypersensitivity reaction to other foreign material (eg, intestinal ascariasis or food particles from a perforated ulcer).

▶ Clinical Findings

Besides abdominal pain, which is often out of proportion to the low-grade fever, there may be nausea and vomiting, ileus, and other systemic complaints. Abdominal tenderness is usually diffuse but mild. Free abdominal fluid, if detectable, should be tapped and inspected for the diagnostic Maltese cross pattern of starch particles.

▶ Treatment

Reoperation achieves little and should be avoided if the diagnosis can be made. Most patients undergo reexploration because they present an erroneous impression of postoperative bowel obstruction or peritoneal sepsis. The diffuse hard, white granulomatous masses studding the peritoneum and omentum are easily mistaken for cancer or tuberculosis unless a biopsy specimen is taken to demonstrate foreign body granulomas.

If granulomatous peritonitis is suspected, the response to treatment with corticosteroids or other anti-inflammatory agents is often so dramatic as to be diagnostic in itself. After clinical improvement, intravenous methylprednisolone can be replaced by oral prednisone for 2-3 weeks. The disease is self-limited and does not predispose to late intestinal obstruction.

ACUTE BACTERIAL SECONDARY PERITONITIS

▶ Pathophysiology

Peritonitis is an inflammatory or suppurative response of the peritoneal lining to direct irritation. Peritonitis can occur after perforating, inflammatory, infectious, or

Table 22–1. Common causes of peritonitis.

Severity	Cause	Mortality Rate (%)
Mild	Appendicitis Perforated gastroduodenal ulcers Acute salpingitis	< 10
Moderate	Diverticulitis (localized perforations) Nonvascular small bowel perforation Gangrenous cholecystitis Multiple trauma	< 20
Severe	Large bowel perforations Ischemic small bowel injuries Acute necrotizing pancreatitis Postoperative complications	20-80

ischemic injuries of the gastrointestinal or genitourinary system. Common examples are listed in Table 22–1. Secondary peritonitis results from bacterial contamination originating from within viscera or from external sources (eg, penetrating injury). It most often follows disruption of a hollow viscus. Extravasated bile and urine, although only mildly irritating when sterile, are markedly toxic if infected and provoke a vigorous peritoneal reaction. Gastric juice from a perforated duodenal ulcer remains mostly sterile for several hours, during which time it produces a chemical peritonitis with large fluid losses; but if left untreated, it evolves within 6-12 hours into bacterial peritonitis. Intraperitoneal fluid dilutes opsonic proteins and impairs phagocytosis. Furthermore, when hemoglobin is present in the peritoneal cavity, *E coli* growing within the cavity can elaborate leukotoxins that reduce bactericidal activity. Limited, localized infection can be eradicated by host defenses, but continued contamination invariably leads to generalized peritonitis and eventually to septicemia with multiple organ failure.

Factors that influence the severity of peritonitis include the type of bacterial or fungal contamination, the nature and duration of the injury, and the host's nutritional and immune status. The grade of peritonitis varies with the cause. Clean (eg, proximal gut perforations) or well-localized (eg, ruptured appendix) contaminations progress to fulminant peritonitis relatively slowly (eg, 12-24 hours). In contrast, bacteria associated with distal gut or infected biliary tract perforations quickly overwhelm host peritoneal defenses. This degree of toxicity is also characteristic of postoperative peritonitis due to anastomotic leakage or contamination. Conditions that ordinarily cause mild peritonitis may produce life-threatening sepsis in an immunocompromised host.

Causative Organisms

Systemic sepsis due to peritonitis occurs in varying degrees depending on the virulence of the pathogens, the bacterial load, and the duration of bacterial proliferation and synergistic interaction. Except for spontaneous bacterial peritonitis, peritonitis is almost invariably polymicrobial; cultures usually contain more than one aerobic and more than two anaerobic species. The microbial picture reflects the bacterial flora of the involved organ. As long as gastric acid secretion and gastric emptying are normal, perforations of the proximal bowel (stomach or duodenum) are generally sterile or associated with relatively small numbers of gram-positive organisms. Perforations or ischemic injuries of the distal small bowel (eg, strangulated hernia) lead to infection with aerobic bacteria in about 30% of cases and anaerobic organisms in about 10% of cases. Fecal spillage, with a bacterial load of 10^{12} or more organisms per gram, is extremely toxic.

Aerobic bacteria account for the majority of bacterial contamination and include both Gram-negative and Gram-positive species. The most frequent Gram-negative organisms encountered include *E coli*, *Klebsiella*, *Enterobacter*, *Proteus mirabilis*, and infrequently *Pseudomonas aeruginosa*. Among the more common Gram-positive organisms seen are *Enterococcus*, *Streptococcus*, and less commonly *Staphylococcus aureus*, and Coagulase-negative *Staphylococcus*. *Bacteroides*, clostridia, and other anaerobes make up the common anaerobic pathogens encountered. Fungi are rarely encountered though may be present in immunocompromised patients, when present, *Candida* are the predominant species.

Intraoperative cultures were obtained frequently in the past if purulence was encountered in the surgical field. Given the polymicrobial nature of peritonitis following intestinal tract perforations these cultures may provide little information that impact postoperative management.

Foo FJ et al: Intra-operative culture swabs in acute appendicitis: a waste of resources. *Surgeon* 2008;6:278.

Montravers P et al: Clinical and microbiological profiles of community-acquired and nosocomial intra-abdominal infections: results of the French prospective, observational EBIIA study. *J Antimicrob Chemother* 2009;63:785.

Theunissen C et al: Management and outcome of high-risk peritonitis: a retrospective survey 2005-2009. *Int J Infect Dis* 2011;15:e769.

Clinical Findings

By estimating the severity of peritonitis from clinical and laboratory findings, the need for specific organ-supportive care and surgery can be determined.

See Chapter 21 for details of radiologic and other investigations.

Symptoms & Signs

The clinical manifestations of peritonitis reflect the severity and duration of infection and the age and general health of the patient. Physical findings can be divided into: (1) abdominal signs arising from the initial injury and (2) manifestations of systemic infection. Acute peritonitis frequently presents as an acute abdomen. Local findings include abdominal pain, tenderness, guarding or rigidity, distention, free peritoneal air, and diminished bowel sounds—signs that reflect parietal peritoneal irritation and resulting ileus. Systemic findings include fever, chills or rigors, tachycardia, sweating, tachypnea, restlessness, dehydration, oliguria, disorientation, and, ultimately, refractory shock. Shock is due to the combined effects of hypovolemia and septicemia with multiple organ dysfunction. Recurrent unexplained shock is highly predictive of serious intraperitoneal sepsis.

The findings in abdominal sepsis are modified by the patient's age and general health. Physical signs of peritonitis are subtle or difficult to interpret in both very young and very old patients as well as in those who are chronically debilitated, immunosuppressed, or receiving corticosteroids and in postoperative patients. Paracentesis or diagnostic peritoneal lavage may be occasionally useful in equivocal cases and in senile or confused patients. A white blood cell count of greater than 200 cells/μL is indicative of peritonitis, with virtually no false-positive and minimal false-negative errors. Delayed recognition is a major cause of the high mortality rate of peritonitis.

Familial Mediterranean fever (periodic peritonitis, familial paroxysmal polyserositis) is a rare genetic condition that affects individuals of Mediterranean genetic background. Its exact cause is unknown. Patients present with recurrent bouts of abdominal pain and tenderness along with pleuritic or joint pain. Fever and leukocytosis are common. Colchicine prevents but does not treat acute attacks. Provocative testing by infusion of metaraminol (10 mg) induces abdominal pain within 2 days.

Laparoscopy has superseded laparotomy in suspect individuals. Free fluid and inflamed peritoneal surfaces are found, but smears and cultures are negative. The appendix should be removed to simplify diagnosis in subsequent episodes. Secondary amyloidosis with renal failure is a late complication that is preventable by a long-term colchicine therapy.

Treatment

A. Preoperative Care

The presentation of patients with peritoneal inflammation following bacterial contamination can range from mild to life threatening. It is necessary to approach each patient with the same goals of diagnosis and prompt treatment in mind. Initial management consists of assessing the patient's resuscitative needs and determining underlying pathology. Once resuscitation is begun, antibiotics administration and other supportive care measures should be pursued followed by imaging and treatment considerations.

1. Antibiotics—Antibiotic administration should be initiated once the diagnosis is made. Antibiotics should be directed against the most likely source and cover the aerobic and anaerobic organisms commonly encountered in gut perforation. Intravenous antibiotics are first line to ensure therapeutic serum levels in the early course of treatment given like ileus and unreliable oral absorption.

While antibiotics are a mainstay in the preoperative treatment of secondary peritonitis, their role in the postoperative period is less clear. Extended postoperative antibiotic courses may offer little benefit when compared with discontinuing antibiotics in the first 24 hours postoperatively in the prevention of intraperitoneal abscess or surgical site infection but can place patients at higher risk for antibiotic related complications and add to resistance in the community.

If the decision is made to continue antibiotics in the postoperative course historically they have been continued until the patient has been afebrile with a normal white blood cell count and a white blood cell count differential with less than 3% band forms. Provided the patient is tolerating a diet there is no added benefit to using intravenous antibiotics over comparable oral agents.

Fraser JD et al: A complete course of intravenous antibiotics vs a combination of intravenous and oral antibiotics for perforated appendicitis in children: a prospective, randomized trial. *J Pediatr Surg* 2010;45:1198.

2. Peritoneal lavage—In diffuse peritoneal contamination, irrigation with copious amounts of warm isotonic crystalloid solution removes gross particulate matter as well as blood and fibrin clots. The addition of antiseptics or antibiotics to the irrigating solution is generally useless or even harmful because of induced adhesions (eg, tetracycline, povidone-iodine). All fluid in the peritoneal cavity should be aspirated because it may hamper local defense mechanisms by diluting opsonins and removing surfaces upon which phagocytes destroy bacteria.

In cases of localized peritoneal contamination irrigation of the peritoneum is not advisable. Recent publications discourage the use of peritoneal irrigation in the surgical bed, favoring the use of suction alone, when encountering collections of purulence and spillage intraoperatively as it is associated with reduced rates of postoperative intraperitoneal abscess and surgical site infections.

Hartwich JE et al: The effects of irrigation on outcomes in cases of perforated appendicitis in children. *J Surg Res* 2013;180(2):222-225.

Moore CB et al: Does use of intraoperative irrigation with open or laparoscopic appendectomy reduce post-operative intra-abdominal abscess? *Am Surg* 2011;77:78.

▶ **Complications**

Postoperative complications are frequent and may be divided into local and systemic problems. Deep wound infections, residual abscesses and intraperitoneal sepsis, anastomotic breakdown, and fistula formation usually become manifest toward the end of the first postoperative week. Persistent high or swinging fever, inability to wean off cardiac inotropes, generalized edema with unexplained continued high fluid requirements, increased abdominal distention, prolonged mental apathy and weakness, or general failure to improve despite intensive treatment may be the sole indicators of residual intra-abdominal infection. This should prompt a thorough examination of the patient for infected catheters and an abdominal CT scan. Percutaneous catheter drainage of localized abscesses or open reexploration is undertaken as needed (see next section).

▶ **Prognosis**

The overall mortality rate of generalized peritonitis is about 40% (Table 22–1). Factors contributing to a high mortality rate include the type of primary disease and its duration, associated multiple organ failure before treatment, and the age and general health of the patient. Mortality rates are consistently below 10% in patients with perforated ulcers or appendicitis, in young patients, in those having less extensive bacterial contamination, and in those diagnosed and operated upon early. Patients with distal small bowel or colonic perforations or postoperative sepsis tend to be older, to have concurrent medical illnesses and greater bacterial contamination, and to have a greater propensity to renal and respiratory failure; their mortality rates are about 50%. Markedly poor physiologic indices (eg, APACHE II or Mannheim Peritonitis Index), reduced cardiac status, and low preoperative albumin levels identify high-risk patients who require intensive treatment to reduce a daunting mortality rate.

INTRAPERITONEAL ABSCESSES

▶ **Pathophysiology**

An intra-abdominal abscess is a collection of infected fluid within the abdominal cavity. Gastrointestinal perforations, postoperative complications, and penetrating injuries are

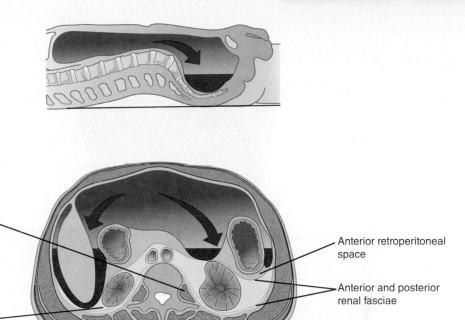

Psoas muscle

Anterior retroperitoneal space

Anterior and posterior renal fasciae

Perinephric space

▲ **Figure 22–1.** Lateral (*top*) and cross-sectional (*bottom*) views of the abdomen, showing fluid gravitating to the dependent areas of the peritoneal cavity. The retroperitoneal compartments are also outlined.

the most common etiologies. An abscess forms by one of two modes. It may develop: (1) adjacent to a diseased viscus (eg, with perforated appendix, Crohn enterocolitis, or diverticulitis) or (2) as a result of external contamination (eg, postoperative subphrenic abscesses). In one-third of cases, the abscess occurs as a sequela of generalized peritonitis. Interloop and pelvic abscesses form if extravasated fluid gravitating into a dependent or localized area becomes secondarily infected (Figure 22–1).

Bacteria-laden fibrin and blood clots and neutrophils contribute to the formation of an abscess. The pathogenic organisms are similar to those responsible for peritonitis, but anaerobic organisms occupy an important role. Experimentally, mixed aerobic (*E coli*) and anaerobic (*Bacteroides fragilis*) infections, especially in conjunction with adjuvants (eg, feces or barium), reduce intraperitoneal O_2 and pH, thereby fostering anaerobic proliferation and abscess formation.

Sites of Abscesses

The areas in which abscesses commonly occur are defined by the configuration of the peritoneal cavity with its dependent lateral and pelvic basins (Figure 22–1), together with the natural divisions created by the transverse mesocolon and

the small bowel mesentery. The supracolic compartment, located above the transverse mesocolon, broadly defines the subphrenic spaces (Figure 22–2A). Within this area, the subdiaphragmatic (suprahepatic) and subhepatic areas of the subphrenic space may be distinguished. The subdiaphragmatic space on each side occupies the concavity between the hemidiaphragms and the domes of the hepatic lobes. The inferior limits of its posterior recess are the attachments of the coronary and triangular ligaments on the dorsal—not superior—aspect of the diaphragm. Anteriorly, the lower limits are defined on the right by the transverse colon and on the left by the anterior stomach surface, omentum, transverse colon, spleen, and phrenicocolic ligament. Although each subdiaphragmatic space is continuous over the convex liver surface, inflammatory adhesions may delimit an abscess in an anterior or posterior position (Figure 22–2B). The falciform ligament separates the right and left subdiaphragmatic divisions.

The right subhepatic division (Figure 22–2B) of the subphrenic space is located between the undersurfaces of the liver and gallbladder superiorly and the right kidney and mesocolon inferiorly. The anterior bulge of the kidney partitions this space into an anterior (gallbladder fossa) and posterior (Morison pouch) section.

The left subhepatic space also has an anterior and posterior part (Figure 22–2C). The smaller anterior subhepatic space

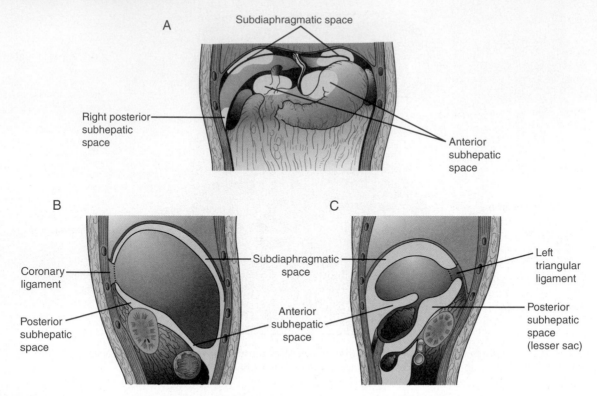

▲ **Figure 22–2.** Subphrenic spaces. **A:** Anterior view. **B:** Right lateral view. **C:** Left lateral view.

lies between the undersurface of the left lobe and the anterior surface of the stomach. Left subdiaphragmatic collections often extend into this anterior subhepatic area. The posterior subhepatic space is the lesser sac, which is situated behind the lesser omentum and stomach and lies anterior to the pancreas, duodenum, transverse mesocolon, and left kidney. It extends posteriorly to the attachment of the left triangular ligament superiorly on to the hemidiaphragm. The lesser sac communicates with both the right subhepatic and right paracolic spaces through the narrow foramen of winslow.

The infracolic compartment, below the transverse mesocolon, includes the pericolic and pelvic areas (Figure 22–3). The diagonally aligned root of the small bowel mesentery divides the mid-abdominal area between the fixed right and left colons into right and left infracolic spaces. Each lateral paracolic gutter and lower quadrant area communicates freely with the pelvic cavity. However, while right paracolic collections may track upward into the subhepatic and subdiaphragmatic spaces, the phrenicocolic ligament hinders fluid migration along the left paracolic gutter into the left subdiaphragmatic area.

The most common abscess sites are in the lower quadrants, followed by the pelvic, subhepatic, and subdiaphragmatic spaces (Table 22–2).

Table 22–2. Common sites and causes of intraperitoneal abscesses.

Site	Cause
Right lower quadrant	Appendicitis, perforated ulcer, regional enteritis
Left lower quadrant	Colorectal perforation (diverticulitis, carcinoma, inflammatory bowel diseases)
Pelvis	Appendicitis, colorectal perforation, gynecologic sepsis, postoperative complications
Subphrenic region	Postoperative complications following gastric or hepatobiliary surgery or splenectomy, perforated ulcer, acute cholecystitis, appendicitis, pancreatitis (lesser sac)
Interloop	Postoperative bowel perforation

▶ **Clinical Findings**

A. Symptoms and Signs

An intraperitoneal abscess should be suspected in any patient with a predisposing condition. Fever, tachycardia, and pain may be mild or absent, especially in patients receiving antibiotics. A deep-seated or posteriorly situated abscess

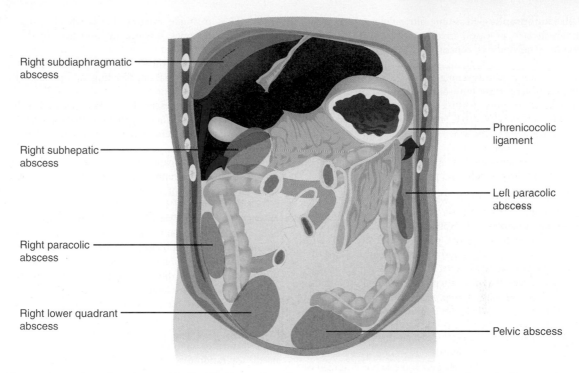

Right subdiaphragmatic abscess

Right subhepatic abscess

Right paracolic abscess

Right lower quadrant abscess

Phrenicocolic ligament

Left paracolic abscess

Pelvic abscess

▲ **Figure 22–3.** The infracolic peritoneal compartment and common abscess sites. Note how paracolic fluid on the right side can migrate up into the subphrenic spaces, whereas collections on the left side are prevented from doing so by the phrenicocolic ligament.

may exist in seemingly well individuals whose only symptom is persistent fever. Not infrequently, prolonged ileus or a sluggish recovery in a patient who has had recent abdominal surgery or peritoneal sepsis, rising leukocytosis, or nonspecific radiologic abnormality provides the initial clue. A mass is seldom felt except late in patients with lower quadrant or pelvic lesions. Irritation of contiguous structures may produce lower chest pain, dyspnea, referred shoulder pain or hiccup, or basilar atelectasis or effusion in subphrenic abscesses; or diarrhea or urinary frequency in pelvic abscesses. The diagnosis is more difficult in postoperative, chronically ill, confused, or diabetic patients and in those receiving immunosuppressive drugs, a group particularly susceptible to septic complications.

Sequential multiple organ failure—principally respiratory, renal, or hepatic failure—or stress-induced gastrointestinal bleeding with disseminated intravascular coagulopathy is highly suggestive of intra-abdominal infection.

B. Laboratory Findings

A raised leukocyte count, abnormal liver or renal function test results, hyperglycemia, and abnormal arterial blood gases are nonspecific signs of infection. Serial post-operative measurement of serum lysozyme (derived from phagocytic cells) is a promising but not widely available test that appears to be highly specific for intra-abdominal pus. Persistently positive blood cultures point strongly to an intra-abdominal focus. A cervical smear demonstrating gonococcal infection is of specific value in diagnosing tubo-ovarian abscess.

C. Imaging Studies

1. X-ray studies—Plain x-rays may suggest an abscess in up to one half of cases. In subphrenic abscesses, the chest x-ray may show pleural effusion, a raised hemidiaphragm, basilar infiltrates, or atelectasis. Abnormalities on plain abdominal films include an ileus pattern, soft tissue mass, air-fluid levels, free or mottled gas pockets, effacement of properitoneal or psoas outlines, and displacement of viscera. Many of these findings are vague or nonspecific, but they may suggest the need for a CT scan. Barium contrast studies interfere with and have been largely superseded by other imaging techniques. A water-soluble upper gastrointestinal series may reveal an unsuspected perforated viscus or outline perigastric and lesser sac abscesses.

2. Ultrasonography—Real-time ultrasonography is sensitive (about 80% of cases) in diagnosing intra-abdominal abscesses. The findings consist of a sonolucent area with well-defined walls containing fluid or debris of variable density. Bowel gas, intervening viscera, skin incisions, and stomas interfere with ultrasound examinations, limiting their efficacy in postoperative patients. Nevertheless, the procedure is readily available, portable, and inexpensive, and the findings are specific when correlated with the clinical picture. Ultrasonography is most useful when an abscess is clinically suspected, especially for lesions in the right upper quadrant and the paracolic and pelvic areas.

3. CT scan—CT scan of the abdomen, the best diagnostic study, is highly sensitive (over 95% of cases) and specific. Neither gas shadows nor exposed wounds interfere with CT scanning in postoperative patients, and the procedure is reliable even in areas poorly seen on ultrasonography. Abscesses appear as cystic collections with density measurements of between 0 and 15 attenuation units. Resolution is increased by contrast media (eg, sodium diatrizoate) injected intravenously or instilled into hollow viscera adjacent to the abscess. One drawback of CT scan is that diagnosis may be difficult in areas with multiple thick-walled bowel loops or if a pleural effusion overlies a subphrenic abscess, so occasionally a very large abscess is missed. CT-guided or ultrasonography-guided needle aspiration can distinguish between sterile and infected collections in uncertain cases.

4. Magnetic resonance imaging—The scanning time, patient inaccessibility during scan acquisition, and upper respiratory motion have limited the usefulness of MRI in the investigation of upper abdominal abscesses. CT scan is generally preferable.

▶ Treatment

Treatment consists of prompt and complete drainage of the abscess, control of the primary cause, and adjunctive use of effective antibiotics. Depending upon the abscess site and the condition of the patient, drainage may be achieved by operative or nonoperative methods. Percutaneous drainage is the preferred method for single, well-localized, superficial bacterial abscesses that do not have fistulous communications or contain solid debris. Following CT scan or ultrasonographic delineation, a needle is guided into the abscess cavity, infected material is aspirated for culture, and a suitably large drainage catheter is inserted.

Postoperative irrigation is vital to remove debris and ensure catheter patency. This technique is not appropriate for multiple or deep (especially pancreatic) abscesses or for patients with ongoing contamination, fungal infections, or thick purulent or necrotic material. Percutaneous drainage can be performed in about 75% of cases. The success rate

exceeds 80% in simple abscesses but is often less than 50% in more complex ones. It is heavily influenced by the availability of appropriate equipment and the experience of the radiologist performing the drainage. Complications include septicemia, fistula formation, bleeding, and peritoneal contamination.

Open drainage is reserved for abscesses for which percutaneous drainage is inappropriate or unsuccessful. These include many cases where there is a persistent focus of infection (eg, diverticulitis or anastomotic dehiscence) that needs to be controlled. In cases without evidence of continued soiling, the direct extraperitoneal route has the advantage of establishing dependent drainage without contaminating the rest of the peritoneal cavity. Only light general anesthesia or even local anesthesia is necessary, and surgical trauma is minimized. Right anterior subphrenic abscesses can be drained by a subcostal incision (Figure 22–4). Posterior subdiaphragmatic and subhepatic lesions can be decompressed posteriorly through the bed of the resected twelfth rib (Figure 22–4) or by a lateral extraperitoneal method. Most lower quadrant and flank abscesses can be drained through a lateral extraperitoneal approach. Pelvic abscesses can often be detected on pelvic or rectal examination as a fluctuant mass distorting the contour of the vagina or rectum. If needle aspiration directly through the vaginal or rectal wall returns pus, the abscess is best drained by making an incision in that area. In all cases, digital or direct exploration must ensure that all loculations are broken down. Penrose and sump drains are used to allow continued drainage postoperatively until the infection has resolved. Serial sono-

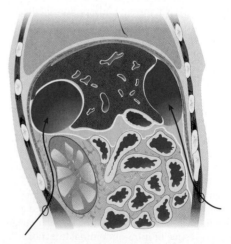

▲ **Figure 22–4.** Extraperitoneal approaches to the right subphrenic spaces. An abscess in the anterior subhepatic space usually requires transperitoneal drainage. Posterior abscesses may also be drained laterally.

grams or imaging studies help document obliteration of the abscess cavity.

Transperitoneal exploration is indicated if the abscess cannot be localized preoperatively, if there are several or deep-lying lesions, if an enterocutaneous fistula or bowel obstruction exists, or if previous drainage attempts have been unsuccessful. This is especially likely in postoperative patients with multiple abscesses and persistent peritoneal soiling. The need to achieve complete drainage fully justifies the greater stress of laparotomy and the small possibility that infection might be spread to other uninvolved areas. Laparoscopy alone is often inadequate, especially in critically toxic patients without a localized focus.

Satisfactory drainage is usually evidenced by improving clinical findings within 3 days after starting treatment. Failure to improve indicates inadequate drainage, another source of (or ongoing) sepsis, or organ dysfunction. Additional localizing studies and repeated percutaneous or operative drainage should be undertaken urgently (ie, within 24-48 hours, depending on the seriousness of the case). Failure to acknowledge adequate progress delays essential studies and incurs higher mortality.

Prognosis

The mortality rate of serious intra-abdominal abscesses is about 30%. Deaths are related to the severity of the underlying cause, delay in diagnosis, multiple organ failure, and incomplete drainage. Right lower quadrant and pelvic abscesses are usually caused by perforated ulcers and appendicitis in younger individuals. They are readily diagnosed and treated, and the mortality rate is less than 5%. Diagnosis is often delayed in older patients; this increases the likelihood of multiple organ failure. Decompensation of two major organ systems is associated with a mortality rate of over 50%. Subphrenic, deep, and multiple abscesses frequently require operative drainage and are associated with a mortality rate of over 40%. An untreated residual abscess is nearly always fatal. Postoperative abscesses, in addition to their deleterious effects on patient's health, add a significant cost to hospitalizations due to extended length of stay, diagnosis, and treatment.

Fike FB et al: The impact of postoperative abscess formation in perforated appendicitis. *J Surg Res* 2011;170:24.

Kaplan M: Negative pressure wound therapy in the management of abdominal compartment syndrome. *Ostomy Wound Manage* 2004;50:20S.

Kim S et al: The perihepatic space: comprehensive anatomy and CT features of pathologic conditions. *Radiographics* 2007;27:129.

Lubner M et al: Blood in the belly: CT findings of hemoperitoneum. *Radiographics* 2007;27:109.

Schimp VL et al: Vacuum-assisted closure in the treatment of gynecologic oncology wound failures. *Gynecol Oncol* 2004;92:586.

RETROPERITONEAL & RETROFASCIAL ABSCESSES

Pathophysiology

The large retroperitoneal space, extending from the diaphragm to the pelvis, is divided into anterior and posterior compartments (Figure 22–1). The anterior portion includes structures between the posterior peritoneum and the perinephric fascia (pancreas, parts of the duodenum, and the ascending and descending colon). The posterior portion contains the adrenals, kidneys, and perinephric spaces. The compartment posterior to the transversalis fascia is involved in retrofascial abscesses.

Abscesses occur less commonly in the retroperitoneum than in the peritoneal cavity. Retroperitoneal abscesses arise chiefly from injuries or infections in adjacent structures: gastrointestinal tract abscesses due to appendicitis, pancreatitis, penetrating posterior ulcers, regional enteritis, diverticulitis, or trauma; genitourinary tract abscesses due to pyelonephritis; and spinal column abscesses due to osteomyelitis or disk space infections.

Psoas abscesses may be primary or secondary. Primary psoas abscesses, which occur without associated disease of other organs, are caused by hematogenous spread of *S aureus* from an occult source and are predominantly seen in children and young adults. They are more common in underdeveloped countries. Secondary psoas abscesses result from spread of infection from adjacent organs, principally from the intestine, and are therefore most often polymicrobial. The most common cause is Crohn disease.

The pyogenic bacteria (*E coli*, *Bacteroides*, *Proteus*, *Klebsiella*) have replaced *Mycobacterium tuberculosis* as the major causative organism. Surprisingly, only a single causative organism is involved in over one-half of cases. A positive blood culture—especially with *Bacteroides*—is an ominous finding.

Clinical Findings

Although they may be symptomless, retroperitoneal abscesses tend to develop in patients with obvious acute illnesses. Fever and abdominal or flank pain are prominent features, sometimes accompanied by anorexia, weight loss, and nausea and vomiting. The clinical findings in patients with psoas abscess consist of hip pain, flexion of the hip with pain on extension, and a positive iliopsoas sign. Abdominal, thigh, and back pain may also occur. The diagnosis is apt to be overlooked when pain in the hip aggravated by walking is the major complaint. The differential diagnosis includes retroperitoneal tumors and hematomas. Radionuclide scanning, bowel contrast studies, and urograms are the common preliminary investigations, but CT scanning most accurately delineates these lesions. Gas bubbles are diagnostic of an abscess. Awareness of the overall clinical picture is essential for CT scanning to differentiate retroperitoneal abscesses from neoplasms or hematomas. Abscesses are confined to specific compartments, whereas malignant lesions, by contrast, frequently violate peritoneal and fascial barriers and can invade bone.

▶ Treatment

Principles of antibiotics and drainage are the mainstay of treating these abscesses as well. Drainage by catheter has a lower success rate for retroperitoneal than intraperitoneal abscesses for the following reasons: (1) retroperitoneal abscesses often dissect along planes, giving a stellate instead of globular shape; (2) they often contain necrotic debris that will not pass through catheters; and (3) they often invade adjacent muscle (eg, psoas abscess). Operation is indicated if there is no clinical improvement following percutaneous drainage. An extraperitoneal approach via the flank is preferred for upper retroperitoneal and perinephric abscesses—and one via the perineum presacrally between the anus and the coccyx for pelvic lesions. Transperitoneal exploration may be unavoidable for deep anterior retroperitoneal abscesses. Resection of necrotic or diseased organs, debridement of the affected compartment, and thorough drainage should be accomplished.

The surgical mortality rate is about 25%. Failure of the fever to subside within 3 days indicates inadequate drainage and persistent sepsis that will prove fatal if not corrected promptly.

▶ Adhesions

Peritoneal adhesions are a frequent and complex problem following intra-abdominal and pelvic surgery. They are a source of major morbidity and significant health care spending, estimated at over a billion dollars annually. Postoperative peritoneal adhesions form in over 90% of open abdominal surgery. Pelvic adhesions account for 12% of infertility cases in women. They can cause pain and are a source of bowel obstructions. They impair operative exposure in future operations, increase operative times as well as intraoperative complications. Peritoneal trauma and ischemia leads to an imbalance between fibrin deposition and the normal fibrinolytic capacity within the peritoneal cavity, favoring the former. Following injury and ischemia, the peritoneum secretes a serosanguinous exudate rich in fibrin, protoglycans, glycosaminoglycans, and hyaluranoic acid. The injured mesothelial cells express tissue factor causing activation of the coagulation cascade which augments fibrin deposition within the secreted exudate. Various chemokines and cytokines attract inflammatory cells to the peritoneum. Hypoxia leads to expression of a fibroblast phenotype that has less fibrinolytic capacity than in the unperturbed state. These fibroblasts infiltrate areas of fibrin deposition and

form collagen to create more organized adhesive bands. Transforming growth factor beta1 (TGF-beta1) is upregulated in peritoneal inflammation and has a significant role in adhesion formation through reduction in fibrinolysis. Plasminogen activator inhibitor (PAI) is secreted by the mesothelium following peritoneal injury and ischemia; it acts to promote fibrin deposition by binding 1:1 with both tissue plasminogen activator (tPA) and urokinase plasminogen activator (uPA). The binding of PAI to uPA and tPA inhibits the conversion of plasminogen to plasmin which is critical for fibrinolysis. Tumor necrosis factor alpha (TNF-alpha) upregulation leads to decreased tPA production and simultaneous increased PAI-1 production by mesothelial cells. VEGF is an angiogenic factor responsible for the neovascularization of peritoneal adhesions, transforming simple adhesions into dense and vascularized fibrous bands that are unable to undergo fibrinolysis. Substance P, a proinflammatory peptide, is upregulated within the peritoneum following peritoneal insult; its interaction with neurokinin-1 receptor leads to a down regulation of metalloproteinases which are integral in fibrinolysis within the peritoneum as well as changes in tPA and PAI-1 expression.

▶ Prevention & Treatment

Current available strategies to minimize adhesions include careful operative technique and barrier methods. Precise surgical technique and gentle tissue handling is critical to minimize peritoneal and serosal damage to limit the inflammatory response responsible for adhesion formation. Minimizing hemorrhage and obtaining complete hemostasis is necessary as activation of the coagulation cascade causes increased fibrin deposition within the peritoneal cavity which further potentiates adhesion formation. It is also important to avoid contaminating the peritoneum with foreign materials such as particles from powdered gloves, fibers from gowns, gauze pads, surgical drapes, and towels which can all promote foreign body reaction and inflammation. Sutures should be minimally reactive as well to limit foreign body reactions. Laparoscopy has been associated with decreased intraperitoneal adhesions through multiple proposed mechanisms including the haemostatic effect of intraperitoneal tamponade during carbon dioxide insufflations of the abdomen and decreased tissue manipulation leading to decreased denudation of the mesothelium.

To date the only commercially available tools used to prevent postoperative adhesions are barrier methods. Barriers exist in solid, liquid, and sprayable forms. They inhibit postoperative adhesion formation by physically separating areas of inflamed and injured peritoneum during the most active early stages of adhesiogensis. Barriers such as hyaluronic acid carboxymethycellulose, Seprafilm Genzyme, are dissolvable and typically remain present within the peritoneal cavity for up to 2 weeks. A large disadvantage of solid barrier methods is that they are only effective at the site the barrier is placed, also they are often difficult to handle and use during laparoscopy. These barriers are associated with the risk of anastomotic leak if wrapped around fresh bowel anastomoses, as well as small increased fistula and peritonitis rates. Liquid barriers have the added benefit of conferring hydro-flotation in between loops of bowel to help prevent adhesions, though this effect is often shortlived depending on the rate of absorption of the liquid by the peritoneum.

There is significant research using pharmacologic agents, by both systemic and by intraperitoneal injection, in adhesion prevention. HMG-CoA reductase inhibitors have been studied for their role in augmenting the profibrinolytic environment of the peritoneum. Angiotensin receptor blocking agents have been shown to downregulate TGF-beta expression and decrease intraperitoneal adhesion formation. Neurokinin-1 receptor antagonists have been shown to decrease adhesion formation in animal models by blocking the actions of Substance P, increasing concentrations of matrix metalloproteinases, and altering tPA and PAI-1 levels within the peritoneum.

Esposito AJ et al: Substance P is an early mediator of peritoneal fibrinolytic pathway genes and promotes intra-abdominal adhesion formation. *J Surg Res* 2012.

Brochhausen C et al: Current strategies and future perspectives for intraperitoneal adhesion prevention. *J Gastrointest Surg* 2012;16:1256.

Brochhausen C et al: Intraperitoneal adhesions–an ongoing challenge between biomedical engineering and the life sciences. *J Biomed Mater Res A* 2011;98.1131

Dinarvand P et al: Novel approach to reduce postsurgical adhesions to a minimum: administration of losartan plus atorvastatin intraperitoneally. *J Surg Res* 2012.

Esposito AJ et al: Substance P is an early mediator of peritoneal fibrinolytic pathway genes and promotes intra-abdominal adhesion formation. *J Surg Res* 2012.

Hellebrekers BW et al: Pathogenesis of postoperative adhesion formation. *Br J Surg* 2011;98:1503.

Lim R et al: Practical limitations of bioresorbable membranes in the prevention of intra-abdominal adhesions. *J Gastrointest Surg* 2009;13:35.

Lim R et al: The efficacy of a hyaluronate-carboxymethylcellulose bioresorbable membrane that reduces postoperative adhesions is increased by the intra-operative co-administration of a neurokinin 1 receptor antagonist in a rat model. *Surgery* 2010;148:991.

Maciver AH et al: Intra-abdominal adhesions: cellular mechanisms and strategies for prevention. *Int J Surg* 2011;9:589.

TUMORS OF THE PERITONEUM AND RETROPERITONEUM

Tumors affecting the peritoneum are of both primary peritoneal origin and more commonly secondary implants from intraperitoneal malignancies. Primary peritoneal malignancies include mesothelial tumors, epithelial tumors, and smooth muscle tumors. Secondary peritoneal tumors can arise from metastatic lesions, infectious origins, and other nonmalignant origins such as endometriosis.

▶ Peritoneal Mesothelioma

Peritoneal mesothelioma is one of few primary peritoneal neoplasms. It arises from the mesothelium which lines the peritoneal cavity. Mesothelioma of the peritoneum can be diffuse or localized, localized having a more favorable prognosis. Four subtypes, epithelioid, sarcomatoid, mixed or biphasic, and well differentiated papillary exist. Well-differentiated papillary is usually found in women of reproductive age, has a high cure rate following resection alone distinguishing it from the others. Epithelioid subtypes have a more favorable prognosis when compared with sarcomatoid, which is rarer and more aggressive. Mixed, or biphasic, subtypes are those with both epithelioid and sarcomatoid components. Its incidence is approximately 300-500 new cases being diagnosed in the United States each year. As with pleural mesothelioma, there is an association with an asbestos exposure history. The peritoneal cavity is the second most common site for malignant mesothelioma accounting for approximately 10%-15% of all new malignant mesothelioma cases. Mean age of presentation is in the fifth decade of life. Men are affected more often than women though the divide is less striking when compared with pleural-based mesothelioma.

▶ Clinical Findings

Presenting symptoms are vague, nonspecific, and frequently cause a delay in diagnosis as patients and practitioners pursue workup and treatment of more benign gastrointestinal tract diseases. Patients most often present with abdominal pain and later increased abdominal girth. Additional presenting signs and symptoms include new hernia, abdominal mass, anorexia, nausea, constipation, and diarrhea. Intestinal obstruction is a late finding in the course of peritoneal mesothelioma.

Diagnosis can be difficult not only given the vague presenting symptoms but also because it can mimic other peritoneal malignancies. Laboratory tests are often unrevealing. CA125 and soluble mesothelin related protein are both commonly elevated, though they have a low specificity. Other tumor markers are not useful in the diagnosis. CT with intravenous contrast typically will demonstrate sheet like thickening of the peritoneum with peritoneal nodules in diffuse cases and distinct masses with peritoneal studding in localized subtypes. In patients who cannot receive iodinated contrast for CT imaging, MRI can be used. Presence of ascites on CT can be variable, ranging from minimal to massive amounts. Laparoscopy with tissue biopsy or CT guided tissue biopsy with immunohistochemical staining for calretinin, cytokeratin 5/6, mesothelin, and Wilms tumor 1 antigen remain the gold standard for diagnosis.

If peritoneal mesothelioma is suspected, laparoscopic tracts should be excised at the time of operation given its propensity to seed port sites. Cytology is of little use in making the diagnosis.

Treatment

Peritoneal mesothelioma is highly malignant neoplasm; mean time from diagnosis to death is less than 1 year without treatment. Current advances in the past decade with debulking surgery and intraperitoneal chemotherapy has extended survival in many patients though these treatments are not yet standardized. At laparotomy the goal is cytoreduction with excision of all tumor deposits greater than 2.5 mm. A midline laparotomy is used for adequate exposure of the abdomen and pelvic contents. Right and left upper peritoneal quadrants, splenectomy, antrectomy, greater omentectomy, lesser omentum stripping, cholecystectomy, sigmoid colectomy, and pelvic peritoneal resection are performed as required to eliminate all tumor deposits larger than 2.5 mm. Completeness of cytoreduction is the most important factor influencing survival.

Hyperthermic (40.5-43°C) intraperitoneal chemotherapy (HIPEC) is being used as adjuvant therapy and has been associated with median survival times of 54 months. Not yet standardized, common regimens include intraperitoneal mitomycin c, doxorubicin, and cisplatin. No prospective comparisons between cytoreduction with and without HIPEC are available. Factors that are contraindications to undergo cytoreduction and HIPEC include inability to perform adequate cytoreduction, advanced age, poor function status, extra-abdominal metastases, hepatic parenchymal metastases, and bulky retroperitoneal disease.

Chua TC et al: Surgical biology for the clinician: peritoneal mesothelioma: current understanding and management. *Can J Surg* 2009;52:59.

Levy AD et al: From the archives of the AFIP: primary peritoneal tumors: imaging features with pathologic correlation. *Radiographics* 2008;28:583.

Mirarbshahii P et al: Diffuse malignant peritoneal mesothelioma–an update on treatment. *Cancer Treat Rev* 2012;38:605.

DESMOPLASTIC SMALL ROUND CELL TUMOR

Desmoplastic small round cell tumors are rare primary peritoneal tumors which are highly aggressive and confer a poor prognosis when diagnosed. This predominantly affects young men, greater than 90% of cases, in the third and fourth decade of life. As with other peritoneal malignancies the presenting signs and symptoms are nonspecific leading to delays in diagnosis. CT is the main imaging modality; typical findings include peritoneal thickening, nodules, heterogeneous intraperitoneal masses often with calcifications and central, low attenuation foci representing necrotic cores within the masses. Mesenteric lymphadenopathy is often present. Given the rarity of the disease, few consensus guidelines exist for its treatment to date and survival even with resection remains less than 20% at 5 years.

Koniari K et al: Intraabdominal desmoplastic small round cell tumor: report of a case and literature review. *Int J Surg Case Rep* 2011;2:293.

PSEUDOMYXOMA PERITONEI

This unusual disease is caused by a low-grade mucinous cystadenocarcinoma of the appendix or ovary that secretes large amounts of mucus-containing epithelial cells. It should be distinguished from benign appendiceal mucocele, which may also have local mucinous deposits but carries a favorable outlook. Patients seldom complain until advanced stages of disease, at which time they have abdominal distention and pain and, in many instances, intermittent or chronic partial small bowel obstruction. Weight loss and other features of cancer are uncommon. The shed neoplastic cells spread freely to two main areas: the upper abdominal sites of peritoneal fluid resorption (undersurface of diaphragm and omentum) and the dependent peritoneal areas (pelvis and lateral abdominal gutters). Distant metastases and visceral involvement are rare. CT scans show a distinctive peritoneal scalloping of the liver margin, calcified plaques, ascites, and low-density masses. Ultrasound features include anechoic areas in the peritoneum, starburst and scalloped appearance of the liver and mobile echogenic foci in the pelvis.

Treatment

At laparotomy, the surgeon should remove as much of the primary lesion and gelatinous material as possible. The omentum also should be resected. This often necessitates right hemicolectomy. If there is no apparent primary tumor, the appendix, and, in women, both ovaries should be removed. Some surgeons advocate radical peritonectomy (including splenectomy, cholecystectomy, appendectomy, sigmoid colectomy, and hysterectomy) to eliminate potential areas of microscopic spread. Whether the higher morbidity incurred is justified remains debated.

Current therapy favors very early intraperitoneal fluorouracil-based adjuvant chemotherapy. Systemic chemotherapy is generally useless. Adjuvant intracavitary radiotherapy has also been advocated, especially for patients with residual disease. Reexploration should be undertaken either as a planned second-look laparotomy or to debulk residual tumor responsible for recurrent obstruction or debilitating mucous ascites. Recent studies quote 10 and 15 year respective survival rates of 63% and 59% when combining cytoreductive surgery with HIPEC.

Chua TC et al: Early- and long-term outcome data of patients with pseudomyxoma peritonei from appendiceal origin treated by a strategy of cytoreductive surgery and hyperthermic intraperitoneal chemotherapy. *J Clin Oncol* 2012;30:2449.

Que Y et al: Pseudomyxoma peritonei: some different sonographic findings. *Abdom Imaging* 2012.

RETROPERITONEAL FIBROSIS

This uncommon entity, is characterized by extensive fibrotic encasement of retroperitoneal tissues. Over two-thirds of cases are idiopathic and the rest secondary to drugs (eg, methysergide, beta-adrenergic blocking agents), retroperitoneal hemorrhage, perianeurysmal inflammation, irradiation, urinary extravasation, or cancer. The fibrosis represents an allergic reaction to insoluble lipid (ceroid) that has leaked from atheromatous plaques, especially those within the aorta. The urinary tract may be involved with a diagnostic triad of hydronephrosis and hydroureter (usually bilateral), medial deviation of the ureters, and extrinsic ureteric compression near the L4-5 level. Desmoplastic involvement of the small and large bowel may give rise to obstructive symptoms. Most patients are men older than 50 who present with renal failure or obstructive uropathy. Pain in the low back or flank is common. Pyuria is present in most patients. The diagnosis is suggested by a CT scan that shows the fibrotic process and any coexisting aneurysmal changes in the aorta. MRI may distinguish fibrosis from lymphoma or metastatic carcinoma. Withdrawal of suspect drugs is usually followed by gradual improvement.

Severe urinary obstruction should be decompressed by ureteric stents or nephrostomy. Prednisone (30-60 mg daily) and immunosuppression have been tried but with inconclusive benefits. These agents should be started early postoperatively before marked fibrosis develops. Tamoxifen has produced regression of desmoid tumors. If surgery becomes necessary, a thick rubbery or fibrotic plaque containing chronic inflammatory cells is found at exploration. Multiple biopsy specimens should be taken to exclude cancer. Ureterolysis should be attempted, and there may be some advantage to wrapping omentum around the freed ureters to reduce the risk of subsequent entrapment. Laparoscopic ureterolysis may occasionally be feasible. The outlook is good as long as there is no underlying cancer.

THE OMENTUM

The omentum is an organ consisting of highly vascularized tissue containing mostly adipose and some lymphoid tissue, described as milky patches, within folds of peritoneum. It is pliable, mobile, and concentrates itself in areas of inflammation within the peritoneal cavity. Anatomically it consists of both greater and lesser components. The greater omentum drapes from the greater curvature of the stomach anteriorly, descends to cover the small intestines, and turns back on itself inserting onto the transverse colon posteriorly, comprising four layers of peritoneum when fused. During embryology, it derives from the dorsal mesogastrium beginning in the fourth week of gestation. Its blood supply is from the right and left gastroepiploic arteries which arise from the gastroduodenal and splenic arteries respectively and its venous drainage exits to the portal system. The lesser omentum is a much thinner structure and extends from the porta hepatis to the inferior curvature of the stomach. During embryology the lesser omentum derives from the septum transversum. Containing mostly fat and lymphocytes, it has active roles in immune function, inflammation, and infection control within the peritoneal cavity. Its role in maintaining the intraperitoneal cavity is a long known function of the omentum, describe as "the abdominal policeman" by Rutherford Morrison in the early 20th century as he noted it frequently to be in areas of infection and perforation within the peritoneal cavity. Its role in the immune and inflammatory function has grown considerably since that time. If foreign bodies are present in the peritoneal cavity the omentum enlarges in size and mass with expansion of stromal cells rich in tissue and vascular growth factors as well as pleuripotent stem cells. These functions allow it to participate in both tissue regeneration and revascularization in areas of intraperitoneal injury, infection, and inflammation.

Shah S et al: Cellular basis of tissue regeneration by omentum. *PLoS One* 2012;7:e38368.

▶ Torsion & Infarction

Primary (spontaneous) torsion of the omentum may develop if a free portion is fixed by an adhesion or trapped within a hernia. Rotation around the pedicle occludes the blood supply and leads to ischemic necrosis.

Clinically, torsion presents as acute abdominal pain with nausea and vomiting. Tenderness is confined to the involved area, usually on the right side but away from McBurney's point. A mobile, tender mass is noted in one-third of cases. These features may suggest acute appendicitis or cholecystitis but are not typical of those diseases. The clinical findings usually mandate surgical exploration, which reveals serosanguineous fluid, a normal appendix, and the hemorrhagic necrotic segment of omentum. Resection of the affected portion is curative.

▶ Tumors & Cysts

The omentum is frequently involved secondarily by intra-abdominal malignant tumors, especially gastrointestinal and ovarian adenocarcinomas. Primary cysts or vascular anomalies, usually incidentally discovered at laparotomy, are readily resected.

MULTIPLE CHOICE QUESTIONS

1. The peritoneal cavity

   A. Is lined by an epithelial surface
   B. Typically contains 100-200 mL of serous fluid
   C. Has a fluid pH of 6.5-6.9
   D. Is divided anatomically into parietal and visceral components
   E. Includes a parietal peritoneal surface investing the small and large bowel

2. Primary bacterial peritonitis

   A. Is common during pregnancy.
   B. Typically affects peritoneal fluid containing a high concentration of albumin.
   C. Is a complication of hypothyroidism.
   D. Is most frequently associated with cirrhosis and ascites.
   E. None of the above.

3. Secondary peritonitis is bacterial contamination

   A. That typically spreads from a hematogenous source
   B. That often originates from gastrointestinal sources
   C. That can usually be treated by antibiotics alone
   D. That usually is mono-microbial
   E. Of the tissues adjacent to the peritoneal cavity (bladder, kidney) that spreads through lymphatic channels to the peritoneum

Stomach & Duodenum

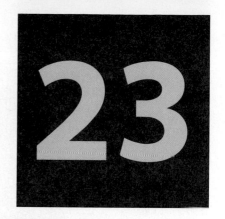

Gerard M. Doherty, MD

▼ I. STOMACH

The stomach receives food from the esophagus and has four functions: (1) it acts as a reservoir that permits eating reasonably large quantities of food at intervals of several hours; (2) food contained in the stomach is mixed, and delivered into the duodenum in amounts regulated by its chemical nature and texture; (3) the first stages of protein and carbohydrate digestion are carried out in the stomach; and (4) a few substances are absorbed across the gastric mucosa.

ANATOMY

The anatomy of the stomach in Figures 23–1, 23-2, and 23-3 illustrates the structure supporting the functions.

The cardia is located at the gastroesophageal junction. The fundus is the portion of the stomach that lies cephalad to the gastroesophageal junction. The corpus is the capacious central part; division of the corpus from the pyloric antrum is marked approximately by the angular incisure, a crease on the lesser curvature just proximal to the "crow's-foot" terminations of the nerves of Latarjet (Figure 23-3). The pylorus is the boundary between the stomach and the duodenum.

The cardiac gland area is the small segment located at the gastroesophageal junction. Histologically, it contains principally mucus-secreting cells, though a few parietal cells are sometimes present. The oxyntic gland area is the portion containing parietal (oxyntic) cells and chief cells (Figure 23-2). The boundary between this region and the adjacent pyloric gland area is reasonably sharp, since the zone of transition spans a segment of only 1–1.5 cm. The pyloric gland area constitutes the distal 30% of the stomach and contains the G cells that manufacture gastrin. Mucous cells are common in the oxyntic and pyloric gland areas.

As in the rest of the gastrointestinal tract, the muscular wall of the stomach is composed of an outer longitudinal and an inner circular layer. An additional incomplete inner layer of obliquely situated fibers is most prominent near the lesser curvature but is of less substance than the other two layers.

▶ Blood Supply

The blood supply of the stomach and duodenum is illustrated in Figure 23-3. The left gastric artery supplies the lesser curvature and connects with the right gastric artery, a branch of the common hepatic artery. In 60% of persons, a posterior gastric artery arises off the middle third of the splenic artery and terminates in branches on the posterior surface of the body and the fundus. The greater curvature is supplied by the right gastroepiploic artery (a branch of the gastroduodenal artery) and the left gastroepiploic artery (a branch of the splenic artery). The mid-portion of the greater curvature corresponds to a point at which the gastric branches of this vascular arcade change direction. The fundus of the stomach along the greater curvature is supplied by the vasa brevia, branches of the splenic and left gastroepiploic arteries.

The blood supply to the duodenum is from the superior and inferior pancreaticoduodenal arteries, which are branches of the gastroduodenal artery and the superior mesenteric artery, respectively. The stomach contains a rich submucosal vascular plexus. Venous blood from the stomach drains into the coronary, gastroepiploic, and splenic veins before entering the portal vein. The lymphatic drainage of the stomach, which largely parallels the arteries, partially determines the direction of spread of gastric neoplasms.

▶ Nerve Supply

The parasympathetic nerves to the stomach are shown in Figure 23-3. As a rule, two major vagal trunks pass through the esophageal hiatus in close approximation to the esophageal muscle. The nerves are originally located to the right and left of the esophagus and stomach during embryonic

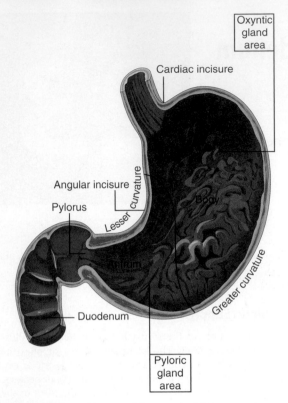

▲ Figure 23–1. Names of the parts of the stomach. The line drawn from the lesser to the greater curvature depicts the approximate boundary between the oxyntic gland area and the pyloric gland area. No prominent landmark exists to distinguish between antrum and body (corpus). The fundus is the portion craniad to the esophagogastric junction.

development. When the foregut rotates, the lesser curvature turns to the right and the greater curvature to the left, and corresponding shifts in location of the vagal trunks follow. Hence, the right vagus supplies the posterior and the left the anterior gastric surface. About 90% of the vagal fibers are sensory afferent; the remaining 10% are efferent.

In the region of the gastroesophageal junction, each trunk bifurcates. The anterior trunk sends to the liver a division that travels in the lesser omentum. The bifurcation of the posterior trunk gives rise to fibers that enter the celiac plexus and supply the parasympathetic innervation to the remainder of the gastrointestinal tract as far as the mid-transverse colon. Both trunks, after giving rise to their extragastric divisions, send some fibers directly onto the surface of the stomach and others along the lesser curvature (anterior and posterior nerves of Latarjet) to supply the

distal part of the organ. As shown in Figure 23–3, a variable number of vagal fibers ascend with the left gastric artery after having passed through the celiac plexus.

The preganglionic motor fibers of the vagal trunks synapse with ganglion cells in the Auerbach plexus (plexus myentericus) between the longitudinal and circular muscle layers. Postganglionic cholinergic fibers are distributed to the cells of the smooth muscle layers and the mucosa.

The adrenergic innervation to the stomach consists of postganglionic fibers that pass along the arterial vessels from the celiac plexus.

PHYSIOLOGY

▶ Motility

Storage, mixing, trituration, and regulated emptying are accomplished by the muscular apparatus of the stomach. Peristaltic waves originate in the body and pass toward the pylorus. The thickness of the smooth muscle increases in the antrum and corresponds to the stronger contractions that can be measured in the distal stomach. The pylorus behaves as a sphincter, though it normally allows a little to-and-fro movement of chyme across the junction.

An electrical pacemaker situated in the fundal musculature near the greater curvature gives rise to regular (3/min) electrical impulses (pacesetter potential, basic electrical rhythm) that pass toward the pylorus in the outer longitudinal layer. Every impulse is not always followed by a peristaltic muscular contraction, but the impulses determine the maximal peristaltic rate. The frequency of peristalsis is governed by a variety of stimuli mentioned below. Each contraction follows sequential depolarization of the underlying circular muscle resulting from arrival of the pacesetter potential.

Peristaltic contractions are more forceful in the antrum than the body and travel faster as they progress distally. Gastric chyme is forced into the funnel-shaped antral chamber by peristalsis; the volume of contents delivered into the duodenum by each peristaltic wave depends on the strength of the advancing wave and the extent to which the pylorus closes. Most of the gastric contents that are pushed into the antral funnel are propelled backward as the pylorus closes and pressure within the antral lumen rises. Five to 15 mL enter the duodenum with each gastric peristaltic wave.

The volume of the empty gastric lumen is only 50 mL. By a process called receptive relaxation, the stomach can accommodate about 1000 mL before intraluminal pressure begins to rise. Receptive relaxation is an active process mediated by vagal reflexes and abolished by vagotomy. Peristalsis is initiated by the stimulus of distention after eating. Various other factors have positive or negative influences on the rate and strength of contractions and the rate of gastric emptying. Vagal reflexes from the stomach have a facilitating

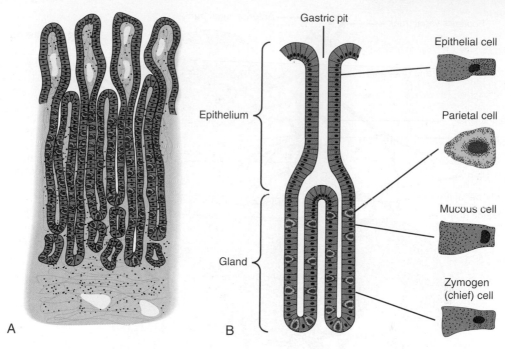

▲ **Figure 23–2.** Histologic features of the mucosa in the oxyntic gland area. Each gastric pit drains three to seven tubular gastric glands. **A:** The neck of the gland contains many mucous cells. Oxyntic (parietal) cells are most numerous in the mid-portion of the glands; peptic (chief) cells predominate in the basal portion. **B:** Drawing from photomicrograph of the gastric mucosa.

influence on peristalsis. The texture and volume of the meal both play a role in the regulation of emptying; small particles are emptied more rapidly than large ones, which the organ attempts to reduce in size (trituration). The osmolality of gastric chyme and its chemical makeup are monitored by duodenal receptors. If osmolality is greater than 200 mosm/L, a long vagal reflex (the enterogastric reflex) is activated, delaying emptying. Gastrin causes delay in emptying. Gastrin is the only circulating gastrointestinal hormone to have a physiologic effect on emptying.

▶ Gastric Juice

The output of gastric juice in a fasting subject varies between 500 and 1500 mL/d. After each meal, about 1000 mL are secreted by the stomach.

The components of gastric juice are as follows.

A. Mucus

Mucus is a heterogeneous mixture of glycoproteins manufactured in the mucous cells of the oxyntic and pyloric gland areas. Mucus provides a weak barrier to the diffusion of H^+ and probably protects the mucosa. It also acts as a lubricant and impedes diffusion of pepsin.

B. Pepsinogen

Pepsinogens are synthesized in the chief cells of the oxyntic gland area (and to a lesser extent in the pyloric area) and are stored as visible granules. Cholinergic stimuli, either vagal or intramural, are the most potent pepsigogues, though gastrin and secretin are also effective. The precursor zymogen is activated when pH falls below 5.00, a process that entails severance of a polypeptide fragment from the larger molecule. Pepsin cleaves peptide bonds, especially those containing phenylalanine, tyrosine, or leucine. Its optimal pH is about 2.00. Pepsin activity is abolished at pH greater than 5.00, and the molecule is irreversibly denatured at pH greater than 8.00.

C. Intrinsic Factor

Intrinsic factor, a mucoprotein secreted by the parietal cells, binds with vitamin B_{12} of dietary origin and greatly enhances absorption of the vitamin. Absorption occurs by an active process in the terminal ileum.

Intrinsic factor secretion is enhanced by stimuli that evoke H^+ output from parietal cells. Pernicious anemia is characterized by atrophy of the parietal cell mucosa, deficiency

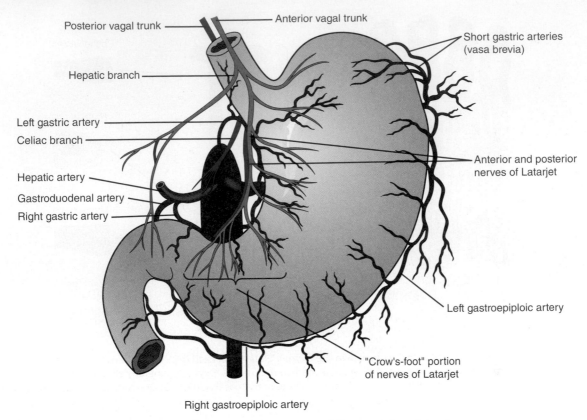

▲ Figure 23–3. Blood supply and parasympathetic innervation of the stomach and duodenum.

in intrinsic factor, and anemia. Subclinical deficiencies in vitamin B_{12} have been described after operations that reduce gastric acid secretion, and abnormal Schilling tests in these patients can be corrected by the administration of intrinsic factor. Total gastrectomy creates a dependence on parenteral administration of vitamin B_{12}.

D. Electrolytes

The unique characteristic of gastric secretion is its high concentration of hydrochloric acid, a product of the parietal cells. As the concentration of H^+ rises during secretion, that of Na^+ drops in a reciprocal fashion. K^+ remains relatively constant at 5–10 mEq/L. Chloride concentration remains near 150 mEq/L, and gastric juice maintains its isotonicity at varying secretory rates.

▶ The Parietal Cell & Acid Secretion

Many of the key events in acid secretion by gastric parietal cells are illustrated in Figure 23–4. The onset of secretion is accompanied by striking morphologic changes in the apical membranes. Resting parietal cells are characterized by

an infolding of the apical membrane, called the secretory canaliculus, which is lined by short microvilli. Multiple membrane-bound tubulovesicles and mitochondria are present in the cytoplasm. With stimulation, the secretory canaliculus expands, the microvilli become long and narrow and filled with microfilaments, and the cytoplasmic tubulovesicles disappear. The proton pump mechanism for acid secretion is located in the tubulovesicles in the resting state and in the secretory canaliculus in the stimulated state.

The basal lateral membrane contains the receptors for secretory stimulants and transfers HCO_3^- out of the cell to balance the H^+ output at the apical membrane. Active uptake of Cl^- and K^+ conduction also occur at the basal lateral membrane. Separate membrane-bound receptors exist for histamine (H_2 receptor), gastrin, and acetylcholine. The intracellular second messengers are cyclic adenosine monophosphate (cAMP) for histamine and Ca^{2+} for gastrin and acetylcholine.

Acid secretion at the apical membrane is accomplished by a membrane-bound H^+/K^+-ATPase (the proton pump); H^+ is secreted into the lumen in exchange for K^+.

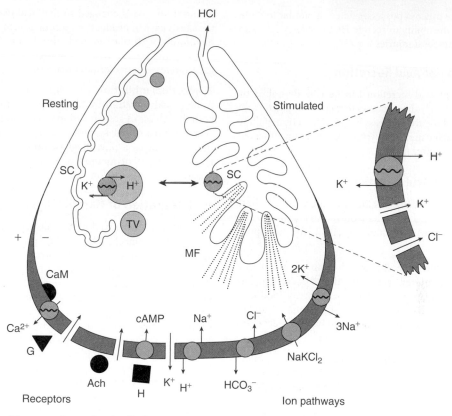

▲ **Figure 23–4.** Diagram of a parietal cell, showing the receptor systems and ion pathways in the basal lateral membrane and the apical membrane transition from a resting to a stimulated state. Ach, acetylcholine; CaM, calmodulin; G, gastrin; H, histamine; MF, microfilaments; SC, secretory canaliculus; TV, tubulovesicles. (Redrawn, with permission, from Malinowska DH, Sachs G: Cellular mechanisms of acid secretion. *Clin Gastroenterol.* 1984;13(2):309–326.)

▶ Mucosal Resistance in the Stomach & Duodenum

The healthy mucosa of the stomach and duodenum is provided with mechanisms that allow it to withstand the potentially injurious effects of high concentrations of luminal acid. Disruption of these mechanisms may contribute to acute or chronic ulceration.

The surface of the gastric mucosa is coated with mucus and secretes HCO_3^- in addition to H^+. Protected by the blanket of mucus, the surface pH is much higher than the luminal pH. HCO_3^- secretion is stimulated by cAMP, prostaglandins, cholinomimetics, glucagon, cholecystokinin, and by as yet unidentified paracrine hormones. Inhibitors of HCO_3^- secretion include nonsteroidal anti-inflammatory agents, alpha-adrenergic agonists, bile acids, ethanol, and acetazolamide. Increases in luminal H^+ result in increased HCO_3^- secretion, probably mediated by tissue prostaglandins.

Gastric mucus is a gel composed of high-molecular-weight glycoproteins and 95% water. Since it forms an unstirred layer, it helps the underlying mucosa to maintain a higher pH than that of gastric juice, and it also acts as a barrier to the diffusion of pepsin. At the surface of the layer of mucus, peptic digestion continuously degrades mucus, while below it is continuously being replenished by mucous cells. Gastric acid is thought to enter the lumen through thin spots in the mucus overlying the gastric glands. Secretion of mucus is stimulated by luminal acid and perhaps by cholinergic stimuli. The layer of mucus is damaged by exposure to nonsteroidal anti-inflammatory agents and is enhanced by topical prostaglandin E_2.

Mucosal defects produced by mechanical or chemical trauma are rapidly repaired by adjacent normal cells that spread to cover the defect, a process that can be enhanced experimentally by adding HCO_3^- to the nutrient side of the mucosa.

The duodenal mucosa possesses defenses similar to those in the stomach: the ability to secrete HCO_3^- and mucus and rapid repair of mucosal injuries.

▶ Regulation of Acid Secretion

The regulation of acid secretion can best be described by considering separately those factors that enhance gastric acid production and those that depress it. The interaction of these forces is what determines the levels of secretion observed during fasting and after meals.

A. Stimulation of Acid Secretion

Acid production is usually described as the result of three phases that are excited simultaneously after a meal. The separation into phases is of value principally for descriptive purposes.

1. Cephalic phase—Stimuli that act upon the brain lead to increased vagal efferent activity and acid secretion. The sight, smell, taste, or even thought of appetizing food may elicit this response. The effect is vagally mediated and is abolished by vagotomy. The vagal stimuli have a direct effect on the parietal cells to increase acid output.

2. Gastric phase—Food in the stomach (principally protein hydrolysates and hydrophobic amino acids) stimulates gastrin release from the antrum. Gastric distention has a similar but less intense effect.

The presence of food in the stomach excites long vagal reflexes, impulses that pass to the central nervous system via vagal afferents and return to stimulate the parietal cells.

A third aspect of the gastric phase involves the sensitizing effect of distention of the parietal cell area to gastrin that is probably mediated through local intramural cholinergic reflexes.

3. Intestinal phase—The role of the intestinal phase in the stimulation of gastric secretion has been incompletely investigated. Various experiments have shown that the presence of food in the small bowel releases a humoral factor, named entero-oxyntin, that evokes acid secretion from the stomach.

B. Inhibition of Acid Secretion

Without systems to limit secretion, unchecked acid production could become a serious clinical problem. Examples can be found (Billroth II gastrectomy with retained antrum) where acid production rose after surgical procedures that interfered with these inhibitory mechanisms.

1. Antral inhibition—pH below 2.50 in the antrum inhibits the release of gastrin regardless of the stimulus. When the pH reaches 1.20, gastrin release is almost completely blocked. If the normal relationship of parietal cell mucosa to antral mucosa is changed so that acid does not flow past the site of gastrin production, serum gastrin may increase to high levels, with marked acid stimulation. Somatostatin in gastric antral cells serves a physiologic role as an inhibitor of gastrin release (a paracrine function).

2. Intestinal inhibition—The intestine participates in controlling acid secretion by liberating hormones that inhibit both the release of gastrin and its effects on the parietal cells. Secretin blocks acid secretion under experimental conditions but not as a physiologic action. Fat in the intestine is the most potent method of inhibition, affecting gastrin release and acid secretion.

▶ Integration of Gastric Physiologic Function

Ingested food is mixed with salivary amylase before it reaches the stomach. The mechanisms stimulating gastric secretion are activated. Serum gastrin levels increase from a mean fasting concentration of about 50 pg/mL to 200 pg/mL, the peak occurring about 30 minutes after the meal. Food in the lumen of the stomach is exposed to high concentrations of acid and pepsin at the mucosal surface. Food settles in layers determined by sequence of arrival, but fat tends to float to the top. The greatest mixing occurs in the antrum. Antral contents therefore become more uniformly acidic than those in the body of the organ, where the central portion of the meal tends to remain alkaline for a considerable time, allowing continued activity of the amylase.

Peptic digestion of protein in the stomach is only about 5%–10% complete. Carbohydrate digestion may reach 30%–40%. A lipase originating from the tongue initiates the first stages of lipolysis in the stomach.

The gastric contents are delivered to the duodenum at a rate determined by the volume and texture of the meal, its osmolality and acidity, and its content of fat. A meal of lean meat, potatoes, and vegetables leaves the stomach within 3 hours. A meal with a very high fat content may remain in the stomach for 6–12 hours.

PEPTIC ULCER

Peptic ulcers result from the corrosive action of acid gastric juice on a vulnerable epithelium. Depending on circumstances, they may occur in the esophagus, the duodenum, the stomach itself, the jejunum after surgical construction of a gastrojejunostomy, or the ileum in relation to ectopic gastric mucosa in Meckel diverticulum. When the term peptic ulcer was first used, it was thought that the most important factor was the peptic activity in gastric juice. Since then, evidence has implicated acid as the chief injurious agent; in fact, it is axiomatic that if gastric juice contains no acid, a (benign) peptic ulcer cannot be present. Appreciation of the role of acid has led to the emphasis on therapy with antacids and H_2 blocking agents for the medical therapy of ulcers and to operations that reduce acid secretion as the major surgical approach. In the case of duodenal and gastric ulcers, *Helicobacter pylori* must colonize and weaken the mucosa before acid is able to do the damage, and therapy directed against this organism has a more definitive effect on the disease.

It has been estimated that about 2% of the adult population in the United States suffers from active peptic ulcer disease, and about 10% of the population will have the disease during their lifetime. Men are affected three times as often as women. Duodenal ulcers are ten times more common than gastric ulcers in young patients, but in the older age groups the frequency is about equal. Probably as a result of a declining prevalence of *H pylori* infection, the incidence has declined to less than half what it was 30 years ago.

In general terms, the ulcerative process can lead to four types of disability: (1) Pain is the most common. (2) Bleeding may occur as a result of erosion of submucosal or extraintestinal vessels as the ulcer becomes deeper. (3) Penetration of the ulcer through all layers of the affected gut results in perforation if other viscera do not seal the ulcer. (4) Obstruction may result from inflammatory swelling and scarring and is most likely to occur with ulcers located at the pylorus or gastroesophageal junction, where the lumen is narrowest.

The clinical features and prognosis of duodenal ulcer and gastric ulcer are sufficiently different to be dealt with separately here.

DUODENAL ULCER

ESSENTIALS OF DIAGNOSIS

- ▶ Epigastric pain often relieved by food or antacids
- ▶ Epigastric tenderness
- ▶ Normal or increased gastric acid secretion
- ▶ Signs of ulcer disease on upper gastrointestinal x-rays or endoscopy
- ▶ Evidence of *H pylori* infection

▶ General Considerations

Duodenal ulcers may occur in any age group but are most common in the young and middle-aged (20–45 years). They appear in men more often than women. About 95% of duodenal ulcers are situated within 2 cm of the pylorus, in the duodenal bulb.

Considerable evidence implicates *H pylori* as the principal cause of duodenal ulcer disease. This microaerophilic gram-negative curved bacillus can be found colonizing patches of gastric metaplasia within the duodenum in 90% of patients with this disease. The bacilli remain on the surface of the mucosa rather than invading it. They are thought to render the duodenum more vulnerable to the injurious effects of acid and pepsin by releasing urease or other toxins.

The epidemiology of peptic ulcer disease reflects the prevalence of *H pylori* infection in different populations. In areas of the world where peptic ulcer is uncommon (eg, rural Africa), human infection is rare. Duodenal ulcer disease has emerged as a major clinical entity in Western society only since the latter part of the 19th century. The incidence reached a peak about 35 years ago and then declined to reach a lower plateau a few years ago. These changes are thought to be explained by variations in *H pylori* infection resulting from public health factors. Within countries like the United States, the distribution of *H pylori* is explainable by a fecal-oral theory of transmission. The prevalence of infection is higher among lower socioeconomic groups. Interestingly, only a minority of infected persons develop ulcers. *H pylori* also has an important role in the etiology of gastric ulcer, gastric cancer, and gastritis. The 10% of duodenal ulcers that are not associated with helicobacter infection are caused by nonsteroidal anti-inflammatory drugs and other agents.

Gastric acid secretion is characteristically higher than normal in patients with duodenal ulcer compared with normal subjects, but only one-sixth of the duodenal ulcer population have secretory levels that exceed the normal range (ie, acid secretion in normal subjects and those with duodenal ulcer overlap considerably), so the disease cannot be explained simply as a manifestation of increased acid production. Whether acid secretion increases in response to helicobacter infection is doubted. One possibility is that the patches of metaplastic gastric epithelium in the duodenum on which helicobacter take up residence result from the action of acid. Then the colonized patches undergo ulceration.

Chronic liver disease, chronic lung disease, and chronic pancreatitis have all been implicated as increasing the possibility of duodenal ulceration.

▶ Clinical Findings

A. Symptoms and Signs

Pain, the presenting symptom in most patients, is usually located in the epigastrium and is variably described as aching, burning, or gnawing. Radiologic survey studies indicate, however, that some patients with active duodenal ulcer have no gastrointestinal complaints.

The daily cycle of the pain is often characteristic. The patient usually has no pain in the morning until an hour or more after breakfast. The pain is relieved by the noon meal, only to recur in the later afternoon. Pain may appear again in the evening, and in about half of cases, it arouses the patient during the night. Food, milk, or antacid preparations give temporary relief.

When the ulcer penetrates the head of the pancreas posteriorly, back pain is noted; concomitantly, the cyclic pattern of pain may change to a more steady discomfort, with less relief from food and antacids.

Varying degrees of nausea and vomiting are common. Vomiting may be a major feature even in the absence of obstruction.

The abdominal examination may reveal localized epigastric tenderness to the right of the midline, but in many instances no tenderness can be elicited.

B. Endoscopy

Gastroduodenoscopy is useful in evaluating patients with an uncertain diagnosis, those with bleeding from the upper intestine, and those who have obstruction of the gastroduodenal segment and for assessing response to therapy.

C. Diagnostic Tests

1. Gastric analysis—A gastric analysis may be indicated in certain cases. The standard gastric analysis consists of the following: (a) Measurement of acid production by the unstimulated stomach under basal fasting conditions; the result is expressed as H^+ secretion in mEq/h and is termed the basal acid output (BAO). (b) Measurement of acid production during stimulation by histamine or pentagastrin given in a dose maximal for this effect. The result is expressed as H^+ secretion in mEq/h and is termed the maximal acid output (MAO).

Interpretation of the results is outlined in Table 23–1.

2. Serum gastrin—Depending on the laboratory, normal basal gastrin levels average 50–100 pg/mL, and levels over 200 pg/mL can almost always be considered high.

Gastrin concentrations may rise in hyposecretory and hypersecretory states. In the former conditions (eg, atrophic gastritis, pernicious anemia, acid-suppressant medications), the cause is higher antral pH with loss of antral inhibition for gastrin release. More important clinically is elevated gastrin levels with concomitant hypersecretion, where the high gastrin level is responsible for the increased acid and resulting peptic ulceration. The best-defined clinical condition in this category is Zollinger–Ellison syndrome (gastrinoma). Antrum attached to the duodenum, but out of continuity with the gastric alimentary flow after gastrectomy (retained antrum), is another cause of elevated gastrin driving excess gastric acid secretion.

A fasting serum gastrin determination should be obtained in patients with peptic ulcer disease that is unusually severe or refractory to therapy.

D. Radiographic Studies

On an upper gastrointestinal series or CT scan with gastrointestinal contrast, the changes induced by duodenal ulcer consist of duodenal deformities and an ulcer niche. Inflammatory swelling and scarring may lead to distortion of the duodenal bulb, eccentricity of the pyloric channel, or pseudodiverticulum formation. The ulcer itself may be seen either in profile or, more commonly, *en face*.

▶ Differential Diagnosis

The most common diseases simulating peptic ulcer are (1) chronic cholecystitis, in which cholecystograms show either nonfunctioning of the gallbladder or stones in a functioning gallbladder; (2) acute pancreatitis, in which the serum amylase is elevated; (3) chronic pancreatitis, in which endoscopic retrograde cholangiopancreatography (ERCP) shows an abnormal pancreatic duct; (4) functional indigestion, in which x-rays are normal; and (5) reflux esophagitis.

▶ Complications

The common complications of duodenal ulcer are hemorrhage, perforation, and duodenal obstruction. Each of these is discussed in a separate section. Less common complications are pancreatitis and biliary obstruction.

▶ Prevention

Prevention of ulcer disease entails avoidance of *H pylori* infection.

▶ Treatment

Acute duodenal ulcer can be controlled by suppressing acid secretion in most patients, but the long-term course of the disease (ie, frequency of relapses and of complications) is unaffected unless *H pylori* infection is eradicated. Surgical therapy is recommended principally for the treatment of complications: bleeding, perforation, or obstruction.

A. Medical Treatment

The goals of medical therapy are: (1) to heal the ulcer and (2) to cure the disease. Treatment in the first category is

Table 23–1. Mean values for acid output during gastric analysis for normals and patients with duodenal ulcer. The upper limits of normal are basal, 5 meq/h; maximal, 30 meq/h.

		Mean Acid Output (meq/h)	
	Sex	**Normal**	**Duodenal Ulcer**
Basal	Male	2.5	5.5
	Female	1.5	3
Maximal (pentagastrin)	Male	30	40
	Female	20	30

aimed at decreasing acid secretion or neutralizing acid. The principal drugs consist of H_2 receptor antagonists (eg, cimetidine, ranitidine) and proton pump blockers (eg, omeprazole, pantoprazole).

After the ulcer has healed, discontinuation of therapy results in an 80% recurrence rate within 1 year, which may be avoided by chronic nighttime administration of a single dose of acid suppressive agent. A better approach is to treat the *H pylori* infection along with the ulcer, since eradication of *H pylori* diminishes recurrent ulceration unless the infection recurs–an uncommon event. The following combination is an effective regimen: lansoprazole, 30 mg twice daily for 14 days; amoxicillin, 1 g twice daily for 14 days; and clarithromycin, 500 mg twice daily for 14 days.

B. Surgical Treatment

If medical treatment has been optimal, a persistent ulcer may be judged intractable, and surgical treatment is indicated. This is now uncommon.

The surgical procedures that can cure peptic ulcer are aimed at reduction of gastric acid secretion. Excision of the ulcer itself is not sufficient for either duodenal or gastric ulcer; recurrence is nearly inevitable with such procedures.

The surgical methods of treating duodenal ulcer are vagotomy (several varieties) and antrectomy plus vagotomy. All of these procedures can be performed laparoscopically. With rare exceptions, one of the vagotomy operations is sufficient (Figure 23–5).

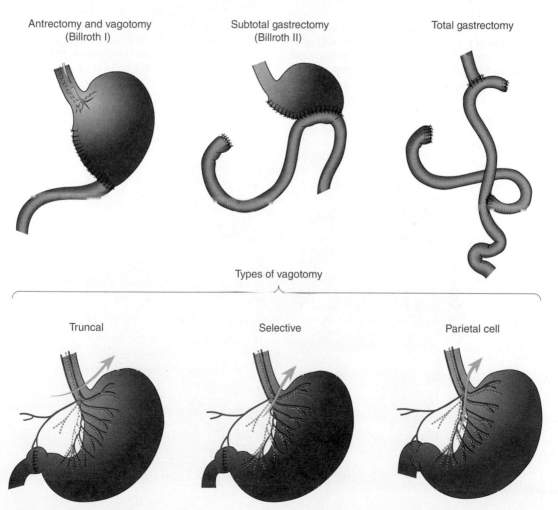

▲ **Figure 23–5.** Various types of operations currently popular for treating duodenal ulcer disease. Total gastrectomy is reserved for Zollinger-Ellison syndrome. The choice among the other procedures should be individualized according to principles discussed in the text.

1. Vagotomy—Truncal vagotomy consists of resection of a 1- or 2-cm segment of each vagal trunk as it enters the abdomen on the distal esophagus. The resulting vagal denervation of the gastric musculature produces delayed emptying of the stomach in many patients unless a drainage procedure is performed. The method of drainage most often selected is pyloroplasty (Heineke–Mikulicz procedure, Figure 23–6); gastrojejunostomy is used less often. Neither procedure gives a superior functional result, and pyloroplasty is less time consuming.

Vagal denervation of just the parietal cell area of the stomach is called parietal cell vagotomy or proximal gastric vagotomy. The technique spares the main nerves of Latarjet (Figures 23–3 and 23–5) but divides all vagal branches that terminate on the proximal two-thirds of the stomach. Since antral innervation is preserved, gastric emptying is relatively normal, and a drainage procedure is unnecessary. Nevertheless, parietal cell vagotomy plus pyloroplasty gives better results (ie, fewer recurrent ulcers) than parietal cell vagotomy alone. Parietal cell vagotomy appears to have about the same effectiveness as truncal or selective vagotomy for curing the ulcer disease, but dumping and diarrhea are much less frequent.

The vagotomy procedures have the advantages of technical simplicity and preservation of the entire gastric reservoir capacity. The principal disadvantage is recurrent ulceration in about 10% of patients. The recurrence rate after parietal cell vagotomy is about twice as high in patients with prepyloric ulcer, and most surgeons use a different operation for an ulcer in this location.

2. Antrectomy and vagotomy—This operation entails a distal gastrectomy of 50% of the stomach, with the line of gastric transection carried high on the lesser curvature to conform with the boundary of the gastrin-producing mucosa.

The terms antrectomy and hemigastrectomy are loosely synonymous. The proximal remnant may be reanastomosed to the duodenum (Billroth I resection) or to the side of the proximal jejunum (Billroth II resection). The Billroth I technique is most popular, but there is no conclusive evidence that the results are superior. When creating a Billroth II

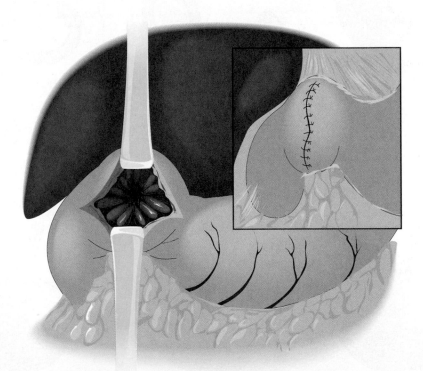

▲ **Figure 23–6.** Heineke-Mikulicz pyloroplasty. A longitudinal incision has been made across the pylorus, revealing an active ulcer in the duodenal bulb. The insert shows the transverse closure of the incision that widens the gastric outlet. The accompanying vagotomy is not shown.

(gastrojejunostomy) reconstruction, the surgeon may bring the jejunal loop up to the gastric remnant either anterior to the transverse colon or posteriorly through a hole in the transverse mesocolon. Since either method is satisfactory, an antecolic anastomosis is elected in most cases because it is simpler. Truncal vagotomy is performed as described in the preceding section; antrectomy by itself will not prevent a high recurrence rate. In most instances, the surgeon will be able to remove the ulcerated portion of duodenum in the course of resection.

Vagotomy and antrectomy is associated with a low incidence of marginal ulceration (2%) and a generally good overall outcome, but the risk of complications is higher than after vagotomy without resection.

3. Subtotal gastrectomy—This operation consists of resection of two-thirds to three-fourths of the distal stomach. After subtotal gastrectomy for duodenal ulcer, a Billroth II reconstruction is preferable. Subtotal gastrectomy is largely of historical interest.

▶ **Complications of Surgery for Peptic Ulcer**

A. Early Complications

Duodenal stump leakage, gastric retention (poor gastric emptying), and hemorrhage may develop in the immediate postoperative period.

B. Late Complications

4. Recurrent ulcer (marginal ulcer, stomal ulcer, anastomotic ulcer)—Recurrent ulcers formed in about 10% of duodenal ulcer patients treated by vagotomy and pyloroplasty or parietal cell vagotomy; and in 2%–3% after vagotomy and antrectomy or subtotal gastrectomy without chronic acid suppression. Recurrent ulcers nearly always develop immediately adjacent to the anastomosis on the intestinal side.

The usual complaint is upper abdominal pain, which is often aggravated by eating and improved by antacids. In some patients, the pain is felt more to the left in the epigastrium, and left axillary or shoulder pain is occasionally reported. About a third of patients with stomal ulcer have major gastrointestinal hemorrhage. Free perforation is less common (5%).

Diagnosis and treatment are essentially the same as for the original ulcer.

5. Gastrojejunocolic and gastrocolic fistula—A deeply eroding ulcer may occasionally produce a fistula between the stomach and colon. Most examples have resulted from recurrent peptic ulcer after an operation that included a gastrojejunal anastomosis.

Severe diarrhea and weight loss are the presenting symptoms in over 90% of cases. Abdominal pain typical of recurrent peptic ulcer often precedes the onset of the diarrhea.

Bowel movements number 8–12 or more a day; they are watery and often contain particles of undigested food.

The degree of malnutrition ranges from mild to very severe. Laboratory studies reveal low serum proteins and manifestations of fluid and electrolyte depletion. Appropriate tests may reflect deficiencies in both water-soluble and fat-soluble vitamins.

An upper gastrointestinal series reveals the marginal ulcer in only 50% of patients and the fistula in only 15%. Barium enema unfailingly demonstrates the fistulous tract.

Initial treatment should replenish fluid and electrolyte deficits. The involved colon and ulcerated gastrojejunal segment should be excised and colonic continuity reestablished. Vagotomy, partial gastrectomy, or both are required to treat the ulcer diathesis and prevent another recurrent ulcer. Results are excellent in benign disease. In general, the outlook for patients with a malignant fistula is poor.

6. Dumping syndrome—Symptoms of the dumping syndrome are noted to some extent by most patients who have an operation that impairs the ability of the stomach to regulate its rate of emptying. Within several months, however, dumping is a clinical problem in only 1%–2% of patients. Symptoms fall into two categories: cardiovascular and gastrointestinal. Shortly after eating, the patient may experience palpitations, sweating, weakness, dyspnea, flushing, nausea, abdominal cramps, belching, vomiting, diarrhea, and, rarely, syncope. The degree of severity varies widely, and not all symptoms are reported by all patients. In severe cases, the patient must lie down for 30–40 minutes until the discomfort passes.

Diet therapy to reduce jejunal osmolality is successful in all but a few cases. The diet should be low in carbohydrate and high in fat and protein content. Sugars and carbohydrates are least well tolerated; some patients are especially sensitive to milk. Meals should be taken dry, with fluids restricted to between meals. This dietary regimen ordinarily suffices, but anticholinergic drugs may be of help in some patients; others have reported improvement with supplemental pectin in the diet, or the use of somatostatin analogs.

7. Alkaline gastritis—Reflux of duodenal juices into the stomach is an invariable and usually innocuous situation after operations that interfere with pyloric function, but in some patients, it may cause marked gastritis. The principal symptom is postprandial pain, and the diagnosis rests on endoscopic and biopsy demonstration of an edematous inflamed gastric mucosa. Since a minor degree of gastritis is found in most patients after Billroth II gastrectomy, the endoscopic findings are to some degree nonspecific. Persistent severe pain is an indication for surgical reconstruction. Roux-en-Y gastrojejunostomy with a 40-cm efferent jejunal limb is the treatment of choice.

8. Anemia—Iron deficiency anemia develops in about 30% of patients within 5 years after partial gastrectomy. It is caused by failure to absorb ingested iron bound in an organic molecule. Before this diagnosis is accepted, the patient should be checked for blood loss, marginal ulcer, or an unsuspected tumor. Inorganic iron—ferrous sulfate or ferrous gluconate—is indicated for treatment and is absorbed normally after gastrectomy.

Vitamin B_{12} deficiency and megaloblastic anemia appear in a few cases after gastrectomy.

9. Postvagotomy diarrhea—About 5%–10% of patients who have had truncal vagotomy require treatment with antidiarrheal agents at some time, and perhaps 1% are seriously troubled by this complication. The diarrhea may be episodic, in which case the onset is unpredictable after symptom-free intervals of weeks to months. An attack may consist of only one or two watery movements or, in severe cases, may last for a few days. Other patients may continually produce 3–5 loose stools per day.

Most cases of postvagotomy diarrhea can be treated satisfactorily with constipating agents.

10. Chronic gastroparesis—Chronic delayed gastric emptying is seen occasionally after gastric surgery. Prokinetic agents (eg, metoclopramide) are often helpful, but some cases are refractory to any therapy except a completion gastrectomy and Roux-en-Y esophagojejunostomy (ie, total gastrectomy).

> Costa F, D'Elios MM. Management of Helicobacter pylori infection. *Expert Rev Anti Infect Ther* 2010 Aug;8(8):887-892.
> Schubert ML, Peura DA. Control of gastric acid secretion in health and disease. *Gastroenterology* 2008;134:1842.

ZOLLINGER-ELLISON SYNDROME (GASTRINOMA)

ESSENTIALS OF DIAGNOSIS

▶ Peptic ulcer disease (often severe) in 95%

▶ Gastric hypersecretion

▶ Elevated serum gastrin

▶ Non-B islet cell tumor of the pancreas or duodenum

▶ General Considerations

Zollinger-Ellison syndrome is manifested by gastric acid hypersecretion caused by a gastrin-producing tumor (gastrinoma). The normal pancreas does not contain appreciable amounts of gastrin. Most gastrinomas occur in the submucosa of the duodenum; others are found in the pancreas and rarely as primary tumors of the liver or ovary. About one-third of patients have the multiple endocrine neoplasia type I syndrome (MEN 1), which is characterized by a family history of endocrinopathy and the presence of tumors in other glands, especially the parathyroid glands and pituitary. Patients with MEN 1 usually have multiple gastrinomas. Those without MEN 1 usually have solitary gastrinomas that are often malignant. The tumors may be as small as 2–3 mm and are often difficult to find.

The diagnosis of cancer can be made only with findings of metastases or blood vessel invasion, because the histologic pattern is similar for benign and malignant tumors.

▶ Clinical Findings

A. Symptoms and Signs

Symptoms associated with gastrinoma are principally a result of acid hypersecretion—usually from peptic ulcer disease. Some patients with gastrinoma have severe diarrhea from the large amounts of acid entering the duodenum, which can destroy pancreatic lipase and produce steatorrhea, damage the small bowel mucosa, and overload the intestine with gastric and pancreatic secretions. About 5% of patients present with diarrhea only.

Ulcer symptoms are often refractory to large doses of antacids or standard doses of H_2 blocking agents. Hemorrhage, perforation, and obstruction are common complications. Marginal ulcers appear after surgical procedures that would cure the ordinary ulcer diathesis.

B. Laboratory Findings

Hypergastrinemia in the presence of acid hypersecretion is necessary for the diagnosis of gastrinoma. Gastrin levels are normally inversely proportionate to gastric acid output; therefore, diseases that result in increased gastric pH may cause a rise in serum gastrin concentration (eg, pernicious anemia, atrophic gastritis, gastric ulcer, postvagotomy state, and acid-suppressing medications). Serum gastrin levels should be measured in any patient with suspected gastrinoma or ulcer disease severe enough to warrant consideration of surgical treatment. H_2 receptor blocking agents, omeprazole, or antacids frequently increase serum gastrin concentrations and should be avoided for several days before gastrin measurements are made. It is often helpful to measure gastric acid secretion to rule out H^+ hyposecretion as a cause of hypergastrinemia.

The normal gastrin value is less than 200 pg/mL. Patients with gastrinoma usually have levels exceeding 500 pg/mL and sometimes 10,000 pg/mL or higher. Patients with borderline gastrin values (eg, 200–500 pg/mL) and acid secretion in the range associated with ordinary duodenal ulcer disease should have a secretin provocative test. Following intravenous administration of secretin (two units/kg as a bolus), a rise in the gastrin level of > 150 pg/mL within 15 minutes is diagnostic.

Marked basal acid hypersecretion (> 15 mEq H^+ per hour) occurs in most Zollinger-Ellison patients who have an intact stomach. In a patient who has previously undergone an acid-reducing operation, a basal acid output of 5 mEq/h or more is suggestive. Since the parietal cells are already under near maximal stimulation from hypergastrinemia, there is little increase in acid secretion following an injection of pentagastrin, and the ratio of basal to maximal acid output (BAO/MAO) characteristically exceeds 0.6.

Hypergastrinemia and gastric acid hypersecretion may occur in patients with gastric outlet obstruction, retained antrum after a Billroth II gastrojejunostomy, and antral gastrin cell hyperactivity (hyperplasia). These conditions are differentiated from gastrinoma by use of the secretin test. Because associated hyperparathyroidism is so common, serum calcium concentrations should be measured in all patients with gastrinoma.

Serum levels of neuron-specific enolase, β-hCG, and chromogranin-A are often elevated in patients with functioning neuroendocrine tumors. Although they are probably of no physiologic importance, the high levels of these peptides may be useful in following the results of therapy.

C. Imaging Studies

A CT or MR scan often demonstrates the pancreatic tumors. Somatostatin-receptor scintigraphy is extremely sensitive for detection of gastrinoma primary and metastatic sites. Transhepatic portal vein blood sampling to find gradients of gastrin production has been supplanted by the intra-arterial secretin test. Infusion of secretin into the artery supplying a functional gastrinoma causes an increase in hepatic vein gastrin levels. This invasive test is usually reserved for difficult situations.

Although used less frequently now with the availability of endoscopy, an upper gastrointestinal series can show ulceration in the duodenal bulb, though ulcers sometimes appear in the distal duodenum or proximal jejunum. The presence of ulcers in these distal ("ectopic") locations is nearly diagnostic of gastrinoma. The stomach contains prominent rugal folds, and secretions are present in the lumen despite overnight fasting. The duodenum may be dilated and exhibit hyperactive peristalsis. Edema may be detected in the small bowel mucosa. The barium flocculates in the intestine, and transit time is accelerated.

▶ Treatment

A. Medical Treatment

Initial treatment should consist of proton pump inhibitor (eg, omeprazole 20–40 mg, once or twice daily) or H_2

blocking agents (eg, cimetidine, 300–600 mg, four times daily; ranitidine, 300–450 mg, four times daily). The dose should be adjusted to keep gastric H^+ output below 5 mEq in the hour preceding the next dose.

B. Surgical Treatment

Resection is the ideal treatment for gastrinoma and is appropriate in all patients with apparently localized disease and no other significant limitations to their survival. Surgical cure may be possible when there are resectable metastases in peripancreatic lymph nodes or the liver. Overall, about 70% of patients have immediate biochemical cure, and about 30% of patients remain disease-free after 5 years.

Every patient with sporadic Zollinger-Ellison syndrome should be considered a candidate for tumor resection. The preoperative workup should include a CT or MR scan of the pancreas and somatostatin-receptor scintigraphy. Regardless of other findings, exploratory laparotomy is then recommended in the absence of evidence of unresectable metastatic disease. If the tumor is found in the pancreas, it is enucleated if possible. Operative ultrasound may help in the examination of the pancreas. Most lesions will be found either in the head of the pancreas or in the duodenum. All patients should have longitudinal duodenotomy and palpation of the duodenal mucosa to identify the frequent primary tumors in this site.

▶ Prognosis

Since H_2 blocking agents become less effective with time, omeprazole is eventually required in medically treated patients. Because it is usually multifocal, the disease can rarely be cured surgically in patients with MEN 1. Malignant gastrinomas can cause death from growth of metastases.

Ito T, Igarashi H, Jensen RT. Zollinger-Ellison syndrome: recent advances and controversies. *Curr Opin Gastroenterol* 2013 Nov;29(6):650-661.

Norton JA, Fraker DL, Alexander HR, Jensen RT. Value of surgery in patients with negative imaging and sporadic Zollinger-Ellison syndrome. *Ann Surg* 2012 Sep;256(3):509-517.

GASTRIC ULCER

ESSENTIALS OF DIAGNOSIS

▶ Epigastric pain

▶ Ulcer demonstrated by x-ray

▶ Acid present on gastric analysis

► General Considerations

The peak incidence of gastric ulcer is in patients aged 40–60 years, or about 10 years older than the average for those with duodenal ulcer. Ninety-five percent of gastric ulcers are located on the lesser curvature, and 60% of these are within 6 cm of the pylorus. The symptoms and complications of gastric ulcer closely resemble those of duodenal ulcer.

Gastric ulcers may be separated into three types with different causes and different treatments. Type I ulcers, the most common variety, are found in patients who on the average are 10 years older than patients with duodenal ulcers and who have no clinical or radiographic evidence of previous duodenal ulcer disease; gastric acid output is normal or low. The ulcers are usually located within 2 cm of the boundary between parietal cell and pyloric mucosa, but always in the latter. As noted above, 95% are on the lesser curvature, usually near the incisura angularis.

Antral gastritis is universally present, being most severe near the pylorus and gradually diminishing. This is associated in most cases with the presence of *H pylori* beneath the mucus layer, on the luminal surface of epithelial cells, and gastric ulcer disease is probably the result of infection with this organism.

Type II ulcers are located close to the pylorus (prepyloric ulcers) and occur in association with (most often following) duodenal ulcers. The risk of cancer is very low in these gastric ulcers. Acid secretion measured by gastric analysis is in the range associated with duodenal ulcer.

Type III ulcers occur in the antrum as a result of chronic use of nonsteroidal anti-inflammatory agents.

Ulcer identified on x-ray or by endoscopy could be an ulcerated malignant tumor rather than a simple benign ulcer. Efforts must be expended during the *initial* stage of the workup to establish this distinction. Despite the generally discouraging results of surgery for gastric adenocarcinoma, those whose tumors are difficult to distinguish from benign ulcer have a 50%–75% chance of cure after gastrectomy.

► Clinical Findings

A. Symptoms and Signs

The principal symptom is epigastric pain relieved by food or antacids, as in duodenal ulcer. Epigastric tenderness is a variable finding. Compared with duodenal ulcer, the pain in gastric ulcer tends to appear earlier after eating, often within 30 minutes. Vomiting, anorexia, and aggravation of pain by eating are also more common with gastric ulcer.

Achlorhydria is defined as no acid (pH > 6.00) after pentagastrin stimulation. Achlorhydria is incompatible with the diagnosis of benign peptic ulcer and suggests a malignant gastric ulcer. About 5% of malignant gastric ulcers will be associated with this finding.

B. Upper Endoscopy and Biopsy

Upper endoscopy should be performed as part of the initial workup to attempt to find malignant lesions. The rolled-up margins of the ulcer that produce the meniscus sign on x-ray can often be distinguished from the flat edges characteristic of a benign ulcer. Multiple (preferably six) biopsy specimens and brush biopsy should be obtained from the edge of the lesion. False positives are rare; false negatives occur in 5%–10% of malignant ulcers.

C. Imaging Studies

Upper gastrointestinal x-rays can show an ulcer, usually on the lesser curvature in the pyloric area. In the absence of a tumor mass, the following suggest that the ulcer is malignant: (1) the deepest penetration of the ulcer is not beyond the expected border of the gastric wall; (2) the meniscus sign is present (ie, a prominent rim of radiolucency surrounding the ulcer), caused by heaped-up edges of tumor; and (3) cancer is more common (10%) in ulcers greater than 2 cm in diameter. Coexistence of duodenal deformity or ulcer favors a diagnosis of benign ulcer in the stomach.

► Differential Diagnosis

The characteristic symptoms of gastric ulcer are often clouded by nonspecific complaints. Uncomplicated hiatal hernia, atrophic gastritis, chronic cholecystitis, irritable colon syndrome, and undifferentiated functional problems are distinguishable from peptic ulcer only after appropriate radiologic studies and sometimes not even then.

Gastroscopy and biopsy of the ulcer should be performed to rule out malignant gastric ulcer.

► Complications

Bleeding, obstruction, and perforation are the principal complications of gastric ulcer. They are discussed separately elsewhere in this chapter.

► Treatment

A. Medical Treatment

Medical management of gastric ulcer is the same as for duodenal ulcer. The patient should be questioned regarding the use of ulcerogenic agents, which should be eliminated as far as possible.

Repeat endoscopy should be obtained to document the rate of healing. After 4–16 weeks (depending on the initial size of the lesion and other factors), healing usually has reached a plateau. In order to cure the disease and avoid recurrent ulcers, *H pylori* must be eradicated. The success of therapy in this regard can be checked by serologic testing for *H pylori* antibodies.

B. Surgical Treatment

Before the significance of *H pylori* in the etiology of gastric ulcer was appreciated, the most effective surgical treatment was distal hemigastrectomy (including the ulcer); somewhat less effective but still useful in high-risk patients was vagotomy and pyloroplasty. Parietal cell vagotomy for prepyloric ulcers was followed by a high (eg, 30%) recurrence rate, but parietal cell vagotomy plus pyloroplasty worked well.

Intractability to medical therapy has now become a rare indication for surgery in gastric ulcer disease, since H_2 receptor antagonists or omeprazole can bring the condition under control, and treatment of *H pylori* infection can almost eliminate the problem of recurrence. Consequently, surgery is needed principally for complications of the disease: bleeding, perforation, or obstruction.

> Lee CW, Sarosi GA Jr. Emergency ulcer surgery. *Surg Clin North Am* 2011 Oct;91(5):1001-1013.

UPPER GASTROINTESTINAL HEMORRHAGE

Upper gastrointestinal hemorrhage may be mild or severe but should always be considered an ominous manifestation that deserves thorough evaluation. Bleeding is the most common serious complication of peptic ulcer, portal hypertension, and gastritis, and these conditions taken together account for most episodes of upper gastrointestinal bleeding in the average hospital population.

The major factors that determine the diagnostic and therapeutic approach are the amount and rate of bleeding. Estimates of both should be made promptly and monitored and revised continuously until the episode has been resolved. It is important to know at the outset that bleeding stops spontaneously in 75% of cases; the remainder includes those who will require surgery, experience complications, or die.

Hematemesis or melena is present except when the rate of blood loss is minimal. Hematemesis of either bright-red or dark blood indicates that the source is proximal to the ligament of Treitz. It is more common from bleeding that originates in the stomach or esophagus. In general, hematemesis denotes a more rapidly bleeding lesion, and a high percentage of patients who vomit blood require surgery. Coffee-ground vomitus is due to vomiting of blood that has been in the stomach long enough for gastric acid to convert hemoglobin to methemoglobin.

Most patients with melena (passage of black or tarry stools) are bleeding from the upper gastrointestinal tract, but melena can be produced by blood entering the bowel at any point from mouth to cecum. The conversion of red blood to dark depends more on the time it resides in the intestine than on the site of origin. The black color of melenic stools is probably caused by hematin, the product of oxidation of heme by intestinal and bacterial enzymes. Melena can be produced by as little as 50–100 mL of blood in the stomach. When 1 L of blood was instilled into the upper intestine of experimental subjects, melena persisted for 3–5 days, which shows that the rate of change in character of the stool is a poor guide to the time bleeding stops after an episode of hemorrhage.

Hematochezia is defined as the passage of bright-red blood from the rectum. Bright-red rectal blood can be produced by bleeding from the colon, rectum, or anus. However, if intestinal transit is rapid during brisk bleeding in the upper intestine, bright-red blood may be passed unchanged in the stool.

▶ Tests for Occult Blood

Normal subjects lose about 2.5 mL of blood per day in their stools, presumably from minor mechanical abrasions of the intestinal epithelium. Between 50 and 100 mL of blood per day will produce melena. Tests for occult blood in the stool should be able to detect amounts between 10 and 50 mL/d. False-positive results may be due to dietary hemoglobin, myoglobin, or peroxidases of plant origin. Iron ingestion does not give positive reactions. The sensitivity of the guaiac slide test (Hemoccult) is in the desired range, and this is the best test available at present.

▶ Initial Management

In an apparently healthy patient, melena of a week or more suggests that the bleeding is slow. In this type of patient, admission to the hospital should be followed by a deliberate but nonemergency workup. However, patients who present with hematemesis or melena of less than 12 hours' duration should be handled as if exsanguination were imminent. The approach entails a simultaneous series of diagnostic and therapeutic steps with the following initial goals: (1) assess the status of the circulatory system and replace blood loss as necessary; (2) determine the amount and rate of bleeding; (3) slow or stop the bleeding by ice-water lavage; and (4) discover the lesion responsible for the episode. The last step may lead to more specific treatment appropriate to the underlying condition.

The patient should be admitted to the hospital and a history and physical examination performed. Experienced clinicians are able to make a correct diagnosis of the cause of bleeding from clinical findings in only 60% of patients. Peptic ulcer, acute gastritis, esophageal varices, esophagitis, and Mallory-Weiss tear account for over 90% of cases (Table 23–2). Questions concerning the symptoms and predisposing factors should be asked. The patient should be questioned about salicylate intake and any history of a bleeding tendency.

Of the diseases commonly responsible for acute upper gastrointestinal bleeding, only portal hypertension is associ-

Table 23–2. Causes of massive upper gastrointestinal hemorrhage. Note that cancer is rarely the cause.

	Relative Incidence (%)	
Common Causes		
Peptic ulcer		45
Duodenal ulcer	25	
Gastric ulcer	20	
Esophageal varices		20
Gastritis		20
Mallory-Weiss syndrome		10
Uncommon Causes		5
Gastric carcinoma		
Esophagitis		
Pancreatitis		
Hemobilia		
Duodenal diverticulum		

ated with diagnostic clues on physical examination. However, gastrointestinal bleeding should not be automatically attributed to esophageal varices in a patient with jaundice, ascites, splenomegaly, spider angiomas, or hepatomegaly; over half of cirrhotic patients who present with acute hemorrhage are bleeding from gastritis or peptic ulcer.

Blood should be drawn for cross-matching, hematocrit, hemoglobin, creatinine, and tests of liver function. An intravenous infusion should be started and, in the presence of massive bleeding, a large-bore nasogastric tube inserted. In cases of melena, the gastric aspirate should be examined to verify the gastroduodenal source of the hemorrhage, but about 25% of patients with bleeding duodenal ulcers have gastric aspirates that test negatively for blood. The tube must be larger than the standard nasogastric tube (16F) so the stomach can be lavaged free of liquid blood and clots. After its contents have been removed, the stomach should be irrigated with copious amounts of ice water or saline solution until blood no longer returns. If the patient was bleeding at the time the nasogastric tube was inserted, iced saline irrigation usually stops it. The large tube can then be exchanged for a standard nasogastric tube attached to continuous suction so further blood loss can be measured.

It is common to give H_2 receptor antagonists or omeprazole, though controlled trials have shown no benefit. If bleeding continues or if tachycardia or hypotension is present, the patient should be monitored and treated as for hemorrhagic shock.

In acute rapid hemorrhage, the hematocrit may be normal or only slightly low. A very low hematocrit without obvious signs of shock indicates more gradual blood loss.

All of the above tests and procedures can be performed within 1 or 2 hours after admission. By this time, in most instances, bleeding is under control, blood volume has been restored to normal, and the patient is being adequately monitored so that recurrent bleeding can be detected promptly. When this stage is reached, additional diagnostic tests should be performed.

▶ **Diagnosis of Cause of Bleeding**

Once the patient is stabilized, endoscopy should be the first study. In general, endoscopy should be performed within 24 hours after admission, and under these circumstances the source of bleeding can be demonstrated in about 80% of cases. Longer delays have a lower diagnostic yield. Two lesions are seen in about 15% of patients. An upper gastrointestinal series should be performed if endoscopy is equivocal or unavailable. Although the diagnostic information provided by endoscopy does not appear to have resulted in decreased blood loss or improved outcome, endoscopic therapy, in the form of sclerosis of varices or injection of a bleeding ulcer, may do so. Having the diagnosis will also help in planning subsequent treatment, including the surgical approach if operation becomes necessary.

Rarely, selective angiography will have diagnostic or therapeutic usefulness. For diagnosis, it is most helpful when other studies fail to demonstrate the cause of bleeding. Infusion through the angiographic catheter of vasoconstrictors (eg, vasopressin) and embolization of the bleeding vessel with Gelfoam may be able to halt the bleeding in special cases.

▶ **Later Management**

Although a precise diagnosis of the cause of the bleeding may be valuable in later management, the patient must not be allowed to slip out of clinical control during the search for definitive diagnostic information. The decision for emergency surgery depends more on the rate and duration of bleeding than on its specific cause.

The need for transfusion should be determined on a continuing basis, and blood volume must be maintained. Blood pressure, pulse, central venous pressure, hematocrit, hourly urinary volume, and amount of blood obtained from the gastric tube or from the rectum all enter into this assessment. Many studies have shown the tendency to underestimate blood loss and inadequately transfuse massively bleeding patients who truly need aggressive therapy. Continued slow bleeding is best monitored by serial determinations of the hematocrit.

Several factors are associated with a worse prognosis with continued medical management of the bleeding episode. These are not absolute indications for laparotomy, but they should alert the clinician that emergency surgery may be required.

High rates of bleeding or amounts of blood loss predict high failure rates with medical treatment. Hematemesis is usually associated with more rapid bleeding and a greater blood volume deficit than melena. The presence of hypotension on admission to the hospital or the need for more than four units of blood to achieve circulatory stability implies a worse prognosis; if bleeding continues and subsequent transfusion requirements exceed one unit every 8 hours, continued medical management is usually unwise.

Total transfusion requirements also correlate with death rates. Death is uncommon when fewer than seven units of blood have been used, and the death rate rises progressively thereafter.

In general, bleeding from a gastric ulcer is more dangerous than bleeding from gastritis or duodenal ulcer, and patients with gastric ulcer should always be considered for early surgery. Regardless of the cause, if bleeding recurs after it has once stopped, the chances of success without operation are lower. Most patients who rebleed in the hospital should have consideration of surgery.

Patients over age 60 years tolerate continued blood loss less well than younger patients, and their bleeding should be stopped before secondary cardiovascular, pulmonary, or renal complications arise.

In 85% of patients, bleeding stops within a few hours of admission. About 25% of patients rebleed once bleeding has stopped. Rebleeding episodes are concentrated within the first 2 days of hospitalization, and if the patient has had no further bleeding for a period of 5 days, the chance of rebleeding is low. Rebleeding is most common in patients with varices, peptic ulcer, anemia, or shock. About 10% of patients require surgery to control bleeding, and most of these patients have bleeding ulcers or, less commonly, esophageal varices. The death rate is 30% among patients who rebleed and 3% among those who do not. The mortality rate is also high in the elderly and in patients who are already hospitalized at the onset of bleeding.

Cheung FK, Lau JY. Management of massive peptic ulcer bleeding. *Gastroenterol Clin North Am* 2009 Jun;38(2):231-243.

Greenspoon J, Barkun A: The pharmacological therapy of non-variceal upper gastrointestinal bleeding. *Gastroenterol Clin North Am* 2010 Sep;39(3):419-432.

HEMORRHAGE FROM PEPTIC ULCER

Approximately 20% of patients with peptic ulcer experience a bleeding episode, and this complication is responsible for about 40% of the deaths from peptic ulcer. Peptic ulcer is the most common cause of massive upper gastrointestinal hemorrhage, accounting for over half of all cases. Chronic gastric and duodenal ulcers have about the same tendency to bleed, but the former produce more severe episodes.

Bleeding ulcers in the duodenum are usually located on the posterior surface of the duodenal bulb. As the ulcer penetrates, the gastroduodenal artery is exposed and may become eroded. Since no major blood vessels lie on the anterior surface of the duodenal bulb, ulcerations at this point are not as prone to bleed. Patients with concomitant bleeding and perforation usually have two ulcers, a bleeding posterior ulcer and a perforated anterior one. Postbulbar ulcers (those in the second portion of the duodenum) bleed frequently, though ulcers are much less common in this site than near the pylorus.

In some patients, the bleeding is sudden and massive, manifested by hematemesis and shock. In others, chronic anemia and weakness due to slow blood loss are the only findings. The diagnosis is unreliable when based on clinical findings, so endoscopy should be performed early (ie, within 24 hours) in most cases.

In the preceding section, the management of acute upper gastrointestinal hemorrhage, the selection of diagnostic tests, and the factors suggesting the need for operation were discussed. Most patients (75%) with bleeding peptic ulcer can be successfully managed by medical means alone. Initial therapeutic efforts usually halt the bleeding. H_2 blockers and proton pump inhibitors decrease the risk of bleeding but have no effect on active bleeding.

After 12-24 hours have passed and the bleeding has clearly stopped, a patient who feels hungry should be fed. Twice-daily hematocrit readings should be ordered as a check on slow continued blood loss. Stools should be tested daily for the presence of blood; they will usually remain guaiac-positive for several days after bleeding stops.

Rebleeding in the hospital has been attended by a death rate of about 30%. Considering early surgery for those who rebleed could improve this figure. Patients who are over age 60 years, present with hematemesis, are actively bleeding at the time of endoscopy, or whose admission hemoglobin is below 8 g/dL have a higher risk of rebleeding. About three times as many patients with gastric ulcer (30%) rebleed compared with those with duodenal ulcer. Most instances of rebleeding occur within 2 days from the time the first episode has stopped. In one study, only 3% of patients who stopped bleeding for this long bled again.

▶ Endoscopic Therapy

Treatments administered through the endoscope may stop active bleeding or prevent rebleeding. Effective methods include injection into the ulcer of epinephrine, epinephrine plus 1% polidocanol (a sclerosing agent), or ethanol; application of clips to bleeding areas; or cautery using the heater probe, monopolar electrocautery, or the Nd:YAG laser. At least two modalities should be available to the endoscopist in the event one is unsuitable for a specific case or fails to work. Except for the laser, all are inexpensive. The indications for treatment are: (1) active bleeding at the time of endoscopy and (2) the presence of a visible vessel in the base of the ulcer. When treatment fails the first time, it may often be repeated with a good chance of success. It is important, however, not to allow the patient to deteriorate during non-operative attempts at halting the bleeding.

Emergency Surgery

Less than 10% of patients bleeding from a peptic ulcer require emergency surgery. Selection of those most likely to survive with surgical compared with medical treatment rests on the rate of blood loss and the other factors associated with a poor prognosis.

The overall death rate is significantly less after vagotomy and pyloroplasty than after gastrectomy for bleeding ulcer, and rebleeding occurs with about equal frequency after either procedure.

During laparotomy, the first step is to make a pyloroplasty incision if the endoscopic diagnosis is a bleeding duodenal ulcer. If a duodenal ulcer is found, the bleeding vessel should be suture-ligated and the duodenum and antrum inspected for additional ulcers. The pyloroplasty incision should then be closed and a truncal vagotomy performed. If the posterior wall of the duodenal bulb has been destroyed by a giant duodenal ulcer, a gastrectomy and Billroth II gastrojejunostomy may be preferable, since this somewhat uncommon ulcer is especially prone to bleed again if left in continuity with the stomach. Gastric ulcers can be handled by either gastrectomy or vagotomy and pyloroplasty. A thorough search should always be made for second ulcers or other causes of bleeding.

Prognosis

The death rate for an acute massive hemorrhage is about 15%. Careful study of the causes of death suggests that this figure could be improved by: (1) more precise blood replacement, since undertransfusion is the cause of some complications and deaths; and (2) earlier surgery in selected patients who fall into serious-risk categories, since the tendency has been to perform surgery on too few patients too late in the illness. Patients who stop bleeding should be treated as outlined in the section on duodenal ulcer.

Cappell MS, Friedel D. Initial management of acute upper gastrointestinal bleeding: from initial evaluation up to gastrointestinal endoscopy. *Med Clin North Am* 2008;92:491.

Cheung FK, Lau JY: Management of massive peptic ulcer bleeding. *Gastroenterol Clin North Am* 2009 Jun;38(2):231-243.

MALLORY-WEISS SYNDROME

Mallory-Weiss syndrome is responsible for about 10% of cases of acute upper gastrointestinal hemorrhage. The lesion consists of a 1- to 4-cm longitudinal tear in the gastric mucosa near the esophagogastric junction; it usually follows a bout of forceful retching. The disruption extends through the mucosa and submucosa but not usually into the muscularis mucosae. About 75% of these lesions are confined to the stomach, 20% straddle the esophagogastric junction, and 5% are entirely within the distal esophagus. Two-thirds of patients have a hiatal hernia.

The majority of patients are alcoholics, but the tear may appear after severe retching for any reason. Several cases have been reported following closed-chest cardiac compression.

Clinical Findings

Typically, the patient first vomits food and gastric contents. This is followed by forceful retching and then bloody vomitus. Rapid increases in gastric pressure, sometimes aggravated by hiatal hernia, cause the tear. Actual rupture of the distal esophagus can also be produced by vomiting (Boerhaave syndrome), but the difference seems to depend on vomiting of food in rupture and nonproductive retching in gastric mucosal tear.

Esophagogastroscopy is the most practical means of making the diagnosis.

Treatment & Prognosis

Initially, the patient is handled according to the general measures prescribed for upper gastrointestinal hemorrhage. In about 90% of patients, the bleeding stops spontaneously after ice-water lavage of the stomach. Patients who are still bleeding vigorously by the time endoscopy is performed are likely to require surgery. The bleeding can sometimes be controlled by endoscopic therapy (eg, electrocautery). If bleeding persists, surgical repair of the tear will be required.

If the diagnosis has been made before laparotomy, the surgeon should make a long, high gastrotomy after the abdomen is opened. The tear may be difficult to expose adequately. The search must be thorough, since in about 25% of patients there are two tears. A running absorbable acid suture should be used to oversew the lesion. Postoperative recurrence is rare.

PYLORIC OBSTRUCTION DUE TO PEPTIC ULCER

The cycles of inflammation and repair in peptic ulcer disease may cause obstruction of the gastroduodenal junction as a result of edema, muscular spasm, and scarring. To the extent that the first two factors are involved, the obstruction may be reversible with medical treatment. Obstruction is usually due to duodenal ulcer and is less common than either bleeding or perforation. The few gastric ulcers that obstruct are close to the pylorus. Obstruction due to peptic ulcer must be differentiated from that caused by a malignant tumor of the antrum or of the pancreas. Malignancy is becoming the more common cause, and it may be difficult to identify.

Clinical Findings

A. Symptoms and Signs

Most patients with obstruction have a long history of symptomatic peptic ulcer, and as many as 30% have been treated for perforation or obstruction in the past. The patient often notes gradually increasing ulcer pains over weeks or months, with the eventual development of anorexia, vomiting, and failure to gain relief from antacids. The vomitus often contains food ingested several hours previously, and absence of bile staining reflects the site of blockage. Weight loss may be marked if the patient has delayed seeking medical care.

Dehydration and malnutrition may be obvious on physical examination but are not always present. A succussion splash can often be elicited from the retained gastric contents. Peristalsis of the distended stomach may be visible on gross inspection of the abdomen, but this sign is relatively rare. Most patients have upper abdominal tenderness. Tetany may appear with advanced alkalosis.

B. Laboratory Findings

Anemia is present in about 25% of patients. Prolonged vomiting leads to metabolic alkalosis with dehydration. Measurement of serum electrolytes shows hypochloremia, hypokalemia, hyponatremia, and increased bicarbonate. Vomiting depletes the patient of Na^+, K^+, and Cl^-; the latter is lost in excess of Na^+ and K^+ as HCl. Gastric HCl loss causes extracellular HCO_3^- to rise, and renal excretion of HCO_3^- increases in an attempt to maintain pH. Large amounts of Na^+ are excreted in the urine with the HCO_3^-. Increasing Na^+ deficit evokes aldosterone secretion, which in turn brings about renal Na^+ conservation at the expense of more renal loss of K^+ and H^+. Glomerular filtration rate may drop and produce a prerenal azotemia. The eventual result of the process is a marked deficit of Na^+, Cl^-, K^+, and H_2O. Treatment involves replacement of water and NaCl until a satisfactory urine flow has been established. KCl replacement should then be started.

C. Saline Load Test

This is a simple means of assessing the degree of pyloric obstruction and is useful in following the patient's progress during the first few days of nasogastric suction.

Through the nasogastric tube, 700 mL of normal saline (at room temperature) is infused over 3–5 minutes, and the tube is clamped. Thirty minutes later, the stomach is aspirated and the residual volume of saline recorded. Recovery of more than 350 mL indicates obstruction. It must be recognized that the results of a saline load test do not predict how well the stomach will handle solid food. Solid emptying can be measured with technetium-99 m-labeled chicken liver.

D. Imaging Studies

Plain abdominal x-rays may show a large gastric fluid level. An upper gastrointestinal series should not be performed until the stomach has been emptied, because dilution of the barium in the retained secretions makes a worthwhile study impossible.

E. Endoscopy

Upper endoscopy is usually indicated to rule out the presence of an obstructing neoplasm.

Treatment

A. Medical Treatment

A large (32F) tube should be passed and the stomach emptied of its contents and lavaged until clean. After the stomach has been completely decompressed, a smaller tube should be inserted and placed on suction for several days to allow pyloric edema and spasm to subside and to permit the gastric musculature to regain its tone. A saline load test may be performed at this point to provide a baseline for later comparison. If chronic obstruction has produced severe malnutrition, total parenteral nutrition should be instituted.

After decompression of the stomach for 48–72 hours, the saline load test should be repeated. If this indicates sufficient improvement, the tube should be withdrawn and a liquid diet may be started. Gradual resumption of solid foods is permitted as tolerated.

B. Surgical Treatment

If 5–7 days of gastric aspiration do not result in relief of the obstruction, the patient should be treated surgically. Persistence of nonoperative effort beyond this point in the absence of progress rarely achieves the result hoped for. Failure of the obstruction to resolve completely (eg, if the patient can take only liquids) and recurrent obstruction of any degree are indications for surgery.

Surgical treatment may consist of a truncal or parietal cell vagotomy and drainage procedure (Figure 23–5). Truncal vagotomy and gastrojejunostomy is the easiest to perform laparoscopically.

Prognosis

About two-thirds of patients with acute obstruction fail to improve sufficiently on medical therapy and require operation to relieve the blockage. Patients who respond to medical treatment should be treated as outlined in the section on duodenal ulcer.

PERFORATED PEPTIC ULCER

Perforation complicates peptic ulcer about half as often as hemorrhage. Most perforated ulcers are located anteriorly, though occasionally gastric ulcers perforate into the lesser sac. The 15% death rate correlates with increased age, female gender, and gastric perforations. The diagnosis is overlooked in about 5% of patients, most of whom do not survive.

Anterior ulcers tend to perforate instead of bleed because of the absence of protective viscera and major blood vessels on this surface. In less than 10% of cases, acute bleeding from a posterior "kissing" ulcer complicates the anterior perforation, an association that carries a high death rate. Immediately after perforation, the peritoneal cavity is flooded with gastroduodenal secretions that elicit a chemical peritonitis. Early cultures show either no growth or a light growth of streptococci or enteric bacilli. Gradually, over 12–24 hours, the process evolves into bacterial peritonitis. Severity of illness and occurrence of death are directly related to the interval between perforation and surgical closure.

In an unknown percentage of cases, the perforation becomes sealed by adherence to the undersurface of the liver. In such patients, the process may be self-limited, but an intraperitoneal abscess develops in many.

▶ Clinical Findings

A. Symptoms and Signs

Perforation usually elicits a sudden, severe upper abdominal pain whose onset can be recalled precisely. The patient may or may not have had preceding chronic symptoms of peptic ulcer disease. Perforation rarely is heralded by nausea or vomiting, and it typically occurs several hours after the last meal. Shoulder pain, if present, reflects diaphragmatic irritation. Back pain is uncommon.

The initial reaction consists of a chemical peritonitis caused by gastric acid or bile and pancreatic enzymes. The peritoneal reaction dilutes these irritants with a thin exudate, and as a result the patient's symptoms may temporarily improve before bacterial peritonitis occurs. The physician who sees the patient for the first time during this symptomatic lull must not be misled into interpreting it as representing bona fide improvement.

The patient appears severely distressed, lying quietly with the knees drawn up and breathing shallowly to minimize abdominal motion. Fever is absent at the start. The abdominal muscles are rigid owing to severe involuntary spasm. Epigastric tenderness may not be as marked as expected because the board-like rigidity protects the abdominal viscera from the palpating hand. Escaped air from the stomach may enter the space between the liver and abdominal wall, and upon percussion the normal dullness over the liver will be tympanitic. Peristaltic sounds are reduced or absent. If delay in treatment allows continued escape of air into the peritoneal cavity, abdominal distention and diffuse tympany may result.

The above description applies to the typical case of perforation with classic findings. In as many as one-third of patients, the presentation is not as dramatic, diagnosis is less obvious, and serious delays in treatment may result from failure to consider this condition and to obtain the appropriate abdominal x-rays. Many of these atypical perforations occur in patients already hospitalized for some unrelated illness, and the significance of the new symptom of abdominal pain is not appreciated.

Lesser degrees of shock with minimal abdominal findings occur if the leak is small or rapidly sealed. A small duodenal perforation may slowly leak fluid that runs down the lateral peritoneal gutter, producing pain and muscular rigidity in the right lower quadrant, and thus raising a problem of confusion with acute appendicitis.

Perforations may be sealed by omentum or by the liver, with the later development of a subhepatic or subdiaphragmatic abscess.

B. Laboratory Findings

A mild leukocytosis in the range of 12,000/μL is common in the early stages. After 12–24 hours, this may rise to 20,000/μL or more if treatment has been inadequate. The mild rise in the serum amylase value that occurs in many patients is probably caused by absorption of the enzyme from duodenal secretions within the peritoneal cavity. Direct measurement of fluid obtained by paracentesis may show very high levels of amylase.

C. Imaging Studies

Plain x-ray or CT scan of the abdomen reveals free subdiaphragmatic air in 85% of patients.

If no free air is demonstrated and the clinical picture suggests perforated ulcer, an emergency CT scan with gastrointestinal contrast, or upper gastrointestinal series should be performed. If the perforation has not sealed, the diagnosis is established by noting escape of the contrast material from the lumen.

▶ Differential Diagnosis

The differential diagnosis includes acute pancreatitis and acute cholecystitis. The former does not have as explosive an onset as perforated ulcer and is usually accompanied by high serum levels of lipase and amylase. Acute cholecystitis with perforated gallbladder could mimic perforated ulcer closely but free air would not be present with ruptured gallbladder. Intestinal obstruction has a more gradual onset and is characterized by less severe pain that is crampy and accompanied by vomiting.

The simultaneous onset of pain and free air in the abdomen in the absence of trauma usually means perforated peptic ulcer. Free perforation of colonic diverticulitis and acute appendicitis are other rare causes.

▶ Treatment

The diagnosis is often suspected before the patient is sent for confirmatory imaging. Whenever a perforated ulcer is considered, the first step should be to pass a nasogastric tube and empty the stomach to limit further contamination of the peritoneal cavity. Blood should be drawn for laboratory studies, and intravenous antibiotics (eg, cefazolin, cefoxitin) should be started. If the patient's overall condition is precarious owing to delay in treatment, fluid resuscitation should precede diagnostic measures. Imaging should be obtained as soon as the clinical status will permit.

The simplest surgical treatment, laparoscopy (or laparotomy) and suture closure of the perforation solves the immediate problem. The closure most often consists of securely plugging the hole with omentum (Graham-Steele closure) sutured into place rather than bringing together the two edges with sutures. All fluid should be aspirated from the peritoneal cavity, but drainage is not indicated. Reperforation is rare in the immediate postoperative period.

About three-fourths of patients whose perforation is the culmination of a history of chronic symptoms continue to have clinically severe ulcer disease after simple closure. This had led to a more aggressive treatment policy involving a definitive ulcer operation for most patients with acute perforation (eg, parietal cell vagotomy plus closure of the perforation or truncal vagotomy and pyloroplasty). Now that ulcer disease can be cured by eradicating *H pylori,* the value of anything more than simple closure is limited.

Concomitant hemorrhage and perforation are most often due to two ulcers, an anterior perforated one and a posterior one that is bleeding. Perforated ulcers that also obstruct cannot be treated by suture closure of the perforation alone. Vagotomy plus gastroenterostomy or pyloroplasty should be performed. Perforated anastomotic ulcers require a vagotomy or gastrectomy, since in the long run, closure alone is nearly always inadequate.

Nonoperative treatment of perforated ulcer consists of continuous gastric suction and the administration of antibiotics in high doses. Although this has been shown to be effective therapy, with a low death rate, it is occasionally accompanied by a peritoneal and subphrenic abscess, and side effects are greater than with laparoscopic closure.

▶ Prognosis

About 15% of patients with perforated ulcer die, and about a third of these are undiagnosed before surgery. The death rate of perforated ulcer seen early is low. Delay in treatment, advanced age, and associated systemic diseases account for most deaths.

STRESS GASTRODUODENITIS, STRESS ULCER, & ACUTE HEMORRHAGIC GASTRITIS

The term stress ulcer has been used to refer to a heterogeneous group of acute gastric or duodenal ulcers that develop following physiologically stressful illnesses. There are four major etiologic factors associated with such lesions: (1) shock, (2) sepsis, (3) burns, and (4) central nervous system tumors or trauma.

▶ Etiology

A. Stress Ulcer

Acute ulcers following major surgery, mechanical ventilation, shock, sepsis, and burns (Curling ulcers) have enough common features to suggest they evolve by a similar pathogenetic mechanism.

Hemorrhage is the major clinical problem, though perforation occurs in about 10% of cases. Despite the predilection of stress ulcers to develop in the parietal cell mucosa, in about 30% of patients the duodenum is affected, and sometimes both stomach and duodenum are involved. Morphologically, the ulcers are shallow, discrete lesions with congestion and edema but little inflammatory reaction at their margins. Gastroduodenal endoscopy performed early in traumatized or burned patients has shown acute gastric erosions in the majority of patients within 72 hours after the injury. Such studies illustrate how frequently the disease process remains subclinical; clinically apparent ulcers develop in about 20% of susceptible patients. Clinically evident bleeding is usually seen 3–5 days after the injury, and massive bleeding generally does not appear until 4–5 days later.

Decreased mucosal resistance is the first step, which may involve the effects of ischemia (with production of toxic superoxide and hydroxyl radicals) and circulating toxins, followed by decreased mucosal renewal, decreased production of endogenous prostanoids, and thinning of the surface mucus layer. Decreased gastric mucosal blood flow also plays a role by decreasing the supply of blood buffers available to neutralize hydrogen ions that are diffusing into the weakened mucosa. Experimental evidence has implicated platelet-activating factor, released by endotoxin, as a possible mediator of gut ulceration in sepsis. The mucosa is thus rendered more vulnerable to acid-pepsin ulceration and lysosomal enzymes. Acid hypersecretion may be involved to some extent, since burn patients who manifest serious bleeding have higher gastric acid output than patients with a more benign course. Disruption of the gastric mucosal barrier to back diffusion of acid has been found in less than half of patients and is now thought to be a manifestation of the disease rather than a cause.

B. Cushing Ulcers

Acute ulcers associated with central nervous system tumors or injuries differ from stress ulcers because they are associated with elevated levels of serum gastrin and increased gastric acid secretion. Morphologically, they are similar to ordinary gastroduodenal peptic ulcers. Cushing ulcers are more prone to perforate than other kinds of stress ulcers.

C. Acute Hemorrhagic Gastritis

This disorder may share some causative factors with the above conditions, but the natural history is different and the response to treatment considerably better. Most of these patients can be controlled medically. When surgery is required for alcoholic gastritis, a high proportion of patients are cured by pyloroplasty and vagotomy.

▶ Clinical Findings

Hemorrhage is nearly always the first manifestation. Pain rarely occurs. Physical examination is not contributory except to reveal gross or occult fecal blood or signs of shock.

▶ Prevention

Acid suppressing medications given prophylactically to critically ill patients decrease the incidence of stress erosions and overt bleeding. Sucralfate is also effective. Patients receiving total parenteral nutrition appear to be protected by this therapy and experience no increased benefit from H_2 antagonists.

▶ Treatment

Initial management should consist of gastric lavage with chilled solutions and measures to combat sepsis if present. H_2 receptor blockers are of no value in the actively bleeding patient, but they probably decrease the rate of rebleeding once bleeding has stopped.

Perform laparotomy if the nonoperative regimen fails to halt the bleeding. Surgical treatment should consist of vagotomy and pyloroplasty, with suture of the bleeding points, or vagotomy and subtotal gastrectomy. There is a trend toward the first of these options, particularly in the sickest patients. When it occurs, rebleeding is nearly always from an ulcer left behind at the initial procedure. Rarely, total gastrectomy has had to be used because of the extent of ulceration and severity of bleeding or because of rebleeding after a lesser operation.

Ali T, Harty RF. Stress-induced ulcer bleeding in critically ill patients. *Gastroenterol Clin North Am* 2009 Jun;38(2):245-265.

GASTRIC CARCINOMA

There are about 21,000 new cases of carcinoma of the stomach in the United States annually. The incidence has dropped to one-third of what it was 40 years ago. This may reflect changes in the prevalence of *H pylori* infection, which has a role in the etiology of this disease. *H pylori* is known to be a cause of chronic atrophic gastritis, which in turn is a recognized precursor of gastric adenocarcinoma. Epidemiologic studies have linked gastric *H pylori* infection with a 3.6-fold to 18-fold (all patients vs. women) increase in the risk of developing carcinoma of the body or antrum (not the cardia), and the risk is proportionate to serum levels of *H pylori* antibodies.

The present incidence in American men is 10 new cases per 100,000 population per year. The highest rate, 63 per 100,000 men, is observed in Costa Rica; in eastern and central European countries, it is about 35 per 100,000 per year. Epidemiologic studies suggest that the incidence of gastric carcinoma is related to low dietary intake of vegetables and fruits and high intake of starches. Carcinoma of the stomach is rare under age 40 years, from which point the risk gradually climbs. The mean age at discovery is 63. It is about twice as common in men as in women.

Gastric epithelial cancers are nearly always adenocarcinomas. Squamous cell tumors of the proximal stomach involve the stomach secondarily from the esophagus. Five morphologic subdivisions correlate loosely with the natural history and outcome.

1. Ulcerating carcinoma (25%)—This consists of a deep, penetrating ulcer-tumor that extends through all layers of the stomach. It may involve adjacent organs in the process. The edges are shallow by contrast with overhanging edges noted in benign ulcers.

2. Polypoid carcinomas (25%)—These are large, bulky intraluminal growths that tend to metastasize late.

3. Superficial spreading carcinoma (15%)—Also known as early gastric cancer, superficial spreading carcinoma is confined to the mucosa and submucosa. Metastases are present in only 30% of cases. Even when metastases are present, the prognosis after gastrectomy is much better than for the more deeply invading lesions of advanced gastric cancer. In Japan, screening programs have been so successful that early gastric cancer now constitutes 30% of surgical cases, and survival rates have improved accordingly.

4. Linitis plastica (10%)—This variety of spreading tumor involves all layers with a marked desmoplastic reaction in which it may be difficult to identify the malignant cells. The stomach loses its pliability. Cure is rare because of early spread.

5. Advanced carcinoma (35%)—This largest category contains the big tumors that are found partly within and partly outside the stomach. They may originally have qualified for inclusion in the preceding groups but have outgrown that early stage.

Gastric adenocarcinomas can also be classified by degree of differentiation of their cells. In general, rate and extent of spread correlate with lack of differentiation. Some tumors are found histologically to excite an inflammatory cell reaction at their borders, and this feature indicates a relatively good prognosis. Tumors whose cells form glandular structures (intestinal type) have a somewhat better prognosis than tumors whose cells do not (diffuse type); the diffuse type is often associated with a substantial stromal component. The intestinal type of tumor accounts for a much larger proportion of cases in countries such as Japan and Finland where gastric cancer is especially common. The gradual decline in incidence in these areas is due principally to decreased occurrence of the intestinal type of tumor. Signet ring carcinomas, which contain more than 50% signet ring cells, have become increasingly more common and now constitute one-third of all cases. They behave as the diffuse type of cancer and occur more frequently in women, in younger patients, and in the distal part of the stomach. Previous *H pylori*—infection is not associated with the development of any specific histologic type of gastric cancer.

Extension occurs by intramural spread, direct extraluminal growth, and lymphatic metastases. Pathologic staging, which correlates closely with survival, is illustrated in Figure 23–7. Three-fourths of patients have metastases when diagnosed. Within the stomach, proximal spread exceeds distal spread. The pylorus acts as a partial barrier, but tumor is found in 25% of cases in the first few centimeters of the bulb.

Early gastric cancer, defined as a primary lesion confined to the mucosa and submucosa with or without lymph node metastases, is associated with an excellent prognosis (5-year survival rate of 90%) after resection. In Japan, mass screening programs detect about 30% of patients with this lesion, whereas in the United States, only 10% of patients have early gastric cancer.

Forty percent of tumors are in the antrum, predominantly on the lesser curvature; 30% arise in the body and fundus, 25% at the cardia, and 5% involve the entire organ. Frequency of location has gradually changed, so that proximal lesions are more common now than 10–20 years ago. Benign ulcers develop at the greater curvature and cardia

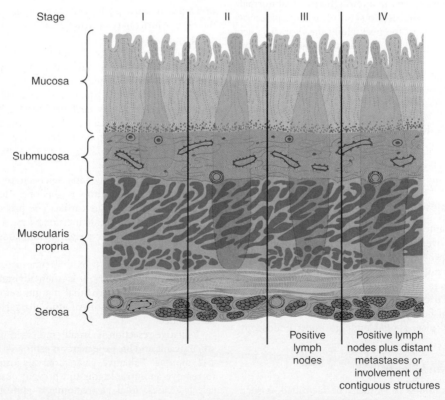

▲ **Figure 23–7.** Staging system for gastric carcinoma. The darkly shadowed areas represent cancers with different depths of mucosal penetration.

less commonly than malignant ones. Ulcers at these points are particularly suspect for neoplasm.

► Clinical Findings

A. Symptoms and Signs

The earliest symptom is usually vague postprandial abdominal heaviness that the patient does not identify as a pain. Sometimes the discomfort is no different from other vague dyspeptic symptoms that have been intermittently present for years, but the frequency and persistence are new.

Anorexia develops early and may be most pronounced for meat. Weight loss, the most common symptom, averages about 6 kg. True postprandial pain suggesting a benign gastric ulcer is relatively uncommon, but if it is present, one may be misled if subsequent x-rays show an ulcer. Vomiting may be present and becomes a major feature if pyloric obstruction occurs. It may have a coffee-ground appearance owing to bleeding by the tumor. Dysphagia may be the presenting symptom of lesions at the cardia.

An epigastric mass can be felt on examination in about one-fourth of cases. Hepatomegaly is present in 10% of cases. The stool will be positive for occult blood in half of patients, and melena is seen in a few. Otherwise, abnormal physical findings are confined to signs of distant spread of the tumor. Metastases to the neck along the thoracic duct may produce a Virchow node. Rectal examination may reveal a Blumer shelf, a solid peritoneal deposit anterior to the rectum. Enlarged ovaries (Krukenberg tumors) may be caused by intraperitoneal metastases. Further dissemination may involve the liver, lungs, brain, or bone.

B. Laboratory Findings

Anemia is present in 40% of patients. Carcinoembryonic antigen levels are elevated in 65%, usually indicating extensive spread of the tumor.

C. Imaging Studies

An upper gastrointestinal series is diagnostic for many tumors, but the overall false-negative rate is about 20%. Major diagnostic problems are posed by ulcerating tumors, a few of which may not be distinguishable radiologically from benign peptic ulcers. The differential features are listed in the section on gastric ulcer, but x-rays alone will not establish a diagnosis of benign ulcer. All patients with a newly discovered gastric ulcer should undergo upper endoscopy and gastric biopsy.

D. Gastroscopy and Biopsy

Large gastric carcinomas can usually be identified as such by their gross appearance at endoscopy. All gastric lesions, whether polypoid or ulcerating, should be examined by taking multiple biopsy and brush cytology specimens during endoscopy. False negative results are seen occasionally as a result of sampling error, and a minimum of six biopsies is necessary for greatest accuracy.

► Treatment

Surgical resection is the only curative treatment. About 85% of patients are operable, and in 50% the lesions are amenable to resection; of the resectable lesions, half are potentially curable (ie, no signs of spread beyond the limits of resection). Preoperative chemotherapy with a multidrug regimen is recommended for most patients.

The surgical objective should be to remove the tumor, an adjacent uninvolved margin of stomach and duodenum, the regional lymph nodes, and, if necessary, portions of involved adjacent organs. The proximal margin should be a minimum of 6 cm from the gross tumor. If the tumor is located in the antrum, a curative resection would entail distal gastrectomy with *en bloc* removal of the omentum, a 3- to 4-cm cuff of duodenum and the subpyloric lymph nodes, and, in some instances, excision of the left gastric artery and nearby lymph nodes. Reconstruction after gastrectomy may be by either a Billroth I or II procedure, but the latter is preferable because postoperative growth of residual tumor near the pylorus may obstruct a gastroduodenal anastomosis early.

Total gastrectomy with splenectomy is required for tumors of the proximal half of the stomach and for extensive tumors (eg, linitis plastica). Whether or not the spleen should be removed in such cases is a subject of debate. Alimentary continuity is most often reestablished by a Roux-en-Y esophagojejunostomy. Construction of an intestinal pouch as a substitute food reservoir (eg, Hunt–Lawrence pouch) is of no nutritional value, and it increases the risks of immediate complications.

Esophagogastrectomy plus splenectomy with intrathoracic esophagogastrostomy is the operation usually performed for tumors of the cardia. The procedure is usually done through two separate incisions: first, a laparotomy for the gastric part, and then a right posterolateral thoracotomy for the anastomosis.

The propensity for proximal submucosal spread must be appreciated at surgery. It is often advisable to perform a frozen section at the proximal margin before constructing the anastomosis. If tumor is found, the gastrectomy should be extended.

Palliative resection is usually indicated if the stomach is still movable and life expectancy is estimated to be more than 1–2 months. Palliative gastrectomy is usually performed to remove an antral lesion and prevent obstruction, but in selected cases, total gastrectomy is appropriate palliative treatment if the operation can be done safely and the amount of extragastric tumor is minimal. Whenever technically feasible, palliative gastrectomy is preferable to palliative gastrojejunostomy.

Adjuvant chemotherapy after curative surgery is recommended, particularly for patients who have undergone preoperative chemotherapy and responded.

▶ Prognosis

In the United States, the overall 5-year survival rate is about 12%. The 5-year survival rate for patients with early gastric cancer is about 90%. The 5-year survival rates in relation to the extent of spread are stage I, 70%; stage II, 30%; stage III, 10%; and stage IV, 0%.

Death from tumor may follow dissemination to other organs or may be the result of progressive gastric obstruction and malnutrition.

Ajani JA, Bentrem DJ, Besh S, et al: Gastric cancer, version 2.2013: featured updates to the NCCN Guidelines. *J Natl Compr Canc Netw* May 1, 2013;11(5):531-546.

GASTRIC POLYPS

Gastric polyps are single or multiple benign tumors that occur predominantly in the elderly. Those located in the distal stomach are more apt to cause symptoms. Whenever gastric polyps are discovered, gastric cancer must be ruled out.

Gastric polyps can be classified histologically as hyperplastic, adenomatous, or inflammatory. Other polypoid lesions, such as leiomyomas and carcinoid tumors, are discussed elsewhere. Hyperplastic polyps, which constitute 80% of cases, consist of an overgrowth of normal epithelium; they are not true neoplasms and have no relationship to gastric cancer. About 30% of adenomatous polyps contain a focus of adenocarcinoma, and adenocarcinoma can be found elsewhere in the stomach in 20% of patients with a benign adenomatous polyp. The incidence of cancer in an adenomatous polyp rises with increasing size. Lesions with a stalk and those less than 2 cm in diameter are usually not malignant. About 10% of benign adenomatous polyps undergo malignant change during prolonged follow-up.

Anemia may develop from chronic blood loss or deficient iron absorption. Over 90% of patients are achlorhydric after maximal stimulation. Vitamin B_{12} absorption is deficient in 25%, although megaloblastic anemia is present in only a few.

Excision with a snare through the endoscope can be performed safely for most polyps. Otherwise, surgical excision is indicated for polyps greater than 1 cm in diameter or when cancer is suspected. Single polyps may be excised through a gastrotomy and a frozen section performed. If the polyp is found to be carcinoma, an appropriate type of gastrectomy is indicated. Partial gastrectomy should be performed for multiple polyps in the distal stomach. If 10–20 polyps are distributed throughout the stomach, the antrum should be removed and the fundic polyps excised. Total gastrectomy may be required for symptomatic diffuse multiple polyposis.

These patients should be followed because they have an increased risk of late development of pernicious anemia or gastric cancer. Recurrent polyps are uncommon.

GASTRIC LYMPHOMA & PSEUDOLYMPHOMA

Lymphoma is the second-most common primary cancer of the stomach but constitutes only 2% of the total number, 95% being adenocarcinomas. Almost all are non-Hodgkin lymphomas and are generally classified as B cell mucosa-associated lymphoid tissue (MALT) lymphomas. They are further subclassified as low-grade or high-grade based on nuclear pattern. About 20% of patients manifest a second primary cancer in another organ.

The principal symptoms are epigastric pain and weight loss, similar to those of carcinoma. Characteristically, the tumor has attained bulky proportions by the time it is discovered; by comparison with adenocarcinoma of the stomach, the symptoms from a gastric lymphoma are usually mild in relation to the size of the lesion. A palpable epigastric mass is present in 50% of patients. Imaging studies will demonstrate the lesion, although it usually is mistaken for adenocarcinoma or benign gastric ulcer. Gastroscopy with biopsy and brush cytology provides the correct diagnosis preoperatively in about 75% of cases. If a pathologic diagnosis has not been made, the surgeon may incorrectly judge the lesion to be inoperable carcinoma because of its large size. Preoperative staging should include a CT scan and bone marrow biopsy.

Treatment of limited extent, low-grade gastric lymphoma consists of antibiotic treatment for *H pylori*, if present. More extensive disease may require therapy with external beam radiation or rituximab.

Gastric pseudolymphoma consists of a mass of lymphoid tissue in the gastric wall, often associated with an overlying mucosal ulcer. It is thought to represent a response to chronic inflammation. The lesion is not malignant, though the presentation, which includes pain, weight loss, and a mass on imaging, cannot be distinguished from a malignant lesion.

Treatment of gastric pseudolymphoma consists of resection. The distinction from lymphoma is made on histologic examination of the specimen, which shows mature germinal centers in pseudolymphoma. No additional therapy is indicated postoperatively.

Zelenetz AD, Wierda WG, Abramson JS, et al. for the National Comprehensive Cancer Network. Non-Hodgkin's lymphomas, version 1.2013. *J Natl Compr Canc Netw* 2013 Mar 1;11(3): 257-272.

GASTRIC LEIOMYOMAS & GASTROINTESTINAL STROMAL TUMOR

Leiomyomas are common submucosal growths that are usually asymptomatic but may cause intestinal bleeding. GIST (previously called leiomyosarcomas) may grow to a large size and most often present with bleeding. Radiologically, the tumor usually contains a central ulceration caused by necrosis from outgrowth of its blood supply. In most cases the tumor arises from the proximal stomach. It may grow into the gastric lumen, remain entirely on the serosal surface, or even become pedunculated within the abdominal cavity. Spread is by direct invasion or blood-borne metastases. CT scans provide useful information on the amount of extragastric extension. Leiomyomas should be removed by enucleation or wedge resection. After the more radical resections required for leiomyosarcomas, the 5-year survival rate is 20%. If technically possible, complete resection of metastases (eg, peritoneal, hepatic) in addition to the primary tumor may improve the outcome. The results are affected by tumor size, DNA ploidy pattern, and tumor grade. Lesions that exhibit 10 or more mitoses in a high-powered field rarely can be cured. Imatinib mesylate is an effective systemic agent used for disseminated disease and as an adjuvant therapy after complete resection.

MÉNÉTRIER DISEASE

Ménétrier disease, a form of hypertrophic gastritis, consists of giant hypertrophy of the gastric rugae; high, normal, or low acid secretion; and excessive loss of protein from the thickened mucosa into the gut, with resulting hypoproteinemia. Clinical manifestations include edema, diarrhea, anorexia, weight loss, and skin rash. Chronic blood loss may also be a problem. Indigestion may respond to antacids, but this treatment does not improve the gastric pathologic process or secondary hypoproteinemia. The hypertrophic rugae present as enormous filling defects on upper gastrointestinal imaging and are frequently misinterpreted as carcinoma. The protein leak from the gastric mucosa may respond to atropine (and other anticholinergic drugs), hexamethonium bromide, eradication of H pylori, or H_2 blocking agents or omeprazole. Rarely, total gastrectomy is indicated for severe intractable hypoproteinemia, anemia, or inability to exclude cancer. Medical management is best for most patients, though the gastric abnormalities and hypoproteinemia may persist. Some cases gradually evolve into atrophic gastritis. In children the disease characteristically is self-limited and benign. There is an increased risk of adenocarcinoma of the stomach in adults with Ménétrier disease.

PROLAPSE OF THE GASTRIC MUCOSA

This uncommon lesion occasionally accompanies small prepyloric gastric ulcers. Episodes of vomiting and abdominal pain simulate peptic ulcer disease. X-ray shows prolapse of antral folds into the duodenum. One must be alert to the presence of gastric or duodenal ulcer as the underlying cause.

Antrectomy with a Billroth I anastomosis is occasionally required. Generally, conservative treatment suffices.

GASTRIC VOLVULUS

The stomach may rotate about its longitudinal axis (organoaxial volvulus) or a line drawn from the mid-lesser to the mid-greater curvature (mesenteroaxial volvulus). The former is more common and is often associated with a paraesophageal hiatal hernia. In other patients, eventration of the left diaphragm allows the colon to rise and twist the stomach by pulling on the gastrocolic ligament.

Acute gastric volvulus produces severe abdominal pain accompanied by a diagnostic triad (Borchardt triad): (1) vomiting followed by retching and then inability to vomit, (2) epigastric distention, and (3) inability to pass a nasogastric tube. The situation calls for immediate laparotomy to prevent death from acute gastric necrosis and shock. Emergency imaging shows blockage at the point of the volvulus. The death rate is high.

Chronic volvulus is more common than acute. It may be asymptomatic or may cause crampy intermittent pain. Cases associated with paraesophageal hiatal hernia should be treated by repair of the hernia and anterior gastropexy. When cases are due to eventration of the diaphragm, the gastrocolic ligament should be divided the entire length of the greater curvature. The colon rises to fill the space caused by the eventration, and the stomach will resume its normal position, to be fastened by a gastropexy.

GASTRIC DIVERTICULA

Gastric diverticula are uncommon and usually asymptomatic. Most are pulsion diverticula consisting of mucosa and submucosa only, located on the lesser curvature within a few centimeters of the esophagogastric junction. Those in the prepyloric region generally possess all layers and are more likely to be symptomatic. A few patients have symptoms from hemorrhage of inflammation within a gastric diverticulum, but for the most part these lesions are incidental findings on imaging or endoscopy. Radiologically, they can be confused with a gastric ulcer.

BEZOAR

Bezoars are concretions formed in the stomach. Trichobezoars are composed of hair and are usually found in young girls who pick at their hair and swallow it. Phytobezoars consist of agglomerated vegetable fibers. Pressure by the mass can create a gastric ulcer that is prone to bleed or perforate.

The postgastrectomy state predisposes to bezoar formation because pepsin and acid secretion are reduced and the triturating function of the antrum is gone. Orange segments or other fruits that contain a large amount of cellulose have been implicated in most cases. Improper mastication of food is a contributing factor that can sometimes be obviated by providing the patient with properly fitted dentures. The fruit may remain in the stomach or pass into the small intestine and cause obstruction.

Large semisolid bezoars of *Candida albicans* have also been found in postgastrectomy patients. Some can be fragmented with the gastroscope. The patient should also be treated with oral nystatin.

Patients with symptomatic gastric bezoars may complain of abdominal pain. Ulceration and bleeding are associated with a death rate of 20%.

Nearly all gastric bezoars can be broken up and dispersed by endoscopy. Neglected lesions with complications (ie, bleeding or perforation) require gastrectomy.

▼ II. DUODENUM

DUODENAL DIVERTICULA

Diverticula of the duodenum are found in 20% of autopsies and 5%–10% of the upper gastrointestinal imaging. Symptoms are uncommon and only 1% of those found by x-ray warrant surgery.

Duodenal pulsion diverticula are acquired outpouchings of the mucosa and submucosa, 90% of which are on the medial aspect of the duodenum. They are rare before age 40. Most are solitary and within 2.5 cm of the ampulla of Vater. There is a high incidence of gallstone disease of the gallbladder in patients with juxtapapillary diverticula. Diverticula do not occur in the first portion of the duodenum, where diverticular configurations are due to scarring by peptic ulceration or cholecystitis.

A few patients have chronic postprandial abdominal pain or dyspepsia caused by a duodenal diverticulum. Treatment is with antacids and anticholinergics.

Serious complications are hemorrhage or perforation from inflammation, pancreatitis, and biliary obstruction. Bile acid-bilirubinate enteroliths are occasionally formed by bile stasis in a diverticulum. Enteroliths can precipitate diverticular inflammation or biliary obstruction and, rarely, have caused bowel obstruction after entering the intestinal lumen.

Surgical treatment is required for complications and, rarely, for persistent symptoms. Excision and a two-layer closure are usually possible after mobilization of the duodenum and dissection of the diverticulum from the pancreas. Removal of the diverticulum and closure of the defect are superior to simple drainage in the case of perforation. If biliary obstruction appears in a patient whose bile duct empties into a diverticulum, excision might be more hazardous than a side-to-side choledochoduodenostomy.

The rare wind sock type of intraluminal diverticulum usually presents with vague epigastric pain and postprandial fullness, though intestinal bleeding or pancreatitis is occasionally observed. The diagnosis can be made by imaging studies. The diverticulum can be excised through a nearby duodenotomy. In some cases, the narrow diverticular outlet can be enlarged endoscopically.

DUODENAL TUMORS

Tumors of the duodenum are rare. Carcinoma of the ampulla of Vater is discussed in Chapter 26.

1. Malignant Duodenal Tumors

Most malignant duodenal tumors are adenocarcinomas, leiomyosarcomas, or lymphomas. They appear in the descending duodenum more often than elsewhere. Pain, obstruction, bleeding, obstructive jaundice, and an abdominal mass are the modes of presentation. Duodenal carcinomas, particularly those in the third and fourth portions of the duodenum, are often missed on barium x-ray studies. Endoscopy and biopsy will usually be diagnostic if the examiner is suspicious enough and can reach the lesion.

If possible, adenocarcinomas and leiomyosarcomas should be resected. Pancreaticoduodenectomy is usually necessary if the tumor is localized. Unresectable lesions should be treated by radiotherapy. Biopsy and radiotherapy are recommended for lymphoma.

After curative resections, the 5-year survival rate is 30%. The overall 5-year survival rate is 18%.

2. Benign Duodenal Tumors

Brunner gland adenomas are small submucosal nodules that have a predilection for the posterior duodenal wall at the junction of the first and second portions. Sessile and pedunculated variants are seen. Symptoms are due to bleeding or obstruction. Leiomyomas may also be found in the duodenum and ordinarily are asymptomatic.

Neuroendocrine tumors of the duodenum are often endocrinologically active, producing gastrin, somatostatin, or serotonin. Simple excision is the treatment of choice.

Heterotopic gastric mucosa, presenting as multiple small mucosal nodules, is an occasional endoscopic finding of no clinical significance.

Villous adenomas of the duodenum may give rise to intestinal bleeding or may obstruct the papilla of Vater and cause jaundice. As in the colon, the risk of malignant change is high—about 50%. Small pedunculated villous adenomas may be snared during endoscopy, but sessile tumors must be locally excised via laparotomy. Tumors that contain malignant tissue should be treated by a Whipple procedure.

SUPERIOR MESENTERIC ARTERY OBSTRUCTION OF THE DUODENUM

Rarely, obstruction of the third portion of the duodenum is produced by compression between the superior mesenteric vessels and the aorta. It most commonly appears after rapid weight loss following injury, including burns. Patients in body casts are particularly susceptible.

The superior mesenteric artery normally leaves the aorta at an angle of 50–60 degrees, and the distance between the two vessels where the duodenum passes between them is 10–20 mm. These measurements in patients with superior mesenteric artery syndrome average 18 degrees and 2.5 mm. Acute loss of mesenteric fat is thought to permit the artery to drop posteriorly, trapping the bowel like a scissors.

Skepticism exists regarding the frequency of this condition in adults who have not experienced acute loss of weight. Most often the patient in question is a thin, nervous person whose complaints of dyspepsia and occasional emesis are more properly explained on a functional basis. When a clear-cut example is encountered, it may actually represent a form of intestinal malrotation with duodenal bands.

The patient complains of epigastric bloating and crampy pain relieved by vomiting. The symptoms may remit in the prone position. Anorexia and postprandial pain lead to additional malnutrition and weight loss.

Upper gastrointestinal imaging demonstrates a widened duodenum proximal to a sharp obstruction at the point where the artery crosses the third portion of the duodenum. When the patient moves to the knee-chest position, the passage of gastrointestinal contrast is suddenly unimpeded.

Many patients whose superior mesenteric artery makes a prominent impression on the duodenum are asymptomatic, and in ambulatory patients one should hesitate to attribute vague chronic complaints to this finding.

Involvement of the duodenum by scleroderma leads to duodenal dilatation and hypomotility and an x-ray and clinical picture highly suggestive of superior mesenteric artery syndrome. In the latter, increased duodenal peristalsis should be demonstrable proximal to the arterial blockage, whereas diminished peristalsis characterizes scleroderma. Patients with duodenal scleroderma usually have dysphagia from concomitant esophageal involvement.

Malrotation with duodenal obstruction by congenital bands can mimic this syndrome.

Postural therapy may suffice. The patient should be placed prone when symptomatic or in anticipation of postprandial difficulties. Ambulatory patients should be instructed to assume the knee-chest position, which allows the viscera and the artery to rotate forward off the duodenum.

Chronic obstruction may require section of the suspensory ligament and mobilization of the duodenum, or a duodenojejunostomy to bypass the obstruction. Patients with various forms of malrotation should be treated by mobilizing the duodenojejunal flexure, which releases the duodenum from entrapment by congenital bands.

REGIONAL ENTERITIS OF THE STOMACH & DUODENUM

The proximal intestine and stomach are rarely involved in regional enteritis, though this disease has now been reported in every part of the gastrointestinal tract from the lips to the anus. Most patients with Crohn disease in the stomach or duodenum have ileal involvement as well.

Pain can in many instances be relieved by antacids. Intermittent vomiting from duodenal stenosis or pyloric obstruction is frequent. The x-ray finding of a cobblestone mucosa or stenosis would be suggestive when associated with typical changes in the ileum. The endoscopic appearance is fairly characteristic, and biopsy with the peroral suction device usually gives an adequate specimen for histologic confirmation of the diagnosis.

Medical treatment is nonspecific and consists principally of corticosteroids during exacerbations. Surgery may be indicated for disabling pain or obstruction. If the disease is localized to the stomach, a partial gastrectomy can be performed. Duodenal involvement most often requires a gastrojejunostomy to bypass the obstruction. Vagotomy should also be performed to prevent development of a marginal ulcer. Recurrent Crohn disease involving the anastomosis is an occasional late complication, but it can usually be managed successfully by reoperation.

Internal fistulas involving the stomach or duodenum usually represent extensions from primary disease in the ileum or colon. Surgical treatment consists of resection of the diseased ileum or colon and closure of the fistulous opening in the upper gut.

Ajani JA, Bentrem DJ, Besh S, et al. Gastric cancer, version 2.2013: featured updates to the NCCN Guidelines. *J Natl Compr Canc Netw* 2013;11(5):531-546.

Ali T, Harty RF. Stress-induced ulcer bleeding in critically ill patients. *Gastroenterol Clin North Am* 2009;38(2):245-265.

Cappell MS, Friedel D. Initial management of acute upper gastrointestinal bleeding: from initial evaluation up to gastrointestinal endoscopy. *Med Clin North Am* 2008;92:491.

Cheung FK, Lau JY. Management of massive peptic ulcer bleeding. *Gastroenterol Clin North Am* 2009;38(2):231-243.

Costa F, D'Elios MM. Management of Helicobacter pylori infection. *Expert Rev Anti Infect Ther* 2010;8(8):887-892.

Greenspoon J, Barkun A. The pharmacological therapy of nonvariceal upper gastrointestinal bleeding. *Gastroenterol Clin North Am* 2010;39(3):419-432.

Ito T, Igarashi H, Jensen RT. Zollinger-Ellison syndrome: recent advances and controversies. *Curr Opin Gastroenterol* 2013;29(6):650-661.

Lee CW, Sarosi GA Jr. Emergency ulcer surgery *Surg Clin North Am* 2011;91(5):1001-1013.

Norton JA, Fraker DL, Alexander HR, Jensen RT. Value of surgery in patients with negative imaging and sporadic Zollinger-Ellison syndrome. *Ann Surg* 2012;256(3):509-517.

Schubert ML, Peura DA. Control of gastric acid secretion in health and disease. *Gastroenterology* 2008;134:1842.

Zelenetz AD, Wierda WG, Abramson JS, et al. The National Comprehensive Cancer Network. Non-Hodgkin's lymphomas, version 1.2013. *J Natl Compr Canc Netw* 2013;11(3): 257-272.

MULTIPLE CHOICE QUESTIONS

1. The blood supply to the stomach

   A. Typically includes direct branches from the celiac axis and superior mesenteric artery
   B. Includes predominant supply of the greater curve of the stomach by the left gastric artery
   C. Includes the right gastroepiploic artery, which is usually a branch of the splenic artery
   D. May include a posterior gastric artery that is typically a branch of the splenic artery
   E. Is anatomically separate from the blood supply to the spleen

2. The four functions of the stomach include all of these except

   A. It mixes the food and controls delivery into the duodenum.
   B. It is the site of the initial stage of protein and carbohydrate digestion.
   C. It acts as a reservoir for food.
   D. It is the site of the assembly of micelles for nutrient absorption.
   E. A few substances are absorbed across the gastric mucosa.

3. Reconstruction of gastrointestinal continuity after resection of portions of the stomach

   A. Usually includes a roux-en-Y reconstruction after distal gastrectomy
   B. Cannot be done by Billroth I reconstruction after total gastrectomy
   C. Includes a gastroduodenostomy for Billroth II reconstruction
   D. Has a risk of duodenal stump leak after Billroth I reconstruction
   E. May require conversion to a Billroth II reconstruction if a patient develops bile gastritis after a Billroth I approach

4. Vagotomy

   A. Can impair the appropriate relaxation of the pylorus
   B. Has several variations, but each denervates the pylorus
   C. Has become more widely applied as ulcer therapy since the introduction of acid-suppressing medications (H2-blockers and proton pump inhibitors)
   D. Impairs gallbladder emptying
   E. Can include division of both the left (posterior) and right (anterior) vagus nerve trunks

5. Management of gastric outlet obstruction

   A. Is typically required for complications due to distal gastric diverticulae or polyps
   B. Should include urgent operation in most patients
   C. Initially includes gastric decompression and acid suppression
   D. Is commonly required in the management of duodenal ulcer disease
   E. Is best managed operatively by distal gastrectomy and Billroth I reconstruction

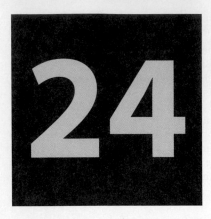

24

Liver & Portal Venous System

Simon Turcotte, MD, MSc

William R. Jarnagin, MD

SURGICAL ANATOMY

▶ Sectors and Segments

The liver develops as an embryologic outpouching from the duodenum. The liver is one of the largest organs in the body, representing up to 2% of the total body weight. The relationship of the liver to the other abdominal organs is shown in Figure 24–1. In classic descriptions, the liver was characterized as having four lobes: right, left, caudate, and quadrate; however, this is an overly simplistic view that fails to consider the more complex segmental anatomy, which is depicted in Figure 24–2.

The anatomical right and left hemilivers are separated by an imaginary line running from the medial aspect of the gallbladder fossa to the inferior vena cava, running parallel with the fissure of the round ligament (Figure 24–3). This division is known as the Cantlie line or the principal plane and marks the course of the middle hepatic vein. The liver is divided into four sectors and eight segments based on the branching of the portal triads and hepatic veins. The structures of the portal triad (hepatic artery, portal vein, and biliary duct) are separate in their extrahepatic course but enter the hepatic hilum ensheathed within a thickened layer of the Glisson capsule.

The three main hepatic veins divide the liver into four sectors, each of which is supplied by a portal pedicle: the right posterior sector (segments VI and VII), the right anterior sector (segments V and VIII), the left medial sector (segment IV), and the left lateral sector (segments II and III) (Figure 24–2). The caudate lobe (segment I) is an exception because its venous drainage is directly into the vena cava and therefore independent of the major hepatic veins. The four sectors delimited by the hepatic veins are called the portal sectors, and these portions of the parenchyma are supplied by independent portal pedicles arising from the right or left main pedicles. The divisions separating the sec-

tors are called portal scissurae, within each of which runs a hepatic vein. Further branching of the pedicles subdivides the sectors into segments. The liver is thus subdivided into eight segments, with the caudate lobe designated as segment I. Segments I-IV comprise the left liver, and segments V-VIII, the right. Each segment is supplied by an independent portal pedicle, which forms the basis of sublobar segmental resections.

▶ Portal Circulation

The portal vein is formed by the confluence of the splenic and superior mesenteric veins at the level of the second lumbar vertebra behind the head of the pancreas (Figure 24–4). It runs for approximately 6-9 cm to the hilum of the liver, where it divides into the main right and left branches. The left gastric vein usually enters the portal vein on its anteromedial aspect just cephalad to the margin of the pancreas, in which case it must be ligated during the surgical construction of a portacaval shunt; in 25% of cases, the left gastric vein joins the splenic vein. Other small venous tributaries from the pancreas and duodenum are less constant but must be anticipated during surgical mobilization of the portal vein.

The inferior mesenteric vein often drains into the splenic vein to the left of its junction with the superior mesenteric vein; alternatively, it may empty directly into the superior mesenteric vein.

In the hepatoduodenal ligament, the portal vein lies dorsal and slightly medial to the common bile duct. Portacaval lymph nodes are encountered along the right lateral aspect of the portal vein, running from the level of the duodenum to the base of the liver and extending posteriorly to the common hepatic artery and celiac axis. These lymph nodes are routinely removed during resections for certain malignancies and must be dissected before a portacaval shunt can be created.

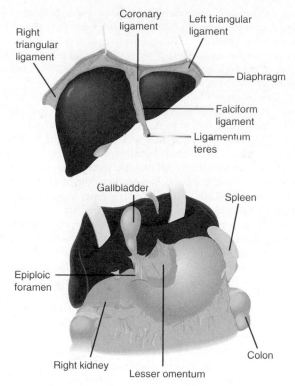

Figure 24–1. Relationships of the liver to adjacent abdominal organs. The liver is invested with peritoneum except on the posterior surface, where the peritoneum reflects onto the diaphragm forming the right and left triangular ligaments.

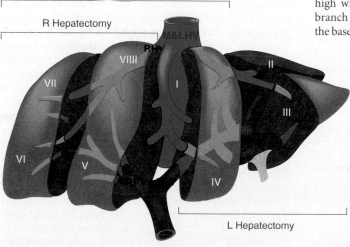

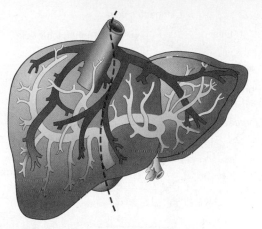

▲ **Figure 24–3.** Anatomy of the veins of the liver. The major lobar fissure, also referred to as the principal plane or Cantlie line, is represented by the dashed line and divides the anatomical right and left liver. Branches of the hepatic artery and biliary ducts follow those of the portal vein. The darker vessels represent the hepatic veins and vena cava; the lighter system represents the portal vein and its branches.

▶ Venous Blood Supply

The anatomy of venous blood supply is shown in Figure 24–2. Both the portal and hepatic venous systems lack valves. The main portal vein terminates in the porta hepatis by dividing into right and left branches. The right branch typically has a short extrahepatic course before subsequently dividing into anterior and posterior sectoral divisions, often high within the porta hepatic or intrahepatically. The left branch has a longer extrahepatic course, running first along the base of segment IV and then entering the umbilical fissure,

▲ **Figure 24–2.** Segmental anatomy of the liver. Each of the eight segments numbered. Segment I (caudate) is not shown but indicated at the back of the liver, posterior to the middle hepatic vein. Segments I–IV comprise the anatomical left liver, and segments V–VIII, the right. The most common major hepatic resections performed and the segments removed with each are indicated. LT, ligamentum teres; LPV, left portal vein; RHV, right hepatic vein; M&LHV, middle and left hepatic veins originating from a common trunk; RPV, right portal vein.

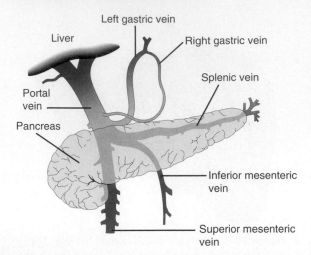

▲ Figure 24–4. Anatomic relationships of portal vein and branches.

Labels in figure: Liver; Left gastric vein; Right gastric vein; Splenic vein; Portal vein; Pancreas; Inferior mesenteric vein; Superior mesenteric vein

where it gives rise to branches to segments II, III, and IV; a large branch to the caudate lobe generally arises from the left portal vein prior to its entry into the umbilical fissure. Variations in the normal portal venous anatomy occur but are less common than aberrancies in the arterial supply or the biliary drainage. The most common anomaly of the portal venous system is separate origins of the right anterior and posterior sectoral branches. The left portal vein may drain primarily into the right anterior pedicle.

The hepatic veins represent the final common pathway for the central veins of the lobules of the liver. There are three major hepatic veins: left, right, and middle. The right hepatic vein drains into the vena cava independently, while the middle and left hepatic veins typically join just outside the liver, forming a common trunk. The middle hepatic vein runs in the principal plane (Cantlie line) and provides drainage for segment IV and the anterior sector of the right liver (segments V and VIII). The left hepatic vein drains segments II and III, while the right hepatic vein drains the posterior sector (segments VI and VII) and provides additional drainage to the anterior sector. A small venous tributary runs within the umbilical fissure, providing accessory drainage of segments III and IV and emptying into the left hepatic vein. Several small accessory veins enter the inferior vena cava directly from the posterior aspect of the right lobe and must be carefully ligated during mobilization and resection of the right liver.

Arterial Blood Supply

The common hepatic artery arises from the celiac axis, ascends in the hepatoduodenal ligament, and gives rise to

the right gastric, gastroduodenal, and proper hepatic arteries; the proper hepatic artery then divides into the right and left hepatic arterial branches in the liver hilum. The hepatic artery supplies approximately 25% of the 1500 mL of blood that enters the liver each minute; the remaining 75% is supplied by the portal vein.

Variations of the standard arterial anatomy of the liver are relatively common, seen in up to 40% of patients. The most common variants involve different origins of the right or left hepatic artery. A replaced right hepatic artery arises entirely from the superior mesenteric artery and courses posteriorly and to the right of the common bile duct within the porta hepatis, which is in contrast to its normal position to the left of the duct. Recognition of this anatomical variant is critical during operations on the extrahepatic biliary tree. An accessory right hepatic artery also arises from the superior mesenteric artery and is found in the same location within the porta hepatis but supplies only a portion of the right liver; in this situation, a separate right branch arising from its normal position off the proper hepatic artery is typically present. An accessory or replaced left hepatic artery arises from the left gastric artery and enters the liver through the gastrohepatic ligament. Up to 25% of patients have a replaced or accessory right hepatic artery, and a similar proportion have a replaced or accessory left hepatic artery. Within the liver, the hepatic arterial branches travel with segmental bile ducts and portal vein branches, and remain as portal triads in subsegmentations, found at each angle of the hexagonal-shape liver lobules.

Biliary Drainage

The biliary tree arises within the liver from bile canaliculi, formed from specialized segments of the hepatocyte membrane. Bile canaliculi join to form progressively larger channels, resulting in segmental bile ducts that drain each segment. The right anterior and right posterior sectoral ducts unite to form the main right hepatic duct, while the union of ducts draining segments II, III, and IV forms the left hepatic duct. The left hepatic duct typically is longer and has a longer extrahepatic course than the right hepatic duct. Drainage of segment I (caudate lobe) is principally into the left hepatic duct, but additional smaller ducts enter the right hepatic duct or drain directly into the hepatic duct confluence, which is formed by the union of the major lobar ducts to form the common hepatic duct. The common hepatic duct descends within the hepatoduodenal ligament for a variable distance to the point of insertion of the cystic duct of the gallbladder to give rise to the common bile duct.

Anatomic variations in the biliary ductal anatomy are seen in approximately 30% of patients and most often involve the right hepatic duct. In approximately 25% of patients, the duct from the right posterior sector joins the common hepatic duct or the left hepatic duct independently. Recognition of this variation is crucial for the surgeon performing a left hepatectomy for avoiding injury of the right posterior biliary drainage. Variations are far less common on the left side.

▶ Lymphatics

Lymphatics draining superficial lobules of the liver follow a subcapsular course to the diaphragm, to the suspensory ligaments of the liver, or to the posterior mediastinum, while others enter the porta hepatis. Lymphatics arising from lobules deep within the liver travel either with the hepatic veins along the vena cava or with the portal veins into the porta hepatis. Most of the lymphatic drainage of the liver is to the hepatoduodenal ligament.

NERVES

The liver and biliary tree are innervated by sympathetic fibers arising from T7 to T10 and by parasympathetic fibers from the right and left vagus nerves. The postganglionic sympathetic nerves arise from the celiac ganglia. Fibers derived from the celiac ganglia and vagus nerves form a plexus of nerves that run along the anterior and posterior aspects of the hepatic artery.

PHYSIOLOGY

Total hepatic blood flow (about 1500 mL/min; 30 mL/min per kg body weight) constitutes 25% of the cardiac output, though the liver accounts for only 2.5% of body weight. About 30% of the hepatic volume is blood (12% of total blood volume). Two-thirds of the flow enters through the portal vein and one-third through the hepatic artery. Pressure in the portal vein is normally low (10-15 cm H_2O [7-11 mm Hg]). The liver derives half of its oxygen from hepatic arterial blood and half from portal venous blood.

Blood flow within the liver is uniform, as demonstrated by an even distribution of microspheres injected into the hepatic artery or portal vein. Hepatic blood flow to the liver is regulated by a number of factors. Muscular sphincters at the inlet and outlet of sinusoids represent a major control point and respond to a number of different stimuli, including the autonomic nervous system, circulating hormones, bile salts, and metabolites. The cells lining the hepatic sinusoids (endothelial cells, Kupffer cells, and stellate cells) can also regulate flow to some extent.

Portal venous and hepatic arterial blood becomes pooled after entering the periphery of the hepatic sinusoid (Figure 24-5). Hepatic arterial flow increases or decreases reciprocally with changes in portal flow; however, portal venous

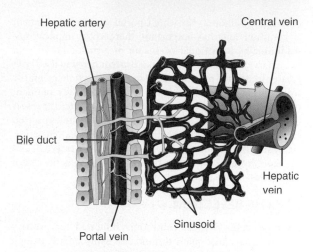

▲ **Figure 24-5.** Vascular anatomy of the liver lobule.

flow does not increase with reductions in arterial flow. This arterial compensatory response is controlled largely by adenosine, which is released into the space of Mall surrounding the hepatic arterial resistance vessels. High concentrations of adenosine dilate the vessels, which increases flow and washes out the adenosine.

Sudden occlusion of the portal vein results in an immediate 60% rise in hepatic arterial flow. The total flow then gradually returns toward normal. On the other hand, sudden reductions in hepatic arterial supply are not immediately met by significant increases in portal vein flow. In both normal subjects and cirrhotics, total hepatic flow, and portal pressure drop following hepatic arterial occlusion. Arterial collaterals develop, and arterial perfusion is ultimately restored.

It is for this reason that interruption of hepatic arterial flow to the right or left liver generally has little impact on hepatic function. The one notable exception is in the setting of biliary obstruction. Decreased hepatic arterial flow to portions of the liver with impaired biliary drainage carries a high risk of hepatic necrosis. Clinically, this is an important consideration in patients undergoing hepatic arterial embolization of liver tumors and in patients undergoing resection of periampullary tumors, where jaundice is common and dissection within the porta hepatic could potentially put the hepatic artery at risk for injury. On the other hand, portal venous flow plays a critical role in maintaining normal hepatic architecture and function. This point is underscored by the observation that occlusion of the right or left portal venous branches results in profound ipsilateral hepatic atrophy and contralateral hypertrophy. Portal vein occlusion is clinically relevant in a number of disease processes, particularly carcinoma of the hepatic duct confluence (hilar cholangiocarcinoma), in which portal venous involvement is common and has important therapeutic implications. Additionally, intentional occlusion of a major portal vein branch (usually the right side) is a procedure being used with greater frequency prior to major hepatic resection, primarily when the regenerative capacity of the future liver remnant (that portion of the liver that remains behind after the resection) is questionable because of either size concerns (too small) or underlying parenchymal disease (steatohepatitis, cirrhosis). By causing atrophy of the liver to be resected, and therefore hypertrophy of the future liver remnant, the risk of postoperative hepatic failure may be reduced.

HEPATIC RESECTION

Liver resection is most commonly indicated for primary and secondary malignant tumors and symptomatic benign tumors; less common indications include traumatic injury, infection/abscesses, and living donor transplantation. Removal of as much as 80% of the normal liver can be performed with the expectation that the liver remnant will regenerate sufficiently for the patient to survive. It must be emphasized, however, that such extensive resections should be considered only in patients with normal hepatic function; those with cirrhosis or significant fibrosis or steatosis (fatty infiltration of the liver) are less likely to tolerate a major hepatic resection. Liver function may be impaired for several weeks after an extensive resection, but the extraordinary regenerative capacity of the liver rapidly provides new functioning hepatocytes. Within 24 hours after partial hepatectomy, cell replication becomes active and continues until the original volume of hepatic tissue is restored. Considerable

regeneration occurs within 10 days, and the process is essentially complete by 4-5 weeks. Excised portions of liver are not re-formed; rather, the growth consists of formation of new lobules and expansion of residual lobules. The stimuli for hepatic regeneration are thought to include the following: hepatocyte growth factor, tumor growth factor (TGF)-α, heparin-binding growth factor, hepatopoietin B, and disinhibition by TGF-β_1 (ie, decreased levels of this inhibitor of hepatic growth).

▶ Preoperative Evaluation

Several different disease-related and patient-related factors must be assessed before deciding to proceed with hepatic resection. Among the most important of these is the preoperative functional status of the liver. Cirrhosis is a relative contraindication for partial hepatectomy because the limited reserve of the residual cirrhotic liver may be insufficient to meet essential metabolic demands, and the cirrhotic liver has a reduced capacity for regeneration. Cirrhosis is a particular concern in patients with hepatocellular carcinoma, which frequently arises in the setting of chronic hepatic parenchymal disease. An increasingly important concern in patients with hepatic colorectal metastases is chemotherapy-induced liver damage, which may also impair regeneration of the liver remnant.

Several tests are available to assess hepatic function prior to operation, none of which is perfect. The Child–Pugh classification is the oldest and most widely employed and remains the most useful assessment. The Child–Pugh system classifies hepatic function on the basis of the amount of ascites, the degree of encephalopathy, albumin and total bilirubin levels, and the prothrombin time (INR) (Table 24–1).

Table 24–1. Child–pugh classification of functional status in liver diseases.

	Points		
	1	2	3
Ascites	Absent	Slight to moderate	Tense, refractory
Encephalopathy[a]	None	Grades I-II	Grades III-IV
Serum albumin (g/dL)	> 3.5	3.0-3.5	< 3.0
Serum bilirubin (mg/dL)	< 2.0	2.0-3.0	> 3.0
Prothrombin time (seconds above control)/INR	< 4.0/< 1.7	4.0-6.0/1.7-2.3	> 6.0/> 2.3
Child–Pugh Classification A (low risk) B (moderate) C (high risk)	Scores 5-6 7-9 10-15		

[a] Grade I, altered mood; Grade II, inappropriate behavior, somnolence; Grade III, markedly confused, stuporous but arousable; Grade IV, unresponsive.

To convert the values for bilirubin to μmol/L, multiply by 17.1.

Originally used to assess mortality related to portosystemic shunts, the Child–Pugh score also predicts mortality in patients with cirrhosis after hepatic resection. In general, only Child–Pugh A and highly selected Child–Pugh B cirrhotics would be candidates for resection. More recently in the United States, to improve allocation of cadaveric liver transplant to cirrhotic patients with the highest risk of death, the Model for End-Stage Liver Disease (MELD) score has been validated. Similar to the Child–Pugh classification, the total bilirubin level, and the INR are accounted for, combined with the serum creatinine level. The MELD score was originally devised to predict mortality of patients awaiting liver transplantation but is also effective for assessing liver function in patients undergoing resection. The indocyanine green clearance test is commonly used in centers outside North America but has not been proven superior to the Child–Pugh scoring system.

Extent of Hepatic Resection

Hepatic resections are classified as anatomical (based on the segmental liver anatomy) or nonanatomical. Wedge resections, enucleations, and resectional debridement of devitalized tissue are examples of the latter. In general, anatomical resections are preferred because they are associated with lower blood loss and, when performed for malignancy, a lower incidence of positive resection margins.

Major resections must be performed in accordance with the segmental anatomy (Figure 24–2). Major resections (right or left hepatectomy or extended hepatectomy) are commonly performed; however, the segmental anatomy of the liver allows smaller resections or bilateral resections to be performed when necessary and appropriate. For example, in selected situations, a resection of the anterior (segments V and VIII) or posterior (segments VI and VII) sectors may be performed rather than sacrificing the entire right liver. Such parenchymal-sparing resections on one side would then allow a resection of part of the contralateral lobe, if necessary. Sequential, two-stage hepatectomy has also proven to benefit patients in the setting of multiple, bilateral liver metastases of colorectal cancer origin, allowing time for the liver remnant to regenerate and compensate for the second resection.

The terminology and extent of the common types of major resections are in Figure 24–2. The operation entails removal of a lobe or segment with its afferent and efferent vessels while avoiding injury to vessels and bile ducts supplying the remnant tissue.

Most elective hepatic resections can be performed through an abdominal incision, although selected situations (very large right lobe tumors) are probably best performed with a thoracoabdominal approach. Laparoscopic resections are being performed with greater frequency, although the open approach is most common and remains the standard. The best perioperative results are obtained by minimizing blood, which is accomplished by: (1) achieving vascular inflow and outflow control prior to parenchymal transaction; (2) performing careful division of the liver with precise control of intrahepatic vascular structures; and (3) using low central venous pressure anesthesia, which reduces hepatic venous blood loss. Clamping of the portal inflow pedicle (Pringle maneuver) for periods of 10-15 minutes is commonly used to minimize blood loss via intrahepatic arterial and portal venous branches, although hepatic venous bleeding is unaffected.

Preoperative Portal Vein Embolization

As discussed previously, preoperative portal vein embolization is a technique that can be used to potentially improve the safety of major hepatic resections. By inducing hypertrophy of the future liver remnant prior to operation, the risk of postoperative liver failure is potentially reduced. The risk of such complications increases significantly with resections that leave behind a liver remnant of less than 25% in patients with normal liver or less than 40% in patients with liver disease.

Postoperative Course

Patients submitted to major resections require close monitoring for the first several postoperative days; however, a prolonged stay in the intensive care unit is unnecessary in most cases. The major concern in the immediate postoperative period is hemorrhage, although in practice, reoperation for bleeding is rarely necessary. Patients without cirrhosis usually exhibit some metabolic changes consistent with mild liver insufficiency, but these quickly normalize, and they are often ready for discharge on the seventh or eighth postoperative day. In the presence of significant hepatic parenchymal disease (ie, cirrhosis, fibrosis, steatosis) or septic complications, postoperative liver function may be significantly impaired.

Many of the postoperative abnormalities can be predicted on the basis of the liver's normal function. The serum bilirubin often increases after major resections but returns to normal as regeneration progresses. A persistent or rising serum bilirubin level should raise concern for a perihepatic fluid collection (biloma) or hepatic failure (especially if other measures of hepatic function are also deteriorating). The serum albumin level usually falls, and the prothrombin time often increases; treatment of the latter with fresh frozen plasma is generally needed only when the INR is markedly elevated (> 2). Some patients may develop ascites, which can be treated with diuresis. Although the liver's glycogen stores are necessarily reduced after a major partial hepatectomy, hypoglycemia is almost never a problem postoperatively; normoglycemia can be easily maintained with 5% dextrose solutions, and profound hypoglycemia should raise concern for liver failure. Serum levels of phosphate, magnesium, and potassium often decrease during the first several postoperative days and require replacement. The liver enzymes (aspartate aminotransferase [AST], alanine aminotransferase [ALT]) are usually increased in the first few days after operation and then normalize. By contrast, the alkaline phosphatase is often initially normal and then increases and can remain elevated for several days to weeks after surgery.

▶ Complications

Complications may occur in up to 40% of patients after major liver resection (≥ 3 segments), but many are relatively minor, and the overwhelming majority are readily managed and resolve without sequelae. Liver-related complications are the most frequent; perihepatic fluid collections requiring drainage occur in approximately 10%-15% of patients. Relative hepatic insufficiency (hyperbilirubinemia, ascites, coagulopathy) is common but resolves in most patients as the liver regenerates; however, hepatic failure is distinctly uncommon in high-volume centers. Pulmonary complications are also seen with some frequency, underscoring the need for aggressive pulmonary toilet postoperatively. The most common pulmonary problems are symptomatic pleural effusions or atelectasis; pneumonia is infrequent. Despite the potential complications associated with major liver resection, mortality rates are low, typically on the order of 1%-3% in high-volume centers. Less extensive liver resections (< 3 segments) are associated with even lower morbidity and mortality rates.

Abdalla EK: Portal vein embolization (prior to major hepatectomy) effects on regeneration, resectability, and outcome. *J Surg Oncol* 2010;102:960.

Chun YS, Laurent A, Mary D, Vauthey JN: Management of chemotherapy-associated hepatotoxicity in colorectal liver metastases. *Lancet Oncol* 2009;10:278.

Covey AM, Brown KT, Jarnagin WR, et al: Combined portal vein embolization and neoadjuvant chemotherapy as a treatment strategy for resectable hepatic colorectal metastases. *Ann Surg* 2008;247:451.

Gold JS, Are C, Kornprat P, et al: Increased use of parenchymal-sparing surgery for bilateral liver metastases from colorectal cancer is associated with improved mortality without change in oncologic outcome: trends in treatment over time in 440 patients. *Ann Surg* 2008;247:109.

Kim WR, Biggins SW, Kremers WK, et al: Hyponatremia and mortality among patients on the liver-transplant waiting list. *N Engl J Med* 2008;359:1018.

Riehle KJ et al: New concepts in liver regeneration. *J Gastroenterol Hepatol* 2011;26-S1:203.

Strasberg SM: Nomenclature of hepatic anatomy and resections: a review of the Brisbane 2000 system. *J Hepatobiliary Pancreat Surg* 2005;12:351-355.

Wicherts DA, Miller R, de Hass RJ, et al: Long-term results of two-stage hepatectomy for irresectable colorectal cancer liver metastases. *Ann Surg* 2008;248:994.

▼ DISEASES & DISORDERS OF THE LIVER

HEPATIC TRAUMA

The liver is injured in approximately 5% of all trauma admissions. Based on the mechanism of injury, liver trauma is classified as penetrating or blunt. Penetrating wounds, constituting more than half of cases, are typically due to projectiles (such as bullets or shrapnel) or knives. In civilian practice, most of these tend to be clean wounds that are dangerous because of intra-abdominal bleeding but do not result in much devitalization of liver tissue. In contrast, high-velocity projectiles, commonly associated with military weapons, are associated with greater energy that is transferred to the abdominal viscera and can shatter the parenchyma, even if the projectile does not enter the liver directly.

Blunt trauma can be inflicted by a direct blow to the upper abdomen or lower right rib cage or can follow sudden deceleration, as occurs with a fall from a great height. Most often a consequence of automobile accidents, direct blunt trauma tends to produce explosive bursting wounds or linear lacerations of the hepatic surface, often with considerable parenchymal destruction. The stellate, bursting type of injury tends to affect the posterior and superior aspect of the right liver (segments VI, VII, and VIII) because of its relatively vulnerable location, convex surface, fixed position, and concentration of hepatic mass. Damage to the left liver is much less common than damage to the right. Injuries that involve shearing forces can tear the hepatic veins where they enter the liver substance, producing an exsanguinating retrohepatic injury in an area difficult to surgically expose and repair.

The improvement in image quality and rapidity of execution of CT scans has transformed the initial management of trauma patients over the past few decades. For patients who can be hemodynamically stabilized with initial resuscitation, CT allows staging of the liver injury, in addition to all other structures from the neck to the pelvis. The staging system described in Table 24–2 is used to categorize liver injuries and provide a common language in order to allow comparisons of results of treatment between institutions. Patients who cannot be stabilized must go directly to the operating room.

There are two main management approaches to traumatic liver injury: nonoperative, which can be combined with angiography and selective embolization, or operative. When angiographic embolization is used as adjuvant to nonoperative management, approximately 85% of patient with blunt hepatic trauma can be successfully managed. A major limitation of arterial embolization is its inability to control bleeding from major venous injuries. Penetrating trauma, however, most often requires surgical intervention. The principal surgical goals are to stop bleeding and debride

Table 24–2. Liver injury scale.[1]

Grade	Type	Description
I	Hematoma	Subcapsular, nonexpanding, < 10% of liver capsule surface area
	Laceration	Capsular tear, nonbleeding; < 1 cm deep in parenchyma
II	Hematoma	Subcapsular, nonexpanding, 10%-50% surface area; intraparenchymal, nonexpanding, < 2 cm in diameter
	Laceration	Capsular tear, active bleeding; 1-3 cm deep into the parenchyma, < 10 cm long
III	Hematoma	Subcapsular, > 50% surface area or expanding; ruptured subcapsular hematoma with active bleeding; intraparenchymal hematoma > 2 cm or expanding
	Laceration	> 3 cm deep into the parenchyma
IV	Hematoma	Ruptured intraparenchymal hematoma with active bleeding
	Laceration	Parenchymal disruption involving > 50% of hepatic lobe
V	Laceration	Parenchymal disruption involving > 50% of hepatic lobe
	Vascular	Juxtahepatic venous injuries; ie, retrohepatic vena cava or major hepatic veins
VI	Vascular	Hepatic avulsion

[1]Increase by one grade when there are two or more injuries to the liver. Grading applied based on best available evidence, whether from x-rays, operative findings, or autopsy findings.

devitalized liver. Because some degree of liver failure is common postoperatively, efforts should be made during each step to maintain adequate oxygenation and perfusion of the liver. Also, when one is debriding liver tissue, care should be taken to avoid injury to the vascular supply of adjacent viable parenchyma.

▶ Clinical Findings

A. Symptoms and Signs

The clinical manifestations of liver injury are those of hypovolemic shock: hypotension, decreased urinary output, low central venous pressure, and, in some cases, abdominal distention. Patients managed nonoperatively are admitted in a monitored setting and closely followed with serial examinations and hematocrit assessments. Patients who develop peritoneal signs on physical examination or the onset of

hemodynamic instability denote the failure of nonoperative management and mandate surgical intervention.

B. Laboratory Findings

With major injuries, particularly those associated with disruption of hepatic veins, the rate of blood loss is usually so rapid that anemia does not develop. Leukocytosis greater than 15,000/μL is common following rupture of the liver from blunt trauma. Polytraumatized patients most often develop acidosis and coagulopathy.

C. Imaging Techniques

Focused abdominal sonography for trauma (FAST) in unstable patients has a sensitivity of 97% for detecting hemoperitoneum larger than 1 L and can direct surgical intervention in patients going directly to surgical management. The exact location of the injury often cannot be reliably identified with FAST. There is no defined role for FAST in stable patients.

High resolution CT scan with intravenous contrast enhancement should be obtained in all stable patients suspected of having a hepatic injury. The CT provides a detailed evaluation of the liver injury and its extent, an estimate of the amount of blood loss, and can demonstrate a contrast blush from the liver parenchyma. The findings are useful for triaging, since minor injuries rarely require surgical treatment, whereas extensive injuries usually do. One must exercise caution, however, in using CT estimates of injury grade, because they correlate poorly (ie, they both understage and overstage) with what is found at surgery. CT scanning is also useful for identifying injuries to other organs, which are not uncommon, particularly in the setting of high velocity blunt trauma.

Angiography is generally not helpful in the acute setting for the diagnosis of liver injury, but may be used as an interventional adjunct in patients who are potential candidates for nonoperative management.

▶ Treatment

Regardless of the grade of blunt liver injury, the hemodynamic stability of patients dictates whether or not a liver trauma should be managed operatively. In contrast, only highly selected patients with penetrating trauma can be managed nonoperatively. In the absence of injury to the spleen and the kidneys, CT findings most often associated with successful nonoperative management include small hemoperitoneum, contained subcapsular or intrahepatic hematoma, unilobar fracture, absence of devitalized liver, minimal intraperitoneal blood, and absence of injuries to other intra-abdominal organs. Failure rate of the nonoperative approach increases with the grade of the liver injury, reaching one out of four patients with grade V blunt injury. Conversely, it should be kept in mind that low-grade injuries can bleed significantly. Drop in hematocrit in stable patients should prompt a CT scan to verify that the lesion is stable rather than expanding, and if a blush of intravenous contrast is associated with the liver injury, often bleeding can be addressed by angiographic embolization.

Most patients with CT or clinical evidence of active bleeding or a major injury, however, require prompt exploration. Most minor parenchymal lacerations have stopped bleeding by the time operation is performed. In the absence of active hemorrhage, these wounds should not be sutured. Active bleeding should be managed by clipping or direct suture of identifiable vessels, if possible, rather than by mass ligatures. Subcapsular hematomas often overlie an active bleeding site or parenchyma in need of debridement and should be explored even though the injury appears to be tamponaded and of limited severity. Blunt injuries associated with substantial amounts of parenchymal destruction may be particularly difficult to manage. Rarely, a very severe pulverizing injury requires formal partial hepatectomy.

Temporary occlusion of the hepatic artery and portal vein can be done quickly by placing a vascular clamp around the entire hepatoduodenal ligament (Pringle maneuver). This can be done for periods of 15-20 minutes and reduce the hemorrhage sufficiently to permit more accurate ligation of bleeding vessels. With major hepatic venous injuries, however, a Pringle maneuver has little effect, and precise repair of the injury may not be possible. Absorbable gauze mesh (eg, polyglycolic acid) can sometimes be wrapped around an injured lobe and sutured in a way that maintains pressure and tamponades the bleeding; this is difficult to accomplish without rendering the involved liver ischemic, however, and such an approach is rarely applicable. In some cases, control of arterial hemorrhage requires ligation of the hepatic artery or one of the accessible major branches (ie, right anterior or right posterior sectoral branches) in the hilum.

The most difficult problems involve lacerations of the major hepatic veins behind the liver. With such injuries, temporary clamping of the inflow vessels has no impact on back-bleeding from the inferior vena cava and does not allow adequate inspection and repair of the injured vessels. For persistent bleeding, the abdominal incision can be extended into a median sternotomy to improve exposure. An ancillary technique, which is used only rarely and has been associated with high mortality rates, is to place a tube through the atrial appendage into the inferior vena cava past the origin of the hepatic veins. Appropriately placed ligatures around the supra- and infra-hepatic vena cava combined with the Pringle maneuver permit total isolation of the liver circulation. Resection of the right liver improves exposure of the retrohepatic vena cava but is difficult to perform in the face of massive hemorrhage.

In many cases, when bleeding is difficult to control, and especially when other injuries must be addressed, damage control is the best strategy and involves packing the liver to achieve hemostasis. The packs are generally left in place for 48-72 hours, during which time the patient remains sedated and intubated in the intensive care unit where adequate resuscitative measures are undertaken to correct hypothermia, acidosis, and coagulopathy. The packs are removed in the operating room; if persistent bleeding is noted, definitive repair of the injury can then be performed in a somewhat more controlled fashion.

The majority of patients who come to operation require little in the way of surgical intervention to control bleeding; drainage of substantial liver lacerations and other injuries is reasonable, since bile leakage can occur. For superficial liver injuries, bleeding can often be controlled with direct compression, topical agents, electrocautery or argon beam coagulation. Suture ligation of bleeding hepatic vessels and debridement of devitalized tissue are indicated in about 30% and 10% of cases, respectively. More extensive procedures are indicated even less often.

Penetrating injuries that also involve the small bowel or colon may result in contamination of perihepatic fluid or devitalized liver tissue, leading to a subhepatic abscess. Placement of drains may help prevent this problem, but a high index of suspicion should be maintained during the postoperative period.

▶ Postoperative Complications

With present techniques, hemorrhage at laparotomy is rarely uncontrollable except with retrohepatic venous injuries. Patients who rebleed early from the liver wound after initial suture ligation should be treated by reexploration and packing, in most cases; rarely is a major resection required. Angiography and CT scanning may provide useful diagnostic information preoperatively in such patients.

Bile leaks can follow both blunt penetrating liver injuries when the biliary system is disrupted. Most bilomas can be treated with image-guided percutaneous drainage. Endoscopic retrograde cholangiopancreatography may help identify the site of injury and may be therapeutic in some cases, since stents can be deployed in selected bile ducts and sphincterotomy of the sphincter of Oddi can relieve pressure in the biliary system. It should be noted, however, that such maneuvers have not been shown to expedite the resolution of biliary injuries, provided that adequate drainage of the biloma has been achieved.

Subhepatic sepsis develops in about 20% of cases; it is more frequent if a major hepatectomy has been performed. Abscess can occur after blunt trauma, especially with concomitant enteric injuries. Most abscess can be managed with percutaneous drainage and antibiotic therapy.

Hemobilia may be responsible for gastrointestinal bleeding in the postoperative period and can be diagnosed by selective angiography. Treatment consists of embolization through the arteriography catheter.

► Prognosis

The death rate of 10%-15% following hepatic trauma depends largely on the type of injury and the extent of associated injury to other organs. About one-third of patients admitted to the emergency department in shock cannot be saved. Only 1% of penetrating civilian wounds are lethal, whereas a 20% death rate attends blunt trauma. The death rate in blunt hepatic injury is 10% when only the liver is injured. If three major organs are damaged, the death rate is close to 70%. Bleeding causes more than half of deaths associated with liver trauma.

Navsaria PH, Nicol AJ, Krige JE, Edu S. Selective nonoperative management of liver gunshot injuries. *Ann Surg* 2009;249:653.

Saltzherr TP, van der Vlies CH, van Lienden KP, et al. Improved outcomes in the non-operative management of liver injuries. *HPB* 2011;13:350.

Yanar H et al. Nonoperative treatment of multiple intra-abdominal solid organ injury after blunt abdominal trauma. *J Trauma* 2008;64:943.

SPONTANEOUS HEPATIC RUPTURE

Spontaneous rupture of the liver is not common. Most cases of ruptured diseased liver are due to hepatic tumors. Approximately 5% of hepatocellular carcinoma can rupture and manifest as hemoperitoneum. Hepatic adenoma larger than 5 cm carries a risk of spontaneous bleeding of approximately 20%-40%.

Many cases of ruptured normal liver occur during or after pregnancy and are related to preeclampsia-eclampsia and/or HELLP syndrome (hemolysis, elevated liver enzymes, low platelet count). Hepatic rupture should be suspected in any pregnant or postpartum patient (especially if hypertensive) who complains of acute discomfort in the upper abdomen.

Spontaneous rupture has also been reported in association with a number of other conditions, including hepatic hemangioma, typhoid fever, malaria, tuberculosis, syphilis, polyarteritis nodosa, and diabetes mellitus. Rupture of the liver in the newborn is related to birth trauma in larger infants after difficult deliveries. The typical progression is intrahepatic hemorrhage expanding to subcapsular hematoma and eventually capsular rupture and free intra-abdominal hemorrhage.

The diagnosis is best made by CT scanning. Angiography and hepatic artery embolization can be quite effective for controlling hemorrhage in the setting of spontaneous rupture. Emergency laparotomy and intraoperative management (as one would for a traumatic liver injury) are reserved for those who fail hepatic artery embolization or are unsuitable for the procedure. Patients who experience hemoperitoneum from spontaneous rupture of hepatocellular carcinoma appear to be at increased risk for peritoneal dissemination of tumor.

Battula N et al. Spontaneous rupture of hepatocellular carcinoma: a Western experience. *Am J Surg* 2009;197:164.

Deneve et al. Liver cell adenoma: a multicenter analysis of risk factors for rupture and malignancy. *Ann Surg Oncol* 2009;16:640.

Stoot JH et al. Life-saving therapy for haemorrhaging liver adenomas using selective arterial embolization. *Br J Surg* 2007;94:1249.

Zeirideen R, Kadir RA. Spontaneous postpartum hepatic rupture. *J Obstet Gynecol* 2009;29:155.

PRIMARY LIVER CANCER

Liver malignancy may arise from hepatocytes (hepatocellular carcinoma [HCC], the most common) or biliary epithelial cells (intrahepatic cholangiocarcinoma). Tumors arising from both cell types (mixed hepatocellular carcinoma/cholangiocarcinoma) have also been described. Neonates may also develop a variant of hepatocellular carcinoma called hepatoblastoma because it is morphologically similar to fetal liver and the occasional presence of hematopoiesis. Primary malignancy arising from other liver cell types (endothelial cells, stellate cells, neuroendocrine cells, or lymphocytes) is exceedingly rare.

Primary hepatic cancer is relatively uncommon in the United States, with an estimated 28,720 new cases in 2012. The incidence of HCC has tripled during the past two decades, largely the result of hepatitis C infection outbreak. The 5-year survival rate of patients with HCC remains under 16%, ranking this tumor amongst the 10 leading cause of cancer related death in both men and women in the United Sates. In Asia and Africa, primary liver cancer is extremely common and in some areas represents the single-most frequent abdominal tumor and the most common cause of cancer-related death. The etiologic factors in these high-risk areas are environmental or cultural, since persons of similar racial background in the United States are at only slightly greater risk than Caucasians.

► Hepatocellular Carcinoma

Chronic hepatitis B and C virus (HBV and HCV) infection is the principal etiologic factor worldwide for HCC. Patients chronically seropositive for HBsAg constitute a high-risk group for development of hepatocellular carcinoma. Hepatitis B virus DNA has been detected integrated into the genome of host hepatocytes and hepatoma cells and has a direct oncogenic effect. Patients with chronic hepatitis B infection may therefore develop hepatocellular carcinoma in the absence of cirrhosis; by contrast, HCC arising in the setting of chronic hepatitis C infection is typically associated with cirrhotic change. Cirrhosis from almost any cause (eg, alcoholism, hemochromatosis, α_1-antitrypsin deficiency, or primary biliary cirrhosis) is associated with an increased risk of hepatocellular carcinoma, and the great majority of these tumors arise in the setting of chronic underlying liver disease. With the increase in obesity in the United States, nonalcoholic fatty liver disease (NAFLD) has become the one of the most common causes of chronic liver disease; a subgroup of these patients with nonalcoholic steatohepatitis (NASH) are at high risk of cirrhosis and malignant transformation. Certain fungal metabolites called aflatoxins have been shown experimentally to be capable of producing liver tumors. These substances are present in staple foods (eg, ground nuts and grain) in some parts of Africa where hepatocellular carcinoma has a high incidence.

HCC constitutes about 85%-95% of primary hepatic cancers. Previously, differences in morphology were used to separate tumors into three types: mass-forming type, characterized by a single predominant mass clearly demarcated from the surrounding liver, occasionally with small satellite nodules; nodular type, composed of multiple nodules, often distributed throughout the liver; and a diffuse type, characterized by infiltration of tumor throughout the remaining parenchyma. A number of staging systems for hepatocellular carcinoma are in current use when considering treatment options for patients with HCC: the Barcelona Clinic Liver Cancer (BCLC), Cancer of the Liver Italian Program (CLIP), Okuda, Chinese University Prognostic Index (CUPI), and Japan Integrated Staging (JIS); these classifications differ on their assessment of tumor burden, related symptoms, and underlying liver dysfunction, and most cannot predict the survival in patients with advanced HCC. The 7th edition of the American Joint Commission on Cancer tumor-node-metastasis (TNM) staging system can be used after pathological examination of the resected liver for determining the prognosis of patients after transplantation. About 50% of resectable tumors are surrounded by a fibrous capsule, which develops as a result of compression of adjacent liver stroma. Encapsulated tumors exhibit a lower incidence of tumor microsatellites and venous permeation compared with non-encapsulated tumors, and the finding is a favorable sign. An uncommon variant, fibrolamellar hepatocellular carcinoma, contains numerous fibrous septa and may resemble focal nodular hyperplasia (FNH). Fibrolamellar hepatoma occurs in a younger age group (average 25 years) and is not associated with cirrhosis or hepatitis virus infection.

A large proportion of patients have intrahepatic or extrahepatic metastases at presentation. Multiple intrahepatic tumors can arise as a result of infiltration of the portal venous system with subsequent dissemination of tumor cells. Vascular invasion is more common with larger tumors (> 5 cm). The extrahepatic sites most commonly involved with metastatic disease include the hilar and celiac lymph nodes and the lungs; metastases to bone and brain are less common, and peritoneal disease (ie, carcinomatosis) is distinctly unusual. Major portal or hepatic veins are often invaded by tumor, and venous occlusion may occur as a result.

Microscopically, there is usually little stroma between the malignant cells, and the tumor has a soft consistency.

The tumor may be highly vascularized, a feature that rarely can result in massive intraperitoneal hemorrhage following spontaneous rupture.

▶ Intrahepatic Cholangiocarcinoma

Cholangiocarcinoma makes up a small fraction of primary liver cancers, although several reports have documented a marked increase in incidence worldwide. Unlike hepatocellular carcinoma, intrahepatic cholangiocarcinoma is less frequently associated with cirrhosis. Primary sclerosing cholangitis is a predisposing condition in a small minority of patients. Widespread infection with liver flukes (*Clonorchis sinensis*) is at least partly responsible for the higher incidence of these tumors in some parts of Asia. Emerging evidence has implicated chronic hepatitis C infection, obesity, diabetes mellitus, chronic liver disease, and cigarette smoking as risk factors for intrahepatic cholangiocarcinoma. In Western centers, the vast majority of intrahepatic cholangiocarcinomas are sporadic. Intrahepatic cholangiocarcinoma generally presents as a large mass within the liver and is therefore clinically distinct from cholangiocarcinoma arising from the extrahepatic biliary tree.

Histologically, these tumors are most often invasive adenocarcinomas, although rare variants have been reported. Intrahepatic or extrahepatic spread of disease is not uncommon by the time the tumor is detected. These tumors infrequently cause symptoms at early stages and therefore often grow to a large size before they become apparent, frequently because of pain. Infrequently, these tumors may contain cells of both cholangiocellular and hepatocellular origin. These mixed tumors are similar to intrahepatic cholangiocarcinoma in that they are infrequently associated with chronic liver disease.

Angiosarcoma of the liver, a rare fatal tumor, has been seen in workers intensively exposed to vinyl chloride for prolonged periods in polymerization plants. Hepatoblastomas are the most common primary hepatic tumors of childhood and is estimated to affect 1 child younger than 15 years in 1 million per year, and approximately 50-70 new cases are reported in the United States yearly.

▶ Clinical Findings

A. Symptoms and Signs

The diagnosis at early and more treatable stages is often difficult, since symptoms are often absent. Screening and surveillance of high-risk patients (with cirrhosis, chronic hepatitis, etc) with ultrasonography of the liver has been recommended. Patients with more advanced tumors may have epigastric or right upper quadrant pain, which may be associated with referred pain in the right shoulder. Weight loss may be present. Jaundice is rare in patients with small tumors and good liver function; the presence of jaundice suggests either very advanced cancer or deteriorating liver function or both.

Hepatomegaly or a mass is palpable in many patients. An arterial bruit or a friction rub may be audible over the liver. Intermittent fever may be a presenting feature. Ascites or gastrointestinal bleeding from varices indicates advanced disease, and ascites fluid with blood should always suggest hepatocellular carcinoma. An acute deterioration in a previously well-compensated cirrhotic patient should also raise the suspicion of hepatocellular carcinoma.

The patterns of presentation can thus be extremely variable and may include: (1) pain with or without hepatomegaly; (2) sudden deterioration of the condition of a cirrhotic patient with the onset of hepatic failure, bleeding varices, or ascites; (3) sudden, massive intraperitoneal hemorrhage; (4) acute illness with fever and abdominal pain; (5) symptoms related to distant metastases; and (6) no clinical findings or symptoms.

B. Laboratory Findings

Depending on the disease extent and underlying hepatic function, laboratory values may range from entirely normal to suggestive of impending liver failure. Serum transaminase levels (AST and ALT) and alkaline phosphatase may be increased but are nonspecific and often seen in patients with chronic liver disease without hepatocellular carcinoma. The presence of a moderate to large liver tumor may bring about an increase in the serum alkaline phosphatase in the absence of underlying liver disease. An elevated serum bilirubin is a more ominous finding and reflects some degree of liver dysfunction, either from the underlying chronic liver disease or from a large volume of cancer within the liver. Tumor extension within the portal venous system is not uncommon, and involvement of the right and left portal trunks or the main portal vein may result in jaundice due to compromised portal venous inflow. Less often, jaundice is the result of tumor involvement of the biliary confluence by direct compression or by intrabiliary tumor extension. Other signs of compromised hepatic function include hypoalbuminemia, coagulopathy, and thrombocytopenia. A large number of patients may be positive for HBsAg or HCV antibody; the proportions of each vary somewhat by geography.

C. Liver Imaging

Liver ultrasound, CT scans, and magnetic resonance imaging (MRI) scans demonstrate the principal lesion in nearly all patients. A triple-phase (no contrast, arterial phase, and portal venous phase), contrast-enhanced helical CT scan of the chest, abdomen, and pelvis generally provides the best images of disease extent within the liver and also assesses for extrahepatic spread. Hepatocellular carcinomas are supplied primarily by the hepatic artery, and the vast majority thus enhance on arterial phase more than the adjacent nontu-morous liver parenchyma (hypervascular). In some cases, the center of the tumor has become necrotic, and only the peripheral areas are hypervascular. Arterial branches supplying the tumor have an irregular appearance compared to the native hepatic artery, and arterial-venous shunting may be seen. Upon venous phase, the arterial contrast typically has washed out, and the HCC bear similar density to the adjacent parenchyma (isodense). In contrast to HCC, cholangiocarcinomas usually appear less vascular than adjacent liver parenchyma, on all phase contrast. As an adjunct to CT, MRI scans with MR angiography or CT angiography may provide more detail regarding vascular involvement and clarify if a tumor is surgically removable.

D. Angiography

Diagnostic angiography was previously used often to assess liver tumors but is now rarely needed for this purpose; it is reserved primarily for treatment (ie, transarterial chemoembolization). Angiography may be equivocal in small HCC, which may be demonstrated with greater certainty by a selective injection of iodized oil (Lipiodol) followed 1-2 weeks later by CT scanning. In a normal liver, the contrast medium is cleared quickly but HCC retains it and remains opacified.

E. Liver Biopsy

The diagnosis can be established by percutaneous core biopsy or aspiration biopsy. Fine-needle aspiration biopsy is associated with an approximately 30% false-negative rate. A negative result therefore does not rule out malignant disease, and a core biopsy should be pursued if the index of suspicion is high. Percutaneous biopsy carries some risk of bleeding, although this is rare in experienced hands; tumor dissemination by seeding resulting from a biopsy can occur in 2%-4%. In patients with cirrhosis, the presence of a hypervascular mass larger than 1 cm with typical imaging features on contrast-enhanced CT or MRI has specificity and predictive positive values of nearly 100% and a biopsy is generally not required in this setting. In other clinical scenario, a diagnostic biopsy is often requested for nonsurgical candidate to guide appropriate liver-directed or systemic treatment.

F. Surveillance

In patients with cirrhosis or chronic hepatitis B, surveillance with biannual liver sonography is recommended since early detection and treatment is the best strategy to achieve long-term survival. The optimal type and timing of imaging studies is the subject of debate, but such programs have proved useful in areas with a high incidence of chronic hepatitis, such as Asia, where a large proportion of patients are now identified with a mass 2 cm in diameter or smaller; other studies in high-risk patients have also proved valuable.

G. Tumor Markers

Alpha fetoprotein (AFP), a glycoprotein normally present only in the fetal circulation, is present in high concentrations in the serum of many patients with hepatocellular carcinoma, testicular tumors, and hepatoblastomas. Increased levels are rarely seen as a product of other tumor types, such as the lung, stomach, pancreas, and biliary tree.

The upper limit of normal in the serum is 20 ng/mL; values above 200 ng/mL are suggestive of HCC, while levels above 400 ng/mL in a cirrhotic patients with a hypervascular liver mass larger than 2 cm in diameter are diagnostic. Levels in the intermediate range are nonspecific and may occur with benign liver diseases, such as cirrhosis and chronic hepatitis, where they represent a manifestation of liver cell proliferation. As imaging methods have improved, the diagnosis of liver cancer is being made earlier, when AFP levels may be normal or only minimally elevated. Additionally, some patients may have normal AFP levels despite the presence of advanced disease. In general, AFP levels correlate with tumor size and vascular invasion, and a number of studies have shown a correlation between high AFP levels and recurrent cancer after resection. AFP levels can also provide a measure of tumor response in patients treated nonoperatively.

▶ Differential Diagnosis

The clinical picture is often nonspecific, and the presenting symptoms may provide little in the way of diagnostic clues. Primary liver cancer may initially be confused with metastatic cancer arising from other abdominal sites. The presence of cirrhosis and findings consistent with chronic liver disease should make hepatocellular carcinoma the leading diagnosis, and this is often confirmed with further testing. In patients without cirrhosis or normal AFP levels (or both), a hypervascular mass in the liver should raise other diagnostic considerations, such as hepatic adenoma, which can be difficult to distinguish from hepatocellular carcinoma on the basis of imaging alone. In addition, certain types of cancer may give rise to hypervascular liver metastases, including melanoma, neuroendocrine carcinoma, and renal cell carcinoma.

When sudden decompensation develops in a cirrhotic patient, the possibility of HCC must always be considered. In rare instances, HCC is associated with metabolic or endocrine abnormalities such as erythrocytosis, hypercalcemia, hypoglycemic attacks, Cushing syndrome, or virilization.

▶ Complications

Sudden intra-abdominal hemorrhage may occur from spontaneous bleeding. Obstruction of the portal vein may produce portal hypertension, and obstruction of the hepatic veins may produce the Budd–Chiari syndrome. Liver failure is a common cause of death in these situations.

▶ Treatment

A. Partial Hepatectomy

Resection is the treatment of choice in selected patients without cirrhosis or in cirrhotics with well-preserved hepatic function. Initial diagnostic laparoscopy, immediately prior to planned laparotomy, may identify previously undetected spread of tumor within the liver or abdominal cavity that would preclude resection; however, with better imaging, the yield of laparoscopy has decreased. The minimal criteria of resectability that must be met are: (1) disease confined to the liver and (2) disease amenable to a complete resection. Multiple tumors in the liver and tumor invasion into major portal or hepatic veins are bad prognostic findings, even if resection is technically feasible; such patients generally are not good candidates for resection. For small and peripherally placed lesions, particularly in cirrhotics, sublobar, segmental resections are preferred if technically feasible. Anatomical segmentectomies are preferred to nonanatomical resections. Larger or more central tumors require more extensive resections. In Western centers, about 25%-30% of patients with hepatocellular carcinoma prove to be candidates for resection; this proportion is over 60% in Japan due largely to widespread surveillance programs.

If gross tumor is left behind or if the margins of resection are involved microscopically, progressive disease is the rule. After a complete resection, the prognosis is best for patients with a solitary, small (< 3 cm), and asymptomatic tumor and well-preserved hepatic function. Several adverse predictors of outcome have been identified, which vary somewhat among studies. However, the presence of vascular invasion (even if microscopic) has been identified in nearly all studies to predict recurrent cancer and poor outcome. Large tumor size (> 5 cm), the presence of satellite tumors, and markedly elevated AFP (> 2000 ng/mL) are also associated with a worse outcome, in part because of their correlation with vascular invasion. Additionally, patients with coexistent hepatocellular disease (ie, cirrhosis) do worse, and this is especially true in the face of significant hepatocellular dysfunction or portal hypertension.

In general, cirrhosis constitutes the major obstacle to resection in patients with hepatocellular carcinoma. Careful patient selection (Child–Pugh A, no portal hypertension) is critical in order to avoid acute liver failure and provide survival benefit to patients. In addition to this immediate perioperative concern, cirrhotic patients have a late risk of death from progression of the underlying liver disease (bleeding esophageal varices or liver failure) and a high rate (> 75%) of new tumors developing in the residual liver. For these reasons, highly selected patients may be better treated with liver transplantation rather than resection.

Overall, the rate of tumor recurrence is approximately 70% at 5 years (although it is higher, as mentioned above, in patients with cirrhosis). Some patients may be candidates for repeat resection or ablative procedures. The 5-year survival rate varies from approximately 40% to 70%, but is lower for patients with cirrhosis.

After the surgery, patients should be followed by periodic physical examinations and blood work to assess liver function. Imaging studies and AFP measurements (if elevated before resection) at regular intervals may help identify early, localized recurrences that may be amenable to repeat resection or palliative therapy.

For intrahepatic cholangiocarcinoma, resection, when possible, is the treatment of choice.

B. Liver Transplantation

Hepatocellular carcinoma is the only solid neoplasm for which transplantation plays a significant role. Liver transplantation has the advantage of treating not only the malignant disease but also the underlying cirrhosis. Previously, the selection criteria for transplanting hepatoma patients were broad and included patients with very advanced disease. Consequently, 5-year survival rates were less than 40%, too low to justify use of a scarce resource. The lessons learned from this early experience have allowed identification of patients most likely to benefit, specifically those with a single tumor no larger than 5 cm in diameter or up to three tumors with none exceeding 3 cm in diameter and no major vascular invasion. Using these strict criteria (the Milan criteria), 5-year survival rates of 70% can be achieved, a survival benefit similar to transplant patients with advanced cirrhosis but without HCC.

It should be emphasized that the benefit of transplantation is realized only when the waiting time for a new graft is under 6 months. Since waiting times can exceed 12 months in many centers, up to 50% of patients develop cancer progression or otherwise become ineligible. This problem has led a number of centers to adopt living donor transplantation as a means of increasing the donor pool, an approach that remains controversial because of donor-related morbidity and mortality. Another approach to this problem has been to increase the number of MELD points for transplantable liver disease, which effectively places eligible patients higher on the priority list.

A major concern of transplantation in cancer patients has been that the immunosuppressive therapy required to support the graft would remove an important defense mechanism against progression of residual microscopic disease. Indeed, calculated tumor doubling times for lesions in transplanted patients have been shown to be greater compared to patients not on immunosuppressive agents. Despite this possibility and although the logistical problems and expense are enormous, transplantation is a reasonable option in patients with cirrhosis who are not candidates for resection and have limited malignant disease burden, as specified in the selection criteria.

At present, transplantation has no role in patients with intrahepatic cholangiocarcinoma outside the controlled clinical trials, since the results to date have been poor.

C. Liver-Directed Therapy

Liver-directed therapies have been the subject of multiple investigations for the treatment of hepatocellular carcinoma. The effectiveness of these approaches for unresectable intrahepatic cholangiocarcinoma is being evaluated.

D. Ethanol Injection

Percutaneous ablative techniques are a reasonable option in patients with small, unresectable hepatocellular carcinoma, of which ethanol injection is the cheapest, easiest, and least morbid. Using ultrasound or CT guidance, 95% ethanol (5-20 mL) is injected through a 22-gauge needle directly into the tumor. This approach can achieve complete necrosis in 90%-100% of tumors smaller than 2 cm, but its efficacy declines rapidly as the tumor size increases. The patient is followed up and retreatment given for residual or new primary tumors. In one multi-institutional series from Italy, survival 1, 2, and 3 years after treatment for patients with solitary, small tumors was 90%, 80%, and 63%, respectively.

E. Radiofrequency Ablation

Radiofrequency ablation (RFA) is another percutaneous ablative approach, useful for treating selected patients with small tumors who are not candidate for surgery or liver transplantation. RFA has generally supplanted ethanol injection as the percutaneous treatment of choice. Under ultrasound or CT guidance, a needle is used to access the lesion; the needle is attached to a radiofrequency generator that generates thermal energy to bring about tumor destruction. RFA can be used percutaneously, laparoscopically, or at laparotomy.

The goal of RFA is the same as that of ethanol injection: to achieve complete tumor necrosis. The efficacy of RFA is limited by tumor size but may be somewhat greater than ethanol injection in this regard; RFA is less effective for tumors adjacent to major vascular structures. A randomized study comparing the two techniques found no differences in survival, although RFA may offer better local tumor control rates. In carefully selected patients, 5-year survival rates of 30%-40% have been reported. RFA has been compared with resection in early HCC in randomized controlled trials, but results have varied. Generally, RFA appear to be as effective as resection in lesions smaller than 2 cm. Ablation techniques, including RFA, have been studied in the context of controlling disease progression while on the waiting list in patients who are candidates for transplantation with some suggestion of benefit.

Microwave ablation and irreversible electroporation are two emerging ablative techniques that may prove to be alternatives to RFA.

F. Arterial Embolization

Hepatic artery embolization is another ablative technique that is more broadly applicable than RFA or ethanol injection. This approach takes advantage of the fact that primary liver cancers derive disproportionately greater blood supply from the hepatic arterial circulation compared to the surrounding liver. The strategy is to combine selective hepatic arterial injection of cancer chemotherapeutic agents with arterial embolization, the latter to produce tumor necrosis and slow the washout of the drugs. Embolization can be used in patients with much larger tumors than can be effectively treated with percutaneous procedures, and the procedure can be staged to treat bilobar disease. Patients must have adequate liver function; those with Child-Pugh C cirrhosis or thrombosis of the portal vein are not suitable candidates.

A variety of techniques have been used. Embolization is often performed with Gelfoam, which dissolves after a few weeks, but other inert agents are also used and are probably more effective for occluding vessels. Some centers use inert particles without chemotherapy (ie, bland emobolization) but most employ a chemotherapeutic component (ie, transarterial chemoembolization or TACE). Doxorubicin, mitomycin, and cisplatin in various combinations are the drugs most often given. Lipiodol, which lodges in the tumor, has occasionally been used as a carrier for the drugs. It remains unclear if the addition of chemotherapeutic agents provides much benefit beyond the necrosis produced by occlusion of the hepatic arterial supply. Many patients require multiple treatments, although the optimal schedule is ill defined. Embolization achieves partial responses in up to 55% of patients. A survival benefit of approximately 10 months has been reported with chemoembolization compared to best supportive care in randomized controlled trials, and 30%-50% of patients are reported to survive at 3 years. Of note, histologic studies of tumors resected shortly after treatment reveal viable neoplastic cells in the tumor capsule, which receives blood from the portal vein as well as the hepatic artery. Recently, a randomized prospective trial showed that the combination of RFA and chemoembolization provided superior disease control rates than either technique alone.

G. Systemic Therapy

Until recently, no systemic treatment was found able to prolong the survival of patients with metastatic hepatocellular carcinoma. The multikinase inhibitor sorafenib, that mainly blocks RAF, VEGF, PDGF, and c-Kit signaling, has however been shown to have antitumor efficacy. In two phase 3, multicenter, randomized, double-blind and placebo-controlled trials, sorafenib improved by 2-3 months the survival of patients with advanced HCC and compensated liver function. The efficacy of combining sorafenib with other biologic and chemotherapeutic agents is being evaluated, as well as its use in less advanced disease status and in the adjuvant setting in an attempt to lessen or delay cancer recurrence.

Gemcitabine-based chemotherapy, in particular with combination with cisplatin, has shown prolongation of survival in patients with metastatic biliary tract cancer.

Cheng AL et al. Efficacy and safety of sorafenib in patients in the Asia-Pacific region with advanced hepatocellular carcinoma: a phase III randomized, double-blind, placebo-controlled trial. *Lancet Oncol* 2009;10:25.

Cheng BQ et al. Chemoembolization combined with radiofrequency ablation for patients with hepatocellular carcinoma larger than 3 cm: a randomized controlled trial. *JAMA* 2008;299:1669.

Clavien PA et al. Recommendation for liver transplantation for hepatocellular carcinoma: an international consensus conference report. *Lancet Oncol* 2012;13:e11-22.

De Jong MC et al. Intrahepatic cholangiocarcinoma: an international multi-institutional analysis of prognostic factors and lymph node assessment. *J Clin Oncol* 2011;29:3140.

El-Serag HB. Hepatocellular carcinoma. *N Engl J Med* 2011;365:1118.

Endo I et al. Intrahepatic cholangiocarcinoma: rising frequency, improved survival, and determinants of survival after resection. *Ann Surg* 2008;247:994.

Forner A, Llovet JM, Bruix J. Hepatocellular carcinoma. *Lancet* 201231;379(9822):1245-1255.

Forner A et al. Diagnosis of hepatic nodules 20 mm or smaller in cirrhosis: porspective validation of the noninvasive diagnostic criteria for hepatocellular carcinoma. *Hepatology* 2008;47:97.

Huitzil-Melendez FD et al. Advanced hepatocellular carcinoma: which staging systems best predict prognosis? *J Clin Oncol* 2010;28:2889.

Llovet JM et al. Sorafenib in advanced hepatocellular carcinoma. *N Engl J Med* 2008;359:378.

Mazzaferro V et al. Liver transplantation for the treatment of small hepatocellular carcinomas in patients with cirrhosis. *N Engl J Med* 1996;334:693.

Park SY et al. Transarterial chemoembolization versus supportive therapy in the palliative treatment of unresectable intrahepatic cholangiocarcinoma. *Clin Radiol* 2011;66:322.

Poustchi H et al. Feasibility of conducting a randomized control trial for liver cancer screening: is a randomized controlled trial for liver cancer screening feasible or still needed? *Hepatology* 2011;54:1998.

Silva MA et al. Needle track seeding following biopsy of liver lesions in the diagnosis of hepatocellular cancer: a systematic review and metas-analysis. *Gut* 2008;57:1592.

Valle J et al. Cisplatin plus gemcitabine versus gemcitabine for biliary tract cancer. *N Engl J Med* 2010;362:1273.

METASTATIC NEOPLASMS OF THE LIVER

In Western countries, metastatic cancer is much more common than primary tumors in the liver. Nearly all solid tumors can potentially give rise to liver metastases; primary cancers of the gastrointestinal tract (colon, pancreas, esophagus, stomach, neuroendocrine), breast, lung, genitourinary system (kidney, adrenal), ovary and uterus, melanoma, and sarcomas account for the overwhelming majority of cases. Spread to the liver may be via the systemic or portal venous circulation. The cirrhotic liver, which often gives rise to primary hepatic tumors, seems to be less susceptible than normal liver to implantation of metastases.

Individual tumor types have characteristic patterns of spread. For example, colorectal cancer spreads to the liver as the first site of metastatic disease in a very high proportion of patients; the lung is the next most common site, but bone, brain, or adrenal metastases are distinctly unusual. By contrast, metastatic lung cancer to the liver typically occurs concomitantly with spread to other sites, with brain, bone, and adrenal among the most common. In general, the vast majority of patients with metastases to the liver also have disease at other sites. A notable exception is colorectal cancer, which in many cases involves the liver only for a prolonged period. In the past, approximately 20% of patients with hepatic metastases had additional tumor deposits in the liver not seen on preoperative imaging studies. As imaging technology has improved, however, this proportion has become increasingly smaller.

▶ Clinical Findings

A. Symptoms and Signs

The signs and symptoms vary with the clinical scenario, the disease extent within the liver, and the presence or absence of metastatic disease to other sites. Patients with an undiagnosed primary tumor may come to attention because of symptoms caused by the metastatic disease. Weight loss, fatigue, pain, and anorexia are the presenting general complaints in many such patients. Signs of liver failure, such as ascites and jaundice, are uncommon and suggestive of very advanced cancer. Fever without demonstrable infection is present in 15% of cases. By contrast, patients with a known history of cancer undergoing routine surveillance often develop liver metastases that cause no symptoms; in a small proportion of cases, liver metastases are found on studies done for unrelated reasons.

Physical examination is frequently unrevealing. Hepatomegaly or a palpable tumor in the upper abdomen may be present, and either may be tender. Portal hypertension may be manifested by abdominal venous collaterals or splenomegaly. A friction rub is sometimes heard over the liver.

B. Laboratory Findings

Laboratory values may be entirely normal or at most reflect only minor nonspecific changes. Patients with advanced cancer can have anemia and hypoalbuminemia. The alkaline phosphatase is increased in most patients. More significant derangements in liver function occur in patients with a large volume of liver disease, although this is uncommon at initial presentation. Tumor marker levels (carcinoembryonic antigen [CEA], carbohydrate antigen [CA] 19-9, CA-125) are often elevated, depending on the tumor type, and may be helpful for monitoring treatment.

The diagnosis can be established in most cases by CT-guided or ultrasound-guided percutaneous liver biopsy or fine-needle aspiration for malignant cells.

C. Imaging Studies

The detection of liver metastases relies on CT and/or MRI scans; ultrasonography identifies tumors in the liver and distinguishes solid from cystic lesions but cannot provide the same degree of anatomical detail. MRI provides useful additional information and may help distinguish benign from malignant disease. However, a high-quality triple phase CT scan with intravenous and oral contrast medium provides excellent assessment of disease extent in the liver and elsewhere in the abdomen. In the past, CT portography was superior to ordinary contrast-enhanced CT and was obtained routinely in patients being considered for hepatic resection, but this is no longer the case. Positron emission tomography using 18-fluorodeoxyglucose (FDG-PET) is a commonly used staging study and may help identify extrahepatic disease, a finding that could change the treatment recommendations. During surgery, intraoperative ultrasound is used to assess the liver for disease not appreciated on imaging studies.

▶ Treatment

For most patients with metastatic liver disease, chemotherapy is the only treatment option, particularly with coexisting metastases outside the liver. Such therapy is usually not curative but rather palliative in most cases. A notable exception is metastatic colorectal cancer, for which resection or other treatments aimed at the liver disease are effective and potentially curative; the recent advent of several active chemotherapeutic agents has further improved the results of treatment. Carefully selected patients with metastases from other primary tumors (sarcoma, breast, ovary, lung, neuroendocrine) may also benefit from resection but represent a small minority of cases.

A. Hepatic Resection

Hepatic resection is most commonly indicated in patients with metastatic colorectal cancer. Of the approximately 130,000 patients diagnosed with colorectal cancer annually in the United States, approximately 50% either have liver metastases at diagnosis or develop liver metastases at some point. In 40% of the latter group, the liver is the only demonstrable site of disease. Hepatic metastases from colorectal cancer thus affect approximately 20,000 patients per year, which is comparable to the annual incidence of pancreatic or esophageal carcinoma.

After a complete resection, the 5-year survival rate has historically been 25%-40%; systemic or regional chemotherapy or both are frequently given after resection and appear to enhance the results of surgery, with more recent series reporting 5-year survival figures of approximately 50%. The presence of extrahepatic metastases and inability to achieve a complete resection are contraindications to resection in most cases. However, as more effective chemotherapeutic options have emerged, the indications for resection have expanded to include selected patients with multiple bilobar tumors and even some with extrahepatic metastatic disease. Extensive use of chemotherapy prior to surgery can cause changes in the liver, particularly steatosis and steatohepatitis, which can impair the liver's normal regenerative response. Caution is therefore needed when considering such patients for major hepatic resections, since operative morbidity and mortality may be increased; preoperative portal vein embolization may reduce the incidence of serious postoperative complications.

The following variables are associated with a worse prognosis after resection: (1) original tumor with involved lymph nodes (stage III or Dukes C); (2) multiple liver lesions; (3) less than 1-year interval between resection of the colon primary and diagnosis of liver disease (disease-free interval); and (4) CEA level higher than 200 ng/mL. Variables that do not influence the outcome include: (1) histologic grade of the tumor; (2) bilateral rather than unilateral disease; (3) site of the primary tumor within the large intestine; and (4) the gender of the patient. The mortality rate for resection of hepatic metastases is 1%-2% in hospitals where this operation is performed frequently.

The liver is the most common site of cancer recurrence after a complete resection. A small proportion of patients with hepatic recurrence may be amenable to a second resection. The use of adjuvant hepatic arterial chemotherapy appears to reduce the risk of intrahepatic recurrence.

The efficacy of liver resection for colorectal cancer has been clearly established and is the most common indication for this procedure. By contrast, for most other tumor types, particularly those arising from the gastrointestinal tract other than the colon or rectum, the benefit of liver resection is much more limited. Rare patients with metastases from renal cell carcinoma, ovarian cancer, adrenocortical carcinoma, or sarcomas appear to derive the most benefit; by contrast, liver resection for metastatic esophageal, gastric, or pancreatic cancer is almost never warranted. In selecting patients with noncolorectal liver metastases for resection, the most important factors are: (1) long disease-free interval; (2) solitary resectable liver tumor; and (3) the absence of extrahepatic metastases.

Neuroendocrine carcinomas (pancreatic islet cell tumors, carcinoids) represent a unique class of tumors that often give rise to liver metastases. Unlike patients with other metastatic tumor types, those with neuroendocrine tumors often survive for many years. Multiple liver metastases are the rule with this disease, so complete resection is usually not possible. However, debulking liver resections are sometimes indicated to palliate tumor-related pain or hormonal symptoms. Partial hepatectomy is also sometimes worthwhile to extirpate a tumor invading directly from a contiguous organ.

B. Radiofrequency Ablation

RFA has been used to treat metastases to the liver from a variety of tumor types. The indications for this procedure remain ill defined. The best candidates are those with a limited number of small liver lesions with no evidence of extrahepatic cancer.

C. Chemotherapy

In a large proportion of patients with metastatic colorectal cancer, the liver is the only evident site of disease. If the lesions cannot be resected, regional intrahepatic chemotherapy can be given by placing a catheter in the gastroduodenal artery (at its origin with the common hepatic artery) connected to an implantable, subcutaneous infusion pump, which allows the delivery of much higher concentrations of drug to the tumor than is possible with systemic administration. This regimen is generally not used for metastases from other kinds of tumors. The pump is primed with floxuridine, which is delivered by continuous infusion (0.1-0.2 mg/kg/d) for 14-day periods alternating with 14-day rests. Systemic chemotherapy is usually given concomitantly. The discovery of extrahepatic lesions at laparotomy for pump placement is a relative contraindication to proceeding with this approach. Treatment is continued until disease progression or excessive toxicity is seen or, rarely, until the response is complete. Toxicity consists mainly of gastroduodenal erosions (caused by unintentional perfusion of these areas), chemical hepatitis, or chemical sclerosing cholangitis. Survival is related principally to the initial amount of liver involvement by tumor, objective response to treatment (which is seen in about 60% of patients), and extent of prior chemotherapy. The median survival of patients with less than 30% of liver replaced by tumor is 24 months, compared with 10 months if the extent of replacement exceeds 30%. Up to 47% of patients with initially unresectable disease may respond enough to become resectable and potentially benefit from surgery. There is a general perception that hepatic artery infusion therapy improves survival, but the objective evidence is inconclusive.

Hepatic artery infusion chemotherapy may be a useful adjunctive therapy after complete tumor resection or RFA. Studies of this option are under way. Systemic chemotherapy (eg, with fluorouracil, irinotecan, or oxaliplatin) after a complete resection of liver metastases has not been proved to improve survival, although it is often prescribed.

D. Miscellaneous

Hepatic artery ligation or angiographic embolization of the tumor has been of benefit in a few patients with hepatic metastases from specific tumor types, particularly neuroendocrine tumors.

▶ Prognosis

Survival varies with the site of origin of the primary tumor and the extent of metastatic disease. Patients with extensive hepatic replacement by multiple lesions have a dismal outlook, with a survival measured in months, compared to perhaps 2–3 years for patients with small solitary lesions. The range of treatment options and effective chemotherapeutic agents is greatest for metastatic colorectal cancer compared to most other tumor types, and survival is generally better in this group.

Brouquet A et al. High survival rate after two-stage resection of advanced colorectal liver metastases: response-based selection and complete resection define outcome. *J Clin Oncol* 2011;29:1083.

Cho CS et al. Histologic grade is correlated with outcome after resection of hepatic neuroendocrine neoplasms. *Cancer* 2008;113:126.

Kemeny NE et al. Conversion to resectability using hepatic artery infusion plus systemic chemotherapy for the treatment of unresectable liver metastases from colorectal carcinoma. *J Clin Oncol* 2009;27:3465.

Nordlinger B et al. Perioperative chemotherapy with FOLFOX4 and surgery versus surgery alone for resectable liver metastases from colon cancer (EORTC Intergroup trial 40983): a randomized controlled trial. *Lancet* 2008;371:1007.

Strasberg SM, Dehdashti F. Role of FDG-PET staging in selecting the optimum patient for hepatic resection of metastatic colorectal cancer. *J Surg Oncol* 2010;102:955.

Tomlinson JS et al. Actual 10-year survival after resection of colorectal liver metastases defines cure. *J Clin Oncol* 2007;25:4575.

Wong SL et al. American Society of Clinical Oncology 2009 clinical evidence review on radiofrequency ablation of hepatic metastases from colorectal cancer. *J Clin Oncol* 2010;28:493.

BENIGN TUMORS & CYSTS OF THE LIVER

▶ Hemangiomas

Hemangioma is the most common benign hepatic tumor and has an incidence of approximately 7%. Except for the skin and mucous membranes, the liver is the most common site of origin. Women are affected more often than men—in some series, up to 75% of patients are female. Histologically, hepatic hemangiomata are of the cavernous type rather than the capillary type. Most are small, solitary subcapsular growths that are found incidentally during laparotomy or autopsy or on imaging studies. Rarely, hemangiomata grow to very large dimensions (giant hemangiomata) and cause abdominal pain or a palpable mass. Most are small to moderate-sized lesions, however; pain is uncommon in tumors smaller than 8-10 cm in diameter.

Rare complications of liver hemangiomata include hemorrhagic shock resulting from spontaneous rupture and the Kasabach–Merritt syndrome, which is usually seen in children and is associated with thrombocytopenia and a consumptive coagulopathy; both of these complications are exceedingly uncommon. Large congenital hemangiomas of the liver may be associated with others in the skin. Large hemangiomata may also give rise to large-volume arteriovenous shunting, resulting in cardiac hypertrophy and congestive heart failure.

Large-bore needle biopsy is hazardous due to bleeding risks; aspiration biopsy with a fine needle is safe but rarely helpful. Fortunately, biopsy is very rarely indicated, since the diagnosis can be made with certainty in most cases by contrast-enhanced CT or MRI scans. The hallmark features of hemangiomata are nodular peripheral enhancement on arterial phase with progressive central enhancement on the more delayed images. MRI is a particularly good study for hemangiomata, which appear very bright on the T2-weighted images, and combined with dynamic intravenous contrast, has a sensitivity and specificity of 98%. Angiography is unnecessary, and nuclear scans lack sufficient sensitivity and specificity.

Irrespective of their size, the only reasons to resect hemangiomata are for symptoms, most commonly pain, or diagnostic uncertainty (rare). Symptomatic hemangiomas should be excised by lobectomy or enucleation. Even large lesions can be safely removed. Radiotherapy or embolization via a catheter in the hepatic artery may be tried in patients who are poor candidates for surgery, but the efficacy of these approaches is limited. The natural history of asymptomatic hemangiomas, whether large or small, is benign. The vast majority of incidentally discovered hemangiomata remain stable in follow-up, do not give rise to symptoms, and therefore do not require resection. Progressive growth of asymptomatic hemangiomata over a relatively short time interval, particularly in young patients, is considered a relative indication for resection.

Concejero AM et al. Giant cavernous hemangioma of the liver with coagulopathy: adult Kasabach-Merritt syndrome. *Surgery* 2009;145:245.

Duxbury MS, Garden OJ. Giant haemangioma of the liver: observation or resection? *Dig Surg* 2010;27:7.

Van den Bos IC et al. Magnetic resonance imaging of liver lesions: exceptions and atypical lesions. *Curr Probl Diagn Radiol* 2008;37:95.

▶ Cysts

A number of different cystic lesions may affect the liver. Simple hepatic cysts, the most common, are unilocular fluid-filled lesions that generally produce no symptoms. The occasionally large cyst may present as an upper abdominal mass or discomfort. Small, simple cysts may be difficult to diagnose on CT and may be confused for metastatic disease; ultrasound and MRI are better modalities to assess the character of cystic lesions. Many patients have multiple simple cysts, which should not be confused with polycystic liver disease, a progressive condition characterized by cystic replacement of virtually the entire liver. Polycystic liver disease is associated in about half of cases with polycystic renal disease. The possibility of echinococcosis should be considered in patients with cystic liver lesions and the appropriate exposure history, although their radiographic appearance is usually quite distinctive.

Most simple cysts have a serous lining and a smooth, thin wall. Intracystic hemorrhage can occur, which can confuse the radiographic appearance. Solitary cysts lined with cuboidal epithelium are classified as cystadenomas and should be resected, since they are premalignant. Cystadenomas are characterized radiographically as complex, with internal septae, an irregular lining, and papillary projections. Complex, multilocular (septated) cysts (if not echinococcal) are often neoplastic and should be resected. However, cystadenomas and cystadenocarcinomas are rare, while internal hemorrhage into a simple cyst is a more common entity and may have a similar appearance. Nevertheless, complex cysts of the liver must be approached with some caution in order to avoid inappropriate interventions. There are few indications for aspirating hepatic cysts—simple cysts reaccumulate fluid quickly, neoplastic cysts must be excised, and parasitic cysts might rupture and the parasite thus be allowed to spread. It is possible to eliminate small cysts by aspiration of the contents followed by an injection into the lumen of 20-100 mL of absolute alcohol; however, small cysts almost never cause symptoms and generally require no treatment.

Large symptomatic cysts are difficult to eradicate with alcohol injections, and serious superinfection of the cyst cavity may occur. The simplest method of treatment consists of laparoscopic cyst fenestration (wide excision of the cyst wall). A tongue of omentum may be fixed so it lies in the residual cyst cavity as an ancillary measure to prevent the edges from coapting. The operation is curative in nearly all patients.

Multiple, small, simple cysts do not usually require treatment, but large polycystic livers that cause discomfort or are associated with obstructive jaundice can be managed by partial resection or surgically unroofing the cysts on the surface of the liver and creating windows between superficial cysts and adjacent deep cysts. The opened cysts are allowed to drain into the abdominal cavity. The results of surgery for polycystic liver disease are often disappointing, with quick return of symptoms in many patients.

Choi HK et al. Differential diagnosis for intrahepatic biliary cytadenoma and hepatic simple cyst: significance of cystic fluid analysis and radiologic findings. *J Clin Gastroenterol* 2010;44:289.
Del Poggio P, Buonacore M. Cystic tumors of the liver: a practical approach. *World J Gastroenterol* 2008;14:3616.
Fukunaga N et al. Hepatobiliary cystadenoma exhibiting morphologic changes from simple hepatic cyst shown by 11-year follow-up imagins. *World J Surg Onc* 2008;6:129.

▶ Hepatic Adenoma

Hepatic adenomas occur predominantly in women of childbearing age and appear to be related to the use of oral contraceptives. Mestranol-containing compounds have been associated with a disproportionate number of cases, but mestranol has been in use longer than the other agents.

The tumors are soft, yellow-tan, well-circumscribed masses that are usually of moderate size (range of 2-15 cm in diameter). Most of those that cause symptoms are in the 8-15 cm range. Two-thirds of hepatic adenomas are solitary; other benign tumors (such as FNH, see next section) are present in some cases. Transition from benign hepatic adenoma to hepatocellular carcinoma is estimated to occur in 5%, with liver cell dysplasia as an intermediate step. Histologically, hepatic adenomas consist of an encapsulated homogeneous mass of normal-appearing hepatocytes without bile ducts or central veins. Intratumoral hemorrhage or central necrosis may be present.

About half of patients are asymptomatic. Most of those with symptoms present with right upper quadrant pain. Spontaneous hemorrhage into the substance of the tumor with subsequent rupture and intraperitoneal bleeding is a well-known potential complication of adenomas estimated to occur in 20%-40% of untreated cases. The true risk of spontaneous hemorrhage is, however, difficult to know with certainty, since the overall incidence of adenomas is unknown. This risk increases with size, and there appears to be a strong association of acute bleeding episodes from adenoma with pregnancy. Patients with this life-threatening problem present with acute pain or even hemorrhagic shock.

Liver function tests and AFP levels are usually normal or minimally deranged. Adenomas typically appear hypervascular compared to the surrounding liver parenchyma, a feature that is apparent on contrast-enhanced CT or MRI scans or angiography. Adenomas can be difficult to distinguish from FNH, another benign tumor often found in young women. Differences in tumor vascularity may be demonstrated on angiography; however, MRI is probably the best study for differentiating these lesions. Adenomas often cannot be distinguished from well-differentiated hepatocellular carcinoma on imaging studies and even on biopsy specimens. Needle biopsy is generally safe but often inconclusive and is associated with a small risk of bleeding.

The general recommendation is that adenomas should be resected because of the risks of malignant change and spontaneous hemorrhage. Unfortunately, the true likelihood of these events is difficult to estimate, since most series include only treated patients. Lesion measuring less than 5 cm can be observed with serial imaging since the risk of malignant transformation or bleeding at this size appears minimal. Symptomatic and large asymptomatic adenomas clearly should be resected. Emergent resection or hepatic artery embolization should be undertaken in patients with evidence of hemorrhage. Small peripheral lesions may be removed with wedge excisions, but larger tumors require more extensive resections. Small adenomas may regress when oral contraceptive agents are discontinued, and close follow-up with imaging studies is not unreasonable in such cases; however, any change in symptoms or imaging characteristics (growth, hemorrhage) should prompt resection. The possibility that a presumed adenoma is actually a well-differentiated hepatocellular carcinoma or contains a focus of malignancy must always be kept in mind; there is no completely reliable means of making the differentiation other than pathologic analysis of the resected specimen.

Most patients recover without sequelae after surgical removal; recurrence is rare. Oral contraceptives should be proscribed permanently in all cases. Radiotherapy and chemotherapy are of no value, but elective hepatic artery embolization may be helpful in patients who are not surgical candidates. Embolization may be particularly helpful in the very rare patient with multiple hepatic adenomas (hepatic adenomatosis), since resection is usually not possible.

▶ Focal Nodular Hyperplasia

FNH accounts for the second most common benign liver process after hemangioma. Like hepatic adenoma, FNH is much more common in young women. The average age is about 40 years, but the tumor can occur at any age. Unlike hepatic adenoma, however, the use of oral contraceptive agents does not appear to predispose to the development of FNH, although it has been suggested that these agents may stimulate growth.

Grossly, the tumor is a well-circumscribed, firm, tan, usually subcapsular mass measuring 2-3 cm in diameter. In patients with symptoms, the lesions are much larger, usually around 10 cm. Multiple tumors can occur; 80% are solitary. The gross appearance on cut section is quite characteristic, consisting of a central stellate scar (which is actually an aggregation of blood vessels) with radiating fibrous septa that compartmentalize the lesion into lobules. Histologically, there are nodular aggregations of normal-appearing hepatocytes without central veins or portal triads. Bile duct proliferation is present in the nodules.

Most patients with FNH are asymptomatic. The few with symptoms present with a right upper quadrant discomfort. Unlike hepatic adenomas, these lesions rarely, if ever, bleed, and the natural history of asymptomatic lesions is benign. Very rare patients with diffuse FNH develop portal hypertension.

Hepatic function tests and AFP levels are usually normal. Hepatic scintiscans usually do not show a filling defect but are of little practical value. CT scans demonstrate the tumor and may also show the central stellate scar. The arteriographic pattern is one of hypervascularity. In most cases, the diagnosis of FNH can be made with noninvasive studies, although distinguishing FNH from hepatic adenomas can be difficult, even for experienced radiologists. MRI scanning is the best modality, but the imaging features of both tumors overlap somewhat, and they occur in similar patient populations. Fine-needle aspiration biopsies are generally not helpful.

Symptomatic lesions should be removed, while asymptomatic tumors (the majority) should be left undisturbed, provided that the diagnosis has been made confidently. In the latter circumstance, a period of observation with imaging studies is recommended to ensure stability. Inability to distinguish FNH from adenoma or malignant disease is an indication for resection in some patients. Discontinuation of oral contraceptives probably has no impact. FNH can be reliably identified on examination of frozen sections.

Cho SW et al. Surgical management of hepatocellular adenoma: take it or leave it. *Ann Surg Oncol* 2008;15:2795.

Dokmak S et al. A single-center surgical experience of 122 patients with single and multiple hepatocellular adenomas. *Gastroenterology* 2009;137:1698.

Grazioli L et al. Hepatocellular adenoma and focal nodular hyperplasia: value of gadoxetic acid-enhanced MR imaging in differential diagnosis. *Radiology* 2012;262:520.

Kim YI, Chung JW, Park JH. Feasibility of transcatheter arterial chemoembolization for hepatic adenoma. *J Vasc Interv Radiol* 2007;18:862.

CIRRHOSIS

Hepatic cirrhosis remains a major public health problem worldwide, with an annual mortality of approximately 23,000 per year in the United States alone. The incidence of cirrhosis is increasing, due in large measure to hepatitis C, and at present is the third-most common cause of death in men in the fifth decade of life. Another contributing factor is the epidemic of obesity, which is associated with NAFLD and progression to cirrhosis in many patients.

Alcohol abuse remains the leading cause of cirrhosis in most Western countries. Alcohol exerts direct toxic effects on the liver that are magnified in the presence of protein and other dietary deficiencies that are often present. Even still, cirrhosis develops in a small minority of patients who abuse alcohol. Alcohol induces a specific cytochrome P450 in the liver (ie, P450 2E1) that participates in its metabolism to acetaldehyde, which has a number of deleterious effects, including antibody formation, decreased DNA repair, enzyme inactivation, and alterations in microtubules, mitochondria, and plasma membranes. Acetaldehyde also promotes glutathione depletion, free radical–mediated toxicity, lipid peroxidation, and hepatic collagen synthesis. Hepatic steatosis and alcoholic hepatitis are stages of alcoholic liver injury that may precede cirrhosis. Alcoholic hyalin, a glycoprotein, accumulates in centrilobular hepatocytes of patients with alcoholic hepatitis. There is some evidence that immunologic responses to alcoholic hyalin may be important in the pathogenesis of cirrhosis.

Regardless of the cause (Table 24–3), collagen deposition in cirrhosis results from increased fibroblastic activity as well as from repair following hepatocellular injury and necrosis. The ultimate result is a liver containing regenerative nodules and connective tissue septa linking portal fields with central canals, which can be graded by severity on pathologic assessment of liver biopsy.

The natural history of cirrhosis is difficult to predict. Once the diagnosis has been established, up to 30% of patients die within a year from hepatic failure or complications of portal hypertension, of which bleeding esophageal varices is the most feared. In newly diagnosed cirrhotics, the chances of dying within the subsequent 2-3 years are influenced by the status of liver function (as reflected by the Child–Pugh classification, [Table 24–1]), the presence of varices, and the portal pressure. A group of cirrhotics with varices followed by the Boston Interhospital Liver Group experienced a 1-year death rate of 66%. Cirrhotics without varices may benefit substantially by abstaining from alcohol. Bleeding episodes occur in up to 40% of all patients with cirrhosis, and the initial episode of variceal hemorrhage is fatal in 50% or more. At least two-thirds of those who survive their initial hemorrhage bleed again, and the risk of dying from the second is similarly high. It is principally for such patients that portal decompressive procedures are recommended.

Other main complications of cirrhosis include ascites, hepatorenal syndrome with hyponatremia and renal insufficiency, coagulopathy, and encephalopathy. Those processes are mainly managed medically to maintain a state of relative physiological compensation. Liver transplantation for appropriate candidates provides the most effective treatment option associated with prolongation of survival.

Ginès P, Schrier RW. Renal failure in cirrhosis. *N Engl J Med* 2009;361:1279.

Rahimi RS, Rockey DC. Complications of cirrhosis. *Curr Opin Gastroenterol* 2012;28:223.

Reuben A. Alcohol and the liver. *Curr Opin Gastroenterol* 2008; 24:328.

Schuppan D, Afdhal NH. Liver cirrhosis. *Lancet* 2008;371:838.

Tripodi A, Mannucci PM. The coagulopathy of chronic liver disease. *N Engl J Med* 2011;365:147.

Wong F. Management of ascites in cirrhosis. *J Gastroenterol Hepatol* 2012;27:11.

▼ PORTAL HYPERTENSION

▶ Etiology

The major causes of portal hypertension are listed in Table 24–4. In all but a few instances, the basic lesion is increased resistance to portal flow. Those associated with increased resistance can be subclassified according to the site of the block as prehepatic, hepatic, and posthepatic; hepatic causes of portal hypertension are further subclassified as presinusoidal, sinusoidal, and postsinusoidal. Cirrhosis accounts for about 85% of cases of portal hypertension in the United States, most commonly from heavy alcohol use. Postnecrotic cirrhosis is next in frequency, followed by biliary cirrhosis. The other intrahepatic causes of portal hypertension are relatively rare in Western countries, although in some parts of the world, hepatic schistosomiasis constitutes the largest single group. Idiopathic portal hypertension occurs with greater frequency in southern Asia.

After cirrhosis, extrahepatic portal venous thrombosis or occlusion is the most common cause of portal hypertension in the United States. Patients with this condition are generally younger than cirrhotics, and many are children. Posthepatic obstruction due to Budd–Chiari syndrome (BCS) or constrictive pericarditis is rare.

Table 24–3. Causes of cirrhosis.

I. Drugs and toxins
Alcohol, Methrotrexate, Isoniazid, Methyldopa, Amiodarone
II. Infections
Viral hepatitis, Schistosomiasis
III. Autoimmune disorders
Autoimmune hepatitis, primary biliary cirrhosis, primary sclerosing cholangitis
IV. Inherited metabolic defects
Hemochromatosis, Wilson disease, alpha1-antitrypsin deficiency, galactosemia, tyrosinemia, glucogen storage disease, hereditary fructose intolerance, urea cycle disorders, alpha/beta lipoproteinemia, progressive familial intrahepatic cholestasis, cystic fibrosis
V. Acquired bile duct disease
Biliary atresia, gallstone obstruction, common bile duct benign stricture
VI. Vascular disorders
Budd-Chiari syndrome, venooclusive disease, congestive heart failure, hereditary hemorrhagic telangiectasia
VII. Miscellaneous
Nonalacoholic streatohepatitis (NASH), total parenteral nutrition, Indian childhood cirrhosis, intestinal bypass surgery, hypervitaminosis A, sarcoidosis, cryptogenic

Modified from Jarnagin WR et al: *Blumgart's Surgery of the Liver, Biliary Tract, and Pancreas*, 5th ed. Philadelphia, PA: Elsevier Saunders, 2012.

Table 24–4. Causes of portal hypertension.

I. Increased resistance to flow
A. Prehepatic (portal vein obstruction)
1. Congenital atresia or stenosis
2. Thrombosis of portal vein
3. Thrombosis of splenic vein
4. Extrinsic compression (eg, tumors)
B. Hepatic
1. Cirrhosis
  a. Portal cirrhosis (nutritional, alcoholic, Laënnec)
  b. Postnecrotic cirrhosis
  c. Biliary cirrhosis
  d. Others (Wilson disease, hemochromatosis)
2. Acute alcoholic liver disease
3. Chronic active hepatitis
4. Congenital hepatic fibrosis
5. Idiopathic portal hypertension (hepatoportal sclerosis)
6. Schistosomiasis
7. Sarcoidosis
C. Posthepatic
1. Budd–Chiari syndrome (hepatic vein thrombosis)
2. Veno-occlusive disease
3. Cardiac disease
  a. Constrictive pericarditis
  b. Valvular heart disease
  c. Right heart failure
II. Increased portal blood flow
A. Arterial-Portal Venous Fistula
B. Increased splenic flow
1. Banti syndrome
2. Splenomegaly (eg, tropical splenomegaly, myeloid metaplasia)

▶ Pathophysiology

Portal hypertension is defined as a hepatic venous pressure gradient (HVPG) (the difference between portal-vein pressure and hepatic-vein pressure) greater than 5 mm Hg, but usually become clinically significant when this gradient reaches 10 mm Hg. Portal venous pressure normally ranges from 7 to 10 mm Hg. In portal hypertension, portal pressure exceeds 10 mm Hg, averaging around 20 mm Hg and occasionally rising as high as 50-60 mm Hg. With those portal pressures, since the venous pressure in the right atrium averages 5 mm Hg, the HVPG can easily become greater than 5 mm Hg.

Since pressure in the portal venous system is determined by the relationship Pressure = Flow × Resistance, portal hypertension could result either from increased volume of portal blood flow or increased resistance to flow. Portal hypertension can be classified by pathophysiologic processes as summarized in Table 24–4.

In practice, however, the liver has tremendous reserve capacity to accommodate increased blood flow, and portal hypertension solely due to this mechanism is extremely uncommon. Increased flow may contribute to portal

hypertension in patients with arterial-portal venous fistulae (traumatic, congenital). When an arteriovenous fistula occurs, portal hypertension and its clinical manifestations usually do not appear for several months, because sinusoidal capacity is so great that the immediate rise in portal pressure is only moderate. With time, however, sinusoidal sclerosis develops, resistance increases, and portal pressure gradually reaches high levels, leading to the formation of varices.

Nearly all clinically relevant cases of portal hypertension result from increased resistance, in itself due to both structural distortion of the liver vascular architecture by fibrosis and dynamic increases in hepatic vascular tone. In addition to increased vascular resistance in the liver, splanchnic vascular bed resistance decreases, a consequence of local production of vasodilators (eg, nitric oxide) and mesenteric angiogenesis, paradoxically worsening the portal hypertension by increasing the splanchnic blood flow to the liver.

The average portal flow in cirrhotic patients with complications of portal hypertension is nonetheless about 30% of normal, ranging from 0 to 700 mL/min. Hepatic arterial flow is usually reduced by a similar proportion. The range of portal flow rates in different patients may vary greatly; in some, blood in the portal vein moves sluggishly or the direction of flow may even be reversed (hepatofugal) so that the portal vein functions as an outflow tract from the liver. These states of low flow predispose to spontaneous thrombosis of the portal vein, a complication of cirrhosis seen in 16% per year in patients with advanced liver disease. Portal thrombosis usually is associated with acute clinical deterioration and renders the portal vein unsuitable for a shunt to decompress the portal venous system.

Fluctuations in the level of portal hypertension may occur in conjunction with changes in blood volume. This is almost never a problem in patients with a normal liver. However, administration of colloid solutions to a patient with underlying liver disease and a normal or expanded blood volume could theoretically aggravate the clinical manifestations of portal hypertension.

A. Disease-Specific Pathophysiology

In alcoholic liver disease, the abnormal resistance is predominantly hepatic and postsinusoidal, as indicated by the results of wedged hepatic vein pressure studies.* The causes of increased resistance in this disease are thought to be: (1) distortion of the hepatic veins by regenerative nodules and

---

*A catheter wedged in a tributary of the hepatic vein permits estimation of the pressure in the afferent veins to the sinusoid. The gradient between the wedged pressure and that in the hepatic vein reflects resistance at any point between the wedged position and the periphery of the sinusoid. The current view holds that the site of principal resistance in normal persons is in reasonably large hepatic veins. In cirrhosis, it is probably in the sinusoids as well as the hepatic veins.

(2) fibrosis of perivascular tissue around the hepatic veins and the sinusoids.

Even in the absence of cirrhosis, acute alcoholic hepatitis can raise portal pressure by producing centrilobular swelling and fibrosis. Sinusoidal resistance to flow is also increased by engorgement of adjacent hepatocytes with fat and resultant distortion and narrowing of vascular channels. Documented cases of normalization or reduction in portal pressure have occurred with resolution of the pathologic changes.

Schistosomiasis can produce a unique form of hepatic presinusoidal obstruction to blood flow from deposition of parasite ova in small portal venules. The subsequent chronic inflammatory reaction leads to fibrosis and cirrhosis. Many patients with schistosomiasis are also at risk for chronic hepatitis, which can exacerbate the liver damage.

BCS (hepatic vein thrombosis) results from obstruction of flow through the hepatic veins. The resulting sinusoidal hypertension produces prominent ascites and hepatomegaly. Conditions (veno-occlusive disease, inferior vena cava obstruction by tumor or congenital webs, right-sided heart failure) that reduce flow through the hepatic veins result in a similar clinical picture.

Banti syndrome was defined as liver disease secondary to primary splenic disease and was incorrectly considered as the cause of portal hypertension now known to result from cirrhosis and other hepatic disorders rather than a consequence of such conditions. Portal hypertension from splenomegaly and increased splenic vein flow has been described in patients with hematologic diseases or tropical splenomegaly and apparently normal liver function. This is extremely uncommon, however, and given the great reserve of the liver to handle increases in portal flow, many such patients probably have some component of liver disease. In cirrhosis, the increased splenic blood flow accompanying "congestive" splenomegaly may occasionally be great enough to warrant splenic artery ligation or splenectomy to decrease portal pressure and improve symptoms, but this situation is rare.

B. Development of Portosystemic Collaterals and Varices

The obstacle to flow through the liver promotes expansion of collateral channels between the portal and systemic venous systems. As the pathologic process develops, portal pressure increases until a level of about 40 cm H_2O (30 mm Hg) is reached. At this point, increasing hepatic resistance, even to the point of occlusion of the portal vein, diverts a greater fraction of portal flow through collaterals without significant increments in portal pressure.

The type of portosystemic collaterals that develops depends partly on the cause of the portal hypertension. In extrahepatic portal vein thrombosis (without liver disease), collaterals in the diaphragm and in the hepatocolic, hepatoduodenal, and gastrohepatic ligaments transport blood into the liver around the occluded vein (hepatopetal). In cirrhosis, collateral vessels circumvent the liver and deliver portal blood directly into the systemic circulation (hepatofugal); these collaterals give rise to esophageal and gastric varices. Other common spontaneous collaterals are through a recanalized umbilical vein to the abdominal wall, from the superior hemorrhoidal vein into the middle and inferior hemorrhoidal veins, and through numerous small veins (of Retzius) connecting the retroperitoneal viscera with the posterior abdominal wall.

Isolated thrombosis of the splenic vein causes localized splenic venous hypertension and gives rise to large collaterals from spleen to gastric fundus (sinistral, or left-sided, portal hypertension). From there, the blood returns to the main portal system through the coronary vein. In this condition, gastric varices are often present without esophageal varices.

Of the many large collaterals that form as a result of portal hypertension, spontaneous bleeding is relatively uncommon except from those at the gastroesophageal junction; spontaneous bleeding from gastric varices can sometimes occur and carries a higher rate of death than gastroesophageal varices. Compared with adjacent areas of the esophagus and stomach, the gastroesophageal junction is especially rich in submucosal veins, which expand disproportionately in patients with portal hypertension. The cause of variceal bleeding is most probably rupture due to sudden increases in hydrostatic pressure. Esophagitis is usually mild or absent.

Garcia-Pagan JC, Valla DC. Portal vein thrombosis: a predictable milestone in cirrhosis? *J Hepatol* 2009;51:632.

Merkel C, Montagese S. Hepatic venous pressure gradient measurement in clinical hepatology. *Dig Liver Dis* 2011;43:762.

Sanyal AJ et al. Portal hypertension and its complications. *Gastroenterology* 2008;134:1715.

Thabut D, Moreau R, Lebrec D. Noninvasive assessment of portal hypertension in patients with cirrhosis. *Hepatology* 2011;53:683.

ACUTELY BLEEDING VARICES

Varices develop in 5%-15% of cirrhotic patients per year. Most patients with cirrhosis develop varices, but only about one-third experience variceal hemorrhage. Each bleeding episode is associated with a mortality rate of up to 25%, and 70% of untreated patients die within a year of the first episode. This high death rate reflects not only the massive hemorrhage but also the frequent presence of severely compromised liver function and other systemic disease that may or may not be related to alcohol abuse. Malnutrition, pulmonary aspiration, infections, and coronary artery disease are frequent coexisting conditions. Additional complicating factors in this patient population include lack of cooperation with treatment and acute alcohol withdrawal, which in its worst manifestation (delirium tremens) adds greatly to the already high mortality rate.

▶ Clinical Findings

A. Symptoms and Signs

If cirrhosis or varices have been documented on previous examinations, hematemesis would strongly suggest bleeding varices as the cause. Patient with significant hemorrhage present with alteration of mental status, hypotension, and tachycardia, often in hypovolemic shock. It must be emphasized that bleeding from varices cannot be accurately diagnosed on clinical grounds alone even though the history or the appearance of the patient may strongly suggest the presence of cirrhosis or portal hypertension. Most patients with bleeding varices have alcoholic cirrhosis, and the diagnosis may seem obvious in a patient with hepatomegaly, jaundice, and vascular spiders who admits to recent binge drinking. Splenomegaly, the most constant physical finding, is present in 80% of patients with portal hypertension regardless of the cause. Ascites is frequently present. Massive ascites and hepatosplenomegaly in a nonalcoholic would suggest the much less common BCS.

B. Laboratory Findings

Most patients with alcoholic liver disease and acute upper gastrointestinal bleeding have compromised liver function. The bilirubin is usually elevated, and the serum albumin is often below 3 g/dL. The leukocyte count may be elevated. Anemia may be a reflection of chronic alcoholic liver disease or hypersplenism as well as acute hemorrhage. The development of a hepatoma by a cirrhotic may first manifest by hemorrhage from varices; CT scan and marked elevation of the serum α-fetoprotein make the diagnosis. Thrombocytopenia and coagulopathy are common.

Table 24–5. First line management of acute bleeding from esophageal varices.

1. Medical–vasoconstrictor
  Somatostatin analogs
  Vasopressin, terlipressin
2. Medical–antibioprophylaxis
  Norfloxacin, ciprofloxacin
  Ceftriaxone (if doubt of quinolone resistance)
3. Interventional, nonsurgical
  Endoscopic variceal ligation
  Transjugular intrahepatic portosystemic shunt (TIPS)
4. Mechanical
  Balloon tamponade (Sengstaken–Blakemore)
5. Surgical
  Emergency portasystemic shunts
  Esophageal transection and reanastomosis
  Esophagogastric devascularization
  Suture ligation of varices

▶ Treatment of Acute Bleeding

The general goal of treatment is to control the bleeding as quickly and reliably as possible using methods with the fewest possible side effects. The methods in use for acute variceal bleeding are listed in Table 24–5 and presented into a current treatment algorithm in Figure 24–6. Over the past decades, improvement in medical, endoscopic, and endovascular technique studied in the setting of randomized control trials has lessened the need for surgical interventions.

The initial management of the patient with massive gastrointestinal hemorrhage is discussed in Chapter 23. Critical initial steps include airway protection, particularly in patients with altered mental status or those with hemodynamic instability, and resuscitation with fluid and blood products. In the cirrhotic patients, correction of coagulopathy and thrombocytopenia should also be initiated early. Patients admitted with variceal hemorrhage are often

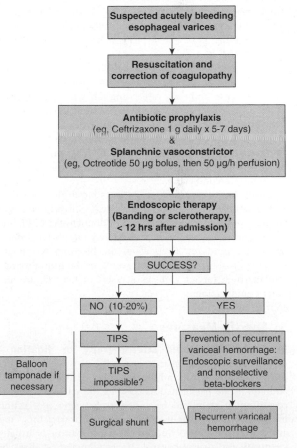

▲ **Figure 24–6.** Algorithm for the management of acute variceal bleeding.

bacteremic as a result of a concomitant infectious process (spontaneous bacterial peritonitis, urinary tract infection, or pneumonia). Clinical trials have shown better outcomes when empiric antibiotic therapy is initiated during an episode of variceal bleed, and usually a third-generation cephalosporin such as ceftriaxone is favored.

Vasoconstrictive drugs which reduce portal pressure (somatostatin and vasopressin analogs) and endoscopic variceal ablation (ligation and sclerotherapy) are the mainstay of initial management. The combined pharmacologic and endoscopic therapy has been shown in single trials and meta-analysis to be more effective in controlling acute bleeding than endoscopic treatment alone. With this initial strategy, control of bleeding can be achieved in 80%-85% of episodes. Endoscopic intervention requires a skilled endoscopist; banding has been shown effective and is considered the treatment of choice, although very profuse bleeding makes ligation a challenge, and sclerotherapy with cyanoacrylate may be useful in this setting if special expertise is available. Balloon tamponade is no longer used routinely but is rather reserved for failure of the pharmacologic/endoscopic therapy for the hemodynamically unstable patients, and when the next line of treatment cannot readily be implemented.

The failure rate of the standard medical therapy for all comers is of 10%-20%, highest in patients with Child-Pugh class C disease, and early rebleeding rate has been reported in up to 30% of patients. Placement of a transjugular intrahepatic portosystemic shunt (TIPS) is currently considered the salvage therapy of choice in this situation. TIPS may not be an option in some cases, for example in face of portal thrombosis, in which situation surgical shunt or devascularization procedures are indicated.

Death rates rise rapidly in patients requiring more than 10 units of blood, and in general, patients still bleeding after 6 units—or those whose bleeding is still unchecked 24 hours after admission—should be considered for portal decompression procedures. Even when the bleeding is brought under control by the initial intervention, the mortality rate remains high (about 35%) as a result of liver failure and other complications.

▶ Specific Measures

1. Acute endoscopic sclerotherapy or ligation— Emergency esophagogastroscopy is the most useful procedure for the diagnosis and the treatment of bleeding varices and should be performed as soon as the patient's general condition is stabilized by blood transfusion, correction of coagulopathy, administration of vasoconstrictors, and antibiotics are given. Endotracheal intubation is usually necessary for airway control. Varices appear as three or four large, tortuous submucosal bluish vessels running lon-

gitudinally in the distal esophagus. The bleeding site may be identified, but in some cases the lumen fills with blood so rapidly that the lesion is obscured. Using fiber-optic endoscopy, 13 mL of sclerosant solution is injected into the lumen of each varix, causing it to become thrombosed. Variations in the type of endoscope or sclerosant solution or whether or not the varices are physically compressed appear to have little influence on the outcome. Endoscopy is usually repeated within 48 hours and then once or twice again at weekly intervals, at which time any residual varices are injected.

Sclerotherapy controls acute bleeding in 80%-85% of patients, and rebleeding during the same hospitalization is about half (25% vs. 50%) the rebleeding rate of patients treated with a combination of vasopressin and balloon tamponade. Even though controlled trials show improvement in the control of bleeding with sclerotherapy, the evidence for increased patient survival is conflicting.

A similar effect is achieved by endoscopic ligation of the varices. The varix is lifted with a suction tip, and a small rubber band is slipped around the base. The varix necroses to leave a superficial ulcer. Several controlled trials have reported rubber band ligation to be more effective in controlling long-term bleeding episodes compared to sclerotherapy, although comparisons in the acute setting are limited. Band ligation is associated with fewer complications and fewer procedures are needed for complete eradication and has thus emerged as the initial endoscopic treatment of choice.

2. Somatostatin and analogs—Octreotide (brand name Sandostatin), is an octapeptide that mimics the hormone somatostatin pharmacologically. Purified somatostatin is not available in the United States. Somatostatin infusion reduces portal pressure without any impact on systemic hemodynamics; this effect may be less pronounced for octreotide. Somatostatin has been shown, in a prospective randomized trial, to effectively control acute bleeding, although other studies have had equivocal results. A meta-analysis of all studies using somatostatin or its analogs did show a significant risk reduction in control of hemorrhage. The efficacy of octreotide remains uncertain, but it appears to reduce the rebleeding rate when used in conjunction with endoscopic therapy. It should be emphasized that no study of somatostatin or octreotide has shown improved survival after an acute bleeding episode. Octreotide is given as an initial bolus of 50 μg followed by a continuous infusion of 50 μg/h for 2-5 days.

3. Vasopressin and analogs—Vasopressin and its analog terlipressin (triglycyl lysine vasopressin) lower portal blood flow and portal pressure by directly constricting splanchnic arterioles, thereby reducing inflow. Vasopressin or terlipressin alone controls acute bleeding in about 80%-85% of patients, and this rate is increased when combined with endoscopic therapy or balloon tamponade. Cardiac output, oxygen delivery to the tissues, hepatic blood flow, and renal blood flow are also decreased—effects that occasionally produce complications such as myocardial infarction, cardiac arrhythmias, and intestinal necrosis. These unwanted side effects may sometimes be prevented without interfering with the decrease in portal pressure by simultaneous administration of nitroglycerin or isoproterenol. Terlipressin has fewer untoward cardiovascular side effects than vasopressin.

Although the results are somewhat contradictory, controlled trials generally indicate that vasopressin plus nitroglycerin is superior to vasopressin alone and that vasopressin alone is superior to placebo in controlling active variceal bleeding. Survival is not increased, however. In fact, while several vasoactive agents effectively stop acute hemorrhage, only terlipressin has been shown to improve survival after an acute event. Vasopressin is given as a peripheral intravenous infusion (at about 0.4 units/min), which is safer than bolus injections. Nitroglycerin can be given intravenously or sublingually. Terlipressin undergoes gradual conversion to vasopressin in the body and is safe to give by intravenous bolus injection (2 mg intravenously every 6 hours); this drug is, however, not available in the United States.

4. Balloon Tamponade—Tubes designed for tamponade have two balloons that can be inflated in the lumen of the gut to compress bleeding varices. There are three or four lumens in the tube, depending on the type: two are for filling balloons within the stomach and the esophagus, and the third permits aspiration of gastric contents. A fourth lumen in the Minnesota tube is used to aspirate the esophagus orad to the esophageal balloon. The main effect results from traction applied to the tube, which forces the gastric balloon, generally inflated first and with 200 mL of air, to compress the collateral veins at the cardia of the stomach. Inflating the esophageal balloon probably contributes little, since barium x-rays suggest that it does not actually compress the varices (Figure 24–7).

The most common serious complication is aspiration of pharyngeal secretions and pneumonitis. Another serious hazard is the occasional instance of esophageal rupture caused by inflation of the esophageal balloon. The esophageal balloon is therefore infrequently used.

About 75% of actively bleeding patients can be controlled by balloon tamponade, usually applied for 6-12 hours. When bleeding has stopped, the balloons are left inflated for another 24 hours. They are then decompressed, leaving the tube in place. If bleeding does not recur, the tube should be withdrawn. The efficacy of other therapies combined with potential complications associated with balloon catheters have led to a marked reduction in the use of the latter approach, which is now reserved as a salvage treatment or

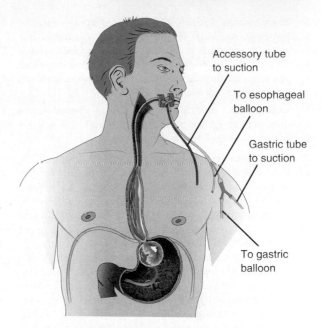

▲ **Figure 24–7.** Sengstaken–Blakemore tube with both gastric and esophageal balloons inflated.

temporary bridge in patients who fail medical and endoscopic therapy.

5. Transjugular Intrahepatic Portosystemic Shunt—TIPS is a minimally invasive means of creating a portosystemic shunt by creating a direct communication between the portal and hepatic venous systems within the liver parenchyma. A catheter is introduced through the jugular vein and, under radiologic control, positioned in the hepatic vein. From this point, the portal vein is accessed through the liver, the tract is dilated, and the channel is kept open by inserting an expandable metal stent, which is left in place. This technique is of great value in controlling portal hypertension and variceal bleeding and is used most commonly as a salvage therapy to stop acute bleeding for the 10%-20% of patients in whom medical and endoscopic therapy fails. TIPS is also indicated to prevent rebleeding in patients with advanced liver disease at high risk for recurrent variceal bleeding. In this latter category of patients, early use of TIPS has been shown in randomized controlled trial to improve survival. The shunt remains open in most patients for up to a year, at which point intimal overgrowth lead to thrombosis and occlusion in many cases. The use of polytetrafluoroethylene (PTFE)-covered stents now appears to have improved the patency rate.

TIPS should not be regarded as definitive therapy, however, even though the shunt usually remains patent for many months. Patients with advanced liver disease are the principal candidates for TIPS, proved most useful as a bridge to transplantation. Patients with less severe cirrhosis should generally be considered for beta-blocker therapy and in some cases for surgical devascularization procedure when transplantation is not a suitable option.

6. Surgery—The operative procedures to control active bleeding are emergency portosystemic shunt and variceal ligation or esophageal transection.

A. Emergency portacaval shunt—Although TIPS, when technically feasible, has largely supplanted more invasive surgical shunts as a salvage procedure for variceal bleed, emergency portacaval shunt success has a success rate of 95% in stopping bleeding in this context. The death rate of the operation is not insignificant, generally related to the status of the patient's liver function (eg, Child–Pugh classification; Table 24–1) as well as the rate and amount of bleeding and its effects on cardiac, renal, and pulmonary function. Some patients with advanced liver disease, especially those with severe encephalopathy and ascites, have an extraordinarily poor survival regardless of the treatment. In such patients, surgery is usually not warranted, even in the face of continued bleeding. On the other hand, patients with good liver function usually recover after an emergency shunt. A controlled trial showed that the death rate in acutely bleeding Child–Pugh C patients was insignificantly lower after endoscopic sclerotherapy (44%) than after emergency portacaval shunt (50%).

For active bleeding, a nonselective end-to-side portacaval shunt is most commonly performed (Figure 24–8C). A side-to-side portacaval shunt might be preferable in an acutely bleeding patient with severe ascites (Figure 24–8B), and this approach (or a variant such as an H-mesocaval shunt) would be required for someone with BCS.

The central splenorenal shunt, in which the portal vein is decompressed via the splenic vein into the left renal vein, is more complicated than portacaval shunts and has no specific advantages. Selective shunts, such as the distal splenorenal (Warren) shunt, in which the gastrosplenic collaterals are decompressed via the splenic vein into the left renal vein, leaving the portal vein intact, are usually too time-consuming for use in emergency operations.

Although the risk of variceal rebleeding is low, approximately 40% of patients develop encephalopathy after portacaval surgical shunting. Hepatic insufficiency is accelerated and liver failure is the cause of death in about two-thirds of those who die after an emergency portacaval shunt. Portacaval shunts can also render liver transplantation more difficult. Renal failure, which is often accompanied by ascites, is another potentially lethal problem. Metabolic alkalosis and delirium tremens are not uncommon postoperatively in alcoholics.

B. Esophageal transection—Varices may be obliterated by firing the end-to-end stapler in the distal esophagus after tucking a full-thickness ring of tissue into the cartridge with a circumferential tie. This procedure has gained popularity in the past decade, and in many surgical units it is considered a last resort therapy when nonsurgical methods fail.

If transection is performed, it must be done as soon as it is recognized that a second attempt at sclerotherapy or band ligation has failed. The results (eg, survival) are better in patients with nonalcoholic cirrhosis. Stapled transection has replaced the older technique of direct suture ligation of the varices. Transection must be viewed as an emergency measure to stop persistent bleeding—not as definitive treatment—since the underlying portal hypertension is not corrected and varices recur months later in many patients.

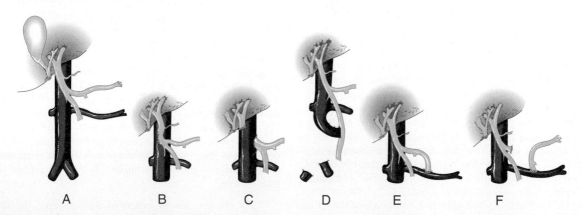

▲ **Figure 24–8.** Types of portacaval anastomoses: **A:** Normal. **B:** Side-to-side. **C:** End-to-side. **D:** Mesocaval. **E:** Central splenorenal. **F:** Distal splenorenal (Warren). The H-mesocaval shunt is not illustrated.

Bambha K et al. Predictors of early re-bleeding and mortality after acute variceal hemorrhage in patients with cirrhosis. *Gut* 2008;57:814.

Bendtsen F, Krag A, Moller S. Treatment of acute variceal bleeding. *Dig Liver Dis* 2008;40:328.

Bosch J et al. Recombinant factor VIIa for variceal bleeding in patients with advanced cirrhosis: a randomized, controlled trial. *Hepatology* 2008;47:1604.

Garcia-Pagan JC et al. Early use of TIPS in patients with cirrhosis and variceal bleeding. *N Engl J Med* 2010;362:2370-2379.

Gonzalez R et al. Combination endoscopic and drug therapy to prevent variceal rebleeding in cirrhosis. *Ann Intern Med* 2008;149:109.

Mercado MA et al. Comparative study of 2 variants of a modified esophageal transection in the Sugiura-Futagawa operation. *Arch Surg* 1998;133:1046.

NONBLEEDING VARICES

Gastroesophageal varices are present in almost half of patients with cirrhosis at the time of diagnosis. Development and growth of esophageal varices each occur at a rate of 7% per year. Patients with varices that have never bled have a 30% chance of bleeding at some point; of those who bleed, 50% die. For patients who do not bleed during the first year after diagnosis of varices, the risk of bleeding subsequently decreases by half and continues to drop thereafter. Patients who have bled once from esophageal varices have a 60%-70% chance of bleeding again, and about two-thirds of repeat bleeding episodes are fatal.

► Evaluation

A. Portal Flow and Pressure Measurements

Measurements of pressure and flow in the splanchnic vasculature have been used for diagnosis and as a guide to therapy and prognosis in portal hypertension. Portal pressure can be measured directly at surgery or preoperatively by any of the following techniques:

1. Wedged hepatic venous pressure (WHVP) accurately reflects free portal pressure when portal hypertension is caused by a postsinusoidal (or sinusoidal) resistance, as in cirrhosis. The portal pressure can be determined with the catheter in the wedged position, corrected by subtracting the free hepatic venous pressure; the HVPG (the pressure gradient from the portal to the hepatic venous systems) can also be determined. This is the most commonly used technique.

2. Direct measurement of splenic pulp pressure is obtained by a percutaneously placed needle.

3. Percutaneous transhepatic catheterization of the intrahepatic branches of the portal vein is the method of choice in patients thought to have presinusoidal block or BCS.

4. Catheterization of the umbilical vein is accomplished through a small incision, and the catheter is threaded into the portal system. With each of these methods, one may also obtain anatomic information by performing angiography through the catheter.

HVPG predicts decompensation and death. Reduction in the HVPG, either spontaneously or after therapy, may help predict the risk of rebleeding in some patients. It has therefore been suggested that HVPG can be used to guide therapy. However, its value currently has been shown primarily in alcoholic liver disease. Also, it is an invasive study that requires special expertise and is not always readily available. Duplex ultrasonography is an accurate noninvasive means of assessing the amount and direction of flow in the portal vein. Preoperatively, duplex ultrasonography is useful to determine patency of the portal vein and direction of flow. Because of spontaneous thrombosis, about 10% of patients with cirrhosis have a portal vein unsuitable for a portacaval shunt. If flow in the portal vein is reversed (hepatofugal), a selective shunt (eg, splenorenal, distal) is not recommended, because it compromises the ability of portal tributaries to serve as an outflow tract for liver blood. Duplex ultrasonography can also be used to follow changes in portal perfusion after shunt operations.

B. Portal Angiography

The portal venous anatomy is often studied preoperatively by angiographic techniques. The objectives are to determine the patency, location, and size of the veins tentatively chosen for a shunt, to demonstrate the presence of varices, and to estimate the degree of prograde portal flow. Some of this information can now be obtained less invasively by duplex ultrasonography. When a splenorenal shunt is contemplated, the left renal vein should be opacified, either by injection of the renal artery or renal vein.

► Treatment

The treatment options consist of expectant management, endoscopic sclerotherapy, nonselective beta-blocker (eg, propranolol, nadolol), portosystemic shunts, devascularization of the esophagogastric junction, and miscellaneous rarely used operations. The treatment of patients with varices that have never bled is usually referred to as prophylactic therapy (eg, prophylactic endoscopic variceal ligation (EVL) or prophylactic propranolol). By convention, procedures performed on patients who have bled previously are referred to as therapeutic (eg, therapeutic shunts).

A. Prophylactic Therapy

Prophylactic therapy is of value, since the mortality rate of variceal bleeding is high (25%), the risk of bleeding in patients with varices is relatively high (30%), and varices can often be diagnosed before the initial episode of bleeding. In patients who have never had a bleeding episode, the following have been shown to be related to the risk of hemorrhage: Child–Pugh classification, the size of the varices, and the presence of red wale markings (longitudinal dilated venules resembling whip marks) on the varices. This information can be used to identify high-risk patients (up to 65% risk of bleeding within a year) who are most likely to benefit from prophylactic treatment.

In cirrhotic patients without varices, treatment with nonselective beta-blockers is not recommended because they do not prevent the development of varices and are associated with side effects. In patients with low-risk varices (small, no red wale marks, no severe liver dysfunction), nonselective beta-blockers may delay variceal growth and thereby prevent hemorrhage. The alternative is to schedule periodic endoscopic screening for detection of variceal growth, at what time medical treatment can be initiated.

In patients who have never bled but have a high risk (medium to large varices or small varices with red wale markings and/or decompensated cirrhosis), EVL, or nonselective beta-blockers are considered equally adequate, as high-quality randomized controlled trial have concluded to similar survival of patients with either approaches. It has been suggested that beta-blocker therapy should be the first-line treatment, with EVL used in patients who cannot tolerate or have contraindications to beta-blockade. Endoscopic sclerotherapy is no longer routinely used as primary prophylaxis. More recently, low-dose carvediol as shown lower rates of first variceal hemorrhage when compared to EVL (10% vs. 23%), but those results needs to be validated in other trials.

B. Therapy of Patients Who Have Bled Previously

As noted earlier, patients who recover from an episode of variceal bleeding have an approximately 60%-70% chance of bleeding again. Much effort has been expended to ascertain the best treatment for these patients. The methods of greatest interest include nonselective beta-blocker therapy, endoscopic band ligation, and portosystemic shunts.

1. Nonselective beta-blocker therapy—As with patients with esophageal varices who have never bled, nonselective beta-adrenergic blocking agents (propranolol, nadolol) effectively reduce the risk of recurrent bleeding episodes. These agents work by decreasing cardiac output and splanchnic blood flow and consequently portal blood pressure. Chronic propranolol therapy, 20-160 mg twice daily (a dose that reduces resting pulse rate by 25%), decreases by about 40% the frequency of rebleeding from esophageal or gastric varices, deaths from rebleeding, and overall mortality. The benefits are greater in Child–Pugh A and

B than in Child–Pugh C cirrhotics. Beta-blocker therapy has been compared to endoscopic sclerotherapy, with no difference in rebleeding or mortality seen but with higher complications in the sclerotherapy group. On the other hand, randomized controlled trials have shown that the combined use of EVL and nonselective beta blockers could further lower the risk of rebleeding. The addition of nitrate drugs to beta-blocker therapy appears to result in a greater reduction of portal pressure compared to beta-blockade alone. This approach is often favored in patients who are not candidates for EVL. Abstinence from alcohol should always be emphasized and may help prevent further bleeding but may not necessarily decrease the mortality related specifically to variceal hemorrhage, as was previously thought.

2. Endoscopic band ligation— Endoscopic band ligation, as described earlier, is an effective means of preventing recurrent bleeding episodes and has been shown to be superior to sclerotherapy in this regard. Both band ligation and beta-blocker therapy appear to be similarly effective in preventing rebleeding. However, the combination of both therapies has been shown to significantly reduce not only the risk of rebleeding but also the recurrence of varices. Thus, combination therapy appears to be the most effective treatment after an initial bleeding episode.

3. Endoscopic sclerotherapy—The technique of endoscopic sclerotherapy was described earlier in this chapter. Sclerotherapy was previously used routinely to reduce the risk of rebleeding but has been replaced by band ligation.

4. Transjugular intrahepatic portosystemic shunt—The TIPS technique is described in the preceding section. TIPS is effective in preventing rebleeding episodes, more so than either endoscopic or pharmacologic therapy alone. However, this advantage is offset by its higher morbidity and mortality rate from the development of hepatic encephalopathy and liver failure. For this reason, as well as the lack of a clear survival or cost-benefit advantage, TIPS is used mainly to salvage patients who fail endoscopic and/or pharmacologic treatment.

TIPS has generally superseded shunt surgery in most patients who fail first-line therapy. A recent large multicenter randomized trial showed that TIPS and surgical shunts had similar rates of rebleeding, encephalopathy, and mortality in Child–Pugh A and B cirrhotic patients. There was a higher incidence of shunt dysfunction in the TIPS patients, perhaps because of the type of stent used, the first generation not being covered with PTFE. The use of TIPS covered with PTFE has significantly lower occlusion rate. The choice between TIPS and surgical shunts therefore currently depends on expertise, anatomical considerations, and patient's preference.

C. Surgical Approaches

The objective of surgical procedures used to treat portal hypertension is either to obliterate the varices or to reduce blood flow and pressure within the varices (Table 24–6). A third option, liver transplantation, can treat both the underlying liver dysfunction and the portal hypertension.

1. Liver transplantation—Any relatively young patient with cirrhosis who has survived an episode of variceal hemorrhage should be considered a candidate for liver transplantation, since any other form of therapy carries a much higher (about 80%) mortality rate within the subsequent 1-2 years as a result of repeat bleeding or complications of hepatic failure. Obviously, continued alcohol use is a contraindication to transplantation in most patients. The good transplantation candidates, however, should not be subjected to portosystemic shunts or other procedures if it appears that they will come to transplantation in the near future. In general, Child-Pugh A patients are candidates for portal decompression; Child-Pugh C patients are candidates for a transplant. A TIPS (see previous section) is an excellent way to control bleeding while the patient is being prepared for a transplant.

2. Portosystemic shunts—The advent of TIPS has resulted in a marked decline in the number of shunt operations performed. However, surgical shunts are durable, and good risk patients appear to benefit from these procedures.

Portosystemic shunts can be grouped into those that shunt the entire portal system (total shunts) and those that selectively shunt blood from the gastrosplenic region while preserving the pressure-flow relationships in the rest of the portal bed (selective shunts). All of the shunt operations commonly used today reduce the incidence of rebleeding to less than 10%, compared with about 75% in unshunted patients. Unfortunately, the price of this achievement is an operative mortality rate of 5%-20% (depending on the Child–Pugh classification), further impairment of liver function, and an increase in encephalopathy (greater with total shunts). Therefore, since shunts have these potential drawbacks, clinical trials are needed to pinpoint their place within an overall treatment strategy.

In one well-designed trial, patients who had bled previously were randomized to chronic sclerotherapy or a distal splenorenal shunt (Warren shunt, Figure 24–8F). Patients randomized to chronic sclerotherapy who had recurrent episodes of bleeding during treatment (ie, treatment failures, which amounted to 30% of the sclerotherapy group) were then treated surgically (ie, shunted). The results showed that 2-year survival was better among those originally randomized to sclerotherapy (90%) than among those originally assigned to the shunt group (60%). This trial supports a general treatment plan consisting initially of endoscopic therapy and reserving portosystemic shunts for the patients in whom the former fails to control bleeding adequately (Figure 24–6).

The choice of shunt has been the subject of much debate and several randomized trials. The principal question in recent years has been whether encephalopathy and survival are better with a selective shunt (eg, a distal splenorenal shunt, Figure 24–8F) than with a total shunt (eg, a mesocaval or an end-to-side portacaval shunt, Figure 24–8 C and 24–8 D). The results are conflicting, but in general they support the contention that there is about half as much severe encephalopathy following selective shunts. None of the trials have shown any particular shunt to be associated with longer survival.

3. Severity of hepatic disease and operative risk—The immediate death rate of an elective shunt procedure can be

Table 24–6. Surgical procedures for esophageal varices.

A. Direct variceal obliteration
  1. Variceal suture ligation
    a. Transthoracic
    b. Transabdominal
  2. Esophageal transection and reanastomosis
    a. Suture technique
    b. Staple technique
  3. Variceal sclerosis
    a. Esophagoscopic
    b. Transhepatic
  4. Variceal resection
    a. Esophagogastrectomy
    b. Subtotal esophagectomy

B. Reduction of variceal blood flow and pressure
  1. Portasystemic shunts
    a. End-to-side
    b. Side-to-side
      1. Side-to-side portacaval
      2. Mesocaval
      3. Central splenorenal
      4. Renosplenic
  2. Selective shunts
    a. Distal splenorenal (Warren)
    b. Left gastric vena caval (Inokuchi)
  3. Reduction of portal blood flow
    a. Splenectomy
    b. Splenic artery ligation
  4. Reduction of proximal gastric blood flow
    a. Esophagogastric devascularization
    b. Gastric transection and reanastomosis (Tanner)
  5. Stimulation of additional portasystemic venous collaterals
    a. Omentopexy
    b. Splenic transposition

C. Measures to preserve hepatic blood flow after portacaval shunt
  1. Arterialization of portal vein stump

predicted from the patient's hepatic function as reflected by the Child–Pugh classification (Table 24–1). In addition to operative death rate, the figures also correlate with the death rate in the first postshunt year. Thereafter, survival curves of the different risk classes become reasonably parallel.

The severity of histopathologic changes in liver biopsies correlates with the immediate surgical death rate, the most ominous findings being hepatocellular necrosis, polymorphonuclear leukocyte infiltration, and the presence of Mallory bodies. The extent of histologic change also correlates with the more easily obtained data in the Child–Pugh classification (ie, severe changes occur in class C patients), so results of biopsies have no independent predictive value.

A. Types of Portosystemic Shunts—Figure 24–8 depicts the various shunts in use currently. Although they differ technically, physiologically there are only three different types: end-to-side, side-to-side, and selective.

1. Total shunts—The end-to-side shunt completely disconnects the liver from the portal system. The portal vein is transected near its bifurcation in the liver hilum and anastomosed to the side of the inferior vena cava. The hepatic stump of the vein is oversewn. Postoperatively, the WHVP (sinusoidal pressure) drops slightly, reflecting the inability of the hepatic artery to compensate fully for the loss of portal inflow. The side-to-side portacaval, mesocaval, mesorenal, and central splenorenal shunts are all physiologically similar, since the shunt preserves continuity between the hepatic limb of the portal vein, the portal system, and the anastomosis. Flow through the hepatic limb of the standard side-to-side shunt is nearly always away from the liver and toward the anastomosis. The extent to which hepatofugal flow is produced by the other types of side-to-side shunts listed previously is not known.

The end-to-side portacaval shunt gives immediate and permanent protection from variceal bleeding and is somewhat easier to perform than a side-to-side portacaval or central splenorenal shunt. Encephalopathy may be slightly more common after side-to-side than end-to-side portacaval shunts. Side-to-side shunts are required in patients with BCS or refractory ascites (when the latter is treated by a portosystemic shunt).

The mesocaval shunt interposes a segment of prosthetic graft or internal jugular vein between the inferior vena cava and the superior mesenteric vein where the latter passes in front of the uncinate process of the pancreas. The mesocaval shunt is particularly useful in the presence of severe scarring in the right upper quadrant or portal vein thrombosis, and in some cases it may be technically easier than a conventional side-to-side portacaval shunt if a side-to-side type of shunt is necessary. In most cases, portal flow to the liver is lost after this shunt. Evidence has been presented, however, that by limiting the diameter of the prosthetic graft to 8 mm

(compared with 12- to 20-mm grafts), prograde flow is preserved in the portal vein, which decreases the incidence of postoperative encephalopathy while still preventing variceal hemorrhage.

2. Selective shunts—Selective shunts lower pressure in the gastroesophageal venous plexus while preserving blood flow through the liver via the portal vein.

The distal splenorenal (Warren) shunt involves anastomosing the distal (splenic) end of the transected splenic vein to the side of the left renal vein, plus ligation of the major collaterals between the remaining portal and isolated gastrosplenic venous system. The latter step involves division of the gastric vein, the right gastroepiploic vein, and the vessels in the splenocolic ligament. The operation is more difficult and time consuming than conventional shunts and except for the experienced operator is probably too complex for emergency portal decompression. If mobilization of the splenic vein is hazardous, the renal vein may be transected and its caval end joined to the side of the undisturbed splenic vein. The segment of splenic vein between the anastomosis and the portal vein is then ligated. Surprisingly, this seems to have little permanent effect on renal function as long as the remaining tributaries are preserved on the oversewn renal vein stump.

In contrast to total shunts, the Warren shunt does not improve ascites and should not be performed in patients whose ascites has been difficult to control. Preoperative angiography should be performed to determine if the splenic vein and left renal vein are large enough and close enough together for performance of this shunt. Recent pancreatitis may preclude safe dissection of the splenic vein from the undersurface of the pancreas.

Another type of selective shunt (Inokuchi shunt) consists of joining the left gastric vein to the inferior vena cava by a short segment of autogenous saphenous vein. The procedure has not become popular, perhaps because of its technical complexity.

Selective shunts tend to become less selective over several years as new collaterals develop between the high-pressure and low-pressure regions of the portal system. This is accompanied by a gradual decrease in portal pressure (measured by WHVP) and evolution of the procedure into a version of side-to-side total shunt. The enlargement postoperatively of small venous tributaries entering the distal splenic vein from the pancreas suggests that this is the path by which nonselectivity develops. It is possible that this can be avoided by mobilizing the splenic vein all the way to the hilum (dividing these small vessels) before performing the splenorenal anastomosis.

B. Choice of Shunt—A reasonable approach to shunt selection is as follows.

The distal splenorenal shunt is the first choice for elective portal decompression. If ascites is present or the anatomy is unfavorable, an end-to-side portacaval shunt is preferred. Side-to-side shunts would be done for patients with severe ascites or BCS. The H-mesocaval and central splenorenal shunts are reserved for special anatomic situations in which the above operations are unsuitable. An end-to-side shunt or H-mesocaval shunt is performed for emergency decompression.

Portacaval and distal splenorenal shunts are often followed by a rise in platelet count in patients with secondary hypersplenism. The response is unpredictable, however, and hypersplenism need not necessarily dictate the type of shunt since it rarely produces clinical manifestations. A central splenorenal shunt, in which splenectomy is performed, should not be considered preferable to other kinds of shunts just because the patient has a low platelet count.

C. RESULTS OF PORTOSYSTEMIC SHUNTS—Over 90% of portosystemic shunts remain patent, and the incidence of recurrent variceal bleeding is less than 10%. The 5-year survival rate after a portacaval shunt for alcoholic liver disease averages 45%. Some degree of encephalopathy develops in 15%-25% of patients. Severe encephalopathy is seen in about 20% of alcoholics following a total shunt; its occurrence is not related to the severity of preshunt encephalopathy.

D. Devascularization Operations

The objective of devascularization is to destroy the venous collaterals that transport blood from the high-pressure portal system into the veins in the submucosa of the esophagus.

The Sugiura-Futugawa procedure initially described in 1973 was done in two stages. The first stage was performed through a thoracotomy and consisted in division of the dilated venous collaterals between esophagus and adjacent structures, transection of the esophagus at the level of the diaphragm, and reanastomosis. The second stage, a laparotomy, was performed immediately after the thoracotomy if the patient was actively bleeding or deferred 4-6 weeks in elective cases. In the second stage of the operation, the upper two-thirds of the stomach was devascularized, and selective vagotomy, pyloroplasty, and splenectomy performed.

More recently, an analogous one-stage operation has been described in many series and performed through laparotomy that consists of splenectomy, devascularization of 8-10 cm of distal esophagus, devascularization of the lesser and greater curvature with ligation of the left gastric and gastroepiploic vessels, transection and end-to-end anastomosis of the lower esophagus 4-5 cm above the gastroesophageal junction (EEA-stapler), pyloroplasty, and insertion of a feeding jejunostomy.

In Eastern and Western series published between 1980 and 1999, the operative mortality ranged from 0% to 36%, up to 80% in Child C patients, the variceal rebleeding rate from 0% to 37%, encephalopathy from 0% to 22%, and esophageal stenosis ranged from 2% to 37%. For cirrhotic patients with extensive portal thrombosis, for who portosystemic shunt cannot be performed, devascularization operations can offer a good alternative.

E. Miscellaneous Operations

Attempts have also been made to decrease portal pressure by decreasing splanchnic inflow through splenectomy or splenic artery ligation. Diseases characterized by marked splenomegaly may rarely be associated with portal hypertension as a consequence of increased splenic blood flow, which has been known to reach levels as high as 1000 mL/min. Splenic blood flow may occasionally be increased enough in patients with cirrhosis to contribute significantly to the portal hypertension. However, splenectomy or splenic artery ligation in cirrhosis most often gives only a transient decrease in portal pressure, and over half of patients having these operations bleed again. Some workers have suggested that the absolute size of the splenic artery (a crude index of splenic flow) correlates with the clinical effectiveness of splenic artery ligation, a good result being predictable if the diameter of the artery is 1 cm or greater.

Berzigotti A, Garcia-Pagan JC. Prevention of recurrent variceal bleeding. *Dig Liv Dis* 2008;40:337.

Garcia-Tsao G, Bosch J. Management of varices and variceal hemorrhage in cirrhosis. *N Engl J Med* 2010;362:823.

Garcia-Tsao G, Bosch J, Groszmann RJ. Portal hypertension and variceal bleeding: unresolved issues. Summary of an AASLD and EASLD single topic conference. *Hepatology* 2008;47:1764.

Gluud LL et al. Banding ligation versus beta-blockers as primary prophylaxis in esophageal varices: systematic review of randomized trials. *Am J Gastroenterol* 2007;102:2842.

Gonzalez R et al. Combination endoscopic and drug therapy to prevent variceal rebleeding in cirrhosis. *Ann Intern Med* 2008;149:109.

Henderson JM et al. Distal splenorenal shunt versus TIPS for refractory variceal bleeding: a prospective randomized controlled trial. *Gastroenterology* 2006;130:1643.

Masson S et al. Hepatic encephalopathy after transjugular intrahepatic portosystemic shunt insertion: a decade of experience. *QJM* 2008;101:493.

Tripathi D et al. Randomized controlled trial of carvediol versus variceal band ligation for the prevention of the first variceal bleed. *Hepatology* 2009;50:825.

Voros D et al. Long-term results with the modified Sugiura procedure for the management of variceal bleeding: standing the test of time in the treatment of bleeding esophageal varices. *Word J Surg* 2012;36:659.

EXTRAHEPATIC PORTAL VENOUS OCCLUSION

Extrahepatic portal vein obstruction is one of many causes of noncirrhotic portal hypertension, the other common cause being noncirrhotic portal fibrosis. These disorders are distinct but appear to share several similar etiological and pathogenetic features, the most notable of which is the clinical manifestation of portal hypertension in the absence of significant hepatic parenchymal dysfunction.

Idiopathic portal vein thrombosis (in the absence of liver disease) is a relatively common cause of portal hypertension in developing countries but is less prevalent in the West. This diagnosis accounts for most cases of portal hypertension in childhood (80%-90%) and for a smaller proportion of cases in adults. Neonatal septicemia, omphalitis, umbilical vein catheterization for exchange transfusion, and dehydration have all been incriminated as possible causes, but collectively they can be implicated in less than half of cases. The causes of portal vein thrombosis in adults include hepatic tumors, cirrhosis, trauma, pancreatitis, pancreatic pseudocyst, myelofibrosis, thrombotic states (eg, protein C deficiency), and sepsis; in particular, cirrhosis and/or hepatocellular carcinoma need to be considered in adult patients. In adult, systemic anticoagulation result in complete portal vein recanalization in approximately 38.3% of cases and partial recanalization in 15%.

Although clinical manifestations may be delayed until adulthood, 80% of patients with idiopathic portal vein thrombosis present between 1 and 6 years of age with variceal bleeding, although hemorrhage from ectopic varices at other locations in the gastrointestinal tract is not uncommon. About 70% of hemorrhages are preceded by a recent upper respiratory tract infection. Some of these children first come to medical attention because of splenomegaly and pancytopenia. Failure to recognize the underlying problem has occasionally led to splenectomy, with the result that portal decompression using the splenic vein is precluded. Ascites is uncommon except transiently after bleeding. Liver function is either normal or only slightly impaired, which probably accounts for the low incidence of overt encephalopathy. There is an increased frequency of neuropsychiatric problems, which may be a subtle form of encephalopathy.

Portal biliopathy refers to abnormalities of the extrahepatic bile ducts, usually the result of bile duct compression from large, dilated venous collaterals within the porta hepatis. These changes result in marked irregularities of the biliary wall that can progress to strictures and even obstructive jaundice and cholangitis in some cases; secondary biliary cirrhosis has been reported. Biliopathy is commonly seen on imaging studies, but most patients remain free of related symptoms.

Because the patient's general condition and liver function are good, the death rate for sudden massive bleeding is below that for other types of portal hypertension. The diagnosis can be confirmed with cross-sectional imaging or direct mesenteric angiography. WHVP is normal to slightly elevated; liver biopsies are normal or may show mild to moderate periportal fibrosis.

Bleeding episodes in children under age 8 years are usually self-limited and often do not require endoscopic sclerotherapy, administration of vasopressin, or balloon tamponade. Even if such interventions are necessary, however, the bleeding episodes are self-limited and uncommonly fatal, so emergency operations are rarely necessary.

Thrombosed portal veins are unsuitable for shunt procedures. Cavomesenteric shunts are best for young children, whose vessels are small. In older individuals, treatment should be started with sclerotherapy; if that fails to control the bleeding, a distal splenorenal shunt is preferred. Splenectomy alone has no permanent effect and sacrifices the splenic vein, which might be needed later for a shunt operation. Shunts in small children have a high rate of spontaneous thrombosis and should be avoided, if possible, until approximately 8-10 years of age, when the vessels are of larger caliber. Even still, using precise technique, some surgeons have obtained a high rate of anastomotic patency in the very young. Encephalopathy and hepatic dysfunction many years after a total shunt may be improved if converted to a selective shunt.

Splenectomy alone is never indicated in this disease, either for hypersplenism or in an attempt to reduce portal pressure, because the rebleeding rate is 90% and fatal postsplenectomy sepsis is not uncommon. If it is not possible to construct an adequate shunt, expectant management is the best strategy. Repeated severe bleeding episodes should be treated by transendoscopic sclerosis. Esophagogastrectomy with colonic interposition may be effective but should be considered a last resort.

Hall TC et al. Management of acute non-cirrhotic and non-malignant portal vein thrombosis: a systematic review. *World J Surg* 2011;35:2510.

Madhu K et al. Non-cirrhotic intrahepatic portal hypertension. *Gut* 2008;57:1529.

SPLENIC VEIN THROMBOSIS

Isolated thrombosis of the splenic vein is a rare cause of variceal bleeding that can be cured by splenectomy. The splenic venous blood, blocked from its normal route, flows through the short gastric vessels to the gastric fundus and then into the left gastric vein, continuing toward the liver. This phenomenon is called left-sided (or sinistral) portal hypertension. As the blood traverses the stomach, large gastric varices are produced that may rupture and bleed. Characteristically, the collateral pattern does not involve the esophagus, so esophageal varices are uncommon.

The principal causes of this syndrome are pancreatitis, pancreatic pseudocyst, neoplasm, and trauma. The mean incidence of splenic vein thrombosis associated with chronic and acute pancreatitis is estimated at 12.4% and 22.6% respectively, with an overall bleeding rate of 12.3%. Splenomegaly is present in two-thirds of patients. Diagnosis can be made by selective splenic arteriography that opacifies the venous phase, but more commonly nowadays on CT scan with portal phase imaging. Splenectomy is curative. Many cases of splenic vein thrombosis are unaccompanied by bleeding varices, and in such cases, no therapy is required. Treatment of acute bleeding from gastric varices is generally endoscopic, and endoscopic variceal obturation with tissue glue appears to be superior to band ligation or sclerotherapy.

Butler JR et al. Natural history of pancreatitis-induced splenic vein thrombosis: a systematic review and meta-analysis of its incidence and rate of gastrointestinal bleeding. *HPB* 2011;13:1477.

Strasberg SM et al. Pattern of venous collateral development after splenic vein occlusion in an extended Whipple procedure: comparison with collateral vein pattern in cases of sinistral portal hypertension. *J Gastrointest Surg* 2011;15:2070.

BUDD–CHIARI SYNDROME

BCS is a rare disorder resulting from obstruction of hepatic venous outflow, which can arise at several different levels, from the small hepatic venous tributaries within the liver parenchyma to the major hepatic venous trunks to the inferior vena cava up to the level of the right atrium. The prevalence of BCS is estimated as 1:100,000, and the largest published series reported on 237 patients treated at four centers in the United States, the Netherlands, and France between 1984 and 2001. Most cases are caused by spontaneous thrombosis of the hepatic veins, often associated with myeloproliferative disorders (polycythemia vera, essential thrombocytosis) or the use of birth control pills. Other common associated conditions include factor V Leiden and factor II gene mutations. Other predisposing factors include protein C and S deficiencies, antiphospholipid syndrome, antithrombin III deficiency, paroxysmal nocturnal hemoglobinuria, Behçet syndrome, and trauma. Some patients present with idiopathic membranous stenosis of the inferior vena cava located between the hepatic veins and right atrium, which is usually associated with secondary thrombosis of the hepatic veins; this condition appears to be more common in Asia than in Western countries. Many patients with BCS are HBsAg-positive, and others have malignancies (eg, hepatocellular carcinoma). Vena caval webs were once thought to be congenital, but more recent evidence suggests that they are the consequence of thrombus formation. Primary BCS originates from within the lumen of the hepatic veins or venules, and occlusion results from thrombosis, webs, or endophlebitis. By contrast, secondary BCS results from extrinsic compression of the venous outflow tract, usually related to a neoplasm or abscess.

Veno-occlusive disease and congestive hepatopathy are two conditions that can cause hepatic venous outflow obstruction, and although the clinical picture of both may be indistinguishable from that of BCS, they differ in the level of obstruction and in predisposing conditions. Veno-occlusive disease is primarily a problem affecting the sinusoids and

terminal venules, while congestive hepatopathy reflects a problem at the level of the heart.

Posthepatic (postsinusoidal) obstruction raises sinusoidal pressure, which is transmitted proximally to cause portal hypertension. Because the parenchyma is relatively free of fibrosis, filtration across the sinusoids and hepatic lymph formation increase greatly, producing marked ascites.

Symptoms usually begin with a mild prodrome consisting of vague right upper quadrant abdominal pain, postprandial bloating, and anorexia. After weeks or months, a more florid picture develops consisting of gross ascites, hepatomegaly, and hepatic failure. At this stage, the AST is usually markedly increased, the serum bilirubin is slightly elevated, and the alkaline phosphatase is inconsistently abnormal.

Except in patients with membranous obstruction of the vena cava, liver scans (CT or MRI) usually demonstrate a marked perfusion abnormality throughout most of the liver except for a small central area representing the caudate lobe, whose venous outflow is spared (it goes directly to the vena cava through multiple small tributaries). CT scans show pooling of intravenous contrast media in the periphery of the liver; patent hepatic veins cannot be seen on ultrasound scans. An enlarged azygos vein may be seen on chest x-rays of patients with caval obstruction. Liver biopsy reveals grossly dilated central veins and sinusoids, pericentral necrosis, and replacement of hepatocytes by red blood cells. Centrilobular fibrosis develops late. The clinical diagnosis should be confirmed by venography, which shows the hepatic veins to be obstructed, usually with a beaklike deformity at their orifice. The inferior vena cava should be opacified to verify its patency, which is a requirement for a successful portacaval shunt. Previously, direct venography was used, but the required information may now be obtained using noninvasive methods, such as CT or MR angiography. The x-rays may show compression of the intrahepatic cava by the congested liver.

Treatment of BCS relies on expert consensus given the low incidence of this disease. Anticoagulation is recommended in the presence of recent or long-standing thrombosis to allow recanalization or to avoid propagation of venous thrombosis. Management of ascites and treatment or prevention of portal hypertension and variceal hemorrhage follows the same algorithms as for cirrhotic patients. Surgical or radiological approaches to relieve sinusoidal pressure have been advocated and are now considered appropriate only for symptomatic patients who do not improve with medical management. In recent years, the development of interventional radiology techniques using thrombolysis and angioplasty has shown possible to insert TIPS in selected patients with recent thrombosis or with short-length stenosis of the IVC or hepatic veins with good outcomes. Portosystemic surgical shunts are considered effective for relieving sinusoidal hypertension with the potential to reverse hepatic necrosis and prevent cirrhosis.

Focal membranous obstruction of the suprahepatic cava may be treated by excision of the lesion with or without the addition of a patch angioplasty. Some cases may be managed nonsurgically by percutaneous transluminal balloon dilation of the stenosis. Occlusion of the inferior vena cava by thrombosis or compression from the liver requires a mesoatrial shunt using a prosthetic vascular graft. Because the incidence of graft thrombosis is relatively high, it may be advisable to perform a second-stage side-to-side portacaval shunt a few months after mesoatrial shunt decompression of the liver in patients with hepatic vein thrombosis whose vena cava was originally blocked by a congested liver. Development of hepatocellular carcinoma is common in patients with membranous obstruction of the vena cava. The postoperative results are excellent in patients without malignant neoplasms.

Liver transplantation is required when medical treatment and portosystemic shunts fail in patients presenting progressive liver failure either from cirrhosis or as part of the acute syndrome. The 1-, 5-, 10-year survival rates with transplantation are of 76%, 71%, and 68%, respectively, and the risk of later hepatocellular carcinoma is eliminated.

Bittencourt PL et al. Portal vein thrombosis and Budd-Chiari syndrome. *Hematol Oncol Clin North Am* 2011;25:1049.

Garcia-Pagan JC et al. TIPS for Budd-Chiari syndrome: long-term results and prognostic factors in 124 patients. *Gastroenterology* 2008;135:808.

Horton JD, San Miguel FL, Ortiz JA. Budd-Chiari syndrome: illustrated review of current management. *Liver Int* 2008;28:455.

Patil P et al. Spectrum of imaging in Budd-Chiari syndrome. *J Med Imaging Radiat Oncol* 2012;569:75.

ASCITES

Ascites is a common manifestation of chronic liver disease, resulting from sinusoidal hypertension as the specific pathophysiologic abnormality. Ascites in hepatic disease results from (1) increased formation of hepatic lymph (from sinusoidal hypertension), (2) increased formation of splanchnic lymph (from splanchnic vasodilatation), (3) hypoalbuminemia, and (4) salt and water retention by the kidneys. Before therapy is started, paracentesis should be performed and the following examinations made on a sample of ascitic fluid: (1) Culture and leukocyte count—spontaneous bacterial peritonitis is common and may be clinically silent. A white count above 250/μL is highly suggestive of infection. (2) LDH levels—a ratio of LDH in ascites to serum that exceeds 0.6 suggests the presence of cancer or infection. (3) Serum amylase—a high level suggests pancreatic disease. (4) Albumin—the ratio of serum to ascites albumin concentrations is above 1.1 in liver disease and below 1.1 in malignant ascites. (5) Cytology—this is pertinent only in patients with a cancer diagnosis or a suspicion of cancer.

Nonhepatic ascites can result from congestive heart failure, chylous leak, peritoneal carcinomatosis, infections such as tuberculosis, coccidiomycosis, and chlamydia, and some autoimmune disease involving the connective tissues, such as systemic lupus erythematosus. Treatments of ascites in these contexts depend on the underlying cause and are not discussed in this chapter.

▶ Medical Treatment

In general, the intensity of medical therapy required to control ascites can be predicted from the pretreatment 24-hour urine Na^+ output as follows: A Na^+ output below 5 mEq/24 h requires strong diuretics; 5-25 mEq/24 h, mild diuretics; and above 25 mEq/24 h, no diuretics. Initial treatment is usually with spironolactone, 200 mg/d. The objective is to stimulate a weight loss of 0.5-0.75 kg/d except in patients with peripheral edema who can mobilize fluid faster. If spironolactone alone is insufficient, another drug such as furosemide should be added. A loop diuretic (eg, furosemide, ethacrynic acid) should be given only in combination with a distally acting diuretic (eg, spironolactone, triamterene). Alternatively, massive ascites may be treated by one or more large volume (eg, 5-L) paracenteses; this is often accompanied by an intravenous infusion of albumin, although the benefits of albumin remain controversial. Caution is required in patients with evidence of renal dysfunction, since aggressive fluid removal can result in renal failure. Close monitoring of serum electrolytes should be done. Because the development of ascites in cirrhosis is a result of renal sodium retention, dietary sodium restriction is a mainstay of treatment. A typical American diet contains 4-6 g of sodium per day. Patients are educated to have a diet of maximum 2 g of sodium per day. Fluid restriction is only indicated in patients with severe hyponatremia, but all should avoid excessive fluid intake.

▶ Surgical Treatment

A. Portacaval Shunt

A history of ascites that has been easy to control need not influence the choice of shunt operation intended to treat variceal bleeding. When ascites has been severe, however, a side-to-side shunt (eg, side-to-side portacaval, H-mesocaval, central splenorenal) may be considered, because it reduces sinusoidal as well as splanchnic venous pressure. A side-to-side portacaval shunt is rarely indicated just to treat ascites (eg, in patients in whom several LeVeen shunts have thrombosed), although the incidence of severe postoperative encephalopathy is high under these circumstances. TIPS is another effective intervention for refractory ascites, probably a better option than repeated paracentesis in good-risk patients, although there is an associated risk of hepatic encephalopathy.

B. Peritoneal-Jugular Shunt (LeVeen Shunt, Denver Shunt)

Refractory ascites can be treated with a LeVeen shunt—a subcutaneous Silastic catheter that transports ascitic fluid from the peritoneal cavity to the jugular vein. A small unidirectional valve sensitive to a pressure gradient of 3-5 cm H_2O prevents backflow of blood. A modification called the Denver shunt contains a small chamber that can be used as a pump to clear the line by external pressure. In practice, Denver shunts become blocked more often than LeVeen shunts.

In patients with ascites due to cirrhosis, use of a LeVeen shunt should be confined to those who fail to respond to high doses of diuretics (eg, 400 mg of spironolactone and 400 mg of furosemide daily) or who repeatedly develop encephalopathy or azotemia during diuretic therapy.

Peritoneovenous shunts may also be used for ascites associated with cancer. The best results occur in patients whose ascitic fluid contains no malignant cells. A LeVeen shunt is of benefit in BCS but is ineffective for chylous ascites. Because the incidence of complications and early shunt thrombosis is high, a LeVeen shunt is relatively contraindicated if the ascitic fluid is grossly bloody, contains many malignant cells, or has a high protein concentration (> 4.5 g/dL). The incidence of tumor embolization is low (5%).

The ascitic fluid should be cultured a few days before the shunt is inserted. Antibiotic coverage should be given for the procedure. The operation can be done with local anesthesia.

Postoperatively, the patient is outfitted with an abdominal binder and instructed to perform respiratory exercises against mild pressure to increase abdominal pressure and flow through the shunt. Dietary salt should not be restricted. A functioning LeVeen shunt alone is unable to fully eliminate the ascites, but it improves symptoms related to distention and renders the patient much more responsive to diuretics. Therefore, furosemide should be administered postoperatively.

An average of 10 kg of weight is lost during the first 10 days after the operation, and eventually the abdomen assumes a normal configuration. Nutrition and serum albumin levels often improve postoperatively. Urinary sodium excretion increases promptly, and renal function may improve in patients with the hepatorenal syndrome. Serious complications and deaths are most common in patients with advanced hepatorenal syndrome or a serum bilirubin level greater than 4 mg/dL. Although some patients eventually bleed from varices following insertion of a LeVeen shunt, the shunt itself does not increase the risk of bleeding and actually decreases portal pressure. Thus, a previous episode of variceal bleeding is not a contraindication for this procedure. Disseminated intravascular coagulation (manifested by increased fibrin split products, decreased platelet count, etc) occurs in more than half of cases but is clinically relevant in only a few. The frequency and severity of disseminated intravascular coagulation may be minimized by emptying most of the ascitic fluid from the abdomen during operation and partially replacing it with Ringer lactate solution. Lethal septicemia may occur if the ascitic fluid is infected at the time the shunt is inserted. In about 10% of cases, the valve becomes thrombosed and must be replaced.

Hydrothorax, usually on the right side, may develop in patients with cirrhosis and ascites. The fluid reaches the chest through a pinhole opening in the membranous portion of the diaphragm, a pathway that can be demonstrated by aspirating the thoracic fluid, injecting technetium [99mTc] colloid into the ascites fluid, and observing rapid accumulation of the label in the chest. Treatment consists of a peritoneovenous shunt and injection of a sclerosing agent into the pleural cavity after it has been tapped dry. If a leak persists, it may be closed surgically by thoracotomy.

Fede G et al. Renal failure and cirrhosis: a systematic review of mortality and prognosis. *J Hepatol* 2012;56:810.

Gines P et al. Management of critically-ill cirrhotic patients. *J Heptaol* 2012;56 suppl 1:S13-S24.

Gordon FD. Ascites. *Clin Liver Dis* 2012;16;285.

White MA et al. Denver peritoneovenous shunts for the management of malignant ascites: a review of the literature in the post LeVeen era. *Am Surg* 2011;77:1070.

HEPATIC ENCEPHALOPATHY

Central nervous system abnormalities may be seen in patients with chronic liver disease and are especially likely after portacaval shunts. Portosystemic encephalopathy, ammonia intoxication, hepatic coma, and meat intoxication are older terms used to refer to this condition. The manifestations range from lethargy to coma—from minor personality changes to psychosis—from asterixis to paraplegia. Hypothermia and hyperventilation may precede coma. The changes may be quite subtle and detectable only with the use of neuropsychological or neurophysiological testing.

▶ Pathogenesis

Hepatic encephalopathy is a reversible metabolic neuropathy that results from the action of chemicals absorbed from the gut on the brain. Increased exposure of the brain to these agents is the result of impaired hepatic metabolism due to cirrhosis or spontaneous or surgically created shunts of portal venous blood around the liver and increased permeability of the blood-brain barrier. The chemical agents responsible for encephalopathy form from the action of colonic bacteria on protein within the gut. Potential aggravating factors include gastrointestinal hemorrhage, constipation, azotemia, hypokalemic alkalosis, infection, excessive dietary protein, and sedatives (Table 24–7). Four main chemical mediators of this syndrome currently attract the most attention.

Table 24–7. Factors contributing to encephalopathy.

A. Increased systemic toxin levels
1. Extent of portal-systemic venous shunt
2. Depressed liver function
3. Intestinal protein load
4. Intestinal flora
5. Azotemia
6. Constipation

B. Increased sensitivity of the central nervous system
1. Age of patient
2. Hypokalemia
3. Alkalosis
4. Diuretics
5. Sedatives, narcotics, tranquilizers
6. Infection
7. Hypoxia, hypoglycemia, myxedema

Low-grade cerebral edema appears to be a major component of the pathophysiologic process.

A. Amino Acid Neurotransmitters

Gamma-aminobutyric acid (GABA), the principal inhibitory neurotransmitter in the brain, produces a state similar to hepatic encephalopathy when given experimentally. It is normally synthesized in the brain and by bacteria within the colon; GABA in the gastrointestinal tract is normally degraded by the liver and is found in increased levels in the serum of patients with hepatic encephalopathy. The passage of GABA across the blood-brain barrier is increased in hepatic encephalopathy. Experiments also indicate the presence of increased numbers of GABA receptors in encephalopathy and increased GABA-ergic tone, perhaps due to a benzodiazepine receptor agonist ligand on the receptor complex (GABA/benzodiazepine receptor). This has raised the possibility of treating encephalopathy with benzodiazepine antagonists, and the drug flumazenil has shown promise in preliminary trials.

B. Ammonia

Ammonia is produced in the colon by bacteria and is absorbed and transported in portal venous blood to the liver, where it is extracted and converted to glutamine. Ammonia concentrations are elevated in the arterial blood and cerebrospinal fluid of patients with encephalopathy, and experimental administration of ammonia produces central nervous system symptoms.

C. False Neurotransmitters

According to this theory, cerebral neurons become depleted of normal neurotransmitters (norepinephrine and dopamine), which are partially replaced by false neurotransmitters (octopamine and phenylethanolamine). The result is inhibition of neural function. Serum levels of branched-chain amino acids (leucine, isoleucine, valine) are decreased, and levels of aromatic amino acids (tryptophan, phenylalanine, tyrosine) are elevated in patients with encephalopathy. Because these two classes of amino acids compete for transport across the blood-brain barrier, the aromatic amino acids have increased access to the central nervous system, where they serve as precursors for false neurotransmitters. Trials of therapy with supplements of branched-chain amino acids have given conflicting results.

D. Synergistic Neurotoxins

This theory postulates that ammonia, mercaptans, and fatty acids, none of which accumulate in the brain in amounts capable of producing encephalopathy, have synergistic effects that produce the full-blown syndrome in patients with liver disease.

▶ Prevention

Encephalopathy is a major side effect of portacaval shunt and is to some extent predictable. Elderly patients are considerably more susceptible. Patients with alcoholic liver disease fare better than those with postnecrotic or cryptogenic cirrhosis, apparently owing to the invariable progression of liver dysfunction in the latter. Good liver function partially protects against encephalopathy. If the liver has adapted to complete or nearly complete diversion of portal blood before operation, a surgical shunt is less apt to depress liver function further. For example, patients with thrombosis of the portal vein (complete diversion and normal liver function) rarely experience encephalopathy after portosystemic shunt. Encephalopathy is less common after a distal splenorenal (Warren) shunt than after other kinds of shunts.

Increased intestinal protein, whether of dietary origin or from intestinal bleeding, aggravates encephalopathy by providing more substrate for intestinal bacteria. Constipation allows more time for bacterial action on colonic contents. Azotemia results in higher concentration of blood urea, which diffuses into the intestine, is converted to ammonia, and is then reabsorbed. Hypokalemia and metabolic alkalosis aggravate encephalopathy by shifting ammonia from extracellular to intracellular sites where the toxic action occurs.

▶ Laboratory Findings

Arterial ammonia levels are usually high, although encephalopathy can certainly be present with a normal ammonia level. The presence of high levels of glutamine in the cerebrospinal fluid may help distinguish hepatic encephalopathy from other causes of coma. Electroencephalography is more sensitive than clinical evaluation in detecting minor involvement. The changes are nonspecific and consist of slower mean frequencies. Studies performed at different times can be compared to assess the effects of therapy.

Treatment

Acute encephalopathy is treated by controlling precipitating factors, halting all dietary protein intake, cleansing the bowel with purgatives and enemas, and administering antibiotics (neomycin or ampicillin) or lactulose. Neomycin may be given orally or by gastric tube (two to four times daily) or rectally as an enema (1% solution one or two times daily). At least 1600 kcal of carbohydrate should be provided daily, along with therapeutic amounts of vitamins. Blood volume must be maintained to avoid prerenal azotemia. After the patient responds to initial therapy, dietary protein may be started at 20 g/d and increased by increments of 10-20 g every 2-5 days as tolerated.

Chronic encephalopathy is treated by restriction of dietary protein, avoidance of constipation, and elimination of sedatives, diuretics, and tranquilizers. To avoid protein depletion, protein intake must not be chronically reduced below 50 g/d. Vegetable protein in the diet is tolerated better than animal protein. Lactulose, a disaccharide unaffected by intestinal enzymes, is the drug of choice for long-term control. When given orally (20-30 g three or four times daily), it reaches the colon, where it stimulates bacterial anabolism (which increases ammonia uptake) and inhibits bacterial enzymes (which decreases the generation of nitrogenous toxins). Its effect is independent of colonic pH. A related compound outside the United States, lactitol (β-galactoside sorbitol), is also effective and appears to work faster. As a powder, it is easier to use than liquid lactulose. Intermittent courses of oral neomycin or metronidazole may be given if lactulose therapy and preventive measures are inadequate.

Haussinger D, Schliess F. Pathogenetic mechanisms of hepatic encephalopathy. *Gut* 2008;57:1156.

Khungar V, Poordad F. Hepatic encephalopathy 2012. *Clin Liver Dis* 2012;16:301.

HEPATIC ABSCESS

Hepatic abscesses may be bacterial, parasitic, or fungal in origin. In the United States, pyogenic abscesses are the most common, followed by amebic abscesses (see Chapter 8). Unless otherwise indicated, the remarks in this section refer to bacterial abscesses.

Cases are about evenly divided between those with a single abscess and those with multiple abscesses. About 90% of right lobe abscesses are solitary, while only 10% of left lobe abscesses are solitary.

In most cases, the development of a hepatic abscess follows a suppurative process elsewhere in the body. Many abscesses are due to direct spread from biliary infections such as empyema of the gallbladder or protracted cholangitis. Abdominal infections such as appendicitis or diverticulitis may spread through the portal vein to involve the liver with abscess formation. About 40% of patients have an underlying malignancy. Other cases develop after generalized sepsis from bacterial endocarditis, renal infection, or pneumonitis. In 25% of cases, no antecedent infection can be documented (cryptogenic abscesses). Rare causes include secondary bacterial infection of an amebic abscess, hydatid cyst, or congenital hepatic cyst.

In most cases, the organism is of enteric origin.

Escherichia coli, Klebsiella pneumoniae, bacteroides, enterococci (eg, *Streptococcus faecalis*), anaerobic streptococci (eg, *Peptostreptococcus*), and microaerophilic streptococci are most common. Staphylococci, hemolytic streptococci, or other gram-positive organisms are usually found if the primary infection is bacterial endocarditis or pneumonitis.

Clinical Findings

A. Symptoms and Signs

When liver abscess develops in the course of another intra-abdominal infection such as diverticulitis, it is accompanied by increasing toxicity, higher fever, jaundice, and a generally deteriorating clinical picture. Right upper quadrant pain and chills may appear.

In other cases, the diagnosis is much less obvious, since the illness develops insidiously in a previously healthy person. In these, the first symptoms are usually malaise and fatigue, followed after several weeks by fever. Epigastric or right upper quadrant pain is present in about half of cases. The pain may be aggravated by motion or may be referred to the right shoulder.

The course of fever is often erratic, and spikes to 40-41°C are common. Chills are present in about 25% of cases. The liver is usually enlarged and may be tender to palpation. If tenderness is severe, the condition may be confused with cholecystitis.

Jaundice is unusual in solitary abscesses unless the patient's condition is worsening. Jaundice is often present in patients with multiple abscesses and primary disease in the biliary tree and in general is a bad prognostic sign.

B. Laboratory Findings

Leukocytosis is present in most cases and is usually over 15,000/μL. A small group of patients, usually the most seriously ill, may fail to develop leukocytosis. Anemia is present in most. The average hematocrit is 33%.

Serum bilirubin is usually normal except in patients with multiple abscesses or biliary obstruction or when hepatic failure has supervened. Alkaline phosphatase is often elevated even in the presence of a normal bilirubin.

C. Imaging Studies

X-ray changes present in the right lung in about one-third of cases consist of basilar atelectasis or pleural effusion. The right diaphragm may be elevated and less mobile than the left.

Plain films of the abdomen are usually normal or show only hepatomegaly. In a few patients, an air-fluid level in the region of the liver reveals the presence and location of the abscess. Distortion of the contour of the stomach on upper gastrointestinal series may be seen with large abscesses involving the left lobe.

Ultrasound and CT scans are the most useful diagnostic tests, providing accurate information regarding the presence, size, number, and location of abscesses within the liver. CT scans have the added advantage of being able to demonstrate abscesses or neoplasms elsewhere in the abdomen. The radioisotope liver scintiscan is able to demonstrate most liver abscesses but is nonspecific, gives little other useful information, and is therefore not helpful.

Differential Diagnosis

In many cases, early findings may be so vague that hepatic abscess is not even considered. The multiple other causes of malaise, weight loss, and anemia would enter into the differential diagnosis. With spiking fevers, one must consider all the causes of fever of unknown origin. Failure to entertain the idea of hepatic abscess and to obtain the necessary scans leads to most errors in diagnosis.

Once imaging tests have demonstrated the abscess, the responsible organisms must be identified. Amebiasis should be considered in cases of a solitary abscess. Compared with amebic abscesses, pyogenic liver abscesses are seen more often in patients older than 50 years and are associated with jaundice, pruritus, sepsis, a palpable mass, and elevated bilirubin and alkaline phosphatase levels. Patients with amebic abscesses more often have been to an endemic area and have abdominal pain and tenderness, diarrhea, hepatomegaly, and positive serologic tests for amebiasis.

Complications

Intrahepatic spread of infection may create multiple additional abscesses and is responsible for some failures after treatment of an apparently solitary abscess. As the untreated abscess expands, rupture may occur in the pleural or peritoneal cavity, usually with catastrophic results. Septicemia and septic shock are common terminal complications of diffuse hepatic infection. Hepatic failure may develop in addition to uncontrolled sepsis, or it may predominate over signs of infection.

Hemobilia may follow bleeding from the vascular wall into the abscess cavity. In this case, hepatic artery embolization or ligation may be required to control bleeding.

Treatment

Antibiotics should be started promptly. Initial coverage, before culture results are available, should be adequate for *E coli, K pneumoniae,* bacteroides, enterococci, and yanaerobic streptococci and consequently would usually include an aminoglycoside, clindamycin or metronidazole, and ampicillin. The regimen may be modified later according to the results of cultures.

About 80% or more of patients with liver abscesses are adequately treated by drainage catheters inserted percutaneously under ultrasound or CT guidance. Whether the patient has a single abscess or multiple abscesses, this is usually the most appropriate initial therapy. The catheters can be removed in 1-2 weeks after output becomes nonpurulent and scant.

In about 40% of patients, the catheters do not drain well following initial placement and must be repositioned. The principal advantage of percutaneous drainage is lower morbidity compared to open drainage, although not necessarily lower mortality. It is easier to provide thorough drainage surgically, so when difficulties are encountered with percutaneous drainage, laparotomy should be performed promptly. Surgical intervention is more often necessary in cases of multiple, loculated collections or when the abscess cavity contains a large amount of necrotic debris. In such cases, open debridement should be considered early. Likewise, early surgical intervention is indicated for patients who are seriously ill (APACHE II score ≥ 15). Rarely, multiple abscesses are confined to a single lobe and can be cured by lobectomy. Biliary obstruction or other causes of sepsis must also be corrected.

Prognosis

The overall mortality rate of 15% is more closely related to the underlying disease than to any other factor. The mortality rate is about 40% in patients with malignant disease. Pleural effusion, leukocytosis over 20,000/µL, hypoalbuminemia, and polymicrobial infection correlate with a poor outcome. In the United States, whether the abscess is solitary or multiple no longer has a major influence on survival, but where benign biliary disease remains a major cause of this disease, multiple hepatic abscesses are associated with a worse prognosis. Death is rare in patients with a cryptogenic liver abscess.

Alasaif HS et al. CT appearance of pyogenic abscesses caused by Klebsiella pneumonia. *Radiology* 2011;260:129.
Reid-Lombardo KM et al. Hepatic cysts and liver abscess. *Surg Clin North Am* 2010;90:679.

MULTIPLE CHOICE QUESTIONS

1. All of the following are true about the blood supply to the liver, except

   A. The portal vein is formed by the confluence of the splenic and superior mesenteric veins at the level of the second lumbar vertebra behind the head of the pancreas.

B. The common hepatic artery arises from the celiac axis, ascends in the hepatoduodenal ligament, and gives rise to the right gastric, gastroduodenal, and proper hepatic arteries.

C. In the hepatoduodenal ligament, the portal vein lies dorsal and slightly medial to the common bile duct.

D. A replaced right hepatic artery typically arises from the inferior mesenteric artery and courses posteriorly and to the right of the common bile duct within the porta hepatis.

E. A replaced left hepatic artery typically arises from the left gastric artery.

2. The Child–Pugh classification of functional status in liver disease does not include

A. Prothrombin time
B. Serum albumin
C. Encephalopathy
D. Serum sodium
E. Serum bilirubin

3. Blunt trauma to the liver

A. Requires operative management in 85% of patients
B. With a laceration 4-cm deep but not affecting the major vasculature is a Grade III lesion
C. Is involved in approximately 20% of all trauma admissions

D. Is more common in the left liver than the right
E. Is best evaluated acutely by MRI to define the ductal anatomy

4. Portal hypertension

A. In the United States, is most often caused by cirrhosis
B. Is defined as a hepatic venous pressure gradient (the difference between portal-vein pressure and hepatic-vein pressure) greater than 25 mm Hg
C. Is caused by Budd-Chiari syndrome in about 25% of cases in the United States
D. Due to hepatic venous thrombosis causes isolated splenic venous hypertension (sinistral or left-sided portal hypertension)
E. Requires operative management in most patients

5. Management of acute bleeding from esophageal varices

A. Can include transecting and anastomosing the mid-esophagus with an end-to-end stapler
B. Should include urgent operation in most patients
C. Should include controlling hemorrhage as expediently and simply as possible
D. Is commonly required in the management of chronic pancreatitis
E. Should reserve invasive procedures for patients who have required more than 15 units blood transfusion

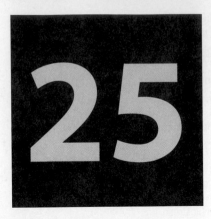

25

Biliary Tract

Gerard M. Doherty, MD

EMBRYOLOGY & ANATOMY

The anlage of the biliary ducts and liver consists of a diverticulum that appears on the ventral aspect of the foregut in 3 mm embryos. The cranial portion becomes the liver; a caudal bud forms the ventral pancreas; and an intermediate bud develops into the gallbladder. Originally hollow, the hepatic diverticulum becomes a solid mass of cells that later recanalizes to form the ducts. The smallest ducts—the bile canaliculi—first appear as a basal network between the primitive hepatocytes that eventually expands throughout the liver (Figure 25–1). Numerous microvilli increase the canalicular surface area. Bile secreted here passes through the interlobular ductules (canals of Hering) and the lobar ducts and then into the hepatic duct in the hilum. In most cases, the common hepatic duct is formed by the union of a single right and left duct, but in 25% of individuals, the anterior and posterior divisions of the right duct join the left duct separately. The origin of the common hepatic duct is close to the liver but always outside its substance. It runs about 4 cm before joining the cystic duct to form the common bile duct. The common duct begins in the hepatoduodenal ligament, passes behind the first portion of the duodenum, and runs in a groove on the posterior surface of the pancreas before entering the duodenum. Its terminal 1 cm is intimately adherent to the duodenal wall. The total length of the common duct is about 9 cm.

In 80%-90% of individuals, the main pancreatic duct joins the common duct to form a common channel about 1-cm long. The intraduodenal segment of the duct is called the hepatopancreatic ampulla, or ampulla of Vater.

The gallbladder is a pear-shaped organ adherent to the undersurface of the liver in a groove separating the right and left lobes. The fundus projects 1-2 cm below the hepatic edge and can often be felt when the cystic or common duct is obstructed. It rarely has a complete peritoneal covering, but when this variation does occur, it predisposes to infarction by torsion. The gallbladder holds about 50 mL of bile when fully distended. The neck of the gallbladder tapers into the narrow cystic duct, which connects with the common duct. The lumen of the cystic duct contains a thin mucosal septum, the spiral valve of Heister that offers mild resistance to bile flow. In 75% of persons, the cystic duct enters the common duct at an angle. In the remainder, it runs parallel to the hepatic duct or winds around it before joining the common duct (Figure 25–2).

In the hepatoduodenal ligament, the hepatic artery is to the left of the common duct and the portal vein is posterior and medial. The right hepatic artery usually passes behind the hepatic duct and then gives off the cystic artery before entering the right lobe of the liver, but variations are common.

The mucosal epithelium of the bile ducts varies from cuboidal in the ductules to columnar in the main ducts. The gallbladder mucosa is thrown into prominent ridges when the organ is collapsed, and these flatten during distention. The tall columnar cells of the gallbladder mucosa are covered by microvilli on their luminal surface. Wide channels, which play an important role in water and electrolyte absorption, separate the individual cells.

The walls of the bile ducts contain only small amounts of smooth muscle, but the termination of the common duct is enveloped by a complex sphincteric muscle. The gallbladder musculature is composed of interdigitated bundles of longitudinal and spirally arranged fibers.

The biliary tree receives parasympathetic and sympathetic innervation. The former contains motor fibers to the gallbladder and secretory fibers to the ductal epithelium. The afferent fibers in the sympathetic nerves mediate the pain of biliary colic.

PHYSIOLOGY

▶ Bile Flow

Bile is produced at a rate of 500-1500 mL/d by the hepatocytes and the cells of the ducts. Active secretion of bile salts into the biliary canaliculus is responsible for most of the

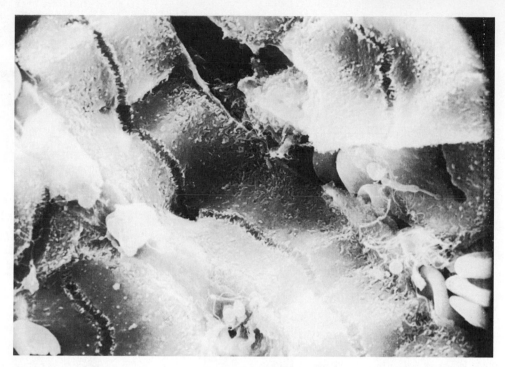

▲ **FIGURE 25–1.** Scanning electron photomicrograph of a hepatic plate with adjacent sinusoids and sinusoidal micro-villi and a bile canaliculus running in the center of the liver cells. Although their boundaries are indistinct, about four hepatocytes constitute the section of the plate in the middle of the photograph. Occasional red cells are present within the sinusoids. (Reduced from × 2000.) (Courtesy of Dr James Boyer.)

volume of bile and its fluctuations. Na^+ and water follow passively to establish isosmolality and electrical neutrality. Lecithin and cholesterol enter the canaliculus at rates that correlate with variations in bile salt output. Bilirubin and a number of other organic anions—estrogens, sulfobromoph-thalein, etc—are actively secreted by the hepatocyte by a different transport system from that which handles bile salts.

The columnar cells of the ducts add a fluid rich in HCO_3^- to that produced in the canaliculus. This involves active secretion of Na^+ and HCO_3^- by a cellular pump stimulated by secretin, VIP, and cholecystokinin (CCK). K^+ and water are distributed passively across the ducts (Figure 25–3).

Between meals, bile is stored in the gallbladder, where it is concentrated at rates of up to 20% per hour. Na^+ and either HCO_3^- or Cl^- are actively transported from its lumen during absorption. The changes in composition brought about by concentration are shown in Figure 25–4.

Three factors regulate bile flow: hepatic secretion, gallbladder contraction, and choledochal sphincteric resistance. In the fasting state, pressure in the common bile duct is 5-10 cm H_2O, and bile produced in the liver is diverted into the gallbladder. After a meal, the gallbladder contracts, the sphincter relaxes, and bile is forced into the duodenum in squirts as ductal pressure intermittently exceeds sphincteric resistance. During contraction, pressure within the gallbladder reaches 25 cm H_2O and that in the common bile duct 15-20 cm H_2O.

CCK is the major physiologic stimulus for postprandial gallbladder contraction and relaxation of the sphincter, but vagal impulses facilitate its action. CCK is released into the bloodstream from the mucosa of the small bowel by fat or lipolytic products in the lumen. Amino acids and small polypeptides are weaker stimuli, and carbohydrates are ineffective. Bile flow during a meal is augmented by turnover of bile salts in the enterohepatic circulation and stimulation of ductal secretion by secretin, VIP, and CCK. Motilin stimulates episodic partial gallbladder emptying in the interdigestive phase.

Bile Salts & the Enterohepatic Circulation

Bile salts, lecithin, and cholesterol comprise about 90% of the solids in bile, the remainder consisting of bilirubin, fatty acids, and inorganic salts. Gallbladder bile contains about 10% solids and has a bile salt concentration between 200 and 300 mmol/L (Figure 25–4).

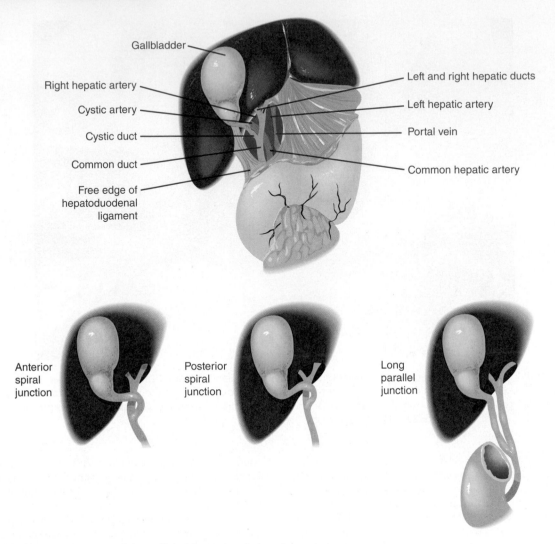

▲ **FIGURE 25–2.** Anatomy of the gallbladder and variations in anatomy.

Bile salts are steroid molecules formed from cholesterol by hepatocytes. The rate of synthesis is under feedback control and can be increased a maximum of about 20-fold. Two primary bile salts—cholate and chenodeoxycholate—are produced by the liver. Before excretion into bile, they are conjugated with either glycine or taurine, which enhances water solubility. Intestinal bacteria alter these compounds to produce the secondary bile salts, deoxycholate and lithocholate. The former is reabsorbed and enters bile, but lithocholate is insoluble and is excreted in the stool. Bile is composed of 40% cholate, 40% chenodeoxycholate, and 20% deoxycholate, conjugated with glycine or taurine in a ratio of 3:1.

The functions of bile salts are: (1) to induce the flow of bile, (2) to transport lipids, and (3) to bind calcium ions in

bile. The importance of the last of these is unknown. Bile acid molecules are amphipathic—that is, they have hydrophilic and hydrophobic poles. In bile, they form multimolecular aggregates called micelles in which the hydrophilic poles become aligned to face the aqueous medium. Water-insoluble lipids, such as cholesterol, can be dissolved within the hydrophobic centers of bile salt micelles. Molecules of lecithin, a water-insoluble but polar lipid, aggregate into hydrated bilayers that form vesicles in bile, and they also become incorporated into bile acid micelles to form mixed micelles. Mixed micelles have an increased lipid-carrying capacity compared with pure bile acid micelles. Cholesterol in bile is transported within the phospholipid vesicles and the bile salt micelles.

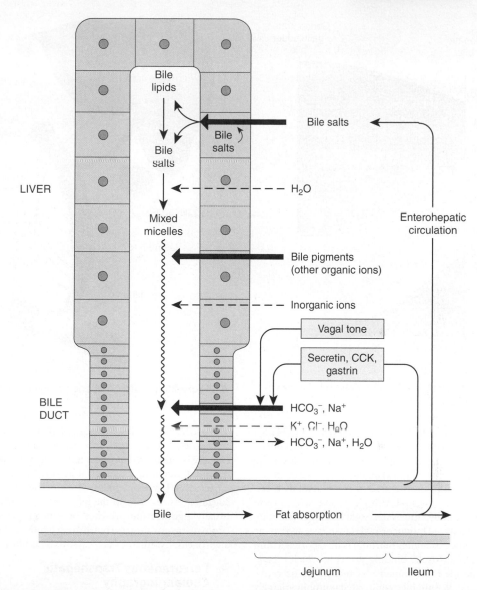

▲ FIGURE 25–3. Bile formation. Solid lines into the ductular lumen indicate active transport; dotted lines represent passive diffusion.

Bile salts remain in the intestinal lumen throughout the jejunum, where they participate in fat digestion and absorption (Figure 25-5). Upon reaching the distal small bowel, they are reabsorbed by an active transport system located in the terminal 200 cm of ileum. More than 95% of bile salts arriving from the jejunum are transferred by this process into portal vein blood; the remainder enters the colon, where they are converted to secondary bile salts. The entire bile salt pool of 2.5-4 g circulates twice through the enterohepatic circulation during each meal, and six to eight cycles are made each day. The normal daily loss of bile salts in the stool amounts to 10%-20% of the pool and is restored by hepatic synthesis.

▶ Bilirubin

About 250-300 mg of bilirubin is excreted each day in the bile, 75% of it from breakdown of red cells in the reticuloendothelial system and 25% from turnover of hepatic heme and hemoproteins. First, heme is liberated from hemoglobin, and the iron and globin are removed for reuse by the organism.

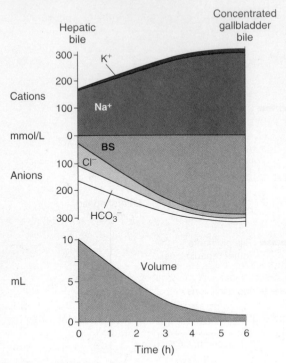

▲ **FIGURE 25–4.** Changes in gallbladder bile composition with time. (Courtesy of J Dietschy.)

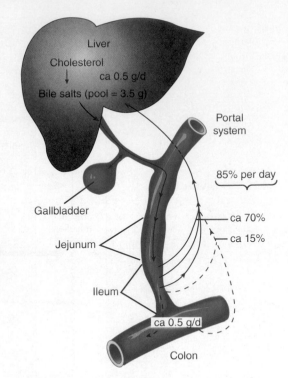

▲ **Figure 25–5.** Enterohepatic circulation of bile salts. (Courtesy of M Tyor.)

Biliverdin, the first pigment formed from heme, is reduced to unconjugated bilirubin, the indirect-reacting bilirubin of the van den Bergh test. Unconjugated bilirubin is insoluble in water and is transported in plasma bound to albumin.

Unconjugated bilirubin is extracted from blood by hepatocytes, where it is conjugated with glucuronic acid to form bilirubin diglucuronide, the water-soluble direct bilirubin. Conjugation is catalyzed by glucuronyl transferase, an enzyme on the endoplasmic reticulum. Bilirubin is transported within the hepatocyte by cytosolic binding proteins, which rapidly deliver the molecule to the canalicular membrane for active secretion into bile. Within bile, conjugated bilirubin is largely transported in association with mixed lipid micelles.

After entering the intestine, bilirubin is reduced by intestinal bacteria to several compounds known as urobilinogens, which are subsequently oxidized and converted to pigmented urobilins. The term urobilinogen is often used to refer to both urobilins and urobilinogens.

DIAGNOSTIC EXAMINATION OF THE BILIARY TREE

▶ Plain Abdominal Film

The posteroanterior supine view of the abdomen will show gallstones in the 10%-15% of cases when they are radiopaque.

The bile itself sometimes contains sufficient calcium (milk of calcium bile) to be seen. An enlarged gallbladder can occasionally be identified as a soft tissue mass in the right upper quadrant indenting an air-filled hepatic flexure.

In several types of biliary disease, the diagnosis may be suggested by air seen in the bile ducts on a plain film. This usually signifies the presence of a biliary-intestinal fistula (from disease or surgery) but also occurs rarely in severe cholangitis, emphysematous cholecystitis, and biliary ascariasis.

▶ Percutaneous Transhepatic Cholangiography

Percutaneous transhepatic cholangiography (THC, PTC) is performed by passing a fine needle through the right-lower rib cage and the hepatic parenchyma and into the lumen of a bile duct. Water-soluble contrast material is injected, and x-ray films are taken.

The technical success is related to the degree of dilatation of the intrahepatic bile ducts. THC is especially valuable in demonstrating the biliary anatomy in patients with benign biliary strictures, malignant lesions of the proximal bile duct, or when endoscopic retrograde cholangiopancreatography (ERCP) (see later) has been unsuccessful. Failure of the contrast medium to enter a duct does not prove that obstruction is absent. Virtually all patients should be premedicated with antibiotics regardless of whether they have cholangitis—septic shock has been produced by sudden inoculation of organisms from bile into the systemic circulation. Otherwise, the contraindications are the same as for percutaneous liver biopsy.

Endoscopic Retrograde Cholangiopancreatography

ERCP involves cannulating the sphincter of Oddi under direct vision through a side-viewing duodenoscope. It requires special training involving more than familiarity with the use of fiberoptic endoscopes. Usually it is possible to opacify the pancreatic as well as the bile ducts. It is the preferred method of examining the biliary tree in patients with presumed choledocholithiasis or obstructing lesions in the periampullary region, and provides access for therapeutic intervention as well.

Ultrasound

Ultrasonography is both sensitive and specific in detecting gallbladder stones and dilatation of bile ducts. In the investigation of gallbladder disease, false-positive diagnoses for stones are rare, and false-negative reports owing to small stones or a contracted gallbladder occur in only 5% of patients examined by real time ultrasound. Ultrasound usually misses stones in the common duct.

Dilatation of bile ducts in a jaundiced patient indicates bile duct obstruction, but it is fairly common for the ducts to be normal in the presence of obstruction. When ultrasound shows dilated ducts, THC will nearly always be technically successful.

The ultrasonographer occasionally reports that the gallbladder contains "sludge." This material is sonographically opaque, does not cast an acoustic shadow, and forms a dependent layer in the gallbladder. On clinical analysis, it is a fine precipitate of calcium bilirubinate. Sludge may accompany gallstone disease or may be a solitary finding. It is observed in a variety of clinical settings, many of which are characterized by gallbladder stasis (eg, prolonged fasting). By itself, sludge is not an indication for cholecystectomy.

Radionuclide Scan (HIDA Scan)

Technetium 99m-labeled derivatives of iminodiacetic acid (IDA) are excreted in high concentration in bile and produce excellent gamma camera images. Following intravenous injection of the radionuclide, imaging of the bile ducts and gallbladder normally appears within 15-30 minutes and of the intestine within 60 minutes. In patients with acute right upper quadrant pain and tenderness, a good image of the bile duct accompanied by no image of the gallbladder indicates cystic duct obstruction and strongly supports a diagnosis of acute cholecystitis. The test is easy to perform

and is occasionally a useful method of confirming this diagnosis.

JAUNDICE

Jaundice is categorized as prehepatic, hepatic, or posthepatic, depending upon the site of the underlying disease. Hemolysis, the most common cause of prehepatic jaundice, involves increased production of bilirubin. Less common causes of prehepatic jaundice are Gilbert disease and the Crigler–Najjar syndrome.

Hepatic parenchymal jaundice is subdivided into hepatocellular and cholestatic types. The former includes acute viral hepatitis and chronic alcoholic cirrhosis. Some cases of intrahepatic cholestasis may be indistinguishable clinically and biochemically from cholestasis due to bile duct obstruction. Primary biliary cirrhosis, toxic drug jaundice, cholestatic jaundice of pregnancy, and postoperative cholestatic jaundice are the most common forms.

Extrahepatic jaundice most often results from biliary obstruction by a malignant tumor, choledocholithiasis, or biliary stricture. Pancreatic pseudocyst, chronic pancreatitis, sclerosing cholangitis, metastatic cancer, and duodenal diverticulitis are less common causes.

The cause of jaundice can be ascertained in the majority of patients from clinical and laboratory findings alone. In the remainder, THC or ERCP and ultrasound or CT scans will be necessary. The indications for these tests are discussed in later sections.

History

The age, gender, and parity of the patient and possible deleterious habits should be noted. Most cases of infectious hepatitis occur in patients under age 30 years. A history of drug addiction may suggest serum hepatitis transmitted by shared hypodermic equipment. Chronic alcoholism can usually be documented in patients with cirrhosis, and acute jaundice in alcoholics usually follows a recent binge. Obstructing gallstones or tumors are more common in older people.

Patients with jaundice due to choledocholithiasis may have associated biliary colic, fever, and chills, and may report previous similar attacks. The pain in malignant obstruction is deep-seated and dull and may be affected by changes in position. Pain in the region of the liver is frequently experienced in the early stages of viral hepatitis and acute alcoholic liver injury. The patient with extrahepatic obstruction may report that stools have become lighter in color and the urine dark.

Cholestatic diseases are often accompanied by pruritus—a source of severe discomfort in some cases. Pruritus may precede jaundice, but usually it appears at about the same time. The itching is most severe on the extremities and is aggravated by warm, humid weather. The cause remains obscure; itching does not correlate with bile salt levels in the skin, as was once believed.

▷ Physical Examination

Hepatomegaly is common in both hepatic and posthepatic jaundice. In some cases, palpation of the liver may suggest cirrhosis or metastatic cancer, but impressions of this kind are unreliable. Secondary stigmata of cirrhosis usually accompany acute alcoholic jaundice; liver palms, spider angiomas, ascites, collateral veins on the abdominal walls, and splenomegaly suggest cirrhosis. A nontender, palpable gallbladder in a jaundiced patient suggests malignant obstruction of the common duct (Courvoisier's sign), but absence of a palpable gallbladder is of little significance in ruling out cancer.

▷ Laboratory Tests

In hemolytic disease, the increased bilirubin is principally in the unconjugated indirect fraction. Since unconjugated bilirubin is insoluble in water, the jaundice in hemolysis is acholuric. The total bilirubin in hemolysis rarely exceeds 4-5 mg/dL, because the rate of excretion increases as the bilirubin concentration rises, and a plateau is quickly reached. Greater values suggest concomitant hepatic parenchymal disease.

Jaundice due to hepatic parenchymal disease is characterized by elevations of both conjugated and unconjugated serum bilirubin. An increase in the conjugated fraction always signifies disease within the hepatobiliary system. The direct bilirubin predominates in about half of cases of hepatic parenchymal disease.

Both intrahepatic cholestasis and extrahepatic obstruction raise the direct bilirubin fraction, though the indirect fraction also increases somewhat. Since direct bilirubin is water-soluble, bilirubinuria develops. With complete extrahepatic obstruction, the total bilirubin rises to a plateau of 25-30 mg/dL, at which point loss in the urine equals the additional daily production. Higher values suggest concomitant hemolysis or decreased renal function. Obstruction of a single hepatic duct does not usually cause jaundice.

In extrahepatic obstruction caused by neoplasms, the serum bilirubin usually exceeds 10 mg/dL, and the average concentration is about 18 mg/dL. Obstructive jaundice due to common duct stones often produces transient bilirubin increases in the range of 2-4 mg/dL, and the level rarely exceeds 15 mg/dL. Serum bilirubin values in patients with alcoholic cirrhosis and acute viral hepatitis vary widely in relation to the severity of the parenchymal damage.

In extrahepatic obstruction, modest rises of AST levels are common, but levels as high as 1000 units/L are seen (though rarely) in patients with common duct stones and cholangitis. In the latter patients, the high values last for only a few days and are associated with increases in LDH concentrations. In general, AST levels above 1000 units/L suggest viral hepatitis.

Serum alkaline phosphatase comes from three sites: liver, bone, and intestine. In normal subjects, liver and bone contribute about equally, and the intestinal contribution is small.

Hepatic alkaline phosphatase is a product of the epithelial cells of the cholangioles, and increased alkaline phosphatase levels associated with liver disease are the result of increased enzyme production. Alkaline phosphatase levels go up with intrahepatic cholestasis, cholangitis, or extrahepatic obstruction. Since the elevation is from overproduction, it may occur with focal hepatic lesions in the absence of jaundice. For example, a solitary hepatic metastasis or pyogenic abscess in one lobe or a tumor obstructing only one hepatic duct may fail to obstruct enough hepatic parenchyma to cause jaundice but usually is associated with increased alkaline phosphatase. In cholangitis with incomplete extrahepatic obstruction, serum bilirubin levels may be normal or mildly elevated, but serum alkaline phosphatase may be very high.

Bone disease may complicate the interpretation of abnormal alkaline phosphatase levels (Figure 25–6). If one suspects that the increased serum enzyme may be from bone, serum calcium, phosphorus, and 5′-nucleotidase or leucine aminopeptidase levels should be determined. These last two enzymes are also produced by cholangioles and are elevated in cholestasis, but their serum concentrations remain unchanged with bone disease.

Changes in serum protein levels may reflect hepatic parenchymal dysfunction. In cirrhosis, the serum albumin falls and the globulins increase. Serum globulins reach high

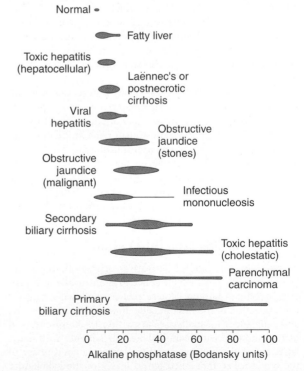

▲ **Figure 25–6.** Range of alkaline phosphatase values in various hepatobiliary disorders.

values in some patients with primary biliary cirrhosis. Biliary obstruction generally produces no changes unless secondary biliary cirrhosis has developed.

▶ Diagnosis

The principal diagnostic objective is to distinguish surgical (obstructive) from nonsurgical jaundice. The history, physical examination, and basic laboratory data allow an accurate diagnosis to be made in most cases without invasive tests (eg, liver biopsy, cholangiograms).

Since most jaundiced patients are not critically ill when first examined, diagnosis and therapy may be conducted in a stepwise fashion, with each test selected according to the information available at that point. Only severe or worsening cholangitis requires urgent intervention. If the jaundice is mild and recent, it often passes within 24-48 hours, at which time an ultrasound scan can be ordered to verify gallstone disease.

In patients with persistent jaundice, the first test is usually an ultrasound scan, which may show dilated intrahepatic bile ducts (indicating ductal obstruction) or gallbladder stones. The lesion may be further delineated by ERCP or THC. ERCP is preferable when the lower end of the duct is believed to be obstructed (eg, suspected carcinoma of the pancreas or other periampullary tumors). THC is usually preferred for proximal lesions (eg, biliary stricture, neoplasm of the bifurcation of the hepatic ducts), because it gives better opacification of the ducts proximal to the obstruction and therefore provides more information that can be used in planning surgery. If the clinical presentation suggests neoplastic obstruction, a CT scan could be selected in preference to an ultrasound scan, because CT gives better definition of mass lesions while also demonstrating the presence and general location of bile duct obstruction.

If ultrasound or CT scans suggest biliary obstruction, a decision must be made about whether cholangiograms are indicated. In general, patients with gallstone disease do not require preoperative cholangiograms, whereas cholangiograms would be routine in patients with neoplastic obstruction, benign biliary stricture, or rare or unknown causes of obstructive jaundice.

PATHOGENESIS OF GALLSTONES

More than 20 million people in the United States have gallstones in their gallbladders; about 300,000 operations are performed annually for this disease, and at least 6000 deaths result from its complications or treatment. The incidence of gallstones rises with age, so that between 50 and 65 years of age about 20% of women and 5% of men are affected (Figure 25–7).

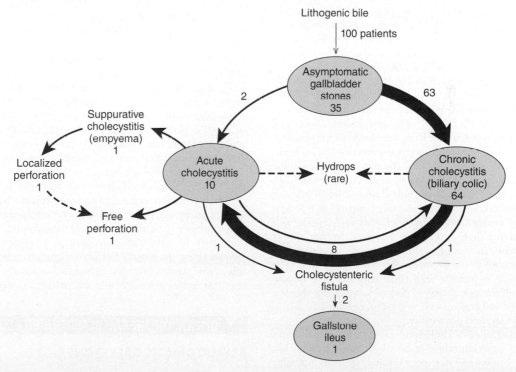

▲ **Figure 25–7.** The natural history of gallbladder stones. The numbers approximate the percentage of patients in each category. Note that most patients with acute cholecystitis have previously had biliary colic.

The gallstones in 75% of patients are composed predominantly (70%-95%) of cholesterol and are called cholesterol stones. The remaining 25% are pigment stones. Regardless of composition, all gallstones give rise to similar clinical sequelae.

Cholesterol Gallstones

Cholesterol gallstones result from secretion by the liver of bile supersaturated with cholesterol. Influenced by various factors present in bile, the cholesterol precipitates from solution and the newly formed crystals grow to macroscopic stones. Except when the common bile duct is dilated or partially obstructed, the stones in this disease form almost exclusively within the gallbladder. Those found in the ducts usually reach that location after passing through the cystic duct.

The incidence of cholesterol gallstone disease is highest in American Indians, lower in Caucasians, and lowest in blacks, with a twofold gradient from one group to the next. More than 75% of American Indian women over age 40 years are affected. Before puberty, the disease is rare but of equal frequency in both sexes. Thereafter, women are more commonly affected than men until after menopause, when the discrepancy lessens. Hormonal effects are also reflected in the increased incidence of gallstones with multiparity and the increased cholesterol saturation of bile and greater incidence of gallstones following ingestion of oral contraceptives. Obesity is the other major risk factor. The relative risk rises proportionately to the extent of overweight due to a progressively increasing output of cholesterol in bile.

As noted previously, cholesterol is insoluble and in bile must be transported within bile salt micelles and phospholipid (lecithin) vesicles. When the amount of cholesterol in bile exceeds the cholesterol holding capacity, cholesterol crystals begin to precipitate from the phospholipid vesicles.

The secretion of bile salt and cholesterol into bile is linked. Bile salt elutes cholesterol from the hepatocyte membrane during passage into the bile canaliculus. At higher bile salt output levels, the amount of cholesterol relative to bile salt entering bile decreases. This means that during low bile flow (eg, during fasting), bile holding capacity for cholesterol is more saturated than during high bile flow. In fact, almost half of persons in Western cultures have bile supersaturated with cholesterol in the morning after an overnight fast. The bile salt pool in patients with cholesterol gallstone disease is about half the size of that of normal subjects, but this is a result of the gallstone disease (eg, gallstones displace bile in the gallbladder) and not a cause.

The occurrence of cholesterol gallstone disease requires cholesterol supersaturation of bile, but that in itself is not sufficient. Cholesterol in supersaturated bile from individuals without gallstone disease precipitates spontaneously at a much slower rate than does the cholesterol in similar bile

from patients with gallstones. Furthermore, among individuals with supersaturated bile, only those with gallstone disease demonstrate cholesterol crystal formation in vivo. These observations are the result of specific bile proteins that either stabilize or destabilize cholesterol-laden phospholipid vesicles. For gallstone formation, the pronucleating factors (eg, immunoglobulin, mucus glycoprotein, fibronectin, orosomucoid) appear to be more important than the antinucleating factors (eg, glycoprotein, apolipoprotein, cytokeratin). Variations in these proteins may be the critical factor determining which of the many individuals with saturated bile develop gallstones.

The fact that gallstones form almost exclusively in the gallbladder even though the composition of hepatic bile is abnormal underscores the important role of the gallbladder in gallstone pathogenesis. This includes concentrating the bile, providing nidi (eg, small grains of pigment) for crystallization of cholesterol, supplying mucoprotein to paste the stones together, and serving as an area of stasis to allow stone formation and growth.

Pigment Stones

Pigment stones account for 25% of gallstones in the United States and 60% of those in Japan. Pigment stones are black to dark brown, 2-5 mm in diameter, and amorphous. They are composed of a mixture of calcium bilirubinate, complex bilirubin polymers, bile acids, and other unidentified substances. About 50% are radiopaque, and in the United States they constitute two-thirds of all radiopaque gallstones. The incidence is similar in men and women and in blacks and whites. Pigment stones are rare in American Indians.

Predisposing factors are cirrhosis, bile stasis (eg, a strictured or markedly dilated common duct), and chronic hemolysis. Some patients with pigment stones have increased concentrations of unconjugated bilirubin in their bile. Scanning electron microscopy demonstrates that about 90% of pigment stones are composed of dense mixtures of bacteria and bacterial glycocalix along with pigment solids. This suggests that bacteria have a primary role in pigment gallstone formation, and it also helps to explain why patients with pigment gallstone disease have sepsis more often than do those with cholesterol gallstone disease. It seems likely that bacterial {b}-glucuronidase is responsible for deconjugating the soluble bilirubin-diglucuronide to insoluble unconjugated bilirubin, which subsequently becomes agglomerated by glycocalix into macroscopic stones.

▼ DISEASES OF THE GALLBLADDER & BILE DUCTS

ASYMPTOMATIC GALLSTONES

Data on the prevalence of gallstones in the United States indicate that only about 30% of people with cholelithiasis come to surgery. Symptoms of gallstone disease generally do not change in severity. Each year, about 2% of patients with asymptomatic gallstones develop symptoms, usually biliary colic rather than one of the complications of gallstone disease. Patients with chronic biliary colic tend to have symptoms of the same level of severity and frequency. The present practice of operating only on symptomatic patients, leaving the millions without symptoms alone, seems appropriate. A question is often raised about what to advise the asymptomatic patient found to have gallstones during the course of unrelated studies. The presence of either of the following portends a more serious course and should probably serve as a reason for prophylactic cholecystectomy: (1) large stones (> 2 cm in diameter), because they produce acute cholecystitis more often than small stones; and (2) a calcified gallbladder, because it so often is associated with carcinoma. However, most asymptomatic patients have no special features. If coexistent cardiopulmonary or other problems increase the risk of surgery, operation should not be considered. For the average asymptomatic patient, it is not reasonable to make a strong recommendation for cholecystectomy. The tendency, however, is to operate on younger patients and temporize in the elderly.

GALLSTONES & CHRONIC CHOLECYSTITIS (BILIARY COLIC)

ESSENTIALS OF DIAGNOSIS

▸ Episodic abdominal pain

▸ Dyspepsia

▸ Gallstones on cholecystography or ultrasound scan

▶ General Considerations

Chronic cholecystitis is the most common form of symptomatic gallbladder disease and is associated with gallstones in nearly every case. In general, the term cholecystitis is applied whenever gallstones are present regardless of the histologic appearance of the gallbladder. Repeated minor episodes of obstruction of the cystic duct cause intermittent biliary colic and contribute to inflammation and subsequent scar formation. Gallbladders from symptomatic patients with gallstones who have never had an attack of acute cholecystitis are of two types: (1) In some, the mucosa may be slightly flattened, but the wall is thin and unscarred and, except for the stones, appears normal. (2) Others exhibit obvious signs of chronic inflammation, with thickening, cellular infiltration, loss of elasticity, and fibrosis. The clinical history in these two groups cannot always be distinguished, and inflammatory changes may also be found in patients with asymptomatic gallstones.

▶ Clinical Findings

A. Symptoms and Signs

Biliary colic, the most characteristic symptom, is caused by transient gallstone obstruction of the cystic duct. The pain usually begins abruptly and subsides gradually, lasting for a few minutes to several hours. The pain of biliary colic is usually steady—not intermittent, like that of intestinal colic. In some patients, attacks occur postprandially; in others, there is no relationship to meals. The frequency of attacks is quite variable, ranging from nearly continuous trouble to episodes many years apart. Nausea and vomiting may accompany the pain.

Biliary colic is usually felt in the right upper quadrant, but epigastric and left abdominal pain are common, and some patients experience precordial pain. The pain may radiate around the costal margin into the back or may be referred to the region of the scapula. Pain on top of the shoulder is unusual and suggests direct diaphragmatic irritation. In a severe attack, the patient usually curls up in bed, changing position frequently in order to be more comfortable.

During an attack, there may be tenderness in the right upper quadrant, and, rarely, the gallbladder is palpable.

Fatty food intolerance, dyspepsia, indigestion, heartburn, flatulence, nausea, and eructations are other symptoms associated with gallstone disease. Because they are also frequent in the general population, their presence in any given patient may only be incidental to the gallstones.

B. Laboratory Findings

An ultrasound scan of the gallbladder should usually be the first test. Gallstones can be demonstrated in about 95% of cases, and a positive reading for gallstones is almost never in error.

About 2% of patients with gallstone disease have normal ultrasound studies. Therefore, if the clinical suspicion of gallbladder disease is high and these two tests are negative, the patient should be studied by ERCP (to opacify the gallbladder in the search for stones) or duodenal intubation and examination of duodenal bile for cholesterol crystals or bilirubinate granules.

▶ Differential Diagnosis

Gallbladder colic may be strongly suggested by the history, but the clinical impression should always be verified by an ultrasound study. Biliary colic may simulate the pain of duodenal ulcer, hiatal hernia, pancreatitis, and myocardial infarction.

An EKG and a chest x-ray should be obtained to investigate cardiopulmonary disease. It has been suggested that biliary colic may sometimes aggravate cardiac disease, but angina pectoris or an abnormal EKG should rarely be indications for cholecystectomy.

Right-sided radicular pain in the T6-T10 dermatomes may be confused with biliary colic. Osteoarthritic spurs, vertebral lesions, or tumors may be shown on x-rays of the spine or may be suggested by hyperesthesia of the abdominal skin.

An upper gastrointestinal series may be indicated to search for esophageal spasm, hiatal hernia, peptic ulcer, or gastric tumors. In some patients, the irritable colon syndrome may be mistaken for gallbladder discomfort. Carcinoma of the cecum or ascending colon may be overlooked on the assumption that postprandial pain in these conditions is due to gallstones.

► Complications

Chronic cholecystitis predisposes to acute cholecystitis, common duct stones, and adenocarcinoma of the gallbladder. The longer the stones have been present, the higher the incidence of all of these complications. Complications are infrequent, however, and the presence of gallstones is not reason enough for prophylactic cholecystectomy in a person with asymptomatic or mildly symptomatic disease.

► Treatment

A. Medical Treatment

Avoidance of offending foods may be helpful.

1. Dissolution—Cholesterol gallstones in the gallbladder can be dissolved in some cases by chronic treatment with ursodiol, which reduces the cholesterol saturation of bile by inhibiting cholesterol secretion. The resulting undersaturated bile slowly dissolves the solid cholesterol in the gallstones.

Unfortunately, bile salt therapy has marginal efficacy. The gallstones must be small (eg, < 5 mm) and devoid of calcium (ie, nonopaque on CT scans), and the gallbladder must opacify on oral cholecystography (an indication of unobstructed flow of bile between bile duct and gallbladder). About 15% of patients with gallstones are candidates for treatment. Dissolution is achieved within 2 years in about 50% of highly selected patients. Stones recur, however, in 50% of cases within 5 years. In general, dissolution therapy—alone or in conjunction with lithotripsy—is used very rarely except in the prevention of gallstones in susceptible populations, such as following weight loss surgery.

B. Surgical Treatment

Cholecystectomy is indicated in most patients with symptoms. The procedure can be scheduled at the patient's convenience, within weeks or months after diagnosis. Active concurrent disease that increases the risk of surgery should be treated before operation. In some chronically ill patients, surgery should be deferred indefinitely.

Cholecystectomy is most often performed laparoscopically, but when the laparoscopic approach is contraindicated (eg, too many adhesions) or unsuccessful, it may be performed through a laparotomy. The difference consists of 4 fewer days in the hospital and fewer weeks off work when done laparoscopically. Regardless of how it is done, operative cholangiography may be included to evaluate for common duct stones. If stones are found, common duct exploration may be performed (see under choledocholithiasis).

► Prognosis

Serious complications and deaths related to the operation itself are rare. The operative death rate is about 0.1% in patients under age 50 and about 0.5% in patients over age 50. Most deaths occur in patients recognized preoperatively to have increased risks. The operation relieves symptoms in 95% of cases.

Gurusamy KS, Koti R, Fusai G, Davidson BR. Early versus delayed laparoscopic cholecystectomy for uncomplicated biliary colic. *Cochrane Database Syst Rev* 2013 Jun 30;6:CD007196.

ACUTE CHOLECYSTITIS

 ESSENTIALS OF DIAGNOSIS

► Acute right upper quadrant pain and tenderness
► Fever and leukocytosis
► Palpable gallbladder in one-third of cases
► Nonopacified gallbladder on radionuclide excretion scan
► Sonographic Murphy sign

► General Considerations

In 80% of cases, acute cholecystitis results from obstruction of the cystic duct by a gallstone impacted in Hartmann's pouch. The gallbladder becomes inflamed and distended, creating abdominal pain and tenderness. The natural history of acute cholecystitis varies, depending on whether the obstruction becomes relieved, the extent of secondary bacterial invasion, the age of the patient, and the presence of other aggravating factors such as diabetes mellitus. Most attacks resolve spontaneously without surgery or other specific therapy, but some progress to abscess formation or free perforation with generalized peritonitis.

The pathologic changes in the gallbladder evolve in a typical pattern. Subserosal edema and hemorrhage and patchy mucosal necrosis are the first changes. Later, PMNs appear. The final stage involves development of fibrosis.

Gangrene and perforation may occur as early as 3 days after onset, but most perforations occur during the second week. In cases that resolve spontaneously, acute inflammation has largely cleared by 4 weeks, but some residual evidence of inflammation may last for several months. About 90% of gallbladders removed during an acute attack show chronic scarring, although many of these patients deny having had any previous symptoms.

The cause of acute cholecystitis is still partially conjectural. Obstruction of the cystic duct is present in most cases, but in experimental animals, cystic duct obstruction does not result in acute cholecystitis unless the gallbladder is filled with concentrated bile or bile saturated with cholesterol. There is also evidence that trauma from gallstones releases phospholipase from the mucosal cells of the gallbladder. This is followed by conversion of lecithin in bile to lysolecithin, which is a toxic compound that may cause more inflammation. Bacteria appear to have a minor role in the early stages of acute cholecystitis, even though most complications of the disease involve suppuration.

About 20% of cases of acute cholecystitis occur in the absence of cholelithiasis (acalculous cholecystitis). Some of these are due to cystic duct obstruction by another process such as a malignant tumor. Rarely, acute acalculous cholecystitis results from cystic artery occlusion or primary bacterial infection by *Escherichia coli*, clostridia, or, occasionally, *Salmonella typhi*. Most cases occur in patients hospitalized with some other illness; acute acalculous cholecystitis is particularly common in trauma victims (civilian or military) and in patients receiving total parenteral nutrition. Small-vessel occlusion occurs early, and unless treatment is given promptly, the disease progresses rapidly to gangrenous cholecystitis and septic complications, at which point the death rate is high.

▶ Clinical Findings

A. Symptoms and Signs

The first symptom is abdominal pain in the right upper quadrant, sometimes associated with referred pain in the region of the right scapula. In 75% of cases, the patient will have had previous attacks of biliary colic, at first indistinguishable from the present illness. However, in acute cholecystitis, the pain persists and becomes associated with abdominal tenderness. Nausea and vomiting are present in about half of patients, but the vomiting is rarely severe. Mild icterus occurs in 10% of cases. The temperature usually ranges from 38°C to 38.5°C. High fever and chills are uncommon and should suggest the possibility of complications or an incorrect diagnosis.

Right upper quadrant tenderness is present, and in about a third of patients the gallbladder is palpable (often in a position lateral to its normal one). Voluntary guarding during examination may prevent detection of an enlarged gallbladder. In others, the gallbladder is not enlarged because scarring of the wall restricts distention. If instructed to breathe deeply during palpation in the right subcostal region, the patient experiences accentuated tenderness and sudden inspiratory arrest (Murphy sign).

B. Laboratory Findings

The leukocyte count is usually elevated to 12,000-15,000/mL. Normal counts are common, but if the count goes much above 15,000, one should suspect complications. A mild elevation of the serum bilirubin (in the range of 2-4 mg/dL) is common, presumably owing to secondary inflammation of the common duct by the contiguous gallbladder. Bilirubin values above this range would most likely indicate the associated presence of common duct stones. A mild increase in alkaline phosphatase may accompany the attack. Occasionally, the serum amylase concentration transiently reaches 1000 units/dL or more.

C. Imaging Studies

A plain x-ray of the abdomen may occasionally show an enlarged gallbladder shadow. In 15% of patients, the gallstones contain enough calcium to be seen on the plain film.

Ultrasound scans show gallstones, sludge, and thickening of the gallbladder wall, and the ultrasonographer can determine even better than the clinician whether the point of maximum tenderness is over the gallbladder (ultrasonographic Murphy sign). This last finding is often absent, however, when the gallbladder is gangrenous. Usually, ultrasound is the only test needed to make the diagnosis of acute cholecystitis.

If additional diagnostic information is desirable (eg, if ultrasound is equivocal or negative), a radionuclide excretion scan (eg, HIDA scan) should be performed. This test cannot demonstrate gallstones, but if the gallbladder is imaged, acute cholecystitis is ruled out except in rare cases of acalculous cholecystitis (the test is positive in most cases of acute acalculous cholecystitis). Imaging of the duct but not the gallbladder supports the diagnosis of acute cholecystitis. A few false positives are seen in advanced gallstone disease without acute inflammation and in acute biliary pancreatitis.

▶ Differential Diagnosis

The differential diagnosis includes other common causes of acute upper abdominal pain and tenderness. An acute peptic ulcer with or without perforation might be suggested by a history of epigastric pain relieved by food or antacids. Most cases of perforated ulcer demonstrate free air under the diaphragm on an x-ray. An emergency upper gastrointestinal series may help.

Acute pancreatitis can be confused with acute cholecystitis, especially if cholecystitis is accompanied by an elevated amylase level. Furthermore, HIDA scans fail to outline the gallbladder in most cases of acute biliary pancreatitis. Sometimes the two diseases coexist, but pancreatitis should not be accepted as a second diagnosis without specific findings.

Acute appendicitis in patients with a high cecum may closely simulate acute cholecystitis.

Severe right upper quadrant pain with high fever and local tenderness may develop in acute gonococcal perihepatitis (Fitz–Hugh–Curtis syndrome). Clues to the proper diagnosis may be found in tenderness in the adnexa, vaginal discharge that shows gonococci on a Gram-stained smear, and a disparity between the patient's high fever and her general lack of toxicity.

▶ **Complications**

The major complications of acute cholecystitis are empyema, gangrene, and perforation.

A. Empyema

In empyema (suppurative cholecystitis), the gallbladder contains frank pus, and the patient becomes more toxic, with high spiking fever (39-40°C, chills, and leukocytosis greater than 15,000/mL. Parenteral antibiotics should be given, and percutaneous cholecystostomy or cholecystectomy should be performed.

B. Perforation

Perforation may take any of three forms: (1) localized perforation with pericholecystic abscess; (2) free perforation with generalized peritonitis; and (3) perforation into an adjacent hollow viscus, with the formation of a fistula. Perforation may occur as early as 3 days after the onset of acute cholecystitis or not until late in the second week. The total incidence of perforation is about 10%.

1. Pericholecystic abscess—Pericholecystic abscess, the most common form of perforation, should be suspected when the signs and symptoms progress, especially when accompanied by the appearance of a palpable mass. The patient often becomes toxic, with fever to 39°C and a leukocyte count above 15,000/mL, but sometimes there is no correlation between the clinical signs and the development of local abscess. Cholecystectomy and drainage of the abscess can be performed safely in many of these patients, but if the patient's condition is unstable, percutaneous cholecystostomy is preferable.

2. Free perforation—Free perforation occurs in only 1%-2% of patients, most often early in the disease when gangrene develops before adhesions wall off the gallbladder. The diagnosis is made preoperatively in less than half of cases. In some patients with localized pain, sudden spread of pain and tenderness to other parts of the abdomen suggests the diagnosis. Whenever it is suspected, free perfora-

tion must be treated by emergency laparotomy. Abdominal paracentesis may be misleading and has proved to be of little diagnostic usefulness. Cholecystectomy should be performed if the patient's condition will permit; otherwise, cholecystostomy is done. The death rate depends partly on whether the cystic duct remains obstructed or the stone becomes dislodged after perforation. The former leads to a purulent peritonitis that is lethal in 20% of cases. In the latter, a true bile peritonitis ensues and over 50% of patients die. The earlier operation is performed, the better the prognosis.

3. Cholecystenteric fistula—If the acutely inflamed gallbladder becomes adherent to adjacent stomach, duodenum, or colon and necrosis develops at the site of one of these adhesions, perforation may occur into the lumen of the gut. The resulting decompression often allows the acute disease to resolve. If the gallbladder stones discharge through the fistula and if they are large enough, they may obstruct the small intestine (gallstone ileus; see below). Rarely, patients vomit gallstones that have entered the stomach through a cholecystogastric fistula. In most patients, the acute attack subsides and the cholecystenteric fistula is clinically unsuspected.

Cholecystenteric fistulas do not usually cause symptoms unless the gallbladder is still partially obstructed by stones or scarring. Neither oral nor intravenous cholangiograms will opacify the gallbladder or the fistula, but the latter may be shown on upper gastrointestinal series, where it must be differentiated from a fistula due to perforated peptic ulcer. Malabsorption and steatorrhea have been reported in isolated cases of cholecystocolonic fistulas. Steatorrhea in this situation could be due either to absence of bile in the proximal bowel following diversion into the colon or, more rarely, to excess bacteria in the upper intestine.

Symptomatic cholecystenteric fistulas should be treated by cholecystectomy and closure of the fistula. The majority is discovered incidentally during cholecystectomy for symptomatic gallbladder disease.

▶ **Treatment**

Intravenous fluids should be given to correct dehydration and electrolyte imbalance, and a nasogastric tube should be inserted. For acute cholecystitis of average severity, parenteral cefazolin (2-4 g daily) should be given. Parenteral penicillin (20 million units daily), clindamycin, and an aminoglycoside should be given for severe disease. Single-drug therapy using imipenem is a good alternative.

There are acute options for the treatment of acute cholecystitis. Since the disease resolves with antibiotics and supportive care in about 60% of cases, one approach is to manage the patient expectantly, with a plan to perform elective cholecystectomy after recovery, reserving surgery during the acute attack for those with severe or worsening disease. This approach is untenable in acute acalculous cholecystitis.

The preferred plan is to perform cholecystectomy in all patients unless there are specific contraindications to operation (eg, serious concomitant disease). Four controlled trials have supported this approach with the following data: (1) the incidence of technical complications is no greater with early surgery; (2) early surgery reduces the total duration of illness by approximately 30 days, length of hospitalization by 5-7 days, and direct medical costs by several thousand dollars; and (3) the death rate is slightly lower with early surgery because of earlier treatment for some patients whose condition would have worsened during expectant management.

The following are the major factors that affect the decision (Figure 25-8): (1) whether the diagnosis is established; (2) the general health of the patient as modified by coexistent disease or the present illness; and (3) signs of local complications of acute cholecystitis. The diagnosis should be clear-cut and the patient optimally prepared; if perforation or empyema is suspected, emergency surgery is indicated.

In about 30% of cases, the diagnosis of acute cholecystitis is established but the general condition of the patient is unsatisfactory. If possible, surgery should be postponed in these cases until the ancillary disease is controlled. Expectant management cannot be rigidly adhered to, however, if the manifestations of cholecystitis worsen.

About 10% of patients require emergency treatment. These are generally clinical situations in which the disease appears to have become complicated or is about to. High fever (39°C), marked leukocytosis (> 15,000/mL), or chills suggest suppurative progression. Acalculous acute cholecystitis should automatically be placed in this category. When the patient's general condition is poor, percutaneous catheter cholecystostomy is the preferable treatment. Patients in better overall health should be treated by cholecystectomy.

The sudden appearance of generalized abdominal pain may indicate free perforation. Appearance of a mass while the patient is under observation may be a sign of local perforation and abscess formation. Changes of this sort are indications for emergency surgery.

Cholecystectomy is the preferable operation in acute cholecystitis, and it can be performed laparoscopically in about 50% of patients. Operative cholangiography should be performed in most cases, and the common bile duct explored if appropriate indications are present (see section on choledocholithiasis). Patients with severe acute cholecystitis who are in poor condition for emergency cholecystectomy should be treated by percutaneous cholecystostomy. Percutaneous cholecystostomy may also be the preferred therapy for acute acalculous cholecystitis. A catheter inserted under ultrasound or CT guidance is allowed to drain the gallbladder of its bile or pus. The resulting decompression controls the acute disease, including any local infection, but the gallstones cannot be removed. Therefore, cholecystectomy should be performed after the patient recovers in order to avoid recurrent attacks. Cholecystectomy is definitive therapy in the patient with acalculous cholecystitis.

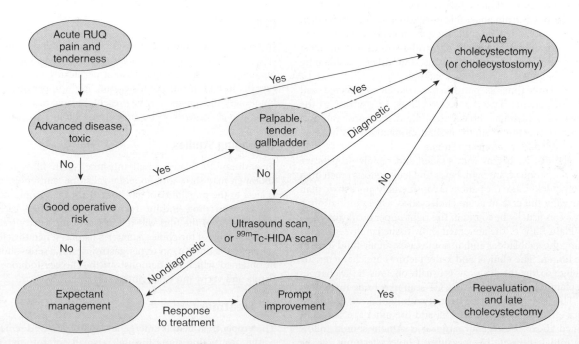

▲ **Figure 25–8.** Scheme for the management of acute cholecystitis.

Prognosis

The overall death rate of acute cholecystitis is about 5%. Nearly all of the deaths are in patients over age 60 or those with diabetes mellitus. In the older age group, secondary cardiovascular or pulmonary complications contribute substantially to the death rate. Uncontrolled sepsis with peritonitis and intrahepatic abscesses are the most important local conditions responsible for death.

Common duct stones are present in about 15% of patients with acute cholecystitis, and some of the more seriously ill patients have simultaneous cholangitis from biliary obstruction. Acute pancreatitis may also complicate acute cholecystitis, and the combination carries a greater risk.

Patients who develop the suppurative forms of gallbladder disease such as empyema or perforation are less likely to recover. Earlier admission to the hospital and early cholecystectomy reduce the chances of these complications.

Gurusamy KS, Koti R, Fusai G, Davidson BR. Early versus delayed laparoscopic cholecystectomy for uncomplicated biliary colic. *Cochrane Database Syst Rev* 2013 Jun 30;6:CD007196.
Gurusamy KS, Rossi M, Davidson BR. Percutaneous cholecystostomy for high-risk surgical patients with acute calculous cholecystitis. *Cochrane Database Syst Rev* 2013 Aug 12;8:CD007088.

EMPHYSEMATOUS CHOLECYSTITIS

Emphysematous cholecystitis is a rare condition in which bubbles of gas from anaerobic infection appear in the lumen of the gallbladder, its wall, the pericholecystic space, and, on occasion, the bile ducts. Clostridia species are the most commonly implicated organisms, but other gas-forming anaerobes such as *E coli* or anaerobic streptococci may be found. Three times as many men as women are affected, and 20% of patients have diabetes mellitus. In contrast to the usual form of acute cholecystitis, the disease probably is a bacterial infection from the earliest moment. In many cases, the gallbladder contains no stones.

The disease begins with sudden and rapidly progressive right upper quadrant pain. Fever and leukocytosis reach high levels quickly, and the patient is considerably more toxic than is usually the case in acute cholecystitis. On examination, a mass can usually be found in the right upper quadrant.

Plain films of the abdomen show tissue emphysema outlining the gallbladder and, in some cases, an air-fluid level in the lumen. The clinical and x-ray pictures are characteristic enough so that the diagnosis is usually obvious. If the changes on plain films are equivocal, a CT scan may bring them out.

The patient should be treated with high doses of antibiotics effective against clostridia and the other species mentioned above. Emergency surgical treatment should follow the initial resuscitative measures. Cholecystectomy can be safely performed in most cases, but the most critically ill

might fare better with cholecystostomy. The types of complications are the same as in other forms of acute cholecystitis, but illness is more severe and death rates are higher.

Gurusamy KS, Rossi M, Davidson BR. Percutaneous cholecystostomy for high-risk surgical patients with acute calculous cholecystitis. *Cochrane Database Syst Rev* 2013 Aug 12;8:CD007088.

GALLSTONE ILEUS

Gallstone ileus is mechanical intestinal obstruction caused by a large gallstone lodged in the lumen. It occurs more often in women, and the average patient age is about 70 years.

Clinical Findings

A. Symptoms

The patient usually presents with obvious small bowel obstruction, either partial or complete. The obstructing gallstone enters the intestine through a cholecystenteric fistula located in the duodenum, colon, or, rarely, the stomach or jejunum. The gallbladder may contain one or several stones, but stones that cause gallstone ileus are almost always 2.5 cm or more in diameter. The lumen in the proximal bowel will allow most of these large calculi to pass caudally until the ileum is reached. Obstruction of the large intestine may follow passage of a gallstone through a fistula at the hepatic flexure or may occur even after the stone has traversed the entire small bowel.

B. Signs

In most patients, the findings on physical examination are typical of distal small bowel obstruction. Obstruction of the duodenum or jejunum may give a perplexing clinical picture because of the lack of distention. Right upper quadrant tenderness and a mass may be present in some cases, but the distended abdomen may be difficult to examine accurately.

C. Imaging Studies

In addition to dilated small intestine, plain films of the abdomen may show a radiopaque gallstone, and unless one is alert to the possibility of gallstone ileus, the ectopic stone can be a puzzling finding. In about 40% of cases, careful examination of the film will reveal gas in the biliary tree, a manifestation of the cholecystenteric fistula. When the clinical picture is unclear, an upper gastrointestinal series should be obtained, which will demonstrate the cholecystoduodenal fistula and verify intestinal obstruction.

Treatment

The proper treatment is emergency laparotomy and removal of the obstructing stone through a small enterotomy. The proximal intestine must be carefully inspected for the presence of a second calculus that might cause a postoperative recurrence. The gallbladder should be left undisturbed at the original operation.

Once the patient has recovered, an elective cholecystectomy should be scheduled if the patient complains of chronic gallbladder symptoms. On this basis, interval cholecystectomy will be required in about 30% of patients. The fistula itself is rarely the source of trouble and closes spontaneously in most patients.

▶ Prognosis

The death rate from gallstone ileus remains about 20%, largely because of the poor general condition of elderly patients at the time of laparotomy. In many cases, the patient has developed cardiac or pulmonary complications during a preoperative delay when the diagnosis was unclear.

CHOLANGITIS (BACTERIAL CHOLANGITIS)

Bacterial infection of the biliary ducts always signifies biliary obstruction, since in the absence of obstruction even heavy bacterial contamination of the ducts fails to produce symptoms or pathologic changes. The block to flow may be partial or, less commonly, complete. The principal causes are choledocholithiasis, biliary stricture, and neoplasm. Less common causes are chronic pancreatitis, ampullary stenosis, pancreatic pseudocyst, duodenal diverticulum, congenital cyst, and parasitic invasion. Iatrogenic cholangitis may complicate transhepatic or T tube cholangiography. Not all obstructing lesions are followed by cholangitis, however. For example, biliary infection develops in only 15% of patients with neoplastic obstruction. The likelihood of cholangitis is greatest when the obstruction occurs after the duct has acquired a resident bacterial population.

With obstruction, ductal pressure rises, and bacteria proliferate and escape into the systemic circulation via the hepatic sinusoids. Experimentally, the incidence of positive blood cultures with ductal infection is directly proportionate to the absolute height of the pressure in the duct.

The symptoms of cholangitis (sometimes referred to as Charcot's triad) are biliary colic, jaundice, and chills and fever, though a complete triad is present in only 70% of cases. Laboratory findings include leukocytosis and elevated serum bilirubin and alkaline phosphatase levels. The predominant organisms in bile (in approximately decreasing frequency) are *E coli*, *Klebsiella*, *Pseudomonas*, *Enterococci*, and *Proteus*. *Bacteroides fragilis* and other anaerobes (eg, *Clostridium perfringens*) can be detected in about 25% of cases, and their presence correlates with multiple previous biliary operations (often including a biliary enteric anastomosis), severe symptoms, and a high incidence of postoperative suppurative complications. Anaerobes are nearly always seen in the company of aerobes. Two species of bacteria can be cultured in about 50% of cases. Bacteremia probably occurs in most cases, and blood cultures obtained at the appropriate time contain the same organisms as the bile. Early in an attack, an ultrasound scan will often give useful diagnostic information. Further workup (THC, ERCP, etc) can proceed later after the acute manifestations are brought under control. Cholangiography is dangerous during active cholangitis.

The term suppurative cholangitis has been used for the most severe form of this disease, when manifestations of sepsis overshadow those of hepatobiliary disease. The diagnostic pentad of suppurative cholangitis consists of abdominal pain, jaundice, fever and chills, mental confusion or lethargy, and shock. The diagnosis is often missed because the signs of biliary disease are overlooked.

Most cases of cholangitis can be controlled with intravenous antibiotics. A cephalosporin antibiotic (eg, cefazolin, cefoxitin) is the drug of choice in the average mild to moderately severe case. If disease is severe or progressively worsens, an aminoglycoside plus clindamycin or metronidazole should be added to the regimen.

For patients with severe cholangitis or unremitting cholangitis despite antibiotic therapy, the bile duct must be promptly decompressed. Most cases of severe acute cholangitis are associated with choledocholithiasis, for which the best treatment consists of emergency endoscopic sphincterotomy. In the uncommon case where this is unsuccessful, laparotomy is indicated in order to decompress the bile duct. Cholangitis accompanying neoplastic obstruction may be managed by insertion of a transhepatic drainage catheter into the bile duct. A cholangiogram should not be obtained because the procedure could worsen sepsis.

Urgent intervention (eg, endoscopic sphincterotomy, percutaneous transhepatic drainage, or operative decompression) is required in about 10% of patients with acute cholangitis. The remaining 90% are eventually treated by elective surgery or endoscopic sphincterotomy following antibiotic therapy and a thorough diagnostic evaluation.

Takada T, Strasberg SM, the Tokyo Guidelines Revision Committee. TG13: updated Tokyo guidelines for the management of acute cholangitis and cholecystitis. *J Hepatobiliary Pancreat Sci* 2013 Jan;20(1):1-7.

CHOLEDOCHOLITHIASIS

 ESSENTIALS OF DIAGNOSIS

▶ Biliary pain

▶ Jaundice

▶ Episodic cholangitis

▶ Stones in gallbladder or previous cholecystectomy

General Considerations

Approximately 15% of patients with stones in the gallbladder harbor calculi within the bile ducts. Common duct stones are usually accompanied by others in the gallbladder, but in 5% of cases, the gallbladder is empty. The number of duct stones may vary from one to more than 100.

There are two possible origins for common duct stones. The evidence suggests that most cholesterol stones develop within the gallbladder and reach the duct after traversing the cystic duct. These are called secondary stones. Pigment stones may have a similar pedigree or, more often, develop de novo within the common duct. These are called primary common duct stones. About 60% of common duct stones are cholesterol stones and 40% are pigment stones. The latter are, on the average, associated with more severe clinical manifestations.

Patients may have one or more of the following principal clinical findings, all of which are caused by obstruction to the flow of bile or pancreatic juice: biliary colic, cholangitis, jaundice, and pancreatitis (Figure 25–9). It seems likely,

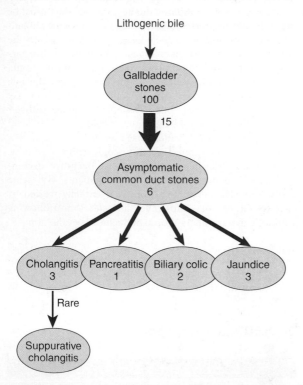

▲ **Figure 25–9.** The natural history of common duct stones. Of every 100 patients with gallbladder stones, 15 will have common duct stones, which will produce the spectrum of syndromes illustrated. Note that the individual syndromes overlap, indicating that they may appear together in various combinations.

however, that as many as 50% of patients with choledocholithiasis remain asymptomatic.

The common duct may dilate to 2-3 cm proximal to an obstructing lesion, and truly huge ducts develop in patients with biliary tumors. In choledocholithiasis or biliary stricture, the inflammatory reaction restricts dilation, so the dilatation is less marked. Dilation of the ductal system within the liver can also be limited by cirrhosis.

Biliary colic is the result of rapid rises in biliary pressure whether the block is in the common duct or neck of the gallbladder. Gradual occlusion of the duct—as in cancer—rarely produces the same kind of pain as gallstone disease.

Clinical Findings

A. Symptoms

Choledocholithiasis may be asymptomatic or may produce sudden toxic cholangitis, leading to a rapid demise. The seriousness of the disease parallels the degree of obstruction, the length of time it has been present, and the extent of secondary bacterial infection (see Cholangitis, above). Biliary colic, jaundice, or pancreatitis may be isolated findings or may occur in any combination along with signs of infection (cholangitis).

Biliary colic from common duct obstruction cannot be distinguished from that caused by stones in the gallbladder. The pain is felt in the right subcostal region, epigastrium, or even the substernal area. Referred pain to the region of the right scapula is common.

Choledocholithiasis should be strongly suspected if intermittent chills, fever, or jaundice accompanies biliary colic. Some patients notice transient darkening of their urine during an attack even though jaundice is not evident.

Pruritus is usually the result of persistent long-standing obstruction. The itching is more intense in warm weather when the patient perspires and is usually worse on the extremities than on the trunk. It is much more common with neoplastic obstruction than with gallstone obstruction.

B. Signs

The patient may be icteric and toxic, with high fever and chills, or may appear to be perfectly healthy. A palpable gallbladder is unusual in patients with obstructive jaundice from common duct stone because the obstruction is transient and partial, and scarring of the gallbladder renders it inelastic and nondistensible. Tenderness may be present in the right upper quadrant but is not often as marked as in acute cholecystitis, perforated peptic ulcer, or acute pancreatitis. Tender hepatic enlargement may occur.

C. Laboratory Findings

In cholangitis, leukocytosis of 15,000/mL is usual, and values above 20,000/mL are common. A rise in serum bilirubin often appears within 24 hours after the onset of symptoms. The absolute level usually remains under 10 mg/dL, and most are in the range of 2-4 mg/dL. The direct fraction exceeds the indirect, but the latter becomes elevated in most cases. Bilirubin levels do not ordinarily reach the high values seen in malignant tumors because the obstruction is usually incomplete and transient. In fact, fluctuating jaundice is so characteristic of choledocholithiasis that it fairly reliably differentiates between benign and malignant obstruction.

The serum alkaline phosphatase level usually rises and may be the only chemical abnormality in patients without jaundice. When the obstruction is relieved, the alkaline phosphatase and bilirubin levels should return to normal within 1-2 weeks, with the exception that the former may remain elevated longer if the obstruction was prolonged.

Mild increases in AST and ALT are often seen with extrahepatic obstruction of the ducts; rarely, AST levels transiently reach 1000 units.

D. Imaging Studies

Radiopaque gallstones may be seen on plain abdominal films or CT scans. Ultrasound scans will usually show gallbladder stones and, depending on the degree of obstruction, dilatation of the bile duct. Ultrasound and CT scans are insensitive in the search for stones in the common duct. ERCP is indicated if the patient has had a previous cholecystectomy. If cholecystectomy has not been performed, cholangiography should be part of operative management. Some clinicians choose preoperative ERCP for patients scheduled for cholecystectomy in order to clear the common bile duct. If ERCP is not technically successful, the surgeon will be forced to convert to open common bile duct exploration to clear the duct of stones.

Bilirubin values above 10 mg/dL are so uncommon in choledocholithiasis that when this finding is present, cholangiography should be performed to rule out the possibility of neoplastic obstruction.

▶ Differential Diagnosis

The workup should consider the same possibilities in differential diagnosis as for cholecystitis.

Serum amylase levels above 500 units/dL can result from acute pancreatitis, acute cholecystitis, or choledocholithiasis. Other manifestations of pancreatic disease should be documented before an unqualified diagnosis of pancreatitis is accepted.

Alcoholic cirrhosis or acute alcoholic hepatitis may present with jaundice, right upper quadrant tenderness, and leukocytosis. The differentiation from cholangitis may be impossible from clinical data. A history of a recent binge suggests acute liver disease. A percutaneous liver biopsy may be specific.

Intrahepatic cholestasis from drugs, pregnancy, chronic active hepatitis, or primary biliary cirrhosis may be difficult to distinguish from extrahepatic obstruction. ERCP would be appropriate to make the distinction, particularly if other studies (eg, ultrasound scan) failed to provide evidence of gallstone disease. If jaundice has persisted for 4-6 weeks, a mechanical cause is probable. Since most patients improve during this interval, persistent jaundice should never be assumed to be the result of parenchymal disease unless a normal cholangiogram rules out obstruction of the major ducts.

Intermittent jaundice and cholangitis after cholecystectomy are compatible with biliary stricture, and the distinction requires ERCP.

Biliary tumors usually produce intense jaundice without biliary colic or fever, and once it begins, the jaundice rarely remits.

▶ Complications

Long-standing ductal infection can produce intrahepatic abscesses. Hepatic failure or secondary biliary cirrhosis may develop in unrelieved obstruction of long duration. Since the obstruction is usually incomplete and intermittent, cirrhosis develops only after several years in untreated disease. Acute pancreatitis, a fairly common complication of calculous biliary disease, is discussed in Chapter 26. Rarely, a stone in the common duct may erode through the ampulla, resulting in gallstone ileus. Hemorrhage (hemobilia) is also a rare complication.

▶ Treatment

Patients with acute cholangitis should be treated with systemic antibiotics and other measures as described in the preceding section; this usually controls the attack within 24-48 hours. If the patient's condition worsens or if marked improvement is not observed within 2-4 days, endoscopic sphincterotomy or surgery and common bile duct exploration should be performed.

The typical patient presents with mild cholangitis and evidence on ultrasound scans of gallbladder stones. Laparoscopic cholecystectomy is indicated and, depending on the experience of the surgeon, laparoscopic exploration of the common duct if an operative cholangiogram or laparoscopic ultrasound demonstrates the expected common duct stones. Laparoscopic common duct exploration is usually accomplished through the cystic duct (which may have to be dilated), but when the common duct is enlarged (> 1.5 cm), it may be accomplished through a choledochotomy incision, just as in open surgery. Eventually, nearly all cases of common duct stones should be manageable by laparoscopic techniques, but at this stage the requisite laparoscopic skills are not available in most hospitals. If the surgeon thinks the common duct stones cannot be removed laparoscopically, it is probably best to remove the gallbladder laparoscopically and the common duct stones by endoscopic sphincterotomy. If the stones cannot be removed by sphincterotomy, a second (open) operation may be necessary.

There is also a lack of consensus regarding the importance of operative cholangiography or ultrasound during cholecystectomy when there are no clues suggesting stones in the duct. In such cases the chances of finding a stone are only 3%-5%, and some consider the effort unwarranted. On the other hand, operative cholangiograms also provide confirmation of the biliary anatomy, which contributes to avoidance of bile duct injuries, and the natural history of the few overlooked stones is worrisome. Therefore, we side with those who perform operative cholangiography liberally in such cases.

When the common duct is explored through the cystic duct and gallstones are removed, the cystic duct must be ligated, but a drainage catheter is not usually left within the common duct. When the common duct is explored through a choledochotomy (either during a laparoscopic or open operation), a T tube is usually left in the duct, and cholangiograms are taken a week or so postoperatively. Any residual stones discovered on these postoperative x-rays can be extracted 4-6 weeks later through the T tube tract.

Patients with common duct stones who have had a previous cholecystectomy are best treated by endoscopic sphincterotomy. Using a side-viewing duodenoscope, the ampulla is cannulated, and a 1-cm incision is made in the sphincter with an electrocautery wire. The opening created in the sphincter permits stones to pass from the duct into the duodenum. Endoscopic sphincterotomy is unlikely to be successful in patients with large stones (eg, > 2 cm), and it is contraindicated in the presence of stenosis of the bile duct proximal to the sphincter. Laparotomy and common duct exploration are required in a few cases.

Stones in the intrahepatic branches of the bile duct can usually be removed without difficulty during common duct exploration. In some cases, however, one or more of the intrahepatic ducts have become packed with stones, and the associated chronic inflammation has produced stenosis of the duct near its junction with the common hepatic duct. It is often impossible in these cases to clear the duct of stones, and if the disease involves only one lobe (usually the left lobe), hepatic lobectomy is indicated.

POSTCHOLECYSTECTOMY SYNDROME

This term has been used to signify the heterogeneous group of disorders affecting patients who continue to complain of symptoms after cholecystectomy. It is not really a syndrome, and the term is confusing.

The usual reason for incomplete relief after cholecystectomy is that the preoperative diagnosis of chronic cholecystitis was incorrect. The only symptom entirely characteristic of chronic cholecystitis is biliary colic. When a calculous gallbladder is removed in the hope that the patient will gain relief from dyspepsia, fatty food intolerance, belching, etc, the operation may leave the symptoms unchanged.

The presenting symptom may be dyspepsia or pain. An organic cause for the symptoms is more likely to be discovered in patients with severe episodic pain than in those with other complaints. Abnormal liver function studies, jaundice, and cholangitis are other manifestations that indicate residual biliary disease. Patients with suspicious findings should be studied by ERCP or THC. Choledocholithiasis, biliary stricture, and chronic pancreatitis are the most common causes of symptoms. Occasionally, there is sufficient evidence to implicate sphincter of Oddi dysmotility as a cause of pain. Relief of pain may follow endoscopic sphincterotomy. Stenosis of the hepatobiliary ampulla, a long cystic duct remnant, and neuromas have been blamed for continued symptoms.

CARCINOMA OF THE GALLBLADDER

Carcinoma of the gallbladder is an uncommon neoplasm that occurs in elderly patients. It is associated with gallstones in 70% of cases, and the risk of malignant degeneration correlates with the length of time gallstones have been present. The tumor is twice as common in women as in men, as one would expect from the association with gallstones.

Most primary tumors of the gallbladder are adenocarcinomas that appear histologically to be scirrhous (60%), papillary (25%), or mucoid (15%). Dissemination of the tumor occurs early by direct invasion of the liver and hilar structures and by metastases to the common duct lymph nodes, liver, and lungs. In an occasional case, where carcinoma is an incidental finding after cholecystectomy for gallstone disease, the tumor is confined to the gallbladder as a carcinoma in situ or an early invasive lesion. Most invasive carcinomas, however, have spread by the time of surgery, and spread is virtually certain if the tumor has progressed to the point where it causes symptoms.

▶ Clinical Findings

A. Symptoms and Signs

The most common presenting complaint is of right upper quadrant pain similar to previous episodes of biliary colic but more persistent. Obstruction of the cystic duct by tumor sometimes initiates an attack of acute cholecystitis. Other cases present with obstructive jaundice and, occasionally, cholangitis due to secondary involvement of the common duct.

Examination usually reveals a mass in the region of the gallbladder, which may not be recognized as a neoplasm if the patient has acute cholecystitis. If cholangitis is the principal symptom, a palpable gallbladder would be an unusual finding with choledocholithiasis alone and should suggest gallbladder carcinoma.

B. Imaging Studies

CT and ultrasound scans may demonstrate the extent of disease, but more often they show only gallstones.

The correct diagnosis is made preoperatively in only 10% of cases.

Complications

Obstruction of the common duct may produce multiple intrahepatic abscesses. Abscesses in or next to the tumor-laden gallbladder are frequent.

Prevention

The incidence of gallbladder cancer has decreased in recent years as the frequency of cholecystectomy has increased. It has been estimated that one case of gallbladder cancer is prevented for every 100 cholecystectomies performed for gallstone disease.

Treatment

If a localized carcinoma of the gallbladder is recognized at laparotomy, cholecystectomy should be performed along with en bloc wedge resection of an adjacent 3-5 cm of normal liver and dissection of the lymph nodes in the hepatoduodenal ligament. If a small invasive carcinoma overlooked during cholecystectomy for gallstone disease is later discovered by the pathologist, reoperation is indicated to perform a wedge resection of the liver bed plus regional lymphadenectomy. Some surgeons also recommend that the common duct be included routinely (ie, even in the absence of gross invasion) in the lymph node dissection for any lesion that involves the full thickness of the gallbladder wall. In the few cases when cancer has not penetrated the muscularis mucosae, cholecystectomy alone should suffice. More extensive hepatectomies (eg, right lobectomy) are not worthwhile. Lesions that invade the bile duct and produce jaundice should be resected if possible. When not, a stent should be inserted endoscopically or percutaneously. There is little that surgery can offer in cases with hepatic metastases or more distant spread.

Prognosis

Radiotherapy and chemotherapy are not effective palliative measures. About 85% of patients are dead within a year after diagnosis.

The 10% of patients who presently survive more than 5 years consist of those whose carcinoma was an incidental finding during cholecystectomy for symptomatic gallstone disease and those in whom an aggressive resection has removed all gross tumor.

Mayo SC, Shore AD, Nathan H, et al. National trends in the management and survival of surgically managed gallbladder adenocarcinoma over 15 years: a population-based analysis. *J Gastrointest Surg* 2010 Oct;14(10):1578-1591.

Wu LM, Jiang XX, Gu HY, et al. Endoscopic ultrasound-guided fine-needle aspiration biopsy in the evaluation of bile duct strictures and gallbladder masses: a systematic review and meta-analysis. *Eur J Gastroenterol Hepatol* 2011 Feb;23(2):113-120.

MALIGNANT TUMORS OF THE BILE DUCT

 ESSENTIALS OF DIAGNOSIS

▶ Intense cholestatic jaundice and pruritus

▶ Anorexia and dull right upper quadrant pain

▶ Dilated intrahepatic bile ducts on ultrasound or CT scan

▶ Focal stricture on transhepatic or retrograde endoscopic cholangiogram

General Considerations

Primary bile duct tumors are not more common in patients with cholelithiasis, and men and women are affected with equal frequency. Tumors appear at an average age of 60 years but may appear at any time between 20 and 80 years of age. More young people have been seen with this disease in recent years. Ulcerative colitis is a common associated condition, and in occasional cases bile duct cancer develops in a patient with ulcerative colitis who has been known to have sclerosing cholangitis for several years. Chronic parasitic infestation of the bile ducts in the Orient may be responsible for the greater incidence of bile duct tumors in that area.

Most malignant biliary tumors are adenocarcinomas located in the hepatic or common bile duct. The histologic pattern varies from typical adenocarcinoma to tumors composed principally of fibrous stroma and few cells. The acellular tumors may be mistaken for benign strictures or sclerosing cholangitis if adequate biopsies are not obtained. About 10% are bulky papillary tumors, which tend to be less invasive and less apt to metastasize.

At presentation, metastases are uncommon, but the tumor has often grown into the portal vein or hepatic artery.

Clinical Findings

A. Symptoms and Signs

The illness presents with gradual onset of jaundice or pruritus. Chills, fever, and biliary colic are usually absent, and except for a deep discomfort in the right upper quadrant the patient feels well. Bilirubinuria is present from the start, and light-colored stools are usual. Anorexia and weight loss develop insidiously with time.

Icterus is the most obvious physical finding. If the tumor is located in the common duct, the gallbladder may distend and become palpable in the right upper quadrant. The tumor itself is never palpable. Patients with tumors of the hepatic duct do not develop palpable gallbladders. Hepatomegaly is common. If obstruction is unrelieved, the liver may eventually become cirrhotic, and splenomegaly, ascites, or bleeding varices become secondary manifestations.

B. Laboratory Findings

Since the duct is often completely obstructed, the serum bilirubin is usually over 15 mg/dL. Serum alkaline phosphatase is also increased. Fever and leukocytosis are not common, since the bile is sterile in most cases. The stool may contain occult blood, but this is more common with tumors of the pancreas or hepatopancreatic ampulla than those of the bile ducts.

C. Imaging Studies

Ultrasound or CT scans usually detect dilated intrahepatic bile ducts. THC or ERCP clearly depicts the lesion, and both are indicated in most cases. THC is of greater value, since it better demonstrates the ductal anatomy on the hepatic side of the lesion. With tumors involving the bifurcation of the common hepatic duct (Klatskin tumors), it is important to determine the proximal extent of the lesion (ie, whether the first branches of the lobar ducts are also involved). ERCP is of value with proximal tumors because if it shows concomitant obstruction of the cystic duct, the diagnosis will most often prove to be gallbladder cancer invading the common duct (not a primary common duct neoplasm). The typical pattern with distal bile duct cancers consists of stenosis of the bile duct with sparing of the pancreatic duct. Adjacent stenoses of both ducts (the double-duct sign) indicate primary cancer of the pancreas. MR cholangiopancreatography may be useful if high-quality studies are available.

Occasionally, bile samples obtained at the time of THC will show malignant cells on cytologic study, but this is not a particularly useful test since the diagnosis of cancer must be presumed from the cholangiographic findings and a negative cytologic study is unreliable. Angiography may suggest invasion of the portal vein or encasement of the hepatic artery. False positives may occur, however.

▶ Differential Diagnosis

The differential diagnosis must consider other causes of extrahepatic and intrahepatic cholestatic jaundice. Choledocholithiasis is characterized by episodes of partial obstruction, pain, and cholangitis, which contrast with the unremitting jaundice of malignant obstruction. Bilirubin concentrations rarely surpass 15 mg/dL and are usually below 10 mg/dL in gallstone obstruction, whereas bilirubin levels almost always exceed 10 mg/dL and are usually above 15 mg/dL in neoplastic obstruction. A rapid rise of the bilirubin level to above 15 mg/dL in a patient with sclerosing cholangitis should suggest superimposed neoplasm. Dilatation of the gallbladder may occur with tumors of the distal common duct but is rare with calculous obstruction.

The combination of an enlarged gallbladder with obstructive jaundice is usually recognized as being due to tumor. If the gallbladder cannot be felt, primary biliary cirrhosis, drug-induced jaundice, chronic active hepatitis, metastatic hepatic cancer, and common duct stone must be ruled out. In general, any patient with cholestatic jaundice of more than 2 weeks' duration whose diagnosis is uncertain should be studied by THC or ERCP. The finding of focal bile duct stenosis in the absence of previous biliary surgery is almost pathognomonic of neoplasm.

▶ Treatment

Patients without evidence of metastases or other signs of advanced cancer (eg, ascites) are candidates for laparotomy. The 30% of patients who do not qualify may be treated by insertion of a tube stent into the bile duct transhepatically under radiologic control or from the duodenum under endoscopic control. The tube is positioned so that holes above and below the tumor reestablish flow of bile into the duodenum. If both lobar ducts are blocked by a tumor at the bifurcation of the common hepatic duct, it is usually necessary to place a transhepatic tube into only one lobar duct. If the lesion blocks the takeoff of the segmental ducts, stents are rarely beneficial.

Laparotomy is indicated in most cases, however, with the objective of removing the tumor. Preoperative decompression of the bile duct with a percutaneous catheter to relieve jaundice does not lower the incidence of postoperative complications. At operation, which may be immediately preceded by diagnostic laparoscopy, the extent of the tumor should be determined by external examination of the bile duct and the adjacent portal vein and hepatic artery.

Tumors of the distal common duct should be treated by radical pancreaticoduodenectomy (Whipple procedure) if it appears that all tumor would be removed. Secondary involvement of the portal vein is the usual reason for unresectability of tumors in this location. Mid-common duct or low-hepatic duct tumors should also be removed if possible. If the tumor cannot be excised, bile flow should be reestablished into the intestine by a cholecystojejunostomy or Roux-en-Y choledochojejunostomy. The choice is based on technical considerations.

Tumors at the hilum of the liver should be resected if possible and a Roux-en-Y hepaticojejunostomy performed. The anastomosis is usually between hilum and bowel rather than between individual bile ducts and bowel. A curative operation nearly always requires resection of either the right or the left lobe of the liver and, in all cases, the caudate lobe. Extension into the lobar and segmental ducts and secondary involvement of the hepatic artery and portal vein are the most common reasons for inability to resect the tumor. Subtotal resections offer little in the way of palliation.

Postoperative radiotherapy is commonly recommended.

▶ Prognosis

The average patient with adenocarcinoma of the bile duct survives less than a year. The overall 5-year survival rate is 15%. Following a thorough radical operation, 5-year survival is about 40%. Biliary cirrhosis, intrahepatic infection, and general debility with terminal pneumonitis are the usual causes of death. Palliative resections and stents may improve the length and quality of survival in this disease even though surgical cure is uncommon. Limited experience with liver transplantation for this disease has been discouraging: tumor has recurred postoperatively in most patients.

American Society for Gastrointestinal Endoscopy (ASGE) Standards of Practice Committee. The role of endoscopy in the evaluation and treatment of patients with biliary neoplasia. *Gastrointest Endosc* 2013 Feb;77(2):167-174.

Kondo S for the Japanese Association of Biliary Surgery; Japanese Society of Hepato-Biliary-Pancreatic Surgery; Japan Society of Clinical Oncology. Guidelines for the management of biliary tract and ampullary carcinomas: surgical treatment. *J Hepatobiliary Pancreat Surg* 2008;15(1):41-54.

BENIGN TUMORS & PSEUDOTUMORS OF THE GALLBLADDER

Various unrelated lesions appear on ultrasound as projections from the gallbladder wall. The differentiation from gallstones is based upon observing whether a shift in position of the projections follows changes in posture of the patient, since stones are not fixed. Cancer should be suspected in any polypoid lesion that exceeds 1 cm in diameter.

▶ Polyps

Most of these are not true neoplasms but cholesterol polyps, a local form of cholesterosis. Histologically, they consist of a cluster of lipid-filled macrophages in the submucosa. They easily become detached from the wall when the gallbladder is handled at surgery. It is not known whether cholesterol polyps are important in the genesis of gallstones. Some patients experience gallbladder pain, but whether this is related to the presence of the polyps *per se* or is a manifestation of functional gallbladder disease has not been established.

Inflammatory polyps have also been reported, but they are quite rare.

▶ Adenomyomatosis

On cholecystography, this entity presents as a slight intraluminal convexity that is often marked by central umbilication. It is usually found in the fundus but may occur elsewhere. It is unclear whether adenomyomatosis is an acquired degenerative lesion or a developmental abnormality (ie, hamartoma). The following synonyms for this lesion appear in the literature: adenomatous hyperplasia, cholecystitis glandularis proliferans, and diverticulosis of the gallbladder. Although the condition is probably asymptomatic in many cases, adenomyomatosis can cause abdominal pain. Cholecystectomy should be performed in such patients.

▶ Adenomas

These appear as pedunculated adenomatous polyps, true neoplasms that may be papillary or nonpapillary histologically. In a few cases they have been found in association with carcinoma in situ of the gallbladder.

BENIGN TUMORS OF THE BILE DUCTS

Benign papillomas and adenomas may arise from the ductal epithelium. Only 90 cases have been reported to date. The neoplastic propensity of the ductal epithelium is widespread, so the tumors are often multiple, and recurrence is common after excision. The affected duct must be radically excised for permanent cure to result.

BILE DUCT INJURIES & STRICTURES

ESSENTIALS OF DIAGNOSIS

▶ Episodic cholangitis

▶ Previous biliary surgery

▶ Transhepatic cholangiogram often diagnostic

▶ General Considerations

Benign biliary injuries and strictures are caused by surgical trauma in about 95% of cases. The remainder result from external abdominal trauma or, rarely, from erosion of the duct by a gallstone. Prevention of injury to the duct depends on a combination of technical skill, experience, and a thorough knowledge of the normal anatomy and its variations in the hilum of the liver. The number of bile duct injuries has risen sharply in the past few years along with the shift from open to laparoscopic cholecystectomy.

The most common lesion consists of excision of a segment of the common duct as a result of mistaking it for the cystic duct. Partial transection, occlusion with metal clips, injury to the right hepatic duct, and leakage from the cystic duct are other examples. A full discussion of how these injuries occur and how they can be prevented is beyond the scope of this text.

A clean incision of the duct without additional damage is best managed by opening the abdomen and suturing the incision with fine absorbable suture material.

▶ Clinical Findings

A. Symptoms

Manifestations of injury to the duct may or may not be evident in the postoperative period. Following laparoscopic surgery, bile ascites, manifested by abdominal distention, bloating, and pain plus mild jaundice, is the usual presentation, since the duct is usually open to the abdomen. The symptoms are relatively mild and may for a time mimic ileus until a worsening picture requires further investigation.

Injuries following open cholecystectomy more often present with intermittent cholangitis or jaundice as a consequence of a biliary stricture. The first clear-cut symptoms may not be evident for weeks or months after surgery.

B. Signs

Findings are not distinctive. Bile ascites produces abdominal distention and ileus and, rarely, true bile peritonitis with toxicity. The right upper quadrant may be tender but usually is not. Jaundice is usually present during an attack of cholangitis.

C. Laboratory Findings

The serum alkaline phosphatase concentration is elevated in cases of stricture. The serum bilirubin fluctuates in relation to symptoms but usually remains well below 10 mg/dL.

Blood cultures are usually positive during acute cholangitis.

D. Imaging Studies

Bile ascites can be suspected on ultrasound or CT scan. Fluid should be aspirated, and if it is bile, the diagnosis is clear. THC and ERCP are necessary to depict the anatomy. After laparoscopic cholecystectomy, the most common pattern is a blocked (by a metal clip) lower duct and an upper duct draining freely into the abdomen. With a stricture, the findings most often consist of focal narrowing of the common hepatic duct within 2 cm of the bifurcation and mild to moderate dilatation of the intrahepatic ducts.

▶ Differential Diagnosis

Choledocholithiasis is the condition that most often must be differentiated from biliary stricture because the clinical and laboratory findings can be identical. A history of trauma to the duct would point toward stricture as the more likely diagnosis. The final distinction must often await radiologic or surgical findings. THC or ERCP should be definitive.

Other causes of cholestatic jaundice may have to be ruled out in some cases.

▶ Complications

Complications develop quickly if the leak is not controlled. Bile peritonitis and abscesses may form. With stricture, persistent cholangitis may progress to multiple intrahepatic abscesses and a septic death.

▶ Treatment

Bile duct injuries should be surgically repaired in all but a few patients who are likely to improve with a nonoperative approach. Excision of the damaged duct and Roux-en-Y hepaticojejunostomy is indicated for most acute and chronic injuries. The entire biliary tree must be outlined by cholangiograms preoperatively. The key to success is the thoroughness of the dissection and the ability ultimately to suture healthy duct to healthy bowel. This, in turn, depends on the experience of the surgeon with this particular operation.

When a definitive repair is technically impossible, the stricture may be dilated with a transhepatic balloon-tipped catheter. This is particularly applicable to patients with portal hypertension, whose hepatic hilum contains numerous venous collaterals that make operation hazardous.

▶ Prognosis

The death rate from biliary injuries is about 5%, and severe illness is frequent. If the stricture is not repaired, episodic cholangitis and secondary liver disease are inevitable.

Surgical correction of the stricture should be successful in about 90% of cases. Experience at centers with a special interest in this problem indicates that good results can be obtained even if several previous attempts did not relieve the obstruction. There is essentially no place for liver transplantation in this disease.

Strasberg SM. A teaching program for the "culture of safety in cholecystectomy" and avoidance of bile duct injury. *J Am Coll Surg* 2013;217(4):751.

UNCOMMON CAUSES OF BILE DUCT OBSTRUCTION

▶ Congenital Choledochal Cysts

About 30% of congenital choledochal cysts produce their first symptoms in adults, usually presenting with jaundice, cholangitis, and a right upper quadrant mass. Diagnosis can be made by THC or ERCP. The optimal surgical procedure is excision of the cyst and construction of a Roux-en-Y hepaticojejunostomy. If this is not technically possible or if the patient's condition will not permit a prolonged operation, the cyst should be emptied of precipitated biliary sludge and a cystenteric anastomosis constructed. Congenital cysts of the biliary tree have a high incidence of malignant degeneration, which is another argument for excision rather than drainage.

▶ Caroli's Disease

Caroli's disease, another form of congenital cystic disease, consists of saccular intrahepatic dilatation of the ducts. In some cases, the biliary abnormality is an isolated finding, but more often it is associated with congenital hepatic fibrosis and medullary sponge kidney. The latter patients often present in childhood or as young adults with complications of portal hypertension. Others have cholangitis and obstructive jaundice as initial manifestations. There is no definitive surgical solution to the problem except in rare cases with isolated involvement of one hepatic lobe, where lobectomy is curative. Intermittent antibiotic therapy for cholangitis is the usual regimen.

Hemobilia

Hemobilia presents with the triad of biliary colic, obstructive jaundice, and occult or gross intestinal bleeding. Most cases in Western cultures follow several weeks after hepatic trauma with bleeding from an intrahepatic branch of the hepatic artery into a duct. It is seen with less frequency now, because the general principles of management of hepatic trauma are better understood. In the Orient, hemobilia usually follows ductal parasitism (*Ascaris lumbricoides*) or Oriental cholangiohepatitis. Other causes are hepatic neoplasms, rupture of a hepatic artery aneurysm, hepatic abscess, and choledocholithiasis. The diagnosis may be suspected from a technetium 99m-labeled red blood cell scan, but an arteriogram is usually required for diagnosis and planning of therapy. Sometimes the bleeding can be stopped by embolizing the lesion with stainless steel coils, Gelfoam, or autologous blood clot infused through a catheter selectively positioned in the hepatic artery. If this is unsuccessful, either direct ligation of the bleeding point in the liver or proximal ligation of an upstream branch of the hepatic artery in the hilum is required.

Pancreatitis

Pancreatitis can cause obstruction of the intrapancreatic portion of the bile duct by inflammatory swelling, encasement with scar, or compression by a pseudocyst. The patient may present with painless jaundice or cholangitis. Occasionally, a distended gallbladder can be felt on abdominal examination. Differentiation from choledocholithiasis and secondary acute pancreatitis depends on biliary x-rays or surgical exploration if the jaundice persists. Jaundice due to inflammation alone rarely lasts more than 2 weeks; persistent jaundice following an attack of acute pancreatitis suggests the development of a pseudocyst, underlying chronic pancreatitis with obstruction by fibrosis, or even an obstructing neoplasm.

Biliary obstruction from chronic pancreatitis may have few or no clinical manifestations. Jaundice is usually present, but the average peak bilirubin level is only 4-5 mg/dL. Some patients with functionally significant stenosis have persistently elevated alkaline phosphatase levels as the only abnormality; when surgical decompression of the bile duct is not performed, these patients often develop secondary biliary cirrhosis within a year or so. Diagnosis of stricture is made by ERCP, which shows a long stenosis of the intrapancreatic portion of the duct, proximal dilatation, and either a gradual or abrupt tapering of the lumen at the pancreatic border, occasionally accompanied by ductal angulation. If cholangiograms show stenosis and if alkaline phosphatase or bilirubin levels remain more than twice normal for longer than 2 months, the stenosis is functionally significant and unlikely to resolve and requires surgical correction. Choledochoduodenostomy is done in most cases. Cholecystoduodenostomy is unreliable because the cystic duct is often too narrow to provide continued biliary decompression.

Patients with obstructive jaundice and pseudocyst usually respond to surgical drainage of the pseudocyst. However, occasionally they do not respond, because chronic scarring—not the cyst—is the cause of obstruction. Procedures to drain both the bile duct and the pseudocyst are indicated if operative cholangiograms demonstrate persistent bile duct obstruction after the cyst has been decompressed.

Ampullary Dysfunction & Stenosis

Stenosis of the hepatopancreatic ampulla (ampullary stenosis) has been implicated as a cause of pain and other manifestations of ampullary obstruction and is often considered as a cause of postcholecystectomy complaints. Some cases are idiopathic, whereas others may be the result of trauma from gallstones. If the patient has secondary manifestations of biliary obstruction (eg, jaundice, increased alkaline phosphatase concentration, and cholangitis) in the absence of gallstones or some other obstructing lesion, and cholangiography shows dilatation of the common duct, ampullary stenosis is a plausible explanation. However, the diagnosis is more often proposed as a reason for upper abdominal pain without these more objective findings. Ampullary dysfunction is postulated in these cases.

Sphincter of Oddi dysfunction may be the cause of biliary-like pain and is often considered in patients who remain uncomfortable after cholecystectomy. The pathogenesis of the symptoms is thought to be similar to that of esophageal dysmotility and the irritable bowel syndrome. The patients typically experience severe, intermittent upper abdominal pain that lasts for 1-3 hours, sometimes following a meal.

Residual gallstone and pancreatic disease must first be ruled out. Ampullary dysfunction can then be diagnosed by sphincter of Oddi manometry. Patients are placed in one of three groups depending on the presence of three objective manifestations of biliary obstruction: abnormal liver function tests, prolonged (> 45 minutes) common bile duct emptying of contrast media after ERCP; and a common duct greater than 12 mm in diameter. Patients in group I have all three findings; patients in group II have one or two findings; and patients in group III have none of the findings. Group I patients are thought to have enough evidence of disease that sphincterotomy should be performed without manometry. Group I patients have abnormal motility so rarely that they should not be considered further for sphincterotomy. Thus, motility studies are most often of value in determining which of the group II patients will improve after sphincterotomy.

The abnormalities sought on the motility studies include an elevated (> 40 mm Hg) basal sphincter pressure and a paradoxic rise in sphincter pressure in response to CCK. The former is most reliable. About 50% of group II patients have elevated sphincter pressures, and these are the ones who benefit from sphincterotomy.

A scintigraphic test may be just as accurate. The patient is given a bolus of CCK followed by ^{99m}Tc-DISIDA. Gamma camera images of the liver and bile duct are obtained for 60 minutes. A scoring system (score: 0-12) is based on the rate of passage of the imaging agent past various relevant points (eg, appearance and clearance through the liver, bile duct, and bowel). The normal range is 0-5; abnormal is 6-12.

Sphincter of Oddi dysfunction is an uncommon explanation for abdominal pain, and it is appropriate to remain skeptical unless the objective findings of biliary obstruction are clear-cut. In well-selected cases, however, endoscopic sphincterotomy is beneficial.

Heetun ZS, Zeb F, Cullen G, Courtney G, Aftab AR. Biliary sphincter of Oddi dysfunction: response rates after ERCP and sphincterotomy in a 5-year ERCP series and proposal for new practical guidelines. *Eur J Gastroenterol Hepatol* 2011;23(4):327-333.

Duodenal Diverticula

Duodenal diverticula usually arise on the medial aspect of the duodenum within 2 cm of the orifice of the bile duct, and in some individuals the duct empties directly into a diverticulum. Even in the latter circumstance, duodenal diverticula are usually innocuous. Occasionally, distortion of the duct entrance or obstruction by enterolith formation in the diverticulum produces symptoms. Either choledochoduodenostomy or Roux-en-Y choledochojejunostomy is usually a safer method of reestablishing biliary drainage than attempts to excise the diverticulum and reimplant the duct.

Ascariasis

When the worms invade the duct from the duodenum, ascariasis can produce symptoms of ductal obstruction. Air may sometimes be seen within the ducts on plain films. Antibiotics should be used until cholangitis is controlled, and anthelmintic therapy (mebendazole, albendazole, or pyrantel pamoate) should then be given. The acute symptoms usually subside with antibiotics, but if they do not, endoscopic sphincterotomy should be performed and attempts made to extricate the worms. If this is unsuccessful and the patient remains acutely ill, the duct should be emptied surgically.

Recurrent Pyogenic Cholangitis (Oriental Cholangiohepatitis)

Oriental cholangiohepatitis is a type of chronic recurrent cholangitis prevalent in coastal areas from Japan to Southeast Asia. In Hong Kong it is the third most common indication for emergency laparotomy and the most frequent type of biliary disease. The disease is currently thought to result from chronic portal bacteremia, with portal phlebitis antedating the biliary disease. *E coli* causes secondary infection of the bile ducts, which initiates pigment stone formation within the ducts.

Biliary obstruction from the stones gives rise to recurrent cholangitis, which, unlike gallstone disease in Western countries, may be unaccompanied by gallbladder stones. The gallbladder is usually distended during an attack and may contain pus.

Chronic recurrent infection often leads to biliary strictures and hepatic abscess formation. The strictures are usually located in the intrahepatic bile ducts, and for some unknown reason the left lobe of the liver is more severely involved. Intrahepatic gallstones are common, and their surgical removal may be difficult or impossible. Acute abdominal pain, chills, and high fever are usually present, and jaundice develops in about half of cases. Right upper quadrant tenderness is usually marked, and in about 80% of cases the gallbladder is palpable. ERCP or THC is the best way to study the biliary tree and can help in determining the need for surgery and the type of procedure.

Systemic antibiotics should be given for acute cholangitis. Surgical treatment consists of cholecystectomy, common duct exploration, and removal of stones. Sphincteroplasty should also be performed to allow any residual or recurrent stones to escape from the duct. A Roux-en-Y choledochojejunostomy is indicated for patients with strictures, markedly dilated ducts (eg, > 3 cm), or recurrent disease after a previous sphincteroplasty. The results of surgery are good in 80% of patients. Chronic intrahepatic stones and infection, which often involve only one lobe, may require hepatic lobectomy.

Although many patients are cured, prolonged illness from repeated infection is almost unavoidable once strictures have appeared or the intrahepatic ducts have become packed with stones.

Sclerosing Cholangitis

Sclerosing cholangitis is a rare chronic disease of unknown cause characterized by nonbacterial inflammatory narrowing of the bile ducts. About 60% of cases occur in patients with ulcerative colitis, and sclerosing cholangitis develops in about 5% of patients with that disorder. Other less commonly associated conditions are thyroiditis, retroperitoneal fibrosis, and mediastinal fibrosis. The disease chiefly affects men 20-50 years of age. In most cases, the entire biliary tree is affected by the inflammatory process, which causes irregular partial obliteration of the lumen of the ducts. The narrowing may be confined, however, to the intrahepatic or extrahepatic ducts, though it is almost never so short as to resemble a posttraumatic or focal malignant stricture. The woody-hard duct walls contain increased collagen and lymphoid elements and are thickened at the expense of the lumen.

The clinical onset usually consists of the gradual appearance of mild jaundice and pruritus. Symptoms of bacterial cholangitis (eg, fever and chills) are uncommon in the absence of previous biliary surgery. Laboratory findings are typical of cholestasis. The total serum bilirubin averages about 4 mg/dL and rarely exceeds 10 mg/dL. ERCP is usually diagnostic, demonstrating ductal stenoses and irregularity, which often gives a beaded appearance. Liver biopsy may show pericholangitis and bile stasis, but the changes are nonspecific.

The complications of sclerosing cholangitis include gallstone disease and adenocarcinoma of the bile duct. The latter is most common in patients with ulcerative colitis. Furthermore, patients with ulcerative colitis and sclerosing cholangitis appear to be at greater risk for colonic mucosal dysplasia and colon cancer than those with ulcerative colitis not associated with sclerosing cholangitis.

Ursodiol (ursodeoxycholic acid), 10 mg/kg/d, improves liver function tests and symptoms. Cholestyramine will give relief from pruritus. Percutaneous transhepatic balloon dilatation can be of value to treat dominant strictures. In cases where the disease is largely confined to the distal extrahepatic duct and the proximal ducts are dilated, a Roux-en-Y hepaticojejunostomy may be indicated. For patients with severe intrahepatic involvement, hepatic transplantation should be considered.

The natural history of sclerosing cholangitis is one of chronicity and unpredictable severity. Some patients seem to obtain nearly complete remission after treatment, but this is not common. Bacterial cholangitis may develop after operation if adequate drainage has not been established. In these cases, antibiotics will be required at intervals. Most patients experience the gradual evolution of secondary biliary cirrhosis after many years of mild to moderate jaundice and pruritus. Liver transplantation is indicated when the disease becomes advanced. The results are good.

MULTIPLE CHOICE QUESTIONS

1. All of the following are current useful imaging modalities for the biliary tree and gallbladder, except

   A. Abdominal ultrasound
   B. Endoscopic retrograde cholangiopancreatography
   C. Abdominal CT scan
   D. Oral cholecystography
   E. Transhepatic cholangiography

2. Serum alkaline phosphatase can come from

   A. Lung
   B. Muscle
   C. Skin
   D. Intestine
   E. Red blood cells

3. Gallstones

   A. Are symptomatic in greater than 50% of people
   B. Are nearly always present in people with chronic cholecystitis
   C. In the gallbladder are not detected by ultrasound in about 50% of cases (false negative)
   D. Are usually detectable by ultrasound if present in the common bile duct
   E. Are comprised of bile pigment in the majority of cases in the United States

4. Acute cholecystitis can be commonly confused with each of the following, except

   A. Diverticulitis
   B. Pancreatitis
   C. Peptic ulcer disease
   D. Acute appendicitis
   E. Fitz–Hugh–Curtis syndrome

5. Management of acute cholangitis

   A. Typically requires emergent operation
   B. Should not include antibiotics until bile cultures are pending
   C. Should usually include draining the biliary tree
   D. Is commonly required in the management of chronic pancreatitis
   E. Should reserve invasive procedures for patients who have required more than 3 days of antibiotics

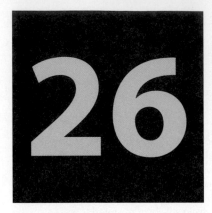

26

Pancreas

Gerard M. Doherty, MD

EMBRYOLOGY

The pancreas appears in the fourth week of fetal life from the caudal part of the foregut as dorsal and ventral pancreatic buds. Both anlagen rotate to the right and fuse near the point of origin of the ventral pancreas. Later, as the duodenum rotates, the pancreas shifts to the left. In the adult, only the caudal portion of the head and the uncinate process are derived from the ventral pancreas. The cranial part of the head and all of the body and tail are derived from the dorsal pancreas. Most of the dorsal pancreatic duct joins with the duct of the ventral pancreas to form the main pancreatic duct (duct of Wirsung); a small part persists as the accessory duct (duct of Santorini). In 5%-10% of people, the ventral and dorsal pancreatic ducts do not fuse, and most regions of the pancreas drain through the duct of Santorini and the orifice of the minor papilla. In this case, only the small ventral pancreas drains with the common bile duct through the papilla of Vater.

ANATOMY

The pancreas is a thin elliptic organ that lies within the retroperitoneum in the upper abdomen (Figures 26–1 and 26–2). In the adult, it is 12-15 cm long and weighs 70-100 g. The gland can be divided into three portions—head, body, and tail. The head of the pancreas is intimately adherent to the medial portion of the duodenum and lies in front of the inferior vena cava and superior mesenteric vessels. A small tongue of tissue called the uncinate process lies behind the superior mesenteric vessels as they emerge from the retroperitoneum. Anteriorly, the stomach and the first portion of the duodenum lie partly in front of the pancreas. The common bile duct passes through a posterior groove in the head of the pancreas adjacent to the duodenum. The body of the pancreas is in contact posteriorly with the aorta, the left crus of the diaphragm, the left adrenal gland, and the left kidney. The tail of the pancreas lies in the hilum of the spleen. The main pancreatic duct (the duct of Wirsung) courses along

the gland from the tail to the head and joins the common bile duct just before entering the duodenum at the ampulla of Vater. The accessory pancreatic duct (the duct of Santorini) enters the duodenum 2-2.5 cm proximal to the ampulla of Vater (Figure 26–1).

The blood supply of the pancreas is derived from branches of the celiac and superior mesenteric arteries (Figure 26–2). The superior pancreaticoduodenal artery arises from the gastroduodenal artery, runs parallel to the duodenum, and eventually meets the inferior pancreaticoduodenal artery, a branch of the superior mesenteric artery, to form an arcade. The splenic artery provides tributaries that supply the body and tail of the pancreas. The main branches are termed the dorsal pancreatic, pancreatica magna, and caudal pancreatic arteries. The venous supply of the gland parallels the arterial supply. Lymphatic drainage is into the peripancreatic nodes located along the veins.

The innervation of the pancreas is derived from the vagal and splanchnic nerves. The efferent fibers pass through the celiac plexus from the celiac branch of the right vagal nerve to terminate in ganglia located in the interlobular septa of the pancreas. Postganglionic fibers from these synapses innervate the acini, the islets, and the ducts. The visceral afferent fibers from the pancreas also travel in the vagal and splanchnic nerves, but those that mediate pain are confined to the latter. Sympathetic fibers to the pancreas pass from the splanchnic nerves through the celiac plexus and innervate the pancreatic vasculature.

PHYSIOLOGY

▶ Exocrine Function

The external secretion of the pancreas consists of a clear, alkaline (pH 7.0-8.3) solution of 1-2 L/d containing digestive enzymes. Secretion is stimulated by the hormones secretin and cholecystokinin (CCK) and by parasympathetic vagal discharge. Secretin and CCK are synthesized, stored, and

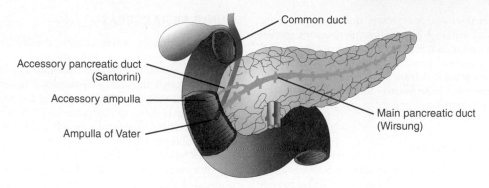

▲ **Figure 26–1.** Anatomic configuration of pancreatic ductal system. Courtesy of W Silen.

released from duodenal mucosal cells in response to specific stimuli. Acid in the lumen of the duodenum causes the release of secretin, and luminal digestion products of fat and protein cause the release of CCK.

The water and electrolyte secretion is formed by the centroacinar and intercalated duct cells principally in response to secretin stimulation. The secretion is modified by exchange processes and active secretion in the ductal collecting system. The cations sodium and potassium are present in the same concentrations as in plasma. The anions bicarbonate and chloride vary in concentration according to the rate of secretion: with increasing rate of secretion, the bicarbonate concentration increases and chloride concentration falls, so that the sum of the two is the same throughout the secretory range. Pancreatic juice helps neutralize gastric

acid in the duodenum and adjusts luminal pH to the level that gives optimal activity of pancreatic enzymes.

Pancreatic enzymes are synthesized, stored (as zymogen granules), and released by the acinar cells of the gland, principally in response to CCK and vagal stimulation. Pancreatic enzymes are proteolytic, lipolytic, and amylolytic. Lipase and amylase are stored and secreted in active forms. The proteolytic enzymes are secreted as inactive precursors and are activated by the duodenal enzyme enterokinase. Other enzymes secreted by the pancreas include ribonucleases and phospholipase A. Phospholipase A is secreted as an inactive proenzyme activated in the duodenum by trypsin. It catalyzes the conversion of biliary lecithin to lysolecithin.

Turnover of protein in the pancreas exceeds that of any other organ in the body. Intravenously injected amino acids

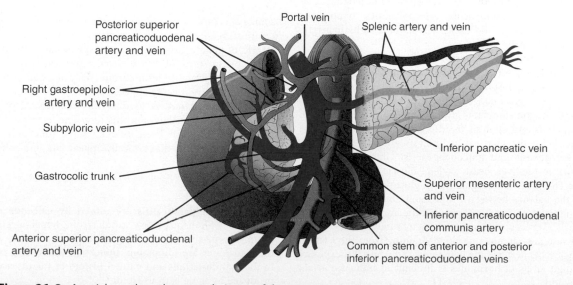

▲ **Figure 26–2.** Arterial supply and venous drainage of the pancreas. Courtesy of W Silen.

are incorporated into enzyme protein and may appear in the pancreatic juice within 1 hour. Three mechanisms prevent autodigestion of the pancreas by its proteolytic enzymes: (1) the enzymes are stored in acinar cells as zymogen granules, where they are separated from other cell proteins; (2) the enzymes are secreted in an inactive form; and (3) inhibitors of proteolytic enzymes are present in pancreatic juice and pancreatic tissue.

▶ Endocrine Function

The function of the endocrine pancreas is to facilitate storage of foodstuffs by release of insulin after a meal and to provide a mechanism for their mobilization by release of glucagon during periods of fasting. Insulin and glucagon, as well as pancreatic polypeptide and somatostatin, are produced by the islets of Langerhans.

Insulin, a polypeptide (MW 5734) consisting of 51 amino acid residues, is formed in the beta cells of the pancreas via the precursor proinsulin. Insulin secretion is stimulated by rising or high serum concentrations of metabolic substrates such as glucose, amino acids, and perhaps short-chain fatty acids. The major normal stimulus for insulin release appears to be glucose. The release and synthesis of insulin are stimulated by activation of specific glucoreceptors located on the surface membrane of the beta cell. Insulin release is also stimulated by calcium, glucagon, secretin, CCK, vasoactive intestinal polypeptide (VIP), and gastrin, all of which sensitize the receptors on the beta cell to glucose. Epinephrine, tolbutamide, and chlorpropamide release insulin by acting on the adenylyl cyclase system.

Glucagon, a polypeptide (MW 3485) consisting of 29 amino acid residues, is formed in the α cells of the pancreas. The release of glucagon is stimulated by a low blood glucose concentration, amino acids, catecholamines, sympathetic nervous discharge, and CCK. It is suppressed by hyperglycemia and insulin.

The principal functions of insulin are to stimulate anabolic reactions involving carbohydrates, fats, proteins, and nucleic acids. Insulin decreases glycogenolysis, lipolysis, proteolysis, gluconeogenesis, ureagenesis, and ketogenesis. Glucagon stimulates glycogenolysis from the liver and proteolysis and lipolysis in adipose tissue as well as in the liver. With the increase in lipolysis, there is an increase in ketogenesis and gluconeogenesis. Glucagon increases cAMP in the liver, heart, skeletal muscle, and adipose tissue. The short-term regulation of gluconeogenesis depends on the balance between insulin and glucagon. Studies on insulin and glucagon suggest that the hormones exert their effects via receptors on the cell membrane. Before entering the systemic circulation, blood draining from the islets of Langerhans perfuses the pancreatic acini, and this exposure to high levels of hormones is thought to influence acinar function.

ANNULAR PANCREAS

Annular pancreas is a rare congenital condition in which a ring of pancreatic tissue from the head of the pancreas surrounds the descending duodenum. The abnormality usually presents in infancy as duodenal obstruction with postprandial vomiting. There is bile in the vomitus if the constriction is distal to the entrance of the common bile duct. X-rays show a dilated stomach and proximal duodenum (double bubble sign) and little or no air in the rest of the small bowel.

After correction of fluid and electrolyte imbalance, the obstructed segment should be bypassed by a duodenojejunostomy or other similar procedure. No attempt should be made to resect the obstructing pancreas, because a pancreatic fistula or acute pancreatitis often develops postoperatively.

Occasionally, annular pancreas will present in adult life with similar symptoms.

PANCREATITIS

Pancreatitis is a common nonbacterial inflammatory disease caused by activation, interstitial liberation, and autodigestion of the pancreas by its own enzymes. The process may or may not be accompanied by permanent morphologic and functional changes in the gland. Much is known about the causes of pancreatitis, but despite the accumulation of much experimental data, understanding of the pathogenesis of this disorder is still incomplete.

In acute pancreatitis, there is sudden upper abdominal pain, nausea and vomiting, and elevated serum amylase. Chronic pancreatitis is characterized by chronic pain, pancreatic calcification on x-ray, and exocrine (steatorrhea) or endocrine (diabetes mellitus) insufficiency. Attacks of acute pancreatitis often occur in patients with chronic pancreatitis. *Acute relapsing pancreatitis* is defined as multiple attacks of pancreatitis without permanent pancreatic scarring, a picture most often associated with biliary pancreatitis. The unsatisfactory term chronic relapsing pancreatitis, denoting recurrent acute attacks superimposed on chronic pancreatitis, will not be used in this chapter. Alcoholic pancreatitis often behaves in this way. The term subacute pancreatitis has also been used by some to denote the minor acute attacks that typically appear late in alcoholic pancreatitis.

▶ Etiology

Most cases of pancreatitis are caused by gallstone disease or alcoholism; a few result from hypercalcemia, trauma, hyperlipidemia, and genetic predisposition; and the remainder are idiopathic. Important differences exist in the manifestations and natural history of the disease as produced by these various factors.

A. Biliary Pancreatitis

About 40% of cases of pancreatitis are associated with gallstone disease, which, if untreated, usually gives rise to additional acute attacks. For unknown reasons, even repeated attacks of acute biliary pancreatitis seldom produce chronic pancreatitis. Eradication of the biliary disease nearly always prevents recurrent pancreatitis. The etiologic mechanism most likely consists of transient obstruction of the ampulla of Vater and pancreatic duct by a gallstone. Choledocholithiasis is found in only 25% of cases, but because over 90% of patients excrete a gallstone in feces passed within 10 days after an acute attack, it is assumed that most attacks are caused by a gallstone or biliary sludge traversing the common duct and ampulla of Vater. Other possible steps in pathogenesis initiated by passage of the gallstone are discussed below.

B. Alcoholic Pancreatitis

In the United States, alcoholism accounts for about 40% of cases of pancreatitis. Characteristically, the patients have been heavy users of hard liquor or wine; the condition is relatively infrequent in countries where beer is the most popular alcoholic beverage. Most commonly, 6 years or more of alcoholic excess precede the initial attack of pancreatitis, and even with the first clinical manifestations, signs of chronic pancreatitis can be detected if the gland is examined microscopically. Thus, alcoholic pancreatitis is often considered to be synonymous with chronic pancreatitis no matter what the clinical findings.

Acute administration of alcohol stimulates pancreatic secretion and induces spasm in the sphincter of Oddi. This has been compared to experiments that produce acute pancreatitis by combining partial ductal obstruction and secretory stimulation. If the patient can be persuaded to stop drinking, acute attacks may be prevented, but parenchymal damage continues to occur owing to persistent ductal obstruction and fibrosis.

C. Hypercalcemia

Hyperparathyroidism and other disorders accompanied by hypercalcemia are occasionally complicated by acute pancreatitis. With time, chronic pancreatitis and ductal calculi appear. The increased calcium concentrations in pancreatic juice that result from hypercalcemia may prematurely activate proteases. They may also facilitate precipitation of calculi in the ducts.

D. Hyperlipidemia

In some patients—especially alcoholics—hyperlipidemia appears transiently during an acute attack of pancreatitis; in others with primary hyperlipidemia (especially those associated with elevated chylomicrons and very low density lipoproteins), pancreatitis seems to be a direct consequence of the metabolic abnormality. Hyperlipidemia during an acute attack of pancreatitis is usually associated with normal serum amylase levels, because the lipid interferes with the chemical determination for amylase; urinary output of amylase may still be high. One should inspect the serum of every patient with acute abdominal pain, because if it is lactescent, pancreatitis will almost always be the correct diagnosis. If a primary lipid abnormality is present, dietary control reduces the chances of additional attacks of pancreatitis as well as other complications.

E. Familial Pancreatitis

In this condition, attacks of abdominal pain usually begin in childhood. Some affected families also have aminoaciduria, but this is not a universal finding. Diabetes mellitus and steatorrhea are uncommon. Chronic calcific pancreatitis develops eventually in most patients, and many patients become candidates for operation for chronic pain. Pancreatic carcinoma is more frequent in patients with familial pancreatitis.

F. Protein Deficiency

In certain populations where dietary protein intake is markedly deficient, the incidence of chronic pancreatitis is high. The reason for this association is obscure, especially in view of the observation that pancreatitis afflicts alcoholics with higher dietary protein and fat intake than those who consume less protein and fat.

G. Postoperative (Iatrogenic) Pancreatitis

Most cases of postoperative pancreatitis follow common bile duct exploration, especially if sphincterotomy was performed. Two practices, now largely abandoned, were often responsible: (1) use of a common duct T tube with a long arm passing through the sphincter of Oddi and (2) dilation of the sphincter to 5-7 mm during common duct exploration. Operations on the pancreas, including pancreatic biopsy, are another cause. A few cases follow gastric surgery or even operations remote from the pancreas. Pancreatitis is particularly common after cardiac surgery with cardiopulmonary bypass, where the risk factors are preoperative renal failure, valve surgery, postoperative hypotension, and (particularly) the perioperative administration of calcium chloride (> 800 mg calcium chloride per square meter of body surface area). Pancreatitis may also complicate endoscopic retrograde pancreatography or endoscopic sphincterotomy.

Rarely, pancreatitis follows Billroth II gastrectomy, owing to acute obstruction of the afferent loop and reflux of duodenal secretions under high pressure into the pancreatic ducts. The condition has been recreated experimentally in dogs (Pfeffer loop preparation).

H. Drug-Induced Pancreatitis

Drugs are probably responsible for more cases of acute pancreatitis than is generally suspected. The most commonly incriminated drugs are corticosteroids, estrogen-containing contraceptives, azathioprine, thiazide diuretics, and tetracyclines. Pancreatitis associated with use of estrogens is usually the result of drug-induced hypertriglyceridemia. The mechanisms involved in the case of other drugs are unknown.

I. Obstructive Pancreatitis

Chronic partial obstruction of the pancreatic duct may be congenital or may follow healing after injury or inflammation. Over time, the parenchyma drained by the obstructed duct is replaced by fibrous tissue, and chronic pancreatitis develops. Sometimes there are episodes of acute pancreatitis as well.

Pancreas divisum may predispose to a kind of obstructive pancreatitis. If this anomaly is present and further narrowing of the opening of the minor papilla occurs (eg, by an inflammatory process), the orifice may be inadequate to handle the flow of pancreatic juice. The diagnosis of pancreas divisum may be made by endoscopic retrograde cholangio-pancreatography (ERCP). If a patient with the anomaly is found to have documented episodes of acute pancreatitis and no other cause is found, it is reasonable to assume that the anomaly is the cause.

Surgical sphincteroplasty of the minor papilla or the insertion of a stent has been proposed as treatment, but results have been suboptimal. This may be due to the presence of irreversible parenchymal changes and the persistence of chronic inflammation. In patients with obvious changes of chronic pancreatitis, surgical treatment should consist of pancreatic resection or drainage.

J. Idiopathic Pancreatitis and Miscellaneous Causes

In about 15% of patients, representing the third largest group after biliary and alcoholic pancreatitis, there is no identifiable cause of the condition. If investigated in greater than usual detail (eg, duodenal drainage examination for cholesterol crystals), many of these patients will be found to have gallstones or biliary sludge undetectable by ultrasound scans. Recent data have linked mutations of the cystic fibrosis gene to idiopathic pancreatitis.

Viral infections and scorpion stings may cause pancreatitis.

▶ Pathogenesis

The concept that pancreatitis is due to enzymatic digestion of the gland is supported by the finding of proteolytic enzymes in ascitic fluid and increased amounts of phospholipase A and lysolecithins in pancreatic tissue from patients with acute pancreatitis. Experimentally, pancreatitis can be created readily if activated enzymes are injected into the pancreatic ducts under pressure. Trypsin has not been found in excessive amounts in pancreatic tissue from affected humans, possibly because of inactivation by trypsin inhibitors. Nevertheless, although the available evidence is inconclusive, the autodigestion theory is almost universally accepted. Other proposed factors are vascular insufficiency, lymphatic congestion, and activation of the kallikrein-kinin system.

For many years, trypsin and other proteases were held to be the principal injurious agents, but recent evidence has emphasized phospholipase A, lipase, and elastase as perhaps of greater importance. Trypsin ordinarily does not attack living cells, and even when trypsin is forced into the interstitial spaces, the resulting pancreatitis does not include coagulation necrosis, which is so prominent in human pancreatitis.

Phospholipase A, in the presence of small amounts of bile salts, attacks free phospholipids (eg, lecithin) and those bound in cellular membranes to produce extremely potent lyso-compounds. Lysolecithin, which would result from the action of phospholipase A on biliary lecithin, or phospholipase A itself, plus bile salts, is capable of producing severe necrotizing pancreatitis. Trypsin is important in this scheme, because small amounts are needed to activate phospholipase A from its inactive precursor.

Elastase, which is both elastolytic and proteolytic, is secreted in an inactive form. Because it can digest the walls of blood vessels, elastase has been thought to be important in the pathogenesis of hemorrhagic pancreatitis.

If autodigestion is the final common pathway in pancreatitis, earlier steps must account for the presence of active enzymes and their reaction products in the ducts and their escape into the interstitium. The following are the most popular theories that attempt to link the known etiologic factors with autodigestion.

A. Obstruction-Secretion

In animals, ligation of the pancreatic duct generally produces mild edema of the pancreas that resolves within a week. Thereafter, atrophy of the secretory apparatus occurs. On the other hand, partial or intermittent ductal obstruction, which more closely mimics what seems to happen in humans, can produce frank pancreatitis if the gland is simultaneously stimulated to secrete. The major shortcoming of these experiments has been the difficulty encountered in attempting to cause severe pancreatitis in this way. However, since the human pancreas manufactures ten times as much phospholipase A as does the dog or rat pancreas, the consequences of obstruction in humans conceivably could be more serious.

B. Common Channel Theory

Flow between the biliary and pancreatic ducts requires a common channel connecting these two systems with the duodenum. Although these ducts converge in 90% of humans, only 10% have a common channel long enough to permit biliary-pancreatic reflux if the ampulla contained a gallstone. Experimentally, pancreatitis produced by pancreatic duct obstruction alone is similar in severity to pancreatitis following obstruction of a common channel, so biliary reflux is discounted as an etiologic factor in this disease.

C. Duodenal Reflux

The above theories do not explain activation of pancreatic enzymes, a process that normally takes place through the action of enterokinase in the duodenum. In experimental animals, if the segment of duodenum into which the pancreatic duct empties is surgically converted to a closed loop, reflux of duodenal juice initiates severe pancreatitis (Pfeffer loop). Pancreatitis associated with acute afferent loop obstruction after Billroth II gastrectomy is probably the result of similar factors. Other than in this specific example, there is no direct evidence for duodenal reflux in the pathogenesis of pancreatitis in humans.

D. Back Diffusion Across the Pancreatic Duct

Just as the gastric mucosa must serve as a barrier to maintain high concentrations of acid, so must the epithelium of the pancreatic duct prevent diffusion of luminal enzymes into the pancreatic parenchyma. Experiments in cats have shown that the barrier function of the pancreatic duct is vulnerable to several injurious agents, including alcohol and bile acids. Furthermore, the effects of alcohol can occur even after oral ingestion, because alcohol is secreted in the pancreatic juice. Injury to the barrier renders the duct permeable to molecules as large as MW 20,000, and enzymes from the lumen may be able to enter the gland and produce pancreatitis.

Some studies have shown that a very early event in several forms of experimental pancreatitis, including that due to pancreatic duct obstruction, consists of zymogen activation within acinar cells by lysosomal hydrolases (eg, cathepsin B). This may represent the long-sought unifying explanation. Other factors must be postulated, however, to account for the variations in severity of the disease. In biliary pancreatitis, transient obstruction of the ampulla of Vater by a gallstone is most likely the first event. Alcoholic pancreatitis probably has several causes, including partial ductal obstruction, secretory stimulation, acute effects on the ductal barrier, and toxic actions of alcohol on parenchymal cells.

E. Systemic Manifestations

Severe acute pancreatitis may be complicated by multiple organ failure, principally respiratory insufficiency (acute respiratory distress syndrome), myocardial depression, renal insufficiency, and gastric stress ulceration. The pathogenesis of these complications is similar in many respects to that of multiple organ failure in sepsis, and in fact, sepsis due to pancreatic abscess formation is a contributing factor in some of the most severe cases of acute pancreatitis. During acute pancreatitis, pancreatic proteases, bacterial endotoxins, and other active agents are liberated into the systemic circulation. The endotoxin probably originates from bacteria that translocate through an abnormally permeable intestinal mucosa. Within the circulation, the proteases and the endotoxin activate the complement system (especially C5) and kinins. Complement activation leads to granulocyte aggregation and accumulation of aggregates in the pulmonary capillaries. The granulocytes release neutrophil elastase, superoxide anion, hydrogen peroxide, and hydroxide radicals, which in concert with bradykinin exert local toxic effects on the pulmonary epithelium that result in increased permeability. Arachidonate metabolites (eg, PGE_2, PGI_2, leukotriene B_4) may also be involved in some way. Analogous events are thought to occur in other organs.

Ceppa EP et al. Hereditary pancreatitis: endoscopic and surgical management. *J Gastrointest Surg* 2013;17(5):847-856.

Spanier BW, Dijkgraaf MG, Bruno MJ. Epidemiology, aetiology and outcome of acute and chronic pancreatitis: an update. *Best Pract Res Clin Gastroenterol* 2008;22(1):45-63.

Working Group IAP/APA Acute Pancreatitis Guidelines. IAP/APA evidence-based guidelines for the management of acute pancreatitis. *Pancreatology* 2013;13(4 suppl 2):e1-e15.

1. Acute Pancreatitis

ESSENTIALS OF DIAGNOSIS

► Abrupt onset of epigastric pain, frequently with back pain

► Nausea and vomiting

► Elevated serum or urinary amylase

► Cholelithiasis or alcoholism (many patients)

► General Considerations

While edematous and hemorrhagic pancreatitis are manifestations of the same pathologic processes and the general principles of treatment are the same, hemorrhagic pancreatitis has more complications and a higher death rate. In edematous pancreatitis, the glandular tissue and surrounding retroperitoneal structures are engorged with interstitial fluid, and the pancreas is infiltrated with inflammatory cells that surround small foci of parenchymal necrosis. Hemorrhagic pancreatitis is characterized by bleeding into the parenchyma and surrounding retroperitoneal structures and extensive pancreatic necrosis. In both forms, the peritoneal surfaces may be studded with small calcifications representing areas of fat necrosis.

▶ Clinical Findings

A. Symptoms and Signs

The acute attack frequently begins with severe epigastric pain that radiates through to the back. The pain is unrelenting and usually associated with vomiting and retching. In severe cases, the patient may collapse from shock.

Depending on the severity of the disease, there may be profound dehydration, tachycardia, and postural hypotension. Myocardial function is depressed in severe pancreatitis, presumably because of circulating factors that affect cardiac performance. Examination of the abdomen reveals decreased or absent bowel sounds and tenderness that may be generalized but more often is localized to the epigastrium. Temperature is usually normal or slightly elevated in uncomplicated pancreatitis. Clinical evidence of pleural effusion may be present, especially on the left. If an abdominal mass is found, it probably represents a swollen pancreas (phlegmon) or, later in the illness, a pseudocyst or abscess. In 1%-2% of patients, bluish discoloration is present in the flank (Grey Turner sign) or periumbilical area (Cullen sign), indicating hemorrhagic pancreatitis with dissection of blood retroperitoneally into these areas.

B. Laboratory Findings

The hematocrit may be elevated as a consequence of dehydration or low as a result of abdominal blood loss in hemorrhagic pancreatitis. There is usually a moderate leukocytosis, but total white blood cell counts over 12,000/mL are unusual in the absence of suppurative complications. Liver function studies are usually normal, but there may be a mild elevation of the serum bilirubin concentration (usually < 2 mg/dL).

The serum amylase concentration rises to more than three times normal within 6 hours after the onset of an acute episode and generally remains elevated for several days. Values in excess of 1000 IU/dL occur early in the attack in 95% of patients with biliary pancreatitis and 85% of patients with acute alcoholic pancreatitis. Those with the most severe disease are more apt to have amylase levels below 1000 IU/dL.

Elevated serum lipase is detectable early and for several days after the acute attack. Since the lipase level tends to be higher in alcoholic pancreatitis and the amylase level higher in gallstone pancreatitis, the lipase/amylase ratio has been suggested as a means to help distinguishing the two.

Elevated amylase levels may occur in other acute abdominal conditions, such as gangrenous cholecystitis, small bowel obstruction, mesenteric infarction, and perforated ulcer, though levels rarely exceed 500 IU/dL. Episodes of acute pancreatitis may occur without rises in serum amylase; this is the rule if hyperlipidemia is present. Furthermore, high levels may return to normal before blood is drawn.

The methods most commonly used for measuring amylase in the serum detect pancreatic amylase, salivary amylase, and macroamylase. However, hyperamylasemia is sometimes present in patients with abdominal pain when the elevated amylase levels consist entirely of salivary amylase or macroamylase and the pancreas is not inflamed.

In severe pancreatitis, the serum calcium concentration may fall as a result of calcium being complexed with fatty acids (liberated from retroperitoneal fat by lipase) and impaired reabsorption from bone owing to the action of calcitonin (liberated by high levels of glucagon). Relative hypoparathyroidism and hypoalbuminemia have also been implicated.

C. Imaging Studies

In about two-thirds of cases, a plain abdominal film is abnormal. The most frequent finding is isolated dilation of a segment of gut (sentinel loop) consisting of jejunum, transverse colon, or duodenum adjacent to the pancreas. Gas distending the right colon that abruptly stops in the mid or left transverse colon (colon cutoff sign) is due to colonic spasm adjacent to the pancreatic inflammation. Both of these findings are relatively nonspecific. Glandular calcification may be evident, signifying chronic pancreatitis. An upper gastrointestinal series may show a widened duodenal loop, swollen ampulla of Vater, and, occasionally, evidence of gastric irritability. Chest films may reveal pleural effusion on the left side. Occasionally, radiopaque gallstones will be apparent on plain x-rays.

Ultrasound study may demonstrate gallstones early in the attack and may be used as a baseline for sequential examinations of the pancreas.

A CT scan of the pancreas using intravenous contrast media should be obtained for one of three reasons: (1) diagnostic uncertainty, (2) confirmation/evaluation of severity based upon other markers or clinical suspicion, or (3) evaluation in the setting of clinical deterioration or failure to respond to therapy. The radiologic findings may be consistent with any of the following: relatively normal appearing pancreas, pancreatic phlegmon, pancreatic phlegmon with extension of the inflammatory process to adjacent extrapancreatic spaces, pancreatic necrosis, or pancreatic pseudocyst, or abscess formation.

Several weeks after the pancreatitis has subsided, ERCP may be of value in patients with a tentative diagnosis of idiopathic pancreatitis (ie, those who have no history of alcoholism and no evidence of gallstones on ultrasound and oral cholecystogram). This examination demonstrates gallstones or changes of chronic pancreatitis in about 40% of such patients.

Differential Diagnosis

To some extent, acute pancreatitis is a diagnosis of exclusion, for other acute upper abdominal conditions such as acute cholecystitis, penetrating or perforated duodenal ulcer, high small bowel obstruction, acute appendicitis, and mesenteric infarction must always be seriously considered. In most cases, the distinction is possible on the basis of the clinical picture, laboratory findings, and CT scans. The critical point is that the diseases with which acute pancreatitis is most likely to be confused are often lethal if not treated surgically.

Chronic hyperamylasemia occurs rarely without any relation to pancreatic disease. Some cases are associated with renal failure, chronic sialadenitis, salivary tumors, ovarian tumors, or liver disease, but often there is no explanation. Analysis of serum amylase isoenzymes is the only way to determine whether the amylase originates from salivary glands or pancreas. Macroamylasemia is a chronic hyperamylasemia in which normal amylase (usually salivary) is bound to a large serum glycoprotein or immunoglobulin molecule and is therefore not excreted into urine. The diagnosis rests on the combination of hyperamylasemia and low urinary amylase. Macroamylasemia has been found in patients with other diseases such as malabsorption, alcoholism, and cancer. Many patients have abdominal pain, but the relationship of the pain and the macroamylasemia is uncertain.

Complications

The principal complications of acute pancreatitis are abscess and pseudocyst formation. These are discussed in separate sections. Gastrointestinal bleeding may occur from adjacent inflamed stomach or duodenum, ruptured pseudocyst, or peptic ulcer. Intraperitoneal bleeding may occur spontaneously from the celiac or splenic artery or from the spleen following acute splenic vein thrombosis. Involvement of the transverse colon or duodenum by the inflammatory process may result in partial obstruction, hemorrhage, necrosis, or fistula formation.

Early identification of patients at greatest risk of complications allows them to be managed more aggressively, which appears to decrease the mortality rate. The criteria of severity that have been found to be reliable are based either on the systemic manifestations of the disease as reflected in the clinical and laboratory findings or on the local changes in the pancreas as reflected by the findings on CT scan. Ranson used the former approach to develop the staging criteria listed in Table 26–1. Just the single finding of fluid sequestration (ie, fluid administered minus urine output) exceeding 2 L/d for more than 2 days is a reasonably accurate dividing line between severe (life-threatening) and mild-to-moderate disease. The local changes in the pancreas as shown on CT scans may be even more revealing. The presence of any of the following indicates a high risk of local infection in the pancreatic bed: involvement of extrapancreatic spaces in the inflammatory

Table 26-1. Ranson criteria of severity of acute pancreatitis.[1]

Criteria Present Initially
Age > 55 years
White blood cell count > 16,000/μL
Blood glucose > 200 mg/dL
SERUM LDH > 350 IU/L
AST (SGOT) > 250 IU/dL

Criteria Developing During First 24 Hours
Hematocrit fall > 10%
BUN rise > 8 mg/dL
Serum Ca^{2+} < 8 mg/dL
Arterial PO_2 < 60 mm Hg
Base deficit > 4 meq/L
Estimated fluid sequestration > 600 mL

[1]Morbidity and mortality rates correlate with the number of criteria present. Mortality rates correlate as follows: 0–2 criteria present = 2%; 3 or 4 = 15%; 5 or 6 = 40%; 7 or 8 = 100%.

process, pancreatic necrosis (areas in the pancreas that do not enhance with intravenous contrast media), and early signs of abscess formation (eg, gas bubbles in the tissue).

Treatment

A. Medical Treatment

The goals of medical therapy are reduction of pancreatic secretory stimuli and correction of fluid and electrolyte derangements.

1. Gastric suction—Oral intake is withheld. A nasogastric tube is often inserted to aspirate gastric secretions, although the latter has no specific therapeutic effect. Oral feeding should be resumed only after the patient appears much improved, appetite has returned, and serum amylase levels have dropped to normal. Premature resumption of eating may result in exacerbation of disease.

2. Fluid replacement—Patients with acute pancreatitis sequester fluid in the retroperitoneum and bowel, and large volumes of intravenous fluids are necessary to maintain circulating blood volume and renal function. In severe hemorrhagic pancreatitis, blood transfusions may also be required. The adequacy of fluid replacement is the single most important aspect of medical therapy. In fact, undertreatment with fluids may actually contribute to the progression of pancreatitis. Fluid replacement may be judged most accurately by monitoring the volume and concentration of the urine.

3. Antibiotics—Antibiotics are not useful in mild cases of acute pancreatitis. However, some studies have shown benefit of antibiotics that penetrate pancreatic tissue for patients with severe pancreatitis. Imipenem is the most commonly used antibiotic, though its use is not universally supported even in patients with severe disease. Antibiotics should also be used for treatment of specific operative complications.

4. Calcium and magnesium—In severe attacks of acute pancreatitis, hypocalcemia may require parenteral calcium replacement in amounts determined by serial calcium measurements. Recognition of hypocalcemia is important because it may produce cardiac dysrhythmias. Hypomagnesemia is also common, especially in alcoholics, and magnesium should also be replaced as indicated by serum levels.

5. Oxygen—Hypoxemia severe enough to require therapy develops in about 30% of patients with acute pancreatitis. It is often insidious, without clinical or x-ray signs, and out of proportion to the severity of the pancreatitis. The most pronounced examples accompany severe pancreatitis, often in association with hypocalcemia. The basic lesion, a form of adult respiratory distress syndrome, is poorly understood. Pulmonary changes include decreased vital capacity and an oxygen diffusion defect.

Hypoxemia must be suspected in every patient, and oxygen saturation should be monitored periodically or continuously for the first few hospital days. An occasional patient requires endotracheal intubation and mechanical ventilation. Diuretics may be useful in decreasing lung water and improving arterial oxygen saturation.

6. Nutrition—Enteral feeding should be used to support nutritional goals during the acute episode. Total parenteral nutrition avoids pancreatic stimulation and should be used for nutritional support only if enteral feeding is not practical for 5 or more days. Neither form of nutrition directly affects recovery of the pancreas.

7. Other drugs—Octreotide, H2 receptor blockers, anticholinergic drugs, glucagon, and aprotinin have shown no beneficial effects in controlled trials.

B. Endoscopic Sphincterotomy

Biliary pancreatitis is caused by a gallstone becoming lodged in the ampulla of Vater. In most cases, the stone passes into the intestine but occasionally it becomes impacted in the ampulla, which results in more severe disease. Less than 10% of cases of biliary pancreatitis are severe (ie, three or more Ranson criteria), but in severe cases, endoscopic sphincterotomy performed within 72 hours of the onset of the disease has been shown to decrease the incidence of concomitant biliary sepsis and lower the mortality rate from the pancreatitis.

C. Surgical Treatment

Surgery is generally contraindicated in uncomplicated acute pancreatitis. However, when the diagnosis is uncertain

in a patient with severe abdominal pain, diagnostic laparoscopy or laparotomy is not thought to aggravate pancreatitis.

When operative evaluation has been performed for diagnosis and mild to moderate pancreatitis is found, cholecystectomy should be performed if gallstones are present, but the pancreas should be left undisturbed. Although some surgeons place drains and irrigating catheters in the region of the pancreas, we prefer to keep foreign bodies out of this area.

The diagnosis of biliary pancreatitis can usually be suspected on the basis of ultrasound studies of the gallbladder early in the acute attack. Cholecystectomy should be performed on these patients during hospitalization for the acute attack soon after the attack resolves. A longer delay (even a few weeks) is associated with a high incidence (80%) of recurrent pancreatitis. Since life-threatening attacks are uncommon in gallstone pancreatitis, operation or endoscopic therapy early in an attack is rarely justified. However, when the attack is especially severe, elective cholecystectomy should be deferred up to several months to allow complete recovery from pancreatitis.

It is currently thought that debridement of dead peripancreatic tissue, which is often (40% of cases) colonized by bacteria, reduces the mortality rate of acute severe necrotizing pancreatitis. Historical controls place the mortality rate at 50%-80% in the absence of operative treatment and 10%-40% among patients subjected to necrosectomy. The diagnosis of necrotizing pancreatitis is suspected from the clinical findings; patients treated surgically have three or more Ranson criteria and average about 4½ criteria. Contrast-enhanced CT scans obtained early in the course of the disease are studied for the presence of nonenhancing areas, which indicate lack of vascular perfusion and reflect the presence of necrotic peripancreatic fat or pancreatic parenchyma. Percutaneous needle aspiration of these areas is used to detect the presence of bacterial colonization. A distinction is made between these cases of "infected necrotizing pancreatitis" and "pancreatic abscess," which may appear later in the course of the disease. Patients with infected necrotizing pancreatitis and severe clinical findings benefit most from surgical therapy, but laparotomy may be undertaken just because of a deteriorating condition in patients with necrotizing pancreatitis in the absence of bacterial colonization. At surgery, all peripancreatic spaces are opened and any necrotic tissue is removed by gentle blunt dissection. This can be accomplished with less invasive videoscopic techniques. Other than CT evidence of necrotic tissue with or without infection, there are presently no other criteria in general use that call for pancreatic surgery in patients with severe pancreatitis.

Surgery for complications of acute pancreatitis, such as abscess, pseudocyst, and pancreatic ascites, is discussed below.

▶ Prognosis

The death rate associated with acute pancreatitis is about 10%, and nearly all deaths occur in a first attack and among patients with three or more Ranson criteria of severity. Respiratory insufficiency and hypocalcemia indicate a poor prognosis. The death rate associated with severe necrotizing pancreatitis is 50% or more, but surgical therapy lowers the figure to about 20%. Persistent fever or hyperamylasemia 3 weeks or longer after an attack of pancreatitis usually indicates the presence of a pancreatic abscess or pseudocyst.

Freeman ML et al. International Multidisciplinary Panel of Speakers and Moderators. Interventions for necrotizing pancreatitis: summary of a multidisciplinary consensus conference. *Pancreas* 2012;41(8):1176-1194.

van Santvoort HC et al. Dutch Pancreatitis Study Group. A step-up approach or open necrosectomy for necrotizing pancreatitis. *N Engl J Med* 2010;362(16):1491-1502.

Working Group IAP/APA Acute Pancreatitis Guidelines. IAP/APA evidence-based guidelines for the management of acute pancreatitis. *Pancreatology* 2013:13(4 suppl 2):e1-e15.

2. Pancreatic Pseudocyst

 ### ESSENTIALS OF DIAGNOSIS

- ▶ Epigastric mass and pain
- ▶ Mild fever and leukocytosis
- ▶ Persistent serum amylase elevation
- ▶ Pancreatic cyst demonstrated by ultrasound or CT scan

▶ General Considerations

Pancreatic pseudocysts are encapsulated collections of fluid with high enzyme concentrations that arise from the pancreas. They are usually located either within or adjacent to the pancreas in the lesser sac. The walls of a pseudocyst are formed by inflammatory fibrosis of the peritoneal, mesenteric, and serosal membranes, which limits spread of the pancreatic juice as the lesion develops. The term pseudocyst denotes absence of an epithelial lining, whereas true cysts are lined by epithelium.

Two different processes are involved in the pathogenesis of pancreatic pseudocysts. Many occur as complications of severe acute pancreatitis, where extravasation of pancreatic juice and glandular necrosis form a sterile pocket of fluid that is not reabsorbed as inflammation subsides. Superinfection of such collections leads to pancreatic abscess

instead of pseudocyst. In other patients, usually alcoholics or trauma victims, pseudocysts appear without preceding acute pancreatitis. The mechanism in these cases consists of ductal obstruction and formation of a retention cyst that loses its epithelial lining as it grows beyond the confines of the gland. In posttraumatic pseudocyst, symptoms usually do not appear until several weeks after the injury. Some are iatrogenic, eg, occurring during splenectomy; others follow an external blow to the abdomen.

Pseudocysts develop in about 2% of cases of acute pancreatitis. The cysts are single in 85% of cases and multiple in the remainder.

▶ Clinical Findings

A. Symptoms and Signs

A pseudocyst should be suspected when a patient with acute pancreatitis fails to recover after a week of treatment or when, after improving for a time, symptoms return. Since it is now fairly routine to obtain a CT scan early in an attack of severe acute pancreatitis, the early stages of pseudocyst formation are often demonstrated radiographically before specific clinical findings appear. The first clinical manifestation is usually a palpable tender mass in the epigastrium, consisting of a swollen pancreas and contiguous viscera (a phlegmon). With time, the mass may subside, but if it persists it most likely represents a pseudocyst.

In other cases, the pseudocyst develops insidiously without an obvious attack of acute pancreatitis.

Regardless of the type of prodromal phase, pain is the most common finding. Fever, weight loss, tenderness, and a palpable mass are present in about half of patients. A few have jaundice, a manifestation of obstruction of the intrapancreatic segment of the bile duct.

B. Laboratory Findings

An elevated serum amylase and leukocytosis are present in about half of patients. When present, elevated bilirubin levels reflect biliary obstruction. Of those patients with acute pancreatitis whose serum amylase remains elevated for as long as 3 weeks, about half will have a pseudocyst.

C. Imaging Studies

CT scan (Figure 26-3) is the diagnostic study of choice. The size and shape of the cyst and its relationship to other viscera can be seen. Acute pseudocysts are often irregular in shape; chronic pseudocysts are most often circular or nearly so. An enlarged pancreatic duct may be demonstrated in patients with chronic pancreatitis. A dilated common bile duct would suggest biliary obstruction, either from the cyst or from underlying chronic pancreatitis.

The gallbladder should be studied by ultrasound to look for stones, especially in patients with acute pancreatitis.

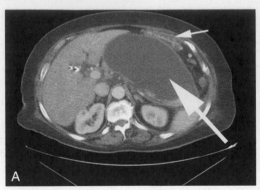
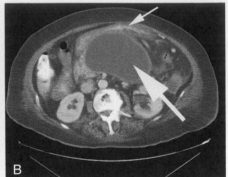

▲ **Figure 26–3.** CT scan of a large pancreatic pseudocyst impinging on the posterior wall of the stomach. The large arrow indicates the pseudocyst; the smaller area indicates the stomach. **A** : More cephalad in the abdomen, the pseudocyst abuts the stomach and liver. **B** : More caudad in the abdomen, the pseudocyst is immediately posterior to the gastric antrum. The stomach is compressed against the anterior wall of the abdomen, and the duodenum is stretched over the pseudocyst, causing early satiety. A cyst in this location is usually best drained into the stomach.

Although ultrasound can also demonstrate pseudocysts, the amount of important detail obtained is limited compared to CT scan, and consequently the role of ultrasound is mainly to follow changes in size of an acute pseudocyst already imaged by CT scan, so the amount of x-ray exposure can be minimized.

MRCP and/or ERCP should be performed if there is concern about significant abnormalities of the bile or pancreatic duct as suggested by CT scans or the results of liver function tests. Either duct may be dilated and in need of surgical drainage in conjunction with drainage of the pseudocyst. ERCP usually opacifies the pseudocyst as well, but the information is not usually of major value in planning treatment, so ERCP is not obtained routinely.

An upper gastrointestinal series will often reveal a mass in the lesser sac that distorts the stomach or duodenum, but this is not particularly useful information. The principal indication for an upper gastrointestinal series is to search for a site of gastric or duodenal obstruction in patients who are vomiting.

With wide use of sensitive imaging studies in the diagnosis of pancreatic disease, small asymptomatic pseudocysts are often demonstrated. The natural history of these subclinical lesions is benign, and there is no indication for prophylactic surgical treatment.

▶ Differential Diagnosis

Pancreatic pseudocysts must be distinguished from pancreatic abscess and acute pancreatic phlegmon. Patients with an abscess exhibit signs of infection.

Rarely, patients with pseudocyst present with weight loss, jaundice, and a nontender palpable gallbladder and are first thought to have pancreatic carcinoma. CT scans show

that the lesion is fluid-filled, which suggests the correct diagnosis.

Neoplastic cysts—either cystadenoma or cystadenocarcinoma—account for about 5% of all cases of cystic pancreatic masses and may be indistinguishable preoperatively from pseudocyst. The correct diagnosis can be made from the gross appearance supplemented by a biopsy obtained at operation.

▶ Complications

A. Infection

Infection is a rare complication resulting in high fever, chills, and leukocytosis. Drainage is required as soon as the diagnosis is suspected. Some lesions can be drained externally via a catheter placed percutaneously using ultrasound guidance. Internal drainage of infected pseudocysts adherent to the stomach can be achieved surgically by cystogastrostomy; otherwise, drainage should be external, because the suture line of a Roux-en-Y cystojejunostomy may not heal.

B. Rupture

Sudden perforation into the free peritoneal cavity produces severe chemical peritonitis, with abdominal rigidity and severe pain. Rapid enlargement of the pseudocyst is sometimes noted before it ruptures. The treatment is emergency surgery with irrigation of the peritoneal cavity and a drainage procedure for the pseudocyst. The wall of a ruptured pseudocyst is usually too flimsy to hold sutures securely, so most ruptured cysts must be drained externally. Rupture of a pseudocyst occurs in less than 5% of cases, and even with prompt treatment it may be fatal.

C. Hemorrhage

Bleeding may occur into the cyst cavity or an adjacent viscus into which the cyst has eroded. Intracystic bleeding may present as an enlarging abdominal mass with anemia resulting from blood loss. If the cyst has eroded into the stomach, there may be hematemesis, melena, and blood in the nasogastric aspirate. The rapidity of the blood loss often produces hemorrhagic shock, which may preclude arteriography. If time permits, however, emergency arteriography should be performed to delineate the site of bleeding, which is usually a false aneurysm of an artery in the cyst wall, and to embolize it if possible. If embolization successfully occludes the bleeding vessel, several weeks should elapse to ensure that bleeding will not recur, and at that point the pseudocyst should be drained surgically in the same fashion as a nonbleeding pseudocyst. If the bleeding cannot be stopped by embolization, emergency surgery should be performed. Usually all that can be done is to open the cyst and suture ligate the bleeding vessel in the cyst wall, followed by external or internal drainage of the cyst. Sometimes it is possible to excise the cyst, which is desirable because doing so more certainly avoids the risk of recurrent hemorrhage.

▶ Treatment

The principal indications for treating pancreatic pseudocysts are to improve symptoms and to prevent complications. Recent data indicate that the natural history of these lesions is more benign than previously thought—that in the absence of symptoms or radiographic evidence of enlargement (and irrespective of cyst size), expectant management is not unreasonable, and that a few untreated cysts resolve spontaneously even after being stable for months. Expectant management is especially important in the first 6-12 weeks of existence of cysts that have arisen during an attack of acute pancreatitis. The chances of spontaneous resolution are about 40%; catheter drainage at this stage is meddlesome; and internal drainage of the cyst by surgery may be difficult or even impossible. Thereafter, for cysts greater than 5 cm, treatment is usually recommended over expectant management (in the absence of contraindications, such as serious concomitant disease), because most cysts can be promptly eliminated by percutaneous catheter drainage or surgical drainage into the stomach or intestine. This obviates the need for prolonged follow-up with repeated ultrasound or CT scans and avoids the risks, albeit low, of complications. Patients who present with a symptomatic pseudocyst and no history of recent acute pancreatitis may be treated without the 6- to 12-week delay, because their cyst wall is tough (mature) enough to hold sutures and allow an anastomosis with the gut. Jaundice in a patient with a pseudocyst is usually caused by pressure from the cyst on the bile duct. Draining the pseudocyst usually relieves the obstruction, but an operative cholangiogram should be obtained to make sure.

A. Excision

Excision is the most definitive treatment but is usually confined to chronic pseudocysts in the tail of the gland. This approach is recommended especially for cysts that follow trauma, where the head and body of the gland are normal. Most cysts should be drained either externally or internally into the gut.

B. External Drainage

External drainage is best for critically ill patients or when the cyst wall has not matured sufficiently for anastomosis to other organs. A large tube is sewn into the cyst lumen, and its end is brought out through the abdominal wall. External drainage is complicated in a third of patients by a pancreatic fistula that sometimes requires surgical drainage but on the average closes spontaneously in several months. The incidence of recurrent pseudocyst is about four times greater after external drainage than after drainage into the gut.

C. Internal Drainage

The preferred method of treatment is internal drainage, where the cyst is anastomosed to a Roux-en-Y limb of jejunum (cystojejunostomy), to the posterior wall of the stomach (cystogastrostomy), or to the duodenum (cystoduodenostomy). The interior of the cyst should be inspected for evidence of a tumor and biopsy performed as appropriate. Cystogastrostomy is preferable for cysts behind and densely adherent to the stomach. This may well be done laparoscopically in the future. To accomplish free, dependent drainage, Roux-en-Y cystojejunostomy provides better drainage of cysts in various other locations. Cystoduodenostomy is indicated for cysts deep within the head of the gland and adjacent to the medial wall of the duodenum—lesions that would be difficult to drain by any other technique. The procedure consists of making a lateral duodenotomy, opening into the cyst through the medial wall of the duodenum, and then closing the lateral duodenotomy. Following internal drainage, the cyst cavity becomes obliterated within a few weeks. Even after cystogastrostomy, an unrestricted diet can be allowed within a week after surgery, and x-rays taken at this time usually show only a small residual cyst cavity.

D. Nonsurgical Drainage

External drainage can be established by a percutaneous catheter placed into the cyst under radiographic or ultrasound control. This is the preferred method for infected pseudocysts. In some centers, it is also used for the majority of uncomplicated pseudocysts as the primary mode of therapy. About two-thirds of cysts so treated are permanently eradicated. It may also be useful to shrink a truly huge pseudocyst (eg, one that occupies half of the abdominal cavity), because it is technically difficult to obtain adequate internal drainage of these lesions into the gut. Occasionally, a sterile cyst may become infected when a narrow catheter is inserted into it. This is more likely when the cyst lumen contains debris that is not drained effectively by this technique. Chronic external pancreatic fistula is a potential complication of this method.

Two other drainage techniques have been tried: (1) passing a catheter percutaneously through the anterior abdominal wall, the anterior wall of the stomach, and through the posterior stomach into the cyst. After several weeks, the catheter is removed, and a chronic tract remains from cyst to gastric lumen. (2) Using a fiberoptic gastroscope to make a small incision through the back wall of the stomach into the cyst.

▶ Prognosis

The recurrence rate for pancreatic pseudocyst is about 10%, and recurrence is more frequent after treatment by external drainage. Serious postoperative hemorrhage from the cyst occurs rarely—most often after cystogastrostomy. In most cases, however, surgical treatment of pseudocysts is uncomplicated and definitively solves the immediate problem. Many patients later experience chronic pain as a manifestation of underlying chronic pancreatitis.

Martin RF, Hein AR. Operative management of acute pancreatitis. *Surg Clin North Am* 2013;93(3):595-610.
Varadarajulu S, Bang JY, Sutton BS, et al. Failure to comply with NCCN guidelines for the management of pancreatic cancer compromises outcomes. *HPB (Oxford)* 2012;14(8):539-547.

3. Pancreatic Abscess

Pancreatic abscess, which complicates about 5% of cases of acute pancreatitis, is invariably fatal if it is not treated surgically. It tends to develop in severe cases accompanied by hypovolemic shock and pancreatic necrosis and is an especially frequent complication of postoperative pancreatitis. Abscess formation follows secondary bacterial contamination of necrotic pancreatic debris and hemorrhagic exudate. The organisms may spread to the pancreas hematogenously as well as directly through the wall of the transverse colon. It is unknown whether prophylactic antibiotics given early in the course of severe acute pancreatitis decrease the incidence of abscess.

▶ Clinical Findings

An abscess should be suspected when a patient with severe acute pancreatitis fails to improve and develops rising fever or when symptoms return after a period of recovery. In most cases, there is improvement for a while before signs of infection appear 2-4 weeks after the attack began. Epigastric pain and tenderness and a palpable tender mass are clues to diagnosis. In many cases, the findings are not especially striking—ie, the temperature is only modestly elevated and the patient does not appear septic. Vomiting or jaundice may be present, but in some cases fever and leukocytosis are the only findings. The serum amylase may be elevated but usually is normal. Characteristically, the serum albumin is below 2.5 g/dL and the alkaline phosphatase is elevated. Pleural fluid and diaphragmatic paralysis may be evident on chest x-rays. An upper gastrointestinal series may show deformity of the stomach or duodenum by a mass, but it usually does not, and the changes are nonspecific in any case. Diagnostic CT scans will usually indicate the presence of a fluid collection in the area of the pancreas. Gas in the collection on plain films or CT scans is virtually diagnostic. Percutaneous CT scan-guided aspiration may be used to aid in diagnosis and obtain a specimen for Gram stain and culture.

In general, the diagnosis is difficult, treatment is often instituted late, illness is severe, and death rates are high.

▶ Treatment

The infected collection must be drained. Percutaneous catheter drainage may be helpful as a first step in order to decrease toxicity or to obtain a specimen for culture. In some cases, catheter drainage will prove to be definitive, but most often the infected retroperitoneal space is honeycombed and contains necrotic debris that cannot pass through the catheter, so surgical debridement is necessary. It is best to consider catheter drainage as a preparatory step for surgery rather than a curative treatment, for that is the usual relationship. Otherwise, there may be a tendency to delay surgery for too long as futile efforts are repeatedly made to manipulate the catheters into better positions. In fact, the two measures—surgical debridement and catheter drainage—are complementary.

Preoperatively, the patient should be given broad-spectrum antibiotics, since the organisms are usually a mixed flora, most often *Escherichia coli, Bacteroides, Staphylococcus, Klebsiella, Proteus, Candida albicans,* etc. Necrotic debris should be removed and external drainage instituted.

Postoperative hemorrhage (immediate or delayed) from the abscess cavity occurs occasionally.

▶ Prognosis

The death rate is about 20%, a consequence of the severity of the condition, incomplete surgical drainage, and the inability in some cases to make the diagnosis.

Martin RF, Hein AR. Operative management of acute pancreatitis. *Surg Clin North Am* 2013;93(3):595-610.

4. Pancreatic Ascites & Pancreatic Pleural Effusion

Pancreatic ascites consists of accumulated pancreatic fluid in the abdomen without peritonitis or severe pain. Since many of these patients are alcoholic, they are often thought at first to have cirrhotic ascites. The syndrome is most often due to chronic leakage of a pseudocyst, but a few cases are due to disruption of a pancreatic duct. The principal causative factors are alcoholic pancreatitis in adults and traumatic pancreatitis in children. Marked recent weight loss is a major clinical manifestation, and unresponsiveness of the ascites to diuretics is an additional diagnostic clue. The ascitic fluid, which ranges in appearance from straw-colored to blood-tinged, contains elevated protein (> 2.9 g/dL) and amylase levels. Once this condition is suspected, definitive diagnosis is based on chemical analysis of the ascitic fluid and endoscopic retrograde pancreatography. The latter procedure frequently demonstrates the point of fluid leak and allows a rational surgical approach if operation is required.

Initial therapy should consist of a period of intravenous hyperalimentation and somatostatin. This often cures the problem. If considerable improvement has not occurred within 2-3 weeks, surgery should be performed. A preoperative ERCP is essential to demonstrate the site of the leak. If it is not entirely obvious from the films taken during ERCP, a CT scan should be performed immediately afterward, while contrast media is still in the pancreatic duct. The greater sensitivity of the CT scan will be enough to reveal the tiny trickle from the pancreatic duct into the abdomen. The operation involves suturing a Roux-en-Y limb of jejunum to the site of the leak on the surface of the pancreas or a pancreatic pseudocyst. With appropriate therapy, the outlook is excellent. The death rate is low in patients treated before debilitation becomes severe.

Chronic pleural effusions of pancreatic origin represent a variant in which the pancreatic fistula drains into the chest. The diagnosis is made by measuring high concentrations of amylase (usually > 3000 IU/dL) in the fluid. A CT scan of the pancreas and retrograde pancreatogram should be obtained. Medical therapy consists of draining the fluid with a chest tube, somatostatin, and total parenteral nutrition. If after several weeks the fistula persists or if it recurs after the tube has been removed, the source of the leak on the pancreas should either be drained into a Roux-en-Y limb of jejunum or excised as part of a distal pancreatectomy.

Martin RF, Hein AR. Operative management of acute pancreatitis. *Surg Clin North Am* 2003;93(3):595-610.

5. Chronic Pancreatitis

ESSENTIALS OF DIAGNOSIS

▸ Persistent or recurrent abdominal pain

▸ Pancreatic calcification on x-ray in 50%

▸ Pancreatic insufficiency in 30%; malabsorption and diabetes mellitus

▸ Most often due to alcoholism

▸ General Considerations

Chronic alcoholism causes most cases of chronic pancreatitis, but a few are due to gallstones, hypercalcemia, hyperlipidemia, duct obstruction from any cause, or inherited predisposition (familial pancreatitis). Direct trauma to the gland, either from an external blow or from surgical injury, can produce chronic pancreatitis if a ductal stricture develops during the healing process. In such cases, disease is often localized to the segment of gland drained by the obstructed duct. Although gallstone disease may cause repeated attacks of acute pancreatitis, this uncommonly leads to chronic pancreatitis.

Pressure within the duct is increased in patients with chronic pancreatitis (about 40 cm H_2O) compared with normal subjects (about 15 cm H_2O). This is a result of increased viscosity of pancreatic juice, partial obstruction by calculi, and impaired distensibility of the gland because of diffuse fibrosis. Sphincteric pressure remains in the normal range. The increased pressure causes dilation of the duct in the patient whose pancreas has not yet become fixed by scarring. It may also impair nutrient blood flow, causing further functional damage. Pathologic changes in the gland include destruction of parenchyma, fibrosis, dedifferentiation of acini, calculi, and ductal dilation.

▸ Clinical Findings
A. Symptoms and Signs

Chronic pancreatitis may be asymptomatic, or it may produce abdominal pain, malabsorption, diabetes mellitus, or (usually) all three manifestations. The pain is typically felt deep in the upper abdomen and radiating through to the back, and it waxes and wanes from day to day. Early in the course of the disease, the pain may be episodic, lasting for days to weeks and then vanishing for several months before returning again. Attacks of acute pancreatitis may occur, superimposed on the pattern of chronic pain. Many patients become addicted to the narcotics prescribed for pain.

B. Laboratory Findings

Abnormal laboratory findings may result from: (1) pancreatic inflammation, (2) pancreatic exocrine insufficiency, (3) diabetes mellitus, (4) bile duct obstruction, or (5) other complications such as pseudocyst formation or splenic vein thrombosis.

1. Amylase—In acute exacerbations, serum and urinary amylase levels may be elevated, but most often they are not, perhaps because pancreatic fibrosis has destroyed so much of the enzyme-forming capacity of the parenchyma.

2. Tests of exocrine pancreatic function—The secretin and CCK stimulation tests are the most sensitive tests to detect exocrine malfunction but are difficult to perform.

3. Diabetes mellitus—About 75% of patients with calcific pancreatitis and 30% of those with noncalcific pancreatitis have insulin-dependent diabetes. Most of the rest have either abnormal glucose tolerance curves or abnormally low serum insulin levels after a test meal. The margin of reserve is such that partial pancreatectomy is quite likely to convert a patient who does not require insulin into one who does require it postoperatively.

4. Biliary obstruction—Elevated bilirubin or alkaline phosphatase levels may result from fibrotic entrapment of the lower end of the bile duct. The differential diagnosis of biliary obstruction in these patients must consider acute pancreatic inflammation, pseudocyst, or pancreatic neoplasm.

5. Miscellaneous—Splenic vein thrombosis may produce secondary hypersplenism or gastric varices.

A. Imaging Studies

MRCP or endoscopic retrograde pancreatography is helpful in establishing the diagnosis of chronic pancreatitis, in ruling out pancreatic pseudocyst and neoplasm, and in preoperative planning for patients thought to be candidates for surgery. The typical findings are ductal stones and irregularity, with dilation and stenoses and, occasionally, ductal occlusion. The discovery of small, unsuspected pseudocysts is common. Retrograde cholangiography should be performed simultaneously to determine whether the common bile duct is narrowed by the pancreatitis, to determine whether biliary calculi are present, and to aid the surgeon in avoiding injury to the bile duct during operation.

▶ Complications

The principal complications of chronic pancreatitis are pancreatic pseudocyst, biliary obstruction, duodenal obstruction, malnutrition, and diabetes mellitus. Adenocarcinoma of the pancreas occurs with greater frequency in patients with familial chronic pancreatitis than in the general population.

▶ Treatment

Medical Treatment

Malabsorption and steatorrhea are managed with support and measures. Controlled trials have shown that administering pancreatic enzymes has little effect on the pain.

Patients with chronic pancreatitis should be urged to discontinue the use of alcohol. Abstention from alcohol will reduce chronic or episodic pain in more than half of cases even though damage to the pancreas is irreversible. Psychiatric treatment may be beneficial. Diabetes in these patients usually requires insulin.

B. Surgical Treatment

Surgical therapy is principally of value to relieve chronic intractable pain. It is essential that every effort be made to eliminate alcohol abuse. The best surgical candidates are those whose pain persists after alcohol has been abandoned.

Surgical treatment in most cases involves a procedure that facilitates drainage of the pancreatic duct or resects diseased pancreas or that serves both purposes. The choice of operation can usually be made preoperatively based on the findings of a retrograde pancreatogram and CT scans. Coincidental bile duct obstruction is common and should be treated by simultaneous choledochoduodenostomy.

1. Drainage procedures—A dilated ductal system reflects obstruction, and when dilation is present, procedures to improve ductal drainage usually relieve pain. Calcific alcoholic pancreatitis most often falls into this category.

The usual finding is an irregular, widely dilated duct (1-2 cm in diameter) with points of stenosis ("chain of lakes" appearance) and ductal calculi. For such patients, a longitudinal pancreaticojejunostomy (Puestow procedure) is appropriate (Figure 26–4). The duct is opened anteriorly from the tail into the head of the gland and anastomosed side-to-side to a Roux-en-Y segment of proximal jejunum. Pain improves postoperatively in about 80% of patients, but improvement of pancreatic insufficiency is uncommon. This procedure, however, has a low rate of success when the pancreatic duct is narrow (ie, < 8 mm).

Sphincteroplasty and distal (caudal) pancreaticojejunostomy (DuVal procedure) are other drainage techniques that were used more often in the past. The latter is only of historical interest, but surgical sphincteroplasty plus extraction of pancreatic ductal calculi continues in use, more are responsible for occasional deaths. For this reason, total pancreatectomy is contraindicated in unreformed alcoholics. For chronic alcoholic pancreatitis, resections from the left of the gland—eg, distal subtotal pancreatectomy—are much less successful than resections of the head and are rarely performed nowadays. The most common indication is chronic focal posttraumatic pancreatitis, in which the head may be normal.

3. Celiac plexus block—Celiac plexus block may be used in an attempt to obtain pain relief before proceeding with a major pancreatic resection in small duct pancreatitis.

▶ Prognosis

Longitudinal pancreaticojejunostomy relieves pain in about 80% of patients with a dilated duct. Weight gain is common but less predictable. The results of pancreaticoduodenectomy are good in 80% of patients, but removal of the distal pancreas is less successful. Total pancreatectomy, which is principally reserved for failures of other operations, gives satisfying relief in 30%-90% of patients depending on the series. The reasons for these widely differing results are not known. Celiac plexus block is of lasting benefit to no more than 30% of patients. In some patients, pain subsides with advancing pancreatic insufficiency.

Except in advanced cases with continuous pain, alcoholics who can be persuaded to stop drinking often experience relief from pain and recurrent attacks of pancreatitis. In familial pancreatitis, the progress of the disease is inexorable, and many of these patients require surgery. The results of longitudinal pancreaticojejunostomy are excellent in familial pancreatitis. Narcotic addiction, diabetes, and malnutrition are serious problems in many patients.

Bachmann K et al. Is the Whipple procedure harmful for long-term outcome in treatment of chronic pancreatitis? 15-years follow-up comparing the outcome after pylorus-preserving pancreatoduodenectomy and Frey procedure in chronic pancreatitis. *Ann Surg* 2013;258(5):815-820.

Familiari P, Boškoski I, Bove V, Costamagna G. ERCP for biliary strictures associated with chronic pancreatitis. *Gastrointest Endosc Clin N Am* 2013;23(4):833-845.

Issa Y, van Santvoort HC, van Goor H, et al. Surgical and endoscopic treatment of pain in chronic pancreatitis: a multidisciplinary update. *Dig Surg* 2013;30(1):35-50.

PANCREATIC INSUFFICIENCY (STEATORRHEA; MALABSORPTION)

Pancreatic exocrine insufficiency may follow pancreatectomy or pancreatic disease, especially chronic pancreatitis. Many patients with varying degrees of pancreatic insufficiency have no symptoms and require no treatment, whereas others may benefit greatly from a rational medical regimen.

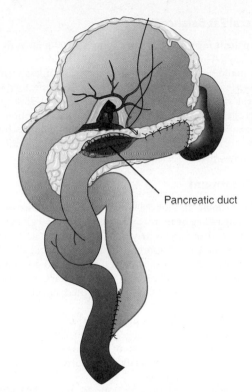

▲ **Figure 26–4.** Longitudinal pancreaticojejunostomy (Puestow) for chronic pancreatitis.

Pancreatic duct

often now through endoscopic access to the pancreatic duct.

2. Pancreatectomy—In the absence of a dilated duct, pancreatectomy is the best procedure, and the extent of resection can often be determined from a CT scan and pancreatogram. In patients with small ducts, the most severe disease is usually located in the head of the gland, and pancreaticoduodenectomy (Whipple procedure) is the operation of choice. A variant of this procedure involves resection of the head of the gland while preserving the duodenum. A Roux-en-Y limb of jejunum is anastomosed to both cut surfaces of the pancreas. If the duct is also dilated in the body and tail, resection of the head can also be combined with longitudinal pancreaticojejunostomy in that part of the gland. Pain relief is satisfactory in about 80% of patients treated by these operations. Total pancreatectomy is indicated when a previous pancreaticoduodenectomy or distal pancreatectomy has failed to give satisfactory pain relief. The reported results are contradictory; pain relief has been excellent in reports from the United Kingdom but less than excellent in reports from the United States. Difficulties in controlling diabetes mellitus occur in 30%-40% of patients who have had total pancreatectomy and

Malabsorption and steatorrhea do not appear until more than 90% of pancreatic exocrine function is lost; with 2%-10% of normal function, steatorrhea is mild to moderate; with less than 2% of normal function, steatorrhea is severe. On a diet containing 100 g of fat/d, normal subjects excrete 5-7 g/d, and the efficiency of assimilation is similar over a wide range of fat intake. Total pancreatectomy causes about 70% fat malabsorption. If the pancreatic remnant is normal, subtotal resections may have little effect on absorption.

Pancreatic insufficiency affects fat absorption more than that of protein or carbohydrate, because protein digestion is aided by gastric pepsin and carbohydrate digestion by salivary and intestinal amylase. Malabsorption of vitamins is rarely a significant problem. Water-soluble B vitamins are absorbed throughout the small intestine, and fat-soluble vitamins, although dependent on micellar solubilization by bile salts, do not require pancreatic enzymes for absorption. Vitamin B_{12} malabsorption has been detected in some patients with pancreatic insufficiency, but it is rarely a clinical problem, and vitamin B_{12} replacement is unnecessary.

Thus, the principal problem in otherwise uncomplicated pancreatic insufficiency is fat malabsorption and accompanying caloric malnutrition.

▶ Tests of Pancreatic Exocrine Function

A. Secretin or Cholecystokinin Test

Pancreatic juice is obtained by peroral duodenal intubation, and the response to an intravenous injection of secretin or CCK is measured. The results vary, depending on the dose and preparation of hormone used. Both tests (using purified hormones or the synthetic octapeptide of CCK) seem to be reliable. Pancreatic fluid should normally have a bicarbonate concentration greater than 80 mEq/L and bicarbonate output above 15 mEq/30 min.

B. Pancreolauryl Test

Fluorescein dilaurate is given orally with breakfast, and urinary fluorescein excretion is measured. Release and absorption of fluorescein depend on the action of pancreatic esterase. The test is relatively specific, but considerable exocrine insufficiency is required for a positive result. It is currently the most widely used test of exocrine function because it is inexpensive and easy to do.

C. PABA Excretion (Bentiromide) Test

The patient ingests 1 g of the synthetic peptide bentiromide (Bz-Ty-PABA), and urinary excretion of aromatic amines (PABA) is measured. Cleavage of the peptide to liberate PABA depends on intraluminal chymotrypsin activity. Patients with chronic pancreatitis excrete about 50% of the normal amount of PABA.

D. Fecal Fat Balance Test

The patient ingests a diet containing 75-100 g fat each day for 5 days. The amounts of dietary fat should be measured and should be the same each day. Excretion of less than 7% of ingested fat is normal. Clinically significant steatorrhea is present when fat malabsorption exceeds about 25%. Total pancreatectomy results in about 70% fat malabsorption.

Examination of a stool specimen for fat globules (obviously much simpler than the fat balance test) is specific and relatively sensitive for fat malabsorption.

▶ Treatment

The diet should aim for 3000-6000 kcal/d, emphasizing carbohydrate (400 g or more) and protein (100-150 g). Patients with steatorrhea may or may not have diarrhea, and dietary restriction of fat is important mainly to control diarrhea. Patients with diarrhea may be restricted to 50 g of fat and the amount increased until diarrhea appears. Permissible fat intake averages 100 g/d distributed equally among four meals.

Pancrelipase replacement may be accomplished with pancreatic extracts containing 30,000-50,000 units of lipase distributed throughout each of four daily meals. Lesser amounts are much less effective; an hourly dosage regimen probably has no advantages.

If enzymes alone do not improve the malabsorption enough, the problem is probably due to destruction of lipase by gastric acid. This can be largely alleviated by adding an H_2 receptor blocking agent to the enzyme regimen. A preparation of enzymes as enteric-coated microspheres (Pancrease) is less vulnerable to low pH and may be more effective in refractory cases.

Medium-chain triglycerides (MCT), which can be obtained as a powder or an oil, may be used as a caloric supplement. This product is more rapidly hydrolyzed and the fatty acids more readily absorbed than are long-chain triglycerides, which make up 98% of the fat in a normal diet. Unfortunately, MCT oil is relatively unpalatable and is frequently associated with nausea and vomiting, bloating, and diarrhea, which limit patient acceptance.

ADENOCARCINOMA OF THE PANCREAS

An estimated 46,420 patients will develop pancreatic cancer in the United States in 2014, and 39,590 will die of the disease. These nearly equal numbers illustrate the dismal prognosis generally associated with pancreatic carcinoma. The death rate per 100,000 people has been basically unchanged since the mid 1960s at about 10/100,000 for men and 27/100,000 for women. After tumors of the lung, prostate and colon, pancreatic carcinoma is the fourth leading cause of death due to cancer in men, and trails lung, breast and colon in women. Factors associated with an increased risk of pancreatic cancer are cigarette smoking, dietary consumption of meat (especially fried meat) and fat, previous gastrectomy (> 20 years earlier), and race.

The peak incidence is in the fifth and sixth decades. In two-thirds of cases, the tumor is located in the head of the gland; the remainder occurs in the body or tail. Ductal adenocarcinoma, mainly of a poorly differentiated cell pattern, accounts for 80% of the cancers; the remainder is islet cell tumors and cystadenocarcinomas, tumors that are discussed later in this chapter. Pancreatic adenocarcinoma is characterized by early local extension to contiguous structures and metastases to regional lymph nodes and the liver. Pulmonary, peritoneal, and distant nodal metastases occur later.

▶ Clinical Findings

A. Symptoms and Signs

1. Carcinoma of the head of the pancreas—About 75% of patients with carcinoma of the head of the pancreas present with weight loss, obstructive jaundice, and deep-seated abdominal pain. Back pain occurs in 25% of patients and is associated with a worse prognosis. In general, smaller tumors confined to the pancreas are associated with less pain. Weight loss averages about 20 lb (44 kg). Hepatomegaly is present in half of patients but does not necessarily indicate spread to the liver. A palpable mass, which is found in 20%, nearly always signifies surgical incurability. Jaundice is unrelenting in most patients but fluctuates in about 10%. Cholangitis occurs in only 10% of patients with bile duct obstruction. A palpable nontender gallbladder in a jaundiced patient suggests neoplastic obstruction of the common duct (Courvoisier sign), most often due to pancreatic cancer; this finding is present in about half of cases. Jaundice is often accompanied by pruritus, especially of the hands and feet.

2. Carcinoma of the body and tail of the pancreas— Since carcinomas of the body and tail of the pancreas are remote from the bile duct, less than 10% of patients are jaundiced. The presenting complaints are weight loss and pain, which sometimes occurs in excruciating paroxysms. In the few patients with jaundice or hepatomegaly, metastatic involvement has usually occurred. Migratory thrombophlebitis develops in 10% of cases. Once considered relatively specific as a clue to pancreatic cancer, this complication is now known to affect patients with other types of malignant disease.

The diagnosis of pancreatic carcinoma can be extremely difficult. The typical patient who presents with abdominal pain, weight loss, and obstructive jaundice rarely presents a problem, but those with just weight loss, vague abdominal pain, and nondiagnostic x-rays are occasionally labeled psychoneurotics until the existence of cancer becomes

obvious. If back pain predominates, orthopedic or neurosurgical causes may be sought at first. One characteristic feature is the tendency for the patient to seek relief of pain by assuming a sitting position with the spine flexed. Recumbency, on the other hand, aggravates the discomfort and sometimes makes sleeping in bed impossible. Sudden onset of diabetes mellitus is an early manifestation in 25% of patients.

B. Laboratory Findings

Elevated alkaline phosphatase and bilirubin levels reflect either common duct obstruction or hepatic metastases. The bilirubin level with neoplastic obstruction averages 18 mg/dL, much higher than that generally seen with benign disease of the bile ducts. Only rarely are serum aminotransferase levels markedly elevated. Repeated examination of stool specimens for occult blood gives a positive reaction in many cases.

Serum levels of the tumor marker CA 19-9 are elevated in most patients with pancreatic cancer, but the sensitivity in resectable (< 4 cm) lesions is too low (50%) for this to serve as a screening tool. Elevated levels also occur with other gastrointestinal cancers. The greatest usefulness of CA 19-9 measurements may be in following the results of treatments. After complete resection of a tumor, elevated levels drop to normal, but they rise again with recurrence.

C. Imaging Studies

Nearly all patients should have a CT scan.

1. CT scan—CT scans show a pancreatic mass in 95% of cases, usually with a central zone of diminished attenuation, and in over 90% of patients with a mass there are signs of extension beyond the boundaries of the pancreas. The upstream pancreatic duct is noted to be dilated in 70% of patients, and the bile duct is dilated in 60% (principally in those with jaundice). The presence of both bile duct and pancreatic duct dilation is strong evidence for pancreatic cancer even in the absence of a mass. Findings suggesting unresectability include local tumor extension (eg, behind the pancreas; into the liver hilum), contiguous organ invasion (eg, duodenum, stomach), distant metastases, involvement of the superior mesenteric or portal vessels, or ascites. In general, size of the mass is only loosely related to resectability. CT scans using modern dynamic scanning techniques are as accurate as angiography in assessing vascular involvement.

2. ERCP—In patients with a typical clinical history and a pancreatic mass on CT, ERCP is unnecessary. In the absence of a mass, an ERCP is indicated. It is the most sensitive test (95%) for detecting pancreatic cancer, though specificity in differentiating between cancer and pancreatitis is low. Consequently, a pancreatogram should be obtained early in cases where the existence of a pancreatic lesion is suspected but unproved. The findings consist of stenosis or obstruction of the pancreatic duct. Adjacent lesions of the bile duct and pancreatic duct (double-duct sign) are highly suggestive of neoplastic disease, especially if the biliary involvement is focal. Although ERCP is useful to distinguish between the various kinds of periampullary tumors, that information rarely alters management.

1. Upper gastrointestinal series—An upper gastrointestinal series is not sensitive in detecting pancreatic cancer, but it provides information about patency of the duodenum that may be useful in deciding whether a gastrojejunostomy will have to be performed. The classic findings consist of widening of the duodenal sweep, narrowing of the lumen, and the "reversed-3 sign," named for the duodenal configuration.

2. Other studies—Angiography has not proved reliable in detecting or staging pancreatic neoplasms, and ultrasound is a poor second to CT scans for imaging.

D. Aspiration Biopsy

Percutaneous aspiration biopsy of pancreatic mass lesions is positive in 85% of malignant tumors. The procedure is relatively safe, but there is a risk of spreading a localized (resectable) tumor, so it is contraindicated in patients who are candidates for surgery. Percutaneous aspiration biopsy is principally of value to verify a presumptive diagnosis of adenocarcinoma of the pancreas in patients with radiographic evidence of unresectability. In these cases, cytologic proof is important, for treatment decisions should not be made solely on the basis of the indirect evidence provided by CT scans and other imaging tests. There is too great a risk of misdiagnosing something unusual, such as a retroperitoneal lymphoma or sarcoma, and administering inappropriate treatment.

▶ Differential Diagnosis

The other periampullary neoplasms—carcinoma of the ampulla of Vater, distal common bile duct, or duodenum—may also present with pain, weight loss, obstructive jaundice, and a palpable gallbladder. Preoperative cholangiography and gastrointestinal x-rays may suggest the correct diagnosis, but laparotomy is sometimes required.

▶ Complications

Obstruction of the splenic vein by tumor may cause splenomegaly and segmental portal hypertension with bleeding gastric or esophageal varices.

▶ Treatment

Pancreatic resection for pancreatic cancer is appropriate only if all gross tumor can be removed with a standard resection. The lesion is considered resectable if the following areas are free of tumor: (1) the hepatic artery near the origin of the gastroduodenal artery; (2) the superior mesenteric artery where it courses under the body of the pancreas; and (3) the liver and regional lymph nodes. Since the pancreas is so close to the portal vein and the superior mesenteric vessels, these structures may be involved early. About 20% of cancers of the head of the pancreas can be resected, but because of local and distant spread, this is rarely possible for lesions of the body and tail.

A histologic diagnosis can usually be made at operation by aspiration biopsy. With small lesions of the head of the gland, it may be difficult to obtain a specimen for histologic diagnosis because much of the palpable mass may consist of inflamed pancreatic tissue. Occasionally, histologic diagnosis is impossible, and clinical decisions must rest on indirect evidence.

For curable lesions of the head, pancreaticoduodenectomy (Whipple procedure) is required (Figure 26–5). This involves resection of the common bile duct, the gallbladder, the duodenum, and the pancreas to the mid body. There is an increasing tendency to preserve the antrum and pylorus. Involvement of a short (< 1.5 cm) segment of the portal vein is not a contraindication to a curative resection. This is managed by a partial or circumferential resection of the affected area.

When the procedure is performed by surgeons who do it frequently, the operative mortality rate is less than 5%. When it is performed by less experienced surgeons, the mortality rate is as high as 20%-30%. Postoperative deaths are due to complications such as pancreatic and biliary fistulas, hemorrhage, and infection.

For unresectable lesions, cholecystojejunostomy or choledochojejunostomy provides relief of jaundice and pruritus. A cholangiogram should be obtained to verify patency between the cystic and common bile ducts unless it is grossly obvious. Percutaneous or endoscopically placed biliary stents may also provide effective palliation and are preferable to surgical biliary decompression if the lesion is known to be unresectable. Gastrojejunostomy is required if the tumor blocks the duodenum. If laparotomy has been performed, gastrojejunostomy should be considered regardless of the presence of duodenal obstruction, because with time this often develops before other life-threatening complications.

Laparoscopy is a useful first step in patients scheduled for a possible Whipple procedure. If metastases are seen that militate against a curative resection, laparoscopic gastrojejunostomy or cholecystojejunostomy (or both) can be performed. If not, one should proceed with the laparotomy. About 15% of patients thought to have localized disease from preoperative studies are found to be unresectable at laparoscopy.

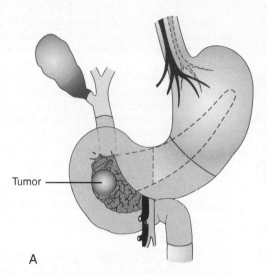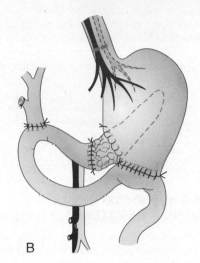

Tumor

A B

▲ **Figure 26–5.** Pancreaticoduodenectomy (Whipple procedure). **A** : Preoperative anatomic relationships showing a tumor in the head of the pancreas. **B:** Postoperative reconstruction showing pancreatic, biliary, and gastric anastomoses. A cholecystectomy and bilateral truncal vagotomy are also part of the procedure. In many cases, the distal stomach and pylorus can be preserved, and vagotomy is then unnecessary.

Gemcitabine-based chemotherapy has clear benefits in patients with metastatic disease. Its utility in combination with radiation therapy and as adjuvant therapy is being defined.

► Prognosis

The mean survival following palliative therapy is 7 months. Following a Whipple procedure, survival averages about 18 months. Factors associated with tumor recurrence and shorter survival include lymph node involvement, tumor size over 2.5 cm, blood vessel invasion, and amount of blood transfused. If tumor cells extend to the margins of the resected specimen, long-term survival is rare. If the margins are clear, about 20% of patients live more than 5 years. Overall 5-year survival is about 10%, but only 60% of these patients are actually free of tumor.

Tempero MA et al. National Comprehensive Cancer Networks. Pancreatic adenocarcinoma, version 2.2012: featured updates to the NCCN Guidelines. *J Natl Compr Canc Netw* 2012;10(6):703-713.
Visser BC, Ma Y, Zak Y, et al. Failure to comply with NCCN guidelines for the management of pancreatic cancer compromises outcomes. *HPB (Oxford)* 2012;14(8):539-547.

CYSTIC NEOPLASMS

Cystic neoplasms of the pancreas usually present with abdominal pain, a mass, or jaundice and are diagnosed from the findings on CT scans.

Cystadenomas can be classified as serous or mucinous. Serous cystadenomas, which are usually microcystic adenomas, are well-circumscribed lesions consisting of multiple small cysts ranging in size from microscopic to about 2 cm. The cut surface has the appearance of a sponge. The multicystic nature of the lesion is usually—but not always—evident on CT scans, which may also show a few calcifications. The epithelium, which is flat to cuboidal, has no malignant potential. Treatment usually entails excision, but in the rare case where this is too hazardous, the lesion may be left in place with the knowledge that complications are rare. An occasional serous cystadenoma will consist of one or more large cysts (ie, macrocystic).

Mucinous cystadenomas (macrocystic adenomas), which are much more common in women than in men, are unilocular or, more often, multilocular lesions that have a smooth lining with papillary projections. The septate appearance on CT scans is characteristic. The cystic spaces measure 2-20 cm in diameter and contain mucus. The lining consists of tall columnar and goblet cells, which are often arranged in a papillary pattern. In time, most mucinous cystadenomas will evolve into cystadenocarcinomas, so total excision is the required treatment.

Cystadenocarcinomas invariably present as a focus of malignancy within an existing mucinous cystadenoma. The tumors are often quite large (eg, 10-20 cm) at the time of diagnosis. Metastases occur in about 25% of cases. Complete excision results in a 5-year survival rate of 70%.

An uncommon lesion, referred to as solid and papillary or papillary-cystic neoplasm of the pancreas, occurs almost exclusively in young women (under age 25 years). The tumor is usually large. It may be locally invasive, but metastases are uncommon, and cure is to be expected after resection.

Farrell JJ, Fernández-del Castillo C. Pancreatic cystic neoplasms: management and unanswered questions. *Gastroenterology* 2013;144(6):1303-1315.

Lee LS, Clancy T, Kadiyala V, Suleiman S, Conwell DL. Interdisciplinary management of cystic neoplasms of the pancreas. *Gastroenterol Res Pract* 2012; 2012:513163.

ADENOMA & ADENOCARCINOMA OF THE AMPULLA OF VATER

Adenoma and adenocarcinoma of the ampulla of Vater account for about 10% of neoplasms that obstruct the distal bile duct. One-third are adenomas and two-thirds adenocarcinomas. Since a remnant of benign adenoma can be found in a majority of adenocarcinomas, it is suspected that malignant change in an adenoma gives rise to most carcinomas. The presenting symptom is most often jaundice or occasionally gastrointestinal bleeding. Weight loss and pain are more common with carcinoma than with adenoma, but the differences are not great enough to allow a distinction to be made on this basis alone.

CT and ultrasound scans reveal dilation of the biliary tree and pancreatic duct. Gallstones are an incidental finding in 20% of patients, and when common duct stones are present, they may incorrectly be held responsible for the biliary obstruction. ERCP can be an important diagnostic study. In 75% of cases, tumor is visible on duodenoscopy as an exophytic papillary lesion, an ulcerated tumor, or an infiltrating mass. An adequate biopsy usually can be obtained of these lesions. In 25% of cases, there is no intraduodenal growth, and endoscopic sphincterotomy is necessary to display the tumor. It is best to wait 10-14 days to biopsy these tumors because of transient artifacts that result from the sphincterotomy. ERCP also demonstrates dilation of the biliary and pancreatic ducts. It has become common to perform a sphincterotomy whenever possible, not only to facilitate performance of a biopsy but also to decompress the biliary tree and allow jaundice to subside in anticipation of subsequent surgical therapy. The value of this step has not been established.

Although some adenomas have been successfully treated by snare excision or, preferably, by neodymium:YAG laser destruction, local resection, or pancreaticoduodenectomy is preferable because of the significant chance that an invasive carcinoma will be undertreated at a time that it is curable. These nonsurgical methods should be reserved for patients who are poor candidates for resection.

Treatment of adenocarcinoma consists of pancreaticoduodenectomy as for pancreatic carcinoma. The operative mortality rate is less than 5%, and the 5-year survival rate is about 50%. The presence of metastases in resectable peripancreatic lymph nodes is not a contraindication to pancreaticoduodenectomy, for the 5-year survival rate under these circumstances is still a respectable 25%. Local excision is an alternative for noninfiltrating papillary adenocarcinomas in patients who are too poor a risk for pancreaticoduodenectomy, but this operation is not as successful as pancreaticoduodenectomy. Endoscopic sphincterotomy alone or with retrograde stent placement (the combination is usually required) is indicated when there is definite evidence (eg, hepatic metastases) that the tumor is incurable. Survival averages less than a year with this approach, however.

Tempero MA et al. National Comprehensive Cancer Networks. Pancreatic Adenocarcinoma, version 2.2012: featured updates to the NCCN Guidelines. *J Natl Compr Canc Netw* 2012;10(6):703-713.

PANCREATIC ISLET CELL TUMORS

Islet cell tumors may be functioning (ie, hormone-producing) or nonfunctioning, malignant or nonmalignant. More than half are functioning; less than half are malignant. Insulinoma, the most common functioning islet cell neoplasm, arises from beta cells and produces insulin and symptoms of hypoglycemia. Tumors of the {d} or {a}$_1$ cells produce gastrin and the Zollinger–Ellison syndrome. Alpha$_2$ cell neoplasms may produce excess glucagon and hyperglycemia. Non-beta islet cell tumors may secrete serotonin, ACTH, MSH, and kinins (and evoke the carcinoid syndrome). Some produce pancreatic cholera, a severe diarrheal illness.

1. Nonfunctioning Islet Cell Tumors

Most of these lesions are malignant tumors of the head of the gland, which present with abdominal and back pain, weight loss, and, in many cases, a palpable abdominal mass. Jaundice is encountered occasionally. CT scans reveal a pancreatic mass, and angiography typically shows it to be hypervascular. The histologic pattern on biopsy specimens is diagnostic of islet cell tumor, but whether or not the lesion is malignant rests on evidence of invasiveness or metastases, not the appearance of the cells. Immunohistochemical staining of the tissue is positive for chromogranin and neuron-specific enolase (markers of APUD tumors). Metastases are present at the time of diagnosis in 80% of patients. Resection of all gross tumor (eg, by a Whipple procedure), the preferred treatment, is possible in less than half of patients because of local extension or distant metastases. A combination of streptozocin and doxorubicin is the most effective chemotherapeutic regimen. The 5-year disease-free survival rate is about 15%.

Kulke MH et al. National Comprehensive Cancer Networks. Neuroendocrine tumors. *J Natl Compr Canc Netw* 2012;10(6):724-764.

Oberstein PE, Remotti H, Saif MW, Libutti SK. Pancreatic neuro-endocrine tumors: entering a new era. *JOP* 2012;13(2):169-173.

2. Insulinoma

Insulinomas have been reported in all age groups. About 75% are solitary and benign. About 10% are malignant, and metastases are usually evident at the time of diagnosis. The remaining 15% are manifestations of multifocal pancreatic disease—either adenomatosis, nesidioblastosis, or islet cell hyperplasia.

The symptoms (related to cerebral glucose deprivation) are bizarre behavior, memory lapse, or unconsciousness. Patients may be mistakenly treated for psychiatric illness. There may be profuse sympathetic discharge, with palpitations, sweating, and tremulousness. Hypoglycemic episodes are usually precipitated by fasting and are relieved by food, so weight gain is common. The classic diagnostic criteria (Whipple triad) are present in most cases: (1) hypoglycemic symptoms produced by fasting, (2) blood glucose below 50 mg/dL during symptomatic episodes, and (3) relief of symptoms by intravenous administration of glucose.

The most useful diagnostic test and the only one indicated in all but a few patients is demonstration of fasting hypoglycemia in the presence of inappropriately high levels of insulin. The patient is fasted, and blood samples are obtained every 6 hours for glucose and insulin measurements. The fast is continued until hypoglycemia or symptoms appear or for a maximum of 72 hours (some investigators truncate the test at 48 hours). Although insulin levels are not always elevated in patients with insulinoma, they will be high relative to the blood glucose concentration. A ratio of plasma insulin to serum glucose greater than 0.3 is diagnostic. Ratios should be calculated before and during the fast. Proinsulin, which constitutes more than 25% of total insulin (the upper limit of normal) in about 85% of patients with insulinomas, should also be measured. Proinsulin levels greater than 40% suggest a malignant islet cell tumor.

Drugs that release insulin (tolbutamide, glucagon, leucine, arginine, calcium) were used in the past as provocative tests. No provocative tests are currently used.

Localization of the tumor is important but may be difficult. In about 10% of cases, the tumor is so small or located so deeply that it is difficult or impossible to find at laparotomy. High-resolution CT and MR scans are successful in demonstrating about 40% of tumors. Endoscopic ultrasound examination of the pancreas may be able to show a much higher percentage. The most important examination is intraoperative ultrasound, which can identify a pancreatic tumor in nearly all cases. It is more sensitive than any preoperative test.

In patients who have had previous resection or significant upper abdominal surgery, exploration with intraoperative ultrasound may be difficult. Invasive preoperative testing may then be useful. Angiography gives a yield of about 50%. Transhepatic portal venous sampling has proved an accurate preoperative localizing method, demonstrating the position in the pancreas in about 95% of lesions. However, this test is time-consuming and somewhat invasive, involving entering the portal vein with a catheter passed percutaneously through the liver and testing blood at various sites within the portal, superior mesenteric, and splenic veins for insulin levels. The point where insulin concentrations rise sharply indicates the site of the tumor. An alternative invasive localizing test uses arteriography with selective calcium infusion into arteries supplying the pancreas. Blood samples from the hepatic veins reveal an increase in insulin level when calcium is infused into an artery supplying the tumor.

▶ Differential Diagnosis

Fasting hypoglycemia may be a manifestation of some nonpancreatic, nonislet cell tumors. Clinically, the condition is identical to that resulting from insulinoma, but the cause is rarely secretion of insulin by the tumors, as serum insulin levels are normal. Most nonislet cell tumors associated with hypoglycemia are large and readily detected on physical examination. The majority are of mesenchymal origin (eg, hemangiopericytoma, fibrosarcoma, leiomyosarcoma) and are located in the abdomen or thorax, but hepatoma, adrenocortical carcinoma, and a variety of other lesions may also produce hypoglycemia. The principal means by which these tumors produce hypoglycemia are the following: (1) secretion by the tumor of insulin-like growth factor II (IGF-II), an insulin-like peptide that normally mediates the effects of growth hormone; and (2) inhibition of glycogenolysis or gluconeogenesis. Rapid utilization of glucose by the tumor, replacement of liver tissue by metastases, and secretion of insulin are other postulated mechanisms that are probably uncommon.

Surreptitious self-administration of insulin is seen occasionally, most often in an individual with access to insulin on the job. If insulin injections have been given for as long as 2 months, insulin antibodies will be detectable in the patient's serum. Circulating C peptide levels are normal in these patients but elevated in most patients with insulinoma. Sulfonylurea ingestion can be detected by measuring the drug in plasma.

▶ **Treatment**

Surgery should be done promptly, because with repeated hypoglycemic attacks, permanent cerebral damage occurs and the patient becomes progressively more obese. Moreover, the tumor may be malignant. Medical treatment is reserved for surgically incurable lesions.

A. Medical Treatment

Diazoxide is administered to suppress insulin release. For incurable islet cell carcinomas, streptozocin is the best chemotherapeutic agent. Sixty percent of patients live up to 2 additional years. Toxicity is considerable; streptozocin is not recommended as a routine adjunct to surgical therapy.

B. Surgical Treatment

At operation, the entire pancreas must be palpated carefully because the tumors are usually small and difficult to find. The gland should also be examined intraoperatively with ultrasound, which may be able to locate a tumor that cannot be felt, or to demonstrate signs of invasion (ie, irregular borders) that indicate malignancy—something that cannot be detected by palpation. When the tumor is found, it may be enucleated if it is superficial or resected as part of a partial pancreatectomy if it is deep-seated or invasive. Insulinomas in the head of the gland can nearly always be enucleated.

Tumors that can be localized preoperatively, and that are placed in favorable anatomic locations, can sometimes be resected using a laparoscopic approach. The same principles of local, complete resection should be followed. Laparoscopic ultrasound is often useful to guide this exploration.

In the past, the tumor could not be detected in about 5% of cases by these methods. The traditional recommendation was to resect the distal half of the pancreas and have the pathologist slice the specimen into thin sections and look for the tumor. If the tumor was found, the operation was concluded; if it was not found, additional pancreas would be resected until an 80% distal pancreatectomy had been performed. Since the tumors are evenly distributed, this strategy is 80% successful in removing the tumor. Intraoperative monitoring of blood glucose is often done as a means of determining if the tumor has been excised, but it is unreliable. With the use of operative ultrasound scanning, however, no more than 1%-2% of insulinomas remain occult, and blind distal pancreatectomy is rarely even considered.

Patients with insulinoma associated with MEN-1 usually have multiple (average of three) lesions. Because persistence of the disease is much more likely in this condition following the standard surgical approach, the operation recommended

here is distal pancreatectomy plus enucleation of any lesions found in the head of the gland.

For islet cell hyperplasia, nesidioblastosis, or multiple benign adenomas, distal subtotal pancreatectomy usually decreases insulin levels enough that medical management is simplified. For islet cell carcinomas, resection of both primary and metastatic lesions is warranted if technically feasible.

Patients with sporadic insulinomas lead a normal life after the tumor has been removed. The outcome is less predictable in patients with MEN-1, who may have several insulin-producing tumors.

Kulke MH et al. National Comprehensive Cancer Networks. Neuroendocrine tumors. *J Natl Compr Canc Netw* 2012;10(6):724-64.

3. Pancreatic Cholera (WDHA Syndrome: Watery Diarrhea, Hypokalemia, & Achlorhydria)

Most cases of pancreatic cholera are caused by a non-beta islet cell tumor of the pancreas that secretes VIP and peptide histidine isoleucine. The syndrome is characterized by profuse watery diarrhea, massive fecal loss of potassium, low serum potassium, and extreme weakness. Gastric acid secretion is usually low or absent even after stimulation with betazole or pentagastrin. Stool volume averages about 5 L/d during acute episodes and contains over 300 mEq of potassium (20 times normal). Severe metabolic acidosis frequently results from loss of bicarbonate in the stool. Many patients are hypercalcemic, possibly from secretion by the tumor of a parathyroid hormone-like substance. Abnormal glucose tolerance may result from hypokalemia and altered sensitivity to insulin. Patients who complain of severe diarrhea must be studied carefully for other causes before the diagnosis of WDHA syndrome is entertained seriously. Chronic laxative abuse is a frequent explanation.

CT scan is the best initial imaging test; somatostatin receptor scintigraphy is also very useful for localization. Approximately 80% of the tumors are solitary, located in the body or tail, and can be removed easily. About half of the lesions are malignant, and three-fourths of those have metastasized by the time of exploration. Even if all of the tumor cannot be removed, resection of most of it alleviates symptoms in about 40% of patients even though the average survival is only 1 year. Streptozocin has produced remissions in several cases, but nephrotoxicity may limit its effectiveness. Treatment with long-acting somatostatin analogues decreases VIP levels, controls diarrhea, and may even reduce tumor size. The effect persists indefinitely in most patients, but in a few it is transient.

Kulke MH et al. National Comprehensive Cancer Networks. Neuroendocrine tumors. *J Natl Compr Canc Netw* 2012;10(6):724-764.

4. Glucagonoma

Glucagonoma syndrome is characterized by migratory necrolytic dermatitis (usually involving the legs and perineum), weight loss, stomatitis, hypoaminoacidemia, anemia, and mild to moderate diabetes mellitus. Scotomas and changes in visual acuity have been reported in some cases. The age range is 20-70 years, and the condition is more common in women. The diagnosis may be suspected from the distinctive skin lesion; in fact, the presence of a prominent rash in a patient with diabetes mellitus should be enough to raise suspicions. Glucagonoma should also be suspected in any patient with new onset of diabetes after the age of 60. Confirmation of the diagnosis depends on measuring elevated serum glucagon levels. CT scans demonstrate the tumor and sites of spread. Angiography is not essential but reveals a hypervascular lesion.

Glucagonomas arise from {a}$_2$ cells in the pancreatic islets. Most are large at the time of diagnosis. About 25% are benign and confined to the pancreas. The remainder has metastasized by the time of diagnosis, most often to the liver, lymph nodes, adrenal gland, or vertebrae. A few cases have been the result of islet cell hyperplasia.

Severe malnutrition should be corrected preoperatively with a period of total parenteral nutrition and treatment with somatostatin analogues. Surgical removal of the primary lesion and resectable secondaries is indicated if technically feasible. If the tumor is confined to the pancreas, cure is possible. Even if it is not possible to remove all the tumor deposits, considerable palliation may result from subtotal removal, so surgery is indicated in almost every case. Low-dose heparin therapy should be administered pre- and postoperatively because of a high risk of deep venous thrombosis and pulmonary embolism. Streptozocin and dacarbazine are the most effective chemotherapeutic agents for unresectable lesions. Somatostatin therapy normalizes serum glucagon and amino acid levels, clears the rash, and promotes weight gain. The clinical course generally parallels changes in serum levels of glucagon in response to therapy.

Kulke MH et al. National Comprehensive Cancer Networks. Neuroendocrine tumors. *J Natl Compr Canc Netw* 2012;10(6):724-764.

5. Somatostatinoma

Somatostatinomas are characterized by diabetes mellitus (usually mild), diarrhea and malabsorption, and dilation of the gallbladder (usually with cholelithiasis). Serum calcitonin and IgM concentrations may be elevated. The syndrome results from secretion of somatostatin by an islet cell tumor of the pancreas, half of which are malignant and accompanied by hepatic metastases. The lesion is usually large and readily demonstrated by CT scan. The diagnosis may be made by recognizing the clinical syndrome and measuring increased concentrations of somatostatin in the serum. Often, however, the somatostatin syndrome is unsuspected until histologic evidence of metastatic islet cell carcinoma has been obtained. When the disease is localized, resection is able to cure about 50% of cases. Enucleation is inappropriate for these tumors. Chemotherapy with streptozocin, dacarbazine, or doxorubicin is the best treatment for unresectable tumors. Small somatostatin-rich tumors of the duodenum or ampulla of Vater have also been reported, but none of these lesions have been associated with high serum levels of somatostatin or the clinical syndrome.

Kulke MH et al. National Comprehensive Cancer Networks. Neuroendocrine tumors. *J Natl Compr Canc Netw* 2012;10(6):724-764.

MULTIPLE CHOICE QUESTIONS

1. All of the following are true about the anatomy of the pancreas, except

    A. The head is adherent to the medial duodenum.
    B. The body is in contact posteriorly with the left crus of the diaphragm and the left adrenal gland.
    C. The common bile duct passes through a groove in the posterior aspect of the head.
    D. The uncinate process lies anterior to the superior mesenteric artery.
    E. The main pancreatic duct is also known as the duct of Wirsung.

2. Serum amylase can come from

    A. Lung
    B. Muscle
    C. Skin
    D. Parotid gland
    E. Red blood cells

3. Acute pancreatitis

    A. Is usually caused by acute cholecystitis
    B. Can be complicated by pancreatic abscess
    C. Causes inflammation of the pancreas that is usually not discernible by CT scan

D. Is associated with common bile duct stones in more than 80% of patients

E. Progresses to chronic pancreatitis in about 40% of those affected

4. Pancreatic adenocarcinoma

A. Is unresectable at the time of diagnosis in most people

B. Is smaller at diagnosis, on average, for tumors in the tail of the pancreas than those in the head

C. Can be resected by pancreaticoduodenectomy for those tumors limited to the tail

D. Has a similar prognosis as malignant pancreatic neuroendocrine tumor

E. Should generally be managed by operative enucleation

5. Management of insulinoma

A. Typically requires emergent operation

B. Should not include preoperative imaging

C. Should usually include resection of the primary tumor

D. Is commonly required in the management of chronic pancreatitis

E. Is a palliative approach to an incurable problem for most people

Spleen

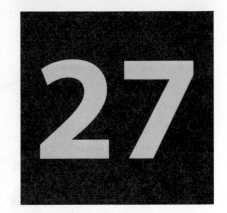

27

Gerard M. Doherty, MD

ANATOMY

The spleen is a dark purplish, highly vascular, coffee bean-shaped organ of mesodermal origin situated in the left upper quadrant of the abdomen at the level of the eighth to eleventh ribs between the fundus of the stomach, the diaphragm, the splenic flexure of the colon, and the left kidney (Figure 27–1). The adult spleen weighs 100-150 g, measures about $12 \times 7 \times 4$ cm, and usually cannot be palpated. It is attached to adjacent viscera, the abdominal wall, and the diaphragm by peritoneal folds or "ligaments." The gastrosplenic ligament carries the short gastric vessels. The other ligaments are avascular except in patients with portal hypertension or myelofibrosis.

The splenic capsule consists of peritoneum overlying a 1- to 2-mm fibroelastic layer that contains a few smooth muscle cells. The fibroelastic layer sends into the pulp numerous fibrous bands (trabeculae) that form the framework of the spleen. Corrosion cast studies demonstrate that the spleen consists of specific segments based on arterial supply numbering between two and six separated by an avascular plane.

The splenic artery enters the hilum of the spleen, branches into the trabecular arteries, and then branches into the central arteries that course through the surrounding white pulp and send radial branches to the peripheral marginal zone and the more distant red pulp. The white pulp consists of lymphatic tissue including T cells adjacent to the central artery (periarteriolar lymphoid sheets [PALS]), with a surrounding area containing lymphoid follicles rich in B cells interspersed with dendritic and reticular cells important in antigen presentation. The vascular spaces of the marginal zone between the red and white pulp channel blood into the splenic Billroth cords and out to the associated sinuses. The red pulp vascular structures have a noncontiguous basement membrane that filters cells such as senescent erythrocytes into the macrophage-lined sinuses.

Accessory spleens (spleniculi) are seen in 10%-15% of the normal population and are located primarily in the gastrosplenic, gastrocolic, and lienorenal ligaments, but they can also be found throughout the peritoneal cavity in the omentum, bowel mesentery, and pelvis. Accessory spleens probably result from a failure of infusion of splenic embryologic tissues. Ordinarily of no significance, they may play a role in recurrence of certain hematologic disorders for which splenectomy is performed. Removal of accessory spleens may lead to remission of disease in these patients. Accessory spleens are more difficult to identify with laparoscopic procedures, but the use of a hand port has allowed identification and resection of accessory spleens with a minimally invasive approach. Patients who fail to respond to initial splenectomy should undergo scanning with technetium 99m-labeled red cells or indium 111-labeled platelets to identify potential sites of missed accessory spleens and can be identified intraoperatively with a hand-held gamma counter.

Ectopic spleen (wandering spleen) is an unusual condition in which a long splenic pedicle allows the spleen to move within the peritoneum. It often resides in the lower abdomen or pelvis, where even a normal-sized spleen can be felt as a mass. The condition is 13 times more common in women than in men. Diagnostic radionuclide scan can diagnose the mass as a spleen. Acute torsion of the pedicle occurs occasionally, necessitating emergency splenectomy, and elective removal of wandering spleens in the pelvis is recommended.

PHYSIOLOGY

The spleen has a dual function as a secondary lymphoid organ important in host immunity, and as a large filter for blood removing senescent erythrocytes and recycling iron. The anatomy of the spleen provides an ideal environment for these two functions with the immune activity in the white pulp and the hematologic function in the red pulp.

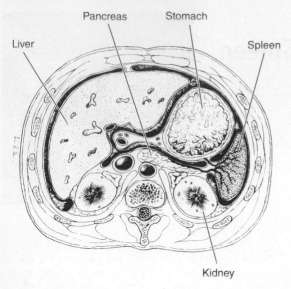

Pancreas   Stomach

Liver   Spleen

Kidney

▲ **Figure 27-1.** Normal anatomic relations of the spleen.

The spleen receives 5% of the total cardiac output, or approximately 150-300 mL/min, such that each red cell averages 1000 passes through the spleen each day. Normal blood cells pass rapidly through the spleen, while abnormal and senescent cells are slowed and entrapped. As they travel through the hypoxic, acidotic, glucose-deprived splenic cords and sinuses of the red pulp, senescent erythrocytes pass into the vascular spaces and are phagocytosed by macrophages in a process called "culling." Part of the membrane of erythrocytes can be removed through the gaps between endothelial cells lining the vascular spaces in a similar process called pitting. In the presence of splenomegaly and other disease states, the flow patterns of the spleen become more circuitous as the red pulp volume expands, so that even normal cells may be trapped.

The spleen is considered to be a secondary organ of the immune system and represents the largest single collection of lymphoid tissue in the body. The white pulp of the spleen contains the various cellular components needed to generate an immune response, with structural and functional relationships similar to those of lymph nodes. Lymphocytes and circulating antigen-presenting cells enter the white pulp via the marginal zone capillaries and traverse the T cell-rich PALS before passing through bridging channels into the red pulp. Primary follicles or germinal centers with secondary follicles at the periphery of the white pulp are sites of B cell expansion and immunoglobulin production. Blood passing through the spleen is exposed to all the key cellular components necessary for both humoral and cellular immune responses. Tissue macrophages in the spleen are key components of generating an immune response particularly

in encapsulated organs. Moreover, the concentration of macrophages in the red pulp vascular spaces facilitates opsonization of particles coated with IgG and plays an important role in the filtration and removal of senescent erythrocytes, the autoimmune hematologic diseases as well as explaining the increased risk of sepsis that follows splenectomy in children under 2 years of age. Even in adults, splenectomy leads to a slight but definite reduction in immune function.

Normally, about 30% of the total platelet pool is sequestered in the spleen. Splenomegaly typically involves expansion of the red pulp, which increases this sequestration to between 80% and 95% of the platelet cell mass. Storage of erythrocytes and granulocytes in the spleen is limited in humans, but newly formed reticulocytes released from the bone marrow concentrate in the spleen to undergo a maturational process.

Scandella JT et al. Form follows function: lymphoid tissue microarchitecture in antimicrobial immune defence. Nature Reviews. *Immunology* 2008;8:764-775.

▼ OPERATIVE INDICATIONS FOR SPLENECTOMY

To better describe and understand operative indications in surgery of the spleen, one could categorize the indications for splenectomy or procedures of the spleen into eight general areas:

1. Hypersplenism is characterized by diffuse enlargement of the spleen by neoplastic disorders, hematopoietic disorders of the bone marrow, and metabolic or storage disorders. These various disease processes result in diffuse enlargement of the spleen and amplify the normal function of elimination of circulating blood cells resulting in general pancytopenia. Erythrocytes and platelets are most commonly affected. Hypersplenism also may cause symptoms of early satiety due to the splenic size.

2. **Autoimmune/erythrocyte disorders** Specific cytopenias are related either to antibodies targeting platelets, erythrocytes, or neutrophils. A second category of diseases relates to intrinsic structural changes within the erythrocyte that lead to a shortened red blood cell half-life with accelerated splenic clearance. There is nothing intrinsically wrong with the spleen, and splenic size is typically normal.

3. Trauma or injury to the spleen.

4. **Vascular diseases** Splenic vein thrombosis and splenic artery aneurysm may require splenectomy for treatment.

5. Cysts, abscesses, and primary splenic tumors are mass lesions of the spleen. This would include treatment of simple cysts, echinococcal cysts, splenic abscess, and various benign neoplasms including hamartomas,

hemangiomas, lymphangiomas, and rare malignant lesions.

6. **Diagnostic procedures** This category of splenectomy occurs when the spleen is removed primarily to make a clinical diagnosis when none is available. A subcategory of this would be staging laparotomy for Hodgkin disease, which has all but been eliminated based on alternative imaging techniques and current treatment regimens.

7. **Iatrogenic splenectomy** Splenectomy that is performed due to an incidental injury to the spleen during surgery within the general abdominal cavity or specifically, the left upper quadrant, can be categorized as iatrogenic splenectomy. This category is likely underreported and may be considered a subcategory of trauma.

8. **Incidental splenectomy** The spleen may be removed as part of a standard operation to remove the distal pancreas most commonly, and also for gastric cancers, left-sided renal cell carcinomas, adrenal cancers, and retroperitoneal sarcomas in the left upper quadrant. The spleen is removed in these instances due to direct tumor extension, vascular involvement, or the need for excision of splenic hilum lymph nodes.

With the increase in splenic preservation for trauma, many institutional series list medical conditions as the most indications for splenectomy. Most recent series report 40%-50% for hematologic conditions, 35%-40% for trauma, and 20%-30% for neoplastic disease. Within the category, idiopathic thrombocytopenia purpura has the highest incidence of splenectomy. Each of these categories of disease will be discussed including the etiology and pathophysiology of the disorder, the specific indications for splenectomy, alternative treatments, and the results of splenectomy.

Bickenbach KA, Gonen M, Labow DM, et al. Indications for and efficacy of splenectomy for haematological disorders. *Br J Surg* 2013;100(6):794-800.

Harbrecht BG et al. Is splenectomy after trauma an endangered species? *Am Surg* 2008;74:410-412.

Musallam KM et al. Postoperative outcomes after laparoscopic splenectomy compared with open splenectomy. *Ann Surg* 2013;257(6):1116-1123.

HYPERSPLENISM

In the past, the term hypersplenism or increased splenic function has been used to denote the syndrome characterized by splenic enlargement, deficiency of one or more blood cell lines, normal or hyperplastic cellularity of deficient cell lines in the marrow, and increased turnover of affected cells. Increased understanding of the pathophysiology of specific disorders has shown that hypersplenism is not synonymous with splenomegaly. Some disorders in which there

is spleen-dependent destruction of blood elements do not manifest all features of hypersplenism. For example, splenomegaly is rarely a feature of immune thrombocytopenic purpura, and splenectomy is not always curative. Conversely, other conditions that enlarge the spleen may not result in destruction or sequestration of blood elements with resultant cytopenias. In disorders with known pathogenesis, the trend has been to classify them as separate disease entities rather than as hypersplenic conditions.

The defects in hypersplenism are exaggerations of normal splenic functions primarily associated with the red pulp. The principal cause of cytopenias in hypersplenism is increased sequestration and destruction of blood cells in the spleen, which is hypertrophied or increased in volume in a variety of diseases. Etiologic factors include: (1) neoplastic infiltration, (2) disease of the bone marrow in which the spleen becomes a site of extramedullary hematopoiesis, or (3) metabolic/genetic disorders such as Gaucher disease. The hyperplastic spleen is not selective in its hyperfunction in most of these disorders. The splenomegaly can lead to an increased turnover in erythrocytes and platelets, with a lesser effect on leukocytes. For example, about 60% of patients with cirrhosis develop splenomegaly and 15% develop hypersplenism. The hypersplenism of cirrhosis is seldom of clinical significance; the anemia and thrombocytopenia are usually mild and rarely are indications for splenectomy.

▶ Clinical Findings

A. Symptoms and Signs

The clinical findings depend largely on the underlying disorder or are secondary to the depletion of circulating blood elements caused by the hypersplenism (Table 27–1). Manifestations of hypersplenism usually develop gradually, and the diagnosis often follows a routine physical or laboratory examination. Some patients experience left upper quadrant fullness, discomfort (can be severe), or early satiety. Others have hematemesis due to gastroesophageal varices.

Table 27-1. Disorders associated with secondary hypersplenism.

Congestive splenomegaly (cirrhosis, portal or splenic vein obstruction)
Neoplasm (leukemia, metastatic carcinoma)
Inflammatory disease (sarcoid, lupus erythematosus, Felty syndrome)
Acute infections with splenomegaly
Chronic infection (tuberculosis, brucellosis, malaria)
Storage diseases (Gaucher disease, Letterer–Siwe disease, amyloidosis)
Chronic hemolytic diseases (spherocytosis, thalassemia, glucose-6-phosphate dehydrogenase deficiency, ellipto-cytosis)
Myeloproliferative disorders (myelofibrosis with myeloid metaplasia)

Purpura, bruising, and diffuse mucous membrane bleeding are unusual symptoms despite the presence of thrombocytopenia. Anemia may produce significant fatigue that may be the chief complaint in this patient population. Recurrent infections may be seen in patients with severe leukopenia.

B. Laboratory Findings

Patients with primary hypersplenism usually exhibit pancytopenia of moderate degree and generalized marrow hyperplasia. Anemia is most prominent, reflecting the destruction of erythrocytes in the hypertrophied red pulp of the spleen. Thrombocytopenia occurs due to sequestration of platelets but also possibly due to increased turnover. In most cases more immature cell types such as reticulocytes are present, reflecting the overactivity of the bone marrow to compensate for the pancytopenias. One exception is myeloid metaplasia, in which dysfunction of the bone marrow is the primary defect.

C. Evaluation of Splenic Size

Before it becomes palpable, an enlarged spleen may cause dullness to percussion above the left costal margin. Splenomegaly is manifested on supine x-rays of the abdomen by medial displacement of the stomach and downward displacement of the transverse colon and splenic flexure. CT scan is useful for differentiating the spleen from other abdominal masses and for demonstrating splenic enlargement or intrasplenic lesions. Some of the largest massive spleens (spleen weight > 1500 g) occur in these types of disease. Finding the edge of the spleen below the iliac crest and crossing the abdominal midline are frequently seen.

▶ Differential Diagnosis

Leukemia and lymphoma are diagnosed by marrow aspiration, lymph node biopsy, and examination of the peripheral blood (white count and differential). In hereditary spherocytosis there are spherocytes, osmotic fragility is increased, and platelets and white cells are normal. The hemoglobinopathies with splenomegaly are differentiated on the basis of hemoglobin electrophoresis or the demonstration of an unstable hemoglobin level. Thalassemia major becomes apparent in early childhood, and the blood smear morphology is characteristic. In myelofibrosis, the bone marrow shows proliferation of fibroblasts and replacement of normal elements. In idiopathic thrombocytopenic purpura (ITP), the spleen is normal or only slightly enlarged. In aplastic anemia, the spleen is not enlarged and the marrow is fatty.

▶ Treatment & Prognosis

The course, response to treatment, and prognosis of the hypersplenic syndromes differ widely depending on the underlying disease and its response to treatment and will be discussed for each particular disorder below. The indications for splenectomy are given in Table 27–2.

Splenectomy may decrease transfusion requirements, decrease the incidence and number of infections, prevent hemorrhage, and reduce pain. The course of congestive splenomegaly due to portal hypertension depends upon the degree of venous obstruction and liver damage. The hypersplenism is rarely a major problem and is almost always overshadowed by variceal bleeding or liver dysfunction.

Table 27–2. Indications for splenectomy.

Splenectomy Always Indicated
Primary splenic tumor (rare)
Hereditary spherocytosis (congenital hemolytic anemia)
Splenectomy Usually Indicated
Primary hypersplenism
Chronic immune thrombocytopenic purpura
Splenic vein thrombosis causing gastric varices
Splenic abscess (rare)
Splenectomy Sometimes Indicated
Splenic injury
Autoimmune hemolytic disease
Elliptocytosis with hemolysis
Nonspherocytic congenital hemolytic anemias
Hodgkin disease (for staging)
Thrombotic thrombocytopenic purpura
Idiopathic myelofibrosis
Splenic artery aneurysm
Wiscott–Aldrich syndrome
Gaucher disease
Mastocytosis-aggressive disease
Splenectomy Rarely Indicated
Chronic leukemia
Splenic lymphoma
Macroglobulinemia
Thalassemia major
Sickle cell anemia
Congestive splenomegaly and hypersplenism due to portal hypertension
Felty syndrome
Hairy cell leukemia
Chédiak–Higashi syndrome
Sarcoidosis
Splenectomy Not Indicated
Asymptomatic hypersplenism
Splenomegaly with infection
Splenomegaly associated with elevated IgM
Hereditary hemolytic anemia of moderate degree
Acute leukemia
Agranulocytosis

NEOPLASTIC DISEASES

Neoplastic diseases in which splenectomy may play a role in the management of hypersplenism include chronic lymphocytic leukemia (CLL), hairy cell leukemia, and non-Hodgkin lymphoma. Lymphoma is discussed in detail in Chapter 44. Related neoplastic disorders of idiopathic myelofibrosis and mastocytosis are also discussed as precursors or variants of neoplastic diseases in which splenectomy are occasionally indicated.

1. Chronic Lymphocytic Leukemia

CLL is a low-grade neoplasm of B cell lineage characterized by accumulations of populations of lymphocytes that are mature morphologically but functionally incompetent. In the United States, CLL occurs as 25%-30% of all leukemias with mean age at diagnosis of 72. The clinical manifestations and natural history are variable, but initially the disease tends to be indolent. In more advanced stages, splenomegaly, which is frequently massive, is a common characteristic of CLL. Most symptoms related to the spleen are from thrombocytopenia and anemia due to secondary hypersplenism (80%-90% of splenic symptoms). Ten to 20% of patients may have symptoms primarily related to pressure from the size of the enlarged spleen.

Other causes of cytopenia in CLL relate to decreased cellular production from the bone marrow. Bone marrow failure can be due to replacement with leukemic cells or to depletion of the bone marrow as a toxic effect of prior antitumor chemotherapy.

Splenectomy in patients with CLL corrects thrombocytopenia in 70%-85% of cases, neutropenia in 60%-70%, and anemia in 50%-60% of cases. The median duration of benefit for both platelets and red cell populations is well over 1 year. Patients with smaller spleens preoperatively, lower preoperative platelet counts, and extensive prior chemotherapy are less likely to respond to splenectomy. However, a positive bone marrow aspirate for leukemic cells is not a contraindication to splenectomy in CLL. Patients who do not have a good performance status should not undergo splenectomy, since patients in terminal stages have unacceptable operative morbidity.

2. Hairy Cell Leukemia

Hairy cell leukemia is a low-grade lymphoproliferative disorder with characteristic "hairy cells"—ie, B lymphocytes with irregular cytoplasmic protrusions positive for tartrate reaction acid phosphatase—which infiltrate the bone marrow and spleen. Patients are typically male, and onset of the disease is in the fifth or sixth decade of life. Symptoms relate to pancytopenia, with anemia requiring transfusions; and to neutropenia, characterized by increased susceptibility to infections and increased bleeding tendencies. Some patients may have symptoms from splenomegaly, which is present in

80% of patients at the time of diagnosis of hairy cell leukemia. The cytopenias are due to a combination of bone marrow replacement and secondary hypersplenism.

The standard therapy for hairy cell leukemia between 1960 and 1995 was splenectomy, but recent advances in pharmacotherapy have superseded this surgical approach. First-line therapy is now treatment with purine nucleoside analogues primarily cladribine, with a complete response rate of 80%-90%. It has never been shown that splenectomy offers survival benefit in this indolent disease, and the operation should be reserved for palliation of splenomegaly in patients who have failed treatment with cladribine and second line agent rituxamib and alpha interferon.

3. Myelodysplastic Syndrome

Myelodysplastic syndromes are a heterogeneous group of clinical hematopoietic stem cell disorders manifested by pancytopenias, and dysplasia of the bone marrow. Pathologic changes include extensive bone marrow fibrosis, extramedullary hematopoiesis in the spleen and liver, and a leukoerythroblastic blood reaction that may evolve into acute myeloid leukemia over time.

The bone marrow is usually almost completely replaced by fibrous tissue, although in some cases it is hyperplastic and fibrosis is minimal. Extramedullary hematopoiesis develops mainly in the spleen, liver, and long bones. Symptoms are attributable to anemia (weakness, fatigue, dyspnea) and to splenomegaly (abdominal fullness and pain which may be severe). Pain over the spleen from splenic infarcts is common. Spontaneous bleeding, fatigue, secondary infection, bone pain, and a hypermetabolic state are frequent. Portal hypertension develops in some cases as a result of fibrosis of the liver, greatly increased splenic blood flow, or both.

Hepatomegaly is present in 75% of cases and splenomegaly with a firm and irregular spleen in all cases. Striking changes in the peripheral blood are referable to the combination of extramedullary hematopoiesis and hypersplenism. Patients are uniformly anemic, and red cells vary greatly in size and shape, many of them distorted and fragmented. The white count is usually high (20,000-50,000/mL). The platelet count may be elevated, but values less than 100,000/mL are seen in 30% of cases due to secondary hypersplenism. Bone marrow aspirates frequently result in a dry tap because marrow is replaced with fibrosis. It was once incorrectly thought that the spleen performed a crucial function of extramedullary hematopoiesis in this disease and that splenectomy could be lethal. In fact, many patients with myeloid metaplasia feel better if the massive spleen is removed, and their hypersplenism is often corrected.

About 30% of patients are asymptomatic at the time of initial diagnosis and require no therapy. When cytopenias and splenomegaly produce symptoms, treatment is primarily supportive using transfusions, androgenic steroids, antimetabolites, and hematopoietic growth factors are indicated. Newer therapies include treatment with immuno-modulatory drugs such as thalidomide or antibodies to VEGF and TNF. A subset of patients with myeloid metapla-sia has a component of autoimmune hemolytic anemia, and in this group of patients immunosuppressive therapy may be beneficial. Splenectomy is indicated in the following situa-tions: (1) major hemolysis unresponsive to medical manage-ment, (2) severe symptoms of massive splenomegaly with mass effect of the spleen, (3) life-threatening thrombocyto-penia, and (4) portal hypertension with variceal hemorrhage. This is one of the rare occasions when portal hypertension may be cured by splenectomy.

Splenectomy in myeloid metaplasia is associated with a 7%-10% death rate and frequent complications often related to postsplenectomy hepatic morbidity. Splenectomy best relieves symptoms of splenomegaly and portal hypertension, but only about 75% of patients get relief from anemia and thrombocytopenia. Younger patients with normal platelet counts and symptoms are the best candidates for splenec-tomy in idiopathic myelofibrosis.

4. Systemic Mast Cell Disease

Systemic mast cell disease, or mastocytosis, is a rare condi-tion characterized by mast cell infiltration of a number of tis-sues, including the spleen. There are two types: indolent and aggressive. In indolent systemic mass cell disease, there is no need for consideration of splenectomy. The aggressive type is associated with hematologic diseases with characteristics of lymphoma. Splenomegaly may occur, with the predomi-nant symptoms resulting from thrombocytopenia due to hypersplenism. In this subgroup of patients with aggressive disease, splenectomy improves platelet counts and is asso-ciated with longer median survival time than for patients with aggressive disease who do not undergo splenectomy, although systemic therapy including alpha interferon has been shown to be effective.

METABOLIC DISORDERS

Metabolic disorders amenable to splenectomy are rare inher-ited diseases that include as a component splenic enlargement due to the pathologic deposition of material within the spleen. In Gaucher disease, excess sphingolipid is deposited in the spleen. In sarcoidosis, the spleen becomes involved with non-caseating granulomas as can be seen in lymph nodes. Inherited disorders also include disease in which there is a specific immunologic target with associated destruction in the spleen.

1. Gaucher Disease

Gaucher disease is an autosomal recessive disorder char-acterized by a deficiency in beta-glucosidase, a lysosomal enzyme that degrades the sphingolipid glucocerebroside.

There is an increased incidence of this disorder in Ashkenazi Jews. Three types of this disease exist, and the one amenable to splenectomy is type I, or the adult type. Pathologically, Gaucher disease results in lipid accumulation within the white pulp of the spleen, the liver, or the bone marrow. Predominant symptoms relate to massive splenomegaly from either the direct effects of the size of the spleen or sec-ondary to cytopenias from hypersplenism.

▶ Treatment & Prognosis

Treatment by total splenectomy alleviates the symptoms but results in accelerated hepatic and bone disease as well as a significant increased risk of postsplenectomy infec-tions. Treatment with partial or subtotal splenectomy has been studied over the past 10 years for both adults and children with Gaucher disease. Removing most of the spleen corrects the symptoms of splenomegaly, but leaving a splenic remnant provides a site for further deposition of lipid that protects the liver and bone. The major problem with partial splenectomy is the eventual recurrence and enlargement of the splenic remnant accompanied by recurrent symptoms. As with hereditary spherocytosis, there is an increase incidence of pigmented gallstones occurring in up to two-thirds of female patients and one-third of male patients. The goal of subtotal splenectomy in Gaucher disease is to leave a small fragment approximately the size of the fist of the patient. Replacement therapy with recombinant glucocerebrosidase enzyme has recently become available, but the cost of chronic treatment is prohibitive.

2. Wiskott–Aldrich Syndrome

Wiskott–Aldrich syndrome is an X-linked disease char-acterized by thrombocytopenia, combined B and T cell immunodeficiency, eczema, and a propensity to develop malignancies. Thrombocytopenia is the major feature of this rare disorder, with most patients presenting with bloody diarrhea, epistaxis, and petechiae at a young age. Platelet counts typically range between 20,000/mL and 40,000/mL, and the platelets that are present are between one-fourth and one-half of normal size. The spleen sequesters and destroys platelets in this disease, releasing "microplatelets" back into the circulation. The genetic defect in this disorder may be related to an abnormal adhesion molecule affecting immune as well as platelet cell-to-cell interaction.

▶ Treatment & Prognosis

Splenectomy in Wiskott–Aldrich syndrome was at one time withheld, since the postoperative course was character-ized by severe and fatal infections due to the underlying immune defect of this disorder combined with loss of the immune function of the spleen. However, splenectomy does normalize platelet shape, size, and numbers, and the use of prophylactic antibiotics after splenectomy has significantly increased survival rates. The optimal treatment of Wiskott-Aldrich syndrome is an HLA-matched sibling bone marrow transplantation. However, splenectomy with antibiotics results in better survival than an unmatched bone marrow transplantation. Patients who do not undergo bone marrow transplantation or splenectomy typically do not survive past the age of 5 years.

3. Chédiak–Higashi Syndrome

Chédiak–Higashi syndrome is a rare autosomal recessive disease characterized by immunodeficiency that increases the susceptibility to bacterial and viral infections and is manifested by recurrent fever, nystagmus, and photophobia. Most patients experience widespread infiltration of tissues with histiocytes similar to a lymphoma. Secondary hepatosplenomegaly with lymphadenopathy, leukopenia, and bleeding complications occur in the accelerated phase of Chédiak-Higashi syndrome. Standard treatment includes chemotherapy, steroids, and ascorbic acid, but these patients have a poor prognosis. Splenectomy has been used in the accelerated phase with beneficial results.

4. Sarcoidosis

Sarcoidosis is a granulomatous disease of unknown origin that can involve virtually any organ or area of the body. Pulmonary disease is most common, but autopsy studies have shown that the spleen is the second most common site, with enlargement by noncaseating granulomas in 50%-60% of patients. However, most patients do not have massive splenomegaly. When this does occur, patients can have significant cytopenias related to hypersplenism as well as the constitutional symptoms and hypercalcemia of sarcoidosis. In this subgroup of patients, splenectomy is indicated as a potential curative procedure for each of these symptoms.

ERYTHROCYTE DISORDERS

In this category of diseases there is generally no intrinsic abnormality of the spleen, as opposed to hypersplenism, in which the spleen is primarily infiltrated by neoplasia or storage products and causes cytopenias due to increased volume of splenic tissue. In the autoimmune disorders, there is a humoral antibody response against proteins on circulating blood cells, resulting in depletion primarily within the spleen. Disorders involving platelets, erythrocytes, and neutrophils are listed in decreasing order of incidence. Erythrocyte disorders are genetic defects in structural components or hemoglobin that increase the clearance of red cells in the spleen, causing a significant decrease in erythrocyte half-life.

1. Hereditary Spherocytosis

ESSENTIALS OF DIAGNOSIS

▶ Malaise, abdominal discomfort.

▶ Jaundice, anemia, splenomegaly.

▶ Spherocytosis, increased osmotic fragility of red cells, negative Coombs test.

▶ General Considerations

Hereditary spherocytosis (congenital hemolytic jaundice, familial hemolytic anemia), the most common congenital hemolytic anemia (affecting 1:5000 individuals), is transmitted as an autosomal dominant trait. It is caused by a variety of genetic defects related to abnormal cellular structural proteins, primarily ankyrin band 3, alpha and beta spectrum and protein 4-2 all, which alter binding of the cytoskeleton to the cellular membrane, causing a decreased cellular plasticity with membrane loss. The normal shape of the erythrocyte is changed from a biconcave disk into a sphere, and the decreased membrane-to-cell volume ratio causes a lack of deformability that delays passage through the channels of the splenic red pulp. Significant cell destruction occurs only in the presence of the spleen. Hemolysis is largely relieved by splenectomy.

The condition is seen in all races but is more frequent in whites than in blacks. When discovered early in infancy, it may resemble hemolytic disease of the newborn due to ABO incompatibility. In occasional instances the diagnosis is not made until later in adult life, but it is usually discovered in the first three decades.

▶ Clinical Findings

A. Symptoms and Signs

The principal manifestations are splenomegaly, mild to moderate anemia, and jaundice. The patient may complain of easy fatigability. The spleen is almost always enlarged and may cause fullness and discomfort in the left upper quadrant. However, most patients are diagnosed during a family survey at a time when they are asymptomatic.

Periodic exacerbations of hemolysis can occur. The rare hypoplastic crises, which often follow acute viral illnesses, may be associated with profound anemia, headache, nausea, abdominal pain, pancytopenia, and hypoactive marrow.

B. Laboratory Findings

The red cell count and hemoglobin are moderately reduced. Some of the asymptomatic patients detected by family surveys have normal red cell counts when first seen. The red cells are usually normocytic, but microcytosis may occur. Macrocytosis may present during periods of marked reticulocytosis. Spherocytes in varying numbers, sizes, and shapes are seen on a Wright-stained smear. The reticulocyte count is increased to 5%-20%.

The indirect serum bilirubin and stool urobilinogen are usually elevated, and serum haptoglobin is usually decreased to absent. The Coombs test is negative. Osmotic fragility is increased; hemolysis of 5%-10% of cells may be observed at saline concentrations of 0.6%. A more accurate reflector of fragility is the cryohemolysis test, which has a sensitivity and specificity of almost 95% for spherocytosis. Occasionally, the osmotic fragility is normal but the incubated fragility test (defibrinated blood incubated at 37°C for 24 hours) will show increased hemolysis. Autohemolysis of defibrinated blood incubated under sterile conditions for 48 hours is usually greatly increased (10%-20%, compared to a normal value of < 5%). The addition of 10% glucose before incubation will decrease the abnormal osmotic fragility and autohemolysis. Infusion of the patient's own blood labeled with ^{51}Cr shows a greatly shortened red cell life span and sequestration in the spleen. Normal red cells labeled with ^{51}Cr have a normal life span when transfused into a spherocytotic patient, indicating that splenic function is normal.

Differential Diagnosis

At present there is no pathognomonic test for hereditary spherocytosis. Spherocytes in large numbers may occur in autoimmune hemolytic anemias, in which osmotic fragility and autohemolysis may be increased but are usually not improved by incubation with glucose. The positive Coombs test, negative family history, and sharply reduced survival of normal donor red cells are diagnostic of autoimmune hemolysis. Spherocytes are also seen in hemoglobin C disease, in some alcoholics, and in some severe burns.

Complications

Pigment gallstones occur in about 85% of adults with spherocytosis but are uncommon under age 10. On the other hand, gallstones in a child should suggest congenital spherocytosis.

Chronic leg ulcers unrelated to varicosities are a rare complication but, when present, will heal only after the spleen is removed.

Treatment

Splenectomy is the sole treatment for hereditary spherocytosis and is indicated even when the anemia is fully compensated and the patient is asymptomatic. The longer the hemolytic process persists, the greater the potential risk of complications such as hypoplastic crises and cholelithiasis. At operation, the gallbladder should be inspected

for stones and accessory spleens should be sought. When there is associated cholelithiasis, cholecystectomy should be performed along with the splenectomy. Unless the clinical manifestations are severe, splenectomy should be delayed in children until age 6 to avoid the risk of increased infection due to loss of reticuloendothelial function. For children under age 5 with severe disease and high transfusion requirements, a partial (80%) splenectomy may correct symptoms while maintaining the normal immune functions of the spleen.

Prognosis

Splenectomy cures the anemia and jaundice in all patients. The membrane abnormality, spherocytosis, and increased osmotic fragility persist, but red cell life span becomes almost normal. An overlooked accessory spleen is an occasional cause of failure of splenectomy. The presence of Howell–Jolly bodies in red cells makes the presence of accessory spleens unlikely.

Gallagher PG. Abnormalities of the erythrocyte membrane. *Pediatr Clin North Am* 2013;60(6):1349-1362.
Perrotta S. Hereditary spherocytosis. *Lancet* 2008;372:1411-1426.

2. Hereditary Elliptocytosis

This autosomal dominant genetic disorder, also known as ovalocytosis, is usually of little clinical significance. Normally, up to 15% oval or elliptic red blood cells can be seen on a peripheral blood smear. In elliptocytosis, at least 25% and up to 90% of circulating erythrocytes are elliptic. As with hereditary spherocytosis, this disease is due to a variety of genetic defects in cytoskeletal proteins such as spectrin. The predominant abnormality is that this structural protein exists as a dimer instead of a tetramer, leading to change in the erythrocyte's shape, decreased plasticity, and a shortened life span of the cell.

Most affected individuals are asymptomatic; about 10% have clinical manifestations consisting of moderate anemia, slight jaundice, and a palpable spleen.

Symptomatic patients should have splenectomy, and cholecystectomy if gallstones are present. The red cell defect persists after splenectomy, but the hemolysis and anemia are cured.

Gallagher PG. Abnormalities of the erythrocyte membrane. *Pediatr Clin North Am* 2013;60(6):1349-1362.

3. Hereditary Nonspherocytic Hemolytic Anemia

This is a heterogeneous group of rare hemolytic anemias caused by inherited intrinsic red cell defects that lead to oxidative hemolysis. Included in the group are pyruvate kinase deficiency and glucose 6-phosphate dehydrogenase (G6PD) deficiency. They are usually manifested in early childhood with anemia, jaundice, reticulocytosis, erythroid hyperplasia of the marrow, and normal osmotic fragility. As with other hemolytic anemias, there may be associated cholelithiasis.

Multiple blood transfusions are often required. Splenectomy, while not curative, may ameliorate some of these conditions, especially pyruvate kinase deficiency. In G6PD deficiency, splenectomy is not beneficial, and treatment consists of avoidance of dietary oxidants.

4. Thalassemia Major (Mediterranean Anemia; Cooley Anemia)

In the most common form of this autosomal dominant disorder, a structural defect in the β-globin chain causes excess α chains to precipitate on the inner surface of the membrane of the erythrocyte and produces abnormal red cells (eg, target cells). Heterozygotes usually have mild anemia (thalassemia minor); however, starting early in infancy, homozygotes have severe chronic anemia accompanied by jaundice, hepatosplenomegaly (often massive), retarded body growth, and enlargement of the head. The peripheral blood smear reveals target cells, nucleated red cells, and a hypochromic microcytic anemia. Gallstones are present in about 25% of patients. A characteristic feature is the persistence of fetal hemoglobin (Hb F).

Since the anemia of thalassemia is due to both increased destruction of red cells and decreased hemoglobin production, splenectomy does not cure the anemia, as in spherocytosis, but it may reduce transfusion requirements by removing an enlarged, uncomfortable spleen. Treatment is by iron chelation and transfusion.

AUTOIMMUNE DISORDERS

The production of IgG autoantibodies specific for cell membrane proteins on erythrocytes causes autoimmune hemolytic anemia; on platelets, it causes ITP and may cause neutropenia in Felty syndrome. Macrophages express Fc receptors for IgG, and antibody-coated cells that pass through the splenic sinuses of the red pulp come into contact with these phagocytic cells. Furthermore, the microenvironment of the red pulp with slow flow of blood with a high cellular content through circuitous spaces facilitates opsonization of cells in the spleen. Production of autoantibodies in the white pulp germinal centers may also enhance cellular destruction, particularly in ITP. Understanding this pathophysiologic mechanism is important, since autoimmune hemolytic anemia caused by IgM autoantibodies (ie, cold agglutinin hemolytic anemia) does not respond to splenectomy because macrophages do not have Fc receptors for IgM. This mechanism also explains why treatment with high-dose intravenous immune globulin is beneficial in these diseases because it blocks the macrophage Fc receptor.

1. Acquired Hemolytic Anemia

ESSENTIALS OF DIAGNOSIS

▶ Fatigue, pallor, jaundice.

▶ Splenomegaly.

▶ Persistent anemia and reticulocytosis.

▶ General Considerations

The autoimmune hemolytic anemias have also been classified according to the optimal temperature at which autoantibodies react with the red cell surface (warm or cold antibodies). This classification is particularly useful, since patients with cold antibodies will not benefit from splenectomy but those with warm antibodies may.

Although hemolysis without demonstrable antibody (Coombs test-negative) may occur in uremia, cirrhosis of the liver, cancer, and certain infections, in most cases the red cell membranes are coated with either immunoglobulin or complement (Coombs test-positive). The antibody in IgG autoimmune hemolytic anemia is specifically directed against the Rh locus on the erythrocyte. Initiation of this disease is either idiopathic (40%-50%) or secondary to drug exposure, connective tissue disorders, or lymphoproliferative disorders. Hemolytic anemia due to cold antibodies is less common and always a secondary immune response. Cold agglutinin hemolytic anemia is due typically to an IgM directed against the I red cell antigen, and hemolysis occurs intravascularly by complement fixation and not within the spleen making splenectomy not beneficial in the setting of cold antibodies.

About 20% of cases of secondary immune hemolytic anemia are due to drug use, and hemolysis is usually mediated by warm antibodies. Penicillin, quinidine, hydralazine, and methyldopa have been most commonly implicated in this syndrome (Table 27–3).

Table 27–3. Disorders associated with immune hemolysis.

Immune drug reaction (penicillin, quinidine, hydralazine, methylodopa, cimetidine)
Collagen vascular disease (lupus erythematosus, rheumatoid arthritis)
Tumors (lymphoma, myeloma, leukemia, dermoid cysts, ovarian teratoma)
Infection (*Mycoplasma*, malaria, syphilis, viremia)

Clinical Findings

A. Symptoms and Signs

Autoimmune hemolytic anemia may be encountered at any age but is most common after age 50; it occurs twice as often in women. The onset is usually acute, consisting of anemia, mild jaundice, and sometimes fever. The spleen is palpably enlarged in over 50% of patients, and pigment gallstones are present in about 25%. Rarely, a sudden severe onset produces hemoglobinuria, renal tubular necrosis, and a 40%-50% death rate.

B. Laboratory Findings

Hemolytic anemia is diagnosed by demonstrating a normocytic normochromic anemia, reticulocytosis (over 10%), erythroid hyperplasia of the marrow, and elevation of serum indirect bilirubin. Stool urobilinogen may be greatly increased, but there is no bile in the urine. Serum haptoglobin is usually low or absent. The direct Coombs test is positive because the red cells are coated with immunoglobulins or complement (or both).

Treatment

Associated diseases must be carefully sought and appropriately treated. For drug-induced secondary hemolytic anemia, further exposure to the offending agent must be terminated. Corticosteroids produce a remission in about 75% of patients, but only 25% of remissions are permanent. Transfusion should be avoided if possible, since cross-matching may be extremely difficult, requiring washed red cells and saline-active antisera. Rituximab is an effective second line therapy now producing durable responses 40% of steroid resistant cases.

Splenectomy is indicated for patients with warm-antibody hemolysis who fail to respond to 4-6 weeks of high-dose corticosteroid therapy, for patients who relapse after an initial response when steroids are withdrawn, and for patients in whom steroid therapy is contraindicated (eg, those with active pulmonary tuberculosis). Patients who require chronic high-dose steroid therapy should also be considered for splenectomy, since the risks of long-term steroid administration are substantial.

Splenectomy is effective because it removes the principal site of red cell destruction. Occasionally, splenectomy identifies the presence of an underlying disorder such as lymphoma. About half of patients who fail to respond to splenectomy will respond to azathioprine or cyclophosphamide. Plasmapheresis has been employed as salvage therapy in patients with refractory hemolytic anemia.

Prognosis

Relapses may occur after splenectomy but are less frequent if the initial response was good. The ultimate prognosis in the secondary cases depends upon the underlying disorder.

Packman CH et al. Hemolytic anemia due to warm autoantibodies. *Blood Reviews* 2008;22:17-31.
Valent P et al. Diagnosis and treatment of autoimmune haemolytic aneaemias in adults: a clinical review. *Wien Klin Wochenschr* 2008;120:136-151.

2. Immune Thrombocytopenic Purpura (Idiopathic Thrombocytopenic Purpura)

 ESSENTIALS OF DIAGNOSIS

► Petechiae, ecchymoses, epistaxis, and easy bruising.
► No splenomegaly.
► Decreased platelet count, prolonged bleeding time, poor clot retraction, normal coagulation time.

General Considerations

Immune thrombocytopenic purpura is a hemorrhagic syndrome with diverse causes that can occur in an acute or chronic form and is characterized by marked reduction in the number of circulating platelets, abundant megakaryocytes in the bone marrow, and a shortened platelet life span. It may be idiopathic or secondary to a lymphoproliferative disorder, drugs or toxins, bacterial or viral infection (especially in children), systemic lupus erythematosus, or other conditions. Although responses to corticosteroids and to splenectomy in these patients are comparable to the responses observed in other patients with immune thrombocytopenic purpura, splenectomy should be reserved for those with signs of blood loss, since surgical complications are high and survival may be short. However, due to the incidence of ITP, this disease is typically the most common indication for splenectomy in most institutional series.

The pathogenesis of both primary and secondary disorders involves a circulating antiplatelet IgG autoantibody usually directed against a membrane protein which is the fibrinogen receptor (glycoprotein IIb/IIIa). In this disorder, the spleen is primarily the site of platelet destruction and may also be a significant source of autoantibody production. Splenomegaly, present in only 2% of cases, is usually a manifestation of another underlying disease such as lymphoma or lupus erythematosus. Five to 15% of HIV-positive patients have thrombocytopenia independent of the immunologic state of their disease that is clinically indistinguishable from typical chronic ITP. The precise pathophysiologic mechanism in relation to HIV infection is not known.

Clinical Findings

A. Symptoms and Signs

The onset may be acute, with ecchymoses or showers of petechiae, and may be accompanied by bleeding gums, vaginal bleeding, gastrointestinal bleeding, and hematuria. Central nervous system bleeding occurs in 3% of patients. The acute form is most common in children, usually occurring before 8 years of age, and often begins 1-3 weeks after a viral upper respiratory illness.

The chronic form, which may start at any age, is more common in women. It characteristically has an insidious onset, often with a long history of easy bruisability and menorrhagia. Showers of petechiae may occur, especially over pressure areas. Cyclic remissions and exacerbations may continue for several years.

B. Laboratory Findings

The platelet count is moderately to severely decreased (always below 100,000/mL), and platelets may be absent from the peripheral blood smear. Although white and red cell counts are usually normal, iron deficiency anemia may be present as a result of bleeding. The bone marrow shows increased numbers of large megakaryocytes without platelet budding.

The bleeding time is prolonged, capillary fragility (Rumpel–Leede test) greatly increased, and clot retraction poor. Partial thromboplastin time, prothrombin time, and coagulation time are normal. Specific determinations of antiplatelet antibody titers can now be routinely assessed to aid in diagnosis. Reduced red cell or platelet survival can be measured by labeling the patient's cells with ^{51}Cr or the platelets with indium-111 and measuring the rate of disappearance of radioactivity from the blood. The spleen's role in producing the anemia or thrombocytopenia can be determined by measuring the ratio of radioactivity that accumulates in the liver and spleen during destruction of the tagged cells; a spleen/liver ratio greater than 2:1 indicates significant splenic pooling and suggests that splenectomy would be beneficial.

Differential Diagnosis

Other causes of nonimmunologic thrombocytopenia must be ruled out, such as leukemia, aplastic anemia, and macroglobulinemia. Thrombocytopenia and purpura may be caused by ineffective thrombocytopoiesis (eg, pernicious anemia, preleukemic states) or by nonimmune platelet destruction (eg, septicemia, disseminated intravascular coagulation, or other causes of hypersplenism).

Treatment

Treatment of immune thrombocytopenic purpura depends on the age of the patient, the severity of the disease, the duration of the thrombocytopenia, and the clinical variant. Secondary immune thrombocytopenias are best managed by treating the underlying primary disorder (eg, if it is drug-induced, the drug should be stopped).

Patients with mild or no symptoms need no specific therapy but should avoid contact sports, elective surgery, and all unessential medications. Corticosteroids are indicated in patients with moderate to severe purpura of short duration. Usually, 60 mg of prednisone (or equivalent) is required daily; this is continued until the platelet count returns to normal and then is gradually tapered after 4-6 weeks. Corticosteroids produce a response in 70%-80%, but sustained remissions in only 20% of adults. Second line therapy with Rituximab improves platelet counts in 30%-40% of patients and sustained complete response in 10%-20%. New agents to stimulate platelet production such as thrombopoietin (TPO) against AMG531 and eltrambopag are being studied as third line medical therapies.

Splenectomy is the most effective form of therapy and is indicated for patients who do not respond to corticosteroids, for those who relapse after an initial remission on steroids, and for steroid-dependent patients. Corticosteroid therapy is not necessary in the immediate preoperative period unless bleeding is severe or the patient was receiving steroids before the operation. If indicated, platelet transfusions are given intraoperatively only after ligation of the splenic artery or removal of the spleen, since platelets from earlier transfusion would be rapidly sequestered in the spleen. For temporary treatment of the thrombocytopenia, intravenous immunoglobulin is effective.

Splenectomy produces a sustained remission in about 68% of patients. As with corticosteroids, success rates are better with acute than chronic immune thrombocytopenic purpura. Two factors associated with better outcomes are shorter duration of disease and younger age. The platelet count usually rises promptly following splenectomy (eg, it may double in 24 hours) and reaches a peak after 1-2 weeks. If the platelet count remains elevated after 2 months, the patient can be considered cured. When corticosteroids and splenectomy have failed, immunosuppressive drugs (azathioprine, vincristine) achieve remission in 25% of cases.

The benefit of splenectomy for HIV-associated ITP has been less clear. The risk of infection and the overall shortened survival in this population argue against splenectomy. However, in HIV patients without AIDS, clinically significant thrombocytopenia responds completely in 70% and there is partial improvement in 20% following splenectomy. Splenectomy does not appear to alter the overall natural history of HIV infection.

Prognosis

Acute immune thrombocytopenic purpura in children under age 16 has an excellent prognosis; approximately 80% of patients have a complete and permanent spontaneous remission. This occurs rarely in adults. Splenectomy is successful in about 80% of patients, but more often in idiopathic cases than in those secondary to another disorder. The proportion of patients undergoing splenectomy for ITP has decreased due to medical treatment other than steroids that have efficacy, although the incidence of chronic TP has increased. Agents to stimulate TPO may have significant benefit for patients who have no improvement in platelet count after splenectomy.

Auger S, Duny Y, Rossi JF, Quittet P. Rituximab before splenectomy in adults with primary idiopathic thrombocytopenic purpura: a meta-analysis. *Br J Haematol* 2012;158(3):386-398.

Dolan JP et al. Splenectomy for immune thrombocytopenic purpura. *Am J Hematol* 2008;83:93-96.

Kuter DJ et al. Efficacy of romiplostim in patients with chronic immune thrombocytopenic purpura: a double-blind randomized controlled trial. *Lancet* 2008;371:395-403.

Newland W et al. Emerging strategies to treat chronic immune thrombocytopenic purpura. *Eur J Haematol* 2008;69:27-33.

Rodeghiero F et al: First-line therapies for immune thrombocytopenic purpura: re-evaluating the need to treat. *Eur J Haematol* 2008;69:19-26.

Shojaiefard A et al: Prediction of response to splenectomy in patients with idiopathic thrombocytopenic purpura. *World J Surg* 2008;32:488-493.

Stasi R et al: Idiopathic thrombocytopenic purpura: current concents in pathophysiology and management. *Thromb Haemost* 2008;99:4-13.

3. Felty's Syndrome

Approximately 1% of patients with rheumatoid arthritis have splenomegaly and neutropenia—a triad known as Felty's syndrome. High levels of IgG have been identified on the surface of neutrophils with evidence of increased of granulopoiesis in the bone marrow. Pathologic analysis of the spleen in Felty's syndrome patients shows a larger proportionate increase in the white pulp as opposed to most conditions of splenomegaly. There is evidence of excess accumulation of neutrophils in both the T cell zone of the white pulp as well as the cord and sinuses of the red pulp.

Patients with severe neutropenia have clinical symptoms of recurring infections in Felty syndrome. Symptomatic patients who have evidence of IgG on the surface of neutrophils should be considered for splenectomy. Neutropenia will improve in 60%-70% of these patients, but relapse of neutropenia as well as recurrent infections in the presence of normal neutrophil counts may occur, and these untoward events have dampened enthusiasm for splenectomy in this disease.

4. Thrombotic Thrombocytopenic Purpura

Thrombotic thrombocytopenic purpura is a rare disease with a pentad of clinical features: (1) fever, (2) thrombocytopenic purpura, (3) hemolytic anemia, (4) neurologic manifestations, and (5) renal failure. The cause is unknown, but autoimmunity to endothelial cells or a primary platelet defect has been implicated, and its occurrence in patients with AIDS has been reported. It is most common between ages 10 and 40 years.

The thrombocytopenia is probably due to a shortened platelet life span. The microangiopathic hemolytic anemia is produced by passage of red cells over damaged small blood vessels containing fibrin strands. Rigid red cells are trapped and fragmented in the spleen, whereas those that escape the spleen may be more vulnerable to damage and destruction in the abnormal microvasculature. The anemia is often severe, and it may be aggravated by hemorrhage secondary to thrombocytopenia. Hepatomegaly and splenomegaly occur in 35% of cases.

▶ Treatment & Prognosis

Until recently, there was no effective therapy for this disorder, and mortality rates as high as 95% were reported. Most patients died of renal failure or cerebral bleeding. Plasmapheresis with plasma exchange has recently emerged as an effective form of treatment that is superior to simple plasma infusion with complete response rate of 55%-65%. Plasma exchange failure can be salvaged with splenectomy with 60% having a substantial response and a 20%-30% relapse rate.

VASCULAR DISORDERS OF THE SPLEEN

Vascular disease of the spleen treated by splenectomy can occur both with the arterial inflow and the venous outflow. The most common disease is splenic vein thrombosis; this can be treated in a straightforward manner by splenectomy. Splenic artery aneurysms are one of the most common sites of visceral aneurysms and may require splenectomy (discussed in Chapter 34).

1. Splenic Vein Thrombosis

▶ Etiology

Thrombosis of the splenic vein can occur as an isolated event not due to any pathologic findings in the spleen but due to diseases that impact on the splenic vein as it travels along the superior border of the pancreas. The most common cause is acute or chronic pancreatitis or a pseudocyst of the body/tail of the pancreas, with the general inflammatory reaction in the pancreas resulting in thrombosis of the splenic vein in 20% of patients. Inflammation from a posterior gastric ulcer is another cause. Direct extension of carcinoma of the pancreas or stomach into the lesser sac may cause splenic vein thrombosis, but the diagnosis is generally not subtle because of other manifestations of these malignancies. Idiopathic retroperitoneal fibrosis may be an alternative cause of splenic vein thrombosis.

Splenic vein thrombosis presents as upper gastrointestinal hemorrhage due to isolated gastric varices. With occlusion of the splenic vein, outflow of blood from the spleen is diverted into the short gastric veins as the remaining collateral vessels. These veins dilate and become varices primarily in the fundus of the stomach, resulting in bleeding in 15%-20% of patients.

▶ **Diagnosis**

Splenic vein thrombosis is suspected when there are isolated varices of the stomach particularly in the proximal greater curvature without any esophageal varices. Since there is no portal hypertension, there are no associated signs or symptoms of cirrhosis. Definitive diagnosis is made by confirming that there is no blood flow in the main splenic vein. Invasive venography is no longer needed because this diagnosis can be confirmed by CT or MRI scans with contrast material or by high-resolution ultrasound. CT or MRI is preferred because the splenic vein may be hidden from ultrasound by bowel gas and CT or MRI allows characterization of the surrounding structures (pancreas, stomach) to assess for causative pathology.

▶ **Treatment & Prognosis**

Splenectomy is curative in patients with splenic vein thrombosis. All of the symptoms relate to increased splenic blood flow through collateral vessels; eliminating that blood flow is curative. If a splenic vein thrombosis is diagnosed—even if the patients have not had an episode of upper gastrointestinal hemorrhage—an elective or prophylactic splenectomy is indicated if the patients are otherwise healthy. In patients with portal vein thrombosis, the magnitude of the disease and associated problems is greatly amplified, and splenectomy is almost never indicated because it is not curative.

Agarwal AK et al. Significance of splenic vein thrombosis in chronic pancreatitis. *Am J Surg* 2008;196:149-154.

2. Cysts & Tumors of the Spleen

Parasitic cysts are almost always echinococcal (see Chapter 8). They may be asymptomatic, but usually the patient notices splenomegaly. Calcification of the cyst wall may be seen on x-ray. Eosinophilia may be found, and serologic tests may confirm the diagnosis. The treatment of choice is splenectomy.

Other cysts are dermoid, epidermoid, endothelial, and pseudocysts. The latter are thought to be late results of infarction or trauma. Splenectomy may be indicated to exclude tumor; however, partial splenectomy or observation has been advocated.

The rare primary tumors of the spleen include lymphoma, sarcoma, hemangioma, and hamartoma. Hamartomas may be confused grossly with splenic lymphoma at laparotomy.

These lesions are usually asymptomatic until splenomegaly causes abdominal discomfort or a palpable mass. The benign vascular tumors of the spleen (angiomas) can produce hypersplenism. Spontaneous rupture with massive hemorrhage can occur. Splenectomy is indicated if the tumor appears to be limited to the spleen. Inflammatory pseudotumors are benign lesions composed of a mixture of inflammatory cells and a granulomatous reaction that can occur in a variety of organs, including the spleen. Constitutional symptoms of lethargy, weight loss, and fatigue occur and can be alleviated by splenectomy.

The spleen is a common site for metastases in advanced cancers, especially of the lung and breast, and melanoma. Splenic metastases are common autopsy findings but are rarely clinically significant.

INFECTIONS OF THE SPLEEN (SPLENIC ABSCESS)

Splenic abscesses are uncommon but are important because the death rate ranges between 40% and 100%. They may be caused by hematogenous seeding of the spleen with bacteria from remote sepsis such as endocarditis, by direct spread of infection from adjacent structures, or by splenic trauma resulting in a secondarily infected splenic hematoma. Splenic abscess is a complication of intravenous drug abuse. In 80% of cases, one or more abscesses exist in organs other than the spleen, and the splenic abscess develops as a terminal manifestation of uncontrolled sepsis in other organs. Enteric organisms are found in over two-thirds of splenic abscesses, with staphylococci and nonenteric streptococci comprising the majority of the remainder. In some patients, unexplained sepsis, progressive splenic enlargement, and abdominal pain are the presenting manifestations. The spleen may not be palpable, because of left upper quadrant tenderness and guarding. A left pleural effusion combined with unexplained leukocytosis in a septic patient suggests a splenic abscess. The finding of gas in the spleen on plain abdominal x-ray is pathognomonic of splenic abscess, but CT scan is the optimal way to define and diagnose a splenic abscess.

Most splenic abscesses remain localized, periodically seeding the bloodstream with bacteria, but spontaneous rupture and peritonitis may occur. Splenectomy is essential for cure if sepsis is localized to the spleen. Percutaneous drainage of large, solitary juxtacapsular abscesses may occasionally be feasible but is associated with an extremely high mortality rate and should be reserved for patients unable to withstand an operation.

DIAGNOSTIC SPLENECTOMY

One indication for splenectomy is for diagnosis in an otherwise asymptomatic patient. Splenectomy may be needed to make a diagnosis when an asymptomatic mass lesion is seen within the spleen on CT scan, ultrasound, or MRI scan for which a definitive diagnosis cannot be made radiographically. Another example is when a patient has either a palpable spleen on physical examination or an enlarged spleen by scan, and otherwise has no clear diagnostic disorder.

Splenic Mass Lesions

For the patients who have an isolated splenic mass, 60% turned out to be malignant lesions and 40% turned out to be benign lesions. Most malignant lesions are lymphoma; next most common is metastatic carcinomas, including some in which the primary diagnosis had not been made previously. In patients with benign lesions, more than half were cysts, and there were also splenic hamartomas and splenic hemangiomas.

In diagnosing an isolated splenic mass, most of these lesions can be diagnosed by doing a fine-needle aspiration biopsy. Certain lesions—such as the cystic lesions or hemangioma—would have classic appearance on gadolinium-enhanced MRI scan, and these scans are another imaging modality that could be utilized to sort out mass lesions without tissue biopsy. PET scans will reliably identify high grade lymphoma and metastatic tumors but may miss low-grade or mantle-zone lymphoma. The risk of bleeding is significant in patients with hemangiomas. These benign tumors of endothelial cells can be definitively diagnosed with gadolinium-enhanced MRI, and this imaging test is optimal for characterizing an isolated splenic mass.

Splenomegaly Without a Diagnosis

The second diagnostic indication for splenectomy is unexplained splenomegaly. Most of these enlarged spleens will be shown to have lymphoma. The minority will have benign diagnoses including benign lymphoid proliferation, benign vascular lesions, and granulomatous disease, as well as splenic infarction and hemorrhage. The role of the fine-needle aspiration and other percutaneous biopsies for nondiagnosed splenomegaly is quite limited with no distinct mass to biopsy; there would be very low yield in terms of being able to make that diagnosis by that form of biopsy.

Staging Laparotomy for Hodgkin Disease

Another type of diagnostic procedure would be a staging laparotomy for Hodgkin disease. Discussion of this procedure is more of a historical note because it has limited use in today's current practice in treating this form of lymphoma.

A standard practice for pathologic staging between 1960 and 1990 was performance of a staging laparotomy in most patients with Hodgkin disease. The reason for performing this invasive procedure was based on reports that laparotomy altered the clinical stage of disease in approximately 35% of patients. There are several reasons why the incidence of performing staging laparotomy has decreased over the past 10-15 years. The primary reason is that it does not alter treatment of Hodgkin disease based on results of recent clinical series. Since systemic chemotherapy treats the whole patient, accurate pathologic staging makes no impact on the treatment outcome or treatment decisions.

IATROGENIC SPLENECTOMY

Procedures in which mobilization of the left upper quadrant is done (such as reflection of the spleen and pancreas medially to expose retroperitoneal tissue, left adrenalectomy, and left nephrectomy) put the spleen at risk for injury during the dissection. Simple mobilization of the splenic flexure of the colon can lead to bleeding from the inferior pole of the spleen that may be difficult to control. The ligaments that go directly from the omentum to the capsule of the spleen may be the most common cause of iatrogenic splenic trauma, as it is a common practice to aggressively retract the omentum as needed for exposure. If there are direct branches that sometimes may be sizable from the omentum to the splenic capsule, this could lead to capsular disruption and troublesome bleeding. A national database on antireflux procedures of 86,411 patients reported an incidence of iatrogenic splenectomy of 2.3%, which translates into 1987 iatrogenic splenectomies for that indication alone over a 6-year period. An outcome study for colon cancer of 42,000 reported iatrogenic splenectomy in less than 1% of all patients but 6% of colon cancers at the splenic flexure. Splenectomy had a significant increase in length of stay and a 40% increase in morbidity.

A recent series listed 73 iatrogenic splenectomies over a 10-year period, or an average of 7 per year. This comprised 8.1% of all splenectomies performed during that time interval. There are probably several times that number of minor or moderate injuries to the spleen during unrelated operations in which the spleen was not removed but was repaired or salvaged. Just as in trauma to the spleen, the techniques of splenorrhaphy can be employed to preserve the spleen. A recent report indicates that use of a mesh wrap splenorrhaphy even in the setting of bowel surgery does not lead to an increased incidence of infection. For minor capsular disruption, the use of the argon beam coagulator for surface cautery is a helpful technique.

The primary teaching point regarding iatrogenic injuries is that the best way to preserve the spleen is to not damage it in the first place. This requires caution in mobilizing tissue in and around the spleen as well as visual inspection of the attachments of the spleen prior to blunt mobilization. Whenever possible, the spleen should be attempted to be preserved to decrease the risk of postsplenectomy sepsis.

Masoomi H, Carmichael JC, Mills S, et al. Predictive factors of splenic injury in colorectal surgery: data from the Nationwide Inpatient Sample, 2006-2008. *Arch Surg* 2012;147(4):324-329.

INCIDENTAL SPLENECTOMY

In a recent large series evaluating reasons for splenectomy from tertiary institutions, the single most common indication for splenectomy was as an incidental procedure on operations on an adjacent organ. In these situations, the spleen needs to be removed either for completeness of resection or because of division of the splenic vasculature The actual primary treatments of those various disease entities in adjacent organs are subjects of multiple other chapters within this textbook, but a few comments need to be made regarding the reasons for splenectomy and whether splenic preservation procedures are possible.

One common indication for an incidental splenectomy is to remove tumors located in the distal pancreas. For decades, it was standard practice to remove the spleen when removing the body and tail of the pancreas because the splenic vein is intimately associated with the distal pancreas. Because of the interest in splenic preservation due to the incidence of post-splenectomy infection, operations have been developed to remove the distal pancreas without removing the spleen. The more technically challenging operation is a distal pancreatectomy with preservation of the splenic artery and vein. A second spleen-preserving distal pancreatectomy involves ligation of the splenic artery and vein but preservation of short gastric vessels and utilizing those vessels as collateral inflow and outflow to maintain splenic viability. Removal of the distal pancreas with splenic preservation has also been recently reported as a laparoscopic procedure. For patients with tumors that mandate removal of the lymph nodes of the splenic hilum or with direct association of the tumor with splenic parenchyma, certainly it is more appropriate to do an operation based on neoplastic principles and perform a distal pancreatectomy/splenectomy. In other indications, if the anatomy is appropriate and the completeness of tumor resection is not compromised, splenic preservation is certainly possible.

Additional procedures in which it is common to perform a splenectomy include proximal gastric cancers. The importance of complete nodal dissection in long-term results in gastric resections has been debated for several decades. Level X lymph nodes are located in the splenic hilum, and for 20%-25% of proximal gastric cancers these nodes will have metastatic cancer mandating removal. A randomized trial showed increased morbidity with a splenectomy and a marginal improvement in survival. Other tumors of the left upper quadrant and retroperitoneum may require splenectomy, including large renal cell carcinomas, left adrenal tumors, and retroperitoneal sarcomas that may infiltrate upward into the spleen. Although the asplenic state does make patients susceptible to infections (see Hyposplenism above), the spleen should be viewed as an expendable organ if necessary to accomplish complete resection of malignancies, and there should be no

hesitation to remove the spleen in these situations to do an appropriate cancer operation.

SPLENOSIS (SPLENIC AUTOTRANSPLANTATION)

In splenosis, multiple small implants of splenic tissue grow in scattered areas on the peritoneal surfaces throughout the abdomen. They arise from dissemination and autotransplantation of splenic fragments following traumatic rupture of the spleen. Splenic implants or intentional autotransplants are capable of cell culling, and some immunologic function appears to be exhibited in cases of intentional autotransplantation. Aggressive attempts at surgical excision are not warranted. Splenosis is usually an incidental finding discovered much later during laparotomy for an unrelated problem. However, the implants stimulate formation of adhesions and may be a cause of intestinal obstruction. They must be distinguished from peritoneal nodules of metastatic carcinoma and from accessory spleens. Histologically, they differ from accessory spleens by the absence of elastic or smooth muscle fibers in the delicate capsule.

▼ SPLENECTOMY

Preoperative preparation of patients undergoing elective splenectomy should correct coagulation abnormalities and deficits in red cell mass, treat infections, and control immune reactions. Because platelets are removed so rapidly from the circulation, they usually are not given for thrombocytopenia until after the splenic artery has been ligated. Antibodies in the patient's serum may complicate cross-matching of blood. Many patients with autoimmune disorders require corticosteroid coverage in the perioperative period. For emergency splenectomy, hypovolemia should be corrected by whole blood transfusions. For elective cases, prophylactic vaccination with a polyvalent pneumococcal vaccine that protects against a common encapsulated offending organism in postsplenectomy infection is recommended. Elective splenectomy is now most commonly performed as a laparoscopic procedure. This reduces the recovery period and is significantly better tolerated by most patients.

Details of surgical technique are not within the scope of this text, but it should be noted that there are two approaches to open splenectomy (Figure 27–2). In one, which is of value chiefly in traumatic rupture of the spleen, the organ is immediately mobilized and the splenic artery is secured from behind as it enters the hilum. In the other, which is of vital importance in the removal of massively enlarged spleens, the organ is left *in situ*. The gastrocolic ligament is opened, and the splenic artery is ligated as it courses along the upper edge of the pancreas. This permits blood to leave the spleen through the splenic vein while all

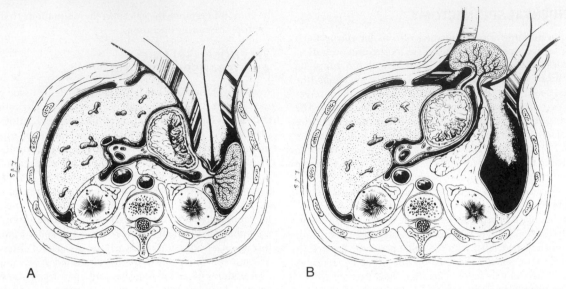

▲ **Figure 27-2.** **A**: Anterior approach to splenic artery. **B**: Mobilization of spleen with posterior exposure of splenic artery.

other attachments (ie, the short gastric vessels and colic attachments) are divided before the spleen is delivered. This method permits the removal of massively enlarged vascular spleens with practically no loss of blood.

Splenorrhaphy is operative repair of the spleen following trauma. The principles of splenorrhaphy are to debride the devitalized tissue and to attempt to approximate the normal contour of the spleen with capsular sutures or external wraps of material. Partial splenic resections may be performed for trauma or for disease states in which splenic debulking is indicated but may be unsuccessful with a higher immediate complication rate. Partial splenectomy for Gaucher disease, large cysts, or benign tumors has been reported using automatic stapling devices as well as microwave coagulators. On the other hand, for autoimmune disorders, it is absolutely essential for cure to remove the spleen completely including excision of accessory spleens. There may be some benefit to obtaining a preoperative nuclear scan and intraoperative identification with a handheld gamma counter.

Massive splenomegaly is defined as a spleen weight of greater than 1500 g or 8 to 10 times the normal size. Disease processes leading to massive splenomegaly include lymphoma, leukemia, and metabolic storage diseases. The morbidity and mortality rates of splenectomy for massive splenomegaly are increased primarily as a result of the risk of severe and rapid intraoperative blood loss. The operative approach in these cases is initial ligation of the splenic artery through the lesser sac at the superior border of the

pancreas. Next, ligation of the short gastric vessels along the greater curvature all the way to the gastroesophageal junction is performed, allowing the stomach and left lobe of the liver to be retracted away from the spleen. Only after decreasing the splenic arterial inflow by the above maneuvers should mobilization of the lateral and superior attachments be performed, leading to removal of the massive spleen.

Laparoscopic splenectomy is now the standard of care in most major centers with high volumes of splenic surgery. Virtually any indication for elective splenectomy qualifies for a laparoscopic approach, including patients with severe thrombocytopenia, patients with massive splenomegaly, patients needing partial splenectomy, and for the removal of accessory spleens and the wandering spleen. Contraindications to laparoscopic splenectomy include portal hypertension and severe co-morbid disease. With improved techniques, laparoscopic partial splenectomy has now been reported for focal mass lesions and hereditary hematologic diseases.

Laparoscopic splenectomy is performed typically using four ports. Midline ports for the cannula as well as for retraction of the stomach away from the splenic hilum are placed. Left subcostal ports are used as operating sites for dissection of the splenic hilum. An angled laparoscope is required for visualization of the superior and lateral attachments of the spleen. Vessels are divided with clips, sutures, or stapling devices. Precise exposure of the hilum with gentle upward traction on the spleen to stretch and expose the vessels is preferred to blind stapling of the hilum. Clinical conditions such as ITP and hereditary spherocytosis are the most common indications for laparoscopic splenectomy as the spleen is of normal size. Search via the laparoscope for accessory spleens is important in these procedures for a successful outcome, and this may be facilitated by the use of a hand port for palpation.

HEMATOLOGIC EFFECTS OF SPLENECTOMY

Absence of the spleen in a normal adult usually has few clinical consequences. Red cell count and indices do not change, but red cells with cytoplasmic inclusions may appear, eg, Heinz bodies, Howell–Jolly bodies, and siderocytes. Granulocytosis occurs immediately after splenectomy but is replaced in several weeks by lymphocytosis and monocytosis. Platelets are usually increased, occasionally markedly so, and may stay at levels of 400,000-500,000/mL for over a year. Even more striking thrombocytosis (eg, 200,000-300,000/mL) may develop after splenectomy for hemolytic anemia. A platelet count of over a million is not an indication for anticoagulants, but antiplatelet agents such as aspirin may help prevent thrombosis.

Davies JM et al. British Committee for Standards in Haematology. Review of guidelines for the prevention and treatment of infection in patients with an absent or dysfunctional spleen. *Br J Haematol* 2011;155(3):308-317.

POSTSPLENECTOMY SEPSIS & OTHER POSTSPLENECTOMY PROBLEMS

Complications related to splenectomy per se are relatively few, with atelectasis, pancreatitis, and postoperative hemorrhage being the most common. If splenectomy is done for thrombocytopenia, secondary bleeding may occur even though the platelet count usually rises promptly. Platelet transfusions should be given if primary hemostasis is abnormal (ie, oozing occurs) and the platelet count remains low. Thromboembolic complications may be more common following splenectomy, but this complication does not correlate with the degree of thrombocytosis. The risk of portal vein thrombosis is 3% and occurs most commonly after splenectomy for massive spleens hemolytic anemia and not after trauma or splenectomy for thrombocytopenia. Symptoms include fever, abdominal pain, diarrhea, and abnormal liver function tests. Treatment consists of anticoagulation plus antibiotics.

Individuals are more susceptible to fulminant bacteremia after splenectomy and have been reported between 1 week and greater than 20 years after splenectomy. This is a result of the following changes that occur after splenectomy: (1) decreased clearance of bacteria from the blood, (2) decreased levels of IgM, and (3) decreased opsonic activity. The risk is greatest in young children, especially in the first 2 years after surgery (80% of cases) and when the disorder for which splenectomy was required was a disease of the reticuloendothelial system. In general, the younger the patient undergoing splenectomy and the more severe the underlying condition, the greater the risk for developing overwhelming postsplenectomy infection. There is a low but significant risk of infection even in otherwise normal adults following splenectomy. Most of these infections occur after the first year, and nearly half occur more than 5 years after splenectomy. Lethal sepsis is very rare in adults. There is a distinct clinical syndrome: mild, nonspecific symptoms are followed by high fever and shock from sepsis, which may rapidly lead to death. *Streptococcus pneumoniae, Haemophilus influenzae*, and meningococci are the most common pathogens. Disseminated intravascular coagulation is a common complication. Awareness of this fatal complication has led to efforts to avoid splenectomy or to perform partial splenectomy or splenic repair for ruptured spleens (analogous to surgical management of liver trauma) to maintain adequate splenic function. Splenic autotransplantation may also achieve partial restoration of splenic function after splenectomy.

The risk of fatal sepsis is less after splenectomy for trauma than for hematologic disorders, probably due to splenic autotransplantation. Prophylactic vaccination against pneumococcal sepsis should be used in all surgically or functionally asplenic patients. Since splenic function may be important in the immune response to vaccine, early administration of polyvalent pneumococcal vaccine (Pneumovax) is advisable. The vaccine provides protection in adults and older children for 4-5 years, after which revaccination is advisable. Since the vaccine is only effective against about 80% of organisms, some authorities have recommended a 2-year course, treatment until age 16, or lifelong prophylaxis with penicillin following splenectomy. Others have advocated use of ampicillin to provide coverage for *Haemophilus influenzae* as well as pneumococci. Antibiotic prophylaxis is essential in children under 2 years of age and should be continued until at least age 6. In general, splenectomy should be deferred until age 6 unless the hematologic problem is especially severe.

Davies JM et al. British Committee for Standards in Haematology. Review of guidelines for the prevention and treatment of infection in patients with an absent or dysfunctional spleen. *Br J Haematol* 2011;155(3):308-317.

Spelman D et al. Guidelines for the prevention of sepsis in asplenic and hyposplenic patients. *Intern Med J* 2008;38:349-356.

MULTIPLE CHOICE QUESTIONS

1. Which of the following is true about the spleen?

   A. The red pulp of the spleen is normally a significant contributor to red blood cell hematopoiesis.
   B. The spleen's venous drainage is evenly divided between the splenic vein and direct branches of the left renal vein.
   C. The outer capsule of the spleen is a continuous sheet of smooth muscle.
   D. The gastrosplenic ligament carries the short gastric vessels.
   E. Normally 80% of the platelet cell mass is sequestered in the spleen.

2. Indications for splenectomy can include

   A. Vascular disease
   B. Splenomegaly associated with infection
   C. Hereditary spherocytosis
   D. Both A and C
   E. A, B, and C

3. Postsplenectomy sepsis

   A. Only occurs within 1 year of operation
   B. Is at greatest risk in young children
   C. Is associated with residual accessory splenules
   D. Is more often lethal in adults than children
   E. Is more common after splenectomy for trauma than for other indications

Appendix

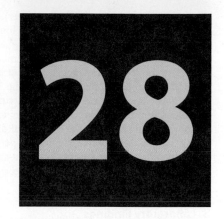

Elliot C. Pennington, MD

Peter A. Burke, MD

ANATOMY & PHYSIOLOGY

In infants, the appendix is a conical diverticulum at the apex of the cecum, but with differential growth and distention of the cecum, the appendix ultimately arises on the left and dorsally approximately 2.5 cm below the ileocecal valve. The taeniae of the colon converge at the base of the appendix, an arrangement that helps in locating this structure at operation. The appendix is freely mobile in the majority and is fixed retrocecally in 16% of adults.

The appendix in children is characterized by a large concentration of lymphoid follicles that appear 2 weeks after birth and number about 200 or more at age 15 years. Thereafter, progressive atrophy of lymphoid tissue proceeds with fibrosis of the wall and partial or total obliteration of the lumen. If the appendix has a physiologic function, it is probably related to the presence of lymphoid follicles.

ACUTE APPENDICITIS

General Considerations

Approximately 7% of people in Western countries have appendicitis at some time during their lives. With more than 250,000 appendectomies for acute appendicitis performed annually in the United States, it is the most common surgical emergency encountered by the general surgeon and accounts for about 1% of all surgical operations.

Obstruction of the proximal lumen by fibrous bands, lymphoid hyperplasia, fecaliths, calculi, or parasites has long been considered to be the major cause of acute appendicitis. A fecalith or calculus is found in only 10% of acutely inflamed appendices. Though evidence of temporal and geographic clustering of cases has suggested a primary infectious etiology this remains to be proven.

As appendicitis progresses, the blood supply is impaired by bacterial infection in the wall and distention of the lumen; gangrene and perforation occur at about 24 hours, though the timing is highly variable. Gangrene implies microscopic perforation, bacterial contamination of the peritoneum, and peritonitis. This process may be effectively localized by adhesions from nearby viscera.

Clinical Findings

Acute appendicitis may simulate almost any other acute abdominal illness, and in turn may be mimicked by a variety of conditions. Progression of symptoms and signs is the rule—in contrast to the fluctuating course of some other diseases.

A. Signs and Symptoms

Typically, the illness begins with vague midabdominal or periumbilical discomfort followed by nausea, anorexia, and indigestion. The pain is continuous but not severe, with occasional mild cramping. The patient may feel constipated or may vomit. Importantly, within several hours of the onset of symptoms the pain shifts to the right-lower quadrant, becoming localized and causing discomfort on moving, walking, or coughing.

Physical examination shows localized tenderness to palpation and perhaps slight muscular guarding. Rebound or percussion tenderness (the latter provides the same information more humanely) may be elicited in the right-lower quadrant. Rectal and pelvic examinations are likely to be negative; if positive, these more often point to another etiology. The temperature is only slightly elevated in the absence of perforation. Administration of narcotic pain medications does not affect the accuracy of the physical examination.

A common misconception is that inflammation of a retrocecal appendix produces an atypical syndrome. This is incorrect; the clinical findings in this situation are the same as for ordinary (antececal) appendicitis. Acute appendicitis may mimic other surgical diseases if the appendix is located outside the right-lower quadrant (ie, sigmoid diverticulitis, acute cholecystisis, or a perforated ulcer). Even when the cecum is normally situated, however, a long appendix may reach to other parts of the abdomen.

Three general points are worth remembering: (1) people with early (nonperforated) appendicitis often do not appear ill. Finding localized tenderness over the McBurney point is the cornerstone of diagnosis. (2) A rule that will help considerably with atypical cases is never to place appendicitis lower than second in the differential diagnosis of acute abdominal pain in a previously healthy person. (3) Patients with appendicitis most commonly have a history of generalized abdominal that over time becomes focused in the right-lower quadrant.

B. Laboratory Findings

The average leukocyte count is 15,000/μL, and 90% of patients have counts over 10,000/μL. In three-fourths of patients, the differential white count shows more than 75% neutrophils. It must be emphasized, however, that 1 patient in 10 with acute appendicitis has a normal leukocyte count, and many have normal differential cell counts. Appendicitis in HIV-positive patients, while up to three times more common, produces the same syndrome as in healthy adults but the white blood cell count is usually normal.

Urinalysis is typically normal, but a few leukocytes and erythrocytes and occasionally even gross hematuria may be noted, particularly in retrocecal or pelvic appendicitis.

C. Imaging Studies

On plain radiographs localized air-fluid levels, localized ileus, or increased soft tissue density in the right-lower quadrant is present in 50% of patients with early acute appendicitis. Less common findings are a calculus, an altered right psoas shadow, an abnormal right flank stripe, or free peritoneal air (from perforated appendicitis). In general, the findings on plain films rarely aid in diagnosis.

A CT examination of the abdomen may be of help in diagnosis. An enlarged appendix with wall thickening, enhancement, or periappendiceal fat stranding is the most useful CT findings of acute appendicitis. Other findings may be present, including focal cecal thickening, appendicoliths, extraluminal or intramural air, and pericecal phlegmon, but are less reliable. Oral contrast administration is not. CT scans are of greatest value in patients with less than typical clinical and laboratory findings, where a positive study would be an indication for appendectomy. In young adults, low-dose CT is noninferior to standard-dose CT. In the face of typical time course of disease, right-lower quadrant pain and tenderness plus signs of inflammation (eg, fever, leukocytosis), a CT scan would be superfluous and, if negative, even misleading. Ultrasound imaging is generally less reliable than CT, though may become more reliable when done using a combined transabdominal and transvaginal approach. When appendicitis is accompanied by a right-lower quadrant mass, an ultrasound or CT scan should be obtained to differentiate between a periappendiceal phlegmon and an abscess or tumor.

D. Appendicitis During Pregnancy

Appendicitis is the most common nonobstetric surgical disease of the abdomen during pregnancy affecting between 1 in 1400 and 1 in 6600 live births, with cases equally distributed through all three trimesters. By far the most common presentation is right-lower quadrant pain, tenderness, and leukocytosis—the classic syndrome—but the enlarged uterus occasionally will have pushed the appendix into the right-upper quadrant, which gives rise to pain in this location. Some symptoms, such as nausea and vomiting, occur in normal pregnancy, which may obscure accurate diagnosis. Fever is less common than with appendicitis in the absence of pregnancy. The main problem is to recognize appendicitis and perform appendectomy promptly. Both CT and MRI are highly sensitive and specific for the diagnosis of acute appendicitis during pregnancy. Delay in operation runs a higher than usual risk of perforation and diffuse peritonitis, because the omentum is less available to wall off the infection. The mother is in greater jeopardy of serious abdominal infection, and the fetus is more vulnerable to premature labor with complications. Laparoscopic appendectomy is well tolerated by the mother and fetus, but the frequency of technical complications is higher than with the open approach. Appendectomy during pregnancy is often followed by preterm labor but rarely by preterm delivery. Early appendectomy in pregnancy has decreased the maternal death rate to under 0.5% and the fetal death rate to less than 10%. Appendectomy in general does not increase a woman's risk for infertility later in life.

▶ Diagnosis & Differential Diagnosis

The clinical diagnosis of appendicitis rests on a combination of localized pain and tenderness accompanied by signs of inflammation, such as fever, leukocytosis, and elevated C-reactive protein levels. Migration of pain from the periumbilical area to the right-lower quadrant is also diagnostically significant. In the absence of signs of inflammation the diagnosis is less certain, and in this situation a CT scan may be of value. The best strategy in equivocal cases is to observe the patient for a period of 6 hours or more. During this time, patients with appendicitis experience increasing pain and signs of inflammation, while those without appendicitis generally improve. False-positive diagnoses often involve cases where the surgeon has accorded more significance to the patient's pain than to the presence or absence of inflammatory signs. Over the past 20 years, the overall false-positive rate for the diagnosis of appendicitis has dropped from 15% to 10% without an accompanying rise in the number of perforations. Thus, diagnostic accuracy appears to be improving. Some patients experience chronic appendicitis, which involves pain lasting 3 weeks or more, and typically includes an acute illness in the recent past compatible with acute appendicitis that was managed nonoperatively.

The diagnosis of acute appendicitis may be difficult in patients at the extremities of age, and it is in these groups that diagnosis is most often delayed. Infants display only lethargy, irritability, and anorexia in the early stages, but may develop vomiting, fever, and pain as the disease progresses. The elderly may not display any classic symptoms, even though the course of appendicitis is more virulent in this age group.

The highest incidence of false-positive diagnosis (20%) is in women between ages 20 and 40 and is attributable to gynecologic conditions such as pelvic inflammatory disease. Compared with appendicitis, pelvic inflammatory disease is more often associated with bilateral lower quadrant tenderness, left adnexal tenderness, onset of illness within 5 days of the last menstrual period, and a history that does not include nausea and vomiting.

Clinical scoring systems can be effective in the diagnosis of acute appendicitis. For example, the Alvarado Score, which uses both physical examination (anorexia, migration of pain, nausea, right-lower quadrant tenderness, rebound pain, and elevated temperature) and laboratory findings (leukocytosis, shift of WBC count to the left) has excellent negative predictive value, with a sensitivity of 99%.

▶ Complications

The complications of acute appendicitis include perforation, peritonitis, abscess, and pylephlebitis.

A. Perforation

Perforation follows the natural history of acute appendicitis, and most likely appears because of delay in seeking treatment. Perforation is accompanied by more severe pain and higher fever (average, 38.3°C) than in simple appendicitis. It is unusual for the acutely inflamed appendix to perforate within the first 12 hours. Appendicitis has progressed to perforation by the time of appendectomy in about 50% of patients under age 10 or over age 50. Perforation in young women increases the subsequent risk of tubal infertility about fourfold.

B. Peritonitis

Localized peritonitis results from microscopic perforation of a gangrenous appendix, while spreading or generalized peritonitis usually implies gross perforation into the free peritoneal cavity. Increasing tenderness and rigidity, abdominal distention, and adynamic ileus are obvious in these patients. High fever and severe toxicity mark progression of this catastrophic illness.

C. Appendiceal Abscess

Localized perforation occurs when the periappendiceal infection becomes walled off by omentum and adjacent viscera. Clinical presentation consists of the usual findings in appendicitis, and may include a right-lower quadrant mass. An ultrasound or CT scan should be performed; if an abscess is found, it is best treated by percutaneous imaging-guided aspiration. Opinion differs about how small abscesses and phlegmons should be handled. Some surgeons prefer a regimen consisting of antibiotics and expectant management followed by elective appendectomy 6 weeks later, so as to avoid spreading the localized infection and the need for a more extensive operation. This strategy is associated with lower rates of overall complications, abscess formation, bowel obstruction, and reoperation. Other surgeons recommend immediate appendectomy, which some believe shortens the duration of illness.

When an unsuspected abscess is encountered during appendectomy, it is usually best to proceed and remove the appendix. If the abscess is large and further dissection would be hazardous, drainage alone is appropriate.

Appendicitis recurs in only 10% of patients whose initial treatment consisted of antibiotics with or without drainage of an abscess. Therefore, when the presence of ancillary conditions increases the risks of surgery, interval appendectomy may be postponed unless symptoms recur.

D. Pylephlebitis

Pylephlebitis is suppurative thrombophlebitis of the portal venous system. Chills, high fever, low-grade jaundice, and, later, hepatic abscesses are the hallmarks of this grave but fortunately rare condition, which affects less than 1% of patients. Prompt surgery and antibiotic therapy is indicated.

▶ Prevention

There is no effective prevention strategy for appendicitis. In the past it was common to perform an incidental appendectomy in young people during the course of an abdominal operation for another illness—as long as the exposure was adequate and there were no specific contraindications. The declining lifetime risk of appendicitis now calls this practice into question. A related question concerns the appropriate course when a laparoscopy is performed for presumptive appendicitis and the appendix looks normal. There is no consensus on these cases, with some surgeons preferring to remove the appendix and some electing to leave it in place. In children, it is not necessary to remove the appendix after an incidentally diagnosed appendicolith.

▶ Treatment

With few exceptions, the treatment of appendicitis is surgical (ie, appendectomy). The operation can be done open

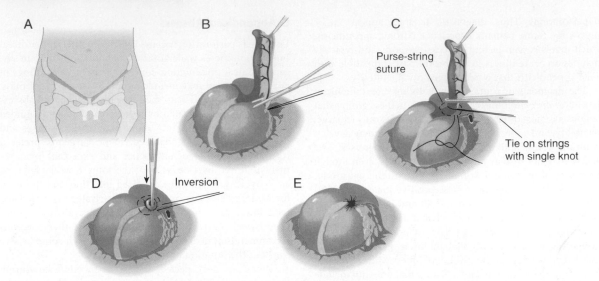

▲ **Figure 28–1.** Technique of open appendectomy. **A:** Incision. **B:** After delivery of the tip of the cecum, the mesoappendix is divided. **C:** The base is clamped and ligated with a simple throw of the knot. The next step—inversion of the stump—is optional. **D:** A clamp is placed to hold the knot during inversion with a purse-string suture of fine silk. **E:** The loosely tied inner knot on the stump assures that there is no closed space for the development of a stump abscess.

(Figure 28–1) or laparoscopically. A laparoscopic approach is desirable when the preoperative diagnosis is uncertain. In select patients, outpatient laparoscopic appendectomy may be possible.

Prophylactic antibiotics are indicated preoperatively with a single-drug regimen, usually a cephalosporin. Culturing abdominal fluid is not indicated even when the appendix has perforated, as the organisms obtained are the typical fecal flora. Abdominal drains are called for only to treat established abscesses.

If a patient with appendicitis cannot be taken to a modern surgical facility for care, treatment should consist of antibiotics alone. The complication-free success rate of this approach is above 93%, though acute appendicitis may recur in this population. Success rates of greater than 60% have been reported at 1 year.

A. Laparoscopic Versus Open Appendectomy

The laparoscopic approach to appendectomy was first described by Kurt Semm in 1983. There has been much debate over the appropriate role of laparoscopy in the treatment of appendicitis since that initial report, with an increasing majority of cases in this country performed laparoscopically. In one large study, patients treated laparoscopically had lower overall morbidity (except organ space surgical site infections in patients with complicated appendicitis), but similar serious morbidity, mortality, and length

of stay. Generally, patients undergoing laparoscopic appendectomy have less postoperative pain and a shorter length of stay by 1 day. However, laparoscopic appendectomy may be associated with increased overall hospital costs and longer operative times. Conversion rates from laparoscopic to open approach range from 0% to 27%, and should be based on surgeon experience, judgment, and ability to safely perform the procedure. Currently most patients in the United States undergo laparoscopic treatment, and this approach is safe for both uncomplicated and complicated appendicitis. In select patients, the appendix can be removed using a single-port technique.

B. Outcomes

Although a death rate of zero is theoretically attainable in acute appendicitis, deaths still occur, some of which are avoidable. The mortality rate in simple acute appendicitis is approximately 0.1% and has not changed significantly since 1930. Progress in preoperative and postoperative care has reduced mortality from perforation to about 5%. Nonetheless, postoperative infections still occur in 30% of cases of gangrenous or perforated appendicitis. While the cases may be more technically challenging, obese patients have similar rates of complication, length of stay, and readmission. The substantial increase in tubal infertility that follows perforation in young women is avoidable by early appendectomy. If the entirety of the appendix is not removed, stump appendicitis can occur in the residual appendix.

C. Controversies

Many controversies exist regarding the treatment of acute appendicitis. Some surgeons routinely irrigate all four quadrants in all appendectomies, while others do not. Irrigation has been shown to reduce postoperative abscess rates in perforated appendicitis only. There is emerging evidence that antibiotics alone may be a preferable initial treatment of uncomplicated acute appendicitis. While it is clear that postoperative antibiotics are not beneficial for nonperforated appendicitis after appendectomy, no consensus exists on the drug regimen or duration of antibiotics for perforated disease.

Amoli HA et al. Morphine analgesia in patients with acute appendicitis: a randomised double-blind clinical trial. *Emerg Med J* 2008;25(9):586-589.

Basaran A, Basaran M. Diagnosis of acute appendicitis during pregnancy: a systematic review. *Obstet Gynecol Surv* 2009;64(7):481-488.

Bondi M et al. Improving the diagnostic accuracy of ultrasonography in suspected acute appendicitis by the combined transabdominal and transvaginal approach. *Am Surg* 2012;78(1):98-103.

Cardenas-Salomon CM et al. Hospitalization costs of open vs. laparoscopic appendectomy: 5-year experience. *Cir Cir* 2011;79(6):534-539.

Cash CL et al. A prospective treatment protocol for outpatient laparoscopic appendectomy for acute appendicitis *J Am Coll Surg* 2012;215(1):101-105.

Coakley BA et al. Postoperative antibiotics correlate with worse outcomes after appendectomy for nonperforated appendicitis. *J Am Coll Surg* 2011;213(6):778-783.

Deugarte DA et al. Obesity does not impact outcomes for appendicitis. *Am Surg* 2012;78(2):254-257.

Gilo NB et al. Appendicitis and cholecystitis in pregnancy. *Clin Obstet Gynecol* 2009;52(4):586-596.

Hekimoglu K et al. Comparison of combined oral and i.v. contrast-enhanced versus single i.v. contrast-enhanced mdct for the detection of acute appendicitis. *JBR-BTR* 2011;94(5):278-282.

Hussain A et al. Prevention of intra-abdominal abscess following laparoscopic appendicectomy for perforated appendicitis: a prospective study. *Int J Surg* 6(5):374-377.

Ingraham AM et al. Comparison of outcomes after laparoscopic versus open appendectomy for acute appendicitis at 222 ACS NSQIP hospitals. *Surgery* 2010;148(4):625-635; discussion 635-627.

Kim K et al. Low-dose abdominal CT for evaluating suspected appendicitis. *N Engl J Med* 2012;366(17):1596-1605.

Klein DB et al. Increased rates of appendicitis in HIV-infected men: 1991-2005. *J Acquir Immune Defic Syndr* 2009;52(1):139-140.

Korndorffer JR et al. SAGES guideline for laparoscopic appendectomy. *Surg Endosc* 2010;24(4):757-761.

Liu K, Fogg L. Use of antibiotics alone for treatment of uncomplicated acute appendicitis: a systematic review and meta-analysis. *Surgery* 2011;150(4):673-683.

Ohle R et al. The Alvarado score for predicting acute appendicitis: a systematic review. *BMC Med* 2011;9:139.

Parks NA, Schroeppel TJ. Update on imaging for acute appendicitis. *Surg Clin North Am* 2011;91(1):141-154.

Rollins MD et al. Prophylactic appendectomy: unnecessary in children with incidental appendicoliths detected by computed tomographic scan. *J Pediatr Surg* 2010;45(12):2377-2380.

Sauerland S et al. Laparoscopic versus open surgery for suspected appendicitis. *Cochrane Database Syst Rev* 2010;(10):CD001546.

Sieren LM et al. The incidence of benign and malignant neoplasia presenting as acute appendicitis. *Am Surg* 2010;76(8):808-811.

Simillis C et al. A meta-analysis comparing conservative treatment versus acute appendectomy for complicated appendicitis (abscess or phlegmon). *Surgery* 2010;147(6):818-829.

St Peter SD et al. Single incision versus standard 3-port laparoscopic appendectomy: a prospective randomized trial. *Ann Surg* 2011;254(4):586-590.

Subramanian A, Liang MK. A 60-year literature review of stump appendicitis: the need for a critical view. *Am J Surg* 2012;203(4):503-507.

Varadhan KK et al. Safety and efficacy of antibiotics compared with appendicectomy for treatment of uncomplicated acute appendicitis: meta-analysis of randomised controlled trials. *BMJ* 2012;344:e2156.

TUMORS OF THE APPENDIX

Benign tumors, including carcinoids, were found in 4.6% of 71,000 human appendix specimens examined microscopically, typically as incidental findings.

Malignant Tumors

Primary malignant tumors were found in 1.4% of appendices in the same large series. Carcinoid and neuroendocrine tumors comprise the majority of appendiceal cancers, and the appendix is the commonest location of carcinoid tumors of the gastrointestinal tract. Carcinoid tumors of the appendix are most commonly found at the tip and are usually benign, but tumors over 2 cm in diameter may exhibit malignant behavior. About half of these tumors are discovered during an appendectomy for acute appendicitis, with the remainder identified incidentally. Lesions less than 2 cm in diameter invade the appendiceal wall in 25% of cases, but only 3% metastasize to lymph nodes. Hepatic metastases and the carcinoid syndrome are truly rare. Appendectomy alone is adequate treatment unless the lymph nodes are visibly involved, the tumor is more than 2 cm in diameter, mucinous elements are present in the tumor (adenocarcinoid), or the mesoappendix or base of the cecum is invaded; in these cases, right hemicolectomy is recommended. The recurrence rate after surgical treatment is near zero.

Colonic adenocarcinoma can arise in the appendix and spread rapidly to regional lymph nodes or implant on other peritoneal surfaces. Most patients present with advanced disease. Adenocarcinoma is virtually never diagnosed preoperatively, and about half of cases present as acute appendicitis. Right hemicolectomy should be performed if disease is localized to the appendix and/or regional lymph nodes. The 5-year survival rate is 60% after right hemicolectomy and only 20% after appendectomy alone, but the latter group includes patients with distant metastases at diagnosis.

▶ Mucocele and Pseudomyxoma Peritonei

An appendiceal mucocele is a cystic, dilated appendix filled with mucin. Simple mucocele is not a neoplasm and results from chronic obstruction of the proximal lumen, usually by fibrous tissue. Rarely, mucocele is caused by a neoplasm—cystadenoma, or adenocarcinoma grade 1 in the older terminology, now often called a mucinous appendix neoplasm (MAN). This lesion may arise de novo or (perhaps) in a preceding simple mucocele. Appendectomy is adequate treatment in either case. If a MAN ruptures, it can lead to a condition known as pseudomyxoma peritonei, characterized by diffuse mucin production throughout the peritoneal cavity, with variable amounts of tumor cellularity. Patients can be treated with either simple appendectomy or right hemicolectomy.

Foster JM et al. Right hemicolectomy is not routinely indicated in pseudomyxoma peritonei. *Am Surg* 2012;78(2):171-177.

Guraya SY, Almaramhy HH. Clinicopathological features and the outcome of surgical management for adenocarcinoma of the appendix. *World J Gastrointest Surg* 2011;3(1):7-12.

Shapiro R et al. Appendiceal carcinoid at a large tertiary center: pathologic findings and long-term follow-up evaluation. *Am J Surg* 2011;201(6):805-808.

MULTIPLE CHOICE QUESTIONS

1. All of the following are true about the appendix, except

   A. The appendix in children is characterized by a large concentration of lymphoid follicles that appear 2 weeks after birth and number about 200 or more at age 15 years.
   B. The taeniae of the colon converge at the base of the appendix.
   C. A fecalith or calculus is found in only 10% of acutely inflamed appendices.
   D. The appendix is fixed retrocecally in 65% of adults.
   E. Acute appendicitis may simulate almost any other acute abdominal illness.

2. Helpful tests in the diagnosis of acute appendicitis include

   A. Abdominal CT
   B. Transvaginal ultrasound
   C. Encephalopathy
   D. A, B, and C
   E. A and C

3. Primary malignant tumors of the appendix

   A. Should prompt right colectomy in nearly all patients
   B. Are most commonly neuroendocrine (carcinoid) tumors
   C. Is the most common etiology of appendicitis
   D. Usually presents due to liver metastases
   E. Are usually found at the base of the appendix

Small Bowel

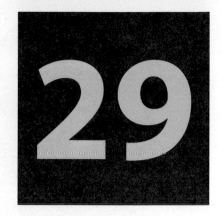

Marco E. Allaix, MD

Mukta Krane, MD

Alessandro Fichera, MD

ANATOMY

▶ Gross Anatomy

The small intestine is the portion of the alimentary tract extending from the pylorus to the ileocecal valve and it consists of three segments—the duodenum, the jejunum (upper two-fifths), and the ileum (lower three-fifths). The anatomy, physiology, and pathology of the duodenum are discussed in Chapter 23.

The jejunum begins at the ligament of Treitz. The jejunum and ileum are suspended on a mobile mesentery covered by a visceral peritoneal lining that extends onto the external surface of the bowel to form the serosa. There is no sharp demarcation between the jejunum and the ileum; as the intestine proceeds distally, the lumen narrows, the mesenteric vascular arcades become more complex, and the circular mucosal folds become shorter and fewer.

The mesentery contains fat, blood vessels, lymphatic channels and nodes, and nerves. The jejunum and ileum are supplied by the superior mesenteric artery (SMA). Branches within the mesentery anastomose to form arcades, and small straight arteries from these arcades enter the mesenteric border of the gut. Venous blood is drained through the superior mesenteric vein (SMV), which then joins the splenic vein behind the pancreas to form the portal vein.

Lymphatic drainage is abundant. Elliptical, lymphoid aggregates (Peyer's patches) are present in the submucosa on the antimesenteric border along the distal ileum, and smaller follicles are evident throughout the remainder of the small intestine. Regional lymph nodes follow vascular arcades and drain toward the cisterna chyli.

The nerve supply for the small bowel is both sympathetic (fibers from the greater and lesser splanchnic nerves) and parasympathetic (from the right vagus nerve). Although both types of autonomic nerves contain efferent and afferent fibers, only the sympathetic afferents appear to mediate intestinal pain.

▶ Microscopic Anatomy

The wall of the small intestine consists of four layers—mucosa (innermost), submucosa, muscularis, and serosa (outermost).

The *mucosa* is characterized by circular folds about 10 mm high, named *valvulae conniventes*, that are taller and more numerous in the proximal jejunum and project into the lumen (Figure 29–1). These folds, combined with the presence of villi on the surface of the valvulae conniventes, increase the absorptive surface area about eight times. There are approximately 20-40 villi/mm^2. They are about 0.5-1 mm long and their walls are made up of epithelial cells with tiny projections named microvilli. The epithelial cells enclose a central axis that contains an arteriole surrounded by blood and lymphatic capillaries, known as a *lacteal*, and fibers from the muscularis mucosae. The microvilli (1 μm in height) amplify the potential absorptive surface area up to 200-500 m^2 (Figure 29–2).

The mucosa is microscopically subdivided into three different layers: (1) the muscularis mucosae, the outermost, consists of a thin sheet of smooth muscle cells; (2) the lamina propria consists of connective tissue that extends from the base of the crypts up into the intestinal villi; and (3) the epithelium which is the innermost layer.

Intestinal epithelium in composed of multiple cell types that rest on a thin basement membrane overlying the lamina propria. There are two major compartments to the intestinal epithelium, the crypt and the villus, each with distinct function and cellular composition. The crypt is populated by cells that are predominantly secretory and which derive from a pluripotent stem cell located above the base of the crypts of Lieberkühn. Paneth cells stay at the base of the crypts; their function is still unknown but may be secretory, as resembling zymogen-secreting cells of the pancreas.

Most of the crypt cells are undifferentiated; some mature into mucus-secreting goblet cells and enteroendocrine

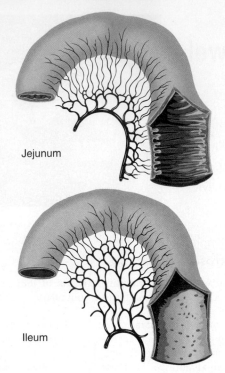

▲ **Figure 29–1.** Blood supply and luminal surface of the small bowel. The arterial arcades of the small intestine increase in number from one or two in the proximal jejunum to four or five in the distal ileum, a finding that helps to distinguish proximal from distal bowel at operation. Plicae circulares are more prominent in the jejunum.

cells, but the majority become absorptive enterocytes. Enteroendocrine cells include enterochromaffin cells (the most common), N cells that contain neurotensin, L cells (glucagon), and motilin and cholecystokinin (CCK) containing cells. Finally, M cells and T lymphocytes play a major role in mucosal cell-mediated immunity.

The villus compartment is nonproliferative. Factors that affect enterocyte differentiation include growth factors, hormones, matrix proteins, and luminal nutrients. The life span of enterocytes is 3-6 days.

The *submucosa* is a dense connective tissue layer populated by different cell types, including fibroblasts, mast cells, lymphocytes, macrophages, eosinophils, and plasma cells. It contains blood vessels, lymphatics, and nerves. Meissner's submucosal neural plexus interconnects with neural elements from Auerbach's plexus. The submucosa is the strongest layer of small bowel wall. The *muscularis* consists of two layers of smooth muscle, a thicker inner circular layer and a thinner outer longitudinal layer. Specialized intercellular junctional structures called *gap junctions* electrically couple

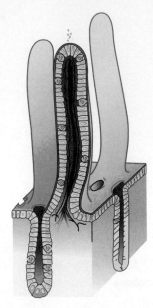

▲ **Figure 29–2.** Schematic representation of villi and crypts of Lieberkühn.

adjacent smooth muscle cells and allow efficient propagation of peristalsis. Ganglion cells and nerve fibers of Auerbach's myenteric plexus interdigitate between layers and communicate with smaller neural elements between cells. The *serosa* consists of a single layer of flattened mesothelial cells that covers the small bowel.

Johansson ME et al. Composition and functional role of the mucus layers in the intestine. *Cell Mol Life Sci* 2011 Nov;68(22): 3635-3641.
Simons BD et al. Stem cell self-renewal in intestinal crypt. *Exp Cell Res* 2011 Nov 15;317(19):2719-2724.

PHYSIOLOGY

▶ Motility

Intestinal motility consists of propulsion of luminal contents (peristalsis) combined with mixing action through segmentation. These functions are accomplished by both the outer longitudinal and inner circular muscle layers of the intestinal wall, mainly under the direct control of the myenteric nervous plexus. The submucosal nervous plexus is primarily involved in the regulation of secretion and absorption. The extrinsic sympathetic input is excitatory and the peptidergic input likely inhibitory. Intestinal motility is also under positive control by local hormones such as motilin and CCK. Smooth muscles of the small intestine undergo spontaneous oscillations of membrane potentials, known as pacesetter potentials, with progressively decreasing frequency from the duodenum to the ileum. The frequency of pacesetter potentials for the entire small intestine is determined by the duodenum, where they originate. A nerve-related cell type known as the interstitial cell of Cajal appears to play a key role in the generation of pacemaker activity. Small bowel motility varies with the fasted and fed state. During the interdigestive or fasting period, a cyclical pattern of motor activity consisting of three phases is observed. Phase I is resting and lasts for about 80% of the cycle. Phase II, about 15%, consists of random contractions of moderate amplitude. Phase III, about 5%, is a series of brief high pressure waves. This three phase cycle results in a pattern called the migrating motor complex, which is abolished by ingestion of food. In the fed state, the pattern of contraction is more frequent and consistent over time. Rather than beginning from a proximal site and propagating distally, contractions begin at all levels along the small bowel and spread distally.

Barrier Function

The intestinal epithelium selectively limits the permeation of potentially harmful luminal substances. The anatomical barrier is the intercellular junction complex, a three-level structure that forms a circumferential seal between adjacent cells: the tight junction faces the lumen, the intermediate junction lies deep to the tight junction, and the desmosome is the innermost element of this complex. Several pathological conditions can alter the barrier function. Certain bacterial toxins, such as *Clostridium difficile*, directly perturb the barrier function through disruption of cytoskeletal-junctional interactions, and various cytokines and proinflammatory mediators can also modulate intestinal permeability.

Digestion & Absorption

Digestion begins in the stomach with the action of gastric acid and pepsin. In the proximal duodenum, ingested food is broken down by pancreatic enzymes such as trypsin, elastase, chymotrypsin, and carboxypeptidases. The activity of intestinal hydrolases and olygopeptidases then accomplishes terminal protein and carbohydrate digestion, and the resulting monosaccharides, amino acids, or di- and tripeptides then serve as substrates for Na^+- or H^+-coupled transporters in the apical membrane of absorptive enterocytes. Fat digestion and absorption occur in the proximal small bowel, where pancreatic lipase partially hydrolyzes triglycerides into two fatty acids and a monoglyceride. These substances are solubilized by bile salts to form micelles that diffuse into enterocytes releasing fatty acid and monoglyceride. Triglycerides are transported intracellularly and incorporated along with cellular protein, phospholipid, and cholesterol to form chylomicrons. They then exit the cell to be absorbed by the lymphatic system. Bile salts are reabsorbed into the enterohepatic circulation in the distal ileum by an ileal Na^+ coupled bile acid transporter.

The small bowel receives about 1-1.5 L/day of ingested fluids and about 8 L of salivary, gastric, and pancreaticobiliary secretions. Most of this fluid is reabsorbed before reaching the colon. Water movement is driven by the active transcellular absorption of Na^+ and Cl^- and by absorption of nutrients such as glucose and amino acids. The energy for many of these processes derives from the activity of a Na^+-K^+ ATPase, that maintains the low Na^+ internal environment that drives uptake via coupled ion exchangers (Na^+/H^+ and Cl^-/HCO_3^-) and Na^+-coupled nutrient transporters.

Secretion

Intestinal crypt cells secrete an isotonic fluid through the active transcellular transport of Cl^-. This process lubricates the mucosal surface and facilitates the luminal extrusion of other secrete substances. Diarrhea results when secretion exceeds intestinal absorptive capacity.

Immune Function

The mucosal immune system is extremely important in defense against toxic and pathogenic threats from the luminal environment. The lamina propria contains numerous immune cells including plasma cells, mast cells, and lymphocytes that produce both immunoglobulins and cytokine mediators.

Plasma cells produce IgA in response to food antigens and microbes. IgA and IgM are secreted into the lumen by a mechanism that involves transcytosis through epithelial cells after binding to the polymeric immunoglobulin receptor on the basolateral membrane. Secretory IgA prevents microbial pathogens from penetrating the epithelial layer. IgA-antigen interactions also occur within the intraepithelial and subepithelial compartments. Intestinal epithelial cells themselves may also contribute to the immune function of the bowel. These cells express major histocompatibility class I and class II molecules on their surface and may function as weak antigen-presenting cells. The epithelial cell layer may transmit important immunoregulatory signals to the underlying lymphocytic population.

Specialized cells known as M cells are found overlying Peyer's patches and act as the major portal of entry for foreign bodies. Specialized membrane invaginations in these cells create a pocket in which lymphocytes and macrophages gather. Luminal substances are immediately delivered to these antigen-presenting cells, and this information is directly conveyed to the underlying follicles. Intraepithelial lymphocytes (IEL) are specialized T cells that reside in the paracellular space between absorptive enterocytes. The precise role of IELs is still uncertain, but they may mediate cross-talk between epithelial cells and the underlying immune and nonimmune cells of the lamina propria. Within the lamina propria and submucosa, mature T cells, B cells, and macrophages carry out traditional cell-mediated immune response including phagocytosis, cell killing, and cytokine secretion. Mucosal and connective tissue mast cells produce numerous mediators that contribute to overall immune response and modulate the many functions of the epithelial cells.

▶ Neuroendocrine Function

The small bowel is a rich source of regulatory peptides that control various aspects of gut function. These substances, released in response to luminal or neural stimuli, exert their biological actions either at distant sites or locally.

Secretin is a 27-amino-acid peptide released by entero-endocrine cells in the proximal small bowel in response to luminal acidification, bile salts, and fat. Its major function is to stimulate pancreatic ductal alkaline secretion. Secretin inhibits gastric acid secretion, and gastrointestinal motility. In addition, it stimulates bile flow by stimulating fluid secretion from cholangiocytes. Other members of the secretin family that share substantial sequence homology and interact with similar receptors include vasoactive intestinal polypeptide (VIP), glucagon, gastric inhibitory polypeptide (GIP), and enteroglucagon. Enteroglucagon and glucagon-like peptides are secreted by neuroendocrine cells in the colon and small bowel and may play an important role in gut adaptation and glucose homeostasis.

CCK is released by specialized enteroendocrine cells in response to luminal amino acids and medium- to long-chain fatty acids. CCK release is inhibited by intraluminal trypsin and bile salts. Two major targets of CCK are the gallbladder and the sphincter of Oddi, where it causes coordinated contraction and relaxation, respectively, to enhance luminal mixing of bile with ingested food. Furthermore, CCK stimulates pancreatic enzyme secretion and cell growth in intestinal mucosa and the pancreas, insulin release and intestinal motility.

Somatostatin is a 14-amino-acid peptide that exerts a wide variety of inhibitory functions in the gastrointestinal tract. It is released from specialized enteroendocrine cells and it acts in paracrine fashion to inhibit intestinal, gastric, and pancreatico-biliary secretion and cell growth. Synthetic forms of somatostatin are used in the clinical practice in patients with enterocutaneous and pancreatico-biliary fistulae.

Peptide YY is a 36-amino-acid peptide secreted by the distal small bowel and it inhibits gastric acid and pancreatic secretion, as well as several intestinal hormones, and decreases intestinal motility.

Motilin is secreted by the duodenum and the proximal jejunum, where it acts to enhance contractility and accelerate gastric emptying.

Neurotensin is produced in the ileum and enteric nerves; it appears to affect a variety of enteric functions including gastric acid secretion, gastric emptying, intestinal motility, and secretion.

Other peptides (VIP, calcitonin-related peptide, galanin, bombesin, neuropeptide Y, gastrin-releasing peptides, and substance P) are released from enteric nerves, but their precise role has not been fully clarified.

Crenn P, Messing B, Cynober L. Citrulline as a biomarker of intestinal failure due to enterocyte mass reduction. *Clin Nutr* 2008;27:328.

Edholm T et al. The incretin hormones GIP and GLP-1 in diabetic rats: effects on insulin secretion and small bowel motility. *Neurogastroenterol Motil* 2009 Mar;21(3):313-321.

Jones MP, Bratten JR. Small intestinal motility. *Curr Opin Gastroenterol* 2008;24:164.

SMALL BOWEL OBSTRUCTION

▶ General Considerations

Small bowel obstruction (SBO) is one of the most common disorders affecting the small bowel. It is characterized by impairment in the normal flow of intraluminal contents and can be divided into mechanical obstruction and paralytic ileus.

Mechanical obstruction implies an extrinsic or intrinsic obstacle that prevents the aboral progression of intestinal contents and it may be complete or partial. Simple obstruction occludes the lumen only; obstruction with strangulation impairs the blood supply also and leads to necrosis of the intestinal wall. Paralytic (or adynamic) ileus is due to a neurogenic failure of peristalsis to propel intestinal contents with no mechanical obstruction.

A. Etiology

The causes of mechanical obstruction can be divided into three groups according to the relationship to the intestinal wall: (1) intraluminal; (2) intramural; and (3) extrinsic. The three most common etiologies are intra-abdominal adhesions, hernias, and neoplasms (Table 29–1).

Table 29–1. Causes of obstruction of the small intestine in adults.

Causes	Relative Incidence (%)
Adhesions	60
External hernia	10
Neoplasms	20
Intrinsic	3
Extrinsic	17
Miscellaneous	10

1. **Adhesions** Sixty to 75% of cases of mechanical SBO are secondary to adhesions related to prior abdominal surgery. Lower abdominal and pelvic surgery appears to be associated with a higher incidence of adhesions compared to upper abdominal surgery. Congenital bands are rarely seen in children.

2. **Hernia** The most common cause of SBO in patients with no history of prior abdominal surgery is a hernia. A careful search for inguinal, femoral, and umbilical hernias must be made during evaluation of every patient presenting with symptoms consistent with obstruction. Internal hernias into the obturator foramen, the foramen of Winslow, or other anatomic defects must also be considered. In patients who have undergone previous surgery, incisional hernias represent another potential cause of SBO especially after laparotomy, in overweight or obese patients, in patients on steroid therapy or with wound infections.

3. **Neoplasms** Intrinsic small bowel neoplasms can progressively occlude the lumen or serve as a leading point in intussusception. Symptoms may be intermittent, onset of obstruction is slow, and signs of chronic anemia may be present. Peritoneal carcinomatosis from several tumors is an extrinsic cause of SBO due to adhesions of small bowel loops to neoplastic nodules.

Other causes of SBO include Crohn disease (CD), intussusception which is most often seen in children without an organic lesion and rarely in adults with a neoplastic intraluminal lesion; volvulus as a consequence of intestinal malrotation in children, or of adhesions in adults; and foreign bodies including bezoars, ingested foreign bodies, and gallstones through a cholecysto-duodenal fistula. Gallstone ileus is discussed in Chapter 25.

B. Pathophysiology

With the onset of obstruction, gas and fluid accumulate and distend the intestinal loops proximal to the site of obstruction. Fluid from the extracellular space also fills the lumen proximal to the obstruction, due to the impaired bidirectional flow of salt and water and fluid secretion enhanced by substances (endotoxins, prostaglandins) released from proliferating bacteria in the intestinal lumen. As a consequence, intraluminal and intramural pressures rise until microvascular perfusion to the intestine is impaired, leading to intestinal wall ischemia, and ultimately necrosis.

Activity of the smooth muscle of the small bowel is increased in an attempt to propel its contents past the obstruction consuming all energy sources. At this point the intestine becomes atonic and enlarges further. Emesis could be feculent due to bacterial overgrowth—particularly with distal obstruction—as the intestinal dilation progresses proximally (Figure 29–3). Bacterial translocation from the lumen to the mesenteric nodes and the bloodstream occurs and abdominal distention elevates the diaphragm and impairs respiration resulting in potential pulmonary complications such as pneumonia, and atelectasis.

When full thickness necrosis of the intestinal wall occurs, luminal content with an elevated bacterial load enters the peritoneal cavity, is absorbed by the peritoneum causing septic shock.

The progression of pathophysiologic events when the bowel is strangulated occurs more rapidly than with simple obstruction and is characterized by an acute impairment of venous return initially followed by arterial flow with subsequent ischemia, necrosis, and perforation of the intestinal wall.

▶ Clinical Findings

Diagnostic evaluation should distinguish mechanical bowel obstruction from ileus, determine the cause of the obstruction, and recognize simple from strangulating obstruction.

Accurate diagnosis requires obtaining a detailed history paying particular attention to medications known to affect intestinal physiology, previous cancer, inflammatory bowel disease, and abdominal surgery and a meticulous physical examination.

A. Signs and Symptoms

Patients usually present with nausea, vomiting, colicky abdominal pain, and obstipation, although residual gas and stool distal to the obstruction may be expelled. With proximal SBO, emesis is usually profuse, containing undigested food in close temporal association with oral intake; abdominal pain is more often described as upper abdominal discomfort associated with epigastric distension. Distal SBO is characterized by diffuse and poorly localized crampy abdominal pain. Feculent vomiting present in cases of longstanding distal SBO is the consequence of bacterial overgrowth and is pathognomonic for a complete mechanical obstruction. In the presence of strangulation, fever often develops, and previously crampy abdominal pain becomes peritonitis.

Initially, vital signs may be normal, but tachycardia and hypotension usually develop as a result of progressive dehydration. Fever is often present with bowel ischemia or perforation. Inspection of the abdomen usually reveals distension that varies based on the site of obstruction and may be absent in cases of proximal obstruction. Peristalsis is usually tremendously increased in the early phases of mechanical SBO, as a result of intensive intestinal muscular contractions. This so-called "peristaltic rush" progressively decreases until it disappears in the late phase of obstruction. The presence of either surgical scars or hernias should be noted, indicating a possible cause of SBO. Rectal examination is essential to detect rectal lesions and to check for the presence of stool.

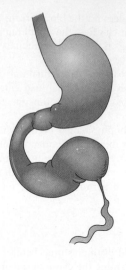
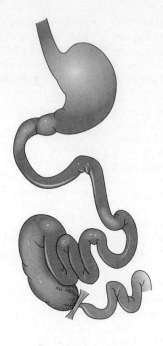
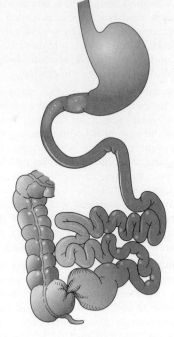

High

Frequent vomiting.
No distention. Intermittent
pain but not classic
crescendo type.

Middle

Moderate vomiting.
Moderate distention. Intermittent
pain (crescendo, colicky)
with free intervals.

Low

Vomiting late, feculent.
Marked distention. Variable
pain; may not be classic
crescendo type.

▲ **Figure 29–3.** Small bowel obstruction. Variable manifestations of obstruction depend on the level of blockage of the small bowel.

B. Laboratory Findings

Laboratory findings reflect intravascular volume depletion and dehydration. An elevated hematocrit is indicative of hemoconcentration. Leukocytosis is often the result of dehydration and an acute stress response rather than an underlying infection. Blood chemistries may reveal elevated serum creatinine levels, indicating hypovolemia with prerenal failure.

Features of strangulated obstruction or perforation include marked leukocytosis and metabolic acidosis.

C. Imaging Studies

Plain x-rays of the abdomen with the patient in supine and upright position can confirm the clinical diagnosis of SBO. They reveal dilated small bowel loops with air-fluid levels in a ladder-like appearance, and a paucity of air in the colon. These features may be minimal or absent in early or high grade obstructions.

Computed tomographic (CT) scan of the abdomen and pelvis with both intravenous and oral contrast is widely used. CT scan can visualize the specific location of the obstruction, showing a discrepancy in the caliber between distended proximal bowel loops and collapsed distal intestine. Moreover, CT scan can also reveal the etiology of SBO and demonstrate signs of strangulation including thickening of the bowel wall, air in the bowel wall or portal venous system, and poor uptake of intravenous contrast by the affected bowel wall. Ascites between dilated bowel loops and in the pelvis is often reported in both simple and strangulated obstruction. Intraperitoneal free air indicates perforation.

▶ Differential Diagnosis

Pain in patients with paralytic ileus is usually not severe but is constant and diffuse, and the abdomen is often distended and mildly tender. If ileus has resulted from an acute intraperitoneal inflammatory process, there should be symptoms and signs of the primary disease as well as the ileus. Abdominal x-rays show the presence of gas in both the colon and in the small bowel.

A postoperative ileus may be caused by several factors, including drugs used for anesthesia and analgesia, and intraoperative manipulation of intestinal loops and the mesentery. Usually, it is temporary; but if it persists for more than 3-5 days, diagnostic evaluation to rule out mechanical causes of obstruction is mandatory.

Colonic obstruction is usually diagnosed by abdominal x-rays that show colonic dilation proximal to the obstructing lesion. In the presence of competent ileocecal valve, a closed loop obstruction occurs with an elevated risk of perforation of the colon. If the ileocecal valve is incompetent, the distal small bowel will be dilated, and patients will exhibit abdominal distension, nausea and vomiting.

Acute gastroenteritis, acute appendicitis, and acute pancreatitis can mimic simple intestinal obstruction, while acute mesenteric ischemia (AMI) must be considered in the differential of small bowel strangulation.

Intestinal pseudo-obstruction comprises a spectrum of specific disorders associated with irreversible intestinal dysmotility, in which there are symptoms and signs of intestinal obstruction without evidence for an obstructing lesion. Acute pseudo-obstruction of the colon carries the risk of cecal perforation and is discussed in Chapter 30. Chronic pseudo-obstruction affecting the small bowel with or without colonic involvement can be idiopathic, or secondary to several (sporadic and familial) visceral myopathies and neuropathies that affect intestinal smooth muscle, and the intra- and extraintestinal nervous system. Systemic disorders such as scleroderma, myxedema, lupus erythematosus, amyloidosis, drug abuse (phenothiazine ingestion), radiation injury, or progressive systemic sclerosis can be complicated by chronic intestinal pseudo-obstruction. In addition, cytomegalovirus and Epstein–Barr viral infections can cause chronic intestinal pseudo-obstruction.

The clinical manifestations of chronic intestinal pseudo-obstruction include recurrent episodes of vomiting, crampy abdominal pain, and abdominal distention. The diagnosis is suggested by clinical findings and medical history, and confirmed by radiologic and manometric studies. Diagnostic laparoscopic full-thickness biopsy of the small bowel may be required to establish the specific cause of the disease. Therapy focuses on palliation of symptoms and nutritional issues.

▶ Treatment

SBO is associated with a marked depletion of liquids caused by decreased oral intake, vomiting, and sequestration of fluid in the bowel lumen. Therefore, vigorous fluid resuscitation and correction of electrolyte disorders (hypochloremic, hypokalemic metabolic alkalosis) is mandatory. A urinary catheter should be placed to monitor urinary output. Gastrointestinal decompression with a nasogastric tube provides relief of symptoms, prevents further gas and fluid accumulation proximally, and decreases the risk of aspiration.

Obstruction that occurs in the early postoperative period is usually partial and only rarely associated with strangulation. Therefore, a period of prolonged total parenteral nutrition and hydration is warranted. Patients who have undergone numerous abdominal operations should initially be conservatively treated with decompression, bowel rest, and serial abdominal exams in hopes of avoiding reentering a hostile abdomen. Patients with CD rarely present with a complete bowel obstruction and these patients often benefit from steroids or other immunosuppressive therapy. However, if signs suggestive of ischemia are detected surgery should be promptly undertaken.

Finally, management of patients with diffuse carcinomatosis is often challenging and in most of cases limited to conservative and palliative treatment.

A. Surgery

The surgical procedure performed varies according to the etiology of the obstruction. However, regardless of the cause of obstruction all small bowel loops must be examined and nonviable segments resected. Criteria suggesting viability include normal pink color, presence of peristalsis, and arterial pulsation.

Laparoscopic adhesiolysis may be performed in carefully selected patients by surgeons skilled in this procedure. Generally, however, an open procedure is performed through an incision that is partly dictated by the location of scars from previous operations.

If the cause of the obstruction cannot be removed, as in case with infiltration of vital structures by cancer or in the case of diffuse carcinomatosis, an anastomosis between proximal small bowel and small or large bowel distal to the obstruction (bypass) may be the best procedure in these patients. In some cases, a stoma can be the only choice of treatment.

▶ Prognosis

Vast majority (more than 80%) of patients with adhesive SBO do not need an operation, since they improve with medical therapy. Among patients who require surgery, perioperative mortality rate for nonstrangulating obstruction is less than 5%; most of these deaths occur in elderly patients with significant comorbidities. Strangulating obstruction has a mortality rate of approximately 8% if surgery is performed within 36 hours of the onset of symptoms and 25% if operation is delayed beyond 36 hours.

Arung W et al. Pathophysiology and prevention of postoperative peritoneal adhesions. *World J Gastroenterol* 2011 Nov 7;17(41):4545-4553.

Branco BC et al. Systematic review and meta-analysis of the diagnostic and therapeutic role of water-soluble contrast agent in adhesive small bowel obstruction. *Br J Surg* 2010 Apr;97(4):470-478.

Ezer A et al. Clinical outcomes of manual bowel decompression (milking) in the mechanical small bowel obstruction: a prospective randomized clinical trial. *Am J Surg* 2012 Jan;203(1): 95-100.

Mullan CP et al. Small bowel obstruction. *AJR Am J Roentgenol* 2012 Feb;198(2):W105-W117.

O'Connor DB et al. The role of laparoscopy in the management of acute small-bowel obstruction: a review of over 2,000 cases. *Surg Endosc* 2012 Jan;26(1):12-17.

van der Wal JB et al. Adhesion prevention during laparotomy: long-term follow-up of a randomized clinical trial. *Ann Surg* 2011 Jun;253(6):1118-1121.

Xin L et al. Indications, detectability, positive findings, total enteroscopy, and complications of diagnostic double-balloon endoscopy: a systematic review of data over the first decade of use. *Gastrointest Endosc* 2011 Sep;74(3):563-570.

Zielinski MD et al. Small bowel obstruction-who needs an operation? A multivariate prediction model. *World J Surg* 2010 May;34(5):910-919.

REGIONAL ENTERITIS

▶ General Considerations

Crohn disease is a chronic inflammatory disease that commonly affects the small bowel, colon, rectum, and anus, but it can also involve the stomach, esophagus, and mouth. CD is a panintestinal condition which may affect any area from the mouth to the anus. The most commonly affected location is the terminal ileum and one-fifth of all patients have more than one intestinal segment affected simultaneously.

The United States, Canada, and Europe have the highest incidence of CD. The current estimated incidence of CD in the United States is approximately four new cases per year for every 100,000 persons, while the prevalence is much higher, between 80 and 150 cases per 100,000.

It is much less common in Asia, South America, and Japan, while accurate data regarding its incidence in Africa are lacking. The peak age for contracting CD is between 15 and 25 years. Familial clusters of disease are not uncommon, with a six- to tenfold increase in the risk of CD in first-degree relatives of those affected by CD or its sister ailment, ulcerative colitis. Although familial aggregations are common, the distribution within families does not indicate a pattern of simple Mendelian inheritance.

A. Etiology

The etiology of CD is not known. CD is an altered immune response that results in inflammation and destruction of intestinal tissues. If this altered immune response is the result of a primary dysfunction in the gut-related immune system or whether an unknown pathological trigger induces an otherwise normal immune system to overreact is still unclear. CD may occur in individuals with a genetic predisposition, while environmental triggers may start the pathological sequence that ultimately manifests as CD.

To date, even though an increase in intestinal permeability in both CD patients and their symptom-free first-degree relatives has been demonstrated no specific primary defect in the systemic or mucosal immune system has been identified. This may lead to an altered mucosal barrier function with abnormal interactions between the multitude of antigenic substrates normally found in the gut lumen and the immunocompetent tissue of the submucosa.

Concerning genetic predisposition, the *CARD15/NOD2* gene has been linked to susceptibility to CD. CARD15 is a gene product related to innate immunity and it is preferentially expressed to Paneth cells of the ileum. Nevertheless, the known mutations of CARD15 are neither necessary nor sufficient to contract the disease. Hence, it appears that the genetic relationship of *CARD15/NOD2* to CD is complex and still poorly understood.

The hypothesis that infectious agents may play a role, either directly as a primary cause of CD, or indirectly as a trigger to stimulate a defective immune system, has always found strength in the identification of noncaseating granulomas as the characteristic histopathologic lesion found in Crohn specimens, and in the isolation of *Mycobacterium paratuberculosis* from resected CD specimens. Nevertheless, even sensitive preliminary chain reaction studies have been unable to provide definitive evidence for the presence of *Mycobacterium paratuberculosis*-specific DNA in CD-affected segments of the bowel. Other infectious agents, including measles virus, non-pylori *Helicobacter* species, *Pseudomonas*, and *Listeria monocytogenes* have been studied, but none of them has been consistently associated with CD.

Although diet modification can ameliorate the symptoms of CD, no dietary factor has been identified as a cause of CD. Smoking, however, has been associated with the development of CD. In addition, smoking is known to exacerbate existing CD and can accelerate the recurrence of disease after resection.

B. Pathology

Histopathologic examination of CD typically demonstrates transmural inflammation characterized by multiple lymphoid aggregates in a thickened and edematous submucosa that can be found within the muscularis propria. Another typical microscopic feature of CD is the noncaseating granuloma. However, it is demonstrated in only 50% of resected specimens and is rarely detected on endoscopic biopsies. Additionally, the presence of granulomas does not correlate with disease activity.

Small mucosal ulcerations, called *aphthous ulcers*, are the earliest gross manifestations of CD. They appear as red spots or focal mucosal depressions, typically directly over submucosal lymphoid aggregates. As the inflammation progresses, the aphthous ulcers enlarge and become stellate. They then coalesce to form longitudinal mucosal ulcerations always along the mesenteric aspect of the bowel lumen. Further progression leads to a serpiginous network of linear ulcerations that surround islands of edematous mucosa producing the classic "cobblestone" appearance. Mucosal ulcerations may penetrate through the submucosa to form intramural channels that can bore deeply into the bowel wall and create sinuses, abscesses, or fistulas.

The inflammation of CD also involves the mesentery and regional lymph nodes such that the mesentery may become massively thickened. With early acute intestinal inflammation, the bowel wall is hyperemic and boggy. As the inflammation becomes chronic, fibrotic scarring develops and the bowel wall becomes thickened and leathery in texture.

▶ Clinical Findings

A. Symptoms and Signs

The clinical presentation and symptoms of CD depend on the involved segment, the pattern and the severity of disease, and the associated complications. The onset of CD is often insidious and many patients will experience some symptoms for months or even years before the diagnosis is made. The most common complaints are intermittent abdominal pain, bloating, diarrhea, nausea, vomiting, weight loss, and fever. Abdominal pain occurs in 90% of cases: when related to partial obstruction it is mostly postprandial and crampy in nature, while when it is from septic complications it is typically steady and associated with fever. Weight loss is usually related to food avoidance, but in severe cases weight loss may be the result of malabsorption. Symptoms can also be related to complications including abdominal mass, pneumaturia, perianal pain and swelling, or skin rash. Rarely some patients can experience a more sudden onset of pain in the right-lower quadrant, mimicking an acute appendicitis.

In patients suspected of having CD, a complete physical exam should include a thorough abdominal evaluation. In cases of ileal CD, tenderness is typically present in the right-lower quadrant and occasionally a palpable mass is present. The oral cavity should be examined for aphthous ulcers, while the presence of fistulas, abscesses, or enlarged skin tags should be assessed in the perianal area. A digital rectal examination should assess for the presence of anal strictures, fissures, and rectal mucosal ulcerations. The skin in the extremities should be examined for the presence of erythema nodosum and pyoderma gangrenosum.

▶ Patterns of Disease

Even though CD can be categorized into three general manifestations, such as stricturing, perforating, and inflammatory disease, these three classes do not represent truly distinct forms of the disease. It is typical that the same patient can present with more than one pattern even in the same segment of bowel. Nevertheless, one pattern tends to be predominant in most cases, determining the clinical presentation and affecting the therapeutic options.

A. Stricturing Pattern

Fibrotic scar tissue is the result of chronic inflammation of CD, and it constricts the intestinal lumen with cicatricial strictures often referred to as "fibrostenotic lesions." Patients with a stricturing pattern of disease generally develop partial or complete intestinal obstruction, and hence their symptoms are primarily obstructive in nature. Being the result of scar tissue, these strictures are not reversible with medical therapy and surgical intervention is often required.

B. Perforating Pattern

Perforating CD is characterized by the development of sinus tracts, fistulae, and abscesses. The sinus tracts penetrate through the muscularis propria and give rise to abscesses or to fistulas if they penetrate into surrounding structures. Inflammatory response around the advancing sinus tract typically results in adhesion to surrounding structures, therefore, free perforation with spillage of intestinal contents into the abdominal cavity is uncommon. Typically, perforating disease is accompanied by a degree of stricture formation, but the fistula or abscess generated by the perforating component of the disease dominates the clinical picture.

C. Inflammatory Pattern

The inflammatory pattern of CD is characterized by mucosal ulceration and bowel wall thickening. The edema that results from inflammation can lead to an adynamic segment of intestine and luminal narrowing. This pattern often gives rise to obstructive symptoms. Of the three patterns of disease, the inflammatory pattern is much more likely to respond to medical therapy.

Other common symptoms and findings include anorexia and weight loss. Patients may develop a palpable mass, usually located in the right-lower quadrant, related to an abscess or phlegmon in perforating disease or a thickened loop of intestine in obstructive disease. Evidence of fistulization to the skin, urinary bladder, or vagina may also be elicited with an accurate history and physical exam.

▶ Laboratory Findings

There is no specific laboratory test that is diagnostic for CD. The diagnosis is made by a thorough history and physical examination along with intestinal radiography and endoscopy. Advanced imaging studies such as CT scan or magnetic resonance imaging (MRI) can assess or detect some of the complications and manifestations of CD, but they are generally not useful in making the initial diagnosis of CD.

A. Imaging Studies

Small bowel follow-through or enteroclysis are the best means for assessing the small bowel for CD. The radiographic abnormalities are often distinctive. Mucosal granulations with ulceration and nodularity can be identified in the early stages of the disease. Thickening of the mucosal folds and edema of the bowel wall can be demonstrated as the disease progresses. With more advanced disease, cobblestoning becomes radiographically apparent. Small bowel contrast studies can also provide information regarding enlargement of the mesentery, as well as formation of an inflammatory mass or abscess demonstrated by a general mass effect separating and displacing contrast-filled loops of small intestine. Even though small bowel contrast studies can demonstrate some of the complications of CD, including high-grade strictures and fistulas, they may not identify all such lesions, including ileosigmoid and ileovesical fistulas. Additionally, small bowel studies may not demonstrate all the areas of disease with significant strictures. Small bowel radiographs can also help in assessing the extent of the disease by identifying the location and length of involved and uninvolved small bowel, and by recognizing whether the disease is continuous or discontinuous with skip lesions separated by areas of normal intestine. Experienced radiologists can also assess areas of luminal narrowing and determine if they are the result of acute inflammatory swelling or are the result of fibrostenotic scar tissue. Such a distinction provides valuable information regarding the value of medical therapy versus early surgical intervention, as inflammatory stenoses are likely to respond to medical therapy while fibrotic strictures are best treated with surgery.

Computed tomography findings of uncomplicated CD are nonspecific and routine CT is not necessary for the diagnosis of CD. CT, however, is very useful in identifying the complications associated with CD—thickened and dilated intestinal loops, inflammatory masses, abscesses, and hydronephrosis resulting from retroperitoneal fibrosis and ureteral narrowing (Figure 29–4). CT is also the most sensitive indicator of an enterovesical fistula as suggested by the presence of air within the urinary bladder. More recently cross-sectional imaging techniques have assumed an increasing role in the imaging of patients with CD. Computed tomography enterography (CTE) has been shown to have a higher sensitivity than barium small-bowel follow through. Based on these findings, CTE is often used combined with ileocolonoscopy as a first-line test for the diagnosis and staging of CD. CTE has several potential advantages over barium studies in the identification of fistulizing disease. CTE does not suffer from superimposition of bowel loops, and it displays the mesentery, retroperitoneum, and abdominal wall

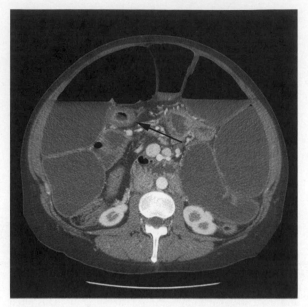

▲ **Figure 29–4.** CT scan showing a markedly thickened loop of distal ileum (arrow) causing obstruction of the more proximal small bowel in regional enteritis.

musculature, typically involved by fistulas. CTE can also readily identify sinus tracts and abscesses. However, recent concerns about radiation-induced cancer arising from medically related CT in young CD patients have encouraged the use of magnetic resonance enterography (MRE). MRE has the same advantages of CTE but does not require ionizing radiation.

B. Endoscopy

While upper endoscopy is useful in the diagnosis of mucosal lesions of the esophagus, stomach, and duodenum a colonoscopy often allows the evaluation of the terminal ileum.

C. Capsule Endoscopy

Capsule endoscopy can detect subtle mucosal lesions that may not be apparent on small bowel x-rays. The value of capsule endoscopy in the diagnosis of CD has been recently evaluated: the rate of abnormalities detected on capsule endoscopy is higher than that of CTE only for the subgroup of patients with known CD. The need for a preliminary small bowel contrast study to detect asymptomatic partial small-bowel obstruction before the capsule endoscopy and the lack of a clear advantage over other imaging studies, limits the utility of capsule endoscopy as a first-line test in CD, and perhaps reserve this study for those cases in which there is a substantial diagnostic uncertainty.

▶ Differential Diagnosis

The differential diagnosis includes irritable bowel syndrome, acute appendicitis, intestinal ischemia, pelvic inflammatory disease, endometriosis, and gynecological malignancies. Other disorders are radiation enteritis, *Yersinia* infections, intestinal injury from nonsteroidal anti-inflammatory agents, intestinal tuberculosis, and small bowel tumors.

When malignancy is suspected, resection should be undertaken to make the diagnosis certain. The exclusion of intestinal tuberculosis can be difficult, as the inflammation and strictures of the terminal ileum can occur very similarly to CD. A previous exposure to tuberculosis should be evaluated and purified protein derivative skin test should be performed, along with chest radiography. Even when the diagnosis of CD is certain, patients who coincidentally are found to also have latent tuberculosis should be treated in accordance with the American Thoracic Society guidelines prior to the initiation of immunosuppressive therapy for management of CD.

Intestinal injury from nonsteroidal anti-inflammatory drugs (NSAIDs) can result in focal enteritis with ulcerations and strictures. These manifestations can be very difficult to distinguish from CD of the small bowel, and often require resection or biopsy to confirm the diagnosis.

▶ Treatment

A. Medical

Long-lasting symptomatic relief while avoiding excessive morbidity is the goal of medical treatment of CD. Even though CD cannot be cured by medical treatment long periods of disease control can be obtained avoiding a surgical intervention. Medical treatment for each individual is based on the course of the disease, the clinical presentation and associated complications.

Corticosteroids are the most effective agents for controlling acute exacerbations of CD, but their use is limited due to the risk of serious side effects, including diabetes, osteoporosis, cataracts, osteonecrosis, myopathy, psychosis, opportunistic infections, and adrenal suppression, that are related to both the dose and the duration of steroid therapy. The majority of patients with active small bowel CD will experience clinical remission with a short course of oral prednisone given in a dose between 0.25 and 0.5 mg/kg/d. For patients unable to take oral medications, methylprednisolone can be administered in the adult at doses of 40-60 mg given as a daily infusion.

The *aminosalicylates* include sulfasalazine and 5-aminosalicylic acid (5-ASA) derivatives. They inhibit leukotriene production by inhibiting 5-lipooxygenase activity and the production of inter-leukin-1 and tumor necrosis factor (TNF). Aminosalicylates are effective in the treatment of mild to moderate CD. 5-ASA given in a controlled-release preparation is also effective as maintenance therapy to prevent recurrence after a flare of disease has been effectively managed either medically or surgically.

Aminosalicylates come in a variety of preparations, each designed to deliver the drug in a topical fashion to the affected bowel segments. For instance, Asacol is 5-aminosalicylic acid contained within a pH-dependent resin that releases the drug in the terminal ileum and colon where the pH is greater than 7.0. Pentasa is 5-aminosalicylic acid contained within ethylcellulose-coated microgranules that slowly releases the active compound throughout the entire small bowel and colon. *Azathioprine* and *6 mercaptopurine* (6-MP) are immunosuppressive agents that inhibit cytotoxic T-cell and natural killer cell function. These agents are effective in treating mild to moderate CD. Azathioprine given at 2.0-2.5 mg/kg/d or 6-MP in doses of 1.0-1.5 mg/kg/d will result in a 50%-60% response rate in patients with active CD. Both 6-MP and azathioprine are also effective in maintaining remission following surgery or successful medical management.

Infliximab is a chimeric mouse-human monoclonal antibody to TNF that is a proinflammatory cytokine that may be important in the pathophysiology of CD. Infliximab binds to both free and membrane-bound TNF, and prevents TNF from binding to its cell surface receptors. Clinical trials have demonstrated an 80% response rate with a single dose of infliximab. It is important to note that the doses and dosing intervals of infliximab must be individualized, but a typical regimen would include 5 mg/kg of infliximab given IV at weeks 0, 2, and 6, with a dose of 5 mg/kg every 8 weeks thereafter. Because Infliximab is a potent immunosuppressive agent concerns have been raised about the risk for poor wound healing and postoperative septic complications. Nevertheless, current available data on the perioperative risks associated with infliximab does not seem to support this hypothesis.

Other agents that are used with varying success in the treatment of CD include methotrexate, metronidazole, cyclosporine, tacrolimus, and thalidomide.

B. Surgical Therapy

Similarly to medical treatment, the goal of surgical treatment of CD is to provide long-lasting symptomatic relief while avoiding excessive morbidity. Like medical treatment, surgery should be considered palliative. Therefore, treatment of complications and palliation of symptoms while avoiding excessive resection of small bowel should be the main aims of surgical treatment.

To avoid excessive loss of small bowel, nonresectional techniques such as strictureplasty may be required. In addition, optimal surgical therapy should be the resection of the only areas of severe and symptomatic CD, leaving behind segments of small bowel affected by mild but asymptomatic CD based on the high risks of recurrence and repeated operations.

C. Indications for Surgery

1. Failure of medical treatment—The failure to respond to medical treatment, the inability to tolerate effective therapy are the most common indications for surgical treatment of CD, as the occurrence of complications related to the medical treatment or the progression of disease while on maximal medical treatment. Some patients may respond to the initial medical therapy only to rapidly relapse with tapering of the medical treatment. For example, some patients respond well to steroid therapy, but become steroid-dependent as tapering of the steroid dose results in recurrent symptoms. Due to the severe complications that are virtually inevitable with prolonged steroid treatment, surgery is warranted if the patient cannot be weaned from systemic steroids within 3-6 months.

2. Intestinal obstruction—Partial or complete intestinal obstruction is a common indication for operation. The clinical presentation of chronic partial SBO is much more typical than complete obstruction, and postprandial cramps, abdominal distension, borborygmi, and weight loss are common symptoms. To avoid them, many patients restrict the diet to soft foods or even liquids. In case of partial obstruction primarily due to acute inflammation and bowel wall thickening, initial medical therapy is warranted. If, however, the obstructive symptoms are secondary to high-grade fibrostenotic lesions, surgery is indicated because medical treatment will not reverse these lesions.

When complete intestinal obstruction occurs, initial conservative treatment consists of nasogastric decompression and intravenous hydration along with administration of intravenous steroids. This treatment leads to decompression of acutely distended and edematous bowel, and in most cases, to resolution of the complete obstruction. However, even patients with complete resolution of the acute obstruction after the initial conservative treatment are at high risk for recurrent episodes of obstruction and are best managed with elective surgery once adequate decompression and resuscitation is achieved. If the obstruction fails to respond to appropriate conservative treatment, then surgery is required. In these situations, a high index of suspicion for small bowel cancer as the cause of the obstruction is mandatory, as obstructions from cancers do not respond to bowel decompression and steroid treatment.

3. Fistulas—Intestinal fistulas occur in one third of CD patients. However, the presence of an intestinal fistula is not in and of itself an indication for surgery. In general, it is the primary indication for surgery if the fistula is in connection with the genitourinary tract, or if their drainage causes personal embarrassment and discomfort (enterocutaneous and enterovaginal fistulas), or if a bypass causing intestinal malabsorption is created.

Fistulas can be classified according to anatomic site, characteristics of the tract (simple vs. complex), and volume of output (high vs. low). A low volume output is less than 200 mL/24 h, while a high volume output is more than 500 mL/24 h.

4. Ileosigmoid fistulas—Ileosigmoid fistula is a common complication of perforating CD of the terminal ileum. Typically, the inflamed terminal ileum adheres to the sigmoid colon that is otherwise healthy. Most ileosigmoid fistulas are small and asymptomatic. These ileosigmoid fistulas do not in and of themselves require operative management. On the other hand, large ileosigmoid fistulas can result in bypass of the intestinal contents from the terminal ileum to the distal colon and thus give rise to debilitating diarrhea. Such symptomatic fistulas should be managed surgically, as they often fail to respond to medical therapy.

More than half of the ileosigmoid fistulas from CD are recognized intraoperatively. Ileosigmoid fistulas can be managed by simple division of the fistulous adhesion and resection of the ileal disease. The defect in the sigmoid colon is then debrided and simple closure is undertaken. In about 25% of cases, resection of the sigmoid colon is needed, particularly when primary closure of the fistula is at risk for poor healing. This is the case when either the sigmoid is also involved in CD, when the fistulous opening is particularly large, or when there is extensive fibrosis extending along the sigmoid colon. Also, fistulous tracts that enter the sigmoid colon in proximity to the mesentery can be difficult to close and often require resection and primary anastomosis.

5. Ileovesical fistula—Ileovesical fistulae occur in approximately 5% of CD patients. Although hematuria and fecaluria are virtually diagnostic of ileovesical fistula, these symptoms are absent in almost 30% of cases. Air within the bladder, as noted on CT scan, is often the best indirect evidence for the presence of an enterovesical fistula, while small bowel x-rays, cystogram, and cystoscopy often do not detect the fistula. An ileovesical fistula is an indicator of complex fistulizing disease, as most ileovesical fistulas occur along with other enteric fistulae.

The necessity for surgery for ileovesical fistula is controversial. While it is not mandatory to operate on all cases of enterovesical fistulas, surgery is warranted to avoid deterioration of renal function with recurrent infections or if symptoms persist in spite of appropriate medical therapy.

Surgical treatment of ileovesical fistulae requires resection of the ileal disease with closure of the bladder defect. Most ileovesical fistulas involve the dome of the bladder, and thus debridement and primary closure can be accomplished without risk of injury to the trigone. Decompression of the bladder with an indwelling Foley catheter should be continued postoperatively until the bladder is confidently healed without leaks. A cystogram taken postoperatively is useful to confirm the seal of the bladder repair, before removing the Foley catheter.

6. Enterovaginal and enterocutaneous fistulas—These are rare fistulas caused by perforating small bowel disease draining through the vaginal stump in a female who has previously undergone a hysterectomy or through the abdominal wall, usually at the site of a previous scar. These fistulas often require surgical intervention because they cause physical discomfort and personal embarrassment. Surgical treatment requires resection of the small bowel disease. The vaginal cuff does not need to be closed; the chronic infection along the abdominal wall fistulous tract requires debridement and wide drainage to allow healing by secondary intention.

7. Abscess—Intra-abdominal CD abscesses tend to have an indolent course with modest fever, abdominal pain, and leukocytosis. In up to 30% of cases preoperative clinical signs of localized infection are absent and the abscesses are discovered only at the time of operation. When an abscess is suspected or an abdominal mass is palpated, a CT scan should be obtained, as 50% of tender intra-abdominal masses will harbor an abscess collection within. The CT scan can detect most chronic abscesses and can also delineate the size and location of the abscess as well as the relationship of the abscess to critical structures such as the ureters, duodenum, and the inferior vena cava.

In the majority of cases, abscesses are very small collections contained within the area of diseased small bowel and its mesentery. In the case of small intraloop or intramesenteric abscesses, resection of the involved bowel segment and its mesentery often extirpates the abscess such that drains are not necessary and primary anastomosis can be performed without risk.

Large abscesses are best managed with CT-guided percutaneous drainage. However, abscess drained percutaneously is very likely to recur or result in an enterocutaneous fistula, and surgical resection is often advised even after successful drainage. Such a fistula may spontaneously close or it may persist and the intestine may continue to be a source of sepsis. With successful drainage of the abscess, the sepsis often clears well enough that it can be tempting to try to manage the disease without subsequent surgery. In the absence of symptoms, initial non-operative management after successful percutaneous drainage can be undertaken in carefully selected patients. If drainage through the fistula continues, surgical resection of the affected segment of intestine becomes necessary.

8. Perforation—Free perforation is a rare complication of CD occurring in less than 1% of patients because the chronic progressive inflammation of CD usually leads to adhesions with adjacent structures, and it is an obvious indication for urgent operation with resection of the diseased segment and exteriorization of the proximal bowel as an end ileostomy. The diagnosis of free perforation is made by detecting a sudden change in the patient's symptoms along with the development of the physical findings of peritonitis or the identification of free intraperitoneal air as demonstrated on plain x-rays or CT scan. The use of immunosuppressants and glucocorticosteroids can blunt many of the physical findings of acute perforation; therefore the index of suspicion for perforation must be higher in immunocompromised patients.

Creation of a primary anastomosis even with a proximal protecting loop ileostomy carries a high risk of anastomotic breakdown and should be avoided. Primary closure of the perforation should never be attempted, as sutures will not be able to approximate the edges of the perforated, edematous, and diseased bowel in a satisfactory and tension-free way and the presence of a distal intestinal stenosis or partial obstruction will cause an increase in the intraluminal pressure at the level of the local repair with subsequent dehiscence.

9. Hemorrhage—Hemorrhage is an uncommon complication from small bowel CD. Angiography in the presence of brisk bleeding leads to localization of the site of bleeding. Bleeding from small bowel tends to be indolent with episodic or chronic bleeding requiring intermittent transfusions, but rarely requires emergent surgery. However, because the risk of recurrent bleeding is high, elective resection of the areas of CD is recommended. Finally, risk for bleeding from peptic ulcer disease is increased in patients, particularly in those receiving corticosteroids.

10. Cancer or suspicion of cancer—The presence of CD increases the risk of adenocarcinoma of the small bowel. The diagnosis of adenocarcinoma of the small bowel is difficult because symptoms and radiographic findings can be similar to those of the underlying CD. Male patients, patients with long-standing disease and patients with defunctionalized segments of bowel appear to be at increased risk for small bowel adenocarcinoma. For this reason, bypass surgery should be avoided for CD of the small intestine and defunctionalized rectal stumps should either be restored to their function or excised.

Adenocarcinoma of the small intestine should be suspected in any patient with long-standing disease whose symptoms of obstruction progress after a lengthy quiescent period.

11. Growth retardation—Growth retardation occurs in a quarter of children affected by CD. Although steroid treatment may delay growth in children, the major cause of growth retardation in CD patients is due to the malnutrition associated with active intestinal disease.

D. Surgical Options

1. Intestinal resection—Intestinal resection with anastomosis is the most common surgical procedure performed for the treatment of small bowel CD. In most cases of CD only limited resections are required with no risk for short bowel syndrome. Only grossly apparent disease should be resected, as wider resections do not improve the surgical outcomes. Grossly normal resection margins with microscopic evidence for CD activity are not associated with early recurrence or other complications. Therefore, intraoperative frozen section of the resection margins is not necessary.

The extent of mesenteric dissection does not affect the long-term results. Division of the thickened mesentery of small bowel CD can be the most challenging aspect of the procedure, as identification and dissection of individual mesenteric vessels is often not feasible. A common technique consists of the application of overlapping clamps on either side of the intended line of transection. The mesentery is then divided between the clamps and the tissue contained within the clamps is suture ligated. In severe cases, a vascular clamp may be used at the root of the small bowel mesentery to obtain proximal control: mattress sutures may then be need to be applied to the cut edge of the mesentery to control bleeding. Even when tissue welding devices such as the LigaSure device are used, mattress sutures in the mesentery are commonly needed for complete hemostasis.

2. Anastomosis—There is no consensus regarding the optimal technique for intestinal anastomosis in CD. Recurrent CD after resection of terminal ileum is most likely to occur at the ileocolonic anastomosis or at the pre-anastomotic ileum. It has been proposed that large caliber anastomoses require a longer period to stricture down to a critical diameter that becomes symptomatic. The argument is made that a longer side-to-side anastomosis may be beneficial over an end-to-end or end-to-side anastomosis. To date, however, clinical data do not indicate a benefit for one particular intestinal configuration over another. Intestinal anastomosis for CD cases can be fashioned with a stapling device or may be hand sutured. Under selective conditions, small bowel anastomotic dehiscence rates is under 1%. In the presence of sepsis, severe scarring, malnutrition, or recent treatment with methotrexate or infliximab, it may be wise to protect the anastomosis with a proximal loop stoma or to forego the anastomosis altogether and bring out an end stoma at the point of resection.

3. Bypass Procedures—Initially conceived to bypass an area of stricture or obstruction, the use of bypass procedures was eventually extended to CD complicated by septic complications. Increased experience with bypass procedures revealed that patients with persistent disease are at higher risk of persistent sepsis, and eventually neoplastic transformation. Therefore, bypass procedures were supplanted by limited intestinal resection as the main surgical option in the late 1960s in all intestinal districts except the duodenum, where a simple side-to-side retrocolic gastrojejunostomy adequately relieves the obstructive symptoms. With increased experience in the performance of strictureplasty, duodenal disease is nowadays more and more commonly handled with strictureplasties.

4. Strictureplasty—Strictureplasties are best performed when resection would otherwise result in loss of a long segment of bowel with an increased risk for short bowel syndrome, including cases of stricturing disease involving long segments of bowel and patients with multiple prior resections. They are also indicated as a simpler alternative to resection in case of short recurrent disease at a previous ileocolic or enteroenteric anastomosis.

There is increased evidence that the acuity of the disease decreases at the site of the strictureplasty and the disease becomes quiescent, maybe in correlation with a simultaneous restoration of absorptive function.

The most commonly performed strictureplasty is the Heinecke–Mikulicz strictureplasty, that is appropriate for short segment strictures of 2-5 cm in length. A longitudinal incision is made along the antimesenteric border of the stricture extending for 1-2 cm into the normal elastic bowel on either side of the stricture. Once the enterotomy is made, the area of the stricture should be closely examined to rule out a malignancy. The longitudinal enterotomy of the Heinecke–Mikulicz strictureplasty is then closed in a transverse fashion with either single- or double-layered sutures.

The Finney strictureplasty can be used for strictures up to 15 cm in length. The strictured segment is folded onto itself in a U-shape, and a row of seromuscular sutures is placed between the two arms of the U. A longitudinal U-shaped enterotomy is then made paralleling the row of sutures. The mucosal surface is examined and biopsies are taken as necessary. In essence, the Finney is a short side-to-side functional anastomosis. A very long Finney strictureplasty may result in a functional bypass with a large lateral diverticulum that, in theory, could be at risk for bacterial overgrowth and the blind loop syndrome. However, this theoretical concern has not been observed in clinical practice.

Repeated Heinecke–Mikulicz or Finney strictureplasties to manage multiple strictures should be separated from each other by at least 5 cm, in order to avoid excessive tension on each suture line.

Patients with long segment stricturing disease and multiple strictures grouped close together are best managed with a side-to-side isoperistaltic strictureplasty, also called Michelassi strictureplasty. The segment of stricturing disease is divided at its midpoint. The proximal and distal ends are then drawn onto each other in a side-to-side fashion. Division of some of the mesenteric vascular arcades facilitates the positioning of the two limbs over each other. The proximal and distal loops are then sutured together with a layer of interrupted seromuscular sutures. A longitudinal enterotomy is then made along both of the loops. The intestinal ends are spatulated to provide a smoothly tailored fit to the ultimate closure of the strictureplasty. The outer suture line is reinforced with an interior row of either inter-rupted or running full-thickness sutures. This inner suture line is continued anteriorly. The anterior closure is then reinforced with an outer layer of interrupted seromuscular sutures to complete the strictureplasty. In appropriately selected patients, perioperative morbidity from stricture-plasty appears to be similar to that of resection and primary anastomosis. Specifically, intestinal suture line dehiscence appears to be uncommon with any of the described stricture-plasty techniques. The most common postoperative com-plication directly related to strictureplasty is hemorrhage from the strictureplasty site, in up to 9% of cases. Usually, the gastrointestinal hemorrhage following strictureplasty is minor and can be managed conservatively with transfusions alone. Rarely, a reoperation to control hemorrhage after strictureplasty is necessary. It is by now also well established that strictureplasty techniques provide excellent long-term symptomatic relief which is comparable to resections with anastomosis.

5. Laparoscopy—Most CD patients are well suited for laparoscopy. They are usually young, otherwise healthy, and interested in undergoing an operation that involves minimal scarring, since they are facing the risk of multiple major abdominal operations in their lifetime.

The indications for laparoscopic surgery for CD should not differ from conventional open surgery as described before. Contraindications to a laparoscopic approach include patients who are critically ill and unable to tolerate the pneumoperitoneum due to hypotension or hypercarbia, patients with extensive intra-abdominal sepsis (abscess, free perforation, or complex fistula), and difficulty in identifying the anatomy (previous surgery, obesity, or adhesions). The same variety of surgical procedures described earlier can be performed laparoscopically.

MANAGEMENT CROHN DISEASE OF THE DUODENUM

Primary CD of the duodenum almost always manifests with stricturing disease that can be managed by strictureplasty or with bypass procedures, while resection of the duodenum for CD is almost never required. When CD fistulas involve the duodenum, it is always the result of disease within a distal segment of the small bowel that fistulizes into an otherwise normal duodenum. Heinecke–Mikulicz stricture-plasties can be safely performed in the first, second, and proximal third portion of the duodenum, while strictures of the last portion of the duodenum are better handled with a Finney strictureplasty constructed by creating an enteroen-terostomy between the fourth portion of the duodenum and the first loop of the jejunum.

If the duodenal stricture is lengthy or the tissues around the stricture are too rigid or unyielding, then a strictureplasty should not be performed and an intestinal bypass procedure

should be undertaken. The most common bypass procedure performed for duodenal CD is a side-to-side retrocolic gastrojejunostomy. This procedure effectively relieves the symptoms of duodenal obstruction related to CD strictures, but carries a high risk for stomal ulcerations. To lessen the likelihood of ulcerations forming at the anastomosis, it has been recommended that a selective vagotomy be performed along with the gastrojejunostomy in order to reduce the risk of vagotomy-related diarrhea. If only the third or fourth por-tions of the duodenum are involved by the structuring CD, a Roux-en-Y duodenojejunostomy to the proximal duodenum is preferred over a gastrojejunostomy, having the Roux-en-Y duodenojejunostomy the advantage of bypassing strictures and eliminating the risk of acid-induced marginal ulceration and the need for vagotomy.

Most of these duodenal fistulas are small in caliber and asymptomatic, but larger fistulas may shunt the duodenal contents to the distal small bowel resulting in malabsorp-tion and diarrhea. In most cases, duodenoenteric fistulas are identified with preoperative small bowel radiography; however, many are discovered only intraoperatively. Most duodenal fistulas are located away from the pancreatico-duodenal margin, and thus these fistulas can be managed by resection of the primary CD with primary closure of the duodenal defect. In case of larger fistulas or fistulas that are involved with a large degree of inflammation closure with a Roux-en-Y duodenojejunostomy or with a jejunal serosal patch may be required.

▶ Prognosis

The risk for recurrence after surgery is high in CD patients. Most cases of histological or endoscopically detected recur-rences, however, do not produce symptoms of CD. For this reason, histological or endoscopic evidence of recurrent dis-ease are not typically used as a guide for clinical management.

The development of symptoms related to recurrent CD activity is the most commonly applied definition of disease recurrence, as it is the recurrence of symptoms that has the most relevance to the patient. The onset of symptoms of recurrent CD is often insidious and the severity of symptoms varies greatly. A CD Activity Index (CDAI) greater than 150 is generally accepted as defining clinical recurrence. Once symptoms suggestive of recurrent disease occur, it is necessary to carry out radiological and endoscopic tests to confirm that the symptoms are in fact related to CD.

The clearest end point as a definition of recurrence is the need for reoperation. While reoperation is the most precise definition of recurrence, even this standard does not allow for accurate and reproducible comparisons between series, as some centers may submit patients to surgery earlier than other centers.

Reported crude and cumulative recurrence rates vary greatly. Symptomatic recurrence occurs in about 60% of patients at 5 years and recurrences increase with time such that at 20 years clinical recurrence can occur in between 75% and 95% of cases. Reports of surgical recurrence rates range from 10% to 30% at 5 years, from 20% to 45% at 10 years, and from 50% to 70% at 20 years. Recurrent CD is most likely to occur in proximity to the location of the previously resected intestinal segment, typically at the anastomosis and preanastomotic bowel, in particular in case of terminal ileal disease. Additionally, the length of small bowel involved with recurrent disease parallels the length of disease originally resected. Also, to a lesser degree of concordance, stenotic disease tends to recur as stenotic disease and perforating disease tends to recur as perforating disease.

While many factors that may influence the risk of recurrence have been studied, the cumulative literature has validated very few as true risk factors. Cigarette smoking has a significant effect on the clinical course of CD. Smoking not only exacerbates existing CD, but also has been identified as a risk factor for the development of CD, and for endoscopic, symptomatic, and surgical recurrence. While the mechanism by which smoking results in exacerbation of CD is not known, the risk from smoking appeared to be dose-related with heavy smokers being at higher risk, and reversible. There is concern that NSAIDs may exacerbate the activity of both ulcerative colitis and CD, but there are not conclusive data.

The risk for recurrent disease can be reduced with postoperative maintenance therapy. The most common agents are controlled-release 5-aminosalicylic acid and 6-mercaptopurine. Maintenance with 5-ASA is associated with few side effects, but up to sixteen pills have to be taken daily. 6-Mercaptopurine is less expensive and is taken on a once-daily basis. Additionally, 6-MP may be more effective in diminishing the risk of recurrence. 6-MP, however, is associated with potential bone marrow suppression, so that patients on 6-MP maintenance must be followed with periodic blood cell counts.

Al-Hawary M et al. A new look at Crohn's disease: novel imaging techniques. *Curr Opin Gastroenterol* 2012 Jul;28(4):334-340. Review.

Campbell L et al. Comparison of conventional and nonconventional strictureplasties in Crohn's disease: a systematic review and meta-analysis. *Dis Colon Rectum* 2012 Jun;55(6):714-726. Review.

Choy PY et al. Stapled versus handsewn methods for ileocolic anastomoses. *Cochrane Database Syst Rev* 2011 Sep 7;(9):CD004320. Review.

Cunningham MF et al. Postsurgical recurrence of ileal Crohn's disease: an update on risk factors and intervention points to a central role for impaired host-microflora homeostasis. *World J Surg* 2010 Jul;34(7):1615-1626. Review.

Danese S. New therapies for inflammatory bowel disease: from the bench to the bedside. *Gut* 2012 Jun;61(6):918-932. Epub 2011 Nov 23. Review.

Fichera A. Crohn's disease: How modern is the management of fistulizing disease? *Nat Rev Gastroenterol Hepatol* 2009 Sep;6(9):511-512.

Fichera A. Laparoscopic treatment of Crohn's disease. *World J Surg* 2011 Jul;35(7):1500-1504.

Kopylov U et al. Anti-tumor necrosis factor and postoperative complications in Crohn's disease: systematic review and meta-analysis. *Inflamm Bowel Dis* 2012 Dec;18(12):2404-2413.

Maggiori L et al. How i do it: side-to-side isoperistaltic strictureplasty for extensive Crohn's disease. *J Gastrointest Surg* 2012 Oct;16(10):1976-1980

Turner D et al. Maintenance of remission in inflammatory bowel disease using omega-3 fatty acids (fish oil): a systematic review and meta-analyses. *Inflamm Bowel Dis* 2011 Jan;17(1):336-345.

SMALL INTESTINE FISTULAS

► General Considerations

Fistulas are an abnormal connection between two epithelial lined organs and while enterocutaneous fistulas (ECF) may form spontaneously as a result of disease, about 80% are complications of surgical procedures (anastomotic dehiscence or injury to bowel during dissection). Fistulas are particularly prone to develop when the surgeon encounters extensive adhesions, inflamed intestine, radiation enteritis, a malnourished patient, or emergency procedures.

► Clinical Findings

A. Symptoms and Signs

Postoperative fistula formation is heralded by fever, abdominal pain, and distention. Frequently a wound infection is recognized and drained 7-10 days postoperatively with subsequent discharge of enteric contents through the abdominal incision. Spontaneous fistulas from neoplasms or inflammatory disease usually develop in a more indolent manner. ECF are often associated with abscesses, which often drain incompletely with fistulization, so that persistent sepsis is a common feature. Intestinal fluid escaping through the fistula may severely excoriate the skin and abdominal wall tissues. Persistent sepsis and difficulty in nourishing the patient contribute to rapid weight loss.

B. Laboratory Findings

Routine laboratory tests reflect the severity of deficits in red cell mass, plasma volume, and electrolytes. Hypokalemia is the most common electrolyte abnormality. Ongoing losses may be significant especially with high output fistulas necessitating serial measurement of serum electrolytes. Leukocytosis due to sepsis and hemo-concentration is common.

C. Imaging Studies

The goals of imaging are to detect concurrent abdominal pathology and to characterize the fistula. Contrast studies with contrast medium administered orally, per rectum, or through the fistula (fistulogram) delineates the abnormal anatomy, including intrinsic bowel disease, and demonstrates the location and number of fistulas, the length and course of fistula tracts, associated abscess cavities, and the presence of distal obstruction. Radiologists can manipulate catheters into tracts and provide detailed diagnostic information; this procedure may also be therapeutic (see later). CT scans, endoscopy, and other special studies may be indicated in certain individuals.

Complications

Fluid and electrolyte losses, malnutrition, and sepsis contribute to multiple-organ failure and death unless effective therapy is instituted promptly.

Treatment

The initial management of an ECF involves recognition of the fistula, control of sepsis, resuscitation, local wound care, and nutritional optimization. A systematic approach combining diagnostic, supportive, and operative procedures is essential in the management of patients with fistulas (Table 29–2). The proper timing of intervention is as critical in few other conditions.

A. Fluid and Electrolyte Resuscitation

Many fistula patients are profoundly depleted of intravascular and interstitial volume especially if the fistula is large, if it is proximal, or if there is partial or complete intestinal obstruction distal to the fistula and correction of hypovolemia and electrolyte imbalances are the first priority. Central venous pressure, urine output, and skin turgor are guides to the progress of volume resuscitation. Fluid and electrolyte resuscitation can usually be accomplished within the first day or two. Subsequent maintenance of homeostasis depends on accurately measuring losses and replacing them.

Table 29–2. Treatment of fistulas.

First
Restore blood volume and begin correction of fluids and electrolyte imbalance.
Drain accessible abscesses.
Control fistula and measure losses.
Begin nutritional support.

Second
Delineate anatomy of fistulas by radiographic studies.

Third
Maintain caloric intake of 2000–3000 kcal or more per day, depending on status of nutrition and energy expenditure.
Drain abscesses as they appear.

Fourth
Operate if fistula fails to close.

B. Control of Fistula

Fistulous effluent must be collected to avoid excoriation of skin and abdominal wall tissues and to record volume losses. An ostomy appliance or pouch should be placed around the fistula and needs to be tailored based on the characteristics of the fistula. Alternatively, a catheter inserted by a radiologist under x-ray guidance may work best. In selected cases, a vacuum-assisted wound management device can be used to control fistula drainage and accelerate closure of the fistula. The assistance of a skilled and experienced wound care and/or enterostomal nurse is indispensable.

C. Control of Sepsis

Abscesses should be drained as soon as they are diagnosed. While therapy with broad-spectrum antibiotics may be necessary to control infection, is not a substitute for proper management of abscesses. Most contained abscesses can be drained percutaneously with CT or ultrasound guidance. Drainage catheters should be left in place until the abscess cavity has resolved which can be confirmed with a drain study once drainage has ceased. A drain study can also demonstrate the presence of persistent communication between the small bowel and the fistula. Free drainage of enteral contents into the abdominal cavity will likely cause peritonitis necessitating an emergent laparotomy.

D. Delineation of Fistula

Radiographic contrast studies (mentioned previously) should be obtained as soon as feasible.

E. Nutrition

Adequate nutrition and control of sepsis make the difference between survival and death for these patients. A useful general rule is to avoid oral intact during the initial stage of treatment. Nasogastric suction may be necessary temporarily. As soon as fluid, electrolytes, and vitamin abnormalities are corrected, parenteral nutrition should be instituted via a central intravenous catheter.

For many patients, total parenteral nutrition is the principal exogenous source of calories and nitrogen until the fistula heals or is closed surgically. For patients with low-output or distal fistulas, the enteral route for nutrition is preferred, and elemental or polymeric diets can be delivered into the distal gut in some patients with proximal fistulas.

F. Other Measures

H_2 receptor antagonists and proton pump inhibitors are useful adjuncts in patients with proximal fistulas. By reducing gastric acid secretion, fistula output is decreased and fluid and electrolyte management is simplified. Somatostatin analogs decrease fistula output and may accelerate fistula closure.

G. Operation

About 30% of fistulas close spontaneously with proper medical management. CD, irradiated bowel, cancer, foreign body, distal obstruction, extensive disruption of intestinal continuity, and a short (< 2 cm) fistula tract are associated with failure of fistulas to heal. Fibrin glue has been effective in some small bowel fistulas; in particular, it may be considered in complicated patients with a history of a hostile abdomen. Treatment may be successful if the fistula is long and the output is low. If they are going to heal spontaneously, fistulas usually close within 5-6 weeks after eradication of infection and institution of adequate nutritional support. Patients who fail 6 weeks of nonoperative management will often require surgical intervention. Serum levels of short-turnover proteins, particularly transferrin, might be useful in predicting which patients are unlikely to close their fistulas. The operation should be postponed, however, until one can predict that the phase of dense adhesions associated with ECFs has resolved and nutrition is optimized typically at least 3 months after the last operation. The fistulous segment should be resected, associated obstruction relieved, and continuity reestablished by a functional end-to-end anastomosis.

► Prognosis

The plan of management outlined earlier results in survival rates of 80%-95% in patients with external fistulas. Uncontrolled sepsis is the chief cause of death.

Coughlin S et al. Somatostatin analogues for the treatment of enterocutaneous fistulas: a systematic review and meta-analysis. *World J Surg* 2012 May;36(5):1016-1029.
Lee Jk et al. Radiographic and endoscopic diagnosis and treatment of enterocutaneous fistulas. *Clin Colon Rectal Surg* 2010 Sep;23(3):149-160.
Martinez JL et al. Factors predictive of recurrence and mortality after surgical repair of enterocutaneous fistula. *J Gastrointest Surg* 2012 Jan;16(1):156-163.
Visschers RG et al. Guided Treatment Improves Outcome of Patients with Enterocutaneous Fistulas. *World J Surg* 2012 Jun 6. [Epub ahead of print]

BLIND LOOP SYNDROME

The normal concentration of bacteria in the small intestine is about 105/mL. Mechanisms that limit bacterial populations include the continual flow of luminal contents, gastric acidity, local effects of immunoglobulins, and the prevention of reflux of colonic contents by the ileocecal valve. Disturbance of any of these mechanisms can lead to bacterial overgrowth and blind loop syndrome. Strictures, diverticula, fistulas, and defunctionalized segments of bowel allow bacterial proliferation.

This entity is rare and clinical manifestations include steatorrhea, diarrhea, abdominal pain, vitamin deficiency, neurologic symptoms, anemia, and weight loss. Steatorrhea is the consequence of bacterial deconjugation and dehydroxylation of bile salts in the proximal small bowel. Deconjugated bile salts have a higher critical micellar concentration, and micelle formation is inadequate to solubilize ingested fat in preparation for absorption. The presence of partially digested triglycerides in the distal ileum inhibits jejunal motility; nevertheless, the unabsorbed fatty acids enter the colon, where they increase net secretion of water and electrolytes, and diarrhea results. Hypocalcemia occurs because calcium is bound to unabsorbed fatty acids in the intestinal lumen. Macrocytic anemia is secondary to malabsorption of vitamin B_{12}, largely because it is consumed by anaerobic bacteria. Vitamin B_{12} deficiency also causes neurologic symptoms due to demyelination of the posterior and lateral spinal columns. Malabsorption of carbohydrate and protein is due partly to bacterial catabolism and partly to impaired absorption of these nutrients because of direct damage to the small intestinal mucosa. All of these mechanisms contribute to malnutrition.

Quantitative culture of upper intestinal aspirates is valuable if properly performed; bacterial counts of more than 10^5/mL are generally abnormal. Endoscopic biopsies of the duodenum can be helpful in patients with suspected small intestinal malabsorption. Laboratory studies reveal impaired absorption of orally administered vitamin B_{12} (Schilling test), D-xylose, and ^{14}C triolein.

Surgical treatment of the underlying disease is carried out whenever possible. If there is no a surgical cause of blind loop syndrome, treatment consists of broad-spectrum antibiotics and medications to control diarrhea. It may be necessary to use different antibiotics in sequence, guided by culture results and response to therapy. Damage to enterocytes appears to be reversible with treatment. Octreotide (somatostatin analog) may reduce bacterial overgrowth and improve abdominal symptoms in patients with scleroderma, according to a recent report.

Bures J et al. Small intestinal bacterial overgrowth syndrome. *World J Gastroenterol* 2010 Jun 28;16(24):2978-2990.
Rana SV, Bhardwaj SB. Small intestinal bacterial overgrowth. *Scand J Gastroenterol* 2008;43:1030.

ACUTE MESENTERIC ISCHEMIA

► General Considerations

Acute mesenteric ischemia (AMI) is a life-threatening clinical condition if not diagnosed promptly and treated adequately. Despite diagnostic and therapeutic advances, morbidity and mortality associated with AMI remains high. A high index of suspicion for this disease is essential since the clinical presentation is often nonspecific. AMI results from four main processes: (1) arterial embolism (50%) most commonly in patients with previous myocardial infarction or atrial fibrillation; (2) acute arterial thrombosis (25%) in patients with diffuse atherosclerosis or less frequently with connective tissue disorders; (3) nonocclusive mesenteric ischemia (20%); and (4) venous thrombosis (5%) associated with portal hypertension, abdominal sepsis, hypercoagulable states, or trauma.

The clinical consequences of acute arterial or venous mesenteric ischemia depend on several factors, including the vessel involved, the level of occlusion, the development of collaterals, and reperfusion. Tissue injury caused by the ischemic event compromises the immune and barrier functions of the small bowel, allowing bacterial translocation, cellular degradation, reactive oxygen species formation in case of reperfusion and intravascular thrombosis. The release of these products into the portal system and the systemic circulation initiates a cascade of events leading to damage of targets organs such as the lungs and kidneys.

A. Symptoms and Signs

The clinical presentation is nonspecific.

Patients with arterial embolism initially present with sudden-onset diffuse abdominal pain that is out of proportion to the clinical examination and often unresponsive to narcotics. The lack of well-developed collaterals causes ischemia which eventually becomes transmural. As ischemia worsens, patients develop nausea and vomiting, bloody diarrhea, and eventually peritonitis.

Patients with acute thrombotic mesenteric occlusion also present with severe abdominal pain, but it is usually chronic postprandial abdominal pain (intestinal angina) accompanied by weight loss.

With cardiogenic or hypovolemic shock, blood is shunted away from the mesenteric circulation and this process is exacerbated by the following local vasoconstriction. Pain in patients with nonocclusive mesenteric ischemia is usually not as sudden as that with embolic or thrombotic occlusion. Moreover, pain is more difficult to assess because many of these patients are hospitalized in intensive care units for life-threatening conditions.

Patients with venous thrombosis commonly complain of nausea, vomiting, diarrhea, and non-localized abdominal pain.

B. Laboratory Findings

There are no laboratory tests that are diagnostic for AMI. In most cases, the white blood cell count is elevated, as are lactic acid, amylase (50% of patients), and creatine kinase (BB isoenzyme) levels correlating with intestinal infarction. Significant metabolic acidosis is usually present.

C. Imaging Studies

Abdominal radiographs are not diagnostic, but can reveal late signs consistent with bowel ischemia, such as gas in the bowel wall or the portal venous system, and free air in the peritoneum.

Duplex ultrasonography plays a limited role in the diagnosis of AMI, given accompanying ileus with air and gas-filled loops of bowel. Moreover, it cannot assess distal mesenteric blood vessel flow and nonocclusive etiology of ischemia.

Angiography is considered the gold standard for diagnosis for acute embolic and acute thrombotic arterial mesenteric ischemia. Angiography should include both AP and lateral views of the celiac artery, the SMA and the inferior mesenteric artery. By selective injection of contrast into the SMA, emboli and thrombi can be identified, whereas patients with nonocclusive mesenteric ischemia typically exhibit evidence of SMA vasospasm. During the same procedure, catheters can be positioned selectively for treatment. Angiography is significantly less useful for the diagnosis of mesenteric venous thrombosis compared to CT scan.

Both CT and magnetic resonance angiography (MRA) have undergone significant advances over the past 10 years. Multislice helical CT scan with three-dimensional spatial resolution of the vascular anatomy allows rapid evaluation of atherosclerosis of the aorta and mesenteric vessels, the status of the small bowel wall, and identifies other causes of abdominal pain, such as pancreatitis, bowel perforation, bowel obstruction, and rupture of abdominal aortic aneurism. Nevertheless, it still has some limitations: while the origins of the main abdominal vessels are well-visualized, secondary, tertiary, and smaller branches are less well defined compared to angiography. On the contrary, CT is diagnostic for venous thrombosis and is the preferred diagnostic imaging modality in patients with a suspected mesenteric venous thrombosis.

One of the main advantages of MRA has is the use of gadolinium which is significantly less nephrotoxic than the contrast utilized for CT scan. However, this diagnostic imaging modality is not widely used due to the lack of access in many institutions.

▶ Differential Diagnosis

Acute pancreatitis, intestinal obstruction, aortic dissection, and cholecystitis are the most frequent pathologies that mimic the clinical presentation of AMI.

▶ Treatment

Once the diagnosis is made, fluid resuscitation, antibiotics, and anticoagulants or drugs that inhibit platelet aggregation should be started.

The treatment consists of nonsurgical and surgical options depending on the underlying cause.

The goals of surgery are to restore blood flow when feasible and resect the segments of bowel that are no longer viable. Because the appearance of ischemic bowel may improve dramatically after restoring blood flow, the small bowel should be observed for at least 30 minutes after reperfusion before any decision for resection is undertaken.

For acute SMA embolism, the standard treatment is a laparotomy and embolectomy, with a catheter passed under direct vision into the arterial segment in order to dislodge and retrieve the embolus. Nonsurgical treatments include catheter-directed thrombolytic therapy to treat early acute embolic occlusion in selected patients who present with a partially occluding embolus in the SMA and do not exhibit peritoneal signs on physical examination.

Surgical treatment of acute thrombotic mesenteric occlusion consists of an antegrade or retrograde bypass because a simple thrombectomy usually leads to reocclusion, Revascularization with saphenous vein or prosthetic graft (in the absence of peritonitis) is the most common procedure. Angioplasty can be performed during diagnostic angiography to dilate stenotic lesions; however, clinical findings suspicious for peritonitis frequently make a laparotomy necessary.

In case of nonocclusive mesenteric ischemia, the treatment requires reversal of the underlying causes of the hypoperfusion. Local infusion of vasodilators using selective catheterization of the SMA may also play a role.

Treatment of mesenteric venous thrombosis is nonsurgical and relies on anticoagulation to reverse the hypercoagulable state. Full anticoagulation with heparin is needed with careful monitoring for gastrointestinal bleeding. Long-term oral or subcutaneous anticoagulation therapy is then begun. Exploratory laparotomy is mandatory when clinical conditions worsen and bowel infarction is suspected.

Finally, second-look laparotomy within 24-48 hours is a key point in the management of patients with AMI who require extensive bowel resection during the first operation or have areas of marginally viable bowel after revascularization.

▶ Prognosis

The prognosis of AMI is poor because diagnosis and treatment are often delayed, infarction is extensive, and arterial reconstruction is difficult. Perioperative mortality rates range from 32% to 69%, and 5-year survival ranges from 18% to 50%. Mortality varies substantially according to the cause of AMI, being lower in cases of venous thrombosis than in cases of arterial origin. The only way to reduce the morbidity and mortality associated with this disease is early diagnosis and treatment, before bowel necrosis develops.

Block TA et al. Endovascular and open surgery for acute occlusion of the superior mesenteric artery. *J Vasc Surg* 2010 Oct;52(4):959-966.

Meng X et al. Indications and procedures for second-look surgery in acute mesenteric ischemia. *Surg Today* 2010 Aug;40(8):700-705.

Menke J. Diagnostic accuracy of multidetector CT in acute mesenteric ischemia: systematic review and meta-analysis. *Radiology* 2010 Jul;256(1):93-101.

Renner P et al. Intestinal ischemia: current treatment concepts. *Langenbecks Arch Surg* 2011 Jan;396(1):3-11.

SHORT BOWEL SYNDROME

▶ General Considerations

Maintenance of adequate nutrition is dependent on the normal digestive and absorptive function of small bowel mucosa. A normal, healthy adult possesses an excess of gut mucosa such that limited resection is well tolerated. However, this depends on the amount of bowel removed and the specific level of resection, the presence or absence of the colon, the absorptive function of the intestinal remnant, adaptation of the remaining bowel, and the nature of the underlying disease process and its complications (Figure 29–5). Symptoms can ensue following surgery, in some cases leading to a condition known as "short bowel syndrome." Because of the important functional capacities of the duodenum in iron and calcium absorption, and of the distal ileum in regard to vitamin B_{12} and bile salts, resections of these specific regions tend to be poorly tolerated. In contrast, up to 40% of the mid-small bowel can be removed with only moderate clinical sequelae. As a general rule, resection of 50% of the small bowel produces significant malabsorption, and if 70% or more of the bowel is resected, survival is threatened. Clinical results in treating short bowel syndrome have improved in recent decades due to recognition of its pathophysiology, improved surgical techniques, and better enteral and parenteral nutritional support.

The most common etiology of short bowel syndrome is a massive resection occurring in the setting of AMI. In children, volvulus of the intestine caused by congenital malrotation can also result in the need for a large resection. Less commonly, patients with neoplasms, trauma, or recurrent Crohn disease develop short bowel syndrome.

The minimal amount of small bowel required to sustain life is variable, but in general survival is threatened in patients with less than 60 cm of intestine beyond the duodenum. Patients with short bowel syndrome have impairment in the absorption of water and electrolytes as well as that of all nutrients (fat, protein, carbohydrates, and vitamins). The colon is vitally important for preventing water loss. In addition, the colon plays an important role in nutrient assimilation by absorbing short-chain fatty acids. The ileocecal valve delays transit of enteric content from the small bowel into the colon, thereby prolonging the contact time between nutrients and the small bowel absorptive mucosa.

Important adaptive changes occur in the remaining intestine following massive resection. In addition to mucosal hyperplasia, there is generally seen to be an increase in the caliber of the remaining small bowel, perhaps adding to the absorptive area. From a functional point of view, the amount of fluid and electrolytes losses following massive resection decrease over time, whereas glucose absorption increases.

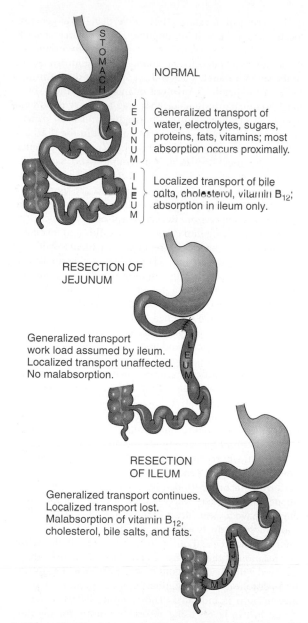

▲ **Figure 29–5.** The consequences of complete resection of jejunum or ileum are predictable in part from the loss of regionally localized transport processes.

NORMAL

Generalized transport of water, electrolytes, sugars, proteins, fats, vitamins; most absorption occurs proximally.

Localized transport of bile salts, cholesterol, vitamin B_{12}; absorption in ileum only.

RESECTION OF JEJUNUM

Generalized transport work load assumed by ileum. Localized transport unaffected. No malabsorption.

RESECTION OF ILEUM

Generalized transport continues. Localized transport lost. Malabsorption of vitamin B_{12}, cholesterol, bile salts, and fats.

Short bowel syndrome is associated with gastric hypersecretion that persists for 1-2 years postoperatively, likely related to loss of the "ileal brake," a mechanism by which luminal fat within the distal small bowel inhibits gastric secretion. The increased acid load delivered to the duodenum inhibits absorption by a variety of mechanisms, including the inhibition of digestive enzymes, most of which function optimally under alkaline conditions. Loss of the terminal ileum also results in impairment in the absorption of conjugated bile salts and fat. With limited ileal resections, an increase in the bile salt load to the colon can cause direct injury to the mucosa and resultant diarrhea. With an ileal resection greater than 100 cm, there is a gradual loss in the total bile salt pool, eventually leading to impairment in fat absorption and the onset of steatorrhea. Ileal resections are also associated with lithogenic bile, such that gallstone formation is seen in approximately 30% of patients who have undergone such surgery. Calcium oxalate urinary tract calculi form in 7%-10% of patients who have extensive ileal resection and an intact colon, due to excessive absorption of oxalate from the colon.

▶ **Treatment**

Initial therapy involves maintenance of fluid and electrolyte balance. Total parental nutrition is often indicated and, depending on the extent of resection, may be required throughout the lifetime of the patient. It is likely that even small amounts of enteral nutrition are beneficial; however, because the luminal nutrients appear to enhance the adaptive response of the remaining gut. Various antidiarrheal and stool-bulking agents have also been used with some benefits. Gastric hypersecretion should be treated with either H2-blockers or proton pump inhibitors. Cholestyramine may be beneficial in patients with limited ileal resections, but if the bile salt pool has been depleted, then cholestyramine is contraindicated. The efficacy of intensive medical management, including maintenance of oral hydration, along with a combination of a high-fiber diet, growth hormone and glutamine is controversial.

The surgical treatment of patients with short bowel syndrome has been disappointing. Various procedures including intestinal lengthening, reversal of short segments, and placation of excessively dilated bowel have been attempted. Although some improvement has been seen in isolated cases, such operations are not widely performed. The results of small bowel transplantation have also been disappointing because of the high rate of rejection. However, more recent experience with small bowel transplantation suggests that this may become a viable surgical alternative in patients with short bowel syndrome.

Thompson JS et al. Current management of the short bowel syndrome. *Surg Clin North Am* 2011 Jun;91(3):493-510.

Ueno T et al. Current status of intestinal transplantation. *Surg Today* 2010 Dec;40(12):1112-1122.

Wales PW et al. Human growth hormone and glutamine for patients with short bowel syndrome. *Cochrane Database Syst Rev* 2010 Jun 16;(6):CD006321.

INTESTINAL DIVERTICULA

▶ General Considerations

Small bowel diverticular disease is an uncommon clinical entity. However, with progressive aging of the general population, small bowel diverticulosis is encountered more often. Overall, the frequency reported in the literature of small bowel diverticula varies with the anatomic location of the disease and the type of investigation used for diagnosis. Clearly, autopsy series report a higher incidence, since small bowel diverticulosis is usually asymptomatic and is found often upon post mortem examination only.

A. Etiology

Diverticular disease of the small bowel is generally classified into two groups: the more common, acquired form and the congenital form which is somewhat rare, other than Meckel's diverticulum in the distal ileum. Primary acquired small bowel diverticula result from the herniation of the mucosa and submucosa through the muscular layer of the bowel wall. These lesions are considered to be false diverticula, with no muscular wall covering. Patients with small bowel diverticula frequently have associated diverticular disease of the colon, diverticula of the esophagus (2%), stomach (2%), or urinary bladder (12%).

In the pathogenesis of small bowel diverticulosis, abnormalities of the myenteric plexus with consequent motor dysfunctions of the small intestine are thought to play a major role. These motility disorders vary in severity and magnitude from localized dysmotility to universal jejunoileal dyskinesia that result in increased intraluminal pressure and ultimately herniation of the mucosa and submucosa through the muscular wall of the small bowel. Usually, diverticula occur where the paired blood vessels penetrate the small bowel wall at the mesenteric site.

In contrast, congenital diverticula are usually considered true diverticula involving the full thickness of the small intestine. Congenital diverticula are often limited to the duodenum (wind-sock diverticulum) and ileum (Meckel diverticulum). Both acquired and congenital diverticula are usually asymptomatic, however, symptoms can originate from small bowel diverticula owing to diverticulitis, perforation, obstruction, or hemorrhage.

B. Duodenal Diverticula

Acquired diverticula are extra-luminal and are a fairly common incidental finding usually visualized either upon esophagogastroduodenoscopy (EGD), endoscopic retrograde cholangiopancreatography (ERCP), or by barium swallow and small bowel follow through. Incidences vary significantly in the literature depending on the diagnostic modality used. In the ERCP literature, incidences up to 23% have been reported, usually increasing with advancing age.

In terms of location, these diverticula are generally located within 2 cm of the ampulla. This is an area of weakening of the duodenal wall mucosa, especially around the papilla of Vater, due to the configuration and orientation of the smooth muscle fiber and the sphincter mechanism of Oddi. If the papilla is involved or included in these diverticula, sphincter dysfunction may lead to biliary dyskinesia, formation of biliary stones, cholangitis, and even pancreatitis. Acquired diverticula are also present in the third and fourth portion of the duodenum with decreasing frequency.

Usually, these diverticula are asymptomatic. Symptoms, when present, often are caused by either dysfunction of the sphincter of Oddi or, when the diverticula are significantly large, by obstruction of the biliary and pancreatic ducts due to external compression. Recurrent episodes of pancreatitis potentially evolving into chronic pancreatitis and formation of biliary stones have been reported in patients with large duodenal diverticula. Furthermore, large diverticula can cause bacterial overgrowth resulting in malabsorption and anemia. Diverticulitis with potential perforation and bleeding from duodenal diverticula has been reported.

Diagnosis is often obtained by EGD or ERCP. An upper GI with a small bowel follow through is also very helpful in localizing the diverticula and in defining the size of it. When a perforation is suspected, CT scan of the abdomen with oral and IV contrast can accurately define the location of the diverticula and the extent of the inflammatory reaction to the diverticular perforation.

Surgical treatment of duodenal diverticula is complicated by significant morbidity and mortality, therefore a prophylactic resection of an asymptomatic duodenal diverticulum is not routinely recommended. In the presence of perforation or bleeding, a generous Kocher maneuver should be performed in order to identify the posterior aspect of the duodenum. It is very important at this stage of the procedure to have a clear idea of the relationship of the biliary and pancreatic ducts with the ampulla in order to avoid an injury that will be extremely difficult to repair in this setting and location. If the pancreatic and biliary structures are not involved with the diverticulum, in the absence of significant retroperitoneal contamination, a primary excision of the diverticulum is indicated. The resulting defect should be closed in two layers using absorbable suture for the inner layer and non-absorbable suture for the outer layer. With a large duodenal defect, a serosal patch technique using a defunctionalized loop of jejunum is a useful alternative. However, in the presence of significant edema and contamination, primary closure around a T-tube with drainage of the surrounding area may be the only solution. In extreme cases, duodenal diverticulization by gastrojejunostomy with a stapled closure of the pylorus may be necessary. A large diverticulum in the third or fourth portion of the duodenum requires mobilization of the distal duodenum with excision and primary closure. In this area, the relationship with the biliary and pancreatic duct is not obviously as crucial and therefore, a more aggressive approach can be undertaken.

C. Jejunoileal Diverticula

The acquired forms of jejunoileal diverticula are usually more common in the proximal jejunum decreasing in frequency throughout the small bowel. Extreme forms of diffuse diverticulosis of the small bowel have been reported. It is a disease of advanced age and is prevalent during the seventh decade of life. These diverticula are located on the anti-mesenteric border of the small bowel. Due to primary motility disturbances of the small intestine, these patients usually present with chronic abdominal pain, early satiety, and different gastrointestinal conditions, such as diarrhea, malabsorption, steatorrhea, Vitamin B_{12} deficiency, and anemia. These patients can present with an acute abdomen in the presence of a free perforation secondary to diverticulitis. Bleeding is also one of the possible complications and localization of the bleeding diverticulum, in the presence of diffuse diverticulosis may present a significant diagnostic challenge to the clinician.

Jejunoileal diverticula are usually identified by small bowel follow-through or enteroclysis. CT scan can help in the diagnosis of large diverticula or in the presence of acute diverticulitis or perforation. More recently, the use of capsule or wireless endoscopy has helped the clinician in diagnosing patients with unclear gastrointestinal symptoms and especially patients with recurrent significant GI bleed secondary to diverticular disease. After the initial experimental papers, several human studies, looking at patients with occult gastrointestinal bleeding, have shown capsule endoscopy to be significantly superior to push enteroscopy and preferred by patients undergoing both procedures. Although small bowel diverticular disease is a rare condition, it may be the cause of a lower GI bleed resulting in a diagnostic dilemma. In the presence of acute significant bleeding, angiography should be attempted for localization of the bleeding diverticulum and possible treatment either by vasopressin injection or, in selected cases by super selective embolization. Injection of methylene-blue to help identifying the bleeding diverticulum at the time of exploration is very helpful technique when the bleeding persists despite medical management.

Asymptomatic jejunoileal diverticula are usually treated conservatively. In the presence of localized segments of multiple diverticula, it has been suggested that a resection, even in the absence of symptomatology, might be indicated because the morbidity from a small bowel resection nowadays is much less than the potential complication from acute diverticulitis. This approach has not been validated by any clinical data thus far. In the presence of diverticulitis and perforation, obviously resection and primary anastomosis is indicated. In the presence of bleeding, if the source is localized by either angiography or capsule endoscopy, the bleeding site should be resected with primary anastomosis. Laparoscopy has been extensively used in the management of this unusual problem.

Woods K et al. Acquired jejunoileal diverticulosis and its complications: a review of the literature. *Am Surg* 2008;74:849.

TUMORS OF THE SMALL BOWEL

▶ General Considerations

Although the small bowel accounts for 75% of the gastrointestinal length and 90% of its absorptive surface, neoplasms of this organ, both benign and malignant, are relatively rare. They represent less than 10% of all gastrointestinal tumors, 1%-3% of gastrointestinal malignancies and 0.4% of all malignancies.

In recent years, the incidence of two small bowel tumors, lymphomas, and gastrointestinal stromal tumors (GIST), have increased substantially. In the case of primary small bowel lymphoma, the incidence in the United States has nearly doubled in the last two decades, due to the increased numbers of immunocompromised patients and immigrants from developing countries. In the case of GIST, the recognition of the KIT protein (CD117) has changed the way spindle cell tumors of the gastrointestinal tract are classified and has led to an increased awareness and recognition.

Several predisposing conditions associated with small bowel malignancies have been identified: CD, familial adenomatous polyposis, hereditary nonpolyposis colorectal cancer, blind loop syndrome, Peutz–Jeghers syndrome, celiac sprue, neurofibromatosis, and IgA deficiency.

The disproportion between the low incidence of malignant tumors of the small bowel and the size of its surface area suggests a significant sparing from or resistance to the development of malignancy. Several hypotheses, based on experimental animal models, have postulated that carcinogens in the enteric content may be in contact with small bowel mucosa over a limited time due to the relatively rapid transit time or may be in a diluted and less carcinogenic form. The preponderance of small bowel adenocarcinomas in the duodenum suggests a role for bile or pancreatic secretions either as primary small bowel carcinogens or even as simple vectors for unknown carcinogens.

Other specific characteristics of the small bowel microscopic and chemical environment might be responsible for the observed cancer resistance. The limited and metabolically inactive bacterial flora of the small bowel is likely unable to transform procarcinogens into their active metabolites especially in an alkaline milieu. In addition, the proximal small bowel secretes a number of enzymes that detoxify carcinogens.

Finally the presence of a high concentration of B cells and lymphocytes and high amounts of secretory IgA in the distal small bowel might constitute an effective local immunosurveillance system that prevents carcinogenesis. This theory seems to be supported by the observation that immunocompromised patients have an increased incidence of lymphoma and Kaposi's sarcoma of the distal small bowel.

Dietary risk factors, such as high caloric dietary intake in general and more specifically consumption of red meat, fat, and salt-cured smoked foods have been shown to increase the incidence of small bowel carcinoma in large population based studies. This similarity in risk factors explains the relatively high risk of synchronous or metachronous colorectal cancer in patients with a known small bowel malignancy.

▶ Pathology

Approximately one-third of primary small bowel neoplasms are benign and two-thirds are malignant. The most common benign tumors are leiomyomas and adenomas; less common lesions include inflammatory polyps, hemangiomas, lipomas, hamartomas (Peutz–Jeghers syndrome), and fibromas. These tumors can occur throughout the small bowel but tend to increase in frequency from proximal to distal, with the exception of adenomas, which occur with the highest frequency in the duodenum.

Adenomas are the most common benign tumors of the small intestine. The duodenum is the most common site of involvement, and the lesion most commonly noted is a villous adenoma. These lesions tend to involve the region of the ampulla of Vater. They may present with obstructive jaundice and are easily diagnosed by upper endoscopy and biopsy. Up to 30 percent of these tumors may have malignant degeneration. The risk of malignant degeneration in a significant proportion of patients poses challenges to treatment planning.

Leiomyomas arise from smooth muscle and can grow both intra- and extraluminally. They can often become very large before causing symptoms. On gross inspection, it is sometimes difficult to distinguish these lesions from their malignant counterparts. This distinction is made histologically with standard criteria including nuclear pleomorphism, increased mitosis and the presence of necrosis although, at times, even histological examination may fail to unequivocally distinguish between benign and malignant histology.

Malignant tumors tend to increase in frequency from proximal to distal, with the exception of adenocarcinomas which are most frequent in the duodenum. Adenocarcinoma is the most common histologic type (45%), followed by carcinoids (30%), lymphomas (15%), sarcomas, and GISTs (10%). Pathologic staging is performed according to the American Joint Committee on Cancer (AJCC) tumor-node-metastasis (TNM) system.

Most small bowel *adenocarcinomas* are solitary, sessile lesions, often appearing in association with adenomas. They are usually moderately to well differentiated and almost always positive for acid mucin. Most arise in the duodenum: within the duodenum, 15% of these tumors are located in the first portion, 40% in the second portion, and 45% in the distal duodenum. Most of these tumors are sporadic with the exception of the ones originating in the context of familial adenomatous polyposis. Presenting symptoms include epigastric and abdominal pain or discomfort, and possibly jaundice and gastric outlet obstruction, depending on the location of the tumor. These symptoms and the accessibility of the duodenum and proximal small bowel to endoscopic modalities allow a relatively high rate of diagnosis and resectability.

Carcinoid tumors are the most common endocrine tumors of the gastrointestinal system.

In the small bowel itself, carcinoids are the most common distal small-bowel neoplasm. These neoplasms arise from enterochromaffin cells and are characterized by the ability to secrete many biologically active substances, including serotonin, bradykinin, dopamine, histamine, and 5-hydroxyindoleacetic acid (5-HIAA). They tend to be small (< 2 cm) and submucosal in location, with a propensity for multicentricity. The most common classification for these tumors is based on embryologic derivation: foregut (stomach and pancreas), midgut (small bowel 90% or more), and hindgut (colon and rectum). Their presentation depends largely on the hormones elaborated and on the site of origin. Up to 40% of small bowel carcinoids are associated with a second gastrointestinal malignancy and 30% present as multiple synchronous lesions.

The gastrointestinal tract is the most frequent site of extra nodal *lymphoma*: the stomach is the most common site followed by the small bowel and the colon, respectively; within the small bowel, lymphomas parallel the distribution of lymphoid follicles, resulting in the ileum being the most common site of involvement. These tumors may be primary or secondary as a manifestation of generalized involvement of systemic lymphoma. For the diagnosis of primary small bowel lymphomas there must be no peripheral or mediastinal lymphadenopathy, with a normal white cell count and differential, and the tumor must be predominantly in the gastrointestinal tract. When primary, they may be multifocal in as many as 15% of cases. Predisposing conditions include immunodeficiency conditions, CD, and celiac disease.

There are five distinct clinical pathologic subtypes of primary small intestinal lymphoma: the adult Western type, the pediatric type, the immunoproliferative or Mediterranean type, enteropathy associated (celiac sprue) T-cell lymphoma, and Hodgkin's lymphoma. The most common is the adult Western type, occurring in the sixth and seventh decade of life with a male predominance.

Sarcomas make up only 10% of small-bowel malignancies. Overall these tumors are located in the jejunum and ileum, are relatively slow growing, and are locally invasive. Their growth pattern is most commonly extramural and therefore, they rarely result in obstruction, but sometimes present with free intra-abdominal bleeding. Due to their insidious nature and growth pattern, greater than three-fourths of these tumors exceed 5 cm in diameter at the time diagnosis. The most common histologic subtypes are GISTs, leiomyosarcomas, fibrosarcomas, liposarcomas, and malignant schwannomas and angiosarcomas. Similarly to sarcomas from other anatomic regions, small-bowel sarcomas rarely metastasize to regional lymph nodes. Hematogenous dissemination tends to be the preferred route of distant spread, primarily to the liver, lungs, and bone. Peritoneal sarcomatosis is noted in later stages of the disease.

Malignant *GIST* is now considered the most common sarcoma of the gastrointestinal tract and accounts for about 5% of all small bowel malignancies. Clinical, histopathological, ultrastructural, and molecular-biological findings have made clear that GIST is a completely separate entity from leiomyoma and leiomyosarcoma. It is currently thought that GISTs originate from stem cells that differentiate towards the interstitial cells of Cajal (ICCs). ICCs arise from precursor mesenchymal cells and are the pacemaker cells of the gastrointestinal tract. Both ICCs and GISTs express KIT protein, have similar ultrastructural features, and express the embryonic form of the heavy chain of smooth muscle myosin.

KIT immunostaining has become the gold standard for the diagnosis of GIST and the term "GIST" should apply only to tumors with KIT immunopositivity. In rare situations a GIST maybe immunohistochemically inert, or, after therapy with imatinib mesylate, KIT immunostaining may become negative. Furthermore a minority of GISTs lacks demonstrable KIT mutations, but KIT is nonetheless strongly activated. Such GISTs might contain KIT mutations, which are not readily detected by conventional screening methods, or alternately, KIT might be activated by non-mutational mechanisms. To better characterize these tumors, other markers have been studied: about 60%-70% of GISTs show immunopositivity for CD34, 30%-40 % for smooth-muscle actin (SMA) and around 5% for S-100 protein. None of the latter antigens are therefore specific for GIST, but can help in the differential diagnosis in KIT negative tumors.

▶ Clinical Findings

A. Symptoms and Signs

The vast majority of patients with benign neoplasms are asymptomatic whereas most of those with malignancies are symptomatic prior to diagnosis. The most common presentation of benign tumors is intermittent episodes of acute crampy abdominal pain associated with intussusception, followed by chronic bleeding with iron deficiency anemia in up to 50% of patients.

Malignant lesions are generally associated with weight loss. Symptoms, when they occur, tend to be vague and nonspecific. In general, most symptoms can be attributed to the location of the tumor, its rate of growth, and its size. For example, tumors in the duodenum tend to be symptomatic at an earlier stage, presenting with pain, gastric outlet obstruction, or obstructive jaundice, whereas those in the jejunum or ileum may present at a later stage with obstructive symptoms. Obstruction in this setting tends to be progressive, compared to benign lesions, whose obstructive symptoms tend to be intermittent as they relate to episodes of intussusception. Bleeding and perforation (in up to 10%) may also occur, predominantly in lymphomatous lesions, but this can also be a feature of any malignant tumor because of ulceration or necrosis.

Carcinoid tumors produce symptoms secondary to hormone production, including hot flashes, bronchospasms, and arrhythmias. This constellation of symptoms, called carcinoid syndrome, occurs when the liver is not able to metabolize the active substances produced by the carcinoid tumor. This is usually the case when tumors are either bulky or metastatic or their venous drainage bypasses the liver.

B. Laboratory Findings

A high index of suspicion is required due to the lack of specificity of these tumor's signs and symptoms. A correct preoperative diagnosis is made in up to only 50% of patients. Biochemical and hematologic studies are often not helpful. Iron deficiency anemia may be detected with chronic blood loss; elevated liver enzymes may be noted with periampullary lesions or hepatic metastases; elevated 24-hour urinary 5-hydroxyindoleacetic acid can be detected in more than 50% of patients with carcinoid tumors.

C. Imaging Studies

Radiographic-contrast imaging modalities tend to be the most useful in the establishment of the diagnosis. Plain films of the abdomen are generally not helpful and at best may demonstrate nonspecific signs of obstruction or a mass effect. Except for the duodenum and the very proximal jejunum, which can often be evaluated by endoscopy, the diagnosis of small intestinal neoplasms depends on contrast studies such as a small-bowel follow-through or preferably enteroclysis. Small bowel follow-through is still the most commonly used method in the evaluation of small bowel pathology although enteroclysis may be a superior imaging modality.

Computed tomography, ultrasonography, and MRI are complementary to barium studies in the detection of small bowel neoplasms. Abdominal CT has a sensitivity of 50%-80% in detecting the primary small bowel tumors and occasionally plays an important role in differentiating benign from malignant tumors. Additionally CT is valuable in staging malignant tumors (presence or absence of hepatic metastases) and in providing important information related to local extent (presence or absence of local invasion, mesenteric implants, and metastatic lymph nodes). More recently, the association of multi-detector CT and MRI with small bowel lumen distension (CTE and MRE) has led to a considerable improvement in the diagnosis of small bowel neoplasms. On CTE, small bowel adenocarcinomas may manifest as a discrete tumor mass, a circumferential narrowing with abrupt concentric or irregular edges, or as an ulcerative lesion with adjacent enlarged lymph nodes. Mucosal ulceration is a suggestive feature, which is well depicted by CTE. Jejunal lesions have a tendency for being annular. Usually, only a short segment of the small bowel is involved. The mass itself usually shows moderate and heterogeneous enhancement after intravenous administration of iodinated contrast material. Rarely, adenocarcinoma may present as an aneurismal dilatation of a small bowel segment, similar to that observed in case of lymphoma. On MR imaging, small bowel adenocarcinomas have morphological features similar to those observed on CT.

On CTE, small GISTs typically present as regular, round, or lobulated masses with homogeneous and relatively marked enhancement after intravenous administration of contrast material, whereas larger tumors are heterogeneous with central necrosis and more prone to extraluminal growth. Due to excellent spatial resolution with multi-detector CT, the submucosal origin of the tumor may be suspected in case of small tumors. The malignant potential of these lesions cannot be stated with certainty on cross-sectional imaging unless metastases are present. In some instances, GISTs may display an aneurysmal pattern similar to that observed in case of lymphoma, so that differentiation between these two entities is difficult. On MR imaging, mesenteric small bowel tumors are usually hyperintense on T2-weighted MR images, with variable degrees of enhancement after intravenous administration of a gadolinium chelate. Because of the lower spatial resolution obtained with MR by comparison with CT, the submucosal origin of the tumor may be difficult to ascertain.

Angiography is rarely helpful in establishing or refining a diagnosis of small-bowel malignancy. In rare cases angiographic demonstration of tumor neovascularity without contrast agent extravasation may be of diagnostic importance in patients with chronic occult bleeding when other diagnostic studies, such as endoscopy and barium contrast have been negative. By contrast, this study is rarely beneficial in localizing bleeding tumors since the vast majority bleeds at a rate considerably below the limit of detection for this technique. Nuclear medicine scan with technetium-labeled red blood cells may identify bleeding sites with blood loss rates as low as 0.1 mL/min.

Fluorodeoxyglucose (labeled with fluorine-18) positron emission tomography (FDG-PET) has been shown to be highly sensitive to assess disease status in patients with GISTs. FDG-PET is used for preoperative staging, but more importantly to assess response to therapy.

D. Endoscopy

Enteroscopy is now available in a fiber optic form, using conventional endoscopes or in a wireless form. Push enteroscopy is currently the most frequently used endoscopic method for small bowel examination. The endoscope is introduced orally. After traversing the curve of the second part of the duodenum, the enteroscope is straightened to reduce any loops formed in the stomach. The enteroscope is then pushed to the maximum length of insertion. Dedicated push enteroscopes are 2-2.5 m in length and offer the opportunity of taking biopsies when the neoplastic lesion has been identified.

The double balloon (push and pull) enteroscopy system consists of a high-resolution video endoscope with a working length of 200 cm, and a flexible overtube 145 cm long. The inflated balloon on the overtube is used to maintain a stable position while the enteroscope is advanced. The overtube balloon is deflated whilst the enteroscope balloon is inflated, and the overtube is advanced along the distal end of the enteroscope (push procedure). This is followed by the "pull procedure:" Both the enteroscope and the overtube are pulled back under endoscopic guidance, with both balloons inflated. This procedure is repeated multiple times to visualize the entire small bowel. Few complications have been reported: post-procedure abdominal pain in up to 20% of patients, pancreatitis, bleeding and small bowel perforation which is more common after polypectomy of large polyps (> 3 cm).

The capsule endoscope is a capsule containing a battery-powered imager, a transmitter, antenna and four light emitting diodes. The imager takes two images per second through the transparent plastic dome of the capsule. The capsule is swallowed and is propelled through the intestine by peristalsis. Images taken by the capsule are transmitted to a battery-powered data recorder worn on a belt. The equipment is removed after 8 hours by which time the capsule has reached the caecum in most of cases. The data from the recorder is then downloaded onto a computer workstation which allows approximately 50,000 images to be viewed as a video. The average reading time of the video images takes between 40 and 60 minutes depending on the experience of the endoscopist. This technique may be affected by two problems: firstly, the presence of dark intestinal contents in the small bowel which may impair visualization of the mucosa, and secondly the rate of gastric emptying and small bowel transit which could lead to the exhaustion of the capsule batteries before the capsule reaches the ileocecal valve. Incomplete examination occurs in 10%-25% of cases.

The main risk is capsule retention. Therefore, this procedure is contraindicated in patients with known strictures or swallowing disorders.

E. Laparoscopy

Limited information is available regarding the efficacy of diagnostic laparoscopy in the diagnosis and work-up of small-bowel neoplasms. At present, its usefulness may reside in obtaining staging information and determining resectability prior to formal laparotomy in the case of tumors of the duodenum, and in obtaining images and potentially tissue diagnoses when other imaging studies have failed to suggest an etiology. It is clear, however, that despite the currently available technology, the diagnosis of these tumors is difficult to establish preoperatively in a significant group of individuals. Laparotomy is often required for definitive diagnosis.

▶ Staging Classification

Radiological staging is mainly based on the use of CT and MRI. Intraoperative assessment plays a role in clinical staging. Metastatic involvement of the liver may be further evaluated by intraoperative ultrasonography. As far as pathologic staging, the TNM staging system has been recently revised by the AJCC, but no major changes have been implemented for small bowel neoplasms. The primary tumor is staged according to its depth of penetration and the involvement of adjacent structures or distant sites. There is no subdivision within the N category based on the number of nodes involved with tumor. Hematogenous metastases or peritoneal metastases are coded as M1. Cancers of the small intestine can metastasize to most organs, especially the liver, or to the peritoneal surfaces. Involvement of the celiac nodes is considered Ml disease.

For small bowel lymphoma the most commonly used staging system is the Ann Arbor system based on lymphatic and extralymphatic involvement on either side of the diaphragm.

▶ Treatment

Treatment of *adenocarcinoma* of the small intestine with localized disease is based on oncologic and anatomic principles. For duodenal lesions the availability of endoscopic ultrasound has allowed better preoperative staging and the availability of endoscopic resection techniques has offered additional therapeutic options. Ultrasound proven benign duodenal or ampullary adenomas can be resected endoscopically with excellent results. Invasive lesions of the first and second portion of the duodenum without major vessel involvement and distant spread are best treated by a pancreaticoduodenectomy (Whipple procedure). For tumors in the third or fourth portion of the duodenum segmental resection with regional lymphadenectomy is indicated. Debate persists about the optimal surgical management of early duodenal cancer. Although early reports suggest that an endoscopic approach could be justified in early favorable lesions,

long-term follow-up is still lacking and surgical resection is to be preferred in the good-risk patients. Palliative options for unresectable or metastatic duodenal carcinoma include gastrojejunostomy and/or biliary enteric bypass or endoscopic/interventional placement of stents to relieve the intestinal and/or biliary obstruction.

Adenocarcinoma of the jejunum and ileum is treated by wide excision, including areas of contiguous spread and the associated mesentery, with negative surgical margins.

Although only small series have been published, these tumors do not seem to respond to the conventional 5-FU based chemotherapy regimens and there is a radiation dose limitation due to small bowel toxicity. However, for palliation of chronic blood loss in patients with locally advanced unresectable duodenal carcinomas radiotherapy may provide short-term benefit.

The mainstay of therapy for *carcinoid* tumors is radical surgical excision. In preparation for surgery a complete assessment of the entire gastrointestinal tract is warranted since up to 40% of midgut carcinoids are associated with a second gastrointestinal malignancy and 30% present with multiple synchronous lesions. In addition, preemptive treatment with octreotide is indicated to prevent carcinoid crisis at the time of surgery. At surgery, wide en block resection including the draining mesentery is the standard approach. This is particularly true for small bowel carcinoid, because these lesions have the propensity to metastasize even when very small. Large lesions near the ampulla may require a pancreaticoduodenectomy for cure, while smaller lesions may be treated with either local excision or endoscopic resection with close endoscopic follow-up. Likewise lesions of the terminal ileum or carcinoid tumors of the appendix larger than 2 cm require a formal right hemicolectomy for oncologic clearance of disease.

Treatment for advanced locoregional and distant disease includes both medical and surgical modalities. Surgery should be indicated in patients with resectable metastatic disease for potential cure or at least meaningful palliation. Orthotopic liver transplantation has been used in the treatment of metastatic neuroendocrine tumors to the liver, with discouraging results.

The role of multimodality therapy, including alpha2b interferon and octreotide, for metastatic carcinoid remains limited. The addition of liver chemoembolization has not been shown to have a significant effect on survival in patients with metastatic disease to the liver but may have a role in controlling or decreasing the symptoms associated with carcinoid crisis. Octreotide has been effective in the treatment of patients with carcinoid syndrome by improving diarrhea in up to 83% of the patients and abolishing flushing and wheezing, but has no effect on survival. In consideration of the slow growth rate of many carcinoid tumors, patients with distant metastatic disease can also undergo resection for debulking and palliation of symptoms. For those patients with extensive unresectable disease, the indications for surgical intervention are limited to the occurrence of obstruction, perforation and bleeding. Radiation therapy has not been proven to be effective in either the adjuvant or palliative setting.

Treatment of small bowel *lymphoma* requires conservative resections with para-aortic and mesenteric lymph node sampling, liver biopsy and bone marrow biopsy performed for staging. Low-grade localized lesions are treated with resection alone, while for intermediate and high-grade lesions resection and chemotherapy is recommended. Radiation is used only for palliation in poor performance patients. This modality is associated with significant side effects, such as bowel necrosis, bleeding and perforation, and is offered for palliation only to patients unfit for surgery or chemotherapy.

Surgical treatment for small bowel *sarcomas* consists of an *en block* resection with tumor free margins. There is no role for extended lymphadenectomy in these tumors. Hematogenous dissemination is the preferred route of metastatic spread to the liver lungs and bones. Carcinomatosis is noted in later stages of the disease. In the presence of metastatic disease, local excision or palliative bypass procedure might be indicated to prevent or ameliorate bleeding and obstruction. Furthermore there is no clear benefit from chemoradiation therapy in the adjuvant setting, since radiation doses are limited due to small bowel toxicity. In the presence of recurrent or metastatic disease partial response rates after palliative chemoradiation therapy have been reported in the 10%-20% range, with minimal improvement in survival at best.

Treatment of localized GISTs is based on surgical resection: the tumor should be removed en block with its pseudocapsule and margins of normal soft tissue or bowel. In the presence of large lesions involving other organs, where an *en block* resection may be associated with significant morbidity, preoperative neoadjuvant use of imatinib mesylate may be entertained.

A significant breakthrough in the management of small bowel tumors and specifically GISTs has come from the understanding of the molecular and genetic makeshift of these lesions. After the discovery that GISTs characteristically express the KIT protein, a transmembrane tyrosine kinase receptor for a stem cell factor, a specific tyrosine kinase inhibitor, imatinib mesylate (Gleevec, Novartis), has been introduced in clinical practice with reduced risks of recurrence.

The role of surgery for recurrent or metastatic disease has been questioned since the introduction of imatinib mesylate. Surgery should still be considered in patients with bleeding and obstructive disease and after partial response to imatinib mesylate if the residual disease is deemed to be resectable.

▶ Prognosis

Prognosis for small bowel *adenocarcinoma* is based on similar variables as for colorectal cancer, including stage, perineural and vascular invasion, grade, resectability, and surgical margins. The majority of tumors have regional spread at time of diagnosis, and up to one-fourth of patients have distant organ disease. Overall, the 5-year survival rate is 20%-30%. For resectable disease of the duodenum, the 5-year survival rate approaches 50%.

The prognosis for *carcinoid* tumors with localized disease is excellent with 5-years survival rates approaching 100% after resection. More than 90% of the symptomatic patients have metastatic disease at the time of surgical exploration. The likelihood of distant disease correlates closely with both the size of the primary lesion and the depth of invasion. For tumors less than 1 cm in size, the risk of lymph node metastases is on the order of 2%; for 1-2 cm lesions, there is an approximate 50% incidence of lymph node involvement; and 80% of tumors greater than 2 cm have positive nodes. Survival rates of up to 68% at 5 years have been reported when all gross metastatic disease, including hepatic metastases, is resected. For extensive unresectable disease, debulking has proven to be of some benefit in terms of symptomatic palliation. The 5-years survival for unresectable disease is approximately 35%-40%, reflecting the relatively indolent growth of these tumors.

Prognostic factors for primary small bowel *lymphomas* include higher grade, greater depth of tumor penetration, lymph node involvement, peritoneal disease and distant metastases. Overall 5-year survival rates range from 20% to 40% for all stages. Five-year survivals of up to 60% have been reported for patients with resected localized low-grade tumors.

Sarcomas tend to have an insidious growth pattern and greater than three-fourths of these tumors are larger than 5 cm at the time of diagnosis and up to 50% of them are not resectable for cure when the diagnosis is established. Prognosis correlates most closely with grade, followed by stage. Five-year survival after curative resection ranges from 60% to 80% for low-grade tumors and is no more than 20% for high-grade lesions.

Assessment of the malignant potential of a primary *GIST* lesion is difficult in many cases unless tumor spread can be documented beyond the organ of origin at the time of diagnosis. Historically, size has been used to assess tumor behavior. While almost all small (< 1 cm) GISTs are clinically benign and tumors larger than 5 cm in diameter are generally malignant, intermediate size GISTs have uncertain malignant potential and no cut-off diameter predicts subsequent malignant behavior with certainty.

Other factors, which have shown prognostic value, include mitotic rate, presence of tumor necrosis, high cellularity, and pronounced pleomorphism; a high S-phase fraction and

DNA aneuploidy in flow or image cytometry; a high Ki-67 score; proliferating-cell nuclear-antigen expression; presence of telomerase activity, incomplete surgical resection, tumor rupture at surgery and invasion of adjacent structures.

Recently *KIT* mutations have been shown to be an independent prognostic factor for patients with GISTs.

The median disease-specific survival is about 5 years for primary disease, and 10-20 months in recurrent or metastatic disease. Most recurrences take place within 5 years of the primary diagnosis, but in the slowly proliferating subset of GISTs and especially after therapy with imatinib mesylate, metastases can appear more than 10 years after the primary diagnosis.

The outcome of patients with *metastatic malignancies* to the small intestine (more commonly ovarian, colon, lung cancers, renal cell carcinoma, and melanoma) is dismal despite palliative therapeutic intervention.

▶ Follow-up

Routine follow-up for small bowel cancers is accomplished with endoscopy and radiologic imaging. The only exception is GIST. As previously discussed, PET scan is used to follow tumor response to imatinib mesylate; to detect recurrence after either complete response to imatinib mesylate or after curative surgery; to identify secondary resistance to imatinib mesylate before tumor progression on treatment.

Appelman HD. Morphology of gastrointestinal stromal tumors: historical perspectives. *J Surg Oncol* 2011 Dec;104(8):874-881.

Bilimoria KY et al. Small bowel cancer in the United States: changes in epidemiology, treatment, and survival over the last 20 years. *Ann Surg* 2009; 249:63-71.

Boudreaux JP et al. The NANETS consensus guideline for the diagnosis and management of neuroendocrine tumors: well-differentiated neuroendocrine tumors of the Jejunum, Ileum, Appendix, and Cecum. *Pancreas* 2010 Aug;39(6):753-766.

Culver EL et al. Sporadic duodenal polyps: classification, investigation, and management. *Endoscopy* 2011 Feb;43(2):144-155.

Fry LC et al. Small-bowel endoscopy. *Endoscopy* 2011 Nov;43(11):978-984.

Ghimire P et al. Primary gastrointestinal lymphoma. *World J Gastroenterol* 2011 Feb 14; 17(6):697-707.

Kamaoui I et al. Value of CT enteroclysis in suspected small-bowel carcinoid tumors. *AJR Am J Roentgenol* 2010 Mar;194(3): 629-633.

Kingham TP et al. Multidisciplinary treatment of gastrointestinal stromal tumors. *Surg Clin North Am* 2009;89:217-233.

Learn PA et al. Randomized clinical trials in gastrointestinal stromal tumors. *Surg Oncol Clin N Am* 2010 Jan;19(1):101-113.

Parc Y et al. Surgical management of the duodenal manifestations of familial adenomatous polyposis. *Br J Surg* 2011 Apr;98(4):480-484.

Poncet G et al. Recent trends in the treatment of well-differentiated endocrine carcinoma of the small bowel. *World J Gastroenterol* 2010 Apr 14;16(14):1696-1706.

Soyer P et al. Imaging of malignant neoplasms of the mesenteric small bowel: new trends and perspectives. *Crit Rev Oncol Hematol* 2011 Oct;80(1):10-30.

Speranza G et al. Adenocarcinoma of the small bowel: changes in the landscape? *Curr Opin Oncol* 2010 Jul; 22(4):387-393.

MULTIPLE CHOICE QUESTIONS

1. The most common cause of small bowel obstruction is

   A. Intra-abdominal adhesions
   B. Neoplasms
   C. Intussusception
   D. Crohn's disease

2. The treatment of small bowel obstruction includes

   A. Nasogastric suction
   B. Fluid and electrolyte resuscitation
   C. Laparoscopic adhesiolysis in highly selected case
   D. All of the above

3. One of the following sentences about acute mesenteric ischemia is wrong:

   A. The most common cause is the arterial embolism.
   B. Thrombosis of mesenteric veins is often associated with portal hypertension.
   C. Deep venous thrombosis can be a cause.
   D. Abdominal pain is the main clinical finding.

4. Which sentence about small bowel tumors is correct?

   A. Adenomas are more common in the distal ileum.
   B. The most common neoplasm is GIST.
   C. Peutz–Jeghers syndrome has a very high malignant potential.
   D. Carcinoid syndrome develops in the presence of liver metastases.

5. Which is the most common intestinal fistula in patients with Crohn's disease:

   A. Ileosigmoid
   B. Ileovesical
   C. Ileocutaneous
   D. Ileovaginal

Large Intestine

Jessica Cohan, MD

Madhulika G. Varma, MD

ANATOMY

The colon begins at the ileocecal valve and ends at the rectum, spanning 140 cm (5 feet) in length. The colon has both intraperitoneal and retroperitoneal components. The cecum, ascending, and descending colon are retroperitoneal, whereas the transverse colon and sigmoid are intraperitoneal (Figure 30–1). The diameter of the lumen is greatest at the cecum (~ 7 cm), and decreases distally. As a result, mass lesions of the cecum are least likely to cause obstruction and the thin wall of the cecum is most vulnerable to ischemic necrosis and perforation from large bowel obstructions. There are four layers of the wall—mucosa, submucosa, muscularis propria, and serosa (Figure 30–2). The mucosa is composed of three layers—a simple columnar epithelium organized to form crypts, lamina propria, and muscularis mucosa. The submucosa is the strength layer of the colon because it has the highest concentration of collagen. Therefore, this layer is especially important to incorporate during anastomoses. The muscularis propria is composed of an inner circular layer and an outer longitudinal layer that thickens into three bands around the circumference to form the taeniae coli. The appendix can be found at the point on the cecum where the taeniae converge. At the rectosigmoid, these bands fan out to form a uniform layer, marking the end of the colon and the beginning of the rectum. The forces of these muscular components of the wall result in shortening of the colon to form sacculations called haustra (Figure 30–3). These are not fixed structures, but can be observed to move longitudinally. The appendices epiploicae are fatty appendages on the serosal surface.

The rectum begins at the sacral promontory and ends at the anorectal ring. It lies between the colon and the anus and is 12-16 cm in length. There are no taeniae as the longitudinal muscle fans out and encompasses the circumference of the rectal wall. The rectum can be further differentiated from the colon by its lack of appendices epiploicae and haustra. The rectum is both an intra- and extraperitoneal organ. Posteriorly, the rectum is only intraperitoneal at the level of the rectosigmoid. However, the anterior and lateral walls of the upper rectum are intraperitoneal. The anterior peritoneal reflection extends low into the pelvis, approximately 5-8 cm above the anal verge and lies between the rectum and the bladder in men and uterus in women (the Pouch of Douglas). Tumors or abscesses in this location can be palpated on digital rectal or vaginal examination. Denonvilliers fascia envelops the anterior wall of the rectum. Beyond the anterior peritoneal reflection lie the seminal vesicles and prostate gland in men. In women, the cervix and rectovaginal septum lie anteriorly and the adnexa anterolaterally. The rectum has three major mucosal folds called the valves of Houston. They are variable in location, but classically occur every 3-4 cm. The superior and inferior folds are on the left and the middle fold is on the right. The middle fold marks the distal extent of the intraperitoneal rectum.

The pelvic floor is made of three muscles—the pubococcygeus, iliococcygeus, and puborectalis collectively known as the *levator ani*. The puborectalis forms a sling at the anorectal junction and is an important component of continence and the defecation mechanism.

▶ Blood Supply & Lymphatic Drainage

The arterial supply of the colon is dictated by its embryological origin. The foregut, which extends to the distal transverse colon, is supplied by the superior mesenteric artery (SMA) through the ileocolic, right colic, and middle colic arteries. The hindgut, which includes the distal transverse colon to the rectum, is supplied by the inferior mesenteric artery (IMA). This gives off the left colic, 2-6 sigmoid branches, and terminates as the superior rectal (hemorrhoidal) artery. The middle and inferior rectal (hemorrhoidal) arteries

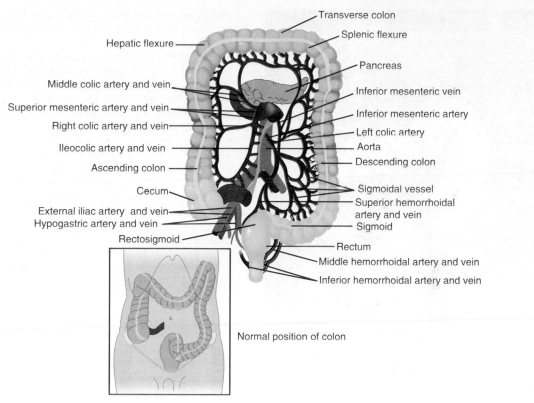

▲ Figure 30–1. The large intestine: anatomic divisions and blood supply. The veins are shown in black. The insert shows the usual configuration of the colon.

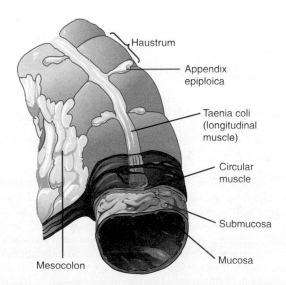

▲ Figure 30–2. Cross-section of colon. The longitudinal muscle encircles the colon but is thickened in the region of the taeniae coli.

originate from the internal iliac artery. There is redundancy in the arterial circulation via the meandering mesenteric artery (Arc of Riolan) as well as the marginal artery of Drummond, which is a network of arterial branches that runs the length of the colon approximately 2.5 cm from the bowel wall. The vasa recta are the terminal arteries arising from the marginal artery. These penetrate the colon wall in multiple areas on the mesenteric side, creating focal areas of weakness that have the potential to form false diverticula. The left colic, sigmoid, and superior rectal branches also originate from the IMA in a variable pattern. The venous drainage generally follows the arterial supply with the exception of the inferior mesenteric vein, which runs lateral to the ligament of Treitz to join the splenic vein. The vascular supply too is highly variable, and "normal" anatomy is found in only 15% of individuals.

The lymphatics drain via continuous plexuses in the submucosal and subserosal layers of the bowel wall. These continue on to the mesenteric lymphatic channels and nodes that accompany the blood vessels, which explain why standard planning for oncologic resections of the colon and rectum is based on the vascular supply.

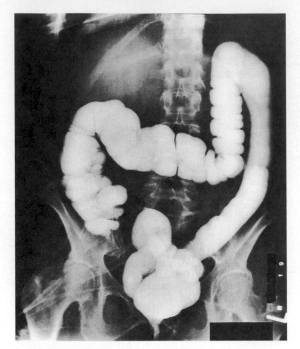

▲ **Figure 30–3.** Barium enema of normal colon. Note the appearance of haustra and the location of the splenic and hepatic flexures.

▶ **Nerve Supply**

The nerve supply to the colon and rectum is autonomic and, like the blood supply, is divided according to embryologic development. Sympathetic nerves to the midgut, including the right and proximal transverse colon, originate in T6-12. These synapse in the superior mesenteric plexus and then follow the SMA and its branches to the right colon. The vagus nerve provides parasympathetic fibers to the midgut. Sympathetic innervation to the hindgut (distal transverse colon to the rectum) arises from L1-3. These sympathetic fibers synapse in the preaortic plexus and then follow the IMA to the bowel wall. Nervous impulses to the bowel wall synapse in the myenteric (Auerbach's) plexus and submucosal (Meissner's) plexus. The myenteric plexus is located in between the circular and longitudinal layers of smooth muscle and is responsible for coordinating motility. The submucosal plexus (Meissner's plexus) is located in the submucosa and regulates secretions, blood flow, and absorption.

The distal rectum and anus is innervated by the hypogastric nerves and the nervi erigentes. The hypogastric nerves are sympathetic fibers that originate from L1-3. These fibers course over the sacral promontory to the hypogastric plexus and form the paired hypogastric nerves near the root of the

IMA. The parasympathetic fibers run in the nervi erigentes, which arise from S2-4 and join the hypogastric nerves near the lateral rectal stalks. The fibers continue anterior and laterally to innervate the rectum, pelvic floor muscles, and bladder, as well as the prostate and seminal vesicles in men. The location of these nerves makes them prone to injury during protectomy. The superior hypogastric plexus is at risk during high ligation of the IMA, the hypogastric nerves are at risk during retrorectal dissection, the inferior hypogastric plexus and nervi erigentes are at risk during mobilization of the lateral stalks, and the periprostatic plexus is at risk during dissection of Denonvillier fascia. Injury to these nerves during proctectomy can cause bladder and sexual dysfunction that is a significant source of postoperative morbidity.

Bleier JI, Maykel JA. Outcomes following proctectomy. *Surg Clin North Am* 2013 Feb;93(1):89-106.

Sakorafas GH, Zouros E, Peros G. Applied vascular anatomy of the colon and rectum: clinical implications for the surgical oncologist. *Surg Oncol* 2006 Dec;15(4):243-255.

PHYSIOLOGY

The primary functions of the colon are absorption, secretion, motility, and intraluminal digestion. These interrelated processes are responsible for converting ileal effluent into semisolid feces. The rectum functions as a capacitance organ, storing feces produced by the colon and allowing defecation at a convenient time. When surgery or disease results in loss of colonic function, there is a significant increase in intestinal losses of water and electrolytes. If the rectum is overloaded by large volume watery stool or its capacity to distend is lost or impaired by surgery or disease, fecal urgency and frequency are noted.

▶ **Intestinal Gas**

Normal volume and composition of intestinal gas has great variation amongst individuals depending on air swallowing, diet, and the composition of the microbial flora. Small amounts of intestinal gas are absorbed through the bowel wall and excreted through the lungs, but the majority (~ 400-1200 mL/d) is discharged as flatus.

Intestinal gas is comprised of nitrogen, oxygen, carbon dioxide, hydrogen, methane, and trace substances such as methyl sulfide, hydrogen sulfide, indole, and skatole. By far, the largest component is nitrogen, which makes up 30%-90% of intestinal gas. Most nitrogen comes from swallowed air, but some also diffuses from the plasma. Fermentation of nonabsorbed carbohydrates such as fiber is responsible for most of the hydrogen and carbon dioxide in gas. In lactase deficient individuals, lactose fermentation contributes as well. Methane is produced by specific hydrogen reducing bacteria (*Methanobrevibacter smithii*) and is only present in 30% of people. Both methane and hydrogen gases are explosive and require caution when using cautery in the bowel lumen.

Patients reporting crampy abdominal pain, bloating, and increased flatus may be suffering from increased gas production. Overproduction may be a result of a malabsorptive state and eliminating lactose, legumes, and/or wheat in the diet may be of help.

▶ Absorption & Secretion

The colon is primarily an absorptive organ. The absorptive capacity is greatest in the cecum and ascending colon and decreases distally. Most nutrients are absorbed in the small bowel; however, when enteric contents reach the colon, they are still rich in water, electrolytes, and some nutrients. Approximately 1-2 L of ileal effluent containing 250 mEq of sodium reaches the cecum every 24 hours. The passive absorption of water and active transportation of sodium allows recovery of more than 90% of the water and sodium content. Every 24 hours, approximately 100-200 mL of water and 2-5 mEq of sodium are excreted in the feces. Table 30-1 gives average values for the composition of ileal effluent and feces. Normal feces are composed of 70% water and 30% solids. Bacteria constitute over half of the solid component. The remaining solids are food waste and desquamated epithelium. Although the absorptive capacity of the colon serves an important role in maintaining homeostasis, it is not essential to life.

This effluent also contains small amounts of nutrients which are absorbed by the colon including fatty acids, amino acids, and vitamin K. Approximately 10% of undigested starch reaches the colon where colonic bacteria fermentation produces short chain fatty acids, which are important both systemically and as a nutrient source for colonocytes.

In addition, the colon is part of the enterohepatic circulation. Bile acids not absorbed in the terminal ileum are passively absorbed in the colon. When this capacity is exceeded, the remaining bile acids are metabolized by colonic bacteria into urobilin and stercobilin. Urobilin, stercobilin, and their metabolites are responsible for giving stool its brown color.

The colon also serves an important secretory function. It secretes hydrogen, bicarbonate, chloride, and potassium ions. The colon is in communication with the circulation and is able to adjust over a wide range as needed. Pathologic states such as inflammatory bowel disease (IBD), shigellosis, cystic fibrosis, and collagenous colitis cause electrolyte and acid-base disturbances by altering colonic secretion.

▶ Motility

Colonic motility serves to maximize absorption and move feces distally in preparation for excretion. There are numerous types of motility and these occur with great variation along the length of the colon. Normal movements are slow, variable, and complex and result in nonorganized flow of the fecal stream. In patients with normal bowel function, enteric contents reach the cecum 4 hours after a meal and the rectosigmoid by 24 hours. However, portions of the fecal stream are mixed so that new effluent may bypass old effluent, and residue from a single meal may pass in bowel movements over 3-4 days.

The enteric nervous system coordinates motility. It is increased by physical activity, stress, and diets high in fiber. In addition, the act of eating stimulates colonic transit. The gastrocolic reflex refers to the activation of colonic motor activity in response to a meal. The magnitude is determined by the fat and caloric composition. This increased activity increases ileal and colonic emptying, causing an urge to defecate.

The colon has three distinct patterns of activity that are under control of the enteric nervous system and a postulated pacemaker in the transverse colon. Retrograde peristalsis consists of annular contractions occurring most commonly in the right colon. These contractions work to keep the stool in the right colon and therefore facilitate absorption. As ileal

Table 30-1. Mean values for electrolyte and water balance in the normal colon. A plus (+) sign indicates absorption from the colonic lumen; a minus (−) sign indicates secretion into the lumen.

	Ileal Effluent		Feces		Net Colonic Absorption (per 24 hours)	
	Concentration (mEq/L)	Quantity (per 24 hours)	Concentration (mEq/L)	Quantity (per 24 hours)	Normal	Maximal Capacity
Na$^+$	120	180 mEq	30	2 mEq	+178 mEq	+400 mEq
K$^+$	6	10 mEq	67	5 mEq	−5 mEq	±45 mEq
Cl$^-$	67	100 mEq	20	1.5 mEq	+98 mEq	+500 mEq
HCO$_3$	40	60 mEq	50	4 mEq	+56 mEq	
H$_2$O		1500 mL		100 mL	+1400 mL	+5000 mL

effluent continues to empty into the cecum, some of the liquid stool flows to the transverse and descending colon, where segmentation predominates. This action consists of random, uncoordinated annular contractions over short segments that propel feces both proximally and distally. Finally, mass movement occurs as a strong coordinated contraction that starts proximally and propels colonic contents distally and occurs in concert with the gastrocolic reflex.

Bowel Habits

There is a broad range of normal bowel habits that varies across cultures. A cross-sectional study of 20,000 men and women across all age groups in Britain showed an average of 1-1.5 bowel movements per day, which increased with fiber and fluid intake and physical activity.

Defecation

The urge to defecate is stimulated by rectal stretch in response to feces. This elicits the rectoanal inhibitory reflex which causes relaxation of the internal anal sphincter and allows the rectal contents to be "sampled" by specialized mucosa in the anorectal transition zone. This mucosa contains sensory fibers that can discriminate between flatus and solid and liquid stool. Immediately following this sensory process, the external sphincter contracts and the contents are moved proximally back into the rectum. Flatus and stool can be discharged, if appropriate. If not, the rectum relaxes and the urge to defecate passes. Normal defecation requires regular colonic function, specifically with regards to stool consistency, in addition to coordinated colonic motility, rectal sensation, sphincter function, and pelvic floor relaxation. When the rectum senses presence of feces and the decision is made to defecate, intra-abdominal pressure is increased and the pelvic floor and anal sphincters relax, allowing the rectum to straighten. After elimination of the stool bolus, the sphincters and pelvic floor resume their tone.

Diarrhea

Diarrhea is defined by the loss of more than 300 mL of fluid per day and chronically affects 5% of the United States population. It can result in severe electrolyte disturbances and dehydration. There are four main etiologies of diarrhea—invasive, secretory, osmotic, and malabsorptive. *Invasive diarrhea* results when enterocytes are destroyed by pathogens such as *Shigella*, *Campylobacter*, and *Entamoeba histolytica*, resulting in low volume loose bowel movements with blood and leukocytes. *Secretory diarrhea* is the result of excessive secretion by colonocytes or enterocytes. This results in high volume, isotonic diarrhea with a low osmotic gap. The primary causes are enterotoxins produced by *E coli* and *Vibrio cholera*, and excessive serotonin secretion in the carcinoid syndrome. *Osmotic diarrhea* occurs when

an osmotically active substance in the bowel lumen draws hypotonic fluid from the circulation. Osmotic diarrhea is characterized by high volume output with a high osmotic gap and no leukocytes. Most commonly, this occurs in patients with disaccharidase deficiencies such as lactose intolerance. *Malabsorptive diarrhea* results from the lack of normal digestive or absorptive processes. Pancreatic insufficiency results in loss of proteolytic and lipase activity causing steatorrhea. Whipple's disease (caused by infection with *Tropheryma whippelii*) and celiac sprue (autoantibodies to gluten) are characterized by inflammatory changes with loss of absorptive capacity of the small bowel. Surgery can also cause malaborption. Extensive small bowel or colonic resections compromise the absorptive capacity and may result in diarrhea. A portion of patients undergoing cholecystectomy will also experience transient diarrhea with fatty meals due to the loss of the bile reservoir capacity of the gallbladder and subsequent steatorrhea.

CONSTIPATION

Epidemiology

Based on an epidemiologic review of the literature, constipation affects 7%-79% of the United States population with a mean of 16%. The wide variation in reports is likely due to broad definitions of constipation including infrequent or hard stools, excessive straining, or incomplete evacuation. Incidence is associated with lower socioeconomic and educational status, non-Caucasian ethnicity, female gender, and increasing age. Low fiber intake is especially important, as it normally bulks stool, triggering colonic motility.

Etiology

Although idiopathic constipation occurs, changes in bowel habits should prompt a search for a cause. Numerous medications cause constipation, such as opiates, antiemetics (ondansetron), antipsychotics (chlorpromazine, haloperidol, risperidone, clozapine), antihypertensives (calcium channel blockers, atenolol, furosemide, clonidine), as well as over the counter medications such as ibuprofen, calcium, and iron supplements. The patient should be asked about previous laxative use, as rebound constipation may occur in patients with a history of laxative abuse. Constipation can be a symptom of a systemic disease such as hypothyroidism, hyperparathyroidism, diabetes, electrolyte disturbance, or connective tissue disorders. It may result from a primary colonic disorder such as Hirschsprung, endometriosis, and benign or malignant strictures. Neurologic disease or injury, psychiatric illness, and physical or sexual abuse may be contributory.

If none of these factors is present, patients may be suffering from a functional constipation syndrome, such as colonic inertia, irritable bowel syndrome, or pelvic floor dysfunction. Patients with colonic inertia report lifelong constipation with laxative dependence. Irritable bowel syndrome (constipation subtype) causes irregular bowel habits, bloating, and abdominal pain classically relieved with bowel movements. Patients with pelvic floor dysfunction or obstructed defecation syndrome report incomplete evacuation and excessive straining that is often improved with digital manipulation. They may have coexistent urinary dysfunction, pelvic organ prolapse, and sexual dysfunction.

Diagnosis

Evaluation for constipation includes a history and physical examination, including review of medications, and digital rectal and anoscopic evaluation. Metabolic etiologies may be ruled out with laboratory tests including TSH, calcium, electrolytes, and blood sugar in the appropriate patient. Anatomic lesions can be identified by colonoscopy. This should be considered in any patient with alarm symptoms (hematochezia, anemia, or weight loss), refractory constipation, and patients who are due for age-appropriate colon cancer screening. Medical therapy with fiber supplementation and laxatives should be tried first. Patients should be encouraged to keep a written record of their bowel habits. In refractory cases, and those in which a functional disorder is suspected, additional testing is indicated.

Anorectal manometry and balloon expulsion test should be considered in severe, refractory cases of constipation where the etiology is not clear and in patients with symptoms of pelvic floor dysfunction. Manometry allows evaluation of the rectoanal inhibitory reflex, sphincter tone, rectal sensation, and coordination. Patients with constipation tend to exhibit a hypertonic internal sphincter with poor squeeze pressures. Electromyography may reveal nonrelaxation or paradoxical contraction of the puborectalis. Balloon expulsion can be performed as an adjunctive study. It involves placing a balloon in the rectum and filling it until the urge to defecate is perceived. The patient is then asked to evacuate the balloon. Normal function is indicated by the ability to evacuate a 50-100 mL balloon in less than 1 minute. This simple test was shown to have 88% sensitivity and 89% specificity for diagnosing defecatory disorders compared with defecography. Defecography (barium, scintigraphic, or magnetic resonance) is useful when the results of manometric testing are not diagnostic.

Colonic transit can be evaluated using radiopaque marker studies. Patients ingest 24 markers and avoid laxatives. An abdominal radiograph is taken on the fifth day with note made of the distribution and number of retained markers. Normal patients will have fewer than five retained markers. In fact, eighty percent of normal patients will have passed all markers by the fifth day. Colonic inertia, a primary disorder of colonic motility, is diagnosed when more than five markers are retained and are scattered throughout the colon.

Obstructed defecation is suggested if markers have accumulated in the rectum. A more detailed examination involves ingestion of radiopaque markers daily for three consecutive days and taking abdominal films on the fourth and seventh days. The number and distribution of retained markers are compared with established normal controls.

Treatment

Initial treatment of constipation should focus on lifestyle and dietary modification. Physical activity, fluid intake, and consumption of fruits, vegetables, and whole grains are increased. A fiber supplement is started in an effort to soften and bulk the stool. A low dose is recommended at first and slowly increased to the desired effect to minimize bloating and flatulence.

Laxatives, stimulants, and enemas should be used only for short periods of time for treatment of acute discomfort. Osmotic laxatives include lactulose, magnesium hydroxide, sodium phosphate, and polyethylene glycol (MiraLAX). These work by increasing the intraluminal osmolarity, creating a gradient that reduces fluid reabsorption. Magnesium hydroxide should be avoided in patients with renal insufficiency. Polyethylene glycol is one of the most commonly recommended laxatives as it is safe and effective, even for use in the long term. Colonic irritants work by increasing motility. Examples include senna, cascara, and bisacodyl. These medications can be limited by crampy abdominal pain. Long-term use of senna and cascara causes melanosis coli (brown discoloration of the mucosa). Stool softeners such as mineral oil and docusate work by increasing stool fluid retention. Enemas stimulate bowel movements by causing direct rectal stretch and irrigation (saline, soap suds), or softening of the stool (mineral oil). Colonic irritants and enemas can cause reduced colon and rectal motility and should not be used for prolonged periods of time. Lubiprostone, linaclotide, and prucalopride are newer agents indicated for the treatment of refractory idiopathic constipation and constipation-predominant irritable bowel syndrome. They cause increased secretion via activation of chloride channels (lubiprostome and linaclotide) and 5-HT4 receptors (prucalopride).

Defecatory disorders, as diagnosed by anorectal manometry, are best managed using biofeedback and pelvic floor retraining. Patients can learn to relax and strengthen the pelvic floor muscles and can develop increased rectal sensation awareness. These techniques have been studied in a randomized fashion and have been shown to be superior to medical management.

Selected patients with constipation benefit from surgery if all functional aspects of defecation have already been addressed. If there is pelvic floor dysfunction, this should be first addressed using biofeedback. Surgery is considered if patients have obstructed defecation from mechanical reasons such as rectal prolapse, rectocele, enterocele, or sigmoidocele may benefit from procedures to address the specific condition. Patients with colonic inertia without pelvic floor dysfunction, irritable bowel syndrome, or diffuse upper gastrointestinal involvement are treated with abdominal colectomy with ileorectal anastomosis. Multiple other approaches, including segmental colectomy and preservation of the cecum have shown conflicting, but overall worse, outcomes. Complications have been reduced with the use of laparoscopic techniques, which have been shown to be safe and effective. The antegrade colonic enema procedure is used more often in pediatric patients. It involves bringing up a piece of bowel (appendix, ileum, cecum, and left colon have been described) to the abdominal wall to allow intermittent catheterization with irrigation of the colon. This technique has been reported in adults with obstructive defecation and neurologic deficits with success. Newer therapies such as sacral nerve stimulation are currently under investigation.

MICROBIOLOGY

The colon of the fetus is sterile but the process of colonization begins immediately after birth. There is marked variation in the composition of the microbial flora between individuals, likely related to genetic, environmental, and dietary factors. Humans have 10 times more bacterial cells in their bodies than human cells, and in fact, bacteria make up 50% of the dry weight of feces. Microbes are present throughout the gastrointestinal tract, and their concentration increases from proximal to distal, with the highest concentrations in the colon and rectum. The majority of colonic organisms are anaerobic, but there is a substantial population of facultative anaerobes. *Bacteroides spp* account for the 60%-70% of the bacterial flora. Other predominant organisms include *Escherichia coli, Lactobacillus bifidus, Kelbsiella, Proteus, Clostridium, Enterobacter, and Enterococcus. Methanobrevibacter smithii* is responsible for methane production.

These bacterial populations are instrumental for the health of the colon. They serve a barrier function and maintain epithelial integrity. Fermentation of undigested polysaccharides creates short chain fatty acids that are an important energy source for colonocytes. In addition, bacteria play an active role in the immune function of the gut. Healthy bacterial populations make it difficult for pathogens to establish infection. In addition, normal microbial flora also serves a role in numerous physiologic processes. They deconjugate unabsorbed bile acids, creating the pigments that give stool its characteristic color, synthesize vitamin K for systemic absorption and use, and recycle colonic nitrogen in the form of urea.

Bharucha AE, Pemberton JH, Locke GR 3rd: American Gastroenterological Association technical review on constipation. *Gastroenterology* 2013 Jan;144(1):218-238.

Mugie SM, Benninga MA, Di Lorenzo C: Epidemiology of constipation in children and adults: a systematic review. *Best Pract Res Clin Gastroenterol* 2011 Feb;25(1):3-18.

Table 30–2. Causes of colonic obstruction in adults.

Cause	Relative Incidence (%)[1]
Carcinoma of colon	65
Diverticulitis	20
Volvulus	5
Miscellaneous	10

[1]Obstruction due to diverticulitis is usually incomplete; volvulus is second to carcinoma as a cause of complete obstruction.

Neish AS: Microbes in gastrointestinal health and disease. *Gastroenterology* 2009 Jan;136(1):65-80.

Vadlamudi HC, Yalavarthi PR, Balambhaigari RY, Vulava J: Receptors and ligands role in colon physiology and pathology. *J Recept Signal Transduct Res* 2013;33(1):1-9.

▼ DISEASES OF THE COLON AND RECTUM

LARGE BOWEL OBSTRUCTION

▶ General Considerations

Fifteen percent of intestinal obstructions in adults occur in the large bowel and the incidence increases with age. Obstruction can result from actual pathology of the bowel wall including malignancy and strictures, mechanical problems such as volvulus, incarcerated hernia, and intussusception, or intraluminal factors such as fecal or foreign body impaction (Table 30–2). Benign strictures are commonly associated with diverticulitis or IBD, but may occur as a result of ischemia, radiation, or as a result of a surgical anastomosis. Acute functional obstruction of the colon (Ogilvie syndrome) can cause the same spectrum of clinical symptoms. It is important to differentiate pseudo-obstruction from mechanical obstruction because the management is different. In contrast to small bowel obstruction, adhesive disease of the large intestine is a very rare cause.

A major factor in the clinical course of large bowel obstruction depends on the competence of the ileocecal valve. Ten to twenty percent of patients have an incompetent ileocecal valve which allows decompression of the large bowel contents into the ileum. However, in the majority of patients, the ileocecal valve does not allow reflux to occur, resulting in a closed loop obstruction with rapidly increasing intraluminal pressure (Figure 30–4). This results in impaired capillary circulation, mucosal ischemia, and subsequent bacterial translocation with systemic toxicity. This process ultimately progresses to gangrene and perforation. This same

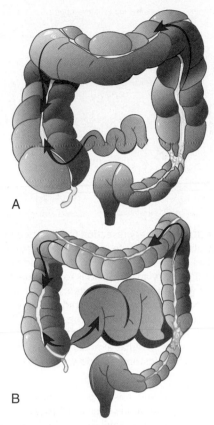

A

B

▲ **Figure 30–4.** The role of the ileocecal valve in obstruction of the colon. The obstruction is in the upper sigmoid. **A:** The ileocecal valve is competent, creating a closed loop between the obstruction and the valve. Tension in the closed loop is increased further by emptying of gas and fluid from the ileum into the colon. **B:** The ileocecal valve is incompetent. Reflux into the ileum is permitted. The colon is relieved of some of its distention, and the small bowel has become distended.

process occurs in volvulus, which by definition is a closed loop obstruction. The cecum has the largest diameter and therefore, by the law of LaPlace, is at greatest risk for perforation. The normal diameter is approximately 7 cm. The risk of perforation is high if the diameter increases acutely or to a size greater than 10-12 cm.

▶ **Clinical Findings**

A. Symptoms and Signs

The history and physical examination can help distinguish a large bowel obstruction from other causes of an acute abdomen and identify those patients requiring urgent therapy.

Obstipation is a universal feature of complete obstruction, though the patient may pass stool and gas located distal to the obstruction after the initial symptoms begin. Classically, the digital rectal examination reveals an empty vault except in cases of distal fecal impaction. Vomiting is a late finding and may not occur at all if the ileocecal valve prevents reflux. If reflux decompresses the cecal contents into the small intestine, the patient may also present with symptoms of small bowel obstruction.

The onset of symptoms maybe acute or gradual, depending on the location and etiology of the obstruction. A patient may report a history of constipation for months preceding any acute obstructive symptoms. Deep, visceral, cramping pain from obstruction of the colon is usually referred to the hypogastrium. Right sided lesions tend to grow to a large size prior to causing obstruction owing to the larger diameter of the lumen and the liquid stool. Therefore, these lesions may be palpable on abdominal examination. If the patient reports repeated episodes of fever and abdominal pain, a diverticular stricture is suspected; a history of hematochezia and weight loss suggests colorectal cancer (CRC). Alternatively, when symptoms occur acutely, volvulus, incarcerated hernia, or intussusception are more likely. A patient with fever, leukocytosis, and peritonitis has likely progressed to develop intestinal ischemia and/or perforation.

B. Imaging Studies

Abdominal films will frequently reveal dilated colon outlining the abdominal cavity. The colon can be distinguished from the small intestine by its haustral markings, which do not cross the entire lumen of the distended colon. Sigmoid volvulus can be identified by a characteristic "coffee bean" appearance which represents a dilated loop of colon starting in the left-lower quadrant extending medially. This finding is seen in 60% of patients. Cecal volvulus tends to appear as a dilated loop originating in the right-lower quadrant extending medially. In patients with other forms of obstruction, the extent of distention is dependent on the competency of the ileocecal valve and its relation to the location of the obstruction. A transition point with no distal colonic gas indicates complete obstruction. If gas is present in the distal rectum, it can represent residual material present prior to the obstruction or the presence of a partial obstruction. In acute pseudo-obstruction, the colon is diffusely dilated with stool and gas throughout (Figure 30–5). A CT scan with rectal contrast is the most useful single test for large bowel obstruction because it can yield information regarding the location and etiology of the bowel obstruction. This has largely replaced contrast enema. A water-soluble contrast medium, such as gastrografin, should be used if strangulation or perforation is suspected. Barium should not be given orally in the presence of suspected colonic obstruction.

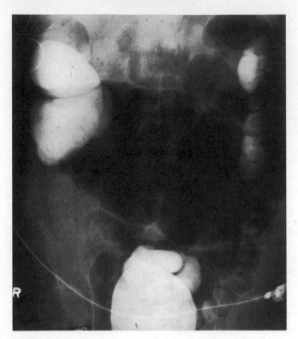

▲ **Figure 30–5.** Plain radiograph demonstrating the dilated colon with pseudo-obstruction (Ogilvie syndrome). (Courtesy of Dr. Santhat Nivatvongs)

▶ **Treatment**

A. Obstruction

An operation is almost always required for mechanical large bowel obstructions. The extent of surgery depends on the patient's acuity and the etiology of the obstruction. The primary goals of treatment are resection of all necrotic bowels and decompression of the obstructed segment. Removal of the obstructing lesion is a secondary goal, but a single operation to accomplish both objectives is preferred whenever possible. Options include resection with primary anastomosis, resection with diversion, diversion alone, and endoscopic stent placement.

Endoscopic stents are being used as a bridge to surgery and as palliative therapy. When used in acutely ill patients with a malignancy, there is no clear advantage of endoscopic stent placement as a bridge to surgery in terms of mortality or complications. However, they do allow decompression of the obstruction and time for physiologic optimization. This can increase the chances of resection with primary anastomosis and reduce the chance for diversion. This comes, however, at the risk of stent-related perforation. Stents may be considered also for palliation in high risk patients whose obstructing cancers are not resectable; however, if the patient will tolerate it, a permanent diverting colostomy is a more durable option.

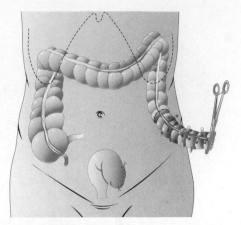

▲ **Figure 30–6.** Primary resection for diverticulitis of the colon, also used in acute large bowel obstructions. The affected segment (shaded) has been divided at its distal end. If primary anastomosis is to be done, the proximal margin (dotted line) is transected, and the bowel is anastomosed end to end. If a two-stage procedure will be used, a colostomy is formed at the proximal margin, and the distal stump is oversewn (Hartmann procedure, as shown) or exteriorized as a mucous fistula. The second stage consists of colostomy takedown and anastomosis.

Generally speaking, obstructing lesions of the right colon can be resected in one stage if the patient's condition is stable. If the patient's condition is precarious or if the colon has perforated, the bowel should be resected and an ileostomy created. Intestinal continuity can be restored at a second operation. Intestinal bypass is sometimes used for unresectable lesions although the relief of the obstruction is not always as effective.

Obstructing lesions of the left colon more commonly require diversion. Ideally the lesion is resected at the initial operation. After resection, anastomosis may be postponed with creation of a temporary end colostomy and Hartmann's pouch (Figure 30–6). If the patient's clinical condition will allow it, a primary anastomosis may be performed with a diverting loop ileostomy if needed to protect the anastomosis. If resection is not possible, the bowel can be decompressed proximally and distally with a loop or double barrel colostomy. These stomas are difficult to manage and are associated with a high rate of prolapse and are thus, avoided if at all possible.

The prognosis depends upon the age and general condition of the patient, the extent of vascular impairment of the bowel, the presence or absence of perforation, the cause of obstruction, and the promptness of surgical management. The overall mortality rate is about 20%. Cecal perforation carries a 40% mortality rate. Obstructing cancer of the colon has a worse prognosis than nonobstructing cancer because it is more likely to be locally invasive or metastatic to nodes or distant sites.

B. Pseudo-Obstruction

Acute pseudo-obstruction of the colon (Ogilvie syndrome) presents with massive colonic distention in the absence of a mechanically obstructing lesion (Figure 30–5). It is a severe form of ileus that occurs most commonly in systemically ill patients and results from an imbalance in the autonomic tone with subsequent absence of peristalsis. Electrolyte disturbances and medications are contributing factors. These patients are usually recovering from major surgery or are hospitalized for other causes, most commonly cardiac disease, trauma, and infection. The mortality rate is 15% overall but increases to 30% in patients who develop ischemia or perforation.

The initial presentation may be missed in critically ill patients. Abdominal distention is the earliest manifestation, but later symptoms include abdominal pain, vomiting, and obstipation and may mimic those of true obstruction; however, 40% of patients will have diarrhea. The differential diagnosis includes toxic megacolon (in patients with ulcerative colitis [UC] and *C difficile* colitis) and mechanical large bowel obstruction. Plain x-rays of the abdomen show marked distention of the colon, often most severe in the right and transverse colon. Contrast enema proves the absence of obstruction, but instillation of radiopaque material should cease as soon as the dilated colon is reached. As opposed to a mechanical bowel obstruction, surgical management in Ogilvie syndrome is reserved for complications including perforation and ischemia.

If the patient has no signs of obstruction or perforation, the initial measures include nasogastric suction, rectal tube placement, fluid resuscitation, and correction of electrolyte imbalances. Systemic illnesses contribute and should be treated appropriately (respiratory failure, cardiac disease, and sepsis). All anticholinergic and narcotic medications should be discontinued. These measures will be effective in 75%-85% of patients. The patient should be followed with serial imaging. The risk of perforation is related to cecal diameter. The highest risk patients have a diameter > 10 cm and should be closely monitored. If there is any sign of clinical deterioration or no improvement in 48 hours, more aggressive treatment is warranted.

The acetylcholinesterase inhibitor neostigmine is an effective treatment for acute colonic pseudo-obstruction in patients without response to conservative measures. It works by acutely increasing acetylcholine levels in the body thereby prompting immediate bowel contraction and decompression. Patients require telemetry monitoring during and after administration as symptomatic bradycardia requiring atropine occurs in 10% of patients. The most common side effects include abdominal cramping and excessive salivation.

It is successful in 90% of patients with a recurrence rate of 7%. If this is unsuccessful, or neostigamine is contraindicated (renal insufficiency, pregnancy, bronchospasm, bradycardia), colonoscopic decompression is the next step in management. Endoscopic decompression carries a risk of perforation but when performed by an experienced team, the risk of perforation is reduced to 2%. This procedure also offers the benefit of visualization of the colonic mucosa for evidence of ischemia. This is initially successful in 80% of patients, but recurrence is common. Ideally a tube is placed into the right colon using fluoroscopic guidance to maintain decompression.

In patients with refractory disease, surgical intervention is required. A percutaneous cecostomy tube is possible in patients who are high risk for surgery. If there is evidence of ischemia or perforation, patients are offered segmental or subtotal colectomy depending on the distribution of disease. This operation carries a high morbidity and mortality, likely related to patient's underlying illness. Primary anastomosis is considered based on the patient's clinical status, but often diversion is performed and intestinal continuity created at during a second procedure months after resolution of disease.

ASGE Standards of Practice Committee, Harrison ME, Anderson MA, et al: The role of endoscopy in the management of patients with known and suspected colonic obstruction and pseudo-obstruction. *Gastrointest Endosc* 2010 Apr;71(4):669-679.

De Giorgio R, Knowles CH: Acute colonic pseudo-obstruction. *Br J Surg* 2009 Mar;96(3):229-239.

Godfrey EM, Addley HC, Shaw AS: The use of computed tomography in the detection and characterization of large bowel obstruction. *N Z Med J* 2009 Oct 30;122(1305):57-73.

Schwenter F, Morel P, Gervaz P: Management of obstructive and perforated colorectal cancer. *Expert Rev Anticancer Ther* 2010 Oct;10(10):1613-1619.

Tan CJ, Dasari BV, Gardiner K: Systematic review and meta-analysis of randomized clinical trials of self-expanding metallic stents as a bridge to surgery versus emergency surgery for malignant left-sided large bowel obstruction. *Br J Surg* 2012 Apr;99(4):469-476.

COLON CANCER AND POLYPS

Background

In the United States, colorectal cancer (CRC) ranks third after prostate and lung cancer in men, and after breast and lung cancer in women in both incidence and mortality. The American Cancer Society predicts that in 2012, more than 143,000 patients will be diagnosed and 51,000 will die as a result of their disease. Men have a higher incidence and mortality than women, and Black Americans have a higher incidence and mortality than other ethnic groups. The overall incidence and mortality from CRC has been decreasing since the early 1980s, likely owing to improved screening.

The frequency of CRCs by location in the colon is shown in Figure 30–7. The average age at diagnosis is 68 years for men and 72 years for women.

The average lifetime incidence of CRC in the United States is more than 5%. Multiple risk factors for CRC have been identified. The most significant are considered non-modifiable. For instance, having a single first degree family member with a diagnosis of CRC increases one's lifetime risk by 2.2. If the relative is diagnosed at an early age, the risk is increased by 3.9 and if there is more than one relative, this risk increases to 4.0. The most significant personal risk factors include IBD, especially with pancolitis, a history of adenomatous polyps, diabetes, and obesity. Modifiable risk factors include increased red and processed meat consumption, smoking, and alcohol. Case control and cohort studies have suggested that protective factors include a high fiber diet, calcium as well as vitamin D supplementation and physical activity. Randomized controlled intervention trials have been unable to demonstrate that these interventions significantly reduce risk for CRCs; however, they are limited by the older age of the study population at the time of intervention, poor adherence, and a relatively short follow up. A large Danish cohort study concluded that 25% of cancers are preventable through a healthy lifestyle.

In addition to lifestyle, chemoprevention in colon cancer has also been suggested as a way to reduce the burden of disease. Celecoxib and low dose aspirin have been shown to reduce the rate of metachronous adenomas in average risk patients found to have adenomas on screening colonoscopy. However, the adverse effects of these medications including cardiovascular events with celecoxib and peptic ulcer disease with aspirin likely outweigh these risks and therefore their use is limited in average risk patients. However, the benefits of celecoxib are more likely to outweigh the risk in patients with familial adenomatous polyposis (FAP), an inherited CRC syndrome, and it has been FDA approved for this indication.

▶ Genetics

CRC develops through a stepwise accumulation of mutations that allow the progression of normal mucosa to adenoma to carcinoma in a pathway known as Loss of Heterozygosity. The inciting event in 85% of sporadic CRCs is the development of chromosomal instability. This allows a cell to accumulate inactivating mutations in tumor suppressors such as adenomatous polyposis coli (APC), P53, deleted in colorectal carcinoma (DCC) and SMAD 4, as well as activating mutations in oncogenes such as K-ras, c-myc, c-src, and BRAF in a stepwise fashion. A less common pathway involves the development of mutations in the genes responsible for DNA mismatch repair and subsequent microsatellite instability. A third mechanism involves the epigenetic silencing of tumor suppressor genes though abnormal methylation. The familial cancer syndromes are caused by germline mutations in these genes, such as APC in familial adenomatous polyposis and mismatch repair genes in Lynch Syndrome, also known as hereditary nonpolyposis colorectal cancer (HNPCC). Approximately 5% of CRCs occur in patients with a hereditary syndrome.

HEREDITARY NONPOLYPOSIS COLORECTAL CANCER

The most common genetic colon cancer syndrome is Lynch syndrome, formerly known as HNPCC. The name of the condition has reverted to Lynch syndrome as these patients may have polyps in addition to cancer. It is an autosomal dominant condition with 80% penetrance whose basis is a mutation in the DNA mismatch repair system clustered on chromosome 2p. Ninety percent of all patients have a mutation in MLH1 or MSH2 which results in microsatellite instability (MSI). Other known mutations include MSH6, PMS2, and PMS1. The lifetime risk of CRC is 66% in men and 43% in women with a median age at diagnosis of 42 and 47 years, but this varies between affected families depending on the mutation. These cancers tend to occur in the ascending colon. A hallmark of the disease is the association with other cancers, including the endometrial, ovarian, gastric, upper urinary tract, biliary, small bowel, and brain.

The diagnosis is usually suspected on clinical grounds using the patient's medical and family history. Four sets of criteria were developed to help make the diagnosis. The Amsterdam criteria were initially developed in 1990 and are based on an accurate, extended family history of colon cancer. They were found to have a sensitivity of 61% and a specificity of 67% for the diagnosis. In 1999 the Amsterdam II criteria were published, which increased the sensitivity by

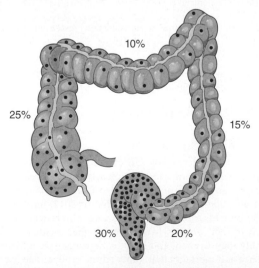

10%

25%

15%

30%   20%

▲ **Figure 30–7.** Distribution of cancer of the colon and rectum.

Table 30–3a. Amsterdam I and II criteria.

Amsterdam I Criteria	
At least three relatives must have histologically verified colorectal cancer.	(1) One must be a first-degree relative of the other two.
	(2) At least two successive generations must be affected.
	(3) At least one of the relatives with colorectal cancer must have received the diagnosis before age 50.
Amsterdam II Criteria	
At least three relatives must have a cancer associated with hereditary nonpolyposis colorectal cancer (HNPCC) (colorectal, endometrial, stomach, ovary, ureter or renal-pelvis, brain, small bowel, hepatobiliary tract, skin [sebaceous tumors])	(1) One must be a first-degree relative of the other two.
	(2) At least two successive generations must be affected.
	(3) At least one of the relatives with HNPCC-associated cancer must have received the diagnosis before age 50.

including extracolonic cancers (Table 30–3a). Patients who meet either of these criteria should be offered genetic testing, which can be used to provide diagnostic and prognostic information for the patient and his or her family. A separate set of criteria, known as the Bethesda Guidelines, was published in 1997 (Table 30–3b). These were designed to have very high sensitivity (94%) at the expense of specificity (49%) and are used to select tumor specimens appropriate for MSI testing. If this test is positive, it is followed by a confirmatory genetic test for the HNPCC mutations, because 15% of sporadic CRC exhibit MSI.

Once a diagnosis has been made, an aggressive screening regimen is initiated including colonoscopy every 1-2 years starting at age 20-25. Women are advised to undergo endometrial cancer screening or hysterectomy if childbearing is complete. In families with a history of upper urinary tract or gastric cancers, screening for renal and ureteral cancer is

Table 30–3b. Revised Bethesda criteria.

1. Colorectal cancer (CRC) diagnosed in individual under age 50 years.
2. Presence of synchronous, metachronous colorectal or other HNPCC-associated tumors, regardless of age.
3. CRC with the microsatellite instability-high (MSI-H) histology (presence of tumor-infiltrating lymphocytes, Crohn-like lymphocytic reaction, mucinous/signet-ring differentiation, or medullary growth pattern) in patient 60 years of age.
4. CRC in one or more first-degree relatives with an HNPCC-related tumor, with one of the cancers being diagnosed under age 50 years.
5. CRC diagnosed in two or more first- or second-degree relatives with HNPCC-related tumors, regardless of age.

initiated at age 30-35 years. A decision analysis model suggested that prophylactic total abdominal colectomy at age 25 would offer a very small survival benefit (1.8 years) and a decreased quality of life compared with colonoscopic surveillance. Therefore, surgical intervention is generally reserved for patients who develop a cancer or polyp that is unable to be removed endoscopically. However, because metachronous tumors occur in 40% of patients at 10 years an aggressive surgical approach is warranted. If a patient presents with a colon cancer, one option would be total abdominal colectomy with ileorectal anastomosis; however, even with this aggressive approach, the risk of developing a future rectal cancer is 6%-20%. Because any rectal remnant left in situ is a risk for developing a future cancer, an aggressive approach is appropriate; however, the decision regarding the specific intervention is multifactorial and depends on the patient's preoperative continence, ability to cope with the change in bowel habits that occur after low anastomoses, and desire to participate in postoperative surveillance. If the patient prefers protectomy or presents with a rectal cancer a restorative proctocolectomy with ileal pouch anal anastomosis (IPAA) (J-pouch) can be offered if safe from an oncologic perspective. However, if the tumor precludes sphincter preservation or the patient is otherwise not a candidate for a J-pouch, a total proctocolectomy with end ileostomy is performed.

FAMILIAL ADENOMATOUS POLYPOSIS AND MYH-ASSOCIATED POLYPOSIS

The second most common CRC syndrome is FAP. This syndrome accounts for less than 1% of all CRCs. Like HNPCC, it is autosomal dominant with nearly 100% penetrance; however, in contrast, these patients are more likely to develop left-sided CRC at an earlier age (> 90% by age 40). Twenty percent of cases of FAP are sporadic. Most are a result of a mutation of the DNA mismatch repair gene APC located on chromosome 5q21. Depending on the location and type of mutation, the phenotypic presentation can range from mild to severe. Individuals with classic FAP typically have more than 100 colonic adenomas but can have more than 1000. These develop at an early age and are present in 50% of patients by age 15. In contrast, patients with attenuated FAP (aFAP) have an average of 30 polyps that develop after age 25. Although most patients with the attenuated form develop colon cancer, the average age is 59 years.

MYH-Associated polyposis (MAP) is clinically similar to FAP and aFAP. Most patients develop a mean of 50 polyps, although cases have been documented with 5-750. However, it is distinguished by family history as it is an autosomal recessive condition caused by mutations in the base excision repair gene MYH.

There are a variety of extracolonic manifestations described in patients affected by the polyposis syndromes. Duodenal neoplasms and desmoid tumors occur in 85% and 15% of patients, respectively. These two manifestations are important because they contribute to increased morbidity and mortality in FAP patients. Esophagogastroduodenoscopy (EGD) is recommended for duodenal screening in these patients beginning at the age of 20. Desmoid tumors are commonly intra-abdominal in FAP patients. They are often found incidentally at surgery but can be aggressive and result in significant GI symptoms. Other manifestations include retinal pigment epithelium hypertrophy, osteomas, and sebaceous cysts. Gardner syndrome is applied to families with the constellation of polyposis, osteoma, dental abnormalities, and soft tissue tumors; Turcot syndrome refers to patients affected by polyposis and medulloblastoma.

Management involves genetic counseling, aggressive screening, and prophylactic colectomy. Patients at risk for FAP should undergo initial colonoscopy at the age of 12, or 20 if suspected to have aFAP. Considering the predominantly left-sided disease in FAP, it has been suggested that these patients can be followed with annual or biannual flexible sigmoidoscopy; however patients with aFAP should be followed with colonoscopy. Prophylactic colectomy is warranted in all patients, especially those with severe polyposis, dysplasia, symptoms, or large adenomas. This can be delayed if there is a mild presentation, but otherwise should be performed as soon as practical. Options are the same as those for HNPCC, and include total proctocolectomy with end ileostomy, restorative proctocolectomy with IPAA, and total abdominal colectomy with ileorectal anastomosis, again depending on preoperative bowel function and patient preference. Abdominal colectomy is reserved for patients with rectal sparing and attenuated disease, which most often occurs in the presence of a specific mutation upstream of c1250. However, the retained rectum is still at risk and these patients still require surveillance proctoscopy with resection or destruction of polyps every 6 months. More commonly, patients elect to undergo restorative proctocolectomy with IPAA. Patients who have a stapled anastomosis will retain about 1 cm of the anal transition zone (ATZ) and due to the predilection for ileal polyps, patients undergoing IPAA require lifelong surveillance. Some surgeons favor mucosectomy to reduce the risk of polyps in the ATZ but the ileal polyps are not affected and the functional outcome of a mucosectomy with handsewn anastomosis is less favorable than for those with a stapled anastomosis. Celecoxib is approved by the FDA for chemoprevention and may be a useful adjunct in these patients. Even with perfect surveillance and appropriate surgical management, FAP patients have an excess mortality related to extracolonic disease including upper GI malignancy and desmoids.

JUVENILE POLYPOSIS

Juvenile polyposis is a rare syndrome characterized by the development of excessive non-adenomatous polyps. It is an autosomal dominant condition, most commonly associated with germline mutations in the SMAD4 or BMPR1A genes. The polyps are a distinct histologic subtype referred to as "juvenile" polyps, which are similar to hamartomas with edematous lamina propria and inflammatory changes. Although the pathway to carcinoma in these patients has not yet been fully elucidated, these patients have an elevated lifetime risk of developing CRC of 39%-68%. It is thought that carcinoma development is a result of neoplastic epithelial changes in the setting of exposure to the inflammatory stromal environment. The syndrome is diagnosed by the presence of five or more juvenile polyps in the gastrointestinal tract or the presence of any number of juvenile polyps with a family history of juvenile polyposis. There are three associated syndromes: Cronkhite–Canada syndrome (juvenile polyposis and ectodermal lesions), Bannayan–Riley–Ruvalcaba syndrome (juvenile polyposis, macrocephaly and genital hyperpigmentation), and Cowden disease (juvenile polyposis, facial trichilemmomas, thyroid cancer, goiter, and breast cancer).

These patients should undergo surveillance of the entire gastrointestinal tract for polyps beginning at the time of diagnosis or the onset of symptoms. This should continue annually in the presence of polyps. However, if the patient is polyp-free, the interval can be extended to 2-3 years. Surgery is reserved for patients with severe diarrhea, bleeding, or intussusception, those who fail endoscopic management of their polyps, exhibit dysplastic changes, and for those patients with a strong family history of CRC.

PEUTZ–JEGHERS SYNDROME

Peutz–Jeghers syndrome is a rare autosomal dominant condition (1/200,000 population) caused by a mutation in the STK11 gene on chromosome 19. The syndrome is defined by multiple hamartomas in the gastrointestinal tract (stomach to the rectum), mucocutaneous pigmentation, and elevated risk of gastrointestinal, breast, pancreatic, cervical, ovarian, and testicular cancers. The lifetime risk of CRC is reported to be 39%. Diagnosis is made in patients with two or more Peutz–Jeghers polyps or a combination of polyps, mucocutaneous pigmentation, or family history. There is insufficient evidence to suggest that the polyps themselves represent a premalignant lesion; however, they do become symptomatic in 50% of patients by the age of 20. Symptoms include anemia secondary to bleeding and abdominal pain secondary to infarction, intussusception, or obstruction. Because of the rarity of the condition, management has not been well defined. Regular endoscopic surveillance (including small bowel capsule endoscopy) is advocated for the early detection of malignancy and resection of symptomatic lesions. This is recommended to begin at age 8, with the frequency determined by the burden of hamartomas. When endoscopic removal is not possible, exploratory surgery with resection and intraoperative small bowel endoscopy is advised. These patients also must undergo appropriate screening for the extra-intestinal malignancies. Optimal regimens are under active study.

COLORECTAL CANCER SCREENING

CRC screening is important for two reasons. The first is the early detection of colorectal carcinomas and the second is preventing CRC through the identification and removal of colorectal adenomas, which are cancer precursors. Trials have shown that the detection of early CRCs by surveillance reduces mortality. Similarly, patients who undergo endoscopic removal of adenomas have a 53% reduction in CRC-specific mortality at 16 years. The benefit is increased in patients with above average risk for CRC.

The most updated guidelines on CRC screening were published in 2008. This includes three separate guidelines from the American College of Gastroenterology (ACG), the United States Preventative Services Task Force (USPSTF), and a joint guideline from the American Cancer Society, the US Multi-Society Task Force on Colorectal Cancer (which includes the American Society of Colon and Rectal Surgeons), and the American College of Radiology (Table 30–4). While they vary in certain recommendations, all agree that screening for average risk patients should begin at age 50 and should occur at regular intervals depending on the method, of which several are available. These include fecal occult blood test (FOBT), fecal immunochemical test (FIT), stool DNA, barium enema, CT colonography, flexible sigmoidoscopy, and colonoscopy. All abnormalities detected

Table 30–4. American Society of Colon and Rectal Surgeons guidelines for colorectal cancer screening.[1]

Risk	Procedure	Onset (Age, y)	Frequency
I. Low Risk			
A. Asymptomatic—no risk factors	Fecal occult blood testing and flex-sig	50	FOBT yearly. Flex-sig every 5 years
B. Colorectal cancer in none of first-degree relatives	Total colon examination (colonoscopy or double-contrast barium enema and proctosigmoidoscopy	50	Every 5-10 years
II. Moderate Risk (20%-30% of people)			
A. Colorectal cancer in first-degree relative, age 55 or younger, or two or more first-degree relatives of any ages	Colonoscopy	40, or 10 years before the youngest case in the family, whichever is earlier	Every 5 years
B. Colorectal cancer in a first-degree relative over age 55	Colonoscopy	50, or 10 years before the age of the case, whichever is earlier	Every 5-10 years
C. Personal history of large (> 1 cm) or multiple colorectal polyps of any size	Colonoscopy	1 year after polypectomy	If recurrent polyps—1 year If normal—5 years
D. Personal history of colorectal malignancy—surveillance after resection for curative intent	Colonoscopy	1 year after resection	If normal—3 years If still normal—5 years If abnormal—as above
III. High Risk (6%-8% of people)			
A. Family history of hereditary adenomatous polyposis	Flex-sig; consider genetic counseling and genetic testing	12-14 (puberty)	Every 1-2 years
B. Family history of hereditary nonpolyposis colon cancer	Colonoscopy; consider genetic counseling and genetic testing	21-40	Every 2 years
		40	Every year
C. Inflammatory bowel disease			
1. Left-side colitis	Colonoscopy	15th	Every 1-2 years
2. Pancolitis	Colonoscopy	8th	Every 1-2 years

[1]Flex-sig, flexible sigmoidoscopy; FOBT, fecal occult blood testing.

by screening tests require a colonoscopy for diagnosis and treatment. The decision of which method to use must be individualized, taking into account several factors, including sensitivity and specificity, risks, costs, patient adherence, and availability. The ACG guidelines suggest that African American men should begin screening at age 45. The USPSTF guidelines recommend screening selectively in patients between ages 75 and 85 years and not screening patients over 85 years. The USPSTF does not recommend the newer stool DNA and CT colonography tests until more performance data are available. All guidelines agree that prevention of colon cancer is the primary goal of screening and that the decision should be made on an individual basis to maximize effectiveness.

All methods have their strengths and weaknesses. Stool tests, like FIT, FOBT, and the stool DNA test are noninvasive with essentially no risks. They are more acceptable to patients as a screening modality; however, there is poor adherence in clinical trials on the part of both the physician and patient with the examination not being performed at the proper intervals or patients not undergoing colonoscopy for positive tests. The sensitivity of FOBT is poor (33%-40%), but this increased to 50%-75% with the development of the SENSA FOBT that is now the standard. Sensitivity and the false positive rate were addressed with the development of the stool DNA test and FIT, although these are substantially more expensive and, as mentioned, the stool DNA test is still undergoing clinical trials. It is important to note that these tests are not designed for prevention, but rather for early detection, as most advanced adenomas are not detected by these tests.

Radiographic options, including barium enema and CT colonography, are more sensitive for the detection of malignant and premalignant lesions. Both require full bowel preparation and have the drawback of radiation exposure; however, procedural risk is low. Barium enema has fallen out of favor as a screening test as it cannot detect small lesions, is unable to provide pathologic information and is very uncomfortable for patients. As CT colonography is still early in its development, its performance and appropriate screening intervals has yet to be defined; however it has been shown to have good sensitivity and specificity. It has a 90% sensitivity and a specificity of 86% for polyps more than 1 cm in size. For polyps more than 6 mm, sensitivity was 78% and specificity 88%. It is likely a poor test for detecting sessile adenomas. Using a cutoff of 6 mm for referral for colonoscopy, 15%-25% of patients would be referred, requiring an additional bowel preparation and the cost of another procedure. In addition, 5%-16% of patients will have an incidental extracolonic finding requiring further evaluation.

Flexible sigmoidoscopy is not often used in the United States for screening purposes. Its utility in preventing CRC is limited because it does not evaluate the proximal colon.

It is therefore combined with a fecal screening test and colonoscopy is recommended if the fecal test is positive. Colonoscopic studies have shown that 30% of patients with advanced adenomas have no distal lesions and would therefore have a normal examination to the splenic flexure. This is more common in women and patients over age 60. This, in combination with the need for bowel preparation, patient discomfort, and poor reimbursement, has made this test infrequently utilized for screening purposes.

Colonoscopy at 10-year intervals is the preferred screening test in the ACG guidelines and is the final common step in every screening program for CRC. Its major drawback is poor adherence, likely related to the need for bowel preparation and sedation, which usually requires a chaperone and a day off work. It is the most expensive screening test and does have a small but real risk of complications (3-5/1000). A concern for missed lesions has prompted the development of tools for measuring quality. However, it is overall a safe and effective screening regimen.

Screening for high risk patients is individualized. Children with possible FAP should begin screening at puberty. Patients in families with HNPCC should begin at age 21. Patients with UC for more than 10 years should begin annual colonoscopy with random biopsies. Patients with a history of early (< age 60) CRC in one first degree relative are offered colonoscopy starting at age 40, or 10 years earlier than the family member's diagnosis. The most recent ACG recommendations state that patients with a family history of CRC occurring in one family member older than age 60 may undergo screening as an average risk patient.

SPORADIC COLORECTAL POLYPS

The term "polyp" is a morphologic term given to tissue that project into the lumen of the gastrointestinal tract and therefore is a broad term encompassing many entities, both benign and malignant. Non-neoplastic polyps account for 90% of all colonic polyps. Subtypes include juvenile, hyperplastic, and inflammatory polyps, as well as hamartomas (Table 30–5). There have been rare reports of carcinoma developing in association with hamartomas, but in general these polyps do not portend an increased risk for cancer. Neoplastic polyps, or adenomas, are the precursor lesions to the vast majority of colorectal adenocarcinomas in a well-studied "polyp to carcinoma" sequence, where colonic mucosa transforms into small tubular adenomas, increases in size, and develops high risk features prior to frank carcinoma. The genetic mechanisms behind this process have been well characterized and are discussed above. An exception to this is the more recently recognized serrated adenoma, which can be difficult to distinguish from hyperplastic polyps. These are found more commonly in the right colon and are thought to progress to carcinoma via MSI.

Table 30–5. Polyps of the large intestine.

Type	Histologic Diagnosis
Neoplastic	Adenoma
	Tubular adenoma (adenomatous polyp)
	Tubulovillous adenoma (villoglandular adenoma)
	Villous adenoma (villous papilloma)
	Carcinoma
Hamartomas	Juvenile polyp
	Peutz–Jeghers polyp
Inflammatory	Inflammatory polyp (pseudopolyp)
	Benign lymphoid polyp
Unclassified	Hyperplastic polyp
Miscellaneous	Lipoma, leiomyoma, carcinoid

Adenomas, while accounting for only 10% of polyps, are common. Screening colonoscopy in asymptomatic patients detects adenomas in 25% of men and 15% of women. In autopsy series, they are detected in up to 60%. They are more common in older age with a prevalence of 30% at age 50 years and 55% at age 80. About 50% of patients with adenomas have more than one lesion, and 15% have more than two. They are predominantly found distal to the transverse colon and approximately half occur in the rectosigmoid area of the colon.

The presence of an adenoma indicates an increased risk for CRC. Further, adenomas themselves may harbor malignancy. The characteristics of the adenoma, including histology, location, shape, and size, significantly influence this risk. Adenomas are subdivided into tubular, tubulovillous, and villous subtypes and these exist on a spectrum. If followed over time, only 5% of tubular adenomas will develop into a malignancy, however, 22% of tubulovillous and 40% of villous adenomas will progress. Further, risk increases with size. Adenomas less than 1 cm harbor carcinoma only 1% of the time, however this risk increases to 10% in adenomas 1-2 cm and 45% of adenomas greater than 2 cm. Other factors include sessile (as opposed to pedunculated) polyps, location in the ascending colon, male sex, age greater than 60, and family history. Overall, the greatest risk factors for both the presence of carcinoma within a polyp and the future development of CRC are size greater than 1 cm and tubulovillous or villous histology. These have been termed "advanced adenomas." Of note, these polyps require surgical resection more often as these features make them less amenable to endoscopic methods.

Adenomas, even in the absence of malignancy, are associated with risk of CRC. Patients found to have adenomas have a risk of developing metachronous cancers twofold to five-fold over patients without them. The risk is estimated to be 5%-10% per year. For these reasons, the consensus guidelines recommend complete excision of the adenoma plus more frequent colonoscopic surveillance. Colonoscopy is repeated at 5-10 years for 1-2 low risk adenomas, at 3 years if 3-10 low-risk or any high-risk adenomas, and less than 3 years if greater than 10 adenomas. Colonoscopy is repeated sooner if there is a question regarding the adequacy of the polypectomy.

Although techniques for endoscopic polypectomy are improving, surgery still remains an important option in the management of colorectal polyps. Surgery is indicated if complete endoscopic resection is not possible. Large polyps, sessile polyps, and those found in the distal rectum are the most challenging to manage endoscopically and result in a higher likelihood of positive margins or incomplete removal. Because up to 20% of these will harbor carcinoma, they require surgical resection. Surgery is also indicated in some completely resected polyps found to contain invasive adenocarcinoma.

Carcinoma is found in 5% of benign appearing endoscopically resected polyps. In 1985, Haggitt reported that depth of invasion was the most important indicator of metastasis and developed a classification system based on depth of invasion (Table 30–6). Level 1, through 4 (limited to proximal two-thirds of submucosa) with favorable histology have a < 1% risk of nodal metastasis and are adequately treated by endoscopic resection with a margin > 2 mm. However, carcinomas exhibiting evidence of vascular or lymphatic invasion, indeterminant margins, a margin < 2 mm, or level 4 with invasion into distal third of submucosa have a 12%-25% chance of lymph node involvement and therefore require formal oncologic resection.

> ## Clinical Findings

A. Signs and Symptoms

The majority of patients with CRC are asymptomatic. Based on a median doubling time of 130 days, it takes at

Table 30–6. Haggitt classification.[1]

Level	Depth
0	Carcinoma *in situ* or intramucosal carcinoma
1	Carcinoma invading through muscularis mucosa into the submucosa but limited to the head of the polyp
2	Carcinoma invading the neck of the polyp
3	Carcinoma invading any part of the stalk
4	Carcinoma invading into the submucosa of the bowel wall below the stalk of the polyp but above the muscularis propria (T1)
Sessile	By definition, equivalent to level 4

[1]From Haggitt RC et al: Prognostic factors in colorectal carcinomas arising in adenomas: implications for lesions removed by endoscopic polypectomy. *Gastroenterology* 1985;89:328.

least 5 years, and often 10-15 years, before a cancer causes symptoms. When symptoms do appear, they are variable, non-specific, and often indicate an advanced lesion or complications. CRCs may cause subclinical bleeding, resulting in an asymptomatic iron deficiency anemia. For this reason, any iron deficiency anemia in a male or nonmenstruating female should prompt a work up to rule out bleeding from the GI tract. However, one-third of patients with CRC have normal hemoglobin at the time of diagnosis. A minority of patients will present emergently with acute obstruction, perforation, or significant bleeding with symptomatic anemia.

Compared with the left colon, tumors of the right colon may reach a more advanced stage before they cause symptoms. Obstruction is rare because the right colon is larger in diameter and has liquid stool. If these tumors bleed, melena, or more commonly occult blood, will be present in the stool. There may be associated vague abdominal pain. Ten percent of patients present with a palpable abdominal mass.

In contrast, the left colon and rectum has a smaller diameter and semisolid feces. Tumors here can cause luminal narrowing and obstruction resulting in narrowing of the stool, constipation, and increased frequency of bowel movements. Rectal cancer can produce tenesmus. When bleeding occurs, it tends to be dark to bright red and may streak or be mixed with the stool. Any patient with ongoing hematochezia, even in the presence of another clinical explanation, such as hemorrhoids, must undergo evaluation for CRC.

Physical examination may help localize and determine the extent of disease. The abdomen should be palpated for masses and the liver examined to rule out enlargement. Auscultation of the lungs is poorly sensitive for metastatic disease. A digital rectal examination may detect a distal rectal cancer. Its location, size, and mobility should be noted. Retrorectal nodes or drop metastases in the Pouch of Douglas (Blumer shelf) may be palpated. Rigid proctoscopic examination gives an accurate location of the tumor, which is important for treatment planning. Lymph node examination may reveal metastasis in the supraclavicular nodes.

The preoperative work up for CRC will determine a clinical stage, allow initial prognostics, and inform the treatment plan. It consists of laboratory tests, radiographic imaging, and endoscopy with biopsies.

B. Laboratory Findings

Useful laboratory tests include a complete blood count, serum chemistries, urine analysis, and liver function tests as clinically indicated. These will detect anemia and other abnormalities that may need to be addressed prior to initiating treatment. The serum marker for CRC is carcinoembryonic antigen (CEA). It is a glycoprotein found throughout the gastrointestinal tract as well as other tissues. It is not sensitive or specific for patients with CRC, specifically for patients without metastatic disease. It is therefore not recommended as a screening test; however, it has been shown to be a useful adjunct to postoperative monitoring for recurrence, specifically in patients with an elevated preoperative CEA that returns to normal after surgery.

C. Colonoscopy

Colonoscopy is the gold standard for the diagnosis of CRC. Complete colonoscopy is indicated in all patients who have suspected or known CRC. It allows tissue diagnosis, localization of the lesion using tattoo, and evaluation for synchronous neoplasms. Three percent of patients with a known colon or rectal cancer have a synchronous lesion. In patients with obstructing lesions, the remaining colon should be evaluated using contrast enema or CT scan. These patients should undergo postoperative surveillance as soon as feasible after their surgery.

D. Mechanisms of Spread

CRC generally grows circumferentially. It takes approximately 1 year for a tumor to encircle three-fourth of the circumference of the bowel wall. This is especially true in the left colon which is smaller in diameter. Submucosal extension through the lymphatic network rarely extends beyond 2 cm from the tumor. As the tumor extends radially, it may penetrate the wall and extend into neighboring structures including the liver, greater curvature of the stomach, duodenum, small bowel, pancreas, spleen, bladder, kidney, ureter, and abdominal wall. Rectal tumors in particular may invade the vaginal wall, bladder, prostate, sacrum, or levators due to the confined space of the pelvis. The inflammatory response incited by extension of the tumor is indistinguishable from frank invasion during gross examination at the time of surgery.

Metastatic disease most often occurs through the lymphatics, although it is also known to occur via seeding, intraluminal spread, or hematogenously. Rectal cancer metastasizes proximally to the mesorectal, iliac, and inferior mesenteric lymph nodes, as well as radially along the pelvic side walls where obturator nodes can become involved. Very distal rectal cancers can also spread to inguinal lymph nodes. Colon cancer spreads along the superior and inferior mesenteric lymph node basins (Figure 30–8). Approximately half of patients undergoing surgery for CRC will have lymph node involvement. Hepatic and pulmonary metastases occur via hematogenous invasion. In colon cancer this may occur through the portal system to the liver, and less commonly the lumbar and vertebral veins to the lungs and other organs. Metastases to ovaries are mostly hematogenous; they are found in 1%-10.3% of women with CRC. Rectal cancer spreads through the systemic circulation via the hypogastric veins.

The "no touch" technique, while never definitively shown to reduce metastatic disease or improve survival, is one of the basic tenets of surgical management of colon cancer. The

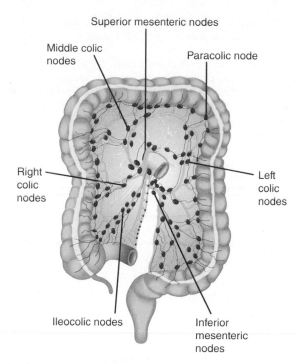

Superior mesenteric nodes

Middle colic nodes

Paracolic node

Right colic nodes

Left colic nodes

Ileocolic nodes

Inferior mesenteric nodes

▲ **Figure 30–8.** Lymphatic drainage of the colon. The lymph nodes (black) are distributed along the blood vessels to the bowel.

concept is to minimize manipulation of the tumor prior to ligation of the blood supply in order to avoid tumor embolus and subsequent metastasis. Transperitoneal metastasis or peritoneal "seeding" may occur when a tumor has extended through the serosa leading to peritoneal implants or generalized carcinomatosis. When found in the Pouch of Douglas, these deposits are palpated on digital rectal examination and referred to as Blumer's shelf.

E. Staging

Accurately staging patients with CRC is important as it allows the development of an adequate treatment plan and determination of prognosis. The clinical stage is determined using preoperative imaging. Pathologic staging is based on imaging and information obtained after resection.

The initial determination required for developing a treatment plan for a patient with colon cancer is whether the tumor is resectable. This can be determined by searching for metastatic disease and determining local invasion. CT of the abdomen and pelvis is used routinely for this purpose. It may reveal lymphadenopathy, hepatic metastases, as well as evidence of obstruction, perforation, or direct extension (Figure 30–9). It has a sensitivity of about 78% for metastatic disease. Metastatic disease to the lungs is most often assessed using a routine preoperative chest x-ray. CT can be used to

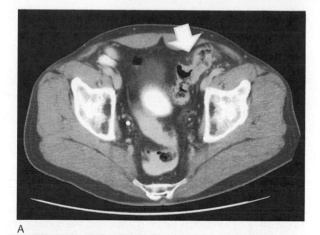

A

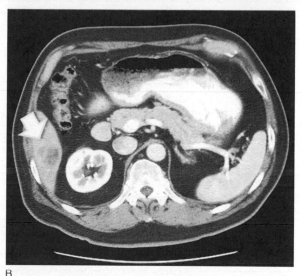

B

▲ **Figure 30–9.** CT scan images. **A:** Primary, circumferential carcinoma of the sigmoid colon (arrow). **B:** Hepatic metastasis (arrow).

further evaluate abnormalities; however, it is not used as an initial test because these patients generally do not develop pulmonary metastases without first developing liver disease. This is because the lymphatic drainage of the colon follows the portal circulation. Positron emission scanning (PET) is not routinely recommended, however it is indicated in patients with suspicious abnormalities on CT that require evaluation for proper treatment planning.

Surgical planning for rectal cancer requires detailed evaluation of the depth of invasion of the rectal wall as well as lymph node involvement and invasion of nearby pelvic structures including the levators, sphincter complex, and genitourinary tract. This information is used to make decisions about neoadjuvant therapy, sphincter sparing procedures, and local excision (LE). Endorectal ultrasound (ERUS) and pelvic magnetic resonance imaging (MRI) are commonly used. ERUS is particularly useful for determining the depth of invasion of the rectal wall and lymph node involvement. MRI is used to detect involvement of the mesorectal fascia and nearby pelvic structures to determine the likelihood of a circumferential resection margin, which is an important predictor of local recurrence. CT and PET CT are often used to assess pulmonary and liver metastasis, although the utility of this imaging modality requires further study.

The standard staging system in the United States is the tumor, node, metastasis (TNM) staging system from the American Joint Committee on Cancer (AJCC). This has replaced the Dukes classification. These are shown in Table 30–7. The clinicopathologic stage is the most important determinant of survival. Stage for stage, patients with colon cancer have a better prognosis than patients with rectal cancer. Similarly, patients with proximal rectal cancers have a better prognosis than those with distal cancers. Poor prognostic factors include complications such as obstruction or perforation, as well as histologic features such as poor differentiation and lymphovascular or perineural invasion.

Table 30–7. TNM classification of cancer of the colon and rectum.[1]

Primary Tumor (T)	
TX	Primary tumor cannot be assessed
T0	No evidence of primary tumor
Tis	Carcinoma *in situ*
T1	Tumor invades submucosa
T2	Tumor invades muscularis propria
T3	Tumor invades through the muscularis propria into the subserosa or into nonperitonealized pericolic or perirectal tissues
T4	Tumor perforates the visceral peritoneum, or directly invades other organs or structures

Regional Lymph Nodes (N)	
NX	Regional lymph nodes cannot be assessed
N0	No regional lymph node metastasis
N1	Metastasis in 1-3 pericolic or perirectal lymph nodes
N2	Metastasis in four or more pericolic or perirectal lymph nodes
N3	Metastasis in any lymph node along the course of a named vascular trunk

Distant Metastasis (M)	
MX	Presence of distant metastasis cannot be assessed
M0	No distant metastasis
M1	Distant metastasis

Stage Grouping				Dukes	Modified Astler–Coller
Stage 0	Tis	N0	M0		
Stage I	T1	N0	M0	A	A
	T2	N0	M0	A	B1
Stage IIA	T3	N0	M0	B	B2
Stage IIB	T4	N0	M0	B	B3
IIIA	T1-2	N1	M0	C	C1
IIIB	T3-4	N1	M0	C2/C3	
IIIC	Any T	N2	M0	C1/C2/C3	
Stage IV	Any T	Any N	M1		

[1]Used with the permission of the American Joint Committee on Cancer (AJCC), Chicago, IL. The original source for this material is *AJCC Cancer Staging Manual*, 6th ed. Lippincott-Raven, Philadelphia, 2002.

TREATMENT OF COLON CANCER

▶ Surgery

Surgical resection of colon tumors is generally performed for patients with curative intent. Patients who are stage I-III or stage IV with resectable metastatic disease in the liver and/or lung are candidates for surgery. However, operative intervention may be necessary in patients with metastatic disease not amenable to complete surgical excision to treat complications of the primary tumor such as obstruction, perforation, or bleeding. Options include resection, diversion, and endoscopic stent placement. Emergency surgery has been associated with significant morbidity (30%) and mortality (10%). For patients specifically with obstruction, a meta-analysis showed no clear advantage of endoscopic stent placement as a bridge to surgery in terms of mortality or complications. In patients with unresectable disease, there is no evidence that prophylactic resection of the primary tumor improves prognosis or outcomes compared with primary chemotherapy treatment. These patients may become resectable after treatment with chemotherapy.

When possible, a laparoscopic approach to colon resection is preferred in most patients as it is associated with decreased hospital stay, postoperative pain, duration of ileus, and better pulmonary function and postoperative quality of life. The long-term oncologic outcomes for the open and laparoscopic approaches have been examined with multiple randomized controlled trials and are equivalent. This approach is not always appropriate for patients with obstructive or perforated lesions and should be abandoned in patients with prohibitive adhesions.

Upon entering the abdomen, the first step is to explore the abdominal cavity to search for metastatic disease not identified on preoperative imaging. If there are no findings that would preclude colectomy, attention is turned to resection. A "no touch" technique minimizes manipulation of the tumor prior to ligation of its blood supply to reduce tumor embolization which has a theoretical risk of causing metastatic disease. Although the extent of resection depends on the necessary lymphadenectomy, a margin of 5 cm on each side of the lesion in the bowel wall is generally considered adequate for clearance of any intramural spread. If there is any invasion into adjacent structures, these must be excised en bloc to achieve negative margins.

An important aspect of the surgical management of colon cancer is the removal of the draining lymph node basin because this allows accurate staging and treatment. Lymph node status is the most sensitive predictor of survival and adjuvant chemotherapy prolongs survival. Sentinel lymph node mapping has been trialed but with poor sensitivity and specificity with both technetium colloid and lymphazurin blue. Therefore, resection of all draining mesenteric lymph nodes remains the standard of care, often necessitating a larger segmental resection than would otherwise be needed for the purpose of margins. An adequate lymphadenectomy contains 12 or more lymph nodes. The extent of resection of the colon and mesocolon for tumors in various locations is shown in Figure 30–10.

A right hemicolectomy is performed for tumors of the cecum and ascending colon. This requires high ligation of the ileocolic, right colic, and right branches of the middle colic artery. If the tumor is at the hepatic flexure or proximal transverse colon, an extended right hemicolectomy is performed with additional ligation of the middle colic artery. During mobilization of the ascending colon and hepatic flexure the surgeon must identify and protect the right ureter, superior mesenteric vessels, and duodenum.

A transverse colectomy with ligation of the middle colic artery is indicated for tumors in the transverse colon. If the tumor is in the splenic flexure or descending colon, a left hemicolectomy is performed with ligation of the IMA at its origin and resection of the distal transverse, descending, and proximal sigmoid colon. Sigmoid tumors are treated with sigmoid colectomy which includes part of the descending colon and proximal rectum. Tumors of the rectosigmoid and upper third of the rectum are removed with an anterior resection, requiring ligation of the sigmoid arteries as well as the middle hemorrhoidal arteries. The extraperitoneal rectum is mobilized and if needed, the splenic flexure may also be mobilized to ensure a tension free anastomosis. With all these resections, attention must be paid to the identification and preservation of the ureters, right kidney, and spleen. Stapled ileocolic anastomoses are associated with a decreased leak rate compared with hand-sewn. However, there does not appear to be a superior type of anastomosis in colocolonic or colorectal anastomoses. Thus, after resection for non-right sided colon cancers, the type of anastomosis is best left to the discretion of the surgeon.

▶ Chemotherapy

Adjuvant chemotherapy is standard of care for patients with stage III (node positive) disease and has been shown to improve survival by 33% and reduce recurrence by 40%. Chemotherapy regimens are based on 5-fluorouracil (5-FU) with levisimole and oxaliplatin (FOLFOX) or capecitabine. Determination of KRAS mutations may also dictate therapy as research shows that two drugs used for CRC, cetuximab (Erbitux) and panitumumab (Vectibix), are not effective in tumors that carry the KRAS mutation. There continues to be debate about the utility of chemotherapy for stage II disease. Without chemotherapy, stage IIb patients have worse 5-year survival than stage III patients likely as a result of routine adjuvant therapy in the stage III patients. However, multiple trials and large database outcomes studies were unable to demonstrate improved survival in stage II patients treated with adjuvant chemotherapy with the exception of QUASAR, a 2007 European randomized trial, which did

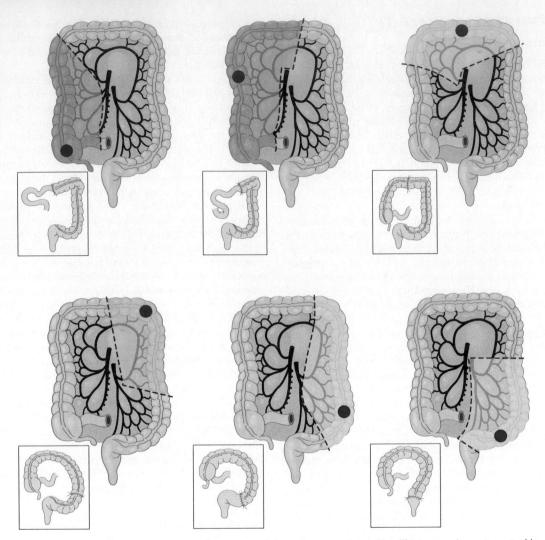

▲ **Figure 30–10.** Extent of surgical resection for cancer of the colon at various sites. The cancer is represented by a black disk. Anastomosis of the bowel remaining after resection is shown in the small insets. The extent of resection is determined by the distribution of the regional lymph nodes along the blood supply. The lymph nodes may contain metastatic cancer.

showed a modest improvement in survival. A Cochrane review including all these patients showed an improved disease free survival but no difference in overall survival. The current thinking is that there is a subset of patients who will benefit from treatment. The NCCN guidelines recommend adjuvant chemotherapy for patients with high risk stage II disease (including T4 tumors, poor differentiation, high grade, perineural or lymphovascular invasion, obstruction, perforation, close or positive margins, or inadequate lymphadenectomy) and consideration of limited treatment of low risk patients. In addition, there is evidence that patients with MSI have a better overall prognosis and are resistant to

5-FU-based chemotherapies. Several trials are in progress to address these areas of uncertainty.

Chemotherapy is the mainstay of treatment for patients with stage IV disease or otherwise unresectable colon cancers. Although a minority of patients with metastatic disease will be candidates for surgical resection, chemotherapy is used in the perioperative period to treat microsocpic foci of disease or in an effort to convert unresectable disease to resectable disease. There is also data to suggest that response to chemotherapy can be used to identify patients who will benefit from surgical metastasectomy. These patients are treated with a chemotherapy regimen similar to patients with stage III disease, with the possible addition of irinotecan and/or a VEG-F inhibitor such as bevacizumab.

TREATMENT OF RECTAL CANCER

▶ Surgery

The choice of operation for rectal cancer depends on many factors. These include the location of the lesion, the depth of penetration and local invasion, histological features such as degree of differentiation and the presence of lymphovascular invasion, and the patient's individual anatomy, general condition, and preoperative bowel function.

A. Local Excision

The surgical management of rectal cancer differs from colon cancer for many reasons, mostly related to its unique anatomy. One aspect of rectal cancer that differentiates it from colon cancer is its accessibility. Very early stage rectal cancers can be treated with LE. This involves resection of a full thickness segment of the rectal wall transanally for distal lesions that are within reach. Transanal endoscopic microsurgery is used for more proximal rectal lesions. This utilizes a specialized proctoscope that allows passage of dissecting instruments and insufflation with carbon dioxide. The resection must involve at least 1 cm margins around the circumference of the tumor and the deep margin must be free. This technique does not sample or treat nodal disease and thus should be limited to a select group of patients at low risk for nodal metastasis. Appropriate patients include those with mobile tumors less than 3 cm in size and that extend less than one-third of the circumference of the rectum. They should be histologically low grade, extend only to the mucosa or submucosa (Tis, T1) and have no radiographic or clinical evidence of nodal metastasis.

The T stage is an important predictor of outcome following local excision (LE). LE was initially offered for all patients with stage I disease, however, the local recurrence rates were found to be unacceptably high (up to 47%) with patients with T2 lesions. Therefore, this therapy is generally reserved for patients with T1 disease, where the local recurrence rate is 5%-18%. There is a newer body of literature suggesting that patients with T1 lesions invading to the outer third of the submucosa have a higher risk for recurrence. If pathological analysis reveals a T2 lesion, positive margins, or high risk features, consideration should be given to radical resection (low anterior resection [LAR] or abdominoperineal resection [APR]) or adjuvant chemoradiation due to the higher risk for lymph node metastases. There is preliminary data that patients who are downstaged using neoadjuvant therapy may be appropriate for this procedure as well but this is not yet standard care.

The initial choice of operation is important, because patients who recur tend to present with advanced disease.

Only 50% of patients with recurrent disease after LE will be candidates for radical resection and their overall survival is poorer than that of patients who initially undergo radical resection. The advantages of LE include decreased morbidity and mortality, short recovery, and in some cases, the opportunity to avoid a colostomy.

B. Radical Excision

When radical excision of a rectal tumor is considered, planning must include assessment of resection for adequate margins, preoperative bowel function, and patient preference while minimizing morbidity. These procedures have a perioperative mortality of 2%. The options include low anterior resection (LAR) or abdominoperineal resection (APR), which includes a permanent colostomy. For cancers in the distal third of the rectum, an ability to achieve a distal margin of 1-2 cm and negative radial margins with complete mesorectal excision is considered the minimum needed to proceed with LAR. Therefore, tumors at the dentate line, with extramural spread to involve the sphincter complex, or direct extension into pelvic structures, require APR. Restoring intestinal continuity is generally considered best when possible from an oncologic standpoint. However, the more distal the anastomosis, the more postoperative bowel function is affected after resection of the rectum. Therefore, a careful evaluation of the patient's preoperative bowel function as well as a discussion with the patient about lifestyle changes is an important aspect of surgical planning.

Historically, recurrence rates were high and survival was low for rectal cancers, however, this has been greatly improved with the technique of total mesorectal excision (TME) and the use of neoadjuvant chemoradiation. TME has dramatically reduced local recurrence rates from 15%-40% to 4%-11% and increased survival in patients without metastatic disease. It generally requires full mobilization of the rectum with en block removal of the mesorectum and bowel wall 5 cm distal to the tumor (tumor-specific TME) if the tumor is in the upper rectum, or completely (TME) if the tumor is in the mid- to distal rectum. It requires dissection posteriorly in the avascular plane between Waldeyer's fascia and the presacral fascia, laterally to encompass the peritoneal reflection but medial to the hypogastric plexus, and anteriorly to include Denonvilliers fascia (Figure 30–11). TME is completed by extending the dissection inferiorly to the levators. This allows removal of the mesorectum *en block* with the rectum and ensures adequate lymph node removal. Further, it removes any tumor that has perineural spread or direct extension outside of the rectum. It is one of the major principles of both LAR and APR.

The laparoscopic approach to rectal tumors is attractive from the standpoint of increasing exposure in the pelvis and minimizing morbidity and length of stay. This approach is associated with earlier return of bowel function and

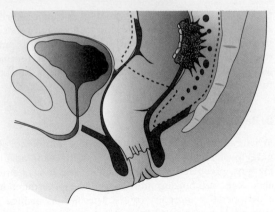

▲ **Figure 30–11.** Total mesorectal excision as depicted in Heald's original publication.

decreased analgesic requirement, although operative time is generally longer. Multiple trials have shown no difference in overall survival or local recurrence rates with follow up extending beyond 5 years.

Because LAR and APR are major operations with extensive pelvic dissection in an often radiated field, the morbidity is higher than colon cancer operations. In addition, LAR includes a technically challenging low anastomosis. Concerns are anastomotic leak, anterior resection syndrome (bowel dysfunction), urinary and sexual dysfunction, wound infection, anastomotic stricture, and injury to the ureters. In cases where identification of the ureters is expected to be difficult, that is, obese patients, those with previous pelvic surgery, and those who have undergoing neoadjuvant chemoradiation, preoperative stent placement can assist with intraoperative identification and preservation of the ureters.

1. Low Anterior Resection—LAR is used when the decision is made to restore intestinal continuity for patients with tumors in the mid- to distal rectum who have good preoperative sphincter function and in whom adequate margins can be achieved. It involves resection of the sigmoid colon and the rectum with the distal transection point being determined by the complete mesorectal excision and attainment of an adequate 1-2 cm distal margin. The operation begins with abdominal exploration to assess metastatic disease. The superior hemorrhoidal artery is ligated at its origin. A higher ligation may be required if there is evidence of lymph node involvement. The rectum is mobilized using the previously described procedure for TME. The rectum elongates after mobilization, potentially adding length to the distal margin. The sigmoid colon is generally resected because its mesentery is removed as part of the vessel ligation. It is also a very muscular segment of the colon and thus, makes for a poor reservoir for bowel function. Furthermore, in patients who have received neoadjuvant chemoradiation,

this segment of the colon has been irradiated and use of the bowel for anastomosis will increase the risk of anastomotic complications such as leak and stricture. The anastomosis is generally performed via a transanal end-to-end stapling device, although a handsewn coloanal anastomosis may be required to achieve an adequate distal margin. There are multiple variations used for low colorectal anastomoses. The most common options are the colonic J pouch, the side-to-end anastomosis and transverse coloplasty. The choice is related to a desire to increase the colonic reservoir without obstructing the outflow. A meta-analysis of 16 trials showed an improvement in bowel function in the colonic J pouch compared to the straight coloanal anastomosis, however, care must be taken to limiting the size of the reservoir to avoid difficulty with complete evacuation.

Temporary diversion of the fecal stream is used to protect the colorectal anastomosis in LAR. This is particularly important in patients who are considered higher risk, including those undergoing neoadjuvant chemoradiation or with a very low anastomosis. Diversion significantly reduces the risk of anastomotic leak and need for reoperation. Both loop ileostomy and colostomy are used. Loop ileostomy is favored as it results in fewer stoma complications including prolapse and sepsis, although this method is associated with a higher risk for dehydration and anastomotic stenosis after closure.

Anastomotic leak occurs in 11% of patients undergoing LAR. Patients at greatest risk for anastomotic leak include elderly patients with low anastomoses and neoadjuvant chemoradiation who were not diverted. Some reports cite patient factors such as male sex, older age, smoking, obesity, and medical comorbidities such as renal failure. The type of anastomosis has not been shown to affect the leak rate. Prophylactic drainage has not been shown to alter the postoperative mortality, clinical or radiological leak rates, wound infection, or need for reoperation.

The Anterior Resection Syndrome occurs in 10%-30% of patients after sphincter preserving operations for rectal cancer and is more pronounced the more distal the anastomosis. Symptoms include clustering (frequent bowel movements in a short period of time), urgency, and incontinence to gas, stool, or both. These symptoms can have a significant impact on quality of life and are likely related to colonic dysmotility, neorectal reservoir dysfunction, sphincter complex damage, and aberrant anal canal sensation. It is worse in patients with a history of pelvic irradiation, rectal prolapse, or anorectal surgery. Most patients have improvement of their symptoms with time, and by 6-9 months after surgery, have a decreased, more manageable number of bowel movements per day. Loperamide, fiber supplementation, and biofeedback are useful adjunctive therapies. Loperamide has the benefit of increasing sphincter tone and slowing stool transit. In patients with intractable incontinence, a permanent stoma may be required.

2. Abdominoperineal Resection—APR is the operation of choice for patients with tumors in the distal third of the rectum in whom achieving negative margins would result in sphincter compromise, as well as those patients who would not tolerate a low anastomosis from a functional standpoint. Resection includes the distal colon, rectum, and anus with creation of an end colostomy. The initial abdominal dissection for APR is similar to that described for LAR. Rectal mobilization is carried down to the levators. The perineal dissection is performed most often with the patient in lithotomy position and can be done by a second team or after the abdominal dissection is complete. For tumors that are anterior in location or to facilitate visualization, a prone positioning after completion of the abdominal portion of the operation is also advocated by some surgeons. An elliptical incision is made around the anus and it is circumferentially dissected in the ischiorectal fat to achieve negative margins with care taken anteriorly in the plane between the anus and the vagina or prostate. This is extended through the levators to reach the inferior aspect of the abdominal dissection. The specimen is removed transanally. The perineal wound is washed out, closed in multiple layers. A drain is placed to prevent wound complications. An effort is made to keep intra-abdominal structures out of the pelvis by closure of the pelvic peritoneum and omental interposition.

Because LAR and APR involve wide dissection in the pelvis, the postoperative complications include those associated with disruption of the pelvic nerves. Urinary dysfunction, specifically urinary retention is reported in 3%-15% of patients, but this is generally transient. Sexual dysfunction tends to become progressively worse with time. In a recent large survey-based analysis, more than half of men experienced erectile dysfunction and two-thirds experienced problems with ejaculation. One-third of women reported dyspareunia. These factors are also likely related to pelvic irradiation.

► Palliative Procedures

If a rectal cancer is unresectable after neoadjuvant therapy, palliative surgery may be indicated to improve symptoms including obstruction, bleeding, or tenesmus. Obstructing cancers can be treated with diversion or endoluminal stents, however, there is a high risk of stent occlusion and perforation. Bleeding and tenesmus may be responsive to fulguration or photocoagulation, although outcomes have been disappointing.

► Chemotherapy and Radiation

Stage I rectal cancers are adequately treated with surgical excision. However, stage II and stage III rectal cancers have high local recurrence rates. Combined-modality therapy including preoperative chemoradiation, surgery, and adjuvant chemotherapy has been shown to increase survival in

these patients. Standard neoadjuvant treatment uses 5-FU as a radiosensitizer. Compared with postoperative chemoradiation, neoadjuvant treatment has been shown to decrease local recurrence and toxicity and increase sphincter preservation. However, it has not been shown to improve overall survival. Twenty percent of patients will have a complete pathologic response which is associated with improved survival. Surgery is planned 4-10 weeks after the completion of treatment. Following resection, adjuvant therapy with FOLFOX or capecitabine is standard, although trials are in progress to determine the optimal duration of treatment.

METASTATIC DISEASE

Metastatic disease is reported in 20% of patients with CRC at presentation and up to 30%-70% of patients will eventually be found to have metastasis. The two most common locations are the liver and the lung. Untreated, these patients have a 5-year survival of 5%. However, selected patients are candidates for surgical resection with curative intent. Surgery results in an improved 5-year survival of 22%-49% for patients with metastatic disease in the liver and 14%-78% for patients with lung disease. If both liver and lung disease are treated surgically, 5-year survival is 30%. After surgery for metastatic disease, 50%-70% of patients have a subsequent recurrence.

Liver and lung metastases are considered resectable if they, and all other sites of disease, including the primary tumor, are amenable to a R0 resection. This is based on the anatomic location as well as leaving an adequate quantity of normal tissue to maintain normal function. Options for patients with extensive disease include preoperative portal vein embolization or staged resection. There are reports of patients being treated with ablative therapies (microwave, radiofrequency) or external beam radiation; however, there are no long-term data available for these procedures. If metastatic disease in the liver initially appears unresectable, induction chemotherapy will result in a clinical response allowing resection in 16% of patients. If metastatic disease recurs after treatment, re-resection is considered in selected patients.

Peritoneal metastasis generally results in poor outcomes with median overall survival of 5-24 months. Current guidelines recommend chemotherapy as the primary treatment. Investigational treatments such as cytoreductive surgery and intraperitoneal chemotherapy show promise in improving survival, however these treatments are associated with significant morbidity and mortality and are not considered standard of care.

POSTOPERATIVE SURVEILLANCE

The goal of postoperative surveillance is to measure the efficacy of treatment and to diagnose recurrences, metastases, and metachronous lesions. After appropriate treatment for

CRC, one-third to one-half of patients will recur. The majority of these (60%-80%) will be in the first 2 years and 90% in the first 5 years after surgery. Three percent will develop a new metachronous tumor by 6 years.

Seventy-five patients with recurrent CRC will have an elevated CEA. Using a cutoff of 6 IU/L yields a sensitivity of 80% and specificity of 42%. It is most sensitive for detection of metastatic disease in the liver, and is elevated months before symptoms appear. Although less sensitive, CT of the abdomen has a similar benefit. Earlier detection improves resectability and survival. If the CEA is elevated, PET scanning is a useful adjunct to the evaluation as it has been shown to have better sensitivity and specificity for recurrent disease than CT.

After many well-designed randomized trials, there is still no consensus on what constitutes appropriate follow up for treated CRC patients. The 2012 NCCN guidelines suggest a history, physical examination, and CEA every 3-6 months. In addition, patients with high risk features such as lymphovascular invasion or poorly differentiated tumors should undergo CT of the chest, abdomen, and pelvis every year for 3-5 years. Colonoscopy should be performed at 1 year, and if normal, subsequent examinations should be scheduled in 3 years, and then every 5 years. For patients with rectal cancer who underwent LAR, proctoscopy should be considered every 6 months for 5 years. Although cost-effectiveness and survival benefit has been suggested for these surveillance strategies, they have not been proven definitively. However, they do increase the possibility of treating recurrences with intent for cure.

▶ Treatment for Recurrent Disease

CRC recurs in up to 50% of patients. In patients with rectal cancer, 35% will have a local recurrence compared with 15% of patients with colon cancer. Otherwise, the most common sites are the liver, lung, and regional lymph nodes. If R0 resection is possible, this can be undertaken in patients who are good surgical candidates in combination with adjuvant chemotherapy. In patients who present with unresectable disease, a combination of palliative chemotherapy and radiation therapy (if appropriate based on location) is administered, although this is unlikely to improve survival. However, the overall prognosis for recurrent CRC is poor. Survival is 35% at 5 years in patients who are candidates for curative surgical resection.

American Cancer Society: *Colorectal Cancer Facts and Figures 2011-2013*. Atlanta, GA: American Cancer Society, 2011.

Beggs AD, Latchford AR, Vasen HF, et al: Peutz-Jeghers syndrome: a systematic review and recommendations for management. *Gut* 2010 Jul;59(7):975-986.

Brosens LA, Langeveld D, van Hattem WA, Giardiello FM, Offerhaus GJ: Juvenile polyposis syndrome. *World J Gastroenterol* 2011 Nov 28;17(44):4839-4844.

Brown CJ, Fenech DS, McLeod RS: Reconstructive techniques after rectal resection for rectal cancer. *Cochrane Database Syst Rev* 2008 Apr 16 (2).

Chen J, Wang DR, Yu HF, et al: Defunctioning stoma in low anterior resection for rectal cancer: a meta-analysis of five recent studies. *Hepatogastroenterology* 2011 Dec 22;59:118.

Den Oudsten BL, Traa MJ, Thong MS, et al: Higher prevalence of sexual dysfunction in colon and rectal cancer survivors compared with the normative population: a population-based study. *Eur J Cancer*. 2012;48(17):3161-3170.

Dominic OG, McGarrity T, Dignan M, Lengerich EJ: American College of Gastroenterology Guidelines for Colorectal Cancer Screening 2008. *Am J Gastroenterol* 2009 Oct;104(10): 2626-2627.

Figueredo A, Coombes ME, Mukherjee S: Adjuvant therapy for completely resected stage II colon cancer. *Cochrane Database of Systematic Reviews* 2008 Jul 16;(3):CD005390

Issa N, Murninkas A, Powsner E, Dreznick Z: Long-term outcome of local excision after complete pathological response to neoadjuvant chemoradiation therapy for rectal cancer. *World J Surg* 2012 Oct;36(10):2481-2487.

Kwak JY, Kim JS, Kim HJ, et al: Diagnostic value of FDG-PET/CT for lymph node metastasis of colorectal cancer. *World J Surg* 2012 Aug;36(8):1898-1905.

Levin B, Lieberman DA, McFarland B, et al: Screening and surveillance for the early detection of colorectal cancer and adenomatous polyps, 2008: a joint guideline from the American Cancer Society, the US Multi-Society Task Force on Colorectal Cancer, and the American College of Radiology. *Gastroenterology* 2008;134:1570.

Lieberman DA, Rex DK, Winawer SJ, et al: Guidelines for colonoscopy surveillance after screening and polypectomy: a consensus update by the US Multi-Society Task Force on Colorectal Cancer. *Gastroenterology* 2012 Sep;143(3):844-857.

Markowitz S, Bertagnolli M: Molecular basis of colorectal cancer. *NEJM* 2009; 361(25):2449-2460.

Marshall JR: Prevention of colorectal cancer: diet, chemoprevention, and lifestyle. *Gastroenterol Clin North Am* 2008;37:73.

Neutzling CB, Lustosa SAS, Proenca IM, da Silva EMK, Matos D: Stapled versus handsewn methods for colorectal anastomosis surgery. *Cochrane Database Syst Rev* 2012 Feb 15;2:CD003144.

Paun BC, Cassie S, MacLean AR, Dixon E, Buie WD: Postoperative complications following surgery for rectal cancer. *Ann Surg* 2010 May;251(5):807-818.

QUASAR Collaborative Group: Adjuvant chemotherapy versus observation in patients with colorectal cancer: a randomized study. *Lancet* 2007;370(9604): 2020-2029.

Sagar J: Colorectal stents for the management of malignant colonic obstructions. *Cochrane Database Syst Rev* 2011 Nov 9;(11):CD007378

Zauber AG, Winawer SJ, O'Brien MJ, et al: Colonoscopic polypectomy and long-term prevention of colorectal-cancer deaths. *NEJM* 2012;366(8):687-696.

OTHER TUMORS OF THE COLON & RECTUM

▶ Neuroendocrine Tumors

Neuroendocrine tumors (NETs), or carcinoids, of the colon and rectum account for approximately 6% of all NETs of the gastrointestinal tract. They are rare, although the incidence is increasing. More than half are found in the rectum. Incidence is increased in patients with IBD. They are rarely symptomatic and are most often diagnosed during screening colonoscopy or incidentally during laparotomy or imaging for other conditions.

Although the prognosis for these tumors is largely undefined because of their rarity, important factors include histologic subtype, tumor size, depth of invasion, and location. They are classified as benign (previously typical carcinoid), low grade malignant (atypical carcinoid), or high grade malignant (small and large cell carcinoma) and are staged according to the tumor, node, metastasis (TNM) system. Survival for rectal carcinoids is better than colon carcinoids, which tend to be associated with colon adenocarcinoma. Benign and low-grade malignant tumors are best managed surgically. There is controversy over the extent of surgery required, but it has been suggested that tumors greater than 1-2 cm or with high-risk histological features are best treated with standard oncologic resection whereas smaller lesions can be managed with local excision. High-grade malignant carcinoids of the large intestine are extremely aggressive and have a poor prognosis even if diagnosed at an early stage. These are best treated with chemotherapy.

▶ Lymphomas

The most common site of extranodal non-Hodgkin lymphoma is the gastrointestinal system; however, the colon and rectum are rarely affected. This disease is more common in middle-aged men and immunosuppressed patients. Symptoms are generally nonspecific, and more than half of patients present with a palpable abdominal mass. On imaging it appears as an infiltrating submucosal lesion with associated mesenteric lymphadenopathy, making it difficult to discern from adenocarcinoma. Another form, lymphomatous polyposis, can mimic familial polyposis coli. Colonoscopy with biopsy is important because depending on the subtype of lymphoma, chemotherapy and/or radiation is the primary treatment. Because the diagnosis is often delayed, patients may need urgent or emergent surgery for acutely symptomatic lesions.

▶ Lipomas

The colon is the most frequent site of gastrointestinal lipomas. They are benign fatty submucosal tumors with an incidence of 1%-4%. They are more common in women and in the right colon. Lipomas are generally asymptomatic, however, they may cause vague abdominal symptoms or intussusception, especially if large in size. Although they can sometimes be difficult to differentiate from colon malignancy, the diagnosis can be made by characteristic findings on endoscopic ultrasound (hyperechoic submucosal lesion). Resection is indicated for symptomatic lipomas or if the diagnosis is not clear by radiographic or endoscopic findings.

GASTROINTESTINAL STROMAL TUMORS

Gastrointestinal stromal tumors (GISTs) are derived from the pluripotential interstitial cells of Cajal and are associated with activating mutations in a specific tyrosine kinase found in the large intestine called KIT or CD 117. Like many of the aforementioned neoplasms, these are submucosal tumors that can grow to a large size before causing symptoms. They are commonly diagnosed radiographically, although occasionally percutaneous or endoscopic biopsy is necessary to confirm or rule out metastatic disease for treatment planning purposes. Surgery is the standard treatment for patients with localized tumors > 2 cm, tumors with high risk features, or symptomatic tumors. Because GISTs spread hematogeneously, local resection with negative margins is adequate. Care must be taken to prevent intraoperative rupture of the tumor pseudocapsule as this is associated with high rates of recurrence. Medical therapy with imatinib mesylate, which selectively inhibits KIT is used for patients with unresectable tumors, metastatic disease, or poor prognostic factors. Sunitinib malate has been introduced as salvage therapy for patients with imatinib-resistant disease. Prognostic factors include location in the GI tract (stomach most favorable), mitotic index, and size. They are associated with generally good overall survival but recurrence is common.

ENDOMETRIOMAS

Endometriosis refers to the presence of endometrial tissue that forms implants in the pelvis and abdomen. Deeply infiltrating endometriosis refers to a subtype with locally invasive implants on the bowel wall. Symptoms include abdominal pain, hematochezia, and pain with defecation. Most patients present with palpable, tender nodules on rectal or vaginal examination. The diagnosis is made endoscopically in most patients. Medical management with NSAIDs, oral contraceptives, and GnRH agonists is generally limited by side effects and does not appear to prevent progression of the disease. Surgery is indicated for persistent symptoms or if malignancy cannot be excluded. The implants are treated with superficial excision, full thickness excision with primary defect closure, and resection with anastomosis. Although early reports cited concern over the development of anastomotic leak and rectovaginal fistulas, these complications have proven to be rare. While the majority of patients experience symptomatic improvement, recurrence is over 10% and long-term follow-up is lacking.

OTHER TUMORS

Other rare tumors of the large intestine have been reported, including neurofibromas, teratomas, rectal duplication cysts, lymphangiomas, and cavernous hemangiomas. Rare malignancies include adenosquamous carcinoma, primary squamous cell carcinoma, and melanoma.

Casali PG, Blay JY, ESMO/CONTICANET/EUROBONET Consensus Panel of Experts: Gastrointestinal stromal tumours: ESMO Clinical Practice Guidelines for diagnosis, treatment and follow-up. *Ann Oncol* 2010 May;21(suppl 5):v98-102. Erratum in *Ann Oncol* 2011 Jan;22(1):243.

Konishi T, Watanabe T, Nagawa H, et al: Treatment of colorectal carcinoids: a new paradigm. *World J Gastrointest Surg* 2010 May 27;2(5):153-156.

Meuleman C, Tomassetti C, D'Hoore A, et al: Surgical treatment of deeply infiltrating endometriosis with colorectal involvement. *Hum Reprod Update* 2011 May-Jun;17(3):311-326.

Nallamothu G, Adler DG: Large colonic lipomas. *Gastroenterol Hepatol* 2011 Jul;7(7):490-492.

Ni SJ, Sheng WQ, Du X: Pathologic research update of colorectal neuroendocrine tumors. *World J Gastroenterol* 2010 Apr 14;16(14):1713-1719.

Stanojevic GZ, Nestorovic MD, Brankovic BR, et al: Primary colorectal lymphoma: an overview. *World J Gastrointest Oncol* 2011 Jan 15;3(1):14-18.

DIVERTICULAR DISEASE OF THE COLON

DIVERTICULOSIS

▶ General Considerations

Diverticula (singular: diverticulum) are more common in the colon than in any other portion of the gastrointestinal tract. Their presence is referred to as diverticulosis. Most colonic diverticula are false, referring to the fact that they consist of mucosa and submucosa that have herniated through the muscular layer of the colon wall. True diverticula, which contain all layers of the bowel wall, are rare in the colon. In the United States, the most common location for diverticula is the sigmoid colon. The descending, transverse, and ascending portions of the colon are involved in decreasing order of frequency. Diverticula form as a result of increased intraluminal pressure acting at areas of relative weakness on the bowel wall caused by the blood supply. The vasa recta extend onto the colon wall, then penetrate the muscular layer between the taenia to supply the mucosa. Therefore, diverticula are most commonly located in the area between the mesenteric taenia and the antimesenteric taenia with a skip area on the antimesenteric border (Figure 30–12).

▶ Epidemiology

In Western countries, 30%-60% of individuals develop diverticula. There is no gender predilection. The prevalence increases with age, although recently there has been an increase in the younger population. Ten percent of patients are affected by age 40 and 65% by age 80. Diverticular disease is more common in Western nations. In Asian countries, there is a predominance of right-sided diverticula. The geologic differences in the incidence of diverticular disease suggest that cultural factors may play an etiologic role. The contribution of a low fiber diet rich in red meat is a commonly cited risk factor but this has not been shown conclusively. Other reported factors include physical inactivity, constipation, increasing age, smoking, obesity, alcohol, and NSAID use. Patients with Ehlers–Danlos and Marfan syndrome, both of which involve abnormal connective tissue, are at increased risk.

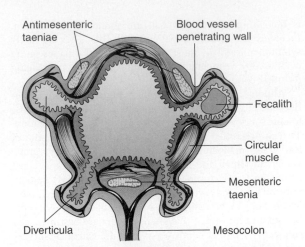

▲ **Figure 30–12.** Cross-section of the colon depicting the sites where diverticula form. Note that the antimeso-colic portion is spared. The longitudinal layer of muscle completely encircles the bowel and is not limited to the taeniae as depicted here.

▶ Symptoms and Signs

Diverticulosis remains asymptomatic in up to 80% of people and is usually detected incidentally on barium enema x-ray, CT scan, or colonoscopy. A history of constipation is often elicited. An abdominal examination may reveal mild tenderness in the left-lower quadrant, and the left colon is sometimes palpable as a firm tubular structure.

▶ Treatment

Asymptomatic patients with diverticulosis may be given a high-fiber diet, although its role is unclear except as a treatment for constipation. There is no evidence to suggest that avoiding nuts, seeds, or popcorn has a protective effect. In fact, no dietary change has been conclusively shown to treat diverticulosis or prevent its complications, although weight loss, smoking cessation, and a diet low in red meat have been suggested as possibilities. Surgery is not indicated for uncomplicated diverticulosis.

▶ Prognosis

The natural history of diverticulosis has not been defined. Complications of diverticulosis including diverticulitis, hemorrhage, stricture, and fistula formation occur in approximately 20% of patients with diverticulosis. Because these estimates rely on patients with known diverticulosis, the incidence of complications in the general population (who have undiagnosed, asymptomatic diverticulosis) may be much lower. About 75% of patients who present with complications of diverticular disease report no prior colonic symptoms.

DIVERTICULITIS

General Considerations

Acute diverticulitis is the result of micro- or macroscopic perforation of a diverticulum resulting in an inflammatory response. The sigmoid colon is the most common location for diverticula and therefore is the most common location of diverticulitis. The severity of disease can range from mild inflammation localized to a segment of the bowel wall (microperforation) to feculent peritonitis (macroperforation). The majority of patients (75%) present with simple, uncomplicated, diverticulitis. This occurs when microperforation is immediately walled off, resulting in localized inflammation. Complicated diverticulitis occurs in 25% of patients and refers to macro- or gross perforation with abscess or peritonitis, as well as those who develop complications including stricture or fistula.

Clinical Findings

A. Symptoms and Signs

Patients with acute diverticulitis classically present with abdominal pain and fullness localized to the left-lower quadrant. The average age of presentation is 62 years. The severity of abdominal pain ranges from mild to severe, often described as steady aching or cramping. It often resembles acute appendicitis except that it is situated in the left-lower quadrant. Occasionally, pain is suprapubic, in the right-lower quadrant, or throughout the lower abdomen depending on the location of the sigmoid and the distribution of disease. Changes in bowel habits, including constipation, diarrhea, or both are common. Dysuria is indicative of inflammation adjacent to the bladder. Nausea and vomiting may be present depending on the location and severity of the inflammation. Physical findings characteristically include low-grade fever, mild abdominal distention, and left-lower quadrant tenderness. There may be a palpable mass. Leukocytosis is common.

Acute diverticulitis can also present with other nontypical symptoms. Small bowel obstruction may occur if a loop of small bowel becomes entrapped in inflammatory tissue. Free perforation of a diverticulum can result in generalized peritonitis rather than localized inflammation. Episodes of recurrent diverticulitis may produce mild symptoms until a complication such as stricture or fistula develops that

prompts the patient to seek medical attention. The course of diverticulitis may be insidious, particularly in the elderly. Patients may present with vague abdominal pain associated with an abscess or recurrent urinary tract infections from a colovesical fistula. In some cases, pain and inflammatory signs are not marked, but a palpable mass and signs of large bowel obstruction are present, so that carcinoma of the left colon seems the more likely. Diagnosing malignancy can be difficult in the setting of inflammation.

B. Imaging Studies

Plain abdominal films are generally not useful unless they show free abdominal air from a diverticulum that has perforated. Other nonspecific findings include ileus, partial colonic obstruction, or left-lower quadrant mass.

CT scan of the abdomen and pelvis with intravenous contrast is the preferred initial imaging study. In most studies, CT has sensitivity, specificity, and accuracy greater than 90%, although 5% of patients will ultimately be found to have cancer as the underlying cause. It is also helpful to rule out other intra-abdominal pathology that may present in a similar fashion. Findings include wall thickening, fat stranding, and diverticula. Complications such as abscess or fistula may be evident (Figure 30–13). Findings on CT scan may also be predictive of the need for surgical intervention or successful nonoperative expectant management. The Hinchey classification was developed in 1978 to help guide clinical decision making for patients with complicated disease and standardize radiographic reporting. These have been updated to reflect improved resolution of CT and currently include the following stages: (0) mild clinical diverticulitis; (1a) pericolic inflammation or

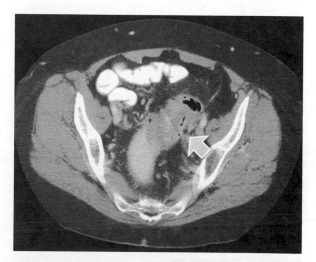

▲ **Figure 30–13.** CT scan showing sigmoid colon involved with diverticulitis. Note the pericolonic stranding, bowel wall thickening, and intramural abscess.

phlegmon; (1b) pericolic or mesocolic abscess; (2) pelvic, intra-abdominal, or retroperitoneal abscess resulting from an extension of a pericolic abscess; (3) purulent peritonitis; and (4) feculent peritonitis.

Colonoscopy is not needed for the evaluation of a patient presenting with classic signs, symptoms, and imaging. However, differentiating acute diverticulitis from other pathology such as IBD, carcinoma, and ischemic colitis can be difficult. If endoscopy is determined to be necessary for appropriate management, a delayed examination after inflammation has subsided is preferred. If timing is critical, then a sigmoidoscopy with low insufflation is recommended over colonscopy to reduce the risk of perforation.

▶ Differential Diagnosis

Acute diverticulitis presents with such variation that the differential diagnosis is broad. It may simulate appendicitis, perforated colonic carcinoma, obstruction with strangulation, colonic ischemia, Crohn disease, cystitis, infectious colitis, and gynecologic disease such as pelvic inflammatory disease, tubal pregnancy, and tubo-ovarian abscess. Differentiation from appendicitis is especially difficult when a redundant sigmoid colon lies in the right-lower quadrant. Free perforation with generalized peritonitis is difficult to differentiate from the other causes of perforation. A thorough history and physical examination as well as imaging studies may be helpful in differentiating these conditions. Colonoscopy is usually deferred upon initial presentation of suspected acute diverticulitis, but may be useful in cases with a high suspicion of carcinoma, vascular insufficiency, or inflammatory disease of the colon. It can be difficult in some cases to rule out carcinoma of the colon, particularly in the more silent forms of diverticulitis that present with a mass or fistula. Occasionally the diagnosis may not be known until the surgical specimen is examined by the pathologist.

▶ Complications

The clinical spectrum of diverticulitis includes complications such as free perforation, abscess, fistula, and obstruction. Fecal peritonitis requires immediate surgery. Abscesses can often be drained percutaneously. Fistulas most commonly involve the bladder or colon, but may also extend to involve the ureter, urethra, vagina, uterus, small bowel, ovaries, fallopian tubes, perineum, and abdominal wall. Colonic obstruction is usually slow in onset and incomplete. Small bowel obstruction may result from inflammatory involvement of the small bowel.

▶ Treatment

A. Medical Management

Approximately 80% of patients with mild acute diverticulitis (Hinchey 0 and Ia) can be managed on an outpatient basis.

However, hospitalization should be considered in patients with mild attacks if they are elderly, immunosuppressed, or have significant comorbidities including diabetes or renal failure. Any patient will need inpatient treatment if there is significant pain, inability to tolerate oral intake, or there is evidence of severe systemic illness. Patients not requiring hospitalization are generally treated with a clear liquid diet, broad spectrum antibiotics (ciprofloxacin and metronidazole or amoxicillin-clavulanate), and close follow up, although this management strategy is largely historical and is being challenged. There is evidence that patients with uncomplicated diverticulitis do not require antibiotics. A recent trial showed no difference in hospital stay, development of complications, or recurrence within 1 year. Patients who were pregnant, immunosuppressed, or septic were excluded.

For those patients requiring hospitalization, treatment depends on the severity of presentation. Generally, patients are managed with bowel rest, intravenous fluids, and systemic broad-spectrum antibiotics. Common regimens cover colonic flora and are chosen based on the patient's allergies and previous antibiotic exposure. Common regimens include a beta-lactam/beta-lactamase inhibitor, a carbapenem, or the combination of a fluoroquinolone plus metronidazole. As clinical manifestations resolve, oral feeding is resumed gradually, initially with a low residue diet. After recovery, a high fiber diet is prescribed if there is no stricture, although this intervention has not been shown conclusively to reduce recurrence. Conservative management is successful in up to 85% of patients. Repeat CT or intervention is indicated when patients fail to improve or if there is clinical deterioration over the initial 48 hours of medical therapy. This often indicates progression to complicated disease that may require surgery.

Over the last decade, more and more patients are being managed conservatively, which has prompted study into strategies to prevent subsequent episodes. Small randomized trials have been conducted on patients who developed diverticulitis twice in 1 year. Mesalamine and rifaximin taken at 1 week intervals every month decreased symptoms and recurrence compared with rifaximin alone. Two small trials of probiotics have shown no significant improvement. However, it has been shown that avoidance of nuts, popcorn and seeds does not reduce the risk of diverticulitis and thus, patients do not need to be counseled to do so.

▶ Interventional Management

Patients with diverticulitis complicated by phlegmon or small abscess without peritonitis (Hinchey Ib) are candidates for conservative treatment. However, large abscesses (> 3 cm) are less likely to resolve with conservative management and should be drained percutaneously if possible. This provides source control and generally results in clinical improvement within days. Percutaneous treatment of an intra-abdominal abscess allows surgical intervention to be performed on an elective basis when there is reduced risk of complications and higher probability of a one-stage operation without a stoma.

▶ Surgical Management

A. Elective Surgery

Recent studies examining the natural history of diverticulitis have demonstrated that over a period of 10 years, recurrent diverticulitis following nonoperative management is expected in 10%-30% of patients. In patients who have a recurrence, a similar proportion will have a third episode. Recurrences tend to occur with similar severity of the previous episode and patients who require urgent surgery usually do so during the first presentation. In other words, it is rare for a patient with a recurrence to require urgent surgery. This indicates a generally benign course for uncomplicated diverticulitis and calls into question the potential benefits of elective prophylactic surgery for patients with a history of acute diverticulitis.

In addition, elective sigmoid colectomy is not without risks. A retrospective review found that 20% of patients experience fecal incontinence, urgency, or incomplete evacuation after sigmoid resection for diverticulitis. The exact indications for surgery have yet to be defined, but overall there has been a general decrease in elective colon resections for diverticulitis in the past 10 years. The American Society of Colon and Rectal Surgeons (ASCRS) guidelines recommend that surgery is offered on an individual basis. Consideration should be given to the patient's previous episodes, frailty, reliability, and access to medical resources. Surgery is generally reserved for complicated disease such as abscess, perforation, stricture, fistula, or high risk patients such as those who are immunologically suppressed. Surgery should also be considered in patients in whom an underlying cancer cannot be excluded.

When interval colectomy is recommended, it is generally delayed by 6-8 weeks to allow resolution of acute inflammation that may add difficulty to the operation. There is evidence that delaying surgery increases the rate of a successful laparoscopic resection with primary anastomosis, which is possible in more than 90% of patients. However, delaying surgery comes with the small but significant risk (2%) of interval development of recurrent severe diverticulitis requiring emergency surgery with high morbidity. Further study is required to determine the optimal timing of surgery.

Definitive resection for sigmoid diverticulitis should include the sigmoid colon distally to the uninvolved rectum. The proximal extent of resection should be the point at which the bowel is soft and appears healthy—this generally includes the entire sigmoid colon. It is unnecessary to resect additional bowel proximally; even if it is involved with diverticula, as they are unlikely to become symptomatic

(Figure 30–6). Laparoscopy has been shown in randomized trials to decrease hospital stay and postoperative pain without increased complications; however, it is a technically challenging operation that should be undertaken only by surgeons comfortable with the technique. In some cases, even in experienced centers, laparoscopy may not be possible due to persistent inflammation and an open approach is required.

A subset of patients will present with colonic stricture as a result of chronic inflammation and scarring. This generally results in symptoms of partial obstruction. If an inflammatory stricture is diagnosed after radiographic and endoscopic evaluation, elective resection is recommended. The distal extent of resection should always include the rectosigmoid junction so that the proximal colon is anastomosed to healthy proximal rectum.

B. Urgent Surgery

Less than 10% of patients will present with complications requiring urgent surgery. Indications include uncontrolled sepsis and failure to improve with medical therapy or percutaneous drainage. There is a lower threshold for surgery for immunocompromised patients given their greater risk of morbidity and mortality with medical management. These are generally features found in patients with Hinchey III or IV disease.

At laparotomy for severe acute diverticulitis, exploration may reveal an inflammatory mass involving large bowel, mesocolon, mesentery, omentum, and sometimes small bowel. Except in cases of free perforation with generalized fecal peritonitis, the diseased diverticulum is not often visible. The type of operation performed is dependent on the extent of colonic inflammation, the amount of peritonitis, the patient's general condition, comorbidities, and nutritional status, the extent of blood loss, and the surgeon's experience and preference.

Ideally, a resection with primary anastomosis is performed as a one-stage procedure. It may not be possible to perform a primary anastomosis if there is gross contamination or infection in the surgical field because of the increased risk of anastomotic leakage. In patients who can tolerate an anastomosis but are still considered high risk, a diverting loop ileostomy is an option.

However, if the risk of an anastomosis is perceived to be too high, two options are available. The standard is the Hartmann procedure, which is a two-stage operation. At the initial operation, the diseased bowel is removed, the proximal end of the colon is brought out as a temporary colostomy, and the distal colonic stump is closed (Figure 30–6). Intestinal continuity is restored in a second operation after the inflammation subsides. There have been reports in the literature of Hinchey III patients having laparoscopic washout and drainage without resection as an alternative to resection. This approach has not been widely adopted and a randomized controlled trial is currently underway to compare this approach with the Hartmann procedure. Increasingly, percutaneous drainage of abscesses avoids the need for staged procedures and allows for primary resection with anastomosis once the inflammation has resolved. However, if percutaneous drainage is unsuccessful, operative drainage is indicated.

A three stage procedure, consisting of diversion and washout followed by resection of the diseased bowel at a second operation, and finally colostomy takedown, is not advised due to the ongoing inflammation of the diseased bowel and associated morbidity despite fecal diversion. However, if the patient will not tolerate a resection, this is an option.

▶ Follow-Up

Colonoscopy is recommended 6-8 weeks after the resolution of symptoms and prior to elective surgical resection to rule out other underlying pathology such as IBD and cancer. Although the presence of malignancy is less than 5% in patients with a radiographic diagnosis of acute diverticulitis, it is especially important to exclude malignancy in the presence of rectal bleeding stricture, or mass. The entire colon should be evaluated prior elective resection for presumed diverticular disease.

▶ Prognosis

The mortality for diverticulitis can be divided by Hinchey stage. Patients with stage I or II disease have a mortality of less than 5%, stage III 13%, and stage IV 43%. Approximately 25% of patients hospitalized with acute diverticulitis require surgical treatment. The operative mortality rate is about 5% in recent reports, compared with 25% historically. Some of this improvement is attributable to the greater use of percutaneous drainage.

Diverticulitis recurs in one-third of patients managed conservatively and in 2%-10% of patients after surgical resection. Most of these recurrences develop within the first 5 years and are most commonly in the rectosigmoid junction due to inadequate resection. More study is required prior to the routine use of mesalamine and probiotics to reduce this risk.

Bachmann K, Krause G, Rawnaq T, et al: Impact of early or delayed elective resection in complicated diverticulitis. *World J Gastroenterol* 2011 Dec 28;17(48):5274-5279.

Chabok A, Påhlman L, Hjern F, et al: Randomized clinical trial of antibiotics in acute uncomplicated diverticulitis. *Br J Surg* 2012 Apr;99(4):532-539.

Klarenbeek BR, de Korte N, van der Peet DL, Cuesta MA: Review of current classifications for diverticular disease and a translation into clinical practice. *Int J Colorectal Dis* 2012 Feb;27(2):207-214.

Levack MM, Savitt LR, Berger DL, et al: Sigmoidectomy syndrome? Patients' perspectives on the functional outcomes following surgery for diverticulitis. *Dis Colon Rectum* 2012 Jan;55(1):10-17.

Peery AF, Barrett PR, Park D, et al: A high-fiber diet does not protect against asymptomatic diverticulosis. *Gastroenterology* 2012 Feb;142(2):266-272.e1.

Rafferty J, Shellito P, Hyman NH, Buie WD: Practice parameters for sigmoid diverticulitis. *Dis Colon Rectum* Jul 2006;49(7):939-944.

Sai VF, Velayos F, Neuhaus J, Westphalen AC: Colonoscopy after CT diagnosis of diverticulitis to exclude colon cancer: a systematic literature review. *Radiology* 2012 May;263(2):383-390.

Strate LL: Lifestyle factors and the course of diverticular disease. *Dig Dis* 2012;30(1):35-45.

Unlü C, Daniels L, Vrouenraets BC, Boermeester MA: Systematic review of medical therapy to prevent recurrent diverticulitis. *Int J Colorectal Dis* 2012 Sep;27(9):1131-1136.

LARGE BOWEL FISTULAE

▶ Colovesical Fistula

Diverticulitis is the etiology of more than half of all colovesical fistulas. This complication occurs in 2%-4% of cases of patients. Other causes include colon cancer, bladder cancer, Crohn colitis, radiation exposure, trauma, and iatrogenic causes. They occur three times more often in men. This predilection is likely anatomical: in women the uterus and adnexa are situated between the colon and the bladder.

The most common presentation is recurrent urinary tract infection. Pneumaturia is reported by up to 70% of patients and fecaluria in up to 50% depending on the size of the fistula. There are no specific physical examination findings, although some patients may have a palpable pelvic mass. There is usually no leukocytosis. Urine analysis is often indicative of urinary tract infection and cultures are polymicrobial. CT of the pelvis with rectal contrast is the most sensitive imaging study and will often show a segment of inflamed colon and bladder wall with air in the bladder. The fistulous connection is rarely seen. Endoscopy and cystoscopy may reveal inflammation at the site of the fistula, but the fistula is rarely visualized. These tests are useful for ruling out malignancy prior to surgical intervention. If the diagnosis is still in question, ingestion of charcoal or poppy seeds with elimination in urine is diagnostic.

The treatment for symptomatic colovesical fistula is elective surgery. The operation should be delayed until any active inflammation (ie, from diverticulitis) has resolved. Up to 50% of colovesical fistulas will undergo spontaneous closure. In these patients, the decision to proceed with surgery depends on the underlying cause of the fistula. In most patients, surgery involves resection of the involved colon with a primary anastomosis. Large bladder fistulas are closed primarily, but most often they do not require closure but are left to close spontaneously with Foley catheter drainage.

However, in malignant fistulas, the tract should be excised en block with the colon and the involved bladder wall, which can be repaired primarily. Omentum is interposed between the anastomosis and the bladder. A urinary catheter is used to decompress the bladder for 5-10 days after surgery. The optimal timing of catheter removal or need for urine cultures or cystogram has not been prospectively validated.

In minimally symptomatic patients at high risk for surgery, conservative management with intermittent antibiotics may be successful. A trial of medical management is also indicated in patients with Crohn colitis, in whom spontaneous closure may be possible.

The prognosis for colovesical fistula is related to the etiology and the general health of the patient. Recurrence is reported to be 4%-5% overall, but is highest in patients with fistulas secondary to radiation therapy and Crohn colitis.

Fiocchi C: Closing fistulas in Crohn's disease–should the accent be on maintenance or safety? *N Engl J Med* Feb 26 2004;350(9): 934-936.

Leicht W, Thomas C, Thüroff J, Roos F: Colovesical fistula caused by diverticulitis of the sigmoid colon : diagnosis and treatment. *Urologe A* 2012 Jul;51(7):971-974. [Translated to English]

Lynn ET, Ranasinghe NE, Dallas KB, Divino CM: Management and outcomes of colovesical fistula repair. *Am Surg* 2012 May;78(5):514-518.

RECTOVAGINAL & COLOVAGINAL FISTULA

Colovaginal fistulae are commonly a complication of diverticulitis, especially in women with a history of hysterectomy. The most common cause of rectovaginal fistula is obstetric injury, followed by Crohn colitis, iatrogenic causes, malignancy, radiation, and trauma. Fistula between the lower third of the rectum and lower half of the vagina are classified as low rectovaginal fistulas, while high fistula are defined as those between the middle to upper third of the rectum and the posterior vaginal fornix. The most common presentation is feculent vaginal discharge, which may be mistaken for fecal incontinence. Patients may also report vaginal flatus, recurrent genitourinary infections, and dyspareunia. There is a significant negative impact on quality of life. A fistula may be observed on anoscopy, rigid sigmoidoscopy, and/or vaginal speculum examination in 85% of patients. Endorectal ultrasound (ERUS), CT with rectal contrast, or barium enema may confirm the diagnosis.

The treatment for recto- and colovaginal fistula is surgical. Colovaginal fistulas are often successfully managed with resection of the involved colon. The vaginal defect may be closed, but will generally close spontaneously if this is technically challenging. The optimal surgical treatment for rectovaginal fistula, on the other hand, is less clear. The treatment is largely based on etiology, individual patient factors and surgeon experience. Numerous procedures have been reported, including direct repair, fibrin glue, endorectal advancement flaps, vaginal advancement flaps, biologic mesh, tissue interposition, and rectal resection. Choice of repair depends on the etiology, size, and location of the fistula. However, the recurrence rate is disappointingly high, especially for patients with Crohn disease who have an ongoing source of inflammation. The optimal approach consists of aggressive medical treatment of the colitis and control of pelvic sepsis followed by surgery. However, reported recurrence rates are 25%-50%. Good results have been reported in patients with multiple recurrences using fecal diversion and repair with a gracilis or omental interposition flap or even proctectomy with permanent stoma.

Ruffolo C, Scarpa M, Bassi N, Angriman I: A systematic review on advancement flaps for rectovaginal fistula in Crohn's disease: transrectal vs transvaginal approach. *Colorectal Dis* 2010 Dec;12(12):1183-1191.

van der Hagen SJ, Soeters PB, Baeten CG, van Gemert WG: Laparoscopic fistula excision and omentoplasty for high rectovaginal fistulas: a prospective study of 40 patients. *Int J Colorectal Dis* 2011 Nov;26(11):1463-1467.

Zhu YF, Tao GQ, Zhou N, Xiang C: Current treatment of rectovaginal fistula in Crohn's disease. *World J Gastroenterol* 2011 Feb 28;17(8):963-967.

ACUTE LOWER GASTROINTESTINAL BLEEDING

▶ Background

Lower gastrointestinal bleeding refers to bleeding originating distal to the ligament of Treitz and involves the small bowel, colon, or rectum. Unlike upper GI bleeds, it occurs in predominantly elderly patients. It accounts for 20% of all GI bleeds and results in over 300,000 hospitalizations in the United States each year. The incidence appears to be increasing with time. Hematochezia refers to the passage of bright red blood, maroon blood, or clots per rectum. Classically, hematochezia indicates a lower GI source of bleeding, however, the color is a function of time spent in the intestinal tract. The black color of melena is the result of the oxidation of iron in hemoglobin. Bright red blood may stem from brisk esophageal variceal bleeding and melena may be the result of slow blood loss from a right-sided colon cancer.

▶ Etiology

Lower GI bleeding can originate from numerous sources. In elderly patients common causes include diverticula, angiodysplasia, malignancy, and ischemia. Younger patients are more commonly affected by IBD, solitary rectal ulcer, and infection. In the appropriate patient, bleeding may be related to coagulopathy, radiation injury, chemotherapy, or a recent procedure such as polypectomy. Chronic, low volume bleeding is seen in patients with malignancy, polyps, hemorrhoids, and fissures. The small intestine can be the source of bleeding in 5% of patients. Other more unusual causes include Meckel's diverticulum (especially with ulceration from ectopic gastric mucosa), and aorto-enteric fistula.

Diverticulosis is the most common source of acute lower GI bleeding. Although bleeding occurs in only 5% of patients with diverticulosis, this presentation is common because of the high prevalence of diverticula in the general population. Diverticula form in areas of weakness where vasa recta penetrate the bowel wall. Structural changes in the bowel wall causes damage to the artery, which can lead to rupture. Diverticular bleeding often presents with painless and massive, but self-limited, hemorrhage. There is a dose-related increase in risk in patients who use NSAIDs. The long-term recurrence rate after the first episode is 25%, however, this increases to 50% after the second episode. Therefore surgery is commonly recommended in the elective setting after a patient presents with recurrent bleeding.

Angiodysplasia, or vascular ectasia, is found in 2% of asymptomatic patients on screening colonoscopy. They are generally located in the right colon in elderly patients and the jejunum in younger patients. These lesions are composed of dilated submucosal vessels with a central feeding vein that have a propensity to bleed spontaneously. Bleeding is typically intermittent and low volume. These patients often present in the outpatient setting with iron deficiency anemia and heme-positive stool. The diagnosis is made in some cases by colonoscopy, and colonoscopic therapy is often successful. There is no need to treat incidentally identified ectasias, as it is estimated that only 15% will cause clinically significant bleeding. Surgery is rarely indicated.

Colitis resulting from IBD, ischemia, radiation, or infection is a third cause of hematochezia. These tend to cause mild blood loss rarely requiring transfusion. These should be suspected in patients with abdominal pain and diarrhea. Acute ischemia may be caused by an acute decrease in blood supply from embolism, hypotension, or spasm. The watershed areas, including the splenic flexure and rectosigmoid junction, are most commonly affected. Infectious colitis can be diagnosed by stool culture. The most common organisms causing bloody diarrhea are *E coli* 0157-H7, *Campylobacter*, and *Shigella*. UC and Crohn colitis can also cause hematochezia during periods of acute inflammation. UC is more commonly associated with bleeding, although it can sometimes be difficult to distinguish between these two entities during an initial colonoscopy. However, the management in this setting is the same. Treatment with steroids and immunomodulators depends on the severity of the disease. This is discussed further in the section on colitis.

▶ **Management**

Chronic rectal bleeding, as seen in patients with colorectal polyps or cancer, and anorectal conditions can be evaluated electively. It is important to include colonoscopy in the evaluation, even if the bleeding can be explained by a benign condition such as hemorrhoids. This is especially true for patients who are more than 50 years of age or have a family history of CRC as it ensures that there is not a more proximal lesion that needs to be addressed.

Acute severe hemorrhage, however, is a potentially life-threatening problem, and prompt evaluation and treatment are critical. The first step in the management of these patients is to evaluate and manage the airway, breathing, and circulation (ABCs). A significant portion of these patients present with hemorrhagic shock. Resuscitation with intravenous fluids and blood products takes priority over initiation of diagnostic procedures. Large bore intravenous catheters should be placed and efforts made to keep the patient warm. Strong consideration should be given to transferring the patient to the intensive care unit or other closely monitored setting. Labs are checked for a coagulation profile, platelet count, and hematocrit. Any coagulation abnormalities should be corrected. Patients should be asked about the recent use of antiplatelet agents and blood thinners. Associated medical conditions should be identified and treated as soon as possible. Digital rectal and anoscopic examinations are performed first to look for an obvious source of bleeding and consideration should be given to the possibility of an upper source. A nasogastric aspirate should be examined to rule out an upper source in most patients. While this is not a perfect test, it can provide quick and useful information in a patient with a life threatening upper GI bleed. If blood is aspirated, there is confirmation of an upper source and EGD should be performed. If bile is aspirated, the source is more likely from the lower GI tract and the diagnostic work up should continue. The next step is determined by patient stability and availability.

A plan of management of acute lower gastrointestinal hemorrhage is outlined in Figure 30–14. Many decisions depend on the rate of bleeding, which is difficult to include in an algorithm. Bleeding stops spontaneously in 90% of patients before transfusion requirements exceed two units, but there are no reliable methods to predict who these patients are or who will have recurrent bleeding. Therefore all brisk GI bleeding must be taken seriously.

There are a wide range of procedures that can be used for both diagnostic and treatment purposes in the acute setting. These include endoscopy, angiography, and radiographic techniques including radionuclide scintigraphy and CT angiography. There is no current gold standard and prospective trials are lacking.

Colonoscopy can be a very useful first test to localize the bleeding in stable patients in whom the colon is the suspected source. It has the advantages of being able to visualize the entire colon and any potential bleeding lesions, even after active hemorrhage has ceased. The sensitivity is 74%-100% and is limited by the fact that there is often no active hemorrhage at the time of the examination and stigmata of recent bleeding are seen in only 8%-43% of cases.

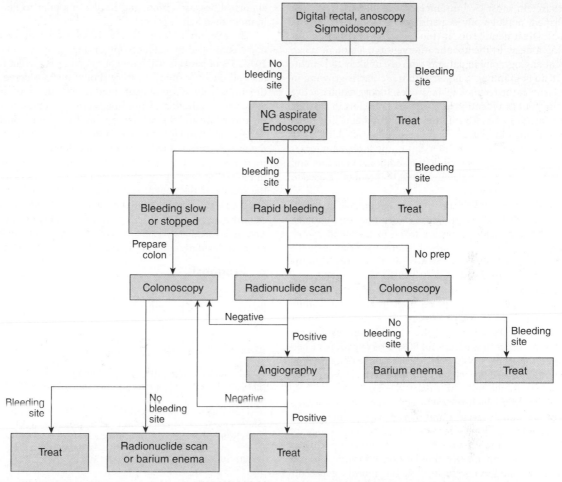

▲ **Figure 30–14.** Plan for diagnosis and treatment of acute lower gastrointestinal hemorrhage. (NG = nasogastric)

This limits the utility of preventative treatment in cases with multiple possible sources, such as diverticular bleeding. Depending on the lesion, clips, electrocautery, and/or sclerotherapy may be used. If there is a neoplastic lesion, it can be biopsied or removed. From an efficiency standpoint, colonoscopy makes sense as a first step because it is required at some point in all patients with hematochezia. The disadvantages, including availability of the procedure, need for sedation, and bowel preparation, often preclude its use. It is a generally safe procedure with complication rates of 0%-2%. In order to maximize the utility of colonoscopy, it should be done urgently versus electively. Prospective studies show that lesion identification is more common if colonoscopy is performed urgently versus electively (42% versus 22%), which facilitates the use of directed methods to control and prevent recurrent hemorrhage. In addition, early colonoscopy reduces length of stay and overall cost. Although this

has not been shown to improve other outcomes, the power of these trials is limited by small sample size. If the patient is stable and EGD and colonoscopy are both normal, a capsule endoscopy or double balloon enteroscopy may be performed to evaluate for a small bowel source.

If there is ongoing active hemorrhage, a radionuclide scan may be considered. It is used as a screening examination to identify patients in whom angiography may be useful. It utilizes 99mTc-labeled red blood cells. The accuracy increases with increased bleeding rates, but has been reported to detect hemorrhage as low as 0.1 mL/min. Radionuclide imaging is particularly useful in patients with intermittent bleeding owing to the long half-life of the tracer. This allows patients to be scanned on multiple occasions during symptomatic periods. In patients with active bleeding, scans are sensitive and specific for identifying the presence of hemorrhage into the GI tract, however they are unable to precisely localize the source in most circumstances. Once bleeding has been confirmed, angiography is performed for localization and possible treatment. This method has been criticized for causing a delay in therapeutic intervention, although it can prevent angiography in patients who are unlikely to benefit.

CT angiography is a newer technique that is growing in popularity as the technology improves. It does require active bleeding, but can identify the location of bleeding in patients with a rate as low as 0.3 mL/min. Unlike radionuclide scanning, CT angiography can localize bleeding, making for a more accurate and timely intervention by formal angiography. The disadvantages include the additional radiation and contrast exposure for a diagnostic test that cannot be used to treat any identified lesion.

If the radionuclide scan or CT angiogram is positive, it can be followed by selective mesenteric angiography, especially if the source appears to be in the small bowel. Angiography requires ongoing hemorrhage of at least 0.5 mL/min and will likely be of no use if the imaging tests are negative. During angiography, if the site of bleeding is demonstrated, which occurs in 40%-86% of patients, vasopressin or embolization can be used to treat the feeding vessel. Embolism is used if possible because re-bleeding is observed in up to 50% of patients treated with vasopressin alone. Embolization is successful 80%-90% of patients when followed for 30 days. Vascular ectasias can be diagnosed by angiography based on a characteristic pattern of an early filling vein, a vascular tuft, and a delayed emptying vein. These lesions should not be treated if bleeding is not demonstrated as they are quite prevalent and usually asymptomatic. The risks of angiography have decreased with the development of super-selective embolization, however, minor complications occur in 26% and major complications (including death and need for surgery) occur in 17%. One must be especially careful in patients with pre-existing renal insufficiency or diabetes, where the combination of hypovolemia and a large dye load creates a high risk for renal failure. In addition, angiography can rarely provide details about the cause of the bleeding and further work up is required after successful treatment.

In patients who have ongoing hemorrhage and a negative the radionuclide scan, colonoscopy should be considered. This can sometimes be performed successfully in the actively bleeding patient without a bowel preparation because blood acts as a cathartic. Even so, colonoscopy in this situation is difficult. However, a complete examination to the cecum is possible in 55%-70% of patients and there is suggestion that the risk of perforation is increased. Endoscopic therapeutic measures can be applied in up to 40% of patients, with success in half of them. Some gastroenterologists favor performing a bowel preparation under urgent conditions. There are multiple regimens, but usually these consist of a large volume preparation (6-8 L) over a short period of time (4 hours) which increases the chances of electrolyte abnormalities, aspiration, and results in a poor to fair prep in more than half of patients.

The majority of lower GI bleeds will stop spontaneously or be controlled by colonoscopy or angiography. However, 10%-25% of patients will have continued or recurrent bleeding and ongoing shock. Surgery should be considered once the transfusion requirement exceeds six units of blood. However, localization of bleeding is critical to the success of the procedure and the reduction of morbidity and mortality. Rarely, the bleeding site has been localized conclusively and the procedure is limited to segmental colonic resection. The mortality rate is less than 10%. When the source is unclear, intraoperative endoscopy can be performed to try to localize the source. If the patient continues to be unstable and the bleeding is suspected to be in the colon, a total abdominal colectomy may be required. This carries a mortality of 10%-30%. This is a fortunately rare occurrence today with improvements in imaging, endoscopy, and interventional techniques.

▶ Prognosis

Up to 90% of lower GI bleeds will stop spontaneously; however, 25% of patients will experience recurrent bleeding. Mortality has been reported in up to 3.6% of patients.

Geffroy Y, Rodallec MH, Boulay-Coletta I, et al: Multidetector CT angiography in acute gastrointestinal bleeding: why, when, and how. *Radiographics* 2011 May-Jun;31(3):E35-E46.

Lhewa DY, Strate LL: Pros and cons of colonoscopy in management of acute lower gastrointestinal bleeding. *World J Gastroenterol* 2012 Mar 21;18(11):1185-1190.

Strate LL, Liu YL, Huang ES, Giovannucci EL, Chan AT: Use of aspirin or nonsteroidal anti-inflammatory drugs increases risk for diverticulitis and diverticular bleeding. *Gastroenterology* 2011 May;140(5):1427-1433.

VOLVULUS

▶ General Considerations

Volvulus involves rotation of a segment of the intestine on an axis formed by its mesentery (Figure 30–15). This results in a closed-loop obstruction and is therefore a surgical emergency. Luminal obstruction occurs when the bowel rotates 180 degrees. If the bowel rotates 360 degrees, the veins are occluded and arterial flow is interrupted. This leads to ischemia, followed by necrosis and perforation if prompt treatment is not instituted. Sigmoid volvulus can be complicated by the additional development of cecal perforation in patients with a competent ileocecal valve. Physiologically this forms a second closed loop obstruction because the proximal colon is unable to decompress into the small bowel. In this situation, the cecum is at greatest risk of perforation by the law of LaPlace because it has the largest diameter.

Most cases of volvulus in the United States involve the cecum or sigmoid colon. A minority of patients present with volvulus of the transverse colon or splenic flexure. Volvulus treatment these patients are still at risk of gangrene and perforation as a result of the closed loop obstruction.

▶ Clinical Findings

A. Cecal Volvulus

The cecum and terminal ileum are involved in the rotation, so the symptoms generally include those of distal small bowel obstruction. Severe intermittent colicky pain begins in the right abdomen. Pain eventually becomes continuous, and the patient will experience the classic symptoms of obstruction: vomiting, distention, and obstipation. Patients may report a history of similar but milder attacks.

Imaging studies are the key to diagnosis. In the early stages, a plain film of the abdomen may show single fluid level that may be mistaken for gastric dilation. In later stages there may be a hugely dilated ovoid cecum that favors the epigastrium or left-upper quadrant. It is classically described as the "coffee bean" sign. In cecal volvulus, the dilated loop points toward the right-lower abdominal quadrant. If a film is taken later in the course, the x-ray may show classic findings of small bowel obstruction superimposed on the cecal volvulus. The distal colon will be decompressed. The success rate of diagnosis based on plain abdominal films is extremely variable, ranging from 5% to 90%. CT shows a distended cecum, often with a mesenteric swirl sign, indicating the rotation of the mesentery. Ischemia and necrosis can be identified by a lack of bowel wall enhancement.

B. Sigmoid Volvulus

Sigmoid volvulus presents in a similar fashion to cecal volvulus. Symptoms include intestinal colic, nausea, and obstipation. Distention tends to be more pronounced in sigmoid volvulus. There may be a history of chronic constipation and dysmotility or transient attacks in which spontaneous reduction of the volvulus has occurred. Abdominal x-rays show a markedly distended loop of bowel like a "bent inner tube" that has lost its haustral markings rising up out of the pelvis extending towards the diaphragm. Barium enema reveals a pathognomonic "bird's beak" deformity with spiral narrowing of the upper end of the lower segment (Figure 30–16). CT should be performed in cases where the diagnosis is unclear as it can demonstrate a dilated sigmoid loop with a mesenteric swirl sign, indicating the mesenteric twist. As with cecal volvulus, the pattern of bowel wall enhancement may help identify patients with ischemia and necrosis of the bowel wall.

▶ Differential Diagnosis

Cecal volvulus must be differentiated from colonic pseudo-obstruction and from other causes of small bowel and colonic obstruction. Sigmoid volvulus mimics other types of large bowel obstruction. Although x-ray examinations can be helpful, they are often not diagnostic for volvulus, and

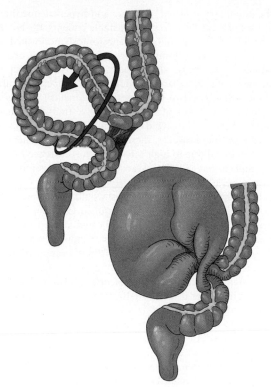

▲ **Figure 30-15.** Volvulus of the sigmoid colon. The twist is counterclockwise in most cases of sigmoid volvulus.

accounts for 5% of all cases of large bowel obstruction in the United States. In pregnant women, volvulus accounts for 25% of intestinal obstructions; most commonly in the third trimester. This may be secondary to the displacement of the colon by the enlarging uterus.

Cecal volvulus often occurs in patients with a hypermobile cecum as a result of incomplete embryologic fixation. The average age of presentation is 53 years. This is in contrast to sigmoid volvulus, which tends to occur in elderly or institutionalized patients who experience high rates of constipation and associated motility disorders. It is thought that a long sigmoid colon with an associated narrow-based mesentery is a risk factor. In parts of Africa and the Middle East, sigmoid volvulus accounts for about 50% of bowel obstructions and tends to effect younger, healthy, male patients. In South America, it is seen in association with megacolon in patients with Chagas disease.

Cecal bascule accounts for 10% of cecal volvulus. It involves anterior-superior movement of the cecum, causing obstruction at the site of the transverse fold in the ascending colon. Patients may describe intermittent bloating, pain, and obstructive symptoms improved by lying down and massaging the abdomen. Mesenteric blood flow is not compromised because there is no twist in the mesentery. However, without

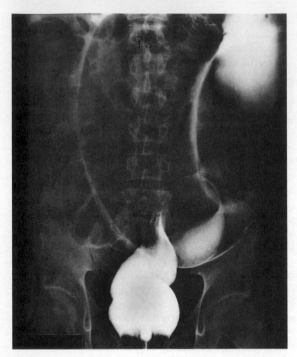

▲ **Figure 30–16.** Volvulus of the sigmoid colon. Barium enema taken with the patient in the supine position. Note the massively dilated sigmoid colon. The distinct vertical crease, which represents juxtaposition of adjacent walls of the dilated loop, points toward the site of torsion. The barium column resembles a "bird's beak" or "ace of spades" because of the way in which the lumen tapers toward the volvulus.

often a CT is performed which eliminates other causes of the abdominal pain and can provide additional information about the presence of complications.

▶ Treatment

Early diagnosis and treatment are imperative because the involved segment of colon is at risk of gangrene and perforation. The first step in the management of these patients is fluid resuscitation and correction of electrolyte imbalances. Vital signs and urine output should be monitored and a nasogastric tube placed. If there is evidence of ischemia, necrosis, or perforation, antibiotics should be administered as the patient is prepared for emergency surgery.

Many techniques have been described for managing patients with cecal volvulus and cecal bascule, but the recommended treatment is ileocecectomy. This can be done via the laparoscopic or open technique depending on the clinical scenario and surgeon preference. If there is necrotic bowel, the blood supply is ideally controlled prior to releasing the volvulus in an attempt to reduce the systemic release of the potentially infected, acidic, and hyperkalemic fluid that can cause cardiac arrest. In unstable patients, the bowel can be left in discontinuity and anastomosis performed at a second look laparotomy. However, a primary ileocolic anastomosis is almost always possible. This approach is associated with less than 5% mortality. Cecopexy (suture fixation of the bowel to the parietal peritoneum) and tube cecostomy (placement of a decompressive transabdominal drain) has been used to avoid a resection and anastomosis in the acute setting, however, these techniques have generally been abandoned due to high rates of both recurrence (30%) and complications (50%). Colonoscopic decompression may be attempted if an expert is available, especially in patients who have serious comorbidities that would make operation hazardous. However, this is successful in less than half of patients. This treatment is contraindicated in patients with suspected strangulation, which occurs in about 20% of cases.

In contrast, sigmoid volvulus without strangulation is more commonly treated initially by urgent endoscopy. A flexible sigmoidoscope or colonoscope is advanced to the obstruction. Under direct visualization, the colon is insufflated and the tip of the scope is used to apply gentle pressure. In 70%-90% of patients, decompression is achieved with the immediate release of gas and stool. The mucosa can then be inspected for signs of ischemia. If there is no evidence of ischemia, the patients is ideally scheduled for resection of the affected bowel with primary anastomosis during the same admission. Half of patients managed with decompression alone will have a recurrence within the first year. However, in patients with severe comorbidities, surgery may need to be delayed or may not be an option. Urgent surgery is indicated if strangulation or perforation is suspected or if endoscopic decompression is unsuccessful. In this case, primary anastomosis is not usually possible and a Hartmann's procedure with washout is performed.

▶ Prognosis

The outcome for patients with volvulus depends on comorbidities, the urgency of the surgery, and the presence of strangulation or perforation. The mortality rate for patients with cecal and sigmoid volvulus is less than 10%, but this increases to 30%-50% if strangulation or perforation has occurred. Patients who undergo semi-elective resection after endoscopic decompression have a mortality rate less than 10%.

Akinkuotu A, Samuel JC, Msiska N, Mvula C, Charles AG: The role of the anatomy of the sigmoid colon in developing sigmoid volvulus: a case-control study. *Clin Anat* 2011;24:634-637.

Swenson BR, Kwaan MR, Burkart NE, et al: Colonic volvulus: presentation and management in metropolitan Minnesota, United States. *Dis Colon Rectum* 2012;55:444-449.

Yassaie O, Thompson-Fawcett M, Rossaak J: Management of sigmoid volvulus: is early surgery justifiable? *ANZ J Surg* 2013 Jan;83(1-2):74-78.

INFLAMMATORY BOWEL DISEASE

Inflammatory bowel disease (IBD) refers to UC, Crohn disease (CD), and indeterminate colitis. The cause of IBD is not known. The disease is likely the result of a combination of genetic, environmental, and host immune response factors.

There is a positive family history of IBD in 15%-40% of patients. Crohn disease seems to have a stronger genetic link than UC. Genome-wide association studies initially identified normal variants of multiple loci associated with the development of IBD; however, these associations are still poorly understood. These genetic associations are heterogeneous and have precluded the development of a useful screening test.

It is postulated that the interplay between the immune system, normal microflora, and colonic epithelium is a factor in the development of IBD, but this is still being investigated. Patients with UC are known to have an increased concentration of normal bacterial flora compared to healthy controls; however, it is not known if this contributes to the disease process. The mucosal immune system has been implicated by the finding that patients with CD have a predominantly Th1 mucosal population, whereas patients with UC have a Th2 predominance. An autoimmune component is suggested by circulating perinuclear antineutrophil cytoplasmic antibody (pANCA) and abnormally high levels of auto-IgG1 antibodies. These antibodies cross react with the epithelium of the colon, biliary tract, skin, eye, and cartilage and have been hypothesized to contribute to extraintestinal manifestations.

Environmental factors are also important. The use of NSAIDs has been associated with flares in patients with CD. Smoking has been shown to be a protective factor for UC. Smokers are less likely to develop the disease, and smoking cessation leads to worsening of disease in smokers with UC. For unclear reasons, this disease is also less common in patients who have undergone appendectomy.

ULCERATIVE COLITIS

▶ General Considerations

UC has a bimodal age distribution, with the first peak between ages 15 and 30 years and a second, smaller peak in the sixth to eighth decades. The annual incidence varies from 1 to 20 per 100,000, and the prevalence is 8-246 per 100,000. UC is more common than CD in adults but less common in children. The disease is found worldwide but is more common in Western countries and the incidence is increasing in Asia. This finding has also contributed to the theory of bacterial flora contributing to the development of the disease.

UC is a diffuse but contiguous mucosal inflammatory disease. Abscesses form in the crypts of Lieberkühn and penetrate the superficial submucosa. In the acute setting, neutrophils predominate whereas in the chronic setting, the infiltrate is largely composed of lymphocytes and plasma cells. There are no granulomas. The overlying mucosa sloughs as the inflammation spreads. Vascular congestion and hemorrhage are prominent, and there is often diffuse thickening of the muscularis mucosa. The normal tissues surrounding the ulcerated areas appear endoscopically protruberant and thus are called pseudopolyps. Except in the most severe forms, the muscular layers are spared. In fulminant disease, the full thickness of the colon wall can be involved, which leads to dilation and ultimately perforation. In patients with long standing or severe disease, the colon becomes shortened and loses its normal haustral markings.

UC classically starts at the rectum and extends proximally without skip lesions. The disease is confined to the rectum (proctitis) or up to the rectosigmoid region (proctosigmoiditis) in at least half of patients. The disease is classified as left-sided colitis if it involves the descending colon, extensive colitis if it extends proximal to the splenic flexure, and pancolitis if the cecum is involved. In patients with pancolitis, a few centimeters of terminal ileum may be involved by proximity in patients with an incompetent ileocecal valve. This is termed backwash ileitis and can make the differentiation of UC from CD challenging. There are no strict diagnostic criteria, but generally a clinical and histologic appearance of UC without evidence of CD is enough to establish a diagnosis and initiate treatment.

▶ Clinical Findings

A. Symptoms and Signs

Patients commonly report frequent, small volume watery stools mixed with blood, pus, and mucus accompanied by tenesmus, rectal urgency, and even fecal incontinence. Many patients will report crampy abdominal pain and variable degrees of fever, vomiting, weight loss, malaise, and dehydration. The symptoms can be episodic with periods of spontaneous improvement or severe and unrelenting. Mild disease may be manifested only by loose or frequent stools, or occasionally constipation. In isolated instances, the only symptoms may be from extraintestinal manifestations such as arthropathy or pyoderma.

If the disease is mild, physical examination may be normal, but in severe disease the abdomen is tender and distended. Severe rectal inflammation may result in considerable tenderness and spasticity of the anus during digital rectal examination. The examining finger may be covered with blood, mucus, or pus. Perianal disease can occur in UC patients as they do in the general population, but signs of anal disease should prompt a workup for CD.

A simple classification of the severity of an attack was devised by Truelove and Witt in 1955. The assessment of disease severity is based on six simple clinical signs including

Table 30–8. Ulcerative colitis disease severity (based on the Truelove and Witt classification).

Symptoms	Mild	Severe	Fulminant
Stools (per day)	< 4	> 6	> 10
Hematochezia	Intermittent	Frequent	Continuous
Temperature	Normal	> 37.5°C	
Pulse (beats/min)	Normal	> 90	
Hemoglobin	Normal	< 75% of normal	Requires transfusion
ESR	< 30 mm/h	> 30 mm/h	

stool frequency, hematochezia, pulse, temperature, hemoglobin, and erythrocyte sedimentation rate (Table 30–8).

B. Laboratory Findings

There is no single diagnostic test for UC, although in unclear cases, serum antibody tests can help differentiate UC from CD. Serum pANCA are found in 60%-70% of patients with UC but also are found in up to 40% of patients with CD. In patients with IBD for whom the differentiation between UC and CD is unclear, the combination of a positive pANCA and negative anti-saccharomyces cerevisiae antibodies (ASCA) has a specificity of 97%, sensitivity of 48%, and a positive predictive value of 75% for UC. A negative pANCA and positive ASCA has a positive predictive value of 86% for CD. Thus serologic testing in patients with IBD may be helpful when considered in the context of other clinical factors.

During an acute flare, basic laboratory tests are used to assist in determining the severity of disease. Anemia, leukocytosis, and an elevated sedimentation rate or C reactive protein is usually present. Severe disease leads to hypoalbuminemia, dehydration, and electrolyte abnormalities. There is often evidence of steatorrhea. To look for signs of superinfection, the stool should be sent for ova and parasite examination, culture (*E. coli* 0157:H7 and *Campylobacter*), and *C difficile* toxin assay.

C. Imaging Studies

In the acute setting, colonoscopy and barium enema should be avoided due to the risk of perforation. If needed for diagnosis, biopsies obtained by proctoscopy should be sufficient. Abdominal x-rays may show dilation of the colon, and can be used to detect free air when perforation is suspected. CT scan has become the most common imaging modality during an acute episode. CT will often show thickened rectum and colon with associated inflammatory changes, however, it does not often lend much to the clinical management of these patients.

Barium enema, which is now infrequently used, shows mucosal irregularity that varies from fine serrations to extensive ulceration with pseudopolyps. As the disease progresses,

haustrations are gradually effaced, and the colon narrows and shortens because of muscular rigidity (Figure 30–17). Widening of the space between the sacrum and rectum is due either to periproctitis or to shortening of the bowel. The presence of a stricture should always arouse suspicion of cancer or CD.

In cases where the diagnosis is unclear, a small bowel series or CT enterography may be performed to look for involvement suggestive of CD.

D. Colonoscopic Findings

Colonoscopy is an essential part of diagnosis and surveillance. The characteristic mucosal changes include loss of

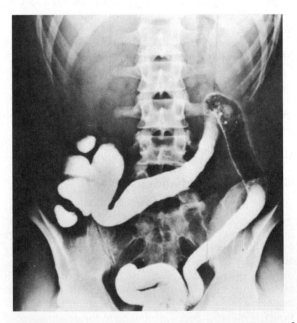

▲ **Figure 30–17.** Ulcerative colitis. Barium enema x-ray of colon. Note shortening of colon, loss of haustral markings ("lead pipe" appearance), and fine serrations at the edges of the bowel wall that represent multiple small ulcers.

vascular pattern, granularity, friability, hyperemia, and ulceration. Pseudopolyps represent islands of normal mucosa against a background of inflamed, denuded bowel wall. These findings begin in the distal rectum and proceed proximally in a continuous fashion. In more advanced disease, the mucosa is purplish-red, velvety, and extremely friable. Blood mixed with mucus is evident in the lumen. If the mucosa is not grossly diseased, biopsy may be helpful to confirm the diagnosis. In the recovery phase, mucosal hyperemia and edema subside. The healing mucosa is typically dull and granular and has a neovascular pattern of telangiectatic vessels that differs from the normal pink mucosa. Patients with disease distal to the splenic flexure may have a "cecal patch," an inflammatory lesion at the appendiceal orifice, that can be misidentified as a skip lesion associated with CD. In the acute setting, colonoscopy is important in determining the severity of disease and response to treatment. These patients are at increased risk for CRC. Screening colonoscopy begins 8-10 years after the initial diagnosis of pancolitis and 12 years after left-sided colitis. Surveillance for dysplasia should be done every 1-2 years. At least 30 random biopsies should be taken throughout the colon to detect dysplasia.

Differential Diagnosis

The differential diagnosis of patients presenting with new onset UC is extremely broad and includes all forms of colitis. Cancer and diverticulitis should also be considered. Infectious colitis can mimic UC but can also be superimposed on patients with underlying UC. Salmonellosis and other bacillary dysenteries are diagnosed by repeated stool cultures. Shigellosis may be suspected on the basis of a positive methylene blue stain for fecal leukocytes. *Campylobacter jejuni* is a common cause of bloody diarrhea; the organisms can be cultured from the stool, and serum antibody titers rise during the illness. Hemorrhagic colitis—a syndrome of bloody diarrhea and abdominal cramps but no fever—is associated with infection by *E coli* O157:H7. Legionella infections can mimic UC. Gonococcal proctitis is detected by culture of rectal swabs. Herpes simplex virus is the most common cause of nongonococcal proctitis in homosexual men. In patients with suspected amoebiasis, corticosteroids should be held until amebiasis is excluded by microscopic examination of stool, rectal swabs, rectal biopsies, or serologic tests.

Cases of histoplasmosis, tuberculosis, cytomegalovirus disease, schistosomiasis, amyloidosis, or Behçet disease may be very difficult to diagnose. Drug-induced colitis may be suspected based on the patient's history. NSAIDs can cause mucosal inflammation and even strictures in the large intestine. Collagenous colitis may or may not be related to NSAID use. Watery diarrhea is the main symptom of this syndrome, endoscopy is grossly normal, and biopsies show a thickened band of collagen just beneath the mucosa. Ischemic colitis has a segmental pattern of involvement quite unlike the contiguous distribution of UC. Functional diarrhea can mimic colitis, but organic disease must be excluded before it can be concluded that the diarrhea is functional. Diversion colitis refers to inflammation of a previously normal segment of colon or rectum following construction of a temporary colostomy. Deficiency of mucosal nutrients may be responsible, and inflammation may be treated with topical application of short-chain fatty acids or restoration of intestinal continuity.

The most difficult differential diagnosis is between mucosal UC and Crohn colitis (Table 30–9). None of the features are specific for one disease, and often the differentiation can be made only after all the data have been assembled. Luckily, in the acute phase, the medical treatment is similar, however, the differentiation is important because it can dictate appropriate surgical therapy. About 10% of cases cannot be classified (indeterminate colitis).

► Complications

A. Extraintestinal Manifestations

Extraintestinal manifestations (EM) occur in approximately 21% of patients with UC. They are more common in women and patients with pancolitis. The pathogenesis is unknown, but it is thought that they may be a result of a systemic autoimmune process. A genetic component is suggested by the fact that they tend to cluster in families. Nearly 80% of patients who develop EM do so after the development of colonic symptoms, but a minority will present with EM prior to symptomatic colonic disease that may lead to a diagnosis of UC. The most common EMs are musculoskeletal (arthralgias, arthritis, ankylosing spondylitis), anterior ocular chamber inflammation (uveitis, iritis, scleritis, and conjunctivitis), skin (erythema nodosum, pyoderma gangrenosum), and primary sclerosing cholangitis (PSC) in order of decreasing frequency. PSC can lead to cirrhosis requiring liver transplant and puts the patient at increased risk for cholangiocarcinoma. For unclear reasons, patients with PSC also develop colorectal cancer at an increased rate. PSC is not improved with treatment of the colonic disease and may develop or progress after curative proctocolectomy. However, arthritis, ocular disease, and skin manifestations are known for paralleling disease activity. Most patients will develop only one EM, but a subset will develop multiple.

Patients with UC also develop symptoms as a result of the disease process in the colon, including iron deficiency anemia and malnutrition. They are at high risk for thrombosis, especially during flares. Patients are also at risk of developing complications from medical treatment using long-term corticosteroids such as diabetes, osteoporosis, cataracts, and adrenal insufficiency.

Table 30–9. Comparison of various features of ulcerative colitis with those of Crohn colitis.

	Ulcerative (Mucosal) Colitis	Crohn Colitis
Signs and symptoms		
Diarrhea	Marked	Present; less severe
Gross bleeding	Characteristic	Infrequent
Perianal lesions	Infrequent, mild	Frequent, complex; may precede diagnosis of intestinal disease
Toxic dilatation	Yes (3%-10%)	Yes (2%-5%)
Perforation	Free	Localized
Systemic manifestations (arthritis, uveitis, pyoderma, hepatitis)	Common	Common
X-ray studies	Confluent, diffuse	Skip areas. Longitudinal ulcers, transverse ridges, "cobblestone" appearance
	Tiny serrations, coarse mucosa, mucosal tags	
	Concentric involvement	Eccentric involvement
	Internal fistulas very rare	Internal fistula common
	Colon only except in backwash ileitis; may be limited to left side	Any portion of intestinal tract may be involved; may be limited to ileum and right colon
Morphology		
Gross	Confluent involvement	Segmental involvement with or without skip areas
	Rectum usually involved	Rectum often not involved
	Mesocolon not involved; nodes enlarged	Thickened mesocolon; pronounced lymph node enlargement
	Widespread, ragged, superficial ulceration	Large longitudinal ulcers or transverse fissures
	Inflammatory polyps (pseudopolyps) common	Inflammatory polyps not prominent
	No thickening of bowel wall	Thickened bowel wall
Microscopic	Inflammatory reaction usually limited to mucosa and submucosa; only in severe disease are muscle coats involved; no fibrosis	Chronic inflammation of all layers of bowel wall; damage to muscle layers usual; submucosal fibrosis
	Granulomas rare	Granulomas frequent
Natural history	Exacerbations, remissions; may be explosive, lethal	Indolent, recurrent
Treatment		
Response to medical treatment	Good response in 85% of cases	Difficult to evaluate; less well controlled over long term
Type of surgical treatment and response	Colectomy with ileoanal anastomosis; proctocolectomy with ileostomy	Segmental colectomy; total colectomy with ileorectal anastomosis; proctocolectomy if rectum severely diseased
	No recurrence	Recurrence common

B. Hemorrhage

Gross hematochezia is common during acute flares of UC. In the chronic setting, patients frequently develop a chronic iron deficiency anemia. Ten percent of patients will require blood transfusion for bleeding during a flare. Massive hemorrhage is a potentially life threatening complication that occurs in up to 5% of patients. This is an indication for urgent colectomy and accounts for approximately 10% of all urgent colectomies in patients with UC.

C. Fulminant Colitis

Fulminant colitis occurs in less than 10% of all patients with UC, but in up to 50% of these patients, it develops during their initial presentation. This represents the most severe, acute form of the disease. Patients are systemically ill and develop inflammation extending into the muscular layer of the bowel. Electrolyte disturbances, especially hypokalemia, may contribute to toxicity and should be treated aggressively. Opioids and anticholinergics should be avoided.

These patients should be fluid resuscitated and treated with broad spectrum antibiotics. Electrolyte disturbances should be corrected. A nasogastric tube is placed for patients with significant signs of distension. A CT scan can detect perforation or ischemia, as well as other causes of abdominal sepsis. Serial abdominal x-rays can trend colonic distention. However, if there is clinical deterioration or no improvement with maximal medical therapy over the course of 48-72 hours, surgery should be considered. Although barium enema is no longer used to diagnose toxic colon, one can see the classic findings in Figure 30–18. These include a thickened bowel wall and dilation of the lumen greater than 6 cm. Luminal air can be seen outlining irregular nodular pseudopolyps. However, patients do not need to have colonic dilatation to have toxic colitis.

D. Perforation

Colonic perforation is the most dreaded complication of severe acute UC and occurs in 3% of hospitalized patients. It is responsible for more deaths than any other complication. The risk of perforation is highest during the initial attack of the disease and correlates well with its extent and severity. It may also occur as a complication of endoscopy or barium enema in acutely ill patients. Patients with toxic colitis are especially vulnerable. Perforation is most common in the sigmoid or splenic flexure and may result in a localized

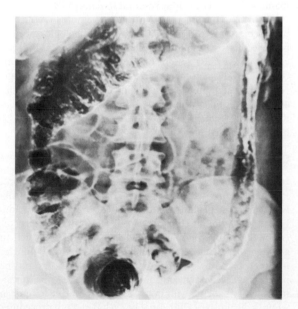

▲ **Figure 30–18.** Barium enema showing acute colonic dilation in ulcerative colitis. Note dilation of the transverse colon, the multiple irregular densities in the lumen that represent pseudopolyps, and the loss of haustral markings.

abscess or generalized fecal peritonitis. Systemic therapy (corticosteroids and antibiotics) may mask the development of this complication. Therefore, serial abdominal examinations, laboratory tests, and abdominal imaging are important in detecting this complication.

E. Malignancy

Colorectal cancer risk increases above that of the general population 10 years after the onset of UC, although the rates vary widely between studies. The risk increases with the duration and severity of disease, and is higher in patients with a family history of CRC, extensive colitis, and PSC. Decreased risk in recent reports may be associated with improved medical treatment of colitis. Cancers in UC tend to be multicentric and broadly infiltrating. They are difficult to recognize endoscopically because they arise from small, flat areas of dysplasia located in a background of ulceration and inflammation. They do not follow the typical adenoma-carcinoma sequence seen in sporadic CRC in the general population. Newer techniques, including narrow-band imaging and chromoendoscopy may improve detection.

Colonoscopic surveillance is recommended beginning 8-12 years after the onset of colitis and continues at 1-2 year intervals. Ideally, approximately 48 random biopsies are taken throughout the colon and rectum to screen for dysplasia. Synchronous CRC is found in 20% of patients undergoing proctocolectomy for low-grade dysplasia, 40%-60% of patients with high-grade dysplasia, and 40%-85% of patients with dysplasia-associated lesion or mass (DALM) regardless of the degree of dysplasia. Low-grade dysplasia places the patient at a ninefold increased risk of developing CRC compared to UC patients without dysplasia. In addition, low-grade dysplasia has been reported to progress to carcinoma without progressing to high-grade dyplasia. IBD-associated cancers account for 1%-2% of all CRCs but occur in younger patients and confer a poorer prognosis. High-grade dysplasia and DALM are clear indications for proctocolectomy, and consideration should be given to patients with low-grade dysplasia. Intensive study is ongoing to identify more sensitive screening methods.

▶ Treatment

A. Medical Therapy

The goals of medical therapy are to stop an acute flare as rapidly as possible and to maintain remission of mucosal inflammation. Traditionally, medical management has been approached in a "step up" fashion, with treatment depending on the severity of disease (classified as mild, moderate, severe, or fulminant), the extent of colonic involvement, and history of previous response to treatment. However, a new paradigm of "top down" treatment has evolved for patients with severe disease as research has shown improved outcomes with more aggressive treatment. The endpoints of therapy have shifted away from symptomatic improvement to objective mucosal healing and steroid free remission. Mild to moderate disease usually can be treated on an outpatient basis. If the disease flare is refractory or progressive, hospitalization may be required. Patients with severe or fulminant disease may require inpatient treatment for supportive therapy (IV hydration, antibiotics, blood transfusion, and monitoring).

Mild to moderate disease is treated with sulfasalazine or 5-aminosalicylates, such as mesalamine, olsalazine, or balsalazide. Sulfasalazine is cheaper, but associated with more side effects and should not be given to sulfa-allergic patients. These drugs can be administered orally or topically in the form of suppositories or enemas in patients with disease limited to the rectum or sigmoid. Seventy percent of patients will respond to this regimen within 1 month. The remaining 30% are started on prednisone 40-60 mg/d. In patients who do not exhibit objective evidence of response or who remain steroid dependent, azathioprine, 6 mercaptopurine, infliximab, and adalimumab are additional options to induce and maintain remission.

In patients with severe disease, these initial steps are bypassed and treatment with intravenous glucocorticoids is initiated. In addition, biologic agents or immunomodulators are added. Infliximab, an anti-TNF antibody, tacrolimus and cyclosporine have been shown in randomized controlled trials to be effective for treatment of severe flares.

If these regimens are not successful, additional medications or surgery are considered. Multiple new drugs show promise in the treatment of patients with refractory disease. Newer biologic agents, such as certolizumab and natilizumab, as well as Tofacitinib, an oral Janus kinase inhibitor have been shown to be effective in inducing remission in patients with steroid refractory moderate to severe UC. Other treatments, such as stem cells and fecal transplants, are currently under investigation.

Once remission has been obtained, a maintenance regimen is required to prevent relapse in most patients. These regimens should be individualized based on the response to the induction regimen and revised as clinically indicated. For mild disease, mesalamine is commonly used. Patients unable to wean from steroids require intensified treatment. Azathioprine, 6 mercaptopurine, methotrexate, infliximab, adalimumab, or newer immunomodulators may be needed to successfully wean patients off steroids.

B. Surgical Therapy

1. Indications—Indications for surgery fall under three broad categories: patients who require urgent or emergency surgery due to severe illness or complications during a flare, patients who have chronic intractable disease or medication intolerance, and those who require treatment for dysplasia or carcinoma. Twenty percent of patients who present with

fulminant colitis will go on to require surgery. There have been no trials comparing medical therapy to surgery for any of these indications. Crohn disease should be ruled out in any patient in whom surgery is being considered, as a proctocolectomy, especially with J-pouch reconstruction, is inappropriate for these patients.

In the acute setting, emergency surgery is indicated for colonic perforation. Other complications, such as toxic megacolon, fulminant colitis, or uncontrolled hemorrhage are initially managed medically. However, if there is no improvement with aggressive medical therapy, surgery is warranted. There are no firm guidelines for how long patients should be treated medically prior to considering surgery. These patients are monitored closely for 48-72 hours. If there is clinical deterioration or no improvement, surgery is indicated.

Another group of patients in whom surgery is considered are those with intractable disease despite maximal medical therapy or those who cannot wean off steroids due to worsening symptoms. In children this may present with growth retardation. Adults may become physically debilitated, psychosocially limited, and experience poor quality of life. There may be medication intolerance, especially in those patients who are steroid dependent. Surgery is also considered for patients with severe extraintestinal manifestations that have developed in parallel with the UC flares such as peripheral arthritis, pyoderma gangrenosum, and ocular manifestations. These may respond to colectomy.

Patients who have biopsy-proven carcinoma are offered proctocolectomy as opposed to standard oncologic resection because this treats both the UC and the cancer. Further, colitis-related CRC tends to be widely infiltrative, multicentric, and difficult to visualize making standard oncologic resection dangerous. Patients with dysplasia or dysplasia-associated lesion or mass are also candidates for surgery as the risk for a synchronous or metachronous malignancy is high as discussed previously.

C. Surgical Procedures

In the elective setting there are two surgical options. Proctocolectomy with ileal pouch-anal anastomosis (IPAA) is the operation of choice in most patients because it provides intestinal continuity (Figure 30–19). However, total proctocolectomy with a permanent end ileostomy is indicated in a subset of patients. Factors include preoperative sphincter function, presence of carcinoma low rectal cancer, and the patient's age, general health, and preferences. IPAA is contraindicated in patients with poor baseline sphincter tone or in whom a diagnosis of CD cannot be excluded. Both procedures are now increasingly performed laparoscopically with equivalent functional results and improved short-term outcomes.

A permanent end ileostomy may be desired by patients who have concerns about the postoperative complications or

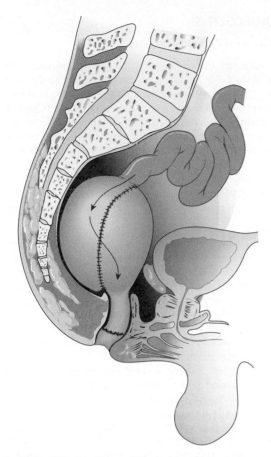

▲ **Figure 30–19.** View of the pelvis after colectomy and ileoanal anastomosis in a male. The J-pouch, shown here, is one of several types of reservoirs and is most commonly utilized. The pouch is anastomosed to the anal canal just above the dentate line.

anticipate difficulty managing the changes in bowel function associated with the ileoanal pouch. Patients frequently experience greater than 10 bowel movements per day during the first 3 months. This eventually decreases to an average of 5-7 bowel movements per day. Twenty percent of patients experience nocturnal seepage or incontinence 1 year after surgery. The most common complications after surgery include small bowel obstruction, infertility, sexual dysfunction, and pelvic sepsis as a result of anastomotic or pouch leaks. Pelvic sepsis occurs in 25% of patients and is the most common cause of pouch failure. Pouchitis affects 40% of patients in the first 10 years after surgery. This is an idiopathic inflammation of the ileoanal pouch that causes abdominal pain, increased bowel movements, and bleeding. It is treated with antibiotics.

Proctocolectomy with IPAA can be performed as a one-, two-, or three-stage procedure. In the elective setting, a two stage procedure is most common, involving proctocolectomy with IPAA and diverting loop ileostomy at the first surgery followed by ileostomy reversal as a second surgery. A single stage operation (without diverting loop ileostomy) is performed only in the most ideal candidates. This approach eliminates the ileostomy-associated complications and avoids a second surgery at the increased risk of the potentially significant consequences of pelvic sepsis from an undiverted anastomotic leak. The three stage procedure is reserved for ill patients who would not tolerate the IPAA during the first surgery secondary to malnutrition or severe active disease. It is also useful in patients with indeterminate colitis in whom confirmation of UC may be made after pathologic evaluation of the surgical specimen allowing the safe formation of the IPAA. The first procedure is a subtotal colectomy with end ileostomy, followed by completion proctectomy, and IPAA. At the time of this procedure, an ileostomy may be avoided in selected patients, otherwise the ileostomy is reversed at a third operation. In the interval between subtotal colectomy and proctectomy, the residual disease in the rectal remnant improves with fecal diversion and if symptoms persist, it can be treated locally with suppositories or enemas.

Proctocolectomy involves mobilizing and resecting the entire colon and rectum. If IPAA is planned, the anal sphincter complex is left in place. The ileum is made into a reservoir most commonly with a "J" configuration (although multiple configurations have been described) and an anastomosis is created just above the dentate line (Figure 30–19). A diverting loop ileostomy is used to protect the anastomosis if there is any intraoperative concern about the anastomosis or if the patient has risk factors for impaired healing such as steroid exposure, anemia, diabetes, or malnutrition. Most of these patients will have been treated with immunosuppressants or immunomodulators in the preoperative period. Although these medications theoretically impact healing, there is no clear evidence to suggest that they increase surgical complications in the setting of diversion.

The continent ileostomy, which was first reported by Kock in 1969 is plagued by complications requiring reoperation in 50% of patients. It has largely been replaced with the IPAA and is mainly mentioned for historical purposes.

D. Prognosis

The mortality rate of UC has dropped sharply in the past two decades. First attacks are seldom fatal when treated by specialists. In one large series, emergency colectomy was required in 25% of patients with severe first attacks; 60% responded rapidly to medical therapy; and 15% improved slowly on medications alone. Overall, the colitis-related mortality rate during the year after onset is about 1%. Emergency colectomy has a mortality rate of 6%; most of these deaths occur in patients with preoperative perforation, a complication that has a fatal outcome in 40% of cases.

Compared to pancolitis, the long-term prognosis of ulcerative proctitis is excellent; only 10% of patients will develop colonic disease by 10 years, and the mortality rate is very low. In patients with pancolitis, the likelihood of operation during the first year is about 25% and the mortality rate is 5% over 10 years. Colorectal cancer in UC is more often diagnosed at an advanced stage than is sporadic cancer, but the stage-for-stage prognosis is the same. Screening with colonoscopy and biopsies seems to have reduced the cancer mortality rate, but there are still many patients who escape detection until the malignancy has progressed to an advanced stage. The operative mortality rate is less than 1% for elective colectomy.

Ahluwalia JP: Immunotherapy in inflammatory bowel disease. *Med Clin North Am* 2012 May;96(3):525-544.

Andersen V, Halfvarson J, Vogel U: Colorectal cancer in patients with inflammatory bowel disease: can we predict risk? *World J Gastroenterol* 2012 Aug 21;18(31):4091-4094.

Causey MW, Stoddard D, Johnson EK, et al: Laparoscopy impacts outcomes favorably following colectomy for ulcerative colitis: a critical analysis of the ACS-NSQIP database. *Surg Endosc* 2013 Feb;27(2):603-609.

Danese S, Fiocchi C: Ulcerative colitis. *N Engl J Med* 2011 Nov 3;365(18):1713-1725.

Devlin SM, Panaccione R: Evolving inflammatory bowel disease treatment paradigms: top-down versus step-up. *Gastroenterol Clin North Am* 2009 Dec;38(4):577-594.

Kornbluth A, Sachar DB, Practice Parameters Committee of the American College of Gastroenterology: Ulcerative colitis practice guidelines in adults: American College Of Gastroenterology, Practice Parameters Committee. *Am J Gastroenterol* 2010 Mar;105(3):501-523.

Ogata H, Kato J, Hirai F, et al: Double-blind, placebo-controlled trial of oral tacrolimus (FK506) in the management of hospitalized patients with steroid-refractory ulcerative colitis. *Inflamm Bowel Dis* 2012 May;18(5):803-808.

Ordás I, Eckmann L, Talamini M, Baumgart DC, Sandborn WJ: Ulcerative colitis. *Lancet* 2012 Nov 3;380(9853):1606-1619.

Pardi DS, D'Haens G, Shen B, Campbell S, Gionchetti P: Clinical guidelines for the management of pouchitis. *Inflamm Bowel Dis* 2009 Sep;15(9):1424-1431.

Reinisch, W, Sandborn WJ, Hommes DW, et al: Adalimumab for induction of clinical remission in moderately to severely active ulcerative colitis: results of a randomised controlled trial. *Gut* 2011;Jun;60(6):780-787.

Sagar PM, Pemberton JH: Intraoperative, postoperative and reoperative problems with ileoanal pouches. *Br J Surg* 2012 Apr;99(4):454-468.

Sandborn WJ, Ghosh S, Panes J, et al: Study A3921063 investigators. Tofacitinib, an oral Janus kinase inhibitor, in active ulcerative colitis. *N Engl J Med* Aug 2012;367(7):616-624.

Sandborn WJ, van Assche G, Reinisch W, et al: Adalimumab induces and maintains clinical remission in patients with moderate-to-severe ulcerative colitis. *Gastroenterology* 2012 Feb;142(2):257-65.e1-3.

Subramanian V, Pollok RC, Kang JY, Kumar D: Systematic review of postoperative complications in patients with inflammatory bowel disease treated with immunomodulators. *Br J Surg* 2006 Jul;93(7):793-799.

CROHN COLITIS

▶ General Considerations

Approximately 45% of patients with CD have diffuse involvement of the GI tract; 30% have disease limited to the small bowel, 20% have disease limited to the colon, and another 5% have isolated anorectal involvement. Symptoms, including diarrhea, abdominal pain, constitutional effects, and extraintestinal manifestations are approximately the same in colonic and enteric disease. Fistulas, abscesses, and intestinal obstruction are more often complications of small bowel disease. Anorectal complications such as anal fistula, fissure, abscess, rectal stricture, as well as hemorrhage occur more commonly in patients with disease affecting the large bowel.

▶ Clinical Findings

Patients present with abdominal pain, diarrhea, and systemic signs such as low-grade fevers, weight loss, and malaise. Symptoms are generally dictated by the distribution of disease, but patients with Crohn colitis may report urgency or mucous, blood, or pus per rectum. Patients with perianal disease may present with perianal pain or discharge. If the inflammatory process has caused structuring, partial obstructive symptoms may be present.

Radiographic features include sparing of the rectum, right colonic and ileal involvement, skip areas, transverse fissures, longitudinal ulcers, strictures, and fistulas. Typical anal lesions of CD include fissures, abscesses or fistulas. Large external skin tags are also common. The differential diagnosis is broad and includes all forms of colitis including UC, infectious and ischemic. Features differentiating CD from UC are summarized in Table 30–9.

▶ Colonoscopy

Colonoscopy is indicated for diagnosis, evaluation for severity of disease, determining response to treatment, and screening for colorectal cancer. Colonoscopy with biopsy is a mainstay in diagnosis. Patients with Crohn colitis have rectal sparing about 50% of the time. Skip lesions are common, with irregular ulcerations separated by edematous or even normal-appearing mucosa. Patients with pancolitis appear to have similar risk profile for cancer as their UC counterparts. The risk of colorectal cancer in Crohn colitis patients is 4 to 20 times that of the general population. The 25-year risk of dysplasia in patients with Crohn colitis is 12%-25%. Data to support surveillance and management strategies for patients with Crohn colitis are limited and often extrapolated from UC patients. Routine annual colonoscopy with random biopsies is recommended beginning 8 years after the diagnosis. Surveillence should include high risk areas, such as segments of intestine excluded from the fecal stream, strictures, and fistulas with focused biopsies performed as needed.

Treatment

A. Medical Therapy

Steroids are effective for acute attacks in up to 70% of patients, but they are not used for maintenance therapy because of the associated side effects and complications. Up to 45% of patients who initially improve with steroids will relapse upon tapering or withdrawal. Oral 5-aminosalicylates (sulfasalazine, 4 g/d; or mesalamine, 2-5 g/d) are effective treatment for Crohn colitis. Topical 5-aminosalicylates are beneficial for disease of the rectum and sigmoid and are often used to wean patients off steroids. Anal abscesses and fistulas require surgical drainage and seton placement to treat local sepsis, but healing is improved with biologic agents.

Immunosuppressants (azathioprine, mercaptopurine, methotrexate) are steroid-sparing drugs that seem to control Crohn colitis well enough that surgery is delayed or avoided. Biologic agents including infliximab and other anti-TNF therapies are effective for inflammatory CD and also specifically indicated for fistulizing or refractory disease. Patients who respond to infliximab induction should receive maintenance therapy. Adalimumab is an effective therapy for patients who are refractory or intolerant to infliximab. Newer human monoclonal antibodies, such as the anti-TNF natalizumab and anti-interleukin ustekinumab have shown promising results in preliminary clinical trials and are now being used more frequently for patients who initially responded to other agents.

B. Surgical Therapy

Failure of medical therapy, neoplasia, and complications of CD are indications for surgery. Patients whose symptoms do not respond to medical treatment, are unable to achieve remission, have intractable weight loss, or have unmanageable side effects should be considered. The choice of operation depends on the severity and distribution of disease, but the general principle is bowel preservation, with resection of only diseased, actively symptomatic areas. In contrast to UC, CD is not cured surgically, and procedures are performed with palliation in mind. However, patients who have distal colon and rectal disease or multiple segments of disease often do better with a proctocolectomy. Disease tends to recur, especially at areas of intestinal anastomosis and short bowel syndrome is a major concern. Cigarette smoking is an independent risk factor for recurrence of CD after resection.

Strictures are more common in patients with longstanding disease. The use of CT or MR enterography is useful to localize the lesion. If the lesion is symptomatic and unresponsive to medical therapy, resection is indicated. If the lesion is asymptomatic, malignancy should be ruled out with biopsies or brushings. Lesions not amenable to surveillance should be considered for resection, as 7% are malignant.

Intra-abdominal abscesses may be managed with percutaneous drainage and antibiotics. Those who do not respond to conservative management may need an operation. Patients with CD are at risk of developing enterocutaneous and enteroenteric fistulas spontaneously or after surgical intervention, and if diagnosed, nutritional optimization and control of sepsis are of utmost importance.

Five percent of patients will develop severe or fulminant colitis. These patients should be treated in a similar fashion as patients with UC including bowel rest, intravenous fluids, broad spectrum antibiotics, and aggressive CD therapy. They should be closely monitored with serial abdominal examinations, laboratory tests, and imaging as indicated. Patients with CD more commonly respond to medical management than patients with UC. When patients require surgery, total abdominal colectomy with end ileostomy is the most common operation performed in the acute setting, although if by operative inspection the disease is limited to a specific part of the large bowel, this can be resected with creation of a colostomy and Hartmann's pouch or mucous fistula. Isolated perforation without toxic megacolon is preferentially treated with segmental resection, as simple closure is associated with a higher mortality rate. Diversion is commonly performed in colonic perforations and occasionally for perforation of small bowel depending on the clinical status of the patient and the intraoperative findings.

Perianal complications include perianal abscess, fistula, ulcer, and fissure. These processes are treated using the same methods as are used in non-IBD patients, although these problems tend to be more complicated and chronic, requiring dedicated surgical follow-up. The key elements to treatment are elimination of sepsis and protection of the anal sphincter.

Dysplasia or cancer of the colon requires surgical treatment. Depending on the location and extent of disease, proctocolectomy or segmental resection is performed for high-grade dysplasia, dysplasia-associated lesions or mass lesions. Twenty percent of patients with high grade dysplasia are found to have carcinoma in the surgical specimen, and half of patients known to have cancer preoperatively are found to have remote dysplasia upon pathologic review. For this reason, total proctocolectomy with end ileostomy should be considered in patients found to have cancer or high grade dysplasia on surveillance colonoscopy.

Prognosis

Surgical procedures—like medical therapy—should be regarded as palliative, not curative, in patients with CD. Although recurrence rates are high and chronic disease is common, a productive life is usually possible with the aid of combined medical and surgical management. The mortality rate is about 15% over 30 years.

Kiran RP, Nisar PJ, Goldblum JR, et al: Dysplasia associated with Crohn's colitis: segmental colectomy or more extended resection? *Ann Surg* 2012 Aug;256(2):221-226.

Masselli G, Gualdi G: MR imaging of the small bowel. *Radiology* 2012 Aug;264(2):333-348.

Sandborn WJ, Gasink C, Gao LL, et al: Ustekinumab induction and maintenance therapy in refractory Crohn's disease. *N Engl J Med* 2012 Oct 18;367(16):1519-1528.

Strong SA et al: Practice parameters for the surgical management of Crohn's disease. *Dis Colon Rectum* 2007;50:1735.

PSEUDOMEMBRANOUS COLITIS

Pseudomembranous colitis is caused by *C difficile*. *C. difficile* colitis was first reported in 1978 but the incidence and severity of infection is increasing with time. Of particular concern is the increasing virulence, with reports of antibiotic resistance and mutant strains with uncontrolled toxin production. Infection causes a range of illness from mild diarrhea to fulminant, life threatening colitis and is particularly dangerous in frail or immunocompromised patients.

► Microbiology

Clostridium difficile is a spore-forming organism that is ubiquitous in the environment. It is a commensal gut organism that exists in 5%-15% of the general population and up to 57% of patients in long-term care facilities. The spores are dormant and extremely resistant to disinfectants and extreme environments. Spread by health care practitioners is reduced significantly by the use of standard contact precautions including disposable gowns and gloves and hand washing with water and soap. Alcohol-based hand sanitizers are not effective. Once ingested, the spore is reactivated after contact with bile salts in the small intestine.

The bacterium exists in both toxin-producing and non-producing forms. Only the toxin-producing bacterium is capable of causing colitis. Toxins A, B, and binary toxin induce apoptosis and provoke inflammation. The epidemic-associated 027 strain is thought to have a mutation causing increased production of toxins A and B, as well as enhanced sporulation making it particularly virulent and transmittable. These toxins as well as a variety of nontoxin virulence factors cause pseudomembranous colitis.

Although *C. difficile* is commensal and the spores are easily transmitted, the presence of normal colonic flora is usually enough to prevent infection. Symptoms generally only occur when the normal flora is disrupted. Therefore, pseudomembranous colitis most often occurs in patients taking antibiotics. Clindamycin is historically the most common cause, but all antibiotics that alter the gut flora have the potential to cause infection. Pseudomembranous colitis may develop as early as 2 days after exposure to antibiotics but has been reported many weeks after they are discontinued. Other risk factors include surgery of the gastrointestinal tract, immunosuppression, and use of proton pump inhibitors and H2 blockers.

► Symptoms and Signs

The most common symptom is diarrhea, which is usually watery, occasionally bloody, and has a characteristic foul odor. Other symptoms include colicky abdominal pain, vomiting, and fever. *C. difficile* infection may also cause a paralytic ileus and therefore, can present without diarrhea. Depending on the severity, patients may present with abdominal distention, tenderness, dehydration, and sepsis. The stool is usually positive for leukocytes. Radiographic studies may reveal colonic wall thickening due to submucosal edema. On abdominal films, this may appear as a "target sign." CT scanning is reserved for patients with complicated disease. It may show colonic wall thickening, ascites, colonic dilation, or perforation.

Changes in the colonic mucosa depend on the severity of the infection. Endoscopy performed for mild to moderate cases will show erythema and edema of the mucosa, with occasional hemorrhage. In severe cases, findings include elevated whitish-green or yellow plaques like "pseudomembranes" overlying inflamed mucosa. The pseudomembrane is made up of leukocytes, necrotic epithelial cells, and fibrin. The rectum is spared in about one-fourth of cases.

► Diagnosis

The gold standard for diagnosis of *C. difficile* colitis was a cytotoxin neutralization assay. This has largely been abandoned owing to its technical difficulty and length of time required to obtain a result (24-48 hours). Instead, the 2013 American College of Gastroenterology (ACG) guidelines recommends using PCR amplification of the genes for toxins A and B from a stool sample. This test has high sensitivity (87%) and specificity (97%) and is cost effective. It can be used as a sole diagnostic test or as part of a two-step approach using a glutamine dehydrogenase (GDH) screening assay, and if positive, following with the PCR confirmatory test. The guidelines recommend against the popular enzyme-linked immunoassay for toxins A and B owing to a cited lack of sensitivity and specificity (75%-95% and 83%-98% respectively); however, the test is still widely used for its ease of performance, low cost, and some studies show similar effectiveness. Stool culture is limited to use in epidemiologic studies. Finally, retesting stool for cure is not recommended because there is a high rate of positive tests after clinical cure, which may lead to prolonged and unnecessary treatment.

► Treatment

A. Medical

After discontinuing the inciting antibiotic agent, which is the first step in treatment for any patient, management is determined by severity of disease. In the United States, vancomycin and metronidazole are the drugs of choice. ACG guidelines recommend treatment of mild to moderate infections with Metronidazole 500 mg three times daily for 10 days. If there is no clinical improvement by day 5, vancomycin is started at a dose of 125 mg orally four times daily for 10 days. Both antibiotics have similar efficacy in patients with mild to moderate disease, but metronidazole is cheaper ($2/d vs. $71-$143/d). A third agent, fidaxomicin, was FDA approved for treatment in 2011 after phase III trials showed non-inferiority for clinical cure and decreased rates of relapse compared to vancomycin in mild-moderate disease. However, this drug is more expensive than vancomyin ($280/d) and post-marketing clinical trials are still underway. There is some evidence that teicoplanin, a bacteriocidal antibiotic, is more effective than vancomycin. However, its use is limited as it is extremely expensive and not available in the United States.

Severe infections (serum albumin < 3 with either a WBC > 15,000 or abdominal tenderness) are treated initially with vancomycin, 125 mg orally four times daily for 10 days, which has been shown to be more effective in patients with severe disease. Patients with complicated disease (admission to ICU, hypotension, fever > 38.5, abdominal distention, altered mental status, WBC > 35,000 or < 2000, lactate > 2.2, or organ failure) are treated with combination therapy consisting of vancomycin 500 mg orally four times daily, vancomycin enemas, and metronidazole 500 mg IV every 8 hours.

Recurrent disease is less well studied, however, ACG guidelines recommend standard treatment if symptoms are mild to moderate. If the patient has more severe illness, treatment should be stepped up as indicated. Oral vancomycin should be administered as a first line treatment and there is some evidence to suggest that pulsed vancomycin can be helpful in patients with multiple recurrences. There is mounting evidence, including a small randomized clinical trial, showing superior clinical efficacy in patients treated with vancomycin plus fecal transplant as opposed to vancomycin alone.

B. Surgical

Although most patients will respond to initial medical management, a subset will develop complicated or "fulminant" colitis. Risk factors include patients with IBD, recent gastrointestinal surgery, and WBC greater than 16,000. These patients are critically ill and have a mortality rate of 35%-80%. An abdominal CT scan is indicated to look for complications of *C. difficile* colitis, such as toxic megacolon and perforation, and exclude other intra-abdominal pathology. Surgical evaluation is recommended for patients with shock (altered mental status, organ dysfunction, lactic acidosis) peritonitis, significant leukocytosis, or failure to improve on medical therapy for 5 days. Although there have been

no randomized controls, timely surgery for these patients provides a substantial decrease in mortality. Given the diffuse involvement of the colon and the severity of the illness, a subtotal colectomy with end ileostomy is recommended. Residual rectal disease may be treated with vancomycin enemas if needed. Intestinal continuity is restored at a later operation.

Bartlett JG, Gerding DN: Clinical recognition and diagnosis of *Clostridium difficile* infection. *Clin Infect Dis* 2008;46(suppl 1):S12.

Butala P, Divino CM: Surgical aspects of fulminant *Clostridium difficile* colitis. *Am J Surg* 2010 Jul;200(1):131-135.

Hall JF, Berger D: Outcome of colectomy for *Clostridium difficile* colitis: a plea for early surgical management. *Am J Surg* 2008;196:384.

Nelson RL, Kelsey P, Leeman H, et al: Antibiotic treatment for Clostridium difficile-associated diarrhea in adults. *Cochrane Database Syst Rev* 2011 Sep 7;(9):CD004610.

Surawicz CM, Brandt LJ, Binion DG, et al: Guidelines for diagnosis, treatment, and prevention of Clostridium difficile infections. *Am J Gastroenterol* 2013 Apr;108(4):478-498.

van Nood E, Vrieze A, Nieuwdorp M: Duodenal infusion of donor feces for recurrent Clostridium difficile. *N Engl J Med* 2013 Jan 31;368(5):407-415.

Vedantam G, Clark A, Chu M, et al: Clostridium difficile infection: toxins and non-toxin virulence factors, and their contributions to disease establishment and host response. *Gut Microbes* 2012 Mar-Apr;3(2):121-134.

ISCHEMIC COLITIS

Ischemic colitis refers to colonic inflammation caused by inadequate perfusion. It is more common in elderly patients and has a mortality of 13%. It occurs as a result of an occlusive or non-occlusive insult. Examples of occlusive ischemic colitis include embolism, thrombosis (arterial or venous), atherosclerosis, trauma, and postsurgical causes such as patients with loss of inferior mesenteric blood supply after aortic aneurysm repair and those with inadequate perfusion to colonic anastomoses. Nonocclusive injury may occur as a result of shock, vasopressors, vasospasm, mechanical obstruction of the lumen, or systemic vasculitides.

An important clinical distinction that must be made when evaluating patients is assessing the colon for gangrenous and non-gangrenous ischemic colitis. Patients with gangrenous forms have transmural, nonreversible injury that is rapidly fatal without surgery. The non-gangrenous type is divided into transient reversible and chronic forms. The chronic form involves the muscularis propria and is prone to stricture development. Transient reversible ischemia involves the submucosa and heals without sequelae. Most cases of ischemic colitis are idiopathic and attributed to a nonocclusive state.

Patients with ischemic colitis present with diarrhea (90%), hematochezia (65%), and abdominal pain (58%). A history of atrial fibrillation, thrombophilia, atherosclerotic arterial disease, recent trauma or surgery, or systemic vasculitis should be sought. Recent severe systemic illness with shock is a common suspected cause. There may be localized or diffuse peritonitis. Blood tests may reveal leukocytosis, hyperamylasemia, and acidosis, as well as electrolyte derangements. The most common location is the sigmoid colon (40%) followed by the transverse colon (17%), splenic flexure (11%), ascending colon (12%), and the rectum (6%).

The most useful diagnostic tests are endoscopy and abdominal CT. Colonoscopy is the diagnostic modality of choice (although contraindicated in critically ill patients with peritonitis) as it allows diagnostic confirmation, determination of severity, and can rule out other types of colitis. The mucosa of the involved segment is edematous, hemorrhagic, friable, and sometimes ulcerated. A grayish membrane may be present, resembling pseudomembranous colitis, but the presence of hyalinized, hemorrhagic lamina on biopsy will differentiate colonic ischemia from *C difficile* colitis. Serial endoscopy can be used to identify patients with progression of mucosal lesions who require surgery. Abdominal CT with contrast shows a thickened colonic wall, decreased wall enhancement, pneumatosis, and occasionally a disruption in the arterial circulation. It is also useful to exclude other conditions.

Initial treatment for patients without gangrene suspected to have reversible ischemic colitis consists of intravenous fluids, bowel rest, broad spectrum antibiotics, and observation with serial abdominal examinations. Approximately 20% of patients will have irreversible disease, whether gangrenous from the beginning, becoming more severe over several days, or just failing to resolve after treatment. These patients need surgery. The extent of the resection is based on the amount of necrotic or severely diseased colon. Most commonly a segmental resection is required, although a subtotal or total colectomy is performed in 20% of patients. Depending on the etiology of the ischemia and the appearance of the remaining bowel, a second-look laparotomy may be planned 12-24 hours later. Primary anastomosis is rarely performed and intestinal continuity is restored during a subsequent operation.

O'Neill S, Yalamarthi S: Systematic review of the management of ischaemic colitis. *Colorectal Dis* 2012 Nov;14(11):e751-e763.

NEUTROPENIC COLITIS

Neutropenic colitis, also referred to as neutropenic enterocolitis, necrotizing enteropathy, ileocecal syndrome, and typhlitis, is a syndrome of colonic necrosis occurring in neutropenic patients. The cause is poorly understood, but likely involves mucosal injury and unimpeded bacterial translocation as a result of profound immunosuppression. Neutropenic colitis should be on the differential diagnosis for any immunosuppressed patient with abdominal pain; however, it is most common in neutropenic patients

undergoing chemotherapy with cytotoxic agents such as the vinca alkaloids and doxorubicin. There are reports in patients with acquired immunodeficiency syndrome (AIDS), aplastic anemia, cyclic neutropenia, and those being treated with a variety of immunosuppressants for other conditions.

The clinical presentation ranges from mild to life-threatening and overall mortality is 30%-50%. Symptoms include fever, nausea, abdominal pain, distention, and watery or bloody diarrhea. These patients often present late and with deceptively benign findings on physical examination owing to the inability to mount a normal inflammatory response. The cecum and right colon are most often affected; however, any part of the small or large bowel, including the appendix, can be involved. Patients are commonly bacteremic and/or fungemic. Causative organisms include gram-negative rods, gram positive cocci, anaerobes, and candida.

Diagnosis is confirmed using abdominal CT scan, which demonstrates bowel wall thickening, distention, and may show pneumatosis or perforation. Initial management consists of bowel rest, intravenous fluids, and broad spectrum antibiotics. Antifungals are started if there is evidence of fungemia or persistent fevers on antibiotics. Resolution of neutropenia is an important prognostic factor, therefore, discontinuation of immunosuppressants, chemotherapeutics, and administration of granulocyte colony stimulating factor (G-CSF) should be considered. Surgery is recommended for patients with perforation, persistent bleeding, or who do not improve with medical management. Most patients undergo segmental resection with proximal diversion.

Badgwell BD et al: Challenges in surgical management of abdominal pain in the neutropenic cancer patient. *Ann Surg* 2008;248:104.
Morgan C, Tillett T, Braybrooke J, Ajithkumar T: Management of uncommon chemotherapy-induced emergencies. *Lancet Oncol* 2011 Aug;12(8):806-814.
Ullery BW, Pieracci FM, Rodney JR, Barie PS: Neutropenic enterocolitis. *Surg Infect* 2009 Jun;10(3):307-314.

▼ INTESTINAL STOMAS: ILEOSTOMY AND COLOSTOMY

Creating an intestinal stoma involves exteriorizing a part of the bowel wall onto the surface of the abdomen. This section will focus on the two most common stomas created in colon and rectal surgery–those made from the ileum (ileostomy) and colon (colostomy).

▶ Indications

Stomas are generally created to protect a distal anastomosis temporarily or as a permanent route for enteric contents when the colon and/or rectum has been resected. There are two configurations for a stoma. The end ileostomy or colostomy is created by fixing the end of the ileum or colon to the abdominal wall. The loop ileostomy or colostomy involves bringing a segment of ileum or colon to the abdominal wall and opening the side of the bowel leaving both a proximal and distal opening. In general, very little, if any, stool passes through the distal limb if the stoma is well constructed. This allows retrograde decompression of the distal bowel and has the benefit of being easier to reverse as both limbs are at the abdominal wall.

In the elective setting, loop ileostomies are commonly used to protect ileoanal anastomoses and low pelvic colorectal or colo-anal anastomoses. These ileostomies are temporary, and divert most of the fecal stream away from the anastomosis. End ileostomies (Figure 30–20) are used in the elective setting for patients who require proctocolectomy and do not desire or are not candidates for IPAA reconstruction. They are also commonly used in patients who require emergency subtotal colectomies and will not tolerate an anastomosis due to severe illness.

The Kock pouch, or continent ileostomy, involved an ileal reservoir and construction of a valve at skin level to allow the patient to catheterize the stoma multiple times per day. This allowed patients not to wear a stoma appliance and to control the timing of stool output. However, this procedure is associated with a high rate of complications and failure. It has largely been replaced with the IPAA.

Colostomies (Figure 30–21) are used in patients with low rectal cancers requiring APR or LAR who are not candidates for a low anastomosis. In addition, they are useful in patients who require diversion for chronic fistula disease or in the emergency setting for patients with a large bowel obstruction, perforation, or trauma where an anastomosis is unlikely to heal or the patient is too ill to tolerate it. Loop colostomies are infrequently used as they are associated with a higher complication rate, particularly prolapse, although they are easier to reverse.

▶ Technical Aspects

When possible, patients should meet with their enterostomal therapist or surgeon prior to their operation for education, counseling, and stoma marking. Preoperative stoma marking has been shown to reduce complications and improve postoperative quality of life. Ileostomies are typically placed in the right-lower quadrant and colostomies in the left-lower

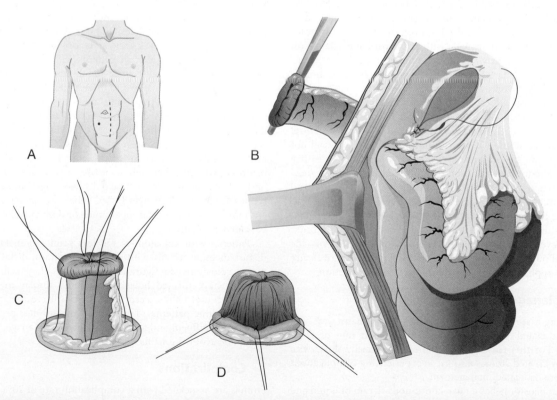

▲ **Figure 30–20.** Ileostomy after colectomy. **A:** A midline incision for colectomy is indicated by the dotted line and the site of the ileostomy by the black dot. **B:** The ileum has been brought through the abdominal wall. **C and D:** The ileostomy stoma has been everted and its margins sutured to the edges of the wound.

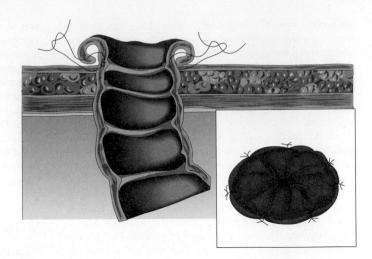

▲ **Figure 30–21.** End colostomy. The margins of the stoma are fixed to the skin with sutures.

quadrant. The placement should avoid wrinkles, folds, scars, and hernias on the abdominal wall. It should be at least 2 inches from the surgical incision and have a clear area extending 2-3 inches around it. It must be visible to the patient. Ideally, it is situated below the patient's belt line in the lateral rectus. The patient should be evaluated in the sitting, standing, and lying positions with and without clothing. The mark is made with active patient participation and it is ideal to provide a stoma appliance for the patient to wear over the mark for several days prior to the operation to ensure it is the optimal position.

There are several key steps during the operation that when followed, can reduce the chance of complications. The first step is to ensure adequate mobilization of the bowel so that the stoma will lie without any tension and will not retract into the abdominal wall. The second step is to pay close attention to the blood supply and preserve the mesentery and associated vessels during mobilization to avoid ischemic injury and subsequent stenosis. The third step is to create a defect in the rectus that is as small as possible that will still allow the stoma to pass without ischemia in order to prevent herniation. Lastly, when maturing the stoma, the aim should be to create 2-3 cm of bowel protrusion to ensure good appliance adhesion and improve skin protection.

▶ Management

Having a stoma changes a patient's life in many ways and is associated with an overall complication rate of 20%-70%. For this reason, these patients, especially those with newly created stomas and those experiencing complications require dedicated management.

An ileostomy has a near-continuous stream of liquid and semi-solid material whereas a colostomy tends to produce more formed stool. Both generally require an appliance to be worn at all times. Some patients choose to irrigate their colostomies to avoid stool output during the day. The sound and timing of flatus cannot be controlled by patients.

After ileostomy creation, there are significant changes in water and electrolyte absorption owing to the loss of the colon (Table 30–1). The small bowel adapts over the first 2 months after surgery. Output increases over the first week up to 1-2 L per day, stabilizes, and over the next 2 months steadily decreases to a steady state of 500-800 mL per day. Output can be higher in patients with diseased small bowel or more proximal stomas. Sodium excretion averages 60 mEq per day, which is two to three times that of patients with intact colons. These patients are at risk for developing salt depletion and dehydration, especially during times of illness or exposure to hot weather. They must take care to stay hydrated and to consume enough salt and potassium in their diets to make up for this. Generally, switching to a bland, constipating diet high in breads, cereals, dairy, peanut butter, bananas, and rice will help decrease high output and reduce fluid and electrolyte losses. Fiber supplements and antimotility agents such as loperamide or diphenoxylate can be added as needed.

Patients with colostomies are less prone to metabolic disturbances, especially with the more common distal (sigmoid) colostomy configuration. Generally, they will continue to have formed bowel movements similar to their previous bowel habits. Fecal impaction will require irrigation in some patients. Transverse colostomies produce semi-liquid effluent and tend to be difficult to manage. They should be avoided for this reason.

▶ Complications

Stomas are associated with a complication rate of 20%-70%. Ileostomies and colostomies are associated with similar complication rates. There is an association of loop colostomy and transverse colostomy with higher complication rates; however, this has never been studied in a randomized fashion and the data are conflicting. The complications seen in ileostomies are different than those seen with colostomies. Ileostomies are more likely to cause high output and dermatitis, whereas colostomies are more likely to develop hernia and odor.

A parastomal hernia refers to herniation of intra-abdominal contents through the defect in the fascia created for the stoma. In the chronic setting, parastomal hernias cause pain, difficulty with stoma appliance fitting, obstruction, and changes in stooling patterns. In the acute setting, there is a risk of incarceration and strangulation. Herniation is more common in patients with end-stomas as opposed to loop-stomas and more common in colostomies than ileostomies. The risk is minimized by creating a fascial defect that is just large enough to accommodate the bowel without ischemia. Some studies have shown a decreased risk of hernias in stomas placed through the rectus muscle, with fascial fixation, and when the preoperative marking is performed by an enterostomal therapist. Other risk factors for hernia development include obesity, COPD, poor nutritional status, and immunosuppression. There is also an increased risk of hernia with time. Conservative management is successful in 70% of patients and includes abdominal binders and restriction on heavy lifting. Flexible ostomy appliances may decrease leaking. Up to 30% of patients will require surgical revision either for failure of conservative management or for presentation with incarceration or strangulation. Surgical treatments vary depending on individual patient factors Options include stoma relocation and mesh repair. Mesh repairs can be local or intraperitoneal, open or laparoscopic. Intraperitoneal synthetic mesh repairs have the lowest recurrent rates, although this approach involves more surgical risk as well as the risk of mesh erosion or infection. Some small studies have shown prophylactic mesh placement to reduce the incidence of parastomal hernia without increasing surgical morbidity, although it is unclear if this approach is cost effective or if the effect is long term.

Stoma prolapse occurs in up to 42% of patients and is associated with similar risk factors as parastomal hernia. In fact, these two complications frequently coexist. It is more common in colostomies and specifically the distal limb of loop colostomies owing to defunctionalization and atrophy from non-use. Symptoms include pain, poor fitting of the stoma appliance, and may progress to obstruction, incarceration, or strangulation. Indications for repair include intractable symptoms or an acute presentation with impending bowel compromise. Incarcerated prolapsed stomas can often be reduced using topical sugar, which draws edema fluid out of the bowel wall allowing reduction. Surgical treatment depends on individual patient factors and options include resection, revision, and relocation.

High volume stoma output is defined as effluent greater than 2 L or any volume leading to dehydration. It is the most common cause of hospital readmission in patients with ileostomies. Patients with intrinsic small bowel disease (such as CD) or proximal stomas are at particularly high risk. Symptoms include dark urine, fatigue, irritability, muscle cramps, and headache. Patients develop dehydration and hyponatremia, which can result in secondary hyperaldosteronism and urinary potassium and magnesium wasting. Treatment is through rehydration, correction of electrolyte abnormalities, and antimotility medications. In the acute setting, intravenous fluids and electrolyte repletion are used, with some patients requiring total parenteral nutrition for a period of time. For marginally dehydrated patients, an isotonic glucose and sodium oral rehydration solution is effective. Long term, patients can use elemental, high carbohydrate, low fat diets to slow output. Helpful foods include breads, cereals, peanut butter, bananas, and rice. Medications such as loperamide, diphenoxylate, and tincture of opium can be used as adjunctive therapy. In refractory cases, the addition of H2 antagonists or proton pump inhibitors as well as octreotide have been shown to be effective.

Skin complications are common in patients with ileostomies. It is associated with parastomal henrniation, retraction, and prolapse, which contribute to poor appliance adherence, and high volume output, which increases leaking. Obese and diabetic patients are more commonly affected. It is most commonly a chemical dermatitis but can result from underlying Candida infection or even pyoderma gangrenosum in patients with IDD. Skin irritation can be avoided with dedicated skin care, reducing the number of appliance changes as much as possible (with a goal of one to two times per week), and surgical correction of contributing factors such as hernia or prolapse. Candida infections are treated with topical antifungals. Pyoderma gangrenosum is a notoriously difficult condition to treat, but may be responsive to local wound care, tacrolimus ointment, and intralesional steroid injections. Occasionally systemic tacrolimus or steroids are required.

Stoma retraction affects 1%-6% of patients with colostomies and 3%-17% of patients with ileostomies. This generally occurs in the immediate postoperative period as a result of tension on the bowel or poor wound healing and occurs more often in obese patients. It causes poor fitting of the stoma appliance and may lead to severe skin irritation. Some patients will be adequately treated with convex appliances, however, many will require surgery. Local revision is a reasonable first step. However, because this does not address tension on the bowel, some patients will progress to require laparoscopic or open revision.

Stenosis is uncommon, affecting 1%-10% of patients. Patients present with obstructive symptoms, or intermittent periods of no stoma output and crampy abdominal pain followed by a sudden large volume discharge. Most commonly, they are a result of ischemic injury, although in rarer cases they may be due to a technical error (fascia or skin is too tight) or underlying disease of the small bowel such as CD or malignancy. Diagnosis should be made by inspection and digital exploration. Hegar dilation in multiple sessions may be effective, but patients often require stoma revision either locally or by a laparoscopic or open intra-abdominal approach.

ASCRS: Stoma siting Procedure. Available at http://www.fascrs.org/physicians/position_statements/stoma_siting/. Accessed 26 April 2013.

Bafford AC, Irani JL: Management and complications of stomas. *Surg Clin North Am* 2013 Feb;93(1):145-166.

Hansson BM, Slater NJ, van der Velden AS, et al: Surgical techniques for parastomal hernia repair: a systematic review of the literature. *Ann Surg* 2012;255(4):685-695.

Person B, Ifargan R, Lachter J, et al: The impact of preoperative stoma site marking on the incidence of complications, quality of life, and patient's independence. *Dis Colon Rectum* 2012 Jul;55(7):783-787.

Rondelli F, Reboldi P, Rulli A, et al: Loop ileostomy versus loop colostomy for fecal diversion after colorectal or colo-anal anastomosis: a meta-analysis. *Int J Colorectal Dis* 2009 May;24(5):479-488.

PERIOPERATIVE MANAGEMENT

BOWEL PREPARATION

Because of the high bacterial load of the large intestine, elective colorectal surgery without prophylaxis carries a 40% risk of wound infection. This has also been reported as a cause for anastomotic dehiscence. It was previously believed that mechanical lavage (bowel prep) of the gastrointestinal tract would prevent these complications by removing fecal waste and the associated bacterial flora. This involves administration of a large volume of unabsorbed fluid, such as polyethylene glycol or alternatively small volume sodium phosphate, which induces an osmotic diarrhea. Retrograde enemas have been used in distal colon and rectal surgery. Healthy patients usually tolerate these preparations well. However, osmotic agents can lead to dehydration and electrolyte disturbances in more fragile patients.

Although mechanical bowel preparation used to be routine for colorectal surgery, there is debate about its safety and utility. Multiple randomized controlled trials have been completed, with few suggestions of adverse outcomes in both bowel prepped and non-prepped patients. Meta-analyses have shown no differences in outcomes. Specifically, mortality, anastomotic leaks (colo-colonic and colo-rectal), and wound infection rates are similar between the two groups. When a leak occurs, the clinical severity is also not influenced by bowel preparation. There is also no difference between patients treated with preoperative enema versus bowel preparation. This suggests that mechanical bowel preparation can be safely omitted before surgery, especially in patients at risk for prep-related complications.

PERIOPERATIVE ANTIBIOTICS

The use of preoperative parenteral antibiotics significantly reduces surgical wound infection by 75% and should be used routinely. There is no evidence to suggest that infection rates are further reduced by continuing antibiotics postoperatively. Ertapenem has been shown to be superior to cefotetan in preventing surgical site infections in a large randomized controlled trial of 1002 patients undergoing elective colorectal surgery. Parenteral antibiotics are superior to oral antibiotics alone in preventing wound infections, although there is evidence that in patients undergoing bowel preparation those who receive oral antibiotics in combination with parenteral antibiotics have decreased infectious complications compared to those patients who are treated with parenteral antibiotics alone. However, oral antibiotic regimens are poorly tolerated and this is less likely to be important as the use of routine bowel preparation decreases.

DEEP VENOUS THROMBOSIS PROPHYLAXIS

Colorectal surgery patients are at higher risk than general surgery patients for the development of perioperative thromboembolism. In historical series, deep venous thrombosis was diagnosed in 20% of general surgery patients and 30% of colorectal patients without prophylaxis. The rate of symptomatic pulmonary embolism is fourfold higher (0.8% vs. 3.1%). This is related to a variety of factors, including the prevalence of IBD and malignancy in this patient population. Extended operative times, pelvic dissection, and modified lithotomy may also be contributing factors. Subcutaneous heparin and low-molecular-weight heparin are equivalent in reducing both deep venous thrombosis and pulmonary embolism. Low-molecular-weight heparin has a simplified dosing regimen and a decreased incidence of heparin induced thrombocytopenia, however, it is more expensive and there seems to be a dose-related increased risk of bleeding complications. Fondaparinux is a newer Xa inhibitor that has also shown efficacy as a prophylactic agent. There is insufficient evidence to recommend one medication over the other at this time. Sequential compression devices are a useful adjunct.

PAIN MANAGEMENT

There is debate about the most useful postoperative analgesia for colorectal surgery patients. The three most commonly used methods are epidural, spinal, and patient controlled analgesia. Multiple studies have shown decreased subjective pain in patients managed with epidurals, however, this does not translate into better outcomes, and in fact, may lead to increased length of stay. This may be related to the increased use of laparoscopy in colorectal surgery. However, fast track programs to reduce length of stay for colorectal surgery have used short-term epidurals for 24-48 hours with some success. Further study is required to define the impact of these regimens on return of bowel function, pulmonary complications, and mortality.

POSTOPERATIVE NUTRITION

Early initiation of nutrition postoperatively has become the standard of care for patients undergoing colorectal operations. The most studied regimen includes initiating a liquid diet within 24 hours after surgery and advancing as tolerated to a regular diet as opposed to older protocols, which mandated fasting until there was evidence of bowel function in the form of flatus or defecation. Initiating feeding early leads to decreased hospital stay but doesn't seem to impact other clinical indicators. However, early feeding must be initiated with other interventions such as minimizing fluids and early ambulation.

Bretagnol F, Panis Y, Rullier E, et al: Rectal cancer surgery with or without bowel preparation: the French GRECCAR III multicenter single-blinded randomized trial. *Ann Surg* 2010 Nov;252(5):863-868.

Cao F, Li J, Li F: Mechanical bowel preparation for elective colorectal surgery: updated systematic review and meta-analysis. *Int J Colorectal Dis.* 2012 Jun;27(6):803-810.

Dag A, Colak T, Turkmenoglu O, Gundogdu R, Aydin S: A randomized controlled trial evaluating early versus traditional oral feeding after colorectal surgery. *Clinics (Sao Paulo)* 2011;66(12):2001-2005.

Lassen K, Soop M, Nygren J, et al: Consensus review of optimal perioperative care in colorectal surgery: Enhanced Recovery After Surgery (ERAS) Group recommendations. *Arch Surg* 2009;144(10):961-969.

Levy BF, Scott MJ, Fawcett W, Fry C, Rockall TA: Randomized clinical trial of epidural, spinal or patient-controlled analgesia for patients undergoing laparoscopic colorectal surgery. *Br J Surg* 2011 Aug;98(8):1068-1078.

Lewis SJ, Andersen HK, Thomas S: Early enteral nutrition within 24 h of intestinal surgery versus later commencement of feeding: a systematic review and meta-analysis. *J Gastrointest Surg* 2009 Mar;13(3):569-575.

McNally MP, Burns CJ: Venous thromboembolic disease in colorectal patients. *Clin Colon Rectal Surg* 2009 Feb;22(1):34-40.

Nelson RL, Gladman E, Barbateskovic M: Antimicrobial prophylaxis for colorectal surgery. *Cochrane Database Syst Rev* 2014 May 9;5:CD001181.

MULTIPLE CHOICE QUESTIONS

1. Protectomy requires pelvic dissection and has the potential to cause injury to the nerves that supply the rectum, pelvic floor muscles, and bladder, as well as the prostate and seminal vesicles in men. Which of the following associations is incorrect regarding the nerves at risk at different points in the operation?

   A. Superior hypogastric plexus near root of IMA
   B. Hypogastric nerves in the retrorectal space
   C. Nervi erigentes near lateral stalks
   D. Inferior hypogastric plexus near Denonvillier fascia

2. A 60-year-old man presents with abdominal pain, fevers, and nausea. He is febrile, focally tender in the LLQ, and has a WBC of 18,000. CT shows sigmoid diverticulitis with a 4 cm pericolonic abscess. What is the optimal management strategy for this patient?

   A. Bowel rest, intravenous fluids, broad spectrum antibiotics
   B. Bowel rest, intravenous fluids, and broad spectrum antibiotics
   C. Bowel rest, intravenous fluids, broad spectrum antibiotics, and percutaneous drainage
   D. Urgent exploratory laparotomy

3. An otherwise healthy 60-year-old man presents with abdominal pain. His CT shows an obstructing mass in the sigmoid colon with dilation of the cecum to 13 cm. After fluid resuscitation, what is the next step in management?

   A. Nasogastric decompression and observation
   B. NPO, antibiotics, and observation
   C. Flexible sigmoidoscopy with biopsies to further evaluate the mass
   D. Exploratory laparotomy

4. A 65-year-old, asymptomatic, woman is found to have a 3 cm sessile polyp in the ascending colon on screening colonoscopy. It was biopsied but could not be resected. Pathology shows tubulovillous adenoma. What is next step in management?

   A. Colonoscopy in 1 year
   B. Colonoscopy in 3 years
   C. Local excision
   D. Right hemicolectomy

5. What is the most common symptom patients experience after removal of the colon?

   A. Vitamin K deficiency
   B. Renal stones
   C. Dehydration
   D. Hyponatremia
   E. Short chain fatty acid deficiency

Anorectum

Cary B. Aarons, MD

Stephen M. Sentovich, MD

ANORECTAL ANATOMY

The anatomy of the anus and rectum dictates the clinical evaluation and treatment of patients with anorectal disorders (Figure 31–1).

From external to internal, the surface anatomy of the anorectum is comprised of gluteal skin, anoderm, the anal transitional zone, and proximally the rectal mucosa. The gluteal skin includes hair, sebaceous glands, and sweat glands. This area, particularly 3-5 cm of anal margin skin circumferentially around the anus, can commonly become infected with the human papilloma virus resulting in anal condyloma. Anal condyloma can also affect more proximal tissue in the anoderm and lower rectal mucosa. Perianal hidradenitis is also relatively common and develops in the apocrine sweat glands of the perianal skin. Unlike anal condyloma, perianal hidradenitis can only occur in the gluteal skin as there are no sweat glands in the anoderm.

The anoderm begins at the anal verge and ends at the dentate line. Unlike the gluteal skin, the anoderm is devoid of hair and sweat glands. Anal fissures occur in the anoderm and can be associated with a sentinel tag externally and a hypertrophied anal papilla internally (Figure 31–2). Surgical excision of too much anoderm during hemorrhoidectomy or other anorectal surgery can result in anal stenosis.

The anal transitional zone lies between the squamous anoderm and the rectal mucosa. In this zone, squamous, cuboidal, transitional, and columnar epithelium exist with longitudinal ridges called the columns of Morgagni. Between the columns of Morgagni are anal crypts with associated anal glands that open into their bases. Clinically, the anal transitional zone is important for two main reasons. First, the anal transitional zone is the crossover from somatic to visceral innervation and for lymphatic drainage from the inguinal to the pelvic nodes. Lymphatics from the anal canal above the dentate line drain via the superior rectal lymphatics to the inferior mesenteric lymph nodes and laterally to the

internal iliac nodes. Below the dentate line, drainage occurs to the inguinal lymph nodes but can occur to the inferior or superior rectal lymph nodes. Second, the anal glands in the crypts are the site of anorectal abscesses and anal fistulas. Anatomically the anal glands in the crypts extend to a variable depth resulting in perianal, intersphincteric, or ischiorectal abscesses when these glands become blocked.

Proximal to the anal transitional zone is the rectal mucosa. Above the dentate line and underlying the rectal mucosa are the vessels that, when abnormally engorged, manifest as internal hemorrhoids. Hemorrhoids are not veins but arteriovenous connections that have pulsatile flow. Patients with bleeding from hemorrhoids can have significant blood loss. Further, internal hemorrhoids are covered by mucosa and because they are above the dentate line, they are viscerally innervated. This is the reason rubber-band ligation of internal hemorrhoids is possible without anesthesia. In contrast, external hemorrhoids are below the dentate line, covered by anoderm and skin. Any surgical intervention on external hemorrhoids requires some type of anesthesia.

Hemorrhoidal vessels are anchored by Treitz' muscle. When the Treitz' muscle attachments weaken, internal and external hemorrhoids can prolapse, bleed and cause perianal irritation and discomfort. Internal hemorrhoids can prolapse and can be confused with rectal prolapse. Generally, internal hemorrhoids prolapse in columns occurring in the right anterior, right posterior and left lateral quadrants around the anus. When the anus is examined, these prolapsing columns of internal hemorrhoids appear as radial folds. This is distinguished from the circumferential folds of rectal prolapse.

The rectum extends 12-15 cm proximal to the dentate line. The rectum has three curves that create folds called the valves of Houston. It is supported by the puborectalis and levator muscles that are also called the pelvic floor. In addition, the rectum is fixed posteriorly by presacral (Waldeyer)

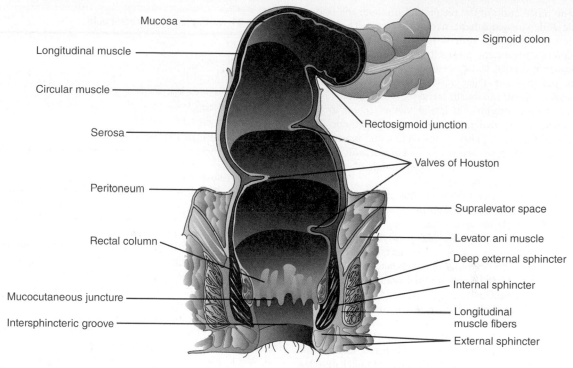

▲ **Figure 31–1.** Anatomy of the anorectal canal.

fascia, laterally by the lateral ligaments, and anteriorly by Denonvilliers fascia. The arterial supply of the anorectum is via the superior, middle and inferior rectal arteries. The superior rectal artery is the terminal branch of the inferior mesenteric artery and descends in the mesorectum. It supplies the upper and middle rectum. The middle rectal arteries arise from the internal iliac arteries and enter the rectum anterolaterally at the level of the pelvic floor musculature. They supply the lower two-thirds of the rectum. Collaterals exist between the middle and superior rectal arteries. The inferior rectal arteries—branches of the internal pudendal arteries—enter posterolaterally, do not anastomose with the blood supply to the middle rectum, and supply the anal sphincters and epithelium.

The venous drainage of the anorectum is via the superior, middle, and inferior rectal veins draining into the portal and systemic systems. The superior rectal veins drain the upper and middle thirds of the rectum and empty into the portal system via the inferior mesenteric vein. The middle rectal veins drain the lower rectum and the upper anal canal into the systemic system via the internal iliac veins. The inferior rectal veins drain the lower anal canal, communicating with the pudendal veins, and draining into the internal iliac veins. Communication between the venous systems allows low rectal cancers to spread via the portal and systemic systems.

Lymphatic drainage of the upper and middle rectum is into the inferior mesenteric nodes. Lymph from the lower rectum may drain into the inferior mesenteric system or into lymphatics around the lower rectum that drain into the inguinal nodes and then into periaortic nodes. Below the dentate line, lymphatic drainage occurs primarily to the inguinal nodes but may drain into the inferior mesenteric lymph nodes.

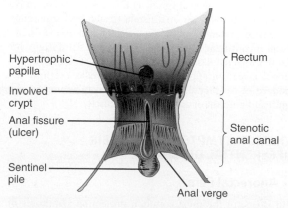

▲ **Figure 31–2.** Diagram of the anorectum showing the fissure or ulcer triad.

The innervation of the rectum is from both the sympathetic and parasympathetic nervous systems. The sympathetic nerves originate from the lumbar segments L1-3, form the inferior mesenteric plexus, travel through the superior hypogastric plexus, and descend as the hypogastric nerves to the pelvic plexus. The parasympathetic nerves arise from the second, third, and fourth sacral roots and join the hypogastric nerves anterior and lateral to the rectum to form the pelvic plexus. Sympathetic and parasympathetic fibers pass from the pelvic plexus to the rectum and internal anal sphincter (IAS) as well as other pelvic viscera. Injury to these nerves can lead to sexual and bladder dysfunction, and loss of normal defecatory mechanisms.

Beneath the surface anatomy of the anus and rectum are the anal sphincter muscles. The IAS muscle is involuntary and is responsible for anal canal resting tone. The IAS is innervated with sympathetic and parasympathetic fibers. Both are inhibitory and keep the sphincter in a basal state of contraction. The external anal sphincter (EAS) muscle is voluntary and responsible for anal canal squeezing tone. The external sphincters are skeletal muscles innervated by the pudendal nerve with fibers that originate from S2-4. The EAS muscle fuses with the pelvic floor muscles to create a bowl-like muscular support of the lower rectum.

While systemic diseases such as diabetes, scleroderma and multiple sclerosis can affect the anal sphincter muscles, far more common is direct injury to the sphincter muscles from vaginal delivery or surgery. Using transanal ultrasound to evaluate the anal sphincter muscles before and after vaginal delivery it has been demonstrated that approximately one-third of women injure their anal sphincter at the time of delivery. Fortunately, only one-third of these women develop fecal incontinence.

Operative intervention for hemorrhoids, anal fissure, and anal fistula can result in anal sphincter injury. Sphincter injury should not occur during hemorrhoid surgery as hemorrhoidal vessels are superficial to the anal sphincter muscles. Division of the anal sphincter is necessary and curative for anal fissure and for anal fistula treated by fistulotomy. While lateral internal sphincterotomy for anal fissure carries a fecal incontinence rate of less than 0.5%, fistulotomy for complex anal fistulas has a rate of over 50%. For this reason, sphincter-sparing approaches to anal fistulas are now the standard of care for patients with anal fistulas involving a significant amount of anal sphincter muscle.

COMMON SYMPTOMS AND THEIR DIFFERENTIAL DIAGNOSIS

▶ Anorectal Pain

Pain is one of the most common presenting symptoms of anorectal disorders. The common causes of anorectal pain are shown in Table 31–1. The vast majority of patients have

Table 31–1. Causes of anorectal pain.

Thrombosed external hemorrhoids
Anorectal abscess
Anal fissure
Anal mass: anal cancer, anal condyloma
Trauma: direct injury, foreign body
Infections: HSV, HIV, CMV, and others
Functional: levator spasm, proctalgia fugax

either thrombosed external hemorrhoid, anal fissure, or anorectal abscess. The other causes of anorectal pain are relatively unusual. The etiology of anorectal pain can often be determined with a careful history that is then confirmed with the physical examination.

For patients with anorectal pain, the most important aspects of the patient history are the nature and onset of the pain and any associated symptoms. If the pain is acute in onset (< 1-3 d) and associated with a lump at the anus, a diagnosis of a thrombosed external hemorrhoid is highly likely. If the pain is acute in onset and associated with fever and swelling at the anus, then an anorectal abscess should be suspected. Finally, if the pain is described as a "cut," "tear," or "sharp as a knife" and associated with bowel movements, then an anal fissure is the probable cause. Inspection alone will usually confirm the suspected diagnosis as an external hemorrhoid, abscess or cellulitis or anal fissure will be present. It is important to efface the anus by pulling the gluteal cheeks apart in order to identify an anterior or posterior anal fissure that occurs just inside the anal canal. Most patients with anorectal pain cannot tolerate a digital examination and anoscopy but fortunately these evaluations are often unnecessary. If after obtaining a history and carefully inspecting the anus and the diagnosis is still in doubt, an examination under anesthesia may be indicated as small number of patients may have an intersphincteric or supralevator abscess that usually cannot be diagnosed by inspection alone.

▶ Anorectal Bleeding

Bleeding is the most common presenting symptom in patients with anorectal disorders. Common causes of anorectal bleeding are shown in Table 31–2. While a careful history may suggest the etiology of bleeding, patients can tolerate and require a thorough physical examination as well as anoscopy and lower endoscopy. Even if anorectal pathology is identified on physical examination or anoscopy, endoscopic evaluation is always necessary in order to rule out proximal pathology such as polyps or cancer.

In patients with anorectal bleeding, the history can help identify the source of the bleeding by fully characterizing the amount, timing and location of the bleeding. Blood seen just on the toilet paper suggests anal canal pathology whereas

Table 31–2. Causes of rectal bleeding.

Hemorrhoids
Anal fissure
Proctitis
Anal fistula
Cancer
Ulceration/infection
Rectal prolapsed/solitary rectal ulcer

blood seen mixed with the stool suggests a more proximal bleeding source. Inspection of the anus may reveal prolapsing hemorrhoids, an anal fissure, an anal fistula, or anal ulcer. Anoscopy is necessary to evaluate for possible internal hemorrhoids and distal proctitis. Flexible sigmoidoscopy is typically recommended for younger patients (< 40 years old) who do not have a family history of colon cancer. Colonoscopy is recommended for patients over age 40 with anorectal bleeding or patients under age 40 who have a family history of colon cancer. While these general guidelines are appropriate for most patients, the choice between flexible sigmoidoscopy and colonoscopy is individualized to each patient's clinical scenario.

Anorectal Mass

Most anorectal mass lesions are either anal skin tags, a thrombosed external hemorrhoid or a sentinel pile associated with an anal fissure (Table 31–3). In addition to the history, physical examination and anoscopy, most patients with mass lesions need either flexible sigmoidoscopy or colonoscopy depending on their age, diagnosis, and whether or not there is a family history of colon cancer. The unusual tumors such as lipoma and GIST that occur deep to the skin, anoderm, and rectal mucosa are difficult to diagnose preoperatively. These tumors often require additional preoperative anatomic evaluation with transanal ultrasonography and/or pelvic MRI to determine their extent and relationship to the anal sphincter muscles.

Table 31–3. Causes of anorectal mass.

Thrombosed external hemorrhoids
Sentinel tag
Anal skin tag
Anal condyloma
Anorectal abscess
Hypertrophied anal papilla
Internal hemorrhoids
Rectal polyp
Anal or rectal cancer
Unusual tumors: GIST, lipoma, endometriosis

Table 31–4. Causes of anorectal discharge.

Prolapsing internal hemorrhoids
Anal fistula
Proctitis
Rectal polyp (villous adenoma)
Anal or rectal cancer
Anal warts
Mucosal/rectal prolapsed
Fecal incontinence/leakage (multiple etiologies)
Post-surgical: keyhole deformity

Anorectal Discharge

Discharge from the anus is a relatively common complaint and has a wide range of possible etiologies (Table 31–4). The most common causes of anorectal discharge are mucosal prolapse, anal fistula, and fecal leakage. Patients with anal fistula often have a history of perirectal abscess. On examination, the patient should be asked to strain in order to identify mucosal and rectal prolapse. Anal sphincter tone should be assessed during the digital examination. In patients with previous anorectal surgery, careful inspection of the anus is important to identify any anal contour abnormalities (keyhole deformities). In addition to anoscopy, most patients will require lower endoscopy. Patients with fecal leakage or incontinence often require further functional and anatomic studies.

HEMORRHOIDS

Hemorrhoids are blood vessels in the lower rectum and anal canal. They are not veins but rather arteriovenous connections with pulsatile flow. External hemorrhoids are located below the dentate line and anatomically identified by the presence of anoderm or skin overlying the hemorrhoidal vessel. Due to either diarrhea, constipation, or straining, a hemorrhoidal vessel can become thrombosed with a clot resulting in a painful lump and possibly some bleeding if the clot ruptures through the anoderm. External hemorrhoids typically cause symptoms when they thrombose, prolapse, or cause irritation/hygiene difficulties. Internal hemorrhoids originate from above the dentate line and are covered by mucosa. These blood vessels can become enlarged/engorged (eg, pregnancy) and/or their anchoring muscle, the Treitz muscle, can become weakened (eg, straining, constipation). When either one or both of these circumstances occur, the hemorrhoidal vessels can prolapse into the lumen of the anal canal as well as can prolapse externally. This mechanical prolapse of hemorrhoidal vessels can cause bleeding, irritation, and pressure-like pain.

Internal hemorrhoids can be classified as grade I-IV by their symptoms and degree of prolapse. Grade I hemorrhoids are prominent but do not prolapse. Grade II hemorrhoids prolapse but spontaneously reduce. Grade III hemorrhoids prolapse but require manual reduction. Grade IV hemorrhoids prolapse and cannot be manually reduced. The four-level grading system helps guide the choice of treatment of hemorrhoids.

Signs & Symptoms

Patients with thrombosed external hemorrhoids complain of acute pain and swelling or lump at the anus. Patients with external hemorrhoid skin tags will have more chronic symptoms of prolapsed, "extra skin," irritation, and difficulty with hygiene after bowel movements. Patients with internal hemorrhoids complain of bleeding, pressure-like pain and prolapse. Patients with bleeding internal hemorrhoids can have significant blood loss and become anemic acutely or chronically. Other than thrombosed external hemorrhoids, patients with hemorrhoids do not complain of sharp pain but rather bleeding, prolapse, irritation, and sometimes a pressure-like pain due to the prolapse. Both external and internal hemorrhoids can become incarcerated and gangrenous resulting in necrosis of skin and mucosa as well as bleeding.

Examination of the patient with a thrombosed external hemorrhoid reveals a purple swelling at the anus consistent with a clot in an external hemorrhoid vessel. Patients with external prolapse and tags reveal chronic protrusion and lumps without acute pain and discoloration. Patients with internal hemorrhoids may reveal nothing externally unless the internal hemorrhoids prolapse externally. Digital evaluation of the rectum can rule out any mass lesions or malignancy but internal hemorrhoids cannot be assessed adequately using digital rectal examination. Anoscopy is necessary to properly evaluate internal hemorrhoids. The examiner asks the patient to push or strain while visualizing each of the three common hemorrhoidal piles in the right anterior, right posterior and left lateral positions within the anal canal. Internal hemorrhoids are present if prolapse or bleeding occurs in any of the three locations visualized during anoscopy. Physical examination alone establishes a diagnosis of hemorrhoids. Further evaluation with laboratory or imaging studies is unnecessary unless there has been significant hemorrhage. All patients should also undergo evaluation of the more proximal colon with flexible sigmoidoscopy or colonoscopy as indicated.

Differential Diagnosis

Since patients and many primary care providers identify any anorectal symptom as being due to hemorrhoids, nearly all patients complain of "hemorrhoids" or will have been told that they have "hemorrhoids."

Patients with rectal bleeding need to be carefully evaluated not only with anoscopy but also with flexible endoscopy to rule out proximal pathology such as colitis, polyps or cancer. Patients with rectal bleeding, under age 40 and without a family history of colon cancer, can undergo anoscopy and flexible sigmoidoscopy. Patients with rectal bleeding between 40 and 50 years of age need evaluation with anoscopy and flexible sigmoidoscopy or colonoscopy with colonoscopy preferred for most patients. Patients over age 50 with bleeding need to be evaluated with anoscopy and colonoscopy. Finally, all patients with a significant family history of colon cancer should undergo anoscopy and colonoscopy regardless of age. Thus, it is very important in patients with rectal bleeding to evaluate the whole colon in most circumstances in order to rule out malignancy.

In patients with symptoms of prolapse, the surgeon must differentiate hemorrhoidal prolapse from true rectal prolapse. Patients with hemorrhoidal prolapse have prolapsing hemorrhoids in one or more of the standard hemorrhoid locations—right anterior, right posterior, and/or left lateral position. Because the hemorrhoids prolapse in these specific locations, the examiner sees prolapsing mucosa and underlying hemorrhoidal vessels with radial folds between the various prolapsing hemorrhoids. Patients with true rectal prolapse have circumferential prolapse of mucosa and full-thickness rectal wall that results in concentric folds. Patients with full-thickness rectal prolapse have decreased sphincter tone whereas patients with prolapsing hemorrhoids typically have normal to increased sphincter tone.

Treatment of External Hemorrhoids

Patients with chronic tags and external hemorrhoids are treated with reassurance particularly if the tags are small and minimally symptomatic. If they have symptoms of irritation, topical hydrocortisone cream can be helpful. If the external hemorrhoids are causing recurring symptoms of irritation, discomfort, and difficulty with anal hygiene then simple surgical excision may resolve them. If a patient with a thrombosed external hemorrhoid is seen within 3 days of the onset of symptoms then excision of the clot may be beneficial. Excision of the clot in these patients who present early to the surgeon allows for faster resolution of their symptoms. Simple incision of the clot is associated with a higher recurrence rate so if surgical intervention is undertaken it should be complete excision of the hemorrhoidal vessel and clot. Most patients with thrombosed external hemorrhoids seek medical attention after 3 days of symptoms. Surgical excision will not hasten resolution of symptoms in these patients, and management is topical and oral pain medications, stool softeners and laxatives. The clot typically resolves in 2 weeks-2 months. After resolution of their clot, occasionally patients are left with a residual skin tag. Hemorrhoidal disease is common during pregnancy and can be treated postpartum if symptoms persist.

Treatment of Internal Hemorrhoids

Patients with mild to moderate internal hemorrhoids (grades I-II) and constipation are treated with fiber, fluids, and possibly laxatives to improve their bowel habits. For most of these patients this medical treatment to improve their bowel function will resolve their hemorrhoidal symptoms. For patients with "hemorrhoids" and hyperactive bowel function, treatment should be directed at the cause of the diarrhea/multiple bowel movements. These patients should not undergo hemorrhoid surgery. Patients with normal bowel habits and persistent hemorrhoidal symptoms are candidates for a surgical approach.

Surgical Treatment of Hemorrhoids in the Office Setting

Internal hemorrhoids can be treated with in-office procedures such as rubber band ligation, sclerotherapy, and infrared coagulation. Most patients with grades I-III hemorrhoids can be successfully treated with office-based procedures. Of the office-based procedures, rubber band ligation is typically the most effective option.

A. Rubber Band Ligation of Hemorrhoids

Small to moderate-sized symptomatic internal hemorrhoids (grades I-III) can be treated with rubber band ligation. This in-office treatment involves placement of an anoscope then grasping the largest hemorrhoidal pile above the dentate line with a clamp and then using a rubber band ligator to place a rubber band around the "neck" of the hemorrhoid. Because the rubber band is placed above the dentate line, patients can tolerate this procedure without anesthesia and usually do not have significant postprocedure pain. After banding patients have either no symptoms or a mild to moderate pressure sensation that resolves in hours to a day or two. The rubber band is a noose around the hemorrhoid's "neck," and the hemorrhoid and rubber band will fall off within 5-10 days resulting in a scar that reduces the hemorrhoid size and degree of prolapse. When this sloughing of the hemorrhoid and rubber band occurs, the patient may experience bleeding that occasionally is severe enough to require an emergent visit. Patients are banded without antibiotics as sepsis after banding is exceedingly uncommon. Since postbanding sepsis presents with urinary retention, fever and increasing pain, any rubber band ligation patient with this constellation of symptoms needs to be evaluated urgently. Treatment of post-banding sepsis requires intravenous antibiotics, band removal, debridement of necrotic tissue and supportive care in an intensive care unit. Banding is usually performed one "pile" at a time but placement of multiple bands at one setting is possible. Postbanding instructions include keeping the stools soft, using pain

medication as needed and returning for urgent reevaluation if signs and symptoms of sepsis develop. Rubber band ligation is well-tolerated and quite successful for patients with grades I-III internal hemorrhoids.

B. Sclerotherapy

Sclerotherapy involves using anoscopy to inject a sclerosing agent into the apex of grades I- II internal hemorrhoids. A variety of sclerosing agents have been used with a commonly used option being phenol in oil. Typically, 3-5 mL of sclerosing solution is injected. While the initial success rate approaches that of rubber band ligation, recurrences are common. Complications are unusual but necrosis, rectal perforation, and sepsis have all been reported.

C. Infrared Coagulation

Infrared coagulation involves application of infrared energy directly to the internal hemorrhoids with an infrared coagulation probe. Using anoscopy, the probe is placed on the hemorrhoid for 1-2 seconds which results in coagulation of the hemorrhoid with a decrease in size and blood flow through the hemorrhoid. Recent studies have shown that infrared coagulation is as good as rubber band ligation for patients with grades I-II internal hemorrhoids. Complications are unusual but include bleeding, necrosis, and sepsis.

Surgical Treatment of Internal Hemorrhoids in the Operating Room

Patients with persistent symptoms despite in-office treatment of their hemorrhoids are candidates for surgery in the operating room. Surgery is usually performed only for patients with grades III-IV internal hemorrhoids. In the operating room, surgical treatment of internal hemorrhoids can be by surgical excision, stapled hemorrhoidopexy or doppler-guided ligation.

A. Excisional Hemorrhoidectomy

Classic excisional hemorrhoidectomy is performed either in the lithotomy or prone position. After the induction of anesthesia the hemorrhoidal piles are excised with scissors, cautery or harmonic scalpel. The resulting wounds are closed, partially-closed or left open depending on surgeon preference. Care is taken to excise just the mucosa, submucosa, and hemorrhoids and to avoid injury to the underlying anal sphincter muscle. In addition, care is taken not to excise too much mucosa and anoderm as this could result in anal stenosis. The procedure takes less than an hour and is scheduled as outpatient surgery. Given that the incisions start externally and end in the anal canal/lower rectum, patients can have significant discomfort postoperatively. Adequate pain control, keeping the bowel movements soft and avoiding constipation are all important postoperatively.

Early complications after excisional hemorrhoidectomy include bleeding, infection, and urinary retention. The rate of urinary retention can be reduced by limiting the amount of intravenous fluids during surgery. Late complications include anal stenosis and mucosal ectropion and whitehead deformity (circumferential mucosal ectropion). Given its high success rate and low recurrence rate, all other surgical interventions are compared to excisional hemorrhoidectomy to determine their efficacy.

B. Stapled Hemorrhoidopexy

A stapled hemorrhoidopexy is useful for patients with circumferential grade II-III hemorrhoids who fail in-office treatment. The technique involves placement of a purse-string suture 3-4 cm above the dentate line in the submucosal plane. The circular stapler's anvil is then placed proximal to the purse string suture and the suture is tied drawing the internal hemorrhoids into the circular stapler. The stapler is then closed and fired removing a circumferential strip of internal hemorrhoids. The staple line, 1-2 cm above the dentate line, is inspected and any bleeding oversewn. Thus, the procedure removes a strip of internal hemorrhoids and creates a hemorrhoidopexy at the staple line that reduces hemorrhoidal prolapse. The procedure does not address external hemorrhoids and thus would not be useful for patients with significant external hemorrhoidal disease. Because the procedure's incision (at the staple line) is above the dentate line, stapled hemorrhoidopexy is associated with less pain and discomfort than traditional excisional hemorrhoidectomy. The results of stapled hemorrhoidopexy have been good and are comparable to excisional hemorrhoidectomy. Complications from stapled hemorrhoidopexy are also comparable to excisional hemorrhoidectomy with the exception of including some unique complications such as rectovaginal fistula and rectal obstruction. Appropriate patient selection and meticulous surgical technique are required to achieve the best results with stapled hemorrhoidopexy. Thus, stapled hemorrhoidopexy is a good option for grade II-III internal hemorrhoids that are not associated with significant external hemorrhoids.

C. Doppler-Guided Hemorrhoidectomy

Doppler-guided hemorrhoidectomy involves the use of a specially designed anoscope with a doppler probe that allows for precise identification and ligation of the hemorrhoidal vessels. Six to eight hemorrhoidal vessels are identified and suture ligated using the doppler probe to identify the vessels and then confirm the interruption of blood flow after suture ligation. Early results have demonstrated that this technique is comparable to excisional hemorrhoidectomy for grade II-III internal hemorrhoids. The complication profile is also favorable. More experience with the doppler-guided hemor-

rhoidectomy is necessary in order to adequately evaluate the long-term effectiveness of the procedure.

▶ Prognosis

The successful treatment of external and internal hemorrhoids is related to changing the patient's bowel habits. Increasing dietary fiber, decreasing constipating foods, introducing exercise, and decreasing time spent on the toilet all decrease the amount of time spent straining in the squatting position. These behavioral modifications are the most important steps in preventing recurrence.

El Nakeeb AM, Fikry AA, Omar WH, et al: Rubber band ligation for 750 cases of symptomatic hemorrhoids out of 2200 cases. *World J Gastroenterol* 2008;14:6525-6530.

Giordano P, Overton J, Madeddu F, Zaman S, Gravante G: Transanal hemorrhoidal dearterialization: a systematic review. *Dis Colon Rectum* 2009;52:1665-1671.

Ratto C, Donisi L, Parello A, Litta F, Doglietto GB: Evaluation of transanal hemorrhoidal dearterialization as a minimally invasive therapeutic approach to hemorrhoids. *Dis Colon Rectum* 2010;53:803-811.

Rivadeneira DE, Steele SR, Ternent C, Chalasani S, Buie WD, Rafferty JL, Standards Practice Task Force of The American Society of Colon and Rectal Surgeons: Practice parameters for the management of hemorrhoids (revised 2010). *Dis Colon Rectum* 2011 Sep;54(9):1059-1064.

Sim HL, Tan KY, Poon PL, Chen A, Mak K: Life-threatening perineal sepsis after rubber band ligation of haemorrhoids. *Tech Coloproctol* 2009;13:161-164.

Wong JC, Chung CC, Yau KK, et al: Stapled technique for acute thrombosed hemorrhoids: a randomized, controlled trial with long-term results. *Dis Colon Rectum* 2008;51:397-403.

ANAL FISSURE

An anal fissure is a tear in the anoderm usually located in the posterior or anterior midline of the anal canal. An anal fissure may be associated with a sentinel tag located at the distal aspect of the anal fissure (anal verge) and/or a hypertrophied anal papilla at the proximal aspect of the fissure. The inciting event causing an anal fissure is thought to be trauma to the anal canal from a hard bowel movement or other cause. This trauma results in a tear that leads to pain and spasm of the internal anal sphincter muscle particularly during and after bowel movements. The spasm results in elevated anal resting pressures that can unfortunately lead to a vicious cycle of further spasm and pain. With elevated resting pressures, the blood flow to the posterior and anterior midline decreases inhibiting healing of the fissure. Fissures are usually classified as either acute with symptoms occurring just over the past month or chronic with symptoms present for greater than 2-3 months. Over 90% of fissures are located in the posterior midline with the rest located in the anterior midline. Given their etiology of spasm and elevated resting pressures resulting in decreased blood flow, chronic anal fissures can be considered "ischemic ulcers" of the anal canal.

Clinical Findings

Patients with an anal fissure complain of sharp pain with or immediately after bowel movements. They may also complain of rectal bleeding and a "hemorrhoid" or sentinel tag. Patients often describe moderate to severe pain like a "knife" or "razor blade" during defecation. Due to the pain, patients fear going to the bathroom that can result in delaying defecation, hardened stool, and additional pain. On inspection of the external anus, there may be a sentinel tag in either the posterior or anterior midline. To visualize the fissure, the examiner needs to evert the anus by pulling the right and left anal margin skin laterally. As the anus is everted, the examiner can carefully inspect the anoderm in the posterior and anterior midline for a tear in the anoderm. Patients with significant pain and spasm may not even tolerate this maneuver. In these patients it is helpful to gently expose the anus and ask the patient to strain to defecate to see if during straining self-eversion of the anus occurs. Due to pain, digital rectal examination, and anoscopy are not performed immediately, but reserved for when the symptoms resolve or the patient is in the operating room. Laboratory and imaging studies are not necessary but flexible endoscopy of some type should be scheduled if it has not been performed recently.

Differential Diagnosis

Classic anal fissures occur in either the posterior (90% +) or anterior (1%-10%) midline. Not all posterior and anterior anal canal tears are anal fissures. Anal canal ulcers can occur from Crohn disease, leukemia, HIV, cancer and infections such as herpes, syphilis, cytomegalovirus, and tuberculosis. These anal canal ulcers mimic anal fissures. A careful history can help identify possible etiologies of an anal ulcer. On the other hand, typical anal fissures are associated with increased sphincter tone so any patient with decreased sphincter tone should be suspected of having an anal canal ulcer rather than a fissure. Further, whenever a "fissure" is located laterally rather than in the posterior or anterior midline, an anal canal ulcer should be suspected. There should be a low threshold to suspect an anal ulcer rather than fissure. In these patients, an examination under anesthesia with biopsy of the ulcer is necessary to rule out an infectious or malignant etiology.

Complications

In addition to causing pain and bleeding, anal fissures can become infected and develop a fissure-fistula complex. This relatively unusual complication is easily treated with a posterior intersphincteric fistulotomy.

Medical Treatment

The pathogenesis of an anal fissure is pain and spasm resulting in increased internal anal sphincter (IAS) muscle pressures, decreased blood flow, and a nonhealing fissure in the anoderm of the anal canal. Treatment is directed at breaking this pain and spasm cycle to relax the internal sphincter muscle, increase blood flow, and allow the fissure to heal. To do this, patients should keep their stools soft with stool softeners and laxatives to avoid further anal canal trauma. In addition, warm baths are recommended to relax the sphincter muscle and allow the fissure to heal. Stool softeners, bulking agents, and sitz baths will heal 90% of anal fissures. Topical ointments can also be prescribed to decrease the anal sphincter pressure. Nitroglycerin ointment (0.2% or 0.4%) or calcium channel blocker ointment (0.2% diltiazem gel) can be used to chemically relax the IAS muscle. Side effects include headache which occurs more frequently after nitroglycerin ointment. Patients who fail this regimen and have a persistent fissure are candidates for surgery or treatment with botulinum toxin. Botulinium toxin injection into the anal sphincter can be successful but is costly and has a higher recurrence rate than surgery. Thus, medical treatment of anal fissures includes stool softeners, bulking agents, warm baths, topical nitroglycerin ointment or diltiazem gel, and possibly botulinum toxin injection. Most patients with acute anal fissures and over 50% of patients with chronic anal fissures are successfully treated without surgery. Patients who fail medical management of their anal fissure should undergo surgical intervention.

Surgical Treatment

Surgical treatment of an anal fissure involves performing a lateral internal sphincterotomy. While the fissure may be biopsied and a sentinel tag or hypertrophied anal papilla excised, the most important part of an operation for anal fissure is directed via a lateral incision at the IAS muscle. In the operating room, a lateral incision is made in the intersphincteric groove between the internal and EAS muscles and a submucosal and intersphincteric dissection is performed in order to clearly identify the IAS muscle. The IAS muscle is then cut the length of the fissure in order to permanently relax the anal canal. After sphincterotomy, relaxation of the anal canal is readily appreciated by the surgeon. This short, outpatient operation has over a 90% success rate and a recurrence rate of less than 10%. Patients often have less pain after surgery. Complications include bleeding, infection, and rarely fecal incontinence (< 0.5%).

Patients who have preexisting fecal leakage or lack increased anal sphincter muscle pressures are poor candidates for lateral internal sphincterotomy which could result in worsening bowel control. These relatively rare patients are better treated with an anal advancement flap that does not involve dividing any sphincter muscle. For a description of the anal advancement flap, see the section on anal stenosis.

Baraza W, Boereboom C, Shorthouse A, et al: The long-term efficacy of fissurectomy and botulinum toxin injection for chronic anal fissure in females. *Dis Colon Rectum* 2008;51:236-243.

Lindsey I: To cut or to daub? An algorithmic approach to anal fissure. *Colorectal Dis* 2012 Jun;14(6):657.

Mentes BB, Guner MK, Leventoglu S, et al: Fine-tuning of the extent of lateral internal sphincterotomy: spasm-controlled vs. up to the fissure apex. *Dis Colon Rectum* 2008;51:128-133.

Nelson RL, Thomas K, Morgan J, Jones A: Non-surgical therapy for anal fissure. *Cochrane Database Syst Rev* 2012 Feb 15;2:CD003431.

Pérez-Legaz J, Arroyo A, Moya P, et al: Perianal versus endoanal application of glyceryl trinitrate 0.4% ointment in the treatment of chronic anal fissure: results of a randomized controlled trial. Is this the solution to the headaches? *Dis Colon Rectum* 2012 Aug;55(8):893-899.

Perry WB, Dykes SL, Buie WD, Rafferty JF, Standards Practice Task Force of the American Society of Colon and Rectal Surgeons: Practice parameters for the management of anal fissures (3rd revision). *Dis Colon Rectum* 2010 Aug;53(8):1110-1115.

ANORECTAL ABSCESS & FISTULA

An anorectal abscess is one of the three common causes of anorectal pain and is the only cause that usually requires urgent surgical treatment. Most anorectal abscesses have a cryptoglandular etiology. When the anal glands in the crypts of the dentate line become blocked, an anorectal abscess can develop. Because these glands extend a variable depth, the developing abscess can track in various anatomic planes. Abscesses are classified by their anatomic location:—perianal, ischiorectal, intersphincteric, and supralevator (Figure 31–3). Fortunately, most abscesses are perianal or ischiorectal and can be relatively easily identified on physical examination. Intersphincteric and supralevator abscesses are unusual and often are only identified by MRI/CT or examination under anesthesia. Most abscesses are cryptoglandular in etiology but some patients develop abscesses related to another disease process such as Crohn, tuberculosis, and cancer. While many abscesses will heal with simple incision and drainage, some 30%-60% of abscesses will not heal and patients will complain of persistent drainage and recurrent inflammation related to an anal fistula. In these patients, the cryptoglandular source and external surgical drainage site remain connected allowing for passage of mucus and stool through this tract. The location of the abscess, thus, determines the location and tract of the resulting anal fistula. Anal fistulas are classified by their relationship with the anal sphincter muscle—intersphincteric, transsphincteric, suprasphincteric, and extrasphincteric. Due to the frequency of the abscesses that created them, intersphincteric and transsphincteric fistulas are the most common anal fistulas.

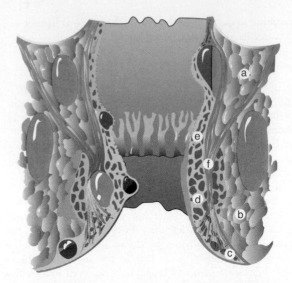

▲ **Figure 31–3.** Composite diagram of acute anorectal abscesses and spaces. (a) Pelvirectal (supralevator) space. (b) Ischiorectal space. (c) Perianal (subcutaneous) space. (d) Marginal (mucocutaneous) space. (e) Submucous space. (f) Intermuscular space.

Suprasphincteric and extrasphincteric fistulas are exceedingly rare. Due to their relationship with the anal sphincter muscle, treatment of anal fistulas should be evaluated and treated by highly specialized surgeons familiar with sphincter-saving techniques in order to avoid complications such as fecal incontinence. Since fistulas occur in 30%-60% of patients after anorectal abscess drainage, patients undergoing abscess drainage should be warned about the possibility of a fistula and should be given appropriate follow-up to insure healing and absence of a persistent fistula tract.

▶ Clinical Findings

Patients with an anorectal abscess complain of acute pain, swelling, and possibly a fever. An occasional patient may complain of leakage of mucus and pus related to the spontaneous drainage of the abscess. For patients with perianal and ischiorectal abscesses, physical examination often reveals erythema, fluctuance, and asymmetry between the right and left perirectal tissues. An occasional patient will present with a symmetric horseshoe abscess cavity circling half or more of the circumference and may have no left-right asymmetry. If a patient has an intersphincteric or supralevator anorectal abscess, there is often none of the above findings on physical examination. Thus, patients with a suspicion of an abscess but no obvious physical examination findings should either be imaged with MRI or taken to the operating room for an examination under anesthesia. Laboratory testing is usually not helpful in patients with an anorectal abscess although frequently these patients will have an elevated white blood cell count. Radiologic studies are also not necessary as the vast majority of anorectal abscesses are obvious on the basis of history and physical examination alone. Some patients with symptoms of an abscess and no physical examination findings may benefit from imaging studies as well as patients with recurrent or complex abscesses such as some patients with Crohn disease. Potential imaging studies include CT, MRI, and anorectal ultrasound. Anorectal ultrasound is not well tolerated in patients with an acute abscess and CT will miss some abscesses. Thus, if an imaging study is necessary, an MRI is the imaging test of choice being able to readily identify complex abscesses and their anatomic extensions.

Patients with an anorectal fistula complain of chronic drainage of mucus and blood, irritation, and usually have an antecedent history of an anorectal abscess. If a patient has persistent drainage 6-8 weeks after abscess drainage, then a fistula should be suspected, and evaluation and treatment for an anal fistula should be initiated. Some patients with anal fistulas will have a relatively remote or no history of an abscess. Physical examination reveals the external opening and often there is a palpable subcutaneous tract between the external opening and the anus. It is important to remember that any nonhealing wound or opening around the anus should be presumed to be a fistula until proven otherwise. Laboratory testing is not necessary in patients with anal fistulas but imaging studies may be useful for recurrent and complex anal fistulas. MRI is the imaging procedure of choice to identify anal fistula tracts, side tracts, and the relationship of the tracts to the anal sphincter muscle. Transanal ultrasonography can also be useful and can be performed intraoperatively using hydrogen peroxide enhancement to highlight the fistula tract.

Differential Diagnosis

The differential diagnosis for patients with anorectal abscess or fistula includes perianal hidradenitis, pilonidal disease, and rarely bartholin gland cyst. On physical examination, it may be difficult to differentiate an anorectal abscess/fistula from complex hidradenitis or pilonidal disease. Further, hidradenitis or pilonidal disease can occur concurrently with an anorectal abscess or fistula. Careful evaluation in the operating room is necessary to determine if an abscess is communicating only with the skin (hidradenitis), only with the midline gluteal cleft (pilonidal disease) or with the anus (fistula). Rare causes of anorectal abscesses and fistulas include tuberculosis, actinomycosis, cancer, and diverticulitis.

Complications

Abscesses can enlarge and spread along various anatomic planes around the anus. Abscesses can form a posteriorly based horseshoe around the anus usually just sparing the anterior perirectal space. Abscesses can also track around

just one side of the anus (1/2 horseshoe). While it may be unusual for a single abscess to destroy a significant amount of anorectal tissue and diminish anorectal function, multiple recurrent abscesses can result in destruction of anorectal anatomy and muscle function resulting in a deterioration of anorectal function.

In rare circumstances, an anorectal abscess can result in systemic sepsis. Treatment should include adequate drainage of the abscess, intravenous antibiotics, and supportive intensive care unit care.

Anorectal abscesses can recur after treatment. The reasons for recurrence include inadequate initial drainage (often because deep postanal space was not drained), the presence of a fistula, and Crohn disease. Nearly all patients with recurrent or complex abscesses should be evaluated for Crohn disease.

Anal fistulas should be treated when identified because although they may be minimally symptomatic they can develop into an acute anorectal abscess. Fistulas, too, may recur after treatment due to undiagnosed side tracts or Crohn disease. Crohn disease should be ruled out in all patients with complicated or recurrent anal fistulas.

▶ Treatment of Anorectal Abscesses

Anorectal abscesses are treated by incision and drainage. For the common perianal and ischiorectal abscesses, a cruciate incision is made over the area of fluctuance as close to the anal verge as possible to decrease the length of a fistula tract if one should develop. Frequently it is useful to excise the skin tips of the cruciate incision in order to allow for adequate drainage and insure that the abscess heals from the inside out as premature skin healing could result in a recurrent abscess. When draining an acute abscess, it is very unlikely to be able to identify an internal opening and the course of the fistula tract if one is present. Thus, when draining an abscess either in the office or the operating room, it is important to concentrate effort at insuring that the abscess is adequately drained and worry about a fistula later if it should develop. For the relative rare intersphincteric abscess, transanal drainage is performed. In the operating room, the intersphinteric abscess is palpated within the anal canal and via an anoscope a longitudinal incision is made to drain the abscess internally into the rectum. Supralevator abscesses can also be treated in this way. Alternatively, supralevator abscesses can be drained in the interventional radiology suite using CT-guidance but this may result in an extrasphincteric fistula if the etiology of the abscess is cryptoglandular.

After surgical drainage, only immunocompromised patients or patients with associated sepsis are treated with antibiotics. For large abscesses, placement of a penrose or mushroom-catheter drain may be necessary to insure adequate drainage. After draining a horseshoe abscess posteriorly, it is useful to make counter incisions at the anterior extent of the abscess on both sides of the anus and put looped penrose or vessel-loop drains from the posterior opening to the anterior opening. These drains are left for at least 2-3 weeks and will allow for better drainage of the entire abscess cavity. Finally, follow-up of patients after abscess drainage is important to insure that the abscess completely heals and does not evolve into a persistently draining fistula tract.

▶ Treatment of Anorectal Fistula

Traditionally, anorectal fistulas have been treated by fistulotomy. Fistulotomy is performed one of three ways. The simplest fistulotomy is a single-stage procedure laying open the fistula tract. A two-stage approach is used for fistulas that involve a significant amount of sphincter muscle. The two-stage approach uses a seton which is a suture or vessel loop drain that is tied to itself after placement in the fistula tract. With the two-stage approach, the first step is a partial fistulotomy and seton placement. After healing from this first step, the second step is a completion fistulotomy. A final method of fistulotomy involves placement of a cutting seton and then gradual division of the fistula tract and involved sphincter muscle by tightening of the cutting seton over time. While fistulotomy may still be utilized for subcutaneous, intersphincteric, and low transphincter fistulas (all have little or no muscle involvement), fistulotomy has fallen into disfavor because division of the sphincter muscle during fistulotomy as well as contour deformities associated with fistulotomy can result in fecal incontinence and leakage. Thus, while fistulotomy is a highly successful way to treat subcutaneous and intersphincteric fistulas that involve minimal to no anal sphincter muscle, transsphincteric fistulas are better treated with a sphincter-sparing approach to avoid the complication of fecal incontinence.

Sphincter-sparing treatment approaches for transphincteric anal fistulas include fibrin glue, anal fistula plug, the ligation of the intersphincteric fistula tract (LIFT) procedure, and the rectal advancement flap. Prior to any of these sphincter-sparing procedures, a vessel loop draining seton is placed into the fistula tract, and the tract is allowed to heal around the seton for 3 months. While this seton placement procedure step can be omitted, studies have shown that the success rate of the subsequent definitive sphincter-sparing procedure is higher after seton placement. For the fibrin glue procedure, the seton is removed, the internal opening suture closed and then fibrin glue is instilled via the external opening to seal the tract. The anal fistula plug procedure is done in a similar fashion just using the plug rather than the glue. No incisions are made with either of these procedures which tend to be very well-tolerated by patients. Unfortunately, the success rate is only 60%-70% for fibrin glue and probably even lower for the anal fistula plug. Thus, a number

of patients (30%-40%) will fail glue or plug at which time further treatment by repeating the glue or plug or by opting for the more invasive LIFT procedure or rectal advancement flap. The main complications for glue/plug are recurrence and abscess (rare).

The relatively new procedure is called LIFT because it involves ligation of the intersphincteric fistula tract. During this outpatient operation after removal of the seton (if placed previously), an interphincteric groove incision is made and the fistula tract in the intersphincteric space is identified and circumferentially dissected free. This dissection allows for proximal and distal suture ligation and division of the fistula tract within the intersphincteric space. This procedure is well-tolerated, spares the sphincter muscle, and is successful 80% of the time. Complications include recurrence of a simpler intersphincteric fistula and rarely abscess formation.

If the previously mentioned sphincter-sparing techniques are unsuccessful in healing an anal fistula, an anorectal advancement flap can be performed. For patients, this is a significantly more involved operation than the above options as it involves much larger incisions, longer operative time, and longer healing time. In the operating room, patients are placed prone for an anterior internal opening or placed in lithotomy position for a posterior internal opening. A U-shaped flap of mucosa, submucosa, and some underlying sphincter muscle is dissected proximally with the base of the "U" just distal to the internal opening. Once the flap is completely mobilized, the internal opening in the underlying sphincter muscle is closed with one or two figure of eight sutures. The tip of the flap is then excised and the flap is advanced distally to cover the suture closure of the internal opening in the sphincter muscle. The flap is then sutured into place providing a double layer closure of the internal opening. The external opening is enlarged and left open for drainage. Patients undergoing anorectal advancement flap are typically observed overnight to control pain and monitor for anorectal bleeding. If the flap remains in place and heals, the internal opening will be closed, and the rest of the fistula tract will heal. The success rate for the rectal advancement flap procedure is 85%-95% with the higher success rates associated with preoperative seton drainage.

▶ Prognosis

With the exception of Crohn patients who can develop recurring anal abscesses and fistulas, the prognosis with anorectal abscesses and fistulas is excellent. The new sphincter-sparing techniques for anal fistulas do require multiple operations, but that is a small price to pay in order to minimize the occurrence of fecal incontinence which can be over 50% in patients after traditional fistulotomy.

Bleier JL, Moloo H, Goldberg SM: Ligation of the intersphincteric fistula tract: an effective new technique for complex fistulas. *Dis Colon Rectum* 2010;53:43-46.

Christoforidis D, Etzioni DA, Goldberg SM, Madoff RD, Mellgren A: Treatment of complex anal fistulas with the collagen fistula plug. *Dis Colon Rectum* 2008;51:1482-1487.

Guidi L, Ratto C, Semeraro S, et al: Combined therapy with inflix-imab and seton drainage for perianal fistulizing Crohn's disease with anal endosonographic monitoring: a single-centre experi-ence. *Tech Coloproctol* 2008;12:1111 1117.

Malik AI, Nelson RL, Tou S: Incision and drainage of perianal abscess with or without treatment of anal fistula. *Cochrane Database Syst Rev* 2010 Jul 7.

O'Riordan JM, Datta I, Johnston C, Baxter NN: A systematic review of the anal fistula plug for patients with Crohn's and non-Crohn's related fistula-in-ano. *Dis Colon Rectum* 2012 Mar;55(3):351-358.

Siddiqui MR, Ashrafian H, Tozer P, et al: A diagnostic accuracy meta-analysis of endoanal ultrasound and MRI for perianal fistula assessment. *Dis Colon Rectum* 2012 May;55(5):576-585.

Steele SR, Kumar R, Feingold DL, Rafferty JL, Buie WD, Standards Practice Task Force of the American Society of Colon and Rectal Surgeons: Practice parameters for the management of perianal abscess and fistula-in-ano. *Dis Colon Rectum* 2011 Dec;54(12):1465-1474.

Subhas G, Singh Bhullar J, Al-Omari A, Unawane A, Mittal VK, Pearlman R: Setons in the treatment of anal fistula: review of variations in materials and techniques. *Dig Surg* 2012 Aug 31;29(4):292-300.

CONDYLOMATA ACUMINATA

Condylomata acuminata are caused by the human papil-lomavirus (HPV) and are transmitted primarily by sexual contact. In the United States, condylomata acuminatum is the most common sexually transmitted viral disease. It is the most common anorectal infection of men who have sex with men (MSM) and is particularly prevalent in HIV-positive patients. The disease is not limited to men or women who practice anoreceptive intercourse. In women, the virus may track down from the vagina, and in men, it may track from the base of the scrotum. A recent study found that 16% of asymptomatic heterosexual men tested positive for anal HPV. In addition to causing anal warts, HPV infection is the primary cause of anal dysplasia and anal squamous cell cancer. While HPV strains HPV-6 and HPV-11 cause benign warts, HPV-16 and HPV-18 are the two HPV strains with the highest risk of anal cancer. Despite the high preva-lence of HPV infection, most HPV-infected individuals will not develop cancer due to the response of the immune system against the virus. Immunocompromised individuals such as patients with HIV or transplant recipients have an increased HPV-related cancer risk. Recently a vaccine has been developed that prevents cancer, precancer, and most types of warts.

Clinical Findings

Patients with condylomata acuminata present with wart-like growth around the anus and in the anal canal. The presence of warts is associated with discomfort, irritation, and pos-sibly some occasional rectal bleeding. Due to HPV's high prevalence in MSM and its risk of causing cancer, primary care physicians, infectious disease clinics, and HIV clinics often screen for HPV with anal pap smears. Patients with positive anal pap smears are referred for further evalua-tion. The appearance of condylomata acuminata and HPV disease can be quite variable. Wart-like growths are typical but flat patches of warty growth can also be seen. Other HPV changes cannot be seen without the assistance of high-resolution anoscopy (HRA). HRA involves applying acetic acid to the anal canal and using a colposcope to look for HPV-related changes in the anoderm and rectal mucosa. Laboratory and radiographic studies are rarely utilized in the evaluation of patients with condylomata acuminata. Thus, evaluation of patients with HPV-related condylomata acu-minata requires careful external examination, anoscopy, and possibly HRA to determine the extent of disease.

Differential Diagnosis

Because of the variable appearance of condyloma acuminata, hemorrhoids, skin tags, and fibroepithelial polyps among many other anal skin conditions can mimic condylomata acuminata. Due to the large differential diagnosis for peri-anal and anal canal skin changes, it is important that a biopsy is taken of all anal canal lesions in order to make an accurate diagnosis.

Prevention

A quadrivalent HPV vaccine against HPV-6, -11, -16, and -18 has been recently developed and has been shown to pre-vent cancer, precancer, and most types of warts. The vaccine is best given prior to any sexual activity but also has efficacy after the initiation of sexual activity. In uninfected individu-als, the efficacy of the vaccine against the development anal dysplasia and anal cancer was 75% whereas in patients with known HPV infections the efficacy was 50%.

Treatment

Condylomata acuminata are treated in the office or the operating room. Significant external disease or any internal anal canal disease is probably best treated in the operating room. Isolated external disease can be safely treated in the office. Condylomata acuminata are treated using a variety of excisional and destructive methods. In the office, anal warts can be excised after injecting local anesthesia or destroyed with bichloroacetic acid, podophyllin, liquid nitrogen, infra-red coagulation, or electrocautery. In the operating room, excision and destruction using electrocautery is commonly used. All excised specimens are sent for pathologic analysis. If highly suspicious lesions are excised during an operation, their location should be specified in the case that the pathology is unfavorable, and re-excision is required. Unless a patient has a significant burden of disease, all lesions are either excised or destroyed in the operating room. Some surgeons will use HRA in the office and operating room in order to identify and treat all HPV-related changes. After surgery pain medication and stool softeners are prescribed, and patients are given appropriate follow-up.

▶ Complications and Prognosis

While some bleeding, pain, and rarely infection may occur after excision of condylomata, the most common complication is recurrence. Patients should be informed prior to surgery that the recurrence rate is high (30%-80%) but that often small areas of recurrence can be treated in the office. Patients should also understand that close follow-up is necessary for early detection of recurrence. This close follow-up is important in order to avoid reoperation and the development of malignancy.

A relatively rare variant of condylomata acuminatum is the locally aggressive but benign giant condylomata acuminatum known as a Buschke–Lowenstein tumor. Treatment is radical excision for palliation or cure. In some patients, surgery has been combined with adjuvant chemotherapy and radiation therapy with success.

After excision of condylomata acuminatum patients should be informed of their pathology results. If an area of squamous cell cancer has been excised on the anal margin, re-excision of this area may need to be performed if the margins were positive. If squamous cell cancer has been identified in the anal canal or from an unknown location around the anus, then the patient should be treated with chemoradiation (Nigro protocol). On the other hand, pathologic analysis may not reveal cancer but rather anal intraepithelial neoplasia (AIN). Anal intraepithelial neoplasia is graded from I (most benign) to III (most ominous and closest to cancer). Many surgeons would return to the operating room to reevaluate and excise areas of AIN-III if there is any question about the completeness of excision at the initial operation. In HIV-positive patients, some grade of AIN is a very common finding. Most surgeons would follow patients with higher grades of AIN at more frequent intervals.

The prognosis of patients with condylomata acuminata is excellent as despite the presence of anal warts and HPV, anal cancer is still quite rare. Further, the prognosis of anal cancer is excellent if located on the anal margin and completely excised. Prognosis of anal canal squamous cell cancer is also good as treatment with chemoradiation is very successful for most localized anal canal squamous cell cancers. Salvage

abdominoperineal resection for recurrence of squamous cell cancer after chemoradiation is unusual.

Centers for Disease Control and Prevention (CDC): Recommendations on the use of quadrivalent human papillomavirus vaccine in males—Advisory Committee on Immunization Practices (ACIP), 2011. *MMWR Morb Mortal Wkly Rep* 2011 Dec 23;60(50):1705-1708.

Giuliano AR, Palefsky JM, Goldstone S, et al: Efficacy of quadrivalent HPV vaccine against HPV Infection and disease in males. *N Engl J Med* 2011 Feb 3;364(5):401-411. Erratum in: *N Engl J Med* 2011 Apr 14;364(15):1481.

Goldstone SE, Moshier E: Detection of oncogenic human papillomavirus impacts anal screening guidelines in men who have sex with men. *Dis Colon Rectum* 2010 Aug;53(8):1135-1142.

Marks DK, Goldstone SE: Electrocautery ablation of high-grade anal squamous intraepithelial lesions in HIV-negative and HIV-positive men who have sex with men. *J Acquir Immune Defic Syndr* 2012 Mar 1;59(3):259-265.

Salit IE, Lytwyn A, Raboud J, et al: The role of cytology (Pap tests) and human papillomavirus testing in anal cancer screening. *AIDS* 2010 Jun 1;24(9):1307-1313.

Swedish KA, Lee EQ, Goldstone SE: The changing picture of high-grade anal intraepithelial neoplasia in men who have sex with men: the effects of 10 years of experience performing high-resolution anoscopy. *Dis Colon Rectum* 2011 Aug;54(8):1003-1007.

Weis SE, Vecino I, Pogoda JM, et al: Prevalence of anal intraepithelial neoplasia defined by anal cytology screening and high-resolution anoscopy in a primary care population of HIV-infected men and women. *Dis Colon Rectum* 2011 Apr;54(4):433-441.

PILONIDAL DISEASE

Pilonidal disease is a chronic gland infection in the depths of the gluteal cleft. While the glands and resulting pits can occur anywhere along the gluteal cleft, they occur most often in the superior gluteal cleft over the sacrum. The pathogenesis of pilonidal disease is thought to be a process in which the follicles in the midline gluteal cleft get blocked, infected, and then drain leaving open midline pits. In the depths of the gluteal cleft these pits have a vacuum effect on loose hair and hair is literally sucked into these pits. During surgery, tufts of hair can be found in the pits and chronic abscess cavity. Thus, while the hair does not cause pilonidal disease, the presence of hair in the pits and glands acts as a foreign body and causes the infection and drainage to persist. Pilonidal disease usually occurs in men (3:1 male to female ratio) between the ages of 15 and 40 with the peak incidence between 16 and 20 years. Although pilonidal disease is typically chronic with recurrent drainage and inflammation, it often regresses with time and is rare after 40 years of age. The pathogenesis and natural history of pilonidal disease is important to remember when recommending treatment. Given its natural history that involves disease regression with time, conservative treatment, and minimal surgery is recommended for most patients.

Clinical Findings

Patients with pilonidal disease present in three main ways—acute abscess, chronic draining pits or complex, recurrent disease after previous surgery. Patients with an acute pilonidal abscess will have pain and possibly swelling in or along the gluteal cleft. Given the relatively fixed nature of the tissues in this region and how deep a typical pilonidal abscess is located, swelling and cellulitis are often absent, and physical examination often underestimates the size of the abscess. Patients with chronically draining midline pits will have one or more pits in the midline with drainage and recurrent inflammation. Often hair will be seen protruding from the pits. Patients with complex disease after previous surgery such as pilonidal cystectomy will have chronic, nonhealing wounds in the midline of the gluteal cleft. History and physical examination are sufficient to make the diagnosis of pilonidal disease regardless of the type of presentation. Laboratory and imaging studies play no role in the evaluation of patients with pilonidal disease.

Differential Diagnosis

Pilonidal disease occurs in the superior gluteal cleft and is usually relatively easy to diagnose. Pilonidal disease occurring inferior in the gluteal cleft and close to the anus may be difficult to distinguish from an anal fistula. An examination under anesthesia may be required in order to differentiate pilonidal pit and cyst from an anal fistula. Further, pilonidal disease off the midline may mimic hidradenitis. Usually, hidradenitis will occur elsewhere and will not be just limited to the gluteal cleft like pilonidal disease.

Treatment

Patients with an acute abscess related to pilonidal disease should undergo incision and drainage of their abscess. Antibiotics are not necessary unless the patient has significant infection, sepsis, or is immunocompromised. The abscess is nearly always located deep to the midline gluteal cleft. Because incisions in the midline heal poorly, an acute abscess should be drained through a lateral incision at least 2 cm off midline. A generous lateral incision allows for adequate drainage of pus and hair from the pilonidal cyst. Shaving a wide area around the gluteal cleft is important to help prevent further accumulation of hair in the cyst. After abscess drainage, patient should be followed to insure healing, but further operative intervention is usually not necessary.

Patients with chronically draining pilonidal pits should be treated conservatively. The whole gluteal cleft and surrounding gluteal skin should be shaved, and all hair in the pits removed. Patients are instructed to bend over in the shower and allow the water to blast the gluteal cleft to help prevent accumulation of hair in the pits. Patients should undergo repeat shaving and hair removed from the pits every week or 2 until resolution of symptoms. If symptoms recur, conservative treatment with shaving and removal of pit hair should be resumed. Patients with persistent drainage and inflammation despite 2-3 months of conservative treatment are candidates for surgery. Traditionally, surgical treatment of pilonidal disease involved pilonidal cystectomy which meant complete removal of the midline chronic abscess cavity. This procedure is associated with wound breakdown and possible development of a nonhealing midline wound that may in fact be more debilitating than the disease prior to surgery. Given this possibility, midline incisions are absolutely avoided. Rather, a minimally invasive operation entitled lateral incision and pit closure is performed. After a lateral incision is made, the abscess cavity in the midline is accessed via this lateral incision to remove all pus, hair, and granulation tissue. Next, the pits in the midline are excised and the minimal 2-3 mm wounds closed with nylon suture. The lateral incision is left open for drainage. If the excised midline pit wounds heal, the pilonidal disease is eliminated, and the lateral incision will heal readily over 2-4 weeks.

Patients with complex, recurrent pilonidal disease with large, nonhealing midline wounds need complex flap surgery to resolve their symptoms. Many types of flaps have been used to close these wounds and all flaps involving incisions in the midline or that cross the midline are plagued by poor healing in the midline. Due to poor midline healing, the Bascom cleft closure flap procedure that not only avoids the midline but eliminates the gluteal cleft is a very good option for these patients. In this procedure, the open wound is excised and the excision is extended laterally off the midline on one side leaving an asymmetric wound. The skin and subcutaneous tissues of the gluteal cleft and cheek of the opposite side are then mobilized and advanced across the midline to the side with the lateral excision. This flap accomplishes two important goals—the flap closure incision is off the midline facilitating healing (and there is no midline portion of the incision) and the gluteal cleft is eliminated as the cleft is mobilized and advanced to the opposite side. Without a gluteal cleft, further pilonidal disease is unheard of.

Complications & Prognosis

Patients with pilonidal disease are young, active adults, and often desire a quick fix for their symptoms. It is important to counsel patients regarding the natural history of the disease. Patients need to understand the chronic nature of the disease but also that it naturally regresses with time. With understanding, patients will more readily participate in conservative treatment and understand the goals of minimally invasive surgery such as lateral incision and pit closure. Overall, the prognosis of patients with pilonidal disease is excellent.

Al-Khamis A, McCallum I, King PM, Bruce J: Healing by primary versus secondary intention after surgical treatment for pilonidal sinus. *Cochrane Database Syst Rev* 2010 Jan;20.

Humphries AE, Duncan JE: Evaluation and management of pilonidal disease. *Surg Clin North Am* 2010 Feb;90(1):113-124.

Loganathan A, Arsalani Zadeh R, Hartley J: Pilonidal disease: time to reevaluate a common pain in the rear! *Dis Colon Rectum* 2012 Apr;55(4):491-493.

Maghsoudi H, Nezami N, Ghamari AA: Ambulatory treatment of chronic pilonidal sinuses with lateral incision and primary suture. *Can J Surg* 2011 Apr;54(2):78-82.

Nordon IM, Senapati A, Cripps NP: A prospective randomized controlled trial of simple Bascom's technique versus Bascom's cleft closure for the treatment of chronic pilonidal disease. *Am J Surg* 2009 Feb;197(2):189-192. [Epub 2008 Jul 17.]

Thompson MR, Senapati A, Kitchen P: Simple day-case surgery for pilonidal sinus disease. *Br J Surg* 2011 Feb;98(2):198-209.

ANAL STENOSIS

Anal stenosis is a relatively unusual condition that is most commonly associated with either previous surgery, malignancy, or Crohn disease. Patients often are successful at self-treating their stenosis by keeping their stools soft with stool softeners and laxatives. Complete anal canal obstruction is rare. Identification of the etiology of the anal stenosis is key to successful treatment.

▶ Clinical Findings

Patients with anal stenosis complain of difficult evacuation and possibly rectal bleeding. The history is important to determine the etiology of their symptoms. The most common cause of anal stenois is previous anorectal surgery particularly hemorrhoid surgery. Since stenosis often occurs years to decades after hemorrhoid surgery, patients should be specifically questioned regarding prior anorectal surgery. Patients with anal stenosis related to Crohn disease usually have a relatively long history of anorectal Crohn disease. This may include treatment of abscesses, fistulas, and anal canal ulcers. Patients with malignancy may have a history of anal condyloma but often will have no antecedent history. Physical examination reveals a narrowed anal canal. Digital examination is still possible in patients with a mild anal stenosis. Moderate to severe anal canal stenosis does not allow digital examination. Due to the severity of stenosis, it may be difficult to determine if the stenosis is due to a mass or tumor. Laboratory and imaging studies play no role in the evaluation of patients with anal stenosis. Flexible endoscopy is important in all patients with anal stenosis. In those patients with moderate to severe stenosis, flexible endoscopic evaluation may be impossible prior to treatment and is done after the stenosis is corrected.

▶ Treatment

Mild anal stenosis can be treated with stool softeners and laxatives with good results. Patients with persistent symptoms despite treatment and those patients with moderate to severe stenosis require endoscopic or surgical intervention. Because malignancy is always a possibility even after hemorrhoid surgery or in patients with Crohn disease, a biopsy of the anal canal stenosis is mandatory. Of course any patient diagnosed with malignancy needs treatment specific for the malignancy which usually involves chemoradiation (anal cancer) and possibly surgery (if rectal cancer). For patients without malignancy, the choice of a surgical procedure is dictated by the etiology of the anal stenosis.

Patients with Crohn disease can undergo endoscopic balloon dilatation of their anal stricture or operative anal stricturoplasty. During anal stricturoplasty, longitudinal incisions are made through the stricture at one to three locations around the anal canal. Recurrent stricture can be treated with repeat balloon dilatation or operative anal stricturoplasty.

Patients with postsurgical anal stenosis have a deficiency of anoderm related to their previous operation and subsequent scarring. Due to their deficiency of anoderm, these patients are not appropriate candidates for stricturoplasty but rather are better served with a local advancement flap into the anal canal to correct their anoderm deficiency. Many local advancement flaps have been described and used successfully such as the V-Y, Y-V, and the anal houseflap. During the anal houseflap operation the patient is placed in the prone position and the anal canal is visualized. Standard operative anoscopes will not fit into the anal canal of patients with moderate to severe stenosis and thus use of a nasal speculum is necessary. With the anal canal visualized, the anoderm is divided longitudinally for the length of the strictured anal canal. Transverse incisions are then made at the proximal and distal aspects of this incision converting the incision wound into a rectangular defect. A house-shaped flap of anal margin skin and subcutaneous tissue is developed and advanced into the anal canal. The flap is then sutured into place, and the donor site closed. In some cases, two or three separate houseflaps around the anus are necessary to adequately correct the anal stenosis. Thus, the advancement of anal margin skin into the anal canal corrects the deficiency of anoderm and relieves the anal stenosis.

The results following anal advancement flap treatment of anal canal stenosis are very good. Potential complications include bleeding, infection, flap necrosis, and flap retraction. If an advancement flap fails it can be repeated in another quadrant around the anus.

Brisinda G, Vanella S, Cadeddu F, et al: Surgical treatment of anal stenosis. *World J Gastroenterol* 2009 Apr 28;15(16):1921-1928.

Farid M, Youssef M, El Nakeeb A, Fikry A, El Awady S, Morshed M: Comparative study of the house advancement flap, rhomboid flap, and y-v anoplasty in treatment of anal stenosis: a prospective randomized study. *Dis Colon Rectum* 2010 May;53(5):790-797.

Katdare MV, Ricciardi R: Anal stenosis. *Surg Clin North Am* 2010 Feb;90(1):137-145.

PRURITUS ANI

Pruritus ani is a challenging dermatologic disorder characterized by intense itching of the perianal skin. Diagnosis of this problem is typically not straightforward and, subsequently, patients are seen by a variety of specialists including, gastroenterologists, dermatologists, and colorectal surgeons. The incidence of pruritus ani ranges from 1% to 5% in adults and typically has a male predominance (ratio 4:1).

Pruritus ani is broadly classified either as primary (idiopathic) or secondary. Up to 90% of cases are considered idiopathic while the remaining secondary cases are caused by a variety of local and systemic conditions.

▶ Clinical Findings

Patients typically present with complaints of an unpleasant perianal burning, which usually starts insidiously. As the condition becomes more chronic, this burning is replaced by varying degrees of itching that can become intolerable. Careful history uncovers that symptoms are often more pronounced at night.

Physical findings on examination can be varied. In the early stages the skin may appear normal; however, as the patient continues to scratch, the local inflammation worsens, resulting in erythematous, excoriated, and macerated skin. In the chronic stage, the skin is often lichenified with coarse ridges and ulcerations.

▶ Differential Diagnosis

Identifying the primary etiology of pruritus ani can be very challenging; therefore, a careful history and physical examination is required. Information on diet, medications, synchronous skin conditions, common anorectal disorders, bowel function and stool consistency, as well as prior anorectal procedures should be ascertained. A thorough examination of the perianal skin and anoscopy are essential. Skin scrapings, cultures, and biopsy of suspicious lesions are important adjuncts to elucidate the underlying etiology. The routine use of endoscopy and radiologic studies is unnecessary unless there is a high index of suspicion for a colorectal cause. Some of the established causes of secondary pruritus ani are summarized in Table 31–5.

▶ Treatment

The goal of treatment should be directed toward establishing clean and dry perianal skin that is free of ulcerations. If pruritus is found to be secondary to one of the aforementioned causes then treatment should be directed towards that specific pathology. The management of idiopathic pruritus is more challenging, often requiring intensive patient education and behavior modification. A high-fiber diet should be encouraged while eliminating foods that may precipitate pruritus. If symptoms improve, then these foods

Table 31–5. Common causes of secondary pruritus ani.

Diet	Dermatologic Conditions
Coffee, tea, caffeinated beverages, alcohol, chocolate, spicy foods, tomatoes (ketchup), dairy products	Psoriasis, contact dermatitis, lichen sclerosus/planus
Local Irritants	**Local Malignancies**
Topical medications, soaps, detergents, fabric	Bowen disease, Paget disease, squamous cell cancer
Anorectal Diseases	**Perianal Infections**
Hemorrhoids, fistula, rectal prolapse, fecal incontinence/soiling, skin tags	Bacterial (*Staphylococcus* or *Streptococcus*), fungal, viral (eg, herpes simplex, HPV), parasitic
Systemic Diseases	**Psychological**
Diabetes mellitus, liver disease, thyroid disorder, renal disease, leukemia	Anxiety, depression, stress

may be slowly reintroduced in order to identify the offending product.

Meticulous perianal hygiene should be stressed as the first step in management. Patients should discontinue use of all topical medications and should clean the perineum only with water, avoiding soaps and other potential irritants. In cases of more severe skin excoriation, skin barrier creams may provide symptomatic relief. A brief trial of topical steroids (hydrocortisone 0.5%-1%) is also often a useful adjunct but should not be used for prolonged periods as it results in thinning of the perianal skin. Topical hydrocortisone 1% has been shown in a double-blinded, randomized, placebo-controlled to reduce daily visual analog score (VAS) for severity of itch by 68% and weekly Dermatology Life Quality Index (DLQI) scores by 75%.

In patients with refractory symptoms, topical capsaicin can be considered. A randomized, placebo-controlled, trial comparing topical capsaicin (0.006%) with placebo (1% menthol) in patients with chronic pruritus ani found that of 44 patients, 31 (70%) had relief of their symptoms. Intradermal injection of methylene blue (1%) has also been described with limited success. Skin necrosis from inappropriate infiltration has been described.

▶ Prognosis

The successful identification and treatment of secondary causes of pruritus ani often yields good results. However, relapses can be common with idiopathic pruritus. Every attempt should be made to continue to reinforce patient education.

Asgeirsson T, Nunoo R, Luchtefeld MA: Hidradenitis suppurativa and pruritus ani. *Clin Colon Rectal Surg* 2011;24 (1):71-80.

Gooding SM, Canter PH, Coelho HF, Boddy K, Ernst E: Systematic review of topical capsaicin in the treatment of pruritus. *Int J Dermatol* 2010;49 (8):858-865.

Lacy BE, Weiser K: Common anorectal disorders: diagnosis and treatment. *Curr Gastroenterol Rep* 2009;11 (5):413-419.

Markell KW, Billingham RP: Pruritus ani: etiology and management. *Surg Clin North Am* 2010;90 (1):125-135.

Samalavicius NE, Poskus T, Gupta RK, Lunevicius R: Long-term results of single intradermal 1% methylene blue injection for intractable idiopathic pruritus ani: a prospective study. *Tech Coloproctol* 2012;16 (4):295-299.

Schubert MC: What every gastroenterologist needs to know about common anorectal disorders. *WJG* 2009;15 (26):3201.

Siddiqi S, Vijay V, Ward M, Mahendran R, Warren S: Pruritus ani. *Ann R Coll Surg Engl* 2008;90(6):457-463.

Sutherland AD, Faragher IG, Frizelle FA: Intradermal injection of methylene blue for the treatment of refractory pruritus ani. *Colorectal Dis* 2009;11(3):282-287.

PROCTITIS & ANUSITIS

Proctitis and anusitis are general terms referring to inflammation within the anal canal or rectum secondary to infectious pathogens or inflammatory causes. Sexually transmitted diseases are an increasingly common cause of proctitis with an incidence exceeding 15 million new cases annually in the United States. The differential diagnosis can be quite broad with a variety of bacteria and viruses; therefore, a systematic approach is important. The diagnosis and management of these conditions depends primarily on the underlying etiology.

1. Herpes proctitis—The Herpes Simplex Virus (HSV) is a DNA virus that is the most prevalent STD in the United States. The majority of anogenital infections are caused by the HSV-2 serotype, accounting for approximately 80%-90% of infections. Anorectal infections typically result from auto-inoculation or direct contact with infected partners. The virus travels along peripheral nerves and has a variable incubation period (days to weeks). Prodromal symptoms may consist of burning, irritation, fever, and myalgia. This typically escalates to more intense, painful proctitis, and tenesmus. The characteristic lesions are small vesicles with surrounding erythema, which eventually coalesce and rupture forming painful ulcerations. Additionally, patients may develop tender inguinal adenopathy.

Evaluation of the rectum with a proctoscope will demonstrate erythematous and friable mucosa with ulcerations and mucopurulent discharge. Tzank smear of the discharge reveals the characteristic multinucleated giants cells with intranuclear inclusion bodies. Viral cultures of the discharge from these vesicles are also highly positive in acute infections.

HSV infections are usually self-limited in the absence of superimposed bacterial infections; therefore, initial treatments, such as sitz baths and oral analgesics are aimed at controlling symptoms. There is no cure for active infections but Acyclovir, Valacyclovir, and Famciclovir will shorten the duration of symptoms and may be used for suppressive therapy in patients with frequent recurrences.

2. Anorectal syphilis—Syphilis is caused by the spirochete, *Treponema pallidum,* which typically has an incubation period of 2-6 weeks. This disease was once on the verge of elimination but the incidence has been increasing steadily, especially young black men.

Acute anorectal infection is characterized by a small papule (chancre) on the anal margin or within the anal canal, which eventually ulcerates and may be mistaken for a routine anal fissure. This eventually regresses spontaneously in 3-4 weeks and is followed by a secondary stage 2-10 weeks later. Secondary syphilis may consist of fever, malaise, arthralgia, a maculopapular rash on the palms and soles of the feet, tenesmus, mucoid discharge, rectal pain, and inguinal adenopathy.

There are several methods for diagnosis. Dark-field microscopy will reveal the spirochetes, which have a corkscrew-shaped appearance. Biopsy shows spirochetes on a Warthin–Starry silver stain. There are also two serologic tests, RPR and VDRL.

Treatment consists of a single dose of penicillin intramuscularly in the early phase. If identified later, three doses are given 2 weeks apart.

3. Gonococcal proctitis—Gonococcal proctitis is caused by the organism, *Neisseria gonorrhoeae,* which is an intracellular gram-negative diplococcus. It is estimated that there are approximately 3 million people infected yearly worldwide; however, there is a large population of asymptomatic carriers. Anorectal infection results from contiguous spread from the genital area in women and from receptive anal intercourse in men.

The incubation period varies but can last up to 2 weeks. Symptoms then include pruritus, tenesmus and a thick, purulent discharge, which can be expressed from the anal crypts. Proctitis of the mid to distal rectum can be identified on proctoscopy. Standard Gram stains of the discharge are generally unreliable; however, culture on Thayer–Martin medium increases the positive yield.

The first-line treatment of anorectal gonorrhea includes a single intramuscular dose of ceftriaxone. Penicillin is no longer recommended given the high rate of resistance. Infected patients and partners should also be treated for concomitant Chlamydia infection, which is very common.

4. Chlamydial proctitis and lymphogranuloma venereum—*Chlamydia trachomatis* is the most common sexually transmitted infection worldwide and the most frequently reported

STD in the United States. This intracellular bacteria has several serotypes that have an incubation period up to 2 weeks. Serotypes D-K are responsible for proctitis and genital infections while serotypes L1-L3 are responsible for lymphogranuloma venereum (LGV).

A large portion of patients will be asymptomatic; however, when present, symptoms of an active anorectal infection include rectal pain, tenesmus, and fever. Similar anorectal complaints are present in patients with LGV but the inguinal adenopathy is often more prominent with large matted nodes with overlying erythema.

Diagnosis of active infections can be challenging with routine culture given the intracellular location of the bacteria. Often patients with suggestive symptoms of proctitis that have a Gram stain demonstrating leukocytes without detectable gonococci are presumed to have a Chlamydia infection and treated accordingly. Cell culture is also possible using a sucrose phosphate media. Treatment consists of a single oral dose of Azithromycin or Doxycycline twice daily for 7 days. Treatment with Doxycycline is extended to 21 days for LGV. Sexual partners should be treated as well to prevent reinfection.

5. Condyloma acuminata—*Condyloma acuminata*, caused by the human papilloma virus, have a recognizable raised, cauliflower-like appearance and are located on the anal margin, within the anal canal, or surrounding the genitalia. This presents one of the most common STDs in the United States for which consultation with a colorectal surgeon is sought. There are more than 60 subtypes of this latent virus with types 6 and 11 producing benign exophytic lesions. Types 16 and 18 are noted to be more aggressive, often causing lesions with high-grade dysplasia that may progress to cancer if left untreated.

Patients are often asymptomatic but may present with complaints of bleeding, itching, or anal discomfort due to the growths. Once present, there is no way to eradicate the infection surgically. The goal of treatment is to remove the macroscopic burden of disease with excisional biopsies and electrocautery. Recurrences are common; therefore, surveillance of these patients is extremely important. Bichloracetic acid, trichloracetic acid, and Imiquimod are topical agents that have been used with reasonable success.

6. Chancroid—Chancroid is a rare sexually transmitted disease in the United States caused by the gram-negative bacteria, *Haemophilus ducreyi*. Globally, the incidence is higher in developing countries.

The infection manifests itself days after transmission with painful inguinal adenopathy and erythematous papules around the genitalia that eventually ulcerate. Diagnosis is typically made with routine culture of the fluid from the ulcers. Treatment consists of single doses of Azithromycin (orally) or Ceftriaxone (intramuscularly).

7. Inflammatory proctitis—Inflammatory proctitis refers to a general mild to moderate inflammation of the rectum that is unrelated to an underlying infection or sexually transmitted disease. Symptoms include rectal bleeding, urgency, tenesmus, and often diarrhea. Examination of the rectum is characterized by a continuous erythematous, friable mucosal surface. If applicable, cultures should be taken to elucidate any infectious etiology and biopsies should be taken to rule out Crohn disease.

This condition can be self-limited but persistent cases typically respond to short courses of steroid enemas. Additionally, mesalamine enemas are efficacious. If there is no improvement after a few weeks of treatment, the patient should be reevaluated.

8. Radiation proctitis—Radiation proctitis is an unfortunate byproduct of pelvic irradiation that typically occurs in two phases. Acute injury occurs during or shortly after the administration of pelvic radiation. This is characterized by vascular congestion and friable mucosa. Symptoms include rectal bleeding, urgency, tenesmus, and diarrhea. The late phase of injury occurs months to years after the completion of treatment and is characterized histologically by fibrosis that can manifest clinically with strictures, fistulas to the urinary tract or vagina, and telangiectasias. Symptoms include bleeding, change in bowel habits, recurrent urinary tract infections, and vaginal discharge. Evaluation should include flexible sigmoidoscopy or colonoscopy and biopsy to make the diagnosis and rule out malignancy.

The initial treatment of acute radiation proctitis incorporates medications that manage symptoms, including bulking agents, antidiarrheals, and antispasmodics. Enemas of steroids, mesalamine, or short-chain fatty acids have been shown to improve proctitis as well. Refractory cases can be treated topical application of 4% formalin to the rectal mucosa. Radiation proctitis complicated by fistulas is best managed surgically with interposition of normal, healthy tissues.

Bennett MH, Feldmeier J, Hampson N, Smee R, Milross C: Hyperbaric oxygen therapy for late radiation tissue injury. *Cochrane Database Syst Rev* 2012;5:CD005005.

Felt-Bersma RJ, Bartelsman JF: Haemorrhoids, rectal prolapse, anal fissure, peri-anal fistulae and sexually transmitted diseases. *Best Pract Res Clin Gastroenterol* 2009;23(4):575-592.

Fleshner PR, Chalasani S, Chang GJ, Levien DH, Hyman NH, Buie WD: Practice parameters for anal squamous neoplasms. *Dis Colon Rectum* 2008;51(1):2-9.

Lee PK, Wilkins KB: Condyloma and other infections including human immunodeficiency virus. *Surg Clin North Am* 2010;90 (1):99-112.

Mansour M, Weston LA: Perianal infections: a primer for nonsurgeons. *Curr Gastroenterol Rep* 2010;12(4):270-279.

Workowski KA, Berman SM: Centers for Disease Control and Prevention Sexually Transmitted Disease Treatment Guidelines. *Clin Infect Dis* 2011;53(Suppl 3):S59-S63.

RECTOVAGINAL FISTULA

Rectovaginal fistulas can be congenital or acquired and are generally characterized by their abnormal connection between the epithelialized mucosal surfaces of the rectum and the vagina. Distal fistulas arising from the anal canal are appropriately termed, anovaginal fistulas. Acquired rectovaginal fistulas are generally caused by obstetric injuries, inflammatory bowel disease, trauma, or infection.

▶ Clinical Findings

A. Symptoms and Signs

The diagnosis of a rectovaginal fistula is typically straightforward based on an accurate history; however, in some instances, patients can be asymptomatic. Commonly, patients will present with complaints of the passage of air or feces from the vagina. The degree of distress often depends of the size of the fistulous opening. With smaller fistulas, more subtle complaints of a foul vaginal discharge, recurrent vaginitis, or dyspareunia may be more common while the feculent drainage from larger fistulas may be confused with fecal incontinence. If the etiology of the fistula is due to inflammatory bowel disease then rectal complaints such as tenesmus or bloody diarrhea may predominate.

On digital rectal examination, the fistula can often be identified as a dimpling or pit in the anterior rectal mucosa, which can be easily be confirmed by anoscopy. Inspection of the vagina will reveal staining of the mucosa with stool and the hyperemic mucosa of the fistula opening contrasting with the normal pink background of the vaginal mucosa. Occasionally, the identification of the fistula can be more challenging despite very suggestive symptoms. In these instances, a thorough examination under anesthesia may be indicated. With a saline-filled vagina, air can be instilled per rectum via a proctoscope. Air bubbles may help identify fistulas that are not readily apparent. Alternatively, diluted methylene blue can be instilled per rectum with a tampon in place in the vagina. Staining of the tampon with methylene blue will confirm the presence of a fistula.

B. Laboratory Studies and Imaging

Adjunct studies are sometimes necessary to identify the fistula location and to determine the quality of the surrounding tissue. Retrograde contrast enemas and CT scans with rectal contrast may identify contrast extravasation into the vagina. CT scans have the added benefit of identifying any associated inflammatory changes. MRI and endorectal ultrasound have also been used with varying results. Endoscopy is a valuable diagnostic tool to assess any underlying inflammatory conditions such as Crohn disease and to exclude underlying malignancy. Biopsies should be performed on any abnormal mucosa in the rectum or around the fistula orifice.

▶ Differential Diagnosis

The most common cause of rectovaginal fistulas is obstetrical trauma accounting for 70%-80% of cases. These fistulas may present immediately but more frequently they manifest weeks after delivery, typically after third- and fourth-degree lacerations. In the Western hemisphere, the incidence has been estimated at up to 0.1% of all vaginal deliveries. Other etiologies include—inflammatory bowel disease—primarily Crohn disease, postoperative trauma, radiation, malignancy, and infection.

▶ Treatment

The management of rectovaginal fistulas primarily depends on its complexity, as determined by the location, etiology, and the quality of the surrounding tissue. Simple fistulas are typically small in diameter, low on the rectovaginal septum, and are secondary to either traumatic injury or infection. On the other hand, complex fistulas are larger in diameter, higher on the rectovaginal septum, and are associated with underlying inflammatory bowel disease, radiation, neoplasm, or previous failed repairs. There are several well-described operative approaches that can generally be divided into transanal, transvaginal, transperineal, and transabdominal repairs.

Common transanal repairs include fistula excision with layered closure, endorectal advancement flap, and rectal sleeve advancement. The mucosal advancement flap is appropriate for simple, low fistulas. During this procedure, a flap composed of mucosa, submucosa, and a portion of internal sphincter muscle is mobilized proximally and used to cover the fistula defect. The base of the flap should be wider than the apex in order to ensure adequate perfusion of the flap. The muscle is then reapproximated in the midline—closing the fistula. The flap is then advanced into the anal canal and secured with absorbable sutures. Success rate are varied in literature, ranging from 50% to 100%.

Rectal sleeve advancement is a reasonable approach for rectovaginal fistulas with extensive stenosis and anal ulcerations due to Crohn disease. Starting at the dentate line, a circumferential incision is made and extended cephalad. The dissection becomes full thickness above the anorectal ring and is extended until the distal rectum is adequately mobilized. The rectum is then pulled down through the anal canal and the diseased rectum is transected. The fistula opening in the vaginal is closed and the rectum is sutured to the dentate line. This repair is often done with a protective diverting ostomy.

Perineoproctectomy is a perineal technique that essentially converts a RVF into a fourth-degree laceration. The vaginal mucosa, sphincter muscles, and the rectum are divided between the fistula openings and reapproximated in layers, ultimately obliterating the fistula tract.

Tissue interpositions are also typically performed through the perineal approach and include the gracilis muscle flap and the Martius (bulbocavernosus muscle) flap. The fundamental concept in these procedures is that normal, healthy tissue is placed between the fistula openings after dissecting the plane between the rectum and the vagina. Successful closure with these procedures has been reported as high as 80% and is an ideal repair for RVF that have failed previous repairs or with abnormal surrounding tissues.

Rectovaginal fistulas that are higher in the rectovaginal septum are usually approached through an abdominal approach. There are several potential procedures, ranging from simple fistula division and closure with interposition of pedicled omentum, to proctectomy with colorectal or coloanal anastomosis. The choice of procedure depends on the quality of surrounding tissues, location, and the etiology of the fistula.

Finally, the last decade has seen increasing use of bioprosthetic plugs and sheets in the management of RVFs. Small series have shown promising results but there is still a paucity of long-term data.

Prognosis

The prognosis for rectovaginal fistulas relates to its overall complexity. Simple, low fistulas can be approached with relatively straightforward transanal or perineal techniques with good results. Fistulas that are higher or associated with inflammatory bowel disease, radiation, or neoplasm are understandably more challenging, often requiring multiple repairs.

Champagne BJ, McGee MF: Rectovaginal fistula. *Surg Clin North Am* 2010;90(1):69-82.

Debeche-Adams TH, Bohl JL: Rectovaginal fistulas. *Clin Colon Rectal Surg* 2010;23(2):99-103.

Ellis CN: Outcomes after repair of rectovaginal fistulas using bioprosthetics. *Dis Colon Rectum* 2008;51(7):1084-1088.

Gosselink MP, Oom DM, Zimmerman DD, Schouten RW: Martius flap: an adjunct for repair of complex, low rectovaginal fistula. *Am J Surg* 2009;197(6):833-834.

Hannaway CD, Hull TL: Current considerations in the management of rectovaginal fistula from Crohn's disease. *Colorectal Dis* 2008;10(8):747-55; discussion 755-756.

Schwandner O, Fuerst A, Kunstreich K, Scherer R: Innovative technique for the closure of rectovaginal fistula using Surgisis mesh. *Tech Coloproctol* 2009;13(2):135-140.

Zhu YF, Tao GQ, Zhou N, Xiang C: Current treatment of rectovaginal fistula in Crohn's disease. *World J Gastroenterol* 2011;17(8):963-967.

Zimmermann MS, Hoffmann M, Hildebrand P, et al: Surgical repair of rectovaginal fistulas—a challenge. *Int J Colorectal Dis* 2011;26(6):817-819.

ANAL & PERIANAL NEOPLASMS

General Considerations

Neoplasms of the anus and surrounding skin are uncommon—accounting for only about 3% of all colorectal malignancies. Approximately 5200 cases are diagnosed annually in the United States, resulting in more than 700 deaths. The overall management of these lesions depends primarily on the histology, the size, and location of the lesion. While the definitions can be confusing, the anal canal is commonly defined, by surgeons, as the region extending from the anal verge to the anorectal ring at the top of the sphincter complex. The lymphatic drainage in this area is variable but clinically important. Proximal to the dentate line, the lymphatic system drains to the internal iliac and inferior mesenteric nodes while distal to the dentate line, drainage is typically to the inguinal nodes. It is important to realize that lesions in this area may not be completely visualized on routine inspection of the perineum. The anal margin is generally defined as the perianal skin extending circumferentially within 5 cm of the anal verge. Lesions in this area are easily visible on examination.

Tumors of the Anal Margin

A. Squamous Cell Carcinoma

The majority of malignant neoplasms of the anal margin are squamous cell cancers (SCC). They have similar presentation to SCCs that occur elsewhere on the skin and are subsequently staged similarly based on size, which has been shown to correlate with lymph node positivity. The American Joint Committee on Cancer (AJCC) staging system is summarized in Table 31–6. The overall incidence of anal margin cancers is low and the prognosis is often more favorable than squamous cell carcinoma of the anal canal. These lesions are typically well differentiated, indolent, and are rarely associated with distant metastasis.

Lesions in this location may present with pain, bleeding, pruritus, tenesmus, or incontinence if locally advanced. On examination, there are rolled, everted edges often with central ulceration. Palpable lymph nodes may be identified in the inguinal region.

The management of anal margin SCC consists of wide local excision for T1 and early T2 lesions that can be easily resected with a 1-cm margin without compromising sphincter function. Poorly differentiated tumors, T3, or T4 cancers should be treated with chemoradiation, including the inguinal and pelvic nodes in the field of treatment. Abdominoperineal resection (APR) should be reserved for recurrent disease, residual disease after radiation, or bulky tumors that are invading the sphincter complex.

B. Basal Cell Carcinoma

Basal cell cancers (BCC) of the anal margin are exceedingly rare, accounting for 0.2% of anorectal cancers. They typically present in older men and approximately one-third of patients will have a history of BCC or a synchronous lesion

Table 31–6. American joint committee on cancer (AJCC) TNM staging of squamous cell cancer.

	Anal Margin	Anal Canal
Tumor (T)		
Tis	Carcinoma *in situ*	Carcinoma *in situ*
T1	Tumor ≤ 2 cm in greatest dimension	Tumor ≤ 2 cm in greatest dimension
T2	Tumor 2-5 cm in greatest dimension	Tumor 2-5 cm in greatest dimension
T3	Tumor > 5 cm in greatest dimension	Tumor > 5 cm in greatest dimension
T4	Tumor invades deep structures	Tumor invades deep structures (not including the sphincters)
Nodal Status (N)		
N0	No regional lymph node metastasis	No regional lymph node metastasis
N1	Regional lymph node metastasis present	Perirectal lymph node metastasis present
N2		Unilateral internal iliac or inguinal lymph node metastasis present
N3		N1 and N2 and/or bilateral internal iliac or inguinal lymph node metastasis present
Distant Metastasis (M)		
M0	No distant metastasis	No distant metastasis
M1	Distant metastasis present	Distant metastasis present

elsewhere. The appearance of these lesions is similar to that of other areas of the body with irregular, raised, pearly edges with superficial plaques or ulcers. Local I invasion and metastatic potential are both typically low.

Wide local excision with an adequate margin is the treatment of choice for small lesions. Local recurrence is fairly uncommon and can usually be re-excised. Larger, bulky lesions can be treated with abdominoperineal resection or radiation.

C. Bowen Disease

Historically, the term Bowen disease referred to squamous cell carcinoma *in situ*. This term as well as anal intraepithelial neoplasia (AIN) II and III have largely been replaced by the classification of high-grade squamous intraepithelial lesion (HSIL), which has similar histologic features. Human papilloma virus infection is common. Patients may complain of itching or pain and examination reveals scaly, erythematous, and sometimes pigmented lesions.

Traditionally, these lesions have been treated wide local excision, often with complex reconstructions for larger lesions. This approach has been plagued by high recurrence rates and generally very morbid. More recent data suggest that HSIL can be adequately treated with targeted biopsy with high-resolution anoscopy, ablation, and close surveillance every 3-6 months. The application of topical Imiquimod (Aldara) or topical 5-FU have been proposed to minimize recurrence, but are generally limited by local skin irritation.

D. Verrucous Carcinoma

Perianal verrucous carcinoma is often referred to as a Buschke-Lowenstein tumor or Giant Condyloma, given its exophytic, cauliflower-like appearance. These lesions can vary in size but are generally slow growing and locally invasive. Histologically, they are considered benign but larger lesions may certainly encompass underlying malignancy—usually invasive squamous cell carcinoma. Patients frequently present with complaints of an anal mass but may also describe pain, fistulas, or abscesses. Wide local excision is recommended for the majority of these lesions and, if large, the resulting defects may require more complex closure with plastic surgeons. More advanced cases with invasion into the sphincter complex may require APR.

E. Paget Disease

Paget disease is a rare condition characterized by an intraepithelial adenocarcinoma of the perianal skin. The most common presenting complaint is intolerable pruritus and examination typically reveals a well-demarcated, erythematous, eczematous rash. Diagnosis is made after a full-thickness biopsy, which shows the pathognomonic Paget cell with a pale vacuolated cytoplasm and peripheral nucleus. These lesions often are associated with synchronous gastrointestinal malignancies, so a complete evaluation of the intestinal tract should be performed.

In the absence of invasive disease, wide local excision is the treatment of choice. It is important to obtain intraoperative frozen sections to ensure negative margins. Large defects can be covered with skin grafts or adjacent tissue transfers. Patients with invasive disease have a poor prognosis and should be considered for radical resection with abdominoperineal resection. Inguinal lymphadenectomy should be added for clinically positive nodal involvement. The role of chemoradiation is not well defined but has been used as an adjunct in invasive and recurrent disease.

Edge SBB, Byrd DR, Compton CC, Fritz AG, Greene FL, Trotti A, ed. AJCC Cancer Staging Manual. Springer, New York, 2010.

Fleshner PR, Chalasani S, Chang GJ, Levien DH, Hyman NH, Buie WD: Practice parameters for anal squamous neoplasms. Dis Colon Rectum 2008;51(1):2-9.

Garrett K, Kalady MF: Anal neoplasms. Surg Clin North Am 2010;90(1):147-161.

Jiang Y, Ajani JA: Anal margin cancer: current situation and ongoing trials. Curr Opin Oncol 2012;24(4):448-453.

Kyriazanos ID, Stamos NP, Miliadis L, Noussis G, Stoidis CN: Extra-mammary Paget's disease of the perianal region: a review of the literature emphasizing the operative management technique. Surg Oncol 2011;20(2):e61-e71.

Minicozzi A, Borzellino G, Momo R, Steccanella F, Pitoni F, de Manzoni G: Perianal Paget's disease: presentation of six cases and literature review. Int J Colorectal Dis 2010;25(1):1-7.

TUMORS OF THE ANAL CANAL

1. Epidermoid Carcinoma

▶ Clinical Findings

Tumors of the anal canal are rare, accounting for about 2% of all colorectal malignancies. Of these, epidermoid carcinomas are the most common. The term epidermoid carcinoma encompasses several histological subtypes including squamous cell, basaloid, mucoepidermoid, and transitional cancers.

The clinical manifestation of anal canal tumors can be quite variable and many patients are initially diagnosed with benign anorectal conditions. They are typically slow growing and the resulting mass commonly causes pain and bleeding. Digital rectal examination and anoscopy are important tools for an accurate diagnosis, during which the size, location, consistency, and degree of fixation should be noted. Additionally, the presence of any palpable inguinal adenopathy should be documented. A biopsy of the lesion confirms the diagnosis and provides the specific subtype. The staging of anal tumors is summarized in Table 31–6. Endoanal ultrasound, MRI, and PET/CT are important adjuncts that aid in defining that degree of distant spread, local invasion, and surrounding adenopathy.

▶ Treatment

Since its introduction in 1974, radiation and chemotherapy with 5FU and mitomycin C (Nigro Protocol) have largely replaced surgery in the treatment of anal cancer. There is ample data that demonstrates equivalent local control, survival rates with preservation of sphincter function. Approximately 30% of patients have persistent or recurrent disease after chemoradiation for anal SCC. Salvage abdominoperineal resection is reserved for recurrent or residual pelvic disease after chemoradiation.

The management of inguinal node disease is variable. Due to the high morbidity rate, prophylactic groin dissection is not recommended. Clinically significant inguinal adenopathy can be included in the field of radiation.

The overall response to chemoradiation should be assessed clinically at about 8 weeks after the completion of treatment. At this point, up to 85% of patients will have complete clinical response. Those with good partial response may be observed closely to ensure that complete response does occur. Any lesions suspicious for residual disease or progression of disease should be biopsied at that time. For those patients with complete clinical response, surveillance entails DRE and examination of inguinal nodes every 3-6 months for the first 2 years and annually thereafter up to 5 years. There is no consensus on the routine use of imaging in surveillance, but it is often practiced.

▶ Prognosis

Complete response rates approach 90% for smaller tumors with 5-year survival that ranges between 70% and 90%. Residual or recurrent disease confers a poorer prognosis with 5-year survival rates between 24% and 58% after salvage APR.

2. Melanoma of the Anal Canal

The anorectum is the third most common site overall for melanoma, but it is the most common site of primary melanoma of the gastrointestinal tract—making it an exceedingly rare condition. It accounts for up to 2% of all melanomas and 2%-4% of all anorectal tumors.

▶ Clinical Findings

Pain, bleeding, and a palpable mass are the most consistent clinical findings with melanoma of the anal canal. Patients may also present with tenesmus, change in the caliber of stools, and weight loss. Like its cutaneous counterpart, anal melanoma are raised and pigmented; however, it is important to note that these lesions may be amelanotic, which may mimic more benign disease.

▶ Treatment

For localized disease, surgery offers the only chance for cure, as there has been no proven benefit for chemotherapy or radiation. Both radical resection with APR and wide local excision have been advocated. Abdominoperineal resection does not confer a survival advantage and is associated with high morbidity rates, subsequently, wide local excision is recommended as the initial surgical approach for localized disease. Large, bulky tumors that involve the sphincter complex will require radical resection.

▶ Prognosis

The prognosis for anorectal melanoma is universally poor because many patients present with advanced disease.

Survival rates generally range from 6% to 28% in the literature. The overall 5-year survival for large, deeply invading, or metastatic disease is less than 10% with a median survival of 12-18 months.

Fleshner PR, Chalasani S, Chang GJ, Levien DH, Hyman NH, Buie WD: Practice parameters for anal squamous neoplasms. Dis Colon Rectum 2008;51(1):2-9.

Glynne-Jones R, Northover J, Oliveira J: Anal cancer: ESMO clinical recommendations for diagnosis, treatment and follow-up. Ann Oncol 2009;20(Suppl 4):57-60.

Heeney A, Mulsow J, Hyland JM: Treatment and outcomes of anorectal melanoma. Surgeon 2011;9(1):27-32.

Meguerditchian AN, Meterissian SH, Dunn KB: Anorectal melanoma: diagnosis and treatment. Dis Colon Rectum 2011;54(5):638-644.

Meyer J, Willett C, Czito B: Current and emerging treatment strategies for anal cancer. Curr Oncol Rep 2010;12(3):168-174.

NORMAL FUNCTION OF THE ANORECTUM

Anorectal physiology is very complex. It requires coordination between the pelvic nerves, pelvic floor muscles, the rectum, and the sphincter complex that results in normal, controlled evacuation of intestinal waste.

Like the colon, the rectum is comprised of two layers of smooth muscle—an inner circular layer and an outer longitudinal layer. It varies in length between 12 and 18 cm and is predominantly confined within the bony pelvis. The peritoneum covers the upper two-thirds of the rectum anteriorly, the upper third laterally, and the lower third of the rectum is extraperitoneal. The rectum is very distensible and, as such, has the capacity to hold large volumes, which is ideal since it primarily functions as a reservoir for stool prior to defecation. Alterations in rectal sensation or compliance by infection, inflammation, or fibrosis will result in urgency.

The anal canal begins at the anal verge, extending cephalad to the anorectal ring, and is surrounded by the levator ani muscles as well as the internal and external sphincter complex. The internal anal sphincter (IAS) muscle, which accounts for approximately 85% of the resting anal pressure, is an involuntary muscle that is the downward continuation of the circular, smooth muscle of the rectum. The IAS is approximately 3 cm in length and supplied by both sympathetic and parasympathetic nerves (S2-4). It is a constant state of contraction due to intrinsic slow-wave impulses. The IAS muscle is surrounded by the striated muscles of the external anal sphincter (EAS), which is a voluntary muscle but also contributes in small part to the overall resting tone. The EAS is supplied by the pudendal nerves.

The pelvic floor (levator ani muscles) is composed of symmetrical sheets of striated muscles with a central ligamentous attachment—the pubococcygeus, the iliococcygeus, and the puborectalis. These muscles surround and support the rectum, vagina, and urethra as they pass through to the perineum. The puborectalis, which wraps around the anorectal junction posteriorly and inserts on the pubic ramus anteriorly, is particularly important to overall continence by increasing the acute angle between the rectum and anal canal, known as the anorectal angle.

Normal defecation is an intricate sequence of events that relies on proper relaxation of these muscles and a few key anorectal reflexes. The stimulus for initiating defecation is distention of the rectum, which stimulates pressure receptors in the pelvic floor muscles, also known as accommodation. This in turn triggers two key reflexes: (1) relaxation of the internal sphincter, the rectoanal inhibitory reflex (RAIR) and (2) contraction of the external sphincter, the rectoanal excitatory reflex. This process allows sampling of the rectal contents that come into contact with the upper anal canal. This allows us to discriminate between gas, liquid, or solid stools. Once the decision has been made to evacuate the rectum, the puborectalis muscle relaxes, allowing straightening of the anorectal angle. Intra-abdominal pressure increases and the EAS relaxes allowing passage of contents through the anus.

In conjunction with a careful history, there are several useful modalities that are employed to investigate evacuation dysfunction. Anal manometry, defecography, endorectal ultrasound, and pudendal nerve terminal motor latency testing can be integral in the diagnosis of fecal incontinence, pelvic dyssynergia, constipation, rectocele, and intussusception, to name a few. A thorough understanding of the anatomy and the available testing modalities is imperative for diagnosis and treatment.

Bajwa A, Emmanuel A: The physiology of continence and evacuation. Best Pract Res Clin Gastroenterol 2009;23(4):477-485.

Barleben A, Mills S: Anorectal anatomy and physiology. Surg Clin North Am 2010;90(1):1-15.

Cho HM: Anorectal physiology: test and clinical application. J Korean Soc Coloproctol 2010;26(5):311-315.

Raizada V, Mittal RK: Pelvic floor anatomy and applied physiology. Gastroenterol Clin North Am 2008;37(3):493-509, vii.

Stoker J: Anorectal and pelvic floor anatomy. Best Pract Res Clin Gastroenterol 2009;23(4):463-475.

FECAL INCONTINENCE

▶ General Considerations

Complete anal continence results from the complex interactions between stool consistency, rectal capacity and compliance, the sphincter complex, and underlying neurological function. Impairment in one or all of these components results in varying degrees of fecal incontinence, which is generally defined as the recurrent, involuntary loss feces or gas through the anus.

The true incidence of fecal incontinence is difficult to determine due to lack of standard definitions and underreporting; however, rates up to 20% have been reported in literature, depending on the study population. Female patients predominate in most series of major incontinence but men and women are affected equally with minor incontinence. Higher rates have been reported in the elderly and patients with certain neurologic disorders.

There are numerous causes of fecal incontinence; however, the most common is related to obstetric injury. The incidence of obstetric tears with vaginal deliveries has been reported in up to 10% of cases. Additionally, occult injuries have identified by ultrasound in up to 35% of cases; therefore presentation with symptoms of incontinence or leakage may be delayed. Other causes include—congenital anomalies, neurologic disorder (eg, spinal cord injury), pelvic floor denervation (stretch-induced injury of the pudendal nerves), conditions causing poor rectal compliance (eg, Crohn disease, ulcerative colitis, radiation proctitis), functional bowel disorders (diarrhea or fecal impaction with overflow incontinence), and iatrogenic injuries (eg, anorectal surgeries).

▶ Clinical Findings

A. Symptoms and Signs

A detailed history of the presenting symptoms is required to differentiate the patient's ability to control gas, liquid and solid stools. Frank incontinence must be differentiated from fecal urgency or soiling which may be associated with other treatable anorectal disorders. Information on diet, activity, medications, obstetric and anorectal surgical history should also be gathered to provide more complete picture. This is understandably and potentially devastating disorder, so attempts should also be made to ascertain the overall level of impact of these symptoms on the patient's daily activities. To aid in this characterization, there are several validated scoring systems, including the Fecal Incontinence Severity Index score, the Cleveland Clinic Florida Incontinence score, and the Fecal Incontinence Quality of Life score, which can provide an objective baseline of these symptoms and can be used to track progress throughout treatment.

Physical evaluation should begin with inspection of the anus and perineum, to document any scars from previous obstetric or anorectal procedures. Benign anorectal conditions, such as fistulas, prolapse, and hemorrhoids may also be readily excluded. Perineal descent during straining is another important finding which indicates an abnormal laxity of the pelvic floor muscles. Finally, digital rectal examination provides useful initial information on the resting sphincter tone and maximum squeeze pressure.

B. Imaging Studies

Further testing for fecal incontinence often require an integrated approach. Anal manometry, endoanal ultrasound, MRI, defecography, and pudendal nerve latency studies have all been employed in the evaluation of the patient with fecal incontinence.

Anal manometry provides an objective assessment of resting sphincter pressure, maximum squeeze pressure, inherent anorectal reflexes, as well as anorectal sensation and compliance. Resting pressure is in large part a reflection of internal sphincter muscle function while maximum squeeze pressure reflects external sphincter function.

While it may be limited by the operator, endoanal ultrasound is an extremely useful tool in the evaluation of these patients. It is an inexpensive office-based procedure that allows visualization of the length and width of the sphincter complex as well as any defects that may be present.

Defecography has a more limited role in the evaluation of incontinence. The study allows visualization of the process of defecation, including the anorectal angle, pelvic floor descent, and internal intussusception.

Pudendal nerve motor latency testing provides information about potential nerve damage to the pelvic floor. It measures the time from nerve stimulation to the onset of response of the pelvic floor muscles. Prolonged times are indicative neuropathy. The degree of denervation does not influence the severity of incontinence but does seem to provide some prognostic information about the outcomes of surgical repairs.

▶ Treatment

The initial management of patients with fecal incontinence should include nonoperative measures. These include diet modification, fiber supplementation, and biofeedback training. If these measures fail, then consideration should be given to surgical repair. Options include sphincteroplasty, sacral nerve stimulation, injectable bulking agents, artificial bowel sphincter, and fecal diversion.

Anterior sphincteroplasty involves direct repair, either in an overlapping or end-to-end fashion, of the external sphincter muscle if a segmental defect is identified on preoperative evaluation. This technique has good short-term with up to 80% of patients experiencing improvement in function; however, at 5-10 years of follow up, function does tend to deteriorate. In literature, diminished success rates have been associated with age, duration of symptoms, and pudendal neuropathy.

Sacral nerve stimulation has recently been approved for the treatment of fecal incontinence and has been shown to be safe and effective. It provides the unique advantage of a temporary evaluation phase before permanent implantation. A temporary electrode is placed with the aid of fluoroscopy into the sacral foramen (usually the third) and the patient is subsequently stimulated for 2-3 weeks. If there is at least a 50% reduction in symptoms then a permanent stimulator is implanted. The precise mechanism of action of SNS is still unknown, but the short-term results have been promising. In many series more than 75% of study participants report greater than 50% improvement in continence episodes and 41%-75% of patients reported complete continence to liquid and solid stool. A recent randomized trial demonstrated that SNS was significantly better than best supportive measures including pelvic floor exercises, bulking agent, and dietary manipulation. Data with long-term follow up is still evolving.

The artificial bowel sphincter is another modality that is approved for treatment of incontinence but is not widely used. The device, which is surgically placed around the sphincter complex, is connected to a tunneled reservoir and pump that inflates and deflates the cuff to allow controlled defecation. This procedure has been limited by infectious complications and device erosion; therefore, is typically reserved for end-stage incontinence in patients without other alternatives except colostomy.

Passive fecal incontinence caused by internal sphincter dysfunction has been shown to respond favorably to injection of bulking agents. Small series have reported the injection of silicone biomaterial into the intersphincteric plane or submucosa with short-term improvement in continence.

If conservative and other surgical options have failed then a diverting colostomy becomes a reasonable solution that can restore a patient's quality of life.

Prognosis

Fecal incontinence is a treatable condition; however, appropriate management requires careful evaluation and proper patient selection. Surgical intervention should be preceded by an initial trial of conservative measures if indicated. Sphincteroplasty has good short-term results with initial success rates of approximately 75%; however, success diminishes over time. Sacral nerve stimulation has been an exciting new surgical development for fecal incontinence with greater than 80% of patients maintaining more than 50% reduction of symptoms after 1-2 years of permanent implantation. Complications requiring explantation of the device are uncommon.

Brown SR, Wadhawan H, Nelson RL: Surgery for faecal incontinence in adults. Cochrane Database Syst Rev 2013 Jul 2;7:CD001757.

Farrell SA: Overlapping compared with end-to-end repair of third and fourth degree obstetric anal sphincter tears. Curr Opin Obstet Gynecol 2011;23(5):386-390.

Glasgow SC, Lowry AC: Long-term outcomes of anal sphincter repair for fecal incontinence: a systematic review. Dis Colon Rectum 2012;55(4):482-490.

Halland M, Talley NJ: Fecal incontinence: mechanisms and management. Curr Opin Gastroenterol 2012;28(1):57-62.

Hannaway CD, Hull TL: Fecal incontinence. Obstet Gynecol Clin North Am 2008;35(2):249-69, viii.

Leung FW, Rao SS: Fecal incontinence in the elderly. Gastroenterol Clin North Am 2009;38(3):503-511.

Luo C, Samaranayake CB, Plank LD, Bissett IP: Systematic review on the efficacy and safety of injectable bulking agents for passive faecal incontinence. Colorectal Dis 2010;12(4):296-303.

Maeda Y, Laurberg S, Norton C: Perianal injectable bulking agents as treatment for faecal incontinence in adults. Cochrane Database Syst Rev 2013 Feb 28;2:CD007959.

Mathis KL, Cima RR, Pemberton JH: New developments in colorectal surgery. Curr Opin Gastroenterol 2011;27(1):48-53.

Mellgren A: Fecal incontinence. Surg Clin North Am 2010;90(1):185-194.

Mowatt G, Glazener C, Jarrett M: Sacral nerve stimulation for fecal incontinence and constipation in adults: a short version Cochrane review. Neurourol Urodyn 2008;27(3):155-161.

Norton C, Cody JD: Biofeedback and/or sphincter exercises for the treatment of faecal incontinence in adults. Cochrane Database Syst Rev 2012;7:CD002111.

Tjandra JJ, Chan MK, Yeh CH, Murray-Green C: Sacral nerve stimulation is more effective than optimal medical therapy for severe fecal incontinence: a randomized, controlled study. Dis Colon Rectum 2008;51(5):494-502.

PELVIC FLOOR DYSFUNCTION

General Considerations

Pelvic floor dysfunction is a global term that can encapsulate several presentations including dysfunctional urinary and bowel evacuation symptoms, sexual dysfunction, as well as pain syndromes. Alternative terms, such as pelvic dyssynergia, obstructed defecation, and paradoxic puborectalis, have also been used further confounding the understanding of the topic. Functional disorders of the pelvic floor are marked by symptoms of obstructed defecation without an anatomic abnormality in the surrounding muscles. As outlined earlier, the process of defecation is intricate. It requires coordination of the pelvic nerves, the rectum, and the surrounding muscles, including the puborectalis and the remaining levator muscles. During normal defecation these muscles relax, allowing the rectum to empty; however, patients with pelvic floor dysfunction have uncoordinated activity that impairs evacuation of intestinal waste.

Understandably, this is can be a debilitating problem affecting a large number of patients, which are predominantly women. In the United States, approximately 24% of women report at least one pelvic floor disorder, which seems to increase with age, parity, and obesity.

Clinical Findings

A. Symptoms and Signs

Symptoms of pelvic floor dysfunction tend to develop slowly and insidiously; therefore, a careful history is paramount to establishing a working diagnosis and developing a strategy for diagnostic testing. Patients commonly describe constipation, straining with bowel movements, or the sense of incomplete evacuation. The residual soft stool in the rectal vault may cause soiling of the anoderm triggering the feeling of incontinence. Attention should be paid to diet as well as obstetric, urologic, and surgical histories. While these symptoms do not impose risk to the patient's health, they do interfere with the overall quality of life. At the time of presentation patients have often tried a plethora of medications and laxatives.

A focused physical examination should start with inspection of the anus and perineum. Profound perineal descent with straining is an indication of laxity of the pelvic floor, which is common with increasing age and multiparity. Digital rectal examination is important and should be performed to rule out rectal masses, to assess pain with palpation of the puborectalis, assess sphincter tone, and contraction/relaxation of the levator muscles. Specifically, paradoxic contraction of the puborectalis with simulated straining should be assessed.

B. Laboratory and Imaging Studies

A colonoscopy and colon transit study should generally be performed to exclude an underlying malignancy and slow-transit constipation, respectively. Additional adjuncts include anal manometry with balloon expulsion and defecography. Anal manometry should assess resting and maximum squeeze pressure as well as the presence of the RAIR. Patients with pelvic floor dysfunction will typically be unable to expel a balloon, which is inserted into the rectum.

Defecography offers a more dynamic view of the rectum, pelvic floor muscles, and anal sphincters. During this examination, the rectum is filled with contrast and the patient is asked to simulate defecation. Vaginal and oral contrast materials are also usually given to provide additional information about the neighboring structures. Defecography is useful in identifying rectoceles, internal and external rectal prolapse, enteroceles, as well as a nonrelaxing pelvic floor.

▶ Differential Diagnosis

Symptoms of constipation and defecation problems are quite common and may be due to a myriad of causes. Anatomic disorders, such as anal or rectal cancers, rectoceles, rectal prolapse, internal intussusception, and enteroceles, should be distinguished from functional disorders like a non-relaxing puborectalis.

▶ Treatment

A. Medical Treatment

Patients with pelvic floor dysfunction due to a nonrelaxing puborectalis should be referred for pelvic floor retraining, also known as biofeedback, which has become an integral part of treatment. During these sessions with the physical therapist, patients are instructed on how to properly relax the pelvic muscles with the aid of visual feedback. This neuromuscular training program is typically instrument-based employing manometry-, or electromyography-based biofeedback.

B. Surgical Treatment

Patients with obstructed defecation due to anatomic causes are candidates for surgery if they have failed initial conservative therapy with fiber supplementation and laxatives.

Rectocele repair is indicated for large rectoceles that have demonstrated failure to empty on defecography. Several approaches have been employed with varying success, including transvaginal, transrectal, and transperineal. A newer technique that has shown some initial short-term success is the stapled Trans-Anal Rectal Resection (STARR) procedure, which uses two circular staplers to produce a circumferential transanal full-thickness resection of the lower rectum. Its widespread use is limited by the lack of data on long-term outcomes and the potential for devastating complications such as pelvic sepsis and fistulas.

Internal rectal prolapse (intussusception) can be present in up to 50% of asymptomatic individuals; therefore, the surgical treatment of internal prolapse associated with obstructed defecation symptoms remains controversial. Rectopexy without concomitant resection has been advocated by some and the STARR procedure has been used by others. Results have been varied in the literature.

▶ Prognosis

Biofeedback has been the mainstay of treatment for nonrelaxing pelvic floor dysfunction. It is minimally invasive and repeatable with good results for those that complete the program. Improvement in symptoms has varied between 40% and 90% in several trials.

Bove A, Pucciani F, Bellini M et al: Consensus statement AIGO/SICCR: diagnosis and treatment of chronic constipation and obstructed defecation (part I: diagnosis). *World J Gastroenterol* 2012;18(14):1555-1564.

Faubion SS, Shuster LT, Bharucha AE: Recognition and management of nonrelaxing pelvic floor dysfunction. *Mayo Clin Proc* 2012;87(2):187-193.

McNevin MS: Overview of pelvic floor disorders. *Surg Clin North Am* 2010;90(1):195-205.

Nygaard I, Barber MD, Burgio KL, et al: Prevalence of symptomatic pelvic floor disorders in US women. *JAMA* 2008;300(11):1311-1316.

Rao SS: Dyssynergic defecation and biofeedback therapy. *Gastroenterol Clin North Am* 2008;37(3):569-86, viii.

ABNORMAL RECTAL FIXATION

▶ General Considerations

Abnormal rectal fixation is a general term for a group of diseases in which the attachment of the rectum to its surrounding structures has developed more laxity, allowing the rectum to, completely or incompletely, protrude through the anal canal. The exact pathophysiology is unknown but, in large part, this is related to chronic straining with defecation. Common anatomic variations may include a patulous anus, redundant sigmoid colon, diastasis of the levator ani muscles, and a deep cul-de-sac.

Rectal prolapse is characterized by an intussusception of the rectum. There are three general categories that ultimately influence symptoms and overall management: (1) internal prolapse (intussusception), which does not extend beyond the anal canal, (2) mucosal prolapse, and (3) complete prolapse, which involves full-thickness protrusion of the rectum through the anus.

In adults, older women are six times more likely to develop rectal prolapse, accounting for 80% to 90% of the patient populations. The peak incidence is after the fifth decade.

► Clinical Findings

A. Symptoms and Signs

Symptoms can vary with the degree of rectal prolapse, but typical complaints include a perianal mass that protrudes with straining, mucoid or bloody discharge, incomplete evacuation, incontinence, pain if the rectum becomes incarcerated.

On examination, a patulous anus or exaggerated perineal descent may be initial clues to the diagnosis if prolapsing rectal tissue is not evident. Digital rectal may reveal diminished or absent tone with complete prolapse but may suggest a mass with straining for internal intussusception. The diagnosis is most easily made with the patient straining in the seated position, which should reproduce the rectal prolapse, identified by the concentric folds of mucosa.

B. Laboratory and Imaging Studies

If the diagnosis remains elusive, defecography should be able to clearly demonstrate either internal or complete prolapse as well as other associated abnormalities such as cystoceles, enteroceles, and rectoceles. In patients who also present with complaints of longstanding constipation, anorectal manometry, and colon transit studies are also crucial. Prior to any surgical intervention, these patients should also undergo colonoscopy.

► Differential Diagnosis

Complete rectal prolapse is often confused with prolapsing internal hemorrhoids; however, the two can easily be separated by close examination of the mucosa. Prolapsing internal hemorrhoids produce radials folds in the visible rectal mucosa, which contrasts with the concentric folds seen with rectal prolapse.

► Complications

The most dreaded complication for rectal prolapse is incarceration, which may lead to tissue ischemia and necrosis. Chronic reducible rectal prolapse may also impair fecal continence due to the repeated stretching of the sphincter muscles.

► Treatment

A. Medical Treatment

A trial of fiber supplementation and diet modification may prove to be beneficial for mild cases of internal intussusception. Biofeedback, rectopexy, and the STARR procedure have been reported in refractory cases but their use remains controversial.

B. Surgical Treatment

Surgical treatment is indicated in patients with full-thickness rectal prolapse. Surgical treatment is broadly divided into abdominal and perineal approaches, which are dictated by the patient's age and comorbidities as well as surgeon preference and experience. Perineal approaches generally results in reduced length of hospital stay and less perioperative morbidity and pain; however, they are plagued by higher recurrence rates.

Rectopexy, resection rectopexy, and mesh rectopexy are the three abdominal procedures that are most widely practiced. The principle component of each of these procedures is the posterior mobilization of the rectum down to the level of the levator muscles. The rectum is elevated from the deep pelvis and sutured to the presacral fascia at the level of the sacral promontory. The lateral ligaments are preserved, as this has been shown to decrease postoperative constipation. Sigmoid resection with tension-free anastomosis to the rectum is performed if excessive redundancy is encountered or if there has been a longstanding history of constipation. Mesh has also been used to fix the rectum to the presacral fascia and should be performed without a concomitant resection. Complications include bowel obstruction, erosion of the mesh, and fistulas. All of these abdominal procedures have been approached laparoscopically with similar results, while maintaining the benefits of a minimally invasive technique.

Perineal proctosigmoidectomy, also known as the Altemeier procedure, combines a perineal proctosigmoidectomy with an anterior levatoroplasty. A full-thickness, circumferential incision is made 1 cm proximal to the dentate line. The mesentery of the rectum and sigmoid colon is sequentially divided until no redundant bowel remains. The colon is transected at this level and an anastomosis is created between the colon and the anal canal with either sutures or a circular stapler. An anterior levatoroplasty is usually added to correct the laxity in the levator muscles commonly associated with this condition.

The Delorme procedure is ideal for short segment mucosal prolapse since it entails a mucosal sleeve resection starting at the dentate line. The excess mucosa is transected and the proximal and distal edges of the mucosa are approximated while the muscle is plicated with interrupted sutures placed circumferentially.

▶ Prognosis

The described abdominal approaches have been shown to be safe and efficacious with approximately a 10% recurrence rate. Perineal approaches are also well tolerated but are associated with higher recurrence rates of 20%-30%.

Cadeddu F, Sileri P, Grande M, De Luca E, Franceschilli L, Milito G: Focus on abdominal rectopexy for full-thickness rectal prolapse: meta-analysis of literature. *Tech Coloproctol* 2012;16(1):37-53.

Felt-Bersma RJ, Tiersma ES, Cuesta MA: Rectal prolapse, rectal intussusception, rectocele, solitary rectal ulcer syndrome, and enterocele. *Gastroenterol Clin North Am* 2008;37(3):645-668, ix.

Goldstein SD, Maxwell PJt: Rectal prolapse. *Clin Colon Rectal Surg* 2011;24(1):39-45.

Jones OM, Cunningham C, Lindsey I: The assessment and management of rectal prolapse, rectal intussusception, rectocoele, and enterocoele in adults. *BMJ* 2011 Feb 1;342:c7099.

Sajid MS, Siddiqui MR, Baig MK: Open vs laparoscopic repair of full-thickness rectal prolapse: a re-meta-analysis. *Colorectal Dis* 2010;12(6):515-525.

Tou S, Brown SR, Malik AI, Nelson RL: Surgery for complete rectal prolapse in adults. *Cochrane Database Syst Rev* 2008(4):CD001758.

Varma M, Rafferty J, Buie WD: Practice parameters for the management of rectal prolapse. *Dis Colon Rectum* 2011;54(11): 1339-1346.

MULTIPLE CHOICE QUESTIONS

1. All of the following are sites of perirectal abscesses, except

   A. Ischiorectal
   B. Perianal
   C. Intermuscular
   D. Infralevator
   E. Submucous

2. Anal bleeding can be commonly caused by

   A. Diverticulitis
   B. Anal condyloma
   C. Anorectal abscess (undrained)
   D. Anal fissure
   E. Thrombosed external hemorrhoids

3. Rectal prolapse

   A. Can be distinguished from prolapsed hemorrhoids based upon imaging
   B. Is an intussusception of the rectum
   C. Cannot involve the muscular layers of the rectum due to fixation to the pelvic sidewalls
   D. Is best evaluated by MRI
   E. Is more common in men than women

4. Epidermoid tumors of the anal canal

   A. Are typically treated with a regimen of chemotherapy and radiation therapy after diagnosis
   B. Are about as common as rectal cancers
   C. Have a 25% response rate to initial therapy regimens
   D. Typically require abdominoperineal resection for complete treatment
   E. Rarely metastasize to regional lymph nodes

5. Management of condyloma acuminata

   A. Are rarely transmitted by sexual contact
   B. Are often treated with antiviral therapy as first line treatment
   C. Can include palliation of macroscopic lesions my operation
   D. Do not carry any risk of dysplasia
   E. Are asymptomatic

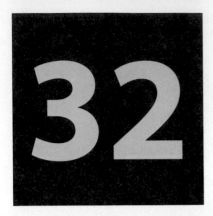

Hernias & Other Lesions of the Abdominal Wall*

Karen E. Deveney, MD

▼ I. HERNIAS

An external hernia is an abnormal protrusion of intra-abdominal tissue through a fascial defect in the abdominal wall. Although most hernias (75%) occur in the groin, incisional hernias represent an increasing proportion (15%-20%), with umbilical and other ventral hernias comprising the remainder. Generally, a hernial mass is composed of covering tissues (skin, subcutaneous tissues, etc), a peritoneal sac, and any contained viscera. Particularly if the neck of the sac is narrow where it emerges from the abdomen, bowel protruding into the hernia may become obstructed or strangulated. If the hernia is not repaired early, the defect may enlarge and operative repair may become more complicated. The definitive treatment of hernia is operative repair.

A *reducible hernia* is one in which the contents of the sac return to the abdomen spontaneously or with manual pressure when the patient is recumbent.

An *irreducible (incarcerated) hernia* is one whose contents cannot be returned to the abdomen, usually because they are trapped by a narrow neck. The term "incarceration" does not imply obstruction, inflammation, or ischemia of the herniated organs, though incarceration is necessary for obstruction or strangulation to occur.

Though the lumen of a segment of bowel within the hernia sac may become obstructed, there may initially be no interference with blood supply. Compromise to the blood supply of the contents of the sac (eg, omentum or intestine) results in a *strangulated hernia,* in which gangrene of the contents of the sac has occurred. The incidence of strangulation is higher in femoral than in inguinal hernias, but strangulation may occur in any hernia.

An uncommon and dangerous type of hernia, a *Richter hernia,* occurs when only part of the circumference of the

bowel becomes incarcerated or strangulated in the fascial defect. A strangulated Richter hernia may spontaneously reduce and the gangrenous piece of intestine be overlooked at operation. The bowel may subsequently perforate, with resultant peritonitis.

HERNIAS OF THE GROIN

▶ Anatomy

All groin hernias protrude through the myopectineal orifice of Fruchaud, a weakness or defect in the transversalis fascia, an aponeurosis located just outside the peritoneum. External to the transversalis fascia are found the transversus abdominis, internal oblique, and external oblique muscles, which are fleshy laterally and aponeurotic medially. Their aponeuroses form investing layers of the strong rectus abdominis muscles above the semilunar line. Below this line, the aponeurosis lies entirely in front of the muscle. Between the two vertical rectus muscles, the aponeuroses meet again to form the linea alba, which is well defined only above the umbilicus. The subcutaneous fat contains the Scarpa fascia—a misnomer, since it is only a condensation of connective tissue with no substantial strength.

In the groin, an indirect inguinal hernia results when obliteration of the processus vaginalis, the peritoneal extension accompanying the testis in its descent into the scrotum, fails to occur. The resultant hernia sac passes through the internal inguinal ring, a defect in the transversalis fascia halfway between the anterior iliac spine and the pubic tubercle. The sac is located anteromedially within the spermatic cord and may extend partway along the inguinal canal or accompany the cord out through the subcutaneous (external) inguinal ring, a defect medially in the external oblique muscle just above the pubic tubercle. A hernia that passes fully into the scrotum is known as a *complete hernia.* The sac and the spermatic cord are invested by the cremaster muscle, an extension of fibers of the internal oblique muscle.

*See Chapter 43 for further discussion of hernias in the pediatric age group and Chapter 21 for a discussion of internal hernias.

Other anatomic structures of the groin that are important in understanding the formation of hernias and types of hernia repairs include the *conjoined tendon,* a fusion of the medial aponeurotic transversus abdominis and internal oblique muscles that passes along the inferolateral edge of the rectus abdominis muscle and attaches to the pubic tubercle. Between the pubic tubercle and the anterior iliac spine passes the inguinal (Poupart) ligament, formed by the lowermost border of the external oblique aponeurosis as it rolls on itself and thickens into a cord.

Just deep and parallel to the inguinal ligament runs the iliopubic tract, a band of connective tissue that extends from the iliopsoas fascia, crosses below the deep inguinal ring, forms the superior border of the femoral sheath, and inserts into the superior pubic ramus to form the lacunar (Gimbernat) ligament. The lacunar ligament is about 1.25 cm long and triangular in shape. The sharp, crescentic lateral border of this ligament is the unyielding noose for the strangulation of a femoral hernia.

The Cooper ligament is a strong, fibrous band that extends laterally for about 2.5 cm along the iliopectineal line on the superior aspect of the superior pubic ramus, starting at the lateral base of the lacunar ligament.

The Hesselbach triangle is bounded by the inguinal ligament, the inferior epigastric vessels, and the lateral border of the rectus muscle. A weakness or defect in the transversalis fascia, which forms the floor of this triangle, results in a direct inguinal hernia. In most direct hernias, the transversalis fascia is diffusely attenuated, though a discrete defect in the fascia may occasionally occur. This funicular type of direct inguinal hernia is more likely to become incarcerated, since it has distinct borders.

A femoral hernia passes beneath the iliopubic tract and inguinal ligament into the upper thigh. The predisposing anatomic feature for femoral hernias is a small empty space between the lacunar ligament medially and the femoral vein laterally—the femoral canal. Because its borders are distinct and unyielding, a femoral hernia has the highest risk of incarceration and strangulation of groin hernias.

Surgeons must be familiar with the pathways of the nerves and blood vessels of the inguinal region to avoid injuring them when repairing groin hernias. The iliohypogastric nerve (T12, L1) emerges from the lateral edge of the psoas muscle and travels inside the external oblique muscle, emerging medial to the external inguinal ring to innervate the suprapubic skin. The ilioinguinal nerve (L1) parallels the iliohypogastric nerve and travels on the surface of the spermatic cord to innervate the base of the penis (or mons pubis), the scrotum (or labia majora), and the medial thigh. This nerve is the most frequently injured in anterior open inguinal hernia repairs. The genitofemoral (L1, L2) and lateral femoral cutaneous nerves (L2, L3) travel on and lateral to the psoas muscle and provide sensation to the scrotum and anteromedial thigh and to the lateral thigh, respectively.

These nerves are subject to injury during laparoscopic hernia repairs. The femoral nerve (L2-L4) travels from the lateral edge of the psoas and extends lateral to the femoral vessels. It can be injured during laparoscopic or femoral hernia repairs.

The external iliac artery travels along the medial aspect of the psoas muscle and beneath the inguinal ligament, giving off the inferior epigastric artery, which borders the medial aspect of the internal inguinal ring. The corresponding veins accompany the arteries. These vessels can be injured during hernia repairs of all types.

▶ Causes

Nearly all inguinal hernias in infants, children, and young adults are indirect inguinal hernias. Although these "congenital" hernias most often present during the first year of life, the first clinical evidence of hernia may not appear until middle or old age, when increased intra-abdominal pressure and dilation of the internal inguinal ring allow abdominal contents to enter the previously empty peritoneal diverticulum. An untreated indirect hernia will inevitably dilate the internal ring and displace or attenuate the inguinal floor. The peritoneum may protrude on either side of the inferior epigastric vessels to give a combined direct and indirect hernia, called a pantaloon hernia.

In contrast, direct inguinal hernias are acquired as the result of a developed weakness of the transversalis fascia in the Hesselbach area. There is some evidence that direct inguinal hernias may be related to hereditary or acquired defects in collagen synthesis or turnover. Femoral hernias involve an acquired protrusion of a peritoneal sac through the femoral ring. In women, the ring may become dilated by physical and biochemical changes during pregnancy.

Any condition that chronically increases intra-abdominal pressure may contribute to the appearance and progression of a hernia. Marked obesity, abdominal strain from heavy exercise or lifting, cough, constipation with straining at stool, and prostatism with straining on micturition are often implicated. Cirrhosis with ascites, pregnancy, chronic ambulatory peritoneal dialysis, and chronically enlarged pelvic organs or pelvic tumors may also contribute. Loss of tissue turgor in the Hesselbach area, associated with a weakening of the transversalis fascia, occurs with advancing age and in chronic debilitating disease.

INDIRECT & DIRECT INGUINAL HERNIAS

▶ Clinical Findings

A. Symptoms

Most hernias produce no symptoms until the patient notices a lump or swelling in the groin, though some patients may describe a sudden pain and bulge that occurred while lifting or straining. Frequently, hernias are detected in the course of routine physical examinations such as preemployment examinations. Some patients complain of a dragging sensation and, particularly with indirect inguinal hernias, radiation of pain into the scrotum. As a hernia enlarges, it is likely to produce a sense of discomfort or aching pain, and the patient must lie down to reduce the hernia.

In general, direct hernias produce fewer symptoms than indirect inguinal hernias and are less likely to become incarcerated or strangulated.

B. Signs

Examination of the groin reveals a mass that may or may not be reducible. The patient should be examined both supine and standing and also with coughing and straining, since small hernias may be difficult to demonstrate. The external ring can be identified by invaginating the scrotum and palpating with the index finger just above and lateral to the pubic tubercle (Figure 32–1). If the external ring is very small, the examiner's finger may not enter the inguinal canal, and it may be difficult to be sure that a pulsation felt on coughing is truly a hernia. At the other extreme, a widely patent external ring does not by itself constitute hernia. Tissue must be felt protruding into the inguinal canal during coughing in order for a hernia to be diagnosed.

Differentiating between direct and indirect inguinal hernia on examination is difficult and is of little importance, since most groin hernias should be repaired regardless of type. Nevertheless, each type of inguinal hernia has specific features more common to it. A hernia that descends into the scrotum is almost certainly indirect. On inspection with the patient erect and straining, a direct hernia more commonly appears as a symmetric, circular swelling at the external ring; the swelling disappears when the patient lies down. An indirect hernia appears as an elliptic swelling that may not reduce easily.

On palpation, the posterior wall of the inguinal canal is firm and resistant in an indirect hernia but relaxed or absent in a direct hernia. If the patient is asked to cough or strain while the examining finger is directed laterally and upward into the inguinal canal, a direct hernia protrudes against the side of the finger, whereas an indirect hernia is felt at the tip of the finger.

Compression over the internal ring when the patient strains may also help to differentiate between indirect and direct hernias. A direct hernia bulges forward through Hesselbach triangle, but the opposite hand can maintain reduction of an indirect hernia at the internal ring.

These distinctions are obscured as a hernia enlarges and distorts the anatomic relationships of the inguinal rings and canal. In most patients, the type of inguinal hernia cannot be established accurately before surgery.

▶ Differential Diagnosis

Groin pain of musculoskeletal or obscure origin occurs primarily with vigorous physical exertion (so-called "sports hernia") and may be difficult to distinguish from a true hernia, even with thorough physical examination. MRI may be helpful in identifying the problem as inflammation, edema, or a muscle or tendon tear or strain.

Herniation of preperitoneal fat through the inguinal ring into the spermatic cord (lipoma of the cord) is commonly misinterpreted as a hernia sac. Its true nature may only be confirmed at operation. Occasionally, a femoral hernia that has extended above the inguinal ligament after passing through the fossa ovalis femoris may be confused with an inguinal hernia. If the examining finger is placed on the pubic tubercle, the neck of the sac of a femoral hernia lies lateral and below, while that of an inguinal hernia lies above.

Inguinal hernia must be differentiated from hydrocele of the spermatic cord, lymphadenopathy or abscesses of the groin, varicocele, and residual hematoma following trauma or spontaneous hemorrhage in patients taking anticoagulants. An undescended testis in the inguinal canal must also be considered when the testis cannot be felt in the scrotum.

The presence of an impulse in the mass with coughing, bowel sounds in the mass, and failure to transilluminate are features that indicate that an irreducible mass in the groin is a hernia.

▶ Treatment

Although inguinal hernias have traditionally been repaired electively to avoid the risks of incarceration, obstruction, and strangulation, asymptomatic or mildly symptomatic hernias may be safely observed in elderly, sedentary patients or those with high morbidity for operation. The annual risk

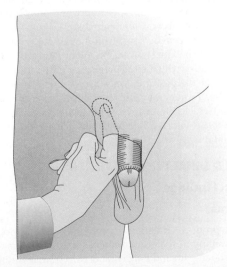

▲ **Figure 32–1.** Insertion of finger through upper scrotum into the external inguinal ring.

of hernia incarceration is not precisely known but has been estimated at fewer than 2/1000 patients per year. However, a high percentage of patients become symptomatic while being observed expectantly. All symptomatic groin hernias should be repaired if the patient can tolerate surgery.

Even elderly patients tolerate elective repair of a groin hernia very well when other medical problems are optimally controlled and local anesthetic is used. Emergency operation carries a much greater risk for the elderly than carefully planned elective operation.

If the patient has significant prostatic hyperplasia, it is prudent to solve this problem first, since the risks of urinary retention and urinary tract infection are high following hernia repair in patients with significant prostatic obstruction.

Although most direct hernias do not carry as high a risk of incarceration as indirect hernias, the difficulty in reliably differentiating them from indirect hernias makes the repair of all symptomatic inguinal hernias advisable. Direct hernias of the funicular type, which are particularly likely to incarcerate, should always be repaired.

Because of the possibility of strangulation, an incarcerated, painful, or tender hernia usually requires an emergency operation. Nonoperative reduction of an incarcerated hernia may first be attempted. The patient is placed with hips elevated and given analgesics and sedation sufficient to promote muscle relaxation. Repair of the hernia may be deferred if the hernia mass reduces with gentle manipulation and if there is no clinical evidence of strangulated bowel. Though strangulation is usually clinically evident, gangrenous tissue can occasionally be reduced into the abdomen by manual or spontaneous reduction. It is therefore safest to repair the reduced hernia at the earliest opportunity. At surgery, one must decide whether to explore the abdomen to make certain that the intestine is viable. If the patient has leukocytosis or clinical signs of peritonitis or if the hernia sac contains dark or bloody fluid, the abdomen should be explored.

A. Principles of Operative Treatment of Inguinal Hernia

1. Durable repair requires that any correctable aggravating factors be identified and treated (chronic cough, prostatic obstruction, colonic tumor, ascites, etc) and that the defect be reconstructed without tension.

2. An indirect hernia sac should be anatomically isolated, dissected to its origin from the peritoneum, and ligated (Figure 32–2). In infants and young adults in whom the inguinal anatomy is normal, repair can usually be limited to high ligation, removal of the sac, and reduction of the internal ring to an appropriate size. For most adult hernias, the inguinal floor should also be reconstructed. The internal ring should be reduced to a size just adequate to allow egress of the cord structures.

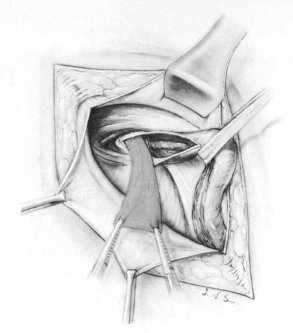

▲ **Figure 32–2.** Indirect inguinal hernia. Inguinal canal opened, showing spermatic cord retracted medially and indirect hernia peritoneal sac dissected free to above the level of the internal inguinal ring.

In women, the internal ring can be totally closed to prevent recurrence through that site.

3. In direct inguinal hernia (Figure 32–3), the inguinal floor is usually so weak that a primary repair using the patient's own tissues would be under tension. Although a vertical relaxing incision in the anterior rectus abdominis sheath was traditionally used, most hernia repairs are now performed using mesh so that a tension-free repair can be accomplished.

4. Even though a direct hernia is found, the cord should always be carefully searched for a possible indirect hernia as well.

5. In patients with large hernias, bilateral repair has traditionally been discouraged under the assumption that greater tension on the repair would result and therefore would increase the recurrence rate and surgical complications. If open mesh repair or laparoscopic methods are used, however, bilateral repairs can be done with low risk of recurrence. In children and young adults with small hernias, bilateral hernia repair is usually recommended because it spares the patient a second anesthetic.

6. Recurrent hernia within a few months or a year of operation usually indicates an inadequate repair, such as

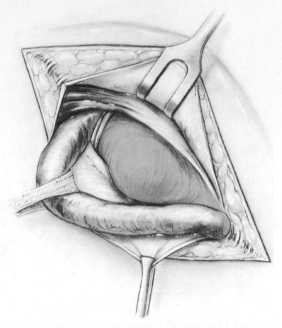

▲ **Figure 32–3.** Direct inguinal hernia. Inguinal canal opened and spermatic cord retracted inferiorly and laterally to reveal the hernia bulging through the floor of the Hesselbach triangle.

overlooking an indirect sac, missing a femoral hernia, or failing to repair the fascial defect securely. Any repair completed under tension is subject to early recurrence. Recurrences 2 or more years after repair are more likely to be caused by progressive weakening of the patient's fascia. Repeated recurrence after careful repair by an experienced surgeon suggests a defect in collagen synthesis. Because the fascial defect is often small, firm, and unyielding, recurrent hernias are much more likely than unoperated inguinal hernias to develop incarceration or strangulation, and they should nearly always be repaired again.

If recurrence is due to an overlooked indirect sac, the posterior wall is often solid and removal of the sac may be all that is required. Occasionally, a recurrence is discovered to consist of a small, sharply circumscribed defect in the previous hernioplasty, in which case closure of the defect suffices.

B. Types of Operations for Inguinal Hernia

The goal of all hernia repairs is to reduce the contents of the hernia into the abdomen and to close the fascial defect in the inguinal floor. Traditional repairs approximated native tissues using permanent sutures. More recently, synthetic mesh has supplanted tissue repairs because multiple prospective,

randomized studies have shown lower recurrence with tension-free mesh repairs than traditional primary tissue repair.

Over the past 20 years, increased experience has been gained with minimally invasive techniques for hernia repair. Laparoscopic approaches offer less pain and more rapid return to work or normal activities. Multiple randomized trials have compared open and laparoscopic hernia repairs. Although details of specific studies vary, long-term recurrence rates of open and laparoscopic repairs are similar. The success of laparoscopic approaches is dependent on experience of the surgeon, as is also true for open repair.

Although repairs today overwhelmingly employ prosthetic material, the presence of infection or need to resect gangrenous bowel may make use of nonbiologic mesh unwise. In these situations, primary tissue repairs may still be a preferable option. For this reason, surgeons need to know the traditional techniques even though they are rarely used today.

Among the traditional autologous tissue repairs, the Bassini repair is the most widely used method. In this repair, the conjoined tendon is approximated to the Poupart ligament, and the spermatic cord remains in its normal anatomic position under the external oblique aponeurosis. The Halsted repair places the external oblique beneath the cord but otherwise resembles the Bassini repair. Cooper ligament (Lotheissen–McVay) repair brings the conjoined tendon farther posteriorly and inferiorly to the Cooper ligament. Unlike the Bassini and Halsted methods, McVay repair is effective for femoral hernia but always requires a relaxing incision to relieve tension. Recurrence rates after these open nonmesh repairs vary widely according to skill and experience of the surgeon but population studies show them to range from as low as 5%-10% to as high as 33%. Though the Shouldice repair has a lower reported recurrence rate, it is not widely used, perhaps because of the more extensive dissection required and a belief that the skill of the surgeons may be as important as the method itself. In the Shouldice repair, the transversalis fascia is first divided and then imbricated to the Poupart ligament. Finally, the conjoined tendon and internal oblique muscle are also approximated in layers to the inguinal ligament.

The open preperitoneal approach exposes the groin from between the transversalis fascia and peritoneum via a lower abdominal incision to effect closure of the fascial defect. Because it requires more initial dissection and is associated with higher morbidity and recurrence rates in less experienced hands, it has not been widely used. For recurrent or large bilateral hernias, a preperitoneal approach using a large piece of mesh to span all areas of potential herniation has been described by Stoppa.

A desire to decrease the recurrence rate of hernias prompted the increased use of prosthetic materials in repair of both recurrent and first-time hernias. Methods include "plugs" of mesh inserted into the internal ring and sheets of mesh to create a tension-free repair. The most widely used technique is that of Lichtenstein, an open mesh repair that allows an early return to normal activities and a low complication and recurrence rate.

Virtually all laparoscopic approaches utilize mesh in the repair. Several methods have been explored, with two methods having emerged as most frequently employed—the transabdominal preperitoneal mesh technique (TAPP) and total extraperitoneal (preperitoneal) mesh placement (TEP). The high incidence of complications that occurred in early studies prompted revisions in the operative technique to avoid injury to lateral nerves. Several prospective randomized trials have subsequently been conducted comparing open with minimally invasive techniques and one type of minimally invasive technique with another. These studies have reported decreased pain and faster return to work with the minimally invasive techniques but increased operative time and cost. Laparoscopic procedures also require general anesthesia and therefore are not appropriate for all patients. Long-term hernia recurrence is equivalent with open and laparoscopic mesh repairs at approximately 4%. Specific situations in which laparoscopic procedures often lower recurrence include the repair of recurrent hernias after anterior open repairs, repair of bilateral hernias simultaneously, and repair in patients who must return to work particularly quickly. Although the percentage of hernias repaired laparoscopically has increased, its use varies considerably across different locales and still represents a minority of groin hernia repairs. The success of both open and laparoscopic repair of groin hernias is highly dependent upon the surgeon's skill and experience with the technique.

C. Nonsurgical Management (Use of a Truss)

The surgeon is occasionally called upon to prescribe a truss when a patient refuses operative repair or when there are absolute contraindications to operation. A truss should be fitted to provide adequate external compression over the defect in the abdominal wall. It should be taken off at night and put on in the morning before the patient arises. The use of a truss does not preclude later repair of a hernia, although it may cause fibrosis of the anatomic structures, so that subsequent repair may be more difficult.

▶ Preoperative & Postoperative Course

Although groin hernia repair is usually an outpatient procedure, a thorough preoperative evaluation should be completed before the day of surgery. The anesthetic may be general, spinal, or local. Local anesthetic is effective for most patients, and the incidence of urinary retention and pulmonary complications is lowest with local anesthesia. Recurrent hernias are more easily repaired with the patient under spinal or general anesthesia, since local anesthetic does not readily diffuse through scar tissue. A sedentary worker may return to work within a few days; heavy manual labor has traditionally not been performed for up to 4-6 weeks after hernia repair, though recent studies document no increase in recurrence when full activity is resumed as early as 2 weeks after surgery, particularly when mesh has been used in the repair.

▶ Prognosis

In addition to chronic cough, prostatism, and constipation, poor tissue quality and poor operative technique may contribute to recurrence of inguinal hernia. Because tissue is often more attenuated in direct hernias, recurrence rates are slightly higher than for indirect hernias. Placing the repair under tension leads to recurrence. Failure to find an indirect hernia, to dissect the sac high enough, or to adequately close the internal ring may lead to recurrence of indirect hernia. Postoperative wound infection is associated with increased recurrence. The recurrence rate is considerably increased in patients receiving chronic peritoneal dialysis, cirrhotics with ascites, smokers, and patients on steroids or who are malnourished.

The current recurrence rate after hernia repair in adults is reported at best to be 4%. Reasons for recurrence include failure to identify a femoral or indirect hernia.

An underappreciated sequela of groin hernia repair is chronic groin pain, which may occur in as high as 10% of patients and is usually attributed to nerve entrapment or neuroma. Laparoscopic repair or prophylactic division of the ilioinguinal nerve in open repairs has been shown to decrease the incidence of chronic groin pain.

Dedemadi G et al: Laparoscopic versus open mesh repair for recurrent inguinal hernia: a meta-analysis of outcomes. Am J Surg 2010;200:291-297.

Eker H et al: Randomized clinical trial of total extraperitoneal inguinal hernioplasty vs Lichtenstein repair. Arch Surg 2012;147:256-260.

Franz M: The biology of hernia formation. Surg Clin N Am 2008;88:1-15.

Gass M et al: Bilateral total extraperitoneal inguinal hernia repair (TEP) has outcomes similar to those for unilateral TEP: population-based analysis of prospective data of 6,505 patients. Surg Endosc 2012;26:1364-1368.

Hallén M et al: Laparoscopic extraperitoneal inguinal hernia repair versus open mesh repair: long-term follow-up of a randomized controlled trial. Surgery 2008;143:313-317.

Itani K et al: Management of recurrent inguinal hernias. J Am Coll Surg 2009;209:653-658.

Matthews RD et al: Inguinal hernia in the 21st century: an evidence-based review. Curr Probl Surg 2008;45:261-312.

Mizrahi H et al: Management of asymptomatic inguinal hernia. Arch Surg 2012;147:277-281.

Nam A et al: Management and therapy for sports hernia. J Am Coll Surg 2008;206:154-164.

O'Reilly E et al: A meta-analysis of surgical morbidity and recurrence after laparoscopic and open repair of primary unilateral inguinal hernia. Ann Surg 2012;255:846-853.

Stylianidis G et al: Management of the hernia sac in inguinal hernia repair. *Brit J Surg* 2010;97:415-419.

Zendejas B et al: Simulation-based mastery learning improves patient outcomes in laparoscopic inguinal hernia repair. *Ann Surg* 2011;254:502-511.

SLIDING INGUINAL HERNIA

A sliding inguinal hernia (Figure 32–4) is an indirect inguinal hernia in which the wall of a viscus forms a portion of the wall of the hernia sac. On the right side, the cecum is most commonly involved, and on the left side, the sigmoid colon. The development of a sliding hernia is related to the variable degree of posterior fixation of the large bowel or other sliding components (eg, bladder, ovary) and their proximity to the internal inguinal ring.

▶ Clinical Findings

Though sliding hernias have no special signs that distinguish them from other inguinal hernias, they should be suspected in any large hernia that cannot be completely reduced. Finding a segment of colon in the scrotum on contrast radiograph strongly suggests a sliding hernia. Recognition of this variation is of great importance at operation, since failure to recognize it may result in inadvertent entry into the lumen of the bowel or bladder.

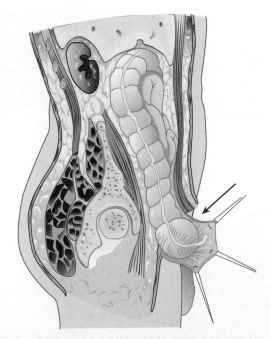

▲ **Figure 32–4.** Right-sided sliding hernia seen in sagittal section. At arrow, the wall of the cecum forms a portion of the hernia sac.

▶ Treatment

It is essential to recognize the entity at an early stage of operation. As is true of all indirect inguinal hernias, the sac will lie anteriorly, but the posterior wall of the sac will be formed by colon, bladder, or retroperitoneal ileum.

After the cord has been dissected free from the hernia sac, most sliding hernias can be reduced by a series of inverting sutures (Bevan technique) and one of the standard types of inguinal repair performed. Very large sliding hernias may have to be reduced by entering the peritoneal cavity through a separate incision (La Roque technique), pulling the bowel back into the abdomen, and fixing it to the posterior abdominal wall. The hernia is then repaired in the usual fashion. Sliding hernias can also be repaired successfully by laparoscopic (TAPP or TEP) techniques in experienced hands.

▶ Prognosis

Sliding hernias have a higher recurrence rate than uncomplicated indirect hernias.

The surgical complication most often encountered during repair of a sliding hernia is entry into the bowel or bladder, usually due to failure to recognize that the hernia is a sliding hernia.

Adams R et al: Outcome of sliding inguinal hernia repair. *Hernia* 2010;14:47-49.

Freundlich R et al: Laparoscopic repair of an incarcerated right indirect sliding inguinal hernia involving a retroperitoneal ileum. *Hernia* 2011;15:225-227.

FEMORAL HERNIA

A femoral hernia descends through the femoral canal beneath the inguinal ligament. Because of its narrow neck, it is prone to incarceration and strangulation. Femoral hernia is much more common in women than in men, but in both sexes femoral hernia is less common than inguinal hernia. Femoral hernias comprise about one-third of groin hernias in women and about 2% of groin hernias in men.

▶ Clinical Findings

A. Symptoms

Femoral hernias are notoriously asymptomatic until incarceration or strangulation occurs. Even with obstruction or strangulation, the patient may feel discomfort more in the abdomen than in the femoral area. Thus, colicky abdominal pain and signs of intestinal obstruction frequently are the presenting manifestations of a strangulated femoral hernia, without discomfort, pain, or tenderness in the femoral region. The patient often has a history of previous repair of an inguinal hernia, lending credence to the concept that a femoral hernia may be overlooked if a thorough search for a femoral hernia is not conducted during an operation for an inguinal hernia.

B. Signs

A femoral hernia may present in a variety of ways. If it is small and uncomplicated, it usually appears as a small bulge in the upper medial thigh just below the level of the inguinal ligament. Because it may be deflected anteriorly through the fossa ovalis femoris to present as a visible or palpable mass at or above the inguinal ligament, it can be confused with an inguinal hernia.

▶ Differential Diagnosis

Femoral hernia must be distinguished from inguinal hernia, a saphenous varix, and femoral adenopathy. A saphenous varix transmits a distinct thrill when a patient coughs, and it appears and disappears instantly when the patient stands or lies down—in contrast to femoral hernias, which are either irreducible or reduce gradually on pressure.

▶ Treatment

A femoral hernia can be repaired through an open or laparoscopic approach, with mesh or primary tissue repair. The traditional primary repair was the McVay (Cooper ligament) repair that employed a relaxing incision in the anterior rectus sheath. More recently, open repair with mesh or laparoscopic preperitoneal repair (TEP) have been used. No matter what the approach, the hernia is often difficult to reduce. Reduction may be facilitated by carefully incising the iliopubic tract, Gimbernat ligament, or even the inguinal ligament. Occasionally, a counterincision in the thigh is required to free attachments below the inguinal ligament. Irrespective of the approach used, successful femoral hernia repair must close the femoral canal.

If the hernia sac and mass reduce when the patient is given opiates or anesthesia and if bloody fluid appears in the hernia sac when it is exposed and opened, one must strongly suspect the possibility of nonviable bowel in the peritoneal cavity. In such cases, it is mandatory to explore the abdomen, an advantage of the laparoscopic approach.

▶ Prognosis

Recurrence rates are equivalent to that of inguinal hernia at 4%-5%.

Chan G: Longterm results of a prospective study of 225 femoral hernia repairs: indications for tissue and mesh repair. *J Am Coll Surg* 2008;207:360-367.

Putnis S: Synchronous femoral hernias diagnosed during endoscopic inguinal hernia repair. *Surg Endosc* 2011;25: 3752-3754.

OTHER TYPES OF HERNIAS

UMBILICAL HERNIAS IN ADULTS

Umbilical hernia in adults occurs long after closure of the umbilical ring and is due to a gradual yielding of the cicatricial tissue closing the ring. It is more common in women than in men.

Predisposing factors include: (1) multiple pregnancies with prolonged labor, (2) ascites, (3) obesity, and (4) large intra-abdominal tumors.

▶ Clinical Findings

In adults, umbilical hernia does not usually obliterate spontaneously, as in children, but instead increases steadily in size. The hernia sac may have multiple loculations. Umbilical hernias usually contain omentum, but small and large bowel may be present. Emergency repair is often necessary, because the neck of the hernia is usually quite narrow compared to the size of the herniated mass and incarceration and strangulation are common.

Umbilical hernias with tight rings are often associated with sharp pain on coughing or straining. Very large umbilical hernias more commonly produce a dragging or aching sensation.

▶ Treatment

Umbilical hernia in an adult should be repaired expeditiously to avoid incarceration and strangulation. Repairs utilizing mesh result in the lowest recurrence rate. The laparoscopic approach is associated with less postoperative pain and faster recovery than open techniques. Mesh should be used for all but the smallest umbilical hernias.

The presence of cirrhosis and ascites does not contraindicate repair of an umbilical hernia, since incarceration, strangulation, and rupture are particularly dangerous in patients with these disorders. If significant ascites exists, however, it should first be controlled medically or by transjugular intrahepatic portosystemic shunt (TIPS) if necessary, since mortality, morbidity, and recurrence are higher after hernia repair in patients with ascites, when the procedure must be performed as an emergency. Preoperative correction of fluid and electrolyte imbalance and improvement of nutrition also improve the outcome in these patients.

▶ Prognosis

Factors that lead to a high rate of complication and recurrence after surgical repair include large size of the hernia, old age or debility of the patient, obesity, and the presence of related intra-abdominal disease. In healthy individuals, surgical repair of the umbilical defects gives good results with a low rate of recurrence.

Aslani N et al: Does mesh offer an advantage over tissue in the open repair of umbilical hernias? A systematic review and meta-analysis. *Hernia* 2010;14:455-462.

Farrow B et al: More than 150 consecutive open umbilical hernia repairs in a major Veterans Administration Medical Center. *Am J Surg* 2008;196:647-651.

Gray S et al: Umbilical herniorrhapy in cirrhosis: improved outcomes with elective repair. *J Gastrointest Surg* 2008;12: 675-681.

McKay A et al: Umbilical hernia repair in the presence of cirrhosis and ascites: results of a survey and review of the literature. *Hernia* 2009;13:461-468.

EPIGASTRIC HERNIA

An epigastric hernia (Figure 32–5) protrudes through the linea alba above the level of the umbilicus. The hernia may develop through one of the foramina of egress of the small paramidline nerves and vessels or through an area of congenital weakness in the linea alba.

About 3%-5% of the population have epigastric hernias. They are more common in men than in women and most common between the ages of 20 and 50. About 20% of epigastric hernias are multiple, and about 80% occur just off the midline.

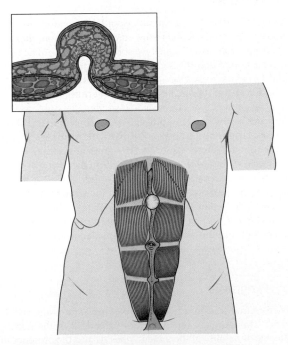

▲ **Figure 32–5.** Epigastric hernia. Note closeness to midline and the presence in upper abdomen. The herniation is through the linea alba.

▶ **Clinical Findings**

A. Symptoms

Most epigastric hernias are painless and are found on routine abdominal examination. If symptomatic, their presentation ranges from mild epigastric pain and tenderness to deep, burning epigastric pain with radiation to the back or the lower abdominal quadrants. The pain may be accompanied by abdominal bloating, nausea, or vomiting. The symptoms often occur after a large meal and on occasion may be relieved by reclining, probably because the supine position causes the herniated mass to drop away from the anterior abdominal wall. The smaller masses most frequently contain only preperitoneal fat and are especially prone to incarceration and strangulation. These smaller hernias are often tender. Larger hernias seldom strangulate and may contain, in addition to preperitoneal fat, a portion of the nearby omentum and, occasionally, a loop of small or large bowel.

B. Signs

If a mass is palpable, the diagnosis can often be confirmed by any maneuver that will increase intra-abdominal pressure and thereby cause the mass to bulge anteriorly. The diagnosis is difficult to make when the patient is obese, since a mass is hard to palpate; ultrasound, CT, or tangential radiographs may be needed in the very obese patient.

▶ **Differential Diagnosis**

Differential diagnosis includes peptic ulcer, gallbladder disease, hiatal hernia, pancreatitis, and upper small bowel obstruction. On occasion, it may be impossible to distinguish the hernial mass from a subcutaneous lipoma, fibroma, or neurofibroma.

Another condition that must be distinguished from an epigastric hernia is diastasis recti, a diffuse widening and attenuation of the linea alba without a fascial defect. On examination, this condition appears as a fusiform, linear bulge between the two rectus abdominis muscles without a discrete fascial defect. Although this condition may be unsightly, repair should be avoided since there is no risk of incarceration, the fascial layer is weak, and the recurrence rate is high. If it is painful or unsightly, a diastasis is best repaired using a laparoscopic plication technique.

▶ **Treatment**

Most epigastric hernias should be repaired, since small ones likely to become incarcerated and large ones are often symptomatic and unsightly. Small defects can usually be closed primarily, although mesh should be used for large hernias. Herniated fat contents are usually dissected free and removed. Intraperitoneal herniating structures are reduced, but no attempt is made to close the peritoneal sac.

Prognosis

The recurrence rate is 10%-20%, a higher incidence than with the routine inguinal or femoral hernia repair. This high recurrence rate may be partly due to failure to recognize and repair multiple small defects.

Palanivelu C et al: Laparoscopic repair of diastasis recti using the "Venetian blinds" technique of plication with prosthetic reinforcement: a retrospective study. *Hernia* 2009;13:287-292.

INCISIONAL HERNIA (VENTRAL HERNIA)

About 10% of abdominal operations result in incisional hernias. The incidence of this iatrogenic type of hernia is not diminishing in spite of an awareness of the many causative factors.

Etiology

The factors most often responsible for incisional hernia are listed below. When more than one factor coexists in the same patient, the likelihood of postoperative wound failure is greatly increased.

1. Poor surgical technique. Inadequate fascial bites, tension on the fascial edges, or too tight a closure are most often responsible for incisional failure.

2. Postoperative wound infection. An infection in the wound increases the risk of hernia formation to as high as 80%, the greatest single risk factor for hernia.

3. Age. Wound healing is usually slower and the closure less solid in older patients.

4. General debility. Cirrhosis, carcinoma, and chronic wasting diseases are factors that affect wound healing adversely. Any condition that compromises nutrition increases the likelihood of incision breakdown.

5. Obesity. Obese patients frequently have increased intra-abdominal pressure. The presence of fat in the abdominal wound masks tissue layers and increases the incidence of seromas and hematomas in wounds.

6. Postoperative pulmonary complications that stress the repair as a result of vigorous coughing. Smokers and patients with chronic pulmonary disease are therefore at increased risk of fascial disruption.

7. Placement of drains or stomas through the primary operative fascial defect.

8. Intraoperative blood loss greater than 1000 mL.

9. Failure to close the fascia of laparoscopic trocar sites over 10 mm in size.

10. Defects in collagen or matrix metalloprotease.

Treatment

Small incisional hernias should be treated by early repair since they may cause bowel obstruction. If the patient is unwilling to undergo surgery or is a poor surgical risk, symptoms may be controlled by an elastic binder.

Defects too large to close easily may be left without surgical repair if they are asymptomatic, since they are less likely to incarcerate bowel than smaller defects.

For only the very smallest incisional hernias (< 2 cm in diameter) should a direct fascia-to-fascia repair be considered. Interrupted or continuous closure may be used, but the sutures should be nonabsorbable. Sutures tied too tightly or tension on the repair will predispose to recurrence.

Although no specific diameter distinguishes a small from a large hernia, a hernia can be considered large when the fascial edges cannot be approximated without tension. Primary closure of a large defect is not advisable, since tension on the closure increases the risk of hernia recurrence. Increasingly, repair of large or recurrent defects is performed using nonabsorbable mesh. Although a variety of techniques exist for placement of the mesh, a retrorectus underlay achieves a lower recurrence rate than an edge-to-edge or onlay placement. If a large dead space persists, a closed drainage system is usually employed in the space above the fascia. The lowest recurrence is achieved if native tissues can be approximated over the mesh underlay.

Laparoscopic techniques are increasingly being used to repair incisional hernias and perform adhesiolysis electively. A sheet of synthetic material is secured to the abdominal wall as an underlay graft; the intraperitoneal placement of the graft enhances the durability of the repair, though it also increases the risk of bowel adhesions or fistula formation.

Alternative methods to repair very large hernias that close the fascial defect using the patient's native tissue include component separation techniques that allow primary closure in the midline (Figure 32-6). These techniques are especially indicated when the procedure is infected or contaminated, making synthetic mesh an unwise choice. In a contaminated or infected field biologic mesh of human or animal origin is increasingly used as an underlay since infection risk is high with synthetic mesh. Best results are seen, when native tissue can be brought together over the biologic mesh.

Prognosis

Results of randomized clinical trials show that mesh repair is superior to primary suture repair, even for small incisional hernias. Despite the increasing use of both open and laparoscopic mesh repairs, however, population-based studies show that incisional hernias continue to recur at a high rate after repair, and the recurrence rate increases with each subsequent reoperation for recurrence, reaching almost 40% on average after the third recurrence. Factors shown to increase risk of hernia recurrence include wound infection,

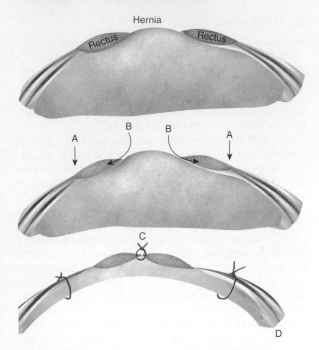

Hernia

Rectus   Rectus

A   B   B   A

C

D

▲ **Figure 32–6.** Component separation technique to allow primary closure in the midline, usually over a mesh underlay. **A.** Division of the external oblique aponeurosis. **B.** Release of the rectus from the posterior rectus sheath. **C.** Closure of the rectus in the midline. **D.** Mesh underlay.

the presence of abdominal aneurysms, smoking, and poor nutrition. Recurrence rates are so high in smokers that many surgeons require patients to stop smoking for a month before the operation. If patients are able to stop smoking, complications and recurrence are cut in half. In all techniques employing mesh, the underlay technique with at least 3-4 cm of underlay of the mesh leads to the lowest recurrence rates. In addition to a high recurrence rate after operations, complications such as infected mesh, bleeding, seroma, and erosion of mesh into bowel causing a fistula occur in a small percentage of cases. Mesh infection is more likely after repair of a hernia occurring in a wound with a previous infection.

Albright E et al: The component separation technique for hernia repair: a comparison of open and endoscopic techniques. *Am Surg* 2011;77:839-843.

Breuing K et al: Incisional ventral hernias: review of the literature and recommendations regarding the grading and technique of repair. *Surgery* 2010;148:544-558.

den Hartog D et al: Open surgical procedures for incisional hernias. *Cochrane Database Syst Rev* 2008 Jul 16;(3): CD006438

Itani KMF et al: Comparison of laparoscopic and open repair with mesh for the treatment of ventral incisional hernia. *Arch Surg* 2010;145:322-328.

Jin J et al: Laparoscopic versus open ventral hernia repair. *Surg Clin N Am* 2008;88:1083-1100.

Lindström D et al: Effects of a perioperative smoking cessation intervention on postoperative complications. *Ann Surg* 2008;248:739-745.

Melvin WS et al: Laparoscopic ventral hernia repair. *World J Surg* 2011;35:1496-1499.

Sauerland S et al: Laparoscopic versus open surgical techniques for ventral or incisional hernia repair. *Cochrane Database of Systematic Reviews* 2011 Mar 16;(3):CD007781.

PARASTOMAL HERNIA

A parastomal hernia is a particularly troublesome hernia to repair successfully, since the stoma's course through the abdominal wall is, by its very nature, a hernia. Studies cite an incidence of up to 50% for this type of hernia. Traditional teaching advises that a stoma be placed through the rectus muscle rather than more laterally, but even perfect stoma placement can result in hernia formation when the fascial opening stretches and allows additional loops of intestine to protrude. Causes include collagen defects and anything that increases intra-abdominal pressure such as straining, heavy lifting, or obesity.

Parastomal hernias should be repaired if they interfere with stoma function or are difficult to reduce, as they can incarcerate and strangulate. If the hernia is asymptomatic or very large, repair is not mandatory. Many options for repair of a parastomal hernia are described. Primary repair and moving the stoma have particularly poor results. The lowest recurrence is found with mesh repair by open or laparoscopic approach, placing the mesh beneath the rectus or intraperitoneally in a keyhole fashion. Because of the high risk of this hernia's occurrence, some even advocate the prophylactic use of mesh when the stoma is placed, though this practice has not gained widespread acceptance.

Israelsson L: Parastomal hernias. *Surg Clin N Am* 2008;88:113-125.

Tam KW: Systematic review of the use of a mesh to prevent parastomal hernia. *World J Surg* 2010;34:2723-2729.

VARIOUS RARE HERNIATIONS THROUGH THE ABDOMINAL WALL

▶ Littre Hernia

A Littre hernia is a hernia that contains a Meckel diverticulum in the hernia sac. Although Littre first described the condition in relation to a femoral hernia, the relative distribution of Littre hernias is as follows—inguinal, 50%; femoral, 20%; umbilical, 20%; and miscellaneous, 10%. Littre hernias of the groin are more common in men and on the right side. The clinical findings are similar to those of Richter hernia; when strangulation is present, pain, fever, and manifestations of small bowel obstruction occur late.

Treatment consists of repair of the hernia plus, if possible, excision of the diverticulum. If acute Meckel diverticulitis is present, the acute inflammatory mass may have to be treated through a separate abdominal incision.

► Amyand Hernia

An Amyand hernia is a groin hernia that contains the appendix. If the appendix is inflamed, it should be removed and the hernia repaired using native tissues or biologic mesh. If the appendix is normal and only an incidental finding in the hernia, it should be returned to the abdomen and a mesh repair employed.

Sharma H et al: Amyand's hernia: a report of 18 consecutive patients over a 15-year period. *Hernia* 2007;11:31-35.

► Spigelian Hernia

Spigelian hernia is an acquired ventral hernia through the linea semilunaris, the line where the sheaths of the lateral abdominal muscles fuse to form the lateral rectus sheath. Spigelian hernias are nearly always found above the level of the inferior epigastric vessels. They most commonly occur where the semicircular line (fold of Douglas) crosses the linea semilunaris.

The presenting symptom is pain that is usually localized to the hernia site and may be aggravated by any maneuver that increases intra-abdominal pressure. With time, the pain may become more dull, constant, and diffuse, making diagnosis more difficult.

If a mass can be demonstrated, the diagnosis presents little difficulty. The diagnosis is most easily made with the patient standing and straining; a bulge then presents in the lower abdominal area and disappears with a gurgling sound on pressure. Following reduction of the mass, the hernia orifice can usually be palpated.

Diagnosis is often made more difficult because the hernial defect may lie beneath an intact external oblique layer and therefore not be palpable. The hernia often dissects within the layers of the abdominal wall and may not present a distinct mass, or the mass may be located at a distance from the linea semilunaris. Patients with spigelian hernias should have a tender point over the hernia orifice, though tenderness alone is not sufficient to make the diagnosis. Both ultrasound and CT scan may help to confirm the diagnosis.

Spigelian hernias have a high incidence of incarceration and should be repaired. Small hernias may be repaired by primary aponeurotic closure though fascial defects larger than 2-3 cm should be repaired using mesh, preferable in an underlay, preperitoneal technique. Open or laparoscopic approach may be used according to the surgeon's experience, with laparoscopy affording an advantage in allowing the evaluation and treatment of bilateral hernia.

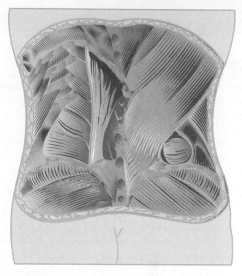

▲ **Figure 32–7.** Anatomic relationships of lumbar or dorsal hernia. On the left, lumbar or dorsal hernia into space of Grynfeltt. On the right, hernia into the Petit triangle (inferior lumbar space).

Bittner J et al: Mesh-free laparoscopic spigelian hernia repair. *Am Surg* 2008;74:713-720.
Saber A et al: Laparoscopic spigelian hernia repair: the scroll technique. *Am Surg* 2008;74:108-112.

► Lumbar or Dorsal Hernia

Lumbar or dorsal hernias (Figure 32–7) are hernias through the posterior abdominal wall at some level in the lumbar region. The most common sites (95%) are the superior (Grynfeltt) and inferior (Petit) lumbar triangles. A "lump in the flank" is the common complaint, associated with a dull, heavy, pulling feeling. With the patient erect, the presence of a reducible, often tympanitic mass in the flank usually makes the diagnosis. Incarceration and strangulation occur in about 10% of cases. Hernias in the inferior lumbar triangle are most often small and occur in young, athletic women. They present as tender masses producing backache and usually contain fat. Lumbar hernia must be differentiated from abscesses, hematomas, soft tissue tumors, renal tumors, and muscle strain.

Acquired hernias may be traumatic or nontraumatic. Severe direct trauma, penetrating wounds, abscesses, and poor healing of flank incisions are the usual causes. Congenital hernias occur in infants and are usually isolated unilateral congenital defects.

Lumbar hernias increase in size and should be repaired when found. Repair is by mobilization of the nearby fascia and obliteration of the hernia defect by precise fascia-to-fascia closure. The recurrence rate is very low.

Stamatiou D et al: Lumbar hernia: surgical anatomy, embryology, and technique of repair. *Am Surg* 2009;75:202-207.

Obturator Hernia

Herniation through the obturator canal is more frequent in elderly women and is difficult to diagnose preoperatively. The mortality rate (13%-40%) of these hernias makes them the most lethal of all abdominal hernias. These hernias most commonly present as small bowel obstruction with cramping abdominal pain and vomiting. The hernia is rarely palpable in the groin, though a mass may be felt on pelvic or rectal examination. The most specific finding is a positive Howship–Romberg sign, in which pain extends down the medial aspect of the thigh with abduction, extension, or internal rotation of the knee. Since this sign is present in fewer than half of cases, diagnosis should be suspected in any elderly debilitated woman without previous abdominal operations who presents with a small bowel obstruction. Though diagnosis can be confirmed by CT scan, operation should not be unduly delayed if complete bowel obstruction is present.

The abdominal approach gives the best exposure; these hernias should not be repaired from the thigh approach. The Cheatle–Henry approach (retropubic) may also be used. Simple repair is most often possible, though bladder wall, pectineal muscle, peritoneum, or mesh has been used when the defect cannot be approximated primarily.

Petrie A et al: Obturator hernia: anatomy, embryology, diagnosis, and treatment. *Clin Anat* 2011;24:562-569.
Stamatiou D et al: Obturator hernia revisited: surgical anatomy, embryology, diagnosis, and technique of repair. *Am Surg* 2011;77:1147-1157.

Perineal Hernia

A perineal hernia protrudes through the muscles and fascia of the perineal floor. It may be primary but is usually acquired following perineal prostatectomy, abdominoperineal resection of the rectum, or pelvic exenteration.

These hernias present as easily reducible perineal bulges and usually are asymptomatic but may present with pain, dysuria, bowel obstruction, or perineal skin breakdown.

Repair is usually done by an abdominal approach, with an adequate fascial and muscular perineal repair. Occasionally, polypropylene (Marlex) mesh or flaps using the gracilis, rectus abdominis, or gluteus may be necessary, when the available tissues are too attenuated for adequate primary repair.

Interparietal Hernia

Interparietal hernias, in which the sac insinuates itself between the layers of the abdominal wall, are usually of an indirect inguinal type but, rarely, may be direct or ventral hernias. Although interparietal hernias are rare, it is essential to recognize them, because strangulation is common and the mass is easily mistaken for a tumor or abscess. The lesion usually can be suspected on the basis of the physical examination provided it is kept in mind. In most cases, extensive studies for intra-abdominal tumors have preceded diagnosis. A lateral film of the abdomen will usually show bowel within the layers of the abdominal wall in cases with intestinal incarceration or strangulation, and an ultrasound or CT scan may be diagnostic.

As soon as the diagnosis is established, operation should be performed, usually through the standard inguinal approach.

Sciatic Hernia

Sciatic hernia is the rarest of abdominal hernias and consists of an outpouching of intra-abdominal contents through the greater sciatic foramen. The diagnosis is made after incarceration or strangulation of the bowel occurs. The repair is usually made through the abdominal approach. The hernia sac and contents are reduced, and the weak area is closed by making a fascial flap from the superficial fascia of the piriformis muscle.

TRAUMATIC HERNIA

Abdominal wall hernias occur rarely as a direct consequence of direct blunt abdominal injury. The patient presents with abdominal pain. On examination, ecchymosis of the abdominal wall and a bulge are usually present. The existence of a hernia may not be obvious, however, and the patient may require CT scan to confirm it. Because of the high incidence of associated intra-abdominal injuries, laparotomy is usually required. The defect should be repaired primarily if possible.

II. OTHER LESIONS OF THE ABDOMINAL WALL

CONGENITAL DEFECTS

Congenital defects of the abdominal wall other than hernias or lesions of the urachus and umbilicus are rare. The important ones involving the urachus and umbilicus are discussed in Chapter 43.

TRAUMA TO THE ABDOMINAL WALL

Rectus Sheath Hematoma

This is a rare but important entity that may follow mild trauma to the abdominal wall or may occur spontaneously in patients with disorders of coagulation, blood dyscrasia, or degenerative vascular diseases.

Abdominal pain localized to the rectus muscle is the presenting symptom. The pain may be sudden and severe in onset or slowly progressive. The key to diagnosis is the physical examination. Careful palpation will reveal a tender mass within the abdominal wall. When the patient tenses the rectus muscles by raising the head or body, the swelling becomes more tender and distinct on palpation, in contrast to an intra-abdominal mass or tenderness that disappears when the rectus muscles are contracted (Fothergill sign). In addition, there may be detectable discoloration or ecchymosis. If the physical signs are not diagnostic, ultrasound or CT scan will demonstrate the hematoma in the abdominal wall.

The condition does not commonly require operation. Coagulation abnormalities should be corrected if possible. The acute pain and discomfort usually disappear within 2-3 days, although a residual mass may persist for several weeks. Rarely bleeding persists, requiring embolization by interventional radiology.

PAIN IN THE ABDOMINAL WALL

A number of conditions are characterized by pain in the abdominal wall without a demonstrable organic lesion. Pain from a diaphragmatic, supradiaphragmatic, or spinal cord lesion may be referred to the abdomen. Herpes zoster (shingles) may present as abdominal pain, in which case it will follow a dermatomal distribution.

Scars may be sensitive or painful, particularly in the first 6 months after surgery.

Entrapment of a nerve by a nonabsorbable suture may cause persistent incisional pain, sometimes quite severe. Hyperesthesia of the skin over the involved dermatome may provide a clue to the cause. If local anesthetic nerve block relieves the pain, nerve block with alcohol or nerve excision may be performed.

In all cases of localized pain in the abdominal wall, careful search should be made for a small hernia—MRI or CT scan may be helpful to rule out a hernia.

ABDOMINAL WALL TUMORS

Tumors of the abdominal wall are not unusual, but most are benign, eg, lipomas, hemangiomas, and fibromas. Musculoaponeurotic fibromatoses (desmoid tumors), which often occur in abdominal wall scars or after parturition in women, are discussed in more detail in Chapter 44.

Endometriomas may also occur in the abdominal wall, particularly in the scars from gynecologic procedures and Caesarian sections. Most malignant tumors of the abdominal wall are metastatic. Metastases may appear by direct invasion from intra-abdominal lesions or by vascular dissemination. The sudden appearance of a sensitive nodule anywhere in the abdominal wall that is clearly not a hernia should arouse suspicion of an occult cancer, the lung and pancreas being the more likely primary sites.

MULTIPLE CHOICE QUESTIONS

1. The most important principle for successful repair of a groin hernia in an adult is

   A. Approximation of the conjoined tendon and inguinal ligament
   B. High ligation of the hernia sac
   C. A vertical relaxing incision in the anterior rectus sheath
   D. A tension free repair
   E. Reduction in the size of the internal inguinal ring

2. All of the following are features of a femoral hernia repair *except*

   A. Complete excision of the hernia sac
   B. Use of a relaxing incision in the anterior rectus sheath when a tissue repair is done
   C. Elimination of the defect in the transversalis fascia
   D. Use of Cooper's ligament or iliopubic tract
   E. Use of the inguinal ligament in the repair

3. Randomized trials of groin hernia repair show

   A. Equivalent recurrence rate of open and laparoscopic hernia repairs with mesh in the hands of experienced surgeons
   B. Lower operative complication rate with a laparoscopic extraperitoneal repair
   C. A greater rate of recurrence with open mesh repairs than laparoscopic repairs
   D. Less chronic pain and numbness with open mesh repairs than laparoscopic repairs
   E. Laparoscopic extraperitoneal repair had the lowest recurrence rate

4. Of the following, the greatest risk for incisional hernia after an abdominal operation is found in patients who

   A. Are more than 65 years old
   B. Have coronary artery disease
   C. Develop a wound infection
   D. Have diabetes
   E. Have COPD

5. Of the following, the most durable method of repairing a large incarcerated incisional hernia containing strangulated bowel is

   A. Open primary repair
   B. Open inlay synthetic mesh
   C. Open biologic mesh inlay
   D. Laparoscopic synthetic mesh
   E. Underlay of biologic mesh with primary tissue brought to midline

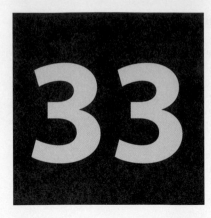

33

Adrenals

Quan-Yang Duh, MD

Chienying Liu, MD

J. Blake Tyrrell, MD

Operations on the adrenal glands are performed for primary hyperaldosteronism, pheochromocytoma, hypercortisolism (Cushing disease or Cushing syndrome), and adrenocortical carcinoma. These conditions are usually characterized by hypersecretion of one or more of the adrenal hormones. Less commonly, surgery may also be performed for nonfunctioning tumors or metastases.

ANATOMY & SURGICAL PRINCIPLES

The normal combined weight of the adrenals is 7-12 g. The right gland lies posterior and lateral to the vena cava and superior to the kidney (Figure 33–1). The left gland lies medial to the superior pole of the kidney, just lateral to the aorta and immediately posterior to the superior border of the pancreas. An important surgical feature is the remarkable constancy of the adrenal veins. The right adrenal vein, 2-5 mm long and several millimeters wide, connects the anteromedial aspect of the adrenal gland with the posterolateral aspect of the vena cava. The left adrenal vein is several centimeters long and travels inferiorly from the lower pole of the gland, joining the left renal vein after receiving the inferior phrenic vein. Variant venous drainage (multiple or anomalous veins) occurs in about 5% of glands and are more common for pheochromocytomas and larger tumors. The adrenal arteries are small, multiple, and inconstant. They usually come from the inferior phrenic artery, the aorta, and the upper pole branch of renal artery.

With the exception of rare nonsecreting cancers, indications for adrenal surgery result from hypersecretory states. Diagnosis and treatment begin with confirmation of a hypersecretory state (ie, measurement of excess cortisol, aldosterone, or catecholamines in blood or urine). In order to determine whether the problem originates in the adrenal, levels of the trophic hormone in question (ie, adrenocorticotropic hormone [ACTH] or renin) must be measured. If levels of the trophic hormone are suppressed but hormone secretion is excessive, autonomous secretion is proved. The next step, except in pheochromocytoma, is to determine the degree of autonomy, a process that usually distinguishes hyperplasias (which respond to most but not all controlling mechanisms) from adenomas and adenomas from cancers. In general, cancers are under little if any feedback control. If the primary problem is not in the adrenal, as in Cushing disease, treatment must be directed elsewhere when possible.

The major principles of adrenal surgery are as follows:

- Whenever possible, the surgeon must be certain of the diagnosis and the location of the lesion before undertaking the operation.

- The patient must be thoroughly prepared so he or she can withstand any metabolic problems caused by the disease or by the operation.

- The surgeon and consultants must be able to detect and treat any metabolic crisis that occurs during or after operation.

SURGICAL APPROACHES

Currently, almost all adrenal tumors are identified preoperatively by localization studies such as CT and MRI, so very few operations require general exploration of the abdomen. This permits the use of minimally invasive surgery. Almost all adrenal tumors can be removed laparoscopically. Traditional open adrenalectomy is necessary only when the tumor is especially large (eg, > 8-10 cm, depending on the surgeon's experience) or for locally invasive adrenocortical cancer where resection of lymph nodes or adjacent organs may be required.

Laparoscopic adrenalectomy can be performed using a transabdominal or retroperitoneal approach. Transabdominal laparoscopic adrenalectomy involves medial rotation of the spleen and pancreas (on the left) or

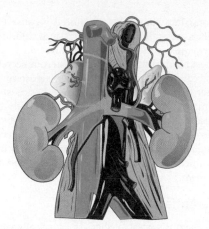

▲ **Figure 33–1.** Anatomy of the adrenals, showing venous return.

the liver (on the right), using gravity to drop the viscera away from the adrenal. Retroperitoneal adrenalectomy involved the use of high insufflation pressure to maintain the space for dissection and to decrease bleeding during dissection. Although transabdominal approach is more suitable for larger tumors and the retroperitoneal approach better for bilateral adrenalectomy and for patients with abdominal adhesions, surgeon preference usually dictate the choice of surgical approach.

The traditional open surgical approach is used when laparoscopic expertise is not available or when required by the size and invasiveness of the tumor. The advantages of laparoscopic operation are so great that it is strongly preferred.

The open anterior approach (midline, subcostal, or "L" incision) allows wide exposure for large tumors but causes more pain and wound complications, and it requires longer hospitalization. The open posterior approach through the bed of the 11th or 12th rib has been superseded by the laparoscopic approach. Thoracoabdominal incision may be used for large or invasive tumors.

DISEASES OF THE ADRENALS

PRIMARY ALDOSTERONISM

 ESSENTIALS OF DIAGNOSIS

▶ Hypertension with or without hypokalemia.

▶ Elevated aldosterone secretion and suppressed plasma renin activity.

▶ Metabolic alkalosis, relative hypernatremia.

▶ Weakness, polyuria, paresthesias, tetany, cramps due to hypokalemia.

▶ General Considerations

Aldosterone, the most potent mineralocorticoid secreted by the adrenal cortex, regulates the body's electrolyte composition, fluid volume, and blood pressure. Excess aldosterone increases total body sodium, decreases potassium levels, increases extracellular fluid volume (without edema), and increases blood pressure. Under normal conditions, aldosterone secretion is regulated by the renin-angiotensin system in a feedback fashion and is also stimulated transiently by ACTH.

In primary aldosteronism, aldosterone levels are elevated and renin levels are suppressed. In secondary hyperaldosteronism, increased aldosterone is due to increased renin secretion. Examples of secondary hyperaldosteronism include renovascular disease, renin-secreting tumors, and cirrhosis with low intravascular volume or diuretic use. Among the subtypes of primary aldosteronism, aldosterone-producing adenoma (APA, aldosteronoma) and idiopathic hyperaldosteronism (IHA) with adrenal hyperplasia are the most common types. Unilateral primary adrenal hyperplasia, aldosterone-producing adrenocortical carcinoma, and familial hyperaldosteronism (FH) (eg, FH type I-glucocorticoid-remediable hyperaldosteronism and FH type II) are rare. Surgery is beneficial only in patients with APAs and in patients with unilateral primary adrenal hyperplasia.

Primary aldosteronism in its classic form is characterized by hypertension, hypokalemia, increased aldosterone secretion, and suppressed plasma renin activity (PRA). However, hypokalemia is not required to make the diagnosis; recent studies have shown that many patients have a normal potassium level. Primary aldosteronism was once thought to be present in about 1% of patients with hypertension, but its prevalence has increased to 5%-13% based on various studies when plasma aldosterone concentration (PAC)-to-PRA was used to screen for hyperaldosteronism in patients with hypertension who were not hypokalemic. Although rare, normotensive primary aldosteronism has been described.

Aldosteronomas are usually solitary and small (0.5-2 cm). They have a characteristic golden-yellow color when sectioned. Tumor cells typically have heterogeneous cytomorphology, resembling those of all three zones of the adrenal cortex, including hybrid cells having cytologic features of the zona glomerulosa and zona fasciculata. Hyperplasia is also often seen in glands harboring adenomas.

▶ Clinical Findings

Aldosterone facilitates the exchange of sodium for potassium and hydrogen ions in the distal nephron. Therefore, when aldosterone secretion is chronically increased, serum potassium and hydrogen ion concentrations fall (hypokalemia and alkalosis), total body sodium rises, and hypertension results.

A. Symptoms and Signs

Symptoms, if present, are usually those of hypokalemia and depend on the severity of potassium depletion. Patients complain of a sense of malaise, muscle weakness, polyuria, polydipsia, cramps, and paresthesias. Tetany and hypokalemic paralysis occur rarely. Headaches are common. Hypertension is usually moderate to severe and may be refractory to medical therapy, but advanced retinopathy is rare. Although extracellular fluid volume is increased, edema is not seen unless renal failure occurs.

B. Laboratory Findings

1. Screening test—Primary aldosteronism should be suspected in patients with hypertension and hypokalemia—either spontaneous or following the administration of diuretics—and in patients with refractory hypertension. The diagnostic evaluation should start with screening tests. A simple ambulatory test determines the ratio of PAC, in nanograms per deciliter, to PRA, in nanograms per milliliter per hour, performed in the morning in a seated ambulant patient. A ratio greater than 20 with a PAC greater than 15 ng/dL suggests primary aldosteronism and warrants confirmatory biochemical studies. Hypertensive individuals without primary aldosteronism usually have ratios of less than 20. If the patient is taking an aldosterone receptor antagonist spironolactone or eplerenone, the data are uninterpretable, and estrogens increase PACs by increasing angiotensinogen. These agents should be discontinued for 6 weeks before the workup.

Many medications affect PAC and PRA. For example, PAC is decreased by angiotensin-converting enzyme inhibitors (ACE inhibitors), angiotensin receptor blockers (ARBs), central alpha-2 agonists such as clonidine, dihydropyridine (DHP) calcium channel antagonists such as amlodipine, and beta-blockers. PRA is increased by ACE inhibitors, ARBs, and DHP-calcium channel antagonists. These medications should be discontinued for 2 weeks if necessary. Peripheral α-adrenergic blockers such as doxazosin, terazosin, prazosin, hydralazine, and non-DHP calcium channel blocker such as verapamil are the preferred antihypertensive agents during evaluation. In many patients, it is unwise to withdraw antihypertensive medications, and one must be content with imperfect data.

2. Confirmatory test—If the screening test is positive, failure to suppress aldosterone secretion with sodium loading will confirm the diagnosis of primary aldosteronism in most patients. Normally aldosterone can be suppressed by oral salt loading or intravenous sodium chloride infusion. The patient should consume a high-sodium diet (5000 mg of sodium for 3 days) or be supplemented with NaCl tablets (2-3 g with each meal) if necessary. A 24-hour urine sample is collected for aldosterone and sodium on the third day.

Serum potassium should be monitored because the high-salt diet increases kaliuresis, and potassium chloride should be supplemented to avoid hypokalemia, which interferes with the test results by decreasing aldosterone secretion and may cause cardiac arrhythmias. Urinary aldosterone excretion higher than 12-14 μg/24 h distinguishes most patients with primary aldosteronism from those with essential hypertension on a high-salt diet, as confirmed by urinary sodium excretion exceeding 200 mEq/24 h. Alternatively, a PAC higher than 10 ng/mL after an infusion of 2 L of normal saline over 4 hours is also consistent with primary aldosteronism.

▶ Differential Diagnosis

Once the diagnosis is established, the surgically correctable forms—APA (aldosteronoma), constituting approximately 35% of primary aldosteronism, and the rare unilateral primary adrenal hyperplasia—should be distinguished from IHA, comprising approximately 65% of primary aldosteronism, due to bilateral adrenal hyperplasia, for which medical therapy is the best management. Aldosteronoma and IHA are the most common subtypes. Compared with those with IHA, patients with aldosteronoma have more severe hypertension, more severe hypokalemia, higher aldosterone secretion (> 20 ng/dL), higher 18-hydroxycorticosterone concentrations (> 100 ng/dL), and are younger. Interestingly more than one third of aldosteronomas have a somatic KCNJ5 gene mutation.

Glucocorticoid-remediable hyperaldosteronism (FH type I) is inherited in an autosomal dominant fashion. The genetic defect results in a chimeric gene. The mutated gene juxtaposes the promoter for expression of the 11-hydroxylase gene, which is ACTH-responsive, with the coding sequence of the aldosterone synthase gene. This leads to aldosterone production under ACTH stimulation in the zona fasciculata. Glucocorticoid therapy reverses this type of hyperaldosteronism. These patients have a family history of onset of hypertension at an early age. The diagnosis can be established by genetic testing. Measurement of 24-hour urine 18-hydroxycortisol and 18-oxocortisol levels is less reliable. The molecular basis for FH type II is not clear although it is also inherited in an autosomal dominant fashion.

Aldosterone-secreting adrenocortical carcinoma is rare and should be suspected if the tumor is larger than 4 cm, especially if it also secrets cortisol and intermediate metabolites.

▶ Tumor Localization

An APA can frequently be demonstrated by high-resolution CT or MRI scanning. Small aldosteronomas can be missed, and in such cases, a patient with a small aldosteronoma not seen on CT may be misdiagnosed as having adrenal hyperplasia. Aldosteronomas that coexist with nonfunctional adenomas can be mislabeled as adrenal hyperplasia because of multinodularity or bilateral masses on CT. Small abnormalities on CT scans may represent hyperplasia rather than true aldosteronomas. Therefore, unless an unequivocal unilateral tumor, preferably larger than 1 cm, is present on the CT scan and the contralateral gland is normal, the diagnosis and localization of aldosteronoma is not certain. When in doubt, adrenal vein sampling should be done. Blood is sampled from the adrenal veins and the inferior vena cava for aldosterone and cortisol levels at baseline and after ACTH infusion. Proper catheter placement is confirmed by finding high cortisol levels in adrenal venous blood compared with the inferior vena cava. Corrected aldosterone levels are calculated from the ratio of aldosterone to cortisol in each venous sample. A lateralization ratio of the corrected aldosterone level higher than 4 indicates unilateral aldosterone secretion, thereby confirming a diagnosis of aldosteronoma in most patients. Adrenal vein sampling is invasive and requires considerable skill and experience. The success rate for cannulating both adrenal veins is about 90% (60%-95% depending on experience of radiologists). Complication of venous sampling, such as adrenal hemorrhage can occur in 1% of patients. Some recommend adrenal vein sampling to be done routinely regardless of CT findings. Whereas others advocate using it selectively when CT scan findings are uncertain (no tumor, bilateral tumors, or small tumor < 1 cm in diameter).

Complications

Uncontrolled hypertension can lead to renal failure, stroke, and myocardial infarction. Severe hypokalemia can cause weakness, paralysis, and arrhythmia, especially in patients taking digitalis.

Treatment

The goal of therapy is to prevent the complications of hypertension and hypokalemia. Unilateral adrenalectomy is recommended for patients with aldosteronoma and medical therapy for those with IHA or those with aldosteronoma who are poor candidates for surgery.

A. Surgical Treatment

1. Preoperative preparation—Blood pressure and hypokalemia should be controlled before surgery. Spironolactone, a competitive aldosterone antagonist, has been the drug of choice. It blocks the mineralocorticoid receptor, promotes potassium retention, restores normal potassium concentrations, and reduces the extracellular fluid volume, thereby controlling blood pressure. Furthermore, it reactivates the suppressed renin-angiotensin-aldosterone system in the contralateral adrenal gland, reducing the risk of postoperative hypoaldosteronism. The medication should be continued to the day of operation. For additional information and

medical regiments for preoperative preparation, see Medical Treatment section.

2. Surgery—Because aldosteronomas are almost always small and benign, laparoscopic adrenalectomy is the procedure of choice. It can be performed safely and with equally good results by several approaches. The lateral transabdominal approach uses gravity to help medially rotate the viscera (liver on the right and spleen and pancreas on the left) and exposes the adrenal gland. It is the most versatile approach since the anatomy is familiar to most abdominal surgeons. The posterior retroperitoneal approach is best in patients with prior upper abdominal operations, but the working space is more limited. Although some surgeons perform a subtotal resection for aldosteronoma, most excise the whole adrenal gland with the tumor. The surrounding adrenal tissue frequently appears hyperplastic. Small aldosteronomas may not be visible intraoperatively. Bilateral adrenalectomy is not indicated, since hypocortisolism will require steroid-replacement treatment. Patients with IHA should be treated medically.

3. Postoperative care—Occasional patients may develop transient aldosterone deficiency because of suppression of the contralateral adrenal gland by the hyperfunctioning adenoma. This is rare in patients treated with spironolactone preoperatively. Symptoms include postural hypotension and hyperkalemia. Adequate sodium intake is usually sufficient for treatment; rarely, short-term fludrocortisone replacement (0.1 mg/d orally) is required.

B. Medical Treatment

The goal is to control hypertension and hypokalemia. Spironolactone, a competitive aldosterone antagonist, has been the drug of choice. Initial dosages of 200-400 mg/d may be required to control hypokalemia and hypertension. Once blood pressure is normalized and hypokalemia is corrected, the dose can be tapered and maintained at about 100-150 mg/d. Spironolactone may have antiandrogenic side effects, such as impotence, gynecomastia, menstrual irregularity, and gastrointestinal disturbances. These potential side effects may make this medication less desirable for some patients. Unlike spironolactone, which also blocks androgen and progesterone receptors, eplerenone is a selective mineralocorticoid receptor antagonist and has fewer endocrine side effects. It has been approved for treatment of hypertension and for heart failure after myocardial infarction. Eplerenone may become the treatment of choice for primary aldosteronism because of its decreased side effects if it is proven as efficacious as spironolactone, in spite of its increased cost. Amiloride, 20-40 ng/d, a potassium-sparing diuretic, may be used alternatively or as a supplement to spironolactone. Other medications, such as ACE inhibitors, calcium-channel blockers, and diuretics, may be required to control hypertension.

▶ Prognosis

Primary aldosteronism usually follows a prolonged and subtly changing course. Untreated hypertension may cause stroke, myocardial infarction, or renal failure.

Removal of an aldosteronoma normalizes potassium levels in nearly 100% of the patients, but hypertension is cured in about 50% of the patients. Persistent hypertension after operation is more common in overweigh men who preoperatively required more than three antihypertensive medications for more than 6 years, but residual hypertension is usually easier to control than before the operation. Essential hypertension and atherosclerosis due to chronic hypertension are contributing factors. Although patients with IHA should be treated medically, adrenalectomy is indicated for those with aldosteronoma because side effects of the medications and compliance make long-term medical treatment undesirable. The low morbidity, short hospitalization, and high success rate of laparoscopic adrenalectomy have made surgery preferable to long-term medical therapy.

Funder JW et al: Case detection, diagnosis, and treatment of patients with primary aldosteronism: an endocrine society clinical practice guideline. *J Clin Endocrinol Metab* 2008;93:3266.

Monticone S et al: Effect of KCNJ5 mutations on gene expression in aldosterone-producing adenomas and adrenocortical cells. *J Clin Endocrin Metab* 2012;97:1567.

Rossi GP et al: The adrenal vein sampling international study (AVIS) for identifying the major subtypes of primary aldosteronism. *J Clin Endocrin Metab* 2012;97:1606.

Stowasser M et al: Update in primary aldosteronism. *J Clin Endocrin Metab* 2009;94:3623.

Walz MK et al: Retroperitoneoscopic adrenalectomy in Conn's syndrome caused by adrenal adenomas or nodular hyperplasia. *World J Surg* 2008;32:847.

Zarnegar R et al: The aldosteronoma resolution score: predicting complete resolution of hypertension after adrenalectomy for aldosteronoma. *Ann Surg* 2008;247:511.

▼ PHEOCHROMOCYTOMA

ESSENTIALS OF DIAGNOSIS

▶ Hypertension, frequently sustained, with or without paroxysms.

▶ Episodic headache, excessive sweating, palpitation, and visual blurring.

▶ Postural tachycardia and hypotension.

▶ Elevated urinary catecholamines or their metabolites, hypermetabolism, hyperglycemia.

▶ General Considerations

Pheochromocytomas are tumors of the adrenal medulla and related chromaffin tissues elsewhere in the body (paragangliomas) that secrete epinephrine or norepinephrine, resulting in sustained or episodic hypertension and other symptoms of catecholamine excess.

Pheochromocytoma is found in less than 0.1% of patients with hypertension and accounts for about 5% of adrenal tumors incidentally discovered by CT scanning. Most pheochromocytomas occur sporadically without other diseases, but about one third are associated with various familial syndromes such as MEN2, NF1, VHL, and familial paraganglioma syndromes. Patients with multiple endocrine neoplasia (MEN)2A may have medullary thyroid carcinoma, pheochromocytoma, and hyperparathyroidism. Those with MEN2B have medullary thyroid carcinoma, pheochromocytoma, mucosal neuromas, marfanoid habitus, and ganglioneuromatosis. Patients with neurofibromatosis type I have café au lait spots, neurofibromatosis, and pheochromocytoma. Patients with von Hippel–Lindau disease may have retinal hemangioma, hemangioblastoma of the central nervous system, renal cysts and carcinoma, pheochromocytoma, pancreatic cysts or neuroendocrine tumors, and epididymal cystadenoma. Familial paraganglioma syndromes are caused by mutations of the succinate dehydrogenase genes *SDHx* (*SDHB, SDHD, SDHC, SDHA,* and *SDHAF2*). All are associated with extra-adrenal paragangliomas. *SDHB* is particularly associated with malignant pheochromocytomas. These syndromes should be considered especially in young patients and in patients with multifocal, extra-adrenal, malignant, or recurrent tumors. Other genetic mutations associated with pheochromocytomas are *TMEM127* and *MAX*. Because of the higher than previously expected prevalence of hereditary pheochromocytoma, all patients with pheochromocytoma should be considered for genetic counseling and testing. The specific genes tests should depend on clinical and biochemical findings and family history. Family members of patients who have been diagnosed with these syndromes also need screening to determine whether they are gene carriers and are at risk for developing the various tumors, including pheochromocytoma.

On pathologic examination, pheochromocytoma appears reddish-gray and frequently has areas of necrosis, hemorrhage, and sometimes cysts. The usual size is about 100 g, or 5 cm in diameter, but they can be as small as 2-3 cm or as large as 12-16 cm. Cells are pleomorphic, showing prominent nucleoli and frequent mitoses. Cytologic findings cannot be used to determine whether a pheochromocytoma is malignant or benign. The veins and capsules may also be invaded even in clinically benign tumors. Malignancy can only be diagnosed in the presence of metastases in non-chromffin cell bearing tissues or invasion into surrounding tissues.

▶ Clinical Findings

A. Symptoms and Signs

The clinical findings of pheochromocytoma are variable, and almost half of them come to attention because of an incidental finding of an adrenal tumor (incidentaloma) on CT or MRI scans performed to evaluate other diseases. Classically, the patient has episodic hypertension associated with the triad of palpitation, headache, and sweating. The patient may also complain of anxiety, tremors, weight loss, dizziness, nausea and vomiting, abdominal discomfort, constipation, and visual blurring. Rarely pheochromocytomas can secrete VIP causing severe diarrhea or ACTH causing Cushing syndrome. The physical examination may be unremarkable except during an attack, when pallor and excess sweating may be observed. Tachycardia, postural hypotension, and hypertensive retinopathy are other signs.

Hypertension, the most common feature of pheochromocytoma, occurs in 90% of patients. More than half have sustained hypertension, which may be mild to moderate, with or without other signs and symptoms of catecholamine excess, and the diagnosis may be missed. In some cases, basal blood pressure may not be elevated, and severe hypertension occurs only while the patient is under stress, such as general anesthesia or trauma. Patients with diastolic hypertension and postural hypotension who are not receiving antihypertensive medications may have pheochromocytoma. Hyperglycemia may occur because epinephrine raises blood glucose and norepinephrine decreases insulin secretion.

In children, hypertension is less prominent, and about 50% have multiple or extra-adrenal tumors. Paragangliomas due to *SDHB* mutations are more likely to metastasize. Pheochromocytomas occur in 40%-50% of patients with MEN2; they tend to be bilateral and multiple but are rarely extra-adrenal or malignant. Biochemical screening for gene carriers of hereditary pheochromocytoma should be performed routinely. Measurement of plasma free metanephrines (metanephrine and normetanephrine) is the most sensitive test for pheochromocytoma in familial syndromes.

B. Laboratory Findings

The diagnosis of pheochromocytoma is best confirmed either by 24-hour urinary fractionated catecholamines and metanephrines measured in the same collection or by plasma free metanephrines. Both tests have high diagnostic sensitivity and specificity (Figure 33–2). Plasma free metanephrines is more sensitive than the urine test, but it has a higher false-positive rate, especially in elderly patients. Urinary output of metanephrines and/or free catecholamines is elevated in more than 95% of patients with pheochromocytoma. In 80% of patients, the level exceeds twice normal. Measurement of urinary vanillylmandelic acid (VMA) is less sensitive, and this test should no longer be used. Assays using high-performance liquid chromatography (HPLC) reduce interference by drugs and diets, but HPLC assays differ among various testing labs, and many drugs and diets can potentially interfere with certain HPLC assays or affect the secretion and metabolism of catecholamines. Examples

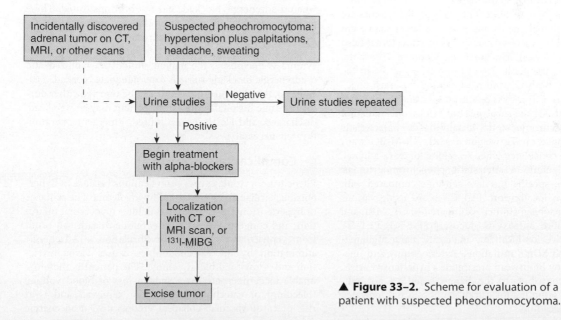

▲ **Figure 33–2.** Scheme for evaluation of a patient with suspected pheochromocytoma.

include acetaminophen, labetalol, vasodilators (nitroglycerin and nitroprusside), nifedipine, theophylline, stimulants (amphetamine, caffeine, nicotine, methylphenidate), many antipsychotics, antidepressants (especially tricyclic antidepressants), buspirone, prochlorperazine, and methyldopa. Interpretation of the study may also be affected by coffee, ethanol, bananas, radiographic dyes, drugs that contain catecholamines, and withdrawal from clonidine. These agents should be discontinued for 2 weeks before measuring urinary catecholamines and metanephrines. The interfering substances vary depending on the specific assays used, so a list and protocol for preparing the patient should be obtained from the specific laboratory. Liquid chromatography-tandem mass spectrometry is a newer assay that has been shown to minimize drug interferences in the measurement of plasma and urinary metanephrines and may improve its diagnostic accuracy.

Overnight urinary collection and short collection periods following a paroxysm, indexed to creatinine, have also been used. Measuring plasma free metanephrines is 96%-100% sensitive and 85%-89% specific. Depending on the particular assay, caffeic acid found in coffee, acetaminophen, phenoxybenzamine, and tricyclic antidepressants may cause false-positive results. Provocative tests—using glucagon, histamine, or tyramine—are not accurate and are potentially dangerous; they are no longer used. Clonidine suppression tests are rarely used.

C. Tumor Localization

Localization studies should be performed only after biochemical studies have confirmed the diagnosis of a catecholamine-secreting tumor. Ninety percent of pheochromocytomas are found in the adrenal glands and most are larger than 3 cm in diameter. Of the extra-adrenal pheochromocytomas (also called paragangliomas), 75% are in the abdomen, 10% in the bladder, 10% in the chest, 2% in the pelvis, and 3% in the head and neck. Both CT and MRI can localize most pheochromocytomas. CT scan is less expensive and gives better anatomic details for the surgeons, but MRI avoids radiation exposure. Pheochromocytoma usually has a characteristic bright appearance on T2-weighted MRI. ^{123}I-MIBG scanning should be considered when searching for extra-adrenal, multiple, malignant, or metastatic pheochromocytomas. MIBG is more specific but less sensitive compared with CT or MRI for localization. PET-CT scans using various PET tracers have been studied. Compared to CT, MRI, and MIBG, 18F-fluoro-2-deoxy-D-glucose (18F-FDG) PET-CT is more sensitive for localizing metastatic paragangliomas in patients with *SDHB* mutations. Arteriography and fine-needle aspiration biopsy can precipitate a hypertensive crisis. They do not contribute to the diagnosis and are not indicated. Venous sampling for catecholamines is not indicated and can be misleading.

▶ Differential Diagnosis

The differential diagnosis includes all causes of hypertension. Hyperthyroidism and pheochromocytoma have many features in common (weight loss, tremor, and tachycardia). The diagnosis of pheochromocytoma is easier if episodic hypertension is present. Acute anxiety attacks mimic the symptoms and may precipitate hypertensive episodes, but anxiety alone rarely produces severe hypertension. Carcinoid syndrome causing episodes of flushing may also be mistaken for pheochromocytoma. Urinary 5-HIAA level is usually markedly elevated, and CT scan may show liver metastases in patients with carcinoid syndrome. Labile essential hypertension is not associated with elevated catecholamine levels.

Pheochromocytoma in pregnancy, if not recognized, will kill half of the fetuses and nearly half of the mothers. Hypertension in pregnancy is usually ascribed to preeclampsia-eclampsia. The diagnosis of pheochromocytoma requires the same biochemical studies; MRI is indicated to localize the tumor when a biochemical diagnosis has been established. CT or MIBG is not used to avoid radiation exposure. α-Adrenergic and β-adrenergic blockers are well tolerated. Timing of the operation is individualized. If recognized early, the tumor is best removed early in the second trimester. Otherwise, α-adrenergic blockade is continued. A planned cesarean section at term is followed by laparoscopic adrenalectomy a few weeks postpartum.

Pheochromocytoma crisis may develop in patients with pheochromocytoma, usually precipitated by trauma, certain medications, surgery, or other procedures. It can also be triggered by glucocorticoids. Crisis usually occurs when α-adrenergic blockade has not been instituted. These patients may develop multisystem failure, especially cardiovascular complications. If pheochromocytomas crisis is not recognized, death is the usual result. Once pheochromocytoma is diagnosed, the patient should be stabilized and α-adrenergic blockade started. After adequate blockade (10-14 days), the pheochromocytoma can be resected either during the same hospitalization or the patient may be stabilized, discharged, and electively readmitted. Emergent operation is rarely necessary.

▶ Complications

Pheochromocytoma causes complications because of hypertension, cardiac arrhythmia, and hypovolemia. The sequelae of hypertension are stroke, renal failure, myocardial infarction, and congestive heart failure. Sudden death can result from ventricular tachycardia or fibrillation. α-Adrenergic stimulation by the catecholamines causes vasoconstriction and a low total blood volume. The patient is therefore unable to compensate for a sudden loss of blood volume (bleeding) or catecholamines (tumor removal) and is at risk of cardiovascular collapse. Preoperative α-adrenergic blockade and restoration of blood volume can prevent these complications.

▶ Treatment

A. Medical Treatment

Treatment with α-adrenergic blocking agents should be started as soon as the biochemical diagnosis is established. The aims of preoperative therapy are (1) to restore the blood volume, which has been depleted by excessive catecholamines; (2) to prevent a severe crisis, with its potential complications; and (3) to allow the patient to recover from cardiomyopathy. Close control of hypertension is necessary in order to keep blood volume normal.

Phenoxybenzamine, a nonselective α-adrenergic antagonist, has a long duration of action and is the preferred drug. It should be started at a dosage of 10 mg/12 h, and the dose should be increased by 10-20 mg every 2-3 days—as postural hypotension allows. Usual doses are 100-160 mg/d; however, dosages as high as 300 mg/d may be necessary. Most patients require 10-14 days of treatment, as judged by stabilization of blood pressure and reduction of symptoms. Nasal stuffiness is usually present when alpha blockade is well established. Calcium-channel blockers and competitive selective α-adrenergic blocking agents such as doxazosin and prazosin may also be effective. Metyrosine inhibits tyrosine hydroxylase and reduces catecholamine synthesis, and can be added to phenoxybenzamine as preoperative therapy.

β-Adrenergic blocking agents are often used to treat arrhythmias and tachycardia but should only be given after alpha blockade has been achieved. Otherwise, a hypertensive crisis may be precipitated because of the unopposed α-adrenergic effect of the catecholamines. Opioids should be avoided because they may stimulate histamine release and precipitate a crisis.

B. Surgical Treatment

The definitive treatment of pheochromocytoma is excision after preoperative localization and alpha-adrenergic blockade.

Smaller (< 5-6 cm) adrenal pheochromocytomas can be safely resected by laparoscopic adrenalectomy. Larger (> 8-10 cm), locally invasive and extra-adrenal tumors are technically more difficult and may require open resection.

During surgery, an arterial line is necessary for continuous blood pressure monitoring. Monitoring of pulmonary artery pressure is usually not necessary in patients who are well blocked.

Nitroprusside should be immediately available to treat sudden hypertension and beta-blockers to treat the cardiac dysrhythmias that may occur when the tumor is manipulated. Manipulation of the gland is less with laparoscopic adrenalectomy, which minimizes fluctuations in plasma catecholamine levels.

Very large malignant tumors may require a thoracoabdominal incision. Malignant pheochromocytomas may invade the adrenal vein or vena cava. Extra-adrenal pheochromocytomas (paragangliomas) are usually found along the abdominal aorta and in the organ of Zuckerkandl near the aortic bifurcation around the inferior mesenteric artery. However, tumors have been found in widely scattered sites such as the bladder, the vagina, the mediastinum, the neck, and even skull base and pericardium. In general, extra-adrenal tumors should be localized with MIBG, CT, MRI, or PET-CT preoperatively to avoid a blind exploration.

In patients with MEN2 or VHL and bilateral pheochromocytomas, cortical-sparing subtotal adrenalectomy on the side of the smaller tumor may avoid postoperative adrenal insufficiency, though it increases the risk for recurrence. In patients with a known hereditary pheochromocytoma syndrome and a unilateral pheochromocytoma, prophylactic resection of the contralateral normal-appearing adrenal gland is not indicated, since bilateral adrenalectomy leads to lifelong hypoadrenalism requiring cortisol replacement. These patients should be followed with biochemical evaluations, and the contralateral adrenal gland should be resected only if pheochromocytoma develops.

Patients undergoing resection of pheochromocytoma who are not adequately prepared preoperatively may have hypertensive crises, cardiac arrhythmia, myocardial infarction, or acute pulmonary edema. In addition, these patients may experience intractable hypotension and die in shock after tumor removal. If the patient has been properly prepared with alpha-blockers, the changes in blood pressure will not be severe. Otherwise, intravenous infusion of large amounts of saline and vasopressors may be necessary to maintain blood pressure after the tumor is removed. Hypoglycemia may develop after tumor removal so blood glucose level should be checked until the patient is eating.

▶ Prognosis

Patients with untreated pheochromocytoma are at high risk for complications from hypertensive crisis and cardiovascular disease, whereas the operative mortality rate is 0%-3%. Mild to moderate essential hypertension may persist after surgery. Second tumors in the remaining adrenal or metastatic tumors can occur years after excision of the primary pheochromocytoma; long-term follow-up is mandatory. Patients with pheochromocytoma should be offered genetic counseling and when appropriate tested for hereditary causes of pheochromocytoma. Long-term prognosis may depend on the mutation present (eg, risk for malignant pheochromocytoma in *SDHB* mutation gene carriers). Metastatic or recurrent malignant pheochromocytoma should be resected if possible to reduce the catecholamine load. Treatment with high-dose ^{131}I-MIBG may be helpful in these patients.

Biggar MA et al: Systematic review of phaeochromocytoma in pregnancy. *Br J Surg* 2013;100:182.

Gimenez-Roqueplo AP et al: An update on the genetics of paraganglioma, pheochromocytoma, and associated hereditary syndromes. *Horm Metab Res* 2012;44:328.

Scholten A et al: Pheochromocytoma crisis is not a surgical emergency. *J Clin Endocrinol Metab* 2013;98:581-91.

Shen WT et al: One hundred two patients with pheochromocytoma treated at a single institution since the introduction of laparoscopic adrenalectomy. *Arch Surg* 2010;145:893.

Walz MK et al: Laparoscopic and retroperitoneoscopic treatment of pheochromocytomas and retroperitoneal paragangliomas: results of 161 tumors in 126 patients. *World J Surg* 2006;30:899.

Wiseman GA et al: Usefulness of 123I-MIBG scintigraphy in the evaluation of patients with known or suspected primary or metastatic pheochromocytoma or paraganglioma: results from a prospective multicenter trial. *J Nucl Med* 2009;50:1448.

HYPERCORTISOLISM (CUSHING DISEASE & CUSHING SYNDROME)

ESSENTIALS OF DIAGNOSIS

▶ Facial plethora, dorsocervical fat pad, supraclavicular fat pad, truncal obesity, easy bruisability, purple striae, acne, hirsutism, impotence or amenorrhea, muscle weakness, and psychosis.

▶ Hypertension, hyperglycemia, and osteopenia or osteoporosis.

General Considerations

Cushing syndrome is due to chronic glucocorticoid excess. It may be caused by excess ACTH stimulation or by adrenocortical tumors that secrete glucocorticoids independently of ACTH stimulation. Excess ACTH may be produced by pituitary adenomas (Cushing disease) or extrapituitary ACTH-producing tumors (ectopic ACTH syndrome). Cushing syndrome not dependent on ACTH is usually caused by primary adrenal diseases such as adrenocortical adenoma and micronodular or macronodular hyperplasia or carcinoma.

The natural history of Cushing syndrome depends on the underlying disease and varies from a mild, indolent disease to rapid progression and death.

Clinical Findings

A. Symptoms and Signs

See Table 33–1. The classic description of Cushing syndrome includes truncal obesity, hirsutism, moon facies, acne, buffalo hump, purple striae, hypertension, and diabetes, but other signs and symptoms are common. Weakness and

Table 33–1. Frequency of manifestations of hypercortisolism.

	Percentage (%)
Obesity	95
Hypertension	70
Glucose tolerance	80
Centripetal distribution of fat	80
Weakness	20
Muscle atrophy in upper and lower extremities	70
Hirsutism	80
Menstrual disturbance or impotence	75
Purple striae	50
Plethoric facies	85
Easy bruisability	35
Acne	40
Psychological symptoms	40
Edema	20
Headache	15
Back pain	60

depression are striking features. Weakness and other features are also seen after prolonged and excessive administration of adrenocortical steroids.

In children, Cushing syndrome is most commonly caused by adrenal cancers, but adenomas and nodular hyperplasia have been described. Cushing syndrome in children also causes growth retardation or arrest.

B. Pathologic Examination

The pathologic features of the adrenal gland depend on the underlying disease. Normal adrenal glands weigh 7-12 g combined. The hyperplastic adrenal glands in patients with Cushing disease weigh less than 25 g combined. In ectopic ACTH syndrome, the combined adrenal weight is greater—from 25 to 100 g.

Adrenal adenomas in Cushing syndrome range in weight from a few grams to over 100 g, usually over 3 cm in diameter, and are larger than APAs. The typical cells usually resemble those of the zona fasciculata. Variable degrees of anaplasia are seen, and differentiation of benign from malignant tumors is often difficult on the basis of cytology alone. These adrenal adenomas occur more frequently in women. Adrenal cancers are frequently very large—almost always over 5 cm in diameter. They are undifferentiated, invade the surrounding tissues, and metastasize via the blood stream.

Rare forms of ACTH-independent Cushing syndrome include ACTH-independent macronodular adrenal hyperplasia, which in some cases is due to aberrant expression of receptors in the adrenals that respond to stimuli other than ACTH. In these cases, the adrenal glands can be massively enlarged. Primary pigmented nodular adrenal disease or micronodular hyperplasia is associated with the syndrome of Carney complex that also includes cardiac myxoma and lentigines.

Rarely, ectopic adrenal tissue can be the source of excessive cortisol secretion. It has been found in various locations, most commonly near the abdominal aorta.

Cushing disease is caused by pituitary adenomas.

Ectopic ACTH syndrome is usually caused by small-cell lung cancer and neuroendocrine tumors (carcinoid tumors) of the pancreas, thymus, thyroid, prostate, esophagus, colon, and ovaries. Pheochromocytoma and malignant melanoma may also secrete ACTH.

C. Laboratory Findings

Since no single test is specific, a combination of tests must be used.

Normal subjects have a circadian rhythm of ACTH secretion that is paralleled by cortisol secretion. Levels are highest in the early morning and decline during the day to their lowest levels in the late evening. In Cushing syndrome, the circadian rhythm is abolished, and total secretion of cortisol is increased. In mild cases, the plasma cortisol and ACTH levels may be within the normal range during much of the day but abnormally high in the evening.

When Cushing syndrome is suspected, the first objective is to establish the diagnosis; the second is to establish the cause. An algorithm for the diagnosis is presented in Figure 33–3. When hypercortisolism is suspected, three tests are available as the initial tests to establish the diagnosis: overnight dexamethasone suppression test, measurement of 24-hour urinary free cortisol, and late night salivary cortisol sampling. Dexamethasone, 1 mg orally will suppress ACTH secretion and stop cortisol production in most healthy individuals. This low-dose dexamethasone, however, will not suppress excessive cortisol production from autonomous adrenocortical tumors or adrenals that are being stimulated by excess ACTH. Since dexamethasone does not cross-react in the assay for plasma cortisol, suppression of endogenous circulating cortisol is easily demonstrated. The test is done as follows: At 11 PM, the patient is given 1 mg of dexamethasone by mouth. A fasting plasma cortisol is measured the following morning between 8 and 9 AM. Suppression of plasma cortisol to 1.8 µg/dL (50 nmol/L) or less excludes Cushing syndrome. Higher cutoff levels have been recommended, but some patients with mild ACTH-dependent Cushing syndrome may be suppressed easily; thus, the response is falsely negative and the diagnosis of Cushing syndrome is missed. On the other hand, this low cutoff level increases the likelihood of a false-positive result. False-positive results are more common in patients with depression, alcoholism,

physiologic stress, marked obesity, obstructive sleep apnea, or renal failure and in those taking estrogens or drugs that accelerate dexamethasone metabolism, such as phenytoin, rifampin, and phenobarbital. Estrogens increase cortisol-binding globulin and elevate total plasma cortisol concentrations. In these situations, measurement of 24-hour urinary free cortisol or salivary cortisol is preferred. Twenty-four-hour urinary cortisol directly measures the physiologically active form of circulating cortisol, integrates the daily variations of cortisol production, and is very sensitive and specific for the diagnosis of Cushing syndrome.

Late night salivary cortisol sampling can also assist in establishing the diagnosis of Cushing syndrome. The procedure involves chewing a cotton tube for 2-3 minutes between 11 PM and 12 AM. Salivary cortisol levels correlate highly with plasma and serum-free cortisol levels. One positive initial screening test result should be confirmed by a second initial screening test to establish the diagnosis. *Once the diagnosis of Cushing syndrome is established,* the next step is to determine the cause. Plasma ACTH measurement by immunoradiometric assay is the most direct method. A normal to elevated ACTH level is diagnostic of hypercortisolism due to pituitary adenoma or ectopic ACTH secretion. Suppressed ACTH levels are diagnostic of hypercortisolism due to a primary adrenal cause such as adenoma, carcinoma, or nodular hyperplasia.

The differential diagnosis of ACTH-dependent Cushing syndrome can be challenging. No test is perfect, and a combination of tests may be necessary. Since 90% of patients have Cushing disease, pituitary MRI is the first test to identify the source of ACTH secretion. However, 10% of normal adults have incidental pituitary lesions 3-6 mm in diameter on MRI, and many patients with Cushing disease have no detectable lesions. Lesions smaller than 3-4 mm are more likely to represent normal variation, artifacts, volume averaging, incidental nonfunctional adenomas, or cysts. An unequivocal pituitary lesion (ie, > 4-5 mm in diameter with decreased signal intensity on gadolinium) strongly suggests Cushing disease.

If the pituitary MRI does not show a definite lesion, the next step is inferior petrosal sinus sampling with corticotropin-releasing hormone (CRH) stimulation. Compared with other biochemical tests, such as high-dose dexamethasone suppression or CRH stimulation, petrosal sinus sampling is the most accurate way to identify an ACTH-secreting pituitary adenoma; the diagnostic accuracy is close to 100%. The test requires simultaneous bilateral venous sampling from the inferior petrosal sinuses. The inferior petrosal sinus connects the cavernous sinus to the jugular bulb and drains the pituitary. A central-to-peripheral ACTH ratio of 2 or greater without CRH stimulation is diagnostic of Cushing disease. CRH, 100 µg given intravenously as a bolus injection, can increase the diagnostic sensitivity to 100%; a peak central-to-peripheral ACTH ratio of 3 or greater is diagnostic of

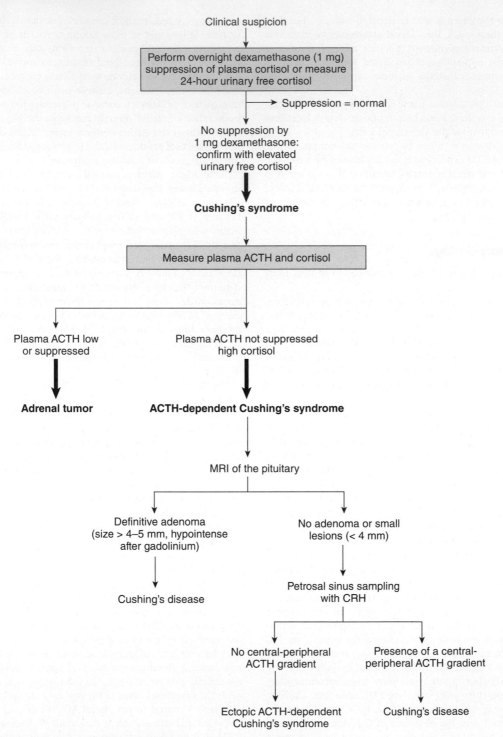

▲ **Figure 33–3.** Cushing syndrome: diagnosis and differential diagnosis.

Cushing disease. The lack of a central-to-peripheral ACTH gradient is diagnostic of an ectopic ACTH-secreting tumor.

In Cushing syndrome caused by primary adrenal diseases, the plasma ACTH level is suppressed. Adenomas are usually 3-5 cm in diameter and secrete only cortisol. Adrenal carcinomas are typically larger than 5 cm in diameter, are usually rapidly progressive, and may cosecrete other hormones, such as adrenal androgens, deoxycorticosterone, aldosterone, and estrogens.

D. Imaging Studies

For Cushing syndrome caused by primary adrenal diseases, thin-section CT or MRI is able to detect virtually all of the adrenal tumors and hyperplasia. MRI of the sella is the imaging study of choice for pituitary adenomas. If a definitive adenoma is not seen, inferior petrosal sinus sampling with CRH stimulation can differentiate Cushing disease from ectopic Cushing syndrome. For ectopic Cushing syndrome, CT or MRI of the chest and abdomen may detect ACTH-secreting tumors. Bronchial carcinoids may be very small and difficult to find; high-resolution thin-cut CT of the chest is indicated. Occasionally, the source of an ectopic ACTH-secreting tumor cannot be determined (occult ectopic ACTH syndrome).

▶ Complications

Severe or lethal complications may result from sustained hypercortisolism, including hypertension, cardiovascular disease, stroke, thromboembolism, infection, severe debilitating muscle wasting, and weakness. Psychosis is common. Death may also be caused by the underlying tumors, such as adrenal carcinoma, small cell lung cancer, and others causing ectopic ACTH syndrome.

The truncal obesity and muscle weakness in patients with Cushing syndrome predispose them to postoperative pulmonary complications. Atrophic skin and easy bruisability also predict poor wound healing.

Nelson syndrome, the progression of an ACTH-secreting pituitary adenoma following bilateral adrenalectomy for Cushing disease, occurred in as many as 30% of patients in the era when bilateral adrenalectomy was used as primary therapy. However, since transsphenoidal resection has become the initial procedure of choice for Cushing disease, and because MRI now allows accurate diagnosis of pituitary adenomas larger than 5 mm, Nelson syndrome occurs in less than 5% of patients.

These tumors in patients with Nelson syndrome are among the most aggressive of pituitary tumors, causing sellar enlargement and extrasellar extension. Plasma ACTH levels are markedly elevated. Patients are frequently hyperpigmented and hypopituitary, with symptoms of mass effects including headaches, visual field deficits, and even blindness from optic nerve compression. Removal of feedback control from hypercortisolism at the pituitary level probably explains the aggressiveness of these tumors.

▶ Treatment

Resection is the best treatment for cortisol-producing adrenal tumors or ACTH-producing tumors. Other treatment options may be necessary to temporarily control hypercortisolism—or for patients not cured by resection or when complete resection is impossible.

A. Excision of Pituitary Adenoma

Patients with Cushing disease are usually treated by transsphenoidal microsurgical excision of the pituitary adenomas. Relief of symptoms is rapid, and the prognosis for adequate residual pituitary-adrenal function is good. Total or subtotal hypophysectomy may be performed in older patients if a discrete tumor is not found. Pituitary procedures fail in about 15%-25% of patients because of failure to find the adenoma, pituitary hyperplasia, or recurrence of adenoma. When pituitary surgery fails, the disease may respond to pituitary irradiation. In some patients, medical therapy or total adrenalectomy will be necessary. Because of the effectiveness of pituitary microsurgery, radiotherapy is usually not recommended as primary treatment for Cushing disease.

B. Adrenalectomy

Compared with patients with other adrenal tumors, those with severe Cushing syndrome are at a higher risk for postoperative complications such as wound infection, hemorrhage, peptic ulceration, and pulmonary embolism. Adrenalectomy, however, is usually successful in reversing the devastating effects of hypercortisolism.

Laparoscopic adrenalectomy causes less morbidity than open adrenalectomy and is preferred for benign hyperplasia or adenomas. Laparoscopic adrenalectomy for adrenocortical carcinoma is technically challenging. If necessary, the operation should be converted to laparotomy to achieve complete tumor resection without breaching the capsule. Local recurrence may be more common after laparoscopic resection for large and invasive cancer, especially if the capsule is breached during dissection.

Unilateral adrenalectomy is indicated for adrenal adenomas or carcinomas that secrete cortisol. The contralateral adrenal gland and the hypothalamic-pituitary-adrenal axis will usually recover from the suppression 1-2 years after the operation. Subtotal resection is not indicated because adenoma and carcinoma may not be readily distinguishable.

Total bilateral adrenalectomy is indicated for selected patients with Cushing disease or ectopic ACTH syndrome in whom the ACTH-secreting tumor cannot be found or resected. It is also indicated for patients with bilateral primary adrenal disease, such as pigmented micronodular hyperplasia or massive macronodular hyperplasia.

Bilateral adrenalectomy can almost always be accomplished by the laparoscopic approach.

Subtotal resection is not recommended in patients with Cushing syndrome, because it usually leaves inadequate adrenocortical reserve initially, and the disease frequently recurs with continuing ACTH stimulation. Total bilateral adrenalectomy with adrenal gland autotransplantation is rarely successful and offers little advantage over pharmacologic replacement.

C. Medical Treatment

Drugs are mainly used as adjuvant therapy. Hypercortisolism may be controlled with ketoconazole, metyrapone, or aminoglutethimide, all of which inhibit steroid biosynthesis. Ketoconazole is usually the first choice. A combination of drugs may be necessary to control hypercortisolism and to decrease dose-related side effects.

Mifepristone (RU 486), a progesterone and glucocorticoid receptor antagonist, is also effective, but it raises cortisol and ACTH levels, making it difficult to monitor the patient. Experience with the medication is still limited.

Mitotane is a dichlorodiphenyltrichloroethane derivative that is toxic to the adrenal cortex. It has been used with modest success in the treatment of adrenal hypersecretory states, especially adrenocortical carcinoma. Unfortunately, serious side effects are common at effective doses.

Pasireotide, a somatostatin analog, and cabergoline, a dopamine receptor (type 2) agonist, may be effective in controlling hypercortisolism in small subsets of patients with Cushing disease. Frequently, a combination of drugs is needed.

D. Postoperative Maintenance Therapy

For patients who require total adrenalectomy, lifelong corticosteroid maintenance therapy becomes necessary after total adrenalectomy. The following schedule is commonly used: no cortisol is given until the adrenals are removed during surgery. On the first day, give 50 mg of hydrocortisone intravenously every 6-8 hours. On the second day, give 25 mg every 6-8 hours. Thereafter, the dose should be tapered as tolerated. The same tapering process is used after excision of a unilateral cortisol-secreting adenoma, because the remaining adrenal may not function normally for months.

As the hydrocortisone dose is reduced below 50 mg/d, it is often necessary to add fludrocortisone (a mineralocorticoid), 0.1 mg daily orally if patients had bilateral adrenalectomy. The usual maintenance doses are about 15-20 mg of hydrocortisone and 0.1 mg of fludrocortisone daily. More than half the hydrocortisone dose is given in the morning.

Patients who have had a total bilateral adrenalectomy and are on maintenance therapy can develop addisonian crisis when under stress, such as general anesthesia or infection. Adrenal insufficiency causes fever, hyperkalemia, abdominal pain, and hypotension, and should be promptly recognized and treated with saline infusion and cortisol.

▶ Prognosis

The prognosis is good after resection of benign adrenal adenomas, pituitary adenomas, or benign ACTH-secreting tumors. Patients with Cushing disease in remission after pituitary surgery have reversal of excess mortality. Symptoms and signs of hypercortisolism resolve, usually over months. Short-term adrenal insufficiency after surgery requires cortisol replacement. Cushing disease can recur after excision of a pituitary adenoma. An occult ACTH-secreting tumor may become apparent later and require removal.

Residual adrenal tissue or embryonic rests are present in up to 10% of patients after total adrenalectomy. Cushing syndrome can then recur if stimulation with ACTH continues.

The prognosis is extremely poor in patients with adrenocortical carcinoma and in those with malignant tumors causing ectopic ACTH syndrome.

Biller BMK et al: Treatment of ACTH dependent Cushing's syndrome: a consensus statement. *J Clin Endocrin Metab* 2008;93:2454.

Feelders RA et al: Stepwise medical treatment of Cushing's disease with pasireotide mono- or combination therapy with cabergoline and low-dose ketoconazole. *N Engl J Med* 2010;362:1846.

Nieman LK et al: The diagnosis of Cushing's syndrome: an Endocrine Society Clinical Practice Guideline. *J Clin Endocrinol Metab* 2008;93:1526.

Sippel RS et al: Waiting for change: symptom resolution after adrenalectomy for Cushing's syndrome. *Surgery* 2008;144:1054.

Toniato A et al: Surgical versus conservative management for subclinical Cushing syndrome in adrenal incidentalomas: a prospective randomized study. *Ann Surg* 2009;249:388.

Tsinberg M et al. Subclinical Cushing's syndrome. *J Surg Oncol* 2012;106:572.

▼ VIRILIZING ADRENAL TUMORS

In adults, hormonally active benign adrenal adenomas usually secrete aldosterone or cortisol. Virilizing tumors in women are more likely to be caused by ovarian tumors. Virilizing adrenal tumors are rare, and virilization is usually due to hypersecretion of adrenal androgens, mainly dehydroepiandrosterone (DHEA), its sulfate derivative (DHEAS), and androstenedione, all of which are converted peripherally to testosterone and 5-dihydrotestosterone. Very rarely, virilizing adrenal tumors secrete only testosterone.

The differentiation of benign from malignant adrenocortical tumors may be difficult when based on histologic features; some patients with histologically benign tumors may develop metastases, and others with histologically malignant tumors may never have recurrent disease. Malignancy is only definitely diagnosed from local or distant spread. Seventy percent of virilizing adrenal tumors exhibit malignant behavior. Adrenocortical carcinomas are usually large tumors with local spread or distant metastases. They often secrete multiple steroids, most commonly cortisol and androgens, leading to Cushing syndrome and virilization.

In children, adrenocortical tumors are rare, but virilization with or without hypercortisolism is the most frequent feature. Virilizing adrenal tumors are less likely to be malignant in children than in adults. Histologic features of malignancy do not always predict malignant behavior. Large tumors (> 100 g) have a worse prognosis.

Signs and symptoms of virilization include hirsutism, male-pattern baldness, acne, deep voice, male musculature, irregular menses or amenorrhea, clitoromegaly, and increased libido. Rapid linear growth with advanced bone age is common in children.

CT and MRI are used to image virilizing adrenal tumors. Resection is the only successful treatment.

Virilization can also be caused by congenital adrenal hyperplasia, an autosomal recessive disorder. The mutated genes encode enzymes essential for cortisol and mineralocorticoid synthesis. 21-Hydroxylase deficiency accounts for 90% of cases. The inhibition of cortisol synthesis leads to stimulated ACTH secretion, accumulation of precursors, and overproduction of androgens. Administration of glucocorticoids is the mainstay of treatment in patients with classic congenital adrenal hyperplasia. Mineralocorticoid replacement is also required. Corrective surgery may be needed in female infants born with ambiguous genitalia. The combination of antiandrogens, aromatase inhibitors, and lower dose glucocorticoid replacement to minimize the effect of excess androgen is being investigated. Adrenalectomy with lifelong steroid replacement is another approach in the most severely affected patients.

FEMINIZING ADRENAL TUMORS

Estrogens are not normally synthesized by the adrenal cortex. Feminizing adrenal tumors are extremely rare and are almost always carcinomas. They are usually seen in men with feminization or in girls with precocious puberty. Vaginal bleeding may be the presenting symptom in adult women. Feminizing adrenal carcinomas frequently hypersecrete other hormones. The diagnosis is based on a finding of increased plasma estrogens. Ovarian tumors and administration of exogenous estrogen should be ruled out.

Definitive treatment is excision of the tumor. The prognosis is guarded.

Cavlan D et al: Androgen- and estrogen-secreting adrenal cancers. *Semin Oncol* 2010;37:638.

ADRENOCORTICAL CARCINOMA

Adrenocortical carcinomas are rare. More than half of patients have symptoms related to hypersecretion of hormones, most commonly Cushing syndrome and virilization. Feminizing and purely aldosterone-secreting carcinomas are rare. In some cases, hormone hypersecretion is subclinical and only found by biochemical studies. The adrenal mass may be palpable. The mean diameter of adrenal carcinoma is 12 cm (range, 3-30 cm). Adrenocortical carcinoma invades the surrounding tissues, and about half of the patients have metastases (lung, liver, and elsewhere) at the time of diagnosis. In those without local spread or distant metastases, a diagnosis of carcinoma based on cytologic features may be wrong.

The median survival is 25 months, and 5-year actuarial survival is 25%. Tumor stage at the initial operation predicts the prognosis. Surgery is the only treatment that potentially provides a cure; however, beneficial outcomes are confined to patients with localized disease. When grossly complete resection is possible, the 5-year survival is 50%. Thus, recurrence is common despite apparent complete resection due to micrometastases at initial presentation. Laparoscopic adrenalectomy is technically more difficult for adrenocortical carcinomas than for other adrenal tumors because the tumor is fragile and adjacent organs may have to be removed. Where the adrenal tumor is small, malignancy is uncertain, and the surgeon is technically capable, starting the operation laparoscopically is acceptable. However, the surgeon should have a low threshold for converting to open or hand-assisted adrenalectomy if a better operation could be accomplished that way. For local recurrent disease, reoperation is indicated and may prolong life. Patients with distant metastases at initial presentation usually die within 1 year. Resecting the adrenal tumor in these patients does not improve survival.

Mitotane, an adrenolytic agent, has been used as an adjuvant to surgery in patients with advanced adrenocortical carcinoma. It controls endocrine symptoms in 50% of patients, and the tumor regresses in some. Some cases of prolonged remission have been reported.

In patients who underwent complete primary resection, older reports of routine adjuvant mitotane therapy postoperatively did not confer definitive benefits. However, a recent large retrospective study showed that mitotane improved recurrence-free survival. Dose-related side effects (eg, gastrointestinal symptoms, weakness, dizziness, and somnolence) may limit its use. A variety of other chemotherapeutic agents has been tried with limited success. A recently completed international multicenter prospective randomized study showed combination chemotherapy of etoposide, doxorubicin, and cisplatin plus mitotane improved the rates of response and progression-free survival over that of mitotane plus streptozocin.

The role of radiation is limited and usually is for palliation, especially for bony metastases.

Fassnacht M et al: Combination chemotherapy in advanced adrenocortical carcinoma. *N Engl J Med* 2012;366:2189.

Gaujoux S et al: Recommendation for standardized surgical management of primary adrenocortical carcinoma. *Surgery* 2012;152:123.

Milgrom SA et al: The role of radiation therapy in the management of adrenal carcinoma and adrenal metastases. *J Surg Oncol* 2012;106:647.

Miller BS et al: Resection of adrenocortical carcinoma is less complete and local recurrence occurs sooner and more often after laparoscopic adrenalectomy than after open adrenalectomy. *Surgery* 2012;152:1150.

Terzolo M et al: Adjuvant mitotane treatment for adrenocortical carcinoma. *N Engl J Med* 2007;356:2372.

▼ INCIDENTALOMAS

Adrenal tumors have traditionally been diagnosed after presentation with clinical symptoms of excess hormone secretion. However, the increased use of ultrasonography, CT, and MRI for various diseases in the abdomen has led to the discovery of what are referred to as adrenal incidentalomas. Most are small nonfunctioning adrenal cortical adenomas; some are functioning adenomas or pheochromocytomas with subclinical secretion of hormones; and some are adrenocortical carcinomas or metastases.

Incidentalomas are found in 4% of CT scans and 6% of random autopsies. The incidence increases with age. Based on a review of 10 studies, subclinical Cushing syndrome and Cushing syndrome account for 6.4% of incidentalomas, pheochromocytoma 3.1%, adrenocortical carcinoma 1.8%, metastatic carcinoma 0.7%, and aldosteronoma for 0.6% (Table 33–2). Thus, 90% of the patients have presumed nonfunctioning cortical adenomas. Simple adrenal cysts, myelolipomas, and adrenal hemorrhages can be identified by the CT characteristics alone. Adrenal cysts can be large but are rarely malignant. Adrenal hemorrhage may occur in preexisting adrenal tumors.

The major issues in managing a patient with an incidentaloma is to determine whether the tumor is hormonally active and whether it is a cancer; either would be an indication for resection. All functioning tumors should be excised. Large nonfunctioning tumors also should be excised because of the increased risk of cancer. Small nonfunctioning tumors are almost always benign adenomas; they can be followed with serial CT scans checking for changes in size. Since most incidentalomas are nonfunctioning adenomas, the workup should be selective to avoid unnecessary expense and procedures.

The workup should include a complete history and physical examination with specific reference to a history of previous malignancy and signs and symptoms of Cushing syndrome or pheochromocytoma. Hyperaldosteronism, pheochromocytoma, and virilizing or feminizing adrenocortical carcinoma should be investigated. Further laboratory studies may be indicated depending on the clinical presentation.

All patients—even those who do not have hypertension—should have a 24-hour urine collection for fractionated catecholamines and metanephrines or plasma free metanephrines to search for pheochromocytoma; the risk of unrecognized pheochromocytoma is high, and the hypertension may be absent or episodic. Most pheochromocytomas are over 2 cm in diameter and characteristically bright on T2-weighted MRI. *Almost half of pheochromocytomas are found incidentally because of CT or MRI scans obtained for other indications.*

Subclinical Cushing syndrome refers to autonomous cortisol secretion in patients without typical signs and symptoms of Cushing syndrome. Autonomous cortisol secretion is best assessed by overnight 1 mg dexamethasone suppression test.

Patients with subclinical Cushing syndrome may experience an addisonian crisis if the tumor is resected and glucocorticoid replacement is not adequate.

Patients who are hypertensive should also have plasma aldosterone and PRA measured to screen for primary hyperaldosteronism.

If the above studies show that the tumor is nonfunctional, the size and imaging characteristics of the tumor and the patient's overall medical condition should determine the appropriate treatment. Nonfunctioning adrenal tumors larger than 5 cm in diameter should usually be removed because of higher risk of cancer. Nonfunctioning adrenal tumors smaller than 3 cm that are homogeneous and have low density on CT or MRI are unlikely to be cancers and can be safely followed. The patient's age and overall medical condition and the CT scan findings will usually determine whether a tumor 3-5 cm in size should be resected. High density, delayed wash out of contrast, irregular borders, and heterogeneity make pheochromocytoma, adrenocortical carcinoma, and metastases more likely.

In patients with a previously treated malignancy such as lung or breast cancer, the chance of an adrenal tumor being

Table 33–2. Adrenal incidentalomas.[1]

Tumor Types	Percentage (%)
Subclinical Cushing/Cushing	6.4
Pheochromocytoma	3.1
Adrenocortical carcinoma	1.9
Metastatic carcinoma	0.7
Aldosterone-producing adenoma	0.6
Presumed nonfunctional adenoma	89.9
Total	100

[1]Based on data reported in Eur J Endocrinol 2009;161:513.

metastatic is greater than 50% and even greater if the adrenal mass is larger than 3 cm. CT-guided fine-needle aspiration biopsy is rarely necessary, but can be used to diagnose metastatic cancer if it will change management of the patient. Fine-needle aspiration of an adrenocortical cancer may not be diagnostic, and breaching the capsule risks local spread of cancer. Needle biopsy of an unexpected pheochromocytoma can precipitate pheochromocytoma crisis. Biochemical screening for pheochromocytoma should be performed prior to biopsy. Resection of a solitary adrenal metastasis from a primary lung cancer may improve long-term survival (to about 25% at 5 years) if there are no other clinically obvious metastases. Patients with a metachronous solitary adrenal metastasis are more likely to benefit from adrenalectomy than are those with a synchronous metastasis. Patients with adrenal metastases from melanoma or renal cell carcinoma also benefit from resection even when there are other foci of metastases. Adrenal metastasis can be resected laparoscopically with minimal risk of local recurrence.

Cawood TJ et al: Recommended evaluation of adrenal incidentalomas is costly, has high false-positive rates and confers a risk of fatal cancer that is similar to the risk of the adrenal lesion becoming malignant; time for a rethink? *Eur J Endocrinol* 2009;161:513.

Iacobone M et al: Adrenalectomy may improve cardiovascular and metabolic impairment and ameliorate quality of life in patients with adrenal incidentalomas and subclinical Cushing's syndrome. *Surgery* 2012;152:991.

Lee JA et al: Adrenal incidentaloma, borderline elevations of urine or plasma metanephrine levels, and the "subclinical" pheochromocytoma. *Arch Surg* 2007;142:870.

Taffel M et al: Adrenal imaging: a comprehensive review. *Radiol Clin North Am* 2012;50:219.

Wang TS et al: A cost-effectiveness analysis of adrenalectomy for nonfunctional adrenal incidentalomas: Is there a size threshold for resection? *Surgery* 2012;152:1125.

MULTIPLE CHOICE QUESTIONS

1. The most common approach to resect a 3-cm functioning adrenal tumor is via

   A. Laparoscopy
   B. Laparotomy
   C. Flank incision
   D. Posterior incision
   E. Thoracoabdominal incision

2. The most sensitive and specific test for diagnosis of pheochromocytoma is

   A. Plasma free catecholamines
   B. 24-hour urinary VMA
   C. 24-hour urinary catecholamines
   D. Plasma free metanephrines
   E. Plasma free VMA

3. The workup of an adrenal incidentaloma includes the following, except

   A. Measurement of 24-hour urinary fractionated metanephrines
   B. Measurement of 24-hour urinary cortisol and creatinine
   C. Fine-needle biopsy of the adrenal tumor
   D. Plasma aldosterone level and renin activity
   E. Obtain family history of adrenal disease

4. Laparoscopic adrenalectomy is usually NOT indicated for

   A. An aldosteronoma
   B. A feminizing tumor
   C. A pheochromocytoma
   D. A metastasis from melanoma
   E. A symptomatic myelolipoma

5. Adrenal tumors can secrete the following, except

   A. Normetanephrine
   B. Aldosterone
   C. Cortisol
   D. DHEAS
   E. 5-HIAA

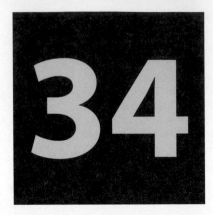

Arteries

34

Joseph H. Rapp, MD

Warren Gasper, MD

Arterial disease can be broadly classified into two categories: occlusive and aneurysmal. The major sequelae of arterial obstruction are tissue ischemia and necrosis, while those of aneurysmal disease are rupture and hemorrhage in the aortic position and thrombosis and embolization in the peripheral arteries.

ARTERIAL OCCLUSIVE DISEASE

Although atherosclerosis is the dominant cause of arterial occlusive disease in Western countries, other etiologies such as congenital and anatomical anomalies, auto immune diseases, and remote thromboembolism can also result in arterial obstruction. Symptoms of occlusive vascular disease primarily are end-organ dysfunction and, in the muscle beds, pain with exercise and tissue necrosis.

ATHEROSCLEROSIS

Atherosclerosis can occur in any artery, with plaques most commonly developing in areas of low shear stress, such as at arterial branch points. Lesions are usually symmetrically distributed, although the rate of progression may vary. Early lesions are confined to the intima. In advanced lesions, both intima and media are involved, but the adventitia is spared. Preservation of the adventitia is essential for the vessel's structural integrity and is the basis for all cardiovascular interventions.

When the hemodynamically significant disease affects a major artery, a parallel system of collateral vessels may preserve flow to the peripheral runoff bed. Collateral vessels are smaller, more circuitous, and always have a higher resistance than the original unobstructed artery. The stimuli for collateral development include abnormal pressure gradients across the collateral system and increased flow velocity through intramuscular channels that connect to reentry vessels. Adequate collateral vessels take time to develop but

often maintain tissue viability in patients with chronic major arterial occlusions.

Generally, arterial insufficiency occurs in medium-sized and large arteries with at least a 50% reduction in arterial diameter. This correlates with a 75% narrowing of cross-sectional area and enough resistance to decrease downstream flow and pressure. Early in the process, compensatory dilation of the vessel wall may preserve lumen diameter as the atherosclerotic lesion develops, but with continued growth, lesions overcome this adaptation and result in flow limiting stenoses. If there is adequate collateral flow, single stenoses or even occlusions are reasonably well-tolerated. Severe ischemia occurs when there are inadequate collaterals or there are multiple levels of disease.

Davì G, Patrono C: Platelet activation and atherothrombosis. N Engl J Med 2008;358:1638.

Libby P, Ridker PM, Hansson GK: Inflammation in atherosclerosis: from pathophysiology to practice. J Am Coll Cardiol 2009;54:2129.

CHRONIC LOWER EXTREMITY OCCLUSIVE DISEASE

General Considerations

Peripheral arterial insufficiency is predominantly a disease of the lower extremities. Upper extremity arterial lesions are uncommon and confined mostly to the subclavian arteries. Even when present, upper extremity atherosclerosis rarely produces symptoms due to abundant collateral pathways. In the lower extremities, however, obstructive lesions are distributed widely, with lesions of the superficial femoral and iliac arteries the most common (Figure 34–1). Symptoms are related to the location and number of obstructions.

Peripheral arterial disease affects at least 20% of individuals older than 70 years with the incidence increasing with

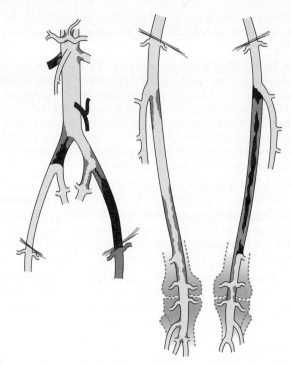

▲ **Figure 34–1.** Common sites of stenosis and occlusion of the visceral and peripheral arterial systems.

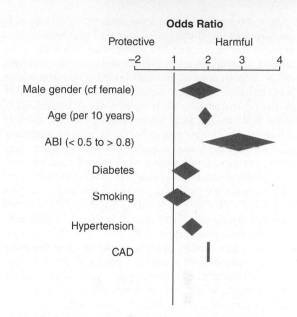

▲ **Figure 34–2.** Odds ratios for risk factors for all-cause mortality. ABI, ankle-brachial index; CAD, coronary artery disease. (Reproduced, with permission, from TASC Working Group: Dormandy JA et al. Management of peripheral arterial disease: epidemiology, natural history, risk factors. *J Vasc Surg.* 2000 Jan;31[1 Pt 2]:S1-S296.)

the increasing incidence of diabetes. Although most patients with this disorder do not develop gangrene or require amputations, adverse outcomes of systemic atherosclerosis, including myocardial infarction and/or stroke, are common. Even after adjustment for known risk factors, individuals with peripheral arterial disease exhibit a several-fold higher risk of mortality than the nonaffected population. A low ankle-brachial index (ABI) is one of the strongest risk factors for all-cause mortality. Peripheral arterial disease is more a marker of a more virulent form of atherosclerosis and early death from cardiovascular or cerebrovascular disease than an indicator of imminent limb loss; thus, identifying and treating associated atherosclerotic risk factors is essential (Figure 34–2).

▶ **Clinical Findings**

A. Symptoms

1. Intermittent claudication—Intermittent claudication refers to pain in muscles of the lower extremity associated with walking and relieved by rest. Because tissue perfusion is adequate at rest, tissue loss is not present and the risk of amputation is low unless there is progression of disease. Claudication is derived from the Latin word meaning "to limp"; therefore, the term should be used only for symptoms in the lower extremities. The pain is a deep-seated ache usu-

ally in the calf muscle, which gradually progresses until the patient is compelled to stop walking. Patients occasionally describe "cramping" or "tiredness" in the muscle. Typically, symptoms are completely relieved after 2–5 minutes of inactivity. Claudication is distinguished from other types of pain in the extremities in that it does not occur at rest and some period of exertion is always required before it appears, it generally occurs after a relatively consistent distance traveled, and it is relieved by cessation of walking. Relief of symptoms is not dependent upon sitting or other positional change. The severity of claudication is traditionally expressed in terms of city blocks.

Regardless of which arterial segment is involved, claudication most commonly involves the calf muscles because of their high workload with the mechanics of normal walking. Occlusions proximal to the origin of the profunda femoris can extend the pain to involve the thigh. Gluteal pain indicates lesions in or proximal to the hypogastric arteries and is often accompanied by impotence. **Leriche syndrome** occurs in men with aortoiliac disease and includes claudication of calf, thigh, and buttock muscles; erectile dysfunction; and diminished or absent femoral pulses. Occasionally, patients describe transient numbness of the extremity accompanying the pain and fatigue of claudication as nerves as well as muscles become ischemic.

The two conditions that most often mimic claudication are osteoarthritis of the hip or knee and neurospinal compression due to congenital or osteophytic narrowing of the lumbar neurospinal canal (spinal stenosis). Osteoarthritis can be differentiated from claudication because pain occurs predominantly in joints, the amount of exercise required to elicit symptoms varies, symptoms are characteristically worse in the morning and upon initiating exercise, rest does not relieve symptoms promptly, the severity of symptoms changes from day to day, and anti-inflammatory agents may relieve the pain. Impingement on the spinal canal or nerve root produces neurospinal compression symptoms; therefore, the pain is typically burning in nature and symptoms may occur with sitting or standing. Neurospinal pain often follows a dermatomal distribution, a key factor in differentiating this from claudication.

Uncommon conditions such as coarctation of the aorta, chronic compartment syndrome, popliteal artery entrapment, and vasculitis can mimic symptoms of atherosclerotic arterial insufficiency. Age at presentation and associated findings may aid in diagnosing these conditions.

The correct diagnosis of vascular claudication should be easily established by determining the location of pain with exercise (calf), the quality of the pain (aching or cramping), the length of time required for relief of symptoms after stopping exercise (immediate), the reproducibility of the distance walked before symptoms begin (initial claudication distance), and most importantly, the reduction or loss of pulses with exercise.

2. Critical limb ischemia—With extensive disease, patients develop ischemic rest pain and/or ulceration. Ischemic rest pain, a grave symptom caused by ischemic neuritis, indicates advanced arterial insufficiency that carries a risk of gangrene and amputation if arterial reconstruction cannot be performed. The pain is severe and burning, usually confined to the forefoot distal to the metatarsals. It may be localized to the vicinity of an ischemic ulcer or pregangrenous toe. It is aggravated by elevation of the extremity or by bringing the leg to the horizontal position. Thus, it appears at bed rest (hence the name) and may prevent sleep. Because gravity aids the delivery of arterial blood, classically, the patient with rest pain can obtain relief by simply hanging the leg over the side of the bed. This simple maneuver will differentiate ischemic rest pain from peripheral neuropathy, which is associated with diabetes and is the most common cause of foot pain at rest. In patients who must keep the foot constantly dependent to relieve pain, the leg and foot may be swollen, causing some confusion in diagnosis. The ischemic neuritis of rest pain is severe and resistant to opioids for relief.

Patients with rest pain may give a history of claudication, but rest pain also may occur de novo in diabetics with distal tibial disease, embolic occlusion of the distal tibial arteries, and patients whose walking is limited by other conditions.

Differentiating ischemic rest pain from neuropathy in diabetics is critical and may require vascular testing to clarify the diagnosis.

3. Nonhealing wounds or ulcers—Patients with severe lower extremity arterial insufficiency often develop ulcers or wounds on the feet even from seemingly trivial trauma. These lesions are most commonly located on the distal foot and toes, but on occasion they can be in the upper foot or ankle. Typically, the wounds are excruciatingly painful, deep, and devoid of any evidence of healing such as contraction or formation of granulation tissue.

4. Erectile dysfunction—Inability to attain or maintain an erection may be produced by lesions that obstruct blood flow through both hypogastric arteries and is commonly found in association with narrowing of the terminal aorta, common iliac, or hypogastric arteries. Vasculogenic erectile dysfunction is less common than that due to other causes.

5. Sensation—Although the patient may report numbness in the extremity, sensory abnormalities are generally absent on examination. If decreased sensation is found in the foot, peripheral neuropathy should be suspected.

B. Signs

Physical examination is of paramount importance in assessing the presence and severity of vascular disease. The physical findings of peripheral atherosclerosis are related to changes in the peripheral arteries and to tissue ischemia.

1. Arterial palpation—Decreased amplitude of the pulse denotes proximal obstructions to flow. The pulse examination can help localize disease. For example, an absent femoral pulse usually signifies aortoiliac disease. It is unusual for collateral flow to be sufficient to produce a pulse distal to an occluded artery.

2. Bruits and thrills—A bruit is the sound produced by dissipation of energy as blood flows through a stenotic arterial segment. With extremely high flows, the energy may vibrate the artery, creating a "thrill." The bruit or thrill is transmitted distally along the course of the artery. Thus, when a bruit is heard through a stethoscope placed over a peripheral artery, stenosis is present at or proximal to that level. The pitch of the bruit rises as the stenosis becomes more marked, until a critical stenosis is reached or the vessel becomes occluded, when the bruit may disappear. Thus, absence of a bruit does not indicate insignificant disease.

3. Response to exercise—Exercise in a normal individual increases the pulse rate without producing arterial bruits or reduction in pulse amplitude. In an individual who complains of claudication, there may be minimal findings at rest, but exercise will produce decreased pulse strength, decreased distal arterial pressure, and possibly an audible bruit unmasking a significant stenosis. Exercise is best used in conjunction with noninvasive vascular testing.

4. Integumentary changes—Chronic ischemia commonly produces loss of hair over the dorsum of the toes and foot and may be associated with thickening of the toenails (ony-chomycosis) due to slowed keratin turnover. With more advanced ischemia, there is atrophy of the skin and sub-cutaneous tissue so that the foot becomes shiny, scaly, and skeletonized.

5. Pallor—Pallor of the foot on elevation of the extremity to approximately 40 cm with a complete absence of capillary refill indicates advanced ischemia. Pallor on elevation does not occur unless advanced ischemia is present. It is always present with ischemic rest pain.

6. Reactive hyperemia—When pallor is produced with elevation, the ischemia results in maximum cutaneous vasodilation. When the extremity is returned to a dependent position, blood returning to the dilated vascular bed pro-duces an intense red or possibly ruborous color in the foot, called reactive hyperemia, and denotes advanced disease. The delay in the appearance of color when the extremi-ties return to a dependent position is proportionate to the impairment in circulation.

7. Rubor—In advanced atherosclerotic disease, the skin of the foot displays a characteristic dark red/cyanotic color on dependency. Because of low inflow, the blood in the capillary network of the foot is relatively stagnant, oxygen extraction is high, and the capillary blood becomes the color of the venous blood. The concurrent vasodilation due to ischemia causes blood to suffuse the cutaneous plexus, imparting a purple color to the skin. The purple discoloration due to severe chronic venous insufficiency does not give way to pallor on elevation.

8. Skin temperature—With chronic ischemia, the temper-ature of the skin of the foot decreases. Coolness can best be detected by palpation with the back of the examiner's hand with comparison to the contralateral foot.

9. Ulceration—Ischemic ulcers are usually very painful and accompanied by rest pain in the foot. They occur in toes or at a site where minor trauma can initiate the injury. The margin of the ulcer is sharply demarcated or punched-out, and the base is devoid of healthy granulation tissue. The surrounding skin is pale and mottled, and signs of chronic ischemia are invariably present.

10. Atrophy—Moderate to severe degrees of chronic ischemia produce gradual soft tissue and muscle atrophy and loss of strength. Joint mobility and gait may be altered due to muscle atrophy. Subsequent changes in foot struc-ture and gait increase the possibility of developing foot ulceration.

11. Necrosis—Severe tissue ischemia may progress to necrosis with minor injuries, infection, or swelling. Necrosis halts proximally at a line where the blood supply is sufficient to maintain viability and results in dry gangrene. If the necrotic portion is infected (wet gangrene), necrosis may extend into tissues that would normally remain viable.

C. Noninvasive Vascular Laboratory Tests

Noninvasive assessment is helpful to determine the severity of hypoperfusion and the sites of hemodynamically signifi-cant stenoses or occlusions.

The **ankle-brachial index** is a quick screening test and the cornerstone of the diagnosis of peripheral vascular dis-ease. The ABI is determined by dividing the systolic pressure obtained by Doppler insonation at the ankle by the brachial arterial pressure. Normally, the ABI is 1.0 or greater; a value below 1.0 indicates occlusive disease proximal to the point of measurement. The ABI correlates roughly with the degree of ischemia (eg, claudication occurs with a value less than 0.7 and rest pain usually appears when the ratio is 0.3 or lower). Elderly patients or patients with diabetic vascular disease may have artificially elevated ABI values due to calci-fied, noncompressible arteries, and toe-to-brachial pressure ratios should be substituted.

Blood pressures can be measured at rest and after exer-cise in the ankle, and the effect of exercise can be monitored. **Exercise testing** confirms and quantitates the diagnosis of claudication. To perform exercise testing, the patient walks on a treadmill at a standard speed and grade until claudica-tion pain is experienced or a time limit is reached. With significant arterial occlusive disease, there will be a decrease in the ABI with exercise, usually measured 1 minute after cessation of walking. If the pain is not due to arterial ste-nosis, no fall in pressure will occur. This test is particularly useful in differentiating neurogenic pain with walking from claudication.

D. Imaging Studies

Color duplex ultrasound imaging is a mainstay of vascu-lar imaging. It is a painless, relatively inexpensive, and (in experienced hands) accurate method for acquiring anatomic and functional information (eg, velocity gradients across stenoses). Although the accuracy of this study is operator dependent, it can supply sufficient information to permit intervention in selected cases.

CT angiography (CTA) is useful for imaging the arterial tree and has the advantage of visualizing cross-sections of the vessel lumen. In many instances, this allows for more accu-rate determination of vessel diameter and stenosis severity than conventional angiography. It does require the adminis-tration of nephrotoxic contrast dye, it is less useful for tibial disease, and its images may be obscured by the presence of calcification or metallic implants. **MR angiography (MRA)**

also can be used to obtain images similar in quality to angiography in most cases. MRA does not show calcifications and gives better visualization of tibial vessels than CTA. MRA also can reveal details of composition of atherosclerotic plaque. Gadolinium-associated nephrogenic fibrosing dermopathy limits its use in patients with renal insufficiency. The integrated use of computer workstations with CT and MR image data can provide three-dimensional (3D) images that can be useful in visualizing patient anatomy and planning interventional procedures.

Conventional arteriography provides detailed anatomic information about peripheral arterial disease. It is reserved for patients warranting invasive intervention such as percutaneous transluminal angioplasty (often shortened to PTA) or vascular surgery. Complications of angiography are related to technique and contrast media. Technical complications such as puncture site hematomas, arteriovenous fistulas, and false aneurysms are rare (1%). Contrast agents may precipitate allergic reactions (0.1%). Patients with renal failure, proteinuria, diabetes, and dehydration are at increased risk for contrast-induced renal failure. Adequate hydration of patients before and after angiography, acetylcysteine, and periprocedural infusions of sodium bicarbonate infusions may reduce the incidence of this complication.

▶ **Treatment & Prognosis**

The objectives of treatment for lower extremity occlusive disease are relief of symptoms, prevention of limb loss, and maintenance of bipedal gait.

A. Nonoperative Treatment

In general, patients with peripheral vascular disease have shortened life expectancies because of their severe atherosclerotic disease. Nondiabetic patients with ischemic disease of the lower extremity have a 5-year survival rate of 70%. The survival rate is 60% in patients with associated ischemic heart disease or cerebrovascular insufficiency. Patients with peripheral vascular disease and renal failure have a 2-year survival rate of less than 50%. Most deaths are due to myocardial infarctions and strokes. Only 20% of deaths are due to nonatherosclerotic causes.

Nonoperative treatment consists of (1) medical management of cardiovascular risk factors, (2) exercise rehabilitation, (3) foot care, and (4) pharmacotherapy.

1. Reduction of cardiovascular risk factors—See Table 34–1. Cigarette smoking is the single most important risk factor for peripheral vascular disease, and all patients should stop smoking. At high levels of consumption, 2-3 packs per day, claudicants will experience immediate improvement in walking distance.

In the past, elevated lipids were not usually associated with peripheral vascular disease. Hyperlipidemia, however, is often present, especially in patients with early onset of disease. Elevated triglyceride levels and low high-density

Table 34–1. Summary of risk factor modification in peripheral vascular disease.

Risk Factor	Therapy	Clinical Effect
Tobacco use	Counseling Pharmacotherapy Nicotine replacement Bupropion, varenicline	Reduced overall mortality Reduced cardiovascular events
Antiplatelet	Aspirin Clopidogrel (Plavix)	Antiplatelet therapy gives > 20% reduction in MI, stroke, or vascular death
Hyperlipidemia	Statin Lipid goals in PAD patients: LDL < 100 mg/dL	20-30% reduction in cardiovascular and all-cause mortality in CAD patients
Hypertension	Target BP < 140/90 in PAD patients Beta-blocker ACE inhibitor	Beta-blocker and ACE inhibitors each associated with > 20% reduction in cardiovascular mortality
Diabetes	Goal hemoglobin Alc < 7%	Benefits in vascular disease unproven
Lifestyle	Daily aerobic exercise Weight loss Healthy, low-fat diet	Reduced lipid levels Reduced cardiovascular events

ACE, angiotensin converting enzyme; BP, blood pressure; CAD, coronary artery disease; LDL, low-density lipoprotein; MI, myocardial infarction; PAD, peripheral artery disease.

lipoprotein (HDL) cholesterol levels are more prevalent than elevated levels of low-density lipoprotein (LDL) cholesterol. Reduction of elevated lipid levels is associated with stabilization or regression of arterial plaques. Statins are extremely effective in reducing LDL cholesterol, and goals of therapy for patients with peripheral vascular disease are to maintain cholesterol levels at less than 100 mg/dL (2.6 mmol/L). Statins have other pleiotropic effects that may reduce inflammation, stabilize plaques, and independently increase walking distance in claudicants. Other antihyperlipidemic medications, including niacin and fibrates (gemfibrozil), may be used to lower hypertriglyceridemia, which can increase HDL cholesterol.

Both type 1 and type 2 diabetes increase the prevalence and severity of cardiovascular disease. Intensive glycemic control reduces the incidence of nephropathy, neuropathy, and retinopathy in diabetes, but it does not correlate with the severity or progression of peripheral arterial disease. In order to reduce all-cause mortality, however, it is recommended that fasting blood sugars should be controlled with hemoglobin A1c levels less than 7%.

2. Exercise rehabilitation—For claudicants, exercise ranging from unsupervised walking to formal supervised exercise on a treadmill significantly improves walking ability. A 21-study meta-analysis of exercise programs showed an average 180% increase in initial claudication distance and a 120% increase in maximal walking distance achieved through exercise. The precise mechanism behind this improvement is not firmly established. Collateral development seems unlikely because ankle pressures and limb flow do not increase substantially. Possible explanations include improved metabolic capacity and conditioning of the muscles.

Since patients with claudication are at a twofold to fourfold greater risk of dying from complications of generalized atherosclerosis than people without claudication, an additional benefit of exercise in these patients is that an improvement in walking distance as part of an aggressive risk factor modification regimen results in an overall decrease in cardiovascular risk.

3. Foot care—The feet of patients with neuropathy or with critical limb ischemia should be inspected and washed daily and kept dry. Mechanical and thermal trauma to the feet should be avoided. Toenails should be trimmed carefully, and corns and calluses should be attended to promptly. Even minor foot infections or injuries should be treated aggressively. Educating the patient to understand neuropathy, peripheral vascular insufficiency, and the importance of foot care is a central aspect of treatment.

4. Pharmacotherapy—The Antiplatelet Trialists Collaboration found an overall 25% decrease in fatal and nonfatal myocardial infarctions, strokes, and vascular deaths in those treated with antiplatelet agents. Aspirin at dosages ranging from 75 to 350 mg/d is the first-line antiplatelet agent recommended, though clopidogrel, which blocks the activation of platelets by adenosine diphosphate (ADP), may be useful in aspirin-intolerant patients. Clopidogrel is also an important adjunctive therapy in reducing thrombogenicity at locations of endovascular arterial treatment. All patients with cardiovascular disease, whether symptomatic or asymptomatic, should be considered for antiplatelet therapy to reduce the risk of cardiovascular morbidity and mortality.

Two drugs have been approved by the FDA for treatment of intermittent claudication. Pentoxifylline produces a small improvement in both initial claudication distance (about 20%) and absolute claudication distance (about 10%). Cilostazol is a phosphodiesterase III inhibitor with vasodilator, antiplatelet, and antilipid activity. Randomized, placebo-controlled, blinded trials have shown an increase of about 50% in absolute claudication distance in patients treated with cilostazol. Quality-of-life assessments also improved

significantly. Gene therapy for cardiovascular disease is being investigated, but conclusions regarding safety and efficacy are premature.

Aboyans V, Criqui MH, Abraham P, Allison MA, Creager MA, et al: Measurement and interpretation of the ankle-brachial index: a scientific statement from the American Heart Association. Circulation 2012;126:2890.

Alonso Coello P, Bellmunt S, McGorrian C, Anand S, Guzman R, et al: Antithrombotic therapy in peripheral artery disease: Antithrombotic Therapy and Prevention of Thrombosis, 9th ed: American College of Chest Physicians Evidence-Based Clinical Practice Guidelines. Chest 2012;141(2 Suppl):e669S.

Critchley JA, Capewell S: Mortality risk reduction associated with smoking cessation in patients with coronary heart disease: a systematic review. JAMA 2003;290:86.

Dormandy JA, Murray GD: The fate of the claudicant—a prospective study of 1969 claudicants. Eur J Vasc Surg 1991;5:131.

Hamburg NM, Balady GJ: Exercise rehabilitation in peripheral artery disease: functional impact and mechanisms of benefits. Circulation 2011;123:87-97.

McCullough PA: Contrast-induced acute kidney injury. J Am Coll Cardiol 2008;51:1419.

Mills EJ, Wu P, Chong G, Ghement I, Singh S, et al: Efficacy and safety of statin treatment for cardiovascular disease: a network meta-analysis of 170,255 patients from 76 randomized trials. QJM 2011;104:109.

Momsen AH, Jensen MB, Norager CB, Madsen MR, Vestersgaard Andersen T, et al: Drug therapy for improving walking distance in intermittent claudication: a systematic review and meta-analysis of robust randomised controlled studies. Eur J Vasc Endovasc Surg 2009;38:463.

Murphy TP, Cutlip DE, Regensteiner JG, Mohler ER, Cohen DJ, et al: Supervised exercise versus primary stenting for claudication resulting from aortoiliac peripheral artery disease: six-month outcomes from the claudication: exercise versus endoluminal revascularization (CLEVER) study. Circulation 2012;125:130.

Rehring TF, Stolcpart RS, Hollis HW Jr: Pharmacologic risk factor management in peripheral arterial disease: a vade mecum for vascular surgeons. Society for Vascular Surgery. J Vasc Surg 2008;47:1108.

B. Operative Treatment

Interventional procedures, open or endovascular, are performed both for limb salvage and for incapacitating claudication. The choice of operative procedure depends on the location and distribution of arterial lesions and the patient's comorbidities. Recognition of coexistent cardiopulmonary disease is particularly relevant, because many patients with peripheral vascular disease also have ischemic heart disease and/or chronic lung disease associated with tobacco use. Preoperative cardiac functional assessment is sometimes necessary, but preoperative myocardial revascularization is not beneficial in patients with reasonable cardiac reserve. All patients undergoing vascular surgery should have preoperative risk assessment. Randomized trials have shown that

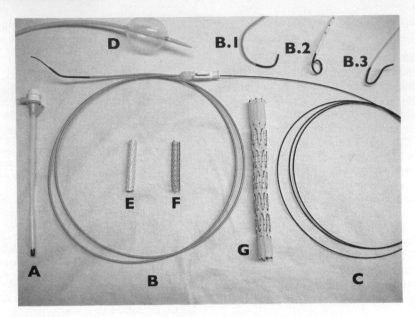

▲ **Figure 34–3.** Endovascular gear. **A:** Sheath. Inserted using Seldinger technique into access vessel. Wires, catheters, and devices pass through the sheath. Sheaths provide stable working access points and protect artery. **B:** Catheter. Variable length, stiffness, coating, and shape (examples: B.1, cobra; B.2, pigtail; B.3, mesenteric selective). Catheters help steer wires through vasculature and also maintain access in vessel. **C:** Guidewire. Variable diameter, length, stiffness, and shape. Used to gain access into vasculature, cross lesions, and deliver devices. **D:** Balloon catheter. **E:** Peripheral stent graft. **F:** Peripheral nitinol self-expanding stent. **G:** Aortoiliac stainless steel/Dacron stent-graft.

perioperative β-blocker, angiotensin-converting enzyme (ACE) inhibitor, and statins may reduce cardiac morbidity in patients undergoing vascular surgery. Evidence is also emerging demonstrating the importance of maintaining statin therapy throughout the perioperative period.

1. Endovascular therapy—Endovascular therapy consists of image-guided techniques to treat diseased arterial segments from within the lumen of the vessel. Access to the arterial system is established by the insertion of valved sheaths, usually percutaneously, into the access vessel, often the common femoral artery. Steerable wires and catheters are then passed through the vasculature under fluoroscopic guidance to the target lesion (Figure 34–3). Once the target lesion is accessed, therapeutic maneuvers, such as angioplasty, or devices, such as stents, can be delivered. In many arterial beds, endovascular therapy is more commonly utilized than open surgical therapy because of its minimally invasive nature and reduction of short-term morbidity and mortality. However, many questions remain concerning the long-term durability of endovascular repairs, and open surgery still plays a major role in the treatment of patients with arterial disease.

2. Percutaneous transluminal angioplasty—with or without placement of an intravascular stent, is often the

treatment of choice when stenoses or even occlusions are relatively short and localized. As the angioplasty balloon expands, it stretches the adventitia, fracturing and compressing plaque, expanding the artery to widen the lumen. Energy losses associated with a stenosis are inversely proportionate to the fourth power of the radius; therefore, even small increases in radius can result in substantial increases in blood flow, although durability of the procedure is improved with the reestablishment of a normal lumen. Concomitant stenting is frequently performed to improve luminal expansion and the arteriographic appearance of the lesion. Stent grafts (stents with fabric covering) may also be used in selected cases or to repair the inadvertent rupture of an artery during angioplasty (Figure 34–4).

Both stents and stent grafts are commonly used from the aortic bifurcation to the distal popliteal artery. Stenting is performed less commonly below the knee, but angioplasty of tibial disease is now common with the use of small catheters and wires. As in the coronaries, drug eluting stents may significantly improve patency rates. Percutaneous mechanical and laser atherectomy are other options in removing obstructing lesions in lower extremity atherosclerotic occlusive disease.

For short, stenotic segments in larger, more proximal vessels, the results of endovascular therapies are good with 1-year success rates of 85% in common iliac disease and 70%

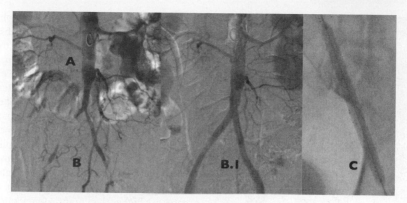

▲ **Figure 34–4.** Aortoiliac occlusive disease. **A:** Aorta. **B:** Severely stenotic/occluded iliac arteries. **B.1:** Widely patent iliac arteries following balloon angioplasty and stenting (**C**).

in external iliac disease. The results with superficial femoral and popliteal lesions are lower (Figure 34–5). The success of endovascular therapy for lower extremity occlusive disease is inversely related to the complexity of the lesion, defined by the number and length of stenoses treated.

Close follow-up of patients post endovascular therapy is required since disease may recur more frequently after angioplasty than after bypass surgery. The patient should be closely followed using noninvasive tests. Repeat angioplasty or stenting may be indicated for recurrent disease, but the improvement in morbidity and mortality of endovascular interventions may be offset by the need for multiple repeat procedures. In general, minimally invasive percutaneous treatment of lower extremity occlusive disease is best used in patients of high operative risk and severe, limb-threatening ischemia (Figure 34–6).

C. Surgical treatment

1. Aortoiliac reconstruction—Open operations are indicated for aortoiliac occlusive disease in younger patients with low operative risk or patients with severe disease not amenable to endovascular therapy. To completely bypass

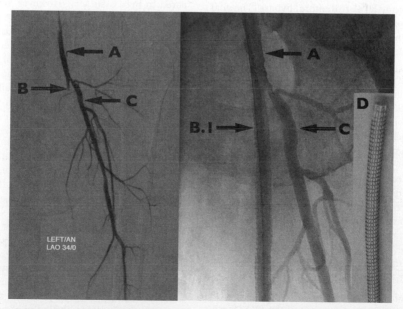

▲ **Figure 34–5.** Superficial femoral artery occlusion, angioplasty, and stent-graft. **A:** Common femoral artery. **B:** Occluded superficial femoral artery. **B.1:** Recannulized, stent-grafted superficial femoral artery. **C:** Profunda femoris artery. **D:** Stent-graft.

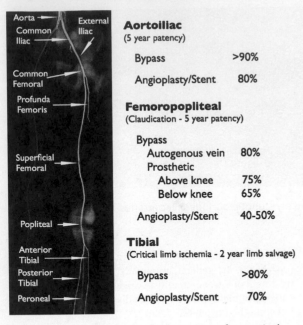

Aortoiliac
(5 year patency)

Bypass	>90%
Angioplasty/Stent	80%

Femoropopliteal
(Claudication - 5 year patency)

Bypass	
Autogenous vein	80%
Prosthetic	
Above knee	75%
Below knee	65%
Angioplasty/Stent	40-50%

Tibial
(Critical limb ischemia - 2 year limb salvage)

Bypass	>80%
Angioplasty/Stent	70%

▲ **Figure 34–6.** Comparison of outcomes for surgical and endovascular intervention in lower extremity occlusive disease.

the aortoiliac segment, an inverted Y-shaped prosthesis is interposed between the infrarenal abdominal aorta and the femoral arteries, creating an **aortofemoral bypass**. The goal of operation is restoration of blood flow to the common femoral artery or, when occlusive disease of the superficial femoral artery is present, to the profunda femoris artery. The clinical results of aortofemoral reconstruction are excellent, although the mortality and morbidity clearly are higher than for endovascular therapy. The operative death rate is 5%; early patency rate, 95%; and late patency rate (5-10 years postoperatively), about 80%. Late complications may be as high as 10% and include graft-intestinal fistula formation, anastomotic aneurysm formation, renal failure, and erectile dysfunction.

Lower risk procedures may be preferable in high-risk patients. If the clinically important lesions are confined to one side, a femoral-femoral or iliofemoral bypass graft can be used. A graft from the axillary to the femoral artery (ie, axillofemoral graft) can be used for bilateral disease. Unfortunately, these "extra-anatomic" methods of arterial reconstruction are more prone to late occlusion than are direct reconstructions.

2. Femoropopliteal reconstruction—When disease is confined to the femoropopliteal segment of the SFA, **femoropopliteal bypass** is used. The principal indication for these operations is limb salvage. In patients with claudication

alone, the indications for femoropopliteal bypass are more difficult to define but must include substantial disability from claudication. For limited lesions of the superficial femoral artery, endovascular therapy is often attempted first, with surgery reserved for extensive disease or angioplasty failure.

The best conduit for femoropopliteal bypass is an autologous greater saphenous vein. The saphenous vein may be left in situ or removed and reversed. Expanded polytetrafluoroethylene (PTFE) may also be used as a conduit, particularly for bypass to the suprageniculate popliteal artery. Below the knee, PTFE conduits produce much lower patency rates than saphenous veins. Operative death rates are low (2%), and 5-year patency rates range from 60% to 80%. Limb salvage rates are higher than graft patency rates.

The profunda femoris artery perfuses the thigh and acts as an important source of collateral flow when the superficial femoral artery is diseased. When there is a stenosis of the profunda, **profundoplasty** alone can be performed for limb salvages with success rates of 80% when the suprageniculate popliteal artery is patent and 40%–50% when the popliteal artery is occluded. Isolated profundoplasty is rarely helpful for treating claudication.

3. Tibioperoneal arterial reconstruction—Reconstruction of tibial arteries (ie, **distal bypass** to the tibial, peroneal, or pedal vessels) is performed only for limb salvage. Advancing technology allows better endovascular therapy in the tibial vessels, with decreased short-term morbidity and mortality, and similar gains in limb salvage when compared to bypass surgery. However, bypass still remains an important mode of therapy for these patients. Autogenous saphenous veins are preferred because prosthetic conduits have high failure rates. Due to smaller vessel size, extensive disease, and probably the length of the bypass conduit, these grafts are not as durable as femoropopliteal bypass, so the limb salvage rate is substantially higher than graft patency. The operative death rate for these procedures is about 5 due to extensive comorbidities.

4. Amputation—Amputation of the limb is necessary within 5-10 years in only 5% of patients presenting with claudication. Amputation is more common if patients continue to smoke cigarettes. Patients with multiple risk factors for atherosclerosis and short-distance claudication are also at increased risk for eventual limb loss. Of patients who present with ischemic rest pain or ulceration, 5%–10% require amputation as initial therapy, and most eventually will require amputation if not revascularized. Successful revascularization results in lower costs than primary amputation and an infinite improvement in quality of life. Occasionally, primary amputation may be preferable to revascularization if the likelihood of successful bypass is low, extensive foot infection is present, or the patient is nonambulatory. Amputation levels, options, and the special needs of amputees are covered in the section on Lower Extremity Amputation.

Bradbury AW, Adam DJ, Bell J, et al: Bypass versus Angioplasty in Severe Ischaemia of the Leg (BASIL) trial: an intention-to-treat analysis of amputation-free and overall survival in patients randomized to a bypass surgery-first or a balloon angioplasty-first revascularization strategy. J Vasc Surg 2010,51:5S-17S.

Hirsch AT, Haskal ZJ, Hertzer NR, et al: ACC/AHA 2005 guidelines for the management of patients with peripheral arterial disease (lower extremity, renal, mesenteric, and abdominal aortic): a collaborative report from the American Association for Vascular Surgery/Society for Vascular Surgery, Society for Cardiovascular Angiography and Interventions, Society for Vascular Medicine and Biology, Society of Interventional Radiology, and the ACC/AHA Task Force on Practice Guidelines (Writing Committee to Develop Guidelines for the Management of Patients with Peripheral Arterial Disease) endorsed by the American Association of Cardiovascular and Pulmonary Rehabilitation; National Heart, Lung, and Blood Institute; Society for Vascular Nursing; TransAtlantic Inter-Society Consensus; and Vascular Disease Foundation. J Am Coll Cardiol 2006;47:1239.

Norgren L, Hiatt WR, Dormandy JA, et al: Inter-Society consensus for the management of peripheral arterial disease (TASC II). TASC II Working Group. J Vasc Surg 2007;45(Suppl S):S5.

Rooke TW, Hirsch AT, Misra S, et al: 2011 ACCF/AHA Focused Update of the Guideline for the Management of Patients With Peripheral Artery Disease (Updating the 2005 Guideline): A Report of the American College of Cardiology Foundation/American Heart Association Task Force on Practice Guidelines. Circulation 2011,124:2020-2045.

ACUTE LOWER EXTREMITY OCCLUSIVE DISEASE

General Considerations

Sudden occlusion of a previously patent artery is a dramatic event characterized by the abrupt onset of severe pain and absent pulses in the involved extremity. Tissue viability depends on the extent to which flow is maintained by collateral circuits. When ischemia persists, motor and sensory paralysis and muscle infarction become irreversible in a matter of hours.

Acute major arterial occlusion may be caused by an embolus, primary arterial thrombosis, trauma, or dissection. The heart is the source of embolus in 80%-90% of episodes, with the remainder from proximal arterial lesions. Aortic aneurysms often contain thrombus, but this material rarely causes symptomatic emboli. In contrast, femoral and particularly popliteal aneurysms embolize frequently. Ulceration in atherosclerotic plaques also can lead to formation of thrombus, which may fragment. Miscellaneous infrequent sources of emboli include cardiac tumors (including cardiac myxoma) and paradoxical emboli (venous thrombi migrating through a patent fora-

men ovale). Up to 5%-10% of spontaneous emboli originate from a source that remains unidentified despite thorough diagnostic interrogation.

It may be difficult to differentiate between sudden thrombosis of an atherosclerotic peripheral artery and embolic occlusion. The former patients usually have pre-existing atherosclerotic stenosis and low blood flow, which predisposes to stagnation and thrombosis. One should also keep in mind the clinical setting and a history of preexisting symptoms such as atrial fibrillation (embolus) or claudication (primary thrombosis).

Clinical Findings

The Five Ps
   Pain
   Pallor
   Pulselessness
   Paresthesias
   Paralysis

Acute arterial occlusion is characterized by the five Ps: pain, pallor, pulselessness, paresthesias, and paralysis. Severe sudden pain is present in 80% of patients, and its onset usually indicates the time of vessel occlusion. Pain is absent in some patients because of prompt onset of anesthesia and paralysis and portends a poor prognosis.

On examination, the key finding is a lack of palpable pulses in a diffusely painful extremity. It is important to determine if sensitivity to light touch is maintained. These fibers are highly susceptible to ischemia, and their dysfunction heralds the beginning of irreversible ischemic changes. The onset of motor paralysis implies impending gangrene. Early intervention is critical. Swelling with acute tenderness of a muscle belly—usually in the calf following acute femoral artery occlusion—generally denotes irreversible muscle infarction. Skin and subcutaneous tissues have greater resistance to hypoxia than nerves and muscles, which may demonstrate irreversible histological changes after 3 hours or less of ischemia.

Treatment & Prognosis

A. Embolism and Thrombosis

Immediate anticoagulation by intravenous heparin slows the propagation of thrombus and allows time for assessment of adequacy of collateral flow and preparation for operation. If light touch is intact, arteriography may be performed to define the anatomy and assist in planning the operation. Diagnosis of acute embolic occlusion is based on an abrupt block of the artery with little accompanying arterial disease; conversely, acute in situ thrombosis is associated with extensive atherosclerosis and a well-established collateral network. The operative treatment for an embolus, embolectomy, differs from that of preexisting atherosclerosis, which may require bypass. Nonoperative management is rarely indicated except in debilitated patients and patients with emboli to major arteries in the upper extremities, which generally have good collateral circulation.

Therapeutic options include catheter-directed thrombolysis, percutaneous mechanical thrombectomy, and surgical embolectomy. For patients with severe acute ischemia, operative therapy is preferable because it is usually associated with the least delay in reestablishing perfusion. Surgical embolectomy may be performed through an arteriotomy at the site of the embolic occlusion or, most commonly, by clot extraction with a balloon (Fogarty) catheter inserted through a remote arteriotomy. Successful embolectomy requires removal of the embolus and the "tail" of thrombus that extends distally or proximally from it. If operation is not performed within the first few hours, the clot may become adherent, and subsequent revascularization is less successful. Intraoperative infusion of thrombolytic agents is often a useful adjunct to embolectomy.

In patients who will tolerate a delay in revascularization (ie, those who do not have neural changes on examination), intra-arterial thrombolysis should be considered. The usual regimen involves selective intra-arterial infusion of low doses of thrombolytic agent (eg, tissue plasminogen activator) directly into the clot. This activates thrombus plasminogen more efficiently, allows high concentrations in the clot while limiting systemic effect, and has acceptable complication rates. In cases of thrombosis on preexisting atherosclerotic lesions, thrombolysis reveals the underlying lesions that will require treatment to prevent recurrent thrombosis.

If revascularization is successful, a reperfusion injury may develop with significant swelling requiring fasciotomy to treat the compartment syndrome that may accompany the reperfusion injury. Renal insufficiency from myoglobin release should be anticipated after reperfusion of ischemic muscle. Treatment consists of vigorous hydration and alkalinization of the urine. Administration of free radical scavengers such as Mannitol may be helpful in this disorder.

Patients with clearly irreversible limb ischemia should undergo amputation without an attempt at revascularization, as revascularization may expose the patient to the serious hazards of reperfusion caused by release of acidic and hyperkalemic venous blood from the dying extremity.

▶ B. Traumatic Arterial Occlusion

Traumatic arterial occlusion must be corrected within a few hours to avoid development of gangrene. Repair of arterial injury is usually performed in conjunction with repair of other injuries. Occasionally, temporary shunts are used to restore flow to the injured extremity while other injuries are addressed and repaired.

▼ PERIPHERAL MICROEMBOLI

Microemboli are most dramatic when they occlude a digital artery perfusing a toe or finger. This causes sudden pain, cyanosis, and coldness or numbness in the affected digit. These changes characteristically improve over several days. If there are multiple emboli, these symptoms may reappear in a different area of the hand or foot. In the lower extremity, this clinical entity has been called **blue toe syndrome** or trash foot. The sudden onset of pain and purple discoloration of a toe in the presence of palpable pulses is recognized as a potentially limb-threatening arterial problem. With each succeeding episode, recovery is slower and less complete.

The most common source of microembolization is cardiac valvular disease. However, if no cardiac valvular lesions are found, a careful examination of the proximal arterial tree must be done to identify an arterial source shedding atheroemboli.

Sudden onset may differentiate peripheral microembolism from other causes of blue toes, such as vasculitis, thromboangiitis obliterans, trauma, or chronic ischemia. If a single toe is affected, it is more likely to be the result of emboli, while multiple cyanotic toes are more likely to be vasculitis or chronic ischemia. It is important to remember that a patent proximal artery is required to serve as a conduit for the embolus, so pulses are intact. Furthermore, a normal blood supply is present in adjacent tissue segments. The appearance of a normally perfused foot with a cyanotic toe is characteristic. However, the waxing and waning symptoms of repeated emboli can make the diagnosis difficult. Unless the syndrome is recognized, alternative diagnoses investigated, and the lesion of origin corrected, survival of the foot or hand may be in peril.

Dean SM: Atypical ischemic lower extremity ulcerations: a differential diagnosis. Vasc Med 2008;13:47.

▼ DIABETIC VASCULAR DISEASE

Atherosclerotic arterial disease in patients with diabetes mellitus is more diffuse and more severe than in nondiabetics. In diabetic patients, the tibioperoneal vessels frequently contain atherosclerotic changes, and the vessels are often heavily calcified. The degree of ischemia may be severe and extensive, and noninvasive tests (ABIs) may be falsely elevated. Fortunately, in many diabetics, the small arteries in the foot are relatively spared, making distal bypass to these arteries possible and allowing foot salvage in cases of threatened limb loss.

Diabetic patients also have a high incidence of neuropathy and are more apt to ignore minor foot injuries, which can develop into ulcerations. Daily foot inspections are essential to avoid progression of minor injuries into limb threatening lesions. Neuropathy is also responsible for loss of tone of intrinsic foot muscles that leads to subluxation of the metatarsal phalangeal joints, resulting in a "rocker-bottom" foot and ultimately producing complete joint destruction termed a Charcot foot. These architectural changes also make skin breakdown more likely to occur and require referral to a foot and ankle clinic.

Conte MS: Diabetic revascularization: endovascular versus open bypass—do we have the answer? Semin Vasc Surg 2012;25:108.
Gibbons GW, Shaw PM: Diabetic vascular disease: characteristics of vascular disease unique to the diabetic patient. Semin Vasc Surg 2012;25:89.
Nehler MR, Whitehill TA, Bowers SP, et al: Intermediate-term outcome of primary digit amputations in patients with diabetes mellitus who have forefoot sepsis requiring hospitalization and presumed adequate circulatory status. J Vasc Surg 1999;30:509.
Prompers L, Schaper N, Apelqvist J, et al: Predictors of outcome in individuals with diabetic foot ulcers. Diabetologia 2008;51:747.

NONATHEROSCLEROTIC DISORDERS CAUSING LOWER LIMB ISCHEMIA

Thromboangiitis Obliterans

Thromboangiitis obliterans (Buerger disease) is characterized by multiple segmental occlusions of obliterating tibial and pedal arteries. The most distal arteries are affected making bypass impossible. Migratory phlebitis may be present. In contrast to atherosclerosis, which involves the intima and media, thromboangiitis obliterans is manifested by infiltration of round cells in all three layers of the arterial wall. The disease occurs almost exclusively in young male smokers. Fortunately, the incidence appears to be decreasing. It is essential that the patient stop smoking to avoid progression of the disease. Patients with Buerger disease may have specific cellular immunity against arterial antigens, specific humoral antiarterial antibodies, and elevated circulatory immune complexes, but a precise diagnosis can be made only by tissue histology. Arteriographic findings are distinctive but not pathognomonic. Sympathectomy decreases arterial spasm and is useful in some patients. Amputation is indicated for persistent pain or gangrene and can be performed adjacent to the line of demarcation with satisfactory primary healing.

The disease may become dormant if the patient can stop smoking. Unfortunately, smoking cessation seems particularly difficult in these patients, and many ultimately require multiple amputations.

Popliteal Artery Entrapment Syndrome

This rare cause of popliteal artery stenosis or occlusion occurs as a result of an anomalous course of the popliteal artery. The popliteal artery normally passes between the two heads of the gastrocnemius muscle as it enters the lower leg. In the entrapment syndrome, the artery passes medial to both heads of the gastrocnemius, causing compression of the popliteal artery when the knee is extended. There are five anatomic variants of popliteal artery entrapment, but all produce similar clinical effects. Fibrous thickening of the intima occurs at the site of compression and gradually progresses to total occlusion. Symptoms vary from calf claudication to those of more severe ischemia depending on lesion severity and embolization. Popliteal artery entrapment should be considered when a young, otherwise healthy patient presents with calf claudication. Until the artery becomes occluded, the only finding is a decrease in strength of the pedal pulses, most evident when using provocative maneuvers like foot dorsiflexion and plantar flexion. MRI and CT studies are most useful in confirmation of the diagnosis. Atherosclerotic changes are notably absent. Treatment consists of returning the popliteal artery to its normal anatomic course or bypass with saphenous vein.

Cystic Degeneration of the Popliteal Artery

Arterial stenosis is produced by a mucoid cyst in the adventitia, usually located in the middle third of the artery. Calf claudication is the most common symptom, and the only finding is a decrease in the strength of the peripheral pulses. Rarely, a mass can be palpated. Arteriography shows a sharply localized zone of popliteal stenosis with a smooth concentric tapering. Ultrasound or CT scans can be used to demonstrate the cyst within the vessel wall. The stenosis may be missed on conventional anteroposterior films and may appear only on lateral exposures. The cyst and the affected artery should be excised and bypassed because of recurrence with evacuation of the cyst only.

Abdominal Aortic Coarctation

Coarctations of the thoracic or abdominal aorta are rare. They may be congenital or may result from an inflammatory large vessel arteritis such as Kawasaki or Takayasu disease. These rare disorders may produce symptoms of lower extremity, mesenteric, or renal ischemia depending on the location of the constriction. The congenital variant of this condition is best managed surgically when it is recognized; autogenous repair may be preferable to the use of prosthetic grafts. Surgical repair in the presence of ongoing inflammation is not recommended because those patients do poorly.

However, if the disease is quiescent with a normal sedimentation rate, standard surgical operations appear to produce satisfactory results.

LOWER EXTREMITY AMPUTATION

General Considerations

More than 90% of the 110,000 amputations performed in the United States each year are for ischemic disease or infective gangrene. More than half of lower extremity amputations are performed for complications of diabetes mellitus, and 15%–50% of diabetic amputees will lose a second leg within 5 years. This risk is about two times higher for men than for women. Other indications for amputations are nondiabetic infection with ischemia (15%–25%); ischemia without infection (5%–10%); osteomyelitis (3%–5%); trauma (2%–5%); and frostbite, tumors, neuromas, and other miscellaneous causes (5%–10%).

Many patients facing amputation are near the end of life because of systemic cardiovascular disease. Approximately 20%–30% of patients undergoing major amputation (below-knee or above-knee) will be dead within 2 years. The prevalence of many comorbidities in this population is also reflected in the perioperative mortality rates for major amputation, ranging from 5% to 10% for below-knee amputations to 10% or higher for above-knee amputations.

The level of amputation is determined by assessing the likelihood of healing of the limb in association with the functional potential of the patient. Compared with normal walking, energy expenditure is increased 10%–40% with a below-knee prosthesis, 50%–70% with an above-knee prosthesis, and 60% with crutches. The clinical conundrum in patients with limb ischemia is twofold: (1) determining which limbs have adequate blood supply to heal at the below-knee level and (2) determining which patients with vascular disease have reasonable rehabilitation potential. The best predictions are based on clinical assessment by an experienced surgeon, assisted by one of the several techniques such as Laser Doppler or transcutaneous measurement of oxygen tension.

Lower Extremity Amputation Levels

Lower extremity amputations are done most commonly at one of the following levels: toe (called digit amputations, which may be extended to include resection of the metatarsal and called ray amputations), transmetatarsal, below-knee, and above-knee. Amputations at other levels (Syme amputation, Chopart amputation, knee disarticulation, and hip disarticulation) are infrequently performed, usually to treat conditions other than vascular disease.

1. Toe and ray amputations—Toe amputations are the most frequently performed amputation (Figure 34–7). Over two thirds of amputations in diabetics involve the toes and

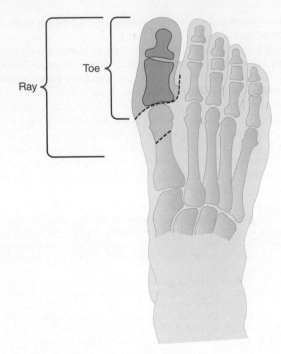

▲ **Figure 34–7.** Toe and ray amputations.

forefoot. A guiding principle is midphalangeal or metatarsal resection to ensure that all cartilaginous articular surfaces are removed because this material has no blood supply. The indications include gangrene, infection, neuropathic ulceration, frostbite, and osteomyelitis limited to the middle or distal phalanx. Good blood flow is required. Contraindications to digit amputation include indistinct demarcation, infection at the metatarsal level, pallor on elevation, or dependent rubor indicating ischemia of the forefoot.

For dry, uninfected gangrene of one or more toes, autoamputation may be allowed to occur. During this process, epithelialization occurs beneath the eschar, and the toe spontaneously detaches, leaving a clean residual limb at the most distal site. Although preferable in many patients (and especially frostbit patients), autoamputation sometimes requires months to complete.

Ray, or wedge, amputation includes removal of the toe and metatarsal head; occasionally, two adjacent toes may be amputated by this method. As with toe amputation, there is modest cosmetic deformity and a prosthesis is not required. Ray amputation of the great toe leads to unstable weight bearing and some difficulty with ambulation resulting from loss of the first metatarsal head.

Complications that may require amputation at higher levels include infection, osteomyelitis of remaining bone, and nonhealing of the incision. These complications have been reported in up to one third of diabetic patients.

2. Transmetatarsal amputation—Transmetatarsal forefoot amputations preserve normal weight bearing. The principal indication is gangrene of several toes or the great toe, with or without soft tissue infection or osteomyelitis. Good blood supply is needed because the incision creates a generous plantar flap. There is no dorsal flap. On the plantar surface, the incision is continued medially to laterally just proximal to the metatarsophalangeal crease. The metatarsal bones are divided with the medial and lateral shafts cut shorter than those in the middle to preserve the normal architecture of the foot and assist with orthotic fitting postoperatively, and the tendons are pulled down and transected as high as possible.

Transmetatarsal amputation produces an excellent functional result. Walking requires no increase in energy expenditure, and the gait is usually smooth. A prosthesis is not mandatory, but to achieve optimal gait, the shoes must be modified.

3. Major leg amputations—An attempt at performing a below-knee amputation is warranted in almost any patient who appears to be a potential candidate for rehabilitation. This may explain why up to one third of patients having below-knee amputations require reamputation.

A. Below-knee amputation—The most common procedure for below-knee amputation is the Burgess technique, which utilizes a long posterior flap (Figure 34–8). The blood supply to a posterior flap is generally better than the supply to an anterior flap or to sagittal flaps, because the sural arteries (which supply the gastrocnemius and soleus muscles) arise high on the popliteal artery, an area not often diseased. The use of rigid dressings and immediate postoperative prostheses has proved advantageous. Application of a rigid cast bandage has several potential advantages: (1) it controls postoperative edema, which may reduce pain; (2) it protects the stump from trauma, particularly when a patient falls during attempts at mobilization; and (3) it allows the patient to be ambulatory with a temporary prosthesis much sooner.

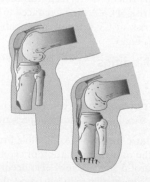

▲ **Figure 34–8.** Below knee amputation.

B. Above-knee amputation—Absolute indications for primary above-knee amputation include contracture at the knee joint (observed in debilitated patients with longstanding extremity pain who have been in a prolonged withdrawal posture with the knee flexed) and nonviable calf muscle or skin for creation of the below-knee flap. The frequent failure of healing of below-knee amputation, the higher perioperative morbidity and mortality in this population (making secondary operations more dangerous), and the modest functional benefit of preserving the knee joint are the major arguments in favor of primary above-knee procedures in nonambulatory patients.

Above-knee amputation may be performed at several levels, including knee disarticulation. Although it is advantageous to preserve as long a lever arm as possible, knee disarticulation is technically more demanding than transfemoral amputation at a higher level. The technique is straightforward. Short anterior and posterior flaps, sagittal flaps, or a circular incision may be used. The bone is divided substantially higher than the skin and soft tissue to avoid tension when the wound is closed and later when the muscles of the thigh atrophy. A simple dressing is then applied.

▼ SPECIAL PROBLEMS OF AMPUTEES

▶ Thromboembolism

The amputee is at great risk for deep venous thrombosis (15%) and pulmonary embolism (2%) postoperatively because (1) amputation often follows prolonged immobilization during treatment of the primary disease and (2) the operation involves ligation of large veins, causing stagnation of blood, a situation that predisposes to thrombosis. If immediate-fit prosthetic techniques are not employed, an additional period of inactivity follows the operation, further increasing the risk of thromboembolism.

▶ Rehabilitation After Amputation

The rehabilitation goals following amputation are highly variable. Younger patients universally want to regain ambulatory status and frequently return to work. Elderly patients with significant comorbid conditions may remain wheelchair-bound, and much of their rehabilitation is focused on providing wheelchair access in their living situations and working on independent transfers. It is important to understand that amputation in an elderly patient is frequently an event that occurs near the end of life. For these people, relief of pain and provision for modest function may be the most appropriate outcome in the limited amount of time they have left.

The length of the residual limb correlates well with regaining the ability to walk. Cardiopulmonary disease and physical weakness make walking an overwhelming effort for some patients; this emphasizes the importance of preserving a below-knee amputation if possible, so that walking will require the least possible amount of energy.

Pain & Flexion Contracture

Physical Therapy consultation is an important adjunct to prevent flexion contractures of the knee or hip occur rapidly in the painful limb because of the natural tendency to assume a flexed posture. Measures to prevent contracture are indicated preoperatively, and application of a rigid dressing postoperatively decreases the incidence of this complication.

Phantom Pain

Persistent sensations in a residual limb are almost universal. Unfortunately, phantom limb pain also is common. Treatment is difficult; improvement has been reported using tricyclic antidepressants, transcutaneous electrical nerve stimulation (TENS), and calcitonin. The incidence and severity of phantom limb pain are increased if there was prolonged ischemia before amputation and decreased if postoperative rehabilitation is rapid.

Ischemia in the Residual Limb

Progressive vascular disease results in ischemia of about 8% of above-knee amputations and 1% of below-knee amputations. Operations are often required to improve arterial flow when gangrene develops in a residual limb. The mortality rate of this condition is high.

Brown BJ, Crone CG, Attinger CE: Amputation in the diabetic to maximize function. Semin Vasc Surg 2012;25:115.

Fleury AM, Salih SA, Peel NM: Rehabilitation of the older vascular amputee: a review of the literature. Geriatr Gerontol Int 2013;13:264.

Jones WS, Patel MR, Dai D, Subherwal S, Stafford J, et al: Temporal trends and geographic variation of lower-extremity amputation in patients with peripheral artery disease: results from US Medicare 2000–2008. J Am Coll Cardiol 2012;60:2230.

Landry GJ, Silverman DA, Liem TK, Mitchell EL, Moneta GL: Predictors of healing and functional outcome following transmetatarsal amputations. Arch Surg 2011;146:1005.

van Eijk MS, van der Linde H, Buijck B, Geurts A, Zuidema S, et al: Predicting prosthetic use in elderly patients after major lower limb amputation. Prosthet Orthot Int 2012;36:45.

▼ CEREBROVASCULAR DISEASE

General Considerations

Unlike in the other vascular beds, symptoms of extracranial carotid disease are most often caused by embolization. Arterial emboli account for approximately one quarter of strokes in Europe and North America, and 80% of these originate from atherosclerotic lesions in a surgically accessible artery in the neck. The most common lesion is at the bifurcation of the carotid artery. Transcranial Doppler studies have shown that emboli are seen in approximately 20% of patients with moderate (> 50% stenosis) lesions at the carotid bifurcation and even higher rates with more than 70% stenoses. The incidence and frequency of emboli is increased in recently symptomatic patients. It would appear that transient deficits and strokes from emboli may not be single events but the result of multiple small emboli that temporarily or permanently obliterate the collateral reserve of the cerebral cortex.

The neurologic dysfunction associated with microemboli may appear as sudden "short-lived," or transient, neurologic symptoms that may include unilateral motor and sensory loss, aphasia (difficulty finding words), or dysarthria (difficulty speaking due to motor dysfunction). These are termed **transient ischemic attacks** (TIA). Most TIAs are brief (minutes). By convention, 24 hours is the arbitrary limit of a TIA. If the symptoms persist, it is a stroke, or **cerebrovascular accident** (CVA). An embolus to the ophthalmic artery, the first branch of the internal carotid artery, produces a temporary monocular loss of vision called amaurosis fugax or permanent blindness. Atherosclerotic emboli may be visible as small bright flecks (Hollenhorst plaques) lodged in arterial bifurcations in the retina.

Characteristically, lesions of atherosclerosis in the internal carotid artery occur along the wall of the carotid bulb opposite to the external carotid artery origin (Figure 34–9). The enlargement of the bulb just distal to this major branch point creates an area of low wall shear stress, flow separation, and loss of unidirectional flow. Presumably, this allows greater interaction of atherogenic particles and the vessel walls at this site and accounts for the localized plaque at the carotid bifurcation.

The accessibility of this localized atheroma allows effective removal of the plaque and a dramatic reduction in stroke risk. Without treatment, 26% of patients with TIAs and more than 70% with carotid stenosis will develop permanent neurologic impairment (CVA) from continued embolization at 2 years. The risk of CVA can be reduced to 9% with plaque removal. The risk of CVA is lower for patients presenting with amaurosis fugax.

Clinical Findings

A. Symptoms

Patients with cerebrovascular disease can be grouped into five categories based on symptoms at presentation.

1. Asymptomatic disease—An audible bruit heard in the neck may be the only manifestation of cerebrovascular disease. Severe carotid stenosis may also occur in the absence of a bruit with markedly reduced blood flow. Ultrasound screening also can identify these patients.

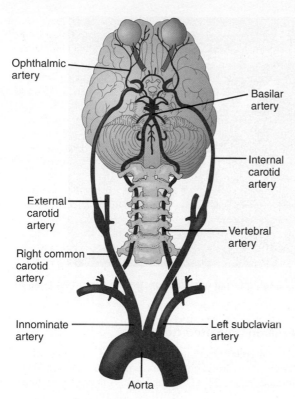

Ophthalmic artery

Basilar artery

Internal carotid artery

External carotid artery

Vertebral artery

Right common carotid artery

Innominate artery

Left subclavian artery

Aorta

▲ **Figure 34–9.** Cerebrovascular circulation anatomy.

2. Transient neurologic episodes—Sudden onset of a neurologic deficit in the distribution of the anterior or middle cerebral arteries requires investigation of the carotid arteries. Symptoms depend on the ischemic area of the brain, the size of the embolus, and the condition of collaterals to the affected area. Hypoperfusion rarely causes transient neurologic and visual attacks. In symptomatic patients, stroke risk after TIA correlates with the severity of internal carotid artery stenosis.

3. Acute unstable neurologic deficits—Patients in this category have multiple (crescendo) TIAs, stroke in evolution, or waxing and waning neurologic deficits and high-grade stenoses. These patients must be treated urgently, because even with anticoagulation, their deficits may become permanent within hours.

4. Stroke (CVA)—Intervention is indicated for patients after stroke that have either complete recovery or mild to moderate deficits, because up to one half will suffer another stroke with further loss of neural function. The timing of intervention is controversial. If the infarct is large and the stenosis severe, a healing period prior to revascularization may be advisable to prevent hemorrhage into the necrotic area with restoration of systemic pressure. In stroke patients, the perioperative risk of additional neurologic deficit is higher than in patients post-TIA.

5. Vertebrobasilar disease—In the posterior circulation, emboli are less common and hypoperfusion is the dominant pathology. Reduction of flow in the vertebral and basilar arteries may cause drop attacks, clumsiness, and a variety of sensory phenomena. Frequently, the symptoms are bilateral. Vertigo, diplopia, or dysequilibrium occurring individually is rarely due to vertebrobasilar disease, but when these symptoms occur in combination, the diagnosis becomes more likely. It is unusual for dizziness alone to be due to cerebrovascular disease.

B. Signs

Auscultation of the carotid and subclavian arteries may delineate the sites of hemodynamically significant disease. However, bruits are nonspecific findings correlating more with overall risk for cardiovascular disease than with stroke.

C. Imaging

1. Doppler ultrasound—The most useful test for the diagnosis of extracranial carotid artery disease is the duplex ultrasound. As the stenosis encroaches on the lumen of the vessel, the velocity of blood increases in the area of the stenosis to maintain distal flow. Doppler spectral velocity analysis determines the flow rate rapidly and with reasonable accurately and thereby gives an estimate of the degree of stenosis. Ultrasound can also display plaque morphology but with less reproducibility than stenosis.

2. CTA and MRA—CTA and MRA are often used for confirmation of duplex findings and planning interventional procedures (Figure 34–10). Both types of angiography can assess the degree of stenosis at the carotid bifurcation, providing information on the configuration of the aortic arch and identifying additional disease in the proximal supra-aortic trunk and intracerebral vessels. These studies also delineate regions of ischemic damage in the brain. Diffusion-weighted MRI of the brain is particularly sensitive and will define areas of injury as well as areas of infarction.

3. Arteriography—Cerebral arteriography is occasionally performed in patients with symptomatic or asymptomatic cerebrovascular disease. It is most useful for cases in which noninvasive studies are in disagreement or in those patients who are candidates for carotid angioplasty and stenting (CAS). Cerebral diagnostic arteriography is invasive and has a low but significant risk of stroke (0.5%–1.0%).

▶ Treatment

Stroke risk is highest immediately after a TIA, returning to baseline at approximately 6 months. Consequently, in symptomatic patients with carotid stenosis, early intervention is mandatory. Antiplatelet therapy, usually in the form of aspirin or clopidogrel, is particularly important in cerebrovascular patients, although clopidogrel should not be initiated in

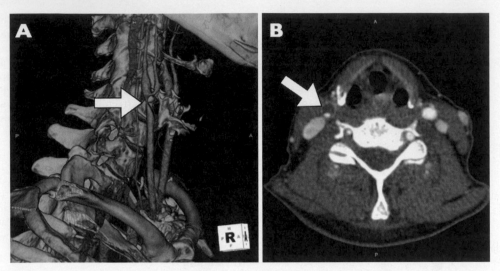

▲ **Figure 34–10.** Carotid bifurcation occlusive disease. **A:** 3D CT angiogram of neck demonstrating carotid bifurcation stenosis. **B:** Axial CT view demonstrating the lesion.

a patient who is scheduled to have a carotid endarterectomy because of the increased risk of bleeding. Cardiovascular risk factor modification is also imperative in reducing stroke and overall mortality. After a completed stroke, caution must be exercised when planning an intervention.

A. Carotid Endarterectomy

Carotid endarterectomy, the removal of the atherosclerotic lesion at the carotid bifurcation, is the primary operation performed (Figure 34–11). In the North American Symptomatic

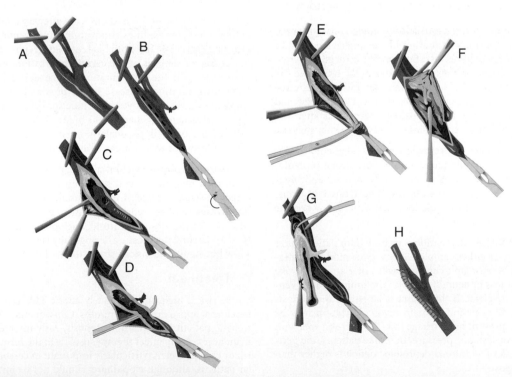

▲ **Figure 34–11.** Technique of carotid endarterectomy.

Carotid Endarterectomy Trial (NASCET), carotid endarterectomy was shown to reduce incidence of ipsilateral stroke from 26% to 9% at 2 years in patients presenting with either TIA or stroke and carotid lesions of 70% stenosis or greater. The results also favored surgery in patients with moderate carotid stenosis (50%–69%), but less dramatically. The 5-year risk of ipsilateral stroke was 15.7% among patients treated surgically ($n = 1108$) and 22.2% among those treated medically ($n = 1118$; $P = .045$). Patients with stenoses of less than 50% did not significantly benefit from surgery.

Large clinical trials have also shown a benefit of surgery for asymptomatic carotid stenosis. Both the Asymptomatic Carotid Atherosclerosis Study (ACAS) in North America and the Asymptomatic Carotid Surgery Trial (ACST) in Europe showed that stroke incidence is halved (12%–6%) by carotid endarterectomy versus best medical therapy, which included antiplatelet agents and statins in the ACST, in patients with substantial carotid narrowing at 5 years of follow-up. While ACAS did not show a benefit for endarterectomy in women, the larger European study did.

Carotid endarterectomy cannot be performed when the internal carotid artery is completely occluded, because complete thrombectomy is difficult and residual clot may embolize, creating additional lesions.

B. Carotid Angioplasty and Stenting

Early studies of carotid angioplasty and stenting (CAS) (Figure 34–12) suggested similar morbidity and mortality rates to carotid endarterectomy. Because of the higher rate of emboli with stenting, cerebral protection devices, either filters placed in the internal carotid or devices that allow a washout of atherosclerotic debris, should always be used. Poststenting, clopidogrel is prescribed for 6 weeks to limit late embolization from the stent.

Two large randomized studies found more strokes after CAS than after endarterectomy, the International Carotid Stent Study (ICSS) and the Carotid Revascularization Endarterectomy versus Stenting Trial (CREST). Conversely, there were more myocardial infarctions after endarterectomy. All women and men over age 70 did worse with CAS. Younger men did well with CAS. Current practice reserves CAS for occlusive lesions of the origins of the arch vessels and for recurrent stenosis after treatment. It is also chosen over endarterectomy in patients with hostile neck anatomy due to prior radiation or "high" lesions not accessible via a neck incision and in patients pre-op for CABG as they are at prohibitive risk for surgery.

C. Treatment Results

The main complication of cerebrovascular interventions is stroke, which occurs in 2%–7% of patients depending on the operative indications and cerebrovascular anatomy. Higher stroke rates occur in the setting of symptomatic stenosis or contralateral carotid occlusion. Lower stroke rates occur with asymptomatic stenosis. The operative death rate for all extracranial cerebrovascular interventions is less than 1%.

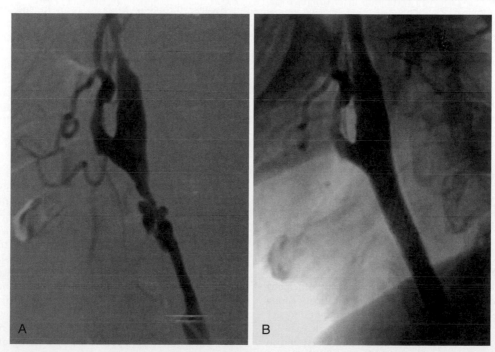

▲ **Figure 34–12.** Carotid angioplasty and stenting. **A:** Conventional arteriogram demonstrating diffuse occlusive disease of common and internal carotid arteries. **B:** Completion arteriogram following angioplasty and stenting of the lesions.

Transient cranial nerve injury occurs in about 10% of cases after endarterectomy and may cause tongue weakness, hoarseness, mouth asymmetry, earlobe numbness, and dysphagia. Less than 2% of peripheral nerve deficits are permanent, although this number goes up with surgery for recurrent disease, making stenting attractive for this indication.

Restenosis or occlusion is uncommon after carotid endarterectomy (5%–10% at 5 years) and appears to be equally uncommon after carotid stenting. For endarterectomy, using a prosthetic patch for closure of the arteriotomy can reduce restenosis.

▶ Subclavian Steal Syndrome

The subclavian steal syndrome is characterized by reversal of flow through the vertebral artery due to a more proximal occlusion or stenosis of the subclavian artery (ie, the vertebral artery serves as a collateral to supply blood to the arm). While this anatomic arrangement is often demonstrated on angiograms, clinical sequelae are rare. Symptoms of effort fatigue in the involved extremity are more common than neurologic complaints. When necessary, treatment consists of bypass grafting from the common carotid to the subclavian artery distal to the lesion or transposition of the subclavian artery beyond the lesion to the side of the nearby common carotid artery.

▶ Concomitant Coronary & Cerebrovascular Disease

When patients have coexistent severe coronary and carotid atherosclerosis requiring treatment, there has been controversy as to which lesion should be addressed first. Since most strokes during cardiac procedures are from atheromatous emboli from the aortic arch, not from low flow through a carotid stenosis, our policy has been to perform combined procedures only in patients with simultaneous symptomatic carotid and coronary disease, with critical bilateral asymptomatic stenoses, or with extremely high-grade (99%) unilateral stenosis. We have initiated a program of stenting the carotid stenoses 1 day prior to coronary artery bypass graft and have found this to be quite satisfactory.

▶ Other Causes of Cerebrovascular Symptoms

Other than atherosclerosis, primary disease of the extracranial arteries is rare.

A. Takayasu (Giant Cell) Arteritis

Takayasu arteritis is an obliterative arteriopathy principally involving the aortic arch vessels that often affects young women. The pararenal abdominal aorta and pulmonary arteries also may be affected. High-dose corticosteroids and cyclophosphamide have been shown to arrest and in some cases reverse the progress of the disease. Operative treatment of nonspecific arteritis should be avoided when the arteritis is active, but it may be successful in quiescent disease.

B. Dissecting Aortic Aneurysms

Dissecting aortic aneurysms may extend into the arch branches, producing obstruction and cerebral symptoms. These are discussed in Chapter 19, Part I.

C. Internal Carotid Dissection

Classically occurring in exercising young adults, dissection originating in the internal carotid artery and localized to its extracranial segment occurs as an acute event that may narrow or obliterate the internal carotid lumen. The primary lesion is an intimal tear at the distal end of the carotid bulb. It may also follow various types of neck trauma or severe hypertension.

Cerebral symptoms are the result of ischemia in the ipsilateral hemisphere. Acute neck pain in association with localized cervical tenderness adjacent to the angle of the mandible is a frequent finding.

Arteriography shows a characteristic pattern of tapered narrowing at or just beyond the distal portion of the carotid bulb. The lumen beyond this point may be obliterated or may persist as a barely visible narrow shadow. If the lumen persists, it resumes a normal caliber beyond the bony foramen.

Because thrombus tends to form in and around the dissected vessel, anticoagulation is the treatment of choice for this disorder. In many patients, the intramural clot will be resorbed, restoring a normal lumen. Intervention is indicated for patients with recurrent TIAs. Stenting is the procedure of choice and will restore the normal carotid contour. If stenting is not successful and symptoms persist, ligation can be performed if the carotid back-pressure exceeds 65 mm Hg. Extracranial to intracranial bypass will be needed if the pressure is low.

D. Fibromuscular Dysplasia

Fibromuscular dysplasia is a nonatherosclerotic angiopathy of unknown cause that affects specific arteries chiefly in young women. Symptoms of cerebrovascular disease can occur when the carotid artery is affected. It is usually bilateral and involves primarily the middle third of the extracranial portions of the internal carotid artery. Several pathologic variants of the disease have been described, but in most of them, the primary lesion is overgrowth of the media in a segmental distribution, producing irregular zones of arterial narrowing. The most common result is a series of concentric rings, producing the radiologic appearance of a string of beads in a long internal carotid artery. Approximately one third of patients are also hypertensive due to renal artery involvement.

The prevalence of fibromuscular dysplasia and the portion of patients who develop symptoms are not known. Once symptoms develop, transient neurologic events are the most common manifestation. However, more than 20% of patients have had a stroke by the time of presentation. Because of the high incidence of neurologic disability, the lesion should be corrected by angioplasty with distal protection when patients develop symptoms. Surgery with dilation of the carotid with graduated dilators or balloon dilation has given excellent results.

Brott TG, Hobson RW, Howard G, Roubin GS, Clark WM, et al: Stenting versus endarterectomy for treatment of carotid-artery stenosis. N Engl J Med 2010;363:11.

Ederle J, Dobson J, Featherstone RL, Bonati LH, van der Worp H B, et al: Carotid artery stenting compared with endarterectomy in patients with symptomatic carotid stenosis (International Carotid Stenting Study): an interim analysis of a randomised controlled trial. Lancet 2010;375:985.

Executive Committee for the Asymptomatic Carotid Atherosclerosis Study (ACAS): Endarterectomy for asymptomatic carotid artery stenosis. JAMA 1995;273:1421.

Fairman R, Gray WA, Scicli AP, Wilburn O, Verta P, et al: The CAPTURE registry: analysis of strokes resulting from carotid artery stenting in the post approval setting: timing, location, severity, and type. Ann Surg 2007;246:551-6.

Ferguson GG, Eliasziw M, Barr HW, et al: The North American Symptomatic Carotid Endarterectomy Trial: surgical results in 1415 patients. Stroke 1999;30:1751.

Fusco MR, Harrigan MR: Cerebrovascular dissections—a review part I: spontaneous dissections. Neurosurgery 2011;68(1):242-57.

Halliday A, et al: Prevention of disabling and fatal strokes by successful carotid endarterectomy in patients without recent neurological symptoms: randomized controlled trial. Lancet 2004;363:1491.

Rothwell PM, Mansfield A, Marro J, et al: Prediction and prevention of stroke in patients with carotid stenosis. Eur J Vasc Endovasc Surg 2008;35:255.

Yadav JS, Wholey MH, Kuntz RE, et al: Stenting and angioplasty with protection in patients at high risk for endarterectomy investigators. Protected carotid-artery stenting versus endarterectomy in high-risk patients. N Engl J Med 2004;351:1493.

RENOVASCULAR HYPERTENSION

General Considerations

More than 23 million people in the United States have hypertension, and renovascular disease is a causative factor in 2%–7% of cases. Atherosclerosis of the aorta and renal artery (two thirds of cases) and fibromuscular dysplasia are the two primary causes of renovascular hypertension. Less common causes of hypertension include renal artery emboli, renal artery aneurysms, renal artery dissection, hypoplasia of the renal arteries, and stenosis of the suprarenal aorta.

Atherosclerosis characteristically produces stenosis at the orifice of the main renal artery. The lesion usually consists of aortic atheroma that protrudes over the renal artery orifice. Less commonly, the atheroma arises in the renal artery itself. Renal artery stenosis is more common in men over age 45 years and is bilateral in about 95% of cases.

Fibromuscular dysplasia usually involves the middle and distal thirds of the main renal artery and may extend into the branches. Medial fibroplasia is the most common variety of fibromuscular dysplasia, accounting for 85% of these lesions. It is bilateral in 50% of cases. Concentric rings of hyperplasia that project into the arterial lumen cause the arterial stenoses. Renal artery aneurysms frequently coexist. Fibromuscular dysplasia occurs mainly in young women, with onset of hypertension usually occurring before age 45 years. It is the causative disorder in 10% of children with hypertension. Developmental renal artery hypoplasia, coarctation of the aorta, and Takayasu aortitis are other vascular causes of hypertension in childhood.

Hypertension due to renal artery stenosis results from the kidney's response to reduced blood flow. Cells of the juxtaglomerular complex secrete renin, which acts on circulating angiotensinogen to form angiotensin I, which is rapidly converted to angiotensin II by ACE. This octapeptide constricts arterioles, increases aldosterone secretion, and promotes sodium retention. Due to the excess aldosterone, hypertension becomes volume-dependent. Over time, pathologic changes occur in the uninvolved kidney, and the hypertension may not be sensitive to ACE inhibition. With sodium restriction and volume reduction (diuretics), the hypertension may once again become sensitive to ACE inhibition. If both kidneys have renal artery stenoses, or if the disease exists in a solitary kidney, renal insufficiency may occur with ACE inhibitor administration with a loss of pressure in the glomerulus due to a reduction of angiotensin II constriction of the efferent arteriole.

Clinical Findings

A. Symptoms and Signs

Most patients are asymptomatic, but irritability, headache, and emotional depression are seen in a few. Persistent elevation of the diastolic pressure is usually the only abnormal physical finding. A bruit is frequently audible to one or both sides of the midline in the flank or upper abdomen. Other signs of atherosclerosis may be present when this is the cause of the renal artery disease.

Other clues to the presence of renovascular hypertension include absence of a family history of hypertension, early onset of hypertension (particularly during childhood or during early adulthood), marked acceleration of the degree of hypertension, resistance to control with antihypertensive drugs, and rapid deterioration of renal function.

One should suspect renovascular hypertension if initial diastolic pressure is greater than 115 mm Hg or if renal function deteriorates while a patient is being given ACE inhibitors. Sudden onset of pulmonary edema with severe hypertension also is highly suggestive of renovascular hypertension.

B. Diagnostic Studies

In the past, several diagnostic tests were devised to diagnose renovascular hypertension. Divided urinary excretion studies, selective renin determinations from renal vein samples, and captopril renal scintigraphy are now rarely used.

Noninvasive or minimally invasive imaging of the renal arteries is justified when the patient has a precipitous drop in blood pressure, decreased renal function with an ACE inhibitor, difficult-to-control hypertension, or unexplained deteriorating renal function.

C. Imaging Studies

In experienced hands, duplex ultrasound scanning has an overall agreement with angiography of over 90%. Renal artery stenosis is characterized by peak systolic velocities in the range of 180-200 cm/s, and the ratio of these velocities to those in the aorta approaches 3.5. CTA or MRA may provide high-resolution images of diseased renal arteries, although must be used with caution in patients with renal insufficiency. The contrast required with CTA is nephrotoxic and gadolinium has been associated with systemic nephrogenic fibrosis in patients with reduced renal clearance.

Renal arteriography is the most accepted method for delineating the obstructive lesion. Since atherosclerotic disease most often involves the origins of the renal arteries, a midstream aortogram should be obtained in addition to selective renal artery catheterization. The presence of collateral vessels circumventing a renal artery stenosis suggests a hemodynamically significant renal artery lesion.

Nonionic contrast agents should be used and the patient should be prepared with overnight hydration. Administration of N-acetylcysteine and periprocedural sodium bicarbonate infusion may give added protections but aggressive hydration remains the primary treatment to reduce the incidence of acute tubular necrosis with angiography and should be used routinely.

▶ Treatment

A. Medical Management

Patients with renovascular hypertension require aggressive management of modifiable risk factors. If hypertension responds well to medical therapy and the renal function is stable, no intervention on the renal artery stenosis is needed.

B. Percutaneous Transluminal Angioplasty and Stenting

Percutaneous transluminal angioplasty (PTA) and stenting is the preferred procedure for most patients (Figure 34–13). Although clearly valuable for some patients, the overall results of percutaneous interventions for renal artery stenosis have been mixed, and large randomized clinical trials suggest that medical treatment with angiotensin receptor blockers may be as effective as stenting in most cases. Patients with fibromuscular dysplasia typically respond to angioplasty alone.

C. Surgical Treatment

In the very young, surgery is still the primary mode of treatment due to concern regarding the long-term durability of angioplasty and stenting. Surgical repair also is required for failed angioplasty and stenting, renal revascularization during a procedure on the aorta, and lesions that are in branch vessels. As with any operation, the indications for arterial reconstruction are influenced by the extent of disease, the patient's life expectancy, and the anticipated morbidity associated with operation. Nephrectomy may be considered when arterial repair is impossible or especially hazardous and the disease is unilateral.

Options include endarterectomy, which is most easily accomplished through an incision into the adjacent aorta, or bypass using prosthetic or autogenous conduits. An alternative is "nonanatomic" bypass such as a hepatorenal or splenorenal procedure. The celiac and splenic arteries often have coexistent occlusive atherosclerotic disease that mandates preoperative arteriographic assessment of these vessels.

Extracorporeal techniques have been developed for distal branch aneurysms or extensive fibromuscular dysplasia. These require removal of the kidney from the abdomen (ex vivo arterial reconstruction), continuous cold perfusion of its vascular tree, and microvascular techniques for arterial replacement. The kidney is then either returned to a site near its original position or transplanted to the ipsilateral iliac fossa.

▶ Prognosis

Procedures for revascularization of the renal artery are successful in lowering blood pressure in over 90% of patients with fibromuscular hyperplasia. Operation for atherosclerotic stenosis results in improvement or cure of hypertension in about 60%. The results for angioplasty and stenting are not as good, perhaps because of atheroembolization to the kidney during angioplasty.

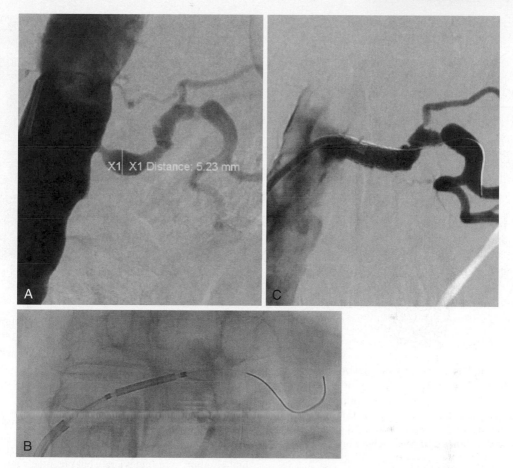

▲ **Figure 34–13.** Renal artery occlusive disease. **A:** Aortogram demonstrating ostial lesion in left renal artery. **B:** Renal stent constrained on delivery catheter over wire positioned across lesion. **C:** Arteriogram demonstrating widely patent renal artery following balloon angioplasty and stent placement.

The results of intervention for salvage of renal function are better than those for treatment of hypertension. The procedural mortality rate of operative renovascular surgery in children is almost nil, whereas it increases to 2%–8% in adults with diffuse atherosclerosis. Stenting of the renal arteries is also very well tolerated.

Herrmann SM, Textor SC: Diagnostic criteria for renovascular disease: where are we now? Nephrol Dial Transplant 2012;27:2657.

Mousa AY, Campbell JE, Stone PA, Broce M, Bates MC, et al: Short- and long-term outcomes of percutaneous transluminal angioplasty/stenting of renal fibromuscular dysplasia over a ten-year period. J Vasc Surg 2012;55:421.

Wheatley K, Ives N, Gray R, Kalra PA, Moss JG, et al: Revascularization versus medical therapy for renal-artery stenosis. N Engl J Med 2009;361:1953.

MESENTERIC ISCHEMIA SYNDROMES

General Considerations

The celiac axis and the superior and inferior mesenteric arteries are the principal sources of blood supply to the stomach and intestines, with the inferior mesenteric artery and internal iliac arteries supplying flow to the distal colon (Figure 34–14). The anatomic collateral interconnections between these arteries are numerous. Single or even multiple visceral artery lesions are generally well tolerated, because collateral flow is readily available (Figure 34–15).

Atherosclerosis is the cause of obstructive lesions in the visceral arteries in the vast majority of cases. Vasculitis (eg, lupus erythematosus, Takayasu disease) is much less common. When atherosclerosis is the cause, the usual lesion

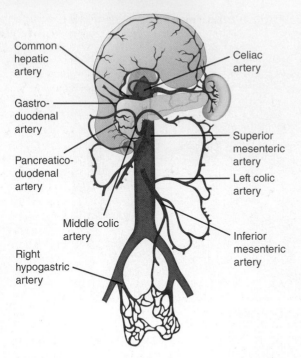

▲ **Figure 34–14.** Visceral arterial circulation and interconnections.

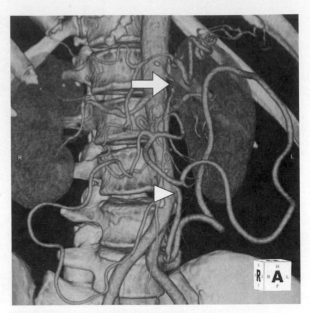

▲ **Figure 34–15.** Three-dimensional CT angiogram demonstrating a critical superior mesenteric artery stenosis (arrow) and collateral vessel enlargement originating at the inferior mesenteric artery (arrowhead).

is a collar of plaque spilling over from the aorta that creates a proximal stenosis or occlusion. Associated atherosclerosis in the aorta and its other branches is common.

CHRONIC MESENTERIC ISCHEMIA

▶ Clinical Findings

The principal complaint is postprandial abdominal pain, which has been labeled abdominal or visceral angina. Pain characteristically appears 15–30 minutes after the beginning of a meal and lasts for an hour or longer. Pain is occasionally so severe and prolonged that opiates are required for relief. Pain occurs as a deep-seated, steady ache in the epigastrium, occasionally radiating to the right or left upper quadrant. Weight loss results from reluctance to eat. Although mild degrees of malabsorption can occur, gastrointestinal absorption studies are not helpful. Diarrhea and vomiting have been described. An upper abdominal bruit may be heard.

Ultrasound can be diagnostic in experienced hands but CTA or arteriography in the anteroposterior and especially the lateral projections demonstrate both the arterial lesion and the patterns of collateral blood flow. Patients should be well hydrated before these procedures because they can precipitate hypercoagulability and osmotic diuresis with dehydration, vascular occlusion, and bowel infarction.

▶ Treatment

Percutaneous transluminal angioplasty (PTA) and stenting has gained acceptance as a first line of therapy for mesenteric ischemia. Results are best for focal, nonorificial stenoses. Embolization to the gut is a rare but potentially fatal complication of instrumentation of these lesions.

Surgical revascularization of the superior mesenteric and celiac axes may be performed by either endarterectomy or graft replacement. During endarterectomy, a sleeve of aortic intima and the orifice lesions in the celiac or superior mesenteric arteries are removed. The operation is performed by a retroperitoneal approach to the aorta through a left thoracoabdominal incision. Alternatively, Dacron grafts may be brought antegrade from the lower thoracic aorta or retrograde from the iliac arteries to the celiac axis or superior mesenteric artery—operations that are performed from within the abdomen.

Operation should be avoided in patients with acute vasculitis as the underlying cause of mesenteric ischemia; high-dose steroids and immunosuppressive agents are indicated instead.

▶ Prognosis

Opening flow to the mesenteric vascular bed almost always results in relief of symptoms. The limited durability of endovascular therapy necessitates close follow-up and reintervention if symptoms recur.

ACUTE MESENTERIC ISCHEMIA

Acute mesenteric ischemia is a highly morbid disorder. Patients classically present with excruciating diffuse abdominal pain with a surprising absence of physical findings such as abdominal tenderness or distention—unless actual bowel perforation produces a surgical abdomen. Symptoms of chronic mesenteric ischemia may precede this catastrophic event, or the onset may be sudden if the cause is embolic occlusion of the superior mesenteric artery. The diagnosis can be difficult, and its recognition is often delayed, resulting in irreversible bowel ischemia. The mortality rate from acute mesenteric ischemia remains high. Patients who require massive bowel resection rarely survive or, if they survive, can develop incapacitating short-gut syndrome. The prognosis improves dramatically if revascularization can be achieved prior to intestinal infarction. This obviously requires early diagnosis, which will only occur if the practitioner has a high index of suspicion.

CELIAC ARTERY COMPRESSION

External compression of the celiac artery, or median arcuate ligament syndrome, is an unusual cause of visceral ischemia. It generally affects young adults, with women more often affected than men, and is commonly associated with rapid weight loss. The classic sign is a loud epigastric bruit with exhalation as the crus of the diaphragm descends to compress the artery. The artery is scarred and must be repaired in conjunction with release of the compressing ligament. The diagnosis is difficult to make with certainty because some compression of the celiac artery by the arcuate ligament is common. Surgery should be advised only after an unsuccessful search for other causes of postprandial pain.

Patients with median arcuate ligament compression respond favorably to operation in most cases; however, some of these patients are not improved even though a technically adequate operation is performed.

Aburahma AF, Campbell JE, Stone PA, Hass SM, Mousa AY, et al: Perioperative and late clinical outcomes of percutaneous transluminal stentings of the celiac and superior mesenteric arteries over the past decade. J Vasc Surg 2013;57:1052.

Tallarita T, Oderich GS, Gloviczki P, Duncan A, Kalra M, et al: Patient survival after open and endovascular mesenteric revascularization for chronic mesenteric ischemia. J Vasc Surg 2013;57:747.

ARTERIAL ANEURYSMS

▶ General Considerations

An aneurysm is defined as a localized dilation of an artery to at least 1.5 times its normal diameter. The expanding vessel elongates as well as dilates. A true aneurysm involves primary dilation of the artery, including all vessel wall layers (intima, media, and adventitia). A false aneurysm, also called pseudoaneurysm, is characterized by a disruption of the artery wall, does not include all layers of the wall, and may actually be a pulsatile hematoma not contained by the artery wall but by a fibrous capsule. A false aneurysm caused by infection is called a mycotic aneurysm.

False aneurysms of the femoral artery secondary to catheterization are the most numerous of all aneurysms. Infrarenal abdominal aortic aneurysms (AAA) are the most common of the true aneurysms. In descending order, other arteries affected are the iliac arteries, the popliteal artery, the arch and descending portions of the thoracic aorta (including dilation after aortic dissection), the common femoral artery, the carotid arteries, and other peripheral arteries. Other rare causes of true aneurysms include Marfan syndrome, Ehlers–Danlos syndrome, Behçet disease, and cystic medial necrosis.

ABDOMINAL AORTIC ANEURYSMS

AAA are found in 2% of the elderly male population, and the incidence may be increasing. In selected groups, the incidence is higher—5% of patients with coronary artery disease and as many as 50% of patients with femoral or popliteal aneurysms have aortic aneurysms. Men are four times as likely to be affected as women. Ruptured aortic aneurysms are a cause of death of men age greater than 65 years in the United States, resulting in 15,000 deaths per year.

Numerous mechanisms have been proposed for the cause of AAA. Structural issues may contribute; reductions in the number of elastic lamellae and virtual absence of vasa vasorum in the media of the distal abdominal aorta compared with the thoracic aorta may favor aneurysmal degeneration. Excessive protease activity or local reductions in the concentration of protease inhibitors have been implicated in aneurysm formation, allowing for the enzymatic destruction of the two principal structural elements of the aorta, elastin, and collagen. There may be hemodynamic factors as well, owing to large pulsatile stresses because of tapering geometry, increased stiffness, and reflected pressure waves from branch vessels in the infrarenal aorta. Genetic factors influencing connective tissue metabolism and structure also have been associated with AAA development. Indeed, a positive family history of aortic aneurysms infers a 20% chance that a first-degree family member will have an aneurysm.

In terms of risk factors, cigarette smoking has a powerful influence on developing an aortic aneurysm, with an 8:1 preponderance of AAA in smokers compared with nonsmokers. The excess prevalence associated with smoking accounted for 78% of all AAA that were 4 cm or larger in the Veterans Administration ADAM study sample.

Hypertension is present in 40% of patients with AAA but did not correlate with enlargement in the ADAM study. Surprisingly, diabetics appear to have a lower incidence of aortic aneurysm formation.

Ninety percent of aneurysms of the abdominal aorta occur between the takeoff of the renal arteries and the aortic bifurcation but may include variable portions of the common iliac arteries. Rupture with exsanguination is the major complication of AAA. Unfortunately, neither the expansion rate nor the rupture risk is predictable. Tension on the aneurysm wall is governed by the law of Laplace. Thus, rupture risk is related to diameter. While relating this to an individual's risk is not possible, population-wide risks have been established. Because most aneurysms cause no symptoms prior to rupture, the number of deaths due to ruptured AAA has not changed significantly in the past 20 years. This has prompted a recommendation for ultrasound screening of smoking males over the age of 65 years.

▶ Clinical Findings

A. Symptoms and Signs

The vast majority of unruptured aneurysms are asymptomatic. Rarely, intact AAAs produce back pain due to pressure on nerves or erosion into vertebral bodies. Severe pain in the absence of rupture characterizes the rare inflammatory aneurysm that is surrounded by 2-4 cm of perianeurysmal retroperitoneal inflammatory reaction.

Eighty percent of 5 cm AAAs are palpable as a **pulsatile abdominal mass** in the mid-abdomen just above and to the left side of the umbilicus. Physical examination for an AAA is less reliable in obese patients. The aneurysm may be slightly tender to palpation. Extreme tenderness suggests a "symptomatic aneurysm" and is found in inflammatory aneurysms or if the aneurysm has recently expanded. A truly noninflammatory, symptomatic (tender) aneurysm demands urgent surgery.

B. Imaging Studies

Plain films of the abdomen reveal calcification in the outer layers of only 20% of abdominal aneurysms.

Ultrasound is the least expensive method for measuring the size of infrarenal aortic aneurysms. Repeated ultrasound examinations are cost effective for observing small AAAs and may be used to follow resolution of the aneurysm after endovascular repair. However, ultrasound examinations do not delineate adjacent structures as well as CT or MR and are less reliable in obese patients.

CT scan or MRI with 3D reconstructions are both accurate methods for assessing aneurysm diameter, although the ADAM trial showed that there can be substantial inter-reader variability in size determinations (Figure 34–16). An important source of error occurs when the course of the aneurysmal aorta is diagonal to the cross-sectional

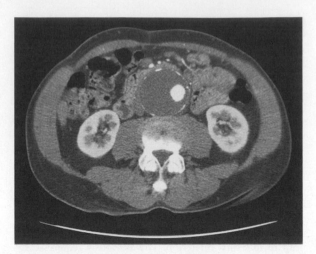

▲ **Figure 34–16.** CT showing the typical position of a 5.5-cm abdominal aortic aneurysm and its proximity to the abdominal wall.

image. This creates an elliptical image of the AAA and a falsely elevated diameter in the larger dimension. CT scans provide valuable information about aneurysm location and size as well as important adjacent structures that affect AAA repair, such as horseshoe kidneys or other renal abnormalities, and venous anomalies, including retroaortic renal veins, circumaortic renal veins, and left-sided or duplicated vena cavae, which may have important surgical implications. If the patient has a multiplanar CT scan, aortograms, once routine studies in planning operative management of AAAs, are not needed.

C. Natural History

Most aneurysms continue to enlarge and will eventually rupture if left untreated. The average expansion rate for an AAA is 0.4 cm per year. The rate of expansion correlates with continued smoking, initial aneurysm diameter, and the degree of obstructive pulmonary disease. An expansion of 0.5 cm in 6 months or 1 cm over 12 months qualifies as rapid enlargement and suggests the aneurysm is unstable and should be repaired.

Aneurysm size is currently the best determinant of rupture risk. About 40% of aneurysms 5.5-6 cm or larger in diameter will rupture within 5 years if untreated, and the average survival of an untreated patient is 17 months. In contrast, the ADAM study found a 0.5% per year rupture rate in AAAs 4-5.4 cm, an overall rate remarkably similar to a comparable trial in the United Kingdom. Thus, *surgery is recommended for aneurysms 5.5 cm or more in size,* but small aortic aneurysms can be safely followed. Regardless of size, repair is mandatory for an aneurysm that is symptomatic or enlarging rapidly.

D. Treatment

1. Endovascular repair—Endovascular repair, introduced in 1991, is achieved with a synthetic graft to which metal stents have been attached (Figure 34–17). Endovascular repair requires that the aorta proximal to the aneurysm have a cylindrical configuration ideally 1.5 cm to allow for adequate sealing and iliac arteries of sufficient size and limited tortuosity so that the device can be introduced from the femoral arteries. Devices for endovascular repair of AAAs are delivered using a system of guidewires and delivery systems with large-bore sheaths. Several devices are available with unique design features. In series of comparable patients, patients with endovascular repair have less operative blood loss, shorter hospital stays, and reduced operative morbidity compared to those undergoing conventional repair.

The most important intermediate or long-term adverse outcome of endovascular repair is persistent perfusion of the aneurysm ("endoleak"). These are divided into types denoting clinical importance. A type 1 endoleak denotes ineffective proximal or distal sealing with pressurization of the aneurysm sac and should be fixed immediately. A type 2 endoleak results in persistent flow through the aneurysm between small aortic branches, usually from the inferior mesenteric artery to a patent lumbar artery. These have relatively low pressures and, unless the aneurysm is enlarging, are not treated. Pressurization of the aneurysm through the graft itself is a type 3 endoleak. The graft should be repaired or replaced if the aneurysm continues to enlarge over time due to a type 2 or type 3 leak.

Rupture has occurred after endovascular aortic aneurysm repair. The rate of late ruptures is low but underscores that patients need extended follow-up to ensure the durability of endovascular aneurysm repair. Endograft repair is more expensive than open repair in spite of the lower periprocedural morbidity and shorter hospital stays. The devices are expensive ($10,000-15,000), and there is further cost due to the extended follow-up with imaging studies to identify graft movement or endoleak.

2. Open repair—Conventional open operative AAA repair consists of replacing the aneurysmal segment with a synthetic fabric graft (Figure 34–18). Tubular or bifurcation grafts of Dacron or PTFE are preferred. The proximal anastomosis is made to the aorta above the aneurysm. The site of the distal anastomosis is determined by the extent of aneurysmal involvement of the iliac arteries. Traditionally, a transperitoneal approach via midline laparotomy has been

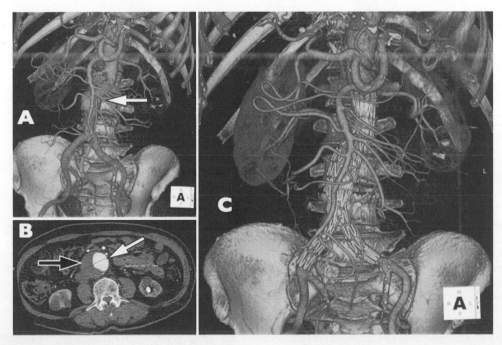

▲ **Figure 34–17.** **A:** Three-dimensional CT angiogram reconstruction of abdominal aortic aneurysm. White arrow points to aortic flow lumen at same level as that in panel B. **B:** Axial CT view. White arrow points to flow lumen, black arrow points to thrombus within aneurysm sac. Notice only aortic flow lumen visualized on CT angiogram, just as in conventional angiography. Total diameter of the aorta, including area containing thrombus, is used in predicting rupture risk and determining need for intervention. **C:** Three-dimensional CT angiogram following aortic stent graft repair.

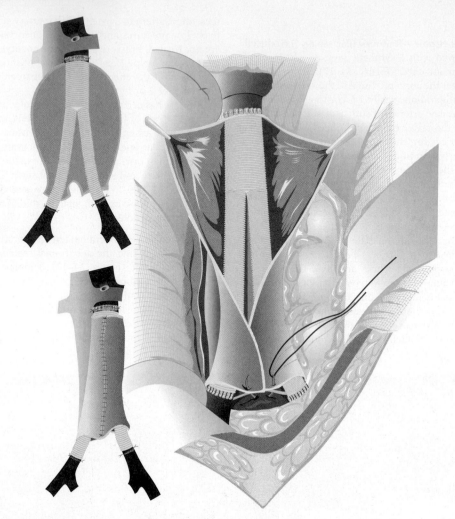

▲ **Figure 34–18.** Replacement of an aortic aneurysm with a synthetic bifurcation graft. The laminated clot within the aneurysm has been removed, and the outer wall is closed over the graft.

used for AAA repair, but retroperitoneal operations via flank incision may decrease perioperative pulmonary and gastrointestinal complications.

Elective infrarenal abdominal aneurysmectomy has a 2%–4% operative death rate and a 5%–10% rate of complications, such as bleeding, renal failure, myocardial infarction, graft infection, limb loss, bowel ischemia, and erectile dysfunction. Paraplegia is a very rare complication due to involvement of an abnormally low artery of Adamkiewicz, a major collateral of the anterior spinal artery. Malignant tumors are encountered unexpectedly in about 4% of cases, although that rate is now dwindling with the routine use of multiplanar CT scans. If gastrointestinal malignancy is encountered during an aneurysm resection, the aneurysm

repair should be done first unless there is impending bowel obstruction.

Long-term results of open aneurysmectomy are excellent: graft failure rate is low and false aneurysm formation at the anastomoses is rare. The long-term survival of these patients is determined principally by their extent of coronary artery disease.

ILIAC ANEURYSMS

Iliac artery aneurysms generally occur in conjunction with AAAs. Isolated iliac aneurysms are unusual, but in some cases, the iliac segment of the aneurysmal artery may enlarge at a greater rate than the aortic segment and is the primary reason for repair. As with aortic aneurysms, most iliac aneurysms are asymptomatic. However, they may present with symptoms related to compression or erosion of surrounding structures, such as obstructive uropathy with ureteral obstruction, neuropathy from compression of local nerves, and unilateral leg swelling from compression of the adjacent iliac vein.

Physical examination can suggest the diagnosis of large (> 4 cm) iliac artery aneurysms if the physician is alert to that possibility. Most symptomatic iliac aneurysms can be palpated as pulsatile masses on abdominal or rectal examinations. However, iliac aneurysms are usually found incidentally on ultrasound or CT.

Similar to aortic aneurysms, iliac aneurysms tend to enlarge and rupture unpredictably, but size is the most important determinant of rupture risk. Iliac aneurysms that are less than 3.5 cm in size should be followed up with serial imaging. Those that enlarge to 4 cm should be repaired in patients without serious operative risk factors.

The challenge of iliac aneurysm repair is in preserving flow to the pelvis through at least one internal iliac artery to prevent pelvic ischemia that can present as buttock claudication, impotence, or ischemia of the distal colon. Open repair of isolated iliac arteries is well tolerated and can be done through a retroperitoneal approach. If the ipsilateral hypogastric artery is also aneurysmal, repair will require opening the sac and ligating the branches from within the aneurysm, taking care not to injure the iliac veins surrounding the aneurysm.

SUPRARENAL AORTIC ANEURYSMS

Aneurysms of the segment of aorta between the diaphragm and the renal arteries account for only 10% of AAAs, with 6% being pararenal and 4% involving the visceral vessels. Resection and graft replacement of the upper abdominal aorta is an operation of far greater magnitude and risk than operations on the infrarenal aorta. Involvement of the renal arteries doubles operative mortality with substantial additional risk for involvement of the visceral vessels. Renal failure and bowel ischemia are much more common after repair of these aneurysms than after repair of infrarenal aortic aneurysms. There is also a risk of paraplegia if flow is interrupted to the artery of Adamkiewicz. An extended incision is usually necessary, and provisions must be made for revascularization of the celiac axis and the superior mesenteric and renal arteries. The use of perfusion catheters for the visceral and renal arteries has improved results, and left heart bypass is used in true thoracoabdominal aneurysms.

Because of the mortality and morbidity of repair of suprarenal aneurysms, there has been considerable interest in endovascular repair of these aneurysms using branched systems. Initial experience from selected centers, including our own, has shown dramatic reduction in morbidity and mortality from these technically demanding endovascular procedures. In patients judged to be high risk for open repair, branched graft repair has equaled the best reported results for open repair.

RUPTURED AORTIC ANEURYSMS

▶ General Considerations

With increasing aneurysm size, lateral pressure within the aneurysm will eventually lead to spontaneous rupture of the aneurysm wall. Although immediate exsanguination may ensue, there is often an interval of several hours between the first episode of bleeding and death from exsanguination when the initial bleed is contained in the retroperitoneal tissues, a "contained rupture." When the periaortic tissue can no longer contain the expanding hematoma, "free rupture" occurs with exsanguination into the free peritoneal cavity.

▶ Clinical Findings

The patient presents with sudden, severe abdominal pain that usually radiates into the back and occasionally into the inguinal region. Lightheadedness or syncope results from blood loss. Pain may lessen and lightheadedness may disappear after the first hemorrhage, only to reappear and progress to shock if bleeding continues. When bleeding remains contained in the periaortic tissue, a discrete, pulsatile abdominal mass may be felt. In contrast with an intact aneurysm, the ruptured aneurysm at this stage is painful to palpation. Signs of an acute abdomen may be present. As bleeding continues, usually into the retroperitoneum, the discrete mass is replaced by a poorly defined mid-abdominal fullness, often extending toward the left flank.

Shock can be profound, manifested by peripheral vasoconstriction, hypotension, and anuria. Unfortunately, the classic triad of pain, a pulsatile abdominal mass, and hypotension is not always present, and precious time may be lost while confirming the diagnosis. An abdominal ultrasound performed in the emergency room will confirm the presence of an aortic aneurysm but may not disclose hemorrhage. CT scans reliably confirm hemorrhage from an aneurysm, but in unstable patients, the delay in progressing to the operating room precludes their use. It is best to follow the adage that a patient with an AAA, signs of an acute abdomen, and hypotension belongs in the operating room.

▶ Treatment & Prognosis

Repair should be performed as soon as intravenous fluids have been started, the airway has been secured, and blood has been sent for cross-matching. Surgical control of the aorta proximal and distal to the aneurysm must be obtained immediately and should be attempted from the abdomen. Attempts to control the proximal aorta through the chest have been associated with poor outcomes. A successful outcome of the operation is related to the patient's condition on arrival, the promptness of diagnosis, and the speed of operative control of bleeding and blood replacement. The operative death rate is between 30% and 80%, with an average of approximately 50%. Because many patients with ruptured aneurysms die before reaching the hospital, the overall death rate approaches 80%. Without operation, the outcome is uniformly fatal. Many centers are now treating ruptured AAA using endovascular stent grafts; morbidity and mortality remain high and abdominal compartment syndrome has been a complication requiring evacuation of the retroperitoneal hematoma.

INFLAMMATORY ANEURYSMS

Inflammatory aneurysms are degenerative aneurysms that elicit a unique inflammatory response adjacent to the external calcified layer of the aneurysm wall. Although similar to retroperitoneal fibrosis, the inflammation is usually confined to the anterior aorta and iliac arteries. The aneurysm may be responsible to chronic abdominal pain and is tender to palpation. One fourth of patients have some degree of ureteral obstruction. CT scanning reliably demonstrates the characteristic thickened wall and confirms the diagnosis. Characteristic pathologic changes include infiltration of the aortic wall by lymphocytes, plasma cells, occasional multinucleated giant cells, and lymphoid follicles with germinal centers. Inflammation resolves in most cases after successful repair. Inflammatory aneurysms are easily recognized at operation by the dense, shiny, white, fibrotic material that envelops the adjacent viscera, especially the duodenum, left renal vein, and inferior vena cava. Those structures are therefore especially vulnerable to operative injury. Endovascular repair is ideal and is the procedure of choice for inflammatory aneurysms. After repair, the inflammatory tissue usually regresses.

INFECTED (MYCOTIC) ANEURYSMS

The confusing term "mycotic aneurysm" is commonly used to denote infected aneurysms in general, which are rarely fungal. The aneurysm is secondary to a microbial aortitis in which virulent bacteria infect the aorta and destroy the aortic wall. Historically, salmonella infection was the most common cause. In the current era, staphylococcus is the more common infection due to intravenous drug use. These organisms may involve every major artery, but aortic involvement predominates.

The typical patient presents with a rapidly enlarging, tender pulsatile mass that may feel warm, if palpable. Fever is present, and half the patients have positive blood cultures. Alternatively, the aneurysm may be discovered late, after successful treatment of the infection. Angiography of these patients may show a saccular false aneurysm. Treatment consists of excision and remote bypass grafting if possible. Liberal application of muscle flap coverage techniques facilitates healing. Direct repair has been successful when done after a course of antibiotics. A prolonged course of antibiotics should be given to guard against recurrence.

PERIPHERAL ARTERIAL ANEURYSMS

General Considerations

Popliteal artery aneurysms account for 70% of peripheral arterial aneurysms. Like aortic aneurysms, they are silent until critically symptomatic. However, unlike aortic aneurysms, they rarely rupture. The presenting manifestations are due to peripheral embolization and thrombosis, possibly due to movement of the artery with knee flexion. Popliteal aneurysms may embolize repetitively over time and occlude distal arteries. Due to the redundant parallel arterial supply to the foot, ischemia does not occur until a final embolus occludes flow to the remaining tibial/peroneal artery. Acute ischemia caused by popliteal aneurysms has a poor prognosis because of the chronicity of the process. The results of both chemical and mechanical thrombolysis may be disappointing because of clot age and adherence to the artery wall. After presentation with acute ischemia, approximately one third of patients will require an amputation. To prevent embolization and thrombosis, popliteal artery aneurysms should be repaired electively if greater than 2 cm in diameter or at any size if lined with thrombus.

Primary aneurysms of the femoral artery are much less common than aneurysms of the popliteal artery. However, pseudoaneurysms of the femoral artery following arterial punctures for arteriography and cardiac catheterization occur with an incidence ranging from 0.05% to 6%. Thrombosis and embolization are the main risks of femoral true or false aneurysms and, like popliteal aneurysms, should be repaired when greater than 2 cm in diameter.

Clinical Findings

A. Symptoms and Signs

Until progressive embolization or thrombosis occurs, peripheral artery aneurysms are usually asymptomatic. The patient may be aware of a pulsatile mass when the aneurysm is in the groin, but popliteal aneurysms are often undetected by the patient and physician. Peripheral aneurysms may produce symptoms by compressing the local vein or nerve, but this is unusual. In most patients, the first symptom is due to ischemia of acute arterial occlusion. The pathologic findings range from rapidly developing gangrene to moderate ischemia that slowly lessens as collateral circulation develops. Symptoms from recurrent embolization to the leg are often transient if they occur at all. Sudden ischemia may appear in a toe or part of the foot, followed by slow resolution, and the true diagnosis may be elusive. The onset of recurrent episodes of pain in the foot, particularly if accompanied by cyanosis, suggests embolization and requires investigation of the heart and proximal arterial tree.

Because popliteal pulses are somewhat difficult to palpate even in normal individuals, a particularly prominent or easily felt pulse is suggestive of aneurysmal dilation and should be investigated by ultrasound. Since popliteal aneurysms are bilateral in 60% of cases, the diagnosis of thrombosis of a popliteal aneurysm is often aided by the palpation of a pulsatile aneurysm in the contralateral popliteal space. Approximately 50% of patients with popliteal aneurysms have an aneurysmal abdominal aorta.

B. Imaging Studies

Duplex color ultrasound is the most efficient investigation to confirm the diagnosis of peripheral aneurysm, to measure its size and configuration, and to demonstrate mural thrombus.

Arteriography may not demonstrate aneurysms accurately, because mural thrombus reduces the apparent diameter of the lumen. Three-dimensional imaging by CTA or MRA is required—especially when operation is considered—to define the anatomy and plan intervention.

C. Treatment

Early operation is indicated for an aneurysm that is greater than 2 cm in size associated with any peripheral embolization or an aneurysm with mural thrombus. Urgent operation is indicated when acute embolization or thrombosis has caused acute ischemia. Intra-arterial thrombolysis may be done in the setting of acute ischemia if examination (light touch) suggests that immediate surgery is not imperative to prevent tissue loss. Bypass with saphenous vein may include either excision or exclusion, depending on location. If exclusion rather than resection is performed, the geniculate "feeder" arteries within the aneurysm should be ligated or progressive enlargement can still occur.

Endovascular repair with covered stents can be used but are less durable than open repair and should be reserved for patients at high operative risk.

Acute pseudoaneurysms of the femoral artery due to arterial punctures can be successfully treated using ultrasound-guided compression and thrombin injections if the aneurysm is not large.

D. Prognosis

The long-term patency of bypass for femoral and popliteal aneurysms is generally excellent but depends on the adequacy of the outflow tract. Late graft occlusion is less common than in similar operations for occlusive disease.

UPPER EXTREMITY ANEURYSMS

▶ Subclavian Artery Aneurysms

Subclavian artery aneurysms are less common than aneurysms of the lower extremity, and most supraclavicular pulsatile masses represent tortuous vessels, not aneurysms. Pseudoaneurysms due to injections by drug addicts are becoming increasingly frequent. An anomaly, the aberrant right subclavian artery (incidence 0.5%), arises from the aorta distal to the left subclavian and courses behind the esophagus. As found in other aberrant arteries, enlargement is common and may compress the esophagus against the trachea, causing difficulty swallowing (termed dysphagia lusoria). This anomaly also is the most common cause of a nonrecurrent laryngeal nerve.

A true subclavian artery aneurysm is usually due to poststenotic dilation in a patient with thoracic outlet syndrome or a large callous from a fractured clavicle. As with popliteal aneurysms, the most common manifestation is embolization with episodic hand ischemia and Raynaud's phenomenon. The diagnosis is often missed. Sudden onset Raynaud's, particularly with a history of waxing and waning digital ischemia, is indication for arterial imaging. Treatment consists of resection of the restricting structures at the time of arterial replacement.

▶ Radial Artery False Aneurysms

The incidence of radial artery false aneurysms has increased as a result of increasing use of radial artery catheters. Occasionally, the aneurysm is infected. If the Allen test is normal and adequate collateralization is confirmed with imaging, treatment consists of excision and ligation. If the ulnar collaterals are insufficient to preserve viability of the hand, excision and replacement with vein should be performed.

Small aneurysms of the palmer arch may be due to repetitive trauma. These aneurysms can be responsible for emboli to the digital arteries. The adage that hand ischemia requires angiography should be applied to ensure that all potentially reversible causes of hand ischemia, including these unusual aneurysms, be identified.

Baxter BT, Terrin MC, Dalman RL: Medical management of small abdominal aortic aneurysms. Circulation 2008;117:1883. Review.

Chuter TA, et al: Endovascular treatment of thoracoabdominal aortic aneurysms. J Vasc Surg 2008;47:6.

Lederle FA, Freischlag JA, Kyriakides TC, Matsumura JS, Padberg FT, et al: Long-term comparison of endovascular and open repair of abdominal aortic aneurysm. N Engl J Med 2012;367:1988.

Lindholt JS, Norman P: Screening for abdominal aortic aneurysm reduces overall mortality in men. A meta-analysis of the mid- and long-term effects of screening for abdominal aortic aneurysms. Eur J Vasc Endovasc Surg 2008;36:167.

Mehta M, Byrne J, Darling RC, Paty PS, Roddy SP, et al: Endovascular repair of ruptured infrarenal abdominal aortic aneurysm is associated with lower 30-day mortality and better 5-year survival rates than open surgical repair. J Vasc Surg 2013;57:368.

Paravastu SC, Ghosh J, Murray D, Farquharson FG, Serracino Inglott F, et al: A systematic review of open versus endovascular repair of inflammatory abdominal aortic aneurysms. Eur J Vasc Endovasc Surg 2009;38:291.

Tsilimparis N, Dayama A, Ricotta J: Open and endovascular repair of popliteal artery aneurysms: tabular review of the literature. Ann Vasc Surg 2013;27:259.

VISCERAL ARTERY ANEURYSMS

General Considerations

The etiology of this interesting group of aneurysms is generally unknown. Most often they occur as single lesions in a younger age group than those at risk for aortic aneurysms. Rupture is the primary danger and is one cause of "abdominal apoplexy."

Splenic Artery Aneurysms

Aneurysms of the splenic artery account for more than 60% of splanchnic artery aneurysms. Women are affected four times more commonly than men and often during childbearing years. Arterial fibrodysplasia and portal hypertension predispose to formation of splenic artery aneurysms. Rupture, the major complication, has been reported in less than 2% of splenic aneurysms; it rarely occurs with lesions smaller than 2-3 cm in diameter. Rupture during pregnancy tends to occur in the third trimester and is associated with a 75% maternal death rate and 90% fetal death rate. Diagnosis is most often made from plain x-ray films of the abdomen, showing concentric calcification in the upper left quadrant.

Intervention is indicated for patients with symptomatic aneurysms, aneurysms in pregnant women, and patients who have a low operative risk profile with aneurysms greater than 3 cm in diameter. Endovascular repair with covered stent grafts is ideal with the use of microcatheters developed for intracranial work, improving the ability to negotiate the often tortuous splenic artery. Laparoscopic ligation of the artery is also feasible.

Hepatic Artery Aneurysms

Hepatic artery aneurysms account for 20% of splanchnic artery aneurysms. There is a 2:1 male-to-female ratio, and the frequency of reported rupture is about 20%. Aneurysm rupture is associated with a 35% mortality rate. Rupture into the biliary tree producing hemobilia is as frequent as intraperitoneal rupture. The symptom triad of intermittent abdominal pain, gastrointestinal bleeding, and jaundice strongly suggests the diagnosis and is present in about one third of patients. Surgery is usually required to control bleeding. If the common hepatic artery is involved, the artery may be safely ligated if collateral flow through the gastroduodenal artery has been demonstrated. Aneurysms in other portions of the artery usually require vascular reconstruction. Endovascular placement with a covered stent is preferred if the anatomy is suitable.

Superior Mesenteric Artery Aneurysms

Aneurysms of the proximal superior mesenteric artery account for 5% of all splanchnic artery aneurysms. Unlike splenic or hepatic aneurysms, 60% of superior mesenteric artery aneurysms are mycotic. The aneurysm may involve the origin or branches of the artery. Symptoms include nonspecific abdominal pain. The diagnosis can be made on CT scan.

Operative therapy for mycotic superior mesenteric artery aneurysms includes ligation if there are adequate collaterals or replacement with a segment of autogenous vessel. Endovascular stent graft placement is not advisable in an acute infection. However, it is valuable for true aneurysms as long as critical branches can be avoided. For distal branch aneurysms, bowel resection may be necessary.

RENAL ARTERY ANEURYSMS

This uncommon aneurysm occurs in less than 0.1% of the population and is often associated with hypertension. The aneurysm is usually saccular and located at a primary or secondary bifurcation of the renal arteries. Women are affected slightly more frequently than men. There are three principal categories: (1) idiopathic, (2) aneurysms associated with medial fibrodysplastic disease, and (3) arteritis-related microaneurysms.

Renovascular hypertension may occur because of distortion of the involved or nearby vessels by the aneurysm. Spontaneous rupture of renal artery aneurysms is rare except during pregnancy. CT scans or digital subtraction angiography should be performed to monitor enlargement. Operation is indicated in women of childbearing age or in patients with associated renal artery disease, uncontrolled hypertension, or large aneurysms. Most renal artery aneurysms can be repaired in situ, but ex vivo repair is occasionally required. Endovascular options are usually limited due to the involved vessel size and the aneurysm's proximity to artery branch points.

VASOCONSTRICTIVE DISORDERS

General Considerations

Vasoconstrictive disorders are characterized by abnormal activity of the sympathetic nervous system that reduces peripheral blood flow, causing tissue ischemia.

Raynaud's Disease/Phenomenon

Raynaud's disease/phenomenon consists of sequential pallor, cyanosis, and rubor of fingers or toes after exposure to cold. Excessive vasoconstriction, sluggish flow, and reflex vasodilation produce the characteristic white-blue-red color changes.

In Raynaud's disease, this response, due to spasm alone without underlying arterial lesions, is quite common and benign.

Sudden onset or progression of symptoms suggests underlying arterial lesions that exaggerate the normal reduction in blood flow caused by vasoconstriction. This is termed Raynaud's phenomenon, a more virulent entity associated primarily with immunologic and connective tissue disorders (eg, scleroderma, systemic lupus erythematosus, polymyositis, or drug-induced vasculitis). However, repeated embolization, occupational trauma (vibration injury, cold injury), and other disorders (cold agglutinins, chronic renal failure, and neoplasia) also have been reported.

Hyperreactivity to cold stimuli may be the initial presentation of arterial pathology. In new onset or severe cases of Raynaud's-type symptoms, a search for underlying pathology is required. All patients with Raynaud syndrome should avoid cold exposure, tobacco, oral contraceptives, β-adrenergic blocking agents, and ergotamine preparations. Calcium-channel blockers are generally prescribed but may cause hypotension. Transdermal prostaglandins, ketanserin, and cilostazol also have been used, with relief of symptoms in some patients. In rare cases, symptoms progress to tissue loss. Finger amputation is necessary once gangrene has developed.

Acrocyanosis

Acrocyanosis is a common, chronic, benign vasoconstrictive disorder related to Raynaud syndrome that is largely restricted to young women. It is characterized by persistent cyanosis of the hands and feet. The changes disappear with exposure to a warm environment. Examination in a cool room shows diffuse symmetric cyanosis, coldness, and occasionally hyperhidrosis of the hands and feet. Cyanosis of the skin of the calf, thigh, or forearm usually displays a reticulated pattern and has been called livedo reticularis and cutis marmorata. The peripheral pulses may diminish in the cold but return to normal with rewarming.

THORACIC OUTLET SYNDROME

General Considerations

Thoracic outlet syndrome refers to the variety of disorders caused by abnormal compression of arterial, venous, or neural structures in the base of the neck. Numerous mechanisms for compression have been described, including cervical rib, anomalous ligaments, hypertrophy of the anterior scalene muscle, and positional changes that alter the normal relation of the first rib to the structures that pass over it. Patients may describe a history of cervical trauma.

Symptoms rarely develop until adulthood. For this reason, it has been assumed that an alteration of normal structural relationships that occurs with advancing years is the primary factor. Even anomalous cervical ribs seem well tolerated during childhood and adolescence.

Transient circulatory changes may occur, but the primary cause of symptoms in most patients is intermittent compression of one or more trunks of the brachial plexus. Thus, neurologic symptoms predominate over those of ischemia or venous compression. When present, compression of the subclavian artery and vein in the thoracic outlet also can produce severe sequelae. Compression of the subclavian artery can produce stenosis and poststenotic dilation of the artery, leading to arterial occlusion or emboli, as discussed earlier. Compression of the vein between the anterior scalene, clavicle, and first rib can produce thrombosis, which can result in severe upper extremity pain and swelling. Compression may be exaggerated with exercise precipitating an occlusion. This syndrome is termed effort thrombosis or **Paget–Schroetter syndrome.**

Clinical Findings

A. Symptoms and Signs

Neural symptoms consist of pain, paresthesias, or numbness in the distribution of one or more trunks of the brachial plexus (usually in the ulnar distribution). Most patients associate their symptoms with certain positions of the shoulder girdle. These may occur from prolonged hyperabduction, as in house painters, hairdressers, and truck drivers. Others may relate their symptoms to the downward traction of the shoulder girdle produced by carrying heavy objects. Numbness of the hands often wakes the patient from sleep. On physical examination, motor deficits are rare and usually indicate severe compression of long duration. Muscular atrophy may be present in the hand. Pulses can be weakened by abduction of the arm with the head rotated to the opposite side (Adson test), though pulse reduction by this maneuver often occurs in completely asymptomatic persons. Light percussion over the brachial plexus in the supraclavicular fossa may reproduce the symptoms in patients with chronic neurologic impingement.

Arterial symptoms are less common and often the result of emboli. A bruit may be heard over the subclavian artery with abduction of the arm, but this is not a specific finding. Venous occlusion results in unilateral arm swelling. There are good collaterals around the shoulder girdle, but symptoms may be debilitating in young active patients, the very patient in whom this is most likely to occur.

B. Diagnosis

Neurogenic thoracic outlet compression must be differentiated from other disorders that mimic this condition (eg, carpal tunnel syndrome and cervical disk disease). Cervical x-rays and peripheral nerve conduction studies are not diagnostic but are valuable to eliminate other possibilities. Unfortunately, there is no recognized objective study to unequivocally confirm the diagnosis of neurogenic thoracic outlet syndrome. Arteriograms may demonstrate subclavian or axillary artery stenosis when the arm is in abduction. This finding is not diagnostic, but poststenotic dilation of the artery is distinctly abnormal and indicates a definite lesion.

Treatment

Most patients with neurogenic TOS benefit from postural correction and a physical therapy program directed toward restoring the normal relation and strength of the structures in the shoulder girdle. Surgical techniques for decompression of the thoracic outlet are reserved for patients who have not responded after 3-6 months of conservative treatment. Some surgeons prefer transaxillary first rib resection, while others prefer a supraclavicular approach. With either operation, the anterior scalene muscle and any associated fibrous bands should be excised. Up to 90% of patients report cure or significant improvement.

Symptomatic arterial stenoses require decompression of the thoracic outlet in combination with arterial reconstruction. Effort thrombosis of the subclavian vein is usually best treated by catheter-directed thrombolysis of the venous occlusion followed by thoracic outlet decompression with or without operative venous reconstruction or angioplasty. Outcomes for these patients with vascular TOS symptoms are excellent with 80%–90% asymptomatic at 6 months.

Sanders RJ, Hammond SL, Rao NM: Diagnosis of thoracic outlet syndrome. J Vasc Surg 2007;46:601. Review.
Schneider DB, Dimuzio PJ, Martin ND, et al: Combination treatment of venous thoracic outlet syndrome: open surgical decompression and intraoperative angioplasty. J Vasc Surg 2004;40:599.

ARTERIOVENOUS FISTULAS

Arteriovenous fistulas may be congenital, often called "malformations," or acquired. Abnormal communications between arteries and veins occur in many diseases and affect vessels of all sizes and in many locations. In congenital fistulas, the systemic effect is often not great, because although the communications may be multiple, they are small. When a limb is involved, extensive arteriovenous communications may exist with increased flow and increased muscle mass and bone length. Surgical correction is rarely successful because of the numerous A-V connections. Massive swelling can be treated with ablation therapy but it also is rarely curative.

Acquired fistulas are usually the result of trauma, violent, or iatrogenic. These communications can have considerable flow, and high-output heart failure can occur. The third class of fistulas is surgically created fistulas for hemodialysis access.

Arteriovenous malformations in the gastrointestinal tract may cause hemorrhage. Osler–Weber–Rendu disease or syndrome (also termed hereditary hemorrhagic telangiectasia) is an autosomal dominant disorder characterized by gastrointestinal bleeding and epistaxis due to large arteriovenous anomalies in the gastrointestinal tract and lungs.

Pulmonary lesions cause recirculation with lower Po_2, polycythemia, clubbing, and cyanosis.

Penetrating injuries either from trauma or iatrogenic ones from arterial punctures are the most common causes of acquired fistulas. Blunt trauma, erosion of an atherosclerotic or mycotic arterial aneurysm into adjacent veins, communication with an arterial prosthetic graft, or neoplastic invasion can all cause arteriovenous fistulas as well. When large vessels are involved, the presentation may be dramatic. For example, if an aortic aneurysm ruptures into the inferior vena cava, the fistula enlarges rapidly and can result in cardiac dilation and failure.

ARTERIOVENOUS FISTULA FOR HEMODIALYSIS

General Considerations

A successful arteriovenous fistula for hemodialysis access requires a large vein (> 5 mm) that lies close to the skin for at least 20 cm. The cephalic vein is ideal for this purpose. A 3-mm vein will usually be able to dilate to 5-6 mm after arterializations. The radial artery to cephalic vein arteriovenous fistula (Cimino fistula) is the classic hemodialysis access fistula. If no suitable vein is available for an autogenous fistula, prosthetic grafts are used, most commonly PTFE. These are most commonly placed in a loop configuration. The poor patency rates of these grafts, 40% at 2 years, and potential for infection have driven national guidelines to encourage a higher rate of autogenous fistula formation. To maximize autogenous vein utilization, current practice includes transposing deep veins such as the basilic vein in the upper arm to the subcutaneous tissue. All veins used for access require dilation and "arterialization" of the wall, which takes at least 6 weeks prior to cannulization for dialysis. Transposed veins may take even longer to mature.

Flow rates of at least 300 cc/min are necessary for efficient dialysis. Patients with a newly created arteriovenous access should be watched carefully for arterial steal and distal extremity ischemia. Diabetics are the most vulnerable to this complication because of calcified proximal arteries or intrinsic arterial lesions of the arm. High-output cardiac failure occurs only rarely.

Clinical Findings

A. Symptoms and Signs

A typical continuous machinery murmur can be heard over the arteriovenous fistulas and is often associated with a palpable thrill and locally increased skin temperature. Proximally, the arteries and veins dilate, and the pulse distal to the lesion diminishes. There may be signs of venous insufficiency, coolness, and hypertrophy distal to the communication on the involved extremity. Tachycardia occurs in some patients as a feature of increased cardiac output. The pulse rate slows (Branham sign) when the fistula is occluded by compression.

In contrast, venous malformations rarely produce hemodynamic effects. In this disorder, the presence of a mass, which may or may not be tender, is the principal finding. Because flow rates are low, bruits and thrills are absent.

B. Imaging Studies

MRI has become the imaging study of choice for the evaluation and follow-up of peripheral arteriovenous malformations, but CTA also gives excellent anatomic information. Precise delineation of arteriovenous fistulas can be done with selective angiography.

▶ Treatment

Not all arteriovenous connections require treatment. Most venous malformations should be treated conservatively. In addition, small peripheral fistulas may be observed and will often remain asymptomatic. Some are surgically inaccessible.

The indications for intervention include hemorrhage, local expansion, severe venous or arterial insufficiency, cosmetic deformity, and, rarely, heart failure. Most fistulas are now managed by embolization under radiographic control. The embolic material used includes blood clot, glass beads, and Gelfoam. Arteriovenous malformations of the head and neck and of the pelvis appear particularly well suited for this form of therapy. Direct injection of sclerosant compounds into venous malformations under fluoroscopic control also has been successful in at least temporarily reducing flow and swelling.

Surgical options are generally reserved for large acquired fistulas. When the fistulous connections involve substantial portions of an extremity, local ligation is invariably followed by recurrence, and only temporary palliation can be expected. Covered stent grafts are now being used for a variety of traumatic fistulas.

▶ Prognosis

The results of therapy vary according to the extent, location, and type of fistula. In general, traumatic fistulas have the most favorable prognosis. Congenital fistulas are more difficult to eradicate because of the numerous arteriovenous connections present.

Sidawy AN, Spergel LM, Besarab A, Allon M, Jennings WC, et al: The Society for Vascular Surgery: clinical practice guidelines for the surgical placement and maintenance of arteriovenous hemodialysis access. J Vasc Surg 2008;48:2S.

MULTIPLE CHOICE QUESTIONS

1. Arterial occlusive disease

    A. Occurs predominantly due to congenital abnormalities or anatomical anomalies

    B. Includes disease caused by atherosclerotic plaques, which typically develop at arterial branch points of high shear stress

    C. Is masked by collateral arterial circulation that typically has a lower resistance than the original unobstructed artery

    D. Typically occurs with at least a 50% reduction in arterial diameter, which correlates with a 75% narrowing of cross-sectional area

    E. Causes symptoms due to high pressure proximal to stenosis

2. Intermittent claudication symptoms include all of these except

    A. "Cramping" in a muscle

    B. Deep-seated ache in the calf

    C. Can be associated with walking

    D. Pain occurs at rest

    E. "Tiredness" in a muscle

3. Acute lower limb ischemia

    A. Usually is caused by increased muscular demand for blood flow in the distribution of an occluded artery

    B. Can be caused by a major arterial dissection

    C. Causes the five Ps: Pain, Petechiae, Pulselessness, Paresthesias, Paralysis

    D. Is generally best managed by initial observation to allow recruitment of collaterals

    E. Threatens skin loss before muscle or nerve damage

4. Carotid endarterectomy

    A. Cannot be performed when the carotid artery is completely occluded

    B. Has not been shown to be beneficial for any patients in prevention of ipsilateral stroke

    C. Is performed through a catheter placed in the ipsilateral femoral artery

    D. Carries a 30% risk of transient cranial nerve injury

    E. Has a restenosis rate of 35% at 5 years

5. Arterial aneurysm

    A. Management requires operative or catheter-based intervention in nearly all patients

    B. Management should include urgent operation in most patients

    C. Is defined as a localized dilation of an artery to at least 1.5 times its normal diameter

    D. Is caused by a disruption of the artery wall and does not include all layers of the wall

    E. Is most commonly a mycotic aneurysm

35

Veins & Lymphatics

Huiting Chen, MD

John R. Rectenwald, MD, MS

Thomas W. Wakefield, MD

I. THE VEINS

VENOUS ANATOMY

Veins of the lower extremity (Figure 35–1) consist of superficial and deep systems joined by venous perforators. The great and small saphenous veins are superficial—veins, the name "saphenous" aptly derived from the Greek word for "manifest, clear," or "visible." They contain many valves and show considerable variation in their location and branching points. The great saphenous vein may be duplicated in up to 10% of patients. Typically, it originates from the superficial arch of the foot and is found anterior to the medial malleolus at the ankle. As it ascends in the calf just beneath the superficial fascia, it is joined by two major tributaries: an anterior vein, which crosses the tibia; and a posterior arch vein, which arises posterior to the medial malleolus beside the posterior tibial artery. The great saphenous vein then enters the fossa ovalis in the groin to empty into the deep femoral vein.

The saphenofemoral junction is marked by four or five prominent branches of the great saphenous vein: the superficial circumflex iliac vein, the external pudendal vein, the superficial epigastric vein, and the medial and lateral accessory saphenous veins. Another important anatomic landmark is the relationship of the great saphenous vein to the saphenous branch of the femoral nerve; as it emerges from the popliteal space, the nerve follows a course parallel to the vein. Injury during saphenous vein harvest for bypass produces neuropathic pain or numbness along the medial calf and foot. The small saphenous vein arises from the superficial dorsal venous arch behind the lateral malleolus at the ankle and curves toward the midline of the posterior calf, ascending to join the popliteal vein behind the knee.

Deep veins of the leg parallel the courses of the arteries. Two or three venae comitantes accompany each tibial artery. At the knee, these paired high-capacitance veins merge to form the popliteal vein, which continues proximally as the femoral vein. At the inguinal ligament, the femoral and deep (profunda) femoral veins join medial to the femoral artery to form the common femoral vein. Proximal to the inguinal ligament, the common femoral vein becomes the external iliac vein. In the pelvis, external and internal iliac veins join to form common iliac veins that empty into the inferior vena cava (IVC). The right common iliac vein ascends almost vertically to the IVC while the left common iliac vein takes a more transverse course. For this reason, the left common iliac vein may be compressed between the right common iliac artery and lumbosacral spine, a condition known as May–Thurner syndrome when thrombosis of the left iliac vein occurs.

Muscular sinusoids represent another component of the deep veins of the leg. These thin-walled, nonvalved venous lakes run longitudinally within soleus muscle bellies and then coalesce to join the posterior tibial and peroneal veins. Blood empties from these sinusoids during muscle contraction; inactivity leads to stasis and may contribute to the development of deep venous thrombosis (DVT).

Blood flow is directed from superficial to deep veins of the leg via valved perforating (communicating) veins. Perforators are located below the medial malleolus (inframalleolar perforator), in the medial calf (Cockett perforators), at the level of the adductor canal (Hunterian perforator), and just above (Dodd perforator) and below (Boyd perforator) the knee.

Delicate bicuspid venous valves prevent reflux and direct the flow of blood from the foot and leg toward the heart and generally against gravity. Valves are more numerous in the distal part of the extremity, decrease in number proximally, and are virtually absent in the IVC itself.

The IVC ascends in the abdomen and ends at the right atrium. It lies to the right of the midline, lateral to the aorta, and receives a number of lumbar veins that connect with the vertebral and paravertebral venous plexuses. The IVC and its tributaries are derived in the 6th to 10th week of life from the fusion and obliteration of several paired embryonic veins:

the anterior and posterior cardinal veins, the subcardinal veins, the supracardinal veins, and the sacrocardinal veins. Because of this complex embryonic development, anomalies in the venous system are not uncommon. The most common abnormality is a circumaortic left renal vein (1.5%-8.7% incidence), followed by a retroaortic left renal vein (1.2%-3.4% incidence), duplication of the IVC (1%-3% incidence), azygos and hemiazygos continuation of the IVC (0.6%), and left-sided IVC (0.2%-0.5% incidence). An unsuspected retroaortic or circumaortic renal vein can be inadvertently injured during aortic cross-clamping. Most unusual is the congenital absence of the suprarenal IVC, which results from failure of the right subcardinal vein branches to join the veins of the embryologic liver. This ultimately results in the infrarenal segment of the IVC joining the azygos-hemiazygos veins to drain into the superior vena cava. The hepatic veins drain directly into the right atrium in patients with this unusual anomaly.

Veins of the upper extremity are also divided into superficial and deep groups, though direction of flow from superficial to deep is not as distinct as in the lower extremity. Dorsal veins of the hand empty into the cephalic vein ("intern vein") on the radial aspect and into the basilic vein on the ulnar aspect of the forearm. The cephalic vein ascends lateral to the biceps muscle into the deltopectoral groove, where it passes through the clavipectoral fascia to join the axillary vein. The cephalic vein is useful for arteriovenous fistulas, both at the wrist and in the upper arm, because it is superficial and lateral in the arm, allowing easy access for hemodialysis needles. The basilic vein, which runs medially in the arm to become the axillary vein, is deeper and thicker walled than the cephalic vein. Its many branches make it tedious to harvest, but it can be used for a bypass conduit or for a laterally tunneled upper-arm dialysis fistula (basilic vein transposition). The median cubital vein links the cephalic and basilic veins in the antecubital space.

Paired brachial veins comprise the deep system of veins. They accompany the brachial artery and join the basilic vein as it becomes the axillary vein. The axillary vein continues medially as the subclavian vein, which passes through a tight space anterior to the first rib and anterior scalene muscle and posterior to the clavicle. The subclavian vein and the internal jugular vein join behind the clavicular head to form the brachiocephalic vein, which empties into the superior vena cava.

Malaki M et al: Congenital anomalies of the inferior vena cava. *Clin Radiol* 2012;67(2):165-171.

Reich-Schupke S, Stücker M: Nomenclature of the veins of the lower limbs—current standards. *J Dtsch Dermatol Ges* 2011;9(3):189-194.

VENOUS PHYSIOLOGY

Knowledge of lower extremity venous anatomy is essential to understanding the physiology of venous flow. The volume of blood in the lower extremities may increase by

one-half liter when an individual moves from a reclining to an erect position (Figure 35–2). Increased blood volume is accommodated by increased venous capacitance, which is regulated by smooth muscle contractility in the vein walls. Erect posture creates a vertical column of blood, exerting a hydrostatic pressure equal to the distance from the toes to the right atrium (about 100-120 mm Hg). The hydrostatic pressure must be overcome to avoid pooling of blood in the legs and to provide venous return to the heart. Several aspects of the venous system make it possible to move blood against the force of gravity. Because the circulation is a closed system, venous return is affected by arterial inflow and by the negative intrathoracic pressure created during inspiration. Functional valves assure unidirectional movement of blood from superficial to deep systems and from

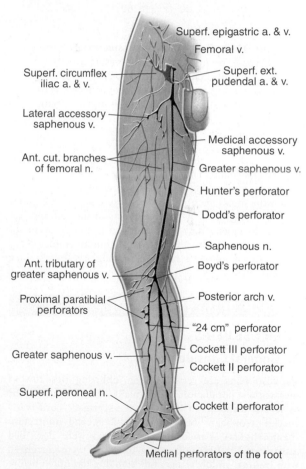

▲ **Figure 35–1.** Anatomy of the superficial and perforating veins of the lower extremity. (Reproduced, with permission, from Mozes G, Gloviczki P et al: Surgical anatomy for endoscopic subfascial division of perforating veins, *J Vasc Surg.* 1996 Nov;24(5):800–808.)

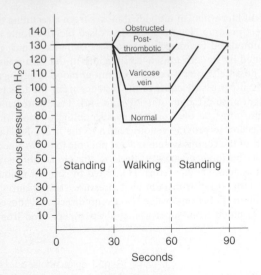

▲ **Figure 35–2.** Pedal venous pressure measurements with exercise. The normal drop in pressure associated with ambulation is impaired by deep vein incompetence and proximal venous obstruction. (Reproduced, with permission, from DeWeese JA: Venous and lymphatic disease. In: *Principles of Surgery*, 4th ed. Schwarz S [editor]. McGraw-Hill, 1983.)

the foot back to the heart. Hydrostatic pressure is dissipated by lack of simultaneous opening of the valves. Soleal venous sinusoids are another central component to the system. When the muscle contracts during exercise, blood empties from the sinusoid into the deep veins of the calf and leg. This high-velocity flow siphons blood from deep veins of the foot upward into the calf, analogous to smoke being drawn up a smokestack by wind blowing past the chimney (Venturi effect).

DISEASES OF THE VENOUS SYSTEM

VARICOSE VEINS

▶ General Considerations

Varicose veins are very common, afflicting 10%-20% of the world's population. Abnormally dilated veins occur in several locations in the body: the spermatic cord (varicocele), esophagus (esophageal varices), and anorectum (hemorrhoids). Varicosities of the legs were described as early as 1550 BC and in the 1600s AD were correlated with trauma, childbearing, and "standing too much before kings." Modern studies identify female sex, pregnancy, family history, prolonged standing, and a history of phlebitis as risk factors for varicose veins. In the Framingham Study, the highest incidence was found in women between 40 and 49 years of age.

Varicose veins are classified as either primary or secondary. Primary varicose veins are thought to be due to genetic or developmental defects in the vein wall that cause diminished elasticity and valvular incompetence. Most cases of isolated superficial venous insufficiency are primary varicose veins. Secondary varicose veins arise from destruction or dysfunction of valves caused by trauma, DVT, arteriovenous fistula, or nontraumatic proximal venous obstruction (pregnancy, pelvic tumor). When valves of the deep and perforating veins are disrupted, chronic venous stasis changes may accompany superficial varicosities. It is important to recognize that untreated, longstanding venous dysfunction from either primary or secondary varicose veins may cause chronic skin changes that lead to infection, nonhealing venous ulceration, and chronic disability. To define the optimal method of treatment, the etiologic factors and distribution of disease must be clearly identified.

▶ Clinical Findings

The clinical presentation of patients with varicose veins can be quite variable. Many varicose veins are asymptomatic and come to medical attention because of aesthetic concerns. If symptomatic, varicose veins may be associated with localized pain, a burning sensation over the vein, a diffuse ache or "heaviness" in the calf (particularly with prolonged standing), or phlebitis. Mild ankle edema may occur. Symptoms generally improve with leg elevation.

The varicosities appear as dilated, tortuous, elongated veins predominantly on the medial aspect of the lower extremity along the course of the great saphenous vein. Overlying skin changes may be absent even in the presence of extensive large varicosities. Smaller flat, blue-green reticular veins, telangiectasias, and spider veins may accompany varicose veins and are further evidence of venous dysfunction. A cluster of telangiectasias below the inframalleolar perforator is termed a corona phlebectatica paraplantaris. Secondary varicose veins can cause symptoms characteristic of chronic venous insufficiency (CVI), including edema, hyperpigmentation, stasis dermatitis, and even venous ulcerations.

Physical examination begins with inspection of all extremities to determine the distribution and severity of the varicosities. Bimanual circumferential palpation of the thighs and calves is helpful. Palpation of a thrill or auscultation of a bruit indicates the presence of an arteriovenous fistula as a possible etiologic factor. Today, tourniquet tests have been virtually replaced by venous duplex ultrasound imaging, which is now used as the primary method with which to map the location and extent of reflux.

▶ Differential Diagnosis

Ulceration, brawny induration, and hyperpigmentation often indicate accompanying chronic deep venous insufficiency. This is important to recognize because the changes generally do not resolve with saphenous vein stripping alone.

Klippel–Trenaunay syndrome (KTS) must be considered if extensive varicose veins are encountered in a young patient, especially if unilateral and in an atypical distribution (lateral leg). The classic triad of KTS is varicose veins, limb hypertrophy, and a cutaneous birthmark (port wine stain or venous malformation). Because the deep veins are often anomalous or absent, saphenous vein stripping can be hazardous. Standard treatment for patients with KTS is graduated support stockings, and a good program of intermittent leg elevation and exercise. Limited stab avulsion of symptomatic varices after thorough duplex ultrasound vein mapping, and occasional surgery for correction of limb length discrepancy may also be indicated.

► Treatment

A. Nonsurgical Treatment

Treatment for both primary and secondary varicose veins initially involves a program directed at management of venous insufficiency, including elastic stocking support, periodic leg elevation, and regular exercise. Prolonged sitting and standing are discouraged. For most patients, knee-high or thigh-high gradient compression stockings of 20-30 mm Hg are sufficient, although some patients require 30-40 mm Hg pressure. The compression stockings are worn all day to diminish venous distention during standing and are removed at night.

B. Surgical Treatment

Traditionally, open surgical approaches have been the mainstay of treatment for saphenous vein disease. The preferred surgical option for saphenous veins remains high ligation with stripping or high ligation alone (Figure 35–3). High ligation and stripping of the saphenous system is performed for patients with an incompetent valve at the saphenofemoral junction and varicosities throughout the length of the great saphenous vein. This was traditionally performed by ligating the saphenofemoral junction and the major proximal saphenous vein branches through a small incision in the groin. Then the saphenous vein was removed to the point of clusters of varicosities. For the small saphenous vein, high ligation alone with short-length phlebectomy with local anesthesia is typically performed to minimize sural nerve injury. Epifascial veins may also be treated in an ambulatory setting, with phlebectomy performed under local anesthesia. Today, most open surgical approaches have been replaced with endovascular techniques (see next paragraph, C). A new treatment strategy called ASVAL (ambulatory selective varices ablation under local anesthesia) embraces the surgical treatment of epifascial veins while sparing the refluxing saphenous vein, minimizing the need to treat

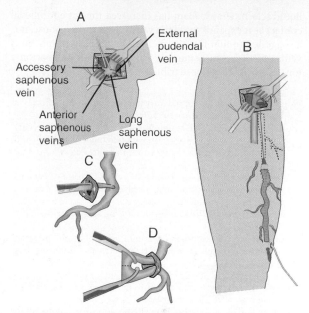

▲ **Figure 35–3.** Technique of varicose vein stripping. (Reproduced, with permission, from Bergan JJ, Kistner RL: *Atlas of Venous Surgery*. Saunders, 1992.)

the saphenous vein in many cases. Although controversial, under the principle of anterograde reflux such that reflux spreads from epifascial to saphenous veins, the treatment of epifascial veins alone is said to correct saphenous reflux. Ongoing research has demonstrated that patients with primary varicose veins or less severe disease have done well with this approach.

C. Endovascular Treatment

In recent years, great advances have been made in endovascular techniques for treatment of varicose veins. Ablation techniques include thermal (radiofrequency and laser) and chemical ablation. Thermal ablation causes treated veins to collapse due to vein wall and lumen fibrosis. Vein reabsorption occurs over the course of several months. Both radiofrequency and laser ablation have been found to be safe and effective in the treatment of incompetent greater saphenous veins (GSVs), and the latest 2011 consensus opinion recommends thermal ablation to surgical or chemical ablation for GSVs. Its use has also been reported in successful treatment of perforator veins, though recent guidelines recommend against selective treatment of incompetent perforating veins in patients with simple varicose veins. However, in patients with "pathologic" perforating veins, subfascial endoscopic perforating vein surgery, ultrasonographically guided sclerotherapy, and thermal ablations remain viable options. Finally, advances have been made in chemical ablation techniques in the form of foam sclerotherapy. Compared to liquid sclerotherapy, foam has increased time of endothelial contact as it expands to fill the vein. Given its ease of use, it is a suggested option for treatment of incompetent saphenous veins and a recommended option along with phlebectomy for treatment of varicose tributaries.

Almeida, JI, Raines JK: Ambulatory phlebectomy in the office. *Pers Vasc Surg Endovasc Ther* 2008;20:348-355.

Bush RG, Shamma HN, Hammond K: Histological changes occurring after endoluminal ablation with two diode lasers (940 and 1319 nm) from acute changes to 4 months. *Lasers Surg Med* 2008;40:676-679.

Gloviczki P, Comerota AJ, Dalsing MC, et al: The care of patients with varicose veins and associated chronic venous diseases: clinical practice guidelines of the Society for Vascular Surgery and the American Venous Forum. *J Vasc Surg* 2011;53(suppl): 25-485.

Mowatt-Larssen E, Shortell C: Truncal vein ablation for laser: radial firing at high wavelength is the key? *J Vasc Endovasc Surg* 2010;17:217-223.

Mowatt-Larssen E, Shortell CK: Treatment of primary varicose veins has changed with the introduction of new techniques. *Semin Vasc Surg* 2012;25(1):18-24.

Pittaluga P, Chastanet S, Rea B, et al: Midterm results of the surgical treatment of varices by phlebectomy with conservation of a refluxing saphenous vein. *J Vasc Surg* 2009;50:107-118.

DEEP VEIN THROMBOSIS

▶ General Considerations

DVT and pulmonary embolism (PE) affect up to 900,000 people per year in the United States, and their incidence increases with age. Treatment is estimated to cost billions of dollars per year, not even including expenditures associated with long-term sequelae of this disease.

The Virchow triad (stasis, vascular injury, and hypercoagulability) should be the cornerstone for assessment of risk factors for DVT. In most cases, the cause is multifactorial.

Acquired risk factors include advanced age, cancer, surgery, trauma, immobilization, hormone replacement therapy, oral contraceptive use, pregnancy, neurologic disease, cardiac disease, and antiphospholipid antibodies. Approximately 30%-40% of patients with a new DVT (both upper and lower extremity) have been found to present with malignancy within 5 years. In men, pancreatic and colorectal cancers are most frequently associated with thrombotic risk, while hematological malignancies carry a lower risk. Cancers of the pancreas, ovary, and brain are mostly associated with thrombotic complications. Breast cancer, especially during its chemotherapy treatment, is also a risk factor. Most of these malignancies are associated with increased fibrinogen or thrombocytosis.

Endothelial injury can result from direct trauma (severed vein, venous cannulation, or transvenous pacing) or local irritation secondary to infusion of chemotherapy, previous

DVT, or phlebitis. Damaged endothelium leads to platelet aggregation, degranulation, and formation of thrombus as well as vasoconstriction and activation of the coagulation cascade. Thrombin activation from release of tissue factor and diminished fibrinolysis mediated by plasminogen activator inhibitor are intraoperative events that may be related to endothelial disruption.

Hypercoagulable states may also be inherited. Genetic causes include deficiencies of natural coagulation inhibitors (antithrombin III, protein C, protein S), factor V Leiden, prothrombin 20210A gene variant, blood group non-O, elevated homocysteine levels, plasminogen abnormalities, elevated levels of coagulation factors (such as factor VIII), and reduced heparin cofactor II activity. Hematologic disorders associated with DVT include disseminated intravascular coagulation, heparin-induced thrombocytopenia, antiphospholipid antibody syndrome, thrombotic thrombocytopenic purpura, hemolytic uremic syndrome, polycythemia vera, and essential thrombocythemia. Inflammatory bowel disease, systemic lupus erythematosus, and obesity are additionally associated with DVT.

DVT occurs most frequently in the calf veins, though it may arise in the femoral or iliac veins. Thrombi originate in soleal sinusoids or in valve sinuses, where there are flow eddies. Treatment of isolated calf vein thrombosis is controversial, as it is associated with a low risk of PE. However, a 2011 meta-analysis of studies spanning nearly 25 years demonstrated significant reductions both in progression to PE and in proximal thrombus propagation in patients treated with anticoagulation compared to patients who not receiving anticoagulation. While the studies were heterogeneous, the summation of the data indicated no statistical increased risk of bleeding in patients who received anticoagulation compared to the control arms. These observations and the improved safety profile of low-molecular-weight heparin (LMWH) are compelling practitioners to treat isolated calf DVTs aggressively. In the latest 2012 ACCP guidelines, it is recommended that "in patients with acute isolated distal DVT of the leg and without severe symptoms or risk factors for extension, we suggest serial imaging of the deep veins for 2 weeks over initial anticoagulation" while "in patients with acute isolated distal DVT of the leg and severe symptoms or risk factors for extension, we suggest initial anticoagulation over serial imaging of the deep veins." The length of anticoagulation recommended is for 3 months.

▶ Clinical Findings

A. Symptoms and Signs

The diagnosis of DVT cannot be made solely on the basis of presenting symptoms and signs, as up to half of patients with acute thromboses have no abnormality detectable in the involved extremity. Homans sign (pain on passive dorsiflexion of the ankle) is nonspecific and positive in only half of cases, and is unreliable. Some patients present with acute PE unaccompanied by leg edema or pain.

Symptomatic patients most often complain of a dull ache or pain in the calf or leg associated with mild edema. With extensive proximal DVT, there can be massive edema, cyanosis, and dilated superficial collateral veins. Low-grade fever and tachycardia occasionally occur. Iliofemoral venous thrombosis can result in phlegmasia. In phlegmasia alba dolens, the leg is pulseless, pale, and cool, which may progress to phlegmasia cerulea dolens, characterized by cyanosis of the limb and a precursor to gangrene.

B. Imaging Studies

Because DVT is difficult to diagnose on the basis of physical signs or symptoms, some objective diagnostic study is required before treatment is started. Historically, the standard for diagnosis was ascending phlebography, accomplished by fluoroscopic imaging during contrast injection into an intravenous line on the dorsum of the foot. The patient stands but is non–weight-bearing on the extremity studied. An abrupt cutoff of the contrast column indicates DVT. The complications of this procedure include risk of contrast allergy, contrast-induced nephropathy, and phlebitis.

Duplex ultrasound is now the best initial test to detect the presence of DVT. It is a noninvasive examination, does not expose the patient to radiation, is easily reproducible, and has specificity and sensitivity of greater than 95%. In this method, the transducer produces a two-dimensional image of the imaged vein and the surrounding tissue. Normally, veins collapse completely when compressed. Vein incompressibility is the primary ultrasonographic diagnostic criterion for acute lower limb DVT. Secondary diagnostic criteria include vein distention, echogenic thrombus within the vein lumen, absence of spectral or color Doppler signal from the vein lumen, and loss of venous flow phasicity and/or loss of response to Valsalva maneuver. Additionally, augmentation is expected in normal, compressible veins. When pressure is applied to the lower extremity distal to the area of evaluation, normally there is increased blood from through the vein with compression. Lack of augmentation is suggestive of an occlusion in the segment of vein between the site of compression and the transducer. It is worth noting that direct thrombus visualization using B-mode imaging is variable depending on the age of the clot: fresh thrombus is anechoic and therefore not visible. Finally, while duplex ultrasound has a high accuracy for proximal DVT, it is less accurate in distal thrombosis and is highly operator dependent. Magnetic resonance venography shows promise as a diagnostic study for this disorder. The sensitivity and specificity of magnetic resonance venography are 100% and 96%, respectively. The injection of gadolinium is useful for determining the age of the thrombus. Advances in magnetic resonance direct thrombus imaging with methemoglobin as an endogenous contrast allows for accurate diagnosis of femoropopliteal DVT with a sensitivity and specificity greater than 100%. This method allows for the paramagnetic properties of methemoglobin to provide a high signal on T1-weighted images against a background of flowing blood and fat. The thrombus may be directly visualized without administration of contrast, making it a viable option for patients with renal insufficiency. CT imaging, especially as part of a PE protocol CT image, may also be a good alternative to establish the diagnosis.

Measurement of D-dimer levels is too nonspecific for use alone and, when combined with a negative risk assessment, may be useful to rule out DVT but not to rule in the diagnosis of DVT. Radiolabeled fibrinogen is too sensitive in the pelvis for use in the acute clinical setting and carries with it a risk of transmission of infectious disease. It is no longer used. Older tests such as impedance plethysmography and venous pressure measurements do not achieve the same accuracy as duplex ultrasound and have been largely abandoned. Recent studies have demonstrated the potential for using soluble P-selectin as a marker for diagnosing DVT. P-selectin is a cell adhesion molecule that is the first upregulated glycoprotein on activated endothelial cells and platelets. As thrombosis and inflammation are interrelated, elevated levels of soluble P-selectin acts as an indicator or biomarker of inflammation. Consequently, a combination of soluble P-selectins with a Wells score has been shown to have a positive predictive value of approximately 90% with a negative predictive value greater than 95% for establishing the diagnosis of DVT.

▶ Differential Diagnosis

A variety of pathologies may mimic the symptoms of DVT. Lymphatic conditions such as adenopathies or lymphangitis can present with lower extremity pain and edema, but without flow on color Doppler images seen with DVTs. Vascular lesions such as hematomas and pseudoaneurysms secondary to catheterization of the common femoral artery may simulate DVTs. These can be differentiated from DVTs under evaluation by gray-scale images showing a delineation of the pseudoaneurysm or hematoma, or by color Doppler imaging which will illustrate the typical "yin-yang" sign of bidirectional flow. Muscular lesions of the thigh such as muscle strains, tears, and contusions may result in pain, stiffness, edema, and a mass. Cellulitis may cause edema, localized pain, and erythema. Unilateral leg swelling can also result from lymphedema, obstruction of the popliteal vein by Baker cyst, or obstruction of the iliac vein by retroperitoneal mass or idiopathic fibrosis. Bilateral leg edema suggests heart, liver, or kidney failure or IVC obstruction by tumor or pregnancy.

Treatment is aimed at reducing the incidence of complications associated with DVT. Short-term complications include recurrent DVT or pulmonary thromboembolism, while long-term complications include the development of varicose veins and chronic venous insufficiency. The primary treatment of DVT is systemic anticoagulation. This reduces the risk of PE and extension of venous thrombosis and also decreases the rate of recurrent DVT by 80%. Systemic anticoagulation does not directly lyse thrombi but stops propagation and allows natural fibrinolysis to occur. Heparin is initiated immediately and dosed to a goal partial thromboplastin time (PTT) of 1.5-2.5 times normal, or, more currently, LMWH, weight-based without monitoring. Achieving therapeutic heparinization within the first 24 hours after diagnosis is shown to reduce the rate of recurrent DVT.

Warfarin is started after therapeutic heparinization. The two therapies should overlap to diminish the possibility of a hypercoagulable state, which can occur during the first few days of warfarin administration, because warfarin also inhibits the synthesis of natural anticoagulant proteins C and S. For both acute lower extremity DVT and acute PE, guidelines recommend starting warfarin the same day as the start of parenteral anticoagulation over delayed initiation, with a continuation of parenteral anticoagulation for a minimum of 5 days until the INR is greater than 2.0 for more than 24 hours. Specifically, in patients with a PE or proximal DVT of the leg provoked by surgery, the recommended treatment is 3 months compared to a longer or shorter time period. Three months of anticoagulation is similarly recommended in patients with (i) PE/proximal DVT of the leg provoked by a nonsurgical transient risk factor, (ii) in patients with PE/an isolated distal DVT of the leg provoked by surgery or by a nonsurgical transient risk factor. In patients who have had an unprovoked PE or DVT of the proximal or distal leg, the recommended treatment is a minimum of 3 months' treatment followed by reevaluation of risk-benefit ratio of extended therapy. After a second episode of DVT, the usual recommendation is prolonged or lifelong warfarin in patients with a low or moderate bleeding risk. In patients with a high bleeding risk, the guidelines recommend 3 months of anticoagulation over extended therapy. The risk for recurrent venous thrombosis is increased markedly in the presence of homozygous factor V Leiden mutations, antiphospholipid antibody, antithrombin III, and protein C or protein S deficiencies, so lifelong anticoagulation is usually recommended for these conditions as well.

LMWH has been shown to be as safe and effective as standard unfractionated heparin (UFH) in the treatment of DVT. It is administered once or twice daily by subcutaneous injection. LMWH does not require monitoring of its anticoagulant effect because of its predictable dose-response relationship, and this feature of the drug has made feasible the outpatient treatment of DVT. Standard UFH inhibits

thrombin because it is large enough to make a three-way complex between thrombin, antithrombin, and itself. LMWHs are much smaller than standard heparin molecules and do not inhibit thrombin; their main therapeutic effect comes from inhibition of factor Xa activity. In patients with acute DVT of the leg or acute PE, the most recent 2012 ACCP guidelines suggest LMWH over both IV and SC forms of UFH. LMWH is suggested over vitamin K antagonist therapy for patients with PE or DVT of the leg and cancer. The advantages of LMWHs over standard heparin preparations include a lower risk of bleeding complications and thrombocytopenia, a lower risk of heparin-induced thrombocytopenia, lower recurrence of VTE, decreased mortality, less interference with proteins C and S, less complement activation, and a lower risk of osteoporosis. Moreover, recent randomized trials have shown regression of thrombus with LMWH. A disadvantage worth noting is that LMWH accumulates in patients with renal failure.

Recent studies evaluating specific factor Xa inhibitors and direct thrombin inhibitors have demonstrated significant promise. Fondaparinux is a synthetic pentasaccharide which binds to antithrombin and catalyzes the inhibition of factor Xa. It has more specific anti-Xa activity than low molecular weight heparin (LMWH), and has a longer half-life than LMWH. It is rapidly and almost completely bioavailable after subcutaneous injection, and does not require coagulation monitoring. However, due to its dependence on renal clearance, its use is contraindicated in patients with renal insufficiency. For the treatment of VTE, fondaparinux is administered at a fixed dose of 7.5 mg for patients weighing 50-100 kg, with the dose adjusted to 5 mg for patients weighing less than 50 kg and 10 mg for those weighing more than 100 kg. In orthopedic patients undergoing total hip or knee arthroplasty or hip fracture surgery (HFS), fondaparinux is among one of the recommended agents for use as prophylaxis by the current 2012 ACCP guidelines (grade 1C). In patients with acute VTE, ACCP guidelines recommend initial treatment with parenteral anticoagulation agents—among those—subcutaneous fondaparinux (grade 1B). For the treatment of VTE, fondaparinux was found to be equal to LMWH for treating DVT, and for PE, it was found as effective as UFH.

Dabigatran etexilate (Pradaxa) is an oral direct thrombin inhibitor. It has been approved for prophylaxis in total hip replacement and total knee replacement in Western Europe and Canada. It demonstrates a low risk for bleeding, offers fixed oral dosing without coagulation monitoring, and does not cause an increase in liver enzymes. When tested against LMWH given twice daily in DVT prophylaxis, it failed to meet the noninferiority target that was achieved when compared with LMWH once daily. Dabigatran was recently found to be as effective as warfarin for the treatment of DVT, and has now been approved by the FDA as an oral anticoagulant for treatment of nonvalvular atrial fibrillation. Another oral agent, Rivaroxaban, has been studied as monotherapy for treatment of DVT and was found noninferior to standard therapy in the primary endpoint of symptomatic recurrent DVT and nonfatal or fatal PE, without any increase in bleeding. Finally, Apixaban is yet awaiting FDA approval, but it has been shown to be superior to warfarin in the treatment of atrial fibrillation in patients with that diagnosis and one additional risk factor for stroke.

The prevention of CVI after DVT can be divided into those measures that are useful with traditional anticoagulant treatment of DVT and measures that involve more aggressive interventions to lyse thrombus. Certain LMWHs decrease indices of CVI compared to standard therapy when used over an extended period of time. Associated with this traditional therapy, the rate and severity of the postthrombotic syndrome (PTS) after proximal DVT can be decreased by approximately 50% by the use of surgical compression stockings and ambulation without increasing the risk of PE.

The clinical outcome after DVT can be thought of as resulting in either valvular reflux, persistent venous obstruction, or their combination. Patients with both obstruction and valvular reflux often have the most severe postthrombotic symptoms. In order to limit these consequences, thrombus removal should be the best solution. The longer a thrombus is in contact with a vein valve, the more likely the valve will no longer function. Additionally, the thrombus initiates an inflammatory response in the vein wall, which may lead to vein wall and valve dysfunction. The most recent guidelines recommend early thrombus removal in patients with limb-threatening venous thrombosis (grade 1A), though recommend that patients with isolated femoropopliteal DVTs to be managed with only conventional anticoagulation therapy (grade 1C).

Techniques for early thrombus removal include catheter-directed thrombolytic therapy and open thrombectomy. In the treatment of acute iliofemoral DVTs, a systematic review and meta-analysis by Casey and colleagues reports that thrombectomy results in significantly decreased risk of developing PTS, venous reflux, and a trend for reduced venous obstruction when compared to systemic anticoagulation. Catheter-directed thrombolysis yielded similar results when compared to systemic anticoagulation, though there were insufficient data to directly compare outcomes of catheter-directed thrombolysis to thrombectomy. Following either therapy, it is currently recommended that patients wear knee-high compression stockings (30-40 mm Hg) for at least 2 years following the procedure.

▶ Prevention of VTE

Surgery increases the risk of DVT 21-fold. This disorder is a reported complication for approximately 20%-25% of patients admitted for a general surgical procedure, 20%-30% of those undergoing an elective neurosurgical procedure,

and 50%-60% of those undergoing hip or knee arthroplasty. These statistics emphasize the need for routine DVT prophylaxis in the surgical patient. The most commonly used measures are elastic stockings, pneumatic sequential compression devices, low-dose UFH (5000 units given by subcutaneous injection), or LMWH given at a prophylactic dose subcutaneously (either once or twice daily).

For general surgical patients, the incidence of DVT is high without prophylaxis, and the risk of PE is 1.6%, 0.9% fatal. Patients have been categorized into levels of risk in the current Chest guidelines based on their risk scoring via the Rogers or Caprini scoring system, placing a very low risk for VTE patient at more than 0.5%, low risk at approximately 1.5%, moderate risk at approximately 3%, and high risk at approximately 6%. In general surgery patients at very low risk for VTE, the recommended prophylaxis is simply early ambulation, with no pharmacologic or mechanical prophylaxis recommended. For patients at low risk, the guidelines suggest mechanical prophylaxis, preferably with intermittent pneumatic compression (IPC). Patients at moderate risk of VTE who are not at high risk for major bleeding complications are suggested LMWH, low-dose unfractionated heparin (LDUH), or mechanical prophylaxis. In those at moderate risk of VTE but at high risk for bleeding, the guidelines suggest mechanical prophylaxis. For high risk VTE patients who are not at high risk for major bleeding, the recommendation is pharmacologic prophylaxis with LMWH or LDUH, with the additional suggestion of mechanical prophylaxis. In the special case of high VTE risk patients with cancer who are not high risk for bleeding complications, the guidelines recommend IPC with LMWH for extended-duration pharmacologic prophylaxis (4 weeks) over a shorter duration.

For orthopedic patients having undergone major surgery including hip fracture surgery (HFS), total hip arthroplasty (THA), or total knee arthroplasty (TKA), an evaluation of the extended postoperative VTE risk (postoperative days 0-35) comparing no prophylaxis with LMWH found the total symptomatic VTE rate decreased from 4.3% to 1.8%, a greater than 60% reduction. These values represent a decrease in rates of PE from 1.5% to 0.55% and a decrease in rates of DVT from 2.8% to 1.25%. Therefore, the current guidelines suggest extending thromboprophylaxis for up to 35 days postoperatively (grade 2B). For patients undergoing THA or TKA, the use of LMWH is suggested over fondaparinux, apixaban, dabigatran, rivaroxaban, LDUH, adjusted-dose VKA, or aspirin. In patients undergoing HFS, LMWH is also the suggested agent, regardless of concomitant use of mechanical prophylaxis. If started preoperatively, LMWH is suggested to be administered ≥12 hours prior to surgery. In patients with increased risk of bleeding or contraindications to both pharmacologic and mechanical thromboprophylaxis, the guidelines suggest against using an IVC filter over no thromboprophylaxis.

For trauma patients, evidence is lacking, and randomized studies are needed. Trauma risk factors include lower extremity or pelvic fractures, surgical procedures, advanced age, femoral vein lines or major venous repairs, prolonged immobility, spinal cord injury, and prolonged duration of hospital stay. In major trauma patients, the guidelines suggest the use of LDUH, LMWH, or mechanical prophylaxis. For these patients at high risk for VTE, such as those with acute spinal cord injury or traumatic brain injury, mechanical prophylaxis is suggested in addition to pharmacologic prophylaxis. Because venous compression ultrasound detection and subsequent treatment of asymptomatic DVT in this population does not reduce the risk of PE or fatal PE, the guidelines do not suggest periodic surveillance with this modality. IVC filters are recommended in patients when anticoagulation is contraindicated, but are not suggested for use as primary prevention.

In neurosurgery, DVT and PE occur equivalent to rates in general surgery patients, and risk factors include intracranial surgery, prolonged surgery, malignant tumors, the presence of leg weakness, and increased age. The recommendations differ between craniotomy and spine surgery patients. In craniotomy patients, the suggested prophylaxis is mechanical or pharmacologic or no prophylaxis. However, in those craniotomy patients who are at very high risk for VTE, such as those with malignant disease, the guidelines suggest pharmacologic prophylaxis in addition to mechanical prophylaxis when it is safe to do so. For spinal surgery patients, mechanical prophylaxis is suggested over no prophylaxis, UFH, or LMWH. Similar to their counterparts, spinal surgery patients at very high risk for VTE are suggested to have both pharmacologic and mechanical prophylaxis when medically safe.

Bauersachs R et al: EINSTEIN investigators (2010) oral rivaroxaban for symptomatic venous thromboembolism. *N Engl J Med* 363(26):2499-2510.

Bozzato S et al: Thromboprophylaxis in surgical and medical patients. *Semin Resp Crit Care Med* 2012;33(2):163-175.

Casey ET et al: Treatment of acute iliofemoral deep vein thrombosis. *J Vasc Surg* 2012;55(5):1463-1473.

De Martino RR et al: A meta-analysis of anticoagulation for calf deep venous thrombosis. *J Vasc Surg* 2012 Jul;56(1):228-37.e1

Falck-Ytter Y et al: Prevention of VTE in orthopedic surgery patients: antithrombotic therapy and prevention of thrombosis, 9th ed: American College of Chest Physicians evidence-based clinical practice guidelines. *Chest* 2012;141(2 Suppl):e278S-e325S.

Gould MK et al: Prevention of VTE in nonorthopedic surgical patients: antithrombotic therapy and prevention of thrombosis, 9th ed: American College of Chese Physicians evidence-based clinical practice guidelines. *Chest* 2012;141(2 Suppl):e227S-e277S.

Guanella R, Righini M: Serial Limited versus single complete compression ultrasonography for the diagnosis of lower extremity deep vein thrombosis. *Semin Respir Crit Care Med* 2012;33(2):144-150.

Kearon C et al: Antithrombotic therapy for VTE disease: antithrombotic therapy and prevention of thrombosis, 9th ed: American college of chest physicians evidence-based clinical practice guidelines. *Chest* 2012;141(2 Suppl):e419S-e494S.

Meissner MH et al: Early thrombus removal strategies for acute deep venous thrombosis: clinical practice guidelines of the Society for Vascular Surgery and the American Venous Forum. *J Vasc Surg* 2012;55(5):1449-1462.

Ramacciotti E et al: Evaluation of soluble P-selectin as a marker for the diagnosis of deep venous thrombosis. *Clin Appl Thromb Hemost* 2011;17(4):425-431.

Schulman S et al: Dabigatran versus warfarin in the treatment of acute venous thromboembolism. *N Engl J Med* 2009;361(24):2342-2352.

Useche JA et al: Use of US in the evaluation of patients with symptoms of deep venous thrombosis of the lower extremities. *Radiographics* 2008;28(6):1785-1797.

van Langevelde K et al: Magnetic resonance imaging and computed tomography developments in imaging of venous thromboembolism. *J Magn Reson Imaging* 2010;32(6):1302-1312.

AXILLARY-SUBCLAVIAN VENOUS THROMBOSIS

▶ General Considerations

Thrombosis of the axillary or subclavian vein is a relatively uncommon event, accounting for less than 5% of all cases of DVT. Only 12% result in clinically apparent pulmonary thromboembolism, but the incidence is higher if all patients undergo diagnostic testing. Besides PE, the most common consequence of axillary-subclavian vein thrombosis is chronic edema and resultant disability. The effects of postthrombotic syndrome (PTS) and recurrent thrombosis are not uncommon.

There are two major etiologies. Primary axillary-subclavian thrombosis, also known as Paget–Schroetter syndrome or "effort thrombosis," occurs as a result of intermittent transient obstruction of the vein in the costoclavicular space during repetitive or strenuous activities involving the upper extremity (Figure 35–4). This condition was first described in independent reports by Paget and von Schroetter in the late 19th century. During strenuous repetitive movements of the upper extremity, the subclavian vein is compressed between the first rib and the anterior scalene muscle posteriorly and the clavicle—with underlying subclavius muscle and fibrous costocoracoid ligament—anteriorly. In many cases, the costoclavicular ligament congenitally inserts more laterally than normal, subjecting the anatomically tight space to further compression of the subclavian vein. Primary subclavian vein thrombosis can also occur in patients with hypercoagulable states such as antiphospholipid antibody syndrome or factor V Leiden mutation. Secondary subclavian vein thrombosis, which is increasing in incidence, results from venous injury by indwelling central venous catheters, external trauma, or pacemaker wires. These patients are less likely to be symptomatic than patients with primary subclavian vein thrombosis.

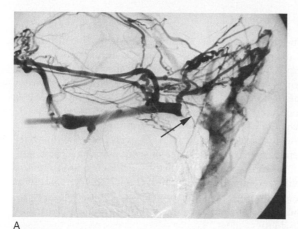

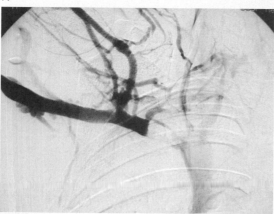

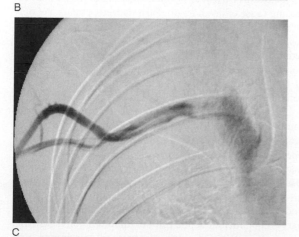

▲ **Figure 35–4. A:** Effort thrombosis in a 13-year-old wrestler. Arrow marks subclavian vein thrombosis refractory to rt-PA thrombolysis. **B:** Arm in abduction. Note disappearance of prominent venous collaterals. **C:** Immediate postoperative venogram following scalenectomy, first rib resection, and thrombectomy.

▶ **Clinical Findings**

A. Symptoms and Signs

Primary axillary-subclavian vein thrombosis usually occurs in healthy young athletes and people who perform repetitive activities that involve hyperabduction of the upper extremities. Most patients present with edema of the affected extremity, diffuse aching pain, and cyanosis of the upper extremity. As venous collaterals develop, dilated veins appear in the chest wall and shoulder region. In less pronounced presentations, patients become symptomatic only when their affected extremity is positioned in a way that predisposes it to vascular occlusion.

Paget–Schroetter syndrome may also be accompanied by symptoms of neurogenic thoracic outlet syndrome, often causing tingling, numbness, and pain in the hand and arm, sometimes in an ulna distribution indicating compression of the C-8/T-1 roots of the brachial plexus between hypertrophied or anomalous anterior and middle scalene muscles.

B. Imaging Studies

Upper extremity venous duplex ultrasound is a sensitive and reliable modality to diagnose axillary-subclavian vein thrombosis.

Magnetic resonance venography has demonstrated promise with greater than 97% sensitivity and specificity for diagnosis, but its cost and limited availability reduce its wide spread use. While computed tomographic venography is widely available, its use exposes the patient to contrast dye. Venography, while invasive, remains the common next step in diagnosis, with a positive venogram indicating subclavian vein compression with the appearance of prominent collateral veins. Obtaining these images allows delivery of catheter-directed thrombolysis and allows for further planning of thoracic outlet decompression surgery.

Chest x-ray should be obtained on all patients to exclude the presence of cervical rib, which can also contribute to compression of the subclavian vein.

▶ **Treatment**

For patients with secondary axillo-subclavian thrombosis, any indwelling central venous lines or pacemaker wires in the thrombosed vein should be removed if possible. If not contraindicated, anticoagulation should be considered as well as arm elevation and pain control.

Patients who have primary venous thrombosis secondary to thoracic outlet compression should be considered for decompression because, if left untreated, the patients have a 35%-65% risk of PTS characterized by recurrent episodes of pain, swelling, and chronic venous insufficiency (CVI) secondary to venous hypertension and valvular damage.

The current standard of care is catheter-directed thrombolysis followed by surgical decompression of the thoracic outlet in the majority of cases. Catheter-directed thrombolysis is beneficial to patients presenting early, and offers therapeutic value without the higher rates of bleeding complications seen in systemic fibrinolysis. As the success of thrombolysis decreases as time from onset of symptoms increases, the early initiation of treatment is paramount. Some have advocated a treatment window of two weeks, as there is progressive fibrosis of the vein and risk of extension of the thrombus distally into the arm with decreased chance of recovery. In patients who are more than six weeks from initial presentation of symptoms, thrombolytic agents were generally ineffective in completely removing the clot. Inflow is typically inadequate by the time patients present with chronic obstruction.

Because the etiology of venous thoracic outlet syndrome is compression of the vein between the first rib–anterior scalene muscle origin and the clavicle, surgery consists of anterior scalenectomy, first rib resection, and venolysis (release of the vein from any externally constricting scar). It is particularly important to resect the entire medial portion of the rib to the sternal junction when an anterior, or subclavicular, approach is used. Some prefer this to the transaxillary approach, as the transaxillary approach prevents full resection of the medial rib, and allows for intact subclavius tendons and costoclavicular ligaments, resulting in kinking of the vein on any of these residual structures. However, others find that the transaxillary dissection minimizes the exposure of the neurovascular structures, minimizing their injury. In either case, for patients presenting with acute occlusion, surgical resection of the anterior scalene and first rib with venolysis is preferred to thrombectomy, balloon venoplasty, and stenting.

For patients with chronic obstruction, Molina and colleagues report successful approaches based on length of the obstructed segment. For patients with short segment chronic obstruction, they have been successful with saphenous vein patch to the subclavian vein. In patients with a long segment of chronic obstruction, they have treated with either long vein patch with upper thigh saphenous vein or implantation of thoracic aortic homografts with subsequent balloon dilation and implantation of a stent for reobstruction. Venous bypass has also been successfully used in patients with residual stenosis after thoracic outlet decompression.

The need for and duration of anticoagulation for patients treated with catheter-directed thrombolysis followed by decompression is unclear. Some authors maintain that no anticoagulation is needed when good surgical outcomes are obtained, while others have anticoagulated for two to three months. All patients who present with primary venous thrombosis should undergo a workup for a hypercoagulable state, the most common of which are mutations in coagulation factor V, protein C and S deficiencies, and antithrombin III. Because of a 40%-60% rate of recurrent thrombosis, these patients are maintained indefinitely on warfarin.

Prognosis

The prognosis after axillary-subclavian vein thrombosis is dependent on the cause of the condition. Most patients experience fairly rapid resolution of their initial presenting symptoms. For patients with secondary forms of this disease, the outcome is dependent on resolution of the underlying condition, such as a malignancy. For patients with Paget–Schroetter syndrome who undergo thoracic outlet decompression, excellent outcomes, characterized by continued venous patency and absence of symptoms of CVI, are typical. In contrast, chronic axillary-subclavian vein thrombosis with symptoms persisting for over 3 months does not often respond to thrombolysis, mechanical thrombolysis, or prolonged anticoagulation and may cause significant long-term disability.

Alla VM et al: Paget-Schroetter syndrome: review of pathogenesis and treatment of effort thrombosis. *West J Emerg Med* 2010;11(4):358-362.

Molina JE et al: Protocols for Paget-Schroetter syndrome and late treatment of chronic subclavian vein obstruction. *Ann Thorac Surg* 2009;87(2):416-422.

Urschel HC Jr, AN Patel: Surgery remains the most effective treatment for Paget-Schroetter syndrome: 50 years' experience. *Ann Thorac Surg* 2008;86(1):254-260; discussion 260.

PULMONARY THROMBOEMBOLISM

General Considerations

Pulmonary thromboembolism is responsible for up to 50,000 deaths each year in the United States. It is the third-leading cause of death among hospitalized patients, yet only 30%-40% of those with pulmonary thromboembolism have suspected DVT at the time of diagnosis. Efforts directed at reduction in the mortality rate of pulmonary thromboembolism demand an aggressive approach to the prevention of DVT and diagnosis of pulmonary thromboembolism in patients identified to be at high risk.

Pulmonary thromboemboli arise from a number of sources. Air embolism can occur during the placement or removal of central venous catheters intraoperatively during operation on large venous vessels. Amniotic fluid emboli may occur during active labor. Fat emboli from long bone fractures cause a syndrome characterized by respiratory insufficiency, coagulopathy, encephalopathy, and an upper body petechial rash. Other less common causes of pulmonary emboli include septic emboli, tumor emboli from atrial myxoma or IVC extension of renal cell carcinoma, and parasitic emboli. However, DVT remains the most common source of pulmonary thromboemboli. Up to 60% of patients with untreated proximal lower extremity DVT may develop pulmonary thromboembolism.

Fewer than 10% of pulmonary thromboemboli will produce pulmonary infarction. The pathophysiology of PE depends on the size and frequency of the emboli as well as the condition of the underlying lung. Obstruction of large pulmonary arteries results in increases in pulmonary artery pressure and acute right-ventricular failure, but many of the clinical manifestations of pulmonary thromboembolism result from release of vasoactive amines that cause severe pulmonary vasoconstriction. Vasoconstriction leads to increased physiologic dead space and systemic hypoxia from a right-to-left shunt. Reflex bronchial vasoconstriction is also common.

▶ Clinical Findings

A. Symptoms and Signs

Signs and symptoms associated with PE are notoriously vague. Dyspnea and chest pain are present in up to 75% of patients with pulmonary thromboembolism. However, these symptoms are nonspecific, especially in patients who may have underlying cardiopulmonary disease. Tachycardia, tachypnea, and altered mental status are highly suggestive findings in an at-risk population. The classic triad of dyspnea, chest pain, and hemoptysis is present in only 15% of patients with pulmonary thromboembolism. Pleural friction rub and the S1Q3T3 morphology on electrocardiography are even less common findings.

B. Imaging and Other Diagnostic Studies

Chest x-ray is most often normal but may show a pleural cap. Electrocardiography may reveal new-onset atrial fibrillation, evidence of right-heart strain, or ischemic changes, but in most cases only acute sinus tachycardia and nonspecific ST and T wave changes are identified. Arterial blood gas determination reveals hypoxia and often a respiratory alkalosis or increased arterial-alveolar oxygen gradient. Plasma D-dimer levels are elevated in the presence of both pulmonary thromboembolism and acute DVT, but this test lacks sufficient specificity to be of primary diagnostic value. In acute massive or submassive PE resulting in hemodynamic instability (systolic blood pressure < 90 mm Hg) and right heart strain leading to myocardial ischemia, cardiac troponins may be elevated. Plasma B-type natriuretic peptide may also be elevated in right heart strain, though it is similarly not specific enough to be used alone for diagnosis of PE.

CT angiography is now the preferred imaging modality used for the diagnosis of PE, due to its wide availability, sensitivity and specificity, characterization of vascular and nonvascular structures, and exceptional speed (Figure 35–5). CT angiograms (CTA) are more accurate than the previously commonly used ventilation-perfusion scan, and when compared to pulmonary angiography, CTAs are less invasive, less time consuming, and less expensive. For CTA, the patient presentation must match the results of the CTA, for the most accurate determination of the diagnosis of PE. For patients in whom massive PE is suspected but

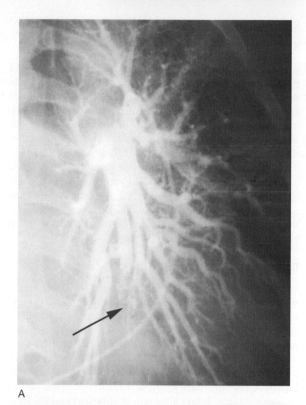

A

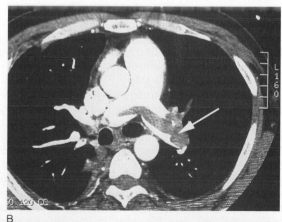

B

▲ **Figure 35–5.** Pulmonary embolism. **A:** Pulmonary angiogram. Arrow marks location of left lower lobe emboli. **B:** Spiral CT. Arrow marks location of large embolus in left main pulmonary artery.

contrast agent administration is undesirable, a bedside echocardiogram may be performed to evaluate for right heart dysfunction as an indication of hemodynamically significant PE. Intravascular ultrasound (IVUS) has also been used for bedside evaluation.

▶ Treatment

A. Anticoagulation

Rapid anticoagulation remains the mainstay of treatment of PE. Heparin, the pentasaccharide fondaparinux, or LMWH anticoagulation is started as soon as the diagnosis is made after initial stabilization with ventilatory support and vasopressor medications. While these drugs are not thrombolytic, they allow the body's fibrinolytic system to function unopposed. Thrombolysis is considered for large clot burden, severe respiratory compromise, hemodynamic instability, or right-heart failure. When compared with heparin alone, thrombolytic therapy speeds the resolution of pulmonary emboli in the first 24 hours. The disadvantages of lytic therapy include its greater cost and higher risk of significant bleeding complications.

B. Inferior Vena Cava Interruption

IVC interruption is considered in patients who have extension of venous thrombus on adequate anticoagulant therapy, patients in whom heparin anticoagulation is contraindicated, patients who have had a complication of anticoagulation, or patients who have had recurrent DVT or PE despite *therapeutic* anticoagulation. More recently, temporary or permanent IVC filters have been placed prophylactically in high-risk patients such as those with unresectable cancer or major trauma. Interestingly, as insertion of an IVC filter does not completely eliminate the risk of a PE, may increases the risk of DVT, and does nothing to prevent postthrombotic syndrome (PTS), the current guidelines suggest that patients who have an IVC filter should receive the standard course of anticoagulation if the contraindication to anticoagulation is no longer applicable.

Historically, IVC interruption was performed as an open surgical procedure, involving ligation or plication of the infrarenal vena cava or placement of a serrated clip to "strain" blood returning to the right atrium. The Greenfield filter, developed in 1973, was initially deployed by venous cutdown. Multiple devices are now available for fluoroscopically guided percutaneous placement through a range of sheath sizes from 6F to 12F and are introduced into the common femoral vein or, in cases of femoral thrombus, into the internal jugular vein. Diagnostic inferior venacavogram is essential prior to placing the filter to exclude the presence of a duplicated IVC because lower extremity DVT might still serve as a source of emboli. The presence of thrombus within the IVC, the diameter of the IVC, and identification of the level of the renal veins are also important to evaluate.

The development and increased use of retrievable IVC filters for both prophylaxis and therapy of VTE is largely driven by the results of the PREPIC study. This study remains the only prospective, randomized clinical trial comparing IVC filters to anticoagulation alone. At 8 years, the study suggested a higher incidence of recurrent DVT in patients who were randomized to the IVC filter arm of the study compared to group who received anticoagulation only. This study suggested that patients with IVC filters in placed had a significantly higher risk of recurrent DVT than patients treated with anticoagulation alone. There was no difference in the incidence of PTS between study groups but patients with IVC filters in place had significantly lower rates of PE over the course of the study compared to the anticoagulation group. While there is a multitude of devices available and many small observational studies that suggest that retrievable filters are safe and effective, no other prospective comparison studies have yet to be performed.

Additionally, alternative imaging modalities (other than venography) are successfully being used to place filters. Specifically, devices are being successfully and safely deployed under ultrasound guidance, both intravascular and transabdominal ultrasound. Kassavin and colleagues recently described the transition from combined use of IVUS-guided and traditional techniques (such as venography) for IVC filter placement to the use of IVUS as the primary road mapping tool had a learning curve of only approximately 20 cases. Compared to traditional placement, the use of IVUS for IVC filter deployment lacks the risks of prolonged radiation exposure and nephrotoxic contrast agents while diminishing the case duration and overall cost.

C. Surgical Treatment

Hemodynamically unstable patients in whom thrombolytic therapy has failed or cannot be instituted require percutaneous or open surgical extraction of the thrombus. Open surgical pulmonary embolectomy is reserved for patients who develop intractable hypotension, those who fail transcatheter pulmonary embolectomy, and those who have tumor or foreign body emboli. Catheter techniques involve mechanical thrombolysis or removal of intact pulmonary emboli using a suction embolectomy device.

▶ Prognosis

PE is one of the most frequent causes of preventable hospital death. Prevention by use of DVT prophylaxis and early diagnosis by selective testing of high-risk patients are essential steps to reducing the morbidity of this disease. The placement of IVC filters in selected patients can aid in prevention of pulmonary embolus but does nothing to treat the underlying disease process (venous thromboembolic disease) or prevent the long-term sequelae of DVT-PTS.

Kassavin DS, Constantinopoulos G: The transition to IVUS-guided IVC filter deployment in the nontrauma patient. *Vasc Endovascular Surg* 2011;45(2):142-145.

Kearon C et al: Antithrombotic therapy for VTE disease: anti-thrombotic therapy and prevention of thrombosis, 9th ed: American College of Chest Physicians evidence-based clinical practice guidelines. *Chest* 2012;141(2 Suppl):e419S-e4194S.

Kuo WT: Endovascular therapy for acute pulmonary embolism. *J Vasc Interv Radiol* 2012;23(2):167-179.e4; quiz 179.

Tapson VF: Acute pulmonary embolism. *N Engl J Med* 2008;358(10);1037-1052.

The PREPIC study group: Eight-year follow-up of patients with permanent vena cava filters in the prevention of pulmonary embolism. *Circulation* 2005;112:416.

SUPERFICIAL THROMBOPHLEBITIS

► General Considerations

Superficial thrombophlebitis (SVT) may appear spontaneously in patients with varicose veins, in pregnant or postpartum women, or in patients with thromboangiitis obliterans or Behçet disease. It may also occur after intravenous therapy or in an area of localized trauma. The presence of superficial phlebitis, particularly if it occurs in a migratory manner, suggests the presence of an abdominal cancer such as carcinoma of the pancreas (Trousseau thrombophlebitis). The most common vein affected is the greater saphenous vein and its branches. In up to 40% of cases, a simultaneous DVT exists, and duplex imaging is a must in these situations. Pulmonary emboli are rare unless extension into the deep venous system occurs.

► Clinical Findings

The patient usually presents complaining of localized extremity pain and redness. Areas of induration, erythema, and tenderness correspond to dilated and often thrombosed superficial veins. Over time, a firm cord may develop. Generalized edema is absent unless the deep veins are involved. The presence of fever and shaking chills suggests septic or suppurative phlebitis, which occurs most commonly as a complication of intravenous cannulation.

► Differential Diagnosis

Superficial thrombophlebitis must be distinguished from ascending lymphangitis, cellulitis, erythema nodosum, erythema induratum, and panniculitis. Unlike these other disorders, superficial phlebitis tends to be well localized over a superficial vein.

► Treatment

The primary treatment of superficial venous thrombophlebitis is the administration of nonsteroidal anti-inflammatory drugs, local heat, elevation, and support stockings or elastic wraps. Ambulation is encouraged. In most cases, symptoms will resolve within 7-10 days. Excision of the involved vein is recommended for symptoms that persist over 2 weeks despite treatment or for recurrent phlebitis in the same vein segment. If there is progressive proximal extension with involvement of the saphenofemoral junction or cephalic-subclavian junction, ligation and resection of the vein at the junction should be performed. More recently, cases in which endovenous thermal ablation was used in the treatment of superficial thrombophlebitis has been reported but not usually during the acute phase of the disease process. Alternatively, LMWH has been studied in the treatment of superficial thrombophlebitis given its anti-inflammatory and antithrombotic effects. In a randomized trial by Rathbun and colleagues comparing daily dalteparin versus ibuprofen three times daily for up to 14 days, dalteparin was found to be superior in preventing extension of superficial thrombophlebitis at 14 days with similar relief of pain.

The approach to treating SVT is variable, as there is no general consensus on ideal treatment. Reports of less than 10% to approximately 40% of presentation of SVT also presents with associated acute DVT. The occurrence of concomitant PE has been reported from 0.5% to 4% in symptomatic patients. Approximately 60%-80% of SVT cases involve the great saphenous vein and 10%-20% of cases involve the small saphenous veins, with involvement of the upper extremity veins occurring next in frequency. The association between SVT and both DVTs and PEs increases as the phlebitis extends toward the saphenofemoral junction. The treatment approach therefore depends on the location, presence of concomitant DVT, and the presence of additional risk factors such as hypercoagulable disorders. Involvement of the junction warrants aggressive treatment with LMWH to prevent further extension into the deep venous system. A recent Cochrane review involving 26 studies and 5521 participants assessed the current approach to patients with superficial thrombophlebitis of the legs. Fondaparinux at a prophylactic dose given for 45 days was associated with lower rates of recurrence and extension of superficial thrombophlebitis compared to placebo. Both NSAIDS and LMWH reduced extension or recurrence when compared to placebo. When comparing LMWH with surgical intervention (saphenofemoral disconnection), both were comparable in reduction of VTE events, though surgery was associated with a statistically insignificant lower risk of extension or recurrence. Alternatively, venous stripping plus elastic stockings demonstrated a lower, non-significant incidence of VTE compared with elastic stockings alone. In general, surgical treatment with ligation of the great saphenous vein at the saphenofemoral junction allows for superior symptomatic relief of pain, while medical management with anticoagulants appears superior for minimizing complications and preventing subsequent DVT/PE.

Septic thrombophlebitis requires treatment with broad-spectrum intravenous antibiotics. If rapid resolution of the cellulitis occurs, no treatment beyond a short course of antibiotics is required. However, if the patient becomes septic, excision of the entire infected vein is required. Catheter removal is required in cases involving central venous catheter infection. In patients refractory to standard medical therapy yet poor candidates for invasive surgical therapy, endovascular treatment using thrombectomy devices, balloon angioplasty, and local intraluminal infusion of antibiotics has been reported. Thrombolytic therapy and mechanical thrombectomy remain options for the treatment of the thrombosed vein segment.

▶ Prognosis

Most episodes of uncomplicated superficial thrombophlebitis respond to conservative management. Cases in which extension into the deep venous system occurs can be associated with thromboembolism.

Di Nisio M et al: Treatment for superficial thrombophlebitis of the leg. *Cochrane Database Syst Rev* 2012;3:CD004982.

Enzler MA et al: Thermal ablation in the management of superficial thrombophlebitis. *Eur J Vasc Endovasc Surg* 2012;43(6): 726-728.

Kar S and Webel R: Septic thrombophlebitis: percutaneous mechanical thrombectomy and thrombolytic therapies. *Am J Ther* 2014 Mar-Apr;21(2):131-136.

Rathbun SW et al: A randomized trial of dalteparin compared with ibuprofen for the treatment of superficial thrombophlebitis. *J Thromb Haemost* 2012;10:833-839.

CHRONIC VENOUS INSUFFICIENCY

CVI can result from congenital venous valvular insufficiency or can result from previous venous thrombosis. In the former circumstance, it is called CVI while in the latter circumstance, it is called the PTS. Varicose veins (also a manifestation of venous insufficiency), CVI, and PTS occur in 76/100,000 person-years, and it has been estimated that 6-7 million Americans suffer from stasis pigmentation changes in the legs with another 400,000-500,000 patients with skin ulceration. Treatment costs are in the billion dollar range. The basic physiologic abnormality in patients with CVI is chronic elevation of venous pressure. The normal venous capacitance can accommodate large-volume changes that occur during exercise with only minimal changes in venous pressure. However, with calf muscle pump dysfunction and valvular reflux, blood pools in the lower extremities and venous hypertension occurs, leading to venous hypertension. Outflow obstruction from proximal obstruction can also produce venous hypertension, resulting in "venous claudication" as the deep venous system fills with blood during exercise. The leg becomes painful, swollen, and heavy (especially with exercise), mimicking arterial insufficiency. Severity of chronic venous disease has been associated with older age and higher body mass index.

Valvular incompetence of the deep veins can be congenital or result from damage following phlebitis, varicose veins, or DVT. The best estimate for the incidence of CVI is approximately 30% after 8-year follow-up. Chronic venous stasis changes are centered in the "gaiter areas" around the ankles. This is the location of the commonly affected perforator veins and is a region with sparse soft tissue support to withstand elevated venous pressures. Brawny edema is produced by extravasation of plasma fluid, red blood cells, and plasma proteins. Lysis of red blood cells results in deposition of hemosiderin, which creates a brownish discoloration. Leukocytes become sequestered in the microcirculation, leading to capillary occlusion and release of superoxide radicals, proteolytic enzymes, and growth factors. Macrophages and T lymphocytes are primary mediators of this inflammatory response, which results in fibroblast activation and scarring and fibrosis of the subcutaneous tissues. Ultimately, this fibrosis results in compromised skin perfusion and ulceration.

▶ Clinical Findings

A. Symptoms and Signs

Both isolated saphenous vein incompetence and deep venous insufficiency can lead to venous varicosities and chronic venous stasis changes. One of the first symptoms to develop is usually ankle and calf edema. Involvement of the foot and toes suggests lymphedema. Typically, the edema is worse at the end of the day and improves with leg elevation. Additional symptoms may include aching, tingling, burning, muscle cramps, heaviness, sensations of throbbing, and leg fatigue. Longstanding disease is characterized by stasis dermatitis, hyperpigmentation, brawny induration, and ulceration. Venous stasis ulcers are large, painful, and irregular in outline. They have a shallow, moist granulation bed, occur in the gaiter area on the medial or lateral aspects of the ankle, and are often accompanied by stasis dermatitis and stasis pigmentation changes.

B. Imaging and Other Diagnostic Studies

Duplex ultrasound can identify the presence and location of incompetent superficial and deep veins and perforating veins and has been used to evaluate the function of individual venous valves. Current guidelines recommend selective scanning of perforating veins in patients with CVI, Duplex imaging has become the most important test of venous pathophysiology today and should be performed in every patient with CVI and PTS. However, it does not easily assess calf muscle pump function or the presence of proximal obstruction. These concerns are addressed with use of other tests, such as air plethysmography, which gives a quantitative assessment of venous reflux (by the venous filling index), calf muscle pump function (by the ejection fraction), and overall venous function (by residual volume function). These measurements help to stratify patients into treatment groups.

Determination of functional outflow obstruction requires venography with or without pressure measurement, although intravascular ultrasound (IVUS) is also very useful to determine the presence or absence of venous obstruction. Descending phlebography involves injection of contrast media into the common femoral vein to test the valves during normal breathing and with a forced Valsalva maneuver. Using this technique, pathologic reflux can be identified in patients with postthrombotic damage. Such testing is reserved in anticipation of surgical correction of the venous pathology if duplex scanning does not provide definite information on pathophysiology.

Differential Diagnosis

Congestive heart failure and chronic liver and kidney disease must be considered in the differential diagnosis of bilateral lower extremity edema. Lymphedema is characterized by nonpitting edema of the dorsum of the foot and toes as well as the calf and generally is not associated with skin pigment changes, dermatitis, or ulceration. Severe arterial insufficiency produces ulcers that are painful, well circumscribed, and located over pressure points on the distal end of the extremity and foot. Ulcers due to autoimmune diseases, erythema nodosum, and fungal infections are distinguished by appearance and distribution.

Treatment

Venous insufficiency is an incurable but manageable problem. Most patients respond well to a conservative treatment program composed of intermittent leg elevation, regular exercise to improve calf muscle pump function, and the use of surgical elastic graduated compression stockings. Although the mechanism by which elastic compression improves the symptoms of CVI has not been clearly established, recent work suggests that external compression may restore competency of dilated valve cusps and affect venoarterial reflex. Most venous ulceration will improve with leg elevation, external compression, and local wound care. Compression can be achieved with an inelastic bandage such as an Unna boot, an occlusive wound dressing covered by elastic bandage wrapping, or surgical support stockings.

Surgery is indicated for a small percentage of patients with nonhealing ulcers or disabling symptoms refractory to conservative management. The three main categories of procedures include those ablative procedures on the superficial venous system in the face of superficial venous reflux, antireflux procedures, and bypass operations for obstruction. If superficial venous reflux is a significant component of the total venous reflux present, then superficial ablation is appropriate. Such ablation has been found successful in preventing recurrent venous ulceration and has also been found to improve patients' symptoms of both varicose veins and venous reflux. Ablation may be performed with traditional open surgical ligation and stripping or the more recent endovenous procedures such as radiofrequency ablation or endovenous laser therapy. The pathology must be accurately

characterized so that an appropriate operative strategy can be developed. The most common abnormality in patients with CVI is incompetence of the popliteal or tibial veins; 50%-60% of patients have incompetent perforators.

Perforating vein interventions are typically performed in patients with recurrent venous ulcers or demonstrated incompetence of perforating veins under the area of ulceration. Since its introduction in the 1980s to the late 2000s, subfascial endoscopic perforator vein surgery (SEPS) was the technique of choice for perforator ablation, as studies revealed that it resulted in a significant lower rate of wound infections and recurrent ulcers compared to the open Linton procedure. However, continued advancements in perforator ablation techniques in more recent years has led to increased use of percutaneous ablation of perforators (PAPS), radiofrequency ablation (RFA), endovenous laser ablation, and sclerotherapy in addition to SEPS. Current guidelines recommend against selective treatment of incompetent perforating veins in patients with simple varicose veins. However, in perforating veins which meet "pathologic" criteria (outward flow ≥500 ms duration, diameter ≥3.5 mm, located beneath healed or open venous ulcer), SEPS, ultrasound-guided sclerotherapy, or thermal ablations are suggested.

While minimally invasive techniques addressing superficial and perforator reflux have advanced, such treatment of deep reflux disease remains challenging. There are both nonthrombotic and postthrombotic etiologies, either of which contributes to the obstructive component of deep reflux disease. Previous surgical options included venous bypass and reconstruction procedures, patch venoplasty, and, specifically in the case of patients for whom iliac-femoral stenosis is confirmed through venography and intravenous ultrasonography (IVUS), venous stenting has been a successful endovascular treatment option. Alhalbouni and colleagues reported the majority of their patients experienced healing of their chronic venous stasis ulcers after stenting of stenotic lesions found by IVUS. Raju et al. describe 5-year continued freedom from venous ulcer after iliac stenting to near 90%, underscoring both the role of obstruction in the pathophysiology and the effectiveness of relieving such obstruction.

Alhalbouni S et al: Iliac-femoral venous stenting for lower extremity venous stasis symptoms. *Ann Vasc Surg* 2012;26(2):185-189.

Gloviczki P et al: The care of patients with varicose veins and associated chronic venous diseases: clinical practice guidelines of the Society for Vascular Surgery and the American Venous Forum. *J Vasc Surg* 2011;53(5 Suppl):2S-48S.

Luebke T et al: Meta-analysis of subfascial endocscopic perforator vein surgery (SEPS) for chronic venous insufficiency. *Phlebology* 2008;24(1):8-16.

Musil D et al: Age, body mass index and severity of primary chronic venous disease. *Biomed Pap Med Fac Univ Palacky Olomouc Czech Repub* 2011;155(4):367-371.

Raju S et al: Unexpected major role for venous stenting in deep reflux disease. *J Vasc Surg* 2010;51(2):401-408; discussion 408.

▼ II. THE LYMPHATICS

LYMPHEDEMA

▶ General Considerations

Much less is known about the fluid dynamics of the lymphatic system than of the venous or arterial system. Most energy for lymph propulsion arises from the intrinsic lymphatic smooth muscle contractions that occur rhythmically. Lymphatic luminal pressures are usually 30-50 mm Hg and can exceed arterial pressure under special circumstances. The lymphatic system carries interstitial fluid and macromolecular proteins lost from the capillaries, as well as infectious agents and foreign material, back into the central circulation. Two to four liters a day of lymph drain into the subclavian vein.

The fundamental mechanism responsible for lymphedema formation is impaired lymph flow out of the extremity. Primary lymphedema includes idiopathic types of lymphedema without an identifiable etiology, and the more commonly recognized type due to abnormal lymphatic development, most often hypoplasia resulting in severe reduction in the number of lymphatics and the lymphatic diameters. It is classified by age at onset of the disease. Congenital lymphedema develops before 1 year of age, is usually bilateral, and affects men more than women; if familial, it is known as Milroy disease. More often, lymphedema develops during adolescence (lymphedema praecox) and is unilateral; there is a 10:1 female predominance. Lymphedema occurring after age 35 is referred to as lymphedema tarda.

Secondary lymphedema results from a wide variety of disease processes that cause obstruction to the lymphatic system. The most common of these is surgical excision and radiation to the axillary or inguinal lymph nodes as part of the treatment of breast cancer, cervical cancer, prostate cancer, melanoma, and soft tissue tumors. Many of these neoplasms tend to develop regional lymphatic metastases before progressing to distant metastatic disease, and their treatment commonly involves complete lymph node dissection of the involved territory. Of note, secondary lymphedema may arise at any time postoperatively, including years and decades after the operation. Less common causes of secondary lymphedema are bacterial and fungal infections, trauma, and lymphoproliferative diseases. In many developing countries, lymphatic obstruction due to filariasis is caused by three different parasites: *Wuchereria bancrofti*, *Brugia malayi*, and *Brugia timori*.

▶ Clinical Manifestations

A. Symptoms, Signs, and Assessment

The history of the disease process will usually define the cause of the lymphedema. Development of painless edema in an adolescent girl with a family history of lymphedema would indicate primary lymphedema as a diagnosis. A history of lymph node dissection, irradiation, or the presence of a parasitic infection suggests secondary lymphedema.

Lymphedema development is usually slowly progressive and painless. In the early stages, the edema is pitting, but as the disease progresses, chronic fibrosis occurs and the edema becomes nonpitting. The distribution of edema is also characteristic. It is usually centered on the ankle (Figure 35–6) and is most pronounced on the dorsum of the foot, producing a buffalo hump appearance. Unlike edema of venous stasis disease, lymphedema also often involves the toes. In the early stages, the skin is normal, but skin thickening and hyperkeratosis occurs with longstanding disease. A chronic eczematous dermatitis may ensue.

Objective assessment is most commonly performed by measuring the circumference of the extremities, with the difference threshold of greater than 2 cm to define lymphedema. Additionally, water displacement is used to assess limb volume. The difference between the two arms before and after surgery of over 200 mL has been used to identify secondary lymphedema.

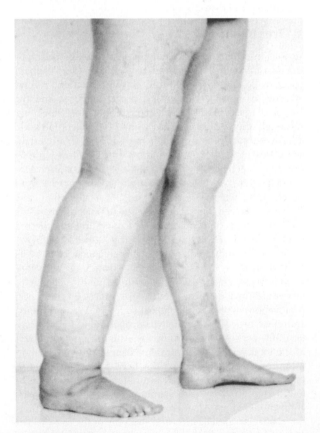

▲ **Figure 35–6.** Acquired lymphedema. Edema is centered at the ankle and involves the foot and toes.

Rarely, lymphangiosarcoma or angiosarcoma may develop as a complication of chronic lymphedema. This neoplastic transformation of blood vessels and lymphatics is called Stewart–Treves syndrome.

B. Imaging Studies

Venous duplex scans are performed to rule out venous insufficiency and exclude venous obstruction. CT and MRI are useful tests in patients with suspected secondary lymphedema from unknown malignancy. Lymphangiography has largely been replaced by radionuclide lymphoscintigraphy, the gold standard for evaluation of lymphatic function. A subcutaneous injection of 99mTc-labeled substance is injected into the first and second web-space of the toes or fingers, and its movement, transition time, and activity are interpreted. Lymphoscintigraphy carries minimal risk, and its use in conjunction with duplex scans permits the detection of lymphatic dysfunction and lymph nodes and provides information on lymph transport and reflux.

▶ Differential Diagnosis

A variety of diseases can result in bilateral lower extremity edema. These include congestive heart failure, pulmonary hypertension, chronic renal or hepatic insufficiency, and hypoproteinemia. In patients with unilateral leg edema, differential diagnosis includes congenital vascular malformations, chronic venous insufficiency, and reflex sympathetic dystrophy.

▶ Treatment

Lymphedema is a chronic disease for which there is no complete cure. However, a variety of conservative measures can substantially reduce the risk of further complications and disability.

No drug therapy is effective. Use of benzopyrones (to increase lymphatic transport by macrophages) has shown some benefit. Diuretics can be useful for acute exacerbation of edema secondary to infection or for coexisting venous stasis disease, but these agents are not recommended for long-term use in lymphedema.

The mainstay of treatment is external compression and meticulous skin care. Mechanical reduction of lymphedema can best be achieved with a program of frequent leg elevation, manual lymphatic drainage massage, low-stretch wrapping techniques, and intermittent pneumatic compression (IPC). Decongestive lymphatic therapy (DLT) is traditionally the first line of treatment regardless of primary or secondary etiology. DLT is composed of manual lymphatic drainage, compression therapy with bandages and IPC, and movement exercises. Many different devices are available for use on the leg, and sleeves can be custom fit for patients with postmastectomy arm lymphedema. Graduated compression

stockings maintain the limb after reduction by pneumatic compression. Good skin care is imperative in order to prevent infection. Moisturizing lotions should be applied regularly, especially after showering or bathing. Drying and cracking of the skin can create portals of entry for bacteria. Infection is difficult to eradicate because of disordered lymphatic drainage and can be limb threatening.

The psychologic impact of chronic lymphedema cannot be underestimated. However, with appropriate patient education that results in the prevention of chronic infection or massive edema, this problem can be manageable.

Operation may be considered in rare cases of severe functional impairment and recurrent lymphangitis. The approaches are either reductive in nature to minimize bulk, or they are reconstructive to rebuild lymphatic channels. Indications for reductive therapies include massive, incapacitating extremities, and the failure of conservative therapy. The Charles procedure involves excision of all skin and subcutaneous tissue from the tibial tuberosity to the lateral head of the fibula and wound coverage by a split thickness skin graft. Due to unpredictable cosmetic outcomes and associated complications such as cellulitis and sepsis, many variations of this procedure now exist with reported decrease in morbidity. More recently, liposuction-circumferential suction-assisted lipectomy has been successful in treating upper-extremity lymphedema secondary to breast cancer therapy. In this scenario, fat is the primary cause of swelling and not fluid, thus lymph reconstruction and conservative measurements are ineffective.

The application of reconstructive techniques is most successful in early disease, when the lymphatics are relatively healthy. Lymphatic channels are rebuilt via microsurgical methods of lympho-venous or lympho-venous-lymphtic bypass anastomosis, lympho-lymphatic segmental interposition, or free lymph node transplantation. Campisi and colleagues present the largest series to date evaluating lymphatic reconstruction, with 1800 patients with primary and secondary lymphedema treated over 30 years with lymphatic-venous anastomoses. Their study demonstrates 87% of their subjects reported subjective improvement and 83% showed significant volume reduction. Notably, more than 90% of these patients were in Campisi stage II and III lymphedema with persistent edema, but still at a relatively early stage before the onset of fibrosis or severe limb deformation. As the disease progresses and irreversible damage inevitably results, there is little success in restoring flow or reducing fibrosclerotic tissue.

Campisi C et al: Microsurgery for lymphedema: clinical research and long-term results. *Microsurgery* 2010;30(4):256-260.

Doscher ME et al: Surgical management of inoperable lymphedema: the re-emergence of abandoned techniques. *J Am Coll Surg* 2012;215(2):278-283.

Murdaca G et al: Current views on diagnostic approach and treatment of lymphedema. *Am J Med* 2012;125(2):134-140.

LYMPHANGITIS

▶ General Considerations

Lymphangitis is usually caused by a hemolytic streptococcal or staphylococcal infection that arises in an area of cellulitis near an open wound. Multiple long red streaks can be seen coursing toward the regional lymph nodes. Severe systemic manifestations include tachycardia, fever, chills, and malaise, which untreated can lead to sepsis and death.

▶ Clinical Findings

A. Symptoms and Signs

Pain at the site of the initial wound is present. High fevers develop rapidly. The streaks may be faint in appearance initially, especially in dark-skinned patients. Regional lymph nodes are often enlarged and tender.

▶ B. Laboratory Findings

An elevated white blood cell count associated with a left shift is almost universally present. Blood and wound cultures should be obtained routinely.

▶ Differential Diagnosis

Lymphangitis should be distinguished from superficial thrombophlebitis, which is usually localized to a single venous segment often with a palpable cord. Patients with thrombophlebitis usually do not appear toxic, as do patients with lymphangitis. Cat-scratch fever should always be considered when lymphadenitis is present. It is also important to differentiate cellulitis and severe soft tissue infections from lymphangitis. In general, lymphangitis is characterized by its superficial location and the linear pattern of erythema.

▶ Treatment

The extremity should be elevated and warm compresses applied. Analgesics and intravenous antibiotics should be instituted immediately. Examination of the wound should be made to determine the need for debridement or incision and drainage of an abscess.

▶ Prognosis

Delayed or inadequate therapy can lead to overwhelming sepsis and death. Aggressive institution of appropriate antibiotic therapy and wound care will usually control the infection within 48-72 hours.

MULTIPLE CHOICE QUESTIONS

1. Which statement regarding the treatment of varicose and perforator veins is true?

   A. Surgical and chemical ablations are preferred compared to thermal ablation of the GSV
   B. Selective treatment of incompetent varicose veins is recommended in patients with simple varicose veins
   C. Thermal ablation is an effective approach to the treatment of saphenous veins
   D. Vein reabsorption after thermal ablation occurs over the course of a few days

2. Three months' anticoagulation is recommended for which of the following?

   A. In patients with PE/an isolated distal DVT of the leg provoked by surgery
   B. In patients with PE/proximal DVT of the leg provoked by a nonsurgical transient risk factor
   C. All patients with DVT
   D. A and B

3. Which imaging study is an appropriate initial evaluation in patients with suspected axillary-subclavian vein thrombosis?

   A. CT angiogram
   B. CT venogram
   C. Chest x-ray
   D. Upper extremity venous duplex ultrasound

4. Which of the following regarding superficial thrombophlebitis is true?

   A. Generalized edema is almost always present
   B. Up to 40% of presentations have associated acute DVT
   C. Ambulation is discouraged due to the painful, inflammatory process
   D. Most episodes of septic thrombophlebitis require surgical excision

5. Lymphedema is a chronic condition for which no definitive cure is currently available. Which of the following is true?

   A. The distribution of edema is exactly the same as that of venous stasis disease
   B. The gold standard for evaluation of lymph function is CT
   C. Venous duplex scans aid in ruling out venous insufficiency and venous obstruction
   D. Diuretics are a mainstay of treatment of minimizing the edema

Neurosurgery

Aditya S. Pandey, MD
B. Gregory Thompson, MD

36

DIAGNOSIS & MANAGEMENT OF ALTERATIONS IN CONSCIOUSNESS

Kyle Sheehan, MD; George A. Mashour , MD, PhD

Alterations of consciousness and the related conditions of delirium, acute confusional state, and acute encephalopathy are among the most common mental disorders encountered in either surgical or medical patients. The prevalence of altered mental status in hospitalized patients is high, with reported rates up to 50%. These conditions are associated with increased mortality rates ranging from 10% to 65%, and excess annual health care expenditures in the billions. Given the high incidence of altered mental states, at least a basic understanding of the pathophysiology, diagnosis, and management of common etiologies is warranted for all medical practitioners.

DEFINITIONS

Consciousness is generally defined as the subjective experience of the environment and the self. It is comprised of two components: arousal, which is the state of wakefulness, and awareness, which is the state of phenomenal perception. This distinction is useful, since the two processes are dissociable. For example, a vegetative state is characterized by a patient that is awake (ie, the cortex is aroused), but not necessarily aware.

Arousal is generated by activity of the ascending reticular activating system, which is composed of neurons within the central mesencephalic brainstem, the lateral hypothalamus, and portions of the thalamus. Widespread projections of these nuclei synapse on neurons in the cerebral cortex and generate an arousal response. Arousal responses define the *level* of consciousness (eg, being awake vs. asleep vs. comatose). **Awareness** is thought to be generated through networks involving the thalamus and association cortices of the frontal, parietal, temporal, and occipital lobes. Processes related to awareness define the *content* of consciousness (eg, seeing a blue circle vs. a red triangle).

Many terms are used to describe the levels of consciousness ranging from alert to comatose. The alert patient is awake and immediately responsive to all stimuli. Stupor is a condition in which the patient is less alert but still responds with stimulation. An obtunded patient appears to be asleep much of the time but still responds to noxious stimuli. A vegetative state is a state of arousal without awareness in which the patient may open his or her eyes, track objects, chew, and swallow, but not respond to auditory stimuli or appear to sense pain (although pain processing is now known to occur in the vegetative state). The comatose patient appears asleep and does not respond to stimuli. Often, terms used to describe states of consciousness lack consistent definitions, and a clear description of a patient's state of arousal and awareness results in more precise communication.

PATHOPHYSIOLOGY OF ALTERED CONSCIOUSNESS

In general, altered states of consciousness can arise from physiologic, pharmacologic, and pathologic causes. Before addressing pathologic causes (which can have structural or nonstructural etiologies), physiologic perturbations such as hypoglycemia, hypoxia, hypercarbia, hyponatremia, and hypothermia should be addressed. Pharmacologic etiologies, such as acute intoxication, overdose, and residual anesthesia from surgery, should also be considered and reversed when possible.

Structural Pathology

The reticular activating system is excited by a wide variety of stimuli, particularly somatosensory stimuli. Given that its nuclei are highly concentrated in the midbrain, it can be damaged by central midbrain lesions, which can result in the loss of arousal and coma.

Less severe dysfunction of the reticular activating system results in an acute confusional state. The cardinal signs of an acute confusional state are somnolence, inattention, and disorientation. Additionally, perceptions may be distorted, leading to hallucinations, and the patient may be unable to organize and interpret a complex stimuli. Disordered perception results in dysfunctional learning, memory, and problem solving. Thought processes can be disorganized and tangential, and the confused patient may develop delusions. In some cases, the acute confusional state presents as delirium, which can, in its hyperactive form, be characterized by heightened arousal, disordered perception, agitation, delusions, hallucinations, and autonomic hyperactivity (diaphoresis, tachycardia, hypertension, and mydriasis). However, it is important to note that hypoactive delirium is the most common type to be manifested in the postoperative setting.

Neurons in the pons, midbrain, and hypothalamus are necessary for regulation of sleep-wake cycles. Therefore, lesions involving the pons may preserve consciousness but disturb sleep. This is in contrast to the typical vegetative state that results from diffuse destruction or injury of the bilateral cerebral cortices, secondary to global cerebral ischemia or anoxia with preservation of the reticular activating system and brainstem sleep centers. This leaves the patient with preserved sleep-wake cycles without the ability to interact with the environment.

Acute confusional states and coma may result from structural or metabolic causes. Structural lesions of the cerebral hemispheres such as hemorrhage (intracerebral, subdural, or epidural), large areas of ischemic infarction, abscesses, or neoplasms can expand over minutes or a few hours and result in significant elevation of the intracranial pressure (ICP).

▶ Nonstructural Pathology

Several nonstructural disorders that diffusely disturb brain function can produce a confusional state or, if severe, coma (Table 36–1). Acute toxic-metabolic encephalopathy (TME), which encompasses delirium and the acute confusional state, is an acute condition of global cerebral dysfunction in the absence of primary structural brain disease. Typically, TME is usually a consequence of systemic disease or secondary to drugs and metabolic toxins that are reversible, thus making prompt recognition and treatment critical.

Additionally, TME is common among critically ill patients and is probably underdiagnosed, especially when it occurs in patients who require mechanical ventilation. Risk factors for the development of TME include admission to an ICU, advanced age, preexisting primary neurodegenerative disease (dementia), nutritional deficiency, infection, temperature dysregulation, and failure of multiple organ systems.

Table 36–1. Etiology of altered state of consciousness.

Physiologic	Pathologic	Pharmacologic
Global cerebral ischemia	Trauma-associated subdural or epidural hematoma	Sedatives
Hepatic encephalopathy	Tumor	Narcotics
Hypoxia/hypercarbia	Infection—meningitis or encephalitis	Alcohol/illicit substances
Hyperosmolar state	Vascular (stroke)	Poisoning
Hypotension	Ischemic stroke (ie, basilar artery thrombosis)	
Hypo/hypercalcemia		
Hypo/hyperthermia	Subarachnoid hemorrhage	
Hypo/hyperglycemia	Intracerebral hemorrhage	
Hypo/hypernatremia	Seizures	
Hypothyroidism	Subclinical status epilepticus	
Thyrotoxicosis	Prolonged post-ictal state	
Uremia		

PATHOPHYSIOLOGY OF ELEVATED INTRACRANIAL PRESSURE

The skull encloses three major components: brain parenchyma, cerebrospinal fluid (CSF), and blood. The volumetric sum of these components is maintained at a constant. Given the nondistensible cranial vault and these three noncompressible substances, an increase in one component must be offset by a decrease in another or pressure will increase. This offset is normally accomplished by displacement of CSF into the contiguous subarachnoid space of the spinal cord, termed "spatial compensation." This delicate balance, however, has physiologic limits. Once these compensatory limits are met, an increase in the volume of any component will lead to an exponential increase in ICP as illustrated by the intracranial elastance curve (Figure 36–1).

Normal ICP in adults is less than 10-15 mm Hg. The presence of tumor or blood, the impedance of CSF drainage (hydrocephalus), cerebral edema, and increased cerebral

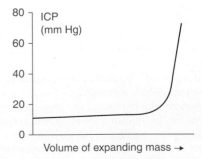

▲ **Figure 36–1.** Intracranial compliance curve demonstrating the approximate relationship between ICP and an expanding intracranial mass.

blood flow (hyperemia as a response to head injury or hypoventilation causing hypercarbia and vasodilation) may raise the ICP to a dangerous level. The increased ICP may lead to reduced cerebral perfusion and ischemia and a mass effect progressing to shifting of the brain parenchyma and devastating herniation.

SIGNS & SYMPTOMS OF INCREASED ICP

Increased ICP is often accompanied by altered mental status, headache, vomiting (without nausea), and papilledema on fundoscopic examination. Cushings triad may be seen in patients with severely increased ICP and consists of hypertension, bradycardia, and respiratory irregularity. Obtundation, focal neurologic findings including unilateral pupillary dilation from pressure or traction exerted on the third cranial nerve (ie, the "blown" pupil), and hemodynamic instability are late findings and indicate pending uncal herniation.

Cerebral Herniation Syndromes

Cerebral herniation occurs when increased ICP results in a portion of the brain shifting from one intracranial compartment to another. These shifts may lead to vascular compromise and infarction of portions of the brain, disruption of white matter pathways, and direct pressure on structures such as cranial nerve III.

Subfalcine Herniation

Occurs in patients with a frontal lobe mass as the cingulate gyrus herniates beneath the falx. Symptoms are often related to the mass or increased ICP.

Lateral Mass Herniation

Occurs in patients with an expanding lateral mass. Symptoms include contralateral hemiparesis, diminished consciousness, and an ipsilateral cranial nerve III palsy. Compression of pupillary fibers also causes a dilation of the pupil and as lateral displacement of the midbrain continues there is ipsilateral hemiplegia. Late in the process, the uncus and hippocampus may herniate transtentorially.

Cerebellar Tonsillar Herniation

Posterior fossa masses cause symptoms by compression of the brainstem and obstructing the flow of CSF (hydrocephalus). As pressure increases, the cerebellar tonsils may be pushed into or through the foramen magnum. As the medulla is compressed, apnea results from dysfunction of the medullary respiratory center.

Upward Transtentorial Herniation

Posterior fossa masses may cause obstructive hydrocephalus. If these patients undergo ventriculostomy, there is a possibility of upward herniation of posterior fossa contents into the region of the thalamus and hypothalamus.

DIAGNOSTIC EVALUATION OF ALTERED CONSCIOUSNESS

The diagnosis of an altered state of consciousness is provided by general physical examination, neuroradiological imaging, drug screens, and certain laboratory studies.

Neurological Examination

The neurologic exam includes assessment of level of consciousness, brainstem reflexes, and motor activity. Rapid, standardized assessment of the level of consciousness is useful for clinical decision-making and communication. The level of alertness reflects the severity of the underlying condition; severely affected patients are comatose. Commonly, the Glasgow Coma Scale (GCS) (Table 36–2) is used to assess level of consciousness in patients with head injury, but is also widely used as assessment of level consciousness regardless of etiology. A patient with a GCS score 8 or less is generally considered to be comatose. The cardinal feature of confusion and delirium is impaired attention. Simple bedside tasks such as serial subtraction or naming the months of the year in reverse can test attention. Marked fluctuations in mental status over time are characteristic. Other common findings include a disturbed sleep-wake cycle, decreased alertness, hypervigilance, hallucinations, sensory misperceptions, impaired memory,

Table 36–2. Glasgow coma scale.

Eye Opening:	
Spontaneous	4
To voice	3
To pain	2
None	1
Verbal Response:	
Oriented	5
Confused, disoriented	4
Inappropriate words	3
Incomprehensible sounds	2
None	1
Best Motor Response:	
Obeys	6
Localizes	5
Withdraws (flexion)	4
Abnormal flexion posturing	3
Extension posturing	2
None	1

and disorientation. The thought process is often disorganized, manifested by confused or rambling conversation.

The cranial nerves and their corresponding brainstem reflexes, including pupillary response to light, corneal reflexes, oculocephalic reflex (doll's eyes), vestibulo-ocular reflex (cold calorics), breathing patterns, cough, and gag reflexes are further used to describe accurately the neurologic status and localize the level of brainstem dysfunction. Generally, the brainstem reflexes are only affected in severe TME. Abnormal patterns of respiration, particularly Cheyne–Stokes respiration, may also occur with significant brainstem dysfunction.

Motor responses may be delineated as spontaneous or induced by noxious stimuli, purposeful or nonpurposeful, unilateral or bilateral, and upper or lower extremity. The patient may display withdrawal from a stimulus, abnormal flexion (decorticate posturing), abnormal extension (decerebrate posturing), or absence of motor activity. A variety of motor abnormalities are also associated with TME: tremor, asterixis, multifocal myoclonus (sudden, nonrhythmic gross muscle twitching), paratonia (increased tone with variable resistance), diffuse brisk deep tendon reflexes, or bilateral extensor plantar responses.

▶ Laboratory Studies

The laboratory investigation of decreased level of consciousness includes a complete blood count, coagulation studies, electrolyte panel, and examination of calcium, magnesium, phosphate, glucose, blood urea nitrogen, creatinine, bilirubin, liver enzymes, ammonia, serum osmolality, and arterial blood gases. Toxicology screening should be performed for suspected intoxications. Blood and CSF cultures should be obtained if infection appears present. Further analysis of CSF with cell counts, protein, glucose, and organism-specific studies such as herpes simplex virus PCR and fungal serology can reveal meningitis, neoplastic cells, or subarachnoid hemorrhage. Thyroid function tests and vitamin B_{12} and serum cortisol concentrations should be assessed if endocrinopathy is considered.

▶ Neuroradiological Studies

Emergent computed tomography (CT) imaging to assess for structural lesions (intracerebral hemorrhage, large territory ischemic stroke, hydrocephalus, neoplasm, and diffuse cerebral edema) is strongly recommended for patients presenting with focal neurological deficits or severe decline in the level of consciousness. Acute ischemic stroke within the first 3-4 hours may be clinically occult on CT imaging. Magnetic resonance imaging (MRI) of the head is generally reserved to further assess for acute ischemic stroke as well as further characterization of neoplastic lesions. MRI should be not relied upon for an emergent diagnosis given the duration of the study.

▶ Electroencephalography

The electroencephalogram (EEG) can both confirm global cerebral dysfunction and exclude subclinical status epilepticus with greater sensitivity than clinical examination alone. After structural lesions have been excluded, EEG should be performed in most patients with altered consciousness at some point during the course of their care. The degree of diffuse slowing of the normal background plus abnormal mixed rhythms in the EEG correlates with the severity of TME. Slowing can be categorized as follows: mild, with a reduction in the normal alpha frequencies (8-13 Hz); moderate, with theta frequencies (4-8 Hz); severe, delta frequencies (less than 4 Hz).

▶ ICP Monitoring

Quantification of ICP is critical for management of patients with large intracerebral lesions resulting in mass effect and shift of midline structures, diffuse cerebral edema, or hydrocephalus. ICP cannot accurately be estimated based on clinical findings or imaging. There are several methods of direct ICP measurement, but the two most commonly employed in clinical practice are ventricular catheters and intraparenchymal microtransducer systems. Other methods such as subarachnoid and epidural devices have much lower accuracy.

The gold standard of ICP monitoring is via an intraventricular catheter connected to a standard pressure transducer. These catheters are usually placed into the lateral ventricle by a small frontal burr hole. The advantages of intraventricular catheters are that they measure global ICP, allow for therapeutic drainage of CSF, and are amenable to external calibration. Disadvantages are risk for infection, hematoma, or difficult insertion.

Microtransducer-tipped ICP monitors are placed in the brain parenchyma or subdural space either through a skull bolt, a burr hole or intraoperatively. They are almost as accurate as intraventricular catheters and have the advantages of lower infection and complication rates. The major disadvantages are an inability to drain CSF, no in vivo calibration and a small zero drift over time.

MANAGEMENT OF ALTERED CONSCIOUSNESS

The initial treatment of a patient with an alteration in consciousness must employ management of the ABCs: airway, breathing, and circulation. Patients who are not responsive enough to protect their own airway require intubation to reduce the risk of aspiration of gastric contents. During intubation, hypoxia and hypotension should be avoided in brain-injured patients and a high suspicion of cervical spine injury should be maintained. A patient presenting with a GCS score 8 or less should be intubated. Mechanical ventilation should be used if necessary to provide adequate oxygenation and ventilation as guided by arterial blood gases. Patients presenting with hypotension and shock must be aggressively treated with fluids and vasopressors to maintain adequate perfusion. Sources of shock (septic, cardiogenic, hypovolemic) should be investigated and treated appropriately.

Regardless of the cause of acute decline of mental status, a number of general measures should be instituted. There should be a discontinuation of all drugs with potential toxicity to the central nervous system, if possible. Antipsychotic medications such as haloperidol or quetiapine can be used for management of severe agitation. Thiamine should be administered to patients with a history of alcoholism, malnutrition, cancer, hyperemesis gravidarum, or renal failure on hemodialysis in order to prevent the development of Wernicke encephalopathy.

In the event that a patient presents with history or examination findings suggestive of elevated ICP, immediate lifesaving measures may be required prior to a more detailed workup with neuroradiological imaging or ICP monitoring. These situations generally rely upon clinical judgment and expert consultation with a neurosurgeon or neurologist is strongly recommended. An examination consistent with a critically elevated ICP (coma with GCS score < 8, unilateral or bilaterally fixed and dilated pupil(s), decorticate or decerebrate posturing and Cushing triad of bradycardia, hypertension, and respiratory depression) warrants immediate intervention while delaying additional diagnostic studies. In addition to standard resuscitation measures, elevation of the head above the heart (usually 30 degrees) to increase intracranial venous outflow, temporary hyperventilation to a goal Paco$_2$ of 26-30 and administration of intravenous hyperosmolar therapy (either mannitol 1-1.5 g/kg or hypertonic saline infusion). Immediately following these measures, rapid evaluation of the underlying diagnosis by the patient history, detailed neurological examination and neuroradiological imaging should be pursued. Neurosurgical consultation should be considered for potential placement of a ventriculostomy as a means to assess ICP and potentially treat with CSF drainage.

If elevated ICP is present, therapy should be directed to maintain ICP less than 20 mm Hg. Interventions should be utilized only when ICP is elevated more than 20 mm Hg for more than 5 minutes. Transient physiologic elevations in ICP may be observed in the setting of coughing, movement, suctioning, or ventilator asynchrony that should not be targeted by therapy. During periods of elevated ICP, it is important to maintain adequate mean arterial pressure to ensure adequate cerebral perfusion pressure (which is mean arterial pressure – ICP).

GENERAL MANAGEMENT OF ELEVATED ICP

1. Blood pressure control—Therapy with vasopressors should be targeted to maintain an adequate cerebral perfusion pressure (CPP = MAP – ICP), typically more than 60 mm Hg. Hypertension should generally only be treated when CPP more than 120 mm Hg. CPP more than 50 mm Hg is associated with cerebral ischemia.

2. Position—Patients with elevated ICP should be positioned with the head elevated 30 degrees above the heart while maintaining the neck in neutral position without excessive flexion or rotation to maximize intracranial venous outflow.

3. Removal of CSF—When hydrocephalus (either obstructive or communicating) is discovered, a ventriculostomy may be utilized to reduce intracranial CSF volume and secondarily ICP. Controlled drainage of CSF at a rate of approximately 1-2 mL/min, at intervals of a few minutes until the goal ICP is reached (ICP < 20 mm Hg) or until CSF is no longer easily obtained is recommended. CSF drainage via an intrathecal lumbar drain is generally contraindicated in the setting of elevated ICP due to the risk of transtentorial herniation.

4. Hyperventilation—The use of mechanical ventilation to lower Paco$_2$ to a goal of 26-30 mm Hg will induce cerebral vasoconstriction, decrease the cerebral blood volume, and rapidly reduce ICP. The effect of hyperventilation on ICP typically lasts for a period of hours prior to metabolic compensation. Therapeutic hyperventilation should be utilized only as an emergent intervention to temporarily control ICP and be replaced by other therapy modalities.

HYPEROSMOTIC THERAPY

1. Mannitol—Osmotic diuretics reduce brain volume by creating an osmotic gradient from the brain parenchyma to the intravascular space, thus drawing free water from the parenchyma. Mannitol, prepared in a 20% solution, can be given as a bolus of 1-1.5 g/kg. Mannitol can be used in serial doses at intervals of every 6-8 hours at a reduced dosage on 0.25-0.5 g/kg as needed for continued elevated ICP. The onset of action is within minutes and the duration of effect varies widely from 4 to 24 hours. Serial measurements of serum sodium, serum osmolality, and renal function are necessary to prevent overdosage. Contraindications to the use of mannitol include serum sodium more than 150 mEq, serum osmolality more than 320 mOsm, or evidence of evolving acute tubular necrosis. In addition, mannitol frequently can induce hypotension and subsequently cerebral perfusion. Mannitol should not be used in patients with acute or chronic renal disease.

2. Hypertonic saline—Bolus dosing of hypertonic saline (tonicity ranging 1.8-23.4 percent) can acutely lower ICP. The typical volume of hypertonic saline varies widely depending on tonicity, ranging from 30 mL of 23.4% to 1 L of 1.8%. Continuous infusion of hypertonic saline (1.8%-3%)

to maintain hypernatremia may also be effective in controlling ICP. A meta-analysis of multiple clinical trials comparing the efficacy of mannitol to hypertonic saline for management of elevated ICP from a variety of causes (traumatic brain injury, stroke, tumors) found that hypertonic saline appeared to have greater efficacy in reducing elevated ICP, but clinical outcomes were not examined. Hypertonic saline should generally not be administered through a peripheral intravenous catheter.

3. Fluid management—Typically, patients with elevated ICP should be kept euvolemic and normo- to hyperosmolar. Administration of free water and hypotonic solutions should be strictly avoided and instead isotonic fluids should be used in all maintenance fluids and infusions. Serum sodium levels should be closely monitored and hyponatremia should be appropriately corrected.

4. Sedation—Maintenance of adequate sedation can decrease ICP by reducing cerebral metabolic demand, ventilator asynchrony, and the sympathetic responses of hypertension and tachycardia. Adequate sedation typically requires the establishment of a secure airway. Infusion of propofol is often the drug of choice for sedation because it can be rapidly titrated, thus allowing for frequent neurologic assessments.

5. Fever—Fever increases brain metabolism, which increases cerebral blood flow and thus elevates ICP. Additionally, fever has been demonstrated to worsen brain injury in animal models. Therefore, aggressive treatment of fever, including acetaminophen and cooling, is recommended in patients with increased ICP.

6. Antiepileptic therapy—Seizures, either convulsive or nonconvulsive, increase cerebral metabolism and result in ICP elevation. Aggressive treatment of seizures with antiepileptic therapy or infusion of anesthetics as well as continuous EEG monitoring is warranted. There is no clear evidence that prophylactic antiepileptic therapy is of any clinical benefit; however, consideration of prophylactic antiepileptic therapy is reasonable when high-risk mass lesions, such as those within supratentorial cortical locations, or lesions adjacent to the cortex, such as subdural hematomas or subarachnoid hemorrhage are present.

7. Glucocorticoids—Glucocorticoids, typically dexamethasone, are reserved for the management of elevated ICP secondary to vasogenic edema secondary to intracranial neoplasm and infection. Typically, dexamethasone is dosed every 6-12 hours at a wide range of dosages. The use of glucocorticoids has been associated with a worse outcome in a large randomized clinical trial in traumatic brain injury and is no longer recommended. Glucocorticoids are not considered to be useful in the management of cerebral infarction or intracranial hemorrhage.

8. Barbiturates—The use of barbiturates to control ICP is based on the drug's ability to dramatically reduce brain metabolism and secondarily cerebral blood flow. Pentobarbital is most commonly used, with a loading dose of 5-20 mg/kg as a bolus, followed by 1-4 mg/kg/h. The barbiturate infusion is titrated based on assessment of ICP, CPP, and the tolerance of side effects. Continuous EEG monitoring is generally used, with titration to an EEG burst suppression pattern indicating appropriate suppression of cerebral metabolism. Barbiturate therapy is complicated and fraught with complications, particularly hypotension, adynamic ileus, reduced mucociliary clearance of the airway, and high risk of infections. In general, the use of barbiturates is reserved for elevated ICP refractory to all other treatment modalities.

9. Therapeutic hypothermia—The use of hypothermia to treat elevated ICP has been controversial for decades, and its use is not recommended as a standard treatment for increased ICP. Hypothermia decreases cerebral metabolism and secondarily reduces cerebral blood volume and ICP. When used, hypothermia is achieved by whole body cooling using surface or intravascular cooling devices to a goal of 32-34°C. Studies have demonstrated significant side effects, including cardiac arrhythmias and severe coagulopathy. Given the multiple uncertainties of the appropriate use of therapeutic hypothermia in patients with elevated ICP, this treatment should be limited to patients with intracranial hypertension refractory to other therapies.

10. Decompressive craniectomy—Decompressive craniectomy is the surgical removal a large portion of the cranial vault to allow for the edematous intracranial contents to expand and subsequently reduce ICP. At the time of the procedure any mass lesion (neoplasm or hematoma) is also removed. Decompressive craniectomy has been considered a last resort; some evidence suggests that it does improve outcomes.

Bhatia A, Gupta AK: Neuromonitoring in the intensive care unit. I. Intracranial pressure and cerebral blood flow monitoring. *Intensive Care Med* 2007;33:1263-1271.

Diedler J, Sykora M, Blatow M, et al: Decompressive surgery for severe brain edema. *J Intensive Care Med* 2009;24:168.

Edwards P, Arango M, Balica L, et al: Final results of MRC CRASH, a randomised placebo-controlled trial of intravenous corticosteroid in adults with head injury-outcomes at 6 months. *Lancet* 2005;365:1957.

Kamel H, Navi BB, Nakagawa K, et al: Hypertonic saline versus mannitol for the treatment of elevated intracranial pressure: a meta-analysis of randomized clinical trials. *Crit Care Med* 2011;39:554.

The Brain Trauma Foundation; American Association of Neurological Surgeons; Congress of Neurological Surgeons; Joint Section on Neurotrauma and Critical Care: Guidelines for the management of severe traumatic brain injury. VI. Indications for intracranial pressure monitoring. *J Neurotrauma* 2007;24:S37-S44.

IMAGING OF THE CENTRAL NERVOUS SYSTEM

Douglas J. Quint Shawn L.A. Hervey-Jumper

INTRODUCTION

Imaging has become central to medical care in the past 25 years and is one of the fastest growing components of medical care expenditures in this country. In no field of medicine has imaging made more of an impact than in the neurosciences. Our ability to demonstrate anatomy and pathology noninvasively and to treat many pathologic central nervous system (CNS) processes utilizing minimally invasive techniques has grown immensely with improvements in imaging technology in the last few years.

Forty years ago, the only way to image the CNS was to replace cerebrospinal fluid (CSF) with contrast material (dye) or air via a lumbar puncture and take x-rays—a painful technique called pneumoencephalography—normal and abnormal CNS structures could be crudely outlined in this manner. Pneumoencephalography was abandoned in the late 1970s with the development of computed tomography (CT). Injecting dye directly into major blood vessels of the neck (cerebral angiography) has been available for three quarters of a century and allows exquisite delineation of intrinsic vascular pathology, but still does little to directly visualize the brain or spinal cord. While angiography is still performed today for both diagnostic and therapeutic purposes, the catheter is now placed via femoral arterial cannulation instead of directly into a neck blood vessel.

With the advent of CT scanning in the early 1970s, direct visualization of the brain was finally possible though resolving different normal brain structures and some pathologic processes remained difficult. Magnetic resonance imaging (MRI) first became available for clinical use in the early 1980s and has been the standard for evaluation of most CNS processes since the mid-1980s.

CT and MRI have continued to mature through the 1990s and into the 21st century. In addition to the introduction of lower radiation dose scanner capabilities on the most recent generation CT scanners, rapid scanning techniques on such scanners ("multislice" or "multidetector" CT scanners) now allow for collection of data reflecting cerebral blood perfusion, which can be collected during a 5-minute study. Similarly, such state-of-the-art scanners can be used to generate models of the major blood vessels of the brain (CT angiograms) lessening the need for more invasive intravascular catheterization in some patients.

MRI advances have been even more dramatic particularly with the release of higher field strength MR scanners (3.0 T) for clinical use in 2005. For example, the sensitivity of some of the newer MRI scanning techniques enables identification of physiologic changes in the brain minutes after ischemia occurs, a time frame that can potentially permit pharmacologic interventions that can affect clinical outcomes (eg, stroke). Functional MRI can assess eloquent areas of the brain near pathologic lesions (eg, tumors) that ideally should be avoided during surgery. MR spectroscopy (MRS) can identify lesion metabolites that can help discriminate among pathologic processes (eg, tumors vs. necrosis vs. ischemia vs. inflammation vs. infections). MRS can also identify metabolites accumulating in the brain in patients with congenital metabolic disorders. MRI can also be used to generate angiographic (MR angiography, MRA) images to evaluate blood vessels without injection of dye or the use of ionizing radiation.

Catheter (endovascular) angiography has been available in various forms for over 80 years, and has also continued to evolve over the last decade. Endovascular surgery—treating blood vessel abnormalities such as aneurysms or arteriovenous malformations (AVMs) through a catheter instead of with open surgery—is now commonly performed and has become the treatment of choice for the management of many lesions. More than half of aneurysms treated in the United States are currently managed endovascularly avoiding the need for craniotomy in the majority of those patients. Similarly, in the setting of an acute stroke due to an obstructing thromboembolus, in an attempt to reopen the involved vessel, a catheter can be placed in the region of the obstructing lesion and a clot mechanically removed through the catheter, or clot-dissolving (eg, thrombolytic) agents injected.

BASIC CENTRAL NERVOUS SYSTEM IMAGING TECHNIQUES

1. Plain radiographs ("x-rays") are relatively inexpensive, universally available and can demonstrate osseous abnormalities such as fractures or gross destructive lesions (Figure 36–2). The main disadvantage of plain x-rays is that essentially all normal soft tissues (eg, all intracranial and spinal canal structures) and pathologic processes (eg, hemorrhage, infarctions, tumors, abscesses, herniated disks, etc) cannot be detected. Even many intrinsic osseous lesions are difficult to delineate. In fact, until 30%-50% of bone marrow trabeculae is replaced by a pathologic process (eg, tumor, infection), no osseous abnormality is seen on a plain radiograph.

   a. Another limitation of plain radiographs is that all structures are superimposed on an single image as the x-ray beam passes through the entire head or spine (as opposed to the "slices" generated on CT and MR scans).

   b. There is little role for plain radiographs for the evaluation of CNS disease as the interior of the head or spinal canal is not imaged. One exception is in patients with suspected child abuse. In these patients, in addition to other cross-sectional imaging (such as CT/MR which are performed to assess for intracranial injuries), plain radiographs should

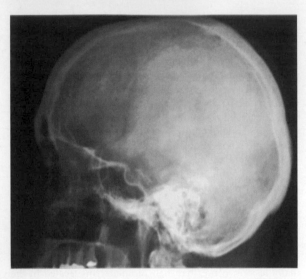

▲ **Figure 36–2.** Lateral plain radiograph (x-ray) of the skull (ionizing radiation). Note the excellent delineation of the osseous structures, but poor delineation of soft tissues; specifically, no portion of the brain is imaged. Also, this study is not tomographic (ie, is not a slice) and therefore both the left and right sides of the head are superimposed.

also be obtained as they may show subtle nondisplaced fractures not readily identified on other imaging tests.

c. Other roles for plain radiographs include assessing spinal motion (ie, lateral flexion/extension radiographs of the cervical or lumbosacral spine to assess spinal stability), localization of foreign bodies, and assessing intracranial or spinal structures where internal fixation hardware and/or other radiodense/ferromagnetic foreign material is present (which can limit the use of CT or MRI scanning).

2. Ultrasound of the CNS, beyond the neonatal period, is predominantly used in the intraoperative setting to evaluate ventricular morphology and underlying parenchymal pathology. Intraoperative ultrasound can be used to help position ventricular catheters during placement of shunts. It can also be used to guide intracranial and intraspinal tumor resections.

a. Outside of the operative setting, ultrasound has growing applications because it is noninvasive, portable, and does not involve radiation. However, an "acoustic window" is necessary for viewing the intracranial/intraspinal tissues meaning that overlying osseous structures usually must be removed before scanning can be performed (ie, portions

of the skull or posterior spinal elements must be removed before the desired regions of the brain or spinal cord, respectively, can be evaluated).

b. Ultrasound has multiple applications in infants (usually such infants still have open fontenelles so no additional "acoustic window" to the brain needs to be created). It has become the imaging study of choice for the evaluation of premature infants to assess for intraventricular hemorrhage and/or hydrocephalus. In adults, intracranial Doppler examinations can be performed by scanning through sutures. For example, scanning through the temporal suture allows access to the circle of Willis. These examinations can be performed at the bedside for assessment of arterial vasospasm (eg, in the setting of subacute subarachnoid hemorrhage). Ultrasound can also be used in younger children to identify the conus medullaris.

3. CT scanning without or with intravenous administration of iodinated contrast material is performed utilizing a thin fan-like band of x-rays (ionizing radiation) that are generated by an x-ray tube that literally moves around the patient in approximately 1 second. The resultant image, which represents a "slice" of tissue, can be obtained with imaging thickness as thin as 1 mm. "Reformatted" submillimeter images can also be generated by the CT computer from the primary axially obtained CT scan data in any plane (sagittal, coronal, off-axis, etc). Three-dimensional images can also be created in this manner.

a. CT demonstrates most osseous abnormalities better than any other imaging test with the possible exception of nondisplaced, nondistracted fractures which are still often better seen on plain x-rays (Figure 36–3). Soft tissue lesions can also be detected with much better sensitivity than plain x-rays. However, resolving some similar, but not identical, normal soft tissues from one another, delineating normal from pathologic soft tissue, and evaluating certain areas of the brain which are limited by scanning artifacts can still be difficult with CT scanning which is why CT remains inferior to MRI for evaluation of most brain and spinal canal abnormalities.

b. When discussing CT images, the terms "density" and "attenuation" refer to the same process, namely, absorption of the x-ray beam. Areas of increased "density" have greater "attenuation" of the x-ray beam and result in more whitish areas on the CT scan image (eg, bones, iodine-based contrast material, acute blood, areas of calcification, and some foreign bodies). Areas of lower density have lower "attenuation" as they absorb less of the x-ray beam as it passes through the patient resulting in darker

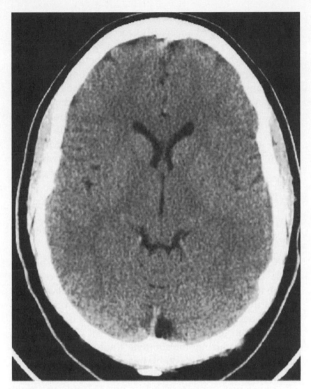

▲ **Figure 36–3.** CT scan (ionizing radiation). This image represents a single section ("slice") through the head (ie, it is a tomographic image; the left and right sides of the head can be separately delineated). The brain is directly imaged though resolving differences in intracranial structures can be difficult (eg, resolving gray and matter structures).

areas on the CT scan image (eg, fluid in the ventricles, gas, and fat).

c. CT image contrast can be adjusted at a workstation after scans have been obtained to highlight differences in the densities of different tissues.

d. Finally, the recent development of new methods of reconstructing CT data has resulted in significant reduction in patient radiation dosage exposure during many CT scans.

4. Myelography involves performing a lumbar subarachnoid puncture (or a lateral C1-2 subarachnoid puncture) and instilling less than an ounce of iodinated contrast material to opacify the spinal canal subarachnoid space which results in outlining cauda equina nerve roots and the spinal cord, and any process that impinges upon (or is within) the subarachnoid space. Such processes include extrathecal tumors, infections, herniated disk material, degenerative spinal changes, and also processes that directly involve the intrathecal structures (spinal cord tumors, vascular malformations, metastases, etc).

a. Myelography is no longer a primary imaging technique for evaluating the spinal canal having been replaced by MRI. It is currently reserved for "problem-solving" such as when the results of an MRI scan are not clear or when MR imaging is not possible (contraindications to MR scanning, internal fixation hardware limits evaluation by MRI, etc).

b. Myelography is essentially always followed immediately (within hours) by CT scanning to better delineate relationships of pathologic processes to the subarachnoid space.

5. MRI is an imaging technique that does not use ionizing radiation.

a. The physics of creating an MR scan are quite complex. Briefly, a patient is placed in a strong magnetic field ($30{,}000 \times$ that of the earth's magnetic field). Radiofrequency pulses are transiently (milliseconds) applied to the patient to briefly perturb the patient's water molecules by raising them to a slightly higher energy level (quantum mechanical model). After turning off the radiofrequency pulse, these water molecules rapidly return to their respective baseline states by giving off their recently absorbed energy. The rate at which these perturbed water molecules return to their respective baseline states can be measured by using extremely sensitive receiver coils in the MR scanner. As the rates at which these molecules return to their respective baseline states varies by local magnetic environment (eg, the local magnetic environment is different in the ventricular system as opposed to the lentiform nucleus, white matter, the eyeball, muscles, tumors, etc), these detectable differences among tissues can be localized in 3-dimensional space and used to create an image.

b. MR images are obtained which highlight different kinds of magnetic field differences between tissues. In general, most MR studies include "T1-weighted" and "T2-weighted" scans as part of the overall evaluation of the patient. MR scans take longer to perform than CT scans in part because T1-weighted (T1w) and T2-weighted (T2w) scans and often additional scans must be obtained separately. T1w images are distinguishable by the black appearance ("absence of MR signal") of the CSF over the surface of the brain and in the ventricles. In contrast, on a T2w scan, the CSF over the surface of the brain and in the ventricles is white (Figure 36–4).

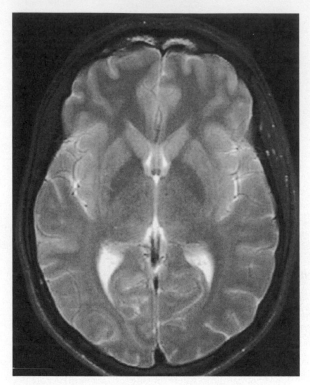

▲ **Figure 36–4.** MR scan (no ionizing radiation). Similar to CT, this image represents a single section ("slice") through the head. The white matter and gray matter structures are more easily resolved that on a CT scan, and even some gray matter structures can be resolved (eg, putamina and globus pallidae).

c. In general, T1w scans are best for delineating anatomy and areas of contrast enhancement. T2w scans are exquisitely sensitive to subtle changes in water concentrations (in both normal and pathologic tissues). These changes are seen in most pathologic processes (eg, strokes, tumors, infections). These subtle changes are manifest as increased signal (more whiteness) on T2w scans.

d. In the past 10 years, most MR studies include "FLAIR" (FLuid Attenuated Inversion Recovery) scans. In general, FLAIR scans can be considered super T2w scans on which normal fluid (eg, in the ventricles and subarachnoid spaces) has no signal (ie, black), and therefore, subtle pathologic process (which still appear white on the FLAIR scans similar to that seen on standard T2w scans) are easier to identify.

e. A gadolinium-based contrast agent can be injected intravenously to enhance the appearance of some pathologic processes such as those outside the blood-brain-barrier (BBB) or are intraaxial but do not have a functioning BBB.

f. MRI best delineates soft tissues both intrinsic and immediately extrinsic to the brain, can be performed in any plane (including nonorthogonal planes), and has no known side effects at the field strengths used for clinical studies. In addition to better demonstrating tissues than CT, MRI is not limited by many of the artifacts that limit evaluation by CT, particularly in the posterior fossa and spinal canal regions where CT can be severely limited. While not ideal for directly visualizing dense osseous structures (where many fractures, cortical erosions, and degenerative changes occur), MR is superb for detecting intrinsic (eg, bone marrow) osseous abnormalities (eg, metastatic disease, discitis/osteomyelitis, etc).

6. Cerebral angiography is performed by directly placing a catheter into the femoral artery, passing it cephalad in a retrograde manner up the aorta to the level of the aortic arch, manipulating it into either a vertebral or carotid artery and then further cephalad into the neck and even intracranially (Figure 36–5). The catheter is moved utilizing intermittent fluoroscopic guidance with small amounts of dye injected at selected intervals to confirm the location of the catheter. When in position, larger amounts of dye are injected and serial plain digital x-rays are rapidly exposed as the dye passes through the intracranial vessels in the distribution of the injected blood vessel. Over 100 images might be obtained during a single 8-second injection of contrast material. This procedure is associated with a 0.1%-0.5% chance of causing a stroke.

a. This technique best delineates intrinsic blood vessel pathology such as atherosclerosis, aneurysms, AVMs, fistulas, vasculitis, blocked vessels, and other intrinsic vascular disorders. It can be used to inject medications into specific blood vessel territories for diagnostic or therapeutic purposes. Catheters can be placed directly into aneurysms, vascular malformations, and recently occluded vessels for definitive therapy.

b. Endovascular (catheter) angiography is risky, expensive, requires complex equipment, and is performed by highly trained personnel. There are currently several alternatives to catheter angiography to evaluate for vascular lesions such as atherosclerotic vascular narrowing and aneurysms. Ultrasound (in the neck), CT angiography, and MR angiography are each useful alternatives in many situations (Figure 36–6).

7. Radionuclide Imaging (Scintigraphy) includes positron emission tomography (PET) and SPECT (single

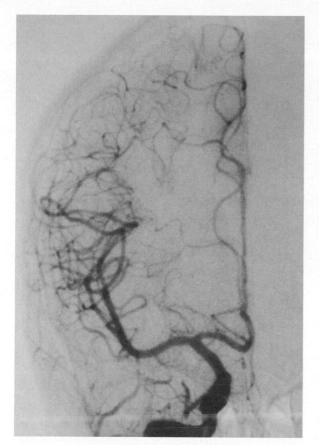

▲ **Figure 36–5.** Angiogram (ionizing radiation). A catheter was placed in the right carotid artery in the neck and dye injected while imaging was performed in a front-to-back projection of the right side of the head. The bones are then digitally "subtracted" from the image. The exquisite delineation of the blood vessels of the right carotid territory are demonstrated, but no intra-axial (ie, brain soft tissues) structures.

photon emission CT) scans which are molecular imaging techniques. Unlike other imaging techniques, these imaging modalities provide information beyond the structural appearance of normal and pathologic tissues. These techniques can provide physiologic information reflecting the functional state of tissues.

a. Low doses of radiotracers (positron emitters for PET scanning and single photon emitting isotopes for SPECT scanning) are used to label molecules or pharmacologic agents to image molecular interactions of biological processes in vivo. The nanomolar concentration of the radiotracer allows in vivo assessment of biologic processes without interfering with the process itself.

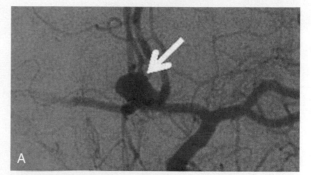

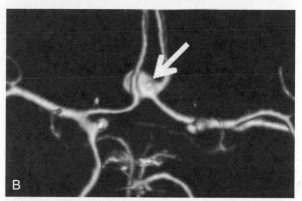

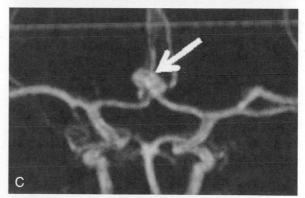

▲ **Figure 36–6.** Aneurysm demonstrated by multiple imaging techniques. **A.** Catheter angiogram (ionizing radiation). **B.** CT angiogram (ionizing radiation). **C.** MR angiogram (no ionizing radiation). Note that the catheter angiogram (A), an imaging modality that is associated with a risk of causing a stroke, best defines this anterior communicating artery region aneurysm (arrow). However, the aneurysm is still well-seen on the CT angiogram (B), an imaging technique that is not associated with any risk of causing a stroke, and is also well-seen on the MR angiogram (C), an imaging technique that is not associated with any risk of causing a stroke and does not employ ionizing radiation.

b. PET and SPECT cameras are able to detect, localize, and quantify regional distribution of radioactivity within the brain. Reconstruction techniques similar to those used in CT (eg, "filtered backprojection" and "iterative reconstruction") yield 2-dimensional and 3-dimensional images of the brain.

c. The main advantage of a PET imaging over SPECT imaging is that PET utilizes "coincidence" detection, which is the ability to detect the simultaneous emission of 2 gamma rays that are generated when positrons annihilate when encountering negative electrons. Practically, this results in the greater spatial resolution of PET compared to SPECT. Both techniques can be used to study the same biologic processes.

d. The biological significance of measured radioactivity on PET and SPECT scans depends on the biological function of the molecule that is attached to the radioisotope. For example, radioligands are available to measure cerebral blood flow, blood brain barrier permeability, neurotransmitter synthesis, enzyme activity, receptor density, glucose metabolic rates, and gene expression, among other physiologic processes. Analysis of regional brain functions can be more specific by performing imaging both before and after specific pharmacological interventions, specialized motor or mental tasks (so-called "activation" studies), or therapeutic interventions, such as stem cell or gene therapy.

e. PET or SPECT imaging can also be used in the clinical arena for localization of epileptogenic foci, diagnosing dementing disorders, distinguishing between tumor recurrence and radionecrosis, and providing a chronologic record of disease progression (or response to therapy).

f. Finally, the same SPECT radioligands that are used for cerebral blood flow imaging (such as Tc-99m HMPAO) can also be used for bedside brain death studies using a standard planar gamma camera. Radioligands such as In-111 DTPA can be used intrathecally for radioisotope cisternograms for the clinical evaluation of patients with hydrocephalus or suspected CSF leaks. Radioisotope studies can also be performed to evaluate patency of CSF shunts.

ADVANCED CENTRAL NERVOUS SYSTEM APPLICATIONS OF MRI, CT, AND ANGIOGRAPHY

▶ **Magnetic Resonance Imaging**

A. MRA

MR data can be collected using software that images only moving tissues (ie, extravascular stationary soft tissue does not generate any MR signal on these studies while moving blood or CSF will generate signal). Using these techniques, images of blood vessels can be created with a sufficient level of detail that, in many cases, formal endovascular catheter angiography can be avoided (eg, demonstration of significant atherosclerotic disease in the region of the carotid artery bifurcation, surveillance imaging of a known aneurysm, etc). CSF flow evaluation can also be performed (eg, at the craniovertebral junction in Chiari patients).

B. Diffusion MRI and Perfusion MRI

Using rapidly applied magnetic field gradients, random molecular motion of water molecules can be converted to images and can be presented as "Diffusion" MR images. Rapidly applied gradients can also be used without or with contrast agent administration to assess cerebral blood perfusion.

Diffusion MR imaging is sensitive to early changes of cerebral ischemia, often on the order of minutes. In the setting of acute cerebral ischemia, MR diffusion imaging changes (which usually reflect acute irreversible ischemic change) and MR perfusion imaging changes (which reflect cerebral blood flow) can be performed. The MR perfusion and diffusion images can then be compared. As diffusion images usually represent permanent injury (infarction) and perfusion (blood flow) deficits are potentially reversible, if an MR perfusion deficit is more extensive than an associated MR diffusion deficit, it is possible that an area of perfusion abnormality without diffusion abnormality represents viable brain that is at risk to go on to permanent injury, but is not yet irreversibly injured (the so-called "ischemic penumbra") and might benefit from aggressive therapy. Alternatively, if a diffusion deficit (representing a region of irreversible brain injury) is similar in extent to a perfusion deficit, then maybe the ischemic changes are permanent and there is no remaining "at risk" penumbra brain, and therefore no aggressive therapy is warranted.

C. MRS

Using standard MR hardware, MRS can be performed to evaluate brain metabolites. Normal brain tissue includes many metabolites the most important of which are *N*-acetyl-aspartate [NAA] (which is found in normally functioning neurons and decreases with neuronal injury), Choline [Cho] (a component of cell membranes which increases in any process that increases cellular turnover such as tumors, acute infections, etc) and Creatine [Cr] (a marker of cellular energy). Lactic acid can also be seen in ischemic cells (as a byproduct of anaerobic glycolysis), but is not present in detectable amounts on MRS in normal brain tissue.

▶ **Computed Tomography**

A. Biopsy

CT can be used for guidance to percutaneously biopsy many lesions that previously required an open surgical procedure.

B. Perfusion CT

While rapidly infusing contrast material through a peripheral vein, using a high-speed multidetector CT scanner, data can be collected that reflects how well different portions of the brain are being perfused. In some patients, there are areas of underperfused brain which may manifest clinically with transient symptoms (eg, transient ischemic attacks); these regions might benefit from revascularization before the patient suffers irreversible injury (ie, a stroke). Evaluations similar to diffusion/perfusion brain MRI to assess for penumbra brain (see above) can also be performed.

C. CT Angiography (CTA)

While rapidly infusing contrast material through a peripheral vein, using a high-speed multidetector CT scanner, data can be collected that can be "reconstructed" with background data removed such that images similar to catheter angiograms can be created without risk of stroke. While intrinsic vascular detail is not as good as endovascular catheter angiography, in many patients, it is adequate to address the relevant clinical issue.

▶ Angiography

A. Endovascular Coiling of Aneurysms

Small wires can be passed through an endovascular (ie, within a blood vessel) catheter and directly deposited into a vascular aneurysm where they form coils after release from the catheter; an aneurysm can be filled with these wire coils resulting in the complete obliteration of the patency of the aneurysm lumen eliminating the chance that such an aneurysm might rupture in the future and obviating the need for a craniotomy for placement of an aneurysm clip.

B. Stenting

Instead of open surgery to address a narrowed atherosclerotic or dissected blood vessel, affected blood vessels can be treated via an intravascular catheter which first uses a balloon to dilate the narrowed portion of the blood vessel and then release a mesh stent to maintain the patency of the newly dilated vessel. Stents can also be placed at the base of wide-necked aneurysms allowing for the endovascular coiling of aneurysms that otherwise would not be technically possible.

C. Treating Intraluminal Thrombus

An acute (within 6-8 hours of onset of symptoms) intraluminal occluding thrombus (clot) or thromboembolus can often be treated with intraarterial catheter placement within the blood clot with off-label (as of 2013) injection of a clot lysing agent (eg, tissue plasminogen activator [t-PA]) to reestablish blood flow to an affected vascular territory

before permanent brain damage occurs. Alternatively, some intravascular clots can be captured and removed from the vascular system using specialized catheters [10].

Brinjikji W, Rabinstein AA, Nasr DM, Lanzino G, Kallmes DF, Cloft HJ: Better outcomes with treatment by coiling relative to clippinf of unruptures intracranial aneurysms in the United States. *AJNR Am J Neuroradiol* 2011;32:1071-1075.

Fleischmann D, Boas FE: Computed tomography—old ideas and new technology. *Eur Rad* 2011;21:510517.

Hacke W, Kaste M, Bluhmki E, et al: thrombolysis with alteplase 3 to 4.5 hours after acute ischemic stroke. *N Eng J Med* 2008;359:1317-1329.

Hopyan J, Ciarallo A, Dowlatshahi D, et al: Certainty of stroke diagnosis: incremental benefit with CT perfusion over non-contrast CT and CT angiography. *Radiology* 2010;255:142-153.

McKinney AM, Palmer CS, Truwit CL, et al: Detection of aneurysms by 64-section multidetector CT angiography in patients acutely suspected of having an intracranial aneurysm and comparison with digital subtraction and 3D rotational angiography. *AJNR* 2008;29:594-602.

Schellinger PD, Bryan RN, Caplan LR, et al: Evidence-based guideline: The role of diffusion and perfusion MRI for the diagnosis of acute ischemic stroke: Report of the Therapeutics and Technology Assessment Subcommittee of the American Academy of Neurology. *Neurology* 2010;75:177-185.

▼ CRANIOCEREBRAL TRAUMA

Hugh J. L. Garton, MD, MHSC Emily Lehmann, MD

OVERVIEW & EPIDEMIOLOGY

Head injury (traumatic brain injury [TBI]) is a leading cause of morbidity and mortality. The incidence of hospitalization for TBI is 75-200/100,000 population. TBI occurs among all ages, peaking in 15- to 24-year-old males. Head injury is very frequent in poly trauma patients managed by trauma surgeons or emergency physicians. Thorough familiarity of the basics of care is therefore highly desirable.

Motor vehicle accidents are the most frequent cause of TBI in the developed world, accounting for 30%-50% of all serious head injuries. Falls and recreational injuries account for about 10%-15% of TBI. Inflicted injury (assault) accounts for about 10%-20% of injuries in adult patients. Age and mechanism or injury are related, as assaults occur mostly to very young infants (child abuse) and to young adults ages 18-24. Falls are the most common source of head injury in patients over 80 years of age. Response to injury also appears to be age dependent. Young people, particularly young men, are more likely to suffer a brain injury, but the chances of dying from that injury are much higher in the elderly. Head injury is the leading cause of death among all patients suffering traumatic injury.

Head injury can be divided on clinical grounds into mild, moderate, and severe forms. About 80% of injuries are mild, including most concussions. Many patients with these injuries do not require hospitalization. Moderate and severe injuries account for about 10% each of the total injury burden and all of these patients are hospitalized. The death rate from head injury is estimated as 20-30/100,000.

Because recovery from moderate and severe injury is often incomplete, survivors of head injury and their care providers often must manage life-long disability.

PATHOPHYSIOLOGY

▶ Classifications/Definitions

Brain injury literature groups injury in several different and unrelated ways which may cause confusion. First, injury can be divided into primary versus secondary types. Primary injury occurs at the time of the brain injury or immediately thereafter. It includes the immediate deformative or concussive forces applied to the brain. Clinically, *primary* injuries include skull fractures, lacerations of the brain, and hemorrhage in and around the brain (which may take some time to fully accumulate). In contrast to *primary* brain injury, *secondary* brain injury denotes the brain's response to injury, including, for example, loss of regulation of cerebral blood flow, cellular ischemic injury, and brain edema. Most of head injury research involves identification and interruption of these secondary injury pathways. Primary injuries can be induced by either *focal* or *diffuse* force application and by either *linear* or *angular* changes in momentum. The brain is much more sensitive to a diffuse, angular application of force than a focal, linear one. Experimentally, concussions occur at much lower total acceleration when an angular force is applied compared to a linear one.

Penetrating injury to the brain results in trauma both from the direct disruption of the brain cause by the projectile, as well as compression/decompression injury due to the passage of the bullet or other device. The energy that a projectile imparts to the head is directly proportional to the projectile mass and to the square of the velocity. Velocity therefore is usually the stronger determinant of the extent of projectile injury and the distinction between low- and high-velocity injuries is important.

Secondary brain injury describes the processes that occur in the brain in response to the primary brain injury. These occur from the sub-cellular to the macroscopic level. Calcium-dependent mechanisms, oxidative stresses from free radicals, and apoptotic mechanisms are all likely involved. Tissue ischemia clearly occurs after severe TBI, and in most cases cerebral blood flow (a marker for tissue perfusion) drops considerably in the early phases after severe TBI. The consequence of the microscopic injury cascade at a more macroscopic level is an increase in brain water content: cerebral edema. This occurs both through cytotoxic (cell injury and cell swelling) and vasogenic (incompetent vasculature) mechanisms, although likely the former mechanism is the

more important. Brain edema acts as additional mass within the cranial vault that must be accommodated in managing intracranial pressure. The skull forms a rigid, protective covering for the brain. Any increase in the amount of material within the skull, such as a hematoma or edema, must be accommodated within the fixed volume of the skull, and will generally increase the intracranial pressure (ICP) (Figure 36–1). The intracranial compartment is subdivided into compartments by folds in the dura. The tentorium divides the cranial vault into a supra and infratentorial compartment while the falx cerebri divides the supratentorial compartment into right and left halves. This compartmentalization is of benefit after trauma by helping restrict the consequences of injury from impacting the other compartments. However, the compartmentalization and the protections that occur because of it are incomplete and in severe injuries, brain material will herniated out from its compartment of origin often producing specific clinical herniation syndromes.

▶ Clinical Assessment

The basics of management for patients with brain injury can be divided into initial resuscitation, primary neurologic survey, a search for lesions requiring immediate surgical management, and finally, identification and management of cerebral edema and increased ICP. These steps are often applied recursively as the patient condition may change frequently during injury course. The processes required to resuscitate, triage, and manage a concussion are less involved than for a severe brain injury, but the basic steps are similar.

Initial resuscitation for patients suffering brain injury is similar to that for all trauma victims. Management of the airway, breathing, and circulation (the ABCs) is paramount. While patients sustaining isolated mild TBI will usually maintain these functions, patients with multiple injuries, or patients with severe brain injuries often cannot maintain these critical functions without assistance. For example, hypoxia occurs in 30% of patients presenting with severe TBI, who often, because of their injury, cannot protect their airway. In addition to its obvious primary deleterious effects on the brain, hypoxia is also a strong stimulus to increase cerebral blood flow through vasodilatation of the cerebral vasculature. The additional volume of blood in the cerebral vasculature then adds measurably to the ICP after injury. Early endotracheal intubation to secure an airway and provide adequate ventilation is essential. All patients with severe brain injuries and many patients with more serious moderate brain injuries may require intubation, purely on the basis of a reduced ability to protect the airway and maintain ventilation. Intubation of a brain-injured patient should be performed with short acting pharmacologic agents. It is best to avoid the use of long-acting sedating medications and even the reflexive repetitive use of shorter acting agents

Table 36–3. Common brainstem reflexes evaluated in patients with traumatic brain injury.

Reflex	Afferent	Brainstem Level	Efferent	How Tested
Pupillary	CN II	Midbrain	CN III	Light shined in the eye, observed for pupillary constriction
Corneal	CN V	Pontine	CN VII	Saline droped into the eye, observed for blink
Gag	CN IX	Medulla	CN XI	Pharynx stimulated with ET tube or probe, observed for swallow/cough or aversion

in the prehospital and trauma bay settings. The loss of the neurological exam that results can impair or delay critical management decisions. Adequate analgesia and sedation are necessary for many trauma patients at intubation and during early resuscitation but the goal should be use the minimum necessary with repeated doses based on reassessment of patient status.

Restoring and maintaining an adequate blood pressure is also of critical importance. This should be accomplished by using intravenous fluids and blood as needed to restore a normal circulating blood volume, and by control of active hemorrhage. The use of pressor agents to support blood pressure may also be appropriate if hypotension persists despite an adequate circulating blood volume. Brain injury, unless it has progressed past a herniation event, is rarely the cause of hypotension, so that a standard search for the source of hemorrhage should accompany resuscitation as for any traumatic injury. Scalp injuries, which often accompany TBI, can be significant source of blood loss especially in children. Database research demonstrates that a single episode of hypotension following a brain injury doubles the risk of dying compared to patients who never have such an episode.

▶ **The Glasgow Coma Scale**

Once the ABCs have been addressed, the goal of the primary neurologic survey is a rapid, accurate categorization of the severity of the brain injury and a search for clinical evidence of large intracerebral hematomas that could require immediate evacuation. The Glasgow Coma Scale is a three component scoring system that is the main tool of the primary neurological survey (Table 36–1). To apply the scale, a patient is asked to give their name or description of what happened and to follow a simple command. Patients who are unresponsive to verbal requests should receive a brief, firm, noxious stimuli. An effective approach is to apply digital pressure to the trapezius muscle and observe for the response. Additional stimuli may be needed elsewhere to confirm the motor response. A patient can localize when their actions are purposeful and they attend specifically to a noxious stimuli, in an attempt to remove it. A patient is withdrawing when they do not attend to stimuli, but do act to move away from noxious stimuli in a nonstereotypic fashion. Decorticate and decerebrate posturing are stereotypic

movements. The possible scores range from 3 to 15. Patients receive the better score when the left and right sides are different. Intubated patients may be given a score of "T" or their verbal score may be estimated from other communicative efforts that they make. The power of this grading scheme is that it is quick and accurate in terms of long term prognosis, assuming the examination is not clouded by sedatives or other confounding factors. Patients who score between 3 and 8 have severe TBI, 9-12 are categorized as moderate and 13-15 as mild closed head injury.

In addition to the determination of the GCS scale, the primary neurological survey includes an assessment of the pupils and gross motor function to assess for the presence of lateralizing signs of a large intracranial hemorrhage. These exams can also alert to the potential presence of a concomitant spinal cord injury. The mass of hematoma, depending on size and location, may produce uncal herniation with unilateral pupillary dilation and contralateral hemiparesis. These findings may indicate that a life threatening intracranial hemorrhage is present, which can be amenable to urgent evacuation. Depending on the situation it may be appropriate to assess other brainstem responses during the primary survey, but more often these are deferred until after an initial head CT scan is obtained. These brainstem reflexes can help to localization injuries (Table 36–3). Two additional brainstem reflexes, the Oculocephalic (doll's eyes) and Oculovestibular (caloric testing) are not usually tested initial in traumatic settings because of potential exacerbation of cervical spine injuries (doll's eyes) or basilar skull fractures (caloric testing).

▶ **Diagnostic Imaging**

Once the patient's airway, breathing, and circulation are safe, the severity of the head injury is determined and the primary neurological survey is completed, all patients with moderate and severe brain injuries should have a CT scan of the head. Rapid use of the head CT is also appropriate in many cases of mild closed head injury, especially when other risk factors, such as the use of anticoagulants, are present. Though the presence of a skull fracture significantly increases the chances of finding a lesion on a head CT, plain skull x-rays are not advised as a substitute to the head CT. MRI may at some point replace CT as the primary imaging tool for

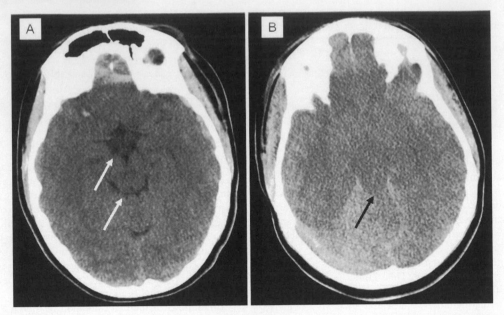

▲ **Figure 36–7.** **A.** Normal head CT demonstrating normal basal cisterns (white arrows). **B.** A head CT demonstrating effacement of basal cisterns (black arrow) and global edema after head trauma.

TBI, but this has not yet occurred. CT is quicker, safer for management of uncooperative patients, and safer for the environmental issues of loose ferromagnetic materials near, on or in the patient. MRI may be useful in assessing cervical and intracranial vasculature, and it may be helpful in more accurate prognostication of injury outcome.

The head CT is reviewed for the presence of surgically significant intracranial hemorrhage. In addition, there are specific radiographic markers that predict increased ICP (Figure 36–7). These include effacement of the basal and convexity subarachnoid spaces (so-called "cisternal effacement"), mass effect (compression/deformation of adjacent brain structures), and shifting of the brain contents from one side to the other causing "midline shift." Patients with certain facial, skull base, and cervical fractures are at risk for cervical intracranial vascular injury and dedicated vascular imaging may be indicated. Conventional angiography, CT, and MRI-based angiography are all potential considerations in these situations. Conventional angiography is the gold standard for injury detection and offers the option of endovascular treatment; however, it is also time intensive and may separate the patient from the optimal critical care environment for a protracted period. CT angiography is convenient and rapid, but may miss some injuries. MRI angiography may be more sensitive but has the same downsides as MRI in other trauma settings. No highly regarded predictive tool exists, but risk factors that should prompt consideration of a vascular injury and subsequent vascular imaging include an unexplained neurological deficit, massive facial bleeding, or epistaxis, fracture involving the foraman lacerum of the skull base or foramen transversarium of the cervical vertebrae.

At the conclusion of the of the head CT scan, the clinical and radiographic information should be synthesized to formulate a plan either to operate to evacuate an intracranial lesion, to evaluate for intracranial hypertension with monitoring technology and clinical examination, or to observe clinically for worsening of neurological status with clinical examinations alone. Radiographic assessments, similar to clinical assessments, are often iterative with repeat imaging used regularly to assess for an alteration in status and optimal management plan.

CLINICAL INJURY PATTERNS/ HERNIATION SYNDROMES

There are several important clinical syndromes that herald herniation events within the brain. Each has both an imaging and clinical correlate. Immediate recognition and treatment of these is essential for patient survival. Herniation is the decompensated response to an increasingly large intracranial mass or unchecked cerebral edema. When the ICP or regional compartment pressure reaches a sufficiently high level, the brain tissue is displaced out of the compartment into the adjacent one. If all the intracranial compartments are under equally high pressure, the brain seeks to exit the calvarium through the foramen magnum. **Subfalcine** herniation occurs when part of the cerebrum is forced from one side to the other under the falx cerebri. This is evident radiographically by the degree of *midline shift* present on head CT or MRI. Usually the falx itself is shifted to some extent with the brain. In trauma, there is a general correlation between the degree of midline shift, the depression in the level of consciousness, and the severity of the injury. Rarely, the anterior cerebral artery can be pinched by the falx when there is subfalcine herniation. **Uncal herniation** occurs when the uncus (latin for "hook") of the temporal lobe is shifted medially by a mass or swelling in the ipsilateral hemisphere. This is most likely to happen with temporal lobe masses because of the close proximity of the mass or swelling to the uncus. Anatomically, the uncus compresses the adjacent subarachnoid space, wherein lies cranial nerve III (oculomotor), resulting in loss of its parasympathetic fiber function to the ipsilateral eye and pupillary dilatation from unopposed sympathetic tone. With more severe or prolonged compression the extraocular muscle function of CN III is lost also, leading to a eye that is deviated interiorly and laterally (unopposed lateral rectus and superior oblique function). If the uncus is forced further medially, it compresses the cerebral peduncle producing contralateral hemiparesis. The clinical syndrome associated with these events therefore is an initial restlessness, then somnolence followed by a dilated ipsilateral pupil, and then contralateral hemiparesis. A somewhat confusing variation is the *Kernohan's notch phenomenon*, wherein the entire brainstem is shifted by the uncus and the contralateral peduncle comes into contact with the opposite tentorial edge, leading to weakness that appears clinically on the same side as the pupillary dilation. This is relevant clinically, because if faced with the clinical contradiction of left pupillary dilatation and left hemiparesis, the left pupillary dilation is a stronger predictor of the ipsilateral nature of the cranial problem, than the left hemiparesis which would otherwise predict a right sided problem. Uncal hernation can have the secondary complication of compression of the posterior cerebral artery which runs near CN III. Patients are at risk for a PCA distribution stroke. **Tonsillar herniation** occurs when the intracranial contents, particular the contents of the posterior fossa, are forced out of the foramen magnum at the base of the skull. The tonsils of the cerebellum are pushed downward and compress the medulla oblongata, leading to respiratory depression and death. Radiographically, this is identified by the loss of CSF spaces around the brainstem and foramen magnum, as brain tissue is pushed into these spaces.

Cushing triad is the constellation of bradycardia, hypertension, and respiratory irregularity that often occupies a herniation event clinically. It is likely due to brainstem compression. The hypertension can be conceptualized as an attempt to protect the brain's perfusion pressure from the high ICP. Intubation and mechanical ventilation often obscure the respiratory part of the triad, but the other two are observed regularly.

SPECIFIC INJURIES AND SURGICAL MANAGEMENT

Skull fractures are the usually the result of focal application of force to the head. These are usually categorized as open or closed, depressed or nondepressed, and basilar or convexity varieties. Depressed fractures can tear the dura or lacerate the cortex of the brain. Depressed fractures greater than the width of the bone are usually considered for operative repair, particularly if there is an associated laceration of the skin. Skull fractures that are not depressed usually do not usually require repair. *Basilar skull fractures* (those fractures involving the bones at the base of the brain (parts of the sphenoid, temporal, occipital bones, and clivus) can damage the vasculature and cranial nerves, and can lead to a CSF leak and meningitis. Clinically, one may suspect a basilar skull fracture in the presence of Battles sign, which is retroauricular ecchymosis, or "raccoon eyes," which is bilateral periorbital ecchymosis. Basilar and nondepressed calvarial vault fractures are usually managed conservatively, although their presence should prompt consideration of vascular and cranial nerve injury. Controversy exists as to the best management of fractures involving the inner table of the frontal sinus, or extending from the skull base into the ethmoid or other skull base sinus. There is the potential for the spread of infection through sinus communication with the epidural space. However, many such fractures heal spontaneously without complications, and management must be individualized.

An **Epidural Hematoma (EDH)** can occur with a skull fracture that lacerates an artery in the dura (Figure 36–8). The classic example is laceration of the middle meningeal artery by the temporal bone. The bleeding occurs on the outside of the dura and collects in and expands the potential epidural space between bone and dura. Because the source of bleeding is an artery, the hematoma can compress the adjacent brain to the point of serious injury or death. Not all epidural hematomas are caused by an arterial injury in the dura. Bleeding from a skull fracture or dural venous sinus can sometimes collect in the epidural space. These "venous epidural hematomas" are much less likely to produce life-threatening compression of the brain. Distinguishing between the two types is largely a matter of location (temporal vs. nontemporal), size (small vs. large), and rate of change (slow vs. fast). Because the primary injury in an isolated epidural hematoma does not involve the brain, the neurological outcome is excellent if the diagnosis and treatment are prompt. The classic presentation of a temporal epidural hematoma is a patient suffering a blow to the temple, and a brief loss of consciousness. This is followed by a lucid interval during which the patient it is considered safe to observe patients with EDH of modest size (about 1-cm deep) when the diagnosis is made in a delayed fashion. The hematomas in many of these cases will reabsorb spontaneously. In contrast, a 1-cm-thick temporal epidural hematoma in a patient only 30 minutes out from injury should be strongly considered for emergent surgical removal of the hematoma prior to care of other injuries not immediately threatening to the airway, breathing, or circulation. The operative approach involves positioning the patient to gain access to the site of the hematoma. For a temporal epidural hematoma, a skin incision is made from the root of the zygoma extending into the ipsilateral frontal region in a reverse question mark fashion. As circumstances dictate, a burr hole can be placed in the temporal region, after incising the temporalis muscle before the skin incision is completed to allow blood to escape from the epidural space. However, in most instances, the blood is clotted and rapid completion of craniotomy must follow. The temporalis muscle is elevated and retracted anteriorly. Additional burr holes are placed as needed and a bone flap is elevated. The hematoma is removed. Lacerated dural vessels can be controlled with bipolar cautery or suture depending on size. The dural surface is inspected for an associated subdural hematoma, and intraoperative ultrasound may be useful as needed. The dura is then sutured to the bony margins of the craniotomy to prevent reaccumulation. When a hematoma has collected in the vicinity of a major dural venous sinus, such as the transverse or sigmoid, the sinus itself may be torn and the resulting hemorrhage that is very difficult to control. The outcome for a patient suffering even from a large EDH can be quite good if managed promptly.

Acute Subdural Hematomas (ASDH) are the result of trauma to the brain causing rupture of veins over the surface of the brain that transit from the cortical surface to the inner surface of the dura to reach the dural sinuses. When these vessels are injured, the blood collects between the dura matter and the arachnoid membrane, in the potential subdural space. The force required to shear vessels in this fashion can occur with a focal blow to the head, but is likely more common with diffuse, rotational force applications to the brain, as often occur in motor vehicle accidents. Except in the elderly, ASDH generally occurs in conjunction with fairly severe associated brain injury. Focal bruising of the brain is often present beneath the subdural hematoma. Most patients present with a significantly depressed level of consciousness and may have other findings related to the compressive mass of the hematoma. A subdural hematoma has more of a crescent shape to it on imaging studies, because there is no barrier to it spreading over the hemispheric surface of the brain. Associated intracerebral hemorrhage and edema is often evident beneath the ASDH (Figure 36–9).

Management of the acute subdural hematoma involves emergent operative removal by craniotomy for lesions more than 1-cm thick. A large craniotomy is generally required,

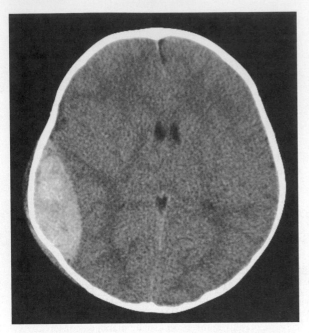

▲ **Figure 36–8.** Acute epidural hematoma after head trauma in a 5-year-old patient.

appears to be neurologically well, as there has been little primary brain injury. During this time, the epidural hematoma either expands slowly enough for the compensatory mechanisms of the brain to maintain consciousness, or the hemorrhage stops temporarily. Subsequently, either due to rebleeding or exhaustion of the compensatory mechanisms, a rapid decline in level of consciousness follows from the mass of hematoma associated with the other elements of uncal herniation, including an ipsilateral CN III Palsy and contralateral hemiparesis. However, this classic sequence is only present in about 25% of patients with EDH. Many patients have no loss of consciousness with injury while conversely, about 20% decline after injury without the lucid interval. Epidural hematomas are usually diagnosed from CT imaging and have a lens-shaped (lentiform) appearance, as the dura is attached firmly to the skull at nearby sutures, tapering each end of the hematoma. CT images are also helpful to judge the impact on the hematoma on the brain, such as the degree of shift of the midline, or compression of adjacent structures. Management of an EDH is determined by lesion size, location, and time from injury to diagnosis. Generally, an EDH more than 1 cm in depth is considered for surgical removal, as are lesions in the temporal fossa where there is less room for further expansion before brain injury occurs. In some cases, an EDH is diagnosed two or more days after the injury that caused it. Since the bulk of hematoma expansion occurs within the first 24-36 hours,

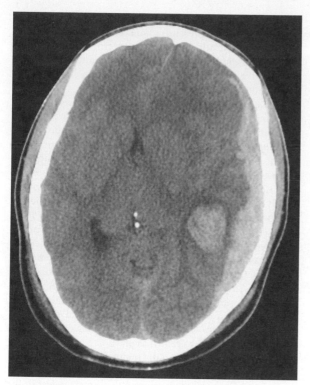

▲ **Figure 36-9.** Acute subdural hematoma with an associated intraparenchymal hemorrhage after head trauma in a 25-year-old patient.

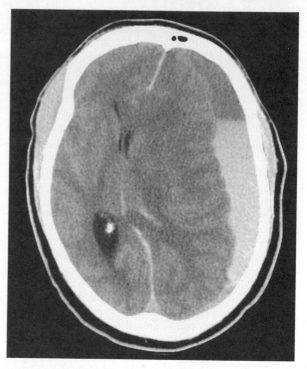

▲ **Figure 36–10.** Chronic subdural hematoma with acute blood layering in fluid in a 55-year-old patient.

and acute brain swelling during the surgical procedure must be expected. Unlike the situation in an EDH, the bleeding source in an ASDH is often difficult to discern. Diffuse hemorrhage arising from under the margins of the bone flap adjacent to dural venous sinuses, is often best managed with gentle packing of hemostatic materials rather than aggressive exploration. Medical management of elevated ICP and the underlying brain injury (see below) is an essential part of the patient's care. Outcomes are often poor, with a mortality of 50%-90%. Survivors often have significant disabilities. Outcomes can be predicted by the admission Glasgow Coma Scale score and in certain cases medical care is likely to be futile and offered only with reservations.

In the elderly, the atrophy of the brain places the transiting veins under stretch and injury can occur with much less force. Subdural hematomas can present more chronically in such elderly patients, even several months after injury, with a several centimeter thick collection. Such **chronic subdural hematomas** should be thought of as a different injury from the ASDH (Figure 36–10).

In cases of chronic subdural hematoma, drainage of the hematoma either through a burr hole in the skull or via a craniotomy is indicated. Outcomes are much better than for ASDH, although recurrence and reoperation are common.

Coagulapathy, whether from anticoagulant medications, or as a complication of severe trauma, presents a special risk to TBI patients who are prone to sudden deterioration from hematoma expansion. Immediate, aggressive correction of coagulapathy is indicated for such patients.

Intraparenchymal contusions are common after trauma. These are hemorrhage mixed with brain and usually occur either at the site of a direct blow to the head, or at a point opposite the point of impact. This later phenomena is called a *contra-coup* injury and is the result of the pressure wave of force moving through the brain and impacting and rebounding from the skull opposite the impact site. Contusions often occur in anterior temporal lobes after frontal impact as the temporal lobes impact into the sphenoid wing anteriorly. The base of the frontal and temporal lobes is also a common site for contusions caused by the brain moving roughly over the irregular bony surfaces of the frontal and middle fossas. Posteriorly, this does not occur as the brain is moving over the smoother tentorium. The clinical presentation of such contusions is specific to their location in the brain, but they can also produce more widespread symptoms through their mass effect as discussed below in secondary brain injury. Intraparenchymal contusions should be distinguished from smaller hemorrhages associated with **diffuse axonal injury (DIA)** discussed below. There is certainly overlap in terms of size and location, but the typical intraparenchymal hemorrhages are more than 0.5 cm in diameter, and relate to either bony anatomy or force vector as described above. Management for these lesions is generally as conservative as the situation will allow because the hematoma is often intimately mixed with brain, some of which may still be functional. Lesions more than 25 cc are often considered for resection, but the relative eloquence of brain and the response to attempted medical management are often important considerations.

Penetrating brain injury usually produces a focal injury pattern specific to the site of penetration. High-velocity injuries such as those from a gunshot produce, in addition to the focal injury, a large area of cavitation, and hemorrhagic injury from the blast effect. Gunshot wounds that pass through the ventricular system, as a marker for the "middle" of the brain, are most often fatal. Management of less-severe penetrating injury revolves around managing the potential infectious complications of injury and repairing the breach to the skull.

DIFFUSE BRAIN INJURY DIAGNOSES NOT TYPICALLY REQUIRING IMMEDIATE SURGICAL MANAGEMENT

Concussion is an immediate and transient loss of consciousness or normal mentation after head trauma, often associated with a period of amnesia. It is a very common injury. Sport injuries are a common source of concussions and young patients appear to be at highest risk. Concussion is most easily induced by sudden rotation of the head. The presumption is that the cerebral cortex is rotating around the more fixed midbrain and dienchephalon, producing disruption of input and outflow from the reticular activating system. Presentation after concussion can be surprisingly varied, with some patients displaying no loss of consciousness, but rather confusion and amnesia. The severity of concussion appears to be proportional to the duration of amnesia, particularly the anterograde (since injury) amnesia. Relying on consensus/expert opinion, several different criteria for diagnosis and grading systems for severity have been proposed. These systems use the duration of the confusion or amnesia and the presence or absence of a loss of consciousness to form a three-tiered scale of severity and are primarily designed to assist with return-to-play decisions for athletes. To the surgeon, the more typical concern is to decide whether a patient presenting with a concussion needs a CT scan of the head. Validated clinical decision rules stress that all patients with a Glasgow Coma Score of less than 15, those that are vomiting and those that are older than 60-65 years

are at high enough risk to warrant a CT scan. Other factors warranting a CT for presenting concussed patients are severe headache, intoxication, persistent anterograde amnesia, a seizure with the injury, evidence of trauma to bone or soft tissue above the clavicle, and severe mechanism of injury such as autopedestrian or ejection injury.

Management for isolated concussions presenting for emergency room evaluation usually includes a period of observation for at least 2 hours, assuming the individual is neurologically normal. Dependent on any other injuries, the patient may be discharged to a responsible adult with written instructions to return for specific symptoms as listed for obtaining a head CT. Patient with abnormal CT scans are usually admitted for care. Long-term outcome is generally good with the majority of patients experiencing no long-term sequellae. However, up to 25% of patients report an increased incidence of headaches and memory difficulties even several months later. **Postconcussive syndrome** is a more severe version of this phenomenon that includes these and other symptoms such as depression, anxiety, emotional liability, insomnia, and fatigue. Treatment is largely one of reassurance and management of individual symptoms. Because athletes are often concussed, questions arise around when it is reasonable to return to play.

Traumatic Subarachnoid Hemorrhage is a relatively common finding in patients suffering severe TBI. Following injury, a relatively small amount of blood may collect in the subarachnoid space, often over the convexities of the brain, but also in the basal cisternal arachnoid spaces. Trauma is the most common cause of subarachnoid hemorrhage, not rupture of an aneurysm, so the report of subarachnoid hemorrhage after trauma should not automatically prompt a search for a ruptured aneurysm. A history of a neurological collapse before the trauma or more dense blood collecting in the basal cisterns or around the larger intracranial vasculature should prompt more concern for a cerebral aneurysm.

Diffuse Axonal Injury occurs when axons become sheared off at the boundary between gray and white matter during rapid brain acceleration or deceleration. The substance of the cerebral cortex is organized in to a series of alternating layers of gray and white matter (gray cortical mantel, subcortical white matter, deep gray matter nuclei of the basal ganglia, and white matter of the internal capsule). These layers have different tissue densities and when subjected to force in trauma, behave differently. The border between these two tissues is often a site of injury as these two layers accelerate or decelerate at rates according to their tissue properties. DIA is a common finding in severe injury, occurring in up to 50% of pts. Clinically, DIA can occur in varying degrees of severity. In minimal cases, a prolonged mildly concussive state of confusion and memory loss might occur. In more severe cases, the presentation is a depressed level of consciousness. Focal findings can occur if there are DIA hemorrhages in specific locations such as the internal capsule or brainstem. The appearance on head CT is one of multiple small (< 1 cm) hemorrhages, scattered throughout the brain at the junction of gray and white matter. Grading schemes that relate the severity of the CT findings to the eventual neurological outcome exist. Effacement of the basal cisterns and midline shift are examples of radiographic prognosticators of poor outcome after DIA. Management for patients suffering from DIA is primarily medical and focuses on prevention and management of secondary brain injury discussed below.

MEDICAL MANAGEMENT AFTER TBI

The medical management is largely directed at detecting and preventing secondary brain injury from seizures, systemic phenomena such as hypotension and hypoxia and intracranial hypertension.

▶ Seizure Management

The incidence of seizures following TBI is estimated at between 5% and 15%. The majority of these events occur within the first 7 days after trauma. A seizure has the possibility of increasing brain demand for oxygen and nutrients, at a point when the injury may limit the ability of the brain to respond in this fashion. Prophylactic anticonvulsants, usually phenytoin (dilantin), or more recently levetiracetam (Keppra), are reasonably used to prevent seizures after a moderate and severe TBI, when there is evidence of non-trivial brain injury on CT scans. However, experimental evidence only supports their use for the first 7 days after a TBI, and there does not appear to be benefit to continuing the prophylaxis beyond 7 days. Patients experiencing seizures outside of the immediate point of impact are candidates for therapeutic anticonvulsant use extending beyond the 7 day time frame, usually for several months or more, depending on whether the seizures recur.

▶ Homeostatsis

Just as in the initial resuscitation, ongoing care of acute brain injury requires careful protection against hypoxia, hypotension, and hyperthermia. Each of these has the potential to increase ICP or further deprive the brain of adequate glucose or oxygen, or both.

▶ Physiology of Increased Intracranial Pressure

Other than its impact on the neurological examination, secondary brain injury manifests itself clinically as cerebral edema and an increase in ICP. **The Monroe–Kelly Doctrine** states that given a fixed intracranial volume, consisting of brain, cerebrospinal fluid, and arterial and venous blood, any additional material must be accommodated by a decline in the amounts of the others, or a rise in pressure due to

the increase in total intracranial material (Figure 36–1). When a mass is introduced into the cranial vault, CSF and later venous blood are displaced to make room for the mass while initially allowing relatively normal ICPs. However, these mechanisms are overcome and eventually the rise in pressure with increasing volume becomes exponential. The compensatory phase is very important clinically, as a patient may harbor a clinically important lesion while showing only modest symptoms of increased pressure in the brain. This model works well in trauma but is overly simplistic and does not explain clinical phenomena that occur over a longer time frame, such as might occur with chronic hydrocephalus or a brain tumor. In such cases, the compressibility of the brain, usually described as its compliance (change in volume for a given change in pressure) matters a great deal and brain pressures may be normal even in the face of a mass that, if it occurred acutely, would overwhelm the compensatory mechanisms mentioned above. Despite these limitations, the compartment model is very useful for managing cerebral edema and increased ICP. Left unchecked, these consequences of secondary injury lead to increased cerebral edema, increased ICP, compression and finally injury of adjacent brain and its vasculature, producing additional brain ischemia and tissue injury, cyclically generating more brain edema and further increased ICP. ICP is both a surrogate measure of the presence of cerebral edema and also a primary actor in ongoing secondary brain injury. Increased ICP, like hypoxia and hypotension, is a strong predictor of mortality and morbidity after head injury.

The concept of **cerebral perfusion pressure (CPP)** highlights the ability of elevations in ICP to reduce tissue perfusion:

$$CPP = MAP - ICP,$$

where MAP is mean arterial pressure.

In adult patients, CPP of less than 70 mm HG is associated with worsened outcome. The equation also illustrates the importance of maintaining an adequate blood pressure in TBI management. Hypotension is among the strongest predictors of poor neurological outcome after TBI.

Detection of cerebral edema and intracranial hypertension is based on suspicion, radiographic features, and direct measurement of ICP. In severe head injury, as measured by the GCS score, the incidence of increased ICP is 50%-60%. Radiographic findings of concern include the presence of mass effect, midline shift, the loss of the evident pattern of sulci and gyri from displacement of CSF, the loss of distinction of the gray/white matter junction, and the effacement of the basal CSF cisterns. Increased ICP can occur in the absence of any of these findings, so in severely head injured patients, direct measurement of the ICP can still be indicated without concerning radiographic features. At present, it is unproven whether treatment directed by ICP is preferable to one based on CT and clinical examination. Nevertheless current guidelines from the Brain Trauma Foundation recommend ICP monitoring for:

1. All patients with GCS 3-8 and abnormal head CT;

2. GCS 3-8 with normal head CT but with hypotension or age more than 40;

3. Patients in whom the neurological exam cannot be assessed because of sedation or need for general anesthesia, if the suspicion of increased ICP is high.

ICP is measured in trauma by either introduction of a transducer into the brain parenchyma or placement of a catheter into the ventricles of the brain to measure the pressure of the cerebrospinal fluid in a minor surgical procedure. Complication rates of intracranial hemorrhage (2% vs. < 1%) and infection (10% vs. 2%) are higher for catheter-based measurement systems over parenchymal transducers, but only a catheter based system can drain CSF, a distinct treatment advantage. Parenchymal monitors are subject to drift in accuracy and may be inaccurate by 3-4 mm HG after 4-5 days. Catheter-based systems may occlude or be unreliable in the face of very compressed ventricles. In trauma, ICP is not measured by lumbar puncture as there is a risk of brain herniation from higher cranial versus lumbar pressures. Normal ICPs range between about 5 and 15 mm Hg at rest and vary with position and activity. Treatment thresholds after brain injury are typically more than 20 mm HG in adult patients, while children and infants likely require treatment at a lower ICP, although the precise numbers are not yet established. Measurement of the ICP allows calculation of the CPP. Managing brain injury patients based on CPP rather than ICP holds interest as a sufficiently high blood pressure should be able to perfuse the brain despite the ICP. However, clinical research suggests that while CPPs less than 70 mm HG in adult patients are associated with poor outcome, artificially raising blood pressure to supraphysiologic levels in an effort to overcome an increase in ICP, worsens, rather than improves outcomes. CPP measurements currently focus care on avoiding relative hypotension during management.

Treatment options for intracranial hypertension and cerebral edema are most easily understood with reference to the four compartment model of the brain noted above (brain, venous, arterial blood, and CSF). When patients present with elevated ICP, treatments available manipulate the volume of one of these compartments. At present, the selection and style of intracranial hypertension management is as much art as science. Few well-designed studies exist to directly compare different management strategies. Each treatment has risks associated with its use. General strategies include employment of less-risky strategies first and escalation as needed, and to apply methods directed at each of the compartments before applying multiple methods to the same compartment, although many therapies work on multiple parts of the model. The following section covers the treatment options in general but not rigid order of preference. A therapy from the end of the list would very rarely be used before one at the beginning, but that adjacent items in the list might be interchanged.

A. Improve Venous Drainage

If blood is restricted from exiting the central nervous system, ICP increases as the venous compartment size is larger. In trauma patients, tight fitting cervical collars, a supine body position, and fighting against the ventilator all increase venous pressures. Loosening collars, elevating the head of the bed 30 degrees and minimizing ventilator pressures all improve venous drainage and lower ICPs. These measures have very little risk and can be employed widely.

B. CSF Drainage

Reducing the size of the CSF space can make more room for brain edema and lower ICP. This is done by draining CSF from the same ventricular catheter used to measure ICP. The risks of this therapy are infection and hemorrhage, and a capable surgeon must be available to place the catheter.

Sedation/Paralysis

Besides caring for the patient's comfort after an injury, sedation and/or chemical paralysis are important in reducing excessive brain metabolism that accompanies agitation from brain injury. This metabolism can be directly toxic in an injured brain, and obligates increased arterial and venous blood volume to supply the tissue with nutrients. In addition, sedatives/paralytic agents reduce fighting against the ventilator, reducing venous congestion. However, these agents reduce the ability to follow the neurological exam and have the side effect of hypotension when given in excess. Typically, agents such as morphine and ativan are used for analgesia and sedation, while muscular paralytics such as vecuronium are used to facilitate ventilation, but there is little evidence supporting the use of specific regimens with the exception of propofol, which should not be used in children. In general, shorter acting agents are preferable to long acting ones because of the desire to periodically examine the patient without their influence.

Osmotic Agents and Diuretics

In theory, excessive brain water can be removed directly in some cases by establishing a favorable osmotic gradient for diffusion of fluid back into the blood stream. Mannitol, a sugar, and concentrated saline solutions (3% NaCl), do not cross the blood brain barrier and therefore provide such a gradient. Their effect appears to require an intact blood brain barrier. Experimentally, they draw water from less injured areas of the brain, rather than from the more injured areas.

This reduces the overall brain volume, and can decrease the ICP, in the four-compartment model. In addition, experimental evidence suggests that a significant part of the ICP reducing effect of osmotic agents comes from reducing the viscosity of blood by altering RBC morphology. This allows delivery of more blood through smaller channels, permitting safe reduction in vessel caliber and, therefore, total intracranial blood volume. The adverse effects of these therapies include dehydration (and hypotension) in the case of mannitol, and nephrotoxicity from increased osmlolarity for all agents. In addition, some of the osmolar particles do make it across the blood brain barrier, and can pull water back into the brain if the therapy is withdrawn too quickly. Dosing regimens for these agents are variable but mannitol is usually used at 0.5-1 gm/kg per dose as often as every 2-3 hours. Dose of 1 gm/kg are given for impending herniation. NaCl 3% may be dosed either continuously at 1-3 cc/kg/h or as bolus doses of similar amounts. Serum sodium and osmolarity measurements should be assessed frequently. For mannitol, a serum osmolarity more than 320 mOsm/L appears to threaten toxicity and limit efficacy, while for hypertonic saline, serum osmolarities of 360 mOsm/dL or more have been reported without renal injury. In this area, the medical literature is limited.

Hyperventilation

The autoregulatory mechanisms of the brain rely in part on CO_2 (or perhaps pH) concentrations in the blood. A high metabolic rate leads to increased $CO2$ production and acidosis. The natural response to this is vasodilatation, to remove waste products and increase the supply of metabolites. Clinically, artificially increasing the respiratory rate (and dropping the $CO2$) significantly decreases the intracranial blood volume by vasoconstriction. The downside risk is that if done to excess, the vasoconstriction produces ischemia. While hyperventilation was once widely practiced, it is now reserved for situations in which the brain injury has produced an excessive, as opposed to reduced degree of blood flow. This is relatively rare. However, it is import to manage ventilator settings to avoiding elevated $CO2$ levels (and reduced $O2$ levels). This avoids unnecessary vasodilation and the increased ICP that results. Arterial $CO2$ levels of 35 mm HG and $O2$ levels of 100 mm HG are the common therapy targets.

Barbiturates

High doses of barbiturates reduce cerebral metabolism and experimentally protect against brain injury from the regional ischemia common in secondary brain injury ("the induced coma"). This reduced demand for metabolites decreases the blood flow requirements for adequate cell nutrition, and thus can decrease ICP. However, no clinical experiment has clearly shown that barbiturates improve outcome. The risk is that these agents can profoundly lower blood pressure. They must be used very carefully if at all.

Hypothemia

In experimental settings, hypothermia appears to slow the destructive secondary injury pathways at a cellular level. This reduces the edema that comes from cell death. However, randomized trials in adult head injury have not shown benefit while pediatric trials are ongoing. In the published trial protocols, cooling is typically begun early in the hospital course, if not immediately, with target temperatures of 32-33°C maintained for several days after the initial injury. Complications associated with the therapy in the adult clinical trials have been an increase in infection rate, and serious electrolyte disturbances, particularly hyperkalemia.

Surgical Decompression

Surgical management of cerebral edema involves enlarging the space available for swelling by removing a portion of the calvarium. The surgical technique is to remove a large portion of the skull over the more effected side (hemicraniectomy) or removal of large portions of both frontal bones (bifrontal craniectomy). The dura is generally opened and patched with either allograft or native periosteum. Clinical studies suggest that surgical decompression is effective in lowering ICP, but data regarding neurological outcomes are varied.

OUTCOMES AFTER TRAUMATIC BRAIN INJURY

While many patients with mild traumatic brain injury return to their preinjury level of function, a significant number develop chronic symptoms of fatigue, memory impairment, headaches, and difficulty with concentration. In one study of prospectively followed injury victims, Thornhill, Teasdale, and colleagues reported that over 50% had some identifiable disability one year after injury, including both physical and mental impairments. These were severe enough to impact activities of daily living in one-third to one-fourth of patients. Predictors for poor outcome included age less than 40, and preinjury disability. The medical literature is mixed with regard to the longer term outcome. In a separate study by the Whitnall and coauthors, the overall rates of disability were similar at 1 year and 5 years from injury, but about 25% of patients had exchanged categories from good to disabled and vice-versa. Changes in depression, anxiety, and reported stress appeared to correlate strongly with category change, and only 7% reported the use of rehabilitation services by the 5 year postinjury point. Patients with moderate closed head injuries have more varied outcomes. Most recover to maintain their activities of daily living and even return to work or school. Detailed neurocognitive testing, however, often reveals deficits in executive function and memory. There are more consistent reports of chronic fatigue and headaches. Severe TBI is often a life altering event for both patient and family event. The prognostic implications of injury are often vitally important for family members making decisions about what degree of aggressive care to provide. As an average, perhaps 15%-20% of all patients with severe injury will make a good recovery, while more than 50% will either die or be severely disabled. Sadly, for some patients, the degree of injury and the poor likelihood of meaningful recovery make the provision of aggressive care an exercise in futility. Elderly patients, those more than 80 years old, with severe head injuries have a very poor prognosis. For patients with the worst prognostic features, such as older age, very low GCS or 3-5 without improvement with resuscitation, lack of pupillary response to light and associated chest or abdominal injuries with hypotension, the prognosis for meaningful recovery is very poor. Once the diagnosis and injury severity are confirmed by examination and imaging studies and the condition is unchanged despite resuscitation and withdrawal of all pharmacologic agents likely to be affecting the examination, a gentle but frank discussion of the situation is necessary and appropriate. However, generally, the younger the patient is, and the higher the presenting GCS score, particularly the motor GCS scores, even within the severe injury group, the better the chances of some degree of recovery. The physician would do well to remember that prognostic information represents a probability of an outcome not a certainty of it. While some families may appreciate knowing these details, others will more appreciate whatever kernels of hope can be provided under the circumstances.

Bullock MR, et al: Surgical management of traumatic parenchymal lesions. *Neurosurgery* 2006;58(3 Suppl):S25-S46; discussion Si-iv.

Guidelines for the management of severe traumatic brain injury. *J Neurotrauma* 2007;24(Suppl):1.

Thornhill S, Teasdale GM, Murray GD, McEwen J, Roy CW, Penny KI: Disability in young people and adults one year after head injury: prospective cohort study. *BMJ* 2000;320(7250):1631-1635.

Timofeev I, Czosnyka M, Nortje J, Smielewski P, Kirkpatrick P, Gupta A, Hutchinson P: Effect of decompressive craniectomy on intracranial pressure and cerebrospinal compensation following traumatic brain injury. *J Neurosurg* 2008;108(1):66-73.

Wakai A, McCabe A, Roberts I, Schierhout G: Mannitol for acute traumatic brain injury. *Cochrane Database Syst Rev* 2013 Aug 5;8:CD001049.

Whitnall L, McMillan TM, Murray GD, Teasdale GM: Disability in young people and adults after head injury: 5-7 year follow up of a prospective cohort study. *J Neurol Neurosurg Psychiatry* 2006;77(5):640-645.

Wood RL: Long-term outcome of serious traumatic brain injury. *Eur J Anaesthesiol* 2008;42(Suppl):115-122.

▼ SPINAL CORD INJURY

John Ziewacz, Frank La Marca

▶ General Considerations

Traumatic spinal cord injury (SCI) is devastating. It primarily affects young people, and often results in significant disability or death. The median age at diagnosis of SCI is 37.6 years. The main causes in order of incidence are: motor vehicle collision, fall, violence, and sports injuries. Despite maximal medical and surgical therapy, the prognosis for significant recovery of a complete lesion is poor. Recent research into stem cell technology and other new modalities of therapy have not yet been effective in human clinical trials.

The cost to the healthcare system and to society is significant. A 25 years old with a high cervical cord injury (C1-4) is estimated to incur $741,425 in medical costs in the first year following SCI, and $132,807 for each year survived thereafter. In addition, the loss of wages and productivity for SCI patients averages $57,000 annually. With 12,000-14,000 Americans suffering SCI per year, the social and economic costs are significant.

The demographics of SCI have changed in the last 30 years. The median age of 37.6 years has increased from 28.7 years in the 1970s. This is a largely due to an increase in the incidence of falls causing SCI in patients more than 60 years of age. Though the relative incidence of both sports injuries and violent injuries has declined over the last 30 years, the larger decrease in sports injuries has placed it below violent injuries as a cause of SCI.

Treatment for SCI consists of acute and chronic management. Acutely, the ABCs (airway, breathing, circulation) must be secured, and the spine immobilized to prevent extension of injuries. Compressive lesions must be identified and the need for urgent surgical management determined. Methylprednisolone is currently a treatment option used widely in the initial phases of SCI, though it is associated with side-effects which may sometimes outweigh the potential benefits of its use. Other acute nonsurgical treatment options aimed primarily at minimizing secondary injury are modest induced hypothermia and hyperbaric therapy. The first would be based on the neuroprotective properties of hypothermia in brain injury but has not yet shown to have proven beneficial effects in humans with traumatic SCI. The second has shown to increase speed of neurological recovery but not an overall improvement in final outcome. Chronic management includes physical, and occupational therapy designed to maximize functionality. Specific therapy and improvement depends on the level and completeness of the injury.

▶ Clinical Findings

Clinical findings in SCI depend on the level, mechanism, and severity of injury. Injuries can be classified as either complete or incomplete. A complete SCI refers to the lack of motor or sensory function below the level of the lesion. Incomplete lesions spare some degree of sensory and/or motor function below the level of the lesion. Incomplete lesions often result in recognized SCI syndromes based on the region of the spinal cord affected. The American Spinal Injury Association publishes a scale to further classify the severity of SCI (Table 36–4).

Table 36–4. The ASIA classification of spinal cord injury.[1]

A = Complete: No sensory or motor function preserved in the lowest sacral segments (S4/5).

B = Sensory incomplete: Sensory but no motor function preserved below the neurologic level including the sacral segments S4/5.

C = Motor incomplete: Motor function is preserved below the neurologic level, and more than half of the key muscles below the neurologic level have a muscle grade less than 3. There must be some sparing of sensory and/or motor function in the segments S4/5.

D = Motor incomplete: Motor function is preserved below the neurologic level, and more than half the key muscles below the neurologic level have a muscle grade greater than or equal to 3. There must be some sparing of sensory and/or motor function in the segments S4/5.

E = Normal: Sensory and motor functions are normal. Patient may have abnormalities on reflex examination.

[1]Adapted from: American Spinal Injury Association. Standards for neurological classification of spinal cord injury (revised 2000). Chicago: ASIA; 2002.

Initial clinical findings include motor deficit, sensory deficit, and hyporeflexia. Initially, all reflexes below the lesion are lost including the bulbocavernosus, cremasteric, and abdominal cutaneous reflex. Over time, these reflexes may return, and the deep tendon reflexes become hyperreflexive due to the loss of descending tonic inhibition of the reflex arc. Initially, paralysis is flaccid, but eventually upper motor neuron signs develop, and a spastic paralysis results. If the lesion is in the high cervical region (C1-5), respiratory effort may be compromised due to the loss of innervation to the phrenic nerve. Loss of bowel or bladder function often occurs, and loss of rectal tone and sensation, as well as priapism may result. The loss of bladder control manifests as urinary retention, and developing urinary incontinence is typically overflow incontinence. Loss of anal sphincter tone and sensation results in leakage of stool and lack of awareness of bowel movements.

An important early finding that can occur in SCI is "spinal shock." This refers to a drop in the systolic blood pressure with accompanying bradycardia, often to a level of 80 mm Hg systolic following SCI. This is due to the loss of sympathetic tone to the regions below the lesion and causes venous pooling and decreased venous return to the heart.

Chronic clinical findings in SCI are related to the long-term need for ventilatory support, immobilization, and need for catheterization. Pneumonia, urinary tract infections, and decubitus ulcers are common findings, and are often the cause of death in spinal cord injured patients.

Incomplete SCIs may demonstrate a variable pattern of sensory or motor preservation, though they can often be categorized into recognizable clinical syndromes, depending on the mechanism of injury and the portion of the cord affected.

A. Central Cord Syndrome

Central cord syndrome (CCS) refers to a pattern of injury that affects the motor strength in the upper extremities more severely than the lower extremities. Sensory function is variable below the level of the lesion, and sphincter control is often affected. This usually occurs in older patients with spinal stenosis following a hyperextension injury. The central cervical cord is a watershed vascular territory that is thought to be disrupted in this syndrome. The spinal cord is somatotopically organized such that cervical fibers are more medial compared to fibers traveling to the lower extremities, resulting in the more severely affected upper extremities.

B. Anterior Cord Syndrome

Anterior cord syndrome (ACS) results from the compression of the anterior portion of the cord by a herniated disk, bone fragment, or from occlusion of the anterior spinal artery. The corticospinal tracts and spinothalamic tracts are preferentially affected due to their more anterior location. The posterior columns are relatively spared. This results in loss of motor function and loss of pain and temperature sensation below the level of the lesion, with preserved proprioception, vibration, and pressure sensation. It is important to distinguish surgical from nonsurgical (ie, anterior spinal artery occlusion) etiologies in this condition.

C. Brown–Séquard Syndrome

Brown–Séquard syndrome occurs after spinal cord hemisection. It is usually the result of penetrating trauma occurring in 2%-4% of spinal cord injuries. Motor function and posterior column function (proprioception, vibration sense) is disrupted on the side of the lesion. Pain and temperature sensation is diminished on the contralateral side due to the crossing of the spino-thalamic tract in the spinal cord at or one or two levels above the entrance of the fibers into the cord.

D. Conus Medullaris Syndrome

Conus medullaris syndrome (CMS) results from injury to the sacral spinal cord. Symptoms include saddle anesthesia, loss of bowel/bladder function, and lower extremity weakness. It includes a combination of both upper and motor neuron signs.

E. Cauda–Equina Syndrome

Cauda–Equina syndrome refers to compression and dysfunction of the lumbo-sacral nerve roots. It is not a true SCI as it only affects the nerve roots and not the cord itself. The clinical syndrome is similar to CMS with saddle anesthesia, loss of bowel/bladder function, and lower extremity weakness, but findings are all lower motor neuron.

Physical Examination

Initial physical examination in SCI focuses on the ABCs (airway, breathing, circulation). The spine should be immobilized to prevent further injury. Special attention must be focused on the airway in high cervical injuries as patients may require endotracheal intubation given injury to the nervous supply to the diaphragm. Blood pressure must be closely monitored given the possibility of spinal shock. This manifests as a drop in the systolic blood pressure and must be addressed immediately in order to prevent further cord ischemia.

In the awake patient after the ABCs have been attended to, a history focusing on mechanism of injury and detailed neurologic examination is undertaken in order to determine the level and completeness of the injury. Motor strength should be tested in all muscle groups and sensation should be tested with pinprick, and proprioception. Rectal tone and sensation should be tested with digital examination. Reflexes should be examined including the bulbocavernosus, cremasteric, and abdominal cutaneous reflexes. Careful palpation of the spine is important to evaluate for obvious step-offs or tenderness to palpation at all levels. The examination must be carefully documented and a neurologic level and evaluation of completeness of the lesion determined.

In the comatose patient, a complete neurologic examination is often difficult. In this situation, observation of spontaneous movements or movements to painful stimuli is important. Deep tendon reflexes should be examined and palpation of the spine should be undertaken to observe for obvious step-offs. Radiologic imaging is often required to adequately determine a level of injury and its etiology.

Differential Diagnosis

After a complete history and physical examination is performed, with the addition of radiographic imaging, the diagnosis of SCI is usually apparent. Radiographic imaging can help determine the mechanism of the injury, which is usually due to a fracture or subluxation of the bony spinal elements.

Some peripheral nerve lesions may resemble SCI, but these can usually be distinguished after careful examination and knowledge of the anatomy of the spinal cord and the peripheral nervous system. Peripheral injuries are typically unilateral and affect only lower motor neurons. Sometimes malingering and conversion disorders may mimic SCI. Serial examinations and inconsistencies in examination, in the setting of unremarkable imaging usually permits differentiation.

Radiologic Examination

In the asymptomatic patient with no spinal tenderness, no distracting injury (eg, long-bone fracture), and no evidence of disturbed consciousness or intoxication, no radiographic imaging is necessary. Patients with spine tenderness, numbness, tingling, or obvious signs of SCI (eg, weakness, loss of bowel/bladder control) require radiographic imaging. The hallmark of radiographic imaging has been three-view cervical spine x-rays with AP/Lateral films of the thoracic and lumbar spine. Current recommendations of the American Association of Neurological Surgeons/Congress of Neurological Surgeons (AANS/CNS) recommend three-view cervical spine x-rays in conjunction with CT scanning of the cervical spine in patients with suspected SCI. With the advent of CT scanning with detailed coronal and sagittal reconstructions, CT scanning alone has replaced x-ray examination as the initial diagnostic study of choice in many centers (Figure 36–11). This obviates the need for multiple

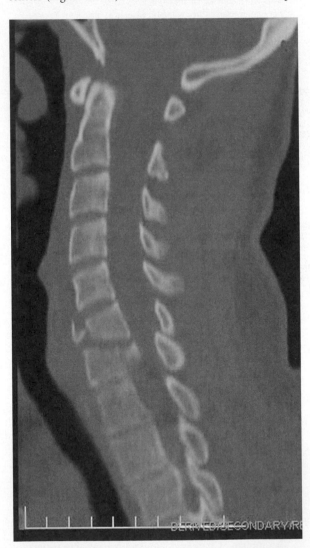

▲ **Figure 36–11.** Sagittal reconstruction of a cervical computed tomography (CT) scan demonstrating a C6-7 traumatic fracture.

x-rays and diagnostic/treatment delay in the case of inadequate plain films. MRI is listed as an option in the diagnosis of SCI by the AANS/CNS as it can better detect ligamentous/soft tissue injury, though it often "overcalls" injuries that do not cause instability and may lead to prolonged and unnecessary immobilization. MRI is often reserved for patients for whom SCI signs and symptoms are present and no clear evidence is found on x-ray imaging or CT, or a herniated disk or other soft-tissue abnormality is suspected. MRI (particularly T2-weighted sequences) also clearly demonstrates compression of and/or signal change within the spinal cord (Figure 36–12).

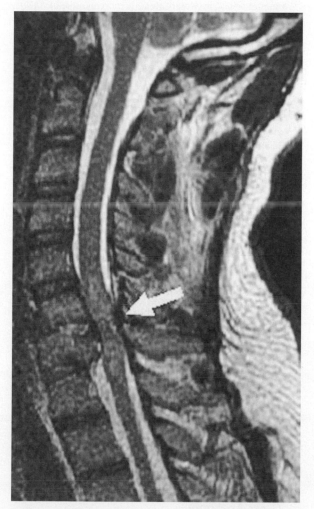

▲ Figure 36–12. Sagittal T2-weighted magnetic resonance image of a C6-7 traumatic fracture demonstrating spinal cord compression and signal change within the spinal cord (arrow).

In awake patients, clearance of the cervical spine consists of normal x-rays (or CT w/reconstructions), CT scan, and flexion/extension views or MRI obtained within 48 hours of injury. At this point, cervical immobilization may be discontinued.

Under current recommendations in obtunded patients, cervical spine clearance may be obtained following normal x-rays, CT, and dynamic flexion/extension films performed under fluoroscopic guidance, normal MRI obtained within 48 hours of injury, or at the discretion of the treating physician. However, with the advent of CT with sagittal and coronal reconstruction providing greater sensitivity for the detection of injury, and the propensity of MRI to "overcall" injuries, some centers clear the cervical spine in obtunded patient with normal x-rays and CT scans. Clearance of the cervical spine in this population is still cause for debate and recommendations are in flux. Further studies will elucidate the necessary and sufficient studies to definitively clear the cervical spine in this population.

In the patient with SCI the combination of x-rays with CT scanning has high sensitivity and identifies the vast majority of lesions causing SCI.

▶ Treatment

Initial treatment of SCI consists of securing the ABCs and immobilizing the spinal column. In the case of high cervical spine injury, the need for endotracheal intubation must be identified and if it is not immediately necessary serial arterial blood gas assessments should be monitored to evaluate for hypocapnia and progressive ventilatory failure. Spinal shock and the resultant decrease in blood pressure must be treated aggressively if it occurs. Volume expansion should be initiated promptly and decreased systolic blood pressure refractory to volume expansion should be treated with pressor therapy. The choice of pressors has not been conclusively defined, but typically a beta-agonist is followed by an alpha-agonist given the possibility of bradycardia in spinal shock.

Patients should be placed in a hard cervical collar and cervical immobilization should be ensured until clearance of the cervical spine, or definitive treatment has occurred. Patients should be placed on a board for transfers and log-rolled for movement until the thoracic and lumbar spine is cleared.

Other initial management considerations include placement of an arterial line to monitor blood pressure on a constant basis, and placement of a Foley catheter to decompress the bladder.

Methylprednisolone has been used in the acute phase of SCI based on studies that demonstrated motor improvement in patient groups that received methylprednisolone in the early period after SCI. However, due to the lack of demonstrated clinical significance of any improvement, and studies demonstrating side-effects of high-dose methylprednisolone, it is offered as an option by the AANS/CNS current guidelines with the knowledge that "evidence suggesting harmful side-effects is more consistent than any suggestion of clinical benefit."

Following initial stabilization and imaging studies, the need for surgical intervention is assessed. Surgery has two main goals: decompression and stabilization. Surgery is employed on an emergent basis for incomplete lesions in the hopes of preserving or improving neurologic function, and on a nonemergent basis for complete lesions, as there is no demonstrated improvement in neurologic function for emergent surgery for complete lesions. Goals of surgery in this setting are to prevent cranial extension of injury, and to prevent progressive deformity. Choice of surgical approach for SCI is not standardized and is dependent on the location of the pathology. Current stabilization procedures typically involve instrumented fusion techniques, and may be approached via an anterior, posterior, or combined approach.

Cervical traction may be employed either alone, or as an adjunct to surgical therapy to attempt realignment of the spinal column. This is accomplished by fixing a halo ring, or specialized devices (ie, Gardner–Wells tongs) to the head, connecting this to a rope and pulley system, and adding weight to adjust the spine in the desired vector.

Chronic treatment of SCI focuses on rehabilitation and adaptation to permanent injury. Rehabilitation can often result in improved neurologic function in incomplete lesions and can help those with complete injuries become as functional as possible. Patients may require ventilatory support, tracheostomy, intermittent catheterization, frequent turning (to prevent decubitus ulcers), and functional accommodations such as wheelchairs and other devices aimed at improving functionality. Attention to long-term care issues can prolong the life and productivity of SCI patients.

Prognosis/Outcome

Despite exciting research into novel treatments, SCI remains a devastating injury. Death in the acute trauma setting from SCI is 20%. Complete lesions that remain so at 72 hours are unlikely to improve beyond one level above the lesion in the long term. Patients with quadriplegia who have initial ventilator dependency have 5-year survival rates of approximately 33%. Incomplete lesions have a more favorable outcome. Among recognized SCI syndromes, CCS and BSS have the most favorable outcomes, with up to 90% of BSS and CCS patients being able to ambulate independently at 1 year. ACS patients have a worse prognosis, with 10%-20% recovering functional motor control. Causes of death in long-term SCI patients are usually due to cardiac, respiratory, or infectious causes—often related to the sequelae of SCI.

Current multidisciplinary approaches to SCI, including emergency department, medical, surgical, and rehabilitation staff provide the best therapy for patients with SCI. Despite this, SCI remains a devastating injury with high rates of mortality and permanent disability. Novel research and innovations will hopefully provide better outcomes for SCI in the future.

American Spinal Injury Association: Standards for neurological classification of spinal cord injury (revised 2000). Chicago: ASIA; 2002.

Kwon BK, Mann C, Sohn HM, et al: Hypothermia for spinal cord injury. *Spine J* 2008 Nov-Dec;8(6):859-874.

Ho CH, Wuermser LA, Priebe MM, Chiodo AE, Scelza WM, Kirshblum SC: Spinal cord injury medicine. 1. Epidemiology and classification. *Arch Phys Med Rehabil* 2007;88(Suppl 1):S49-S54.

McKinley W, Santos K, Meade M, Brooke K: Incidence and outcomes of spinal cord injury clinical syndromes. *J Spinal Cord Med* 2007;30:215-224.

Priebe MM, Chiodo AE, Scelza WM, Kirshblum SC, Wuermser LA, Ho CH: Spinal cord injury medicine 6. Economic and societal issues in spinal cord injury. *Arch Phys Med Rehabil* 2007;88(Suppl 1):S84-S88.

▼ PERIPHERAL NERVE LESIONS

Cheerag Upadhyaya, MD Linda Yang, MD John McGillicuddy, MD

▶ General Considerations

Familiarity with the pertinent aspects of peripheral nerve anatomy and physiology combined with focused history and physical examination aids in the management of peripheral nerve lesions. The history and physical examination may then be complimented by electrodiagnostic and radiographic studies.

▶ Microscopic Anatomy

Peripheral nerves are composed of varying combinations of sensory and motor axons. An axon is a long projection from a nerve cell body that is bounded by a cell membrane as well as a basement membrane. Some axons are surrounded by sheaths of myelin, a fatty substance secreted by Schwann cells. Myelin insulates the axon, thereby increasing the velocity of neurotransmission. The axon is, in turn, surrounded by a layer of connective tissue called endoneurium. Axons travel together in bundles called fascicles, each of which is covered by another layer of connective tissue called perineurium. Fascicles are grouped together to form a peripheral nerve, which is surrounded by a final layer of connective tissue called epineurium.

▶ Gross Anatomy

A peripheral nerve is comprised of fibers from more than one spinal nerve root and each spinal nerve root contributes fibers to more than one peripheral nerve. Spinal nerve lesions manifest as radiculopathies with blurred sensory disturbances, while peripheral nerve lesions demonstrate sharply demarcated sensory disturbances. Spinal nerve lesions results in mild to moderate weakness in muscles supplied by one spinal nerve, but by more than one peripheral nerve. Peripheral nerve lesions manifest more severe muscle atrophy and weakness in muscles supplied solely by the peripheral nerve.

ACUTE PERIPHERAL NERVE INJURIES

▶ General Considerations

Common etiologics of acute peripheral nerve injury include penetrating trauma, blunt trauma, traction, fractured bones, or compression from hematomas. Minor peripheral nerve injuries arise from blunt trauma that temporarily compresses or stretches a nerve, but leaves its axons intact (neurapraxia). In such cases, axonal transport may be temporarily impaired, but Wallerian degeneration, or the death of axons distal to the point of injury, does not occur. These injuries generally recover spontaneously over the course of days to weeks. Slightly more severe injuries may interrupt axons and their myelin sheaths while leaving endoneurium intact (axonotmesis). In these cases, Wallerian degeneration inevitably follows. Axonal regeneration may occur spontaneously, however, guided to areas of previous innervation by intact endoneurial tubes. With this type of injury, there is a good prognosis for spontaneous functional recovery, with axonal regeneration occurring at a rate of about 1 mm/d or 1 inch/mo.

Peripheral nerves may be severed cleanly (neurotmesis), as in the case of iatrogenic scalpel injuries during surgery. If the divided ends of the nerve remain in proximity, regeneration can occur via axonal sprouting from the proximal stump. These axonal sprouts may bridge the gap to the distal stump, propagating through preserved endoneurial tubes at a rate of 1 mm/d. Severe crush injuries may create internal damage to a peripheral nerve without completely transecting it. Such injuries disrupt axons and their endoneurium and disturb the organization of fascicles within the nerve. In these cases, fibrous scar tissue may form within the macerated nerve which can block the regeneration of axonal sprouts. A tangle of axonal sprouts contained in fibrous scar tissue is called a neuroma. Neuroma formation acts as a barrier to spontaneous peripheral nerve regeneration.

▶ Clinical Findings

A careful clinical history and a meticulous neurological examination are paramount in determining which peripheral nerves have been injured and the type of injury present. The type of trauma will generally suggest whether or not the nerve is in continuity. A penetrating injury with a sharp object, such as a knife, suggests a clean transection that is amenable to immediate surgical repair. Nonpenetrating trauma or a stretch injury is more suggestive of nerve continuity.

Determine the timing of motor and sensory deficits may also aid in the assessment of the nerve injury. For example, in the setting of a penetrating sharp injury, an immediate deficit at the time of the injury would suggest direct involvement of the peripheral. However, a delayed deficit would suggest an enlarging adjacent lesion such as a hematoma or pseudoaneurysm.

The physical examination includes inspection, observation, evaluation of the relevant vasculature, range of motion assessment, and neurological examination. A laceration, fracture, or bruising/abrasions may suggest the site of an underlying nerve injury. A Horner's sign (ptosis, meiosis, anhydrosis) is suggestive of a proximal T1/lower trunk brachial plexus lesion. An impaired range of motion can make assessment of strength difficult to evaluate accurately. An elevated hemidiaphragm is suggestive of a phrenic nerve injury.

The sensory and motor findings associated with acute peripheral nerve injury vary widely, depending on which particular nerve is injured. Pain may also be a symptom, but it usually develops in a delayed fashion. Pain can occur as a result of neuroma formation, where it is often associated with a tender lump in the area of injury. Neurogenic pain may also develop because of a disturbance in the processing of pain signals. This type of pain, when associated with autonomic hyperfunction, is referred to as complex region pain syndrome (formally known as causalgia or reflex sympathetic dystrophy); it is notoriously difficult to treat. When neurogenic pain is associated with nerve root avulsion it is known as deafferentation pain. Deafferentation pain often responds well to surgical intervention via dorsal root entry zone ablation.

In the diagnosis of acute peripheral nerve injury, EMG and nerve conduction studies are generally not useful until at least three weeks after injury. Nevertheless, it is important to obtain baseline electrodiagnostic studies as they are important for monitoring recovery. In the case of brachial plexus injury, it is useful to obtain an MRI scan or CT myelogram to look for pseudomeningocoeles in the vicinity of the nerve roots, which would indicate nerve root avulsion.

Certain peripheral nerve injuries are associated with traumatic fractures of specific bones. For example, the radial nerve is particularly vulnerable to injury from fractures of the humerus. Traumatic injuries of the radial nerve classically occur with fractures of the shaft of the humerus, at the level of the spiral groove. Such injuries result in weakness of wrist extension, finger extension, and thumb extension, as well as numbness over the radial aspect of the dorsal surface of the hand. In this type of injury, elbow extension is not affected, since muscular branches to the triceps are given off proximal to the spiral groove.

Trauma to the brachial plexus can cause a wide array of neurological signs and symptoms. Clinical manifestations are determined by the location of the lesion within the brachial plexus as well as the severity of the injury. Erb-Duchenne palsy is a well-described condition involving injury primarily to the upper trunk of the brachial plexus (derived from C5 and C6 nerve roots). It typically results from a stretch injury such as traction on the arm at the time of birth, or a fall that forcefully separates the head from the shoulder. The resulting deficits to the deltoid, biceps, rhomboids, brachioradialis, supraspinatus, and infraspinatus, leave the arm hanging to the side, internally rotated and extended at the elbow. This posture is often called the "waiter's tip position."

▶ Differential Diagnosis

In acute trauma, when unilateral limb findings are present, it is important to differentiate acute radiculopathy from peripheral nerve injury. A thorough neurological exam is critical. Several general principles should be considered. Radiculopathy is often accompanied by neck or back pain, which tends to radiate down an arm or a leg. Also, the sensory findings of radiculopathy tend to be blurred, reflecting the overlapping nature of dermatomes, while sensory findings in peripheral nerve injuries are sharply demarcated. Weakness from radiculopathy occurs in muscles innervated by one spinal nerve, but by more than one peripheral nerve. Thus, it is often only partial weakness, since nearly all muscles are innervated by more than one spinal nerve.

One crucial task in diagnosing acute peripheral nerve trauma is to rule out ongoing neural compression. Acute trauma to a peripheral nerve usually results in maximal deficits at the time of injury. A peripheral nerve deficit that progresses should raise a red flag and initiate further workup. Immediate surgical exploration should be considered in order to address compressive lesions such as expanding hematomas or growing traumatic pseudoaneurysms. Sources of ongoing neurologic compression should be removed as soon as possible.

▶ Treatment and Prognosis

Sharp nerve transections with clean ends (knife wounds, for example) should be repaired within three days. The repair should be performed in an end-to-end fashion, with no tension across the repair site. Transections from penetrating trauma that do not have clean edges or where significant tissue loss is present, should be repaired in a delayed fashion. During exploration of the wound, transected nerve stumps should be identified and tagged. The tagged nerves ends should be attached to fascia to reduce the possibility of retraction. After three weeks, the lesion should be reexplored and the injured nerve repaired. At that time, areas of axonal damage and neuroma formation are easier to visualize.

Better visualization of damaged axons reduces the possibility of subsequent neuroma formation at the site of repair.

In the case of nonpenetrating injury, where stretch or temporary compression is the likely etiology of the problem, recovery often occurs spontaneously, without the need for surgery. In these cases, nonoperative management with serial neurological examinations, including electrophysiologic testing, should be the initial treatment modality. If, after three months, there is no sign of clinical recovery, the injured nerve should be explored. Intraoperative electrophysiologic nerve mapping should be performed to determine if there is conduction across the site of injury. If there is no conduction of evoked potentials, the neuroma should be resected. The stubs should be trimmed and brought together primarily if it can be done without creating tension. If primary anastamoses of the two nerve ends would result in tension across the repair, then a nerve graft should be employed (usually the sural nerve). If intraoperative stimulation reveals conduction across an area of injury, than the nerve should be left intact and allowed to regenerate on its own. A well-known mnemonic for remembering the appropriate timing of operative repair for traumatic nerve injuries is "the rule of threes": three days for a sharp transection, three weeks for a open ragged transection, and three months for a closed stretch injury.

Peripheral nerve repair is generally performed under the microscope using 8-0 or 9-0 suture for coaptation. Many surgeons now use tissue glue, rather than suture, to coapt the nerve endings. In the case of nerve root avulsions, which cannot be repaired directly, nerve-transfer procedures may be employed, such as coapting a fascicle from an intact ulnar nerve to a nonfunctioning musculocutaneous nerve in order to restore elbow flexion.

Prognosis for recovery depends on the type of injury as well as the treatment. Axonal regeneration occurs at a rate of one inch per month, proximally to distally. Thus, clinical recovery may proceed slowly. Maximal recovery occurs over the course of approximately one to two years. Rehabilitation and physical therapy is important for avoiding the development of muscle contractures that may limit mobility when nerve function has returned. Tendon transfers may be of assistance if neural function does not completely recover.

PERIPHERAL ENTRAPMENT NEUROPATHIES

▶ General Considerations

Peripheral nerves are subjected to chronic mechanical forces, such as compression, stretching, and friction. These forces, when applied over time, may lead to peripheral nerve entrapment syndromes, such as carpal tunnel syndrome, or ulnar nerve entrapment. Both static and dynamic factors may contribute to chronic peripheral nerve injury. Static factors include musculotendinous anomalies or inflexible anatomic tunnels that compress peripheral nerves. Dynamic factors include mobile joints, muscular contraction, or nerve mobility that leads to stretching of a peripheral nerve or increased friction along its course during movement. Peripheral entrapment neuropathies occur more frequently in upper rather than lower limbs, probably because of the greater mobility of the arms.

▶ Clinical Findings

Entrapment neuropathies are characterized by weakened muscles as well as sensory disturbances in the distribution of a single peripheral nerve. In general, any given individual muscle is supplied by one peripheral nerve. Thus, entrapment of a peripheral nerve can lead to severe motor findings in a muscle it innervates. Muscle atrophy and fasciculations are not uncommon in peripheral nerve entrapment. Marked atrophy on clinical examination should raise the surgeon's suspicion that a peripheral nerve lesion is present. Sensory complaints associated with entrapment neuropathy generally include parasthesias, rather than pain, in the distribution of the involved nerve. Percussion over the nerve may result in an electric sensation radiating along the nerve and its territory. In the clinical setting, this is known as Tinel's sign. Electrodiagnostic testing is also useful in the diagnosis of peripheral nerve entrapment. The finding of a nerve conduction delay at the site of compression on nerve conduction studies is common to all compression neuropathies.

The most common peripheral nerve entrapment syndrome is median nerve entrapment at the wrist. This condition generally arises from compression of the median nerve by the transverse carpal ligament, and is therefore referred to as carpal tunnel syndrome. Carpal tunnel syndrome occurs with higher frequency in patients with conditions leading to connective tissue thickening: rheumatoid arthritis, acromegaly, hypothyroidism, pregnancy, and may be related to repetitive hand or wrist movements. Common presenting symptoms include dysesthetic pain in the hands that is worse at night, often awaking the patient from sleep. This occurs because many people sleep with flexed wrists, a position which exacerbates median nerve compression at the wrist. The pain sometimes radiates upward, into the forearm. Patients also complain of numbness on the palmer side of the hand as well as the first three to three and a half digits, including the thumb. When the ring finger is involved, the sensory disturbance "splits" the finger, involving the radial side of the digit only. The intrinsic hand muscles innervated by the median nerve in the hand are sometimes referred to as the "LOAF" muscles, stemming from a commonly used mnemonic device: Lumbricals (first and second only), Opponens pollicus, Abductor pollicis brevis, and Flexor pollicis brevis. Patients with carpal tunnel syndrome may complain of decreased grip strength, or difficulty grasping small objects. Atrophy of the abductor pollicus brevis, at

the lateral base of the thumb may be present. There is often a positive Tinel's sign at the wrist. Phalen's test is a clinical maneuver that is sometimes used in the diagnosis of carpal tunnel syndrome. The patient's wrists are held in forced flexion for at least thirty seconds. The test is considered positive if this maneuver produces symptoms of median neuropathy in the hand.

Ulnar nerve entrapment is the second most common peripheral nerve entrapment syndrome, behind carpal tunnel syndrome. The most common site of ulnar nerve entrapment is at the elbow. Patients typically present with upper extremity pain that localizes to the medial aspect of the elbow. Paresthesias and numbness of the small finger and the ulnar half of the ring finger are also common. A Tinel's sign is often present at the medial aspect of the elbow: tapping the patient over this area sends electric sensations into the fourth and fifth digits. The ulnar nerve innervates most of the intrinsic hand muscles, including the adductor pollicis, the first dorsal interosseous, and the hypothenar muscles. Patients complain of hand weakness, leading to reduced grip strength and pinch strength. They complain of dropping things, or of trouble opening jars. Atrophy of hand intrinsic muscles may be marked, particularly the first dorsal interosseous and the muscles of the hypothenar eminence. When nerve dysfunction is severe, the hand may take on a "claw hand" appearance. The patient may also exhibit a Froment sign: when asked to hold a piece of paper between the thumb and index finger, the distal interphalangeal joint will flex because the patient fires the flexor pollicis longus muscle, innervated by the median nerve, to compensate for lack of abductor pollicis function.

▶ Differential Diagnosis

The differential diagnosis for peripheral nerve dysfunction includes neuropathies of infectious origin (both bacterial and viral), hereditary conditions (such as Charcot–Marie–Tooth disease), neuropathy associated with nutritional deficiency (such as vitamin B_{12} deficiency), metabolic or endocrinologic conditions (such as diabetes), inflammatory or immune-mediated conditions (such as polyarteritis nodosa), and toxic conditions (such as lead poisoning.) When more than one peripheral nerve is involved, the surgeon should be wary of the diagnosis of generalized neuropathy, which is typically symmetrical and bilateral. Decreased amplitude on electrodiagnostic studies (which suggests axonal loss) is characteristic of neuropathy of hereditary or metabolic origin. Peripheral nerve entrapment, on the other hand, causes damage to the myelin surrounding an axon, thereby slowing conduction velocity but not affecting amplitude.

Chronic cervical or lumbar radiculopathy must also be ruled out. Several features that separate radiculopathy from peripheral nerve dysfunction were outlined in the section on acute peripheral nerve injuries. It is important to recognize that sensory changes that "split" the ring finger suggest ulnar nerve dysfunction, rather than C8 radiculopathy.

Treatment and Prognosis

Surgical management of peripheral nerve entrapment generally involves decompressing the involved nerve. In the case of carpal tunnel syndrome, the transverse carpal ligament is divided, thus relieving compression on the median nerve as it passes from the wrist into the hand. In the case of ulnar neuropathy, simply freeing the nerve from surrounding scar tissue or hypertrophied connective tissue (external neurolysis) is usually sufficient.

Surgical management of peripheral nerve entrapment should be strongly considered when patients present with significant motor weakness or muscle atrophy. Surgical intervention should also be considered when patients fail to improve with medical treatments. Nonoperative management strategies include avoidance of repetitive activities that precipitate symptoms, or the use of immobilization braces that hold joints in positions that avoid compression.

Carpal tunnel release results in excellent relief of symptoms in 80% of patients and partial relief in another 10%. Similar results are observed for surgical management of ulnar neuropathy.

PERIPHERAL NERVE TUMORS

General Considerations

Peripheral nerve tumors can be divided into non-neoplastic masses, benign masses, and malignant masses. The non-neoplastic masses include traumatic neuromas, morton neuromas, and nerve sheath ganglion cysts. Benign masses include neurofibromas, schwannomas (also know as neurilemmoma), perineuriomas, lipofibromatous hamartoma (also know as neural fibrolipoma), nerve sheath myxoma, and finally granular cell tumors. Malignant masses include the malignant peripheral nerve sheath tumor (MPNST).

Neurofibromas can be subdivided into solitary, diffuse, and plexiform varieties. The solitary neurofibroma is the most common benign peripheral nerve tumor. Axons are incorporated within the neurofibroma along with Schwann cells, collagen matrix, perineurial cells, and fibroblasts. Because the axons are intermixed within the tumor, the tumor cannot be excised without resecting a portion of the involved nerve. Diffuse neurofibromas and plexiform neurofibromas are less common than the solitary variety. The diffuse neurofibroma typically involves the skin and subcutaneous tissues. Plexiform neurofibromas are large, irregular expansions of nerves ranging from small cutaneous nerves to large trunks. Neurofibromas are commonly found in patients with neurofibromatosis Type 1 (NF1/von Recklinghausen's disease).

Schwannomas are slowly growing lesions made up of Schwann cells in a collagen matrix. Differentiating schwannomas from neurofibromas is that the nerve fascicles run alongside the tumor, rather than through the tumor as in neurofibromas. Schwannomas are the second most common peripheral nerve tumor. Generally, only mild neurologic deficits occur, and operative resection can be considered in the setting of pain, paresthesias, or weakness in the distribution of the nerve.

MPNST is the most common malignant peripheral nerve tumor. Nearly two-thirds arise from neurofibromas in the setting of NF1. The remainder arise either de novo or in patients with history of prior external beam radiation.

Clinical Findings

The symptoms of peripheral nerve tumors are generally related to the nerve involved and include weakness, numbness, paresthesias, and pain. MRI with gadolinium contrast can be useful in imaging the tumors.

Differential Diagnosis

The differential diagnosis of peripheral nerve tumors include entrapment neuropathies, non-neoplastic masses, radiculopathies, and neuropathies associated with infection, malnutrition, metabolic, endocrinologic, inflammatory, immune-mediated, and toxic conditions. Generally, a symptomatic peripheral nerve tumor will be palpable. Further, the peripheral nerve tumor can occur anywhere along the course of the nerve, whereas entrapment neuropathies typically occur in defined locations and the various other neuropathies listed are often diffuse processes. Finally, a radiculopathy will be symptomatic in the distribution of the nerve root, likely involving several peripheral nerves.

Treatment & Prognosis

Schwannomas can generally be resected without any neurologic deficit since the nerve fascicles run alongside the tumor. The fascicles can generally be dissected free. Operative resection is curative. Neurofibromas generally cannot be resected without neurologic deficit since the axons run within the substance of the tumor. Indications for surgical resection of solitary neurofibromas are large tumor mass, accelerated growth, neurologic deficit, and pain. Plexiform neurofibromas (excluding superficial ones) can rarely be totally resected and should generally be followed.

Generally, the prognosis for benign peripheral nerve sheath tumors is very good with improvement in pain, weakness, and paresthesias noted after resection of solitary lesions. MPNST require aggressive surgical treatment. The expected 5 year survival is 15%-20% in patients with NF-1 and 56% in patients with de novo disease.

O'Brien M on behalf of the Guarantors of Brain: Aids to the Examination of the Peripheral Nervous System. 5th Ed. Edinburgh: Saunders Elsevier; 2010.

Song JW, Waljee JF, Burns PB, et al: An outcome study for ulnar neuropathy at the elbow: a multicenter study by the surgery for ulnar nerve (SUN) study group. *Neurosurgery* 2013;72(6):971-981.

▼ BRAIN TUMORS

Daniel Orringer, MD Shawn Hervey-Jumper, MD

▶ Clinical Presentation

Whenever possible, the evaluation of a brain tumor patient begins with a detailed history focusing on the most common symptoms observed in patients bearing intracranial mass lesions. Headaches are the most common symptom in brain tumor patients, occurring in at least 50% of patients at some point. Classically, brain tumor patients present with headaches that are worse upon waking in the morning and may often be severe enough to wake a patient from sleep. This type of headache is thought to occur as a result of temporary increases in intracranial pressure caused by physiologic elevations in PCO_2 common during sleep. Normally, transient increases in PCO_2 that occur during sleep do not result in headache. However, in the brain tumor patient, during sleep, the combination of elevated intracranial pressure due to mass effect from the presence of the tumor and cerebral vasodilation due to increased PCO_2, causes an additive increases in intracranial pressure, ultimately resulting in headache. Headaches related to elevated intracranial pressure can also occur throughout the day as a result of maneuvers that raise intracranial pressure, such as straining, coughing, or bending over.

More commonly, headaches seen in brain tumor patients are not related to elevations in intracranial pressure. Headaches typically caused by brain tumors occur as the neoplastic process involves intracranial structures containing pain fibers. Unlike the brain parenchyma, the dura is richly innervated with pain fibers and is likely the most common source of headaches in brain tumor patients. Dural irritation is also involved in the pathogenesis of other types of headaches. This pathophysiologic overlap may explain the clinical observation that brain tumor-associated headaches may lack any distinguishing characteristics. Brain tumor patients often describe their headaches as deep and aching but these features are highly variable. These may have been previously misdiagnosed as sinus, tension, or migraine headaches. Headaches in brain tumor patients may also be due to visual difficulties in the setting of direct or indirect (through elevated intracranial pressure) tumor effects on the optic pathways and oculomotor nerves.

A number of attributes of the headaches associated with brain tumors can provide useful diagnostic information.

First, brain tumors in patients who present with headaches are more likely to be found in noneloquent or functionally silent areas of the central nervous system. Second, headaches occur more frequently in patients with rapidly growing brain tumors. Rapidly growing brain tumors commonly cause severe headaches from meningeal irritation, hemorrhage within the tumor, and/or obstructive hydrocephalus. Obstructive hydrocephalus is a neurosurgical emergency that must be considered in any brain tumor patient presenting with the acute onset of severe headache. In addition, the location of headaches in brain tumor patients commonly provides localizing information. Brain tumors are usually located ipsilateral to the most severe pain.

Seizures are another common presenting finding in patients with brain tumors. Interestingly, seizures are more common with low-grade gliomas than high-grade gliomas. The incidence of seizures in patients with low-grade glioma is estimated as high as 85%. Seizures are the initial presenting symptom in 9% of patients with metastatic brain tumors and 18% of patients with high-grade glioma. Moreover, 25%-50% of all patients with brain tumors experience seizures at some point in their disease course. While seizures associated with brain tumors can be disabling, they can also lead to early diagnosis, and, therefore early treatment.

The nature of seizure activity may hold diagnostic significance. Subcortical and cortical tumors are more likely to cause seizures than those of deeper structures. Focal seizures with primarily motor phenomena, such as tonic-clonic seizures, often occur as a result of involvement of tumor with the primary motor cortex within the frontal lobe. Temporal tumors resulting in temporal lobe seizures typically have variable manifestations that may make localization difficult. Focal seizures due to parietal lesions may present with language disturbance, somatosensory abnormalities, or vestibular symptoms. Focal seizures caused by brain tumors may be secondarily generalized and may ultimately affect multiple cortical regions, causing variable symptomatology. Status epilepticus also can occur as a presentation of brain tumors.

Syncope, another common presentation of brain tumor, must be distinguished from seizure. There are multiple pathophysiologic mechanisms underlying syncope in brain tumor patients. In patients with tumor burden resulting in chronically elevated intracranial pressure and decreased brain compliance, a sudden additional rise in intracranial pressure may compromise cerebral blood flow, resulting in syncope. Transient increases in intracranial pressure that may result from sneezing, coughing, vomiting, or straining are tolerated in patients with normal physiology but may cause syncope in brain tumor patients. Syncope caused by transient increases in intracranial pressure may represent impending herniation and requires urgent neurosurgical attention.

In addition, there are a number of symptoms that commonly present in association with headache, seizure, or syncope. Nausea and vomiting are present at the initial encounter with at least 40% of patients with brain tumors. Nausea and vomiting may be caused by elevations in intracranial pressure and/or direct tumor involvement of the area postrema in the dorsal surface of the fourth ventricle.

Cognitive decline is common especially in the elderly patient and is often misdiagnosed as Alzheimer's disease. Cognitive decline may easily be confused with depression and is thought to result from generalized fatigue, loss of appetite, and interest in everyday activities. Frontal tumors frontal masses are commonly associated with cognitive decline. Frontal masses, especially those affecting both frontal lobes may also result in apraxia and urinary retention.

A key component of the interview of the brain tumor patient the past medical and family history. The incidence of central nervous system metastases is increasing due to improved survival in patients with the most common types of solid organ cancers. A family history of brain tumors may suggest a familial cancer syndrome. Among the most common familial syndromes predisposing to brain tumor occurrence include von Hippel–Lindau syndrome, tuberous sclerosis, neurofibromatosis 1 and 2, Turcot syndrome (familial adenomatous polyposis), and Lynch syndrome (hereditary nonpolyposis colorectal cancer).

▶ Physical Findings

Physical findings are highly variable depending on tumor location and extent of disease. Nonspecific physical findings can occur with elevated intracranial pressure including papilledema (edema of the head of the optic nerve associated with engorgement of retinal veins) and oculomotor palsy (due to uncal herniation). However, the most helpful physical findings are those that assist in localizing the lesion (Table 36–5). Focal neurologic signs such as muscle weakness are common and when caused by peritumoral edema may be rapidly reversible with the administration of steroids.

Aphasia suggests involvement with cortical language centers located in the dominant frontal or parietal lobe. Aphasic patients may be misdiagnosed with dementia or psychiatric disorders. The diagnosis of brain tumor should be considered in, patients without psychiatric history who develop a psychiatric disorder.

▶ Imaging

Radiographic imaging is performed to confirm the clinical diagnosis of brain tumor. Imaging provides information regarding localization, tumor type and the effect of a lesion on surrounding structures. Due to its wide availability, speed, and affordability, noncontrast CT is commonly the initial screening test for patients with brain tumors. CT is also the test of choice for evaluating the extent of tumor invasion into adjacent bony structures. CT angiography can

Table 36–5. Brain tumor-localizing signs and symptoms.

Location	Sign(s)
Frontal lobe[a]	Impaired intellectual function
	Language impairment,[b] specifically abulia
	Impaired gait
	Personality changes
	Hemiparesis[c]
Dominant temporal lobe	Aphasia
	Impaired auditory discrimination
	Memory loss
	Contralateral superior quadrantanopia
Nondominant temporal lobe	Seizures
	Visual, auditory, olfactory hallucinations
	Contralateral superior quadrantanopia
Uncus	CN III palsy
Parietal lobe	Impaired sensory perception
	Contralateral inferior quadrantanopia
	Aphasia
	Anosoagnosia[d]
Occipital lobe	Visual deficits
Posterior fossa	Posterior hcadahcc
	Neck stiffness
	Opisthotonos
Brainstem	Cranial nerve palsies
	Long-tract signs
Cerebellopontine angle	Unilateral hearing loss
	Tinnitus
	Vertigo
	Facial palsy
	Facial anesthesia
	Cerebellar signs
Sellar region	Endocrine abnormalities
	Bitemporal hemianopsia
	CN III palsy
Pineal region	Parinaud syndrome:
	Upgaze palsy
	Ptosis
	Loss of pupillary light reflex
	Retraction-convergence nystagmus
Meningeal infiltration	Cranial nerve palsies
	Diffuse headache
	Meningeal reaction

[a]usually occurs only if both frontal lobes involved.
[b]occurs only when dominant hemisphere is involved.
[c]when motor cortex is involved.
[d]when nondominant temporal lobe is involved.

be helpful in evaluating blood supply to tumors or in evaluating the relationship of blood vessels to the tumor.

Whenever possible MRI of the brain with and without gadolinium-based contrast is performed in the brain tumor patient. Traditional morphologic MRI is performed to assess tumor location, size, cellularity, associated cystic components, associated edema or hemorrhage, necrosis, margins, and invasion into surrounding structures, vascularity, and enhancement. Morphologic data can be used to estimate the WHO grade and suggest the tissue diagnosis of a lesion. However, the gold standard for brain tumor diagnosis remains tissue histology. High-quality contrast MRI images are vital for defining the relationship of tumor tissue to eloquent cortical areas and, consequently an operative plan. In addition, MRI images can be reconstructed to create three-dimensional models that can be used during surgery.

Metabolic MRI or magnetic resonance spectroscopy (MRS) can be used to supplement information obtained from traditional morphologic MRI. MRS is used to compare the small molecule content of tumor tissue and normal surrounding brain tissue. MRS improves the accuracy of brain tumor diagnosis by differentiating brain tumors from lesions that appear similar on routine MRI such as abscesses. In addition MRS detects subtle changes in small molecule content that correlate with tumor grade. In treated brain tumors, MRS enables differentiation between radiation necrosis and residual tumor.

A number of alternative magnetic resonance techniques have clinical application in the imaging of brain tumors. These can enable clinicians to make more accurate preoperative diagnoses and provide information about interaction of tumor tissue with adjacent functional cortical structures. Diffusion MRI characterizes brain tumors based on measurement of molecular mobility and is useful in differentiating tumors from similar-appearing lesions, estimating cellularity, and measuring response to treatment. Perfusion MRI is useful for evaluating tumor angiogenesis, endothelial permeability, and response to treatment. Functional MRI maps functional cortical areas and can be used to create an operative corridor or plan for resection that minimizes risk to eloquent surrounding structures. Similarly diffusion tensor imaging defines the integrity of white matter tracts surrounding a tumor and is commonly used in the planning of both surgical and radiation therapy.

Traditional catheter-based cerebral angiography has both historical and contemporary significance in brain tumor imaging. Cerebral angiography was once used to infer tumor location and morphology by measuring displacement of blood vessels by a tumor. Currently, angiography is used in the context of highly vascular lesions, including some meningiomas and hemangiomas, for preoperative embolization. Embolization of vascular tumors diminishes operative risk and difficulty.

▶ Tumor Types

A. Gliomas

Fifty percent of newly diagnosed brain tumors are primary tumors of glial origin (astrocytes and oligodendrocytes). Glial tumors are stratified in a scale of increasing aggressiveness. Grades one and two are classified as low-grade gliomas whereas, grades three and four are high grade. High-grade gliomas are faster growing and consequently carry a worse prognosis than low-grade gliomas.

Low-Grade Gliomas: Astrocytes, Oligodendrogliomas, and Mixed Gliomas—Approximately 26% of newly diagnosed glial tumors are astrocytomas and 2% are oligodendrogliomas. Between 1500 and 1800 new low-grade gliomas are diagnosed in the United States each year. WHO grade 1 gliomas are reserved for pilocytic tumors. Pilocytic astrocytomas represent 5.2% of all primary intracranial tumors in adults and 20% of all brain tumors in children younger than 15 years. WHO grade 2 lesions are diagnosed based on their infiltration and tendency to progress to higher grade lesions over time. The most common subtypes of low-grade gliomas include juvenile astrocytomas, diffuse astrocytomas, oligodendrogliomas (representing 6.5%), and mixed gliomas.

The etiology of low-grade gliomas is unknown. Genetic studies suggest that mutation or deletion of the tumor suppressor gene TP53 plays a role in the tumorigenesis of low-grade gliomas. Known oncogenic signaling pathways have consequences on tumor metabolism promoting a cellular switch to aerobic glycolysis. Isocitrate dehydrogenase 1 and 2 (IDH 1 and 2) catalyze the decarboxyation of isocitrate into alpha ketoglutarate. IDH1 and IDH2 mutations are found in 40% glioma (70% of low grade, 50% of grade III, and 5%-10% of primary glioblastoma). The impact of these mutations on low-grade diffuse gliomas remains unclear; however, they offer a robust and independent survival benefit in all tumor grades.

Low-grade astrocytomas occur with peak incidence in the young adult population (most commonly in 20-40s). They originate in white matter regions within the CNS, grow slowly and distort surrounding brain structures. Histologically, there is a modest increase in cellularity, disruption of the normal orderly pattern of glial cells, and elongated nuclei. There is no endothelial proliferation or tissue necrosis. Three histologic subtypes of low-grade astrocytomas include fibrillary, gemistocytic, and protoplasmic.

Oligodendrogliomas occur predominantly within the gray matter of the cerebral hemispheres, are well-circumscribed, calcified, and have a slight predominance for the frontal lobes. Like astrocytomas, they occur predominantly in younger patients with most frequent diagnosis in the third decade of life. Histologically, oligodendrogliomas are characterized by uniform cell density and round nuclei with

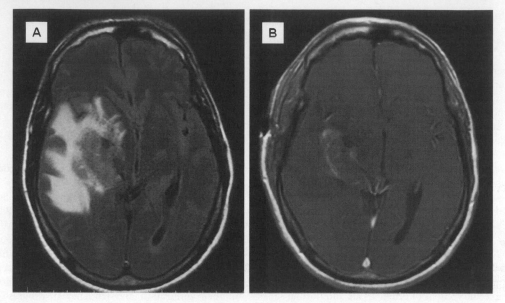

▲ **Figure 36–13.** Magnetic resonance imaging of a deep right temporal mass proven to be a high-grade glioma. (A) FLAIR imaging demonstrating a mass with significant surrounding white matter edema. (B) T1-weighted contrast enchanced image demonstrating smaller enhancing portion of the mass.

perinuclear halos appearing as a classic "fried egg" appearance. Oligodendrogliomas rarely show a mutation in *TP53*. In 1994 a codeletion in the long arm of chromosome 1p36 and the short arm of chromosome 19q13 was shown to predict chemosensitivity and better prognosis.

Radiographically, low-grade gliomas are iso- or hypodense to brain on CT scan and do not enhance with contrast. Calcification is common in oligodendrogliomas. On MRI, low-grade glioma are iso- to hypointense on T1-weighted imaging (T1WI) and typically hyperintense on T2-weighted imaging (T2WI) and are not contrast-enhancing.

High-Grade Gliomas—The term malignant glioma includes anaplastic astrocytoma (AA), glioblastoma multiforme (GBM), gliosarcoma, and malignant oligodendroglioma (Figure 36–13). There is wide difference in the prognosis, aggressiveness, and response to therapy between the different tumors in this group.

Malignant astrocytoma, the most common type of adult brain tumor, makes up 15% of all intracranial tumors and 50%-60% of primary brain tumors. While relatively rare, malignant astrocytoma is the fourth most common cause of cancer-related deaths. The incidence of AAs and GBM increases with increasing age. There is little difference in incidence from nation to nation, however, in the United States these tumors are less common among Africans and African Americans.

The majority of malignant gliomas occur sporadically. However, patients with the autosomal recessively inherited, Turcot syndrome have a high rate of malignant glioma (usually medulloblastomas and astrocytomas) in combination with familial adenomatous polyposis. Similarly, patients with tuberous sclerosis and neurofibromatosis type 1 and 2 often develop brain tumors including gliomas.

The most significantly mutated genes in glioblastoma include TP53 (seen in 42% of patients), PTEN (seen in 33%), neurofibromatosis 1 (NF1) (21%), EGFR (18%), PIK3R1 (10%), and PIK3CA (7%). Mutations of *TP53* have been identified in the autosomally dominantly inherited Li–Fraumeni syndrome, which results in malignant gliomas in addition to tumors involving breast, blood, bone, and the adrenal cortex. It has recently been suggested that a subpopulation of cells with stem-like properties (cancer stem cells) are present in glioblastoma offering resistance to chemotherapy and radiation.

A hallmark of malignant gliomas is the propensity to invade and migrate along white matter tracts. Invasion increases with increased grade and growth factors such as epidermal growth factor increase this invasion. Autopsy studies show that malignant glioma cells spread through the CSF and extend into and beyond areas on MRI with T2 signal change. Histologically, grade 3 gliomas show mitotic activity and nuclear atypia but no necrosis, while grade 4 tumors have nuclear atypia, mitoses, endothelial proliferation, and areas of necrosis. The radiologic hallmarks of GBM are ring enhancement and areas of central necrosis detected on CT and MRI.

Gangliogliomas—Gangliogliomas are rare tumors found most commonly in patients between the ages of 15 and 20 with a history of seizures. They represent 1% of CNS neoplasms in adults, 7.6% in children. They can be found in any region of the central nervous system, but seem to occur predominantly in the temporal lobes. Gangliogliomas are distinguished histologically from pure gliomas by their mixture of neuronal and glial elements. Calcification is common. Macroscopically, they may appear solid or cystic. They are generally well-circumscribed, cystic tumors that may display a mural nodule projecting into the cyst cavity. Imaging characteristics vary in their enhancement and signal qualities on MRI. Lesions can exhibit cystic or solid components or a combination of both. Tumor calcification is a common imaging feature. Gangliogliomas are typically benign WHO I or II tumors with indolent behavior offering a 93%-98% 5-year survival. Five percent of gangliogliomas, however, are aggressive anaplastic or malignant gangliogliomas WHO grade III-IV based on the presence of increased cellularity, microvascular proliferation, and areas of necrosis.

Brainstem Gliomas—Brainstem gliomas represent 10%-20% of all CNS tumors in children. Brainstem gliomas are a heterogeneous group with diverse clinical presentations, prognoses, and patterns of growth. They are described as focal, diffuse, cervicomedullary, and dorsally exophytic. Focal tumors are less than 2 cm in size with a well-circumscribed appearance on MRI and no surrounding edema. They are most prevalent in the midbrain and medulla, but can occur at any level in the brainstem. These children typically present with focal cranial nerve deficits and contralateral hemiparesis. Diffuse tumors (diffuse intrinsic pontine gliomas) account for the majority of brainstem gliomas (80%) and commonly arise in the pons. These patients typically present with bilateral cranial nerve deficits, ataxia, and long tract signs. Cervicomedullary brainstem gliomas take their origin from the upper cervical cord and extend rostrally into the cervicomedullary junction and often present with lower cranial nerve deficits and long tract signs. Dorsal exophytic tumors account for 20% of brainstem gliomas and arise from the floor of the fourth ventricle. They are typically sharply delineated from surrounding structures. These patients present with cranial nerve deficits, elevated intracranial pressure, and failure to thrive.

MRI scan has allowed for the recognition of the four classes of brainstem glioma. Even though MRI contrast signal poorly correlates with histologic grade, MRI provides adequate anatomic visualization. Focal tumors are classically well circumscribed and small without infiltration or a significant amount of surrounding edema. Dorsal exophytic tumors arise in the floor of the fourth ventricle and are

typically hypointense on T1-weighted imaging, hyperintense on T2-weighted imaging, and homogenously enhance with gadalinium contrast. Diffuse brainstem tumors are hypointense on T1-weighted images and hyperintense on T2 sequences. Because MRI characteristics for diffuse tumors are highly specific an accurate diagnosis can be made in the majority of cases. Recent literature has shown that the mortality associated with biopsy of brainstem tumors may have been modestly exaggerated. Biopsy is therefore considered in cases of abnormal clinical presentation or imaging.

B. Primitive Neuroectodermal Tumors

Primitive neuroectodermal tumors (PNET) are thought to originate in cells from primitive neural crest. PNET includes medulloblastomas, pinealoblastomas, ependymoblastomas, esthesioneuroblastomas, and neuroblastomas. PNET are more common in children than adults. Medulloblastomas are PNETs within the posterior fossa and account for 20% of childhood brain tumors and 1% of all adult tumors. Medulloblastomas are the most common primary central nervous system tumor in children younger than 18 years old.

Several syndromes result in an increased incidence of medulloblastomas, including tuberous sclerosis, neurofibromatosis, Gorlin syndrome, and Turcot syndrome. Loss of portions of chromosome 17 either through deletions or unbalanced translocation is associated with over 50% of medulloblastomas. Over the past decade, transcriptional profiling of medulloblastomas revealed the existence of 4 distinct subgroups, WNT, SHH, Group 3, and Group 4. WNT medulloblastomas have a classic histology, WNT gene expression signature, and the best prognosis with more than 95% in 5 years. These patients tend to be the least common (10% of cases) and are rarely metastatic. SHH-driven medulloblastomas exhibit a desmoplastic histology (although occasionally large cell or anaplastic are seen). Patients SHH tumors represent an intermediate prognosis with survival ranging from 60% to 80%. Group 3 medulloblastoma have the worst prognosis with 50% metastatic at the time of diagnosis. These tumors exhibit aberrant MYC expression with focal high-level amplifications. Group 4 medulloblastomas account for 40% of cases with an intermediate prognosis similar to the SHH subgroup. Group 4 tumors are driven by the oncogenes MYCN and CDK6 (cyclin-dependent kinase 6). Unlike other subgroups group 4 medulloblastoma predominantly affect men and metastases are seen in 30% of cases. These subgroups have reestablished what was previously considered a single tumor entity but are now requiring different therapeutic approaches.

Grossly, medulloblastomas typically occur within the cerebellar vermis and are poorly demarcated, purplish, soft, and friable. Histologically, these tumors are highly cellular, composed of homogenous fields of small, round, blue-cell tumors with hyperchromatic nuclei, minimal cytoplasm, and occasional calcification. Other histologic characteristics of these tumors include varying degrees of neuronal and glial differentiation, Homer Wright rosettes (nuclei surround a clear central area of cell processes indicative of neuroblastic differentiation) are often present and mitotic figures are numerous.

Meduloblastomas are PNET within the posterior fossa. Histologically similar tumors within the pineal gland are pinealoblastomas, and within the supratentorial space are neuroblastomas. Retinoblastomas are histologically similar tumors within the eye, PNET originating from olfactory epithelium are termed *esthesioneuroblastomas*, and intraventricular PNET are ependymoblastomas.

On CT, medulloblastomas are typically hyperdense, homogenously enhancing, and occasionally cystic. Small areas of calcification can be appreciated on CT. Scattered areas of hemorrhage, necrosis, and calcification can occur. On MRI, medullolastomas are isointense or hyopintense to brain on T1WI, hyperintense to brain on T2WI and intensely contrast enhancing. If medulloblastoma is suspected, MRI of the spine is obtained to rule out metastases. Lumbar puncture should be performed with extreme caution because the majority of children have associated obstructive hydrocephalus.

C. Pineal Tumors

The pineal gland is bounded ventrally by the quadrigeminal plate and midbrain tectum, dorsally by the splenium of corpus callosum, rostrally by the posterior aspect of the third ventricle, and caudally by the cerebellar vermis. Tumors in this region are usually found incidentally on MRI and are most common in children, making up 3%-8% of pediatric brain tumors. The pineal region has several diverse cell types including glial cells, arachnoid cells, pineal glandular tissue, ependymal lining, sympathetic nerves, germ cells, and remnants of ectoderm. Tumors within this area can therefore be grouped into 4 categories: germ cell tumors, pineal parenchymal cell tumors, glial cell tumors, and other miscellaneous tumors and cysts. In the pediatric population germinomas and astrocytomas are the most common tumor type. Germ cell tumors and pineal cell tumors occur primarily during childhood. In the adult population, pineal tumors are more commonly gliomas and meningiomas.

Germ cell tumors, ependymomas, and pineal cell tumors can metastasize through the CSF causing myelopathic or radiculopathic symptoms. Pineal tumors typically present with symptoms of increased intracranial pressure from obstructive hydrocephalus, direct brainstem and cerebellar compression and endocrine dysfunction. In addition, Parinaud syndrome (upgaze paralysis, convergence-retraction nystagmus, pseudo-Argyll Robertson pupils, eyelid retraction, and conjugate downgaze in the primary position) is associated with pineal tumors.

MRI is the primary diagnostic imaging modality for pineal tumors, but it does not reliably predict tumor histology. In contrast, tumor markers may be useful in the diagnostic process, to determine response to treatment, or as an indicator of early recurrence. Elevation of serum or CSF alpha-fetoprotein (AFP) or human chorionic gonadotropin (HCG) suggests a germ cell tumor. Mildly elevated AFP suggests the presence of a fetal yolk sac tumor. Marked elevation of AFP suggests endodermal sinus tumors while smaller elevations are suggestive of embryonal cell carcinoma or immature teratoma. HCG is often markedly elevated with choriocarcinomas.

D. Ependymoma

Ependymomas were previously thought to arise from the ependymal cells lining the ventricles and central canal of the spinal cord; however, they have recently been shown that radial glial cells are the cells of origin. They occur in both children and adults and 65% occur within the posterior fossa (most commonly in children). Ependymomas are quite rare representing only 6% of all gliomas in adults. However, they are the third most common brain tumor in children (behind pilocytic astrocytomas and medulloblastomas). Three cases per 100,000 children younger than 15 are diagnosed each year with this tumor type.

The etiology of posterior fossa ependymomas is unknown however significant advancements have been made over the past decade on their biological profile allowing the identification of different molecular subgroups. Group A patients have laterally located tumors and younger patients with more than 50% recurrence rate (independent of extent of surgical resection). Group B patients have a slightly more favorable prognosis and older age at diagnosis. Familial cases have also been identified. As with several other primary CNS tumors, these tumors often have loss of heterozygosity of chromosome 22q, which contains the neurofibromatosis 2 (*NF2*) gene. Patients with neurofibromatosis have an increased incidence of gliomas including ependymomas.

A histologic grading system that correlates with tumor aggressiveness is used to classify ependymomas. Histologically, ependymomas are often characterized by, epithelium-like cells in a rosette pattern, formed by a ring of polygonal cells surrounding a central cavity. Tumors may also exhibit perivascular pseudorosettes, intranuclear inclusions, calcifications, and papillary clusters.

The imaging characteristics of ependymomas are variable, but they are typically isodense to cerebral cortex on noncontrast head CT. Calcifications and cystic components within the tumor are frequent. On MRI the solid portion is typically isointense to gray matter on T1WI and isointense to hyperintense on T2WI.

E. Cerebral Lymphoma

Cerebral lymphoma involving the brain, spinal cord, or ocular structures can occur either primarily or as a metastasis. The source of premalignant lymphocytes is controversial because the CNS lacks lymphoid tissue. CNS lymphoma occurs most commonly in severely immuno-compromised patients where it is commonly associated with Epstein–Barr virus infections. CNS lymphoma represents 1% of intracranial tumors with a steady increase in prevalence over the past 20 years. The increase in CNS lymphoma is likely secondary to the increased number and longer lifespan of patients with acquired immunode-ficiency syndrome (AIDS) and immunosuppression after organ transplantation. Interestingly, the incidence of CNS lymphoma has steadily increased in immunocompetent patients with an increase from 2.5 to 30 cases per 10 million. Deletions of *DKN2A* are frequently reported in CNS lymphoma.

Macroscopically, primary CNS lymphomas occur within the parenchyma, subependyma, or meninges and can be either circumscribed or irregular. Microscopically, they exhibit diffuse perivascular distribution and infiltrate the walls of blood vessels (perivascular cuffing). The tumor cells are similar in histology to systemic non-Hodgkins lymphoma cells. Primary CNS lymphomas are monoclonal B-cell lymphomas of diffuse large cell or large cell immuno-blastic variant. Anti-CD45 antibody staining differentiates CNS lymphoma from other tumor types.

On CT, CNS lymphomas are typically hyper- or isodense to brain with strong contrast enhancement. On MRI, these tumors are usually isointense or hypointense on T1WI, hyperintense on T2WI and display varying degrees of gadalinium enhancement. Low-volume lumbar puncture performed during the workup of CNS lymphoma may reveal high protein, low glucose pleocytosis. While CSF cytology may be diagnostic, stereotactic brain biopsy is often needed for definitive diagnosis.

F. Choroid Plexus Tumors

The most common tumors of the choroid plexus include choroid plexus papillomas. Choroid plexus carcinomas are rare. Choroid plexus papillomas are most prevalent in patients less then 2 years old and account for less than 1% of all intracranial tumors. Presenting symptoms result from elevated intracranial pressure due to hydrocephalus, and mass effect from tumor growth.

G. Meningiomas

Meningiomas are typically benign, slow growing extra-axial tumors arising from the arachnoid cap cells of the meninges (Figure 36–14). They can originate wherever arachnoid is present. They are characterized by either their location, or histopathology, and are commonly located along the falx, cortical convexity, and sphenoid bone.

Menigniomas account for 15%-19% of primary brain tumors and as many as 3% of the population older than 60 years have an intracranial meningioma on autopsy.

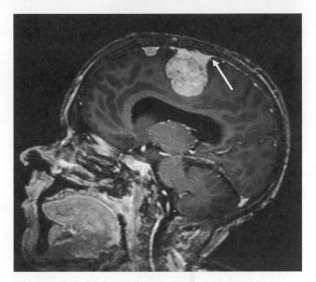

▲ **Figure 36–14.** Sagittal MRI image demonstrating a contrast enhancing dural-based lesion (arrow) proven to be a meningioma at time of resection.

Their incidence increases with age and peaks by 45 years of age. There is a female-to-male ratio of 2:1.

Inactivation of the NF2 gene found on the long arm of chromosome 22 (22q12.3) is the main genetic event associated with the development of meningiomas. Loss of one copy, truncated, or mutations toward the 5′ end of the NF2 gene occurs in up to 80% of sporadic meningiomas and all patients with neurofibromatosis type 2. Consequently, NF2 patients are more likely to develop intracranial meningioma of varying types. Chromosome 22q contains the *NF2* tumor suppressor gene, Merlin.

There are multiple histologic subtypes of meningioma, but they are typically characterized by the presence of densely packed sheets of cells (similar to appearance of normal arachnoid cells), psammoma bodies (whorls of calcium and collagen), intranuclear cytoplasmic pseudoinclusions, and Orphan Annie nuclei (nuclei with central clearing from peripheral migration of chromatin). Radiographically, meningiomas are hyperdense to brain and a broad dural attachment can often be identified. On T2-weighted MRI, most meningiomas are hyperintense and are typically contrast enhancing on both CT and MRI.

H. Nerve Sheath Tumors and Acoustic Neuromas

Nerve sheath tumors are benign tumors of Schwann cell origin that involve predominantly the fifth, seventh, eighth, and tenth cranial nerves. The most common, vestibular schwannomas (aka acoustic neuromas, AN) originate in the internal auditory canal from the inferior or superior portion of the vestibular nerve at the junction of the central and peripheral myelin. The three most common presenting symptoms include insidious hearing loss, high-pitched tinnitus, and disequilibrium.

AN account for 8%-10% of all intracranial tumors in adults. Most ANs are unilateral, however, patient with neurofibromatosis type 2 commonly have bilateral AN. AN is believed to result from the loss of a tumor suppressor gene located on the long arm of chromosome of 22.

Macroscopically, ANs are lobular, encapsulated, and solid with grayish colored material. Surrounding cranial nerves are often stretched over the capsule of the tumor. Microscopically, these tumors are identical to peripheral schwannomas. They are comprised of Antoni A and Antoni B fibers. Antoni A fibers are dense, narrow, elongated bipolar cells with numerous nuclei and firm cytoplasm. Antoni B fibers are a loose reticulated semi-palisading arrangement of Schwann cells.

CT is useful for distinguishing tumor extension into the bony internal auditory canal. On MRI, ANs are isointense on T1WI without contrast. With gadalinium enhancement they are often homogenously enhancing. The lack of a dural tail, differentiates AN from cerebellopontine angle meningiomas.

I. Pituitary Tumors

Pituitary adenomas are benign tumors originating from the anterior pituitary gland and represent 10% of intracranial tumors diagnosed. They are most commonly diagnosed between 40 and 50 years of age. They are classified according to their endocrine function or histological staining. Secreting tumors release supraphysiologic levels of hormones that result in distinct clinical syndromes. Hypersecretion of prolactin causes amenorrhea-galactorrhea syndrome in women and impotence in men. Hypersecretion of adrenocorticotropic hormone (ACTH) causes Cushings disease. Hypersecretion of growth hormone causes acromegaly in adults and gigantism in children. Pituitary adenomas can hypersecrete thyrotropin (producing hyperthyroidism) or gonadotropins (leutinizing hormone and follicle stimulating hormone).

Pituitary tumors may exert mass effect on adjacent structures. Optic chiasm compression results in bitemporal hemianopsia. Compression of the pituitary gland itself results in varying degrees of hypopituitarism. Compression upon the cavernous sinus causes ptosis, facial pain, and diplopia from pressure upon cranial nerves III, IV, V1, V2, and VI. Occlusion of the cavernous sinus may cause proptosis and chemosis.

J. Metastatic Brain Tumors

Metastatic brain tumors originate in from malignancies outside of the CNS that have spread to the brain or spinal cord (Figure 36–15). They are most common brain tumor

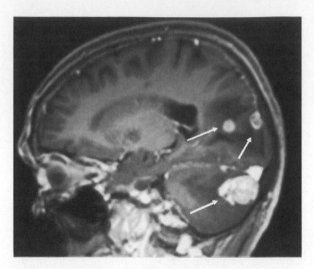

▲ **Figure 36–15.** Sagittal MRI image demonstrating multiple contrast enhancing lesions (arrows) in the infra- and supratentorial spaces. Biopsy demonstrated metastatic adenocarcinoma.

with a yearly incidence of 100,000-200,000 cases per year in the United States. Autopsy studies show that 20%-25% of patients with cancer have brain metastasis. Metastases occur more frequently in adults in their fifth to seventh decades of life. The most common primary tumors in adults giving rise to CNS metastases are lung, breast, skin, renal, and colon cancers. In children, leukemia and lymphoma, osteogenic sarcoma, and rhabdomyosarcoma are the most common primary tumors that spread to the CNS.

Histopathology of metastases mirrors that of the primary tumor. MRI is more sensitive than CT in detecting metastases. Metastases are typically seen at the gray-white junction and show varying degrees of contrast enhancement.

▶ Differential Diagnosis

The differential diagnosis of intracranial masses is narrowed through a detailed history and physical exam. Important considerations include patient demographics, chronology of symptoms, past medical history, and specific neurologic deficits. Once imaging is obtained, the list of possible diagnoses can be further refined, as the location of a lesion can suggest its nature. For example, the three most common posterior fossa tumors of childhood include astrocytoma, medulloblastoma, and ependymoma. The most common tumors of the cerebellopontine angle include meningioma, acoustic neuroma, and epidermoid cyst. In addition the pattern of contrast enhancement and whether the lesion appears to arise from within the brain parenchyma or meninges are important considerations in generating an accurate differential diagnosis.

▶ Treatment

A. Preoperative Medical Management

With few exceptions, surgery is the backbone of the current treatment of brain tumors. The success of surgical intervention depends on adequate preoperative medical management and surgical planning. Steroids are commonly used preoperatively to reduce the symptoms of mass effect and edema caused by the tumor. The timing and dose of steroids varies based on surgeon preference. A common regimen for adults is dexamethasone 6 mg IV or PO every six hours. If mass effect is profound, doses as high as 20 mg every four hours may be considered. Some surgeons believe that it is easier to resect a tumor when peritumoral edema is minimized by preoperative decadron administration.

The use of anticonvulsants in brain tumor patients at presentation, preoperatively, and postoperatively is somewhat controversial. Without question, patients presenting with seizures attributed to a brain tumor should be initiated on an anticonvulsant. However, with few exceptions, there is no data to suggest prophylactic use of anticonvulsants reduces the risk of new onset seizures in brain tumor patients. Among the exceptions are: (1) tumor involvement in highly epileptogenic areas such as the motor cortex, (2) low-grade gliomas, which carry a high risk of seizures, (3) patients with metastatic lesions that commonly invade the cortex, and (4) patients with both metastases and leptomeningeal spread.

Because of a favorable toxicity profile and cost, phenytoin is the first line antiepileptic agent. Phenytoin may cause GI upset and should be administered with a H_2 blocker or proton-pump inhibitor. Phenytoin levels must be monitored to ensure a therapeutic serum drug concentration. Leviteracetam is an alternative used for patients if there is potential for drug interactions related to induction of the P450 system by phenytoin. In contrast to phenytoin, levels of leviteracetam need not be monitored.

B. Surgical Considerations

The surgeon must decide whether the goal of intervention is obtaining biopsy only, subtotal resection, or attempting gross total resection. With few exceptions, gross total resection offers the best chance of survival and is the preferred treatment. Tumor resection requires careful consideration of a number of key factors including: (1) tumor size, (2) location, (3) gross, radiographic, and pathologic characteristics, (4) sensitivity to radiation, and importantly, (5) the medical and neurologic status of the patient.

The timing of surgery is important in preoperative planning. Patients who present with rapid deterioration due to elevated intracranial pressure typically require prompt intervention. Tumor growth can be brisk in patients with large, high-grade tumors and small increases in tumor volume can cause a profound increase in intracranial pressure. Rapid intervention may also be necessary in the setting of obstructive hydrocephalus. Cerebrospinal fluid diversion (typically via ventriculostomy) is an alternative to urgent tumor resection in patients with obstructive hydrocephalus secondary to tumor growth. In cases where tumor burden is not causing profound neurologic deficit or elevated intracranial pressure, resection can be arranged as a semi-elective procedure.

Once in the operating room for brain tumor resection, a number of important principles of positioning are vital to a successful resection. Most tumor resections require immobilization of patient's head in a Mayfield head holder. The position should be selected create the most direct access to the lesion while avoiding risk to other bodily structures. Positioning should promote venous drainage from the lesion and the cranial compartment by ensuring the jugular veins are not compressed and that the head is elevated. In most cases, surgeons prefer to position the patient with the operative corridor perpendicular to the floor. This approach generally minimizes brain retraction and is the most ergonomic for the surgeon. Pressure points of the remainder of the patient should be padded especially thoroughly given the lengthy nature of some tumor resections.

The shape of the skin incision and bone flap is dependent on the desired approach, size of the lesion, and surgeon preference. Small tumors can be adequately exposed and resected via linear or curvilnear incisions with a small bone flap. Resection of deep lesions, especially those involving the skull base, often require creation of a sizable scalp flap and removal of a large window of bone. Whenever possible, incisions should be planned behind the hairline, minimizing the amount of hair removal in deference to cosmetic concerns. The placement of the incision is largely determined by the location of the lesion. Frameless stereotaxy, a technology that relies on a three-dimensional rendering of the patient's preoperative MRI, can enable accurate tumor localization based on preoperative imaging and can be helpful in minimizing the size of the incision. Standard approaches to intracranial lesions minimize the morbidity of exposure by limiting the risk to key neural and vascular structures.

The central goal of brain tumor surgery is maximizing the removal of neoplastic tissue while minimizing collateral damage to surrounding normal brain and vascular structures. Standards for achieving this goal vary based on tumor type. For example, the goal of the resection of a high-grade glioma is to remove all enhancing portions of the tumor, in contrast to the goal for the resection of a low-grade glioma to remove the tissue that appears abnormal on T2-weighted MRI. Several large retrospective studies published in the last decade suggest that duration of survival is directly related to extent of resection or the proportion of tumor removed at the time of surgery. The goal for resection of meningioma is to remove both the tumor and its dural origin. Metastatic tumors are typically well demarcated and often encapsulated and the goal is to remove the entire tumor.

One of the central challenges in brain tumor surgery is that neoplastic tissue that is easily detected on MRI is often virtually indistinguishable from normal brain. Several studies evaluating the extent of brain tumor resection highlight the fact that in many cases, especially in diffusely invasive brain tumors, a significant amount of residual tumor remains even after gross total resection. Moreover, surgeons have a limited ability to predict when all resectable tumor has indeed been removed. Consequently, a variety of technologies have been developed to improve surgical outcomes. Stereotactic navigation is utilized to improve extent of resection but there is little evidence that it can improve extent of resection. Retrospective analyses suggest that intraoperative MRI, an approach in which brain tumor resection is performed in a highly specialized surgical suite containing an MRI machine, improves extent of resection. Fluorescent and visible dyes have been proposed as a means of identifying tumor margins intraoperatively for more than 60 years. Recently a phase III clinical trial has demonstrated that the fluorescent dye 5-ALA may improve the extent of resection and six-month progression-free survival in glioblastoma patients. A number of efforts are underway to use dye-based and label-free intraoperative microscopy to improve the surgeon's ability to distinguish tumor-infiltrated brain from noninfiltrated tissue.

Intraoperative electrophysiologic monitoring of brain activity is often used in tumors within eloquent cortex to determine a safe route for exposure of tumor and the safe limits for extent of resection. Electrophysiologic motor mapping can be performed with the patient under general anesthesia or awake. In asleep motor mapping, specific regions of the motor cortex or corticospinal tract are stimulated with electrical current while the electromyographic response in target muscles is recorded. In awake motor mapping direct electrical stimulation of motor cortex or corticospinal tracts is performed while a patient is asked to perform specific tasks. An arrest of motor activity with direct electrical stimulation suggests that the portion of brain being stimulated is involved in motor function. Similarly, in awake language mapping specific regions of the brain, commonly the dominant frontal and temporal lobes are stimulated to look for speech arrest. Awake language mapping of brain tumor patients has broadened our understanding of the organization of the human language cortex and circuits.

Following resection, meticulous attention is paid to achieving hemostasis in the operative corridor to minimize the risk of postoperative hemorrhage. Whenever possible, to diminish the risk of cerebrospinal fluid leak, a watertight dural closure is performed. The bone flap is replaced and the galea is reapproximated. Scalp closure that omits closure of the galea provides little strength and raises the risk of dehiscence.

C. Postoperative Management

Following resection patients are observed closely in an ICU setting, typically for overnight, where serial neurological examinations are carried out. Depending on the extent of resection, steroids may be tapered over the days following surgery. Anticonvulsants are continued in patients who have a history of seizures and, when there has been extensive brain dissection, they may be continued for 1-4 weeks following surgery. Given the prognostic significance of extent of resection for glioma patients and the difficulty in detecting residual tumor during surgery, it is becoming standard practice for surgeons to obtain postoperative MRI imaging with contrast to evaluate for residual tumor within 24 hours of resection. When there is a low suspicion of residual tumor or when further surgery is not possible, postoperative imaging may be deferred.

D. Adjuvant Therapies

Surgical resection is cornerstone of brain tumor therapy but it is rarely capable of eradicating all tumor cells. Furthermore, resection may not be favored when eloquent structures are likely to be damaged. Adjuvant radiation and chemotherapy regimens have been developed to address the inability of current surgical techniques to reliably eradicate residual or unresectable tumor.

1. Radiation—Radiation kills tumor cells by directly damaging cellular structures, inducing lethal mutations in cellular DNA and by activating pathways for programmed cell death. Radiation can be delivered to brain tumors in a fractionated manner, which allows normal tissue repair between treatments and increases the toxicity of the radiation to tumor tissue.

Regimens for radiation therapy of brain tumors vary with tumor type. The optimal dose and timing of adjuvant radiation therapy for low-grade glioma is controversial. Typically, radiation is reserved in low-grade glioma until there is evidence of tumor progression or neurologic deterioration. Early radiation therapy is suggested in elderly patients, for tumors that have crossed the midline and in the setting of intractable seizures. Because of the cognitive consequences of radiation therapy, it may be delayed in younger patients until there is suspicion of recurrence

For high-grade glioma, the findings of a study conducted by the Brain Tumor Cooperative Group (BTCG) demonstrated an increase in survival in HGG patient undergoing radiation therapy plus surgery compared to surgery alone from 14 to 31 weeks. A landmark study on the use of radiation in conjunction with temozolomide has defined the current standard for radiation therapy in glioblastoma patients: 2 Gy given 5 days per week for 6 weeks, totaling 60Gy.

Two important clinical trials have established the standard therapy for metastatic lesions. Currently, acceptable care of patients with brain metastases consists of resection followed by whole brain radiation therapy, or stereotactic radiosurgery (SRS), in which a high dose of radiation is administered to the tumor bed, in addition to whole brain radiation therapy. The use of radiation therapy has been extensively investigated. Currently, radiation therapy is indicated as an adjunct to surgery in the setting of recurrent meningioma or subtotal resection. Occasionally in a poor surgical candidate or if a meningioma is in a location carrying high surgical risk, radiation therapy may be used in isolation.

2. Chemotherapy—Clinical trials of chemotherapy for low-grade glioma have been limited and the use of chemotherapy for this remains experimental. The one exception is low-grade gliomas, typically those with 1p deletion and oligodendroglial lineage, which are particularly sensitive to PCV (procarbizine, carmustine, and vincristine) or temozolomide. In contrast, a recent clinical trial in patients with proven GBM comparing radiation alone to radiation in combination with the oral alkylating agent temozolomide demonstrated a modest but significant increase in survival from 12.1 to 14.6 months. The current standard of care for patients with GBM combines radiation therapy with oral temozolomide. Chemotherapy has not shown any benefit in the treatment of brain metastases and meningiomas. Future efforts in the development of novel chemotherapeutic agents are focused on developing novel inhibitors of signaling pathways that are active only in brain tumor cells. Developing novel methods for the delivery of traditional chemotherapeutic agents is also an area of active research.

▶ Complications

Patients with primary and metastatic brain tumors are at risk of developing postoperative medical as well as surgical complications. Sawaya proposed the most common classification scheme for complications associated with brain tumor surgery in 1998. In a case series of 400 craniotomies for treatment of brain tumors, complications were classified as neurological, regional, and systemic. Neurologic complications are outcomes that produce visual field, motor, sensory, or language deficits. Neurologic complications are the result of injury to normal brain structures, cerebral edema, hematoma, or vascular injury. In most series, the risk of a new neurologic deficit after craniotomy for resection of an intrinsic brain tumor ranges from 10% to 25%. The risk factors for adverse neurologic outcomes include older age (greater than 60 years), deep tumor location, tumor proximity to eloquent regions, and low functional performance score (Karnofsky score less than 60%). Neurologic complications can be minimized by individualizing the surgical approach for each patient, cortical mapping techniques, minimizing excessive brain retraction, meticulous hemostasis, and early identification of major venous structures.

Regional complications are those related to the surgical wound or brain parenchyma, without neurologic deficit. They occur in 1%-5% of patients undergoing craniotomy for resection of an intrinsic brain tumor. Regional complications include wound infections, pneumocephalus, Cerebrospinal fluid fistula, hydrocephalus, seizure, brain abscess/cerebritis, meningitis, and pseudomeningocele. These complications occur more readily in the elderly. Posterior fossa location and reoperations are associated with a higher rate of pseudomeningocele, CSF fistula, hydrocephalus, and wound infections. Postoperative wound infections and cellulitis occur in 1%-2% of patients after supratentorial craniotomy. They typically result from skin bacterial contamination (*Staphylococcus aureus* and *Staphylococcus* epidermidis). The risk of postoperative seizures following supratentorial craniotomy is 0.5%-5%. Prophylactic antiepileptic drugs can be routinely used in the postoperative period; however, their dose and duration is an area of controversy.

Systemic complications include all generalized adverse events, including deep vein thrombosis (DVT), pulmonary embolus, pneumonia, urinary tract infections, myocardial infarction, and sepsis. These medical complications occur in 5%-10% of patients undergoing craniotomy for removal of an intrinsic brain tumor and are more prevalent in older patients (greater than 60 years) and neurologically impaired patients (Karnofsky score less than 60%). DVT is the most common complication occurring in 1%-10% of patients within the first month after a craniotomy. Patients with systemic cancer, glioblastoma multiforme, meningiomas, lower extremity paralysis, bed rest, and prolonged surgery are at particularly increased risk of developing a DVT or pulmonary embolus. Early postoperative mobilization, intermittent compression devices, and postoperative anticoagulation with low-molecular-weight heparin have decreased the incidence of postoperative DVT.

Craniotomy for resection of brain tumor can be performed safely and most complications can be prevented with careful preoperative planning, meticulous surgical technique, and attentive postoperative care.

▶ Prognosis

The prognosis of brain tumor patients varies based on a number of factors, including, but not limited to, general functional status at the time of diagnosis, tumor type, location, and age.

A. Glioma

The prognosis of glioma patients is determined by tumor grade, age, extent of resection, Karnofsky performance status, and treatment response. Improvement in survival when radiographically complete resection is achieved is greatest for those with low-grade lesions. While more modest, high-grade glioma patients with radiographically complete resection also have survival improvement compared to incomplete resection. Achieving gross total resection improves survival by lowering the risk of recurrence and reducing tumor cell burden to levels that can be eradicated or controlled with adjuvant therapy.

B. Meningioma

In general, the prognosis of meningioma patients is more favorable than that of glioma patients. The prognosis of meningioma patients is determined by the extent of resection and tumor grade. The Simpson classification system stratifies meningioma patients into outcome groups based on extent of resection. Patient age, extent of surrounding structure invasion, male gender, genetic factors, and tumor grade are among the factors that are linked to prognosis. Recurrence has been estimated to occur in approximately 20% of patients with benign meningiomas but is much more common in higher grade lesions.

▶ Metastases

The survival of patients with untreated brain metastasis is quite poor (1-2 months), but survival can be prolonged by 4 or more months with optimal surgical and radiation therapies. Extent of extracranial disease is a key prognostic factor in patients with brain metastases. Age and Karnofsky performance status have an important bearing on overall survival.

Kool M, Korshunov A, Remke M, et al: Molecular subgroups of medulloblastoma: an international meta-analysis of transptome, genetic aberrations, and clinical data of WNT, SHH, Group 3, nad Group 4 medulloblastomas. *Acta Neuropathol* 2012;123:473-484.

Prabhu VC, Khaldi A, Barton KP, Melian E, Schneck MJ, Primeau MJ, Lee JM: Management of diffuse low-grade cerebral gliomas. *Neurol Clin* 2010 Nov;28(4):1037-1959.

Taylor MD, et al: Molecular subgroups of medulloblastoma: the current consensus. *Acta Neuropathol* 2012;123:465-472.

▼ TUMORS OF THE SPINE AND SPINAL CORD

Anthony C. Wang, MD Khoi D. Than, MD Paul Park, MD

INTRODUCTION

Neoplastic pathology affecting the spinal cord is uncommon in the general population but it is an important consideration in the evaluation of patients presenting with neck and/or back pain with or without associated radicular symptoms, sensorimotor deficits, and bowel or bladder dysfunction. An estimated 15% of primary CNS tumors are intraspinal, and most of these are benign. Since the first resection of a spinal cord tumor was reported in 1888, surgery has remained a mainstay of treatment in the majority of spinal tumors, though radiotherapy and chemotherapy have demonstrated benefit in a growing number of instances.

Spinal tumors are differentiated based upon their locations relative to three anatomic compartments. Extradural tumors are located outside of the thecal sac, and arise either from the osseous spine or epidural space. Intradural-extramedullary tumors occur within the thecal sac but are outside of the neural tissues of the spinal cord. These tumors most commonly develop from the leptomeninges or nerve roots. Intramedullary tumors are found within the spinal cord and originate from either the spinal cord parenchyma or pia mater.

In addition to gender and age of presentation, localization of the lesion to the cervical, thoracic, lumbar, or sacrococcygeal spine aids in refining the differential diagnosis as certain tumors demonstrate a predilection for particular regions of the spinal column.

▶ Clinical Presentation

Symptoms experienced by patients presenting with spinal tumors are more commonly produced by compression than direct invasion of the spinal cord or nerve roots. Classically, the pain associated with neoplasms is unremitting, worse in the supine position, and more noticeable at rest or in bed. Hence, the patient may wake up at night due to pain. Although the progression of symptoms can be insidious, radicular pain, motor weakness, paresthesias, or anesthesia can frequently occur as a result of nerve compression. Long tract myelopathic findings such as ataxia, hyperreflexia, spasticity, fasciculations, sensorimotor loss, or sphincter dysfunction can be caused by spinal cord compression. Recognized unusual findings include muscle wasting or hyporeflexia, referred pain, autonomic changes such as in Horner's syndrome, and Brown–Séquard hemicord syndrome. Fracture and deformity causing axial pain often occur as well, and may be the presenting complaint.

Extradural tumors frequently involve the osseous spine, and so most typically present with axial pain, often increased by motion or Valsalva maneuver. Signs and symptoms of neural compression occur secondarily. Intradural-extramedullary tumors present most commonly with motor deficits and other long tract disturbances. Intramedullary tumors can demonstrate an insidious succession of symptoms including neuralgic pain that can progress to myelopathy.

▶ Diagnosis

A. Radiographic Evaluation

MRI is currently the primary mode of assessment of spinal tumors (Figure 36–16). Contrast-enhanced T1-weighted sequences are the standard initial imaging modality for the evaluation of suspected extradural, intradural-extramedullary, and intramedullary lesions. Nearly all intramedullary lesions demonstrate contrast uptake, and the resolution

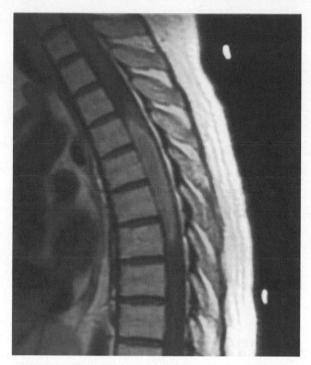

▲ **Figure 36–16.** Sagittal T1-weighted image with contrast of the upper thoracic spinal cord demonstrating an intradural, intramedullary lesion found on biopsy to be a high-grade glioma.

that MRI provides is typically sufficient for determination of margins and infiltration. The addition of angiography is indicated for the suspicion of a vascular pathology.

If MRI is not obtainable, then more invasive methods are used. Myelography, which was once the modality of choice for imaging the spinal canal, provides excellent structural detail. Fusiform cord widening, a dumbbell-shaped deformity, or complete blockage are classic findings suggesting the presence of a mass lesion. Plain, contrast-enhanced, and postmyelography CT imaging can aid in the assessment of bony spine anatomy. Nuclear scintigraphy is used primarily in the identification of skeletal metastases. Catheter angiography can be employed in the evaluation of suspected vascular lesions. Plain x-rays of the spine have limited utility in the initial assessment of spinal tumors. Findings such as enlarged intervertebral foramina and interpedicular spaces, or bone erosion with scalloped edges suggest the presence of an enlarging mass.

B. Laboratory Analysis

Lumbar puncture can provide additional clues to the presence of a spinal cord tumor. Elevated CSF protein is present in approximately 95% of cases, though CSF glucose is normal. Xanthochromia and the presence of fibrinogen causing clotting can also occur. Specific CSF and serum immunocytochemical tests can aid the diagnosis of specific neoplasms.

C. Differential Diagnosis

Among all spinal tumors, extradural lesions are discovered with the greatest frequency, comprising an estimated 55%-60%. A vast majority of these are metastatic lesions via hematogenous dissemination along Batson's venous plexus. The most common primary sources of vertebral metastases are lung, breast, and prostate.

Benign spine tumors of the osseous spine are very rare, and may be incidental findings, or cause pain, radiculopathy, myelopathy, spinal instability, or deformity. Biopsy is utilized at times, and appropriate management may be observational, as is common in the case of eosinophilic granuloma, ablative, as can be performed for osteoid osteoma, or surgical. Primary benign spine tumors can be classified using the Enneking system.

Approximately 5% of bone malignancies involve the spine, the four most common being osteosarcoma, chondrosarcoma, Ewing's sarcoma, and chordoma. Survival varies significantly by pathology. The high rates of recurrence, limited survival duration, and functional morbidity associated with these tumors support the aggressive multimodal strategies typically employed in treatment of these tumors. In some cases, complete resection with negative margins, or even en bloc resection, is possible. In other cases, surgical resection may serve to decrease tumor burden, thereby improving the efficacy of adjuvant treatments such as chemotherapy and radiotherapy. At times, surgical intervention is necessary for functional indications, either for neural decompression or spinal stabilization.

Only 0.5% of tumors involving the spinal column are primary neoplasms. Of the intradural tumors, an estimated 70% are extramedullary. Schwannoma, neurofibroma, and meningioma comprise the bulk of these cases. The nerve sheath tumors, schwannoma and neurofibroma, are usually benign, and can demonstrate a typical dumbbell-shaped appearance, caused by the neuroforamina through which they sometimes pass. They are an important consideration when deviation of the pleural reflection on x-ray suggests a posterior mediastinal mass. Schwannomas are well-differentiated and typically grossly resectable; however, neurofibromas cannot be resected completely from its parent nerve. In the setting of type-1 neurofibromatosis, suspicion of multiple neurofibromas, meningioma, and ependymoma should be heightened. Schwannoma, neurofibroma, and meningioma multiplicity is associated with type-2 neurofibromatosis. Meningiomas are seen most often in the thoracic spines of middle-aged women, and arise from persistent arachnoid cap cells.

Intramedullary tumors comprise only approximately 10% of all spinal tumors, and arise most commonly in the cervical segment of the spinal cord. Glial tumors are the most common of these, with ependymomas occurring twice as frequently as astrocytomas in adults. In children, the relationship is reversed, with astrocytomas being twice as common as ependymomas. Myxopapillary ependymomas form at the conus medullaris and filum terminale, and are a very common tumor to be found at this location.

▶ Treatment

Treatment options are tailored to the patient. Some patients present with axial pain absent of radiculopathy while others present with mild or stable evidence of spinal cord compression causing myelopathy. Still others present with rapidly progressive course of neurologic deterioration.

Generally, primary tumors of the spinal column are best treated by complete resection, if possible. In the vertebral column, en bloc resection is frequently the goal of surgery, whereas with any involvement of the spinal cord, gross total resection is the desired treatment. Symptomatic deformity or spinal instability warrants consideration for surgical fixation, as functional deterioration profoundly affects survival.

Extradural metastases are the most frequently seen tumors of the spinal column, and their treatment is complicated by many factors. Decompression of the spinal cord is the initial surgical consideration. Resection followed by adjuvant radiation has shown promising oncologic results. Spine stability must then be addressed depending on the patient's overall prognosis.

In 2007, the WHO updated a comprehensive classification of neoplasms affecting the CNS based upon the specific cell type from which each tumor arises, which guides therapy and prognosis in cases of most intramedullary tumors. Overall, functional outcome depends heavily on the severity and duration of neurologic symptoms at the time of presentation, while survival outcome depends largely on the pathology in question, and less so, on the ability to gain adequate surgical resection.

Intradural-extramedullary tumors are generally best treated by surgical resection; outcomes appear to depend heavily upon extent of resection, though preservation of preexisting neurologic function remains the primary objective in surgery. Determination of a dissection plane between tumor and spinal cord is the initial aim of any resection procedure. Overall, prognosis is excellent in nearly all cases of spinal intradural-extramedullary neoplasms, unless paraplegia is the presenting condition. In contrast, recurrence of infiltrative neoplasms is very common, and progression to paralysis is common. Progressive neurologic deterioration demands particular focus on facilitating appropriate surgical therapy.

Binning M, Klimo P Jr, Gluf W, Goumnerova L: Spinal tumors in children. *Neurosurg Clin N Am* 2007;18(4):631-658.

Louis DN, Ohgaki H, Wiestler OD: The 2007 WHO classification of tumours of the central nervous system. *Acta Neuropathol* 2007;114(2):97-109.

Mukherjee D, Chaichana KL, Parker SL, Gokaslan ZL, McGirt MJ: Association of surgical resection and survival in patients with malignant primary osseous spinal neoplasms from the Surveillance, Epidemiology, and End Results (SEER) database. *Eur Spine J* 2013 Jun;22(6):1375-82.

Ozawa H, Kokubun S, Aizawa T, Hoshikawa T, Kawahara C: Spinal dumbbell tumors: an analysis of a series of 118 cases. *J Neurosurg Spine* 2007;7(6):587-593.

Thakur NA, Daniels AH, Schiller J, Valdes MA: Benign tumors of the spine. *J Am Acad Orthop Surg* 2012;20(11):715-724.

Zadnik PL, Gokaslan ZL, Burger PC, Bettegowda C: Spinal cord tumours: advances in genetics and their implications for treatment. *Nat Rev Neurol* 2013 May;9(5):257-266.

▼ PITUITARY TUMORS

Wajd N. Al-Holou, John E. Ziewacz, Ariel Barkan, William F. Chandler, Stephen E. Sullivan

▶ Clinical Considerations

The pituitary gland, involved in the regulation of the major hormonal axes of the body, is located in the sella turcica ("Turkish Saddle") of the sphenoid bone and is comprised of the anterior pituitary (adenohypophysis), posterior pituitary (neurohypophysis), and functionally insignificant pars intermedia separating the two lobes. The anterior pituitary secretes Prolactin, ACTH, TSH, LH, FSH, and GH. The posterior lobe is a repository of the hypothalamic hormones Oxytocin and Anti-Diuretic hormone (ADH, vasopressin).

Pituitary tumors are typically benign adenomas that arise from the anterior lobe of the pituitary gland. They comprise approximately 10% of CNS tumors. With the increasing use of brain MRI, there has been an increase in the diagnosis of incidentally discovered pituitary adenomas, known as incidentalomas, with nearly a 23% imaging prevalence. Pituitary adenomas are classified by both their secretory status (secreting vs. nonsecreting), and their size. Microadenomas have diameters up to 1 cm, while tumors greater than 1 cm are termed macroadenomas (Figure 36–17). Secreting (endocrine-active) tumors are further classified by which hormone is being hypersecreted and the resulting clinical syndrome.

▶ Clinical Findings

Clinical findings in patients with pituitary adenomas are caused by compression of surrounding structures, decrease in pituitary function, hypersecretion of pituitary hormones, and rarely, acute pituitary failure (apoplexy). Pituitary tumors can also be asymptomatic, and discovered incidentally.

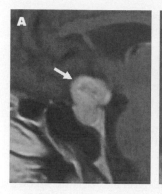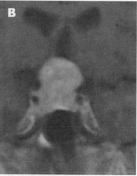

▲ **Figure 36–17.** Magnetic resonance imaging **A.** sagittal plain and **B.** coronal plain of a pituitary macroadenoma.

A. Compression

Compression caused by slowly expanding adenomas causes a variety of findings which include headache, bitemporal hemianopsia (decreased perception of the lateral visual fields), diplopia, and hypopituitarism (decreased secretion of pituitary hormone).

Bitemporal hemianopsia results from the upward extension of the tumor with associated compression of the decussating nasal fibers of the optic chiasm, which lie directly above the pituitary gland. This can be detected on examination as red color desaturation in the temporal visual fields. Without treatment, visual findings can progress to loss of visual acuity and eventual blindness.

Hypopituitarism results from compression and injury of the normal pituitary cells by the expanding mass. Diminished secretion of GH, LH, and FSH occurs early, while diminished secretion of TSH and ACTH occurs later.

Symptoms related to decreased production of LH and FSH manifest as hypogonadism: loss of libido and erections in men and amenorrhea in women. In men, this is often overlooked and only recognized in retrospect. The decreased production of LH and FSH can be due to either direct compression of the gland, or to compression of the stalk, which releases the tonic inhibition of prolactin secretion by dopamine from the hypothalamus. This results in a mild increase in prolactin (usually less than 150 ng/mL) which inhibits *gonadotropin* release. This can cause galactorrhea as well, and is the mechanism of the amenorrhea/galactorrhea syndrome.

Decreased production of TSH causes classic findings of hypothyroidism, including cold intolerance, weight gain, fatigue, coarse hair, and myxedema. Decreased production of ACTH causes hypocortisolism resulting in fatigue, slow return to health after minor illness and orthostatic hypotension. As the body's intrinsic stress response is diminished with the loss of ACTH production, in rare circumstances, this can result in cardiovascular collapse when the individual is under extreme stress.

B. Hypersecretion

Functional adenomas produce symptoms related to hypersecretion of a specific hormone. They can also produce findings related to compression, but this is less common than in nonfunctional tumors, given that they are often discovered at an earlier stage because of the clinical findings caused by hypersecretion.

Prolactinomas are the most common functional pituitary tumor, accounting for nearly 30%-40% of pituitary tumors. Prolactinomas cause hypersecretion of prolactin. Interruption of the pituitary stalk can cause hyperprolactinemia as well, but levels are typically more modest (150 ng/mL or less). Levels greater than 300 ng/mL are virtually always associated with prolactin secreting tumors. Symptoms of hyperprolactinemia are gender-dependent and may include galactorrhea, amenorrhea (via suppression of gonadotropins), diminished libido, and infertility.

Growth hormone-secreting tumors are the next most common endocrine active tumors. They cause gigantism in children and acromegaly in adults. Acromegaly is characterized by classic physical changes such as soft tissue and skeletal overgrowth, prognathism, widely spaced teeth, macroglossia, as well as nerve entrapment syndromes and arthropathy. It also results in conditions associated with increased morbidity and mortality including cardiomyopathy, sleep apnea, and glucose intolerance. Acromegaly is insidious in onset and is often not noticed by the patient's friends or family. Patients often note a change in shoe size as an adult, an inability to wear a wedding ring, or recognize a striking physical change when comparing a recent to a past photograph.

Tumors that secrete ACTH are the cause of Cushing disease, which refers specifically to hypercortisolism caused by a functional, ACTH-producing, pituitary tumor. The resultant signs and symptoms of hypercortisolism from any etiology are termed Cushing syndrome. Characteristic findings include weight gain (with centripetal fat distribution), "buffalo hump," that is, redistribution of fat to the posterior neck, purple abdominal striae, thin skin with easy bruising, round "moon" face, glucose intolerance, hypertension, osteoporosis, poor wound healing, psychiatric disturbance (depression, mood lability), amenorrhea, impotence, and hyperpigmentation (only with elevated ACTH). These patients have a significant increase in morbidity and mortality if left untreated, with reports of a fourfold to fivefold increase in mortality in some studies. Gonadotropin producing tumors are rare and result in the hypersecretion of LH and FSH. They are often clinically silent, and usually behave like nonfunctioning tumors. In women, they can produce amenorrhea and infertility.

TSH-producing tumors are very rare, accounting for less than 1% of secretory tumors. Clinical findings are those of classic hyperthyroidism including weight loss, tachycardia, heat intolerance, anxiety, and tremor. As opposed to classical thyrotoxicosis (multinodular goiter, Graves' disease, and iatrogenic causes) in which plasma TSH concentrations are undetectably low, in patients with thyrotropinomas TSH levels are "normal" or frankly elevated despite high free T4 and T3 concentrations.

C. Acute Pituitary Failure (Apoplexy)

Acute pituitary failure is usually the result of hemorrhage and/or necrosis in a preexisting adenoma. Symptoms are abrupt and may result in severe headache, visual disturbance, ophthalmoplegia, and change in mental status. Pituitary apoplexy is often considered a neurosurgical emergency, especially in the setting of visual loss. Urgent decompression is warranted for acute or continuing neurologic decline, in order to prevent untoward neurologic consequences, especially blindness. Pituitary hormonal failure almost always accompanies an apoplectic event, and rapid administration of corticosteroids is necessary to avoid cardiovascular collapse.

D. Stalk Compression

Symptoms related to stalk compression are rare in the setting of pituitary adenomas and consist of prolactin elevation and loss of antidiuretic hormone (ADH). Diabetes insipidus results from impairment of hypothalamic input and the resultant diminished release of ADH. This causes an inability to concentrate the urine and resulting dehydration and hypernatremia. Symptoms include frequent high-volume urination and excessive thirst. This can be very dangerous in the setting of a patient with an impaired thirst mechanism. Stalk compression is more common with tumors directly involving the stalk such as craniopharyngioma and Langerhans cell histiocytosis.

Mild prolactin elevation results from blocking hypothalamic dopamine from accessing the pituitary prolactin-producing cells. This release of tonic inhibition results in a modest elevation of prolactin (usually less than 150 ng/mL). This is called the "stalk effect" and may result in amenorrhea and galactorrhea.

▶ Differential Diagnosis

The differential diagnosis for sellar and parasellar masses is broad. The hallmarks of distinguishing among the multiple possibilities are a detailed history and physical examination, MRI scan, and pituitary hormone testing. The history and physical examination should be aimed at symptoms related to pituitary hyper- or hyposecretion, and compression of surrounding structures. A detailed visual field examination should be included in the evaluation of any potential pituitary mass. Often, formal visual field testing by an Ophthalmologist is warranted. MRI should be obtained with and without contrast, with thin cuts through the sellar region in coronal and sagittal planes. This will identify the size, configuration, and extent of invasion of a pituitary tumor. Laboratory testing should include evaluation of anterior pituitary hormones, directly or indirectly, in order to establish a hyper- or hyposecretory state. These include prolactin, 8:00 AM cortisol, free T4, TSH, IGF-1, GH, LH, FSH, and testosterone (in men). If symptoms of diabetes insipidus are present, serum sodium and osmolality, and urine osmolality should be obtained to confirm the diagnosis. An overnight water deprivation test may be warranted to evaluate if the patient is able to concentrate urine appropriately.

If a hypersecretory state is not detected on detailed laboratory testing, the lesion is likely a nonfunctional pituitary adenoma or other entity. Other possibilities include craniopharyngioma, Rathke's cleft cyst, or meningioma. A number of other less common lesions are in the differential including metastasis, epidermoid, dermoid, germinoma, abscess, Langerhans histiocytosis, choristoma, chondrosarcoma and chordoma. Rarely, a giant aneurysm can mimic a pituitary tumor.

If a hypersecretory state is discovered, the diagnosis depends on the hormone that is being hypersecreted. It is important to distinguish a primary pituitary lesion causing hypersecretion from a lesion in another location, such as an ACTH-secreting carcinoid lung tumor.

Prolactin levels greater than 200 ng/mL indicate the presence of a prolactinoma. Modest elevations in prolactin, less than 150 ng/mL, can be caused by compression of the pituitary stalk, antidopaminergic drugs, estrogen excess (usually from oral contraceptives), chest wall lesions, primary hypothyroidism, and hypothalamic damage. In evaluating prolactin in patients with giant adenomas (> 3.5 cm), it is important to include serial dilutions up to 1:1000 in addition to the undiluted serum value. The purpose of this is to obviate a false negative value in cases of extremely elevated prolactin levels caused by the so-called "hook effect." This results from excess prolactin binding to both antibodies of the laboratory assay, causing a lack of formation of the complexes identified in the current assays. If the diluted level is still elevated, one can conclude there is a truly elevated prolactin level.

If there is concern for hypercortisolism, a 24-hour urinary free cortisol should be obtained to diagnose hypercortisolism. This should always be repeated for confirmation of the abnormal elevation. If this value is clearly elevated then hypercortisolism is definite and search is initiated to find the etiology of the hypercortisolism. If the level is equivocal and suspicion of hypercortisolism is still strong, then a low- and high-dose dexamethasone suppression test may be employed.

Once hypercortisolism is confirmed, the location of the pathology must be identified. Identification of an adenoma on MRI will obviate the need for further endocrinological studies. Endogenous hypercortisolism is either ACTH-dependent, most commonly from a pituitary adenoma or ectopic ACTH from a pulmonary malignancy, or ACTH-independent, resulting from an adrenal source (adrenal adenoma or carcinoma). Tests useful in confirming an ACTH-dependent tumor include a 4 PM erum ACTH. If ACTH level is elevated, then the source needs to be identified. The low- and high-dose dexamethasone suppression test (Liddle test) can also help to confirm a pituitary etiology. In Cushing disease serum cortisol is not suppressed with the low dose of 0.5-mg dexamethasone q 6 hours for 2 days, but does suppress with the higher dose of 2.0 mg q 6 hours for 2 days. In patients with ectopic sources of ACTH production, cortisol level is not suppressed even with the high-dose dexamethasone suppression test. In cases of proven ACTH-dependent hypercortisolism in which a pituitary tumor is not seen on MRI, inferior petrosal sinus sampling (IPSS) is required to confirm a pituitary etiology, as well as to help localize the side of the tumor. IPSS can identify a pituitary source of hypercortisolism in 98%, but it is not very effective in identification of laterality, being correct in no more than 69% of cases.

Laboratory diagnosis of GH secreting tumors is often indirect. This is because the secretion of GH is pulsatile and levels in patients without a hypersecreting tumor can often be elevated at certain times during the day. Patients with active acromegaly may have completely normal random GH levels. IGF-1 (somatomedin-C) is the gold standard for diagnosing GH secreting tumors. IGF-1 is produced in the liver and other organs and is dependent on GH for its production. Serum levels of IGF-1 are relatively stable and provide a better confirmatory test than the more volatile GH.

LH and FSH secreting tumors are diagnosed by serum elevated levels in the setting of a pituitary mass diagnosed on MRI.

TSH secreting tumors are rare and must be distinguished from other pathologic entities on the hypothalamic-pituitary-thyroid axis. Secondary hyperthyroidism (that produced by a pituitary tumor) is diagnosed by an elevated TSH level as well as an elevated free T4 level. In primary hyperthyroidism, free T4 would be elevated and TSH would be suppressed via a negative feedback mechanism.

▶ Treatment

Treatment of pituitary tumors depends on their size, hormonal characteristics, and level of invasiveness. Micro- or macroadenomas that are nonsecreting and are not causing symptoms of compression may be treated conservatively, and followed with serial imaging. The natural history of nonsecreting microadenomas is often benign.

Nonsecreting macroadenomas that cause signs of compression are currently treated surgically. The typical surgical approach is a transsphenoidal route. This is generally performed transnasally, using the operating microscope and/or the endoscope. Recent advances in frameless stereotactic guidance and endoscopic techniques have allowed a greater ability to localize lesions intraoperatively and provide a more minimally invasive approach to treatment of pituitary adenomas. The use of endonasal endoscopic approaches has increased in recent years and provides wider intraoperative visualization, but may be associated with increased intranasal morbidity. Nonetheless, both endoscopic and microscopic endonasal approaches are effective surgical treatment modalities, and the choice of technique is often surgeon-dependent.

Occasionally, if an adenoma has an unusual amount of suprasellar extension, or lateral extension a craniotomy may be necessary. In some cases, lesions that invade the cavernous sinus or have a significant amount of extrasellar extension are not surgically accessible by any approach and radiation therapy is often necessary to provide tumor control.

Patients with hypopituitarism due to compression who do not experience return of pituitary function postoperatively require hormone replacement on a chronic basis. If chronic steroid replacement is necessary, it is important that patients be provided with a medic-alert bracelet for the possibility of trauma or illness. These patients have a loss of intrinsic cortisol production, and can suffer from cardiovascular collapse if their cortisol deficiency is not recognized and supplemented with stress-dose steroids.

Treatment for hypersecreting tumors depends on the hormone being secreted. It is very important to establish the hormonal profile of a tumor prior to treatment for this reason. Currently, prolactinomas are treated first with a dopamine agonist. The most common medications used to treat prolactinomas are cabergoline and bromocriptine. Cabergoline is a selective D-2 dopamine receptor agonist that is widely considered first-line therapy for prolactinomas. It is favored over bromocriptine because of its selectivity, twice weekly dosing, better tumor control, effective lowering of prolactin levels, greater return of gonadal function/menstrual cycles, and possibility of obviating the need for life-long therapy. Two randomized trials showed better prolactin normalization with cabergoline as compared to bromocriptine. Recently, association of cabergoline with cardiac valvular disease has prompted a reexamination of the initial treatment of prolactinoma, but currently medical treatment as first line is still favored. Cardiac complications are generally seen with much higher doses than required to treat a prolactinoma. Most prolactinomas respond well to medical treatment, but 10%-20% of patients do not. If medical therapy fails to reduce the tumor size or its mass effect, or sufficiently control prolactin levels, surgery via transsphenoidal approach may be offered. Surgical management occasionally may be indicated in patients with rapidly worsening visual loss, and can be considered in patients attempting pregnancy, although cabergoline is still the first-line intervention in these patients.

Other hypersecreting tumors are treated via transsphenoidal approach, as with nonsecreting adenomas. Postoperative laboratory testing confirms the efficacy of therapy. As with nonsecreting tumors, craniotomy and/or radiation are sometimes necessary, depending on the extent and location of tumor growth. Pituitary replacement may be necessary postoperatively as well.

In the case of pituitary apoplexy, treatment often consists of urgent transsphenoidal decompression to prevent further visual deficit, and prompt initiation of stress dose steroid replacement in order to avoid a pituitary crisis.

▶ Summary

Pituitary adenomas are largely benign tumors that are either secreting or nonsecreting. Diagnosis is established with history, physical examination, MRI, and hormonal testing. Treatment consists of conservative therapy for nonsecreting micro/macroadenomas without symptoms of compression, medical therapy for prolactinomas, and transsphenoidal surgery for symptomatic macroadenomas and other hypersecreting tumors. Occasionally, craniotomy and/or radiation may be necessary for further tumor control. Depending on hormonal status, chronic pituitary replacement may be necessary postoperatively. Successful treatment of pituitary tumors can often be achieved with the combined effort of a medical endocrinologist and pituitary neurosurgeon.

Chandler WF: Treatment of disorders of the pituitary gland: pearls and pitfalls from 30 years of experience. *Clin Neurosurg* 2009;56:18-22.

Fernández-Balsells MM, Murad MH, Barwise A, Gallegos-Orozco JF, Paul A, Lane MA, Lampropulos JF, Natividad I, Perestelo-Pérez L, Ponce de León-Lovatón PG, Erwin PJ, Carey J, Montori VM: Natural history of nonfunctioning pituitary adenomas and incidentalomas: a systematic review and metaanalysis. *J Clin Endocrinol Metab* 2011 Apr;96(4):905-912.

Lania A, Beck-Peccoz P: Pituitary incidentalomas. *Best Pract Res Clin Endocrinol Metab* 2012 Aug;26(4):395-403.

Lucas JW, Zada G: Endoscopic surgery for pituitary tumors. *Neurosurg Clin N Am* 2012 Oct;23(4):555-569.

Oh MC, Kunwar S, Blevins L, Aghi MK: Medical versus surgical management of prolactinomas. *Neurosurg Clin N Am* 2012 Oct;23(4):669-678.

Sarwar K, Huda M, Van de Velde V, Hopkins L, Luck S, Preston R, McGowan B, Carroll P, Powrie J: The prevalence and natural history of pituitary haemorrhage in prolactinoma. *J Clin Endocrinol Metab* 2013 Jun;98(6):2362-2367.

Sheth SA, Bourne SK, Tritos NA, Swearingen B: Neurosurgical treatment of Cushing disease. *Neurosurg Clin N Am* 2012 Oct;23(4):639-651.

Steffensen C, Maegbaek ML, Laurberg P, Andersen M, Kistorp CM, Norrelund H, Sørensen HT, Jorgensen JO: Heart valve disease among patients with hyperprolactinemia: a nationwide population-based cohort study. *J Clin Endocrinol Metab* 2012 May;97(5):1629-1634.

Wind JJ, Lonser RR, Nieman LK, Devroom HL, Chang R, Oldfield EH: The lateralization accuracy of inferior petrosal sinus sampling in 501 patients with Cushing's disease. *J Clin Endocrinol Metab* 2013 Jun;98(6):2285-2293.

▼ PEDIATRIC NEUROSURGERY

Debbie K Song, MD Cormac O. Maher, MD Karin M. Muraszko, MD

CONGENITAL MALFORMATIONS

▶ Craniospinal Dysraphism

Craniospinal dysraphism results from improper formation and closure of the neural tube during development. These may be classified based on whether they are open or closed neural tube defects, the location of the lesion, or the embryological basis for the malformation. Open neural tube defects are those in which neural elements are exposed or covered by a dysplastic membrane, while closed neural tube defects are skin covered.

Myelomeningocele, the most common type of spinal dysraphism compatible with life, occurs with an incidence of 1 in every 1200-1400 live births. It is due to a local failure of neural tube closure during primary neurulation. Fusion of the lateral cutaneous ectoderm and the process of disjunction also fail to occur in myelomeningocele, resulting in a midline cutaneous defect over exposed neural tissue called the neural placode. Therefore, myelomeningoceles are considered open neural tube defects. Myelomeningoceles occur most commonly in the lumbar spine, and the anatomic level of the spinal cord lesion approximates the patient's neurologic deficits. The diagnosis of a neural tube defect can be suspected prenatally with an elevated maternal serum alpha-fetoprotein and confirmed by in utero imaging such as a maternal-fetal MRI or ultrasound. Pregnant mothers who have inadequate folate intake or who have other children with neural tube defects are at increased risk for giving birth to a child with a myelomeningocele. A Chiari II malformation is found in most patients with myelomeningocele. Eighty percent of patients with myelomeningocele have associated hydrocephalus. Other CNS abnormalities that can be found with increased incidence among patients with myelomeningocele include lipomas, syringomyelia, and diastematomyelia. Patients with myelomeningocele commonly have orthopedic problems that include scoliosis, hip dislocation, knee, and foot deformities. Besides a neurogenic bladder, patients with myelomeningocele are at increased risk of genitourinary abnormalities, as well as intestinal, cardiac, esophageal, and renal abnormalities. Workup for the newborn child with myelomeningocele includes a cranial and spinal ultrasound, and orthopedic and urology consults. The neonate should be placed in the prone position, with pressure off of the myelomeningocele. The myelomeningocele should be covered in moist. Surgical closure of the myelomeningocele is performed soon after birth. The Management of Myelomeningocele Study is an ongoing trial examining the utility of in utero myelomeningocele repair.

Closed neural tube defects, also referred to as occult spinal dysraphisms, can arise from problems with disjunction, secondary neurulation, or postneurulation events. Types of closed neural tube defects include dermal sinus tracts, spinal lipomas, neurenteric cysts, sacral dysgenesis, and diastematomyelia. Spina bifida occulta, which is characterized by a defect in the posterior elements of the spine, is often a harbinger of an underlying closed neural tube defect. These malformations can tether the spinal cord in an abnormally low position and produce excessive tension on the neural elements. Neuronal dysfunction may ensue with symptoms of a clinical tethered cord syndrome such as back or leg pain, worsening lower extremity motor and sensory function, decline in bladder and bowel function, worsening lower extremity orthopedic deformities, and progressive scoliosis. Early surgical repair of occult spinal dysraphisms is often recommended at the time of diagnosis in order to prevent the onset or halt the progression of neurological symptoms.

Dermal sinus tracts are epithelial-lined tracts that originate in the midline skin, usually in the caudal lumbosacral region above the S2 level. The sinus tract extends from a pinhole opening in the skin, through bifid spinous processes, and extends into the dura to communicate with the spinal cord. The lining of the dermal sinus tract contains normal skin appendages which can shed and communicate with the intradural space, and recurrent episodes of meningitis and arachnoiditis may ensue. They appear as dimples above the gluteal crease and must be differentiated from pilonidal cysts, which are closer to the anus. Both entities may drain from the skin. The skin around the ostium of a dermal sinus tract may be discolored or have a hairy tuft. Dermal sinuses can be associated with lipomas, dermoid tumors, or epidermoid cysts at any point along the tract or within the spinal canal. Examination of the child with a suspected dermal sinus tract should include assessment of sphincter function, lower extremity reflexes, and motor and sensory function. Treatment should be performed in an expeditious fashion after diagnosis in order to reduce the risk of CNS infection and prevent the development of neurological deficit. Less commonly, dermal sinus tracts can occur in the cranial region. The most common cranial locations are in the occipital or nasal region. Children may present with a midline dimple at the tip of the nose or in the occipital region and a history of recurrent meningitis. Cranial dermal sinus tracts can be associated with intracranial dermoid cysts.

Spinal lipomas are the most common closed neural tube defects and include three separate entities: intradural lipomas, lipomyelomeningoceles, and lipomas derived from the caudal cell mass including fibrolipomas of the filum terminale. A lipomyelomeningocele consists of an intradural lipoma that is attached to the spinal cord and extends through defects in the dura, bony spine, and fascia to become continuous with the subcutaneous fat. Seventy percent of lipomyelomeningoceles are associated with subcutaneous fatty masses. Lipomyelomeningoceles present as skin-covered lumbosacral masses above the gluteal crease. The overlying skin may be discolored from a port-wine stain or hemangioma, have a hairy tuft, or contain an ostium of a dermal sinus tract. The caudal end of the spinal cord is usually tethered in a low-lying position in cases of lipomyelomeningocele, with the conus medullaris positioned below the normal L1-2 level. Filum terminale fibrolipomas and distal conus lipomas, in contrast to lipomyelomeningocles, are malformations of secondary neurulation. Intradural lipomas, lipomyelomeningoceles, and filum terminale lipomas can all tether the spinal cord. The neurological examination in such children may be normal, or patients may present with symptoms of a clinical tethered cord syndrome. Symptoms may become more prominent and neurological deficits can worsen during growth spurts. As a child gains weight, intraspinal lipomas will also undergo fat deposition which can compress or tether neural elements. Treatment of lipomyelomeningoceles includes cord untethering with resection or debulking of the intraspinal lipoma.

Diastematomyelia, also known as a split cord malformation, occurs when the spinal cord is split into 2 hemicords. The hemicords may be contained within separate dural sleeves separated by a bony septum, or both hemicords may be contained within a single dural sac and separated by a fibrous septum. The 2 hemicords reunite below the level of the lesion. Diastematomyelia is most commonly found in the lumbar spine and has a gender predilection for women. Children with diastematomyelia often have cutaneous stigmata such as a nevus or a hairy tuft (hypertrichosis) at the level of the malformation. Bony anomalies, including spina bifida occulta, hemivertebrae, butterfly vertebrae, bony spurs at the level of the lesion, scoliosis, and orthopedic foot deformities are associated with split cord malformations. Clinically, diastematomyelia presents with symptoms of a tethered cord. Surgical treatment involves resection of any bony spurs and/or septum, untethering of the spinal cord, and reconstitution of a single dural sac.

Encephaloceles occur when there is a herniation of brain tissue and meninges through defects in the cranial vault. The tissue contained within an encephalocele consists of dysplastic and nonfunctional neural tissue with variable amounts of blood vessels, choroid plexus, dura, and ventricular tissue. The prognosis in children with encephaloceles is dependent on the amount of neural tissue contained within the encephalocele. Encephaloceles can be categorized as either posterior or anterior cranial fossa malformations depending on their location, and they are further classified according to the bone through which the herniation of tissue occurs. Posterior encephaloceles are associated with other midline congential anomalies, including myelomeningocele, Dandy–Walker malformation, Klippel–Feil anomaly, dorsal interhemispheric cysts, abnormalities of the corpus callosum, and neuronal migration disorders. For occipital and parietal encephaloceles, it is important to delineate the relationship of the lesion with adjacent venous sinuses. The goals of operative repair include removal of the encephalocele sac, preservation of any possible functional neural tissues, and closure of the dura in a water-tight fashion and of the wound with nondysplastic skin. Up to 50% of infants will develop hydrocephalus within 1 month of encephalocele repair; thus, surveillance with serial cranial ultrasounds is warranted in this group.

▶ Arachnoid Cysts

Arachnoid cysts are developmental anomalies that form between separated layers of the arachnoid membrane. The walls of an arachnoid cyst may thicken with collagen deposition over time or hemorrhage. These cysts most commonly occur in the middle cranial fossa and retrocerebellar region. The brain may be shifted by the arachnoid cyst, but the overall brain volume is usually close to normal. Arachnoid cysts are asymptomatic, incidental findings in the vast majority of cases. Occasionally, they may present with symptoms specific to the location of the lesion. The natural history of an arachnoid cyst is usually benign. Most cysts do not change over time, although some may enlarge, shrink, or even disappear completely. Treatment is rarely indicated, and only if the arachnoid cyst is clearly symptomatic. There are various surgical treatment options available including endoscopic or open fenestration of the cyst as well as cystoperitoneal shunting.

▶ Chiari Malformations

Chiari malformations consist of 4 types of congenital hindbrain abnormalities. Only Chiari Malformation Types I and II are commonly seen. Chiari I malformations are defined on imaging when the cerebellar tonsils extend at least 5 mm below the foramen magnum (Figure 36–18). The tonsils may assume a pointed, peg-shape instead of the normal rounded shape, causing crowding at the foramen magnum which limits CSF flow through the craniovertebral junction. Other CNS abnormalities associated with Chiari I malformation include syringomyelia (cavitation within the spinal cord), basilar invagination, platybasia, and Klippel–Feil anomaly. Children with Chiari I malformations are often asymptomatic but may also present with occipital headaches that are exacerbated by straining or coughing. Other symptoms include weakness, numbness, progressive scoliosis, long tract signs, central sleep apnea, or hydrocephalus. The workup should include imaging of the brain and spine to assess for the presence of a syrinx and CSF flow studies to evaluate flow at the foramen magnum. For symptomatic children with a Chiari I malformation and syrinx, surgical treatment

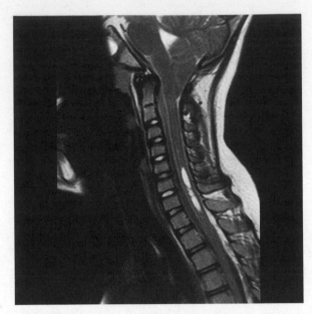

▲ **Figure 36–18.** Sagittal T2-weighted MRI scan of a Chiari showing typical peg-like appearance of cerebellar tonsils and associated syringomyelia.

is recommended. Surgery is never indicated for asymptomatic children with no syrinx. The decision to proceed with surgical intervention in a child with a diagnosis of type I Chiari malformation on imaging, headaches, but no syrinx must be made carefully given the common occurrence of headaches as well as incidental Chiari I in the neurologically normal population. Surgical treatment entails some combination of a suboccipital craniectomy, C1 laminectomy, and duraplasty. Syringomyelia associated with Chiari I malformation usually resolves or improves significantly after posterior fossa decompression.

Chiari II malformations are found in patients with myelomeningocele. On imaging, these patients exhibit a low position of the cerebellar vermis and tonsils below the foramen magnum; elongation, kinking, and displacement of the medulla below the foramen magnum and around the cervical spinal cord; abnormal lamination of the cerebral cortex; and often an upward displacement of the rostral cerebellum through a low-lying tentorium. Additional associated MR imaging characteristics of Chiari II malformations include hydrocephalus, fusion of the inferior colliculi of the brainstem, a large thalamic massa intermedia, a high-riding third ventricle, an elongated fourth ventricle, and a disproportionately small posterior fossa with asymmetric and flattened cerebellar folia. Symptomatic patients may present with apnea and other respiratory abnormalities secondary to compression of the medullary respiratory control center. Long tract signs, headache, ataxia, and gait instability may also be evident. In addition to myelomeningocele, other CNS abnormalities associated with Chiari II malformations include basilar impression, corpus callosum abnormalities, and cortical malformations. For symptomatic patients, surgical treatment consists of a posterior fossa decompression. Chiari III and IV malformations are very rare. Chiari III malformations include features of Chiari II malformation as well as an occipital encephalocele. Chiari IV malformations are characterized by severe cerebellar hypoplasia without an encephalocele.

▶ Craniosynostosis

Craniosynostosis refers to the premature fusion of one or more cranial sutures. When this occurs, bone growth is restricted in a direction perpendicular to the fused suture, and there is compensatory growth at other sites. The result is a misshapen head which may take one of several forms depending on which of the cranial sutures is involved. One or multiple sutures may be affected. The incidence of craniosynostosis is approximately 5 per 10,000 live births, and men are affected more than women.

Sagittal synostosis, the most common type of single suture synostosis, results in an elongated, boat-shaped skull referred to as scaphocephaly. In scaphocephaly, the biparietal diameter is reduced, while the anterior-posterior (AP) diameter is increased. Frontal bossing is common in this condition. Patients with sagittal synostosis have a palpable keel-like prominence over the fused sagittal suture.

Coronal synostosis may be either unilateral or bilateral. Unilateral coronal synostosis produces an asymmetric head shape known as plagiocephaly. The forehead on the affected side is flattened, while the forehead on the unaffected appears to bulge abnormally. Bilateral coronal synostosis results in brachycephaly, characterized by a broad, flattened forehead. The AP diameter is reduced, while the bitemporal and biparietal diameters are increased. When bilateral coronal synostosis occurs in combination with sagittal synostosis, turricephaly results. Turricephaly is characterized by a high, tower-like head shape with a vertical forehead.

Metopic synostosis is associated with trigonocephaly, a head shape that is characterized by a triangular-shaped forehead and hypotelorism. The bitemporal diameter is narrowed, and there is often a bony ridge in the midline of the forehead, over the fused metopic suture.

True unilateral lambdoid craniosynostosis is rare with an incidence of 1 in 300,000 live births, and it must be differentiated from positional posterior plagiocephaly, an increasingly common diagnosis. In unilateral lambdoid synostosis, there may be slight prominence of the forehead on the unaffected side. The ear on the affected side will be posteriorly and inferiorly displaced relative to the contralateral ear of the unaffected side. The head shape is trapezoidal when viewed from above.

While most cases of craniosynostosis are sporadic and involve a single suture, multiple-suture craniosynostosis occurs in certain genetic syndromes. Crouzon's syndrome is an autosomal dominant disorder characterized by the premature fusion of the bilateral coronal, frontosphenoid, and frontoethmoid sutures. Clinically, the condition is characterized by brachycephaly, maxillary hypoplasia, shallow orbits, proptosis, and a beaked nose. Apert's syndrome is an autosomal dominant condition which is characterized by pansynostosis. Clinically, patients have hypertelorism, midface hypoplasia, and shallow orbits in addition to their craniosynostosis. Symmetric syndactyly and short thumbs are also characteristic of Apert's syndrome. Hydrocephalus is common in this condition.

Operative repair of craniosynostosis is often improving cosmesis. Operative approaches vary from endoscopic strip craniectomies of the involved suture to more extensive cranial vault reconstruction.

HYDROCEPHALUS

Disturbances in cerebrospinal fluid (CSF) circulation or absorption result in hydrocephalus. Hydrocephalus can be classified into 2 types: obstructive or communicating. In obstructive hydrocephalus, CSF circulation is blocked within the ventricular system and there is enlargement in the ventricles proximal to the obstruction. In communicating hydrocephalus, CSF absorption is blocked at the level of the arachnoid granulations. Rarely, hydrocephalus may be due to the overproduction of CSF, as is the case in certain choroid plexus tumors.

The incidence of congenital hydrocephalus ranges from 0.9 to 1.8 per 1000 births. Neonatal hemorrhages of the germinal matrix and choroid plexus, as well as infections can cause adhesions to form in the cerebral aqueduct or at the foramen of Magendie and Luschka, interfering with CSF absorption.

Hydrocephalus can cause elevations in intracranial pressure which may manifest in different ways depending on the age of the child. In neonates and infants whose anterior fontanelle is still open, untreated hydrocephalus will present with a tense or bulging fontanelle, apneic and bradycardic episodes, engorgement of the scalp veins, upward gaze palsy, gaps between the cranial sutures, rapid increases in head circumference, irritability, poor head control, and poor oral intake. In children with a closed cranial vault whose fontanelle has closed, untreated hydrocephalus will present with symptoms of intracranial hypertension including lethargy or excessive sleepiness, papilledema, headache, nausea, vomiting, gait disturbance, increased fussiness, or upgaze or lateral gaze palsy.

Several surgical options can be considered in the treatment of hydrocephalus. The most common CSF diversionary procedure is ventriculoperitoneal shunting, creating a shunt between the cerebral ventricles and the peritoneal cavity. Other types of shunts may drain into other locations including the right atrium (ventriculoatrial shunt) or pleural cavity (ventriculopleural shunt). In children with certain types of obstructive hydrocephalus, an endoscopic third ventriculostomy may be considered, which involves fenestration of the floor of the third ventricle, thereby creating an alternative CSF pathway.

Shunt failure or infection may manifest with signs and symptoms of acute intracranial hypertension. Ventricular enlargement may or may not be present in shunt failure. Prompt treatment of acute hydrocephalus and/or shunt failure is indicated to prevent irreversible neurologic injury including herniation, blindness, or death.

PEDIATRIC CENTRAL NERVOUS SYSTEM TUMORS

Brain tumors are the most common solid tumors of childhood. The locations and types of tumors in the pediatric population differ from those in adults. Approximately two-thirds of brain tumors in children between 2 and 12 years of age occur in the infratentorial space. Brain tumors present in varying manners among different age groups. In neonates and infants, brain tumors may manifest with nonspecific findings, and mass effect from a tumor may not be clinically evident initially due to a compliant skull and an open fontanelle. In young children, a primary brain tumor may present with symptoms related to intracranial hypertension such as headache, nausea, and vomiting. Papilledema may be evident on funduscopic examination. Older children more often present with focal neurological signs and symptoms. The most common pediatric posterior fossa brain tumors are medulloblastoma, juvenile pilocytic astrocytoma, and ependymoma. When a posterior fossa brain tumor is diagnosed, preoperative imaging of the entire neuraxis should be performed whenever possible to evaluate for drop metastases in the spinal canal.

▶ Medulloblastoma

Medulloblastomas comprise approximately 20% of all pediatric brain tumors and 30% of all posterior fossa tumors in children. They appear as hyperdense lesions in the region of the fourth ventricle on CT imaging and enhance following contrast administration (Figure 36–19). Complete or near-complete surgical resection is the goal, as the extent of residual tumor is related to prognosis. Patients with medulloblastoma are stratified into either a standard or high-risk group. Those children who are younger than three years, have greater than 1.5 cm² residual tumor on postoperative imaging, or have dissemination of tumor away from the primary site as deemed by either imaging studies or positive CSF cytology have a worse prognosis and are classified as high risk. Postoperative craniospinal radiation with a boost

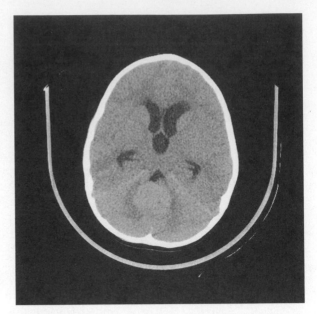

▲ **Figure 36–19.** Head CT demonstrating large mass (medulloblastoma) within the fourth ventricle causing ventricular dilation.

to the posterior fossa is indicated in children older than 3 years. Those patients who are classified as high risk are typically treated with chemotherapy as well. Because of the increased morbidity of radiation in children less than 3 years of age, chemotherapy is used to delay the radiation dose in such young patients. Recurrences, if they occur, typically occur within 3 years. The 5-year survival in standard risk patients is 70%, while that in high-risk patients is approximately 40%. Up to 25% of patients with a posterior fossa medulloblastoma may require a CSF diversionary procedure due to persistent postoperative hydrocephalus.

▶ Cerebellar Astrocytoma

Cerebellar astrocytomas account for approximately 20% of all pediatric brain tumors. The peak age of presentation is 10 years. The characteristic appearance on imaging studies is an enhancing mural nodule with a surrounding cyst. The goal of treatment is complete surgical resection, as patients with a gross total resection have a 90% long-term survival rate without any additional adjuvant therapies.

▶ Ependymoma

Ependymomas can arise anywhere along the neuraxis in relation to an ependymal surface. In the pediatric population, 90% of ependymomas are intracranial, and of these, two-thirds are located in the posterior fossa. Ependymomas commonly arise from the floor of the fourth ventricle in close proximity to the brainstem. When located in the fourth ventricle, ependymomas may extend out the foramina of Luschka and Magendie into the surrounding CSF subarachnoid cisterns. Dissemination of ependymoma tumor cells in the CSF can occur in up to 10% of cases, underscoring the importance of full neuraxis imaging to properly stage the disease. Treatment usually consists of tumor resection and postoperative focal radiation.

▶ Brainstem Glioma

Brainstem gliomas are a heterogeneous group of tumors of varying histology, biological behavior, and prognosis. Brainstem gliomas are typically be subdivided into four groups based on imaging characteristics: diffuse brainstem gliomas, focal brainstem gliomas, dorsally exophytic brainstem gliomas, and cervicomedullary gliomas. Diffuse brainstem gliomas represent up to 80% of all brainstem gliomas and carry the worst prognosis. They most commonly occur in the pons and can extend into the medulla or midbrain. The majority of children who are affected are between 6 and 10 years of age, and they present with a relatively short clinical history of unilateral or bilateral cranial neuropathies, progressive ataxia, gait abnormality, and long tract signs. On MR imaging studies, diffuse brainstem gliomas appear as non-enhancing, hypointense masses that expand the pons (Figure 36–20). They appear hyperintense on T2-weighted sequences, and with disease progression the tumor may completely encase the basilar artery. Histologically, they are

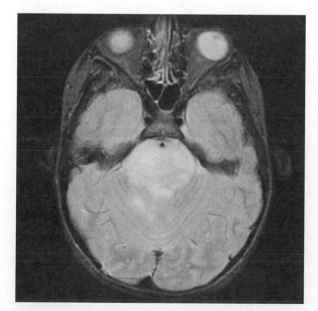

▲ **Figure 36–20.** Magnetic resonance imaging appearance of a diffuse pontine glioma.

malignant (WHO grade III or IV) astrocytomas. Diagnosis of a diffuse brainstem tumor can be made on the basis of imaging alone, and biopsy is usually not recommended. Radiation therapy and steroids may improve symptoms but have not been shown to prolong survival. These tumors are universally fatal, with a median survival of 8-10 months.

Other types of brainstem gliomas are associated with a better prognosis. Dorsally exophytic brainstem tumors grow from the subependymal surface into the fourth ventricle, away from the brainstem. They are characterized by slow growth with gradual onset of symptoms. Eventually they may obstruct CSF outflow from the fourth ventricle and result in hydrocephalus. Surgical excision should be performed when the predicted morbidity is not prohibitive. Histologically, focal intrinsic and dorsally exophytic brainstem gliomas are usually lower grade (WHO grade I or II) lesions. Cervicomedullary brainstem gliomas have similar behavior and histology as intramedullary spinal cord gliomas. These tumors may cause symptoms including weakness and lower cranial neuropathies. They should be resected.

▶ Tumors of Infancy

Brain tumors are present in 1.1 newborns per 100,000 births. Infantile tumors include medulloblastoma, central neuroblastoma, supratentorial primitive neuroectodermal tumor (PNET), pineoblastoma, and atypical teratoid/rhabdoid tumor (AT/RT). These are all high-grade tumors with a propensity to spread throughout the CSF. Medulloblastoma, central neuroblastoma, supratentorial PNET, and pineoblastomas are all considered PNETs with similar histologies. The combination of bilateral retinoblastomas and a midline pineoblastoma is referred to as "trilateral neuroblastoma" and carries a dismal prognosis. Atypical teratoid/rhabdoid tumors are usually found in the posterior fossa and are associated with deletions on chromosome 22 in over 90% of cases. AT/RTs have a poor prognosis, and most children die within 1 year of diagnosis.

▶ Pineal Region Tumors

Tumors arising in the region of the pineal gland comprise 3%-8% of pediatric brain tumors. Histologically, pineal region tumors are most often germ cell tumors such as germinomas, teratomas (mature and immature), embryonal cell carcinomas, choriocarcinomas, and endodermal sinus tumors. Germinomas are the most common pineal region tumors and demonstrate a gender predilection for men. Pineal parenchymal tumors such as pineocytoma or pineoblastomas occur less frequently. Pineal tumors can compress the cerebral aqueduct and cause hydrocephalus. Patients may present with a Parinaud's syndrome consisting of impaired upgaze, convergence-retraction nystagmus, lid retraction, convergence paralysis, pupillary dilatation, and light-near dissociation. Complete neuraxis imaging should be performed as drop metastases can occur via CSF pathways. Serum and CSF should be tested for tumor markers that may be secreted by germ cell tumors including placental alkaline phosphatase, alpha-fetoprotein, and beta-human chorionic gonadootropin (beta-HCG). Radiation therapy with or without chemotherapy is the mainstay of treatment for germ cells tumors.

DNET

Dysembryoplastic neuroepithelial tumor (DNET) is a low-grade cortical based tumor with a median age of presentation of 7 years. They appear as superficial cystic tumors in the temporal or frontal lobes. On MR imaging, they are hypointense on T1-weighted sequences, hyperintense on T2-weighted sequences, and do not enhance. The affected cortical gyrus often has a bubbly appearance. There is no edema or mass effect associated with DNETs. Patients with these tumors typically present with a long history of intractable complex partial seizures and have a normal neurological exam. Gross total resection of the tumor is curative and usually eliminates seizures.

Sellar Tumors

Tumors that arise in the region of the sella turcica and pituitary gland in children include pituitary adenomas and craniopharyngiomas. Pituitary adenomas are relatively rare among children. Craniopharyngiomas, however, represent 6%-9% of all pediatric brain tumors and are the most common nonglial intracranial masses in children. On imaging, craniopharyngiomas appear as cystic tumors which originate from a suprasellar location. Calcification within these tumors is common. Craniopharyngiomas are hyperintense on T1- and T2-weighted sequences due to fat, cholesterol, and proteinaceous contents within the cystic tumor. Craniopharyngiomas may cause symptoms attributable to intracranial hypertension and hydrocephalus or they may present with visual disturbances. Also, craniopharyngiomas may cause endocrine disturbances such as growth failure, diabetes insipidus, hypothyroidism, or menstrual dysfunction. A thorough endocrine workup is warranted in patients with suspected craniopharyngioma. The surgical approach depends on the location and extent of the craniopharyngioma. Potential surgical complications include diabetes insipidus or hypothalamic insufficiency.

Hypothalamic Optic Gliomas

Gliomas of the optic pathway are more common in the pediatric population. Included in this category are optic nerve gliomas and chiasmatic/hypothalamic astrocytomas. Histologically, these tumors are most often pilocytic astrocytomas. Optic nerve gliomas are associated with neurofibromatosis 1 (NF-1). Gliomas of the optic chiasm and

hypothalamus are cystic, globular tumors that enhance and rarely calcify. They may cause hydrocephalus due to compression at the foramen of Monro. Infants with hypothalamic/chiasmal gliomas present with visual loss, macrocephaly, and a diencephalic syndrome consisting of failure to thrive, cachexia, motor hyperactivity, and hyperalertness. Children 2-5 years of age may present with visual loss and endocrine dysfunction including short stature or precocious puberty. Symptoms in older children include visual loss and hypopituitarism. The goals of surgical treatment for chiasmatic/hypothalamic tumors are to obtain a tissue diagnosis and reestablish patent CSF pathways. Radiation has a clear benefit in extending progression-free survival. The 10-year relapse-free rate is approximately 55% with radiation versus 14% with biopsy alone. Chemotherapy is reserved for younger patients less than 5 years of age in order to delay radiation. The 10-year survival following surgical biopsy and radiation for chiasmatic/hypothalamic gliomas ranges from 48% to 55%; however, these tumors and their treatments are associated with significant morbidity, including visual impairment, endocrine dysfunction, obesity, and neurocognitive decline.

Choroid Plexus Tumors

Choroid plexus tumors include choroid plexus papillomas and choroid plexus carcinomas. They represent 2%-4% of all pediatric brain tumors. Choroid plexus papillomas occur in the atrium of the lateral ventricle in children and are attached to normal choroid plexus. These tumors avidly enhance and may calcify. If a gross total resection of the tumor is achieved, no adjuvant therapy is required. Choroid plexus papillomas are WHO grade I or II tumors and have a good prognosis. Choroid plexus carcinomas are malignant tumors for which the average age of diagnosis is 2 years. Like choroid plexus papillomas, these tumors are usually located in the lateral ventricles. Forty-five percent of choroid plexus carcinomas demonstrate dissemination at diagnosis. These tumors contain necrosis and can hemorrhage. Treatment consists of surgical resection, radiation therapy, and possibly chemotherapy. For children younger than 3 years of age, multiagent chemotherapy is used to delay the onset of radiation therapy. The prognosis is poor.

Spinal Cord Tumors

Spinal cord tumors in children account for 15% of all pediatric CNS tumors. Spinal cord tumors typically present with progressive back and leg pain, neurologic deficit, gait instability, torticollis, or bowel and bladder dysfunction. The most common intradural-intramedullary spinal cord tumors are low-grade glial tumors including astrocytomas. Treatment consists of early surgery, as postoperative morbidity is worse if preoperative neurologic deficits exist. Near-total resections of low-grade spinal cord gliomas in children can confer long-term progression-free survival. High-grade gliomas are treated with surgical debulking followed by adjuvant therapies. Intradural-extramedullary tumors in children include dermoid cysts, teratomas, and neurofibromas. Extradural primary spinal tumors that occur in childhood can present with myelopathy and spinal cord compression; such tumors include aneurysmal bone cysts, osteoid osteomas, osteoblastomas, eosinophilic granulomas, and rarely, metastatic disease.

Phakomatoses

Phakomatoses are neurocutaneous syndromes that manifest with skin lesions and central nervous system tumors. Most of the phakomatoses are inherited conditions. NF-1 is an autosomal dominant inherited condition caused by a mutation on chromosome 17. Optic nerve gliomas are associated with NF-1 and, in affected children, usually occur before 6 years of age. Neurofibromatosis 2 (NF-2) is an autosomal dominant syndrome that results from a mutation on chromosome 22. Typical CNS tumors associated with NF-2 include bilateral acoustic neuromas, meningiomas, schwannomas, and intramedullary spinal cord ependymomas.

Tuberous sclerosis (TS) is an autosomal dominant syndrome that arises from mutations in chromosomes 9, 11, or 16. Children with TS can get periventricular hamartomas known as subependymal nodules near the foramen of Monro and adjacent to the caudate nucleus. In 15% of patients with TS, subependymal nodules can transform into a subependymal giant cell astrocytoma, a WHO grade I lesion. These are benign, enhancing tumors that arise at the foramen of Monro and cause obstructive hydrocephalus. These tumors typically occur prior to the end of the second decade of life. They can enlarge with time, and gross total resection of the subependymal giant cell astrocytoma is considered curative. The CNS lesions in TS frequently cause seizures.

Von Hippel–Lindau (VHL) disease is an autosomal dominant disease due to a mutation on chromosome 3. Patients with VHL can get hemangioblastomas, most commonly in the posterior fossa and spinal cord. Although hemangioblastomas are considered benign tumors, they may recur in multiple locations in patients with VHL.

CEREBROVASCULAR DISEASE IN CHILDREN

Aneurysms & Vascular Malformations

Children may present with a variety of intracranial vascular malformations such as arteriovenous malformations (AVMs), venous angiomas, capillary telangiectasias, and cavernous malformations. AVMs may present with seizures or focal deficits from a hemorrhage. Without treatment, patients are at risk for recurrent hemorrhages. AVMs are usually treated with surgery in the pediatric age group but

may occasionally be treated with stereotactic radiation or embolization techniques. In patients with an autosomal dominant inherited cavernous malformation syndrome, the cavernous malformations may be multiple and hemorrhage at an earlier age. Cavernous malformations are treated with surgical resection. Intracranial saccular aneurysm rupture is rare in the pediatric population. Depending on the size and configuration of the aneurysm, these lesions may be treated by surgical clipping, endovascular coiling, or managed conservatively.

Vein of Galen Malformations

Vein of Galen malformations are congenital vascular malformations characterized by extensive arterial feeders draining into an enlarged vein of Galen. Although these malformations are also known as Vein of Galen aneurysms, they represent arteriovenous fistulae. Newborns can present with high-output cardiac failure due to the arteriovenous shunting. Hydrocephalus is common from compression of the cerebral aqueduct by the malformation. Seizures are also associated with these lesions. The extensive arteriovenous shunting can produce a steal effect and result in cerebral ischemia and infarction. The prognosis may be poor for patients diagnosed in early infancy with heart failure. The prognosis is better for those diagnosed later in life. Treatment usually involves endovascular embolization of feeding arteries.

Moyamoya Disease

Moyamoya disease is an idiopathic vasculopathy that leads to progressive occlusion of one or both internal carotid arteries with secondary formation of a collateral capillary network at the base of the brain. The disease can also involve the proximal middle and anterior cerebral arteries. On angiography, the collateral vessels have a characteristic "puff-of-smoke" appearance. Children with Moyamoya disease present with ischemic events that may be provoked by straining or hyperventilation. Refractory headaches, seizures, and alternating hemiplegia are also associated with Moyamoya disease. Moyamoya is treated with surgical revascularization to improve blood flow via direct or indirect bypass procedures.

SPASTICITY

Spasticity in children is most often due to cerebral palsy, and several surgical options are available for treatment. In determining whether a child with hypertonia will benefit from surgical intervention, it is important to assess if dystonia is present as well and its contribution to the hypertonia, the ambulatory potential of the child, and to what extent the underlying spasticity is useful for the child in terms of providing strength and allowing them to support their own weight.

In addition to medication, orthopedic procedures, and periodic injections that are used to treat spasticity, the neurosurgical treatments for spasticity include placement of an intrathecal baclofen pump and selective dorsal rhizotomy (SDR). An intrathecal baclofen pump entails inserting a catheter into the intrathecal space and connecting it to a subcutaneous pump so that the antispasticity drug baclofen may be continuously delivered. Depending on at what spinal level the catheter tip is placed, upper and lower extremity spasticity may be treated. Intrathecal baclofen pumps are useful if the upper extremities are affected by severe hypertonia, if the tone conferred by spasticity is required for standing or walking, or if the lower extremity spasticity in nonambulatory patients is disabling and hinders care of the patients. Those patients who are ambulatory and whose spasticity primarily affects their lower extremities may be candidates for an SDR. It is thought that inputs entering the spinal cord through the dorsal roots have a net excitatory effect on the anterior roots, thus contributing to spasticity. The premise of an SDR is to intraoperatively stimulate lumbosacral dorsal nerve rootlets and record responses from the anterior nerve roots and muscles. This allows for the identification of those nerve rootlets that are relatively more involved into maintaining hypertonia, and such nerve rootlets are sectioned. SDR has been shown to improve ambulation, but the procedure does not confer previously nonambulatory patients the ability to walk.

PEDIATRIC TRAUMA AND BIRTH INJURIES

▶ General Principles

Head injury and its management are discussed elsewhere, and treatment principles used in the management of adult trauma also apply to the pediatric patient. Certain aspects of trauma that are unique to the pediatric population are highlighted. Head injuries are 30 times more common in children than spinal cord injuries, and they represent the most common cause of mortality and morbidity in children. In infants and young children, the brain and head are disproportionately large compared to the trunk and torso, and the neck and paraspinal musculature are incompletely developed. In children younger than 4 years, the skull is soft, unilaminar, and without diploë; as a result, it provides less protection to the brain for absorbing a traumatic impact and is more prone to fracture. Skull fractures in children can be linear, depressed, or ping-pong ball fractures. Ping-pong ball fractures occur in newborns and appear as a focal area of caved in skull that resembles a crushed ping-pong ball. No surgical intervention is required for ping-pong ball fractures in the temporoparietal region, as the growing skull will correct the deformity. Surgical elevation of a frontal ping-pong ball fracture may be considered for cosmetic purposes.

▶ Nonaccidental Trauma

Nonaccidental head trauma is the leading cause of death and morbidity in children less than 2 years of age. In shaken baby syndrome, there may be few signs of external trauma with significant neurological injury. Alternatively, the child may present with lethargy, irritability, poor feeding, apneic episodes, or seizures. Multiple skull fractures that are associated with underlying brain injury, bilateral chronic subdural hematomas or subdural hematomas of varying ages, subarachnoid hemorrhage, and retinal hemorrhages should raise the index of suspicion for child abuse. Subdural hemorrhages commonly occur along the bilateral convexities or in the posterior interhemispheric fissure. MR imaging is best at evaluating subdural hematomas of varying ages, as well as the extent of DIA that occurs with the acceleration-deceleration and rotational forces in shaken baby syndrome. A workup should include imaging of the brain and possibly spine, a skeletal survey to assess for long-bone or rib fractures, a funduscopic examination to check for retinal hemorrhages, and a thorough external exam to assess for bruising. Death from nonaccidental trauma is most often due to refractory intracranial hypertension.

▶ Spine Trauma

Spinal cord injury is relatively rare in the pediatric population and accounts for 5% of all spinal cord injury. The pediatric spine continues to develop throughout the first 2 decades of life. Ligamentous injury is more common than bony injury, owing to ligamentous laxity, immature supporting musculature, and the developing bony joints of the spine. The cervical spine is most commonly injured in children, and in children less than 9 years of age, two-thirds of cervical spine injuries occur between the C1 and C3 levels.

Al-Holou WN, Yew AY, Boomsaad ZE, Garton HJ, Muraszko KM, Maher CO: Prevalence and natural history of arachnoid cysts in children. *J Neurosurg Pediatr* 2010;5(6):578-585.

Cunningham ML, Heike CL: Evaluation of the infant with an abnormal skull shape. *Curr Opin Pediatr* 2007;19:645-651.

Lew SM, Kothbauer KF: Tethered cord syndrome: an updated review. *Pediatr Neurosurg* 2007;43:236-248.

Nield LS, Brunner MD, Kamat D: The infant with a misshapen head. *Clin Pediatr* 2007;46:292-298.

Shu HG, Sall WF, Maity A, et al: Childhood intracranial ependymomas. Twenty-year experience from a single institution. *Cancer* 2007;110:432-441.

Strahle J, Muraszko KM, Kapurch J, Bapuraj JR, Garton HJ, Maher CO: Chiari malformation Type I and syrinx in children undergoing magnetic resonance imaging. *J Neurosurg Pediatr* 2011;8(2):205-213.

Strahle J, Muraszko KM, Kapurch J, Bapuraj JR, Garton HJ, Maher CO: Natural history of Chiari malformation type I following decision for conservative treatment. *J Neurosurg Pediatr* 2011:8(2):214-221.

INTRACRANIAL ANEURYSMS AND ARTERIOVENOUS MALFORMATIONS

Aditya S. Pandey, MD Tristram Horton, MD John A Cowan, Jr, MD Neeraj Chaudhary, MD Joseph G. Gemmete, MD B. Gregory Thompson, MD

INTRACRANIAL ANEURYSMS

▶ General Considerations

Intracranial aneurysms (IAs) represent an abnormal dilation or expansion of an artery within the cranial vault. Autopsy studies suggest that IAs are present within 1%-5% of the population. Most epidemiologic studies suggest that CAAs are more common in women (3:2) and results in the clinical presentation of approximately 30,000-35,000 people annually in the United States. Aneurysms are categorized as saccular, fusiform, or mycotic, and can be ruptured, expanding, or unruptured. Aneurysms can be located anywhere within the cerebral artery tree but are most commonly located in the Circle of Willis. The specific type, status, and location of an IA can drastically affect a patient's clinical presentation, treatment options, and outcome. Intracranial aneurysms can be detected with a variety of imaging modalities, including cerebral angiography (Figure 36–21), computed tomography angiography (CTA), or magnetic resonance angiography (MRA). Patients with intracranial aneurysms should be referred to a neurosurgeon who specializes in the treatment of neurovascular diseases.

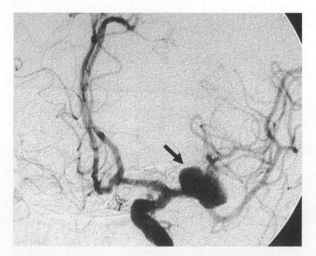

▲ **Figure 36–21.** An anterior view of left carotid artery cerebral angiogram demonstrating a large cerebral artery aneurysm (arrow) at the middle cerebral artery bifurcation.

Table 36–6. Hunt–Hess scale.[1]

Grade	Findings
I	Mild headache or nuchal rigidity
II	Severe headache, nuchal rigidity, possible cranial nerve deficit
III	Lethargic, confused, mild focal deficit
IV	Stuporous, moderate to severe hemiparesis, early decerebrate posturing
V	Deep coma, decerebrate posturing, moribund

[1]Adapted from: Hunt WE, Hess RM: Surgical repair as related to time of intervention in the repair of intracranial aneurysms. *J Neurosurg* 1968;28:14.

▶ Clinical Findings

A ruptured intracranial aneurysm typically presents as a sudden, severe headache associated with nuchal rigidity and lethargy. Patients often describe the headache as the "worst headache of my life," however, sentinel (or smaller) bleeds may not present with such severity. Other features at presentation can include vomiting, seizure, focal neurologic deficit (eg hemiparesis, oculomotor palsy, etc), or coma. The Hunt–Hess grading scale is commonly used to convey the severity of symptoms and is often used to risk-stratify patients (Table 36–6). The Fisher and World Federation of Neurological Surgeons are other grading scales commonly employed for patients presenting with spontaneous subarachnoid hemorrhage (SAH), based radiographically and clinically, respectively. Approximately 10%-20% of patients die prior to reaching a hospital and the overall mortality rate approaches 30%-50%. The peak age of rupture is between 45 and 55 years. The rebleed rate of a ruptured intracranial aneurysm is approximately 25% at two weeks and 50% by 6 months. The mortality of a rebleed approaches 80%.

Since the cerebral arteries course within the subarachnoid space, aneurysm rupture results in SAHs. Subarachnoid hemorrhages have a classic appearance on computed tomography (CT) scans, where the blood fills the normal cerebrospinal fluid (CSF) spaces surround the cortex, brainstem, and cerebellum (Figure 36–22). The differential diagnosis of SAH includes aneurysm rupture, trauma, coagulopathy, pretruncal (or perimesencephalic) venous bleed, cranial/spinal AVM, or dural venous sinus thrombosis. Intracranial aneurysm rupture may cause intracerebral hemorrhage, subdural hemorrhage, and intraventricular hemorrhage.

Expanding IAs may or may present with symptoms of SAH. Patients with an expanding IA may exhibit neurologic symptoms consistent with focal compression. Though often not as dramatic a presentation as with rupture,

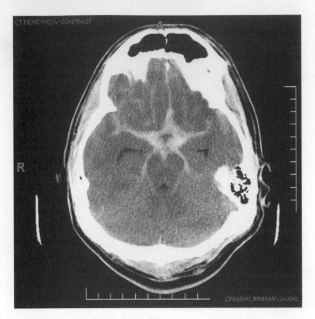

▲ **Figure 36–22.** Classic appearance of a large subarachnoid hemorrhage. Notice the hemorrhage pattern fills the cerebrospinal fluid spaces at the base of the brain and around the brainstem.

expanding CAAs should be treated as emergencies. The specific deficit at presentation is dependent on the location of the aneurysm. Aneurysms along the posterior communicating (PComm) artery, classically present with a third nerve palsy (pupil dilation, eye abducted, and downward in position). Aneurysms along the posterior cerebral artery, although rarer, can have such a presentation. Aneurysms on the anterior communicating (AComm) artery can present with signs of optic apparatus compression. Cavernous internal carotid artery aneurysms can produce oculomotor palsies with retro-orbital pain. Ophthalmic artery aneurysms can lead to unilateral vision loss. Giant aneurysms (> 2.5 cm) can lead to more pronounced symptoms, including hemiparesis, obstructed hydrocephalus, hypothalamic dysfunction, seizures, and brainstem compression due to mass effect.

With the increasing availability and resolution of neuroimaging modalities, the detection of unruptured (and often asymptomatic) aneurysms is increasing. Although controversial, the estimated rupture rate of an unruptured intracranial aneurysms is 0.1%-2% per year. The rupture risk is dependent upon a number of factors, including aneurysm size, shape, and location. Other factors, including the hypertension and smoking history, as well as genetic predisposition (female sex, family history of SAH, certain arteriopathies), also play an important role in estimating the risk of aneurysm growth and rupture. Given the potentially

devastating consequences of IA rupture, however, treatment of an unruptured IA should be considered in most cases.

▶ Treatment

A. Initial Management

A rapid history and physical examination of the patient including determination of the patient's airway, breathing, and circulation ("ABCs") should be performed in patients with a suspected ruptured intracranial aneurysm. Patients with unstable or unprotected airways or poor respiratory effort should be intubated and placed on mechanical ventilation. Maintenance of Pco2 values between 28 and 32 mm Hg can help acutely lower intracranial pressure and this range promotes adequate cerebral perfusion. Blood pressure should be controlled with a ceiling level of 160/90 mm Hg, maintained as needed with intravenous medications. Prophylactic anticonvulsant and gastrointestinal (H$_2$ blocker or proton pump inhibitor) should be given as well. An arterial line and central venous line should be placed to further assist in management. Basic laboratory values needed include blood gas, complete blood count, coagulation function, sodium level, blood urea nitrogen, and creatinine. An electrocardiogram and chest x-ray should also be performed. Occasionally, patients presenting with SAH can exhibit signs and symptoms of pulmonary edema and/or heart failure requiring further intervention. Determination of the type and status of the CAA, via cerebral imaging, is paramount in dictating the remainder of the treatment algorithm. Demonstration of SAH on the initial head CT in patients with suspected CAA should be immediately followed by an assessment of the cerebral vascular tree (conventional angiography, CTA, etc). If the head CT does not demonstrate SAH and suspicion is high, a lumbar puncture can be performed. Typically, in the setting of CT-negative SAH, a lumbar puncture will reveal xanthochromia or high red blood cell counts that do not decrease (or "clear") across serial CSF samples. Cerebrospinal fluid diversion, typically through ventriculostomy, can be performed if the patient presents with hydrocephalus or has concerns for elevated intracranial pressure.

B. Surgical Management

Currently, two (three) main modalities exist for treating CAAs: surgical clip occlusion and endovascular coiling, and more recently, endovascular flow diversion. Surgical clip occlusion requires an open craniotomy and microsurgical dissection to the base of a CAA in order to apply a surgical clip around the neck of the aneurysm. In some cases, the aneurysm may require trapping and bypass (either surgical or endovascular) for treatment. Endovascular coiling utilizes a similar approach as conventional angiography and is thus less invasive. The endovascular surgeon navigates a microcatheter to the aneurismal defect and inserts detachable coils into the aneurysm dome. These coils promote thrombus formation and thus exclude the aneurysm from the native circulation.

The decision between clipping or coiling a CAA is complex and beyond the scope of this text. Factors considered in this decision include a patient's age, overall medical condition, and preference as well as the aneurysm's size, location, and morphology and the ruptured versus unruptured status of the aneurysm. To date, one trial has attempted to compare the two approaches for a very select group of ruptured CAAs. The study concluded that endovascular coiling resulted in slightly less morbidity and mortality at one year follow-up. The three randomized prospective trials comparing clipping and coiling have all found coiling to have lower risk of unfavorable outcome compared to clipping in the treatment of ruptured intracranial aneurysms. One study found clipping to be superior to coiling, with a significantly higher increased risk of death or readmission secondary to rebleeding in patients treated endovascularly. However, this study was limited by its retrospective cohort design. Case series with long-term follow-up have demonstrated some increase in rebleeding and/or the need for further treatment with endovascular coiling as compare to clip occlusion. More recent studies have shown a decrease in the recurrence and rebleeding rate after endovascular treatment of intracranial aneurysms. One study found that rebleeding rate was a function of degree of aneurysm occlusion on initial treatment, rather than the treatment modality itself.

C. Medical Management

The medical management of patients who undergo either surgical clip occlusion or endovascular coiling for a ruptured CAA is particularly challenging. Patients require recovery in an intensive care setting that has particular expertise in neurological conditions. Once an aneurysm has been secured the blood pressure parameters are loosened and "permissive" hypertension is allowed (typically do not treat unless SBP > 200 mm Hg). Early tracheostomy and enteral feeding tubes are placed in patients who have neurologic deficits affecting respiratory or swallowing function. Patients are typically placed on Nimodipine, which has been demonstrated to slightly decrease postoperative vasospasm. Magnesium sulfate infusions are used in some centers for prevention of vasospasm although the data for this, while promising, is emerging.

Vasospasm is an idiopathic response of cerebral blood vessels to subarachnoid blood whereby the vessel constricts thus limiting distal blood flow. The peak time for vasospasm occurs between 4 and 14 days postbleed. Approximately 20%-40% of patients with have symptomatic vasospasm with 30% of those suffering a permanent neurologic deficit. Vasospasm can occur anywhere along a vessel and in vessels distant from the treated aneurysm. Patients can exhibit significant neurologic

sequelae from vasospasm such as hemiparesis, aphasia, visual disturbance, etc depending on the particular vessel affected. Subtle findings including elevation in temperature and mental status changes can be harbingers of vasospasm. Vasospasm is typically treated using a regimen referred to as "triple H" therapy. This therapy involves hypertension (using vasopressors if needed to achieve SBP > 180), hemodilution (achieve hematocrit ~30%), and hypervolemia (using albumin or hypertonic solutions to achieve CVP 8-14 mm Hg). Cerebral angioplasty is an effective means for treating proximal constriction and is a first line treatment for symptomatic patients. Distal or diffuse spasm can respond to injection of calcium-channel blockers (eg, verapamil and nicardipine) papaverine, or milrinone (a phosphodiesterase-3 inhibitor) through a super-selective microcatheter.

▶ Outcomes/Prognosis

For elective surgical clip occlusion or endovascular coiling, mortality rates (1%-2%) and morbidity rates (5%-10%) are relatively low. Risk factors for poor outcome would include aneurysm location, size, and presence of intraoperative rupture as well as other comorbid conditions (eg, coronary artery disease, diabetes, age, etc). In patients presenting with SAH, patient age, comorbid conditions, and Hunt–Hess grade are the strongest predictors of outcome. Overall, for patients stable enough for surgical intervention, mortality rates range from 10% to 20% with morbidity rates of 20%-40%.

Amenta PS, Dalyai RT, Kung D, et al: Stent-assisted coiling of wide-necked aneurysms in the setting of acute subarachnoid hemorrhage: experience in 65 patients. *Neurosurgery* 2012;70(6):1415-1429.

International Subarachnoid Hemorrhage Aneurysm Trial (ISAT) of Neurosurgical Clipping versus Endovascular Coiling in 2143 Patients with Ruptured Intracranial Aneurysms: a randomised trial. *Lancet* 2002;360:1267-1274.

Johnston SC: Rates of delayed rebleeding from intracranial aneurysms are low after surgical and endovascular treatment. *Stroke* 2006;37:1437-1442.

Johnston SC, Dowd CF, Higashida RT, et al: Predictors of rehemorrhage after treatment of ruptured intracranial aneurysms. The Cerebral Aneurysm Rerupture after Treatment (CARAT) Study. *Stroke* 2008;39:120-125.

Molyneux AJ, Kerr RS, Yu L, et al: International Subarachnoid Aneurysm Trial (ISAT) of Neurosurgical Clipping versus Endovascular Coiling in 2143 Patients with Ruptured Intracranial Aneurysms: a randomised comparison of effects on survival, dependency, seizures, rebleeding, subgroups, and aneurysm occlusion. *Lancet* 2005;366:809-817.

McDougall CG, Spetzler RF, Zabramski JM, et al: The barrow ruptured aneurysm trial. *J Neurosurg* 2012;116:135-144.

O'Kelly, CJ, Kulkarni AV, Austin PC, et al: The impact of therapeutic modality on outcomes following repair of ruptured intracranial aneurysms: an Administrative Data Analysis. *J Neurosurgery* 2010;113:795-801.

Arteriovenous Malformations

Key concepts:

1. Congenital, abnormal connections of arteries and veins without intervening capillaries

2. Annual rupture risk of brain AVM's is 2%-4% per year

3. Treatment may be surgical, endovascular, or with radiosurgery and is performed to prevent intracranial hemorrhage

4. In some instances, observant management may be appropriate

General Considerations

AVMs are tangles of congenital abnormal connections between artery and vein with no normal intervening capillary bed. Ninety percent of AVMs are found in the supratentorial space with the remainder found in the brainstem and spine. AVMs can present at any time but are more common in younger patients. Vascular malformations are commonly seen in neurosurgical practice and with modern imaging techniques are increasingly diagnosed in asymptomatic patients being evaluated for headaches or after minor head trauma. Because of this, as well as their risk of rupture and the high morbidity associated with intracranial hemorrhage, it is important that all acute care physicians be aware of their presentation, initial management, and treatment of these lesions.

Epidemiology and Presentation

As many AVMs are asymptomatic, it is difficult to absolutely determine their prevalence. Autopsy data estimate that AVMs occur in less than 1%-4% of the population. A limited number of population-based studies have been conducted to study the natural history and bleeding risks in patients with AVMs. In counseling patients, the following formula has been used to estimate lifetime of intracranial hemorrhage due to AVM rupture:

Lifetime risk (%) = 105 − patient age in years

Hemorrhage is the most common presentation, occurring in over 50% of patients. Because of this, many patients with AVMs are initially evaluated in the emergency department. Seizures and headaches are also frequent, especially with larger lesions. Spinal AVMs may cause back or radicular pain, lower extremity weakness, gait disturbance, or incontinence. Large AVMs with high-volume venous drainage can cause steal phenomena; focal neurologic deficits may result from decreased tissue perfusion of surrounding brain. Increasingly, patients are referred after AVM's are found incidentally by computed tomography (CT) or magnetic resonance imaging (MRI).

Initial Evaluation & Care

The initial evaluation of AVMs depends upon the patient's presentation. Many patients who present with rupture are stable, neurologically and medically. The majority of intracranial bleeding from AVM rupture is intraparenchymal. Although there may be an aspect of subarachnoid hemorrhage, it is rare to see isolated subarachnoid hemorrhage in the setting of AVM rupture. In contrast to aneurysmal subarachnoid hemorrhage, where the presence of clot in the subarachnoid space is often immediately devastating, AVM bleeds are less likely to cause death. Also in contrast to aneurysmal subarachnoid hemorrhage, vasospasm is a relatively rare event with AVM associated hemorrhage. This is not to suggest a ruptured AVM is a minor problem—mortality associated with a single hemorrhage is estimated at 10% and morbidity 30%. However, the heterogeneous nature of presenting complaints in patients with AVMs helps explain why the initial approach to patients with AVM's varies from those with aneurysms, especially in the acute setting.

In ruptured patients, after ensuring the fundamentals of emergency care—airway, breathing, and circulation—are addressed, a complete neurological evaluation should be performed. Neurosurgical consultation is appropriate. Blood pressure should be maintained in the normal range. In any patient with suspected intracranial hemorrhage, a noncontrast head CT should be obtained as soon as possible. Depending upon physician and institutional preferences, CT angiography (CTA) or conventional diagnostic angiography (Figure 36–23) may then be performed to further evaluate the angiographic architecture of the AVM and to guide treatment. MR angiography (MRA) takes longer to obtain than CTA and the angiographic image quality, in our opinion, is suboptimal when compared to CTA; it is not routinely used in the acute setting.

With an initial CT scan that appears consistent with AVM rupture, a standard approach includes conventional angiography. This provides the neuroendovascular team the potential to proceed with AVM embolization during the same procedure as the diagnostic angiogram. Alternatively, for small or deep AVMs, CTA may be appropriate, as these types of lesions are often treated with radiosurgery and the risks of diagnostic angiography may be avoided. In some instances, CTA may not provide a sufficiently clear picture of the AVM and conventional angiography will need to be performed. In this case, it is important to closely monitor renal function due to the multiple contrast dye loads. Adequate hydration with intravenous fluids is important, and in patients with renal insufficiency, bicarbonate infusion and Mucomyst are useful for renal protection. Any patient with intracranial hemorrhage, even those who are neurologically intact, should initially be admitted to the neurosurgical intensive care unit for close monitoring with hourly neurologic examinations.

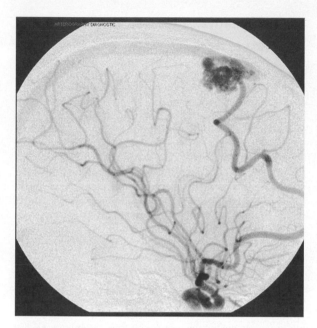

▲ **Figure 36–23.** Cerebral angiogram demonstrating a frontal arteriovenous malformation filling from the left anterior cerebral artery.

Table 36–7 Spetzler–Martin AVM grading scale.

Graded Feature	Points Assigned
Size of AVM	1
< 3 cm	2
3-6 cm	3
> 6 cm	
Eloquence[1] of adjacent brain	
Noneloquent	0
Eloquent	1
Venous drainage	
Superficial	0
Deep	1

[1]Eloquent areas include: visual, language, and sensorimotor cortex; the thalamus and hypothalamus; the internal capsule; the brainstem; the cerebellar peduncles; and the deep cerebellar nuclei.

In patients presenting with seizures or those with large bleeds and mass effect, treatment with antiepileptic medication is appropriate. Phenytoin or Keppra are effective in the acute setting for seizure prophylaxis.

An important concept when discussing brain AVM treatment options and prognosis with patients and the multiple physicians who may care for patients with these lesions is AVM grade. Grading is most often performed using the Spetzler–Martin scale (Table 36–7). Points are assigned based upon size (< 3 cm, 1 point; 3-6 cm, 2 points; or > 6 cm, 3 points), venous drainage (superficial, 0 points; or deep, 1 point), and eloquence (absent, 0 points; present, 1 point) of the surrounding brain, yielding Grades of I-V. The size and venous drainage categories are straightforward; eloquent areas are defined as the sensorimotor, language, and visual cortex; the thalamus and hypothalamus; the internal capsule; the brainstem; the cerebellar peduncles; and the deep cerebellar nuclei. AVM grade correlates with surgical results.

▶ **Treatment**

Four options currently exist for the treatment of AVMs. They are endovascular embolization, microsurgical resection, SRS, and observant management. Treatment often employs a combination of these approaches. AVMs should be treated in referral centers with significant experience. There is no treatment algorithm for these complex lesions.

Multiple variables intrinsic to the AVM or the patient have been implicated as making certain lesions higher risk for bleeding; most of these are controversial. It is important to evaluate each patient individually, preferably with a multidisciplinary team of vascular neurosurgery, interventional neuroradiology, and radiation oncology. Multiple factors must be considered prior to recommending treatment, including AVM grade and location (for surgical safety), angiographic architecture and presence of reachable arterial pedicles (for endovascular safety), and the ability of the patient to safely tolerate an invasive procedure. Patient preference is also important, especially when considering radiosurgery. Treatment is primarily performed because of intracranial hemorrhage—to prevent an initial or recurrent hemorrhage, or to evacuate the intracranial clot that occurs after AVM rupture. Secondary treatment goals include the relief of mass effect causing headache or seizures.

A. Endovascular Embolization

The goal of endovascular embolization for AVMs is usually to reduce the size of the nidus and risk of bleeding during microsurgical resection or to reduce the size of the AVM prior to radiosurgery. However, in some cases (10%-20%) complete cure can be achieved with embolization alone. It is important to appropriately counsel patients prior to AVM embolization that if complete occlusion of the AVM cannot be achieved, further treatment with surgery or radiosurgery is necessary as incompletely embolized AVMs may have a higher risk of bleeding.

B. Microsurgical Resection

As complete obliteration is the only way to cure an AVM, microsurgical resection for small, superficial lesions is the gold standard by which all other treatment modalities are measured. Most neurosurgeons agree that Spetzler–Martin Grade I-III AVMs on the cerebral convexity should be surgically resected. Complication rates associated with these lesions are low, when they are operated on by neurosurgeons with significant experience. Spetzler and Martin retrospectively reported the risk of minor and major neurologic deficit and death in a series of 100 patients with Grade I–V AVMs. For Grade I patients, risk of minor and major deficit was 0%; Grade II AVMs carried a 5% risk of minor deficit and 0% risk of major deficit; Grade III lesions had a 12% risk of minor deficit and 4% risk of major deficit. There were no deaths. Complication rates are higher for Grade IV and V AVMs. Grade IV AVMs carried a 20% risk of minor deficit and 7% risk of major deficit. With Grade V lesions, risks of minor and major deficit were 19% and 12%, respectively. The prospective application of the Spetzler–Martin scale in 120 patients revealed permanent, major neurological deficits in 0% of Grade I-III patients, 21.9% of Grade IV patients, and 16.7% of Grade V patients. The relatively high risk of neurological deficit in Grade IV and V patients make recommending surgery for these lesions a difficult decision. As endovascular technology has improved, however, some of these lesions may be approached endovascularly first, with the goal of attempting to reduce the size of the AVM prior to surgical resection.

C. Stereotactic Radiosurgery

Radiosurgery is an excellent treatment modality for many AVMs, especially those located in deep locations of the cortex or lesions of the basal ganglia, thalamus, or brainstem that are not easily approachable from a microsurgical or endovascular standpoint. SRS is also indicated for patients with significant medical comorbidities and can be used if an AVM is subtotally resected. In general, SRS works best for AVMs less than 3 cm in size. In patients with AVMs larger than 3 cm, preradiosurgical embolization may be used to reduce the size of the nidus. The complete obliteration rate after SRS is 90% with small AVMs. The primary disadvantage of SRS is the 2-3 years it takes for the AVM to involute. During that period, the patient remains at baseline risk of hemorrhage (~4%) from AVM rupture.

D. Observant Management

Although this is not the opinion of the vast majority of neurosurgeons and neurointerventionalists, there are occasions when conservative management is indicated. Older patients with comorbid conditions may not benefit from aggressive management. Because of the risk of complications during open or endovascular operations with Grade IV and V AVMs, and because of the reduced rate of complete obliteration after radiosurgery for large lesions, some surgeons advocate conservative treatment for these AVMs.

▶ Postoperative Care

Patients who have undergone endovascular or open operations should be observed postoperatively in an ICU until it is certain they are neurologically stable. Typically, patients are sent to the ward on postoperative day one from microsurgical resection. Postembolization patients are usually discharged home after an overnight stay. Complications after microsurgical resection include the usual postcraniotomy difficulties such as bleeding and seizures. Hydrocephalus can also occur, especially in patients who present with ventricular blood as part of an initial intracranial hemorrhage. Complications to keep in mind after embolization include stroke, renal insufficiency, and groin hematoma. Creatinine and hematocrit should be monitored. Any patient with unstable vital signs or decreasing hematocrit after embolization should be assumed to have a retroperitoneal hematoma, should undergo abdominal CT scanning and be treated aggressively.

After AVM resection, a phenomenon known as normal perfusion pressure breakthrough can occur. As the pathological shunting of blood through the AVM nidus is removed, relative increases in blood flow to the surrounding blood vessels and brain occurs. As these blood vessels are often chronically dysregulated by the relative lack of blood flow caused by the AVM, hemorrhage can result when blood flow returns to normal. One similarly dangerous potential complication after partial embolization is AVM rupture. In general, endovascular neurosurgeons and interventionalists do not embolize more than 1/3 of an AVM at a time. This is because with larger embolizations, dramatic changes in blood flow to the AVM can occur, effectively overwhelming the pathologic vessels remaining, causing hemorrhage. For these reasons, in both instances, patients must be carefully observed postoperatively. Also, it is critical that blood pressure remain in the normotensive range for at least 24 hours posttreatment.

▶ Spinal Arteriovenous Malformations

Spinal AVMs are divided into 4 types: (1) dural arteriovenous fistulas; (2) glomus AVMs; (3) juvenile intradural AVMs; and (4) intradural, extramedullary arteriovenous fistulas. Types 1 and 4 have high blood flow but low pressure; types 2 and 3 have high blood flow, high pressure and are more likely to hemorrhage. Dural arteriovenous fistulas (type 1) are the most common spinal vascular malformation seen. They typically occur near the thoracolumbar junction and consist of a single transdural arterial feeding vessel that directly connects to an intradural arterialized vein. Embolization of the feeding artery, or clip placement across the artery, is curative. Symptoms from spinal AVMs may be due to hemorrhage or venous congestion. Acute or subacute lower extremity neurological deficit, gait difficulties, myelopathy, or loss of bladder or bowel control may result. Initial diagnostic evaluation should include spinal MRI/

MRA. Patients with spinal vascular malformations should also undergo cranial imaging to ensure vascular abnormalities of the brain are not present. In patients with negative imaging, spinal angiography is performed.

▶ Summary

Arteriorvenous malformations within the central nervous system are rare. However, with advances in imaging, an increasing number of these lesions are being diagnosed. Arteriorvenous malformations are congenital tangles of direct arterial-venous connections that place patients at risk of hemorrhage of approximately 2%-4% per year. The morbidity and mortality associated with intracranial hemorrhage is high and the most patients with AVMs are young. Because of this, treatment is often recommended to prevent intracranial hemorrhage, or to relieve mass effect causing seizures, headaches, or other neurologic deficits. Treatment options include endovascular embolization, surgical resection, SRS, or a combination of these. With an experienced team of neurosurgeons, interventionalists, and radiation oncologists, treatment can be accomplished with minimal risk. In a minority of cases, observant management may be appropriate.

Spetzler RF, Hamilton MG: The prospective application of a grading system for arteriovenous malformations. *Neurosurgery* 1994;34:2-7.

SURGICAL MANAGEMENT OF MEDICALLY INTRACTABLE REFRACTORY EPILEPSY

J. Nicole Bentley Oren Sagher

KEY CONCEPTS

- ▶ Understand the prevalence, varied etiologies, and broad classification of epilepsy
- ▶ Describe the various diagnostic modalities for epilepsy
- ▶ Recognize that focal and lateralizing epilepsy is more amenable to surgery
- ▶ Recognize that mesial temporal sclerosis is highly epileptogenic with very favorable outcomes following surgical resection
- ▶ Appreciate palliative and curative surgical treatments for epilepsy

INTRODUCTION

Epilepsy is a disease affecting 1% of the world's population, and is characterized by a wide range of phenotypes and physical manifestations. The underlying pathology giving rise to epilepsy is equally varied, resulting in a disease that is challenging both to classify and to treat.

Epilepsy is a syndrome of recurrent seizures, the onset of which is due to abnormal neuronal synchronization. The locus of misfiring characterizes a seizure's semiology, or external signs, and may propagate to surrounding areas. Medical management involves pharmacotherapies and occasionally, alternative therapies, such as dietary restrictions, to reduce seizure frequency. However, one-third of patients are refractory to these therapies. Many studies have demonstrated the efficacy of surgery in cases of failed medical management, and have repeatedly shown that early surgery in appropriate candidates provides the greatest benefit. This chapter will focus on the workup and surgical options in these patients.

CLASSIFICATION

Seizures are classified by their association with alteration in consciousness; "simple" seizures are defined as those that occur in the setting of retained awareness, and "complex" seizures result in loss of awareness. Further classification relies on the locus of seizure onset. If focal, the seizure is considered "partial," and may be characterized by a stereotypical movement, such as lip smacking or eye deviation. Primary generalized seizures, on the other hand, are considered to affect the entire brain *at their onset*. Primary generalized epilepsy is usually secondary to a genetic derangement in cell membrane function. A localized group of misfiring neurons may also give rise to *auras*, or sensory forewarnings, heralding an oncoming seizure. Examples of auras include a taste or light perception, or paresthesias. A partial seizure may spread within the brain—a process known as secondary generalization.

DIAGNOSIS

Several modalities are employed in the diagnosis of epilepsy. These include clinical examination, neurophysiology, imaging, and neuropsychologic assesments.

▶ Clinical Examination & Laboratory Assessment

The clinical symptomatology associated with the epilepsy is a critical component of the diagnosis of epilepsy, and is called its semiology. Symptoms during the time of seizure may provide localizing clues to the region of onset. For example, seizures starting with motor twitching of the upper extremity are likely to be caused by a lesion in the vicinity of the primary motor cortex. Past medical history of febrile seizures or encephalitis are associated with risk of epilepsy. In addition, family history of epilepsy appears to be a strong risk factor in the development of epilepsy. Finally serum metabolic studies should be undertaken in order to rule out potentially reversible entities. Such studies include fasting blood glucose, serum electrolyte panel, complete blood count, and erythrocyte sedimentation rate, renal and hepatic functional assays. In patients where historical data and the clinical examination point to an intoxicating entity, applicable urine and serum toxicology assays should be obtained.

▶ Electrophysiology

The standard modality for recording brain activity is the scalp electro-encephalogram (EEG). EEG recordings are usually obtained both between and during seizures. In some instances, patients undergo long-term monitoring with video EEG where seizure semiology can be assessed together with EEG pattern. Generally, the presence of lateralized or localized seizures is suggestive of a focus that may be amenable to surgical resection. In patients whose seizure localization cannot be demonstrated convincingly by scalp EEG, intracranial EEG electrodes may be placed. These electrodes can either be placed on the surface of the brain (subdural electrodes) or within the substance of the brain (depth electrodes). Subdural electrodes register surface cortical activity, while depth electrodes can provide information related to deep structures such as the hippocampus.

▶ Imaging Studies

MRI is the usual imaging study of choice for evaluating patients with epilepsy. Structural lesions such as tumors, vascular malformations, or dysplastic cortex can be easily identified on MRI. Highly epileptogenic entities such as mesial temporal sclerosis with hippocampal atrophy can also be detected with high resolution MRI scans, as demonstrated in Figure 36–24.

Nuclear medicine studies such as positron emission tomography (PET) and single photon emission computed tomography (SPECT) scans can serve as complementary diagnostic tests. These tests are especially useful when the MRI and EEG do not correlate. PET studies demonstrate metabolic activity within the brain, while SPECT studies reflect regional blood flow patterns at the time of tracer injection. SPECT studies performed at the beginning of a seizure often demonstrate increased flow to areas involved in seizure onset. Alternatively, PET studies performed between seizures are more likely to demonstrate hypometabolism within epileptogenic foci. Both studies are useful for patients with focal epilepsy who have normal MRIs, or in whom the site of seizure origin is uncertain.

Magnetoencephalography (MEG) is a functional imaging technique that can accurately provide information on synchronized electrical activity in the brain. MEG detects the magnetic dipole equivalents of electrical current. In addition, it has the advantage of providing a three-dimensional localization of neuronal activity. Finally, there is accumulating data to suggest a high correlation between MEG and intracranial seizure localization.

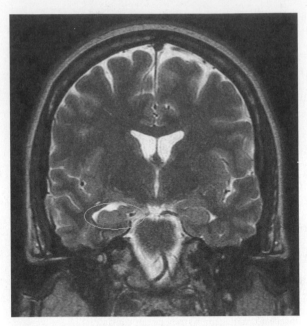

▲ **Figure 36–24.** Coronal MRI of the brain demonstrating right mesial temporal sclerosis with associated atrophy of the right hippocampus and prominence of the temporal horn of the right lateral ventricle.

▶ Neuropsychological Examination

Neuropsychological evaluation is an important component of the epilepsy workup. Patients should undergo a battery of standardized neuropsychological tests assessing verbal and nonverbal intelligence, memory, executive functions, and behavioral functions. These tests often point to subtle deficiencies that accompany the presence of a seizure focus. In addition to these tests, patients may undergo more invasive neuropsychological tests such as the **Wada test**. The Wada test involves selective injection of a fast-acting barbiturate such as amobarbital into each hemisphere via the carotid artery while memory and language functions are tested. The goal of the Wada test is to assess language and memory dominance. If the Wada test suggests that a significant amount of language function is subserved by the diseased hemisphere, then surgical resection may result in significant deficits.

SURGICAL SELECTION

In general, patients with structural lesions such as tumors and vascular malformations should be managed primarily with surgical resection. Additionally, patients for whom medical therapies have failed to produce an adequate response should be considered for surgery. A consensus definition of medical failure has recently been published, and is defined as failure of two or more antiepilpetic drugs to reduce seizures to a clinically meaningful level, assuming that appropriate doses and regimens have been used. The likelihood of attaining seizure-freedom with pharmaco-therapies once two drugs have failed has been shown to be consistently low, less than 5%.

Evidence suggests that early surgical intervention improves outcomes. Delays in surgery may result in enceph-alopathy, psychosocial abnormalities, learning disabilities, and risk of seizure-related injuries. Additionally, a condi-tion known as SUDEP, or sudden unexpected death in epilepsy, affects a significant number of patients suffering from epilepsy, presumably occurring secondary to cardio-respiratory compromise. With surgical success, patients can be gradually weaned off anticonvulsants, thereby sparing them of the deleterious long-term effects of these medica-tions. However, in patients with epileptogenic foci within the eloquent cortex, the risk of postsurgical deficits must be considered against the probability of rendering the patients seizure-free. Ultimately, the decision to recommend surgery is made by a multidisciplinary team consisting of epileptolo-gists, neurosurgeons, radiologists, neuropsychologists, and social workers.

GOALS OF SURGERY

Surgical procedures can be viewed as either curative or palliative. Curative procedures are designed for patients with seizures convincingly localized to a specific cortical region which is safe to remove. The goal in curative surgery therefore is complete resection of the affected cortex, and procedures include anterior temporal lobectomy, selec-tive amygdalohippocampectomy, neocortical resections, and hemispherectomy. Palliative surgery is employed in situa-tions where a seizure focus is either not identified or cannot be safely removed. For example, patients with congenital syndromic epilepsies such as Lennox–Gastaut syndrome experience life-threatening generalized seizures for which there is no identifiable focus. The goal of palliative surgery therefore is reduction in seizure frequency and severity. Common palliative procedures include placement of a vagus nerve stimulator and corpus callosotomy.

SURGICAL TECHNIQUES

Temporal Lobectomy

The most common cause of drug-resistant epilepsy is mesial temporal sclerosis. Among its several radiographic features, this entity is characterized by hippocampal atrophy on MRI, however, the relationship between the presence and timing of MRI abnormalities and pathophysiology remains poorly understood. While abnormalities on MRI are not an absolute necessity for successful temporal lobectomy, rates of seizure-freedom are lower. Consensus guidelines have recommended that patients who are medically refractory

to drug therapy, having failed two or more appropriately prescribed anticonvulsants, should be evaluated by a multi-disciplinary epilepsy surgery center.

The surgical technique involves a temporal craniotomy with en bloc resection of 3.5 cm (dominant) or 4 cm (non-dominant) of the lateral temporal lobe. En bloc resection of the amygdala, parahippocampal gyrus, and hippocampus is also performed. The long-term seizure-free outcomes are around 60%-80%, with strong trends toward improved quality of life in surgical groups. Though studies have been limited by small sample sizes, there are several well-designed trials that continue to support surgery for appropriate can-didates, with a safety profile similar to medically treated groups.

Potential complications include minor visual field defi-cits and deficits with short-term memory.

Selective Amygdalohippocampectomy

As mentioned earlier, the extent of surgical resection is lim-ited in mesial temporal sclerosis of the language-dominant hemisphere. However, minimally invasive techniques have been developed that spare more of the overlying temporal cortex, minimizing damage to the language pathways. This "selective" procedure involves resection of the amygdala and hippocampus via a temporal craniotomy. The approach to these structures is variable, either through a slit in the temporal lobe cortex or through the sylvian fissure. A comparison of the standard anterior temporal lobectomy to selective amygdalohippocampectomy found that seizure freedom was comparable in the two groups, with 85.2% and 93.1% of patients experiencing seizure-freedom at 3-years, respectively. Potential complications are similar to nonselec-tive lobectomies.

Extratemporal Resections

These procedures are performed in patients with focal epilepsy arising outside the temporal lobe. The frontal lobe is the most common location for such resections. In light of the potential overlap with functional areas, resection is often limited and seizure-free outcome is not as favorable as that seen in temporal lobe epilepsy, averaging approxi-mately 50%. Surgery entails a craniotomy with resection of cortex, at times guided by intraoperative EEG recordings. Complications are contingent upon associated eloquent areas involved.

Hemispherectomy

The hemispherectomy or functional hemispherotomy involves surgical resection or disconnection of one hemisphere from the other. The procedure is used in patients with diffuse unilateral hemispheric seizures that typically result in a neurologically devastated or nonfunctional hemisphere. Hemispherectomy can control seizures in about 70%-90% of patients, with the best outcomes being reported in Sturge–Weber syndrome, Rasmussen's Encephalitis, and porencephaly. In properly selected cases, function is preserved with associated improvements in cognitive, behavioral, and motor domains.

As originally described, hemispherectomy entailed complete removal of half of the brain. This was fraught with progressive postoperative neurological deficits secondary to deposition of iron over the brain (superficial cerebral hemosiderosis). In light of these problems, a modified functional hemispherectomy has replaced the anatomic hemispherectomy. This procedure involves disconnecting the corpus callosum and the various interhemispheric commissures. The major risks include hemorrhage, damage to functioning cortex, persistent seizures, disseminated intravascular coagulation, and transient decrease in contralateral muscle tone.

Corpus Callosotomy

This procedure is palliative and is utilized in situations where patients have diffuse epileglonic foci involving both hemispheres. Sectioning the corpus callosum prevents interhemispheric propagation of seizures and is used in both pediatric and adults, with varying extent of sectioning based on patient age and EEG. The procedure typically involves resection of the anterior two-thirds of the corpus callosum, with the option of further resections if seizures persist. Efficacy of the procedure is greatest in drop attacks that cause sudden atonic attacks, with a reported response of 88%. Less responsive seizure types include generalized tonic-clonic, absence, complex partial, and simple partial, with success ranging from 14% to 40%.

Multiple Subpial Transections

This procedure is indicated for patients with seizure foci within functionally important cortex, such as primary motor cortex. The procedure is palliative, with reported efficacy ranging from 33% to 46%. Shallow vertical transections are created across cortical gyri, disrupting the horizontal connections believed to propagate seizures between vertical columns of cells. The procedure is often performed with cortical resections, which has limited the ability to conclusively define outcomes in many studies.

Vagus Nerve Stimulation

The vagus nerve stimulation (VNS) is a relatively low-risk surgical procedure that decreases seizure frequency in patients whose disease is not safely amenable to resection. The exact mechanism by which this technique curbs epilepsy is unknown, but may be due to innervation of the nucleus solitarius which sends fibers to hemispheric regions involved in seizure onset. The stimulator electrode is placed along the vagus nerve in the neck, which is then connected to a generator implanted on the anterior chest wall. In multi-institutional double-blinded, randomized controlled trials, a reduction of seizure frequency of 24%-31% has been reported. A greater response was seen in the pediatric population, with a seizure reduction rate of 50%-90%. Although not considered a curative, intervention, 2% of patients become seizure-free. The main risks of the procedure include injury the vagus nerve, carotid artery, and jugular vein; however, this remains a low-risk intervention in comparison to other surgical modalities.

Stereotactic Radiosurgery

The application of highly focused irradiation to specific brain regions, known as radiosurgery, has been used to treat a wide variety of brain lesions such as tumors and vascular lesions. The role of radiosurgery in seizure control has been fairly limited. However, it has been proposed as a potential treatment of deep-seated seizure foci, such as hypothalamic hamartomas, which are benign malformations in the hypothalamus associated with gelastic epilepsy. Surgical resection in this location is fraught with risk, and it appears that radiosurgery may be used more safely in this subset of patients.

FUTURE DIRECTIONS

Many avenues of surgical treatment for refractory epilepsy are being developed in response to advancements in technology. One example is a closed-loop system implanted into the brain that detects seizure onset and automatically responds by delivering pulsed stimulation to the focus. Preliminary trials have reported seizure reductions of 50%-75%. Stimulation of the anterior nucleus of the thalamus has also been shown to result in seizure reduction, though the mechanism is poorly understood. Stem-cell therapies, gene therapies, and advances in neuronal visualization are also providing tools that increase the understanding and successful treatment of refractory epilepsy.

Anderson WS, Kossoff EH, Bergey GK, Jallo GI: Implantation of a responsive neurostimulator device in patients with refractory epilepsy. *Neurosurg Focus* 2008;25:E12.

Berg AT, Mathern GW, Bronen RA, Fulbright RK, DiMario F, Testa FM, et al: Frequency, prognosis and surgical treatment of structural abnormalities seen with magnetic resonance imaging in childhood epilepsy. *Brain* 2009;132:2785-2797.

Engel J, Jr., McDermott MP, Wiebe S, Langfitt JT, Stern JM, Dewar S, et al: Early surgical therapy for drug-resistant temporal lobe epilepsy: a randomized trial. *JAMA* 2012;307:922-930.

Iida K, et al: Characterizing magnetic spike sources by using magnetoencephalography-guided neuronavigation in epilepsy surgery in pediatric patients. *J Neurosurg* 2005;102(2 Suppl):S187-S196.

Immonen A, Jutila L, Muraja-Murro A, Mervaala E, Lamusuo S, Kuikka J, et al: Long-term epilepsy surgery outcomes in patients with MRI-negative temporal lobe epilepsy. *Epilepsia* 2010;51(11):2260-2269.

Lee KJ, Shon YM, Cho CB: Long-term outcome of anterior thalamic nucleus stimulation for intractable epilepsy. Stereotactic and functional neurosurgery 2012;90:379-385.

Milby AH, Halpern CH, Baltuch GH: Vagus nerve stimulation in the treatment of refractory epilepsy. *Neurotherapeutics* 2009;6:228-237.

Sagher O, Thawani JP, Etame AB, Gomez-Hassan DM: Seizure outcomes and mesial resection volumes following selective. *Neurosurg Focus* 2012 Mar;32(3):E8.

Schachter SC, Guttag J, Schiff SJ, Schomer DL: Advances in the application of technology to epilepsy: the CIMIT/NIO Epilepsy Innovation Summit. Epilepsy Behav: E&B 2009;16:3-46.

Schramm J, Kuczaty S, Sassen R, Elger CE, von Lehe M: Pediatric functional hemispherectomy: outcome in 92 patients. *Acta Neurochir (Wien)* 2012;154:2017-2028.

Sunaga S, Shimizu H, Sugano H: Long-term follow-up of seizure outcomes after corpus callosotomy. *Seizure* 2009;18:124-128.

▼ SURGICAL MANAGEMENT OF PAIN

Arnold Etame Parag G. Patil

The subjective, emotional, and physical components of pain make its management complex. Hence, pain management is an interdisciplinary endeavor encompassing medical, surgical, and psychological treatment modalities. Surgery for pain should be reserved for patients who have been unresponsive to therapies directed toward the inciting processes and to oral pain medications.

Pain may be classified as *nociceptive or neuropathic.* Nociceptive pain results from tissue injury. Common characteristics include constant aching or throbbing and responsiveness to opiate medications. Neuropathic pain is initiated or caused by a primary lesion or dysfunction in the nervous system. Common characteristics include burning, allodynia, and paresthesias. Neuropathic pain responds poorly to opiate medications. Pain surgeons should be familiar with these concepts to assess medical intractability.

The aim of surgery is to interrupt pain signaling pathways. Ablative surgical techniques involve physical interruption through the destruction of neural tissue. Nonablative procedures involve functional interruption through the modulation of pain transduction mechanisms.

ABLATIVE PROCEDURES TO INTERRUPT AFFERENT PAIN PATHWAYS

Neurosurgical procedures to physically interrupt pain signaling have been directed toward the nerves (neurectomy), spinal roots (rhizotomy), dorsal root ganglia (ganglionectomy), dorsal root entry zone (DREZ lesioning), spinal cord (cordotomy, myelotomy), and cerebral cortex (cingulotomy). Ablative surgery for pain is most often utilized in the treatment of cancer-related, nociceptive pain, as long-term analgesia is less commonly observed for these procedures.

▶ Neurectomy

Neurectomy involves cutting an injured nerve or the nerve to a painful region. Target nerves are identified on the basis of local anesthetic blockade. Denervation of joints, distal sensory nerves, and neuroma surgery are examples of peripheral neurectomy. Neurectomy is not typically utilized for cancer-related pain because of the changing pain distribution with tumor growth. Reported success rates for pain control with neurectomy vary widely between 40% and 90%.

▶ Rhizotomy & Ganglionectomy

Rhizotomy and ganglionectomy target the dorsal sensory rootlets or ganglia, respectively. Spinal cord segments are identified through paraspinal local anesthetic blockade, with placebo controls. The procedures are utilized most commonly for cancer-related regional pain or occipital neuralgia. These procedures are rarely utilized in the treatment of extremity pain because of functional impairment resulting from the loss of proprioception. Successful longer term pain control has been reported in 40% to 70% of patients.

▶ Dorsal Root Entry Zone Lesioning

Dorsal root entry zone surgery targets the superficial dorsal horn region, where sensory fibers enter the spinal cord. Levels including and flanking the region of interest, as defined by imaging studies or pain distribution, are typically ablated. A knife or radiofrequency heating is used to make the lesion. Dorsal root entry zone surgery is most effective in the treatment of neuropathic pain following nerve root avulsion and at-level spinal cord injury pain. Risks of surgery include injury to descending motor pathways and decreased sensory function in the territory of the ablated region. In carefully selected patients, rates of successful pain control range from 70% to 90%.

▶ Cordotomy & Myelotomy

Cordotomy is a spinal procedure to interrupt pain transmission along the lateral spinothalamic tract. Cordotomy is most commonly performed in patients with intractable, unilateral, nociceptive cancer pain at the level of the chest or below. The procedure may be performed either with a knife or with radiofrequency heating. Risks of surgery include lower extremity weakness, ataxia, and respiratory or urinary dysfunction. These risks are significantly increased when cordotomy is performed bilaterally.

Midline myelotomy involves destruction of the mesial dorsal columns at a single spinal level to treat midline, bilateral, or visceral pain. The procedure typically preserves dorsal column and spinothalamic signal transmission. Risks include transient lower extremity paresthesias and weakness.

Rates of successful pain control with cordotomy and myelotomy are initially high (> 80%) but decline over time (40% at 2 years).

Cingulotomy

Unlike procedures directed along pathways of pain neurotransmission, cingulotomy is directed toward alteration of the experience of pain. Because the cingulate gyrus is part of the limbic system, radiofrequency ablation of the anterior cingulate gyrus reduces the affective, unpleasant aspects of pain, particularly in patients with obsessive and affective components to their pain. Cingulotomy is performed in relatively few centers and only in carefully selected patients. Following cingulotomy for intractable, cancer-related pain, over 50% of patients have been reported to have moderate to complete pain relief.

PROCEDURES TO MODULATE AFFERENT PAIN PATHWAYS

Intrathecal Analgesic Delivery Pumps

When compared to oral narcotics, intrathecal administration of morphine provides more potent analgesia with reduced side effects, such as nausea, constipation, and sedation. To benefit from intrathecal delivery, patients should have significant reduction in pain level with oral opiates, limited by intolerable side effects.

Analgesics such as morphine are delivered through a catheter placed into the cerebrospinal fluid of the spinal canal. The catheter tubing is then connected to an external or surgically implanted pump. External pumps are utilized in patients with cancer-related pain and expected survival of less than 3 months. Principal complications of intrathecal drug delivery include the side-effects of the medication, mechanical failure of the system, and infection.

Intrathecal drug delivery may be effective in either nociceptive or neuropathic pain syndromes. However, as with oral opiate administration, long-term tolerance to medications can develop. Hence, these devices are most beneficial for patients with cancer-related pain syndromes and limited life expectancy.

Peripheral Nerve & Spinal Cord Stimulation

Peripheral nerve and spinal cord stimulators deliver pulses of electricity to injured nerves or the dorsal columns of the spinal cord, respectively. According to the gate theory of pain, such stimulation blocks the flow of pain signals from the periphery to the brain.

Peripheral nerve stimulation is most effective in neuropathic peripheral nerve syndromes such as occipital neuralgia and complex regional pain syndrome. More recently, peripheral stimulation has been used to treat headaches and fibromyalgia. Spinal cord stimulation is most effective in patients with lumbosacral radiculopathy due to scar tissue formation following back surgery as well as in patients with complex regional pain syndrome.

Patient candidates typically undergo an initial trial with a temporary electrode applied to the spinal cord or nerve. After the 1-week trial, permanent placement is performed if benefit is demonstrated. Benefit is measured as a reduction in pain as well as an increase in daily activities. Complications of the therapy are most commonly stimulating lead migration, breakage, and infection.

Deep Brain Stimulation

Deep brain stimulation involves the precise surgical placement of electrodes into the deep nuclei of the brain. Common targets of deep brain stimulation for pain include the thalamus, which is the sensory relay of the brain, and the periaqueductal gray region, which results in the upregulation of endogenous opiates. Once electrodes are implanted, trial stimulation is performed for 1-2 weeks. A successful trial is characterized by the experience of pain-relieving and tolerable paresthesias in the treated region during thalamic stimulation, a sense of warmth and ocular movement during periaqueductal stimulation, a poststimulatory pain-relieving effect, and the absence of an analgesic effect during sham stimulation. Following the trial, a pulse generator is connected to the wires and implanted in the chest. Long-term results in patients with a successful trial are variable, ranging from 19% to 79%.

Motor Cortex Stimulation

Electrical stimulation of the region of the motor cortex results in analgesia in neuropathic pain syndromes such as hemibody poststroke pain and trigeminal deafferentation pain. The mechanism of motor cortex stimulation is unknown.

The surgical procedure involves placement of a stimulating electrode under the skull in the region of the motor cortex. Patients undergo a trial of stimulation. Stimulus intensity is typically set to 80% of the level needed to produce motor cortical responses. Following a successful trial, the electrodes are connected to an implantable pulse generator in the chest. Motor cortex stimulation has a success rate of 70% in facial pain syndromes and of 50% in central neuropathic pain.

SURGICAL MANAGEMENT OF MOVEMENT DISORDERS

Arnold Etame Parag G. Patil

Neurosurgical procedures for movement disorders have evolved considerably in recent years. Formerly popular stereotactic tissue-destructive procedures, such as pallidotomy and thalamotomy, have been superseded by nonlesional deep-brain stimulation (DBS). Careful, prospective and well-controlled studies have demonstrated significant benefits of DBS in the treatment of Parkinson disease, essential tremor (ET), and dystonia.

PARKINSON DISEASE

▶ Clinical Considerations & Pathophysiology

James Parkinson was the first to describe the "shaking palsy" in 1817. The clinical signs of Parkinson disease (PD) are tremor, bradykinesia (slowness of movement), rigidity (increased muscle tone), and postural instability. The tremor of PD occurs at rest, has a "pill-rolling" character, and typically decreases with voluntary movement. The rigidity of PD has a "cogwheel" ratchet-like quality during passive movement. Postural instability results from a loss of reflexes, leading to impaired balance. Other signs of PD include a shuffling gait, decreased voice volume, slowed reaction time, and dementia. A popular scale for the measurement of Parkinsonism is the Unified Parkinson Disease Rating Scale (UPDRS).

PD is accompanied by a loss of dopaminergic neurons in the substantia nigra pars compacta. According to a well-accepted model of basal-ganglia function, the loss of dopamine results in activation of the subthalamic nucleus and the globus pallidus pars interna (GPi). The GPi inhibits motor regions of the thalamus, resulting in decreased cortical excitation and the symptoms of PD. The central role of the GPi and subthalamic nucleus in this scheme provides the impetus for the surgical therapies for PD.

Idiopathic PD must be distinguished from other Parkinsonian syndromes that have similar signs and symptoms. These syndromes include multiple system atrophy, progressive supranuclear palsy, corticobasal degeneration, and dementia with Lewy bodies. There are no laboratory or blood tests that help in the diagnosis of PD. CT and MRI studies of patients with PD are typically normal. For each patient, the diagnosis is based entirely on the history and physical examination as well as responsiveness to medication. As a result, only 75% of patients with a clinical diagnosis of PD are confirmed at autopsy.

▶ Medical Management

Medical management strategies for the treatment of PD center upon manipulation of the dopaminergic system. l-dopa, which was introduced in 1967, crosses the blood-brain barrier and is converted by dopaminergic neurons into dopamine. l-dopa is often compounded with carbidopa, an inhibitor of dopamine metabolism in the bloodstream, to increase the efficiency of l-dopa delivery to the brain. Other medications that are useful in the treatment of PD include inhibitors of the COMT and MAO-B enzymes, which metabolize dopamine, as well as direct agonists of

dopamine receptors in the brain. Patients with non-PD, atypical Parkinsonian syndromes do not respond well to l-dopa therapy.

Over 5-10 years, PD patients develop several troublesome side effects of l-dopa. Dyskinesias are involuntary writhing movements of the face and extremities that occur at peak dopamine levels. In addition, after chronic therapy, patients may develop on-off fluctuations in which their Parkinsonian symptoms oscillate in an unpredictable manner. Finally, patients may develop involuntary freezing during movement. The presence of such side effects of l-dopa should prompt surgical evaluation.

▶ Surgical Management

Lesional stereotactic surgery for PD has been performed since the 1950s. Principal targets for ablation include the thalamus (thalamotomy) and the GPi (pallidotomy). With the introduction of l-dopa, these lesional surgical therapies declined. However, with the appearance of l-dopa side effects in the 1980s and with the development of DBS techniques in the 1990s, surgery for PD has increased significantly. At present, DBS of the subthalamic nucleus or GPi is favored over lesional surgery because of its heightened safety and reversibility. Since FDA approval in 1997, over 10,000 patients with PD have been treated with DBS.

Surgical indications for the treatment of PD are well established. Guidelines defined by the Core Assessment Program for Surgical Interventional Therapies in PD (CAPSIT-PD) include the following:

- A diagnosis of idiopathic PD for a period of 5 years
- Exclusion by history and MRI of atypical Parkinsonism
- Dopaminergic responsiveness (33% reduction in UPDRS motor score with l-dopa)
- No significant cognitive deterioration or depression

The goal of surgery for PD is an improvement in motor symptoms. DBS results in significant improvements in tremor, rigidity, bradykinesia, postural stability, freezing, and gait, compared to the *off*-l-dopa state. DBS is not expected to provide improvement to patients with PD beyond their best *on*-l-dopa state. However, as doses of l-dopa are typically lowered after DBS surgery, DBS provides relief from the dyskinesias and on-off fluctuations associated with chronic l-dopa therapy.

A recent study has determined that DBS results in a significant improvement in quality of life for patients with PD. Compared to medication alone, DBS provides increased ability to perform activities of daily living, improved emotional well-being, decreased stigma of disease, and reduced bodily discomfort. Benefits are likely to be reduced, however, in patients over 70 or with significant cognitive deficits in whom motor improvements alone are unlikely to alter quality of life significantly.

ESSENTIAL TREMOR

Clinical Considerations & Pathophysiology

ET is the most common movement disorder, affecting an estimated 2% to 4% of the population. ET can be present in adolescence but most often appears in middle age or later life and is slowly progressive. There is a strong genetic component, with 25% to 60% of patients reporting a family history of tremor, typically with an autosomal dominant pattern of inheritance.

The tremor of ET occurs during maintenance of posture against gravity and with action. ET can occur in any part of the body but is most commonly observed in the hand (90%-100%), head (40%-60%), and voice (25%-35%). The tremor of ET is distinguished from rest tremors, which occur when a limb is fully supported against gravity, and from intention tremors, which occur during visually guided movement as the limb approaches the target. However, in severe cases, patients with ET may experience either rest or intention tremor in addition to action tremor.

The pathophysiology of ET is not well understood, though cerebellar function appears to be involved. In addition to tremor, patients with ET may have mildly ataxic or dysmetric gait, oculomotor deficits, and disordered eye-hand movements, reminiscent of cerebellar dysfunction. In addition, PET studies have demonstrated increased cerebellar activity in patients with ET. It is thought that disruption to olivocerebellar rhythmicity may be central to the development of ET.

ET must be differentiated from other tremor disorders. Disease processes resulting in action tremor may include PD, enhanced physiological tremor, dystonia, and Wilson disease. Other tremor disorders may include cerebellar (intention) tremors, Holmes (rubral) tremor, toxic/metabolic disorders, and psychogenic disorders.

Medical Management

In many cases, ET begins late in life, progresses slowly, and is neither physically disabling nor psychologically burdensome. Some patients may experience reduced tremor by restricting or eliminating caffeine from the diet or by wearing small weights about their wrists. Some patients may experience reduced tremor with moderate alcohol consumption. However, alcohol is not typically recommended as a treatment because of risks of resulting chemical dependence in susceptible individuals.

For patients with disabling tremor, first-line therapies include beta-blockers, such as propranolol, and the antiepileptic primidone. Approximately 50%-70% of patients obtain benefit from beta-blockade. Primidone is a medication related to phenobarbital, with similar efficacy to beta-blockade in the treatment of ET. In some patients, the two therapies may be combined for an additive effect. Additional pharmacological agents for ET include gabapentin, topiramate, and long-acting benzodiazepines, such as clonazepam. Finally, a subset of patients with ET may be treated by local botulinum toxin injection.

Surgical Management

As in the treatment of PD, lesional surgery for ET has been largely superseded by DBS. The targets of ablation and DBS are the same, the ventralis intermedius nucleus of the thalamus. The ventralis intermedius nucleus receives inputs from the deep cerebellar nuclei, including the dentate nucleus, which may account for its importance in the treatment of ET. A unilateral procedure is favored for patients with disabling unilateral extremity tremor, while a bilateral procedure may be required to control bilateral or axial tremors.

Thalamotomy of the ventralis intermedius nucleus is highly effective in the treatment of ET, with over 80% of patients experiencing effective long-term tremor suppression. Complications of thalamotomy occur in some 25% of patients and primarily include hemorrhage, weakness, dysarthria, and ataxia.

Ventralis intermedius nucleus DBS has largely replaced thalamotomy in the surgical treatment of ET. In a prospective, randomized study comparing DBS to thalamotomy, both therapies achieve similar tremor control. However, DBS results in fewer adverse effects. DBS may have more favorable effects on patient functional status, including activities of daily living. Complications of thalamotomy and DBS are more pronounced in patients following a bilateral procedure.

PRIMARY DYSTONIA

Clinical Considerations & Pathophysiology

Dystonia is the sustained cocontraction of opposing muscle groups. Patients with dystonia exhibit abnormal and awkward postures, engage in repetitive movements, and often experience significant pain. Dystonia may affect muscles throughout the body (eg, generalized dystonia) or muscles in a region (eg, torticollis), or it may have a specific focus (eg, blepharospasm). Like tremor, dystonia may be an isolated finding or a manifestation of a more generalized neurological condition.

The pathophysiology of dystonia is not known. Some cases of dystonia have been shown to result from dopamine deficiency or disordered function of dopamine receptors in the basal ganglia. One model suggests that decreased or dysregulated activity in GPi results in disinhibition of motor cortical areas.

Dystonia often occurs as an idiopathic condition, without a clear etiology. Alternatively, dystonia may occur as a secondary condition, resulting from birth injury, stroke, drug toxicity, or a hereditary degenerative neurological condition.

Recently, over a dozen hereditary forms of previously idiopathic dystonia have been identified, including mutations of the *DYT1* gene on chromosome 9. The distinction between primary and secondary dystonia is important, as secondary dystonias respond less well to surgical interventions.

▶ Medical Management

Primary dystonia may be treated with anticholinergic drugs such as trihexyphenidyl, benzodiazepine muscle relaxants such as valium, or the injection of botulinum toxin into affected muscle groups. In addition, some dopamine-blocking medications have been utilized in the treatment of dystonia, although use of such medications also may worsen some forms of dystonia. Physical therapy is also an important component of dystonia treatment to prevent the formation of fixed muscle contractures.

▶ Surgical Management

Patients who fail to respond to oral medications and who fail to achieve adequate relief with botulinum toxin injections should be referred for surgical management. Dystonia has been treated with either ablation or stimulation of the GPi. Pallidotomy improves dystonia by 60% to 70% when measured by standard rating scales. Bilateral pallidal DBS is also highly effective in the treatment of primary dystonia. By comparison to sham stimulation, DBS significantly improved motor symptoms, pain, and quality of life. The most common side effect of pallidal DBS is dysarthria.

TECHNIQUES OF STEREOTACTIC NEUROSURGERY

Stereotactic neurosurgery involves the ablation of tissue or the placement of electrodes deep into the brain. Both the clinical efficacy and risks of surgery depend on submillimeter accuracy, requiring specialized techniques. Patients are typically placed in a stereotactic frame. This frame is affixed to the skull, under local anesthetic. The patient then undergoes an MRI or CT scan. Performance of a scan while in the frame allows a precise coordinate system to be defined within the brain.

In the operating room, a small hole is drilled into the skull, allowing the introduction of microelectrodes along a trajectory leading to the target. The microelectrodes record extracellular neuronal activity. Each region of the brain has a specific electrophysiological signature. Depending on the surgery, the patient may be examined for motor or sensory responsiveness of cellular activity.

Once electrophysiology has confirmed the target for surgery, DBS electrodes are placed into the same location along the same trajectory. With the electrode in position, stimulation is applied and the patient is examined for undesirable clinical effects. Once a desirable effect is confirmed,

the electrodes are secured. As a second stage, the electrodes are tunneled under the skin to an implantable stimulation generator placed under the skin, just below the clavicle. This generator may be precisely tuned to the requirements of each patient.

In lesional surgery, a radiofrequency or cryoprobe is placed into the location following microelectrode recording, and a temporary lesion is created. When the absence of undesired effects is confirmed, a permanent lesion is created.

▼ INTERVERTEBRAL DISK DISEASE

D. Andrew Wilkinson Khoi Than Paul Park

▶ General Considerations

The spinal column is composed of 33 longitudinally stacked bone segments called vertebrae: 7 cervical, 12 thoracic, 5 lumbar, 5 sacral (fused), and 2-4 coccygeal (fused). A typical vertebra is composed of a rounded body anteriorly and a protective boney arch posteriorly, which together form a canal through which the spinal cord passes. Vertebral bodies articulate anteriorly via intervertebral discs and posteriorly via synovial joints formed by the articular facets of adjoining vertebrae. They are also connected by several ligaments: the anterior and posterior longitudinal ligaments which traverse the vertebral bodies from top to bottom, the supraspinous and interspinous ligaments which run between the posterior projecting spinous processes of each vertebra, and the ligamentum flavum which connects the lamina (part of the posterior arch) at each vertebral level.

In a normal adult, the spinal cord extends from the cranio-cervical junction to the lumbar level, where it tapers and typically ends at L1-2 as the conus medullaris. Eight sets of nerve roots exit the spine in the cervical region, though there are only seven cervical vertebrae. The C1 nerve root exits above the C1 vertebra, while the C2 nerve root exits between the C1 and C2 vertebrae. The C8 nerve root exits between the C7 and T1 vertebral bodies, and the T1 nerve root exits between the T1 and T2 vertebral bodies. This relationship continues downward to the level of the sacrum. Thus, the nerve root that emerges at the L5-S1 level is the L5 nerve root. In the case of lumbar disk herniation, the affected nerve root is typically the root that is passing by to exit at the next level. As an example, a disk herniation at the L4-5 level would typically compress the L5 nerve root. Conversely, in the cervical spine the nerve that is affected is at the level of the disk herniation. A C5-6 disk herniation would therefore impact the C6 nerve root.

Intervertebral disks act as pads separating the vertebral bodies of the spine. They also function as shock absorbers, helping to cushion and distribute downward forces on the spine. Additionally, intervertebral disks allow a limited amount of movement to occur between different spinal levels so that the spine may bend and rotate. The intervertebral disk is composed of a gel-like, elastic fibrocartilaginous central nucleus (the nucleus pulposis) surrounded by a fibrous outer ring (the annulus fibrosis) composed of 15-25 concentric layers of parallel fibers. Vertebral body end-plates less than 1 mm thick and composed of hyaline cartilage form an interface between the bone of the vertebral bodies and the disk, sandwiching the nucleus pulposis superiorly and inferiorly.

Intervertebral disks degenerate over time. Coupled with degeneration of the facets, this process is termed spondylosis. At birth, the nucleus pulposis contains 80% water. As people age, however, disks gradually lose their water and elasticity, becoming less gel-like. The process of disk degeneration is common and may even be "normal" as people age. About 20% of teenagers have signs of mild disk degeneration, whereas by age 70, approximately 60% of disks are severely degenerated. Degenerated disks do not distribute load in the same way as healthy, well-hydrated disks. They do not maintain their height under load-bearing conditions and, as a consequence, more load is placed on vertebral bodies and adjacent facet joints. This promotes the formation of osteophytes. If osteophytes form in the spinal canal, within the neural foramina, or in the lateral recess, neurologic compression may develop over time. With loss of disk height, the tensional forces on the ligamentum flavum are reduced, causing the ligmentum to remodel, thicken, and bulge into the canal (ligamentous hypertrophy). Degeneration can also lead to spondylolisthesis or subluxation of one vertebral body over another. Degenerative disk disease occurs at all levels of the spine; however, because the lumbar spine and cervical spine have greater mobility, pathology is more common in these regions.

CERVICAL SPINE

► General Considerations

Degeneration of the cervical spine is a process leading to bulging of intervertebral disks, hypertrophy of facet joints, and osteophyte formation. Chronic degeneration initially manifests as neck pain. As osteophytes enlarge and ligamentous hypertrophy progresses, neurologic symptoms may develop. Compression of nerve roots leads to radiculopathy, while compression of the spinal cord itself leads to myelopathy. Alternatively, disk degeneration may occur acutely when the nucleus pulposis of a disk is extruded through a tear in the annulus. If an acute disk herniation occurs centrally, the spinal cord may become compressed, causing severe neurologic injury. This may result in paraplegia or quadriplegia, depending on the level and severity of the herniation. More commonly, however, disk rupture results in compression of a nerve root by the extruded disk fragment as well as local inflammatory changes, causing radiculopathy. This is

typically manifest as pain radiating down the arm, sensory disturbance and, sometimes, weakness in the distribution of the involved nerve root.

► Clinical Findings

A. Symptoms & Signs

Degenerative disease of the cervical spine often presents with a history of neck pain which may either be abrupt, in the case of disk rupture, or slowly progressive. There is often a loss of cervical lordosis (the normal, backward, C-shaped curvature of the neck), which may be related to muscle spasm or to deformity from chronic degeneration. In addition to neck pain, which often abates over time, compression of a single nerve root by an osteophyte or disk fragment (radiculopathy) often causes an aching pain along the medial border of the scapula on the side of the lesion. This scapular pain tends to be longer lasting than the neck pain. The characteristic finding in radiculopathy is a sharp, burning pain that radiates down the arm, following the distribution of the involved spinal nerve. This pain may be exacerbated when the patient tilts the head toward the side of the pain, crowding the neural foramina on the affected side (Spurling maneuver). Indeed, the patient may habitually tilt the head to the opposite side to reduce the pain. Hyperextension of the neck (with or without compression of the head) may worsen the pain. Sensory disturbances (parasthesias, numbness, or decreased sensation) tend to occur in the terminal distribution of the involved dermatome, that is, in the fingers rather than the proximal arm. Hypersensitivity of the skin in the distal distribution of the dermatome is also common. A decrease or loss of deep tendon reflexes is a frequent and early finding in radiculopathy from a herniated disk or a compressive cervical osteophyte. Weakness from radiculopathy occurs in muscles innervated by one spinal nerve (but by more than one peripheral nerve); that is, it is myotome-based. Thus, weakness from radiculopathy is often partial or incomplete, since nearly all muscles are innervated by more than one spinal nerve. Profound weakness, atrophy, and muscle fasciculations are rare in radiculopathy, except in very long-standing cases. The presence of these findings should generate suspicion of a peripheral nerve lesion.

C5 radiculopathy (typically resulting from pathology at the C4-5 level) involves pain radiating into the shoulder, with sensory disturbances crossing over the top of the shoulder and extending to the mid-portion of the upper arm (following the distribution of the C5 dermatome). Patients may exhibit weakness of shoulder abduction (deltoids) and forearm flexion. The biceps reflex may be attenuated. C6 radiculopathy (as from a C5-6 herniated disk) typically involves pain radiating from the neck into the lateral aspect of the arm, with sensory disturbance in the dorsum of the hand and, in particular, the thumb. Patients may present with weakness of forearm flexion (biceps). The biceps reflex as well as the bracheoradialis reflex may be attenuated. C7 nerve root compression (from C6-7 pathology) often involves pain radiating from the neck into the back of the shoulder, the triceps and the dorsolateral surface of the forearm. Sensory disturbance typically involves the index and middle fingers. Weakness of forearm extension (triceps) is generally noticed in a delayed fashion, perhaps because day-to-day extension of the forearm occurs with the assistance of gravity. The triceps reflex is often attenuated.

In advanced cases of degenerative disk disease of the cervical spine, signs of myelopathy may develop, including hyperreflexia, spasticity leading to gait disturbance, and sensory disturbance in the upper and lower extremities. Patients with myelopathy from cervical stenosis often complain of difficulty manipulating objects with their hands (eg, problems buttoning their shirt).

B. Diagnostic Studies

Plain films are useful in determining the degree of degenerative change present in the cervical spine. In cases of cervical deformity, plain films are used for evaluating the alignment of the cervical spine. Flexion-extension plain films are important when there is a question of instability of the cervical spine (eg, when a patient is having positional symptoms). Likewise, computed tomography (CT) scans may offer detailed views of the bony anatomy and are often useful for preoperative planning, especially in cases of severe deformity. CT also offers good resolution of boney anatomy when bone spurs are suspected as the cause of neural compression. The major disadvantage of CT scanning is the lack of resolution of soft tissue structures; it is difficult to detect compression from a herniated disk on a normal CT scan. CT myelography solves the problem of visualizing soft tissue compressive lesions. However, its main disadvantage is its invasiveness: Puncture of the thecal sac (required for dye injection) carries a small risk of neurologic injury. In the era of magnetic resonance imaging (MRI), CT myelography is often reserved for cases where the spine has been previously instrumented, which may cause significant artifact on MR imaging, or if the patient has other metallic devices that preclude magnetic scanning (eg, a cardiac pacemaker).

MR imaging allows the resolution of neural structures in a noninvasive manner and has become the most common imaging method for evaluating potentially compressive pathology of the cervical spine. MRI can detect soft tissue disk herniation and nerve root compression. It is also useful in detecting chronic or acute changes in the spinal cord that may be associated with myelopathy. Findings on MRI should be carefully correlated with clinical findings, as false positives are frequently generated. MR imaging reveals degenerative disk disease of the cervical spine in 25% of asymptomatic people less than 40 years of age and in 60% of people over 40 (Figure 36–25).

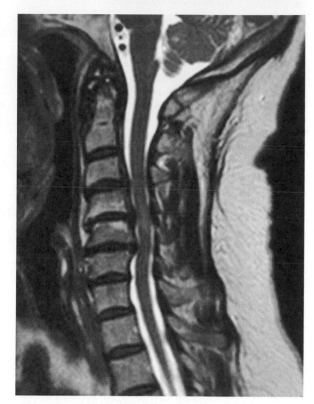

▲ **Figure 36–25.** Sagittal T2 weighted MRI of cervical spine showing multilevel disk protrusions causing central canal stenosis and cord signal change.

Electrodiagnostic studies, particularly EMG, may be useful in diagnosing radiculopathy. Nerve conduction studies alone are of little value in identifying radiculopathy and are generally normal, even with severe compression of a nerve root. EMG, on the other hand, is more sensitive. Classic EMG findings in radiculopathy are fibrillations at rest in muscles supplied by a single nerve root (ie, a myotome) along with denervation in the corresponding paraspinal muscles. Unfortunately, EMG will not reliably detect fibrillations in muscles until at least 3-4 weeks following the onset of radiculopathy. This may lead to false negative studies if the test is performed too soon. Even when performed after an appropriate waiting period, EMG findings may be normal in upward of 50% of cases of spinal nerve compression in patients with radicular symptoms, but no signs of weakness, numbness, or decreased reflexes.

▶ Differential Diagnosis

Neck pain associated with a history of malignancy, unexplained weight loss, pain unrelieved by bed rest, or age more than 50 with cancer risk factors should raise suspicion of a metastatic tumor invading the cervical spine. Similarly, infectious etiologies such as diskitis, osteomyelitis, or abscess should be considered when there is a history of fever, immunosupression, or recent infection. Peripheral nerve entrapment syndromes such as carpal tunnel syndrome or ulnar nerve compression may mimic cervical radiculopathy. In general, severe weakness and muscle atrophy is suggestive of a peripheral nerve lesion, while early loss of a reflex (biceps, triceps) suggests radiculopathy. Other conditions that may mimic cervical degenerative disk disease include myocardial infarction, idiopathic brachial plexitis (Parsonage Turner syndrome), or inflammatory conditions such as ankylosing spondylitis or sarcoidosis. Local conditions affecting the shoulder (rotator cuff tears, acromial bursitis, etc) must also be ruled out.

▶ Treatment & Prognosis

Most conditions that cause pain in the cervical spine (such as exacerbations of degenerative arthritis, muscle spasm, or minor trauma) are self-limiting and ultimately do not require operation. Acute neck pain may be treated with gentle exercise or a mobilization program, moist heat, or a soft collar to help muscle relaxation. Anti-inflammatory medications are also useful in this regard. For persistent neck pain, intermittent traction is sometimes helpful, either through physical therapy or with a home traction kit. Roughly 80%-90% of patients improve with medical management alone, though many continue to have mild symptoms they ultimately learn to manage.

Neck pain itself responds poorly to operative management. Even in cases of radiculopathy where imaging reveals a clear-cut disk herniation compressing a nerve root, surgical management is most likely to improve only arm pain rather than neck pain. Surgical management of cervical degenerative disk disease should be reserved for cases failing medical management and where there is neurologic compression (leading to either myelopathy or radiculopathy). Operative management of the cervical spine involves decompression of the spinal cord or nerve roots, with or without fusion. The cervical spine may be approached either anteriorly or posteriorly. The choice depends on many factors, including the age of the patient, the number of levels involved, whether the compressive lesion is predominantly anterior or posterior, and any concurrent deformity of the cervical spine. Both anterior and posterior approaches may be used to decompress nerve roots and/or the spinal cord. For complicated cases involving extensive degenerative change, particularly with severe deformity, a combined anterior/posterior approach may be employed.

Disk herniations and osteophytes may be addressed anteriorly, either by removing just the disk (anterior cervical discectomy, with or without fusion) or by drilling away the vertebral body (a procedure known as corpectomy). Posterior cervical laminectomy is useful for decompression of multiple levels, as in the case of multilevel cervical stenosis secondary to ligamentous hypertrophy. Because there is a risk of subsequent deformity (progressive kyphosis related to loss of the posterior tension band following operation), some patients who are approached posteriorly may need to be fused. The decision to fuse should be made on a case-by-case basis. Artificial disk replacement (arthroplasty) in lieu of fusion has been shown to maintain segmental mobility and appears to be a viable alternative to fusion, though long-term results are not yet available. Posterior keyhole foraminotomy is ideally suited for soft disk herniations that occur laterally (it cannot be used for central disk bulges) and may be done in a minimally invasive fashion using tubular retractors.

In the case of cervical radiculopathy, symptoms improve in approximately 80% of patients following operative management. Where surgical decompression is performed for myelopathy, neurologic improvement occurs in approximately 70% of cases.

THORACIC DISK DISEASE

Thoracic disk herniations are rare, with an incidence between 0.25% and 0.75% of all disk herniations. The majority of thoracic disk herniations occur below the level of the mid-thoracic spine. Often there is a delay in diagnosis because of poorly defined symptoms and the lack of objective findings on physical exam. If the disk herniation is secondary to trauma and results in severe cord compression, paralysis may be the result. If the disk herniation is secondary to degenerative changes, the cord compression occurs more slowly and is associated with a variety of presentations.

Patients may present with symptoms of axial pain, radiculopathy, myelopathy, or some combination of the three. The axial pain may be described as dull, aching, burning, stabbing, or cramping. Load bearing, activity, or valsalva will often exacerbate the pain. Radicular symptoms generally present in the appropriate dermatomal band. Myelopathy can present as paraparesis, but more often presents with a vague history of lower extremity weakness, heaviness, stiffness, or numbness. Bowel and bladder complaints can occur.

Treatment is surgical and is directed at alleviating pain or preventing progression of a neurologic deficit. There are a variety of surgical options including laminectomy for stenosis as well as a variety of approaches (thoracotomy, costotransversectomy, lateral extracavitary, transpedicular) for pathology that occurs in the anterior spine, such as a disk herniation. In cases of a thoracic disk herniation, a strictly dorsal midline approach (laminectomy) offers poor exposure of the disk and has a high risk of neurologic injury.

LUMBAR SPINE

▶ General Considerations

One must understand the anatomy of the lumbosacral roots to appreciate the clinical syndromes associated with a displaced lumbar intervertebral disk. An extruded lumbar intervertebral disk can lead to loss of reflexes (ankle jerk, patellar reflex), motor loss, sensory loss, and pain in a dermatomal distribution. A central disk herniation can lead to a variety of presentations up to paraplegia below the level of the lesion along with urinary symptoms. A typical disk herniation will usually spare the exiting nerve root, but impinge upon the traversing nerve root of the level below. A rarer far lateral disk herniation, however, will impinge upon the exiting nerve root.

With age, the disk will degenerate. Autopsy specimens have noted disk degeneration starting as early as the second decade of life, and nearly all individuals have some degree of degeneration by the sixth decade. Osteophytes may then form around the disk space and cause stenosis of the spinal canal and neuroforamina.

Ninety-five percent of lumbar disk herniations occur at the L5/S1 and L4/L5 levels. Only 4% of lumbar disk herniations occur at the L3/L4 levels and are infrequent at the upper lumbar levels.

▶ Clinical Findings

A. Symptoms & Signs

The symptoms and signs of lumbar disk herniation are variable. A large central disk herniation can present with cauda equina syndrome. In these cases, patients may present with saddle anesthesia, urinary dysfunction, diminished rectal tone, and leg weakness. Generally, however, patients complain of symptoms of radiating leg pain with a variable component of back pain. Valsalva maneuvers (coughing, sneezing, etc) or movement will generally exacerbate the pain. Alternatively, rest will often improve the pain. The pain itself can be described as a constant burning, aching type pain with an intermittent sharp, shooting pain that radiates down into the legs. Straight leg raise and crossed straight leg raise may support the diagnosis of lumbar disk herniation. The straight leg raise is positive if raising the straightened leg to an angle of 30 degrees causes sciatica in the ipsilateral leg. This test is 80% sensitive but only 40% specific. The crossed straight leg raise is positive if raising the leg to 30 degrees causes sciatica in the contralateral leg, and though this test is only 25% sensitive, it is 90% specific. It should be noted that patients with a high lumbar disk herniation or a far lateral disk herniation may not have these signs. Examination of the paravertebral musculature may reveal tenderness and/or muscle spasm.

Motor findings may be helpful in predicting the involved lumbar level. Compression of the L4 nerve root (L3/4 herniation) may cause weakness of knee extension (quadriceps). Compression of the L5 nerve root (L4/5 herniation) may precipitate weakness of the extensor hallicus longus and ankle dorsiflexion (tibialis anterior). Finally, compression of the S1 nerve root (L5/S1 herniation) may lead to weakness

of ankle plantarflexion (gastrocnemius). Reflexes may also be diminished. The ankle jerk (Achilles) reflex is diminished with S1 nerve root compression and the patellar reflex is diminished with L4 nerve root compression.

Sensory examination is often variable and the least helpful in predicting the involved lumbar level. L4 nerve root compression can be associated with anterior thigh to medial ankle sensory findings. L5 nerve root compression can present with findings along the dorsum of the foot and the first web space. Finally, S1 nerve root compression may present with sensory findings along the lateral and plantar regions of the foot.

B. Imaging Studies

If symptoms are limited to pain and the patient does not have risk factors for other diseases, it is reasonable to delay imaging workup for 4 weeks since improvement in pain over time is not uncommon. Persistent symptoms, however, are an indication for imaging. Plain radiographs have limited utility in the diagnosis of disk herniation. However, they are useful in evaluating trauma, infection, or neoplastic process. Myelography may identify extradural filling defects and can be particularly helpful when combined with CT scanning. Indeed, CT myelography remains useful in the setting when an MRI scan is not possible.

MRI has become the gold standard for the diagnosis of herniated disks (Figure 36–26). MRI is noninvasive and does not involve radiation exposure. MRI provides detailed images of the disk spaces, surrounding soft tissue, and thecal sac. MRI can help exclude tumors, cysts, and postoperative scarring as etiologies of the patient's symptoms. It is important to correlate the patient's symptoms and the imaging findings precisely since MRI imaging can generate a significant number of false positives. For example, nearly 20% of normal individuals under the age of 40 and over 50% of individuals over the age of 40 were noted to have lumbosacral imaging abnormalities.

C. Special Examinations

EMG can be useful diagnosing radiculopathy, but its utility is rather limited. EMG classically has findings of fibrillations at rest in the muscles supplied by a single nerve root and denervation of corresponding paraspinal muscles. Unfortunately, fibrillations require at least 3-4 weeks from the onset of the radiculopathy to be evident on EMG examination. Nerve conductions studies (NCS) are of minimal utility in diagnosing radiculopathy.

▶ Differential Diagnosis

It is important to obtain a complete history and physical, as the differential diagnosis for patients with back pain and radicular

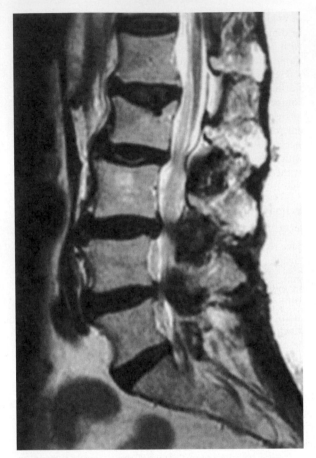

▲ **Figure 36–26.** Sagittal T2-weighted MRI of lumbar spine showing multilevel disk bulges, ligamentum flavum hypertrophy, and retrolisthesis at L2-L3.

symptoms is broad. A history of trauma can point to fractures, especially in the setting of osteoporosis and/or steroid use. Tumors which often metastasize to the spine include prostate, breast, kidney, thyroid, and lung cancer. Patients with metastatic disease often have nocturnal pain and pain that persists even with rest and a supine position. Inflammatory disorders, infections, bony abnormalities (spondylolithesis), peripheral neuropathies, degenerative spinal cord lesions, peripheral vascular occlusive disease, and peripheral nerve lesions should all be considered in the differential diagnosis.

▶ **Treatment**

A. Medical Measures

The natural history of the radicular pain associated with lumbar disk disease is that of improvement over time.

Therefore, conservative measures are recommended for patients who present with a new radiculopathy without neurologic impairment. Conservative measures are directed toward initially limiting physical activity, including a brief period of bed rest followed by a gradual exercise program. It is also important for patients to modify their types of movement, for example to limit heavy lifting, twisting, or bending. Physical therapy can be useful after the acute period for instruction in abdominal and back musculature strengthening exercises.

The core of medical treatment is nonsteroidal anti-inflammatory drugs (NSAIDs). Oral steroids (ie, solumedrol dose pack) also may be useful in the acute setting, and epidural steroid injections and narcotics may be helpful in alleviating pain.

B. Surgical Treatment

Patients who present with acute neurologic motor deterioration warrant immediate surgical attention. Surgery is also indicated in patients who fail the conservative measures outlined above and continue to suffer from debilitating pain.

The microdiskectomy is the "gold standard" surgical intervention for patients with a herniated lumbar disk. A microdiskectomy involves a laminotomy to gain access to the disk space. The nerve root and the thecal sac are protected while the disk fragment is identified and removed. A fusion can sometimes be recommended in the setting of recurrent disk herniations at the same level or pain associated with joint instability.

▶ **Prognosis**

Overall, patients who have symptoms of radicular pain without neurologic deterioration have an excellent prognosis with improvement in symptoms over time. However, if loss of motor strength has already occurred, it is less likely to return even after surgical correction.

Boselie TF, Willems PC, van Mameren H, de Bie R, Benzel EC, van Santbrink H: Arthroplasty versus fusion in single-level cervical degenerative disc disease. *Cochrane Database Syst Rev* 2012;9:CD009173.

Jacobs W, Van der Gaag NA, Tuschel A, et al: Total disc replacement for chronic back pain in the presence of disc degeneration. *Cochrane Database Syst Rev* 2012;9:CD008326.

Kovacs FM, Urrutia G, Alarcon JD: Surgery versus conservative treatment for symptomatic lumbar spinal stenosis: a systematic review of randomized controlled trials. *Spine* 2011;36:E1335-E1351.

Matz PG, Anderson PA, Holly LT, et al: The natural history of cervical spondylotic myelopathy. *J Neurosurg Spine* 2009;11:104-111.

CSF DIVERSION FOR HYDROCEPHALUS

Hugh J. L. Garton, Jason Sack

OVERVIEW, EPIDEMIOLOGY, & PATHOPHYSIOLOGY

Hydrocephalus is a common diagnosis in both adult and pediatric patients. Most often this disease is chronically treated with an implanted catheter system to divert CSF from the brain to an alternative absorptive space such as the pleural or peritoneal space. Children and adults with CSF shunts can require surgical treatment for other associated conditions. The presence of the shunt may thus complicate the surgical management of various intra-abdominal processes. For example, a child with the distal portion of his shunt within the peritoneal may develop appendicitis. What management steps should be taken with regard to the management of the potentially contaminated CSF shunt catheter? In addition, CSF shunt failure is common, occurring in up to 30%-35% of individual within 1 year of initial shunt placement. About 1% of all shunt failures are fatal. Familiarity with the diagnosis and treatment of shunt failure is therefore desirable for providers caring for patients in whom a CSF shunt is present.

In pediatric patients, hydrocephalus is commonly seen in patients with a history of premature birth, intraventricular hemorrhate, after meningitis, in patients with myelomeningocele or other congenital cranial malformations and in patients with brain tumors. In adults, patients suffering from subarachnoid hemorrhage, brain tumor, or head injury may develop hydrocephalus. In older adults, "normal pressure" hydrocephalus is a potentially treatable cause of dementia. CSF shunt management is also used in the management of idiopathic intracranial hypertension (IIH) (also know as pseudotumor cerebri).

Among children, the prevalence of hydrocephalus is estimated at about 1-2 per 1000 children. Among adult patients, the incidence of IIH, and the shunt treatment for it appear to be increasing in accordance with increasing obesity rates.

Pathophysiologically, hydrocephalus results from an interruption in CSF circulation. The choroid plexus of the brain's ventricular system generates about 80% of the total adult CSF production of about 20 cc/h, by an active ion pump dependent process. The remainder is thought to be generated by more general metabolic processes of the brain and arachnoid. Importantly, the production of CSF is independent of the intracranial pressure over a wide range of physiologic values. Thus, the increase in intracranial pressure that typically results from the increasing CSF volumes within the nervous system does not act to check the further production of spinal fluid. Once produced, spinal fluid moves in an oscillatory fashion out of the ventricular system and into the subarachnoid space around the brain. From there, it is reabsorbed by passive, pressure dependent mechanisms into the cerebral venous sinuses and possibly into lymphatic systems adjacent to the dura. The vast majority of hydrocephalus results from interruption of the egress of CSF. Traditionally, hydrocephalus has been classified as either **obstructive**, if the blockage to CSF outflow prevents egress from the ventricular system, or **communicating** if reabsorption is interrupted beyond the ventricular system, at the dural venous and/or lymphatic absorption sites. The determination of the site of obstruction is usually radiographic and may require invasive studies. To the non-neurosurgeon, this distinction is mostly important in determining the safety of lumbar puncture. If a patient has obstructive hydrocephalus, a lumbar puncture (LP) may be unsafe because of the potential for differential pressures between the cranial and spinal spaces after the LP. Radiographically, hydrocephalus is sometimes assumed to be communicating when all four ventricles are dilated, as opposed to only ventricles I-III. However, blockage at the outflow of the fourth ventricle to the subarachnoid space could produce the same CT or MRI picture despite obstructive physiology. Consultation with a neurosurgeon or neurologist may be helpful if the situation is unclear.

CLINICAL PRESENTATION/ASSESSMENT

The relative difference between the volume of CSF produced and reabsorbed, along with the relative compressibility of the brain determine the severity and type of clinical symptoms and signs at presentation. Slower buildup of CSF or a brain more compliant to compression, such as might occur at the extremes of age, produce a more protracted course of symptoms compared to rapid CSF accumulation in a poorly compressible brain. Whether presenting initially or after treatment failure, the symptoms of hydrocephalus can be grouped in to three broad categories: those related to acute increased intracranial pressure, usually seen with a more rapid accumulation of CSF or a poorly compliant brain, those related to more chronic deformation of the nervous system by more slowly accumulating CSF, and those symptoms that are specific to treatment complications, including CSF shunt infection.

Acute, rapidly progressive hydrocephalus presents with headaches, nausea, and vomiting and as it progresses, a deterioration in level of consciousness. The headaches associated with hydrocephalus and/or CSF shunt failure may have morning predominance, or worsen with a valsalva maneuver. Patient may be lethargic, or difficult to arouse or awaken with ordinary stimuli. Some patients may present with a loss of upgaze or Parinaud's syndrome, others with cranial nerve VI palsy from increased intracranial pressure. In young children with an open fontanelle, this area may be tense and raised. Hydrocephalus of a more slowly progressive nature may present with more subtle signs of cognitive impairment. In the elderly, so called **Normal Pressure Hydrocephalus** presents with the triad of dementia, gait disturbance and incontinence. Other signs include papill-edema, and in young children, an inappropriately expanding head size. If the patient has already undergone treatment for hydrocephalus with a CSF shunt, then additional symptoms and signs to consider include those of device infection, including a stiff neck, fever, and redness around the device. If the device has broken or malfunctioned then CSF may accumulation around the shunt. If the distal cavity into which a shunt is placed fails to absorb spinal fluid, there may be symptoms related to this such as abdominal pain with a large intraperitoneal fluid collection (so-called pseudocyst). Some CSF shunt devices possess diagnostic chambers that can be manually compressed and observed for response. However, the utility of such tests is questionable and best left to a neurosurgeon.

Patients presenting with clinical features described above, especially with a history of a CSF shunt in place for prior treatment of hydrocephalus must be promptly evaluated with imaging studies, usually a CT or MRI scan of the brain. In the setting of a possible shunt failure, it is critical to have previous images available for comparison. Patients with working shunts may have ventricles that are smaller than normal; "normal ventricular size" or "no evidence of shunt failure" in a radiology report has been demonstrated to correlate poorly with final diagnosis. Additional studies that can be useful include plain radiographs of the shunt and imaging of the cavity into which the CSF shunt is draining, such as by ultrasound of the abdomen. Other invasive diagnostic studies may be necessary, usually as directed by a neurosurgical consultant. These can include a CSF shunt tap, in which a portion of the shunt that sits under the scalp is accessed percutaneously similar to a vascular access port. It is helpful to know that a high percentage of shunts failures occur within the first 2 years after shunt failure, with a reduction in failure rates following this. In children, young age at presentation also appears to be a risk factor for repeated shunt failure. Similarly, most shunt infections occur within 1 year from shunt placement. However, despite these epidemiologic data, a perfectly predictive clinical decision algorithm remains elusive and a low threshold for obtaining imaging studies and appropriate expert consultations is warranted.

▶ MANAGEMENT

Progressive hydrocephalus must be dealt with in a timely manner to minimize neurologic deterioration. As noted above, the rate of pathologic CSF accumulation may vary and produce different clinical symptoms. However, because of the potential for acute and fatal deterioration from hydrocephalus, the initial presumption should be that rapid intervention is needed, subject to reconsideration after all the data are available.

Medical management of hydrocephalus may be appropriate in the management of IIH (pseudotumor cerebri),

and in some patients after subarachnoid hemorrhage. It is also used in the initial management of hydrocephalus in neonates after an intraventricular hemorrhage. The diuretics acetazolamide and furosemide are used in this context. Both decrease CSF production by inhibiting carbonic anhydrase, albeit by slightly different mechanisms—thus producing an additive effect when used in combination. However, randomized control trials of diuretic therapy in newborns demonstrated no reduction in the need for subsequent shunt placement for patients on diuretic regimens. If diuretics are utilized, patients must be closely monitored for electrolyte imbalances and acetazolamide toxicity (acute gastritis, parasthesias, drowsiness.). It should be noted that with the exception of IIH, protracted use of diuretics to manage hydrocephalus is rarely successful and in most cases, surgical therapy is indicated without a trial of diuretics.

Intraventricular administration of fibrinolytic agents (eg, streptokinase) has also been investigated as a treatment for newborns with posthemorrhagic hydrocephalus. However, a systematic review of randomized trials failed to show any benefit, in terms of reducing shunt requirement or death. Furthermore, secondary intraventricular hemorrhage is a potential complication of this treatment.

Temporary drainage includes serial LPs, ventricular taps, placement of an external ventriculostomy catheter, or implanted reservoir in communication with the ventricular system for periodic aspiration. These techniques are used when natural history suggests possible resolution of the hydrocephalus, as may occur in IVH in the newborn and in SAH. In addition, temporary diversion is appropriate when the patient's condition precludes definitive treatment.

Endoscopic third ventriculostomy (ETV) is an alternative to CSF shunt placement for the treatment of some forms of hydrocephalus. During the endoscopic procedure a perforation is made in the floor of the third ventricle communicating it to the subarachnoid space. ETV is currently used as the initial treatment of choice in cases of obstructive hydrocephalus and is curative in 80% of properly selected patients, avoiding the need for shunt placement. ETV patients may suffer recurrent hydrocephalus if the fenestration closes. The vast majority of such failures have occurred within the first year after the procedure, and failures beyond 5 years are exceedingly rare.

CSF shunt treatment is indicated in most cases of progressive hydrocephalus, when conservative management and ETV are not indicated, or have previously failed. This procedure involves placement of a mechanical shunt as a means to divert excess CSF from the ventricles into other body cavities. CSF shunts have a ventricular catheter, a valve that regulates unidirectional flow, and distal tubing to distribute the CSF to its absorption site. Many shunts also have reservoirs that can be percutaneously tapped for diagnostic purposes, or as a temporizing measure in shunts in which the distal tubing or valve becomes blocked. Most often, the proximal catheter of the shunt system is placed into one of the lateral ventricles, either in the frontal horn via a frontal approach or via the atrium of the lateral ventricle via a parietal approach. Shunt systems are used to treat a variety of other conditions such as intracranial cysts, or chronic subdural hematomas/hygromas. The proximal catheter placement in such cases is dictated by the location of the pathology to be treated. Shunt valve mechanics regulate the amount of drainage. Most are differential pressure systems that respond to increasing fluid pressure by allowing more CSF through the valve. Various shunts are deigned to open in different pressure ranges (eg, low: 4-7 cm H_2O; medium: 8-12 cm H_2O; high: 13-15 cm H_2O), and some valves can be externally adjusted to different performance levels using a magnet. These adjustable ("programmable") valves may be inadvertently reprogrammed by other external magnets and while all systems approved for sale in the United States as of this writing are MRI compatible to 1.5 Telsa, the patient must have the valve setting checked and reset as necessary following an MRI. Alternative systems are designed to produce a constant flow through the valve over a range of physiological intracranial pressures. Valve systems may incorporate devices that prevent excessive drainage from the siphoning effect of a long run of distal tubing running inferiorly when patients assume an upright posture. The distal end of the system is comprised of a catheter that terminates in a body cavity, wherein the fluid can be adequately absorbed. A ventriculoperitoneal (VP) shunt, in which the catheter terminates into the abdominal cavity and fluid is absorbed by the peritoneum, is the most commonly used shunt at present. Other common distal sites include the pleural space (V-Pleural shunt) and the cardiac atria (VA shunt). These two sites are chosen when extensive scarring or adhesions, recent abdominal infection, peritonitis, or morbid obesity preclude peritoneal catheter placement. Other less common options for distal placement of a ventricular shunt include gall bladder, and ureter/bladder. Immediate complications from shunt placement are fortunately rare but include misplacement of the ventricular catheter with inadequate shunt function. Much more rarely a patient may suffer intracranial hemorrhage or perforated abdominal viscus.

Complications that are not encountered intraoperatively, but may nonetheless present in the early postoperative period include: inguinal hernia and/or hydrocele; ascites; pseudocyst formation; septicemia, pulmonary thromboembolism, and cardiac tamponade with VA placement; subcutaneous CSF collections and fistulas; hemorrhage; shunt obstruction/occlusion; and infection (shunt and/or incisional).

CSF SHUNT FAILURE

While the surgical procedure of CSF shunt placement is generally an uncomplicated process, the long-term management of shunted hydrocephalus is more problematic. Multiple clinical studies in both adult and pediatric patients attest to the high rate of device failure, from tubing obstruction, catheter fracture, infection, excessive drainage, and compartmentalization of the ventricular system (with a catheter draining part of the ventricular system, but with another part expanding because of noncommunication). In young children undergoing first shunt placement, roughly 1/3 of shunts will require reoperation in the first year following surgery. Shunt infection rates in these children are as high as 10%-12%. Adult patients fair somewhat better but 20% will still require reoperation within the first year after shunt failure. Analysis of the "shunt survival" curves shows that failure rates for devices drops considerably after the first year or two from surgery, but the threat of failure remains present to some degree as long as the device remains in place.

In evaluating a patient for potential CSF shunt failure, the epidemiological data above provide a baseline estimate of the probability of the diagnosis. Other risk factors for shunt failure include young age at shunt placement and recent previous shunt surgery. A history and physical exam along with images compared to previous findings, as described above, should allow for a reasonably accurate diagnosis. However, several pitfalls deserve mention. First, as has been noted, not all patients with CSF shunt failure will show significant expansion of the ventricular system. Some patients, particularly those with a long history of shunted hydrocephalus may present with the so-called "slit-ventricle" syndrome. The radiographic finding of "slit-ventricles" is relatively common for patients with a functioning shunt. The clinical "slit-ventricle" syndrome presents with episodic severe headaches that appear to be due to intermittent occlusion of the shunt in a small ventricular system that does not dilate despite an increase in CSF pressures because change in ventricular size is too small to be noted on standard radiographs. The diagnosis is often confirmed by direct intracranial pressure measurements obtained from a separately placed ICP monitor.

A second group that deserves special attention is children and adults with myelomeningocele. Given a frequent need for both urological and plastic surgical care, these patients are frequently encountered on surgical services. About 70% of patients with this spinal dysraphism will require treatment for hydrocephalus, most with a CSF shunt. Myelomeningocele is associated with a number of abnormalities of the brain stem and foramen magnum. These abnormalities allow CSF shunt failure to produce a much wider array of clinical symptoms than would otherwise be the case. As intracranial CSF and pressure build because of CSF shunt failure, downward pressure on the brainstem can produce lower cranial nerve palsies, including swallowing and breathing irregularities. The death rate from shunt failure may be higher in this population, and more precipitous, related to the susceptibility of the hindbrain to herniation. In additional, CSF shunt failure may precipitate or exacerbate a preexisting syrinx in these patients, producing symptoms related to spinal cord dysfunction.

Shunt contamination may occur during unrelated intra-abdominal procedures, in the case of a VP shunt, or from repeated bacterema in ventriculoatrial shunts. Infections of this sort can obviously occur at any time, and are not temporally restricted to the year or so following the most recent shunt surgery. Clinically, the presentation of infection may lack an overt inflammatory response with fever and redness around the shunt. Rather, the presentation may be more insidious, with failure of the CSF to absorb and development of a pseudocyst. The presence of a large intra-abdominal fluid collection in a patient with a VP shunt should raise suspicion of shunt infection, although sterile fluid collections are not uncommon.

Abdominal surgical procedures in patients with VP shunts raise the issue of the best management of an intraperitoneal distal shunt catheter during and after the procedure. While no validated guideline exists, the literature and the author's experience suggest that the infection risk is low during clean and clean contaminated cases. If an enterotomy or open bladder procedure is to be performed, it is reasonable to relocate the shunt away from this area once the tubing is identified intraperitoneally, and/or protect it with gause sponges during the procedure. Other than routine preoperative antibiotics, expectant management for shunt infection and failure can be practiced and the shunt does not require externalization. In situations where there is frank contamination of the shunt catheter in the abdomen, externalization of the shunt appears prudent. Laparoscopic procedures have been demonstrated to transiently increase intracranial pressure, but there is no body of literature to suggest that this produces identifiable complications, presumably due to its transient nature. Constipation and ileus, conversely have been suggested to be a source of at least transient shunt dysfunction due to increased abdominal pressure.

Shunt externalization, when necessary, involves palpation of the shunt proximal to its entry into the peritoneum, followed by a sterile prep and, if the patient is awake, local anesthesia. If the shunt has been in place for several years, it may be quite adherent to the surrounding tissues and the procedure is then best performed in the operating room with anesthesia. For recently placed shunts, this is less of an issue and the procedure can be performed at the bedside, assuming a cooperative patient. A cut down is made of over the shunt tract, avoiding laceration of the underlying tubing. The catheter is often encased in a thick sheath of scar that must be teased open to gain access to the catheter. If a specimen of fluid is required from a peritoneal fluid collection, the tubing is withdrawn slightly, then cut and aspirated distally. In a large pseudocyst a liter or more of fluid may be withdrawn. The distal catheter is then withdrawn from the patient and then discarded. The remaining tubing should be observed for CSF drainage and connected to a sterile, enclosed CSF drainage system. Neurosurgical consultation is advisable before embarking on the procedure. Patients with externalized shunts are draining isotonic CSF and may suffer hyponatremia if appropriate fluid and electrolyte replacement are not performed, particularly in young children.

ONGOING CARE

Patients with VP or ventriculopleural shunts do not require prophylactic antibiotics for surgical or dental procedures in which the shunt is outside the operative field. **Prophylactic antiobiotics** may be helpful when the shunt is in the operative field, as described above, or during a planned CSF shunt revision. For patients with ventriculo-atrial CSF shunts in place, an argument can be made for antibiotic prophylaxis before procedures likely to result in bacteremia including dental procedures. Dental practice guidelines suggest this also. American Heart Association guidelines for endocarditis prophylaxis recommend Amoxicillin 2 g 30-60 minutes before the procedure for adults and 50 mg/kg for pediatric patients or Clindamycin 600 mg adult and 20 mg/kg pediatric doses for penicillin allergic patients.

Shunt independence has been reported for children with a prior history of shunt placement. In this situation, a child previously depended on a CSF shunt becomes once again able to drain CSF independently. Clinically, this issue is often raised when a CSF shunt has gone without a revision for many years or even decades, or a CSF shunt is found disconnected in the absence of clinical symptoms. One series reported that 3% of children with hydrocephalus became shunt independent later in life. However, in the setting of a shunt found to be fractured on x-ray without ventricular enlargement or clinical symptoms of shunt failure, it is clinical experience that CSF can often drain between the fractured catheter segments through the tube of scar tissue that forms around the catheter initially after shunt placement. Such a scarred tract can subsequently close over, even several years after the catheter fracture and separation of the fractured tubing ends. Therefore, caution should be exercised in the presumption of shunt independence unless it has been verified by invasive testing. Patients incidentally found to have broken shunt catheters may reasonably be referred to a neurosurgeon for evaluation.

Shunted hydrocephalus during pregnancy frequently raises concerns over management of headaches during pregnancy, mechanism of delivery, and over the potential impact of hydrocephalus on the pregnancy outcome. Pregnancy, particularly in the third trimester, increases intra-abdominal pressures. For patients with VP shunts, this can lead to a relative decrease in CSF shunt function. In cases series of pregnant patients with hydrocephalus, headaches are not uncommonly reported, particularly during the third trimester. These may herald shunt failure, the evaluation of which may be complicated by a desire to avoid radiation administration during pregnancy. MRI may be a useful option in these circumstances. In the absence of radiographic manifestations of shunt failure, or additional clinical symptoms, safe observation of headaches has been successfully practiced, but treatment decisions must be individualized and other diagnoses, particularly eclampsia and preeclampsia must be considered. There is little evidence to suggest that the presence of a CSF shunt is a contraindication to labor and vaginal delivery. It has been argued that patients who are suspected of being symptomatic from increased intracranial pressure may benefit from avoiding protracted labor, but no comparative studies exist to provide a clear answer. Hydrocephalus, and the presence of a CSF shunt does not, per se, appear to impact pregnancy outcome. However, recalling that hydrocephalus is coincident with other diagnoses, such as epilepsy and myelomeningocele that do have a significant impact on the potential for birth defects, the importance of prenatal care can be emphasized.

Whitelaw A and Odd DE: Intraventricular streptokinase after intraventricular hemorrhage in newborn infants. *Cochrane Database Syst Rev* 2007;(4):CD000498.

Li G, Dutta S.: Perioperative management of ventriculoperitoneal shunts during abdominal surgery. *Surg Neurol* 2008;70(5): 492-495.

Wilson W, et al: Prevention of infective endocarditis: guidelines from the American Heart Association: a guideline from the American Heart Association Rheumatic Fever, Endocarditis, and Kawasaki Disease Committee, Council on Cardiovascular Disease in the Young, and the Council on Clinical Cardiology, Council on Cardiovascular Surgery and Anesthesia, and the Quality of Care and Outcomes Research Interdisciplinary Working Group. *Circulation* 2007;116(15):1736-1754.

Wu Y, et al: Ventriculoperitoneal shunt complications in California: 1990 to 2000. *Neurosurgery* 2007;61(3):557-562; discussion 562-563.

CENTRAL NERVOUS SYSTEM INFECTIONS

Khoi D. Than   Anthony C. Wang Jean-Christophe A. Leveque Stephen E. Sullivan

BRAIN ABSCESS

Brain abscesses are an uncommon entity, with approximately 2000 cases reported in the United States each year. There is a higher incidence in developing countries, and men are affected slightly more often than women. Classically, these abscesses arise locally from otorhinolaryngeal infections or hematogenously from distant infections, though opportunistic infections have become an important consideration upon initial presentation as well. The pathogenic organisms most commonly implicated are of the *Streptococcus* family; *Klebsiella*, *Staphylococcus aureus*, and anaerobes are also frequent. In immunocompromised patients, it is important to include *Toxoplasma*, *Listeria*, and *Nocardia* as possible etiologic agents, as well as fungal pathogens.

A patient with a brain abscess can present with nonspecific symptoms. Headache, nausea, vomiting, and altered mental status can occur due to increased intracranial pressure (ICP), while unilateral headache, seizures, and many focal neurological deficits occur due to the presence of a mass lesion. Fever and nuchal rigidity are also seen in many cases. Additional findings in the newborn patient may include cranial enlargement, meningeal signs, irritability, and failure to thrive.

Risk factors for brain abscess include sinus, ear, or dental infections. These sources usually lead to formation of frontal or temporal lobe abscesses through direct spread. Hematogenous spread from intra-abdominal, pelvic, pulmonary, or cardiac seeding occurs most commonly via the middle cerebral artery, leading to microembolic infarcts at the gray-white junction. Risk factors for these types of abscesses include infectious lung processes and congenital cyanotic heart disease. In these conditions, the lungs have a decreased filtering capability, and the associated relative hypoxia promotes abscess formation. Head trauma—blunt, penetrating, or surgical—can introduce a nidus for infection with delayed abscess formation. Parasitic infections such as cysticercosis should be considered more likely in recent foreign travelers.

The differential diagnosis for brain abscess includes subdural empyema, septic emboli, dural sinus thrombosis, mycotic aneurysm, meningitis, focal necrotizing encephalitis (herpes simplex virus), and tumor, as all of these conditions can present with headaches and altered mental status. In the initial evaluation of brain abscess, blood work that should be drawn includes a white blood cell count, cultures, erythrocyte sedimentation rate (ESR), and C-reactive protein (CRP); however, normal test results do not rule out the diagnosis. The key to diagnosing brain abscess is correlating the clinical scenario with an imaging study, such as contrast-enhanced computed tomography (CT) or MRI. The classic finding on CT or MRI is a circular lesion with a strongly contrast-enhancing surround rim. CT images are typically the first obtained on admission, although MRI is the imaging modality of choice as it can provide greater anatomic detail. MRI evaluation for brain abscess should always include diffusion-weighted images (DWI), which can differentiate between ring-enhancing lesions of infectious and neoplastic origin, as abscesses are typically hyperintense on DWI while neoplastic lesions are hypointense.

One general warning is to avoid LP, as cerebrospinal fluid (CSF) results are often nondiagnostic and this procedure is associated with a worsened outcome in patients with brain abscesses. Less than one-quarter of patients have positive CSF cultures, and, with a large enough abscess, there is a real risk for transtentorial or brainstem herniation. CSF sampling should be considered only if parasitic pathogens are suspected. A definitive diagnosis is made by biopsy sampling of the abscess through surgical means.

The treatment of brain abscesses involves both surgical and medical therapy. Treatment should also be aimed at correcting the primary source of infection (ie, draining a pulmonary empyema or repairing a correctable heart defect). Initial surgical treatment usually consists of needle aspiration of the abscess; the abscess can be monitored serially with imaging, and the procedure repeated as necessary. A total excision via a craniotomy can be performed if the abscess is in its chronic, encapsulated form and is located in a surgically amenable region of the brain. It is advisable to perform surgery before starting antibiotics in order to confirm the diagnosis as well as to identify the organisms and their antibiotic sensitivities. Antibiotic therapy typically consists of 6-8 weeks intravenous treatment followed by 4-8 weeks oral treatment. Patients should receive routine follow-up imaging and should also be started on an antiepileptic medication. Glucocorticoids should be considered to counteract symptomatic intracranial hypertension, although their role is less important than in the treatment of brain tumors.

In certain situations, medical therapy can suffice without the need for surgery. These situations include an abscess in its early stages (ie, symptoms for less than 2 weeks), a small (< 2 cm) abscess, or a definite clinical improvement after 1 week of antibiotics only. Medical treatment without surgery should also be considered in poor surgical candidates, patients with multiple abscesses and/or concomitant meningitis, patients with abscesses in eloquent locations, or patients with hydrocephalus and ventricular shunts.

Patients with brain abscess have a reported mortality risk of 0%-30% depending on etiology and presentation. An overall 50% morbidity risk of permanent neurological deficits is conferred, which depends heavily upon the severity of presenting symptoms.

SUBDURAL EMPYEMA

A subdural empyema is a collection of pus that forms in the subdural space. It is less common than brain abscess, but like abscesses, it is more commonly found in men. Subdural empyema is an emergent condition because, unlike the brain parenchyma with abscesses, the subdural space does not pose much of a barrier to prevent the spread of infection. Additionally, antibiotics have poor penetration into the subdural space.

The most common cause of subdural empyema (70%) is paranasal sinusitis, especially in cases involving the frontal sinus. Chronic otitis media accounts for another 15% of cases. As such, the organisms typically cultured from a subdural empyema include *Streptococcus* (aerobic and anaerobic) and *Staphylococcus*. Symptoms present in the majority of patients with subdural empyema include fever, headache, nuchal rigidity, hemiparesis, and altered mental status. Other common symptoms include seizures and sinus tenderness.

Computed tomography or MRI imaging will typically diagnose a subdural empyema. Three-fourths of empyemas are located over the convexity, while 15% are parafalcine (ie, adjacent to the falx cerebri). Just as with brain abscesses, LP should be avoided due to the risk of herniation.

Almost all cases of subdural empyema will require surgical drainage, preferably emergently. The two surgical options are burr-hole drainage and craniotomy. Although burr-hole drainage is less invasive, it is also less effective; thus, craniotomy is the preferred surgical option. Antibiotics are used for a course of 4-6 weeks, and patients are put on therapeutic or prophylactic antiseizure medication. Medical treatment alone can be effective if the empyema is small, there is minimal neurologic involvement, and antibiotics have an early efficaciousness.

Subdural empyema carries a 15% mortality rate. Half of patients have residual neurological deficits at the time of hospital discharge. Factors known to be associated with poor prognosis include age more than 60 years, obtunded or comatose state at presentation, and empyema formation secondary to surgery or trauma.

OSTEOMYELITIS

Osteomyelitis can affect the skull or the vertebrae. Osteomyelitis of the skull usually results from contiguous spread from an infected sinus or from penetrating trauma (ie, postoperative). The infectious agents are typically *S. aureus* or *epidermidis*, and treatment consists of debridement surgery followed by 6-12 weeks of antibiotics (intravenously for the first 1-2 weeks). Surgical treatment is aimed at removing all infected bone. A cranioplasty or other hardware is not placed until several months later in order to minimize the risk of reseeding an infection.

Vertebral osteomyelitis (VO) represents 3% of all cases of osteomyelitis, and is more common than skull osteomyelitis because of the spine's rich vascular supply. Both anterograde arterial seeding as well as retrograde venous plexus spread have been implicated in VO, with *S. aureus* as the most common organism. VO caused by *Mycobacterium tuberculosis* is known as Pott's disease. Those at higher risk for developing VO include intravenous drug users, diabetics, sickle cell patients, patients on hemodialysis, and the elderly.

The most common presentation in patients with VO is that of back pain (> 90%), usually unaffected by activity. Other typical presenting symptoms include fever, weight loss, radicular pain, and myelopathy. The neurologic symptoms are usually a result of destruction of the vertebral body and subsequent retropulsion of bone into the spinal canal or neural foramen. The most commonly affected segment of the spine is the lumbar region followed by, in order, the thoracic, cervical, and sacral segments. Any source of infection can theoretically put one at risk for developing VO, although important sources include infections of the urinary tract, respiratory system, and mouth. VO also develops at sites of previous spine surgeries.

Definitive diagnosis of VO is made with positive cultures, either from biopsy of the tissue itself or via blood cultures in the setting of suggestive radiographic findings. MRI has demonstrated excellent diagnostic accuracy of more than 90% of cases and is the preferred diagnostic modality. When unable to obtain MRI, bone scintigraphy with single photon emission computed tomography has also demonstrated excellent sensitivity.

The treatment of VO is nonsurgical in the vast majority of cases, with disease resolution being accomplished via antibiotic therapy alone. The goal of therapy should be to minimize neurologic involvement, and to maintain structural stability of the spine. Surgical treatment is indicated to obtain a tissue diagnosis if closed needle biopsy is unfeasible. In patients with a worsening neurologic deficit, the onset of structural instability, or a failure of medical management, surgery is warranted for abscess drainage, alleviation of compression, and stabilization.

SPINAL EPIDURAL ABSCESS

Spinal epidural abscesses (SEA) are often associated with VO, with the majority of cases arising from *S. aureus.* *Streptococcus* species are the second most commonly implicated organism (Figure 36–27). SEA are located most often in the thoracic region (50%), followed by the lumbar (35%), and cervical (15%) regions. The vast majority of abscesses (80%) are located posterior to the spinal cord.

The primary infection leading to SEA can be from hematogenous spread or direct extension. Hematogenous spread is more common, with skin infections being the usual

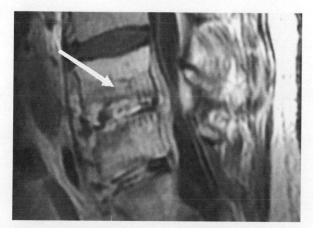

▲ **Figure 36–27.** Sagittal magnetic resonance T1-weighted image with contrast of the lumbar spine demonstrating diskitis/osteomyelitis associated with a spinal epidural abscess.

originating source. Other mechanisms of hematogenous spread include nonsterile intravenous injections, bacterial endocarditis, urinary tract infections, respiratory infections, and oropharyngeal abscesses. SEA caused by direct extension can be from decubitus ulcers or penetrating trauma, including following spinal procedures.

Patients with SEA are typically middle aged. Risk factors for developing SEA include diabetes, intravenous drug use, chronic renal failure, and alcoholism. Patients often present with back pain, spine tenderness, fever, sweats, and rigors. When motor weakness ensues, there is a very rapid progression to paraplegia. Thus, the diagnosis and treatment of SEA is emergent.

The workup of SEA should include a complete blood count, ESR, CRP, and blood cultures. An LP is contraindicated given the potential to spread infection from the epidural to the intradural space. The imaging modality of choice is MRI, although CT and myelography may also be used to arrive at a diagnosis.

The treatment of SEA, as with most infections of the central nervous system, is surgery plus antibiotics. Surgery is used to drain pus, debride any granulation tissue, and provide stability (usually in cases where there is bony destruction secondary to VO). Antibiotics are given intravenously for 3-4 weeks and then orally for another 4 weeks. Nonsurgical management with antibiotics only is rare and reserved only for very poor surgical candidates, abscesses that are very extensive in length, or cases in which complete paralysis has been present for at least 3 days with irreversible neurologic injury.

The overall prognosis for patients with SEA is relatively poor, with a mortality rate of 20%. In patients that survive, restoration of baseline neurological function is rare.

MULTIPLE CHOICE QUESTIONS

1. Intracranial pressure

    A. Is normally between 30 and 40 torr
    B. Is directly (linearly) related to increasing intracranial mass
    C. Cannot be measured directly
    D. Is normally maintained at a stable level by displacement of CSF
    E. Is often affected by changes in the size of the skull after trauma

2. Strategies to reduce intracranial pressure can include all of the following except

    A. Drainage of CSF
    B. Hyperventilation
    C. Treatment with mannitol
    D. Trendelenburg position
    E. Sedation

3. Spinal cord injury

   A. Rarely includes the use of systemic corticosteroid therapy
   B. Is accompanied by initial hyporeflexia
   C. Is termed complete if there is no motor function below the level of injury
   D. Is accompanied by priapism and increased anal sphincter tone
   E. Can cause a Brown–Séquard syndrome, with loss of motor function and loss of pain and temperature sensation below the level of the lesion, with preserved proprioception, vibration, and pressure sensation

4. Peripheral nerve injury recovery

   A. Occurs with axonal regeneration after wallerian degeneration at a rate of 1 mm per day
   B. Is best treated by delayed (3 month) repair is the case of acute sharp injury
   C. Should be treated by segmental resection and nerve graft in cases of apparent stretch injury
   D. Occurs more quickly with systemic corticosteroid therapy
   E. Is likely to be functionally successful if a neuroma forms

5. Pituitary tumors

   A. Are typically adenocarcinomas
   B. Should be treated by urgent operation in most patients
   C. Can cause symptoms related to the compression of the pituitary stalk causing increased prolactin levels
   D. Can cause Cushing syndrome by overproduction of growth hormone
   E. Cause visual symptoms due to hormonal release

The Eye & Ocular Adnexa

Linda M. Tsai, MD

Ian Pitha, MD, PhD

Stephen A. Kamenetzky, MD

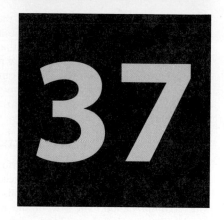

Ophthalmology has evolved substantially over the past decade. Innovations in surgical techniques and tissue banking as well as developments in ophthalmic surgical devices and implants, allow an increasingly sophisticated approach to ophthalmic surgery. Advances in imaging the microanatomy of the eye facilitate diagnosis and guide treatment. Nonetheless, the majority of diagnoses in ophthalmology can be made after a targeted history and careful examination without the need for sophisticated equipment.

EXAMINATION OF THE EYE

Evaluation of the eye and its adnexa requires a good history, assessment of visual function and physical examination of the eyes. Occasionally, special examinations may be required to identify specific ocular disorders or to establish the presence of associated systemic disease.

The basic equipment required for an eye examination by a nonophthalmologist includes the following: (1) a visual acuity chart, (2) a handheld flashlight, (3) an ophthalmoscope, and (4) a tonometer.

The basic medications required for an eye examination are (1) a local anesthetic such as proparacaine 0.5% or tetracaine 0.5%; (2) fluorescein strips; and (3) dilating drops, such as phenylephrine 2.5% or tropicamide 0.5%-1%.

▶ History

In addition to eliciting a chief complaint, determining whether visual loss is monocular or binocular, central or peripheral, and painful or painless is important. Prior ophthalmic history (including known ophthalmic conditions, prior eye surgery or trauma, history of contact lens use, and relevant family history) should be obtained. A review of past medical history and all medications should be included as well.

▶ Visual Acuity Testing

Central visual acuity, using the patient's glasses if available, should be determined in all patients. The Snellen chart is most commonly used. The patient faces the test chart at a distance of 6 m (20 ft). Each eye should be tested separately. Visual acuity corresponds to the smallest line the patient can read. The patient who is unable to read the largest letter on the chart (typically a 20/200 letter) should be moved progressively closer until that character can be read and that distance recorded in the chart. If no letters are recognizable, the patient should be tested for the ability to count fingers, see hand motion or perceive light. If a vision chart is not readily available, the ability to read small print or a name badge can provide useful information. Preschool children or illiterates can be tested with the E chart or Allen picture chart.

▶ Visual Field Testing

Confrontation visual fields can be used to detect gross visual field defects such as quadrantanopia, hemianopia, or severe visual field constriction. With one eye occluded, the patient is asked to fixate on the examiner's face and detect finger count or hand motion in each quadrant. Formal visual field testing (perimetry) is used to more carefully examine the central and peripheral visual fields. The technique is performed separately for each eye and measures the function of the retina, the optic nerve and intracranial visual pathway. Perimetry relies on subjective patient responses so results will depend on the patient's alertness and cooperation. Several methods are used to assess visual field functions, including the tangent screen, Goldmann perimetry, and computerized automated perimetry.

▶ Eye Movements

Ocular motility should be assessed in all positions of gaze. One should also observe the patient for random eye movement and assess the alignment of the eyes when the patient is looking straight ahead. The position of the light reflection from a penlight ("reflex") on the cornea is at the same point in each eye when the eyes are properly aligned. The oculocephalic reflex (doll's head) can be tested. The upward rotation of the cornea in response to resistance to forced eyelid closure (Bell phenomenon) should be noted when clinically appropriate.

Assessment of Pupillary Functions

Examination of the pupils should be performed before any dilating drops are instilled. Both the direct and consensual light reflex should be assessed. The pupils should constrict with accommodation. The size of the pupils should be noted in light and dark conditions and any difference in size (anisocoria) should be recorded. Irregular pupils may indicate traumatic, postsurgical, neurological, or congenital defects. In hospitalized patients and those with neurological disorders requiring monitoring of pupillary reaction to assess clinical status, pupils should be dilated with discretion and only with short-acting mydriatics.

Inspection of Anterior Segment & Adnexa

The eyelids, conjunctiva, cornea, sclera, and lacrimal apparatus should be evaluated. Unusual prominence of the globes (proptosis), abnormal eyelid position and the inability to fully close eyelids are important features that should be documented. Eversion of the upper eyelid to enable inspection of the hidden conjunctival surface should be performed when appropriate. The conjunctiva is inspected for anatomic defects, foreign bodies, lacerations, inflammation, discharge, tearing, dryness, or other abnormalities. In patients who are unconscious, the presence or absence of Bell phenomenon (upward rotation of the cornea during sleep) may be an important measure of neurological function. Corneal sensation should be tested before anesthetic drops are used.

A direct ophthalmoscope focused on the ocular surface can provide magnification for the examination. A magnifying glass and a handheld flashlight can also be used. Shining a light across the eye from the lateral to medial aspects and noting whether or not the nasal iris is shadowed can assess the depth of the anterior chamber. The presence of shadowing may indicate a narrow anterior chamber angle requiring special precautions if dilating drops are to be used.

Ophthalmoscopy

Ophthalmoscopy is important for the diagnosis of both ocular and systemic conditions and can provide critical information in neurologic and neurosurgical contexts. In most instances, the optic nerve head can be clearly seen without dilating the pupils. When describing the optic nerve, it is important to note any nerve head edema and the cup-to-disc ratio. Vessel caliber, tortuosity, arteriovenous nicking, and the presence of retinal hemorrhages are additional findings that can aid in diagnosis. In hospitalized patients with neurologic and neurosurgical disorders, dilation of the pupils should be performed with discretion.

Tonometry

Tonometry measures intraocular pressure (IOP). The most common instruments used are the Tono-Pen and the Goldmann applanation tonometer. The normal intraocular pressure varies between 10 and 20 mm Hg. IOP measurements can vary slightly with corneal thickness.

SYMPTOMS & SIGNS OF OCULAR DISORDERS

Decrease in Visual Acuity

Efforts should be made to determine if the decrease in visual acuity is unilateral or bilateral, painful or painless, persistent or transient, recent or chronic, isolated or associated with other symptoms. Unilateral acute painful loss of vision may be due to angle-closure glaucoma, endophthalmitis, or uveitis. Painless unilateral loss of vision is often caused by ischemic optic neuropathy, optic neuritis, central retinal artery or vein occlusion, retinal detachment, vitreous hemorrhage or retinal hemorrhages. Transient painless unilateral loss may be due to retinal migraine or amaurosis fugax. Hemispheric strokes are often responsible for visual field loss with preservation of the central visual acuity.

Disturbances in Vision

Disturbances in vision include image distortion, light sensitivity (photophobia), color change, spots before the eyes, visual field defects, night blindness, momentary loss of vision, or halos around lights. Distortion of normal shape (metamorphopsia) is most commonly caused by macular lesions. Photophobia can be due to corneal inflammation, iritis, ocular albinism, or aniridia. Toxicity from systemic medications such as digoxin and certain retinal conditions can cause the patient to complain of abnormally colored vision (chromatopsia). Patients with vitreous opacities or intraocular inflammation may report floating spots in their vision, even if retinal tears and detachment have to be ruled out as a cause. Visual field defects may be due to lid edema, retinal and optic nerve lesions, visual pathway lesions, or cortical abnormalities. Night blindness may be genetic (as in patients with retinitis pigmentosa) or acquired. Important causes of acquired night blindness include vitamin A deficiency, glaucoma, optic atrophy, cataract, or retinal degeneration. Transient loss of vision may imply impending cerebrovascular accident or partial occlusion of the internal carotid artery. Colored halos around lights can be caused by elevated intraocular pressure, most commonly due to acute angle-closure glaucoma. Incipient cataract or incorrect refractive error can cause colorless halos around point light sources.

Double Vision (Diplopia)

Diplopia can be constant or intermittent, sudden or gradual, painful or painless, horizontal or vertical. It may occur only in certain gaze positions. It is important to first determine if the diplopia is monocular or binocular. Binocular diplopia is only present when both eyes are open and disappears when either eye is closed. Binocular diplopia is most often due to misalignment of the eyes from extraocular muscle dysfunction or neurologic abnormalities. Monocular diplopia (multiple images in a single eye) occurs with refractive error, lenticular changes, macular lesions, malingering, or conversion reactions.

Ocular & Orbital Pain

Ocular pain may result from corneal lesions, inflammation, rapid increase in intraocular pressure, anterior uveitis, cyclitis, scleritis, or optic neuritis. Other causes of pain include inflammation of the orbital contents, tumors in the orbit and dacryocystitis (lacrimal sac inflammation). Eyelid pain and irritation can also arise from infections of the meibomian glands and the glands of Zeis and Moll.

Redness of the Eye

Acute redness (injection) of the eye not associated with trauma is caused by conjunctivitis, acute anterior uveitis, acute angle-closure glaucoma, corneal infection or corneal abrasion (Table 37–1). Subconjunctival hemorrhage may also present as a red eye but this is usually painless and otherwise asymptomatic. Conjunctivitis from bacterial, chlamydial, viral, or allergic causes is a frequent cause of red eye. Nonspecific irritation from exogenous agents or a foreign body can also cause redness. Chemical and thermal injuries cause similar findings. "Dry eye" or ocular surface anomalies can cause redness, a foreign-body sensation, and variable degrees of decreased vision.

Discharge

Ocular discharge may be described as watery, mucopurulent, purulent, or crusting of the lid margins. When watery discharge is not associated with redness or pain, it may be due to excessive tear production or obstruction of the lacrimal outflow passages. Watery discharge with photophobia, pain, or irritation indicates possible keratitis or keratoconjunctivitis. Purulent or mucopurulent discharge is a sign of bacterial infection, severe inflammation of the conjunctival surface, or bacterial infection of the lacrimal sac or canaliculus. *Pseudomonas* or *Haemophilus* species involvement is common. When the discharge forms mucoid strings, it is characteristic of allergic disorders involving the conjunctiva (vernal conjunctivitis) or dry eye syndrome.

Swelling of the Eyelids

For unilateral swelling, the cause is often a stye or chalazion. Bilateral swelling suggests blepharitis or allergic dermatitis. Systemic diseases associated with water retention, hyper-

Table 37–1. Differential diagnosis of common causes of inflamed eye.

	Acute Conjunctivitis	Acute Iritis[1]	Acute Glaucoma[2]	Corneal Trauma or Infection
Incidence	Extremely common	Common	Uncommon	Common
Discharge	Moderate to copious	None	None	Watery or purulent
Vision	No effect on vision	Slightly blurred	Markedly blurred	Usually blurred
Pain	None	Moderate	Severe	Moderate to severe
Conjunctival injection	Diffuse; more toward fornices	Mainly circumcorneal	Diffuse	Diffuse
Cornea	Clear	Usually clear	Steamy	Change in clarity related to cause
Pupil size	Normal	Small	Moderately dilated and fixed	Normal
Pupillary light response	Normal	Poor	None	Normal
Intraocular pressure	Normal	Normal	Elevated	Normal
Smear	Causative organisms	No organisms	No organisms	Organisms found only in corneal ulcers due to infection

[1]Acute anterior uveitis.
[2]Angle-closure glaucoma.

thyroidism, or hypothyroidism can also cause swelling or puffiness of the eyelids.

Displacement of the Eyes

The most common cause of both unilateral and bilateral exophthalmos (proptosis) is hyperthyroidism. Other etiologies include tumors of the orbit.

Strabismus

Strabismus results from misalignment of the eyes due to muscle imbalance. Ocular deviations may be lateral (exotropia), medial (esotropia), upward (hypertropia), or downward (hypotropia). Binocular diplopia is not a frequent complaint in congenital strabismus. Full ocular motility is intact in the majority of strabismus cases.

Leukocoria

A white pupil in a child indicates a serious eye disorder. The most frequent cause of leukocoria is congenital cataract, which requires urgent management to prevent amblyopia. Other causes include retinoblastoma, retinopathy of prematurity, toxocariasis, persistent hyperplastic primary vitreous, vitreous hemorrhage, retinal detachment, retinal dysplasia, incontinentia pigmenti, Coats disease, and Norrie disease.

Other Symptoms

Patients may present with other symptoms such as burning, itching, gritty, and foreign-body sensations, or a "sandy" feeling. These symptoms in elderly patients are suggestive of dry eye syndrome. Itching is also frequently associated with allergic disorders.

▼ DISEASES OF THE EYE & ADNEXA

DISEASES OF THE OCULAR ADNEXA

ACUTE HORDEOLUM

Acute hordeolum (stye) is a common infection of the glands of the eyelids. External hordeolum involve the glands of Zeis or Moll. Internal hordeolum is an infection of the meibomian glands. The usual causative agent is *Staphylococcus aureus*. Acute hordeolum is characterized by pain, localized swelling, and redness of the eyelid. A large hordeolum is infrequently associated with a preauricular lymph node.

If there is no abscess formation, treatment with warm compresses three times daily and topical broad-spectrum antibiotic drops such as tobramycin or sulfacetamide 10% three or four times daily for 5-7 days usually suffices. Ophthalmic ointments (erythromycin or bacitracin) twice daily for 5-7 days are also effective. Oral antibiotics, especially tetracycline derivatives, can be useful for patients with acne rosacea. If the infection does not resolve and is localized, treatment consists of making a local horizontal (skin) or vertical (conjunctiva) incision.

HERPES ZOSTER

Herpes zoster virus (HZV) is caused by a reactivation of latent varicella virus (chickenpox) dormant in the dorsal root ganglion. Approximately 15% of herpes zoster cases arise from the ophthalmic division of the trigeminal nerve (herpes zoster ophthalmicus [HZO]). Hutchinson sign (involvement of the nasociliary nerve which supplies the tip of the nose) occurs in about one-third of patients with HZO. If present, it suggests intraocular involvement. Reactivation is associated with decreased cell-mediated immunity and patients with HIV, blood dyscrasias, neoplasms, or other forms of immunosuppression are at increased risk.

Clinical Findings

HZO can involve virtually any ocular and adnexal tissues. Reactivation often starts with headache, malaise, fever, and ocular pain without cutaneous findings. Within 24-48 hours, the classic vesicular lesions develop unilaterally in a dermatomal distribution. Corneal involvement presents with the acute event or may follow it by months or years. A corneal pseudodendritic pattern is common. Conjunctivitis, keratitis, episcleritis/scleritis, and uveitis can also occur. Dry eye and poor corneal sensation are common.

Treatment

Treatments of skin lesions include warm compresses and topical antibiotic ointment. Aggressive lubrication is often needed for maintenance of the ocular surface. Oral antiviral medication is the standard of care. Oral acyclovir (800 mg five times a day) or valacyclovir (1000 mg three times a day) initiated within 72 hours of symptoms has been demonstrated to accelerate the resolution of skin rash and the healing of skin lesions, reduce lesion formation and viral shedding and reduce the incidence of episcleritis, keratitis, and iritis. Oral antivirals appear to reduce both acute zoster-associated pain and postherpetic neuralgia. Topical antiviral medication and steroids are used in certain situations to treat corneal lesions or uveitis. The Zostavax vaccine has been approved for the prevention of herpes zoster in the elderly. In patients without known risk factors for HZO (patients under age 50 without chronic immunosuppression) consider HIV testing.

Oxman MN et al: Vaccination against herpes zoster and postherpetic neuralgia. *J Infect Dis* 2008;197(Suppl 2):S228-S236.

DACRYOCYSTITIS

Dacryocystitis is a common infection of the lacrimal sac. Acute or chronic, it occurs most often in infants and in persons older than 40 years. It is usually unilateral and always secondary to obstruction of the nasolacrimal duct. In rare instances, the nasolacrimal duct may be obstructed by a tumor.

In children the nasolacrimal duct opens spontaneously during the first month of life. Failure of canalization leads to obstruction of the sac and secondary dacryocystitis. The cause of acquired nasolacrimal duct obstruction is often unclear, but trauma to the nose or infection may be responsible. In infants, dacryocystitis leading to obstruction may be due to *Haemophilus influenzae*, staphylococci, or streptococci. In patients with trachoma, nasolacrimal and canalicular obstruction is common. The cause of acute dacryocystitis in adults is usually *S. aureus* or β-hemolytic streptococci. In chronic dacryocystitis, *Streptococcus pneumoniae* is a common pathogen.

▶ Clinical Findings

A. Symptoms and Signs

Acute dacryocystitis is characterized by pain, swelling, tenderness, and redness in the tear sac area. In chronic dacryocystitis, tearing and discharge are the principal signs. Purulent material can often be expressed through the puncta.

B. Laboratory Findings

Culture and sensitivity of organisms obtained from cotton swab should be performed.

▶ Treatment

A. Adults

Acute dacryocystitis responds well to systemic antibiotic therapy, but recurrences are common if the obstruction is not surgically relieved.

B. Infants

When ductal obstruction is due to failure of canaliculization in the first month of life, daily vigorous massage of the tear sac is indicated. Topical antibiotics should be instilled in the conjunctival sac four or five times daily. If this is not successful, probing of the nasolacrimal duct is indicated. Most ophthalmologists postpone probing until age 6-9 months to allow sufficient time for the passage to open on its own. Both the upper and the lower canaliculi should be probed. In cases of previous failure or in children older than age 2, balloon dacryocystoplasty at the time of probing may increase chances of success. In recalcitrant cases, stenting of the nasolacrimal system or surgical creation of a new tear drain between the eye and nose (dacryocystorhinostomy) is required.

ORBITAL CELLULITIS

Orbital cellulitis is characterized by an abrupt onset of swelling and redness of the lids, accompanied by proptosis, decreased vision, diplopia, and fever. It is usually caused by staphylococci or streptococci. Immediate treatment with intravenous antibiotics is indicated to prevent abscess formation and rapid increase in the orbital pressure with compromise of the blood supply to the eye. The response to antibiotics is usually excellent, but surgical drainage may be required if an abscess forms. Computerized tomography (CT) is indicated to rule out abscess formation. Preseptal cellulitis is limited to the area anterior to the orbital septum and is treated with oral antibiotics while monitoring closely for progression to full-blown orbital infection.

▼ DISEASES OF THE EYE SURFACE

CONJUNCTIVITIS

Acute conjunctivitis is a common cause of red eye. Infectious causes include bacterial, viral, chlamydial, fungal, and parasitic agents. Noninfectious causes include chemical irritation, allergy, hypersensitivity to topical medications, vitamin A deficiency, dry eye syndrome, floppy eyelid syndrome associated with obstructive sleep apnea and injury.

▶ Clinical Findings

A. Symptoms and Signs

Patients with conjunctivitis complain of redness, irritation, foreign-body sensation, and conjunctival discharge. One or both eyes may be affected. The eyelids are often stuck together in the morning. Bacterial conjunctivitis has conjunctival hyperemia with purulent or mucopurulent discharge and variable degrees of lid swelling. Gonococcal conjunctivitis is characterized by hyperacute onset of copious mucopurulent discharge and can be a vision-threatening infection. In viral conjunctivitis, follicles are present in the inferior conjunctival fornix and preauricular lymph nodes are often involved. The hallmark symptom of allergic conjunctivitis is itching.

B. Laboratory Findings

If bacterial conjunctivitis is suspected, appropriate microbiologic testing should be performed, including blood and chocolate agar plates, Gram and Giemsa stains, and bacterial cultures.

▶ Treatment

For patients with suspected bacterial conjunctivitis, topical broad-spectrum antibacterial agents should be prescribed (eg, sulfacetamide 10% eye drops or ciprofloxacin 0.3% eye drops QID), with the addition of erythromycin or bacitracin ophthalmic ointment at bedtime if clinical indications warrant.

Viral conjunctivitis is usually self-limited and does not require treatment. If the diagnosis is unclear, topical antibiotics are often used. Contact precautions are necessary in all situations of suspected bacterial and viral conjunctivitis because spread of disease occurs through contact with contaminated tears.

Treatment of patients with allergic conjunctivitis consists of topical decongestants (naphazoline 0.1%) and H₁ receptor blocker (levocabastine) or a mast cell stabilizer (cromolyn). Combination mast cell and antihistamine drops such as olopatadine are also available. In severe cases of allergic conjunctivitis, topical corticosteroids or cyclosporine might be required but should be initiated only with the assistance of an ophthalmologist.

CORNEAL ULCERS

Corneal infections leading to ulceration may be due to bacteria, viruses, fungi, or protozoa.

▶ Clinical Findings

A. Symptoms and Signs

Patients with corneal ulcers complain of pain, photophobia, and blurring of vision. Patients develop conjunctival hyperemia and chemosis with ulceration of the cornea and whitish or yellowish infiltrate. Hypopyon (pus in the anterior chamber) may be present in cases caused by bacterial or fungal infections. Contact lens users and people with diminished corneal sensation or incomplete eyelid closure are at increased risk of developing corneal infections.

B. Laboratory Findings

Laboratory studies include culture and cytologic inspection of corneal scrapings.

▶ Treatment

Corneal ulceration is a serious condition requiring careful management to avoid permanent visual loss. The most devastating infection of the cornea is caused by *Pseudomonas aeruginosa*. Topical antibiotics should be given on an empirical basis until the results of culture and sensitivity tests are available. Organism-specific antimicrobial treatment should then be started. Patients using topical corticosteroids should stop using them. Central corneal ulcers may leave corneal scars, causing loss of vision. Patients severely affected may require corneal transplantation.

Patients wearing contact lenses (especially extended-wear contacts) are at higher risk of corneal ulcers. Contact lens wear should be stopped if corneal infection is suspected.

HERPES SIMPLEX

Herpes simplex virus (HSV) is a DNA virus that can affect the eye either in a primary ocular reaction or a reactivated state when latent virus travels down the axon of the sensory nerve to its target tissue. HSV is extremely common, with about 90% of the population seropositive for HSV antibodies. HSV-1 usually causes infection above the waist (face, lips, and eyes); HSV-2 infections are usually below. Rarely, HSV-2 is transmitted during birth to the infant eye through infected genital secretions (Table 37-2).

▶ Clinical Findings

A. Symptoms and Signs

Primary infections usually occur in children between ages 6 months and 5 years, accompanied by generalized symptoms of a viral illness. Ocular HSV is usually self-limited with the most common symptoms being blepharoconjunctivitis and a dendritic keratitis.

B. Laboratory Findings

A clinical diagnosis can be made if there is a classic dendritic presentation. However, definitive diagnosis is made using viral culture or Giemsa-stained smears of corneal scrapings

Table 37–2. Herpes simplex virus (HSV) vs. herpes zoster virus (HZV).

	HSV	**HZV**
Rash	Clear vesicles on erythematous base; crusting	Vesicular rash along dermatomal distribution, not crossing midline; Hutchinson sign (nasociliary branch of V1) may be present
Epithelial lesion	Dendritic epithelial lesions with heaped edges	Pseudodendrites (mucous plaques without true terminal bulbs)
Staining	Edges stain with rose bengal; central ulceration stains with fluorescein	Minimal fluorescein staining
Patient population	Young	Older or immunocompromised

that reveal mononuclear cells, polymorphonuclear neutrophil leukocytes, multinucleated giant epithelial cells, and eosinophilic Lipschütz inclusion bodies in the cell nuclei. Enzyme-linked immunosorbent assay (ELISA) can be used to detect live viral particles.

Treatment

The mainstays of treatment are topical and oral antiviral medications. Antibiotic ointment may be used at night to help prevent bacterial superinfection. Topical trifluorothymidine 1% (Viroptic) or ganciclovir ophthalmic gel 0.15% (Zirgan) is used to treat keratitis. Oral acyclovir (400 mg five times a day) or valacyclovir (500 mg three times a day) is usually added. Topical steroids can be used to treat corneal scarring or uveitis but only with concurrent topical or systemic antiviral therapy. Cost effectiveness of prophylaxis with valacyclovir or acyclovir has been analyzed but currently they are rarely used unless significant visual loss has occurred from previous herpetic episodes.

Kaufman HE et al: Ganciclovir ophthalmic gel 0.15%: safety and efficacy of a new treatment for herpes simplex keratitis. *Curr Eye Res* 2012;37(7):654-660.

DRY EYE

Dry eye is a disorder of the tear film due to either deficiency of production or excess tear evaporation. The tear film is composed of mucin, aqueous, and lipid components. Abnormalities of any layer lead to a wide variety of symptoms. Dry eye has become one of the most common reasons for visits to ophthalmologists. Symptoms are often exacerbated by weather, climate, reading, and computer use (decreased blink rate). Women have a much higher incidence of symptomatic dry eye. Primary lacrimal deficiency from disease such as Riley-Day syndrome and hypoplastic lacrimal glands is rare. Secondary lacrimal deficiency is more common and can be related to prior radiation therapy, lymphoma, sarcoidosis, graft-versus-host disease, HIV, hemochromatosis, and amyloidosis. Systemic medications such as anticholinergics (including antihistamines and antidepressants), antiadrenergics, and diuretics can cause decreased tear production. Dry eye has also been associated with menopause (presumably due to decreased androgens). Evaporative dry eye problems are usually associated with meibomian gland dysfunction. The protective lipid and mucin layers that normally keep the aqueous layer of tears stable are reduced, leading to a poor-quality tear film that breaks up easily. This problem is often associated with acne rosacea and treated conservatively with warm compresses and oral tetracycline if needed. Oral flax or fish oil supplements may help.

Clinical Findings

Symptoms of tear deficiency often include foreign-body sensation, redness, decreased vision, and even reflex tearing. Symptoms are usually worse at the end of the day or after prolonged visual tasks.

Symptoms of evaporative tear loss include a chronic "film" over the vision, redness, burning, and itching of the eyelid margin. These symptoms are often worse in the morning. The quick breakup time of the tear film can cause difficulty with reading.

Post-LASIK (laser-assisted in situ keratomileusis) patients have decreased corneal sensation, lower tear production, and diminished blink rate, which may cause dry eye symptoms for 6-18 months or more postoperatively.

Treatment

Treatment for aqueous deficiency includes tear supplementation. Punctal occlusion may be used in eyes shown to have decreased tear production.

In meibomian gland disease, eyelid hygiene is extremely important. Hot compresses with eyelid scrubs can improve tear quality and prevent evaporative tear loss. Mild topical corticosteroids or systemic tetracycline may also be used, especially if the patient has associated signs of acne rosacea. Topical cyclosporine A, because of its anti-inflammatory action, has been found to dramatically improve dry eye symptoms, although it may take up to 6 weeks for improvement.

PTERYGIUM

Pterygium is a fleshy, triangular conjunctival growth that is usually associated with excessive exposure to wind, sun, sand, and dust. Unilateral or bilateral, it is often on the nasal side of the cornea. There may be a genetic predisposition, but no hereditary pattern has been described.

Treatment is by superficial excision. Excision is indicated if the growth threatens vision by approaching the visual axis. After excising large or recurrent pterygia, autologous conjunctival tissue or amniotic membrane can be used to cover the defect. The conjunctiva is obtained from the upper bulbar conjunctiva and sutured to the denuded area. This leads to rapid restoration of integrity of the epithelial surface and may prevent recurrences. Patients should be advised to wear ultraviolet (UV) protection outdoors. Recurrences can occur. Topical mitomycin eye drops have been used to prevent recurrences of the disease, but serious complications such as scleral thinning and keratitis have been reported.

Zheng K et al: Comparison of pterygium recurrence rates after limbal conjunctival autograft transplantation and other techniques: meta-analysis. *Cornea* 2012 Dec;31(12):1422-1427.

▼ INTRAOCULAR DISEASES

CATARACT

Cataract is opacity of the lens and is the leading cause of curable blindness in the world. There are three types of cataracts: (1) congenital, (2) those associated with other disorders, and (3) age-related. Some cataracts are rapidly progressive, while others may develop more slowly. Surgical removal is indicated when patients have difficulty with daily activities or if visual development is at risk.

1. Congenital Cataract

Congenital cataract may be genetically determined or may be caused by intrauterine factors that interfere with normal development of the lens. Intrauterine viral infections (most commonly rubella) can cause congenital cataracts. Congenital cataract can be unilateral or bilateral and complete or incomplete. Dense cataract present at birth is an indication for urgent surgical management to ensure proper development of visual function.

Phacoemulsification or simple aspiration with central posterior capsulotomy and limited anterior vitrectomy under general anesthesia is recommended for removal of congenital cataracts. Preservation of the peripheral posterior capsule and zonules is important for future implantation of intraocular lenses. If the cataract is aspirated, leaving the posterior capsule intact, the posterior capsule becomes opaque, requiring capsulotomy at a later stage. Correction with soft contact lenses can be started immediately after surgery. Posterior chamber intraocular lenses can be implanted when the child is older, although children as young as 2 years are being treated with primary intraocular lens implants. Restoration of true binocular vision is seldom achieved after removal of unilateral congenital cataracts.

2. Cataracts Associated With Other Disorders

Many systemic conditions are associated with cataracts, including diabetes mellitus, galactosemia, hypocalcemia, myotonic dystrophy, Down syndrome, and cutaneous disorders such as atopic dermatitis. Certain systemic medications and eye drops containing corticosteroids can also cause cataracts. Other disorders of the eye, such as retinal detachment or chronic uveitis, may also be associated with cataracts. Eyes that have undergone retinal surgical procedures, particularly vitrectomy, have increased risk of cataract development. Physical trauma to the lens as well as injury from thermal and ionizing radiation can cause cataract formation.

3. Age-Related (Senile) Cataract

This is the most common type of cataract. The rate of progression is variable. Diagnosis is by slit-lamp examination.

Nuclear changes of the lens produce a brunescent color and often affect distance vision. In advanced cortical cataracts, a white opacity may be seen in the pupillary area upon gross inspection. Monocular diplopia can occur. Posterior subcapsular cataracts are often in younger patients, causing glare and affecting reading.

▶ Treatment

Once the cataract causes visual impairment, treatment is by surgical removal of the lens. Clinical trials of agents that might delay or prevent the formation of cataracts are under way, but no pharmacologic means of prevention is currently available.

Phacoemulsification of the cataract is the procedure of choice in most developed countries. Primary lens implant is preferred unless there is a contraindication to its use. In that situation, optical correction can be achieved with eyeglasses or contact lenses.

A. Intracapsular Lens Extraction

Intracapsular extraction, rarely used today, removes the lens entirely with its capsule either by forceps or a cryoprobe. This procedure cannot be performed on children or young adults because of the adhesion between the lens and the vitreous.

B. Extracapsular Extraction

For standard extracapsular cataract extraction, the anterior capsule of the lens is removed, the nucleus of the cataract is expressed, and the residual cortical material is aspirated from the eye through a 9-11 mm incision. Smaller incision techniques that involve manual fracturing the lens nucleus prior to expression are available. The posterior capsule is left intact and an intraocular lens is placed in the capsular bag. The incision is then sutured with 10-0 nylon. In 25%-35% of patients undergoing extracapsular cataract extraction, the posterior capsule will become opacified. This is treated by Nd:YAG laser capsulotomy. If such a laser is not available, surgical incision of the opaque posterior capsule is required.

C. Phacoemulsification

See Figure 37–1. Phacoemulsification is the most common form of extracapsular cataract extraction and involves technology that fragments the nucleus of the lens using a high-frequency ultrasonic probe while simultaneously aspirating these fragments from the eye. The advantage of phacoemulsification is that incision size is reduced, less astigmatism is induced, and the patient can be more quickly rehabilitated. Remaining cortical material is removed by irrigation and aspiration, and an intraocular lens implanted. The insertion of foldable or injectable intraocular lenses through very small incisions is now possible, and often the wound is self-

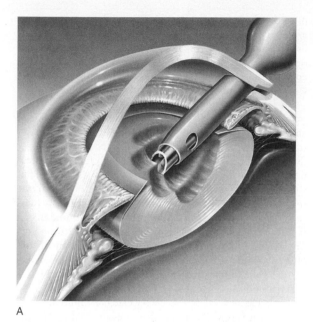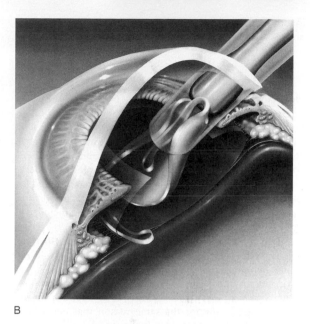

A

B

▲ **Figure 37–1.** Phacoemulsification. **A.** Phacoemulsification probe removing lens nucleus through a clear corneal incision. **B.** Implantation of an injectable intraocular lens implant into the capsular bag through a small incision. (Photos, Courtesy of Alcon Laboratories, Inc.)

sealing. Local anesthesia (either by injection or topically) is used for most adult patients.

D. Laser Assisted

Recently, femtosecond lasers have been utilized to perform multiple steps of cataract surgery including wound creation, opening the anterior lens capsule (capsulotomy), and fragmenting the cataractous lens. Development of this technology for cataract surgery could have a significant impact in the future, but at the present time there is no evidence that this technique (which is more expensive) improves visual outcomes.

Friedman NJ et al: Femtosecond laser capsulotomy. *J Cataract Refract Surg* 2011 Jul;37(7):1189-1198.

Nagy Z et al: Initial clinical evaluation of an intraocular femtosecond laser in cataract surgery. *J Refract Surg* 2009 Dec;25(12):1053-1060.

Venkatesh R et al: Phacoemulsification versus manual small-incision cataract surgery for white cataract. *J Cataract Refract Surg* 2010 Nov;36(11):1849-1854.

ANGLE-CLOSURE GLAUCOMA

About 1% of people over age 35 have anatomically narrow anterior chamber angles. In such patients, if the pupil dilates spontaneously or is dilated with a mydriatic or cycloplegic agent, the angle may close and an attack of acute glaucoma precipitated. For this reason, it is wise to estimate the depth of the anterior chamber angle before instilling these drugs.

Acute angle-closure glaucoma is manifested by sudden onset of pain, headache, blurring of vision, and colored halos around lights. Some patients develop nausea and vomiting. The eye is red, the cornea is hazy, and the pupil is mid-dilated and does not react to light. Intraocular pressure is elevated.

The attack can be aborted by use of topical pilocarpine, beta-blockers, apraclonidine and latanoprost drops, systemic acetazolamide and, if necessary, an intravenous hyperosmotic agent such as Mannitol. Definitive treatment consists of peripheral iridotomy, which establishes a communication between the posterior and anterior chambers and reopens the angle. This is usually done with an argon or Nd:YAG laser. Rarely, surgical peripheral iridectomy is required.

OPEN-ANGLE GLAUCOMA

In open-angle glaucoma, the intraocular pressure is elevated, causing gradual cupping (segmental atrophy) of the optic nerve. The damage to the nerve results in loss of vision, ranging in severity from slight constriction of the upper nasal peripheral visual field to complete blindness (absolute glaucoma). The cause of the decreased rate of aqueous outflow that characterizes open-angle glaucoma has not been fully determined. The disease is bilateral but can be asymmetric and is probably genetically influenced. African Americans are particularly at risk.

▶ Clinical Findings

Open-angle glaucoma is painless, so patients are often unaware of damage until late in the course of the disease. On examination, there may be cupping of the optic disc. There is loss of peripheral visual field, but central vision acuity is usually preserved even when peripheral field loss is quite advanced. Tonometry, evaluation of the optic nerve and visual field testing are the three principal tests used for the diagnosis and continued clinical evaluation of glaucoma. Central corneal thickness should be assessed and included in risk calculations for glaucoma.

The normal intraocular pressure ranges from 10 to 20 mm Hg. Intraocular pressures higher than 21 is considered ocular hypertension, although this diagnosis should never be made on the basis of a single tonometric measurement. Transient elevations of intraocular pressure do not constitute glaucoma for the same reason that periodic or intermittent elevations of blood pressure do not constitute hypertensive disease. All persons over age 20 should have tonometric and ophthalmoscopic examinations every 3-5 years. If there is a family history of glaucoma or other risk factors, annual examination is indicated. Low-tension glaucoma is an uncommon condition characterized by visual field changes and optic nerve cupping in the presence of intraocular pressure that remains in the normal range.

▶ Treatment

See Table 37–3. Most patients can be controlled with topical medications including beta-blockers (eg, timolol maleate 0.25%-0.5%, one drop twice daily), α-adrenergic agonists (eg, brimonidine 0.2%, one drop twice daily), carbonic anhydrase inhibitors (eg, dorzolamide 2%, one drop twice daily), or prostaglandins (eg, latanoprost 0.005%, one drop once daily). Oral carbonic anhydrase inhibitors (eg, acetazolamide) can be used in patients with persistent elevation of intraocular pressures despite topical treatment. Miotics (eg, pilocarpine 1%-4%, one drop four times daily) and epinephrine eye drops (0.5%-2.0%, one drop twice daily) are less commonly used today.

In laser trabeculoplasty, laser energy is applied to the trabecular meshwork. This technique can lead to significant and sustained decreases in intraocular pressure. Argon laser trabeculoplasty (ALT) and selective laser trabeculoplasty (SLT) may be used in place or along with topical medications. SLT produces similar pressure responses to ALT, but studies suggest it can be repeated multiple times in each eye. In those with persistent pressure elevation, surgery is indicated to create an alternate drainage passage for fluid to exit the eye. The most common procedure is trabeculectomy. The success of this procedure has been improved by the use of intraoperative application of mitomycin or 5-fluorouracil to inhibit the fibrosis and closure of the newly created filtering channel.

Drainage devices are also used to facilitate fluid drainage from the eye to lower intraocular pressure. Currently, the most widely used is the Ex-Press glaucoma filtration device. In certain types of glaucoma (such as neovascular glaucoma, aphakic glaucoma or for those with who have failed previous surgery), insertion of a more complex drainage device is required, often referred to as a glaucoma valve or tube shunt. An alternative approach that aims to decrease aqueous production through destruction of ciliary body tissue (diode transscleral cyclophotocoagulation or endophotocoagulation) is also employed in some situations.

de Jong LA: The Ex-PRESS glaucoma shunt versus trabeculectomy in open-angle glaucoma: a prospective randomized study. *Adv Ther* 2009 Mar;26(3):336-345.

de Jong LA et al: Five-year extension of a clinical trial comparing the EX-PRESS glaucoma filtration device and trabeculectomy in primary open-angle glaucoma. *Clin Ophthalmol* 2011;5:527-533.

Table 37–3. Types of glaucoma medications and side effects.

Class	Mechanism	Side Effects	Pregnancy Class
Beta-blockers (eg, timolol)	Decrease aqueous production	Hypotension, bradycardia, asthma exacerbation	C
α₂-adrenergic agonist (eg, brimonidine, Propine)	Decrease aqueous production	Allergy, tachyphylaxis, CNS depression	B
Cholinergics (eg, pilocarpine)	Increase outflow	Brow ache, cataract formation, retinal detachment	C
Carbonic anhydrase inhibitors (eg, acetazolamide, dorzolamide)	Decrease aqueous production	Sulfa allergy, systemic metabolic acidosis, tingling, aplastic anemia, metallic taste	C
Prostaglandin analogues (eg, latanoprost)	Increase outflow	Bitter taste, iris color change, red eye	C

DIABETIC RETINOPATHY

Diabetes is the leading cause of new blindness in most industrialized countries. Diabetic retinopathy eventually develops in almost half of all diabetics and is a major cause of blindness. There are two clinical classifications: (1) **nonproliferative or background diabetic retinopathy** and (2) **proliferative diabetic retinopathy**. The prevalence of retinopathy increases with the duration of diabetes. Patients who have had type 1 diabetes for 5 years or less are at low risk of retinopathy. However, 27% of those with diabetes for 5-10 years and 71%-90% of those with diabetes for longer than 10 years have some form of diabetic retinopathy. After 20-30 years, the prevalence of retinopathy rises to 95%, with 30%-50% of those patients having proliferative changes. The risk for diabetic retinopathy also increases with duration for type 2 diabetes.

Diabetes can have other effects on the eye. Poor corneal healing and decreased corneal sensation have been noted. Neovascular glaucoma caused by iris neovascularization (which blocks the outflow passage in the anterior chamber angle) is seen in some patients with proliferative disease. Optic neuropathy and cranial neuropathies can also occur.

▶ Clinical Findings

Microaneurysms, intraretinal hemorrhages, cotton wool spots, and lipid deposits due to vascular leakage are the retinal changes seen in early diabetic retinopathy. Later stages include retinal ischemia and neovascularization with subsequent vitreous hemorrhage often associated with traction or rhegmatogenous retinal detachment. Diabetic retinopathy may be asymptomatic until vision decreases, usually from macular edema or vitreous hemorrhage. The presence of renal microvascular disease correlates well with the presence of diabetic retinopathy.

▶ Treatment

Careful control of blood sugar and blood pressure appears to reduce the incidence and severity of diabetic retinopathy. Recent epidemiologic studies show that many diabetics fail to have recommended yearly eye examinations. If patients are followed closely and early retinopathy is detected and treated according to the guidelines of the early treatment diabetic retinopathy study (ETDRS), the risk of severe visual loss is less than 5%. Treatment consists of photocoagulation, either of the macula to reduce edema or of the retinal periphery to reduce ischemic neovascular changes. Adjunctive intravitreal injection of triamcinolone with laser treatment has been suggested for macular edema and proliferative retinopathy. Intravitreal injections of agents that neutralize vascular endothelial growth factor (VEGF) now play a central role in treatment of diabetic macular edema. These anti-VEGF agents may also be useful for the treatment of proliferative disease. Rare complications from these injections include endophthalmitis and steroid-induced glaucoma.

Kook D et al: Long-term effect of intravitreal bevacizumab (avastin) in patients with chronic diffuse diabetic macular edema. *Retina* 2008 Oct;28(8):1053-1060.

Nguyen QD et al: Ranibizumab for diabetic macular edema: results from 2 phase III randomized trials: RISE and RIDE. *Ophthalmology* 2012 Apr;119(4):789-801.

AGE-RELATED MACULAR DEGENERATION

Age-related macular degeneration (AMD) is the leading cause of central visual loss among individuals 65 and older. The pathophysiology is not completely understood although there is a strong genetic component that interacts with aging and environmental influences such as tobacco use. Regardless of the mechanism, the disease appears to affect the retinal pigment epithelium at the level of Bruch membrane. Drusen (yellowish deposits in the retina caused by the thickening, hyalinization, and calcification of the retinal pigment epithelium) are characteristic of AMD.

1. Atrophic ("Dry") Macular Degeneration

Atrophic ("dry") macular degeneration is the most common form of AMD, occurring in approximately 80% of those with the disease. Drusen, pigment changes, and atrophy are present, but there is no leakage of fluid into the subretinal space. Usually, only minimal to moderate visual loss is present although patients may complain of distorted vision (metamorphopsia).

2. Exudative ("Wet") Macular Degeneration

Exudative ("wet") macular degeneration is characterized by the development of a choroidal neovascular membrane that leaks fluid and blood. This causes a serous detachment of the central fovea that can lead to profound vision loss.

▶ Clinical Findings

Visual loss is caused by geographical atrophy, serous detachment of the retinal pigment epithelium, or choroidal neovascularization. Central visual acuity is primarily affected with the peripheral vision remaining intact. Metamorphopsia is a classic patient complaint. Patients can follow their own progression of disease with an Amsler grid.

▶ Treatment

The age-related eye disease study (AREDS) is the first large, prospective clinical trial to show the benefit of antioxidant and zinc supplementation on the progression of atrophic AMD and associated visual loss. In evaluating the rate of progression to advanced visual loss, nutritional supplements benefited only patients who had moderate to severe disease. Supplements were not found to prevent the development of AMD or to prevent progression in patients with mild disease. The AREDS2 study started in 2008 and is examining the use of alternate micronutrients including omega-3-fatty acids in preventing the progression of AMD.

Treatment of exudative AMD was revolutionized through the use of intravitreal injections of anti-VEGF agents. Previously established therapeutic strategies such as standard laser photocoagulation or photodynamic therapy (PDT) reduced the rate of vision loss when compared to controls but did not improve acuity. These treatments remain beneficial in certain specific situations. Intravitreal injection of anti-VEGF agents such as ranibizumab (Lucentis) and bevacizumab (Avastin) has led to actual improvements in visual acuity. Intravitreal injection carries a small risk of infection and treatment resistance can be seen.

Smoking cessation is extremely important in AMD patients and should be stressed. Exercise and control of other systemic diseases such as hypertension and hypercholesterolemia may also help.

Comparison of Age-related Macular Degeneration Treatments Trials (CATT) Research Group: Ranibizumab and bevacizumab for treatment of neovascular age-related macular degeneration: two-year results. *Ophthalmology* 2012 Jul;119(7):1388-1398.

Dhoot DS et al: Ranibizumab for age-related macular degeneration. *Expert Opin Biol Ther* 2012 Mar;12(3):371-381.

SanGiovanni JP et al: The relationship of dietary lipid intake and age-related macular degeneration in a case-control study: AREDS Report No. 20. *Arch Ophthalmol* 2007 May;125(5):671-679.

Sparrow JR et al: Complement dysregulation in AMD: RPE-Bruch's membrane-choroid. *Mol Aspects Med* 2012 Aug;33(4):436-445 [Epub 2012 Apr 5].

RETINAL DETACHMENT

Detachment of the retina is usually spontaneous but may be secondary to trauma. Spontaneous detachment occurs most frequently in persons over 50 years of age. Spontaneous detachments are ultimately bilateral in 20%-25% of cases.

▶ Clinical Findings

Retinal tears or holes are the most important predisposing factor. Increased risk of retinal detachment is also associated with cataract surgery and high myopia. In the presence of a retinal tear or hole, fluid from the vitreous cavity enters the defect and transudation from choroidal vessels detaches the retina from the pigment epithelium (rhegmatogenous). These small retinal holes may be sealed prophylactically with laser or cryotherapy to prevent detachment.

The superior temporal retina is the most common site of detachment. The area of detachment can rapidly increase

causing progressive visual loss. Central vision remains intact until the macula becomes detached. On ophthalmoscopic examination, the detached retina is seen as an elevated gray membrane.

▶ Treatment

All cases of retinal detachment should be referred immediately to an ophthalmologist. If the patient must be transported a long distance, the head should be positioned to try to minimize the progression of the detachment. If the upper retina is detached, the head should be kept flat. Patients with an inferior detachment should be kept upright.

Retinal detachment is a true ophthalmic emergency if the macula is threatened. If the macula is detached, permanent loss of central vision may occur even if the retina is successfully reattached by surgery. Treatment consists of drainage of subretinal fluid and closure of retinal tears by cryosurgery, laser, or scleral buckling. This produces an inflammatory reaction that causes the retina to adhere to the choroid. The creation of an inflammatory adhesion between the choroid and the retina helps to prevent future redetachment.

In uncomplicated retinal detachment with a superior retinal tear and healthy vitreous, pneumoretinopexy may be performed. The procedure consists of injection of air or certain gases into the vitreous cavity through the pars plana and positioning the patient to allow the gas bubble to seal the retinal hole and permit spontaneous reabsorption of the subretinal fluid.

About 85% of uncomplicated cases can be reattached with one operation. About 10% will need more than one procedure, and the remainder never reattach. The prognosis is worse if the macula is detached, if the vitreous is not healthy, or if the detachment is of long duration.

Without treatment, retinal detachment almost always becomes total in 1-6 months.

STRABISMUS IN CHILDREN

Any child under age 7 with obvious strabismus should be seen without delay to allow prompt treatment to prevent amblyopia. About 3% of children are born with or develop strabismus. In descending order of frequency, the eyes may deviate inward (esotropia), outward (exotropia), upward (hypertropia), or downward (hypotropia).

▶ Clinical Findings

Children with manifest strabismus suppress the visual image from the deviating eye to avoid diplopia, and the vision in that eye fails to develop normally. This is the first stage of amblyopia. Most cases of strabismus are obvious, but if the angle of deviation is small or if the strabismus is intermittent, the diagnosis can be missed.

Fortunately, amblyopia due to strabismus can be detected by routine visual acuity testing of all preschool children.

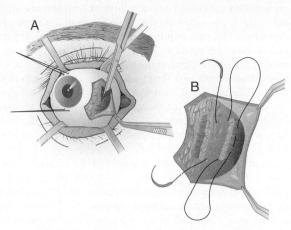

▲ **Figure 37–2. A.** Exposure of an extraocular muscle in surgery for strabismus. **B.** Recession of the muscle behind its original insertion followed by suturing to the sclera with absorbable suture.

Those who cannot be tested with a standard eye chart can use visual acuity testing with an illiterate E card or Allen picture chart.

▶ Treatment

The objectives in the surgical treatment of strabismus in children (Figure 37–2) are to achieve good visual acuity in each eye and align the eyes so that normal binocular vision with fusion can occur. Surgery can be performed in infants, and the earlier the problem is detected and corrected, the better the chance of getting a good result. Correcting the problem in children above age 7-8 often fails to result in visual improvement.

If the child is under age 6 years and has an amblyopic eye and strabismus, patching of the better eye should be instituted to improve the vision before surgery for strabismus is performed. At age 1, patching may be successful within 1 week; at age 6, it may take a year to achieve the same result. Surgery to align the eye is usually performed after the visual acuity has been equalized.

Surgery for correction of strabismus consists of weakening or strengthening the extraocular muscles. To weaken the action of a muscle, it is recessed by detaching it from its insertion site and resuturing it to a more posterior location of the sclera. To strengthen a muscle's action, it is separated at the insertion site from the globe, and a portion of it is resected and then resutured to its original insertion site. Muscles should not be recessed more than 8 mm or resected more than 6 mm.

For correction of exotropia, the lateral rectus muscles in both eyes can be recessed. Alternatively, the lateral rectus muscle can be recessed and the medial rectus muscle

resected in the same eye. The amount of recession and resection and the number of extraocular muscles chosen is determined by the degree of ocular deviation. The decision to involve one or both eyes is influenced by the visual acuity and potential of each eye. In patients with esotropia, the options are to recess the medial recti of both eyes or to recess the medial rectus in combination with resecting the lateral rectus in the same eye.

For vertical deviation, the vertical muscles are recessed, resected, tucked, or weakened by myectomy.

STRABISMUS IN ADULTS

In adults with mature visual systems, development of strabismus usually produces double vision. Strabismus can arise from head trauma, microvascular infarct as in diabetes, intracranial hemorrhage, elevated intracranial pressure, brain tumor, or orbital disease.

▶ Treatment

Surgical management of strabismus is the same as described for children. Since visual pathways have already been formed, the indications for surgery are for cosmetic reasons or because of diplopia. Care must be taken not to induce diplopia after surgery.

OCULAR MIGRAINE

Migraine is a disorder with multiple clinical presentations. Recurrent headaches are classic, and ocular symptoms are often associated. The pathophysiology of migraine is uncertain and there may be a genetic component. The differential diagnosis for migraine headaches includes stress-tension headache, cluster headache, sinus congestion/pathology, elevated intracranial pressures, orbital inflammation, orbital neoplasia, and temporal arteritis. A thorough headache history and neurologic examination are important diagnostic tools.

Patients with ocular migraine present with visual symptoms; headache and nausea, if present at all, follow. The ocular symptoms can mimic retinal disease, and a dilated ocular examination is needed to rule out retinal pathology when the symptoms are atypical. The flashing lights from retinal disease are primarily unilateral, while migraine presents with bilateral visual distortion. Asking the patient to cover each eye and see if the symptoms are unilateral or bilateral may clarify the situation. Prophylaxis to prevent migraine with oral β-adrenergic blockers, calcium-channel blockers, and tricyclic antidepressants may be used. Triptans such as sumatriptan (Imitrex) are often used to treat the acute episodes. Onabotulinum toxin A (Botox) injections are an effective treatment option for debilitating migraine not controlled by other medications. Acephalgic migraine typically is not treated with systemic agents because of the self-limited nature of the disease.

Classical Migraines

Classical migraine is characterized by throbbing headaches preceded by visual auras lasting about 20 minutes. The aura may consist of bright or dark spots, zigzag lines (fortification scotoma), heat haze distortions, scintillating scotomas, and tunnel vision. Homonymous or altitudinal hemianopia may rarely occur. The headaches that follow may vary in intensity.

Retinal Migraine

Retinal migraine is characterized by acute, transient unilateral loss of vision that can be identical to that seen in amaurosis fugax. Vascular etiologies must be ruled out with thorough ocular and medical examination before attributing symptoms to be migraine. Amaurosis is often shorter in duration and has a more "curtain-like" quality.

Ophthalmoplegic Migraine

Ophthalmoplegic migraine is very rare and typically starts before the age of 10 years. It is characterized by a recurrent transient third nerve palsy that is associated with a typical migraine headache.

Complicated Migraine

Complicated migraine is associated with neurologic deficits such as tingling in the extremities, hemisensory disturbance and partial visual loss. Rarely, the deficit persists after the headache has resolved. Antiplatelet therapy with aspirin is often recommended.

Diener HC et al: OnabotulinumtoxinA for treatment of chronic migraine: results from the double-blind, randomized, placebo-controlled phase of the PREEMPT 2 trial. *Cephalalgia* 2010;30(7):804-814.

OCULAR BURNS

CHEMICAL BURNS

Apart from the history, the diagnosis of chemical eye burns is usually based on the presence of swelling of the eyelids and marked conjunctival hyperemia and chemosis. The limbal area may show blanched patchy areas and conjunctival sloughing, especially in the interpalpebral area. There is usually corneal stromal haze and diffuse edema, with wide areas of epithelial cell loss and corneal ulcerations. Defects in the corneal epithelium can be better visualized with the instillation of fluorescein dye.

Alkali burns of the eye are particularly serious because the agents tend to rapidly penetrate intraocularly. Retained particles in the conjunctival fornices may continue to release alkaline material and must be promptly removed. Patients are managed by instilling a topical anesthetic agent and then immediately irrigating copiously (at least several liters) with tap water or any other available solution until a neutral pH is reached. This may require hours of flushing. Double eversion of the upper eyelid should be performed to look for and remove material lodged in the superior fornix. This can be easily done by using a forceps or moist cotton applicator. Topical dilating drops such as atropine 1% or homatropine 5% are instilled, and a topical antibiotic ointment such as ophthalmic erythromycin and bacitracin should be applied. Severe injuries that result in eyelid destruction require hospitalization and specialized care.

Acid burns cause rapid damage but are in general less serious than alkali burns because of lack of intraocular penetration. Irrigation is carried out as described above, the patient is given an analgesic, and the eye is patched for a short time. Close follow-up is needed. Topical antibiotic ointment may also be used.

THERMAL BURNS

The treatment of thermal burns of the eyes is similar to the treatment of burns elsewhere on the body. Adequate systemic analgesia should be provided. A topical anesthetic agent such as proparacaine 0.5% or tetracaine 0.5% is used to minimize pain during manipulation. In cases of burns involving the cornea, topical dilating drops such as atropine 1% or homatropine 5% are instilled. Antibiotic drops are often prescribed for 3-5 days.

BURNS DUE TO ULTRAVIOLET RADIATION

Injuries to the corneal epithelium by UV rays vary in severity. They are described as actinic keratitis, snow blindness, welder's arc burn or flash burn, depending on the source of ultraviolet radiation. Patients present with severe pain, tearing, and photophobia. The examination reveals diffuse punctate staining of the cornea, best seen with fluorescein staining, proper magnification, and a cobalt blue light.

A topical antibiotic such as ophthalmic erythromycin or bacitracin ointment is instilled. Topical nonsteroidal drops such as diclofenac or ketorolac tromethamine can be used for pain.

OCULAR TRAUMA

Eye injuries are common in spite of the protection afforded by the bony orbit. Blunt trauma is the most common injury, but penetrating injuries of the globe, although less frequent, are often more serious. The use of protective eyewear at work helps prevent most serious occupational injuries.

Clinical Evaluation

A careful history should be obtained from the patient or someone who knows what happened. Visual acuity should be checked. The eyelids, conjunctiva, cornea, anterior chamber, iris, lens, vitreous, and fundus should be evaluated. Corneal damage (such as abrasions) can be detected by instilling fluorescein dye and using a cobalt blue light to examine the anterior surface. CT scan or x-ray examination is helpful in looking for fractures of the orbital bones or foreign bodies. Patients with severe injuries should have immediate ophthalmic consultation.

PENETRATING OR PERFORATING INJURIES

Penetrating or perforating ocular injuries require immediate treatment and prompt surgical repair to maximize chances for preservation of vision.

Facial injuries—especially those occurring in automobile accidents can be associated with penetrating ocular trauma. Some injuries may be undetected because of eyelid swelling or because the patient's other injuries have demanded the attention of the emergency room staff. Accurate records and a description of how the injury occurred should be obtained. The eye and ocular adnexa should be examined, including vision testing and testing of ocular motility. *Do not apply pressure on the globe.* X-ray examination and CT scan are performed to rule out fractures of orbital bones or the presence of intraocular foreign bodies. An eye with a penetrating injury should be protected from further injury with a Fox or similar shield and light dressing. Parenteral broad-spectrum antibiotics such as cefazolin or gentamicin should be given. Antiemetics (eg, ondansetron, 4 mg intravenously) should be given to the patient when needed to prevent vomiting, which can lead to extrusion of the intraocular contents.

Careful repair and approximation of corneal and scleral lacerations should be performed in the operating room. Magnetic metallic intraocular foreign bodies can be extracted with a magnet in the operating room. The major objectives in management of ocular penetrating or perforating injuries are to relieve pain, preserve or restore vision, and achieve good cosmetic results. Pain relief may be achieved by the administration of intravenous or subcutaneous morphine or meperidine. Sedatives such as diazepam 5 mg may be given orally as required.

LACERATIONS OF THE OCULAR ADNEXA

Lacerations of the eyelids and the periorbital skin should be carefully evaluated. Small linear skin lacerations can be easily repaired with 6-0 nylon sutures. The sutures can usually be removed in 3-5 days. In cases of deep eyelid lacerations, intraocular or orbital damage should be ruled out before the repair is performed. The skin of the eyelids has good elasticity and in adults is frequently present in surplus quantities. This facilitates the development of flaps and grafts. In deep lacerations of the eyelids, if the wound divides the orbicularis muscle parallel to its fibers, only skin sutures are

Table 37–4. Types of ocular injury associated with blunt trauma.

Eyelids	Ecchymosis, swelling, laceration, abrasions, conjunctival, or subconjunctival hemorrhages
Cornea	Edema, lacerations
Anterior chamber	Hyphema, recession of angle, secondary glaucoma
Iris	Iridodialysis, iridoplegia, rupture of iris sphincter
Ciliary body	Hyposecretion of aqueous humor
Lens	Cataract, dislocation
Vitreous	Vitreous hemorrhage
Ciliary muscle	Paralysis
Retina	Commotio retinae, retinal edema, choroidal breaks in Bruch membrane, choroidal hemorrhage

generally required. When the muscle fibers are transversely divided, they should be approximated with 6-0 absorbable synthetic sutures. The skin can be approximated with nylon sutures. In patients with lacerations resulting in round or oval losses of skin, the skin is undermined and the laceration approximated. For larger defects, reconstruction with flaps may be required. Flaps used in reconstruction of the eyelids are advancement flaps, rotational flaps, transposition flaps, island flaps, and Z-plasty flaps.

When flaps cannot be used, free skin grafts may be obtained from behind the ear or from the skin of the inner upper arm. Special care should be taken with repair of lacerations of the lower lid to be certain that the lid is not closed under tension to prevent eversion and distortion of the lid margin.

BLUNT TRAUMA TO THE OCULAR ADNEXA & ORBIT

Contusions of the eyeball and ocular adnexa may result from blunt trauma (Table 37–4). The extent of damage to the vision may not be obvious upon initial examination. A careful dilated eye examination is needed for all patients with this type of injury.

BLOWOUT FRACTURE OF THE FLOOR OF THE ORBIT

Blowout fracture of the floor of the orbit can be associated with enophthalmos, double vision in primary position or upgaze, restriction of ocular movement, hypotropia, and decreased or absent sensation over the maxillary area in the distribution of the infraorbital nerve. CT scan of the orbit will document the extent of the orbital injury that can involve the medial wall as well as the floor. There may be air noted in the sinuses. Evaluation and management of patients with blowout fractures may involve both an ophthalmologist and an otolaryngologist because of potential associated fractures of the maxilla or zygoma. Patients are usually treated with a systemic antibiotic (cephalothin or amoxicillin/potassium clavulanate), told not to blow their nose and reassessed within 1 week by an ophthalmologist. Many blowout fractures do not require surgical correction. Operative management is recommended if there is significant enophthalmos, continued diplopia in primary gaze or significant instability of the orbital floor.

CORNEAL & CONJUNCTIVAL FOREIGN BODIES

Patients often give a history of working with high-speed tempered steel tools, drilling, or hammering against a hard object. There may be no history of trauma to the eye, and the patient may not be aware of a foreign body. In most cases, however, the patient complains of foreign-body sensation in the eye or under the eyelid with associated pain, tearing, and photophobia.

A corneal foreign body can be seen with the aid of a loupe and diffuse light. Conjunctival foreign bodies often become embedded in the inner surface of the upper lid, which must be everted to facilitate inspection and removal. A topical anesthetic such as proparacaine 0.5% or tetracaine 0.5% is applied. Sterile fluorescein should be instilled to assist in the visualization of small foreign bodies. Some loose foreign bodies can be removed with a moist cotton applicator; others require use of the tip of a hypodermic needle. Topical antibiotic ointment should be instilled (eg, erythromycin or bacitracin) and the eye patched for a few hours if necessary. Patients with continued foreign-body sensation, pain, or decreased vision need to be referred to an ophthalmologist for the possibility of corneal ulceration.

Use of the topical anesthetic by the patient will decrease healing and increase risk of corneal ulceration. Topical anesthetics should be used only for examination purposes, *never* for treatment. If there is any suspicion of penetrating trauma or history consistent with that type of injury, appropriate ultrasound and radiologic tests should be performed.

▼ OCULAR TUMORS

Tumors of the adnexal structures can often be recognized early because they are usually visible and cause local disfigurement, interference with vision or displacement of the globe. Intraocular tumors are more difficult to diagnose, but in children ocular tumors such as retinoblastoma that affect visual function may present with strabismus or leukocoria. Tumors of the eye may be primary (affecting only the ocular or adnexal tissues) or secondary to metastatic tumors. In the eye, the highly vascular choroid is most frequent site of metastasis is the choroid. The tumors that

most frequently metastasize to the eye are carcinoma of the breast and lung.

The history of growth of the lesion is extremely important, as well as recent changes in its size or appearance. Excisional biopsy of lesions of the skin or conjunctiva is indicated if cancer is suspected.

LID TUMORS

▶ Benign Tumors of the Eyelids

The most frequent benign tumors of the eyelids are melanocytic nevi. Excision is indicated primarily for cosmetic reasons (Figure 37–3). Xanthelasma represent lipid deposits in histiocytes in the dermis of the skin of the eyelid. In such patients, a lipid profile is indicated. Treatment is indicated for cosmetic reasons and consists of simple excision. The lesions tend to be larger than the surface size would indicate and recurrences are common. Care must be taken not to foreshorten the eyelid skin and impair eyelid closure.

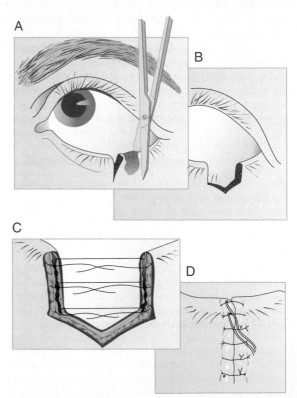

▲ **Figure 37–3.** Tumor of the left lower eyelid involving the lid margin. **A.** Two vertical incisions are made. **B.** The defect after removal of the tumor. **C.** Suturing of the tarsus and orbicularis with absorbable sutures. **D.** Approximation of the eyelid margin. Skin is approximated with 6-0 silk sutures.

Hemangiomas of the eyelids consist of two types: capillary and cavernous. Capillary hemangiomas consist of dilated capillaries and proliferation of endothelial cells. The lesions appear as bright red spots. They may show rapid growth in early childhood but later often undergo involution and subside spontaneously. Treatment of hemangiomas in infancy and early childhood is not indicated unless they cause interference with vision that may lead to amblyopia. Low-dose oral steroids, local injection of steroids, or systemic use of beta-blockers may cause rapid involution. Cavernous hemangiomas are venous channels in the subcutaneous tissue. They appear bluish in color and are distended. Surgical excision may be required. Radiation is not recommended because it leads to excessive scarring of the eyelid.

Other benign tumors of the eyelids include verrucae and molluscum contagiosum. These lesions are caused by viruses.

Missoi TG et al: Oral propranolol for treatment of periocular infantile hemangiomas. *Arch Ophthalmol* 2011 Jul;129(7):899-903.

Malignant Tumors of the Eyelids

Squamous cell carcinoma has a tendency to grow slowly and painlessly. It begins as a small lesion covered by a layer of keratin. The lesion may erode, causing an ulcer with hyperemic edges. It may enlarge to form a fungating mass and invade the orbit. Early excision can result in cure. If early treatment is not provided, squamous cell carcinoma can involve the lymphatic system to the preauricular and submandibular lymph nodes.

Basal cell carcinoma begins as a slowly growing, locally invasive tumor forming the so-called "rodent ulcer" with raised nodular borders. It is the most common malignant eyelid tumor. Inner canthal basal cell carcinoma invades locally and can extend into the orbit. Treatment should include complete excision to prevent recurrence. Mohs is usually performed to assure clean margins prior to eyelid reconstruction. Often, the lesions are more extensive than they appear visually. Systemic metastasis is rare.

Malignant melanomas of the eyelids behave similar to malignant melanomas of the skin.

CONJUNCTIVAL TUMORS

Benign tumors of the conjunctiva include melanocytic nevi (pigmented or nonpigmented), papillomas, granulomas, dermoids, and lymphoid hyperplasia. Malignant tumors of the conjunctiva include carcinoma, malignant melanoma, and lymphoma. Carcinoma of the conjunctiva arises frequently at the limbus or the inner canthus in the exposed area of the bulbar conjunctiva. Early in the course of the disease, the lesion can resemble a pterygium. The tumor is slightly elevated, with a gelatinous surface and may spread over the corneal surface. These grow slowly. Treatment is by wide excisional biopsy and cryotherapy or topical interferon alpha.

Shah SU et al: Topical interferon alfa-2b for management of ocular surface squamous neoplasia in 23 cases: outcomes based on American Joint Committee on Cancer classification. *Arch Ophthalmol* 2012 Feb;130(2):159-164.

INTRAOCULAR TUMORS

Benign Intraocular Tumors

Melanocytic nevi of the iris, ciliary body, or choroid are common. No treatment is required. Retinal angioma may be seen in patients with phacomatoses (eg, Bourneville disease). Choroidal hemangioma is another less frequently encountered benign intraocular tumor.

Malignant Intraocular Tumors

Malignant intraocular tumors include malignant melanoma of the uvea, retinoblastoma, and a rare tumor of the ciliary body known as diktyoma or medulloepithelioma.

Malignant melanoma of the uvea is the most common primary intraocular tumor in adults. It typically occurs in the fifth or sixth decade and is almost always unilateral. The most frequent site is the choroid, but malignant melanoma can occur also in the ciliary body or iris. Malignant melanomas of the choroid often do not cause decrease in vision. Necrosis of the tumor can lead to intraocular inflammation. Histopathologic examination shows spindle-shaped cells with or without prominent nuclei and large epithelioid tumor cells. Intraocular malignant melanomas may spread directly through the sclera by local invasion or directly into the central nervous system via optic nerve extension.

Malignant melanomas can be detected by ophthalmoscopy after pupillary dilation.

Treatment of malignant melanoma consists of enucleation or radiotherapy with radioactive plaques or charged particles. Extension outside the eye may require exenteration of the orbit. Patients with small melanomas—less than 10 mm in diameter—can be followed with serial fundus photos. Similarly, small melanomas of the iris that have not invaded the iris root can be safely followed and observed until growth is documented. If there is growth of the iris tumor, treatment is by local iridectomy. If the iris malignant melanoma invades the root and ciliary body, it can be removed surgically by iridocyclectomy.

Retinoblastoma is a rare but life-threatening condition in childhood. It is the most frequent intraocular malignant tumor in children. It arises from embryonic cone cells of the photoreceptor layer. Most patients with retinoblastoma present in the first or second year of life. Patients present with leukocoria or strabismus. Retinoblastoma may be unilateral or bilateral and is often multifocal. There are both sporadic and inherited forms of the disease. It may grow slowly to fill the intraocular space and undergo necrosis, leading to calcific deposits. Tumor cells may seed on the iris and in the anterior chamber, causing fluffy whitish exudates.

Spontaneous remission of retinoblastoma has been reported. Treatment options include radiotherapy, cryotherapy, chemotherapy, intra-arterial chemotherapy, and enucleation.

Abramson DH: Chemosurgery for retinoblastoma: what we know after 5 years. *Arch Ophthalmol* 2011 Nov;129(11):1492-1494.

ORBITAL TUMORS

Orbital tumors are of two types: primary and secondary. Benign primary orbital tumors include dermoid cysts, hemangiomas, lipomas, fibromas, osteomas, chondromas, neurofibromas, and lacrimal gland tumors. Malignant tumors include rhabdomyosarcoma, adenocarcinoma of the lacrimal gland and lymphomas. In children, rhabdomyosarcoma often presents with acute, painless unilateral proptosis and needs to be evaluated immediately. Secondary tumors include malignant melanoma and retinoblastoma from the intraocular structures and malignant melanomas and carcinomas from the skin of the eyelids and conjunctiva. Metastatic lesions commonly are from the lung or breast. Neuroblastoma can also metastasize to the orbit in children. Meningiomas of the cranial nerves may invade the orbit through the optic canal.

Treatment and prognosis in all cases depend on the type of tumor.

▼ LASER TREATMENTS FOR OCULAR DISEASE

The laser has many useful applications in ophthalmology. Using various gases, a single-wavelength beam can be produced that can be absorbed by specific tissues in the eye.

FOCAL DIABETIC TREATMENT

Macular edema occurs in the preproliferative stage of diabetic retinopathy and is characterized by retinal thickening (with or without exudates) within the central macular area. This procedure is performed with a slit-lamp laser delivery system using a contact lens and is aided by fluorescein angiography. Improvement may not occur for several months. Long-term studies by the National Institutes of Health have shown that treatment with an argon laser may improve visual outcome by as much as 50%.

PANRETINAL PHOTOCOAGULATION

Panretinal photocoagulation is indicated for treatment of proliferative diabetic retinopathy. Using a contact lens and a slit-lamp delivery system, extensive destruction of peripheral retina is undertaken to decrease production of vasoproliferative factors and increase retinal oxygenation, causing regression of abnormal blood vessels.

LASER SURGERY FOR CORRECTION OF REFRACTIVE ERROR

LASIK is a lamellar refractive surgical procedure, which involves creation of a partial-thickness corneal flap under high suction. The flap is then lifted and an ArF (argon-fluoride) excimer beam is used to ablate stromal tissue with minimal thermal effect. The flap is then replaced and allowed to heal. The combination of precision, minimal postoperative discomfort, and quick visual recovery make this the most popular refractive technique. A newer technology of flap creation with femtosecond laser instead of microkeratome blades is becoming more popular.

MULTIPLE CHOICE QUESTIONS

1. A 61-year-old Caucasian woman presents with sudden-onset right-sided head pain, right eye redness, and blurred vision. Examination of the right eye is difficult due to the patient's nausea and vomiting, but reveals visual acuity of 20/400, a mid-dilated, unreactive pupil, a hazy cornea, and an intraocular pressure of 57. What is the best course of action at this time?

   A. Obtain an immediate head CT to rule out orbital abscess.
   B. Arrange for follow-up with an ophthalmologist within the next 1-2 weeks.
   C. Medically manage the patient's pain and nausea and arrange an urgent ophthalmology consult.
   D. Start the patient on oral acyclovir as this is likely herpes simplex-induced uveitis

2. A 42-year-old man with a history of chronic sinusitis presents with worsening left eyelid swelling over the preceding 3 days and intermittent double vision for the past 8 hours. Examination reveals swollen, red, and warm left eyelids. Visual acuity is 20/20 in both eyes and pupillary reactions are normal; however, extraocular motility is limited on lateral gaze in the left eye. What is the best course of action at this time?

   A. Start the patient on a course of oral antibiotics.
   B. Arrange for an outpatient CT scan and endocrine follow-up as this is likely thyroid ophthalmopathy.
   C. Obtain a maxillofacial CT scan and start on IV antibiotics.

D. Start the patient on a course of valacyclovir 1000 mg three times daily.

3. Which statement regarding herpes simplex virus is TRUE?

A. Eye infections are most commonly caused by the HSV-2 virus.

B. If a vesicular lesion is seen on the tip of the nose this suggests intraocular involvement of HSV.

C. Early use of antivirals may help reduce the risk of postherpetic neuralgia.

D. HSV keratitis classically presents with a dendritic corneal lesion.

4. Which of the following conditions is not treated with VEGF (vascular endothelial growth factor)-targeting agents?

A. Diabetic macular edema.

B. Exudative "wet" macular degeneration.

C. Nonexudative "dry" macular degeneration.

D. Neovascular glaucoma.

5. A 25-year-old man reports from his job as a janitor after "ammonia" splashed in his right eye. What is the best course of action at this time?

A. Send out for special ophthalmic solution, perform a complete dilated exam, and call for an ophthalmology consult.

B. Use artificial tears to rinse out remaining ammonia.

C. Instill tetracaine 0.5% and irrigate with ~2 liters of saline (or any other immediately available fluid) immediately.

D. Instill topical dilating drops and antibiotic ointment.

38

Urology

Christopher S. Cooper, MD

Fadi N. Joudi, MD

Mark H. Katz, MD

EMBRYOLOGY OF THE GENITOURINARY TRACT

A basic understanding of genitourinary embryology facilitates learning many aspects of urology. Embryologically, the genital and urinary systems are intimately related. Associated anomalies of the two systems are commonly encountered.

The Kidneys

The kidneys pass through three embryonic phases (Figure 38–1): (1) The **pronephros** is a vestigial structure without function in human embryos that, except for its primary duct, disappears completely by the fourth week. (2) The pronephric duct gains connection to the **mesonephric tubules** and becomes the mesonephric duct. While most of the mesonephric tubules degenerate, the mesonephric duct persists bilaterally; from where it bends to open into the cloaca, the ureteral bud grows cranially to interact with the metanephric blastema. (3) This forms the **metanephros,** which is the final phase. The metanephros develops into the kidney. During cephalad migration and rotation, the metanephric tissue progressively enlarges, with rapid internal differentiation into the nephron and the uriniferous tubules. Simultaneously, the cephalad end of the ureteral bud expands and divides within the metanephros to form the renal pelvis, calices, and collecting tubules.

The Bladder & Urethra

Subdivision of the cloaca (the blind end of the hindgut) into a ventral (urogenital sinus) and a dorsal (rectum) segment is completed during the seventh week and initiates early differentiation of the urinary bladder and urethra. The urogenital sinus receives the mesonephric duct and absorbs its caudal end, so that by the end of the seventh week, the ureteral bud and mesonephric duct have independent openings. The ureteral orifice migrates upward and laterally. The mesonephric duct orifice moves downward and medially, and the structure in between (the trigone) is formed by the absorbed mesodermal tissue, which maintains direct continuity between the two tubes (Figure 38–2).

The fused müllerian ducts also meet the urogenital sinus at Müller's tubercle. The urogenital sinus above Müller's tubercle differentiates to form the bladder and the part of the prostatic urethra proximal to the seminal colliculus in the male or the bladder and the entire urethra in the female (Figure 38–3). Below Müller's tubercle, the urogenital sinus differentiates into the distal part of the prostatic urethra and the membranous urethra in the male or the distal vagina and vaginal vestibule in the female. The rest of the male urethra is formed by fusion of the urethral folds on the ventral surface of the genital tubercle. In the female, the genital folds remain separate and form the labia minora.

The prostate develops at the end of the 11th week as several groups of outgrowths of urethral epithelium both above and below the entrance of the ejaculatory duct (distal vas deferens). The developing glandular element (seminal colliculus) incorporates the differentiating mesenchymal cells surrounding it to form the muscular stroma and capsule of the prostate. The seminal vesicles form as duplicate buds from the distal end of the mesonephric duct (vas deferens).

The Gonads

The potential to differentiate along male or female lines is present in every embryo initially. The development of one set of sex primordia and the gradual involution of the other are determined by the genetic sex of the embryo and differential secretion of numerous hormones. The *SRY* gene—or testis-determining factor—on the Y chromosome drives the gonad to differentiate into a testicle. Gonadal differentiation begins during the seventh week (Figure 38–3). If the gonad develops into a testis, the germinal epithelium progressively grows into radially arranged, cord-like seminiferous tubules. The production of müllerian-inhibiting factor by the testicle

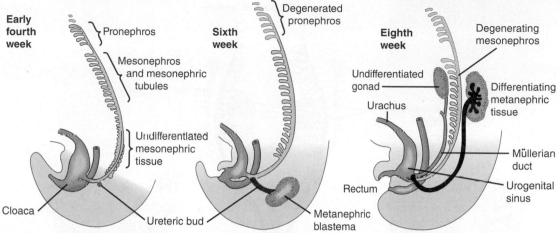

▲ **Figure 38–1.** Schematic of the development of the nephric system. Only a few of the tubules of the pronephros are seen early in the fourth week, while the mesonephric tissue differentiates into mesonephric tubules that progressively join the mesonephric duct. The first sign of the ureteral bud from the mesonephric duct is seen at 4 weeks. At 6 weeks, the pronephros has completely degenerated and the mesonephric tubules start to do so. The ureteral bud grows dorsocranially and has met the metanephric blastema. At the eighth week, there is cranial migration of the differentiating metanephros. The cranial end of the ureteral bud expands and starts to show multiple successive outgrowths (renal calices).

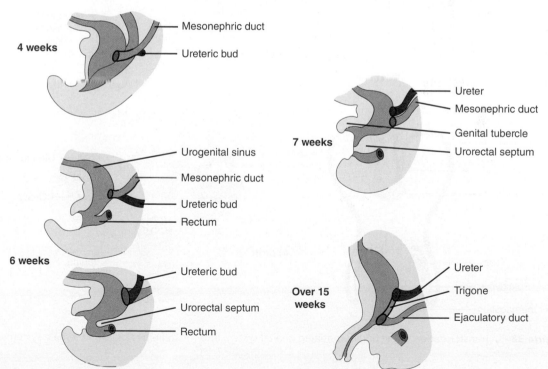

▲ **Figure 38–2.** The development of the ureteral bud from the mesonephric duct and their relationship to the urogenital sinus. The ureteral bud appears at the fourth week. The mesonephric duct distal to this ureteral bud is gradually absorbed into the urogenital sinus, resulting in separate endings for the ureter and the mesonephric duct. The mesonephric tissue that is incorporated into the urogenital sinus expands and forms the trigonal tissue. The mesonephric duct forms the vas deferens in the male and Gartner's duct (if present) in the female.

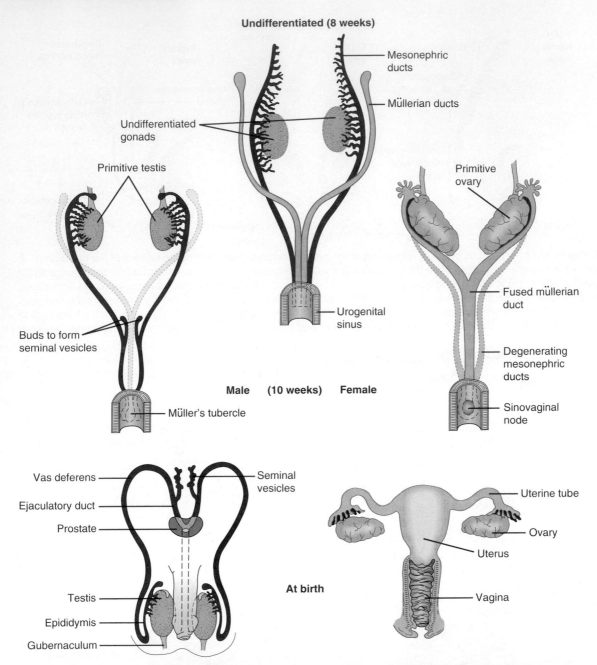

Undifferentiated (8 weeks)

Mesonephric ducts

Müllerian ducts

Undifferentiated gonads

Primitive testis

Primitive ovary

Buds to form seminal vesicles

Fused müllerian duct

Urogenital sinus

Degenerating mesonephric ducts

Male   (10 weeks)   Female

Müller's tubercle

Sinovaginal node

Vas deferens

Seminal vesicles

Ejaculatory duct

Prostate

Uterine tube

Ovary

Uterus

At birth

Testis

Epididymis

Vagina

Gubernaculum

▲ **Figure 38–3.** Transformation of the undifferentiated genital system into the definitive male and female systems.

causes regression of the müllerian duct and acts in a local (paracrine) fashion so that only the ipsilateral müllerian duct is affected. The subsequent production of testosterone by the testicle leads to masculinization of the mesonephric (wolffian) duct structures (ie, epididymides, vas deferens, seminal vesicles, and ejaculatory duct). If the gonad develops into an ovary, it becomes differentiated into a cortex and a medulla; the cortex later differentiates into ovarian follicles containing ova. The lack of testosterone leads to the disappearance of the mesonephric duct.

The testes remain in the abdomen until the seventh month and then pass through the inguinal canal to the scrotum, following the path of the gubernaculum. The mechanism of descent remains uncertain. Lack of complete testicular descent is known as cryptorchidism; descent to an abnormal site beyond the external inguinal ring is known as testicular ectopia.

The ovary, which is attached to ligaments, undergoes internal descent to enter the pelvis.

In the female, the genital duct system develops from the müllerian ducts, which fuse at their caudal ends and differentiate into the uterine tubes, the uterus, and the proximal two-thirds of the vagina.

The external genitalia start to differentiate by the eighth week. The genital tubercle and genital swellings develop into the penis and scrotum in the male and the clitoris and labia majora in the female. The external genitalia are masculinized by dihydrotestosterone (DHT), which is created from testosterone under the influence of 5α-reductase.

With the breakdown of the urogenital membrane in the seventh week, the urogenital sinus achieves a separate opening on the undersurface of the genital tubercle. The expansion of the infratubercular part of the urogenital sinus forms the vaginal vestibule and the distal third of the vagina. The two folds on the undersurface of the genital tubercle unite in the male to form the penile urethra; in the female, they remain separate to form the labia minora.

ANATOMY OF THE GENITOURINARY TRACT: GROSS & MICROSCOPIC

The Kidneys

The kidneys lie retroperitoneally in the posterior abdomen and are separated from the surrounding renal fascia (Gerota's fascia) by perinephric fat. The renal vascular pedicle enters the renal sinus; the vein is anterior to the artery, and both are anterior to the renal pelvis. The renal artery divides just outside the renal sinus into anterior and posterior branches that undergo further subdivisions with variable extents of distribution. They are end arteries and thus result in segmental infarction when occluded. The venous tributaries anastomose freely and usually drain into one renal vein.

The Renal Parenchyma

The renal parenchyma consists of more than 1 million functioning units (nephrons) and is divided into a peripheral cortex containing secretory elements and a central medulla containing excretory elements. The nephron starts as Bowman's capsule, which surrounds the glomerulus and leads to elongated proximal and distal convoluted tubules with the loop of Henle in between, ending in a collecting duct that opens into a minor calix at the tip of a papilla.

The Renal Pelvis & Calices

The renal pelvis and calices are within the renal sinus and function as the main collecting reservoir. The pelvis, which is partly extrarenal and partly intrarenal (but occasionally is totally extrarenal or intrarenal), branches into three major calices that in turn branch into several minor calices. These calices are directly related to the tips of the medullary pyramids (the papillae) and act as a receiving cup to the collecting tubules. The pelvicaliceal system is a highly muscular structure; the fibers run in many directions and are directly continuous from the calices to the pelvis, allowing synchronization of contractile activity.

The Ureter

The ureter connects the renal pelvis to the urinary bladder. It is a muscularized tube; its muscle fibers lie in an irregular helical arrangement and function primarily in peristaltic activity. Ureteral muscle fibers are directly continuous from the renal pelvis cranially to the vesical trigone distally.

The blood supply to the renal pelvis and ureters is segmental, arising from multiple sources, including the renal, gonadal, and vesical arteries, with rich subadventitial anastomoses.

The Bladder

The bladder is primarily a reservoir with a meshwork of muscle bundles that not only change from one plane to another but also branch and join each other to constitute a synchronized organ. Its musculature is directly continuous with the urethral musculature and thus functions as an internal urethral sphincteric mechanism in spite of the lack of a true circular sphincter.

The ureters enter the bladder posteroinferiorly through the ureteral hiatus; after a short intravesical submucosal course, they open into the bladder and become continuous with the trigone, which is superimposed on the bladder base though deeply connected to it.

The Urethra

The adult female urethra is about 4 cm long and is muscular in its proximal four-fifths. This musculature is arranged in an inner longitudinal coat that is continuous with the inner longitudinal fibers of the bladder and an outer circular coat that is continuous with the outer longitudinal coat of the bladder. These outer circular fibers comprise the sphincteric mechanism. The striated external sphincter surrounds the middle third of the urethra.

In the male, the prostatic urethra is heavily muscular and sphincteric. The membranous urethra is within the urogenital diaphragm and is surrounded by the striated external sphincter. The penile urethra is poorly muscularized and traverses the corpus spongiosum to open at the tip of the glans.

The Prostate

The prostate surrounds the proximal portion of the male urethra; it is a fibromuscular, cone-shaped gland about 2.5 cm long and normally weighing about 20 g in the adult. It is traversed from base to apex by the urethra and is pierced posterolaterally by the ejaculatory ducts from the seminal vesicles and vas deferens that converge to open at the verumontanum (seminal colliculus) on the floor of the urethra.

The prostatic glandular elements drain through about 12 paired excretory ducts that open into the floor of the urethra above the verumontanum. The prostate is surrounded by a thin capsule, derived from its stroma, which is rich in musculature, and part of the urethral musculature and the sphincteric mechanism. A rich venous plexus surrounds the prostate, especially anteriorly and laterally. Its lymphatic drainage is into the hypogastric, sacral, obturator, and external iliac lymph nodes.

The Testis, Epididymis, & Vas

The testis is a paired organ surrounded by the tunica albuginea and subdivided into numerous lobules by fibrous septa. The extremely convoluted seminiferous tubules gather to open into the rete testis, where they join the efferent duct and drain into the epididymis. The epididymis drains into the vas deferens, which courses through the inguinal canal into the pelvis and is joined by the duct from the seminal vesicle to form the ejaculatory duct, which opens before opening into the prostatic urethra on either side of the verumontanum.

Arterial supply is via the spermatic, vas deferential, and external cremasteric arteries. Venous drainage is through the pampiniform plexus, which drains into the internal spermatic veins; the right spermatic vein joins the vena cava, and the left joins the renal vein.

Testicular lymphatics drain into the retroperitoneal lymph nodes; the right primarily into the interaortocaval area, the left into the para-aortic area, both just below the renal vessels.

PHYSIOLOGY OF THE GENITOURINARY TRACT

The Kidneys

The kidneys maintain and regulate homeostasis of body fluids by glomerular filtration, tubular reabsorption, and tubular secretion.

A. Glomerular Filtration

This mechanism is dependent on glomerular capillary arterial pressure minus plasma colloid osmotic pressure plus Bowman's capsular resistance. The resultant glomerular filtration pressure (about 8-12 mm Hg) forces protein-free plasma through the capillary filtering surface into Bowman's capsule. Normally, about 130 mL of plasma is filtered every minute through the renal circulation; the entire volume of plasma recirculates through the kidney and is subjected to the filtration process once every 27 minutes.

B. Tubular Reabsorption

About 99% of the filtered volume is reabsorbed through the tubules, together with all the valuable constituents of the filtrate (chlorides, glucose, sodium, potassium, calcium, and amino acids). Urea, uric acid, phosphates, and sulfates are also reabsorbed to varying degrees. The process of reabsorption is a combination of active and passive transport mechanisms. Reabsorption of water and electrolytes is under the control of adrenal, pituitary, and parathyroid hormones.

C. Tubular Secretion

Tubular secretion helps (1) to eliminate certain substances and thus maintain their plasma levels and (2) to exchange valuable ions from the filtrate for less desirable ions in the plasma (eg, a sodium ion from the urine for a hydrogen ion in the plasma). Failure of adequate secretory function leads to the acidosis commonly encountered in chronic renal disease.

The Ureteropelvicaliceal System

This system is one continuous tubular structure with a syncytial type of smooth musculature that is imperceptibly in motion from one segment to the other. Waves of peristaltic contractions start from the calices and are propagated along the smooth muscle cells to the renal pelvis. At normal urine flow rates, many of these contraction waves are terminated at the ureteropelvic junction; however, some are transmitted to the ureter and down toward the urinary bladder. These peristaltic waves occur at a rate of about 5-8/min, involve a 2-cm to 3-cm segment at a time, and usually proceed at the velocity of 3 cm/s. Frequency, amplitude, and velocity are influenced by urine output and flow rate. In a state of diuresis, there may be a 1:1 relationship between caliceal contractions and ureteral contractions. Ureteral filling is primarily passive and occurs by reception of a bolus of urine from a renal pelvis contraction. The ureteropelvic junction closes after passing a bolus of urine, preventing back-pressure and back-flow of urine into the renal pelvis secondary to the elevated ureteral contraction pressure. A contraction ring forms in the proximal ureter, and as it migrates down the ureter, it pushes the bolus of urine antegrade. In states of diuresis, the size of the bolus increases and the pressure in the bolus may be greater than the pressure in the contraction ring ahead of it. In this case, the ureteral walls cannot coapt, and urine is transported as an uninterrupted column of fluid.

The Ureterovesical Junction

The ureterovesical junction allows flow of urine from the ureter to the bladder and at the same time prevents retrograde flow. The continuity and the specific muscular arrangement of the intravesical ureter and the trigone provide a muscularly active valvular mechanism that can efficiently adapt itself to the variable phases of bladder activity during filling and voiding.

The normal resting pressure of the ureterovesical junction (10-15 cm H_2O) is greater than the more cephalad ureteral resting pressure (0-5 cm H_2O). Progressive bladder filling leads to firm occlusion of the intravesical ureter against retrograde urine flow and to increased resistance to antegrade flow resulting from trigonal stretching. During voiding, trigonal contraction completely seals the intravesical ureter against any antegrade or retrograde flow of urine.

The Urinary Bladder

The urinary bladder functions primarily as a reservoir that can accommodate variable volumes without increasing its intraluminal pressure. When the bladder reaches full capacity, the detrusor muscle voluntarily contracts following relaxation of the external sphincter and maintains its contraction until the bladder is completely empty. Funneling of the bladder outlet with progressive downward movement of the dome ensures complete emptying.

The vesical sphincteric mechanism is primarily a smooth muscle sphincter in the bladder neck and male prostatic urethra and in the proximal four-fifths of the female urethra. There is no purely circular sphincteric entity, but there are abundant circularly oriented smooth muscle fibers that are directly continuous with the outer coat of the detrusor muscles. The sphincter has an abundance of alpha receptors that respond to sympathetic neural input from the pelvic nerve to maintain urethral closure. Parasympathetic input from the pelvic nerve facilitates bladder contracture and voiding.

There is a voluntary striated muscle sphincter that is part of the urogenital diaphragm and surrounds the mid urethra in the female and the membranous urethra in the male. It responds to somatic neural input from the pudendal nerve. It is essential for continence when the internal sphincter is nonfunctional. Its pathologic irritability or spasticity can lead to obstructive manifestations.

DEVELOPMENTAL ANOMALIES OF THE GENITOURINARY TRACT

Genitourinary tract anomalies constitute about one-third of all congenital abnormalities and occur in over 10% of the population. The severity varies from lesions incompatible with life to insignificant findings detected during diagnostic studies for unrelated reasons. The anatomic abnormalities are often not intrinsically harmful, yet they may predispose to infection, stone formation, or chronic renal failure.

RENAL ANOMALIES

Bilateral absence of the kidneys is rare and is associated with oligohydramnios, Potter facies, and pulmonary hypoplasia. It occurs more often in males and results in death shortly after birth. Unilateral renal agenesis is seen more often but is not usually associated with illness. **Renal agenesis** is thought to be due to both lack of a ureteral bud and lack of subsequent development of the metanephric blastema. The trigone is absent on the affected side. Because adrenal gland development is unrelated to kidney development, both adrenals are usually present in the normal position. Rarely, more than two kidneys are seen, a condition clearly dissimilar to ureteral duplication, as described later.

Abnormal ascent of the metanephros leads to an **ectopic kidney,** which may be unilateral or bilateral. Lumbar, pelvic, and the less common thoracic and crossed ectopic varieties are seen. Ectopic kidneys are associated with genital anomalies in 10%-20% of cases. Fusion abnormalities are also associated with failure of normal ascent and include fused pelvic kidneys and **horseshoe kidneys** (the most common), which are typically fused at the lower poles. Intravenous urography typically establishes the diagnosis. The relationship of the kidneys to the psoas muscles is abnormal; Instead of an oblique orientation with the medial border of the kidney parallel to the psoas muscle, the kidneys are vertical and the medial border intersects and crosses the psoas muscle. Horseshoe kidneys have an elevated incidence of vesicoureteral reflux and are at increased risk of ureteropelvic junction obstruction (UPJO). The latter may be related to a high ureteral insertion in the renal pelvis, crossing of the ureter over the isthmus, or compression by one of many anomalous arteries. Failure of rotation during ascent results in "malrotated" kidneys and is rarely significant.

Polycystic Kidneys

Parenchymal anomalies include a variety of cystic and dysplastic lesions. Polycystic kidney disease is hereditary and bilateral. The autosomal recessive polycystic kidney disease (ARPKD), previously called infantile PKD, has numerous small cysts that arise only from the collecting ducts and result in bilateral symmetrical enlargement of the kidneys. The autosomal dominant ADPKD, previously called adult PKD, has cysts arising from all areas of the nephron, which are usually larger and more variable in size than the ARPKD cysts. ARPKD occurs in 1 in 40,000 births and may be detected in utero by the presence of enlarged hyperechogenic kidneys and oligohydramnios. Infants usually die of respiratory failure rather than renal problems; however, the 1-year survival probability after the first month is over 85%. These children have declining renal function as well as severe hypertension and hepatic periportal fibrosis with portal hypertension leading to hypersplenism and esophageal varices.

The genes mutated in ADPKD may include the *PKD1* gene (located on chromosome 16p13.3) in 85% of patients or the *PKD2* gene (on chromosome 4q21-23) in 12%-15% of patients. These genes code for the polycystin-1 and polycystin-2 proteins, respectively. ADPKD occurs in 1 in 1000 individuals and is a major cause of end-stage renal disease in adults. Cysts may also be present in the liver, pancreas, and spleen, and cerebral arterial aneurysms may occur. Renal cystic enlargement exerts pressure on normal parenchyma, leading to its gradual destruction and glomerulosclerosis.

The diagnosis is often made during a workup for hypertension or uremia discovered in the third to sixth decades. Hematuria with or without flank pain is a common finding. An intravenous urogram reveals the enlarged kidneys, with marked elongation of the calices, which are compressed by large cysts. Ultrasonography or CT scan readily makes the diagnosis.

Surgery is rarely warranted. Therapy is medical and ultimately includes dialysis. The median age for reaching end-stage renal disease is 54 years in PKD1 and 74 years in PKD2. Renal transplantation is often indicated, though potential family donors must be carefully screened to determine whether they have the same disorder. The leading cause of death in ADPKD is cardiovascular disease, which may relate to early untreated hypertension.

Medullary Sponge Kidney

Medullary sponge kidney results from collecting tubular ectasia (see section on Polycystic Kidneys) and is associated with recurrent urolithiasis and an increased incidence of infection in 50% of patients. The lesion is often bilateral and may involve all of the calices. Intravenous urograms reveal dilated collecting tubules as a "blush" in the renal papilla. Microscopic hematuria is common. Specific antibiotics should be given for documented infections, and prophylactic therapy for renal stones should be recommended on the basis of metabolic stone evaluation.

Simple Renal Cysts

Simple renal cysts are common (approximately 50% after age 50) and are thought to arise from tubular dilation. They may be solitary or bilateral and multiple. They rarely have pathologic significance except in the differentiation from solid renal masses. (See the section on Renal Adenocarcinoma.)

Multicystic Dysplastic Kidney

Multicystic dysplastic kidney is a congenital abnormality consisting of macroscopic cysts of variable sizes compressing dysplastic renal parenchyma. It is usually associated with an atretic proximal ureter. The disorder occurs in about 1 in 3000 live births and is frequently noted on prenatal ultrasound. Rarely, it may occur bilaterally and is associated with oligohydramnios and renal failure. It may be distinguished from other causes of hydronephrosis by the absence of any renal function on renal scan. There is an increased incidence of contralateral UPJO (5%-10%) and reflux (18%-43%), either of which increases the patient's risk of subsequent chronic renal insufficiency.

The chance of developing a malignancy in multicystic dysplastic kidney appears to be no greater than 1 in 2000. There may also be an increased incidence of hypertension. These two factors constitute a rationale for treatment by nephrectomy. However, conservative management with routine ultrasound examinations at intervals of 6-12 months is reasonable practice, since about half involute within 5 years.

Renal Vascular Abnormalities

Multiple renal arteries occur in 15%-20% of patients and are significant only when they cause UPJO. Congenital **renal artery aneurysms** are infrequent; they are differentiated from acquired lesions by their location at the bifurcation of the main renal artery or at a distal branch point. The lesions are usually asymptomatic, but they can cause hypertension. They require surgical treatment only if hypertension is uncontrolled, if they are incompletely calcified, or if they have a diameter of more than 2.5 cm. **Congenital arteriovenous fistulas** are rare but may result in hematuria, hypertension, or cardiac failure necessitating operative treatment.

Renal Pelvis Anomalies

UPJO is the most common cause of antenatal hydronephrosis. The condition may be associated with compression by anomalous renal arteries or intrinsic stenosis of the junction. The diagnosis is not uncommonly made when gross hematuria follows minor trauma. Symptoms include intermittent flank pain, particularly with orally induced diuresis. There is a bimodal age at presentation, with an initial peak in infancy and a secondary presentation in early adulthood. Renal ultrasound provides a safe screening technique in patients suspected of having UPJO. Diuretic renal scan may confirm the diagnosis and suggest functional significance. Intravenous pyelogram or retrograde pyelography may further define the anatomy. Bilaterality is not uncommon, and the condition requires surgical repair if symptomatic or severe. With the advent of laparoscopic and robotic surgery, minimally invasive repair of UPJO with dismemebered pyeloplasty has become standard of care. Success rates with pyeloplasty are superior to endoscopic approaches in the primary setting. Percutaneous or ureteroscopic incision of the obstruction with short-term stenting has been successful in adults, but endoscopic incision is most useful in the setting of recurrent UPJO, when redo pyeloplasty becomes much more difficult, or when patients are poor surgical candidates due to comorbidities.

Buffi NM et al: Robot-assisted, single-site, dismembered pyeloplasty for ureteropelvic junction obstruction with the New da Vinci platform: A Stage 2a Study. *Eur Urol* 2014 Mar 13; pii:S0302-S2838(14)00210-00213. doi: 10.1016/j .eururo.2014.03.001.

URETERAL ANOMALIES

▶ Congenital Obstruction of the Ureter

Congenital obstruction of the ureter may be due to ureterovesical and UPJO or to neurologic deficits such as sacral agenesis or myelomeningocele. Functional ureteral obstruction—also known as **primary obstructive megaureter**—is not uncommon. Symptoms are renal pain during diuresis or resulting from pyelonephritis. Excretory urograms depict dilation above the obstruction. Vesicoureteral reflux is uncommonly associated with megaureter. Milder forms without symptoms or significant hydronephrosis are the rule and do not require treatment if renal function is normal. When treatment is necessary, it consists of division of the ureter proximal to the obstruction and reimplantation of the ureter into the bladder, often involving ureteral tapering or plication.

▶ Duplication of Ureters

Bifurcation of the ureteral bud before it interacts with the metanephric blastema results in incomplete ureteral duplication, commonly in the mid or upper ureter. A second ureteral bud from the metanephric duct leads to complete ureteral duplication (Figure 38–4; right kidney) draining one kidney. This represents the most common ureteral anomaly, occurring in 1 in 125 people. It occurs twice as often in females. The presence of more than two ureters on each side is not common, but bilaterality of ureteral duplication occurs in 40%. Usually, all of the duplicated ureters enter the bladder; the ureter draining the upper pole of the kidney enters closest to the bladder neck (due to its later reabsorption into the bladder). Because of this relationship, the ureter draining the lower pole often has a short intramural tunnel and an inadequate surrounding musculature and is thus prone to vesicoureteral reflux. The ureter draining the upper pole may be ectopic (because of its late absorption) and thus empty into the bladder neck, urethra, or genital structures (vagina or vestibule in the female and seminal vesicle or vas deferens in the male [Figure 38–4; left kidney]). The ureter draining the upper pole is prone to obstruction and may be associated with a ureterocele, which is a common cause of obstruction. Duplication becomes significant when hydronephrosis or pyelonephritis occurs. The diagnosis is

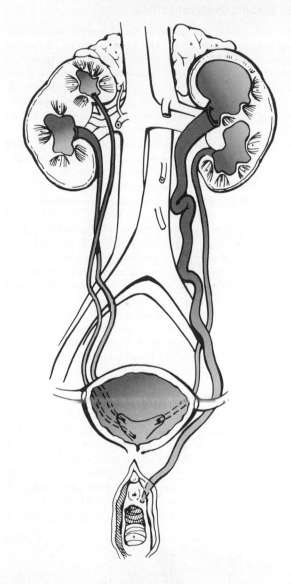

▲ **Figure 38–4.** Duplication of ureters and ectopic ureteral orifice. Complete duplication with obstruction to one ureter with ectopic orifice on left. The ureter with the ectopic opening always drains the upper pole of the kidney.

made by intravenous urography. Ureteral reimplantation to prevent recurrent infection is necessary in some cases. An anastomosis between the upper pole renal pelvis and the lower pole ureter or a low ureteroureterostomy are alternatives in selected cases. The upper pole of the kidney and its ureter may require removal if obstruction is severe and renal function of that segment is poor.

▶ Ectopic Ureteral Orifice

Ureteral ectopia can occur in the absence of duplication and drain into any of the abnormal positions mentioned previously. If the orifice lies proximal to the external urinary sphincter, no incontinence ensues, but vesicoureteral reflux is common. In contradistinction to the female, the ectopic orifice in the male never lies distal to the external sphincter, making incontinence an extremely rare presentation. Should the ectopic orifice in the female drain into the vagina or at the vestibule, there may be continuous leakage of urine apart from voiding. Most ectopic orifices involve the ureter draining the upper pole of a duplicated system, and most are observed in females. Hydroureteronephrosis of the involved segment frequently occurs due to ureteral obstruction as it traverses the muscle of the bladder neck.

An ectopic orifice may be seen beside the urethral orifice or in the roof of the vagina on endoscopy. Renal ultrasound or intravenous urograms often demonstrates hydroureteronephrosis of the upper renal segment. Cystography may show reflux into the ectopic orifice but may require cyclic voiding first to decompress the obstructed segment with bladder neck relaxation and subsequently to permit reflux. In the rare case when there is significant upper pole renal function, the ureter can be divided and reimplanted into the bladder or lower pole ureter. Usually, however, heminephro-ureterectomy is necessary.

▶ Ureterocele

A ureterocele is a ballooning of the distal submucosal ureter into the bladder. This structure commonly has a pinpoint orifice and therefore leads to hydroureteronephrosis. If large enough, it may obstruct the vesical neck or the contralateral ureter. It is most common in females with ureteral duplication and always involves the ureter draining the upper renal pole.

Most ureteroceles are now detected by prenatal ultrasound. Symptoms are usually those of pyelonephritis or obstruction. Intravenous urograms may show a negative shadow in the bladder cast by the ureterocele. The ureter and renal calices may be normal or may reveal marked dilation or no excretory function at all. A cystogram may show reflux into the ipsilateral lower pole ureter.

Treatment of ureteroceles depends on multiple factors, including the presence or absence of reflux in any or all of the ureters as well as whether or not the ureterocele is completely contained within the bladder (intravesical/orthotopic) or if a portion is at the bladder neck or urethra (extravesical/ectopic). A simple method of establishing drainage involves cystoscopy and puncture of the ureterocele. Associated reflux, if present, can be managed with prophylactic antibiotics until the child has grown larger, at which time a technically easier ureteral reimplant may be performed with a decompressed ureter. In the relatively uncommon situation when there is no associated reflux, an upper pole heminephrectomy is considered. Minimally obstructive ureteroceles within the bladder in adults do not require treatment.

Patel MN et al: Robot-assisted management of congenital renal abnormalities in adult patients. *J Endourol* 2010 Apr;24(4):567-570. doi: 10.1089/end.2009.0313.

VESICOURETERAL REFLUX

The main function of the ureterovesical junction is to permit free drainage of the ureter and simultaneously prevent urine from refluxing back from the bladder. Anatomically, the ureterovesical junction is well equipped for this function, because the ureteral musculature continues uninterrupted into the base of the bladder to form the superficial trigone. Additionally, the terminal 4-5 cm of ureter are surrounded by a musculofascial sheath (Waldeyer's sheath) that follows the ureter through the ureteral hiatus and continues in the base of the bladder as the deep trigone (Figure 38–5).

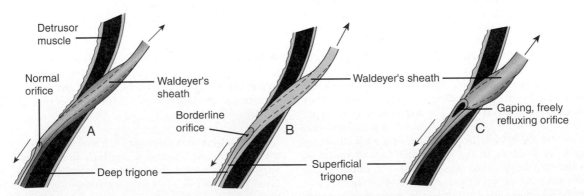

▲ **Figure 38–5.** Vesicoureteral reflux. The length and fixation of the intravesical ureter and the appearance of the ureteral orifice depend on the muscular development and efficiency of the lower ureter and its trigone. **A:** Normal structures. **B:** Moderate muscular deficiency. **C:** Marked deficiency results in a golf hole distortion of the submucosal ureter.

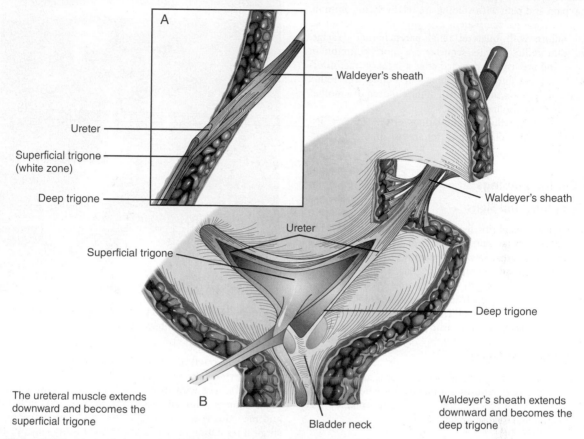

▲ Figure 38–6. Normal ureterotrigonal complex. **A:** Side view of ureterovesical junction. The Waldeyer muscular sheath invests the juxtavesical ureter and continues downward as the deep trigone, which extends to the bladder neck. The ureteral musculature becomes the superficial trigone, which extends to the verumontanum in the male and stops just short of the external meatus in the female. **B:** Waldeyer's sheath is connected by a few fibers to the detrusor muscle in the ureteral hiatus. This muscular sheath, inferior to the ureteral orifices, becomes the deep trigone. The musculature of the ureters continues downward as the superficial trigone. (Adapted, with permission, from Tanagho EA, Pugh RCB: The anatomy and function of the ureterovesical junction. *Br J Urol.* 1963 June;35(2):151–165.)

Direct continuity between the ureter and the trigone offers an efficient, muscularly active, valvular function. Any stretch of the trigone (with bladder filling) or any trigonal contraction (with voiding) leads to firm occlusion of the intravesical ureter, thus increasing resistance to flow from above downward and sealing the intravesical ureter against retrograde flow (Figure 38 6).

▶ **Etiology & Classification**

Vesicoureteral reflux may be classified as primary reflux due to developmental ureterotrigonal weakness or associated with ureteral anomalies such as ectopic orifice or uretero-cele, and secondary reflux due to bladder outlet or urethral obstruction, neuropathic dysfunction, iatrogenic causes, and

inflammation, especially specific infection (eg, tuberculosis). Primary reflux is associated with some degree of congenital muscular deficiency in the trigone and terminal ureter.

Reflux is associated with an increased incidence of pyelonephritis and renal damage. It also allows bacteria free access from the bladder to the kidney.

Reflux is the most common cause of pyelonephritis and is found in 30% to 50% of children presenting with urinary tract infection. It is present in over 75% of patients with radiologic evidence of chronic pyelonephritis and is responsible for end-stage renal disease in a large percentage of patients requiring chronic dialysis or renal transplantation.

In primary reflux, the child (on average, between 2 and 3 years of age) usually presents with symptoms of pyelonephritis or cystitis. Vague abdominal pain is not uncommon. Renal pain and pain with voiding are relatively uncommon. On rare occasions, the patient may present with advanced renal failure with bilateral renal parenchymal damage. Significant reflux and its sequelae are more common in females and are usually detected after a urinary tract infection. About one-third of the siblings of a child with reflux will also have reflux, and one-half of the children of a mother with reflux will also have reflux.

In secondary reflux, manifestations of the primary disease (neuropathic, obstructive, etc) are usually the presenting symptoms.

▶ Clinical Findings

A. Symptoms and Signs

With acute pyelonephritis, fever, chills, and costovertebral angle tenderness may be present. Children usually do not have renal pain but may complain of vague abdominal pain. Occasionally, daytime frequency, incontinence, or enuresis may be caused by infection associated with reflux. In cases of obstruction or neuropathic deficit, a palpable hydronephrotic kidney or a distended bladder may be found. The diagnosis may be elusive in infants who present with ill-defined symptoms.

B. Laboratory Findings

Urinalysis usually reveals evidence of infection (pyuria and bacteriuria). Urine cultures are mandatory when infection is suspected. Renal function tests may be abnormal if reflux and infection have caused renal scarring.

C. Imaging Studies

The most useful study for conclusive diagnosis of reflux continues to be voiding cystourethrography (Figure 38–7). This study demonstrates the grade of reflux as well as the urethral anatomy. Radionuclide voiding studies are extremely sensitive at detecting reflux but do not demonstrate the anatomic detail seen with a voiding cystourethrogram. Radionuclide voiding studies are often performed as follow-up after an initial voiding cystourethrogram because they offer the advantage of decreased radiation exposure.

Radioisotopic renal scanning provides accurate differential renal function data and detection of renal scars. Ultrasound can provide accurate measurement of renal size and may demonstrate the presence of renal scarring and ureteral or caliceal dilation. In many cases, there may be no abnormality visible in the upper urinary tract, or only mild distal ureteral dilation may be seen.

D. Urodynamic Considerations

A significant number of children with dysfunctional voiding present with urinary tract infections and are subsequently

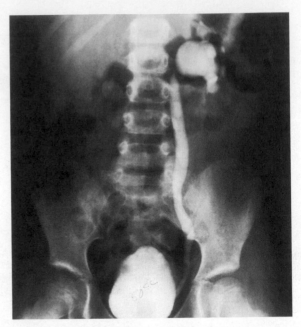

▲ **Figure 38–7.** Voiding cystourethrogram showing total (grade IV) left vesicoureteral reflux.

found to have reflux. These children contract the bladder against a closed external sphincter. Elevated voiding pressures associated with dysfunctional voiding may increase renal damage with an associated urinary tract infection and may also lessen the chance for either spontaneous or surgical resolution of reflux. When the history suggests the possibility of voiding dysfunction (incontinence, frequency, urgency), urodynamic studies are conducted to evaluate the voiding dynamics. Treatment of voiding dysfunction may result in resolution of the reflux.

▶ Treatment

Although some children with lower grades of reflux may not require antibiotics, traditionally any child with reflux was maintained on prophylactic antibiotics to attempt to decrease the incidence of urinary tract infections. Several recent studies suggest that the practice of daily antibiotic prophylaxis in all children with reflux may be of limited benefit in preventing urinary tract infection. Prompt treatment of pyelonephritis prevents renal scar formation. Factors causing secondary reflux—such as dysfunctional voiding or obstruction—should be corrected.

In many children, reflux resolves with time. Reflux is graded as seen on voiding cystourethrography as follows:

Grade I: Contrast enters ureter
Grade II: Contrast enters the renal collecting system
Grade III: Slight dilation of the calices or ureter

Grades IV and V: Progressively increased amounts of caliceal dilation and ureteral dilation or tortuosity

Reflux most likely to resolve is of lower grade or detected at a younger age. Over 70% of children with grades I, II, or unilateral grade III reflux will have resolution within 5 years. Resolution in children with grade V or bilateral grade IV reflux can be anticipated in less than 10% of cases. Other factors that appear to negatively affect the chance for reflux resolution include early reflux during bladder filling, presentation with a febrile urinary tract infection, renal scars, and voiding dysfunction.

In obstructive secondary reflux (eg, posterior urethral valves), release of obstruction may cure reflux. Occasionally, surgical reimplantation is still required. In neuropathic reflux, intermittent catheterization for control of infection may allow return of valvular competence. However, many cases require bladder augmentation for a noncompliant bladder and ureteral reimplantation. In reflux associated with ectopic orifices, duplication with ureterocele, and other congenital malformations, reimplantation is generally required.

The aim of surgery is to correct the reflux. This is accomplished by the creation of a longer submucosal tunnel for the ureter. With bladder filling and increased pressure, the ureter is compressed between the mucosa and underlying detrusor muscle. This flap valve prevents reflux of urine. The necessary length of the tunnel to stop reflux depends on the diameter of the ureter, with a 5:1 length-to-diameter ratio being ideal. One of three methods is used in most cases: (1) in suprahiatal repair (Politano-Leadbetter procedure), a new ureteral hiatus is developed about 2.5 cm above the original one, and the ureter—after passing through a submucosal tunnel—is sutured to the cut edge of the trigone at the level of the original orifice. (2) In the cross-trigonal repair (Cohen procedure), the original hiatus is maintained, and the ureter is advanced through a submucosal tunnel, extending across the trigone to the contralateral bladder wall. (3) A totally extravesical ureteral advancement procedure (extravesical ureteroplasty) achieves results similar to those achieved with the intravesical methods, with a shorter hospital stay and shorter convalescence.

Injections of subureteric bulking agents have also been used to increase submucosal support of the ureter. With proper placement beneath the ureteral orifice under endoscopic vision, these injections act to bolster the deficient antireflux mechanism. Concern regarding late sequelae of Teflon injections (eg, particle migration) has prevented use of this approach in the United States. Currently, hyaluronic acid/dextranomer (NASHA/Dx) gel (Deflux) is the only FDA-approved material for endoscopic injection to manage vesicoureteral reflux in children. Short-term success in stopping reflux with the injection techniques appears to be around 75% overall, with most success with grades I-III reflux. The long-term success rates still need to be evalu-

ated, as many studies only have short term (ie, 3 month) follow up.

Routh JC, Inman BA, Reinberg Y: Dextranomer/hyaluronic acid for pediatric vesicoureteral reflux: systematic review. *Pediatrics* 2010 May;125(5):1010-1019. doi: 10.1542/peds.2009-2225. Epub 2010 Apr 5. Review. PMID: 20368325.

▶ Prognosis

The long-term prognosis is excellent for patients with mild to moderate reflux successfully treated with antibiotic prophylaxis. There are few instances of recurrent infection or renal insufficiency. Patients with more significant reflux or persistent urinary tract infections may benefit from subureteric injection or surgical reimplantation; the success rate is approximately 95% with the open surgical technique (cessation of reflux, clearance of renal infection, and absence of obstruction). Unfortunately, for patients with advanced disease (irreversible ureteral decompensation and severe bilateral scars), the prognosis is less favorable. These patients account for a significant proportion of patients with end-stage renal disease who ultimately require chronic dialysis, renal transplantation, or both.

BLADDER ANOMALIES

Anomalies of the bladder are infrequent and include the following: (1) agenesis, or complete absence, which results in a persistent cloaca; (2) bladder **duplication,** which may be complete, with separate ureteral openings drained by duplicated urethras, or incomplete, with a septum or hourglass deformity; and (3) **urachal anomalies,** which in the most severe forms appear as a patent opening at the umbilicus and are usually associated with some form of bladder outlet obstruction. In less severe forms, a **urachal diverticulum** may be present at the dome of the bladder or a **urachal cyst** along the course of the partially obliterated urachus. These latter conditions may cause abdominal pain and umbilical or bladder infection requiring surgical treatment. Occasionally, adenocarcinoma develops in a urachal remnant (see section on Tumors of the Bladder).

Failure of cloacal division results in a persistent cloaca. Incomplete division is more frequent (though still rare) and results in a rectovesical, rectourethral, or rectovestibular fistula (usually with imperforate anus or anal atresia).

▶ Exstrophy of the Bladder

Exstrophy of the bladder is the most severe bladder anomaly—the result of a complete ventral defect of the urogenital sinus and the overlying inferior abdominal wall musculature and integument. The lower central portion is devoid of skin and muscle. The anterior bladder wall is absent, and the posterior wall is contiguous with surrounding skin. Urine drains onto the abdominal wall, the rami of the pubic bones are widely separated, and the open pelvic ring may affect gait. In males, the penis is shortened and the urethra is epispadiac. The exposed bladder mucosa tends to be chronically inflamed.

Currently, the favored treatment is bladder salvage, which includes closure of the bladder in the newborn period. Urethral closure and penile reconstruction have also been advocated at the time of the initial bladder closure. Ureteral obstruction or vesicoureteral reflux may develop and require ureteral reimplantation. The closed bladder may have a small capacity, and incontinence is often a complication. Patients frequently require multiple operations, including bladder augmentation and bladder neck reconstruction. Good results have been observed in more than half of all patients treated, with preservation of renal function and continence.

▶ Prune Belly Syndrome

Prune belly syndrome consists of a triad of abnormalities: deficient abdominal wall musculature, bilateral cryptorchidism, and variable amounts of dilation of the urogenital tract. The cause is not known. Almost all children with prune belly syndrome have reflux. The incidence of eventual renal failure is 25%-30%. Risk factors for renal failure include bilateral abnormal kidneys on ultrasound or renal scan, a serum creatinine that never falls below 0.7 mg/dL, and clinical pyelonephritis. These children are managed with prophylactic antibiotics and frequent urine cultures, followed by prompt treatment of any urinary tract infections. Abdominoplasty may be performed to help correct the abdominal wall defect.

▶ Congenital Neurovesical Dysfunction

Congenital neurovesical dysfunction frequently accompanies a posterior myelomeningocele or sacral agenesis, with associated spinal abnormalities. Both conditions may result in incontinence and recurrent urinary infection with late sequelae (ureteral reflux, pyelonephritis, and renal failure). These children require frequent evaluation of their kidneys and kidney function because high bladder storage pressures may harm the kidneys.

PENILE & URETHRAL ANOMALIES

▶ Hypospadias

Hypospadias results from failure of fusion of the urethral folds on the undersurface of the genital tubercle. The urethral meatus is ventrally displaced on the glans on the shaft of the penis or more proximal at the level of the scrotum or perineum. With more proximal displacement, chordee (ventral curvature of the penile shaft) frequently occurs and

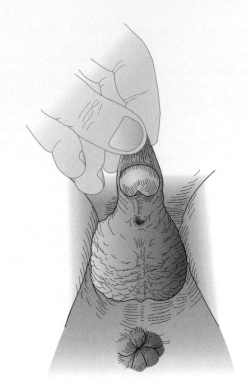

▲ **Figure 38–8.** Hypospadias, penoscrotal type. Redundant dorsal foreskin that is deficient ventrally; ventral chordee.

requires treatment, or it precludes straight erections and normal intercourse (Figure 38–8). The midscrotal hypospadiac penis may resemble female external genitalia with an enlarged clitoris and labia. Sexual assignment in these latter infants requires hormonal and chromosomal analysis.

In hypospadias with the meatus positioned proximal to the corona, the prepuce is abnormal—not forming a complete cylinder due to a ventral defect. Circumcision should not be done in these patients, as the prepuce can be used later in surgical repair.

The degree of hypospadias dictates the need for repair. If the opening is glandular or coronal (85% of patients), the penis is usually functional both for micturition and procreation, and repair is done primarily for cosmetic reasons. Openings that are more proximal on the shaft require correction to allow voiding while standing, normal erection, and proper sperm deposition during intercourse. Surgical plastic repair of hypospadias is currently accomplished by a variety of highly successful one-stage operations and is routinely performed between 6 and 18 months of age. The most common complications of hypospadias surgery include meatal stenosis and fistula formation; however, improved techniques have decreased the incidence of these complications.

Epispadias

Epispadias is a rare congenital anomaly that is commonly associated with bladder exstrophy. When it occurs alone, it is considered a milder degree of the exstrophy complex.

The urethra opens on the dorsum of the penis, with deficient corpus spongiosum and loosely attached corpora cavernosa. If the defect is extensive, it may extend to the bladder neck, causing incontinence because of deficient sphincter muscles. The pubic bones are separated, as in exstrophy. Marked dorsiflexion of the penis is usually present.

Treatment consists of correction of penile curvature, reconstruction of the urethra, and reconstruction of the bladder neck in incontinent patients.

Urethral Strictures

Congenital urethral strictures are rare but when present are most common in the fossa navicularis (just proximal to the meatus) and in the bulbomembranous urethra. Commonly, these strictures are thin diaphragms that may respond to simple dilation or to direct vision internal urethrotomy. Rarely is open surgical repair necessary. Congenital urethral strictures in girls and meatal stenosis in boys are uncommon. When the latter does occur, it appears to be acquired, as it is seen only in circumcised boys.

Urethral Diverticulum

In males, urethral diverticula are nearly always in the pendulous or bulbous urethra. They are often associated with an obstructive flap of the urethral mucosa (anterior urethral valve), thought to represent incomplete closure of the urethral folds. Treatment by endoscopic unroofing is usually successful, though most diverticula are small and require no therapy. In females, they occur in adult life and are usually manifested by irritative symptoms and recurrent infection. The cause is unknown, but the disorder is most likely congenital. Treatment is usually by transvaginal excision. Diverticula may occasionally harbor stones or tumors.

Posterior Urethral Valves

Posterior urethral valves are the most common obstructive urethral lesion in newborn and infant males and the most common cause of end-stage renal disease in boys. They consist of obstructive folds of mucosa, which originate at or are attached at some point to the verumontanum in the prostatic urethra. The embryologic derivation is indefinite. They are partially obstructive and thus lead to variable degrees of back-pressure damage to the urinary bladder and upper urinary tract. Dilation and obstruction of the prostatic urethra are always present. Spontaneous urinary ascites from the kidneys is often seen in neonates. This clears when the obstruction is relieved.

About one-third of children with posterior urethral valves are now diagnosed by prenatal ultrasound. Another one-third are diagnosed in the first year of life, with the remaining third presenting later. Clinical manifestations consist of difficult voiding, a weak urinary stream, and a midline lower abdominal mass that represents a distended bladder. In some cases, the kidneys are palpable and the child may have signs and symptoms of uremia and acidosis. Urinary incontinence and urinary tract infection may occur. Laboratory findings include elevated serum urea nitrogen and creatinine and evidence of urinary infection. Ultrasound shows evidence of bladder thickening and trabeculation, hydroureter, and hydronephrosis. Demonstration of urethral valves on a voiding cystourethrogram establishes the diagnosis, as does endoscopic identification of valves. Up to 70% of children with valves may have vesicoureteral reflux.

Treatment consists of destruction of the valves by endoscopic incision. In a premature infant with a small urethra prohibiting transurethral resection, a temporary cutaneous vesicostomy may be required to provide drainage and improve impaired kidney function.

The prognosis depends on the original degree of kidney damage and the success of efforts to prevent or treat infection. Rates of chronic renal failure or end-stage renal disease range from 25% to 67% of boys with valves. Poor prognostic factors include the presence of bilateral reflux or an elevated nadir serum creatinine in the first year of life. Many of these children have delayed development of urinary continence due to bladder changes and impaired urinary concentration.

SCROTAL & TESTICULAR ANOMALIES

Testicular Torsion

Neonatal testicular torsion (extravaginal torsion) is an extremely rare condition. The entire testicle and the tunica vaginalis are twisted. No trigger mechanism associated with the torsion has been identified. Although the vast majority are necrotic and nonsalvageable, several studies have reported salvage of testicular tissue when torsion is detected immediately following birth. Any scrotal swelling in the neonate requires close follow-up. Intravaginal testicular torsion in adolescents is described later in this chapter.

Scrotal Lesions

Congenital scrotal lesions include hypoplasia of the scrotum (unilateral or bilateral) in association with cryptorchidism and bifid scrotum with extensive hypospadias. Midline inclusion cysts may also occur.

CRYPTORCHIDISM

Etiology & Classification

True undescended testicles stop along the normal path of descent into the scrotum. They may remain in the abdominal cavity (least common), in the inguinal canal (canalicular), or just outside the external ring (suprascrotal, most common). Testes may also pass through the external ring and then be located ectopically, most commonly in a superficial inguinal pouch. The incidence of undescended testicles increases from 3% to 5% in full-term infants to 30% in premature infants. Most undescended testicles descend within the first 6 months of life, and by 1 year of age the prevalence is 1%. The left testicle is affected more often, and 1%-2% of children with cryptorchidism will have both testicles affected. Twenty percent of boys who present with cryptorchidism have one nonpalpable testis. Of nonpalpable testes, 20% are intra-abdominal; 40% are canalicular, scrotal, or ectopic testes; and 40% are atrophic or absent.

Clinical Findings

The diagnosis of cryptorchidism relies on physical examination. Absence of an identifiable testicle with ultrasound, computed tomography, or magnetic resonance imaging (MRI) does not prove testicular agenesis and therefore does not alter the need for surgical exploration. Testicular examination in the infant and young child requires two hands, with the first hand being swept from the anterior iliac spine along the inguinal canal to gently express any retained testicular tissue into the scrotum, which is palpated with the other hand. A true undescended or ectopic inguinal testis may slip or "pop" under the examiner's fingers. To distinguish a retractile testicle, the testicle is brought into the scrotal position, holding it in place for a minute to fatigue the cremaster muscle. After this, a retractile testicle remains in the scrotum, whereas an ectopic or undescended testis immediately snaps back out of the scrotum. If a testis cannot be palpated in the inguinal canal or the scrotum, or in the typical ectopic sites, evaluation for a nonpalpable testis must be performed.

A child with bilateral nonpalpable testes should undergo hormonal evaluation for testicular absence. Elevations in luteinizing hormone (LH) and follicle-stimulating hormone (FSH) and absence of detectable müllerian-inhibiting substance suggest testicular absence. Testicular absence is confirmed by a negative human chorionic gonadotropin (hCG) stimulation test. The hCG stimulation test is performed by the administration of intramuscular hCG (2000 IU/day for 3-4 days). Raised gonadotropin levels (FSH and LH) *and* a lack of a testosterone rise from hCG indicate bilateral absent testes, and a formal surgical exploration is unnecessary. When one or both components are lacking or there is detectable müllerian-inhibiting substance, surgical exploration is warranted.

Surgical Therapy

Treatment of the undescended testicle offers the possibility of improved fertility, correction of patent processus vaginalis, prevention of testis torsion, and improvement in body image. There is controversy whether orchidopexy decreases the risk of malignancy, but placement of an undescended testicle in the scrotum assists physical examination of the testis. Histologic changes related to infertility occur in the undescended testicle as young as 1 year of age, and spontaneous descent rarely occurs after 6 months of age, making this the optimal time for surgical correction.

Almost 90% of undescended testes have an associated patent processus vaginalis, which predisposes to formation of a hydrocele or hernia. Occult inguinal hernia in patients with untreated undescended testis can present at any time with the typical symptoms or complications, including incarceration.

Prior to any surgical intervention, the patient is reexamined while under anesthesia because on occasion a retractile testicle descends under anesthesia or a previously nonpalpable testicle becomes palpable. For a palpable testicle, an open inguinal approach is performed. For the nonpalpable testicle in a child, a laparoscopic approach is preferred, but an open inguinal approach may be performed.

Outcomes

Success rates following orchidopexy are 74% for the abdominal testis, 87% for canalicular, and 92% for those distal to the external ring. The most significant complication is testicular atrophy, which occurs in 1%-2% of cases of orchidopexy, while complete devascularization of the testis is rare. Paternity rates have been reported at 65%, 90%, and 93% in men with bilateral cryptorchidism, unilateral cryptorchidism, and normally descended testicles, respectively. If only one testis is undescended, the sperm count is subnormal in 25%-33% patients, and serum FSH concentration is slightly elevated. These abnormalities suggest that both testes are abnormal, perhaps congenitally, although only one fails to descend. If both testes are undescended, sperm count usually is severely subnormal, and serum testosterone may be reduced.

Alternative Therapy

Hormonal therapy is an option in the treatment of cryptorchidism because the condition may be related to hypogonadotropic hypogonadism. hCG is the only hormone approved for use in the treatment of cryptorchidism in the United States. Side effects of hCG treatment include enlargement of the penis, growth of pubic hair, increased testicular size, and aggressive behavior during administration. The likelihood of success with hormonal therapy is greatest for the most distal undescended testes or for testes that have been previously descended. Some suggest that hormonal therapy is effective only for retractile and not truly undescended testes. Although hormonal therapy may not be effective in achieving testicular descent, it may improve fertility in cryptorchid boys.

ACQUIRED LESIONS OF THE GENITOURINARY TRACT

OBSTRUCTIVE UROPATHY

Obstruction is one of the most important abnormalities of the urinary tract, since it eventually leads to decompensation of the muscular conduits and reservoirs, back-pressure, and atrophy of renal parenchyma. It also invites infection and stone formation, which cause additional damage and can ultimately end in complete unilateral or bilateral destruction of the kidneys.

Both the level and the degree of obstruction are important to an understanding of the pathologic consequences. Any obstruction at or distal to the bladder neck may lead to back-pressure affecting both kidneys. Obstruction at or proximal to the ureteral orifice leads to unilateral damage unless the lesion involves both ureters simultaneously. Complete obstruction leads to rapid decompensation of the system proximal to the site of obstruction. Partial obstruction leads to gradual progressive muscular hypertrophy followed by dilation, decompensation, and hydronephrotic changes.

▶ Etiology

Acquired urinary tract obstruction may be due to inflammatory or traumatic urethral strictures, bladder outlet obstruction (benign prostatic hyperplasia or cancer of the prostate), vesical tumors, neuropathic bladder, extrinsic ureteral compression (tumor, retroperitoneal fibrosis, or enlarged lymph nodes), ureteral or pelvic stones, ureteral strictures, or ureteral or pelvic tumors.

▶ Pathogenesis

Regardless of its cause, acquired obstruction leads to similar changes in the urinary tract, which vary depending on the severity and duration of obstruction.

A. Urethral Changes

Proximal to the obstruction, the urethra dilates and balloons. A urethral diverticulum may develop, and dilation and gaping of the prostatic urethra and ejaculatory ducts may occur.

B. Vesical Changes

Early detrusor and trigonal thickening and hypertrophy compensate for the outlet obstruction, allowing complete bladder emptying. This change leads to progressive development of bladder trabeculation, cellules, saccules, and, finally, diverticula. Subsequently, bladder decompensation occurs and is characterized by the above changes plus incomplete bladder emptying (ie, postvoid residual urine). Trigonal hypertrophy leads to secondary ureteral obstruction owing to increased resistance to flow through the intravesical ureter. With detrusor decompensation and residual urine accumulation, there is stretching of the hypertrophied trigone, which appreciably increases ureteral obstruction. This is the mechanism of back-pressure on the kidney in the presence of vesical outlet obstruction (while the ureterovesical junction maintains its competence). Catheter drainage of the bladder relieves trigonal stretch and improves drainage from the upper tract.

A very late change with persistent obstruction (more frequently encountered with neuropathic dysfunction) is decompensation of the ureterovesical junction, leading to reflux. Reflux aggravates the back-pressure effect on the upper tract by transmitting abnormally high intravesical pressures and favors the onset or persistence of urinary tract infection.

C. Ureteral Changes

The first change noted is a gradual increase in ureteral distention. This increases ureteral caliber and stimulates hyperactive ureteral contraction and ureteral muscular hypertrophy. Because the ureteral musculature runs in an irregular helical pattern, stretching of its muscular elements leads to lengthening as well as widening, causing the dilated ureter to assume a tortuous, serpiginous course, weaving back and forth across the relatively straight course of the ureteral vessels, which are unaffected by the ureteral obstruction. This is the start of ureteral decompensation, where tortuosity and dilation become apparent. These changes progress until the ureter becomes atonic, with infrequent, ineffective, or completely absent peristalsis.

D. Pelvicaliceal Changes

The renal pelvis and calices, subjected to increased volumes of retained urine, distend. The pelvis shows evidence first of hyperactivity and hypertrophy and then of progressive dilation and atony. The calices show similar changes to a variable degree, depending on whether the renal pelvis is intrarenal or extrarenal. In the latter, caliceal dilation may be minimal in spite of marked pelvic dilation. In the intrarenal pelvis, caliceal dilation and renal parenchymal damage are maximal. The successive phases seen with obstruction are rounding of the fornices, followed by flattening of the papillae and finally clubbing of the minor calices.

E. Renal Parenchymal Changes

With continued pelvicaliceal distention, there is parenchymal compression against the renal capsule and, more importantly, compression of the arcuate vessels results in a marked drop in renal blood flow leading to parenchymal ischemic atrophy. With increased intrapelvic pressure, there is progressive dilation of the collecting and distal tubules, with compression and atrophy of tubular cells.

Clinical Findings

A. Symptoms and Signs

The findings vary according to the site of obstruction.

1. **Infravesical obstruction**—Infravesical obstruction (eg, due to urethral stricture, benign prostatic hypertrophy, bladder neck contracture) leads to difficulty in initiation of voiding, a weak stream, and a diminished flow rate with terminal dribbling. Burning and frequency are common associated symptoms. A distended or thickened bladder wall may be palpable. Urethral induration due to stricture, benign prostatic hypertrophy, or cancer of the prostate may be noted on rectal examination. Meatal stenosis and impacted urethral stones are readily diagnosed by physical examination.

2. **Supravesical obstruction**—Renal pain or renal colic and gastrointestinal symptoms are commonly associated. Supravesical obstruction (eg, due to ureteral stone, UPJO) may be completely asymptomatic when it develops gradually over a period of months. An enlarged kidney may be palpable. Costovertebral angle tenderness may be present.

B. Laboratory Findings

Evidence of urinary tract infection, hematuria, or crystalluria may be seen. Impaired renal function may be noted in cases of bilateral obstruction. Postrenal azotemia (serum changes reflecting impaired renal function due primarily to obstruction) is suggested by elevation of serum urea nitrogen and serum creatinine with a ratio greater than 10:1.

C. Imaging Studies

Radiologic examination is usually diagnostic in cases of stasis, tumors, and strictures. Dilation and anatomic changes occur above the level of obstruction, whereas distal to the obstruction, the configuration is usually normal. This helps in localizing the site of obstruction. Combined antegrade imaging by intravenous urograms and retrograde imaging by ureterograms or urethrograms is sometimes needed to demonstrate the obstructed segment. In supravesical obstruction, demonstration of stasis and delayed drainage is essential to establish and quantitate the severity of obstruction.

1. **Ultrasonography**—Ultrasonography reveals the degree of dilation of the renal pelvis and calices and allows for diagnosis of hydronephrosis even in the prenatal period. Color Doppler ultrasound can reveal blood flow and restrictive indices to help determine functional impairment.

2. **Isotope studies**—A technetium-99m DTPA scan or MAG-3 scan portray the degree of hydronephrosis as well as renal function. Use of diuretics during the scan can provide specific data on the significance of the obstruction and the need for treatment. Multiple studies can reveal ongoing functional changes.

3. **CT scan**—CT scan is of particular value in revealing the degree and site of obstruction as well as the cause in many cases. The use of contrast (CT urogram) agents allows estimation of residual renal function.

4. **MR urogram**—MRI provides anatomic images and identification of the site of obstruction. With dynamic contrast-enhanced MR urography, functional information is also obtained without the use of ionizing radiation.

5. **Antegrade urography**—Antegrade urography via percutaneous needle or tube nephrostomy is valuable when the obstructed kidney fails to excrete the radiopaque material on excretory urography. The Whitaker test requires percutaneous catheter access to the collecting system above the site of suspected obstruction. This permits fluid introduction into the renal pelvis and simultaneous measurement of urine flow rate and pressures in the bladder and renal pelvis, thus providing a quantitative assessment of the degree and severity of obstruction. The fluid transport can be measured and the degree of obstruction estimated by the use of a pressure monitor.

Complications

The most important complication of urinary tract obstruction is renal parenchymal atrophy as a result of back-pressure. Obstruction also predisposes to infection and stone formation, and infection occurring with obstruction leads to rapid kidney destruction.

Treatment

The first goal of therapy is relief of the obstruction (eg, catheterization for relief of acute urinary retention). Definitive therapy often requires surgery, but minimally invasive techniques are becoming utilized more often. Simple urethral stricture may be managed by dilation or internal urethrotomy (incision of the stricture under direct vision through the resectoscope). However, urethroplasty (open surgical graft or flap of skin or buccal mucosa to replace urethral diameter) may be required and have better long-term success. Benign prostatic hyperplasia classically requires excision, but laser techniques are providing satisfactory outcomes with less morbidity. Impacted ureteral stones may either be removed or bypassed by a catheter unless it is thought that they may pass spontaneously.

Ureteral or UPJO requires surgical repair; however, endoscopic approaches within the ureter or by laparoscopy may be equal to open repair. Renal stones may be removed instrumentally via retrograde or antegrade percutaneous approach by direct extraction with baskets or by ultrasonic or laser lithotripsy or by irrigation through a tube placed directly into the kidney.

Preliminary drainage above the obstruction is sometimes needed to improve kidney function. Occasionally, intestinal urinary diversion or permanent nephrostomy is required. If damage is advanced, nephrectomy may be indicated.

► Prognosis

The prognosis depends on the cause, site, duration, and degree of kidney damage and renal decompensation. In general, relief of obstruction leads to improvement in kidney function except in seriously damaged kidneys, especially those destroyed by inflammatory scarring.

Padmanabhan P, Nitti VW: Primary bladder neck obstruction in men, women, and children. *Curr Urol Rep* 2007;8:379.

URETEROPELVIC JUNCTION OBSTRUCTION

Stenosis of the renal pelvis outlet is commonly due to congenital narrowing of the junction or compression by anomalous vessels. However, the lesion may be acquired. Presentation in adults often includes the abrupt onset of flank pain usually following ingestion of large amounts of fluids. Presentation in childhood is now most often made following the diagnosis of hydronephrosis by prenatal ultrasonography.

The diagnosis may be confirmed with a diuretic nuclear renal scan or intravenous urography, which reveals hydronephrosis with a dilated renal pelvis and slow drainage of either radiotracer or contrast medium. Occasionally, patients present with intermittent hydronephrosis and normal urograms, except during attacks of pain, when x-rays show typical obstruction. These patients generally have normal renal parenchyma. Retrograde ureteropyelography is usually needed in patients with chronic moderate to severe obstruction to determine the extent of the lesion and to provide assurance that the distal ureter is normal. Marked obstruction may make it difficult to determine whether kidney function is surgically salvageable. In these cases, it may be necessary to perform either (1) differential radioisotope renography with use of a diuretic during the study or (2) percutaneous nephrostomy and creatinine clearance by 24-hour urine collection.

Severe obstruction with minimal remaining renal function is best treated by unilateral nephrectomy. If renal function is adequate (> 10%-15% of total renal function or > 10 mL/min creatinine clearance), surgical repair of the stenosis, either by creation of a renal pelvis flap or by resection of the stenotic area and reanastomosis (dismembered repair), is warranted. Laparoscopic and/or robotic pyeloplasty has emerged as the standard of care in adults for the repair of UPJO. The use of ureteroscopy or percutaneous nephroscopy with endopyelotomy, incising the strictured ureteropelvic junction, offers an alternative method of therapy and is most useful in secondary UPJO, after primary repair has failed. Endoscopic approaches are less successful in the presence of a crossing vessel, poor renal function, and significant hydronephrosis. The surgical results of all the above methods are excellent in terms of functional preservation, improvement of urine flow, and relief of symptoms, but dilation of the calices may persist.

Singh I, Hemal AK: Robot-assisted pyeloplasty: review of the current literature, technique and outcome. *Can J Urol* 2010 Apr;17(2):5099-5108.

URETERAL STENOSIS

Ureteral stenosis can be secondary to congenital or acquired lesions. Congenital causes can include compression by an anomalous vessel such as a lower pole renal artery in UPJO or a retroperitoneal vein or primary megaureter where the distal ureter is partially obstructed. More commonly, the ureter is secondarily obstructed due to acquired conditions such as inflammation from chronic ureteral stones, trauma secondary to gynecologic or vascular surgery, or external penetrating trauma from a knife or gunshot wound. Enlarged pelvic lymph nodes or an iliac artery aneurysm or retroperitoneal fibrosis may obstruct the ureter, as can intrinsic ureteral cancer or bladder cancer infiltrating the ureter at its insertion into the bladder. Finally, infection such as urinary tuberculosis can cause distal ureteral strictures, and bilateral ureteral obstruction can occur from bladder neck obstruction with urinary retention secondary to benign prostatic hyperplasia.

Chronic conditions with slow development may not cause symptoms, whereas acute obstruction such as that from a stone will cause severe flank pain that may radiate to the groin or testes/labia. Diagnosis is most often made by a CT urogram with contrast that will show delayed function and a dilated renal pelvis and ureter down to the site of the obstruction. This is often an unsuspected finding on a CT done for other reasons in an asymptomatic patient.

Treatment depends entirely on the cause. Severe stenosis may require resection of the lesion and spatulated end-to-end anastomosis of the ureter. Less-severe obstruction may be managed by cystoscopy and ureteral or balloon dilation of the narrowed area under direct vision via a ureteroscope. Placement of an indwelling ureteral stent may dilate the stenosis over time and be a useful treatment as well in selected patients.

RETROPERITONEAL FIBROSIS

See also Chapter 22.

One or both ureters may be compressed by a chronic inflammatory process, usually of unknown cause, which involves the retroperitoneal tissues of the lumbosacral area. When the source of fibrosis is unknown, the entity is known as idiopathic retroperitoneal fibrosis. Patients treated for migraine with methysergide may develop this fibrosis. Sclerosing Hodgkin disease and fibrosis from metastatic cancer have also been implicated. Symptoms include flank pain, lower back and abdominal pain (from ureteral obstruction), and those associated with uremia. Some patients present with complete anuria. Urinary infection is unusual. If both ureters are obstructed, the serum creatinine is elevated, but unilateral renal obstruction from fibrosis may present with normal or slightly elevated creatinine levels.

Excretory urograms show hydronephrosis and a dilated ureter down to the point of obstruction. The ureters are displaced medially in the lumbar area. Retrograde ureterograms show a long segment of ureteral stenosis, though a catheter usually passes easily through the ureter. Ultrasound lacks the anatomic specificity to make the diagnosis, but obstruction proximal to the fibrotic mass yields hydronephrosis and hydroureter. Large areas of fibrosis can be identified with ultrasound. CT scans and MRI offer the most diagnostic information about the fibotic mass and both the degree and level of obstruction. If the patient has significant worsening of renal function, indwelling ureteral stent(s) or percutaneous nephrostomy tube(s) should be placed. When the patient's condition has improved, definitive therapy can be accomplished. If methysergide is suspected to be the causative agent, fibrosis may subside when the drug is discontinued. When malignancy is in the differential diagnosis, a percutaneous or laparoscopic biopsy should be considered prior to treatment. These patients may benefit from administration of corticosteroids and/or other immunosuppressive agents. Chronic indwelling ureteral stents have also been used successfully. If these methods fail, ureterolysis must be performed to free the ureter from the fibrous plaque. The involved ureter should be dissected from the plaque, moved to a lateral position, and wrapped with omentum to prevent recurrent entrapment. This has been accomplished quite successfully with laparoscopic and robotic approaches.

Keehn AY et al: Robotic ureterolysis for relief of ureteral obstruction from retroperitoneal fibrosis. *Urology* 2011 Jun;77(6):1370-1374.

BENIGN PROSTATIC HYPERPLASIA

▶ General Considerations

The cause of benign prostatic enlargement is not known but is probably related to hormonal factors. The mechanism for opening and funneling the vesical neck at the time of voiding is altered by hyperplasia of the prostate, which causes increased outflow resistance. Consequently, a higher intra-

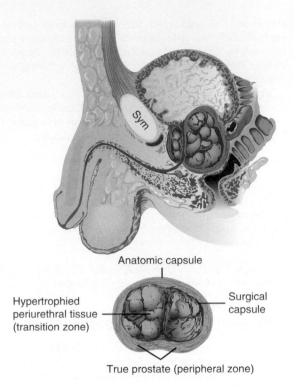

▲ **Figure 38–9.** Benign prostatic hyperplasia. The enlarged periurethral glands are enclosed by the surgical capsule. The true prostate has been compressed.

vesical pressure is required to accomplish voiding, causing hypertrophy of the vesical and trigonal muscles. This may lead to the development of bladder diverticula—outpocketings of vesical mucosa between the detrusor muscle bundles. Hypertrophy of the trigone causes excessive stress on the intravesical ureter, producing functional obstruction and resulting in hydroureteronephrosis in late cases. Stagnation of urine can lead to infection; the onset of cystitis exacerbates the obstructive symptoms. The periurethral and subtrigonal prostate enlargement produces the most significant obstruction.

The prostate in young men has an anatomic capsule like an apple peel. In men with prostatic enlargement, there is a thick "surgical" capsule similar to an orange peel, composed of peripherally compressed true prostatic tissue ("peripheral zone"). The hyperplastic benign periurethral glands correspond to the "transition zone" and are the cause of the obstruction (Figure 38–9).

▶ Clinical Findings

A. Symptoms and Signs

Typically, the patient has lower urinary tract symptoms and notices hesitancy and loss of force and caliber of the stream. The urgent need to void when the bladder is nearly full may be an early sign. He may also be awakened by the urge to void several times at night (nocturia). Postvoid dribbling ("terminal dribbling") is particularly disturbing. The complication of infection increases the degree of obstructive symptoms and is often associated with burning on urination. Acute urinary retention may supervene. This is associated with severe urgency, suprapubic pain, and a distended, palpable bladder.

The size of the prostate rectally is not of primary diagnostic importance, since there is a poor correlation between the size of the gland and the degree of symptoms and amount of residual urine. The American Urological Association (AUA) developed a 7-item, self-administered questionnaire (AUA symptom score) that can assist the patient and physician in evaluating the patient's lower urinary tract symptoms.

B. Laboratory Findings

Urinalysis may reveal evidence of infection. Residual urine is commonly increased (> 50 cc), and a timed urinary flow rate is decreased (< 10-15 cc/s). The serum creatinine may be elevated in cases with prolonged severe obstruction.

C. Imaging Studies

Pelvic ultrasound can easily identify post-void urine residual as well as estimate prostate size and anatomy, in particular, the presence or absence of median lobe tissue. Bladder wall thickness, trabeculation, and diverticula can also be identified with ultrasound. Renal ultrasound can identify hydronephrosis in advanced cases of BPH. Transrectal ultrasound of the prostate provides better imaging of the prostate than the transabdominal approach but is more invasive and typically not required. Computerized tomography (CT), MRI, and excretory urography also provide anatomical information for an enlarged prostate, but are more time consuming and costly and should only be utilized in unusual circumstances (eg, ruling out malignancy).

D. Cystoscopic Examination

Cystourethroscopy reveals secondary vesical changes (eg, trabeculation and diverticula) and enlargement of the prostatic urethra. Lateral lobe hypertrophy (so-called "kissing lobes") as well as median lobe tissue can be easily visualized. Although cystoscopy is not required to make the diagnosis of BPH, it may identify other conditions in the differential diagnosis (eg, urethral stricture, bladder neck contracture, malignancy) as well as complications secondary to BPH (eg, bladder stones).

E. Urodynamic Studies

Simultaneous physiologic monitoring of bladder filling and emptying, urethral sphincter activity, abdominal pressure, and pelvic floor muscle activity (electromyography) can be extremely useful in documenting whether bladder outlet obstruction, poor bladder function, or other causes are responsible for lower urinary tract symptoms. While urodynamic studies are not required for diagnosis in all cases, they are helpful in cases with large postvoid residual volumes or underlying neurologic disease to help determine appropriate management.

▶ Differential Diagnosis

Neurogenic bladder may produce a similar syndrome. A history suggesting a neuropathic etiology, such as diabetes mellitus, stroke, Parkinson's disease, or spinal cord injury or compression, may be obtained. Neurologic deficit involving the spinal nerves S2-4 is particularly significant.

Cancer of the prostate also causes symptoms of vesical neck obstruction. Serum prostate-specific antigen (PSA) may be elevated in patients with benign prostatic hypertrophy, and the level increases as the volume of the prostate increases. Thus, an absolute value is not diagnostic, but in general, if it is over 10 ng/mL, the possibility of cancer should be evaluated.

Acute prostatitis may cause symptoms of obstruction, but the patient is septic and has infected urine. The prostate is exquisitely tender.

Urethral stricture diminishes the caliber of the urinary stream. There is usually a history of gonorrhea or local trauma. A retrograde urethrogram or cystoscopy shows the stenotic area. A stricture blocks the passage of an instrument or catheter.

▶ Complications

Obstruction and residual urine lead to vesical and prostatic infection and occasionally pyelonephritis; these may be difficult to eradicate. Long-term obstruction can lead to renal failure.

The obstruction may lead to the development of bladder diverticula. Infected residual urine may contribute to the formation of calculi.

Functional obstruction of the intravesical ureter, caused by the hypertrophic trigone, may lead to hydroureteronephrosis.

▶ Treatment

The indications for operative management are impairment of or threat to renal function and bothersome symptoms. Because the degree of obstruction progresses slowly in most patients, conservative treatment may be adequate. Drugs that relax the prostatic capsule and internal sphincter (α-adrenergic blocking agents) or decrease the volume of the prostate (5α-reductase inhibitors or antiandrogens) have been tried with considerable success.

A. Conservative Measures

Treatment of chronic prostatitis may reduce symptoms. The resolution of a complicating cystitis usually affords some relief. In order to protect vesical tone, the patient should be cautioned to void as soon as the urge develops. Forcing fluids over a short time causes rapid vesical filling and decreasing vesical tone; this is a common cause of sudden acute urinary retention and thus should be avoided. Patients with urinary obstructive symptoms should avoid the use of cold remedies, including antihistamines and alpha agonists, because they are also a common cause of urinary retention. These conservative measures are of only temporary help—if any—in patients with BPH. There has been recent great interest, particularly by patients, in the use of phytotherapy for treatment of lower urinary tract symptoms, including saw palmetto, pumpkin seeds, and other plant extracts. Despite previous claims of efficacy based on small retrospective studies, a recent large, multicenter randomized trial of 369 men comparing placebo versus saw palmetto showed no improvement in AUA symptom score or secondary outcomes (eg, peak flow and PVR) in the saw palmetto group. Thus, the use of saw palmetto extracts for the treatment of BPH is not recommended.

Barry MJ, et al: Effect of increasing doses of saw palmetto extract on lower urinary tract symptoms: a randomized trial. *JAMA* 2011 Sep 28;306(12):1344-1351.

Controversy surrounds choices in the treatment of benign prostatic hyperplasia. No treatment (watchful waiting) may be appropriate in patients who complain of mild to moderate symptoms and thus have low AUA symptom scores and residual urine less than 70-100 cc. Interest has also focused on nonoperative medical therapy for those with more significant symptoms. α-Adrenergic blocking agents relax the internal (bladder neck) sphincter and prostatic capsule. Selective agents that are long-acting and preferentially work for this purpose include tamsulosin and silodosin. 5α-Reductase inhibitors block conversion of testosterone to DHT (the androgen active in promoting prostate growth) and are useful for large glands, particularly in combination with an alpha-blocker, which has been shown to best prevent urinary retention and other common progressive symptoms of prostatic obstruction. More recently, daily tadalafil, a PDE-5 inhibitor commonly used in the treatment of erectile dysfunction, has been shown to have efficacy in treating symptoms related to BPH.

Catheterization is mandatory for acute urinary retention. Spontaneous voiding may return, but a catheter should be left indwelling for at least a few days and preferably one week while detrusor tone returns. Several studies have documented improved success of voiding trials after retention if α-blockers are initiated for at least 48 hours prior to catheter

removal. If several voiding trials fail, additional treatment is indicated.

Zeif HJ et al: Alpha blockers prior to removal of a catheter for acute urinary retention in adult men. *Cochrane Database Syst Rev* 2009 Oct 7;(4):CD006744.

B. Surgery

Surgery for BPH is offered to men in whom medical therapy fails to provide adequate symptom relief and/or objective parameters such as post-void residual fail to improve. Additionally, men may request surgery because of poor compliance with medical therapy or desire to stop medications. Absolute indications for BPH surgery include recurrent infections, development of bladder stones, renal failure due to BPH, and persistent urinary retention due to obstruction. Men with large amounts of median lobe tissue (intravesical protrusion) tend to have a poor response to medical therapy and benefit most from early surgery.

There are two common approaches used in surgery for BPH: transurethral and transabdominal (open vs. minimally invasive). The transurethral route is by far the most common and preferred in patients with glands weighing less than 100 g because morbidity rates are lower and the hospital stay is shorter. With new technology, even larger glands can be managed with the transurethral approach. Larger glands, however, may require open surgery (suprapubic or retropubic enucleation), depending on the preference and experience of the urologist. Open surgery for BPH is the exception rather than the rule because of increased morbidity.

Transurethral approaches are the least invasive and require the shortest hospital stay (typically ambulatory or one night). The gold standard is the monopolar transurethral resection of the prostate (TURP), by which a resectoscope with a monopolar loop electrode is utilized to remove the obstructing BPH tissue. Hypotonic irrigation solution is required and hyponatremia due to excess systemic absorption ("TURP Syndrome") is a unique complication of this approach. Additional complications of TURP include hematuria, UTI, stress incontinence, impotence, retrograde ejaculation, urethral stricture, and bladder neck contracture. Incontinence and impotence are rare complications in the hands of experienced surgeons (< 5%). TURP has reliably demonstrated improvement in AUA symptom score, flow rate, and PVR in randomized controlled trials. The more recent use of bipolar energy has allowed for the use of saline irrigation during TURP, eliminating the risk of hyponatremia.

Transurethral laser vaporization of the prostate with holmium or KTP (potassium titanyl phosphate) laser technology has demonstrated similar efficacy to TURP in well-selected patients with smaller glands. The major advantage of the laser approaches is less risk of bleeding, and even the ability to perform the procedure while patients remain on anticoagulation. Holmium-laser enucleation of the prostate (HOLEP) utilizes laser energy to enucleate the prostate adenoma (rather than vaporize the tissue). The tissue must then be morecellated to be removed via the resectoscope. HOLEP has similar efficacy to TURP and laser vaporization but may be more technically challenging.

An alternative transurethral approach for the treatment of BPH is transurethral incision of the prostate (TUIP). This procedure consists of a linear incision starting at the bladder neck and ending distally at the verumontanum, allowing expansion of the entire prostatic urethra. Typically two incisions are made with a cutting current at the 5 and 7 O'clock positions. TUIP is typically reserved for men with a steep/high bladder neck or small, obstructive prostates of 30 g or less in size.

Open and robotic enucleation of the prostate for BPH is reserved for larger glands where transurethral approaches would be unable to remove sufficient tissue to provide long-term relief of the obstruction.

▶ Prognosis

Most patients with marked symptoms receive considerable relief and substantial improvement in urine flow following surgical treatment; however, those with milder forms may benefit from drug therapy. Unless absolute indications for surgery exist (see above), most men begin with medical therapy and progress to surgical interventions if substantial symptoms persist.

American Urological Association Guideline: Management Of Benign Prostatic Hyperplasia (BPH). Available at www.auanet .org. Accessed May 10, 2014.

URETHRAL STRICTURE

Acquired urethral strictures in men may be due to external trauma or to prior instrumentation (most common). Strictures may be inflammatory, due to gonorrhea, tuberculous urethritis, or schistosomiasis, or may rarely be a complication of cancer. The common presenting symptoms are dysuria, weak stream, splaying of the urinary stream, urinary retention, and urinary tract infection. Evidence of scarring due to trauma or induration and perineal fistula may be seen. Urethroscopy reveals the degree of narrowing. A retrograde urethrogram delineates the site and degree of stricture.

Urethral stricture must be differentiated from bladder outlet obstruction due to BPH, impacted urethral stones, urethral foreign bodies, and tumors.

Initial treatment consists of transurethral direct-vision internal urethrotomy (incision of the stricture). Successful results are obtained in 75% of patients. For long, dense strictures or those failing to respond to an initial internal urethrotomy, open surgical repair is indicated. This is probably best achieved by the transpubic or perineal route if the lesion involves the membranous urethra. If the bulbar urethra is involved, the perineal approach is indicated; if the distal/penile urethra is involved, the ventral penile approach is appropriate. End-to-end anastomosis is satisfactory for short segment strictures, usually 2 cm or less, with a more than 90% success rate. Longer strictures often require pedicle flaps for distal urethral strictures or onlay grafts (eg, buccal mucosa) for proximal strictures.

Lee YJ et al: Current management of urethral stricture. *Korean J Urol* 2013 Sep;54(9):561-569.

HEMATURIA

Hematuria, gross or microscopic, is a common urologic consult because it can be a presenting sign for underlying urologic malignancies. Red-colored urine may not necessarily include blood, and microscopic examination looking for red blood cells is prudent. Microscopic hematuria is defined as three or more red blood cells per high-powered field on urine microscopy in two of three properly collected specimens. The degree of hematuria bears no relation to the seriousness of the underlying cause. Urine dipstick test is the simplest method to check for blood and has a sensitivity of 91%-100% and a specificity of 65%-99%. Caution should be taken because false positives (menstrual blood, myoglobin, and hemolysis, among others) and false negatives (dipstick exposed to moisture and presence of reducing agents like ascorbic acid) can lead to confusing results. For this reason, further evaluation of microscopic hematuria performed only when microscopic analysis confirms the diagnosis. Knowledge of the medical history and medications can help rule out other causes of colored urine. Beets, rifampin, and phenazopyridine, among other substances, can cause urine discoloration. Anticoagulation at normal therapeutic levels does not predispose to hematuria, and patients should be evaluated for the hematuria, because 13%-45% of these patients may have significant urologic disease.

Ideally, a clean-catch midstream sample should be collected. If that is not possible, a catheterized specimen is indicated. It is important to note that hematuria can be due to urologic or renal parenchymal disease. The differential diagnosis thus includes benign causes like renal or bladder stones, papillary necrosis, urinary tract infections, prostatitis, or instrumentation, and malignant causes like renal, renal pelvis, bladder, prostate, or urethral cancer. Renal parenchymal causes of hematuria include glomerular and interstitial renal disease. These patients may have proteinuria and casts on the urinalysis, and the red blood cells are typically dysmorphic. Nephrology evaluation is required for hematuria associated with glomerular or interstitial renal disease.

Patients with hematuria referred to urology are classified into low-risk and high-risk groups. High-risk groups include smokers, age older than 40 years, history of exposure to pelvic radiation or cyclophosphamide, occupational exposure to chemicals or dyes, and history of urinary tract infections or other urological disorders. It is recommended that a complete workup be performed for all patients with symptomatic hematuria, all patients with gross hematuria, and high-risk patients with microscopic hematuria. The workup includes history and physical examination, serum creatinine, upper tract imaging (typically CT urogram), cystoscopy, and urine cytology. Asymptomatic patients younger than 40 years who have microscopic hematuria and have no risk factors can be evaluated with upper tract imaging and either cystoscopy or voided cytology, as the risk of significant pathology in this population is very low. If the workup is negative, it is recommended that the patient be evaluated with urinalysis, voided cytology, and blood pressure check at 6, 12, 24, and 36 months.

▼ URINARY TRACT INFECTIONS

Urinary tract infection is the second-most common type of infection in humans and is frequently encountered by primary care physicians as well as urologists.

These infections are caused by a variety of pyogenic bacteria that typically produce a nonspecific tissue response. The most common organisms are gram-negative bacteria, particularly *Escherichia coli.* Less common are *Enterobacter aerogenes, Proteus vulgaris, Proteus mirabilis, Pseudomonas aeruginosa,* and *Enterococcus faecalis.*

Owing to the short length of the female urethra and bacterial colonization of the introitus, ascending infection is a common occurrence in young girls and in sexually active women. In men, ascending infection is often a consequence of urethral instrumentation.

Although relatively uncommon, descending or hematogenous urinary tract infection is usually associated with local urinary tract disorders—most commonly, obstruction and stasis; less commonly, trauma, foreign bodies, or tumors.

Lymphatic spread occasionally occurs from the large bowel or from the cervix and adnexa in the female through the perivesical and periureteral lymphatics.

Direct extension to the urinary bladder of nearby inflammatory processes (eg, appendiceal abscess, enterovesical fistula, or pelvic abscess) may occur.

▶ Predisposing Factors

Infection is usually initiated or sustained by predisposing factors. Predisposing systemic factors include diabetes mellitus, immunosuppression, and malnutrition; these disorders likely interfere with normal bladder and body defense mechanisms. Predisposing local factors include incontinence, constipation, organic or functional obstruction, stasis (residual urine), foreign bodies (especially catheters and stones), tumors, or necrotic tissue. Vesicoureteral reflux facilitates transport of bacteria from the bladder to the kidney, which subsequently predisposes to pyelonephritis.

▶ Classification of Urinary Tract Infection

Urinary tract infection is classified as (1) upper urinary tract infection (most commonly acute or chronic pyelonephritis or infection due to renal abscess), (2) lower urinary tract infection (cystitis or urethritis), or (3) genital infection (prostatitis, epididymitis, seminal vesiculitis, or orchitis).

▶ Urologic Instrumentation or Surgery & Urinary Tract Infection

In the absence of urinary tract infection, surgery of the upper urinary tract should require only short-term prophylactic antibacterial therapy. In the presence of infection, one attempts to sterilize the system before operation. If stenting or tube drainage is required and there are no symptoms of infection, colonization does not call for antibacterial therapy until the stent or tube is to be changed or removed. Broad-spectrum antibacterial prophylaxis is started at that time.

With lower urinary tract surgery, antibacterial therapy is advised before operations involving the urethra and the bladder, especially for women in whom contamination from vaginal organisms is likely. Men undergoing prostatectomy for obstructive prostatism often have urinary tract infection, particularly when catheter drainage is used preoperatively. In these cases, antimicrobial therapy is necessary before and after surgery to prevent bacteremia.

In the presence of urinary tract infection, any urethral instrumentation poses a threat of bacteremia, and possibly sepsis—more apt to occur in men than in women. Appropriate antibacterial coverage should be instituted before manipulation.

A. Principles of Catheterization

After a short-term single catheterization, the rate of infection is 1%-5%. However, in certain patients—pregnant women, elderly, or debilitated patients—and in the presence of urologic disease, the risk is much higher. An indwelling catheter often leads to bacterial colonization, especially in women. The incidence is proportionate to the duration of catheterization and reaches approximately 95% after 5 days.

Strict aseptic technique is of critical importance in catheterization. Proper cleansing of the genitalia is essential. Iodophor preparations may be used for cleaning the vaginal introitus or the glans penis. Many common urinary tract pathogens are present in normal colonic flora, and these organisms often gain access to the urinary tract of catheterized patients. Cross-contamination of urinary catheters (passive transmission of bacteria from patient to patient on the hands of hospital personnel) is a frequent mode of transfer of resistant organisms. Measures directed to the prevention of catheter cross-contamination are essential. Closed catheter drainage is probably the best way to reduce cross-contamination.

With sterile technique during catheterization and a closed drainage system, most catheters can be kept sterile for 48-72 hours. In a closed drainage system, an added airlock or one-way valve preventing reflux of urine from the collecting bag to the draining tubes also helps prevent infection. The general principles are as follows: (1) Indwelling catheters should be used only when absolutely necessary. (2) Catheters should be inserted with strict aseptic technique. (3) A closed drainage system, preferably with a one-way valve, is advisable. (4) Nonobstructed dependent drainage is essential. (5) Unnecessary irrigation of the system should be avoided. (6) If the catheter is needed for a prolonged period, it should be changed every 2-4 weeks to minimize encrustation and stone formation. (7) Catheterized patients with asymptomatic catheter colonization should be given antibiotics just before the catheter is changed or removed—not during the period of catheterization unless symptomatic infection occurs.

B. Evaluation

Imaging of the urinary tract is recommended in every febrile infant or young child following the first urinary tract infection. Imaging includes a renal and bladder ultrasound and a voiding cystourethrogram. The renal ultrasound may detect hydronephrosis, duplication anomalies, stones, or abnormalities of the bladder wall and should be obtained at the earliest convenient time. A cystogram may be obtained by instillation of contrast medium with fluoroscopy or by instillation of a radionuclide. Radionuclide cystography has the advantage of decreased radiation, while the contrast-voiding cystourethrogram has the advantage of providing better anatomic detail, which may help detect bladder or urethral abnormalities. Either method should include a voiding phase because reflux is the most likely abnormality to be detected and may only occur with voiding. The cystogram should be obtained once the child is free of infection.

Imaging recommendations in adults with a urinary tract infection vary depending on the patient's past history and present symptoms. Renal/bladder ultrasound is a good initial study to identify upper- (eg, hydronephrosis, stones, or abscess) and lower- (eg, urinary retention or bladder calculi) tract sources of infection. CT scan with intravenous contrast can identify stigmata of pyelonephritis (see below).

C. Antibacterial Therapy

The choice of antibiotics depends on the type of organism and its sensitivity, as determined by urine cultures. For uncomplicated infection, adequate urine concentrations of the antibiotic determine efficacy, but in cases of bacteremia and septic shock, serum concentrations are crucial. Commonly used oral medications are sulfonamides, nitrofurantoin, ampicillin, trimethoprim-sulfamethoxazole, fluoroquinolones, and oxytetracycline. For parenteral therapy, aminoglycosides and cephalosporins are effective against the most common organisms (ie, *P. mirabilis, E. aerogenes,* and *P. aeruginosa*).

ACUTE PYELONEPHRITIS

▶ General Considerations

Except in the presence of stasis, foreign bodies, trauma, or instrumentation, pyelonephritis is an ascending type of infection. Pathogenic organisms usually reach the kidney from the bladder, often via an incompetent ureterovesical junction.

▶ Clinical Findings

A. Symptoms and Signs

In acute attacks, pain is present in one or both flanks. Diagnosis in infants requires a high index of suspicion, since they may present with nonspecific symptoms such as fever and failure to thrive. Young children commonly present with poorly localized abdominal pain; irritative lower urinary tract symptoms may be present. Chills and fever are common. Severe infection may produce hypotension, peripheral vasoconstriction, and acute renal failure. Gross hematuria is not common but can be observed more frequently in women and the elderly.

B. Laboratory Findings

Pyuria and bacteriuria are consistent findings. Leukocytosis with a shift to the left is common. Urine culture identifies the organism.

C. Imaging Studies

In acute attacks, only minimal changes such as delayed visualization and poor concentrating ability are noted on intravenous urography. CT scans may demonstrate zones of decreased enhancement in the renal parenchyma as well as perinephric fat stranding. Renal or ureteral calculi may be seen on plain abdominal x-rays or nonenhanced CT scans. Chest x-ray may show a small ipsilateral pleural effusion.

▶ Differential Diagnosis

Pneumonia, acute cholecystitis, or splenic infarction can be confused with pyelonephritis. Acute appendicitis sometimes causes pyuria and microhematuria. Any acute abdominal illness such as pancreatitis, diverticulitis, or intestinal ischemia can simulate pyelonephritis. Appropriate history, examination, urinalysis and imaging usually make the distinction.

Complications

If the diagnosis is missed in the acute stage, the infection may become chronic. Both acute and chronic pyelonephritis may lead to progressive renal damage and abscess formation.

Treatment

Specific antibiotic therapy should be given for at least 7 days to eradicate the infecting organism after proper identification and sensitivity determination. Symptomatic treatment is indicated for pain and irritative voiding symptoms. Adequate fluid intake to assure optimum urinary output is required. Failure to simultaneously identify and treat predisposing factors (eg, obstruction) is the principal cause of failure to respond to therapy, leading to progressive infection, chronic pyelonephritis, and possibly sepsis. Patients not responding to culture-sensitive antibiotics should be imaged, looking for intrinsic (eg, calculi) or extrinsic obstruction or renal abscess.

Prognosis

The prognosis is good with adequate treatment of both the infection and its predisposing cause, depending on the degree of preexisting renal parenchymal damage.

EMPHYSEMATOUS PYELONEPHRITIS

Emphysematous pyelonephritis is a form of acute necrotizing pyelonephritis secondary to a gas-producing bacteria (*E. coli* in 66% of cases and *Klebsiella* in 26%). It is commonly seen in patients with poorly controlled diabetes (over 90% of cases) or in patients with upper urinary tract obstruction. The diagnosis is made by the usual signs of acute pyelonephritis and by the presence of gas in the renal collecting system and parenchyma seen on plain films, ultrasound, or CT. The condition is life threatening, with a mortality rate of 40%-80% with intravenous antibiotics alone. Obstruction requires drainage either percutaneously or by stent placement. Operative treatment, including nephrectomy and drainage along with antibiotics, decreases the mortality rate to less than 20%.

CHRONIC PYELONEPHRITIS

Chronic pyelonephritis is the result of inadequately treated or recurrent acute pyelonephritis. The diagnosis is primarily made by x-ray, since patients rarely have signs or symptoms until late in the course, when they develop chronic flank pain, hypertension, anemia, or renal failure. Pyuria is not a consistent finding. Because chronic pyelonephritis may be a progressive, localized immune response initiated by bacteria long since eradicated, urine cultures are usually sterile. Early cases may have no findings on intravenous urography, whereas in late cases it may reveal small kidneys with typical caliceal

deformities (clubbing), with evidence of peripheral scarring and a thin cortex. Voiding cystourethrography may document vesicoureteral reflux as the cause. Complications include hypertension, stone formation, and chronic renal failure.

Antibiotic treatment is not helpful in these patients unless ongoing infection can be documented. The prognosis depends on the status of renal function but is generally not good, particularly when the disease is contracted in childhood. Progressive deterioration of renal function usually occurs.

Xanthogranulomatous pyelonephritis is a form of chronic pyelonephritis seen most frequently in middle-aged diabetic women and rarely in children. The disease is usually unilateral and is associated with prolonged obstructing nephrolithiasis. Patients often have nonspecific symptoms similar to those of acute pyelonephritis but have an enlarged kidney with calculi and a mass often indistinguishable from tumor. Proteus species are common causative agents. Nephrectomy is usually the treatment of choice, though a partial nephrectomy may be performed for focal disease. Histologic examination confirms the diagnosis following nephrectomy by the demonstration of foamy lipid-laden macrophages.

PAPILLARY NECROSIS

This disorder consists of ischemic necrosis of the renal papillae or of the entire pyramid. Excessive ingestion of analgesics, sickle cell trait, diabetes, obstruction with infection, and systemic conditions decreasing renal blood flow are common predisposing factors.

The symptoms are usually those of chronic cystitis with recurring exacerbations of pyelonephritis. Renal pain or renal colic may be present. Azotemic manifestations may be the presenting symptoms. In acute attacks, localized flank tenderness and generalized toxemia may occur. Laboratory findings consist of pyuria, hematuria, occasionally glycosuria, and acidosis. Impaired kidney function is shown by elevated serum creatinine and urea nitrogen. Intravenous urography usually shows impaired function and poor visualization in advanced cases. Evidence of ulceration, cavitation, or linear breaks in the base of the papillae and radiolucent defects due to sloughed papillae may be seen; the latter may become calcified. Retrograde urograms may be needed for proper imaging if kidney function is markedly impaired.

Preventive measures consist of proper management of diabetic patients with recurrent infections and avoidance of chronic use of analgesic compounds containing phenacetin and aspirin.

Intensive antibacterial therapy may be needed, though it is commonly unsuccessful in eradicating infection. Little can be done surgically except to remove obstructing papillae and correct predisposing factors (eg, reflux, obstruction) if identified.

In severe cases, the prognosis is poor. Renal transplantation may be required.

RENAL ABSCESS

While renal abscess is occasionally due to hematogenous spread of a distant staphylococcal infection, most abscesses are secondary to chronic nonspecific infection of the kidney, often complicated by stone formation. The onset may be acute, with high fever, but occasionally low-grade fever and general malaise are the presenting symptoms. Localized costovertebral angle tenderness and a palpable flank mass may be present. A mass may be evident on intravenous urograms, DTPA scans, sonograms, CT scans, or renal angiograms. If the abscess is due to hematogenous spread, the urine does not contain bacteria unless the abscess has broken into the pelvicaliceal system. More frequently, gram-negative organisms are found, as would be expected in light of the preponderance of ascending infection.

If organism sensitivity can be established by appropriate tests (blood and urine cultures and sensitivity tests), treatment with the proper antibiotic is indicated. Many infections have responded to percutaneous drainage and irrigation with antibiotic solutions, especially in cases of unilocular abscess cavity seen on either ultrasound or CT examination. In multilocular abscess or persistent bacteremia despite percutaneous drainage, surgical drainage or even heminephrectomy may be necessary.

When the abscess is found to be secondary to chronic renal infection, nephrectomy is usually indicated because of advanced destruction of the kidney.

PERINEPHRIC ABSCESS

Abscess between the renal capsule and the perirenal fascia most often results from rupture of an intrarenal abscess into the perinephric space. *E. coli* is the most common causative organism. The pathogenesis usually begins with severe pyonephrosis secondary to obstruction, as with renal or ureteral calculi. Clinical findings are similar to those of renal abscess. A pleural effusion on the affected side and signs of psoas muscle irritation are common. Abdominal plain films may show obliteration of the psoas muscle shadow, and an intravenous urogram may show poor concentration of contrast medium and hydronephrosis. CT scan is the current study of choice for diagnosis.

Treatment involves prompt drainage of the abscess and use of appropriate systemic antibiotics, including coverage of anaerobes. Percutaneous drainage is often successful; however, open surgical drainage is necessary if percutaneous drainage is incomplete.

CYSTITIS

Cystitis is more common in females and is usually an ascending infection. In males, it usually occurs in association with urethral or prostatic obstruction, prostatitis, foreign bodies, or tumors. The urinary bladder is normally capable of clearing bacterial inoculation unless an underlying pathologic process interferes with its defensive mechanisms.

In the acute phase, the principal symptoms of cystitis are dysuria, frequency, urgency, and hematuria; low-grade fever and suprapubic, perineal, and low back pain may be present. In chronic cystitis, irritative symptoms are usually milder.

Evidence of prostatitis, urethritis, or vaginitis may be present. Laboratory findings, in addition to hematuria, consist of bacteriuria and pyuria. Leukocytosis is not common. Urine culture identifies the organism. Cystoscopy is not advisable in the acute phase. In chronic cystitis, evidence of mucosal irritation may be present.

In any documented recurrent lower urinary tract infection (particularly in males), a complete urologic workup is indicated. Instrumentation is contraindicated in the acute phase, but cystoscopy is essential to identify the predisposing factor in chronic or recurrent bacterial cystitis. Upper tracts should be investigated with renal ultrasound when a lower tract source of infection is not identified.

Specific antibacterial therapy is given according to sensitivity testing of recovered organisms (*E. coli* in > 80% of cases). Sterilization of urine should usually be followed by a variable period of continuous antibiotic therapy (depending on the predisposing factor or the chronicity and recurrence of the disease). Prolonged suppressive medication is usually indicated in cases associated with voiding dysfunction.

In females with recurrent postcoital cystitis, premedication (eg, sulfonamides, nitrofurantoin) on the night of intercourse and the following day in addition to immediate postcoital voiding decreases recurrences.

PROSTATITIS

▶ Acute Bacterial Prostatitis

Acute bacterial prostatitis is a severe acute febrile illness caused by ascending coliform bacteria, which frequently colonize the male urethra. Symptoms include high fever, chills, low back and perineal pain, and urinary frequency and urgency with diminished stream or retention. On examination, the prostate is extremely tender, swollen, and warm to the touch. A fluctuant abscess may be palpable. The prostate must be examined cautiously, because vigorous palpation may cause acute septicemia. Laboratory findings include pyuria, bacteriuria, and leukocytosis.

Transurethral manipulation by catheter or cystoscopy should be avoided if possible; urinary retention should be treated by gently introducing a urethral catheter or introducing a percutaneous suprapubic tube. Treatment with systemic antibiotics (fluoroquinolones or aminoglycosides and ampicillin-cephalosporin) should be started immediately and should be adjusted later when results of urine culture or blood culture (or both) and sensitivity tests are known.

E. coli is found in 80% of cases. Treatment with oral antibiotics for several weeks after the initial phase has subsided is necessary to eradicate the bacteria completely.

Prostate abscess can develop from a smoldering acute prostatitis (typically gram negative bacteria) or from hematogenous seeding, often from gram-positive staphylococcus species. Pelvic imaging (CT, MRI, or ultrasound) identifies a hypodense fluid collection within the prostate parenchyma. Treatment includes a long course of culture-sensitive antibiotics and drainage of the abscess. Transrectal needle drainage and transurethral unroofing of the abscess are both successful modalities. Ultrasound-guided transrectal needle drainage can be done under local anesthesia, with or without intravenous sedation, whereas transurethral unroofing is performed with a resectoscope in the operating room, typically under general anesthesia. Thus, if feasible, it seems reasonable to attempt transrectal drainage first, and if the abscess recurs or persists then proceed to transurethral unroofing.

▶ **Chronic Prostatitis**

Chronic prostatitis is a common and complex problem. With differential diagnosis including urethritis, bacterial and nonbacterial prostatitis, prostatodynia (chronic pelvic pain syndrome [CPPS]), and seminal vesiculitis, assigning the correct diagnosis may challenge even the expert. The symptoms are varied and include suprapubic pain, low back pain, orchialgia, dysuria at the tip of the penis, and urinary frequency and urgency. The urinalysis may be normal. There may be a clear white urethral discharge. Prostate examination may be normal or reveal a soft, boggy prostate.

Expressed prostatic secretions may contain numerous leukocytes (> 10 per high-power field) in clumps as well as macrophages. Cultures of urine are usually sterile, but cultures of expressed prostatic secretions and urine obtained after prostatic massage are usually positive in bacterial prostatitis. *Chlamydia* or *Ureaplasma* may be an offending organism, particularly in men under age 35. Determination of the site of infection may require differential cultures. The first part of the voided urine stream is collected as VB_1 and the midstream specimen as VB_2. The prostate is then massaged to obtain expressed prostatic secretions, and the post-massage urine is collected as VB_3. The differential leukocyte and bacterial counts from each of these specimens can help localize the site of infection. If VB_1 has high levels of leukocytes and bacteria relative to the other specimens, urethritis is likely; if VB_2 has high levels, a site above the bladder neck is likely; and if the expressed prostatic secretions, VB_3, or both have high counts, prostatitis is likely.

For chronic bacterial prostatitis, at least a 4- to 6-week course of a fluoroquinolone or trimethoprim-sulfamethoxazole is often given. Surgical treatment for prostatitis is rarely indicated or helpful. Some patients improve following discontinuation of caffeine and alcohol, and a few respond to repeated prostatic massage. Patients with no evidence of bacterial infection or obstructive findings, and those who have recurrent pelvic pain in association with voiding dysfunction (eg, intermittent or weak urinary stream) may be treated with α-adrenergic blocking agents or biofeedback to decrease the internal and external sphincter tone. 5α-Reductase inhibitors may be helpful.

ACUTE EPIDIDYMITIS

Acute epididymitis is most commonly a disease of young males, caused by bacterial infection ascending from the urethra or prostate. The disease is less common in older males, but when it does occur, it is most often due to infection secondary to urinary tract obstruction or instrumentation.

The symptoms are sudden pain in the scrotum, rapid unilateral scrotal enlargement, and marked tenderness that extends to the spermatic cord in the groin and may be relieved by scrotal elevation **(Prehn's sign)**. Fever is present. An acute hydrocele may result, and secondary orchitis with a swollen, painful testicle may occur. Laboratory studies reveal pyuria, bacteriuria, and marked leukocytosis.

Epididymitis must be differentiated from torsion of the testis, testicular tumor, and tuberculous epididymitis. A technetium-99m pertechnetate scan reveals increased uptake with epididymitis but decreased uptake with torsion. Scrotal ultrasound distinguishes between the solid mass of a testicular tumor and an enlarged, inflamed epididymis and can also identify epididymal or testicular abscess, which requires operative treatment. Increased blood flow on Doppler ultrasound also helps distinguish epididymitis from torsion, though it is not completely reliable.

Cultured aspirates from inflamed epididymides of males under age 35 tend to show gonococci and chlamydiae; in men older than 35, *E. coli* is most common. Epididymal aspiration for culture is not required routinely, however. Pyuria with a negative urine culture suggests the presence of chlamydial infection in both prostate and epididymis. (See also section on Tuberculosis.)

Treatment consists of antibiotics, usually ceftriaxone and doxycycline in males under age 35 and fluoroquinolones in those over age 35. In some patients, pain is relieved by scrotal hypothermia, and consideration should be given to infiltration of the spermatic cord by 1% bupivacaine. Nonsteroidal anti-inflammatory drugs are recommended to aid in pain relief. In most instances, prompt treatment results in rapid resolution of pain, fever, and swelling. Patients must refrain from exertion for 1-3 weeks.

Exacerbations can be controlled by treating the predisposing factor. Chronic epididymitis rarely resolves completely; it has no consequences except, occasionally in bilateral cases, sterility due to scarring and obstruction of the delicate epididymal tubules. Rarely, epididymectomy is necessary for severe and refractory pain.

TUBERCULOSIS

Tuberculosis is a commonly missed genitourinary infection that should be considered in any case of pyuria without bacteriuria or in any case of urinary tract infection that does not respond to treatment.

Genitourinary tuberculosis is always secondary to pulmonary infection, though in many cases, the primary focus has healed or is quiescent. Infection occurs via the hematogenous route. The kidneys and (less commonly) the prostate are the principal sites of urinary tract involvement, though any part of the genitourinary system can be affected.

Pathology

Renal tuberculosis usually starts as a tuberculoma that gradually enlarges, caseates, and finally ulcerates, breaking into the pelvicaliceal system. Caseation and scarring are the principal pathologic features of renal tuberculosis. In the ureter, tuberculosis usually leads to distal strictures, periureteritis, and mural fibrosis.

In the bladder, the infection is characterized by areas of hyperemia and a coalescent group of tubercles, followed by ulcerations. Bladder wall fibrosis and contraction are the end results.

Urethral involvement in the male is uncommon but when present leads to urethral stricture, usually in the bulbous portion. Periurethral abscess and fistula are possible complications.

Genital tuberculosis may involve the prostate, seminal vesicles, and epididymides, either separately or in association with renal involvement. Tubercle formation with later caseation and fibrosis is the basic pathologic feature. The prostate becomes enlarged, with palpable nodules and an irregular consistency. The affected seminal vesicle is fibrotic and distended. Induration and thickening of the epididymis and beading of the vas deferens are characteristic findings. The testicles are rarely involved.

Clinical Findings

A. Symptoms and Signs

The patient commonly presents with lower urinary tract irritation, usually with pyuria. Less common manifestations are hematuria, renal pain, and renal colic.

B. Laboratory Findings

"Sterile" pyuria is the rule, but 15% of cases have secondary bacterial infection (eg, E. coli). Mycobacteria can be identified on an acid fast stain of the centrifuged sediment of the first morning urine collected on three successive days (positive in 90% of cases). Culture of the sediment should yield the mycobacteria, which may then be speciated by niacin and nitrate tests, both of which must be positive for a diagnosis of Mycobacterium tuberculosis.

C. Imaging Studies

Radiologic findings that suggest genitourinary tuberculosis include moth-eaten, caseous renal cavities, or bizarre, irregular calices. Strictures in straight, rigid, moderately dilated ureters and a contracted bladder with vesicoureteral reflux are all suggestive evidence.

Treatment

A. Medical Treatment

Tuberculosis must be treated as a systemic disease. Once the diagnosis is established, medical treatment is indicated regardless of the need for surgery. Whenever possible, medical treatment should be continued for at least 3 months before surgery is considered.

Active medications against tuberculosis include rifampin, isoniazid, pyrazinamide, ethambutol, and streptomycin. Standard initial treatment is with rifampin, isoniazid, and pyrazinamide for 8 weeks. Pyridoxine, 100 mg/d, is given in divided doses to counteract the vitamin B_6 depletion effect of isoniazid. In patients with more severe infections, ethambutol or streptomycin may be added to the initial treatment. Following the initial 8 weeks of therapy, rifampin and isoniazid are continued in combination three times per week for another 8 weeks. Liver function tests must be followed in view of the hepatotoxicity of rifampin, isoniazid, and pyrazinamide.

B. Surgical Measures

If medical therapy fails to cure a unilateral lesion, nephrectomy may be necessary. However, this is rare. In bilateral disease that has seriously damaged one kidney and is in an early stage in the other, unilateral nephrectomy may be considered; in localized polar lesions, partial nephrectomy may be done.

In unilateral epididymal involvement, epididymectomy plus contralateral vasectomy is indicated to prevent descent of the infection to the prostate; bilateral epididymectomy should be done if both sides are involved.

For a severely contracted bladder, augmentation enterocystoplasty increases vesical capacity following eradication of the infection.

Prognosis

In a high percentage of cases, cure is obtained by medical means. Unilateral renal lesions have the best prognosis.

Schneeberger C, Geerlings SE, Middleton P, Crowther CA: Interventions for preventing recurrent urinary tract infection during pregnancy. Cochrane Database Syst Rev 2012 Nov 14;11:CD009279. doi: 10.1002/14651858.CD009279 .pub2. Review. PMID: 23152271.

Williams G, Craig JC: Long-term antibiotics for preventing recurrent urinary tract infection in children. Cochrane Database Syst Rev. 2011 Mar 16;(3):CD001534. doi: 10.1002/14651858 .CD001534.pub3. Review. PMID: 21412872.

Widmer M, Gülmezoglu AM, Mignini L, Roganti A: Duration of treatment for asymptomatic bacteriuria during pregnancy. Cochrane Database Syst Rev 2011 Dec 7;(12):CD000491. doi: 10.1002/14651858.CD000491.pub2. Review. PMID: 22161364.

CALCULI

RENEL STONE

General Considerations

Stone disease is common, with the lifetime risk of stone formation in the United States exceeding 12% in males and 6% in females. Prevalence of stone disease varies by racial background and geographic location within the United States, with older white males and southeastern states having the highest prevalence. Seventy-five percent of most stones are composed of calcium salts (oxalate and phosphate), while uric acid and struvite stones (magnesium-ammonium phosphate stones that form secondary to urea-splitting organisms) constitute 10% each. Formation of calcium stones can be due to one or multiple factors that include hypercalciuria, hypocitraturia, hyperoxaluria, and hyperuricosuria. In patients with hyperparathyroidism or those who ingest large amounts of calcium or vitamin D or in patients who are dehydrated or immobilized, hypercalciuria promotes stone formation.

Uric acid stones form in acidic urine. Cystine stones, which make up 1% of all stones, usually form secondary to impaired renal reabsorption of cystine. Owing to the radiodensity of sulfur, cystine stones are radiopaque (albeit less so than calcium stones), whereas uric acid stones are radiolucent. Stones that obstruct the ureteropelvic junction or ureter lead to hydronephrosis and possibly infection.

Clinical Findings

A. Symptoms and Signs

If the stone acutely obstructs the ureteropelvic junction or a calix, moderate to severe renal pain is noted, often accompanied by nausea, vomiting, and ileus. The pain starts in the upper lateral back and may radiate anteriorly and inferiorly toward the groin. Gross or microscopic hematuria is common. Symptoms of infection, if present, are exacerbated. Nonobstructing calculi are usually painless. This includes staghorn calculi, which may form a cast of all calices and the pelvis. In the symptomatic patient, there may be costovertebral angle tenderness and a quiet abdomen. Infection secondary to obstruction may lead to high fever and a rigid abdomen.

B. Laboratory Findings

With acute infection, leukocytosis is to be expected. Urinalysis may reveal red and white blood cells and bacteria. A pH of 7.6 or higher implies the presence of urea-splitting organisms. A pH consistently below 5.5 is compatible with the formation of uric acid or cystine stones. If the pH is fixed between 6.0 and 7.0, renal tubular acidosis should be considered as a cause of nephrocalcinosis. Crystals of uric acid (rhomboid) or cystine (hexagonal) in the urine are suggestive. A 24-hour urine collection can help identify the metabolic effect that predisposes to stone formation (hypercalciuria, hypocitraturia, hyperoxaluria). Hypercalciuria can be resorptive (due to hyperparathyroidism), absorptive (increased gastrointestinal absorption), or renal (increased urine loss of calcium). Citrate is a stone inhibitor and hypocitraturia predisposes to stone formation.

Increases in urine calcium and phosphate plus hypercalcemia (and hypophosphatemia) suggest the presence of hyperparathyroidism, and measurement of serum parathyroid hormone is helpful. Excessive urinary uric acid is compatible with uric acid stone formation.

A qualitative test for urinary cystine should be part of the routine evaluation. If levels are elevated, a 24-hour quantitative measurement should be made. Hyperchloremic acidosis suggests distal renal tubular acidosis with secondary renal calcifications. Total renal function is impaired only if the stones are bilateral, and particularly if chronic infection complicates the clinical presentation.

C. Imaging Studies

About 90% of calculi are radiopaque; the majority are calcium stones and can be seen on plain x-ray. However, stones smaller than 5 mm can be difficult to see on plain x-ray, and bowel gas may obscure stone visualization as well.

Renal ultrasound can be an excellent initial and follow-up imaging modality to identify renal calculi, although results depend on the quality of the sonographer. Stones are hyperechoic and cast an acoustic shadow. Small stones can be missed on ultrasound and sizing estimates can be poor. Hydronephrosis implies a downstream obstruction in the ureter, possibly from obstructing calculus, but ureteral stones are poorly visualized with ultrasound.

Spiral (helical) CT has become the study of choice, because the entire urinary tract can be scanned rapidly and without contrast injection (Figure 38–10). Calculi can be readily identified and distinguished from clot or tumor. Stones are accurately sized and localized with CT, and the anatomic detail is very helpful prior to operative intervention. CT scans deliver significant doses of ionizing radiation, making ultrasound an attractive initial modality to look for stones or obstruction, followed by CT for confirmation and more anatomic detail.

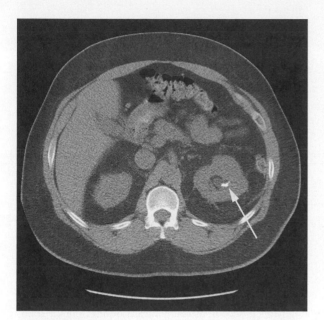

▲ **Figure 38–10.** CT scan without intravenous contrast demonstrating a left renal calculus (arrow).

D. Stone Analysis

If a stone has previously been passed or if one is recovered, its chemical composition should be analyzed. Such information may be useful when planning a preventive program.

▶ Differential Diagnosis

Acute pyelonephritis may begin with acute renal pain mimicking that of renal stone. Urinalysis reveals pyuria, and urograms or CT fails to reveal a calculus.

Renal adenocarcinoma may bleed into the tumor, causing acute pain mimicking that of an obstructing stone. Imaging can make the differentiation.

Transitional cell tumors of the renal pelvis or calices mimic uric acid stone; both are radiolucent. CT scan without contrast or ultrasound reveal the stone by virtue of increased density compared with adjacent soft tissues.

Renal tuberculosis is complicated by stone formation in 10% of cases. Pyuria without bacteriuria is suggestive. Urography reveals the moth-eaten calices typical of tuberculosis.

Papillary necrosis may cause renal colic if a sloughed papilla obstructs the ureteropelvic junction. Imaging (particularly CT) settles the issue.

Renal infarction may cause renal pain and hematuria. Evidence of a cardiac lesion, nonfunction of the kidney on urography, and exclusion of a calculus help in differentiation. Infarction is confirmed by angiography, radioisotopic renography, or color Doppler ultrasound.

Other conditions to be considered in the differential diagnosis include UPJO, obstruction due to blood clots, ureteral strictures or fungal bezoars, and renal abscess.

▶ Complications

Acting as a foreign body, a stone increases the probability of infection. However, primary infection may incite stone formation. A stone lodged in the ureteropelvic junction leads to progressive hydronephrosis. A staghorn calculus, as it grows, may destroy renal tissue by pressure, and the infection that is usually present also contributes to renal damage. The presence of an obstructed renal unit with associated infection should be considered a urologic emergency. Drainage of the kidney should be performed promptly with insertion of a ureteral stent or percutaneous nephrostomy tube. Obstruction without infection can be managed without immediate drainage if renal function is preserved and pain is controlled (see ureteral calculi section below). Persistent obstruction for longer than 2-4 weeks requires intervention because permanent renal damage can ensue.

▶ Prevention

An effective preventive regimen depends on stone analysis and chemical studies of the serum and urine.

A. General Measures

Ensure a high fluid intake (3-4 L/d) to keep solutes well diluted. This measure alone may decrease stone-forming potential by 50%. Treat infection, relieve stasis or obstruction, and advise the patient to avoid prolonged immobilization.

B. Specific Measures

1. Calcium stones—Remove the parathyroid tumor, if present. High dietary sodium promotes renal calcium absorption, and restriction to 100 mEq/d may be helpful. Limitation of proteins and carbohydrates may also reduce hypercalciuria. Recent randomized trials have shown that in men with recurrent calcium oxalate stones and hypercalciuria, restricted intake of animal protein and salt, combined with a normal calcium intake, provides greater protection than the traditional low-calcium diet. Potassium citrate can decrease stone formation by increasing urine levels of citrate, which is a stone inhibitor.

Oral orthophosphates are effective in reducing the stone-forming potential of urine by decreasing urine calcium and increasing inhibitor activity. Thiazide diuretics such as hydrochlorothiazide, 50 mg twice daily, decrease the calcium content in urine by 50%. If hyperuricosuria is coincident with calcium urolithiasis, then allopurinol and urinary alkalinization can reduce the formation of urate crystals, which may act as a nidus for calcium crystallization.

For a patient with primary absorptive hypercalciuria, cellulose sodium phosphate can be given. This substance combines with calcium in the gut to prevent absorption.

2. Oxalate stones (calcium oxalate)—Consider a phosphate or a thiazide diuretic (see above). Elimination of excessive oxalate in coffee, tea, colas, leafy green vegetables, and chocolate may also be helpful. Excess vitamin C can be metabolized to oxalate and thus should be avoided.

3. Magnesium-ammonium-phosphate stones—These stones are usually secondary to urinary tract infection due to bacteria that produce urease (primarily proteus species). Eradication of the infection prevents further stone formation but is impossible when stones are present. Acetohydroxamic acid, a urease inhibitor, can be used for oral chemolysis and can potentiate antibiotic action. After all calculi have been removed, prevention of stone growth is best accomplished by urinary acidification and suppression antibiotic therapy.

4. Metabolic stones (uric acid, cystine)—These substances are most soluble at a pH of 7.0 or higher. Give potassium citrate, 10-20 mEq by mouth three times a day, and monitor the urine pH with a litmus paper indicator or urine dipstick test. For uric acid stone formers, limit purines in the diet and give allopurinol if they have hyperuricemia. Patients with mild cystinuria may need only urinary alkalinization, as described previously. For severe cystinuria, penicillamine, 30 mg/kg/d orally, reduces urinary cystine to safe levels. Penicillamine should be supplemented with pyridoxine, 50 mg/d orally. Tiopronin, which has fewer side effects than D-penicillamine and captopril, can be used as well.

▶ **Treatment**

A. Conservative Measures

Intervention is not required for small, nonobstructive, asymptomatic caliceal stones. Hydration and dietary management may be sufficient to prevent growth of existing or new calcium stones in patients without metabolic abnormalities. Those with identifiable metabolic disorders may benefit from the specific measures described previously. Patients with known uric acid stones can be treated with hydration and urinary alkalinization, which can help dissolve the stone. Patients with active infection, obstruction, or intractable nausea or pain may need definitive treatment. In the acute setting, a ureteral stent or percutaneous nephrostomy tube can be inserted.

B. Ureteroscopic Intervention

Patients with small stones can be managed with ureteronephroscopy and laser lithotripsy or basketing of the stones. The presence of a ureteral stent several days prior helps passively dilate the ureter and facilitates the procedure, but new, smaller caliber ureteroscopes preclude the need for elective preoperative stenting. As described above, stents should be placed emergently in the setting of infection/sepsis with obstructing calculus. After stenting and an appropriate course of antibiotics (typically 10-14 days), the definitive stone surgery is undertaken. Post-operatively, a ureteral stent is often left in place for several days to prevent acute obstruction secondary to edema or small stone fragments.

C. Percutaneous Intervention (Endourology)

In selected patients with symptomatic or large upper tract stones, percutaneous stone removal may be indicated. A percutaneous tract enters the renal collecting system through an appropriate calix (**percutaneous nephrostomy**). The tract is subsequently dilated, and endoscopic extraction of the stones (**percutaneous nephroscopy** and **percutaneous nephrolithotomy [PCNL]**) is done. Pulverization of the fragments is accomplished by means of ultrasonic, electrohydraulic, or laser probes passed through the nephrostomy tract. For cystine and uric acid stones, alkaline or other irrigants that increase the specific crystal solubility may be used (eg, N-acetyl-L-lysine or propionyl glycine for cystine stones). Specific antibiotic treatment for infection must be given before irrigation to prevent sepsis.

Success with these endourologic methods approaches 100%. The advantages over surgical procedures include no incision and rapid recovery and return to full activity. Disadvantages include the occasional need for multiple treatments to completely remove the calculi and the uncommon occurrence of significant hemorrhage, collecting system perforation, or stricture.

D. Extracorporeal Shock Wave Lithotripsy

With this technique, patients are positioned in the path of shock waves focused on the renal calculi with the aid of fluoroscopy or ultrasound. General or regional anesthesia is required in selected patients, but sedation may be sufficient. The shock waves (more than 1500 are usually given) pulverize the stones, and the small particles pass spontaneously in the postoperative period. With appropriate patient selection, results are excellent. Lower pole renal stones have lower success rates because pulverized fragments are less likely to completely pass. In addition, stones greater than 1.5 cm may produce to many fragments to successfully pass. PCNL is the treatment of choice for larger stones greater than 1.5-2.0 cm. Calcium stones and magnesium-ammonium-phosphate stones have been treated successfully. Because of the physical properties of the crystal lattice, extracorporeal shock wave lithotripsy (ESWL) is not as effective in fragmenting cystine stones. Radiolucent uric acid stones, which can be visualized using contrast medium are amenable to ESWL treatment. A variety of ESWL devices now effectively pulverize stones using less energy and thus can be used with only intravenous sedation; an increased number of pulses are required to obtain the same results as with previous higher energy devices. Some instruments use ultrasound instead of x-ray for stone localization. Complications include incomplete fragmentation and need for secondary procedures, ureteral obstruction from stone fragments, and perinephric hematoma.

E. Open and Laparoscopic Surgical Removal of Stones

Endourologic intervention and ESWL have markedly decreased the indications for open surgery. Rarely, both percutaneous nephrolithotomy and ESWL are contraindicated, and open nephrolithotomy is necessary. The goal of any approach is to remove all stone fragments, and the approach chosen must allow for intraoperative localization by radiography or ultrasonography. Incisions into the renal pelvis (pyelolithotomy) or the renal parenchyma (radial nephrotomy or anatrophic nephrolithotomy) may be required for complete stone removal. Instillation of a mixture of thrombin and calcium into the kidney causes the fragments to become trapped in a dense clot, which is removed through a pyelotomy incision (coagulum pyelolithotomy). Operative nephroscopy allows a full view of all the calices and removal of all fragments. "Bench" surgery with autotransplantation of the kidney may be required in very few instances. Rarely, poorly functioning kidneys containing symptomatic stones require nephrectomy, especially in cases of XGP. Laparoscopic and robotic pyelolithotomy have been used with excellent success and decreased morbidity compared with open surgery. This is especially the case in patients undergoing concomitant robotic pyeloplasty for UPJ obstruction.

▶ Prognosis

The recurrence rate of renal stone can be as high as 40% and can be decreased with sufficient attention to measures for prevention of stone formation. The danger of recurrent stones is progressive renal damage due to obstruction and infection.

URETERAL STONE

▶ General Considerations

Ureteral stones originate in the kidney. When symptoms occur, ureteral obstruction is implicit and renal function endangered. Complicating infection may occur. Most ureteral stones pass spontaneously, or with the assistance of medical expulsive therapy, especially if they are less than 0.5 cm in greatest dimension.

▶ Clinical Findings

A. Symptoms and Signs

The onset of pain is usually abrupt. Pain is felt in the costovertebral angle and radiates to the ipsilateral lower abdominal quadrant. Nausea, vomiting, abdominal distention, and gross hematuria are common. When the stone approaches the bladder, symptoms mimic cystitis, with frequency and urgency. If the kidney is infected, acute ureteral obstruction exacerbates the infection.

The patient is usually in such agony that only parenteral opioids and NSAIDS will give relief. Costovertebral angle tenderness and guarding may be evident. Absence of bowel sounds and abdominal distention signify ileus. Fever may occur as a result of complicating renal infection.

B. Laboratory Findings

Laboratory findings are similar to those for renal stone. Unilateral obstruction secondary to ureteral stone may cause acute exacerbation of renal function, but not in all cases.

C. Imaging Studies

CT stone protocol is the gold standard to confirm stone size, location and degree of obstruction (Figure 38–11). Plain films may reveal an opacity in the region of the ureter and ultrasound will demonstrate ipsilateral hydronephrosis. Excretory urograms and retrograde urography reveal a filling defect (lack of dye) at the location of the stone. Almost all

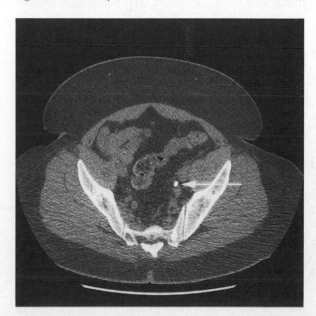

▲ **Figure 38–11.** CT scan without intravenous contrast demonstrating a left ureteral calculus (arrow).

stones are radiopaque on CT scan. The density (hardness) of the stone can be estimated using the Hounsfield Units (HU). Calcium based stones are, on average, more than 1000 HU. Uric acid and struvite (infection) stones have lower HU.

Differential Diagnosis

A tumor of the kidney or renal pelvis may bleed, and passage of a blood clot may cause ureteral colic. Urograms may reveal a radiolucent area in the ureter surrounded by the radiopaque urine. A CT scan with and without contrast agents reveals no radiopacity in the ureter and helps define the renal parenchymal or renal pelvis tumor.

A primary tumor of the ureter may cause obstructing pain and hematuria. The urogram reveals the ureteral filling defect, often with secondary obstruction. A CT scan can differentiate a stone from tumor. Urinary cytologic study may reveal malignant urothelial cells.

Acute pyelonephritis may cause pain as severe as that seen with stone. Pyuria and bacteriuria are found but do not rule out stone. Stone is absent on noncontrast CT or urography.

A sloughed papilla (consequent to conditions such as diabetes mellitus) traversing the ureter may cause colic and produces a urogram compatible with uric acid stone. Papillary sloughs should be evident, however.

▶ Complications

If obstruction from the ureteral stone is prolonged, progressive renal damage may ensue. Bilateral stones may cause oliguria or anuria, requiring immediate drainage of the proximal collecting system with indwelling ureteral stents or percutaneous nephrostomy. Unilateral obstructing stone in patients with a solitary kidney requires immediate drainage.

Infection may supervene, but many renal infections are iatrogenic (ie, introduced at the time of stone manipulation).

▶ Prevention

See Renal Stone.

▶ Treatment

A. General Measures

Most ureteral stones pass spontaneously—particularly those less than 0.5 cm in diameter. Once the diagnosis has been established, analgesics should be given and the patient hydrated. Recent reports have found alpha-antagonist therapy useful in expulsion of distal ureteral stones by relaxing smooth muscle. Randomized controlled trials have confirmed shorter time to stone passage with the use of alpha antagonists when compared with placebo. Periodic plain films should be taken to follow the progress of the stone and interval renal ultrasound studies obtained to assess the degree of hydronephrosis. The urine should be strained until the stone passes in order to recover the calculus for analysis. With larger stones, acute obstruction can be temporarily relieved by inserting an indwelling ureteral stent.

B. Specific Measures

If the stone causes intractable pain, progressive hydronephrosis, or acute infection, it should be removed. Obstructing stones in the upper two-thirds of the ureter can often be successfully treated by ureteroscopy or ESWL, with or without ureteral stent insertion to help facilitate stone passage. Ureteroscopy permits laser fragmentation or stone basket retrieval under direct vision. Open and laparoscopic/robotic surgical removal (ureterolithotomy) is only very rarely required for very large ureteral stones. ESWL has been applied to ureteral stones in the proximal ureter but is more problematic in the distal ureter owing to bone interference by surrounding pelvis, which interferes with imaging and attenuates shock wave force. Ureteral stones which have not spontaneously passed with medical expulsive therapy after 4 weeks should be considered for surgical removal with the above techniques.

▶ Prognosis

About 80% of ureteral stones pass spontaneously. Stones larger than 1 cm rarely pass spontaneously. Periodic clinical evaluation, plain films, and renal ultrasound should be performed to document ureteral stone passage and prevent long-term renal damage from obstruction. Patients often do not witness small stones pass if a strainer is not utilized. If still uncertain about definitive stone passage, repeat CT scan can be obtained with the caveat of additional radiation exposure.

VESICAL STONE

Primary vesical calculi are rare in the United States but are common in Southeast Asia and the Middle East. The cause is probably dietary. Secondary stones usually complicate vesical outlet obstruction with residual urine and infection; 90% of those affected are men. Other causes of bladder stasis such as neurogenic bladder, and bladder diverticula also promote vesical stone formation. They are common in vesical schistosomiasis or in association with radiation cystitis. Foreign bodies in the bladder may act as a nidus for the precipitation of urinary salts. Most stones contain uric acid or struvite (in infected urine).

▶ Clinical Findings

A. Symptoms and Signs

Symptoms of bladder neck obstruction are elicited. There may be sudden interruption of the stream and urethral pain if a stone occludes the bladder neck during voiding.

Hematuria is common. Vesical distention may be noted; evidence of urethral stricture or an enlarged prostate is usually found.

B. Laboratory Findings

Pyuria and hematuria are almost always present.

C. Imaging Studies

Vesical calculi may be missed on plain x-rays due to the high component of radiolucent uric acid. Excretory urograms reveal a filling defect in the bladder and ultrasound reveals a large echogenic shadowing focus. CT scan easily identifies the number and size of the stones. Cystoscopy directly visualizes the stone(s) and also evaluates the entire urethra for stricture and/or prostate hypertrophy.

▶ Differential Diagnosis

A pedunculated vesical tumor may suddenly occlude the vesical neck during voiding. Excretory urograms, pelvic ultrasound, CT scan, or cystoscopy leads to definitive diagnosis.

Extravesical opacifications may simulate stones on a plain film.

▶ Complications

Acting as foreign bodies, bladder stones exacerbate urine infection and can cause obstruction at the level of the bladder neck. Antibiotic therapy for concomitant UTI is often unsuccessful given that the stones harbor persistent bacteria.

▶ Prevention

Prevention requires relief of the primary obstruction, removal of the stones, and sterilization of the urine.

▶ Treatment

A. General Measures

Analgesics should be given for pain and antimicrobials for control of infection until the stones can be removed.

B. Specific Measure

Small stones can be removed or crushed transurethrally (**cystolitholopaxy**). Larger stones are often disintegrated by transurethral electrohydraulic lithotripsy (shock wave–generating probe) or laser destruction, or they may require suprapubic transvesical removal (vesicolithotomy). If the nidus for stone formation is urinary stasis due to BPH, concomitant TURP or suprapubic transvesical prostatectomy should be performed at the time of stone removal.

▶ Prognosis

Recurrent vesical stone is uncommon if the obstruction and infection are treated.

NEPHROCALCINOSIS

Nephrocalcinosis is a precipitation of calcium in the tubules, parenchyma, and, occasionally, the glomeruli. It always causes renal functional impairment, often severe. Stones may be found in the calices and pelvis. The common causes are primary or secondary hyperparathyroidism, excessive milk-alkali or vitamin D intake, or they may be found with severe renal damage associated with renal tubular acidosis, or sarcoidosis. Calcifications may also be seen in the skin, lungs, stomach, spleen, and corneas, or around the joints.

▶ Clinical Findings

A. Symptoms and Signs

There are no specific symptoms. In childhood, the patient may merely fail to thrive. Stones or sand may be passed. The complaints are usually those of the primary disease. Physical examination may reveal an enlarged parathyroid gland, corneal calcifications, and pseudorickets.

B. Laboratory Findings

The urine may be infected. In renal tubular acidosis, the pH is fixed between 6.0 and 7.0. Urinary calcium is high in hyperparathyroidism, both primary and secondary. Tests of renal function are depressed; uremia is common. Hypercalcemia and hypophosphatemia are seen with primary hyperparathyroidism; secondary hyperparathyroidism may be associated with a low serum calcium and an elevated serum phosphate. Hyperchloremic acidosis and hypokalemia accompany renal tubular acidosis.

C. Imaging Studies

A plain x-ray reveals punctate calcifications in the papillae of the kidneys. Caliceal or pelvic stones may also be noted. The pattern of calcification may have to be differentiated from renal tuberculosis and medullary sponge kidney.

▶ Complications

Complications include renal damage caused by the calcifications and renal and ureteral calculi. Chronic renal infection may complicate the primary disease.

▶ Treatment & Prognosis

The primary cause should be treated if possible (eg, parathyroidectomy). Hydration with isotonic saline along with furosemide can help enhance calcium excretion. Discontinue vitamin D and milk-alkali producers if the primary cause was due to excessive intake. With hyperchloremic acidosis, alkalinize the urine with potassium citrate. Osteomalacia requires administration of vitamin D and calcium even though nephrocalcinosis is present.

If nephrocalcinosis is secondary to primary renal disease, the outlook is poor. If the cause is correctable and renal function is fairly good, the prognosis is more favorable.

Aboumarzouk OM, Kata SG, Keeley FX, McClinton S, Nabi G: Extracorporeal shock wave lithotripsy (ESWL) versus ureteroscopic management for ureteric calculi. Cochrane Database Syst Rev 2012 May 16;5:CD006029. doi: 10.1002/14651858 .CD006029.pub4. Review. PMID: 22592707.

GENITOURINARY TRACT TRAUMA

INJURIES TO THE KIDNEY

▶ General Considerations

Renal injury is uncommon but potentially serious and often accompanied by multisystem trauma. The most common causes are athletic, industrial, or automobile accidents. The degree of injury may range from contusion to laceration of the parenchyma or disruption of the renal pedicle.

▶ Clinical Findings

A. Symptoms and Signs

Gross hematuria following trauma means injury to the urinary tract. Pain and tenderness over the renal area may be significant but could be due to musculoskeletal injury. Hemorrhagic shock may result from renal laceration and lead to oliguria. Nausea, vomiting, and abdominal distention (ileus) are the rule. Physical examination may reveal ecchymosis or penetrating injury in the costovertebral angle or flank. Extravasation of blood or urine may produce a palpable flank mass. Other injuries should be sought.

B. Laboratory Findings

Serial hematocrit determinations will give clues to persistent bleeding. Hematuria is to be expected, but the absence of hematuria does not exclude renal injury (as in renal vascular injury).

C. Imaging Studies

A plain film may reveal obliteration of the psoas shadow; this suggests the presence of a retroperitoneal hematoma or urinary extravasation. Bowel gas may be displaced from the area. Evidence of transverse vertebral process or rib fractures may be noted. In the past, the excretory urogram was used for evaluating renal trauma. Excretory urograms may show a normal kidney if it is mildly contused or may show extravasation of contrast medium if the kidney is lacerated. Nonfunction suggests injury to the vascular pedicle. The excretory urogram should demonstrate that the contralateral kidney is normal. CT scan with intravenous contrast medium is now the method of choice for staging a patient with hemodynamically stable renal trauma. CT scans may miss urinary extravasation if performed too rapidly following intravenous contrast administration—before the contrast is excreted into the collecting system and ureter. Therefore, trauma protocol CT scans should include a delayed phase of imaging, allowing time for contrast to be excreted in to the collecting system. If renal vascular damage is suspected and the patient's condition is stable, preoperative renal angiography may facilitate planning of renovascular reconstruction or permit arterial stenting. In special circumstances, selective renal artery embolization may control segmental arterial bleeding. Renal imaging is indicated in any adult with gross hematuria or microscopic hematuria with shock. Imaging is also required with deceleration injuries and is indicated in children with gross or microscopic hematuria in the setting of trauma.

▶ Differential Diagnosis

Bony fractures or contusion of soft tissues in the region of the kidney may cause confusion. Hematuria might be secondary to ureteral or vesical injury. The absence of a perirenal mass (ie, hematoma or urinoma) or contrast extravasation on urograms or CT scan would rule out significant trauma.

▶ Complications

A. Early

The most serious complication is continued perirenal hemorrhage, which may be fatal. Serial hematocrit, blood pressure, and pulse determinations are essential. Serial CT scans may also be useful. Evidence of an enlarging flank mass implies persistent bleeding. In most cases, bleeding stops spontaneously, probably as a result of tamponade by the perirenal fascia. Delayed bleeding 1 or 2 weeks later is rare. Infection of the perirenal hematoma may occur.

B. Late

History, examination, and imaging are recommended 1-3 months after management of renal trauma to look for persistent renal damage from prolonged perinephric hematoma, obstruction, and/or urinary extravasation. Ultrasound is a good imaging modality to evaluate the integrity of the kidney and to assess for residual perinephric fluid collections and/or hydronephrosis. The blood pressure should be checked at regular intervals, because hypertension may be a late sequela.

▶ Treatment

Treat shock and hemorrhage with fluids and transfusion. Most patients with blunt renal trauma stop bleeding and heal spontaneously. Bed rest is indicated until hematuria resolves and blood counts stabilize. If bleeding persists, angiography with possible segmental arterial embolization is an option if the patient is hemodynamically stable. Persistent hemodynamic instability requires laparotomy with renorrhaphy or nephrectomy.

Penetrating renal trauma usually requires exploration. Lacerations may be sutured, the collecting system closed, and urinary extravasation drained. Nephrectomy or partial nephrectomy may be necessary to remove devitalized tissue and secure the collecting system.

Late complications may occur. Perinephric abscess/infected hematoma should be drained. Hypertension may be due to renal ischemia and requires medical or surgical correction.

▶ Prognosis

Most injured kidneys heal spontaneously, though the patient must be examined at intervals for the onset of hypertension due to renal ischemia or progressive hydronephrosis due to secondary ureteral stricture. Many patients with genitourinary trauma have associated injuries. In most cases, death is due to associated injury rather than renal injury.

INJURIES TO THE URETER

▶ General Considerations

Most ureteral injuries are iatrogenic in the course of pelvic surgery. Ureteral injury may occur during transurethral bladder or prostate resection or ureteral manipulation for stone or tumor. Ureteral injury is rarely a consequence of penetrating trauma. Unintentional ureteral ligation during operation on adjacent organs may be asymptomatic, though hydronephrosis and loss of renal function results. Ureteral division leads to extravasation and urinoma.

▶ Clinical Findings

A. Symptoms

If the ureteral injury is not recognized at surgery, the patient may complain of flank and lower abdominal pain on the injured side. Ileus and pyelonephritis may develop. Later, urine may drain through the wound (or through the vagina following transvaginal surgery) or there may be increased output through a surgical drain. Wound drainage may be evaluated by comparing creatinine levels found in the drainage fluid with serum levels; urine exhibits very high creatinine levels when compared with serum. Intravenous administration of 5 mL of indigo carmine causes the urine to appear blue-green; therefore, drainage from a ureterocutaneous fistula becomes blue, compared to serous drainage. Anuria following pelvic surgery not responding to intravenous fluids may rarely signify bilateral ureteral ligation or injury. Peritoneal signs may occur if urine leaks into the peritoneal cavity.

B. Laboratory Findings

Microscopic hematuria is usually found but may be absent. Tests of renal function may be normal unless both ureters are occluded. Drainage fluid will have increased levels of creatinine when compared with serum creatinine.

C. Imaging Studies

Excretory urograms may show evidence of ureteral occlusion. Extravasation of radiopaque fluid may be seen in the region of the ureter. Retrograde ureterography depicts the site and nature (occlusion or division) of the injury.

Ultrasonography may reveal hydroureter and hydronephrosis or a fluid mass representing urinary extravasation. CT urography (including delayed phase imaging) identifies the location of the ureteral injury, surrounding urinary extravasation, and potential urinoma or fistula.

▶ Differential Diagnosis

Ureteral injury may mimic peritonitis if urine leaks into the peritoneal cavity. Excretory urography reveals the ureteral involvement.

Oliguria may be due to dehydration, transfusion reaction, or bilateral incomplete ureteral injury. A survey of fluid and electrolyte intake and output, including serial body weights, should prove helpful in delineating a medical versus surgical etiology for oliguria. Nephrology consultation should be considered. Total anuria may signify bilateral ureteral injury and indicates the need for immediate urologic evaluation.

Vesicovaginal and ureterovaginal fistulas may be confused. Methylene blue solution instilled into the bladder stains the vaginal drainage in the case of vesicovaginal fistula. Cystoscopy may show the vesical defect. Retrograde ureterography should reveal a ureteral fistula. The presence of both injuries occurring simultaneously should also be considered and evaluated.

▶ Complications

These include urinary fistula, ureteral obstruction or stenosis with hydronephrosis, renal infection, peritonitis, and uremia (with bilateral injury).

▶ Prevention

Before operation for large pelvic masses, which may cause displacement of the ureters, catheters should be placed in the ureters to facilitate their identification at surgery. Although the catheters may not prevent injury, they facilitate recognition of a ureteral injury intraoperatively and allow for immediate repair.

▶ **Treatment**

A. Injury Recognized at Surgery

1. Ureteral division—Repair of a ureter inadvertently cut during surgery consists of anastomosis of the ends over an indwelling stent (ureteroureterostomy), reimplanting the ureter into the bladder if the injury is juxtavesical (neoureterocystostomy), or anastomosing the proximal segment of divided ureter to the side of the contralateral ureter (transureteroureterostomy). The anastomosis must be tension free, and the area of repair must be drained. Injuries resulting from cautery must be adequately debrided prior to reanastomosis.

2. Ureteral resection—Repair of a ureter from which a substantial segment has been removed requires interposition of a ureteral substitute or mobilization of the proximal and distal ureter to provide a tension-free anastomosis. With loss of the distal ureter, the bladder may be hitched cephalad to the psoas muscle, or a bladder flap may be created to facilitate a ureteral implant. In extreme cases, autotransplant of the kidney to the pelvis or bowel interposition may be necessary.

B. Injury Discovered After Surgery

Early intervention is recommended as soon as the ureteral injury is recognized. Depending on the findings, any of the procedures noted above may be utilized. If a long segment of ureter is not viable, an intestinal ureter may be constructed. If hydronephrosis is advanced or if sepsis develops, percutaneous nephrostomy should precede repair. When the patient's condition is stable, definitive repair can be accomplished. If the injury is partial or incomplete, attempted ureteral stent placement for 4-6 weeks followed by repeat evaluation may obviate the need for laparotomy and open repair. Delayed nephrectomy may be indicated if the repair is unsuccessful and the contralateral kidney is normal.

▶ **Prognosis**

In cases of iatrogenic injury, the results are best if the injury is recognized at the time of surgery. Late repair, if severe periureteral fibrosis has developed, is less likely to afford a good outcome.

INJURIES TO THE BLADDER

▶ **General Considerations**

The most common cause of vesical injury is an external blow over a full bladder. Rupture of the organ is seen in 15% of patients with pelvic fracture. The bladder may be inadvertently opened during pelvic surgery or injured by cystoscopic maneuvers (eg, transurethral resection of bladder tumor). If the injury is intraperitoneal (40% of all bladder ruptures), blood and urine will extravasate into the peritoneal cavity, producing signs of peritonitis. If it is extraperitoneal (54% of all bladder ruptures), a mass develops in the pelvis. About 6% of all bladder ruptures have a combination of both intraperitoneal and extraperitoneal extravasation.

▶ **Clinical Findings**

A. Symptoms and Signs

There is usually a history of hypogastric or pelvic trauma. Hematuria and suprapubic pain and possible inability to void are expected. Associated injury may cause hemorrhagic shock. There is suprapubic tenderness and guarding. Intraperitoneal extravasation causes peritoneal signs, while extraperitoneal extravasation results in formation of a pelvic urinoma.

B. Laboratory Findings

A falling hematocrit reflects continued bleeding. Hematuria is expected in patients who are able to void. A patient who cannot void should be catheterized unless pelvic fracture (and urethral injury) is suspected or blood is noted at the urethral meatus.

C. Imaging Studies

A plain film may reveal fracture of the pelvis. An extraperitoneal collection of blood and urine may displace the bowel gas laterally or out of the pelvis. If bladder trauma is suspected, cystography should precede excretory urography. Extravasation is most reliably demonstrated by a postdrainage cystogram film showing persistent contrast outside the area of the suspected bladder. If one suspects urethral trauma, a retrograde urethrogram should precede catheter insertion. The excretory urogram may suggest the diagnosis of bladder perforation but by itself is insufficient to exclude bladder injury. A CT cystogram is diagnostic for bladder injury and urinary extravasation. It also reliably distinguishes between intra- and extraperitoneal injury. A catheter is placed, the bladder filled by gravity with diluted contrast (350-400 mL), and subsequently the CT scan is performed.

▶ **Differential Diagnosis**

Renal injury is also associated with bladder trauma and usually presents with hematuria. Imaging shows changes compatible with renal trauma; the cystogram is negative.

Injury to the membranous urethra can mimic extraperitoneal rupture of the bladder. A urethrogram reveals the site of injury. Urethral disruption is a contraindication to urethral catheterization.

▶ **Complications**

Extraperitoneal extravasation may lead to pelvic abscess. Intraperitoneal extravasation causes delayed peritonitis, oliguria, and azotemia.

Treatment

Treat shock, hemorrhage, and other life-threatening injuries. Marked extraperitoneal extravasation should be drained, the bladder decompressed by either a suprapubic or urethral catheter, and appropriate antibiotics administered. Small extraperitoneal extravasations are treated nonoperatively by urethral catheter.

Intraperitoneal extravasation of bladder urine requires exploratory laparotomy, midline cystotomy, bladder closure, and bladder catheter drainage. Penetrating injuries (ie, gunshot, stabbing) require exploration, +/− debridement, and closure of the bladder. The ureters should also be evaluated in all cases of bladder injury by preoperative imaging or intraoperative assessment, which may be done by injecting indigo carmine and looking for ureteral extravasation or by retrograde passage of 5F feeding tubes through the ureteral orifice. A closed surgical drain is left in place.

Prognosis

Early diagnosis minimizes morbidity and mortality rates. The prognosis depends chiefly on the severity of associated injuries.

INJURIES TO THE URETHRA

Membranous Urethra

Injury to the membranous urethra is usually a consequence of pelvic fracture and thus is associated with hemorrhage and multiorgan injury. The mechanism of injury is blunt trauma and deceleration resulting in shearing forces applied to the prostate and urogenital diaphragm. Penetrating injuries result from external missiles or laceration by bone fragments acting as secondary projectiles.

If the urethral disruption is incomplete, the patient may be able to void, and hematuria would be inevitable. Urethral injury is suspected if blood is expressed from the urethral meatus. In cases of complete avulsion, extravasation causes a suprapubic mass. Rectal examination may reveal a nonpalpable or upwardly displaced prostate.

X-ray reveals a fractured pelvis; urethrography delineates any extravasation, and cystography identifies an associated bladder injury. An immediate excretory urogram or CT scan should be obtained in all cases to assess kidney and ureteral function.

Treatment must be coordinated with care of associated injury. Once a membranous urethral injury with urinary extravasation has been identified, suprapubic cystostomy should be performed either at the time of laparotomy or percutaneously before placement of external pelvic fixation. Definitive urethral repair may be delayed until the patient has recovered from the acute injury and pelvic fractures have healed. Occasionally, when urethral disruption is incomplete, late repair is unnecessary. Primary repair may be indicated in cases of severe prostatomembranous dislocation, major bladder neck laceration, or concomitant pelvic vascular or rectal injury.

Late sequelae are urethral stricture, impotence, and incontinence. Urethral stricture must be identified by retrograde urethrography and may be treated by transurethral incision of the stricture or urethroplasty. Impotence due to injury of nerves to the corpora cavernosa that course adjacent to the membranous urethra may resolve without treatment during the year following injury. Vascular injury of the hypogastric or pudendal arteries may cause impotence following trauma. Cavernosometry and arteriography confirms the diagnosis; appropriate treatment may include vascular reconstruction. Incontinence depends on the neurologic status of the patient. Medical or surgical therapy is utilized to increase bladder capacity and bladder outlet resistance.

Bulbous Urethra

The bulbous urethra may be injured as a result of instrumentation or, more commonly, falling astride an object (straddle injury). Urethral contusion may cause a perineal hematoma without injury to the urethral wall. Laceration leads to urinary extravasation.

Perineal pain and some urethral bleeding are to be expected. Sudden swelling in the perineum may develop following attempted urination. Examination reveals a perineal mass; swelling due to extravasation of blood and urine involves the penis and scrotum and may spread onto the abdominal wall.

If the patient can void well and the perineal hematoma is small, no treatment is necessary. If urethrography reveals significant extravasation, suprapubic cystostomy should be performed. Minor injury without extravasation (contusion, compression by hematoma) may be managed by careful insertion of a urethral catheter.

The only serious complication is stricture, which requires subsequent internal urethrotomy or surgical repair.

Pendulous Urethra

External injury to this portion of the urethra is not common, since the penis is so mobile. The erect organ, however, is vulnerable, and pendulous urethral injury often occurs in conjunction with penile fracture (see below). Injury during urethral instrumentation (eg, urethral catheter and urethroscopy) is another common etiology.

Urethral bleeding and penile swelling are to be expected. A urethrogram reveals the site and severity of injury.

If voiding is normal, no treatment is required. A large hematoma may require drainage. If significant injury is present, a suprapubic tube should be inserted and delayed surgical repair performed after swelling and inflammation have resolved.

INJURIES TO THE PENIS

Mechanisms of penile injury include penetration, blunt trauma to the erect penis during sexual activity (eg, fracture of corpora cavernosa), avulsion of skin, and amputation.

Tourniquet injury is also uncommon; the circumferential compression may be due to a rubber band, a steel ring, string, or a hair and may be exacerbated by subsequent erection. The tourniquet may have been applied unintentionally, but child abuse cases have been reported in which the penis has been ligated as punishment for enuresis.

Treatment includes assessment and care of urethral injuries if present. Removal of tourniquet, split-thickness skin grafting of avulsion injuries, and primary closure of corporal lacerations are principles of therapy. Penile fracture is considered a urologic emergency and immediate repair minimizes the inherent risk of future impotence and penile curvature. The penis may be acutely reimplanted up to 16 hours following amputation using microsurgical techniques.

INJURIES TO THE SCROTUM & TESTIS

Avulsion of the scrotal skin may require a meshed split-thickness skin graft. If the avulsion is severe, involving the skin and dartos muscle, then the testes may be implanted in the subcutaneous tissue of the thigh and dressed outside the wound with 0.25% acetic acid–soaked gauze. Scrotal reconstruction is performed at a later time, frequently by using skin grafts.

Penetrating trauma rarely injures the mobile testes. Lacerations should be explored, debrided, and closed primarily. If hemorrhage into the tunica vaginalis is noted, drainage is indicated.

Blunt trauma to the testes may cause contusion or rupture. Rupture of the tunica albuginea may be demonstrated by ultrasonography as abnormal echotexture of the parenchyma. In cases of rupture, scrotal exploration is imperative allows debridement and closure of the tunica albuginea. The testes may ultimately undergo atrophy despite these efforts.

▼ TUMORS OF THE GENITOURINARY TRACT

Tumors of the genitourinary tract are among the most common neoplastic diseases found in adults. Prostate cancer, for example, is the most common cancer in men (33%), and renal and bladder cancer account for nearly 10% of all malignant tumors in men, but only about 3% in women. Even though excellent diagnostic methods are available, one-third of all genitourinary tumors are not found until regional or distant spread has occurred. Advances in diagnosis and treatment of genitourinary tract tumors have occurred in recent years, and the prognosis has improved in conditions such as Wilms tumor, testicular cancer, and bladder cancer. The mainstay of diagnosis continues to be physical examination, complete urinalysis, CT urography and cystoscopy

whenever indicated. Curative treatment of these tumors continues to be surgical in most instances.

RENAL ADENOCARCINOMA (RENAL CELL CARCINOMA)

▶ General Considerations

Malignant tumors of the kidney account for approximately 3% of all tumors in adults. Often, the diagnosis is found incidentally on ultrasound, CT scan, or MRI. Microscopic or gross hematuria evaluation can also identify renal cell carcinoma (RCC). Advanced or metastatic disease can present with flank mass, weight loss, or pathologic fracture. rRisk factors for RCC include cigarette smoking, obesity, and hypertension. The disease occurs in men three times more commonly than in women. A suppressor gene on chromosome 3p has been shown to be present in von Hippel–Lindau renal cancers as well as in most sporadic RCC. The most common cell type is clear cell (also called conventional) carcinoma, accounting for 70%-80% of renal carcinomas. The cell of origin is in the proximal convoluted tubule. Other cell types include papillary (10%-15%), chromophobe (3%-5%), and collecting duct renal carcinoma (1%). The tumor metastasizes commonly to the lungs (50%-60%), adjacent renal hilar lymph nodes (25%), ipsilateral adrenal (12%), opposite kidney (2%), and lytic lesions in mainly long bones (30%-40%).

Numerous conditions predispose to renal cell cancer, including von Hippel–Lindau syndrome (cerebellar hemangioblastomas, retinal angiomatosis, and bilateral RCC), tuberous sclerosis, and acquired renal cystic disease developing in patients with end-stage renal disease. Paraneoplastic syndromes are common in RCC and are often what suggests the diagnosis, yet they rarely have prognostic significance. These syndromes include hypercalcemia, erythrocytosis, hypertension, fever of unknown origin, anemia, and elevated liver enzymes **(Stauffer's syndrome)**. RCC has a predilection for producing occlusive tumor thrombi in the renal vein and the inferior vena cava (particularly from the right kidney), manifested by signs of lower extremity edema and acute scrotal varicocele when occluding the left renal vein. This phenomenon of inferior vena cava thrombus occurs in approximately 5%-10% of patients. Occasionally, the tumor thrombus reaches up to the right atrium.

▶ Clinical Findings

A. Symptoms and Signs

Painless gross or microscopic hematuria throughout the urinary stream ("total hematuria") occurs in some patients. The degree of hematuria is not necessarily related to the size or stage of the tumor. Although a triad of hematuria, flank pain, and a palpable flank mass suggests RCC, fewer than 10% of patients will so present. Both pain and a palpable mass are late events occurring only with tumors that are very large or invade surrounding structures or when hemorrhage into the tumor has occurred. Symptoms due to metastases may be the initial complaint (eg, bone pain, respiratory distress). Localized disease is often identified incidentally on imaging.

B. Laboratory Findings

Microscopic urinalysis reveals hematuria in most patients. The erythrocyte sedimentation rate may be elevated but is nonspecific. Elevation of the hematocrit and levels of serum calcium, alkaline phosphatase, and aminotransferases occur in fewer than 10% of patients. These findings nearly always resolve with curative nephrectomy and thus are not usually signs of metastases. Anemia unrelated to blood loss occurs in 20%-40% of patients, particularly those with advanced disease.

C. Imaging Studies

The diagnosis of RCC is often made by CT (and, less frequently, by intravenous urography) performed as an initial step in the workup of hematuria, an enigmatic metastatic lesion, or suspicious laboratory findings (Figure 38–12). Ultrasonography and CT scan often reveal incidental renal masses, which now account for 50% of the initial diagnoses of RCC in patients without manifestations of renal disease. Plain abdominal x-rays may reveal a calcified renal mass, but only 20% of renal masses contain demonstrable calcification. (Twenty percent of masses with peripheral calcification are malignant; more than 80% with central calcification are malignant.) The initial technique for workup of hematuria is currently CT urography which can accurately identify an enhancing renal mass which is diagnostic for RCC. CT scan is also helpful in local staging and can reveal tumor penetration of perinephric fat; enlargement of local hilar lymph nodes, indicating metastases; or tumor thrombi in the renal vein or inferior vena cava. CT angiography can delineate the renal vasculature, which is helpful in surgical planning for partial nephrectomies.

1. Ultrasonography—Occasionally, some masses detected on CT require further characterization by ultrasound. Abdominal ultrasonography can define the mass as a benign simple cyst or a solid mass in 90%-95% of cases. Abdominal ultrasound can also identify a vena caval tumor thrombus and its cephalad extent in the cava.

2. MRI—MRI is not more accurate than CT and is much more expensive. It is, however, the most accurate noninvasive means of detecting renal vein or vena caval thrombi. With the further refinement of pulse sequencing and the use of paramagnetic contrast agents, MRI has become one

of the primary techniques for staging solid renal masses. Magnetic resonance angiography (MRA) has become particularly useful for mapping the blood supply and the relationship to adjacent structures in candidates for partial nephrectomy.

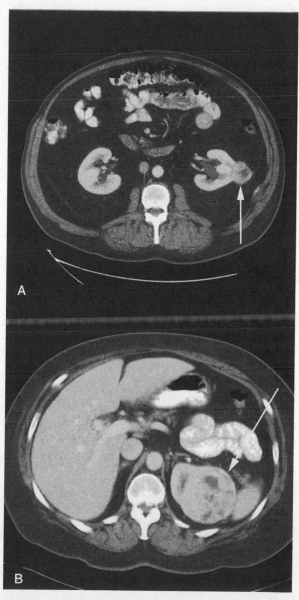

▲ **Figure 38–12.** **A:** Adenocarcinoma of the left kidney. CT scan of the abdomen shows an exophytic lesion from the midpolar kidney (arrow). **B:** CT scan showing a large left renal mass (arrow) incidentally found on imaging done to evaluate nonspecific abdominal pain. Final pathology revealed clear cell renal carcinoma.

D. Other Diagnostic or Staging Techniques

Isotopic bone scanning is useful in patients with bone pain, elevated alkaline phosphatase, or known metastases. Chest x-ray is sufficient if negative, but if equivocal, then CT scan of the chest can be used to detect metastases. Identification of metastatic disease in the thorax warrants consideration of brain imaging to rule out occult disease. There are currently no tumor markers specific for RCC. Occasionally, biopsy of the mass can be useful in when imaging is not definitive, or when metastases from another primary malignancy are a possibility. Previously, such procedures were discouraged because of fear of disseminating the tumor along the needle tract, but this has proved to be rare, and the technique is safe. False negative results and insufficient tissue for diagnosis are limitations of renal mass biopsy. Fortunately, imaging is diagnostic in most cases.

▶ Differential Diagnosis

A variety of lesions in the retroperitoneum and kidney other than renal cysts may simulate renal cancer. These include lesions due to hydronephrosis, adult polycystic kidney disease, tuberculosis, xanthogranulomatous pyelonephritis, metastatic cancer from another primary cancer, angiomyolipoma or other benign renal tumors, or adrenal cancer and retroperitoneal lipomas, sarcomas, or abscesses. In general,

one or more imaging techniques described above should make the differentiation. Percutaneous biopsy is necessary in rare instances when imaging cannot make the diagnosis.

Hematuria may be caused by renal, ureteral, or bladder calculi; renal pelvis, ureteral, or bladder tumors; or many other benign conditions usually delineated by the studies described. Cystoscopy is obligatory in hematuric patients with a normal CT scan or intravenous urogram to rule out disease of the bladder and to determine the source of the hematuria.

▶ Complications

Occasionally, patients may present with acute flank pain secondary to hemorrhage within a tumor or colic secondary to obstructing ureteral clots. Tumor in the renal vein or vena cava may cause an acute left varicocele or lower extremity edema associated with proteinuria. Pathologic fractures are due to osteolytic metastases in long bones. Brain metastases can present with seizure or other neurologic symptoms.

▶ Treatment

Staging is the key to designing the treatment plan (Table 38–1). Patients with disease confined within the renal fascia (Gerota's fascia) or limited to nonadherent renal vein or vena caval tumor thrombi (stages T1, T2, and T3a) are best treated

Table 38–1. TNM staging classification and prognosis of renal cell cancer.

Robson Stage	T	N	M	Five-Year Survival (%)
I. Tumor confined by renal capsule	T1 (< 7.0 cm tumor) T2 (> 7.0 cm tumor)	N0 (nodes negative)	M0 (lack of distant metastases)	80-100
II. Tumor extension to perirenal fat or ipsilateral adrenal but confined by Gerota's fascia	T3a	N0	M0	50-60
IIIa. Renal vein or inferior vena cava involvement	T3b (renal vein involvement) T3c (renal vein and caval involvement below the diaphragm) T4b (caval involvement above the diaphragm)	N0	M0	50-60 (renal vein) 25-35 (vena cava)
IIIb. Lymphatic involvement	T1-3	N1 (single regional node involved) N2 (multiple regional, contralateral, or bilateral nodes involved)	M0	15-35
IIIc. Combination of IIIa and IIIb	T3-4	N1-2	M0	15-35
IVa. Spread to contiguous organs except ipsilateral adrenal	T4	N1-2	M0	0-5
IVb. Distant metastases	T1-4	N0-2	M1	0-5

by surgical extirpation with either radical nephrectomy or partial nephrectomy. Radical nephrectomy traditionally includes en bloc removal of the kidney and surrounding Gerota fascia (including the ipsilateral adrenal), the renal hilar lymph nodes, and the proximal half of the ureter. However, adrenal-sparing radical nephrectomy is routinely performed for mid- and lower-pole renal tumors with equivalent outcomes.

In patients with very large or central tumors and a normal contralateral kidney, radical nephrectomy is recommended. In all other cases, attempts should be made for nephron-sparing surgery. Successful partial nephrectomy with negative surgical margins offers the same survival benefit as radical nephrectomy. Typically hilar-vessel occlusion with bulldog or satinsky clamp(s) is performed to allow for resection in a relatively bloodless field.

Laparoscopic radical or partial nephrectomy has been advocated as a method equal to the open approach with the advantages of less blood loss, shorter hospitalization, and earlier return to normal function. It is the gold standard in institutions with appropriate expertise. Laparoscopic or percutaneous cryoablation of RCC has also shown considerable promise. Alternatively, radiofrequency ablation has been utilized for small renal tumors. These ablative technologies do not provide pathologic diagnosis; so percutaneous biopsy can be performed before the procedure or intraoperatively.

Nephrectomy has not been associated with improved survival rates in patients with multiple distant metastases (stage IV), and the procedure is not recommended unless patients are symptomatic or a promising therapeutic protocol is being studied. Flanigan and others have shown, however, that up to a 6-month improvement in survival can be achieved with nephrectomy—even with soft tissue metastasis—in selected patients who also receive interferon alpha systemic therapy. Patients with solitary pulmonary metastases have benefited from joint surgical removal of both the primary lesion and the metastatic lesion (30% survival at 5 years). Preoperative arterial embolization in patients with or without metastases does not improve survival rates, though it may be helpful as a single treatment measure in patients with symptomatic but nonresectable primary lesions. Radiation therapy is of little benefit except as treatment for symptomatic bone metastases. Medroxyprogesterone for metastatic RCC has given an equivocal 5%-10% response rate of short duration. Vinblastine has also had a response rate of approximately 20%, again of minimal duration. There are no other cytotoxic chemotherapeutic agents of benefit.

Immunotherapy with interferon alpha has had a 15%-20% response rate. Other interferons, alone (interferon beta, interferon gamma) or in combination with chemotherapeutic agents, have been less effective than interferon alpha. Adoptive immunotherapy—using lymphocytes (lymphokine-activated killer cells) from exposure of the patient's own peripheral blood lymphocytes to interleukin-2 (IL-2) *in vitro* followed by reinfusion into the patient along with systemic IL-2 infusion—has shown up to 33% objective response rates. High-dose intravenous IL-2 causes a profound capillary leak syndrome and substantial toxicity. Subsequent studies have shown only a 16% response rate.

Recent advances in research on the von Hippel–Lindau tumor suppressor gene has led to identification of growth factors including vascular endothelial growth factor (VEGF) and platelet-derived growth factor as molecular targets in treating advanced renal cancer. Initial studies using bevacizumab, an anti-VEGF antibody, have shown promising results. Sorafenib, a tyrosine kinase inhibitor that blocks the pathway leading to the production of several growth factors, has been studied in patients with metastatic renal cancer and shown longer median progression-free survival than placebo (24 weeks vs. 6 weeks). Sunitinib, another tyrosine kinase inhibitor, has shown longer progression-free survival and higher response rates than interferon alpha in patients with metastatic renal cancer. These oral agents are currently used as first-line therapy in this group of patients.

Temsirolimus is another targeted agent that is a specific inhibitor of the mammalian target of rapamycin kinase (mTOR inhibitor) and has shown promising results. It is now used as first-line therapy in poor prognosis patients. Many other agents are currently being studied.

▶ Prognosis

Patients with localized RCC (stages T1, T2, and T3a) treated surgically have 5-year survival rates of approximately 70%-80%, whereas rates for those with local nodal extension or distant metastases are 15%-25% and less than 10%, respectively. Most patients who present with multiple distant metastases succumb to disease within 15 months (Table 38–1). The advent of new agents for RCC may improve the outcome in these patients.

RENAL SARCOMA

Renal sarcomas include rhabdomyosarcoma, liposarcoma, fibrosarcoma, and leiomyosarcoma; the latter is the most common, though all are very uncommon. Sarcomas are highly malignant and are usually detected at a late stage and thus have a poor prognosis. The diagnostic approach is similar to that of RCC. The histology of the lesion is rarely suspected preoperatively, although local invasion into surrounding retroperitoneal structures is more common than with RCC. These tumors have a tendency to surround the renal vasculature and do not exhibit neovascularity on MRA.

Treatment is surgical, with wide local excision; however, local recurrence and subsequent distant metastases are the rule. There is no therapy of proved benefit for metastatic disease.

SECONDARY MALIGNANT RENAL TUMORS

Metastatic tumors to the kidney are more common than primary renal tumors and often develop from primary tumors of distant sites, most commonly the lung, stomach, and breast. It is rare for the diagnosis to be made before autopsy; this suggests that renal metastasis is a late event. There are usually no symptoms, though microscopic hematuria occurs in 10%-20% of cases. Imaging reveals a renal mass, often difficult to distinguish from RCC. Contiguous spread of a tumor adjacent to the kidney is not infrequent (eg, tumors of the adrenal, colon, and pancreas and retroperitoneal sarcomas). Tumors such as lymphoma, leukemia, and multiple myeloma may also infiltrate the kidney. Routine radiologic, hematologic, and chemical examinations should demonstrate the primary tumor in most cases. Percutaneous biopsy may be appropriate in certain circumstances.

BENIGN RENAL TUMORS

► Renal Oncocytoma

Renal oncocytomas are benign renal neoplasms. The tumors are generally asymptomatic and not associated with the paraneoplastic syndromes. The finding of a central stellate scar on CT or a spoke-wheel pattern of feeding arteries on angiography may suggest the diagnosis, although these findings have been found to be unreliable. Oncocytomas can coexist with renal carcinoma in the same lesion or in other lesions in the same kidney (7%-30%). This finding, along with difficulty differentiating oncocytoma from clear cell or chromophobe renal cancers on fine-needle aspirates, make it difficult to make a definitive diagnosis preoperatively. Consequently, definitive treatment of these lesions with radical or partial nephrectomy, or with ablation (cryoablation or RFA) has been recommended.

► Mesoblastic Nephroma

Mesoblastic nephroma is a benign congenital renal tumor seen in early childhood, which must be distinguished from the highly malignant nephroblastoma, or Wilms tumor. Unlike Wilms tumor, mesoblastic nephroma is commonly diagnosed within the first few months of life. Histologically, it is distinguished from Wilms tumor by cells resembling fibroblasts or smooth muscle cells and by the lack of epithelial elements. The prognosis is excellent; complete surgical resection is curative, and neither chemotherapy nor radiotherapy is required.

► Angiomyolipoma

Angiomyolipoma is a benign hamartoma seen most often bilaterally in adults with tuberous sclerosis (which also includes adenoma sebaceum, epilepsy, and mental retardation). The tumor is also common in middle-aged women, but only unilaterally. These tumors can be detected following spontaneous retroperitoneal hemorrhage, though 50% of these lesions are currently diagnosed incidentally. CT scan can be diagnostic, with negative Hounsfield units detected in the fat-containing area of the tumor. Occasionally, an angiomyolipoma eludes diagnosis preoperatively and requires resection (especially the lipid-poor angiomyolipoma). Asymptomatic patients with small (< 4 cm) tumors and typical findings on CT scan of fat within the tumor do not require surgery, as the prognosis is excellent without treatment. These patients can be followed with serial imaging. Those presenting with a retroperitoneal hemorrhage or a size greater than 4 cm should have the tumor removed surgically with partial nephrectomy or embolized via angioinfarction, which has been shown to be effective.

► Other Benign Renal Tumors

Other benign renal tumors include (1) **fibroma,** a renal parenchymal capsular or perinephric fibrous mass; (2) **lipoma,** an adipose deposit within or around the kidney, often perihilar or within the renal sinus; (3) **leiomyoma,** a common retroperitoneal tumor that may arise from the renal capsule or renal vascular walls; and (4) **hemangioma,** which is occasionally found to be the elusive cause of hematuria. Hemangiomas are generally quite small, and the diagnosis can be confirmed by direct vision of the lesion in the renal collecting system on ureteroscopy.

Hudes G et al: Temsirolimus, interferon alfa, or both for advanced renal-cell carcinoma. *N Engl J Med* 2007;356:2271.

Motzer RJ et al: Sunitinib versus interferon alfa in metastatic renal-cell carcinoma. *N Engl J Med* 2007;356:115.

Nabi G, Cleves A, Shelley M: Surgical management of localised renal cell carcinoma. *Cochrane Database Syst Rev* 2010 Mar 17;(3):CD006579. doi: 10.1002/14651858.CD006579 .pub2. Review. PMID: 20238346.

TUMORS OF THE RENAL PELVIS & CALICES

► General Considerations

In over 90% of cases, tumors involving the collecting system of the kidney are urothelial (or transitional cell) carcinomas. Fewer than 5% of tumors in this location are squamous carcinomas (often in association with chronic inflammation and stone formation) or adenocarcinomas. The cause of urothelial carcinoma of the upper urinary tract is similar to that of epithelial tumors in the ureter or bladder; there is a strong association with cigarette smoking and exposure to industrial chemicals. Excessive use of phenacetin-containing analgesics and the presence of Balkan nephritis are also predisposing factors.

► Clinical Findings

A. Symptoms and Signs

Gross or microscopic painless hematuria occurs in over 70% of patients. The lesions are usually asymptomatic unless bleeding causes acute flank pain secondary to obstructing clots. Presenting symptoms can often be due to metastases to bone, the liver, or the lungs. Physical examination is usually negative for any positive findings.

B. Laboratory Findings

Microscopic hematuria on urinalysis is the rule. Pyuria is not seen. Cytologic examination of voided urine specimens may be diagnostic in high-grade tumors. Urine obtained from the ureter by retrograde catheterization or by brushing with specialized ureteral instruments can improve the diagnostic accuracy of cytologic examinations. Direct biopsy during ureteroscopy is the most accurate. There are no commonly associated paraneoplastic syndromes or diagnostic serum tumor markers in urothelial carcinoma. A large number of urine markers are currently being studied, but only *in situ* hybridization studies identifying abnormalities in chromosomes 3, 7, 17, and 9p21 can be recommended at present.

C. Imaging Studies

The diagnosis is commonly made on CT urography or intravenous urography and confirmed by retrograde pyelography and ureteroscopy with biopsy. Renal ultrasound or CT scan can be used to rule out calculus. CT scan is also useful in local staging of the tumor. The tumors metastasize to the lungs, liver, and bone, so chest x-ray, CT scan of the lungs and liver, and a bone scan are useful to determine the presence of metastases. Urothelial carcinoma tends to be multifocal in the urinary tract, involving the opposite kidney (1%-2%), ipsilateral ureter, or bladder (38%-50%). Surveillance of these potential sites is important.

D. Endoscopic Findings

Cystoscopy is necessary when gross hematuria is present to determine the location of the bleeding. Lateralizing hematuria can be identified with cystoscopy (bloody efflux from one ureteral orifice). Retrograde pyelography and ureteral cytologic studies or brushing, as described previously, can be useful, though mildly abnormal cytologic findings may occur in patients with upper tract inflammation or calculi. Rigid or flexible ureteroscopes can be used to view the upper ureter and renal pelvis directly. Biopsy of upper tract lesions is possible through these instruments. Although percutaneous approaches to the renal collecting system have been perfected, their use for diagnosis or treatment of suspected urothelial carcinoma in routine cases is not recommended, because of the possibility of spreading tumor cells outside the kidney.

► Differential Diagnosis

A variety of conditions may mimic transitional cell carcinoma of the renal pelvis, including calculi, sloughed renal papillae, tuberculosis, and RCC with pelvic extension of the tumor. These can usually be ruled out by the diagnostic studies described previously.

► Complications

Occasionally, bleeding may be severe enough to require immediate nephrectomy. Infection may develop, particularly when there is obstruction and hydronephrosis, requiring prompt use of systemic antibiotics.

► Treatment

Renal urothelial carcinoma is treated by nephroureterectomy (perifascial nephrectomy and removal of the entire ureter, down to and including the ureteral orifice within the bladder). Transureteral or percutaneous endoscopic techniques for resection of selected low-grade lesions have been successful, particularly in patient with significant chronic kidney disease and/or solitary renal units. Upper tract instillation of bacille Calmette-Guérin (BCG) or mitomycin C has been reported with modest results. High recurrence rates and the potential for local tumor spread would argue against this approach in high-grade or extensive lesions. Laparoscopic nephroureterectomy has become common practice, but management of the distal ureter and bladder cuff by this technique has been the subject of controversy. Regional lymph node dissections have not been traditionally performed, although recent reports have shown some benefit for patients with aggressive disease. Because 50% of these patients will develop urothelial carcinoma of the bladder, cystourethroscopy must be performed postoperatively; it is usually done quarterly during the first year, twice the second year, and then annually.

► Prognosis

Because most of these tumors are low grade and noninvasive, the 5-year tumor-free survival rate is higher than 90% for lesions treated with complete removal of the ipsilateral upper urinary tract. Survival rates are much lower for lesions that invade the renal parenchyma or are of high histologic grade. A poor prognosis is associated with tumors having histologic features of squamous carcinoma or adenocarcinoma. These tumors are mildly radiosensitive, but preoperative or postoperative radiotherapy has not been particularly helpful. Metastatic lesions are particularly problematic, and survivors are rare. Chemotherapy combinations, which have shown benefit in urothelial carcinoma of the bladder (methotrexate, vinblastine, Adriamycin, and cisplatin [MVAC] or gemcitabine and cisplatin), are also efficacious in urothelial carcinoma of the upper urinary tract.

TUMORS OF THE URETER

▶ General Considerations

Ureteral tumors are rarely benign, but benign fibroepithelial polyps do occasionally occur within the ureter. More than 90% of ureteral tumors are urothelial carcinomas. The cause is unknown, but tobacco smoking and exposure to industrial chemicals are known to be associated. Ureteral urothelial carcinoma is often found in association with renal pelvis urothelial carcinoma and slightly less often with bladder urothelial carcinoma. The lesions develop in persons aged 60-70 years and are twice as common in men as in women. More than 60% of these tumors occur in the lower ureter.

▶ Clinical Findings

A. Symptoms and Signs

Gross or microscopic hematuria is the rule (80% of cases). Because ureteral tumors grow slowly, they may not cause symptoms even though they completely obstruct the kidney. Occasionally, gross hematuria may cause acute obstruction because of clots. The initial presentation may be due to symptomatic metastases to bone, lungs, or liver.

B. Laboratory Findings

Urinalysis commonly reveals hematuria. There are no biochemical markers specific to the diagnosis, though patients with metastases may have abnormal liver function tests or anemia. Serum creatinine levels may be elevated with complete unilateral obstruction in elderly patients. Cytologic studies of voided urine or ureteral urine or brush biopsy studies may be diagnostic.

C. Imaging Studies

The diagnosis may be made on CT or intravenous urography, though the tumor often obstructs the ureter completely, so that cystoscopy and retrograde pyelography are required for definition of the lesion. These studies often reveal a filling defect in the ureter (classically described as a goblet sign). The ureter is dilated proximal to the lesion. CT scan is useful in ruling out nonopaque calculi and in abdominal tumor staging. Chest x-ray, CT scans, and bone scans are helpful in determining the presence of metastases.

D. Endoscopic Findings

Cystoscopy is necessary when gross hematuria is present to determine the site of bleeding. Retrograde pyelography may then be necessary. Ureteroscopy may provide a direct view of the tumor and access for biopsy.

▶ Differential Diagnosis

Nonopaque calculi, sloughed renal papillae, blood clots, or extrinsic compression by retroperitoneal masses or nodes may all produce signs, symptoms, and x-ray findings similar to those with ureteral tumors. The radiographic, cytologic, and endourologic studies listed above should make the distinction, but surgical exploration is required occasionally.

▶ Treatment

Most ureteral transitional cell carcinomas are not associated with metastases and can be definitively treated with nephroureterectomy. Selected patients with noninvasive low-grade lesions may be treated by segmental ureteral resection with end-to-end anastomosis (ureteroureterostomy), or ureteral reimplantation for lesions in the distal one-third of the ureter. In some patients carefully selected with low-grade noninvasive tumors, resection or laser ablation can be considered. Regional lymph node dissections have not been traditionally performed, although recent reports have shown some benefit. Preoperative or postoperative radiation therapy appears to be of no benefit. As with renal pelvis and bladder urothelial carcinoma, cystoscopy should be performed periodically postoperatively. Patients with metastases are rarely helped by removal of the primary tumor. These tumors are responsive to chemotherapy. Traditional agents that have been used include cisplatin with gemcitabine or MVAC. These have shown reasonable response rates but poor long-term outcomes.

▶ Prognosis

The 5-year survival rate for patients with low-grade noninvasive lesions treated surgically approaches 100%. Those with high-grade or invasive lesions have a poorer prognosis, and those with metastases have a 5-year survival rate of less than 10%.

TUMORS OF THE BLADDER

▶ General Considerations

Vesical neoplasms account for nearly 6% of all cancers in men and are the second-most common cancer of the genitourinary tract in men. In women, these tumors account for 2% of all cancers and are the most common cancer of the genitourinary tract. Men are affected twice as often as women. More than 90% of tumors are urothelial carcinomas, while a few are squamous cell carcinomas (associated with chronic inflammation, as in bilharziasis) or adenocarcinomas (often seen at the dome of the bladder in patients with a urachal remnant).

Most urothelial carcinomas (70%-80%) are nonmuscle invasive (not invasive into the bladder detrusor musculature) when recognized. Only 10%-15% of recurrent tumors become invasive.

The cause of urothelial carcinoma is unknown; there is a strong association with chronic cigarette smoking and exposure to chemicals prevalent in dye, rubber, leather, paint, and other chemical industries.

Table 38–2. Treatment and prognosis of tumors related to stage of disease.

Conventional Stage	TNM Stage	Tumor Involvement	Treatment	Five-Year Survival (%)
0	Ta	Mucosa only	Transurethral resection	85-90
A	T1	Submucosal invasion (lamina propria)	Transurethral resection and intravesical chemoimmunotherapy	60-80
B1	T2a	Superficial muscle invasion	Total cystectomy and pelvic lymphadenectomy	50-55
B2	T2b	Deep muscle invasion		30-50
C	T3	Perivesical fat invasion		30-40
D1	T3-4N+	Regional lymph node invasion	Systemic chemotherapy	6-35
D2	T3-4M1	Distant metastases		0-10

The treatment and prognosis depend entirely on the degree of anaplasia (grade) and the depth of penetration of the bladder wall or beyond (Table 38–2). Most of these tumors develop on the trigone and the adjacent posterolateral wall; thus, ureteral involvement with obstruction is a possibility. Tumors tend to be multifocal within the bladder. Approximately 5% of patients develop upper urinary tract urothelial carcinoma as well.

▶ Clinical Findings

A. Symptoms and Signs

Gross or microscopic hematuria is a common finding that leads to the diagnosis. Patients with diffuse noninvasive tumors, particularly carcinoma *in situ*, may have urinary frequency and urgency. Occasionally, large necrotic tumors become secondarily infected, and patients exhibit symptoms of cystitis. Pain secondary to clot retention, tumor extension into the bony pelvis, or ureteral obstruction may occur but are not frequent presenting complaints. When both ureters are obstructed, azotemia with attendant secondary symptoms may be the finding that requires diagnostic studies.

External physical examination is not generally revealing, though occasionally a suprapubic mass may be palpable. Rectal examination may reveal large tumors, particularly when they have invaded the pelvic sidewalls. Thus, bimanual examination is a necessary part of staging evaluation.

B. Laboratory Findings

Microscopic hematuria is the only consistent diagnostic finding. Patients with bilateral ureteral obstruction may have azotemia and anemia. Liver metastases may cause elevation of serum transaminases and alkaline phosphatase. There are no paraneoplastic syndromes or tumor markers consistently present in patients with urothelial carcinoma. Urinary markers currently being studied are various tumor-associated antigens, growth factors, and nuclear matrix proteins, but none are proved to be accurate enough to obviate cystoscopy for diagnosis.

C. Imaging Studies

Small bladder tumors are not seen on intravenous urography but may be seen on CT. Larger tumors usually produce filling defects in the bladder on both urography or CT (Figure 38–13). Ureteral obstruction with hydroureteronephrosis may occur as well. Invasion of the bladder wall may be predicted in patients with asymmetry or marked irregularity of the bladder wall. Noninvasive lesions seen on CT or intravenous urography tend to be exophytic within the bladder, without evidence of bladder wall distortion.

Ultrasonography by external, transrectal, or transurethral routes can accurately define moderate-sized bladder tumors and can often depict deep invasion.

CT scan can be useful for staging, but the depth of bladder wall penetration and delineation of tumor deposits

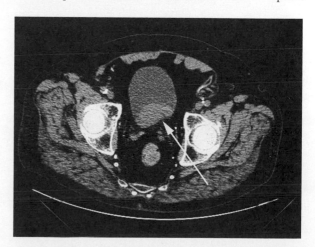

▲ **Figure 38–13.** Noncontrast CT scan showing space-occupying lesion (transitional cell carcinoma) on the posteroinferior of the bladder (arrow).

in adjacent nonenlarged lymph nodes are not accurately defined. In patients with nodal metastases suspected on CT scans, fine-needle aspiration and cytologic studies may confirm the diagnosis and eliminate the need for surgical exploration. MRI is helpful in the pelvis, where motion artifacts are minor and the scant pelvic fat is just enough to provide organ differentiation. However, the information is not superior to that obtained with CT.

D. Urinary Cytologic Studies

Urothelial tumors shed neoplastic cells into the urine in large numbers. Low-grade tumor cells may not appear abnormal on cytologic examination, but higher-grade tumor cells can be detected by cytologic study with high specificity. These studies are most useful in checking for recurrence of urothelial carcinoma. Flow cytometry (differential staining of DNA and RNA within urine cells to measure the amount of nuclear protein and thus the relative number of aneuploid [abnormal] cells) has been used to screen patients with some success. This technique may be useful for early diagnosis of recurrence. The urinary fluorescence *in situ* hybridization assay is more sensitive and comparably specific for bladder cancer cells as compared to cytology.

E. Endoscopic Findings

Cystoscopy is mandatory in any adult patient with unexplained hematuria and a normal upper-tract imaging study. Many urothelial carcinomas are not identified on CT or intravenous urography. Cystoscopic examination should detect nearly all tumors in the bladder (Figure 38–14). Only a few patients will have carcinoma *in situ* (high-grade noninvasive tumor) that is not visible. Any tumor seen should be biopsied and preferably resected to completion if the patient

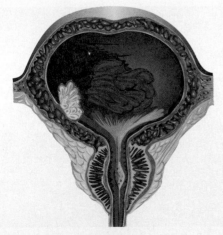

▲ **Figure 38–14.** Transitional cell (papillary) carcinoma of the bladder with minimal invasion of the bladder wall.

is under anesthesia. The entire bladder, including the bladder neck, should be routinely scrutinized in all patients with microscopic hematuria. In patients without visible tumor and no other causes of hematuria, random biopsies may be diagnostic of carcinoma *in situ*. A bimanual examination should be done during cystoscopy in all patients with urothelial carcinoma to be certain that the bladder is not fixed, signifying extensive extravesical extension.

F. Staging

Therapy depends on the stage of the tumor as seen on histologic sections and examinations for metastases. Table 38–2 sets forth the stage, treatment, and prognosis of patients with urothelial carcinoma of the bladder. The histologic grade of the tumor is also important in determining treatment and prognosis, but in general, low- and high-grade histologic characteristics tend to occur in low- and high-stage tumors, respectively.

As previously discussed, CT scan, MRI, or both may be helpful in predicting the stage of the tumor. Isotope bone scanning, chest x-ray, and chest CT scan evaluate the possibility of bone or pulmonary metastases and should be done before determining therapy in patients with invasive lesions.

▶ Treatment

A. Transurethral Resection, Fulguration, and Laser Therapy

Endoscopic transurethral resection of superficial and submucosally invasive low-grade tumors can be curative. Nevertheless, because the tumor recurs in more than 50% of patients, cystoscopy should be performed periodically. Quarterly examinations are recommended during the first year following tumor resection, every 6 months during the second year, and annually thereafter. Periodic urinary cytologic examinations can be helpful as well. Upper tract surveillance with CT urography is recommended for high-grade tumors, typically every 2 years. Low-grade tumors do not require upper tract surveillance unless hematuria recurs without evidence for tumor recurrence in the bladder. Recurrent small tumors without obvious invasion may be treated by fulguration only, though biopsy is recommended to document the stage and grade.

Neodymium:YAG lasers have been used for desiccation of low-grade, low-stage tumors. There is as yet no proven advantage to this approach except that patients can be treated under local anesthesia as outpatients and perhaps that tumor cells are rendered nonviable and thus incapable of reimplantation elsewhere in the bladder or urethra. Biopsies for diagnosis and staging are still required.

B. Intravesical Therapy

A variety of chemotherapeutic agents have been used in patients with recurrent low-grade, low-stage tumors.

Mitomycin C is instilled into the bladder by catheter (40 mg in 40 mL of water) and left indwelling for 1-2 hours. Patients are treated once a week for 6 weeks and may undergo a less frequent maintenance regimen. Treatment results in decreased frequency of recurrence or no recurrence in nearly 50% of patients. Other agents include thiotepa and doxorubicin.

Immunotherapeutic drugs, which include BCG, are effective in prophylaxis (60%) of recurrent papillary tumors and curative (70%) in carcinoma *in situ*, a highly malignant lesion less responsive to the cytotoxic agents described earlier. Intravesical BCG is the gold-standard first line therapy for carcinoma *in situ* of the bladder. Side effects of BCG include vesical irritability (90%), low-grade fever, and systemic BCG-osis (1%). Although the mechanism of action of BCG is not entirely known, it is suspected to induce T-cell recruitment and subsequent cytokine release locally at the tumor site. It is the most effective agent currently used. Interferon alpha has also been studied and is effective (nearly 50% of cases) for carcinoma *in situ*, with less toxicity than BCG; however, its durability as a single agent is poor. The combination of BCG and interferon alpha has shown nearly 50% response rates and is occasionally used in patients who have failed BCG. BCG is contraindicated in immunocompromised patients due to risk of systemic BCG infection and the likely decreased efficacy.

Immediate instillation of Mitomycin C after transurethral resection has shown a substantial decrease in recurrence rates and is now standard of care.

C. Radiation Therapy

Definitive radiation therapy should be reserved for patients who have inoperable muscle-invasive bladder cancer localized to the pelvis or who refuse surgical treatment, as the 5-year survival rate is only 30%. In some patients with recurrence after radiation therapy, salvage cystectomy can be curative (in at least 30% of cases), though surgical morbidity rates are high. Radiation, when used, is combined with systemic chemotherapy.

D. Surgical Therapy

Occasional patients are seen with muscle-invasive lesions (T2) localized to an area in the bladder well away from the bladder base or orifices and without tumor in other sites of the bladder (proved by multiple biopsies) or beyond. Partial cystectomy (removal of the tumor with a cuff of normal bladder) may be appropriate in these patients. Such tumors are rare, and patients must be selected carefully for partial cystectomy. All other patients with high-grade or invasive (T2 and T3) lesions without distant spread or a fixed pelvis on bimanual examination are best treated by radical cystectomy and pelvic lymph node dissection. This includes removal of the bladder and the prostate in men. Removal of the entire urethra may be necessary in selected patients with tumors at the bladder neck or in the prostate or in those with diffuse carcinoma *in situ* in the bladder. In women, the uterus, ovaries, fallopian tubes, urethra, and the anterior vaginal wall are usually removed *en bloc* with the bladder. Vaginal-sparing cystectomy can be performed as well.

Urinary diversion is required and is accomplished with the use of intestinal conduits, pouches or neobladders. Ileal conduit urinary diversion creates a urostomy on the skin and requires continuous bag drainage. This is the most common urinary diversion with the lowest complication rates. Continent cutaneous urinary diversions requiring intermittent cutaneous catheterization rather than cutaneous bag drainage became popular in the late 1980s. The basic principles are large-volume reservoirs with detubularization of bowel to maintain low intrapouch pressures and construction of an intussuscepted or plicated ileal segment to provide cutaneous continence. Orthotopic neobladder reservoirs also have been devised using bowel configurations similar to those described above to connect directly to the membranous urethra in men and in the distal two thirds of the female urethra, permitting the patient to void normally. These procedures are appropriate in both men and women and have been shown to be safe, with minimal increase in morbidity over cutaneous diversions.

Robotic cystectomy has been done in large numbers at select centers in the United States and Europe. With short-term follow up, oncologic outcomes appear equivalent to open surgery with potentially less blood loss and faster convalescence postoperatively. In most cases, the urinary diversion is done via open surgery, but more recently, ileal conduit and neobladder urinary diversions have been performed intracorporeally with robotic assistance.

E. Systemic Chemotherapy

Chemotherapy in the form of CMV (cisplatin, methotrexate, and vinblastine) or MVAC (CMV plus doxorubicin [Adriamycin]) has been used precystectomy (neoadjuvant) or postcystectomy (adjuvant) for muscle-invasive tumors or as treatment of metastatic urothelial cancer. More recently, gemcitabine and cisplatin have become standard of care after a randomized trial showed similar efficacy to MVAC with fewer side effects. A recent randomized trial showed improved survival in patients with locally advanced bladder cancer who received neoadjuvant chemotherapy and cystectomy compared to those who underwent cystectomy alone. Adjuvant chemotherapy has been shown in randomized trials to help patients with locoregional disease but not patients with localized disease (stage T1-T2). Several reports of efficacy with either CMV or MVAC for treatment of metastatic disease have shown a 60% overall objective response rate with a 30% complete response rate. A few long-term survivors with apparent cure have been reported (10%-15%), and either of these regimens thus appears to be a definite advance in the treatment of urothelial cancer. Other chemotherapeutic agents used in urothelial cancer include paclitaxel and carboplatin in various regimens that appear to have similar efficacy with less toxicity.

▶ Prognosis

Approximately half of the low-grade superficial tumors are controlled by transurethral surgery or intracavitary use of chemotherapeutic agents (Table 38–2). Following radical cystectomy, the 5-year survival rate varies with the extent, stage, and grade of the tumor, but with T2N0M0 tumors averages about 50%-70%. The complications of urinary diversion (ureteral obstruction with hydronephrosis, pyelonephritis, and nephrolithiasis) also influence the outcome.

CARCINOMA OF THE PROSTATE

▶ General Considerations

In adult men, prostate cancer is the most common neoplasm (after skin cancer) and the second-most common (after lung cancer) cause of death due to cancer. The tumor is more prevalent in black men than in any other group in the United States. The tumor rarely occurs before age 40, and the incidence increases with age such that more than 75% of men older than age 85 have prostate cancer on autopsy. In most of these older men, however, the disease is not clinically apparent; only 10% of men over age 65 develop clinical evidence of the disease. Ninety-five percent of tumors are adenocarcinomas. The tumor arises primarily in the peripheral zone (85%), an area that differs in embryologic derivation from the periurethral (transition) zone, which is the site of formation of benign prostatic hyperplasia. The cause of prostate cancer is unknown, but many factors appear to be involved, including genetic, hormonal, dietary (particular high-fat diets), and perhaps environmental carcinogenic influences.

▶ Screening

Screening with PSA monitoring and digital rectal examination (DRE) has been controversial due to conflicting evidence regarding a decrease in mortality. Two very large randomized controlled trials examining the effects of PSA screening on mortality have recently been completed, one in the United States and one in Europe. The US trial did not show a survival benefit in the screening group, although the control group was significant contaminated with men who had some previous PSA testing. The European study showed a relative survival benefit of 20% in the screening group after 10 years of follow-up, and the data will be reanalyzed with longer follow-up.

Based on all available evidence, the US Preventive Services Task Force released a recommendation against routine screening for prostate cancer in 2011. The American Urological Association recommends a shared decision making discussion about prostate cancer screening with men between the ages 55-69, and at a younger age for those men with a positive family history in a first degree relative or for African Americans. If screening is agreed upon, serum PSA level and DRE are performed annually or every two years based on the clinician's discretion.

▶ Clinical Findings

A. Symptoms and Signs

Nonpalpable (T1) carcinoma of the prostate presents without physical signs and is only diagnosed by the pathologist when prostate tissue is removed as treatment for symptomatic bladder outlet obstruction presumed to be caused by benign prostatic hyperplasia or is found by an elevated PSA (T1c). Patients T2 or higher disease have a hard nodule on the prostate that can be felt during rectal examination (Table 38–3). T3 disease is palpable (or visible by imaging) beyond the capsule of the prostate or demonstrates seminal vesicle involvement. T4 disease invades adjacent organs including the rectum and pelvic sidewall. Previously, 50% of patients presented with evidence of metastases, including weight loss, anemia, bone pain (commonly in the lumbosacral area), or acute neurologic deficit in the lower limbs. Today, however, fewer than 20% of patients present in this way because of earlier diagnosis due to wide use of PSA screening (stage migration).

B. Laboratory Findings

Patients with extensive metastases may have anemia due to bone marrow replacement by tumor. Those with bilateral ureteral obstruction secondary to trigonal compression by tumor may exhibit azotemia and uremia. Serum alkaline phosphatase is often elevated in patients with bone metastases but not in those with localized disease.

PSA is elevated in the serum of most men with prostate cancer, but high-grade (Gleason 8-10) cancers and ductal variant adenocarcinomas can present with normal PSA levels. Values above 4 ng/mL are considered abnormal but rise normally with age and significant benign prostatic hypertrophy. PSA can also be falsely elevated due to cystoscopy, prostate biopsy, urethral catheterization, and urinary tract infection. Routine DRE does not usually affect PSA levels.

Methods for enhancing PSA specificity include the following: (1) age-specific PSA (younger men [< age 50 years], normal < 2.5 ng/mL; older men [> age 70 years], normal > 6.5 ng/mL); (2) PSA density (PSA divided by prostate volume), where less than 0.15 ng/mL suggests cancer; (3) percent-free PSA (total PSA minus complexed PSA), where lower values signify an increased risk of cancer (useful for total PSA levels between 4 and 10). While total PSA is useful for staging, it is not absolute. PSA appears to be most helpful

Table 38–3. Treatment and prognosis of prostate cancer related to tumor stage.

Conventional Stage	TNM Stage 1997	Clinical Findings	Treatment	Fifteen-Year Recurrence-Free Survival (%)
A1	T1a	Nonpalpable tumor; incidental finding at transurethral prostatectomy (low-grade cancer seen in < 5% of prostate)	Observation	100
A2	T1b	Same as above except tumor is high-grade, or > 5% of prostate is involved, or both	Radical prostatectomy with pelvic lymphadenectomy	70-80
B1	T2a	Tumor involves one lobe or less	External beam radiation	85
B2	T2b	Tumor involves more than one lobe	Brachytherapy	60-70
C	T3a	Unilateral extraprostatic extension	Radiation with or without pelvic lymphadenectomy	20-60
C2	T3b T3c T4a T4b	Bilateral extraprostatic extension Seminal vesicle invasion Invades bladder neck or rectum Invades levator muscle and/or fixed to pelvic sidewall	Hormonal therapy (orchiectomy or LHRH/ antiandrogen) when symptomatic Irradiation for isolated bone pain	0-10
D	N+ or M+	Pelvic lymph node involvement or distant metastases	Hormonal therapy (orchiectomy or LHRH/ antiandrogen) when symptomatic Irradiation for isolated bone pain	0-10

in following up on patients after treatment, as levels fall to undetectable after surgery and decrease dramatically after radiation therapy when there is a complete response. There are several new prostate cancer markers currently being investigated, but none have become widely used to date. PCA3 urinary assay shows promise in men with persistently elevated PSA levels and previous negative biopsies.

C. Imaging Studies

Transrectal ultrasound has become very useful for evaluating prostate volume and guiding biopsy needles into the peripheral zone and other specific areas, such as the base, the apex, and the transition zone of the prostate. The study can also reveal typical hypoechoic peripheral zone lesions in 70% of patients with palpable lesions. Because many prostate cancers are not hypoechoic and not all hypoechoic lesions are cancer, transrectal ultrasound alone for screening for prostate cancer is not recommended. CT scan may reveal urinary retention, distal ureteral obstruction with resultant hydronephrosis, and pelvic lymphadenopathy. Locally advanced disease and bony metastases can also be visualized on CT scan. A chest x-ray or CT may help in identifying the uncommon lung metastases but more often shows typical osteoblastic metastases in the thoracic spine or ribs. An abdominal x-ray may reveal metastases in the lumbosacral spine or ilium. Abdominopelvic CT is not usually recom-

mended unless the disease is palpable, Gleason score is 7 or more, or PSA level is more than 20 ng/mL.

Endorectal MRI (eMRI) appears to be more helpful than CT scan in the staging of prostate cancer. This study allows for localization of malignant lesions within the prostate as well as assessment for extracapsular extension, seminal vesical invasion, involvement of adjacent organs, and lymph node involvement. eMRI is useful for clinical staging and preoperative planning but is reliant upon having a radiologist with expertise in this field.

Positron emission tomography is not typically utilized for prostate cancer staging.

D. Biopsy

The diagnosis is established by transrectal ultrasound–guided biopsies in most instances. Because the great majority of patients have biopsies due to an elevated serum PSA (stage T1c) and no abnormal findings on exam or imaging, biopsies of the base, middle, and apex of the prostate—concentrating on the peripheral zone, with 6 biopsies per side of the prostate—are required for accurate diagnosis.

Differentiation of the tumor is graded by the pathologist using the Gleason score, which assigns a grade of 1-5 (low to high grade) for both the primary and secondary forms of the tumor. The two numbers are added, and the cancer can thus be Gleason sum 2-10, with 10 being the most poorly differentiated cancer. Gleason score is an independent predictor of disease recurrence. Typically, pathologists give Gleason scores between 6 and 10.

E. Staging

Rectal examination can provide initial staging in patients with palpable tumors (Table 38–3). Needle biopsy is confirmatory, and histologic grading (Gleason score) can fairly accurately predict the metastatic potential of the tumor. Imaging as described above can be useful for staging of the primary tumor (eMRI) and to rule out metastatic disease (eMRI, bone scan).

▶ Differential Diagnosis

Nodules caused by benign prostatic hyperplasia may be difficult to distinguish from cancer; benign nodules are usually rubbery, whereas cancerous nodules have a much harder consistency. Fibrosis following a prior prostatectomy for benign disease or secondary to chronic prostatitis or prior biopsies may be associated with lesions indistinguishable from cancerous nodules and require biopsy for definition. Occasionally, phleboliths or prostatic calculi on the surface of the prostate may be confusing; however, transrectal ultrasound can be helpful in the differentiation and for biopsy guidance.

▶ Treatment

A. Curative Therapy

Curative treatment for localized prostate cancer includes radical prostatectomy and various forms of radiation therapy (external beam radiation therapy, transperineal radioactive seed placement [brachytherapy with ^{125}I, ^{103}Pd, or ^{192}Ir], and cyberknife). Complete staging is important so that appropriate candidates will be selected. Patients with localized prostate cancer are stratified into three risk groups (Table 38–4). Low-risk patients have similar 5-year recurrence survival rates irrespective of the curative treatment

Table 38–4. Localized prostate cancer risk groups.

Low risk	PSA ≤10 ng/mL Clinical stage T1c-T2a Gleason score 2-6
Intermediate risk	PSA 10-20 ng/mL Clinical stage T2b Gleason score 7
High risk	PSA >20 ng/mL Clinical stage ≥T2c Gleason 8-10

modality. Intermediate-risk and high-risk patients have better recurrence-free rates with prostatectomy or external beam radiation compared to brachytherapy. None of these modalities have been compared in randomized trials. The only reported randomized trial compared watchful waiting to radical prostatectomy and showed improved disease-free as well as overall survival in the prostatectomy group. Studies have shown that compared to external beam radiotherapy alone, combined androgen deprivation (for 6 months to 3 years) and external beam radiation improve survival in patients with localized prostate cancer, especially patients in the intermediate and high-risk groups. Patients with grossly positive pelvic lymph nodes are not candidates for curative therapy. Recent advances in surgical technique have led to a low incidence of incontinence (1%-4%) and preservation of potency in up to 70% of patients. Alternative procedures include external beam pelvic irradiation plus brachytherapy and transperineal cryoablation of the prostate for primary and recurrent disease after radiation.

For the past decade, robotic-assisted radical prostatectomy has increased in popularity and has been shown to have decreased blood loss and length of hospital stay and more rapid return to normal activity than open surgery. Oncological and functional (continence and potency) outcomes are equivalent to open surgery. More than 80% of prostatectomies in the United States are now performed with the da Vinci™ Robot.

B. Palliative Therapy

Patients with metastatic disease cannot be cured, but significant palliation can be offered. Androgen deprivation therapy in the form of luteinizing hormone–releasing hormone (LHRH agonist or bilateral orchiectomy) is effective in 70%-80% of symptomatic patients. Estrogen-based treatments are less commonly used due to the numerous side effects (in about 25% of patients), including congestive heart failure, thrombophlebitis, and myocardial infarction, and thus should not be used except in selected patients. These hormonal treatments are not additive, and use of both treatments simultaneously has no advantages over use of either alone. LHRH agonists have shown efficacy comparable to that of estrogen or orchiectomy, with reduced side effects, and are preferred by patients who find bilateral orchiectomy unacceptable. The drug must be given by injection every 1-6 months (depending on dosage) or via subcutaneous pellet annually. Studies have also shown that if an LHRH agonist is used, concomitant administration of an antiandrogen (flutamide or bicalutamide) may slightly improve survival. Studies to determine if orchiectomy plus an antiandrogen is more effective than orchiectomy alone have not shown an advantage to the combination. Antiandrogens should be administered for at least one week prior to inception of LHRH agonists to prevent the short-term flare that occurs with initiation of LHRH monotherapy. LHRH antagonists have more recently become available and have a faster onset to castration, and do not require pre-treatment with antiandrogens.

Hot flashes, osteoporosis, cardiac disease, and cognitive impairment are all potential long-term side effect of androgen deprivation.

Controversy continues concerning whether to treat asymptomatic patients at the time of diagnosis or to wait until symptoms develop. Because either approach is palliative only and there are no definitive studies showing survival advantages with early treatment, it is recommended that treatment be withheld until PSA is relatively high (> 20 ng/mL) or symptoms occur except in patients who cannot accept a no-treatment philosophy. Recent studies do show that patients who have had a radical prostatectomy and have node-positive disease do have a slight survival advantage with early hormonal treatment.

Patients whose prostate cancer becomes hormone refractory (median of 18 months after starting treatment) can be treated by ketoconazole (which inhibits adrenal androgen production) with oral corticosteroids for short-term response. Radiation therapy for symptomatic bone lesions can be helpful, as can local irradiation for an obstructing or bleeding prostate tumor. On occasion, transurethral prostatectomy is required to relieve bladder outlet obstruction. Chemotherapy with docetaxel and prednisone has shown a slight survival advantage in phase III trials.

▶ **Prostate Cancer Prevention**

Because the etiology of prostate cancer is not known, prevention is difficult to determine. However, there is evidence that a low-fat diet and lycopene (found in processed tomatoes) decrease the growth of prostate cancer cells *in vitro* and *in vivo* in animals. Further large-scale epidemiologic studies suggest a decrease in prostate cancer in humans who consumed vitamin E and selenium. However, these studies were not planned specifically for this purpose, and thus the results were questionable. A current randomized trial comparing selenium and vitamin E (SELECT) was recently halted due to the lack of evidence of prostate cancer prevention. The largest chemoprevention trial (Prostate Cancer Prevention Trial [PCPT]), with over 18,000 men, compared finasteride (5α-reductase) to placebo and found a 25% reduction in prostate cancer with finasteride but also showed an increased risk of high-grade cancer in the finasteride-treated patients. While this is thought to be an artifact of the study, these results have limited enthusiasm for recommending prevention therapy with finasteride routinely.

▶ **Prognosis**

Radical prostatectomy cures 70%-80% of the patients suitable for that operation, but its use should be limited to those with a reasonable life expectancy (Table 38–3). Currently, about 60%-70% of patients with prostatic cancer

are amenable to curative therapy when their disease is discovered.

Andriole GL et al: Mortality results from a randomized prostate-cancer screening trial. *N Engl J Med* 2009;360:1310.
Bill-Axelson A et al: Radical prostatectomy or watchful waiting in early prostate cancer. *N Engl J Med* 2014;370:932-942.
Schroder FH et al: Screening and prostate-cancer mortality and a randomized European study. *N Engl J Med* 2009;360:1320.

TUMORS OF THE URETHRA

Malignant tumors of the urethra are rare. The disease is more common in women than in men (4:1). Squamous cell types are seen most often in both sexes.

In women, urethral bleeding is the most common symptom. Distal urethral lesions of low grade and without extension can be treated by radiotherapy or wide local excision. Advanced disease is best treated by combination radiotherapy, chemotherapy, and surgery to achieve good local and distant disease control. Surgery includes anterior exenteration (removal of the bladder, uterus, adnexa, and urethra with the anterior vaginal wall), including pelvic lymphadenectomy and urinary diversion. The prognosis is excellent for distal lesions without extension, but 5-year survival rates are less than 50% for those with proximal lesions.

In men, the lesion is most commonly in the bulbomembranous urethra and is associated with a history of chronic urethral strictures, often secondary to gonorrheal infection. Patients present with urethral bleeding, a weak urinary stream, and a perineal mass. The diagnosis is made by urethroscopy and biopsy. Distal penile urethral lesions can be treated by partial or total penectomy. Lesions in the bulbous urethra or more proximal lesions require extensive surgical resection, including en bloc removal of the penis, urethra, prostate, bladder, pelvic lymph nodes, and urinary diversion. In both men and women with distal lesions, inguinal lymphatics may be involved, but node dissection is required only when gross disease is palpable. Prophylactic node dissection is controversial. Five-year survival rates are 60% for distal urethral tumors but less than 40% for the more common proximal lesions.

Primary irradiation—other than to distal lesions in the female—is rarely helpful. Patients with metastatic disease may respond to methotrexate or cisplatin alone or in combination, but objective remissions are usually of short duration.

TUMORS OF THE TESTIS

▶ **General Considerations**

Most testicular tumors are malignant germ-cell tumors. Non–germ-cell tumors such as Sertoli cell tumors and

Leydig cell tumors are rare and usually benign. Germ-cell tumors are categorized as either seminomatous (35%) or nonseminomatous (embryonal, 20%; teratocarcinoma, 38%; teratoma, 5%; and choriocarcinoma, 2%). Cryptorchidism predisposes to testicular cancer, with the incidence increasing inversely with the level of testicular descent (ie, testicles remaining in the abdomen have a much higher incidence of cancer). Metastases first develop in the retroperitoneal nodes; right-sided tumors metastasize primarily to the interaortocaval region just below the renal vessels and left-sided tumors primarily to the left para-aortic area at the same level. Distant spread is to supraclavicular areas (left, primarily) and the lungs. Almost 50% of patients have metastases when first evaluated, and this is more common for nonseminomatous tumors.

▶ Clinical Findings

A. Symptoms and Signs

Testicular tumors present as a painless firm mass within the testicular substance. They often have been present for several months before the patient seeks consultation. Occasionally (10%), a hydrocele is present, obscuring palpation of the mass. A few patients have spontaneous bleeding into the mass, causing pain. Patients with high serum levels of hCG may have gynecomastia. Patients with extensive abdominal metastases may present with abdominal pain, anorexia, and weight loss. Examination may reveal palpable retroperitoneal nodes when spread is extensive or palpable supraclavicular nodes, particularly on the left side.

B. Laboratory Findings

In general, testicular tumors do not alter the usual laboratory parameters, but serum tumor markers are diagnostically helpful. Patients with extensive retroperitoneal metastases may have bilateral ureteral obstruction that causes azotemia and anemia.

Serum lactic dehydrogenase, particularly isoenzyme I, is elevated in approximately 60% of patients. β-HCG, a particularly sensitive marker, is a glycoprotein produced by 65% of nonseminomatous testicular tumors but only 10% of seminomas. The alpha-subunit of the molecule is identical to LH, but the beta-subunit is unique to testicular tumors in adult men. There is cross-reactivity in some assays between the alpha- and beta-subunits; treated patients who develop modest elevations should have simultaneous assay of LH to be certain the marker detected is β-hCG.

α-Fetoprotein is elevated in 70% of patients with non-seminomatous testicular cancer but is *not* elevated in patients with seminoma. Patients in whom histologic study has shown seminoma but in whom serum AFP is elevated should be suspected of having nonseminomatous elements in the primary specimen or metastatic lesions.

Approximately 85% of patients demonstrate elevation of one of these markers at presentation. Serum levels decrease when the tumor is completely removed or regresses. Markers are used mainly to follow tumor regression or predict recrudescence, as even minute amounts of tumor may cause serum elevations; however, tumor may be present without elevation of serum markers.

C. Imaging Studies

Abdominal CT scan defines enlarged lymph nodes in approximately 90% of cases when they are present. Chest x-ray and CT scan will detect most pulmonary metastases.

Scrotal ultrasound is useful for identifying the typical hypoechoic lesion in the testicle. Regardless of the findings on ultrasound, however, a young man with an intratesticular mass on palpation requires surgical definition of the mass.

▶ Differential Diagnosis

Testicular masses in men aged 18-40 are frequently malignant and should be treated accordingly. Confusion can occur with scrotal hydroceles, cord hydroceles, epididymal masses or cysts, or epididymitis. Most of these can be differentiated from masses within the testicle by palpation, but if not, scrotal ultrasound is usually helpful.

▶ Treatment

See also Table 38–5.

Inguinal orchiectomy with high ligation of the cord at the internal ring is proper initial treatment for all subtypes of testicular cancer. Rarely is incisional biopsy of the testicle advisable. Recommendations for further therapy (retroperitoneal node dissection, chemotherapy, radiation therapy) are then based on the pathologic findings. A staging workup, including postoperative measurement of serum markers, chest x-ray, and chest and abdominal CT scan, is conducted to determine the extent of disease.

A. Nonseminomatous Tumors

Following orchiectomy, three management options are available: (i) active surveillance, (ii) retroperitoneal lymph node dissection (RPLND), and (iii) systemic chemotherapy. Treatment is based on clinical staging and pathology from the orchiectomy specimen. Patients with no evidence of metastatic disease on imaging and normal serum tumor markers postorchiectomy are candidates for close surveillance with the knowledge that about 20% will relapse and require salvage therapy. This strategy avoids the adverse effects of RPLND and/or systemic chemotherapy. Surveillance, however, is rigorous and should only be offered to motivated and reliable patients.

RPLND is recommended for clinical stage I patients (no evidence of metastatic disease on imaging) or for those with

Table 38–5. Treatment and prognosis of testicular cancer related to tumor stage.

Conventional Stage	TNM Stage	Clinical Findings	Treatment	Five-Year Survival (%)
I	T1	Confined to testicle	Nonseminoma: RPLND vs. surveillance; Seminoma: irradiation	>95
IIA	N1	Regional nodes < 2 cm	Adjuvant chemotherapy Nonseminoma: RPLND or chemotherapy; Seminoma: XRT or chemotherapy	>90
IIB	N2	Nodes 2-5 cm	Adjuvant chemotherapy Nonseminoma; RPLND or adjuvant chemotherapy; Seminoma: XRT or chemotherapy	>85
IIC III	N3 M+	Nodes > 5 cm Distant metastases	Chemotherapy followed by resection of residual disease	~70

All patients undergo inguinal orchiectomy.
RPLND: Retroperitoneal lymph node dissection.

retroperitoneal lymphadenopathy that is not bulky (stage IIA-IIB). The extent of lymphadenectomy depends on the testicle involved but in general includes para-aortic and paracaval nodes from the renal vessels down to the aortic bifurcation and along the external iliac artery to the internal inguinal ring on the involved side. Adverse effects of RPLND include severe hemorrhage from vascular injury to the vena cava, aorta or major branches, chylous ascites, loss of seminal emission, and damage to surrounding structures. If necessary, adjacent organs involved are removed *en bloc* with the lymph node tissue (eg, nephrectomy). Seminal emission can be preserved with modified templates or nerve sparing techniques that prospectively identify and preserve the sympathetic fibers that coalesce near the bifurcation of the aorta.

Patients with any nonseminomatous cell type who have extensive retroperitoneal or chest metastases are best treated after orchiectomy by multiagent chemotherapy—typically bleomycin, etoposide, and cisplatin. Residual masses postchemotherapy are surgically excised. Combination chemotherapy with bleomycin, etoposide, and cisplatin achieves over a 90% cure rate in stage II patients and a 70% cure rate in stage III patients. Patients who do not respond may be treated with ifosfamide, doxorubicin, or both, with some expectation of success.

B. Seminoma

In the absence of extensive distant spread, patients with pure seminoma should be treated with external beam radiation therapy (2500 cGy) to the retroperitoneum following orchiectomy. A recent study showed that one cycle of carboplatin is equivalent to radiation therapy for stage I seminoma. In the presence of bulky abdominal disease or more distant metastases, survival rates are better with multiagent chemotherapy (described earlier) given initially *in lieu* of radiation

therapy. Patients with substantial residual retroperitoneal tumor (> 3 cm) after chemotherapy may benefit from surgical removal of the remaining tumor.

▶ Prognosis

Even in the presence of metastases, many of these patients can be cured, with overall survival rates more than 90%. The only exception is patients with pure choriocarcinoma, who still have a poor survival rate (35% at 5 years) despite extensive chemotherapy.

TUMORS OF THE PENIS

Cancer of the penis is a rare disease occurring in the fifth to sixth decades. The cause is uncertain. The disease is rarely seen in circumcised men. The lesion commonly is on the glans penis or foreskin. Early cases may exhibit a painless red, velvety lesion, but most often the lesion is an exophytic nodular or wart-like growth with secondary infection. The initial diagnosis is made by a generous incisional biopsy of the lesion, which reveals squamous cell carcinoma in over 95% of cases. The tumors tend to metastasize to superficial or deep inguinal nodes, though the attendant infection may cause enlarged, tender nodes, which may be difficult to differentiate from metastatic cancer.

The differential diagnosis includes syphilitic chancre, soft chancre due to *Haemophilus ducreyi* infection, and simple or giant condyloma. Biopsy usually differentiates among these conditions.

Small, noninfiltrating lesions (carcinoma *in situ*) can be treated with fluorouracil cream, external beam radiation, or laser therapy. However, close follow-up is mandatory in patients so treated. Larger lesions not involving deep structures that are limited to the distal penis are treated by partial penile amputation at least 2 cm proximal to the lesion, leaving enough of the penis for adequate direction of the urinary stream. Deeply infiltrating and proximal lesions require total penectomy, with formation of a perineal urethrostomy.

Patients with high-risk features (high T stage, high grade, or presence of lymphovascular invasion) are at risk of inguinal nodal metastases. Prophylactic node dissection has been associated with improved survival.

Palpable inguinal nodes should be treated with antibiotics for 6 weeks following treatment of the primary lesion to eliminate infection. Persistently palpable nodes require bilateral ilioinguinal lymphadenectomy. An alternative would be fine-needle aspiration of the palpable nodes and node dissection if positive for metastases. Even those who undergo delayed node dissection when the nodes become palpable can be cured, though this is a lower percentage. Radiation therapy for palpable nodes or as prophylaxis for nonpalpable nodes has been occasionally effective, but mostly in the palliative setting.

Patients with distant metastases (to the pelvic nodes, lungs, or bone) have a poor prognosis, though cisplatin and methotrexate have shown objective but not durable responses. Five-year survival rates for patients with noninvasive lesions localized to the penis are 80%; for those with inguinal node involvement, 50%; and for those with distant metastases, nil.

Jewett MA, Groll RJ: Nerve-sparing retroperitoneal lymphadenectomy. *Urol Clin North Am* 2007;34:149.

Kondagunta GV, Motzer RJ: Adjuvant chemotherapy for stage II nonseminomatous germ cell tumors. *Urol Clin North Am* 2007;34:179.

Neill M et al: Management of low-stage testicular seminoma. *Urol Clin North Am* 2007;34:127.

Secin FP et al: Evaluation of regional lymph node dissection in patients with upper urinary tract urothelial cancer. *Int J Urol* 2007;14:26.

Sonpavde G, Sternberg CN: Treatment of metastatic urothelial cancer: opportunities for drug discovery and development. *Br J Urol (Int)* 2008;102:1354. Review.

Vaughn DJ: Chemotherapy for good-risk germ cell tumors: current concepts and controversies. *Urol Clin North Am* 2007;34:171.

▼ NEUROPATHIC (NEUROGENIC) BLADDER

A neuropathic bladder has abnormal activity secondary to a neurologic condition. To understand the variety of neuropathic bladder conditions, a basic understanding of the normal innervation and myoneurophysiology is required.

▶ Myoneural Anatomy

The urinary bladder and its involuntary sphincter develop and differentiate from the tubular urogenital sinus. The differentiation of the encasing mesenchymal cells forms the musculature of the detrusor and urethral sphincter.

▶ Innervation

The innervation of the bladder and its involuntary sphincter is via the autonomic nervous system. The parasympathetic supply to the bladder and the sphincter is via the pelvic nerves, which arise from S2-4. These fibers also carry the stretch sensory receptors to the same spinal cord center (S2-4).

The sensory supply for pain, touch, and temperature is carried via the sympathetic fibers arising from the thoracolumbar segments (T11-L2).

Motor and sensory supply of the trigone is via the thoracolumbar sympathetic fibers.

The striated external sphincter, as well as the entire urogenital diaphragm, receives its motor and sensory innervation from the somatic fibers arising from S2-4 (via the pudendal nerve).

It is clear that the S2-4 segment is the origin of the motor supply to the bladder musculature, to the involuntary sphincter, and to the striated external sphincter. The trigone is the only structure that is partly independent in its innervation. This is why segment S2-4 is called the spinal cord center for micturition. It is located at the level of the T12 and L1 vertebral bodies. There are connections between the spinal reflex center and the midbrain and cerebral cortex. Through these connections, inhibition, and control of the spinal cord reflexes can be maintained. The micturition reflex is coordinated in the pontine micturition center.

▶ Myoneurophysiology

The primary functions of the urinary bladder are to store and empty urine at a safe pressure and in a continent fashion. Intact myoneural elements are essential for these functions. The primary reservoir function is possible because of the specialized detrusor muscle arrangement and because of the bladder compliance phenomenon. The normal adult bladder can accommodate volumes up to 400 mL without increasing intravesical pressure. Bladder fullness is perceived through increases in stretching of bladder mechanoreceptors.

Distention and stretch initiate detrusor activity that can be controlled and inhibited by the high cortical centers or can be allowed to progress to active detrusor contraction and voiding. Normally during voiding, detrusor contraction continues until the bladder is completely empty unless voiding is voluntarily interrupted or inhibited.

Before voiding begins, the pelvic floor and the striated external sphincter relax, the bladder base descends, and the bladder outlet assumes a funnel shape. As a result, urethral resistance decreases. This is followed by detrusor muscle contraction and a rise in intravesical pressure to 20-40 cm of water, which results in a urine flow of about 15-30 mL/s. When the bladder is completely empty, the pelvic floor and striated external sphincter contract, elevating the bladder base, increasing urethral pressure, and ending voiding. Intact nerve pathways are essential for these synchronized activities to occur.

Cystometry

Cystometry is a simple method for testing the bladder's storage function and gives the following information: bladder capacity, extent of accommodation or compliance, the ability to sense bladder filling and temperature, and the presence of an appropriate detrusor muscle contraction. In addition, postvoid residual urine can be measured at the same time. A normal cystometrogram is shown in Figure 38–15A.

Uroflowmetry

Uroflowmetry is the measurement of urine flow rate. If detrusor contraction is properly coordinated with sphincter

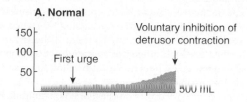

A. Normal

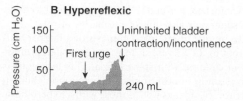

B. Hyperreflexic

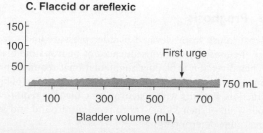

C. Flaccid or areflexic

▲ **Figure 38–15.** Cystometrograms. **A:** Normal cystometrogram. **B:** Cystometrogram in a patient with hyperreflexic bladder caused by transection of the spinal cord above S2. **C:** Cystometrogram in a patient with an areflexic flaccid neuropathic bladder caused by a myelomeningocele.

relaxation, then the outlet resistance falls as the bladder pressure increases, and the flow rate is adequate. Normally, the flow rate changes with age but is more than 20 mL/s in men under 60 and more than 25 mL/s in women under 50 years of age. Any flow rate below 12 mL/s suggests obstruction or detrusor dysfunction. A flow rate under 10 mL/s strongly suggests underlying pathology.

Urodynamics

Urodynamic studies require measurement of bladder pressure during micturition. The pressure measured within the bladder (intravesical pressure) is a combination of the intra-abdominal pressure and the pressure generated by the detrusor. To determine the detrusor pressure, the intra-abdominal pressure is measured with a rectal catheter, and this pressure is subtracted from the total intravesical pressure (measured by the bladder catheter). The urine flow rates may then be assessed in light of the detrusor pressure. No consensus exists on a critical value for pressure and flow that is diagnostic of obstruction. Nomograms have been developed for evaluating the pressure-flow relationship and thus to categorize these values as obstructed, equivocal, or unobstructed.

Electromyographic Recording

Needle or patch electrodes may be employed to record the activity of the external sphincter. This information is useful when obtained during micturition. Increased activity in the sphincter after voiding begins suggests detrusor-sphincter dyssynergia.

Classification & Clinical Findings

Several classification systems exist that describe the variety of pathologic bladder conditions that develop secondary to neuropathies. Many bladder conditions are predictable on the basis of the neurologic lesion. A lesion above the brain stem (ie, stroke) affecting micturition frequently results in involuntary bladder contractions (detrusor hyperreflexia) with coordinated (synergistic) sphincter relaxation. These patients have urge incontinence.

A complete lesion of the spinal cord (ie, trauma) above the T12 vertebral body may leave the spinal reflex center intact. This often leads to what has been categorized as an upper motor neuron lesion. These patients have detrusor hyperreflexia and uncoordinated sphincter activity (detrusor-sphincter dyssynergia). Although detrusor contractions can generate abnormally high intravesical pressure, they are not effective in producing adequate urine flow because of the spastic external sphincter. Thus, there is residual urine. Bladder capacity is reduced. Detrusor contraction and mass reflexes can be initiated from certain trigger areas.

Figure 38–15B is a typical cystometrogram of a hyperreflexic bladder.

An injury to the spinal reflex center or below often leads to what has been categorized as a lower motor neuron lesion. These patients often develop detrusor areflexia. Trauma is the most common cause, but tumors, ruptured intervertebral disks, and meningomyelocele may also cause this type of neuropathic bladder. Both motor and sensory fibers are usually affected, and there is loss of sense of fullness (Figure 38–15C). These contractions are usually weak and unsustained, and bladder emptying is incomplete, resulting in large amounts of residual urine.

The bladder dynamics in a person with a neuropathic bladder often change over time. This may occur secondary to changes in innervation (ie, tethering of spinal cord, multiple sclerosis, recovery from spinal shock) or changes in the bladder. For example, a patient with a hyperreflexic bladder and dyssynergic sphincter often develops a trabeculated, noncompliant bladder over time. These changes require periodic reevaluation of all patients with neuropathic bladders regardless of the initial classification.

► Differential Diagnosis

Cystitis, interstitial cystitis, and organic obstruction (eg, due to BPH or urethral stricture) are occasionally confused with neuropathic bladder, but associated neurologic lesions usually help make the diagnosis of neuropathic bladder. Psychosomatic disturbances can cause spasm of the external sphincter, incomplete voiding, retention, or incontinence.

► Complications

Common complications include urinary tract infection, stone formation, and incontinence. The most serious consequences of these lesions are the hydrodynamic back-pressure on the kidneys, hydronephrosis, infection, decompensation of the ureterovesical junction, and loss of renal function.

► Treatment

Immediately following spinal cord injury, there is a shock phase that may last a few weeks up to 2-3 years. The average time is 2-3 months. The bladder is completely dissociated from nervous control and thus has no sensation and is areflexic.

Treatment is aimed at avoiding the aforementioned complications in the hope of partial or complete recovery. During the shock phase, continuous closed drainage or, preferably, clean intermittent (every 4-6 hours) catheterization should be instituted until bladder activity is restored.

A. Hyperreflexic Bladder

In the hyperreflexic bladder, attaining a functional bladder depends on mobilizing residual urine and increasing the bladder capacity. Residual urine volume can be decreased by reducing urethral resistance by several methods: alpha antagonists, surgery (eg, TURP), or clean intermittent catheterization.

Functional capacity can be increased by decreasing detrusor instability with anticholinergic drugs (eg, oxybutynin), Botox injection into the bladder with cystoscopic guidance, or by operative bladder augmentation. This is often performed with small or large intestine (enterocystoplasty).

Conversion to a flaccid areflexic bladder can be achieved by cord rhizotomy. The storage function of the bladder is preserved, and the patient can be managed by clean intermittent catheterization.

Supravesical urinary diversion may be called for in patients with upper tract deterioration due to elevated storage pressures or female incontinence. Male incontinence may be controlled by a condom catheter.

B. Areflexic Bladder

Function of the flaccid bladder can be improved by measures that facilitate complete emptying; these include voiding by the Credé maneuver (suprapubic pressure), transurethral resection of the bladder neck to reduce outlet resistance, and timed voiding or timed clean intermittent catheterization. An indwelling urethral catheter or suprapubic cystostomy is required in a few cases, but chronic indwelling tubes should be avoided if possible.

Suprapubic urinary diversion (ileal or colon conduit, etc) can circumvent deterioration of upper tracts. Implantable prosthetic sphincters, periurethral bulking agent injections, or urethral slings may also improve urinary control.

A new technique of microanastomosis of a lumbar ventral nerve root to the S3 ventral root has generated promising results in children with spina bifida. This technique is reported to result in improved bladder function in children with an areflexic bladder as well as those with a hyperreflexic bladder.

► Prognosis

Renal injury from elevated bladder pressure and infection are the most serious consequences of neuropathic bladder. When diversion or bladder augmentation is required, proper timing of the operation is essential for preservation of kidney function. Patients with a neuropathic bladder require close follow-up of their kidneys with renal ultrasound and serum creatinine determinations.

Cooper CS et al: Pediatric reconstructive surgery. *Curr Opin Urol* 2000;10:195.

Van Arendonk KJ et al: Improved efficacy of extended release oxybutynin in children with daytime urinary incontinence converted from regular oxybutynin. *Urology* 2006;68:862.

OTHER DISEASES & DISORDERS OF THE GENITOURINARY TRACT

SIMPLE RENAL CYST

A simple renal cyst is usually unilateral and solitary but may be multiple and bilateral. The cause of this disorder is unclear. The cyst can compress and destroy adjacent parenchyma. Cysts contain fluid that resembles (but is not) urine. Most are diagnosed in patients after the fourth decade. Occasionally, what appears to be a simple cyst may in fact be a papillary cystadenocarcinoma—an uncommon form of renal cancer with both solid and cystic components. In those cases, however, ultrasound usually demonstrates a complex mass with both cystic and solid components.

Flank pain may be a presenting symptom, though most renal cysts are found incidentally on imaging for other purposes. CT scan and ultrasound are the most common imaging modalities. A mass may be felt in the flank or upper quadrant and must be distinguished from tumor. Urinalysis and tests of renal function are normal. If the CT scan or ultrasound reveals an equivocal cystic mass, cyst aspiration may be performed, the fluid submitted for cytologic examination, and the cyst filled with contrast material to delineate its wall. A simple cyst must be distinguished from adenocarcinoma of the kidney; ultrasonography or CT scan usually makes that distinction.

Complications are rare, but bleeding into or infection of a cyst may occur.

If the diagnosis of cyst is established, surgery is not necessary unless the lesion causes pain due to mass effect or endangers renal function. Simple percutaneous aspiration with instillation of 95% ethanol may suffice. If sclerosis fails, laparoscopic or open cyst decortication may be performed.

RENAL ARTERY ANEURYSM

Aneurysm of the renal artery is relatively rare. It results from weakening of the artery wall by arteriosclerosis, poststenotic dilation, intimal or perimedial fibroplasia, or trauma. If the aneurysm causes stenosis of the artery, hypertension may ensue secondary to ischemia and activation of the renin-angiotensin system. A plain abdominal x-ray may reveal a ring-like calcification in the wall. Angiography or CT scan is diagnostic.

Surgery is indicated in the following situations: (1) secondary renal ischemia and hypertension, (2) dissecting aneurysm, (3) aneurysm associated with pain or hematuria, (4) anticipation of pregnancy, (5) aneurysm coincident with significant stenosis, (6) radiographic evidence of incomplete calcification or increase in size on serial films, and (7) aneurysm containing thrombus with evidence of distal embolization. If the aneurysm ruptures, emergency nephrectomy may be necessary.

RENAL INFARCTION

The common causes of renal artery occlusion include emboli due to subacute infective endocarditis, atrial or ventricular thrombi, arteriosclerosis, polyarteritis nodosa, trauma, and, in the neonate, umbilical artery catheterization. Multiple emboli are common and lead to patchy renal ischemia. Occlusion of a main renal artery causes renal total infarction.

The patient may suffer from severe flank pain, or the lesion may be silent. Hematuria is common. Excretory urograms may reveal no excretion of radiopaque material or may only opacify a portion of the kidney. With complete acute occlusion of the main renal artery, a ureteral catheter drains no urine, yet the retrograde urogram reveals normal anatomy. Renal angiography, color Doppler ultrasound, or MRA makes the diagnosis by revealing occlusion of the artery or arterioles; a renal scan shows similar findings. CT scan after the intravenous injection of radiopaque medium shows no concentration in the ischemic area. Ureteral stone may mimic renal infarction, but urograms, CT scan, or angiograms distinguish one from the other. Following renal infarction, hypertension may develop secondary to renal ischemia; it may later resolve spontaneously.

If the diagnosis is made promptly (within 5-8 hours), thrombectomy or endarterectomy should be considered. Otherwise, anticoagulation therapy should be instituted (eg, heparin). Thrombolytic therapy (eg, streptokinase) may be used to lyse the clot. If permanent hypertension develops, definitive treatment of the arterial occlusion or nephrectomy (preferably laparoscopic) should be performed.

RENAL VEIN THROMBOSIS

Thrombosis of the renal vein affects both infants and adults and can be either acute or chronic. In children, thrombosis may be caused by severe dehydration (eg, due to ileocolitis and diarrhea or the nephrotic syndrome). In adults, it may be secondary to renal infection, ascending thrombosis of the vena cava, or caval occlusion due to tumor thrombus. There is usually flank pain and a palpable distended kidney. If renal vein thrombosis is secondary to infection, the patient is septic and urinalysis reveals pus cells and bacteria. In noninfectious cases, the urine may reveal microhematuria and mild proteinuria. The patient with bilateral involvement is azotemic. Nephrotic syndrome may develop. Excretory urograms show delayed opacification in an enlarged kidney. The calices are elongated. Later, the kidney may become atrophic. Renal angiography reveals stretching and bowing of arterioles. Selective renal venography demonstrates the thrombus, as does renal ultrasound.

Treatment should attempt to eliminate the underlying cause whenever possible. If the diagnosis of unilateral infected renal vein thrombosis can be established, nephrectomy should be performed. In bilateral disease, anticoagulant or thrombolytic therapy (or both) is required.

VESICAL FISTULAS

Vesical fistulas may be congenital or acquired. Congenital fistulas usually involve the urachus. Acquired fistulas may be iatrogenic or due to trauma, tumor, or inflammation.

The most common types of vesical fistulas are vesicovaginal, vesicointestinal, and vesicocutaneous. Vesicovaginal fistulas are commonly secondary to gynecologic or birth trauma; rarely, they occur as a complication of infiltrating cervical carcinoma. Vesicointestinal fistulas are most often due to inflammatory bowel disease: Crohn disease, diverticulitis, and appendicitis. Cystostomy in the presence of bladder outlet obstruction, bladder cancer, or foreign body may result in vesicocutaneous fistula.

Diagnostic maneuvers include cystoscopy, conventional cystography, barium enema or barium swallow, and CT scan with contrast infusion. Oral charcoal may be useful for detecting a urinary intestinal fistula, as the granules can be seen in spun urine under the microscope.

Therapy for vesicovaginal fistula requires surgical closure, with placement of an omental flap between the bladder and the vagina. For vesicointestinal fistula, the primary intestinal lesion must be resected and the bladder closed. An indwelling urethral catheter is necessary during the healing period.

INTERSTITIAL CYSTITIS

This lesion is most commonly found in middle-aged women. Urinary frequency both day and night is most often accompanied by suprapubic pain with bladder distention. The cause is uncertain, though some suggest an autoimmune collagen disease, while others have documented the presence of mast cells and mast cell mediators (histamine and prostaglandin) in bladder biopsy specimens of affected patients.

The diagnosis is based on the history and the results of cystoscopy under general anesthesia. Cystoscopy reveals a small-capacity bladder and punctate hemorrhage following hydrodistention. (Studies suggest this is a nonspecific finding.) Biopsy may reveal lymphocytic infiltration, mast cell infiltration, and submucosal fibrosis. In patients suspected of having interstitial cystitis, one must rule out carcinoma *in situ* with cystoscopy, urine cytologic study, and possible bladder biopsies of suspicious areas.

Treatment of established cases of interstitial cystitis often fails. First line treatment is with dietary modification of foods that can irritate the bladder mucosa (eg, caffeine, spicy foods). If poorly controlled by diet alone, pharmacotherapy with several different agents has shown utility. Pentosan polysulfate sodium is FDA approved for the treatment of interstitial cystitis. Antidepressants, antihistamines, and anticholinergics have also been utilized with some benefit. Temporary response has been obtained with bladder hydrodistention and intravesical instillations with agents such as dimethylsulfoxide. Systemic corticosteroids have their

proponents as well, and BCG has been tried with limited success. Some patients who are refractory to the above therapies undergo operative intervention. Neuromodulation with Interstim has demonstrated limited success. Finally, the last resorts of therapy include augmentation of bladder capacity by enterocystoplasty or, rarely, cystectomy and permanent urinary diversion.

URINARY STRESS INCONTINENCE

Involuntary loss of urine during stress (coughing, sneezing, or physical strain) is a common complaint of postmenopausal women. The cause is related to pelvic relaxation with age, resulting in descent of the trigone and proximal urethra. There is obliteration of the urethrovesical angle, which normally provides resistance at the bladder outlet. The diagnosis is made by the history and physical examination and urodynamic evaluation. When the bladder is full, the patient should be asked to cough while in both the supine and upright positions, producing incontinence. Digital pressure applied to the paraurethral tissues in an anterior direction through the vagina reestablishes the urethrovesical angle and prevents stress incontinence (Marshall test).

Treatment in patients with normal bladder function and low residual urine is initiated with behavioral therapy and Kegel exercises; if unsuccessful, pharmacologic methods include anticholinergics to minimize any concomitant urge incontinence. Definitive management is surgical. Currently, the most effective surgical approach is a transvaginal sling procedure with a piece of autologous fascia or synthetic mesh placed at the level of the bladder neck or mid-urethra. Other approaches include the use of bulking agents (eg, calcium hydroxylapatite) injected into the periurethral tissues, resulting in increased urethral outflow resistance.

FEMALE URETHRITIS & PERIURETHRITIS

Urethritis in the female may be acute or chronic. Acute urethritis can be gonorrheal in origin. Chemical urethritis is occasionally acquired from exposure to soap or bath oils. Chronic urethritis is a common problem in women, since the female urethra is exposed to pathogenic bacteria because of its anatomic location. Urethral trauma, instrumentation, and increase in the number of pathogenic organisms lead to infection and overt urethritis. Urethritis usually precedes cystitis.

Hormonal changes associated with menopause cause vaginal and urethral mucosal changes, leading to irritative symptoms and increased susceptibility to inflammation.

Urethritis usually causes irritative voiding symptoms similar to those of cystitis and, occasionally, functional obstructive symptoms. Examination may reveal urethral discharge, marked tenderness, or congested everted mucosa at the external meatus. Induration of the urethra may be associated with vaginitis and cervicitis. Endoscopy may reveal obstruction, mucosal congestion, and inflammatory polyps. Urethral calibration rarely reveals obstruction. Spasm of the external sphincter may be noted.

Treatment is directed to the underlying cause. Estrogen cream is indicated for senile vaginitis. Surgical treatment consists of urethral dilation and opening and draining infected periurethral ducts. Alpha-blockers given orally may also help decrease urethral resistance. Correction of vaginitis, cervicitis, and cervical erosions helps in ameliorating symptoms.

FEMALE URETHRAL CARUNCLE

Urethral caruncle, commonly seen after menopause, represents granulomatous overgrowth of the posterior lip of the external meatus. The caruncle is tender and causes pain with intercourse and urination. The primary concern is exclusion of urethral cancer. Treatment is complete excision.

FEMALE URETHRAL DIVERTICULUM

Urethral diverticulum in the female commonly presents as recurrent lower urinary tract infection. It should be suspected whenever urinary infection fails to resolve with treatment. Symptoms are urinary dribbling and cystic swelling in the anterior vaginal wall during voiding. If diverticulum is suspected, it can usually be identified during panendoscopy and opacified by contrast medium on a voiding cystourethrogram while occluding the external meatus. Pelvic MRI provides excellent diagnostic detail. These lesions occasionally contain stones or tumors. Treatment consists of transvaginal diverticulectomy.

SPERMATOCELE

Spermatocele is a retention cyst of a tubule of the rete testis or the head of the epididymis. The cyst is distended with a milky fluid that contains sperm. Located at the superior pole of the testis and caput epididymidis, the spermatocele is soft and fluctuant and can be transilluminated. No treatment is needed unless the spermatocele is painful, in which case surgical excision may be performed.

VARICOCELE

Varicocele is due to incompetent valves in the testicular vein, permitting transmission of hydrostatic venous pressure; distention and tortuosity of the pampiniform plexus results. Varicocele is found in 15% of male adolescents with left-sided predominance (90%), presumably because of venous drainage of the left testes to the left renal vein, causing increased retrograde venous pressure. Bilateral varicoceles are palpable in fewer than 2% of male adults.

Mild varicoceles are commonly asymptomatic, but a dragging scrotal sensation may be noted. Varicocele may lead to infertility in some men.

Asymptomatic varicocele is best untreated unless it is a suspected factor in male infertility. Treatment then consists of operative ligation of the spermatic vein at or above the internal inguinal ring. In recurrent varicocele, transfemoral catheterization and occlusion or ablation of the spermatic vein may be performed with a detachable balloon or sclerosing agents. The technical success rate is high.

TORSION OF THE SPERMATIC CORD

Torsion of the spermatic cord (intravaginal torsion or torsion within the space of the tunica vaginalis) is most common in adolescent boys. A twist in the spermatic cord interferes with testicular blood supply. If torsion is complete, testicular infarction may occur within 4-6 hours. The cause is unknown, but an underlying anatomic abnormality (spacious tunica vaginalis, loose epididymotesticular connection, undescended testis) is usually present.

Clinical findings consist of precipitous onset of lower abdominal and scrotal pain and scrotal swelling. There may be a history of previous trauma in young adolescents. The testis is swollen, tender, and retracted. The pain is not relieved by testicular support. The cord above the swelling is normal. The cremasteric reflex is usually absent on the affected side.

Torsion must be differentiated from orchitis, epididymitis, and pain due to testicular trauma. Technetium 99m pertechnetate scan *may* differentiate orchitis-epididymitis from testicular torsion if performed early in the course of symptoms: The former demonstrates increased blood flow, in contrast to the ischemic pattern of torsion. Color Doppler ultrasound is more definitive and less time consuming and can delineate the lack of testicular blood flow. No radiologic study is completely accurate, and imaging should be used to confirm the clinical decision that the cause of the acute scrotum is not torsion. If the diagnosis cannot be established by examination, history, and imaging, exploration is required.

Torsion of the spermatic cord is a surgical emergency! Contralateral orchiopexy is always necessary because of frequent bilateral involvement (ie, the "bell clapper" deformity: lack of fixation of the cord structures by the testicular mediastinum) and the high incidence of recurrent torsion and infertility in bilateral cases.

TORSION OF TESTICULAR APPENDAGES

The epididymis and the testicle often have a vestigial remnant of embryologic ducts known as an appendix testis or appendix epididymis. These structures can undergo spontaneous infarction usually in young boys, causing acute testicular pain and swelling that may be difficult to differentiate from testicular torsion. With torsion of the appendix testis or epididymis, physical examination often demonstrates point tenderness at the site of the torsed appendage. Occasionally, the infarcted appendage can be seen through the scrotal wall as a "blue dot" sign on the scrotum. This sign is only visible early in the course, prior to hydrocele formation and onset of scrotal edema. Scrotal ultrasound occasionally delineates the enlarged appendage and a normal testicle, establishing the diagnosis. In most cases—and certainly in equivocal ones—immediate scrotal exploration and removal of the infarcted appendage is required to rule out testicular torsion. Although the appendages often occur bilaterally, appendiceal torsion does not; thus, removal of the opposite appendage is not indicated.

MALE INFERTILITY

Male infertility accounts for 30%-50% of infertile couples (10%-15% of marriages). Both partners should be evaluated for causes of infertility.

The causes of male infertility include the following: congenital anomalies (genetic, such as Klinefelter's syndrome, or developmental, such as absent vas deferens); trauma (both testicular, resulting in atrophy, and neurologic, resulting in erectile or ejaculatory dysfunction); infections (either systemic or reproductive organ specific); endocrine disorders (pituitary insufficiency, androgen deficiency); acquired anatomic abnormalities (varicocele, vasectomy); or drug side effects (nitrofurantoin, estrogens, antineoplastic agents).

▶ Diagnosis

The most important aspect of infertility evaluation is the history, which uncovers the cause in many patients. The physical examination is no less important and may reveal small testicles, a varicocele, or absence of the vas deferens.

A. Semen Analysis

Semen analysis is essential in evaluation of male factor infertility. At least two samples should be analyzed, since values may vary over time and with the method of collection. The specimen is produced by masturbation after 3 days of ejaculatory abstinence and collected in a clean wide-mouth container and examined within 2 hours. Determination of the volume, pH, liquefaction, sperm count, viability, abnormal forms, and motility constitutes a complete analysis. Normal values include volume of more than 2.0 mL, concentration greater than 20 million sperm per mL, more than 50% motile sperm, and 75% or more viable sperm (World Health Organization criteria).

B. Hormone Studies

Patients with no sperm in the ejaculate (azoospermia) or very low counts (oligospermia, < 10 million sperm/mL) should have serum FSH, LH, and testosterone levels measured. Patients with low testosterone should have prolactin levels checked and, if elevated, should be investigated for pituitary tumor. A significant elevation of FSH represents a problem with spermatogenesis.

C. Testicular Biopsy

Testicular biopsies are indicated in azoospermic patients to distinguish obstructive versus parenchymal disease. Testicular biopsy should be performed in patients with unexplained oligospermia to establish a histologic diagnosis, to assess prognosis, and to direct treatment. If the serum FSH is more than two times normal, one may presume the presence of severe and irreversible testicular damage without confirmatory testis biopsy.

Vasography requires injection of contrast material into the vas. The purpose of this study is to delineate obstruction of the vas, epididymis, seminal vesicle, or ejaculatory duct. Vasography is used in patients who are azoospermic and have no evidence of retrograde ejaculation while demonstrating normal spermatogenesis on testicular biopsy. Seminal fructose levels should be obtained before operative exposure of the vas. Absence of fructose would indicate obstruction of the ejaculatory duct, and if this diagnosis is confirmed by vasography, the obstructing tissue may be resected by transurethral methods.

D. Other Diagnostic Studies

The **sperm penetration assay,** performed by incubation of sperm with hamster eggs whose zona pellucida has been enzymatically removed, offers an objective method of determining the ability of sperm to penetrate the ovum. The **cervical mucus penetration test** compares sperm motility in cervical mucus with a known standard. Although these two important parameters of sperm function can be evaluated, neither test alone can establish the cause of male factor infertility.

Antisperm antibodies can be measured in the serum of either the male or female partner or in the seminal fluid. This assessment is indicated when spontaneous sperm agglutination or decreased sperm motility is noted on semen analysis. If antisperm antibodies are found, immunosuppressive therapy in the form of steroids may be effective in reducing agglutination (clumping) and increasing motility. Another method of treating antisperm antibodies is *in vitro* sperm washing with immunobeads coated by antihuman antibody. The sperm not bound by antibody remain in the supernatant and can be used for intrauterine insemination.

Studies to detect a nonpalpable varicocele are not recommended except in cases in which the physical examination is inadequate. Physical examination is the most effective method of detecting clinically significant varices. Venography is reserved for patients with recurrent varices, since identification of collateral venous channels would direct choice of therapy.

Transrectal ultrasound is used to support the diagnosis of ejaculatory duct obstruction in the azoospermic patient. Absence of the seminal vesicles or distention due to distal obstruction can be identified. This study should be preceded by measurement of fructose in the ejaculate (lack of fructose suggests obstruction of the ejaculatory duct) and examination of postejaculate urine (to determine the presence of sperm, suggesting retrograde ejaculation).

▶ Treatment

A. Nonoperative Treatment

Primary male infertility may be caused by hypogonadotropic hypogonadism, diagnosed by demonstrating low serum levels of FSH, LH, and testosterone. Spermatogenesis may be stimulated by administration of hCG followed by FSH. Isolated absence of either FSH or LH is rare; the LH deficiency is overcome by administration of testosterone, and lack of FSH is treated by administration of menotropins. Hyperprolactinemia may contribute to male infertility and would be treated with bromocriptine.

Infection of the reproductive organs should be treated when found during evaluation of male infertility. Infection may cause infertility immediately by several mechanisms: decreased spermatogenesis due to hyperthermia, immune interaction with sperm causing agglutination and decreased motility, as well as later sequelae such as obstruction of the ejaculatory tract. Pyospermia suggests the diagnosis, and treatment should be designed to eliminate the common pathogens: *Neisseria gonorrhoeae*, *Chlamydia trachomatis*, and *Ureaplasma urealyticum* (all are sensitive to tetracycline).

If antisperm antibodies are found in either partner, steroids may be used to suppress the immune system. One must use steroids with caution and after thorough discussion of possible side effects with the patient; acne, hypertension, gastrointestinal bleeding, and avascular necrosis of the hip have been reported with steroid administration. Response to treatment is assessed by repeat semen analysis and measurement of antisperm antibodies in the patient's serum. Sperm washing in an attempt to remove cytotoxic antibodies may improve motility and decrease clumping; washed semen may then be instilled into the uterus (artificial insemination of the husband's semen) or used in conjunction with *in vitro* fertilization (IVF) techniques.

Retrograde ejaculation or lack of seminal emission—usually due to spinal cord injury or sympathetic nerve injury during retroperitoneal surgery leading to bladder neck (ie, internal sphincter) incompetence—can be treated with α-adrenergic drugs or antihistamines to reestablish internal sphincter function and antegrade ejaculation. Alternatively, alkalinized postejaculate urine can be collected and centrifuged and the concentrated sperm instilled into the female partner's uterus.

Clomiphene and tamoxifen are antiestrogens that are currently used in patients with idiopathic oligospermia, though the efficacy of these medications has been doubted.

B. Operative Therapy

Ligation of varicocele yields pregnancy in 30%-50% of patients. Several approaches are available, including inguinal and retroperitoneal. Transvenous occlusion of the spermatic vein by balloon is useful especially in cases of recurrent varicocele.

Obstruction of the epididymis-vas system may be amenable to vasovasostomy or vasoepididymostomy. Currently, these procedures are performed with the aid of the operating microscope, and patency is established in 50%-90% of cases.

Obstruction of the ejaculatory ducts is rare. When this diagnosis is made, transurethral resection of the ducts may establish patency.

C. Assisted Reproductive Techniques

These include the following: artificial insemination with husband's sperm (AIH), gamete intrafallopian transfer, and IVF using intracytoplasmic sperm injection after retrieving eggs by transvaginal ultrasound guidance and sperm by testicular aspiration in selected partners. In cases of male factor infertility not amenable to treatment, artificial insemination by donor sperm is also available.

PRIAPISM

Priapism is a rare disorder in which prolonged, painful erection occurs, usually not associated with sexual stimulation. The blood in the corpora cavernosa becomes hyperviscous but not clotted. About 25% of cases are associated with leukemia, metastatic carcinoma, sickle cell anemia, or trauma. In most cases, the cause is uncertain.

If the erection does not subside, needle aspiration of the sludged blood of the corpora followed by lavage with alpha-adrenergic agents such as phenylephrine should be performed. Delayed or unsuccessful treatment may result in impotence. Unsuccessful treatment calls for the Winter procedure, in which a biopsy needle is passed through the glans into one of the corpora, creating a fistula between corpora cavernosa and corpus spongiosum. If this procedure is successful, then potency is usually maintained. Other procedures include excising the tunica albuginea at the tip of the corpora cavernosum, proximal cavernosal-spongiosum shunt, and saphenous vein-cavernous shunt. If priapism persists, impotence results.

In sickle cell anemia, hydration and hypertransfusion often give relief and should constitute initial therapy.

PEYRONIE'S DISEASE

Fibrosis of the dorsal covering sheaths of the corpora cavernosa occasionally occurs without known cause in men over age 45. Trauma to the penis during intercourse has been implicated in the etiology of Peyronie's disease. The fibrosis does not permit the involved surface to lengthen with erection, thus leading to dorsal chordee. The disorder may be due to vasculitis in the connective tissues. Palpation of the penile shaft reveals a raised, firm plaque dorsally. There is an association with Dupuytren contracture.

Controversy exists regarding treatment. Expectant therapy or medical treatment, including vitamin E, para-aminobenzoic acid, colchicine, and intralesional verapamil may limit progression of disease. Operative therapy is necessary for patients who do not respond or for impotent patients. In the potent patient, either plication of the tunica albuginea on the opposite side of the plaque or a Nesbit procedure—excision of an ellipse of the tunica albuginea from the ventral convex aspect of the shaft and suture closure—or plaque excision and dermal grafting have been used successfully. If the patient is impotent, insertion of a penile prosthesis is the procedure of choice.

Taylor FL, Levine LA: Peyronie's disease. *Urol Clin North Am* 2007;34:517.

PHIMOSIS & PARAPHIMOSIS

Phimosis—inability to retract the foreskin to expose the glans—may be congenital but is more often acquired. At birth, the foreskin cannot be easily retracted, but by age 3, the prepuce becomes pliant and the glans can be exposed and cleansed. If the foreskin is then retractable, circumcision is not necessary. Acquired phimosis is usually a result of chronic and recurrent bacterial balanitis (infection of the prepuce), common in patients with diabetes or balanitis xerotica obliterans. These patients are best treated by circumcision.

Paraphimosis is the inability to reduce a previously retracted foreskin. The prepuce becomes fixed in the retracted position proximal to the corona. With prolonged retraction, lymphedema of the prepuce exacerbates the condition and increases the circumferential pressure of the shaft proximal to the glans. Manual reduction can usually be accomplished using the index fingers to pull the prepuce distally while pushing the glans into the prepuce. If this measure fails, the preputial cicatrix may be incised (dorsal slit) and the foreskin reduced with relative ease. Circumcision may be performed as an elective procedure once the edema has subsided.

CONDYLOMATA ACUMINATA

Condylomata acuminata are wart-like lesions that occur on the penis, scrotum, urethra, and perineum in men and the vagina, cervix, and perineum in women. They are caused by human papillomavirus and are usually transmitted by sexual contact. Pain and bleeding are common presenting complaints. Warts outside the urethra can be treated with excision, application of podophyllum resin, liquid nitrogen, or CO_2 laser. Urethroscopy is needed to determine the proximal extent of lesions in the urethra. Intraurethral fulgura-

tion, CO_2 laser treatment, injection of fluorouracil solution, or interferon-α can be therapeutic.

IMPOTENCE

Impotence is the inability to obtain and sustain an erection satisfactory for sexual intercourse.

▶ Causes of Impotence

Causes can be grouped into the following categories: neurologic, vascular, endocrine, systemic, pharmacologic, and psychologic. Treatment is directed accordingly.

A. Neurologic

Reflex erections are mediated by the afferent fibers of the pudendal nerve and efferent fibers of the parasympathetic outflow (S2-4). Psychogenic erections are initiated via cerebral centers. Specific neurologic diseases that may cause impotence may be congenital (spina bifida), acquired (cerebrovascular accident, Alzheimer disease, multiple sclerosis), iatrogenic (electroshock therapy), neoplastic (pituitary or hypothalamic tumors), traumatic (cord compression), infectious (tabes dorsalis), and nutritional (vitamin deficiency).

B. Vascular

Vascular causes of impotence may be cardiac (anginal syndromes, congestive failure), aortoiliac disease (Leriche syndrome, atherosclerosis, and other embolic phenomena), microangiopathy (diabetes, radiation injury), and abnormal venous drainage.

C. Endocrine

The accepted endocrine causes of impotence are hypogonadism, hyperprolactinemia, pituitary tumors, hypothyroidism, Addison disease, Cushing syndrome, acromegaly, and testicular feminizing syndrome.

D. Pharmacologic

Impotence is a common and often unsuspected complication of many therapeutic and illicit drugs. Major groups that may cause sexual dysfunction are the following: tranquilizers, antidepressants, antianxiety agents, anticholinergic drugs, antihypertensives, and many drugs with abuse potential. One should recognize that virtually all antihypertensives (including diuretics) can be associated with impotence or ejaculatory dysfunction. Drugs with abuse potential include alcohol (both as a direct affect and secondary to cirrhosis) and cocaine.

E. Psychogenic

Up to 50% of cases of impotence are related to psychogenic factors. Establishing an organic cause of impotence is important in choosing appropriate therapy. Factors that indicate a psychogenic cause are the following: selective erectile dysfunction (episodic, normal nocturnal erections, normal erections with masturbation), sudden onset, associated anxiety or external stress, affect disturbances (anger, anxiety, guilt, fear), and patient convinced of an organic cause.

▶ Diagnosis

The history and physical examination suggest the cause in most cases. Confirmatory tests are necessary to ensure an appropriate choice of therapy.

In investigating a possible neurologic cause of impotence, the neurologic examination should include review of systems with respect to bladder and bowel function. More invasive studies include a cystometrogram, electromyography of the external urethral sphincter, and bulbosphincteric reflex latency.

Vascular impotence is suggested by signs of peripheral vascular disease as well as a history of atherosclerotic heart disease. Noninvasive diagnostic testing is performed with penile duplex Doppler studies to assess arterial inflow. Venous leak can be evaluated with cavernosography and cavernosometry. Arteriography is rarely required but may be indicated in patients with a history of pelvic trauma and those considering microvascular arterial revascularization.

Endocrine evaluation mandates measurement of serum testosterone and prolactin; many investigators include assessment of FSH and LH. Routine automated chemical screening may suggest other hormonal abnormalities that require additional testing. These studies should also detect systemic disease capable of causing impotence: cirrhosis, renal failure, scleroderma, and diabetes.

Psychogenic impotence may be established by nocturnal penile tumescence monitoring or outpatient snap-gauge cuffs. Additional testing includes one of the following: Minnesota Multiphasic Personality Inventory, DeRogatis Sexual Function Inventory, and Walker Sex Form.

▶ Treatment

A. Nonoperative Treatment

First-line treatment includes oral phosphodiesterase inhibitors (sildenafil, vardenafil, tadalafil). These medications are contraindicated in men with heart disease who are taking nitroglycerin. These medications work in patients who have normal blood flow and neurologic innervation. In patients without arterial-vascular causes of impotence, intracorporal injections of papaverine, phentolamine, or prostaglandin E_1 (or all three) offer a nonoperative means of restoring sexual function. Intractable psychogenic impotence may also respond to this treatment. Intraurethral pellets of alprostadil (prostaglandin E_1) can also be used; however, they often cause pain and are not favored by most patients. Finally, a vacuum erection device can be used to sustain erection.

Endocrine disturbances responsible for impotence include low testosterone and hyperprolactinemia. Testosterone deficiency is treated by replacement therapy using a once-daily topical testosterone gel or depot testosterone intramuscular injection every 2-3 weeks. Hyperprolactinemia is treated by bromocriptine therapy; the patient should be evaluated to assess the presence of a pituitary tumor.

Pharmacologic causes of impotence require altering medical treatment to ameliorate or eliminate secondary impotence. The ability to change medications depends on the severity of the underlying disease.

Psychogenic impotence is treated by a trained sex therapist, and response may be anticipated in most cases. The importance of eliminating organic causes of impotence before embarking on psychological therapy is obvious. The best psychological methods applied to organic impotence do not resolve the dysfunction but serve to frustrate both the therapist and patient.

B. Operative Treatment

Penile prosthesis insertion is currently the most common operative method for treatment of impotence. Two categories of prosthesis are in use: semirigid and inflatable. The semirigid prostheses are composed of a rigid shaft and a flexible hinge at the penile-pubic junction or a malleable soft metal case within the prosthesis; the erection is constant and is satisfactory to effect vaginal penetration, but the penile circumference is not equal to that of a natural erection.

Inflatable prostheses offer erections more similar in size to those experienced by the patient prior to the onset of impotence when compared to those achieved by semirigid prostheses. Two types of inflatable prostheses are available. The standard inflatable prosthesis consists of two corporal inflatable rods, a reservoir situated in the retropubic space, and a pump placed in the scrotum; the new inflatable rods combine the simplicity of two corporal rods with the sophistication of a self-contained pump and reservoir system (FlexiFlate and Hydroflex), permitting the convenience of inflation and deflation without tubing and multiple components.

Satisfactory results are achieved in 85% of patients. Complications common to both types of prostheses are infection and erosion of skin or urethra. The inflatable prostheses are also at risk for mechanical failure of the pump, tubing or reservoir leak, and aneurysm or rupture of the corporal cylinders.

Arterial revascularization of the penile arteries has met with limited success. Aortoiliac reconstruction improves erectile function in only 30% of cases. Microsurgical revascularization of the penile arteries (dorsal artery of the penis or deep corporal arteries) is successful in about 60% of patients. While these methods avoid the risks of prosthetic infection and offer the advantage of reestablishing the natural physiologic mechanisms or erection, the mediocre success rate (when compared with the results of prosthetic insertion) would suggest that microsurgical penile revascularization be reserved for carefully selected cases.

Seftel AD et al: Office evaluation of male sexual dysfunction. *Urol Clin North Am* 2007;34:463.

MULTIPLE CHOICE QUESTIONS

1. During development, the kidneys pass through three embryonic phases, including all of the following except

   A. Prenephros
   B. Pronephros
   C. Mesonephros
   D. Metanephros

2. The most common site for an undescended testis to reside is

   A. Just outside the external ring
   B. Inside the abdomen
   C. In the inguinal canal
   D. In the wall of a sliding hernia sac
   E. None of the above

3. Patients evaluated for hematuria are considered low risk for malignancy based upon all of the following except

   A. Less than 40 years of age
   B. No history of pelvic irradiation or cyclophosphamide exposure
   C. Non-smokers
   D. Have a history of urinary tract infections
   E. Microscopic hematuria

4. Renal stones composed of calcium salts can be promoted by

   A. Hyperoxaluria
   B. Hypercitrauria
   C. Hypocalciuria
   D. Hypouricosuria
   E. All of the above

5. Palliative therapy for prostate cancer can include

   A. LHRH antagonists
   B. Estrogen blockade
   C. Transurethral prostatectomy
   D. Somatostatin agonists
   E. Depot testosterone therapy

Gynecology

R. Kevin Reynolds, MD

PERTINENT HISTORY & PHYSICAL EXAM FOR GYNECOLOGIC DISEASES

Accurate diagnosis and treatment of gynecologic disease begins with obtaining a complete history and physical examination. A thorough history should include

- First day of the most recent menstrual cycle
- Current genital tract symptoms
- Age at first menses (menarche)
- Interval from starting one menses to the next (cycle length)
- Duration and amount of menstrual flow
- Presence or absence of irregular or unexplained bleeding
- Symptoms associated with each menstrual cycle such as cramping before or during menses
- Other genital tract symptoms such as urinary or fecal incontinence, prolapse, dyspareunia, discharge, or pruritus
- Sexual history including assessment of risk factors such as knowledge of safe sex practices, age of first intercourse (coitarche), number and gender of partners, and presence of any history of abuse
- Number of pregnancies and subsequent outcome including term delivery, mode of delivery, preterm delivery, miscarriage, or abortion
- Contraceptive use including type, duration
- History of sexually transmitted disease such as infection with human papillomavirus (HPV), gonorrhea, or Chlamydia
- Adequacy of cervical cancer screening with Pap tests including date of most recent screen and any prior history of abnormal screens
- History of any gynecologic surgery including type, date, and indication
- Age of menopause
- Presence of postmenopausal bleeding regardless of amount of flow
- Hormone therapy of any type including oral contraceptives, postmenopausal estrogen replacement therapy, hormone therapy of breast cancer, etc
- Family history of pertinent cancer sites including ovarian cancer, endometrial cancer, breast cancer, and colorectal cancer. Determine the age at time of cancer diagnosis and relationship of the affected individual to the patient
- Determine the ethnicity of the patient regarding potential for hereditary diseases

Perform a complete pelvic examination. Inspect external genitalia including vulva and urethra for development, symmetry, and visible lesions. Place a vaginal speculum to inspect the vagina and cervix for symmetry, or visible lesions and perform Pap test, cultures, or wet mount tests as indicated to evaluate symptoms or update screening. Bimanual examination is then performed with careful compression of pelvic viscera between the examiner's hand on the abdominal wall and the finger(s) in the vagina. The process is repeated with the rectovaginal examination whereby one finger is placed in the vagina and one is inserted into the rectum. The rectovaginal exam allows the examiner to feel higher into the pelvis and may improve the ability to feel the cardinal and uterosacral ligaments, cul de sac peritoneum, ovaries, rectocele, and sphincter integrity. The rectovaginal exam is particularly important for assessing pelvic masses or malignancies, rectocele, and fecal incontinence.

EMBRYOLOGY & ANATOMY

Development of the reproductive tract in the female fetus results from fusion and differentiation of the Müllerian ducts and the urogenital sinus. Fusion defects may result in duplication, malformation, or absence of genital tract structures.

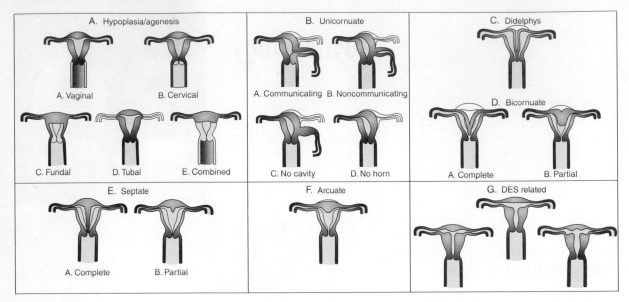

▲ **Figure 39–1.** Classification of müllerian anomalies. DES, diethylstilbestrol. (From Schorge JO, Williams JW: *Williams Gynecology,* New York: McGraw-Hill, 2008.)

The most common defects are imperforate hymen, presence of longitudinal or transverse septae within the vagina, congenital absence of the vagina, and duplication defects of the uterus (Figure 39–1). The etiology of most of these congenital defects is idiopathic, but some cases arise as a result of teratogens such as androgen exposure to the developing fetus during the first and second trimesters.

Careful examination of the newborn is necessary. Cursory examination of the genital structure of the newborn may result in errors of gender assignment. Ultrasound and/or MRI, examination under anesthesia, and possible laparoscopy or hysteroscopy provide information for accurate diagnosis. One-third or more of children diagnosed with genital tract anomalies will have associated with anomalies of the urinary tract such as absent kidney, horseshoe kidney, and duplication of ureters.

The pelvis is a space constrained by bony architecture and filled with gastrointestinal urologic and gynecologic viscera. The blood supply is rich, including the external and internal ileac arteries and veins, and numerous branches within the pelvis. Motor nerves including the sciatic, obturator, and femoral nerves transit the pelvis along the pelvic sidewall. Sensory nerves including the genitofemoral nerve are superficially located and easily injured. The ureter is closely placed to the uterine artery and is at risk for injury during hysterectomy procedures (Figures 39–2A and 39–2B). A pelvic surgeon must be intimately familiar with the close spacing of critical pelvic structures to minimize risk of injury.

▼ THE LOWER GENITAL TRACT: VULVA, VAGINA, & CERVIX

SCREENING & TREATMENT OF PREMALIGNANT LOWER GENITAL TRACT NEOPLASIA

As recently as 1945, cervical cancer and related lower genital tract cancers were the most common cancers in women. With the advent of the Pap test in the 1940s, cervical cancer incidence began to fall with more than an 80% reduction of risk of mortality in the ensuing six decades. It is now understood that virtually all cervical cancers and some vaginal and vulvar cancers are caused by persistent infection with oncogenic strains of the human papillomavirus (HPV). There are more than 75 HPV types identified, with types 6 and 11 most commonly associated with condyloma and types 16 and 18 associated with preinvasive and invasive carcinoma. Prevalence of HPV infection is as high as 80% of the population, but most infections are transient in nature. With appropriate screening and treatment to detect individuals with persistent high-risk HPV infection, the risk of developing invasive cervical cancer is low. In parts of the world without screening, cervical cancer remains prevalent and is the second most common cancer diagnosis for unscreened women. FDA approval of vaccination effective for the prevention of oncogenic HPV strains occurred in 2006 and has the potential to greatly reduce HPV mediated lower genital tract cancers in women.

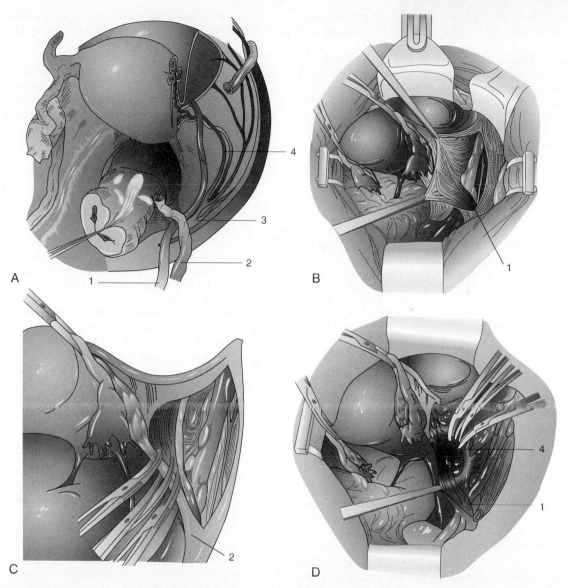

▲ **Figure 39–2.** Pelvic retroperitoneal anatomy. ***A:*** Dissected right retroperitoneal space illustrating the course of the pelvic ureter. The right uterine adnexa are transected adjacent to the uterus, the ovarian vessels are severed just distal to the pelvic brim, and the peritoneum is removed from the right pelvic sidewall and the right portion of the bladder. The ureter (1) enters the pelvis by crossing over the bifurcation of the common iliac artery just medial to the ovarian vessels (2). It then descends medial to the branches of the internal iliac artery (3). The ureter then courses through the cardinal ligament and passes under the uterine artery (4, "water under the bridge") approximately 1–2 cm lateral to the cervix at the level of the internal cervical os. The origin of the uterine artery from the internal iliac artery (3) is shown. The ureter then courses medially toward the base of the bladder. The distal part of the ureter is associated with the upper portion of the anterior vaginal wall. ***B:*** The retroperitoneal space is entered, and the peritoneum is retracted medially to show the ureter (1) crossing over the external and internal iliac artery bifurcation. Note that the ureter remains attached to the peritoneum of the pelvic sidewall and the medial leaf of the broad ligament. ***C:*** The ovarian vessels (2) are clamped and transected after visualization of the ureter. ***D:*** The uterine artery (4) is being clamped and transected. Note the ureter (1) crossing under this vessel lateral to the cervix.

A number of professional groups, including the American Cancer Society, American College of Obstetricians and Gynecologists, American Society for Clinical Pathology, American Society for Colposcopy and Cervical Pathology (ASCCP), and the National Comprehensive Cancer Network have issued consensus guidelines for cervical cancer screening that were updated in 2012. The US Preventive Services Task Force issued nearly identical recommendations in 2012. The guidelines address initiation of screening, screening interval, and discontinuation of screening.

When to initiate screening

Begin at age 21
When to discontinue screening

1. Age > 65 with adequate negative prior screening

2. Hysterectomy

3. Discontinuation of screening should not occur if the patient has a history of CIN2, CIN3, or adenocarcinoma *in situ*. In this case screening should continue for 20 years

Screening interval

1. Women aged 21-29 years

   a. Cytology alone every 3 years
   b. Liquid-based or glass-smear cytology is acceptable

2. Women aged 30-65 years

   a. Cytology with high-risk HPV cotest every 5 years (preferred)
   b. Cytology alone every 3 years (acceptable)

3. Women vaccinated against HPV

Follow age-specific guidelines

If cytology or HPV testing results are abnormal, then further evaluation is warranted. The ASCCP issued guidelines in 2013 that addressed triage and treatment for women with screening test abnormalities. Key points are as follows:

1. Cytologic tests should be reported using standard nomenclature defined by the Bethesda System. Key preinvasive diagnoses with which the clinician should be familiar include

   a. Atypical squamous cells (ASC). The report will indicate either "uncertain significance" (ASC-US), or "cannot rule out high-grade dysplasia" (ASC-H). ASC-US should be further tested by ordering a reflex hybrid capture assay for high-risk HPV DNA unless the patient is an adolescent. ASC-H has a high risk of high-grade dysplasia and must be evaluated with colposcopy

   b. Low-grade squamous intraepithelial lesion (LSIL) is virtually always caused by HPV, and HPV

testing has been shown not to be cost effective. In adolescent patients, a repeat cytology exam in 1 year is recommended. In adults, colposcopy is performed.

   c. High-grade squamous intraepithelial lesion (HSIL) has a high likelihood of high-grade dysplasia on biopsy and invasive cancer will sometimes be detected. Patients with HSIL, regardless of age, are evaluated with colposcopy

   d. Glandular abnormalities refer to disease in the endocervical canal. These lesions are difficult to see and may therefore be detected later. Skip lesions occur in 10%-15% of cases, indicating the importance of evaluating the entire canal with curettage or similar sampling methods. All three glandular lesions reported have a high likelihood of high-grade dysplasia and a moderate likelihood of associated invasive cancer. Colposcopy and endocervical gland sampling with curettage with possible endometrial sampling is required. Cells in this category will be reported as

   i. Atypical glands, not otherwise specified (AGC-NOS)
   ii. Atypical glands, favor neoplasia
   iii. Adenocarcinoma *in situ* (AIS)

2. Adolescents and young adult women, defined as being 24 years of age and younger, have a very high prevalence of HPV infection and a very low likelihood of cervical cancer. Because the disease will often regress in this age range, management guidelines have become progressively more conservative

3. The colposcope is a binocular microscope (Figure 39–3) that allows close inspection of the squamo-columnar junction (SCJ) on the cervix where the majority of squamous cervical cancers arise. High-grade lesions have a characteristic appearance including white light reflection after staining with acetic acid in areas of dysplasia (aceto-white change), abnormal vascular patterns (punctation, mosaic, and atypical vessels), and altered contours. Small biopsies are obtained with colposcopic guidance using cervical biopsy forceps designed for this task. Treatment decisions are based on biopsy results. (Figure 39–4).

4. Biopsy proven low-grade cervical intraepithelial neoplasia (CIN-1) has a high likelihood of spontaneous regression with a median time of 2 years and very little likelihood of progressing to cancer. Management is conservative in order to minimize treatment morbidity that has been shown to adversely affect fertility. Persistence of disease longer than 2 years may either be treated or surveillance may be continued

5. Biopsy-proven high-grade cervical intraepithelial neoplasia (CIN 2-3) has a much higher risk of progressing

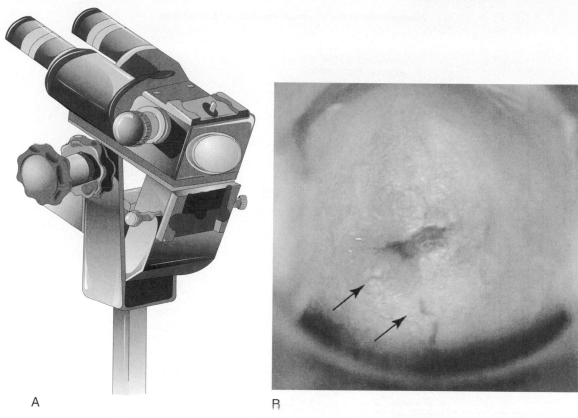

▲ **Figure 39–3.** Colposcopy. **A:** Zeiss colposcope. (From *Current Diagnosis & Treatment Obstetrics and Gynecology,* New York: McGraw-Hill, 2006.) **B:** Mosaic vascular pattern with atypical vessels (arrows). (From Schorge JO, Williams JW: *Williams Gynecology,* New York: McGraw-Hill, 2008.)

to invasive disease if left untreated. Treatment options are discussed in the section on Surgery for Benign Cervical Disease

6. HPV mediated disease may also affect the vagina and vulva. Colposcopic examination and directed biopsies allow triage of lesions into low-grade and high-grade lesions that are managed either by surveillance or removal, respectively

7. A new consensus system of nomenclature for squamous neoplasia of the anogenital tract was published in 2012. In this system, neoplasms of the cervix, vagina, and vulva are now classified as low-grade or high-grade squamous intraepithelial neoplasms (LSIL and HSIL, respectively). This two-tiered classification system was designed to reflect the understanding of the biology of these lesions, and recognizes that LSIL rarely progresses, while HSIL has a significant risk of progression to cancer

Darragh TM, Colgan TJ, Cox JT, et al: The lower anogenital squamous terminology standardization project for HPV-associated lesions: background and consensus recommendations from the College of American Pathologists and the American Society for Colposcopy and Cervical Pathology. *J Low Genit Tract Dis* 2012;16(3):205-242.

Massad LS, Einstein MH, Huh WK, et al: 2012 updated consensus guidelines for the management of abnormal cervical cancer screening tests and cancer precursors. *J Low Genit Tract Dis* 2013;17(5):S1-S27.

Screening for cervical cancer. *Obstet Gynecol* 2012;120:1222-1238.

SURGERY FOR BENIGN VULVAR DISEASE

There are a large number of possible masses and benign neoplasms of the vulva. The clinical approach is to rule out potential malignancy and to treat symptomatic lesions. Biopsy or excision of small masses is usually performed in

Management of the abnormal Pap test in adult women

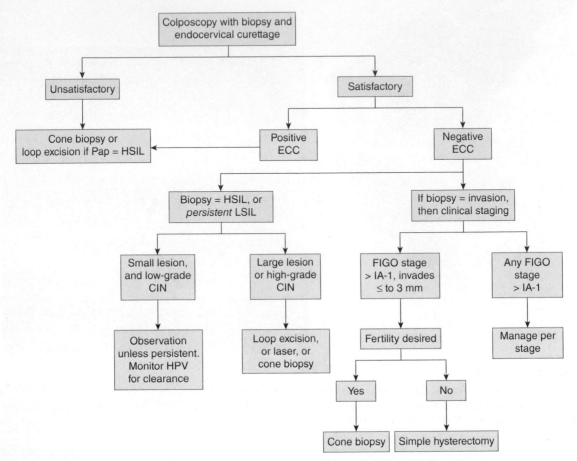

▲ **Figure 39–4.** Colposcopy triage. Satisfactory colposcopy is defined as complete visualization of the squamocolumnar epithelium, which comprises the cervical region most likely to develop invasive disease. ECC refers to endocervical curettage to obtain tissue from the endocervix above the area that may be inspected with the colposcope. Colposcopically directed biopsies are taken. Low-grade dysplasia usually resolves and the preferred treatment is observation with periodic retesting for high-risk HPV DNA on 12-month intervals. Any high-grade CIN in women 25 years and older must be treated. Persistent low-grade cervical intraepithelial neoplasia (CIN) may be treated or surveillance may be continued. New guidelines treat adolescent and young adult patients differently. See text for details.

the office setting under a local anesthetic with either a punch biopsy instrument or scalpel. Punch biopsy sites are usually left open, while elliptical excisions are closed with fine, interrupted, absorbable sutures. The differential diagnosis for benign lesions is as follows:

1. Solid lesions
    a. Leiomyoma
        Natural History: Uncommon on vulva. Benign smooth muscle tumor that arises from deep connective tissues. Occurs at any age, predominating

in fourth and fifth decades. May become very large. Rarely undergoes malignant degeneration
        Appearance: Slowly growing, firm, usually mobile subcutaneous nodule
        Diagnosis: Excisional biopsy
        Treatment: Local complete excision
    b. Lipoma
        Natural History: Uncommon on vulva. Benign tumor of histologically normal appearing adipose cells. Large lesions may ulcerate. Usually asymptomatic.

Rarely associated with family Lipoma syndrome, an autosomal dominant disease. Rarely undergoes malignant degeneration

Appearance: Soft, rounded, slowly growing sessile or pedunculated mass ranging widely in size

Diagnosis: Excisional biopsy if symptomatic

Treatment: Local excision if symptomatic

c. Syringoma

Natural History: Benign tumor of eccrine ductal origin within fibrous stroma. Occurs mostly after puberty

Appearance: Multiple, 1-2 mm, flesh-colored or yellow papules on lateral labia major

Diagnosis: Biopsy

Treatment: Local excision

d. Trichoepithelioma

Natural History: Rare benign tumor on vulva, derived from hair follicle without hair development

Appearance: Single or multiple small pink or flesh colored nodules that can mimic basal cell carcinoma

Diagnosis: Biopsy

Treatment: Local excision

e. Granular cell tumor

Natural History: Rare benign tumor of nerve sheath. Occurs in adults and children. Usually asymptomatic and solitary in 85%

Appearance: Slow growing subcutaneous nodule, usually on labia majora, clitoris, or mons pubis

Diagnosis: Biopsy

Treatment: Wide local excision

f. Neurofibroma

Natural History: Rare on vulva. Benign tumor of nerve sheath. Half occur in patients with von Recklinghausen disease, an autosomal dominant heritable disease affecting skin, nervous system, bone, and endocrine glands. Rare before puberty. Rarely undergoes malignant degeneration

Appearance: Solid, cutaneous nodules usually less than 3 cm, but reported as large as 25 cm.

Diagnosis: Clinical appearance of von Recklinghausen disease or biopsy.

Treatment: In asymptomatic patients with von Recklinghausen disease, no treatment for a vulvar lesion is needed. For symptomatic patients, local excision

g. Schwannoma

Natural History: Rare. Benign tumor of neuroectodermal nerve sheath

Appearance: Usually solitary

Diagnosis: Biopsy

Treatment: Local excision

2. Glandular lesions

a. Papillary hidradenoma

Natural History: Benign tumor of apocrine sweat glands. Contains both glandular and myoepithelial elements. Occurs after puberty. Usually asymptomatic. Virtually always in Caucasian women

Appearance: Hemispherical in shape, measuring less than 2 cm in diameter. Usually located in labia majora or lateral labia minora

Diagnosis: Biopsy

Treatment: Local Excision

b. Nodular hidradenoma

Natural History: Benign tumor of eccrine sweat glands. Probably arises from embryonic rests. Clear cells on biopsy. Rare on vulva

Diagnosis: Biopsy

Treatment: Local Excision

c. Ectopic breast or nipple

Natural History: Rare. May occur on the vulva with or without underlying glands and lactation has been reported. Rarely undergoes malignant degeneration

Appearance: Amorphous swelling of the labia most often detected with pregnancy. Pigmented vestigial nipple may or may not be present

Diagnosis: Biopsy

Treatment: Local excision if symptomatic

d. Endometriosis

Natural History: Rare on vulva. Benign ectopic endometrial tissue. May cause cyclic pain and may ulcerate or bleed

Appearance: Nodule with blue or red-brown appearance. Cyclic tenderness

Diagnosis: Biopsy

Treatment: Local excision

3. Cysts

a. Bartholin cysts or masses

Natural History: Cysts are common, arising in 1%-2% of women. Cysts often occur after gland abscesses, although the duct may become occluded any time. Small cysts usually asymptomatic. Large or infected cysts are painful

Appearance: Spherical cyst or nodule in subcutaneous tissue of posterior labia majora

Diagnosis

i. Incise and drain abscesses

ii. Biopsy recurrent cysts or solid nodules

Treatment

i. Incise and drain abscesses using a small balloon-tip catheter (Word) catheter introduced through a stab incision in the medial aspect of the cyst cephalad to the hymen. The catheter should remain in place for 2 weeks to allow tract epithelialization. In the event of surrounding cellulitis, antibiotic therapy can be added

ii. Marsupialize or resect recurrent cysts

iii. Resect solid nodules since these may be malignant

b. Epithelial inclusion cyst (sebaceous cyst)

Natural History: Common. Usually on labia majora. Can occur at any age and may be solitary or multiple. Usually asymptomatic. Caused by trauma to skin or occlusion of pilosebaceous duct

Appearance: Single or multiple, round cysts usually ranging from 2-3 mm up to 1-2 cm in diameter. Often have yellow color

Diagnosis: Clinical appearance

Treatment: No treatment if asymptomatic. If symptomatic, local excision

c. Wolffian cyst (Mesonephric cyst)

Natural History: Uncommon. Benign, thin-walled cysts on lateral vagina at the introitus

Appearance: Round cysts with thin smooth walls on lateral vagina at the introitus (Diagnosis: Clinical appearance or biopsy

Treatment: No treatment if asymptomatic. If symptomatic, local excision

d. Cyst of canal of Nuck (Mesothelial cyst)

Natural History: Uncommon. Benign cyst

Appearance: Smooth cysts usually located in anterior labia majora or inguinal canal. Thought to be due to peritoneal inclusions. May become large. Differential diagnosis includes inguinal hernia

Diagnosis: Clinical appearance or excisional biopsy

Treatment: No treatment if asymptomatic. If symptomatic, local excision

4. Vascular lesions

a. Angiokeratoma

Natural History: Very common. A clinically insignificant variant of hemangioma that occurs almost exclusively on vulva (and scrotum in men). Occurs during reproductive years. Contains dilated vessels and may have hyperkeratotic overlying epithelium. May resemble Kaposi sarcoma or angiosarcoma. Some forms associated with inborn errors of glycosphingolipid metabolism

Appearance: Red to purple to brown-black 2-5 mm papules usually in large numbers anywhere on the vulva

Diagnosis: Clinical appearance. Occurrence of multifocal lesions in childhood may indicate inborn errors of glycosphingolipid metabolism

Treatment: None, if asymptomatic. Symptomatic lesions treated with laser ablation, electrodessication, or local excision

b. Capillary hemangioma

Natural History: Capillary hemangioma (strawberry hemangioma) occurs in infants and young children. Usually regresses spontaneously over time. May ulcerate or bleed

Appearance: Well demarcated, red, slightly raised lesion

Diagnosis: Clinical appearance

Treatment: None if asymptomatic

c. Cavernous hemangioma

Natural History: Rare on vulva. Dilated vessels that may be associated with underlying pelvic hemangioma. Usually regresses spontaneously over time. May ulcerate or bleed

Appearance: Dilated vessels

Diagnosis: Clinical appearance

Treatment: None if asymptomatic

5. Nevi and pigmented skin lesions

a. Vitiligo

Natural History: Inherited disorder with loss of melanocytes. Asymptomatic

Appearance: Depigmented skin in well-circumscribed macular pattern

Diagnosis: Clinical appearance

Treatment: None

b. Fibroepithelial polyp (skin tag, acrochordon)

Natural History: Very common. Single or multiple. Hormonal factors are implicated in development and lesions are more common in obese or diabetic patients (Fisher, Nucci). Also common in axilla

Appearance: Multiple soft skin colored or pigmented lesions. Usually painless unless inflamed or torsed

Diagnosis: Gross recognition. Biopsy or excision if symptomatic

Treatment: Excise, electrodesiccate or freeze with liquid nitrogen if symptomatic

c. Seborrheic keratosis

Natural History: Common on body but uncommon on vulva. Usually occur after age 30. Probably autosomal dominant inheritance (Fitzpatrick). Multiple lesions occurring over a short period of time may indicate internal malignancy (Leser-Trelat syndrome)

Appearance: Lesions appear "stuck on" and are brown to black in color. Most are asymptomatic but can be pruritic. Occur on hair bearing skin

Diagnosis: Gross appearance, biopsy or excision

Treatment: If asymptomatic, no treatment. If symptomatic, excise, electrodesiccate, curette, or freeze with liquid nitrogen

d. Lentigo simplex

Natural History: Most common hyperpigmentation lesion on vulva. Occurs on skin and mucous membranes

Appearance: Usually small, less than 4 mm, flat, uniformly pigmented. Often resemble junctional nevi

Diagnosis: Clinical appearance. Biopsy only if clinical morphology worrisome. Remember ABCDE criteria: Asymmetry, Border irregularity, Color variegations, Diameter larger than 6 mm, Enlargement or Elevation

Treatment: None required

e. Vulvar melanosis

Natural History: Hyperpigmented macules or freckles are benign and asymptomatic. They are usually acquired, beginning between ages 30 and 40

Appearance: Asymptomatic brown to black irregular macular patches on vulva

Diagnosis: Clinical appearance. Biopsy only if clinical morphology worrisome. Remember ABCDE criteria: Asymmetry, Border irregularity, Color variegations, Diameter larger than 6 mm, Enlargement or Elevation

f. Treatment: None required

Acquired melanocytic nevocellular nevus

Natural History: Common, especially in Caucasians. Tend to develop in childhood and early adulthood, followed by gradual involution by age 60. Lesions are usually asymptomatic

Classification (Fisher)

i. Junctional nevus: melanocytes at the dermal-epidermal junction above the basement membrane. First stage of nevus evolution. Least common type on vulva

ii. Compound nevus: melanocytes in both the dermis and above the basement membrane. Second stage of nevus evolution

iii. Intradermal nevus: melanocytes exclusively in the dermis below the basement membrane. Final stage of evolution after which many nevi involute

iv. Other types include halo nevus, blue nevus

Appearance:

i. Junctional nevus: Pigmented macule with smooth border and uniform tan, brown or dark brown pigmentation

ii. Compound nevus: Papule with dome shape or macule. Dark brown or black color. May have hairs

iii. Intradermal nevus: Papule with dome shape or macule. Skin colored, tan or light brown

Diagnosis: Clinical appearance. Biopsy if clinical morphology worrisome. Remember ABCDE

criteria: Asymmetry, Border irregularity, Color variegations, Diameter larger than 6 mm, Enlargement or Elevation

Treatment: None required if asymptomatic and if ABCD criteria are benign. All others: local excision

g. Dysplastic nevus

Natural History:

i. Rare on the vulva

ii. Lesions arise later in childhood than nevi in general and continue to develop throughout life

iii. Sun exposure contributes to development of these lesions on other areas of the body. Several genetic loci have been implicated for development of melanoma

iv. Risk of melanoma doubles with one dysplastic nevus and increases 12-fold if 10 or more dysplastic nevi are present

v. Dysplastic nevi are sometimes associated with a hereditary propensity for melanoma

Appearance

i. On biopsy, atypical cells are superficial and the deeper cells are without atypia. Pagetoid spread of cells is noted in lower third of epithelium

ii. Tend to be larger in size than nevi (> 10 mm vs < 5 mm, respectively)

iii. Dysplastic nevi are asymmetrical, with variegation of color

Diagnosis: Wood lamp accentuates pigmentation and margins are more easily delineated. Remember ABCDE criteria: Asymmetry, Border irregularity, Color variegations, Diameter larger than 6 mm, Enlargement or Elevation. Excisional biopsy

Treatment: Excisional biopsy. Careful longitudinal skin surveillance exams

SURGERY FOR MALIGNANT VULVAR DISEASE

Vulvar cancer accounts for about 5% of gynecologic malignancies. At least 90% of vulvar cancers are of squamous cell type. Etiology of vulvar carcinoma is grouped into the HPV-associated basaloid-warty histological group and the non-HPV-associated keratinizing squamous cancers. The age distribution is bimodal with younger women more likely to develop HPV-associated disease and older women more likely to develop keratinizing squamous cell carcinoma. The latter group is often associated with lichen sclerosis of the vulva. Vulvar intraepithelial neoplasia (VIN) is a preinvasive form of HPV-associated neoplasia and is often associated with persistent pruritus. Uncommon histological types of vulvar cancer include melanoma (6%), Bartholin gland adenocarcinoma (4%), basal cell carcinoma (< 2%), extramammary Paget disease of the vulva (< 1%), and rare sarcomas, found arising primarily in the soft tissues, or metastases from other tumor sites.

Lesions arise in the labia majora in about 50% of cases and about 25% of cases occur on the labia minora. Clitoral lesions and Bartholin gland adenocarcinomas are less common. The natural history of vulvar carcinoma includes spread to inguinal lymph nodes. Lesion depth and diameter are of prognostic value for assessing risk of metastasis, and to a lesser degree histological type, and presence of lymphatic involvement. Lesions of ≤ 1 mm depth have less than 1% risk of nodal metastasis, and define a category of microinvasive disease that may be treated more conservatively by omitting the inguinal node dissection. Lymph node status is the most significant predictor of survival.

In patients with HPV-mediated disease, multifocal involvement of the vagina and cervix predisposes to a significantly higher risk of cancer at these sites. Smoking is a cofactor for the development of HPV-mediated disease. Smoking cessation may reduce risk of persistent or progressive disease. Women with extramammary Paget disease, in *in situ* apocrine adenocarcinoma related to breast tissue developed along the milk-line *in utero*, there is a significant risk of a second, underlying adenocarcinoma elsewhere. Sites that require evaluation include colon, especially for perianal lesions, Bartholin gland, cervix, endometrium, ovary, and breast.

Cancer of the vulva is staged by International Federation of Gynecology and Obstetrics (FIGO) criteria, which is a surgical staging system. Melanoma is staged using AJCC staging rules.

▶ Appearance

VIN occurs in women 15-20 years before the average age of invasive disease. Incidence has risen strongly and the average age at time of incidence has fallen from 52.7 years in 1961 to 35 years in 1992. One-third of lesions are solitary, and two-thirds are multifocal. Lesions are widely variable in size and may be slightly raised or papillary. Color variation ranges from white, red, or brownish patches on the skin or mucosa. Ulcerated lesions or underlying subcutaneous induration may indicate invasion. Larger lesions have a higher probability of lymph node involvement, but metastatic disease in the lymph nodes may not be palpable. Local spread may involve the urethra, vagina, anus, and rarely the symphysis pubis or other pelvic bones.

▶ Diagnosis

Biopsies are necessary to establish the correct diagnosis. The differential diagnosis is large and includes benign lesions discussed earlier in addition infections that mimic neoplasms and also vulvar dystrophies. Granulomatous infections such as lymphogranuloma venereum and granuloma inguinale of the vulva may be clinically suspicious, and biopsy of the involved may need to be supplemented with

cultures for documentation of infection. These infections are rare unless a patient has traveled internationally. VIN is best diagnosed by colposcopic examination techniques including use if magnification and staining the epithelium with 5% acetic acid. Lesions usually appear acetowhite.

▶ Treatment

Focal VIN may be treated by wide excision or CO_2 laser photoablation. Excision is preferred for lesions in the hair bearing skin and laser is generally less prone to cause scarring in the mucosal surfaces. Laser ablation is contraindicated if there is any suspicion of invasion. A skinning vulvectomy with split-thickness skin grafting is effective for widely multifocal disease. Extramammary Paget disease requires wide but superficial excision as the tumor cells often spread far wider than is visible to the surgeon. Local recurrences are common, but invasion is rare.

Vulvar cancer is staged using the international system developed by the FIGO (Table 39–1). Microinvasive lesions

Table 39–1. FIGO staging for vulva r cancer.

Stage	Revised 2009
I	Tumor confined to vulva
IA	Lesion ≤ 2 cm in size, and stromal invasion of ≤ 1 mm, nodes negative
IB	Lesion > 2 cm in size, or stromal invasion of > 1 mm, nodes negative
II	Tumor of any size extending to adjacent perineal structures: (anus, lower 1/3 of urethra, lower 1/3 of vagina); nodes negative
III	Tumor of any size with or without extension to adjacent perineal structures: (anus, lower 1/3 of urethra, lower 1/3 of vagina); inguinofemoral nodes positive
IIIA(i)	With 1 lymph node metastasis of ≥ 5 mm
IIIA(ii)	1-2 lymph node metastases of < 5 mm
IIIB(i)	With 2 or more lymph node metastases of ≥ 5 mm
IIIB(ii)	3 or more lymph node metastases of < 5 mm
IIIC	Positive nodes with extracapsular spread
IVA(i)	Invades upper urethra or vagina; bladder or rectal mucosa; or fixed to pelvic bone
IVA(ii)	Fixed or ulcerated inguinofemoral nodes
IVB	Any distant mets including pelvic nodes

Depth of invasion measured from epithelial-stromal junction of the adjacent most superficial dermal papilla to the deepest point of invasion. This system applies for all tumor types other than melanoma. Melanoma should be staged using the AJCC melanoma staging system. Staging assessment may require cystoscopy, sigmoidoscopy, and chest x-ray for locally advanced lesions. (Reproduced, with permission, from Pecorelli S: Revised FIGO staging for carcinoma of the vulva, cervix, and endometrium. *Int J Gynecol Obstet.* 2009; May;105(2):103–104) of less than or equal to1 mm invasion are adequately treated by wide and deep local excision with 1 cm margins due to the low likelihood of nodal spread. Stage I lesions are generally treated with radical local excision with a 1-2 cm margin. For lesions greater than 1 mm in depth, sentinel node mapping of inguinal nodes is carried out to assess for spread of disease. Radiation therapy with concurrent chemosensitization is required for inoperable lesions and for patients with positive nodes or involved resection margins.

▶ Prognosis

Following radical resection with negative nodes and margins, a 5-year rate of 90% is anticipated. If nodes are involved, survival is linked to number of nodes involved, unilaterality versus bilaterality, and bulk of disease.

Levenback CF, Ali S, Coleman RL, et al: Lymphatic mapping and sentinel node biopsy in women with squamous cell carcinoma of the vulva: a gynecologic oncology group study. *J Clin Oncol* 2012;30:3786-3791.

SURGERY FOR BENIGN VAGINAL DISEASE

▶ Imperforate Hymen

Diagnosis of imperforate hymen is often delayed until puberty, when either a workup for primary amenorrhea has ensued or the patient presents with menstrual symptoms such as cramping, without associated menses. If the patient has obstructed flow of her menses, defined as hematocolpos, examination will reveal a bulging imperforate hymen. Confirmatory rectal exam will detect a bulging, cystic mass. In younger girls, the finding is more subtle due to the absence of swelling. Delay of diagnosis may result backpressure causing a cystically enlarged uterus (hematometra) and possible retrograde menstruation leading to endometriosis. In the presence of a tightly distended hematocolpos, compression of the bladder and ureters may result in urinary obstruction.

Imperforate hymen is treated with a hymenotomy, where the obstructed hymen is incised or resected with either a scalpel or laser.

▶ Longitudinal Vaginal Septum

Duplication of the vagina resulting in a septum may occur with or without similar defects in the uterus based on where the defect of Müllerian duct fusion occurred. The duplication may take the form of a partial longitudinal septum or complete duplication of the vagina. Patients will occasionally report bleeding despite placing a tampon during menses, indicating the possibility of a second passage for menstrual flow. Excision is performed transvaginally for symptomatic patients including those with dyspareunia, obstruction of labor or similar problems.

▶ Transverse Vaginal Septum

Occasionally, the vagina fails to communicate with the urogenital sinus at the introitus. This may result in formation of a transverse septum, most of which are partial. If the septum is imperforate, hematocolpos will develop following menarche. Marsupialization or excision of the septum restores vaginal patency.

▶ Vaginal Agenesis

Vaginal agenesis, or absence of the vagina, is associated with absence of the uterus in most cases. The lower vagina, derived from the urogenital sinus may be present, but Müllerian ductal structures comprising the upper two-thirds of the vagina and the uterus are absent or deficient. Diagnosis is usually made at time of evaluation for primary amenorrhea.

Vaginal agenesis is treated by reconstruction of a functional vagina. Treatment is usually deferred until the patient wishes to become sexually active. In a motivated patient, the vagina may be created by nonoperative dilation and elongation of the vulvar vestibule or vaginal introitus. This method, called the Frank nonoperative technique, requires up to 2 hours of dilating per day for 4-6 months. Success has been reported with vaginal dilators, vaginal molds, modified bicycle seat, and with intercourse alone. If there is failure to progress, or if the anatomy does not favor dilation alone, surgical construction using a skin graft (McIndoe procedure), interposed bowel, or myocutaneous flaps from the perineum are effective.

▶ Gartner Duct Cyst

Gartner duct cysts are derived from mesonephric (Wolffian) duct remnants and contain a serous fluid. They are usually located in the lateral walls of the upper vagina and are generally asymptomatic. These cysts are detected most often during a routine physical examination. Small asymptomatic cysts require no treatment. Gartner duct cysts may occasionally reach 5-6 cm diameter. Larger or symptomatic cysts should be excised.

SURGERY FOR MALIGNANT & PREMALIGNANT VAGINAL DISEASE

Vaginal intraepithelial neoplasia (VAIN) is the term used to describe the preinvasive neoplastic changes that arise in the vagina. VAIN is frequently present whenever carcinoma *in situ* or invasive carcinoma of the cervix or vulva is present, and it may develop in the vagina years after completion of treatment for cancers of these two sites. Carcinoma *in situ*, or VAIN 3, of the vagina is most often detected with a Pap test. Subsequent evaluation with colposcopy, staining with 5% acetic acid and directed biopsies provide an accurate assessment of grade and location of disease.

▶ Treatment

Low-grade dysplasia (VAIN 1) has a low probability of progression and may be managed with surveillance using the same principles as for management of low-grade cervical dysplasia. High-grade dysplasia (VAIN 2-3) should be treated by local excision of involved areas or with CO_2 laser photoablation. New terminology for these lesions was published in 2012. Low-grade lesions are now referred to as LSIL and high-grade lesions previously called VAIN 2, VAIN 3 and carcinoma *in situ*, are now referred to as HSIL. The irregular surface topography of the vagina caused by rugae makes successful visualization of lesions for treatment challenging. Recurrence rates for dysplasia are higher for vaginal dysplasia than for similarly treated cervical dysplasia, with a failure rate in the 25% range. Intravaginal placement of topical 5-fluorouracil is an off-label indication that has been reported in the literature, and failure rates are higher than for resection or ablation. Topical 5-fluorouracil has been reported to cause painful vaginal ulcers that heal poorly, limiting the utility of this treatment to carefully selected patients. Extensive involvement of the vagina may require subtotal or complete vaginectomy with skin grafting for maintenance of sexual function. For the elderly, sexually inactive patient, colpocleisis, where the vagina is resected and closed permanently is an option.

Invasive carcinoma of the vagina is rare, accounting for less than 2% of gynecologic malignancies. Most vaginal cancers involve extension from either cervical or vulvar cancers, both of which are more common than lesions arising in the vagina. By convention, if the cancer involves cervix or vulva in addition to the vagina, the tumor is categorized as either cervical or vulvar cancer, respectively. True vaginal cancer arises only in the vagina. About 85% of vaginal cancers are of squamous type. The next most common type is adenocarcinoma, usually with clear cell type. Rare primary tumors of the vagina include mixed mesodermal tumors, sarcoma botryoides (embryonal rhabdomyosarcoma), sarcoma, adenocarcinoma arising from Gartner duct or Müllerian duct remnants, embryonal carcinoma, and malignant melanoma.

The most common presenting symptoms of vaginal cancer include postmenopausal bleeding in about 65% of patients and persistent vaginal discharge in about 30%. Most tumors arise in the upper third of the vagina along the anterior and posterior surfaces. These sites are usually covered by the vaginal speculum and can easily be missed unless the physician observes all vaginal surfaces upon insertions and withdrawal of the speculum. Diagnosis is confirmed by biopsy.

Staging of carcinoma of the vagina is defined by FIGO and is clinical rather than surgical (Table 39–2). Squamous cancers are most commonly found in postmenopausal

Table 39–2. FIGO staging for vaginal cancer.

FIGO Stage	Description	TNM Class
Stage 0	Carcinoma *in situ*; intraepithelial neoplasia grade 3	Tis N0 M0
Stage I	The carcinoma is limited to the vaginal wall	T1 N0 M0
Stage II	The carcinoma has involved the subvaginal tissue but has not extended to the pelvic wall	T2 N0 M0
Stage III	The carcinoma has extended to the pelvic wall	T1 N1 M0 T2 N1 M0 T3 N0 M0 T3 N1 M0
Stage IV	The carcinoma has extended beyond the true pelvis or has involved the mucosa of the bladder or rectum. Bullous edema as such does not permit a case to be allotted to stage IV	
IVA	Tumor invades bladder and/or rectal mucosa and/or direct extension beyond the true pelvis	T4 any N M0
IVB	Spread to distant organs	Any T Any N M1

Benedet JL, Hacker NF, Ngan HYS, eds: Staging classifications and clinical practice guidelines of gynaecologic cancers. Int J Gynaecol Obstet 2000;70:207. http://www.figo.org/content/PDF/staging-booklet.pdf.

patients, although they may occur even in adolescent patients. Clear cell adenocarcinoma of the vagina is more likely to occur in women below the age of 25, generally arising in vaginal adenosis. Diethylstilbestrol (DES) has been implicated in increasing the incidence of clear cell carcinoma from 1:50,000 in the unexposed population to 1:1000 in women exposed to DES *in utero*. Although DES is no longer produced or prescribed in this country, DES and similar substances have been detected in the environment and in some food supplies.

Treatment of vaginal cancer is most often a combination of radiation therapy and chemosensitization using treatment plans similar to cervical cancer. Radical surgery such as radical hysterectomy with vaginectomy is possible for selected, small, upper vaginal lesions, favoring lesions on the posterior wall due to the improved likelihood of attaining adequate margins. Surgery is preferred for young patients with clear cell carcinoma as long as negative margins can be attained. In over 50% of patients tumor has penetrated the vaginal wall at the time of the initial examination. Involvement of the bladder and rectum is common. Survival for stage I disease is about 70%, but falls to about 40% for stage II and stage III disease.

Darragh TM, Colgan TJ, Cox JT, et al: The lower anogenital squamous terminology standardization project for HPV-associated lesions: background and consensus recommendations from the College of American Pathologists and the American Society for Colposcopy and Cervical Pathology. *J Low Genit Tract Dis* 2012;16(3):205-242.

SURGERY FOR MALIGNANT CERVICAL DISEASE

Cervical cancer is the twelfth most common cancer of women in the United States, but remains the second most common cancer of women worldwide. Almost all cervical cancers arise because of persistent infection with high-risk human papillomavirus (HPV) types, most commonly types 16 and 18. Low-risk HPV types such as types 6 and 11 are usually associated with condyloma and rarely, if ever, are associated with cancer. Cervical cancer can be considered a sexually transmitted disease since most HPV infections are transmitted via sexual contact. Early sexual debut and multiple partners greatly increase the risk of exposure to high-risk HPV types. HPV infections are common and about 80% of the population will have detectable HPV antibodies indicating prior infection. In most infected individuals, the immune system will mount a successful response, with a median time to regression of infection of about 2 years. Persistent infection with a high-risk HPV type after age 30 increases the relative risk of cervical cancer more than 400-fold for HPV 16 over the population at large. Persistent infections and progression to cancer may be more likely in women who smoke or those with dietary deficiency of folate, and beta-carotene. Progression to cancer is usually gradual, allowing development of effective screening strategies with Pap tests and testing for high-risk HPV DNA in addition to effective triage with colposcopy. Low-grade lesions usually regress, making potentially destructive treatments that have an adverse effect on fertility unnecessary. In 2006, the FDA first approved a vaccine for primary prevention of HPV infection. The vaccine is targeted for adolescents prior to their sexual debut. Widespread vaccination may largely eradicate cervical cancer in the future, although the vaccines are selective only for the most common of high-risk HPV types raising the possibility of shifting prevalence of HPV types.

About 75% of cervical cancers are squamous type; the remainder consist of adenocarcinomas, mixed carcinomas (adenosquamous), and rare sarcomas (mixed mesodermal tumors, lymphosarcomas). The relative prevalence of cervical adenocarcinoma has risen in recent years and now accounts for about 25% of cases.

Most cervical cancers arise from a preinvasive dysplastic lesion through a process that generally lasts for years. Carcinoma *in situ* occurs most frequently in the fourth decade, whereas invasive carcinoma is encountered most often in perimenopausal women between ages 40 and 50. Once invasion occurs, spread is by direct extension to the vagina and the parametrium in addition to lymphatic channels to the iliac and obturator nodes, with occasional direct spread to para-aortic nodes. Staging is clinical, since not all stages will require surgery. The staging system defined by FIGO is used internationally, and is included in Table 39–3. Probability of lymph node metastasis increases according to the extent of the primary lesion, being approximately 12% in stage I, 30% in stage II, and 45% in stage III. About 80% of patients with stage IV cancer have lymph node involvement.

Table 39–3. FIGO staging for cervical cancer.

FIGO Stage	Revised 2009
Stage I	Carcinoma confined to cervix (extension to corpus would be disregarded)
IA	Invasive carcinoma, diagnosed only by microscopy. All macroscopically visible lesions, even with superficial invasion, are Stage IB
IA-1	Measured stromal invasion ≤ 3 mm and < 7 mm in horizontal spread
IA-2	Measured stromal invasion > 3 mm and ≤ 5 mm with a horizontal spread of 7 mm or less
IB	Clearly visible lesion confined to the cervix or microscopic lesion greater than Stage IA
IB-1	Clinically visible lesion ≤ 4 cm in greatest dimension
IB-2	Clinically visible lesion > 4 cm in greatest dimension
Stage II	Tumor invades beyond uterus but not to pelvic wall or to the lower third of vagina
IIA	Tumor without parametrial invasion
IIA-1	Clinically visible lesion ≤ 4 cm in greatest dimension
IIA-2	Clinically visible lesion > 4 cm in greatest dimension
IIB	Tumor with obvious parametrial invasion
Stage III	Tumor extends to the pelvic wall and/or involves lower third of vagina and/or causes hydronephrosis or nonfunctioning kidney. Determination is based on rectal exam with no cancer-free space between tumor and pelvic wall
IIIA	Tumor involves lower third of the vagina, with no extension to pelvic wall
IIIB	Extends to pelvic wall or causes hydronephrosis or nonfunctioning kidney
Stage IV	Carcinoma extends beyond true pelvis or with biopsy proven spread to bladder or rectal mucosa. Bullous edema does not cause case to be allotted to Stage IV
IVA	Spread to adjacent organs
IVB	Spread to distant organs

Reproduced, with permission, from Pecorelli S: Revised FIGO staging for carcinoma of the vulva, cervix, and endometrium. *Int J Gynecol Obstet.* 2009 May;105(2):103–4.

Dysplasia & Carcinoma *In Situ*

Successful screening has greatly reduced the incidence and mortality of cervical cancer and its precursors over the last 50 years. Current screening recommendations for lower genital tract cancers of the vulva, vagina, and cervix have been discussed previously in this chapter. When a neoplastic lesion is detected by screening, proper and timely triage is needed. High-grade squamous intraepithelial lesions are typically asymptomatic.

Colposcopic examination of the cervix is the gold standard for assessing dysplasia, carcinoma *in situ* and early invasive disease. Application of Lugol iodine can be a useful adjunct to the colposcopic exam. Normal mature squamous epithelium of the cervix and vagina contains glycogen and stains a dark brown color, whereas dysplastic cells lack glycogen and stain a light yellow color.

Colposcopically directed biopsy is performed for visible abnormalities including acetowhite change, abnormal vessels, ulceration, and papillary lesions. Biopsy confirmed CIN-1 is managed conservatively since most of these lesions regress spontaneously and there is very little risk of progression to cancer. Biopsy showing a high-grade dysplastic lesion including moderate dysplasia (CIN-2), severe dysplasia (CIN-3), and carcinoma *in situ* (CIN-3), are treated with either ablative therapy or resection using cryotherapy or electrosurgical loop excision, respectively. Treatment is directed to either ablation or removal of the entire transformation zone, defined as the area bounded by the original and current squamocolumnar junction. These two treatment modalities are usually performed in the office setting and are well tolerated. There are some exceptions when treating adolescent and young adult patients under age 25, so the clinician must be familiar with current guidelines. Some dysplastic lesions may extend into the endocervical canal including squamous lesions and most glandular lesions. The preferred treatment for lesions extending out of colposcopic view into the endocervical canal is usually excision with a cold-knife cone biopsy in the operating room. Both electrosurgical loop excision and cold-knife cone biopsy increase future risk of preterm delivery, mandating careful triage of only those individuals truly requiring an excisional therapy.

Invasive Carcinoma

Early stromal defined as microinvasion, is usually asymptomatic. Larger lesions frequently cause postmenopausal bleeding (46%), intermenstrual bleeding (20%), or postcoital bleeding (10%). A watery or malodorous vaginal discharge may be the only symptom. Pain is a manifestation of advanced stage disease typically extending to the pelvic sidewall with entrapment of the sciatic nerve or femoral nerve. Inspection of the cervix typically reveals an ulcerated or papillary lesion of the cervix that bleeds on contact. The cytologic examination almost always demonstrates exfoliated malignant cells, although the false-negative rate for Pap tests approach 50% for invasive lesions due to obscuration of malignant cells by inflammation and necrotic debris.

Differential Diagnosis

Chronic cervicitis may appear similar to cancer of the cervix. Polyps of the cervix are often benign, but malignancy can only be ruled out with biopsy. Nabothian cysts are benign, common, and can appear bizarre to the untrained eye, but are readily distinguished from cancer by biopsy.

Natural History

Spread of cervical cancer into the parametrium may cause obstruction of the ureter, resulting in hydroureter, hydronephrosis, and uremia. Bilateral obstruction of the ureters leads to failure of kidney function and death. Involvement of the iliac and obturator lymph nodes may lead to lymphatic obstruction resulting in lymphedema. Pelvic sidewall nerves, especially the sciatic nerve, may become compressed, causing sciatica or pain in the low back, hip, and leg. Tumor invasion into the bladder or rectum sometime causes vesicovaginal or rectovaginal fistula, especially following radiation therapy. Widespread metastases to lung, liver, brain, and bone may occur.

Treatment

Treatment of cervical cancer is stratified by stage. Microinvasive disease, defined as FIGO stage IA-1, has less than a 1% chance of lymphatic metastasis and may be managed conservatively with cone biopsy for preservation of fertility or with simple hysterectomy when preservation of fertility is not desired or relevant. Radical hysterectomy with bilateral pelvic lymph node dissection is the preferred treatment for FIGO stage IA-2, IB, and IIA lesions. Radical hysterectomy results is resection of much wider margins than is performed with a simple hysterectomy, including removal of cardinal and uterosacral ligaments and the upper third of the vagina, in addition to pelvic, obturator and para-aortic nodes. Radical hysterectomy procedures may be performed either via laparotomy or laparoscopy. The radical hysterectomy is a completely different type of hysterectomy than the simple or total hysterectomy. Procedural details for the most commonly used hysterectomy types are described in Table 39–4.

Complications of radical surgery include hemorrhage, infection, thromboembolism, and less than 1% risk of ureterovaginal, vesicovaginal, or rectovaginal fistula. Early stage lesions may also be treated with radiation therapy and concurrent chemosensitization with cisplatin with equal likelihood of cure but higher potential morbidity.

Table 39–4. Types of hysterectomy.

	Comparison of Hysterectomy Types		
Anatomic Structure	**Extrafascial Type 1**	**Modified Radical Type 2**	**Radical Type 3**
Uterus	Removed	Removed	Removed
Ovaries	Optional removal	Optional removal	Optional removal
Cervix	Removed	Removed	Removed
Vaginal margin	None	1-2 cm margin	Upper 1/3 of vagina
Ureters	Not mobilized	Dissected through broad ligament	Dissected through broad ligament
Cardinal ligaments	Divided at uterine border	Divided where ureter transits the broad ligament	Divided at pelvic sidewall
Uterosacral ligaments	Divided at cervical border	Partially resected	Divided near sacral origin
Bladder	Mobilized to base of cervix	Mobilized to upper vagina	Mobilized to middle vagina
Rectum	Not mobilized	Mobilized below cervix	Mobilized below middle vagina

The recently developed radical trachelectomy with laparoscopic lymphadenectomy offers carefully selected individuals with stage IA-2 or stage IB-1 squamous lesions of ≤ 2 cm diameter a fertility sparing option. The cervix, upper vagina, and supporting ligaments are removed as with a radical hysterectomy, but the uterine corpus is preserved. In the posttrachelectomy pregnancies currently reported, there is a 10% likelihood of second trimester loss, but 72% of patients carry their gestation to 37 weeks or more.

Advanced-stage disease, including FIGO stage IIB and above, requires treatment with external radiation, brachytherapy implants and concurrent chemosensitization. At least five randomized trials have confirmed a survival advantage for cisplatin-based therapy given weekly during radiation therapy. Delayed complications of radiation therapy affect quality of life and include cystitis and proctitis, but are uncommon and usually. Severe radiation cystitis or proctitis may result in hemorrhage, fistula, or strictures, typically arising several years after treatment in about 1%-3% of patients. Radiation necrosis of the cervix and diffuse radiation pelvic fibrosis are rare complications. Radiating the reproductive tract destroys the function of the uterus, and unless the ovaries have been surgically transposed out of the pelvis, ovarian failure is unavoidable. Recurrent or persistent disease in the central pelvis following radiation therapy may potentially be cured with the ultraradical pelvic exenteration procedure.

▶ **Prognosis**

Survival is strongly linked to stage at time of diagnosis. Properly treated stage I disease averages 90% survival at 5 years, and approaches 96% in radical hysterectomy cases with negative margins and negative nodes. For stage II, 5-year survival is about 65%; dropping to about 45% for stage III and to less than 10% for stage IV.

Massad LS, Einstein MH, Huh WK, et al: 2012 updated consensus guidelines for the management of abnormal cervical cancer screening tests and cancer precursors. *J Low Genit Tract Dis* 2013;17(5):S1-S27.

Schneider A, Erdemoglu E, Chiantera V, et al: Clinical recommendation: radical trachelectomy for fertility preservation in patients with early stage cervical cancer. *Int J Gynecol Cancer* 2012;22(4):659-666.

SURGERY FOR PELVIC FLOOR DEFECTS

Cystocele, Rectocele, & Incontinence

An understanding of pelvic support defects requires a thorough knowledge of the anatomic relationship of the pelvic viscera and their supporting tissues. These conditions were originally thought to result from stretching and tearing of the muscles, nerves, and connective tissues of the pelvis during vaginal childbirth. The current understanding is that many pelvic floor defects arise from site-specific tears or breaks of pelvic connective tissue. Causes can include stretching, compression, or tearing during parturition; in addition to behaviors that increase intra-abdominal pressure such as chronic constipation, heavy lifting, obesity, and chronic cough. Smoking, poor nutrition and lack of pelvic floor exercise my exacerbate pelvic floor defects. The symptoms of pelvic floor defects may include: pelvic pressure

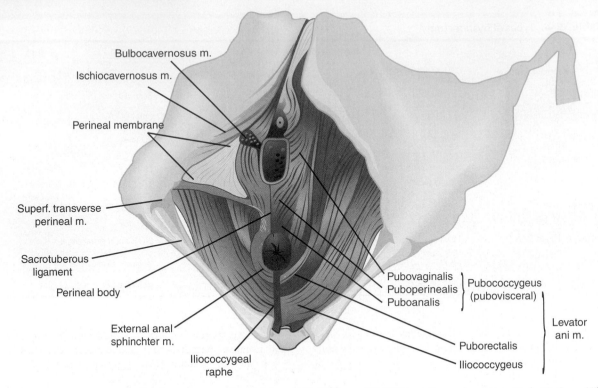

Bulbocavernosus m.

Ischiocavernosus m.

Perineal membrane

Superf. transverse perineal m.

Sacrotuberous ligament

Perineal body

External anal sphinchter m.

Iliococcygeal raphe

Pubovaginalis
Puboperinealis
Puboanalis

Pubococcygeus (pubovisceral)

Puborectalis
Iliococcygeus

Levator ani m.

▲ **Figure 39–5.** Anatomy of pelvic support. (From Schorge JO, Williams JW: *Williams Gynecology,* New York: McGraw-Hill, 2008.)

or a sensation of "falling out" of the pelvic organs, a mass protruding from the vagina (which may be a cystocele, rectocele, cervix, or all of these), stress incontinence, fecal incontinence, and other difficulties with defecation.

Complete examination generally requires evaluating the patient in the lithotomy and standing position, and by asking her to Valsalva or cough. Vaginal support is described with three different levels, illustrated in Figure 39–5. Level I includes the cervix and upper third of the vagina. Level I support is comprised superiorly by uterosacral ligaments, endopelvic fascia, and smooth muscle; laterally by support from the cardinal ligaments; and anteriorly from the pubocervical fascia. Level II defines mid-vaginal support and is comprised laterally by attachments to the arcus tendineus fascia pelvis, anteriorly by the pubocervical fascia, and posteriorly by Denonvillier fascia. Level III refers to support of the lower vagina and urethra. Level III support is provided anteriorly by attachment of the urogenital membrane to the symphysis pubis, laterally to the levator ani muscle and posteriorly to the perineal body. A pelvic organ prolapse quantification profile (POPQ) has been defined by the International Continence Society, the American Urogynecology Society, and the Society of Gynecologic Surgeons (Figure 39–6). Use

of the POPQ quantitates the extent and location of defects such that subsequent therapy is directed more specifically. Descent and bulging of the anterior vagina is usually a cystocele, a paravaginal defect, or an anterior enterocele. An anatomic defect in the posterior vagina is usually a rectocele or enterocele.

Additional testing that may be necessary for elucidation of the site-specific defect include assessment of urethral mobility with the so-called Q-tip test, cystourethroscopy, cystometrogram, anoscopy, colonoscopy, anal manometry, and transanal ultrasound. Chronic urinary tract infections must be ruled out prior to deciding upon surgical repair. For fecal incontinence, gastrointestinal disorders such as irritable bowel syndrome, infections such as *Clostridium difficile* or other causes of diarrhea, or malabsorption must be ruled out before proposing surgery.

Repair of pelvic floor defects is based on the principle of identification of the specific site of injury leading to site-specific repair. Pelvic support defects are often treated non-surgically. For example, postmenopausal woman with mild to moderate defects as determined by the POPQ score may experience improvement of symptoms after the administration of a topical estrogen, initiation of Kegel exercises, or

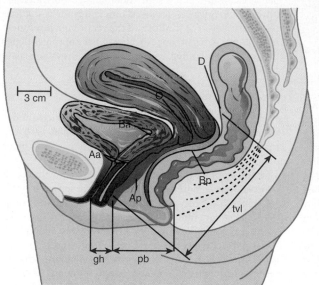

The Nine–Point POPQ and Staging Definitions		
Point	**Description**	**Range**
Aa	Anterior wall 3 cm from hymen	−3 to +3
Ba	Most dependent part of the rest of the anterior wall	−3 to +TVL
C	Cervix or vaginal cuff	+/− TVL
D	Posterior fornix (if no prior total hysterectomy)	+/− TVL
Ap	Posterior wall 3 cm from hymen	−3 to +3
Bp	Most dependent part of the rest of the posterior wall	−3 to +TVL
GH	Genital hiatus (mid-urethra to PB)	No limit

▲ **Figure 39–6.** Pelvic organ prolapse quantification table. Six sites (points Aa, Ba, C, D, Bp, and Ap), genital hiatus (GH), perineal body (PB), and total vaginal length (TVL) are used for quantification of pelvic organ support. Each point is described with respect to position relative to the hymen in centimeters. Positive values represent distance outside the hymen, and negative numbers represent distance superior to the hymen. (Schwartz SI, Brunicardi F: *Schwartz's Principles of Surgery: Self-Assessment and Board Review,* 8th ed. New York: McGraw-Hill, 2007.)

by fitting a pessary to support pelvic structures. Pessaries are inert material manufactured in many different sizes and shapes that can be fitted to the patient. When inserted in the vagina, a pessary mechanically supports pelvic structures resulting in temporary correction of the underlying symptoms. A pessary is a good option for patients choose not to undergo surgery or for those who cannot have surgery.

▶ Differential Diagnosis

Urethral diverticulae may mimic cystocele and produce a bulge of the anterior vaginal wall. A discrete mass is usually palpable. Pressure or massage of the mass may result in turbid or purulent urethral drainage. Vaginal cysts such as Gartner duct or Skene duct cysts are occasionally mistaken for bladder support defects.

▶ Treatment

Categories of pelvic floor defects include anterior compartment, vault prolapse, uterine prolapse, enterocele, posterior compartment, urinary incontinence, and fecal incontinence.

Anterior Compartment

Anterior compartment defects, including cystocele, paravaginal defects often are associated with concurrent urinary incontinence. **Stress incontinence** is involuntary loss of urine. Stress incontinence is associated with leakage caused by increases in intra-abdominal pressure including coughing, heavy lifting, or Valsalva maneuver in the absence of detrusor contraction. Stress incontinence is usually demonstrated during examination by asking the patient to cough. Stress incontinence should be distinguished from other common types of urinary incontinence including urge and overflow incontinence. With **urge incontinence,** the detrusor muscle contracts or spasms resulting in leakage with associated urgency. **Mixed incontinence** is defined as a combination of stress and urges incontinence. **Overflow incontinence** is often a continual slow leak of urine but may present with symptoms of any of the other types of incontinence. It can be ruled out by detecting large residual urine volume following voiding. Surgical correction of stress incontinence occasionally produces urge incontinence that may persist in 10%-15% of patients.

Normally, the proximal urethra is supported above the urogenital diaphragm and is subjected to the same intra-abdominal pressure changes as those applied to the bladder. In patients with anterior vaginal compartment defects, increased intra-abdominal pressure causes the hypermobile proximal urethra and bladder base to descend into the vagina. Pressure in the bladder thereby exceeds the sphincter pressure resulting in leakage of urine. Intrinsic sphincter deficiency is a second mechanism of stress incontinence. Risk factors include previous incontinence surgery, prior radiation therapy, and age over 50.

Site-directed repair of anterior compartment defects may include anterior colporrhaphy, or repair of paravaginal defect. Repair or stress urinary incontinence often involves retropubic colposuspension using either the Burch or Marshall-Marchetti-Krantz procedures. Success of these two procedures is approximately 85% at 5 years. Recurrent or difficult cases of stress urinary incontinence are often surgically treated with use of slings or grafts to augment support. Grafts may be created from endogenous fascia, usually harvested from the rectus fascia, or exogenous sources including allografts, xenografts, or synthetic mesh. Procedures utilizing the grafts may include sling procedures or the tension-free vaginal tape procedure (TVT), which has significantly reduced the morbidity of graft procedures compared to historical controls. For patients with intrinsic sphincter deficiency or for patients who are not candidates for more involved surgical procedures, a minimally invasive treatment involves injection of collagen at the urethrovesical junction as a bulking agent to increase outlet resistance.

Prolapse

Prolapse, where the level I support involving upper vagina or uterus is deficient, results in symptomatic descent of the upper vaginal tissues and/or uterus. Prolapse may also be associated with anterior and posterior compartment defects.

Repair of vaginal prolapse is generally performed with a unilateral sacrospinous ligament suspension (SSLS) procedure performed transvaginally or with an abdominal sacrocolpopexy procedure performed via laparotomy or laparoscopy. In the SSLS procedure, the upper vagina is sutured to the uterosacral ligament. In the abdominal sacrocolpopexy procedure, a retroperitoneal mesh is sutured from the upper vagina to the anterior longitudinal sacral ligament. Treatment of uterine prolapse sometimes involves hysterectomy combined with SSLS or with abdominal sacrocolpopexy procedures. Uterine preservation is permissible, combined with plication of uterosacral ligaments or the other procedures described above. Results of surgical correction of prolapse are not optimal since up to one-third of patients require reoperation for recurrent disease. Sacrocolpopexy outcomes appear to be more durable.

Enterocele

Enterocele is a hernia that develops between the vagina and the rectum. Diagnosis is confirmed by palpation on pelvic exam and can also be documented on transvaginal ultrasound. Surgical repair requires reapproximation of the fascial defect at the apex of the rectovaginal septum via laparotomy, laparoscopy, or by vaginal approach depending on other planned combined procedures such as hysterectomy.

Posterior Compartment

Posterior compartment defects, including rectocele and anal sphincter defects often are associated with concurrent fecal incontinence or difficulty with defecation. Fecal incontinence is involuntary loss of stool or flatus.

Etiology of fecal incontinence is associated with diarrhea; increased bowel motility; neurological disorders such as diabetes, spinal cord injury, or multiple sclerosis; and pelvic support defects including injury to the anal sphincter. Testing includes careful exam of level II and level III structures, anal sphincter tone, and voluntary anal sphincter contraction. Additional test that may be needed to elucidate the etiology of the lesion include anal manometry, transanal ultrasound, MRI, colonoscopy, defecography, and electromyography. Diarrheal illness and gastrointestinal disorders such as irritable bowel syndrome are treated prior to consideration of surgery.

Nonsurgical treatment may include use of medication to slow transit time, bulking agents, biofeedback, and electrical stimulation therapy.

Site-directed repair of posterior compartment defects may include posterior colporrhaphy, where posterior fascial defects are repaired primarily or with grafts, sphincteroplasty, or repair of rectal prolapse.

In patients for whom sexual activity is not an issue, closure (colpocleisis) or removal (colpectomy) of the vagina is an option.

Delancey JO: Why do women have stress urinary incontinence? *Neurourol Urodyn* 2010;29(Suppl 1):S13-S17.

Urinary Tract Fistula

Urinary tract fistulas to the vagina include vesicovaginal, ureterovaginal, and urethrovaginal types. Vesicovaginal fistula is the most common type. In the United States, most urinary tract fistulae occur following pelvic surgery with unrecognized injury or because of ischemia. Potential causes of ischemic change include effects of radiation therapy upon vasculature of pelvic organs. Less common in this country, but much more frequently in other parts of the world is ischemic injury following prolonged or obstructed labor. Fistulas may also occur as a result of tumor invasion, retained foreign bodies, and chronic inflammation.

Most urologic fistulae arise following gynecologic surgery rather than urologic or colorectal surgery. Total abdominal hysterectomy is the procedure most often complicated by the development of vesicovaginal fistula. A skillful surgeon using a technique of careful identification of anatomic structures can greatly minimize the risk of causing fistula formation. Injuries recognized at the time of primary surgery should be repaired immediately. Development of postoperative fistulae may require a waiting period to allow inflammation to subside before undertaking repair.

▶ Symptoms & Signs

Vaginal leakage of urine or constant urinary leakage are symptoms of a urologic fistula. If the fistula involves the distal urethra, the patient may experience vaginal leakage only at the time of voiding. Vesicovaginal and ureterovaginal fistulae almost always develop near the vaginal vault. A urethrovaginal fistula opens into the anterior vagina.

On speculum exam, urine will usually be seen pooling at the vaginal apex. Most fistulae in nonradiated patients are small and may not be readily seen with the naked eye. Confirmation of a suspected vesicovaginal fistula may be demonstrated by instilling dilute methylene blue dye or sterile milk into the bladder with a catheter while inspecting the vaginal vault. A small fistula may leak very little and is often better seen by placing a tampon in the vagina when methylene blue dye is instilled and then removing the tampon to inspect for blue staining after 15-20 minutes. If a vesicovaginal fistula is not detected, IV methylene blue or indigo carmine blue dye will be excreted through the ureters. This is best detected by placement of a tampon for about 30 minutes followed by inspection for staining.

Other useful diagnostic tests include cystoscopy, cystogram, and intravenous pyelogram to assess for the site of injury.

▶ Treatment

In nonradiated, noninfected tissue, many small fistulae will close spontaneously if the bladder is drained with an indwelling catheter. Larger fistulae or small fistulae that fail conservative management must be repaired surgically. Time of the order of 8-12 weeks must be allowed for resolution of edema and inflammatory reactions prior to undertaking repair. Premature repair has a high likelihood of being unsuccessful. Urinary tract infections should be treated and skin integrity should be protected with an occlusive barrier cream before surgical correction is attempted.

Repair of vesicovaginal fistulae involves a number of techniques including layered closure with the Latzko procedure via the vaginal approach, or via laparotomy with omental interposition. Principles of repair include meticulous and atraumatic technique using fine suture material;

approximation without tension; and bladder decompression postoperatively. Ureterovaginal fistulae are repaired with ureteroneocystostomy if the ureteral injury is in the lower pelvis and with ureteroureterostomy for injury sites higher in the pelvis. These are usually performed via laparotomy, but the laparoscopic approach is also used. Fistulae in radiated tissue cannot be repaired primarily due to chronic tissue ischemia. These fistulae require the introduction of a nonradiated blood supply provided by bulbocavernosus or gracilis myocutaneous flaps for successful repair or permanent diversion.

Rectovaginal Fistula

Rectovaginal fistulae may occur following obstetrical injury, pelvic surgery, cervical or rectal cancer, radiation therapy, inflammatory bowel disease, or diverticular disease. The patient will report vaginal passage of flatus or feces, or foul vaginal discharge, sometimes associated with bleeding. The fistula can often be demonstrated upon speculum examination, or by palpation on rectovaginal exam. Diagnostic studies such as barium enema or sigmoidoscopy may be useful for smaller lesions.

To reduce the risk of infection and breakdown of a planned fistula repair, the bowel should be prepared with a low-residue diet, antibiotics, and a cathartic bowel regimen preoperatively. A rectovaginal fistula in the lower third of the vagina should be repaired after the surrounding inflammation and edema have resolved, usually requiring a delay on the order of 12 weeks. Rectovaginal fistulae in the upper two thirds of the vagina are best treated with a preliminary diverting colostomy, followed by fistula repair and subsequent colostomy take down 2-3 months after the repair.

Fistulae caused by inflammatory bowel disease such as Crohn disease have a high likelihood of recurrence unless the disease is clearly in remission. Ileostomy and abdominoperineal resection are necessary in patients whose symptoms are unacceptable despite medical management. Fistulae associated with radiation therapy can rarely be repaired and those associated with cancer are not amenable to surgical repair. A diverting colostomy provides considerable relief of symptoms.

▼ THE UPPER GENITAL TRACT

SURGERY FOR BENIGN UTERINE DISEASE

Congenital Uterine Anomalies

Congenital duplication defects of the uterus are rare, with a reported incidence of 0.4%-1% and are usually diagnosed following investigation for recurrent spontaneous abortions, premature labor, fetal malpresentation, retained placenta, and postpartum hemorrhage. (Figure 39–1) Anomalies include septate uterus, comprised of a simple midline septum; bicornuate uterus, which is a duplication of the uterine horns; and uterus didelphys consisting of complete duplication of the corpus and cervix. These anomalies are often detected with physical examination, especially during or after pregnancies complicated by malpresentation, or preterm labor. Testing with MRI or hysterosalpingogram will usually confirm the diagnosis, and are combined with ultrasonography or laparoscopy if the diagnosis remains uncertain. Combined laparoscopy and hysteroscopy is useful for planning surgical correction.

Surgical correction of uterine anomalies is indicated for prevention of documented or anticipated pregnancy-related complications. A septate uterus is twice as likely to cause spontaneous abortion than a bicornuate uterus, with an overall loss rate of 88% reported for patients with a complete septum. The septate uterus is treated with a septoplasty, completed in most cases by hysteroscopic division or resection of the septum with up to an 86% success rate for subsequent pregnancy. Alternatively, the abdominal metroplasty is indicated for a large or thick septum or for the bicornuate uterus. A wedge of myometrium is resected allowing the two horns of the uterus to be reconstructed. This procedure results in measurable loss of uterine volume. Pregnancies occurring after abdominal metroplasty should be delivered by cesarean section as the risk of uterine rupture is increased.

Abnormal Uterine Bleeding

Abnormal uterine bleeding may occur at any age. It is not unusual for a female infant to have a small amount of self-limited vaginal bleeding attributable to the decline of circulating estrogen from maternal sources after delivery.

Abnormal uterine bleeding during the reproductive years is described according to the chronicity and amount of bleeding because this is often useful in elucidating the etiology. Hypermenorrhea, also referred to as menorrhagia, is defined as excessive or prolonged bleeding at the normal time of menstruation. Polymenorrhea is defined as bleeding that occurs more frequently than every 3 weeks, and metrorrhagia, defines intermenstrual bleeding that occurs in the interval between menses.

Hypermenorrhea may be due to such physical disease of the uterus including uterine leiomyoma, adenomyosis, and endometrial polyp. Dysfunctional uterine bleeding is abnormal uterine bleeding related to functional response of a normal uterus to extrauterine causes such as abnormal cycling of estrogen and progesterone in patients with anovulation, oligo-ovulation, or persistence of the corpus luteum. This condition is seen most often in adolescents and in perimenopausal women. Polymenorrhea is sometimes related to a shortened proliferative phase secondary to hypothyroidism. Causes of metrorrhagia include endometrial polyps, submucous leiomyoma, coagulopathy, granulomatous infections such as tuberculosis, or cancer of the cervix or uterine corpus. Complications of pregnancy should not be overlooked as a cause of abnormal bleeding in women of reproductive age.

Postmenopausal bleeding is defined as any vaginal bleeding occurring a year or more after menopause and is of concern because it may be a symptom of endometrial cancer. When postmenopausal bleeding is fully evaluated including biopsy and hormone studies, the majority will be attributed to benign etiologies such as atrophic change, benign polyp, cervicitis, and physiologic withdrawal from exogenous hormones. Endometrial cancer is detected in about 15% of cases of postmenopausal bleeding, but is also linked to the age of the patient: a 50-year-old woman has about a 2% chance of cancer, while an 80-year-old woman with the same symptom has about a 60% chance of malignancy. Cervical cancer may also present with postmenopausal bleeding. The exogenous administration of estrogenic substances, including hormone replacement therapy, and use of estrogen analogs such as tamoxifen cause postmenopausal bleeding. Much less likely are estrogen-producing tumors of the ovary, coagulopathy, or environmental sources of estrogenic substances. Postmenopausal bleeding in any amount ranging from scant brown vaginal discharge to frank, profuse, bright red bleeding should prompt further workup. Cancer should be considered the likely cause until proven otherwise.

▶ Clinical Findings

Obtain a complete history and perform a careful pelvic examination including a Pap test. The exam will often reveal vaginal, cervical, uterine, or adnexal disease. A complete blood count and measurement of red cell indices will ascertain the degree of chronic blood loss. Additional blood studies including thyroid function testing and testing for coagulopathy may be necessary in some cases.

Abnormal bleeding in women over the age of 35 or with Pap test results showing atypical glandular cells of any type, or in women of any age with a Pap test showing atypical glandular cells, or women with risk factors for gynecologic cancer, endometrial biopsy is required to confirm a diagnosis. The biopsy should be timed at an appropriate time in the menstrual cycle, such as after the sixteenth day of the cycle if anovulatory bleeding is suspected, but may be performed at any time to evaluate for hyperplasia or carcinoma. Endometrial sampling with a disposable suction device can be accomplished in an office setting in most patients. Obese patients or patients with cervical stenosis may require dilatation and curettage in the operating room. Pregnancy should always be ruled out before performing a biopsy in a woman of reproductive age.

Hysteroscopy, involving insertion of a narrow diameter videoscope through the cervix while distending the uterine cavity allows inspection of the endometrium and directed biopsy of suspicious features. Hysteroscopy if very useful for determination of the cause of bleeding and offers the opportunity for simultaneous treatment such as hysteroscopic resection of a polyp. Hysteroscopy can be accomplished in an office or outpatient surgical setting and is recommended when bleeding is recurrent or resistant to therapy or when structural abnormalities of the endometrium such as polyps or submucous leiomyomata are suspected.

Transvaginal ultrasound is useful to measure endometrial thickness and structural abnormalities of the uterus such as a polyp or leiomyoma. In the postmenopausal patient, an endometrial strip of less than or equal to 4 mm virtually excludes the likelihood of cancer. Biopsy is still preferable unless it is unable to be performed for technical reasons. The sonohysterogram, where saline is introduced into the endometrial cavity during ultrasound increases diagnostic accuracy for defects in the endometrial cavity.

▶ Treatment

Dilation and curettage is both diagnostic and therapeutic for many causes of uterine bleeding. Definitive treatment, however, will be targeted toward the etiology of the abnormal uterine bleeding.

Medical management of most nonneoplastic causes of abnormal uterine bleeding is generally prescribed before considering surgery because many symptoms will resolve or managed without surgical intervention. Chronic blood loss due to hypermenorrhea produced by leiomyoma or hyperplasia, can be reduced by the administration of a progestin. A gonadotropin-releasing hormone (GnRH) agonist will result in amenorrhea and is sometimes prescribed prior to planned surgery for leiomyomata. The antiprogestin mifepristone may significantly shrink leiomyomata, but a side effect includes increased risk of endometrial hyperplasia. Dysfunctional bleeding due to chronic anovulation is treated with cyclic progestin therapy, or oral contraceptives. For women who wish to conceive, ovulation induction with drugs such as with clomiphene are prescribed. Control of acute heavy bleeding may be achieved through the use of higher doses of combination oral contraceptives prescribed as one pill four times a day for 3 or 4 days, tapered to one pill a day over one week. Alternatively, intravenous conjugated estrogen, 25 mg every 4 hours, has been used also to control acute bleeding. Such a regimen must be followed by a progestin to prevent additional irregular bleeding at a later time. Following control of acute bleeding, maintenance therapy with an oral contraceptive is recommended. Another strategy for maintenance includes placement of an intrauterine device (IUD) containing levonorgestrel resulting in amenorrhea in about 25% of women and light menses in the remainder. In the absence of identified intrauterine pathology, hypermenorrhea associated with ovulatory cycles can be ameliorated with nonsteroidal anti-inflammatory drugs.

Persistence of symptoms will generally require surgical intervention. Surgical treatment of bleeding caused by uterine leiomyoma is discussed later in this chapter. Severe or intractable dysfunctional uterine bleeding may require hysterectomy. Endometrial ablation by hysteroscopically directed electrosurgery, or use of proprietary endometrial ablation devices may avoid hysterectomy in the premenopausal patient with bleeding that cannot be managed medically. Ablation generally requires normal size and shape of the uterine cavity. Only about 20% of women report amenorrhea following endometrial ablation, and about one-third will undergo eventual hysterectomy. Placement of a levonorgestrel-containing IUD is nearly as effective as hysteroscopic endometrial ablation.

Postmenopausal bleeding due to atrophic changes may resolve with estrogen therapy, administered with progestin in either a cyclic or continuous fashion. Postmenopausal bleeding attributed to physiologic withdrawal bleeding from prescribed estrogen-based therapy is treated by discontinuing therapy or converting to a continuous regimen. Curettage for removal of benign endometrial polyps is often curative, although polyps may recur. Endometrial carcinoma is a relative contraindication to estrogen therapy and is treated surgically with possible postoperative adjuvant radiation or chemotherapy based upon stage and grade of the tumor. Well-differentiated endometrial adenocarcinoma in young women who desire to maintain fertility has been successfully treated using high-dose progestins in about three-fourths of cases.

Adenomyosis

Extension of endometrial glands and stroma into the myometrium is defined as adenomyosis. Symptomatic adenomyosis is most prevalent in the between age 35 and menopause. Symptoms include dysmenorrheal, hypermenorrhea, polymenorrhea, metrorrhagia, and dyspareunia. Concurrent endometriosis is common. Symptoms typically improve after menopause supports.

Upon pelvic examination, the uterus is slightly to moderately enlarged and is frequently tender to palpation, particularly in the secretory phase of the menstrual cycle. Preoperative confirmation of adenomyosis is challenging. Neither ultrasound nor endometrial biopsy is useful for making the diagnosis. The T2 weighted sequences on MRI is more effective, with sensitivity of 70% and specificity of 86%. Definitive diagnosis is confirmed after hysterectomy.

▶ Differential Diagnosis

Leiomyomata of the uterus are common and cause many symptoms similar to adenomyosis. Low-grade endometrial stromal sarcoma is rare, but can be mistaken as adenomyosis. This is an indolent malignancy with a significant likelihood of local recurrence. Distant metastases to the ovary, peritoneal surfaces, and lung are occasionally seen. Tumors of this type should not be morcellated. Subsequent treatment may include pelvic radiation therapy and hormone therapy based on stage at time of diagnosis and presence of estrogen and progesterone receptors.

▶ Treatment

Total hysterectomy with or without bilateral salpingo-oophorectomy is the only clearly effective treatment. Hormonal approaches may be successful in treating symptoms, particularly if the patient is nearing menopause. Menopause causes symptoms to regress.

Leiomyomata

Uterine leiomyomata, or fibroids, are present in 20%-30% of women of reproductive age. The true prevalence is unknown because many fibroids are asymptomatic. Black women have a threefold higher incidence than white, Asian, and Hispanic women. Other risk factors include obesity, nulliparity, and early menarche or infertility. Myomas arise from monoclonal proliferation and are stimulated by estrogen, progesterone, and growth factors. Fibroids increase growth rate during pregnancy and regress after menopause. Fibroids are usually multifocal and vary hugely in size, ranging from a few millimeters to masses that fill the abdomen. Location of leiomyomata can be nearly anywhere within the uterus. Descriptive terms for location include intramural for fibroids arising within the myometrium, subserosal for lesions below the exterior surface of the uterus, and submucosal for fibroids below or adjacent to the endometrium. Other types of leiomyomata include pedunculated lesions connected with a narrow vascular stalk to the uterus, intraligamentous lesions within the broad ligament, and parasitic leiomyomata, detached from the uterus and deriving blood supply from adjacent organs.

▶ Clinical Findings

Symptoms are determined by location, number, and size of the lesions. Common symptoms include hypermenorrhea, prolonged menses, pelvic pressure, increased abdominal girth, urinary frequency, dyspareunia, low back pain, and constipation. Infertility may occur secondary to fibroids, particularly if the uterine cavity is enlarged or distorted by a submucous lesion. Adverse pregnancy outcomes such as abnormal placentation, malpresentation, abruption, and dysfunctional labor are recognized complications associated with fibroids. Degenerative changes may spontaneously occur, potentially causing significant pain that requires treatment. Submucous leiomyomata are more likely to cause hypermenorrhea, polymenorrhea, and metrorrhagia.

Palpation of the uterus during bimanual examination detects a lobular and enlarged structure with a characteristic rubbery consistency. Soft and tender lesions are characteristic of degenerating fibroids. Larger lesions may be felt on abdominal examination.

Anemia may result from acute or chronic abnormal uterine bleeding. Endometrial biopsy should be performed in women with abnormal uterine bleeding to rule out endometrial cancer. Pelvic ultrasound is the most useful study for diagnosis. Sonohysterogram or hysteroscopy are useful for confirmation of submucous leiomyomata. MRI is expensive and should be utilized selectively for evaluation of an atypical lesions that could represent sarcoma or for of lesions prior to a myomectomy. Hydronephrosis may be apparent on imaging studies, arising as a result of external compression of the by the mass.

▶ Differential Diagnosis

Uterine leiomyosarcoma is a rare but aggressive neoplasm. Among women undergoing surgery for fibroids, only 0.23% is found to harbor sarcoma. The rapidly growing leiomyoma, defined as 6 cm growth in 1 year, will be malignant in less than 0.1% of cases. In a postmenopausal woman with an enlarging uterine mass, sarcoma is more likely. Most sarcomas are not detected prior to surgery, although a high T1/high T2 pattern on MRI has been reported to be predictive of sarcoma. On cut section, leiomyomata are well-circumscribed, solid tumors with a pseudocapsule and an off-white, whorled appearance. If a lesion lacks an apparent capsule, appears necrotic, is soft or friable, then a frozen section should be submitted. These findings are likely to represent a sarcoma.

Other potential diagnoses to consider include solid ovarian tumors. Enlargement of the uterus may arise due to adenomyosis or could represent an undiagnosed pregnancy. A pregnancy test should be considered.

▶ Treatment

Asymptomatic fibroids require no therapy. Women with hypermenorrhea or polymenorrhea often benefit from a trial of cyclic or continuous oral contraceptives or progestins. GnRH agonists decrease myoma size and stop menstruation prior to surgery. However, long-term use of GnRH agonists causes osteoporosis. Treatment with the antiprogestin mifepristone may result in significant shrinkage of fibroids, but may cause endometrial hyperplasia. In premenopausal women, leiomyomata grow soon after medication is discontinued.

For women with symptoms unresponsive to medical management, several treatment options are available. Myomectomy is a procedure for removal of leiomyomata with subsequent repair of resultant defects in the uterine wall in order to preserve the uterus. Myomectomy is usually offered to women who desire to retain their fertility. Some women who do not desire pregnancy also choose this option. Myomectomy is performed via laparotomy, laparoscopy, or hysteroscopy depending on the location, number, and size of the leiomyomata. Women who have completed childbearing and desire an alternative to hysterectomy may choose uterine artery embolization or guided focused ultrasound surgery, both of which are designed to decrease the size of lesions. Embolization involves diminishing blood flow to the uterus by occluding vessels to the lesion using angiography. Uterus and fibroids have been reported to decrease in size by one-third to one half. Bleeding and pelvic pressure improve in 80%-90% of women. Hysterectomy is definitive treatment for women with symptomatic myomas. Alternatives to total abdominal hysterectomy include vaginal hysterectomy, supracervical hysterectomy, and laparoscopic hysterectomy.

Prognosis

Myomectomy results in improvement of symptoms in 80% of women. Ten percent of women undergoing myomectomy require additional surgery for recurrent lesions and 50% will develop recurrent leiomyomata.

SURGERY FOR MALIGNANT UTERINE DISEASE

Endometrial Cancer

Endometrial carcinoma is the most common gynecologic malignancy in the United States. It is primarily a disease of postmenopausal women. Tumors are grouped into type I and II categories based on their underlying etiology. The more common type I tumors arise due to prolonged estrogen stimulation of the endometrium. The estrogen is most commonly endogenously produced estrone arising by aromatase conversion of androstenedione in peripheral adipocytes. Obese women produce much more estrogen and are at much higher risk for developing this cancer. Exogenous estrogens prescribed without accompanying progestin in postmenopausal women greatly increases the risk of endometrial cancer as does treatment with other estrogen receptor agonists such as tamoxifen when prescribed for treatment or prevention of breast cancer. Other risk factors for development of endometrial cancer include diabetes, early menarche, late menopause, and low parity. Oral contraceptives are protective against this cancer. Also at risk are premenopausal women with chronic anovulation such as with polycystic ovary syndrome.

Complex hyperplasia with atypia is a precursor lesion for type I endometrial cancer. These tumors usually express estrogen and progesterone receptors. Type II endometrial cancer consists of anaplastic or high-grade, papillary serous, clear cell, and squamous carcinomas. These tumors rarely express estrogen or progesterone receptors and are not thought to arise as a result of estrogen stimulation. Adverse prognostic factors include grade, histology, depth of myometrial invasion, cervical extension, tumor size, and extension beyond the uterus.

Endometrial cancer is staged surgically as shown in Table 39–5.

Clinical Findings

Postmenopausal bleeding is the presenting symptom in about 90% of cases and should be considered to be cancer until proven otherwise. Common etiologies of postmenopausal bleeding include physiologic bleeding from hormone replacement therapy (27%), benign polyps (7%-23%), cervicitis (6%-14%), endometrial carcinoma (13%-16%), atrophy (10%),

Table 39–5. FIGO staging for endometrial cancer.

FIGO Stage	Revised 2009
Stage I	Tumor confined to corpus uteri
IA	No or less than 50% myometrial invasion
IB	Invasion equal or greater than 50% of myometrium
Stage II	Tumor invades cervical stroma but does not extend beyond uterus
Stage III	Local and/or regional spread. Positive cytology has to be reported separately without changing the stage
IIIA	Tumor invades serosa and/or adnexae
IIIB	Vaginal and/or parametrial involvement (direct or metastases)
IIIC	Metastases to pelvic and/or para-aortic lymph nodes
IIIC-1	Positive pelvic nodes
IIIC-2	Positive para-aortic nodes with or without positive pelvic nodes
Stage IVA	Tumor invades bladder or bowel mucosa
Stage IVB	Distant metastases, including intra-abdominal and/or inguinal lymph nodes
Grade 1	
Grade 2	
Grade 3	

Grade of tumor is related to the proportion of nonsquamous, solid growth pattern in the tumor. Grade 1 is comprised of ≤ 5% of nonsquamous solid growth pattern; grade 2 is 6-50% nonsquamous solid growth pattern; and grade 3 is > 50% nonsquamous solid growth pattern. (Reproduced, with permission, from Pecorelli S: Revised FIGO staging for carcinoma of the vulva, cervix, and endometrium. *Int J Gynecol Obstet.* 2009 May;105(2):103–4.)

cervical carcinoma (1%-4%). Despite workup, up to 20%-23% of cases will have no identified etiology. Cervical stenosis with pyometrium or hematometrium is highly suggestive of endometrial carcinoma. Pain is not a common symptom. Vaginal cytology is positive in 40%-80% of cases but is entirely unreliable as a diagnostic tool for endometrial cancer. Endometrial biopsy performed in the office using a disposable biopsy instrument is highly sensitive. If endometrial biopsy fails to provide a definitive diagnosis, dilatation and curettage of endocervix and endometrium, is definitive.

Type II endometrial carcinoma comprised of poorly differentiated, or adverse histological types, may disseminate relatively early in the course of the disease. Metastatic spread may occur to the vagina, regional pelvic and para-aortic lymph nodes, ovaries, lungs, brain, and bone. The most frequent site of recurrence following treatment for endometrial carcinoma is the vaginal vault.

Prevention

Oral contraceptives have been shown to reduce the risk of endometrial cancer by up to 50% depending on duration of treatment. Progestin therapy will reduce the possibility of endometrial carcinoma in the anovulatory patient as well as in postmenopausal women receiving estrogen replacement therapy. Progestins in both OCP and hormone replacement regimens cause downregulation of estrogen receptors and atrophy of endometrium.

Treatment

Endometrial cancer is staged surgically. The route of surgical approach for the staging procedure can be either via laparotomy or laparoscopy. Definitive therapy includes total hysterectomy, bilateral salpingo-oophorectomy, pelvic and para-aortic lymphadenectomy and pelvic washings for type I cancers. For type II lesions, omentectomy is usually added. Lymphadenectomy is sometimes omitted for patients with type I lesions with low-risk such as small, grade-1 cancers without myometrial invasion.

If the cervix is grossly involved, patients may receive preoperative radiation followed by total hysterectomy, bilateral salpingo-oophorectomy, pelvic and para-aortic lymphadenectomy and pelvic washings. Alternatively, a radical hysterectomy bilateral salpingo-oophorectomy, pelvic and para-aortic lymphadenectomy may be performed without preoperative radiation. The radical hysterectomy includes removal of the upper third of the vagina, cardinal, and uterosacral ligaments.

Adjuvant pelvic radiation therapy is administered to patients with cervical extension (stage II); deep myometrial invasion with a grade 3, type I lesion; or vaginal extension (stage IIIB). A randomized clinical trial comparing radiation to chemotherapy with cisplatin and doxorubicin showed a survival benefit for patients with positive nodes (stage IIIC) treated with chemotherapy. Metastatic and type II lesions such as papillary serous carcinomas are very likely to recur after surgery regardless of stage. These tumors are usually treated with multimodal therapy using a combination of radiation and chemotherapy.

Metastatic or recurrent disease is usually treated with multimodal therapy using surgery, radiation and/or chemotherapy based on the location, size, and histology of lesions. Chemotherapy combinations usually include either a doublet of cisplatin with paclitaxel or doxorubicin or a triplet regimen combining all three drugs. Metastatic cancer of type I may be treated with progestin therapy.

Prognosis

Survival at 5 years is about 70%-90% for stage I disease, depending on grade and myometrial invasion. Survival declines to about 60% in stage II. Anaplastic tumors, deep myometrial penetration, and absence of estrogen and progesterone receptors all worsen the prognosis.

Uterine Sarcoma

Uterine sarcomas fall into three histological groups including leiomyosarcoma, endometrial stromal sarcoma, and carcinosarcoma. These tumors are rare, accounting for about 3% of uterine neoplasms. Sarcomas of the uterus spread via hematogenous and lymphatic pathways in addition to direct extension. Lung and liver are frequent sites of metastases and recurrence.

In patients in whom the tumor is confined to the pelvic organs, treatment consists of total hysterectomy, bilateral salpingo-oophorectomy, pelvic and para-aortic lymphadenectomy, omentectomy and pelvic washings. There are no randomized trials documenting survival benefit for adjuvant therapy with either chemotherapy or radiation. However, individualized postoperative radiation and/or chemotherapy may be offered based on the poor prognosis of these tumors. Radiation reduces pelvic recurrences, but does not appear to improve overall survival.

The outlook for patients with uterine sarcoma is dependent on grade and stage of the tumor. Leiomyosarcomas with more than ten mitoses per ten high-power fields carry a poor prognosis, with recurrence within 5 years in about two-thirds of patients. About 40% of patients with carcinosarcoma survive. Isolated, late recurrence of leiomyosarcoma in the lung is treated by resection of the affected lobe with generally good salvage rates of about 50% at 2 years.

Gemcitabine and Taxotere is the combination with the highest likelihood of response for metastatic or recurrent leiomyosarcoma. High-dose progestin therapy is very effective for treatment of metastatic low-grade endometrial sarcoma. Carcinosarcoma is most effectively treated with combination of either cisplatin and ifosfamide or ifosfamide and paclitaxel.

Gestational Trophoblastic Disease

Gestational trophoblastic disease refers to tumors arising from placental tissue. They are unique among all neoplasms in that their genetic complement is provided by the father, thereby resulting in a tumor with genetic material and markers foreign to the patient. Gestational trophoblastic diseases may be divided into preinvasive and invasive types. The preinvasive types include complete and partial hydatidiform moles.

The frequency of hydatidiform mole is about 1:700 to 1:2000 pregnancies in the United States, Canada, and Western Europe and about 1:85 to 1:520 pregnancies in Asia. Hydatidiform mole is more common in women over 40. A prior history of gestational trophoblastic disease significantly increases the risk of recurrence with a future gestation.

The gross appearance of a hydatidiform mole is related to the hydropic villi in the absence of a fetal circulation. The histological appearance reveals varying degrees of trophoblastic proliferation. Hydatidiform moles can be classified as either complete or partial, based on cytogenetics and histopathology. These features are compared in Table 39–6. The majority of complete moles carry a 46XX karyotype, with chromosomes exclusively of paternal origin. Partial moles are typically triploid with 69XXX or 69XXY, where two or three sets of chromosomes are paternal in origin. Complete moles are not associated with a developing fetus, and partial moles may include a fetus that is typically small and with multiple anomalies.

Invasive gestational trophoblastic disease is categorized as invasive mole, choriocarcinoma, or placental site trophoblastic tumor. Invasive mole is diagnosed after 15% of complete moles and 3.5% of partial moles. Metastases occur following 4% of complete moles and 0.6% of partial moles. Choriocarcinoma occurs following 3%-7% of hydatidiform moles and 1:40,000 term pregnancies. Out of all choriocarcinoma cases, 50% are preceded by a mole, 25% by spontaneous abortion, and 25% by term pregnancy. Placental site trophoblast tumor (PSTT) is a very rare variant with only 55 cases reported in the literature by 1991.

Invasive mole is comprised of hyperplastic trophoblasts with villi invading myometrium. Choriocarcinoma involves sheets of syncytiotrophoblasts with no villi and demonstrates invasion into myometrium or other tissues. Necrosis and hemorrhage are common. PSTT is comprised of intermediate cytotrophoblasts.

Human chorionic gonadotropin (β-hCG) is a clinically useful tumor marker for all types of preinvasive and invasive gestational trophoblastic disease except PSTT, where human placental lactogen (hPL) may be elevated.

▶ Clinical Findings

The most common presenting symptom with hydatidiform mole is vaginal bleeding, occurring in 97% of complete moles and 73% of partial moles. On pelvic exam, about 50% of complete moles and 8% of partial moles will reveal uterine size greater than expected for a given estimated gestational age. Theca lutein cysts are physiologic ovarian cysts as a result of hyperstimulation by very high levels of β-hCG produced by 50% of complete moles. These cysts typically resolve once the β-hCG level regresses following appropriate treatment. Preeclampsia may develop in 27% of women with complete moles and virtually never with partial moles. Clinical hyperthyroidism can develop in about 7% of women with complete moles with very high β-hCG levels due to cross reactivity of this hormone with thyroid stimulating hormone. A rare but potentially fatal complication is trophoblastic embolization to the lung during or after evacuation of large complete moles.

Diagnosis is usually confirmed with either ultrasound or β-hCG values. Serum β-hCG levels are above 100,000 mIU/mL in 46% of women with complete moles and these values persist beyond the twelfth week gestation, neither of which should be observed in a normal pregnancy. Ultrasound will usually demonstrate multiple small sonolucencies due to the hydropic villi. In a partial mole, the fetus, if present, will usually be small and afflicted with multiple anomalies.

▶ Differential Diagnosis

Threatened abortion or missed abortion will often present with similar symptoms of bleeding and both are more likely than gestational trophoblastic disease. A multiple gestation must be considered because it may produce unusually high levels of β-hCG in addition to uterine size greater than the gestational date.

▶ Complications

Metastasis is most common with choriocarcinoma, but may occur with any of the invasive types of gestational

Table 39–6. Features of hydatidiform moles.

Characteristic	Complete Mole	Partial Mole
Karyotype	46XX (90%) 46XY (10%) All paternal chromosomes	Triploid (90%) 69XXX or 69XXY Diploid (10%) 46 paternal chromosomes
Fetus	Absent	Often present
Villous edema	Prominent and diffuse	Focal if at all
Fetal RBC	None	Usually present
Proliferation of trophoblast	Prominent	Mild to moderate
Likelihood of local invasion	15%	3.5%
Likelihood of metastasis	4%	0.6%

trophoblastic disease. The most common sites of spread include lung (80%), vagina (30%), pelvis (20%), brain or liver (10%), bowel or kidney or spleen (<5%). Unlike virtually any other tumor, metastatic disease is still potentially curable in many patients.

▶ **Treatment**

Once the diagnosis of a molar pregnancy has been established, the uterus should be evacuated by suction curettage. All specimens are submitted for histology and cytogenetics. Theca lutein cysts of the ovaries regress following treatment of the mole and should not be surgically excised.

Following evacuation of the uterus, weekly serum β-hCG levels should be monitored until normalized for 3 weeks; followed by monthly testing for 6-12 months depending on assessment of pretreatment risk factors. If the β-hCG value plateaus for 3 weeks or rises for 2 weeks, invasive gestational trophoblastic disease including either invasive mole or choriocarcinoma should be suspected. Effective contraception during the surveillance phase is important in order not to complicate interpretation of the β-hCG.

Patients with invasive or persistent gestational trophoblastic disease should be evaluated with a metastatic workup including pelvic examination, CT scan of the head, chest, abdomen, and pelvis, a complete blood count, and renal and liver function tests. Lumber puncture to detect occult central nervous system metastases is sometimes necessary.

Staging of gestational trophoblastic tumors is outlined in Table 39–7. Unlike most neoplasms, gestational trophoblastic disease is staged using a nonanatomic staging system based on prognostic factors. Current FIGO staging combines anatomic staging with the modified WHO prognostic scoring system. For anatomic stage I disease, risk is usually low and for anatomic stage IV disease, risk is usually high. Stage II and III disease is best stratified with the modified WHO prognostic scoring system. Stage is recorded as anatomic stage and FIGO modified WHO score, separated by colon.

Single-agent chemotherapy is the preferred treatment for patients with stage I or low-risk disease who wish to maintain reproductive options. If future childbearing is not an issue, patients with invasive mole may be treated with a hysterectomy and possible adjuvant chemotherapy. Preferred regimens for single-agent therapy include methotrexate or dactinomycin. Both of these regimens can be toxic and should be administered under the guidance of a gynecologic oncologist or medical oncologist. Intermediate and high-risk gestational trophoblastic disease should receive aggressive combination chemotherapy. The most effective regimen reported includes etoposide, methotrexate, dactinomycin, cyclophosphamide, and vincristine (EMACO). There is

Table 39–7. FIGO anatomic staging for gestational trophoblastic disease.

FIGO Staging	Description			
Stage I	Disease confined to the uterus			
Stage II	GTN extends outside of uterus, but is limited to genital structures including adnexa, vagina, broad ligament			
Stage III	GTN extends to lungs with or without genital tract involvement			
Stage IV	All other metastatic sites			
Modified WHO Prognostic Scoring System as adapted by FIGO				
Description	**Score**			
Factor	**0**	**1**	**2**	**4**
Age (years)	< 40	≥40		
Antecedent pregnancy type	Mole	Abortion	Term	
Pregnancy to treatment interval (months)	< 4	4 - < 7	7 - 13	≥ 13
Pretreatment β-hCG (mIU/L)	< 10^3	10^3 - 10^4	10^4 - 10^5	≥ 10^5
Tumor size including uterus (cm)	–	3 - 5	≥ 5	–
Site of metastases	Lung	Spleen Kidney	GI	Brain Liver
Number of metastases	0	1 - 4	5 - 8	> 8
Previous failed chemo regimens			Single	≥ 2

Total: If score is ≥ 7, then patient is high risk and requires intensive, multiagent chemotherapy. Current staging combines anatomic staging with the modified WHO prognostic scoring system. Stage is recorded as anatomic stage and FIGO modified WHO score, separated by colon. Example of format: Stage IV: 8.

occasionally a role for surgery or radiation for selected metastatic disease sites and intrathecal methotrexate is sometimes needed for treatment of central nervous system disease.

Prognosis

The prognosis for cure of gestational trophoblastic tumors is excellent, including cases with pulmonary metastases, which are still considered low risk. Five-year survival of up to 85% is reported in cases with high-risk metastatic disease. The risk of recurrence of gestational trophoblastic disease in a future pregnancy has a relative risk of 20-40, but in absolute terms, this translates to a recurrence risk of less than 5%. During any subsequent pregnancy, ultrasound is recommended. The placenta should be examined after delivery, and β-hCG should be monitored until normalization.

SURGERY FOR BENIGN FALLOPIAN TUBE DISEASE

Infertility Attributed to Fallopian Tube Disease

Infertility is defined as failure to conceive after 1 year of normal coital activity without use of contraceptives. About 15% of couples are infertile within this definition. When the etiology of infertility is evaluated, approximately 40% will be attributable to male factor infertility including low sperm count, impaired motility, or abnormal morphology of sperm. Anatomic abnormality of the pelvic organs is the single most common cause of infertility in women, and tubal factor infertility is the most common cause of infertility.

Common causes for tubal factor infertility include acute and chronic salpingitis, endometriosis, and adhesions from previous appendicitis with rupture or surgery. Chlamydia and gonorrhea infections are the most common causes of tubal damage causing infertility. Desire to reverse previous tubal sterilization may also be a reason for tubal surgery. One-third of infertile couples have more than one problem.

History

It is important to elicit any history of sexually transmitted disease, pelvic inflammatory disease, pelvic surgery, cyclic pain, or dyspareunia.

Clinical Findings

The size and mobility of the uterus should be assessed. Adnexae should be palpated for masses consistent with endometrioma or hydrosalpinx, in particular. Cul de sac or uterosacral ligament nodularity and tenderness suggest endometriosis. Ultrasound may reveal the presence of isoechoic masses suggesting endometriosis or a tubular mass consistent with hydrosalpinx. Hysterosalpingogram, a test that involves fluoroscopic assessment of tubal patency by transcervical injection of the uterus with radiocontrast, may reveal an obstruction including its location. Use of a water-based dye is indicated for the first attempt, and if occlusion is noted, an oil contrast medium may be used subsequently. The oil based hysterosalpingogram is reported to have therapeutic benefit.

Laparoscopy is warranted if the evaluation for anatomic abnormalities is inconclusive. Therapeutic interventions including lysis of adhesions or ablation of endometrial implants may be efficacious. If laparoscopy is performed following a normal hysterosalpingogram 24% will have mild endometriosis and 6% of patients will have adhesions.

Treatment

Tuboplasty procedures may be performed to restore tubal patency. However, in vitro fertilization has become a much more popular intervention in recent years for treatment of infertility attributed to tubal occlusion or when multiple infertility factors affect the couple. Hydrosalpinx is usually treated by salpingectomy in order to optimize subsequent in vitro fertilization. Other factors of prognostic significance include age of the couple, and presence of other causes of infertility including ovulatory dysfunction or male factor infertility.

Heterotopic pregnancies and multiple gestation pregnancies are much more likely than the general population for patients undergoing in vitro fertilization.

Prognosis

Age and severity of tubal disease are predictors of success. Women with mild adhesive disease and age less than 35 have the highest success rates, approaching 70%. For severe tubal disease, success is less than 15%. Ectopic pregnancy is twenty times more likely with a history of Fallopian tube surgery or preexisting scar resulting in a 10% incidence. IVF success rates vary by program and have generally been improving steadily in recent years. Decisions regarding planned tubal surgery versus IVF should take into account the relative costs and success rates.

Ectopic Pregnancy

Ectopic pregnancy is implantation of a viable pregnancy in a location other than within the endometrium lining the uterus. Risk factors for ectopic pregnancy include prior tubal surgery, previous ectopic pregnancy, history of pelvic inflammatory disease or Chlamydia infection, and pregnancy arising from assisted reproduction techniques. Smoking and history of infertility are also associated with increased risk of ectopic pregnancy. Over 95% of ectopic pregnancies occur in the Fallopian tube, generally within the ampullary portion. A less common location includes interstitial pregnancy within the tubal lumen where it passes through the myometrium. Rare sites include cervix, ovary, omentum, pelvis, and abdomen. Heterotopic pregnancy refers to the rare occurrence of an intrauterine pregnancy with a synchronous ectopic pregnancy. The incidence of heterotopic pregnancy has increased from a spontaneous rate of 1:30,000 pregnancies to 0.1%-1% for pregnancies arising from assisted reproductive technology.

The incidence of ectopic pregnancy has been reported to occur in approximately 2% of pregnancies, although the true incidence is difficult to ascertain due to the potential for spontaneous resolution of some ectopic pregnancies resulting in unrecognized disease in addition to under reporting of early ectopic pregnancies treated medically rather than surgically. Pregnant women with pain or bleeding have a fourfold higher incidence of ectopic pregnancy. The primary potential morbidity of ectopic pregnancy is the potential rupture of the Fallopian tube or other implantation site resulting in hemorrhage. Failure to make a timely diagnosis can result in hemorrhagic shock and death.

Symptoms & Signs

Patients will usually present with amenorrhea and a diagnosis of pregnancy. Subsequent irregular bleeding occurs in many but not all cases. In the early evolution of the ectopic pregnancy, patients may be asymptomatic. Presence of pain is also variable. Classic symptoms of a ruptured ectopic include severe abdominal pain, referred pain to the shoulder and hemodynamic instability. Upon pelvic examination an adnexal mass may or may not be present. The uterus is usually slightly enlarged and softened secondary to hormonal influence of the ectopic pregnancy.

Diagnostic Studies

Trophoblastic cells of the blastocyst produce β-hCG that may be detected shortly after implantation. The rise of β-hCG is logarithmic, with a doubling time of about 48 hours. The β-hCG should rise at least 66% every 48 hours in 85% of normal pregnancies and will plateau in normal pregnancy late in the first trimester. Ectopic pregnancies show a slower rise of β-hCG in all but 15% of cases. An absolute β-hCG does not permit distinction between an ectopic and a nonviable intrauterine pregnancy.

Transvaginal ultrasound has almost 100% sensitivity for detection of intrauterine pregnancy as long as care is taken to discriminate between an actual pregnancy and the pseudo sac, defined as intrauterine fluid that can be mistaken for an intrauterine pregnancy. A true gestational sac is located eccentrically in the uterus and should demonstrate a fetal pole. The absence of an intrauterine pregnancy in the setting of a positive β-hCG is strongly suggestive of an ectopic pregnancy if the β-hCG value is above the discriminatory threshold of transvaginal ultrasound to detect a gestational

sac. The discriminatory threshold has been reported to occur with β-hCG values above 1500-3000 mIU/mL, although variables such as body mass index, quality of ultrasound equipment, and experience of the sonographer all impact on the threshold value. Diagnosis of the ectopic pregnancy by direct ultrasound localization of the pregnancy is much less accurate than detection of intrauterine implantation.

Other tests that are of value include obtaining a blood count to assess for anemia in addition to serum progesterone levels. Variability of progesterone values in normal pregnancy limits the utility of this test for diagnosis of ectopic pregnancy.

Treatment

If the β-hCG shows an abnormal rate of rise, including plateau, slow rise, or declining values, then ultrasound is warranted. However, if the β-hCG value is below the discriminatory threshold, suction curettage is useful to distinguish between a nonviable intrauterine pregnancy and an ectopic gestation. The absence of chorionic villi in the curettage specimen in the presence of an elevated hCG is predictive of an ectopic pregnancy, though in early gestation the curettage may be falsely negative for villi.

Treatment of ectopic pregnancy is either surgical or medical depending on several variables. The surgical approach is definitive, but invasive and more costly than medical management. Medical management results in successful treatment for 90% of appropriately selected patients. Methotrexate is utilized for medical management. Appropriate indications for medical management require a hemodynamically stable patient who is compliant and has no medical contraindication to methotrexate. Relative contraindications include a gestational sac > 3.5 cm, presence of fetal cardiac motion, or a β-hCG value of > 15,000 mIU/mL. Administration of a single dose of methotrexate has reported efficacy of 84%. Use of multidose regimens increases the rate of success. Failure of the β-hCG value to fall by at least 15% within 4-7 days after treatment indicates that additional methotrexate or surgery is indicated. Patients who are Rh negative are given $RH_o(D)$ immune globulin whether treated medically or surgically. Other developments in medical management include the use of other agents such as potassium chloride, prostaglandins, and mifepristone, but these have not been studied as well as methotrexate.

Surgical options for treatment of ectopic pregnancy are intended to remove the ectopic gestation and preserve functional Fallopian tube, if possible. If the patient is hemodynamically stable, the laparoscopic approach is usually preferred. If she is in shock or if the abdomen is distended with blood, emergent laparotomy is necessary. If the Fallopian tube is generally healthy, a salpingostomy is possible whereby the involved section of the Fallopian tube is removed through an incision in the antimesenteric portion of the tube, while leaving the remainder of the tube intact. If the tube is more extensively damaged, complete or partial salpingectomy is recommended. If conservative approaches to preserve the Fallopian tube are utilized, the β-hCG value should be monitored postoperatively until normalization occurs.

Expectant management of a documented ectopic pregnancy may be an option in stable patients if the β-hCG value is less than 200 mIU/mL and declining. Patients must be counseled regarding the risks of rupture and hemorrhage, and emergency management must be readily available.

▶ Contraception

Contraception to prevent unwanted pregnancy may be attained using either reversible or permanent methods. Reversible methods include hormonal contraceptives via oral, transcutaneous or subcutaneous routes; injectable long acting progestins; IUD; and condoms, to name a few. Modern IUD contraceptives contain progestational hormones or copper, delivered in low doses to the uterine cavity where they inhibit sperm motility and block fertilization. They are inserted as an office procedure without requiring local anesthetic or cervical dilation in most cases. Both copper and progestin devices are highly effective and long lasting. Contemporary IUD contraceptives do not increase the risk of pelvic infection. Progestin-releasing IUD devices menstrual flow by about 50% and have been shown to be as effective for control of abnormal uterine bleeding, prevention of hyperplasia during estrogen replacement therapy, and treatment of hyperplasia.

Subdermal implant contraception uses low serum concentrations of contraceptive progestins found in birth control pills to thicken cervical mucus and inhibit ovulation. These actions result in failure rates comparable to those reported following sterilization and intrauterine contraception. Their duration of action is FDA approved for 3 years. As with intrauterine contraceptives, the principal side effect is change in menstrual bleeding; the majority of users experience a diminution in blood loss but an increase in number of days of bleeding, sometimes at unpredictable intervals.

Contraceptive implants require subdermal insertion with a disposable trocar with local anesthetic and are removed under local anesthetic through a small incision. These procedures take only a few minutes, and pain and infections are rare. Contemporary systems utilize a single-rod and are easier to use, have a shorter life, and are associated with somewhat more acceptable bleeding patterns than the now-discontinued multirod implants.

Unintended pregnancies result in about one million abortions per year in the United States. Uterine aspiration using either manual or electric vacuum pumps allows safe elective abortion in the first trimester, with a mortality rate of less than 1:200,000 procedures. Morbidity and mortality

of abortion rises substantially as the length of gestation increases.

Permanent sterilization options are available for both men and women. Prior to performing any permanent sterilization procedure, the physician must carefully counsel and determine whether a permanent method of contraception is appropriate for the patient. Reversal of permanent sterilization is costly and often ineffective. Permanent male sterilization via vasectomy is safe, effective with reported failure rates of 1.5 per 1000, and minimally invasive. For women, there are several permanent sterilization options. Most of the procedures for women are designed to occlude or remove the Fallopian tube via laparotomy or laparoscopy. These include Pomeroy, Irving, Uchida, and Madelener laparotomy operations in addition to laparoscopic procedures using unipolar or bipolar electrosurgical coagulation of the Fallopian tubes, application of Silastic bands or proprietary clips (Filshie clips, Hulka clips). Mini laparotomy for Pomeroy-type tubal occlusion is often utilized for postpartum sterilization. There are now a limited number of proprietary methods of transcervical tubal occlusion based on intrauterine access to the tubal ostia using a hysteroscope.

The observed failure rate for tubal ligation procedures ranges from 0.7% to 3.6%, which is comparable to the failure rate of IUD and subdermal implants.

SURGERY FOR MALIGNANT FALLOPIAN TUBE DISEASE

Benign and malignant tumors of the Fallopian tubes are very rare. Adenocarcinoma of the Fallopian tube accounts for less than 1% of female reproductive tract cancers. Women with *BRCA1 and 2* mutations are at increased risk for Fallopian tube cancer concordant with their increased risk for ovarian cancer.

The most common presenting symptoms for cancer of the Fallopian tubes are postmenopausal vaginal bleeding or history of intermittent and profuse, watery vaginal discharge. The latter symptom is referred to as *hydrops tubae perfluens*. An adnexal mass is sometimes, but not always palpable. Tumor markers such as CA-125 are usually elevated, although early stage disease may result in elevation of the CA-125 in less than half of patients with Fallopian tube or ovarian cancers. The diagnosis of the Fallopian tube carcinoma is usually not made preoperatively.

The differential diagnosis for Fallopian tube cancer includes disorders that may result in enlargement or obstruction of the distal Fallopian tube. The most common example would be hydrosalpinx whereby obstruction of the Fallopian tube results in accumulation of fluid within the lumen and causes distension of the tube. Common causes of hydrosalpinx include prior infection or endometriosis. Another potential confounding diagnosis is the presence of paratubal cysts, which are simple cysts arising in the mesosalpinx or loosely attached to the exterior of the tube. Paratubal cysts are nearly always benign and arise from Müllerian and Wolffian duct remnants.

Fallopian tube cancer is staged using the FIGO staging rules for ovarian cancer.

Treatment for Fallopian tube cancer is identical to treatment for ovarian cancer. Multimodal therapy including a primary surgery for staging and debulking of disease is followed by adjuvant chemotherapy based on the stage and grade of the disease. A more detailed discussion of the surgery and postoperative adjuvant therapy considerations is described in the ovarian cancer section of this chapter. If the disease is confined to the tube, the prognosis is good. Like ovarian cancer, most Fallopian tube cancers are of advanced stage at the time of diagnosis, and the subsequent survival is much lower.

SURGERY FOR BENIGN OVARIAN DISEASE

▶ Adnexal Masses

Adnexal masses are abnormal structures arising in the ovary, Fallopian tube, or broad ligament. Preoperative assessment can narrow the differential diagnosis, but definitive diagnosis usually requires surgical resection or biopsy.

The differential diagnosis of adnexal masses is complex (Table 39–8). Every structure native to the pelvis can potentially present as a detectable adnexal mass. The majority is benign, but the probability of malignancy increases with age. About 10% of persistent adnexal masses attributable to the ovary are malignant in premenopausal women rising to nearly 50% in postmenopausal women.

▶ Functional Cysts

Functional cysts are relatively common in reproductive age women, but are also reported in postmenopausal women. These cysts are usually larger than 3 cm in order to be diagnosed and may attain diameters of up to 10 cm. Histological examination reveals no pathologic features such as atypia, necrosis, or invasion. Follicular cysts produce estrogen until resolution of the cyst and the corpus luteum cyst produces progesterone until resolution. Because of the hormone production by these types of cysts, menses may be delayed or irregular, often leading to an incorrect clinical diagnosis of ectopic pregnancy. The least common type of functional cyst is the theca lutein cyst, which arises as a physiologic response to hyperstimulation by elevated β-hCG values produced by complete hydatidiform moles. Functional cysts usually regress spontaneously within 1-3 months, or in the case of theca lutein cysts, when the β-hCG value normalizes following treatment.

Correct identification of functional cysts prevents many unnecessary surgical procedures. The functional cyst is typically a smooth, unilateral cyst on pelvic examination. Transvaginal ultrasound will show a simple, sonolucent

Table 39–8. Differential diagnosis of adnexal masses.

Ovarian Etiology	Fallopian Tube Etiology

Functional ovarian cyst
  Corpus luteum cyst
  Follicular cyst
  Theca lutein cyst
	Non-neoplastic Fallopian tube
	  conditions

	Ectopic pregnancy
	  Tubo-ovarian abscess/PID
	  Hydrosalpinx
	  Paraovarian or paratubal cyst

Endometrioma	
Polycystic ovaries	Malignant Fallopian tube neoplasms
	Uterine Etiology

Benign ovarian neoplasm
  Germ cell
    Mature cystic teratoma
  Epithelial
    Serous cystadenoma
    Mucinous cystadenoma
  Stromal
    Adenofibroma
    Fibroma
    Thecoma
	Benign conditions
	  Pedunculated leiomyoma
	  Uterine anomalies
	  Undiagnosed pregnancy
	
	Malignant neoplasms
	  Endometrial carcinoma
	  Uterine sarcoma

	Nongynecologic Etiology

Malignant ovarian neoplasm
  Germ cell
    Dysgerminoma
    Immature teratoma
    Endodermal sinus (yolk sac)
    Embryonal
    Choriocarcinoma
	Diseases of appendix or colon
	
	Diseases of bladder
	
	Vascular anomalies
	
	Bony deformation

Epithelial
  Invasive
    Papillary serous
    Endometrioid
    Mucinous
    Clear cell
    Transitional cell
  Low malignant potential
    Serous
    Mucinous	

Stromal
  Sertoli-Leydig
  Granulosa cell, adult	

Granulosa cell, juvenile	

morphology and β-hCG is not elevated. Follow-up examination with ultrasound after 4-6 weeks will generally demonstrate resolution without treatment. About 85% of functional cysts smaller than 6 cm regress, but larger masses may be more likely to persist. Feedback inhibition on pituitary gonadotropin production by hormonal suppression with oral contraceptives may prevent development of additional functional cysts and are advocated by some clinicians to assist in the regression of existing cysts. Hormonal suppression is by no means required, however, since the majority of functional cysts will regress without intervention.

The majority of functional cysts remain asymptomatic, but they will occasionally rupture or undergo torsion resulting in acute colicky abdominal or flank pain. Torsion requires prompt surgical intervention, usually with laparoscopy, in order to restore the vascular supply to the ovary by untwisting the pedicle before significant ischemia or necrosis of the ovary can occur. If the functional cyst ruptures pain of varying levels may occur. In rare cases, bleeding from the ovary leads to hemodynamic instability requiring surgery. Hospitalization for observation for 24 hours, allowing serial examinations and blood counts is appropriate for patients with symptomatic cyst rupture.

Persistent Adnexal Masses

Adnexal masses that persist are likely to be neoplasms. Benign masses can generally be removed effectively by the general gynecologic surgeon, while malignancies are more effectively treated by gynecologic oncologists with expertise for surgical staging, debulking, and administration of adjuvant therapies to optimize outcome. Triage of adnexal masses provides the best opportunity to serve the patient's interest by having the correct surgical team involved in care of the patient.

The most useful test for assessment of the newly diagnosed adnexal mass is transvaginal ultrasound. Ultrasound is particularly well suited for delineation of the morphologic features of adnexal masses. Medical literature abounds with description of morphology that correlates with benign and malignant neoplasms of the ovary. Figure 39–7 illustrates the morphologic features used to distinguish possible cancers from likely benign lesions. The reported sensitivity for identifying a malignant ovarian neoplasm is 90%-94%, but specificity is only about 60%. Specificity can be improved to about 85% without reducing sensitivity by evaluating Doppler waveforms in the tumor vessels. Vessels arising in malignant lesions have lower resistance to flow than in normal tissues: the ratio of diastolic to systolic flow is therefore higher than in normal tissue (Figure 39–8) and this can be quantitated by reporting the pulsatility index. This test is more specialized, costly and time consuming, limiting its effective use to selected lesions. MRI appears to have a promising role in the characterization of adnexal masses, but is much more costly than ultrasonography.

In addition to ultrasound, tumor markers can be very useful for triage of the palpable adnexal mass. The ideal tumor marker is elevated only in the presence of cancer and should correlate with the burden of disease. In reality, no marker is perfect. There are identified markers for ovarian malignancies arising from germ cell, epithelial and stromal origin. Optimal use of tumor markers involves ordering markers most likely to be clinically useful based on clinical presentation rather than to order all of them. Commonly used tumor markers are listed in Table 39–9. Many new markers will likely be validated in the next few years, including panels of multiple markers using gene chip technology. For example, malignant germ cell neoplasms usually arise in women younger than 35, are almost always unilateral, and typically demonstrate solid morphology on ultrasound evaluation. In this setting, it would be appropriate to order tumor markers including alpha fetoprotein (AFP), β-hCG, and lactate dehydrogenase (LDH). Epithelial tumors are more often complex cystic and solid, bilateral lesions. In this circumstance CA-125, CA-19-9 and CEA are better markers. Interpretation of CA-125 is difficult in premenopausal women because benign diseases such as endometriosis, which is much more common than ovarian cancer, will cause false positive test results. In addition, many tumor markers are normally elevated in pregnancy, thereby complicating evaluation of masses diagnosed during pregnancy.

The American College of Obstetricians and Gynecologists has issued a committee opinion regarding triage of adnexal masses that recommends referral of individuals with high-risk characteristics to gynecologic oncology subspecialists. For postmenopausal women, referral is warranted for patients with a pelvic mass and at least one of the following: CA-125 above 35 U/mL, ascites, nodular or fixed mass, evidence of abdominal or distant metastasis, or family history of one or more first-degree relatives with ovarian or breast cancer. In premenopausal women, the recommendations are identical except the threshold for CA-125 is raised to > 200 U/mL, to account for diseases such as endometriosis in this age group. Motivation for referral is based upon data showing higher staging accuracy and improved outcome when subspecialists treat ovarian cancer patients.

Low-risk masses thought to be functional cysts are managed expectantly. A mass that persists, or demonstrates worrisome features on exam, imaging studies or tumor marker measurement should be resected. A basic principle of surgical resection for ovarian neoplasms is not to allow spill or rupture of cyst contents into the abdomen. It is never appropriate to needle aspirate an ovarian mass that may harbor malignancy because of the potential to spread disease intra-abdominally. The surgical procedure to be performed is either oophorectomy or ovarian cystectomy for high-risk and low-risk lesions, respectively. The route of surgical approach may be either with laparoscopy or laparotomy. The laparoscopic approach is better suited for cystic masses that are small enough to be placed in a specimen retrieval bag without spill or rupture. Large or solid masses or evidence of metastatic disease such as ascites or omental caking require laparotomy for removal. Ovarian conservation is chosen after a balanced assessment of relative risk for cardiac disease versus ovarian cancer. In women with benign appearing masses under 60, they can expect some cardioprotective benefit even after menopause.

A simple cystic mass of less than 5 cm with normal CA-125 is considered low risk, even in the postmenopausal woman. Conservative management is reasonable.

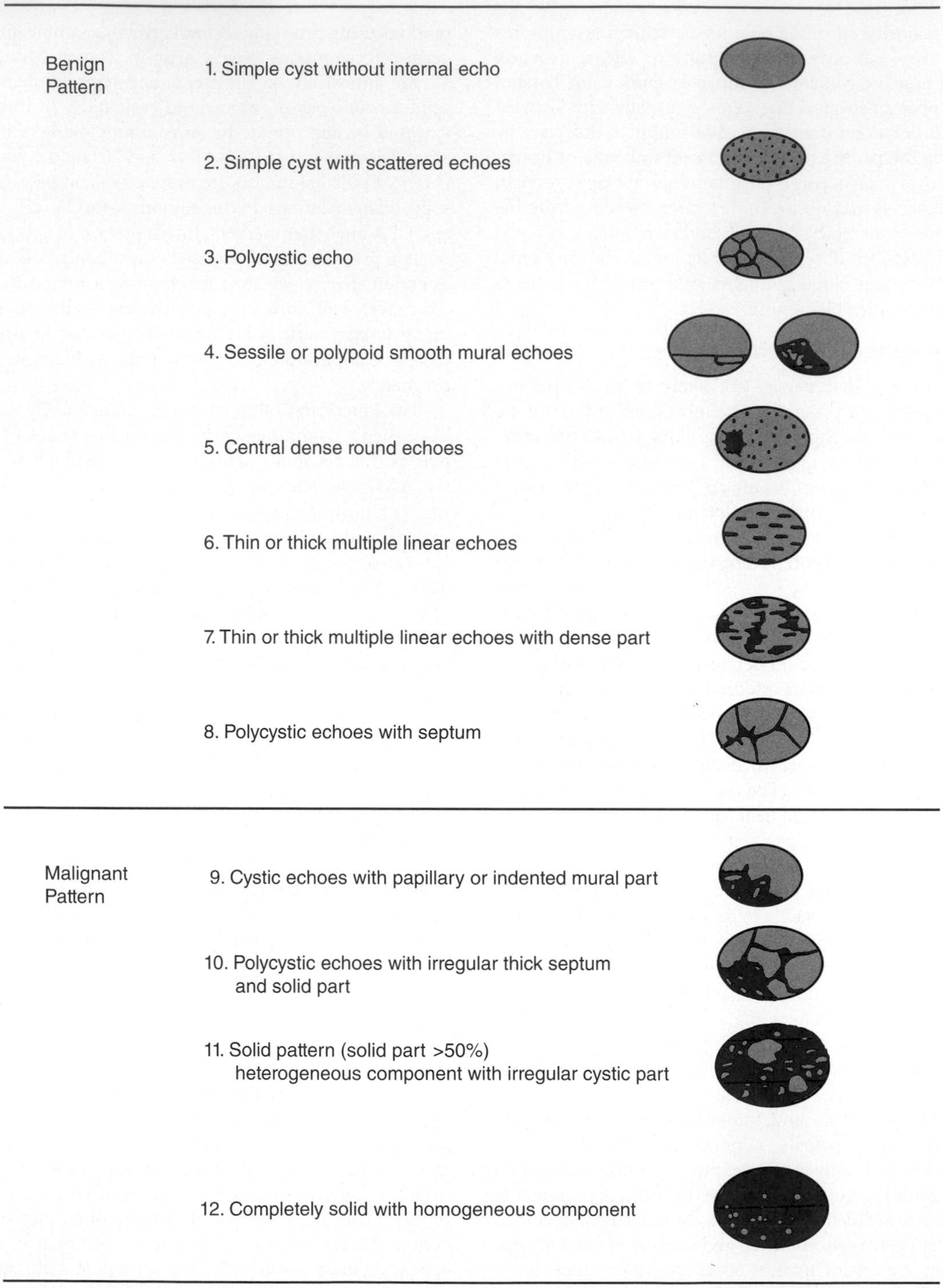

Benign Pattern

1. Simple cyst without internal echo

2. Simple cyst with scattered echoes

3. Polycystic echo

4. Sessile or polypoid smooth mural echoes

5. Central dense round echoes

6. Thin or thick multiple linear echoes

7. Thin or thick multiple linear echoes with dense part

8. Polycystic echoes with septum

Malignant Pattern

9. Cystic echoes with papillary or indented mural part

10. Polycystic echoes with irregular thick septum and solid part

11. Solid pattern (solid part >50%) heterogeneous component with irregular cystic part

12. Completely solid with homogeneous component

▲ **Figure 39–7.** Differential diagnosis of adnexal masses by ultrasound morphology. (From Kawai M et al: Transvaginal Doppler ultrasound with color flow imaging in the diagnosis of ovarian cancer. Obstet Gynecol 1992;79:163.)

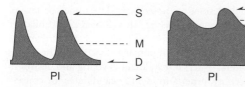

▲ **Figure 39–8.** Doppler waveform and pulsatility index (PI) indicating the objective differences between perfusion in normal versus malignant tissue. If the ratio of 1/PI is greater 0.8, the likelihood of cancer is 96% (*p* < 0.01). The waveform on the right has high diastolic flow, and the pulsatility index is low, consistent with a cancer diagnosis. PI = (peak systolic flow − peak diastolic flow)/mean flow. (From Kawai M et al: Transvaginal Doppler ultrasound with color flow imaging in the diagnosis of ovarian cancer. *Obstet Gynecol* 1992;79:163.)

SURGERY FOR MALIGNANT OVARIAN DISEASE

Ovarian cancer is stratified into three histological groups based on the cellular origin of the tumor. Epithelial tumors, germ cell tumors, and sex cord-stromal tumors comprise the primary lesions, and the fourth category is from disease arising elsewhere that metastasizes to ovary. Epithelial carcinoma accounts for about 85% of ovarian cancers, and about 5% arise from each of the remaining categories of germ cell, sex-cord stromal and metastatic disease from other sites. The peak incidence of epithelial ovarian cancer is in the fifth and sixth decades of life, while malignant germ cell tumors are more likely to occur under the age of 30. Stromal tumors have a bimodal distribution with peaks around ages 25 and 55 years of age. Malignant ovarian disease spreads by primary extension in the peritoneal cavity, in addition to lymphatic and hematogenous spread.

Epithelial ovarian cancer etiology can be either sporadic or hereditary. The sporadic cases appear to be strongly related to number of lifetime ovulations or chronicity of gonadotropin stimulation. There are also data to suggest environmental impact with the observation that tubal ligation results in reduction of risk, and diets with high lipids relative to omega-3 fatty acids increase risk. About 10% of ovarian cancers are hereditary. Three pedigrees account for most hereditary cases, including ovary-site specific, breast-ovary, and hereditary nonpolyposis colorectal cancer (HNPCC). Genetic inheritance of a mutation in the *BRCA1* or *BRCA2* gene imparts up to a 40% or a 25% lifetime risk of developing ovarian cancer, respectively. Ethnic groups including Ashkenazi Jews and Icelandic peoples have increased incidence of founder mutations that increase risk. Other reproductive factors associated with an increased risk include infertility, including use of ovulation induction agents. A recent discovery is that many if not the majority of epithelial cancers may arise in the fallopian tubes and subsequently spread to the ovaries.

Epithelial tumors are divided into invasive and low malignant potential (borderline) types. The invasive type accounts for 80% of epithelial cancer and is usually detected in advanced stages. The low malignant tumors occur in women with an average age 10-15 years younger than for invasive disease and up to 80% are stage I at diagnosis. Destructive stromal invasion is absent in low malignant potential tumors, but they are considered to be malignant and have the potential to metastasize. Epithelial tumors are subcategorized by histology as serous, mucinous, endometrioid, clear cell, transitional cell, or undifferentiated types. Serous tumors are the most common, comprising about 50% of epithelial carcinomas. Endometrioid carcinomas are the second most frequent variety, accounting for 24% of ovarian cancers, and are sometimes associated with endometriosis. Clear cell tumors, accounting for less than 5% of epithelial tumors, are also associated with endometriosis and have a more virulent natural history. Mucinous tumors account for 15% of epithelial cancers, and may become very large. Epithelial ovarian cancer is commonly involves both ovaries.

Germ cell cancer types include dysgerminomas, immature teratoma, endodermal sinus tumor, mixed types, and rare nongestational choriocarcinoma. Germ cell cancers are almost always unilateral and are commonly detected while stage I. Germ cell cancers are three time more common in women of Asian or African descent. A separate entity is adult-type cancer arising in an otherwise benign mature cystic teratoma. This can occur in up to 1% of mature cystic teratomas and is most commonly a squamous carcinoma.

The most common sex-cord stromal tumors include Sertoli-Leydig, adult granulosa, and juvenile granulosa cell tumors. These are frequently hormonally active tumors. Sertoli-Leydig cell tumors occur most often in the third

Table 39–9. Tumor markers for ovarian cancer.

Tumor Histology	Commonly Used Serum Markers
Epithelial Tumors	CA-125, CA-19-9, CEA, HE-4, OVA1
Papillary serous	CA-125
Endometrioid	CA-125, HE-4
Mucinous	CA-19-9, CEA
Germ Cell Tumors	AFP, β-hCG, lactate dehydrogenase (LDH)
Dysgerminoma	LDH
Endodermal sinus	AFP
Immature teratoma	None
Mixed type	AFP, β-hCG, lactate dehydrogenase (LDH)
Choriocarcinoma	β-HCG
Sex-Cord Stromal Tumors	Testosterone, estradiol, inhibin A and B
Sertoli-Leydig	Testosterone
Granulosa cell	Estradiol, inhibin A and B

decade, and arise from Wolffian duct remnants. They are rare and usually produce testosterone, resulting in manifest defeminization (amenorrhea, atrophy of the breast) and virilization (deepening of the voice, hirsutism, clitoral hypertrophy). Adult granulosa cell tumors arise in the sixth decade and are estrogen-producing tumors in most instances. Because of the estrogen production, postmenopausal bleeding is common, and endometrial cancer may arise in up to 15%. Juvenile granulosa cell tumors are similar, but arise in younger patients. Like germ cell tumors, the sex-cord stromal tumors are unilateral in most cases and detection is typically at early stages.

Metastatic carcinoma from other primary sites occurs not infrequently. Common sites include the gastrointestinal tract (Krukenberg tumor), breast, pancreas, lymphoma, and kidney. These tumors are classically solid, and bilateral. Prognosis for these tumors is especially poor.

▶ Clinical Findings

Almost 90% of stage I patients have symptoms and only 5% are asymptomatic. The symptoms usually include gastrointestinal complaints that persist for an average of 12 days per month for 3 months. Less often, pelvic pain or metrorrhagia may be present. On examination, any mass should prompt further evaluation. An ovarian mass should be regarded as potentially malignant until proven otherwise. Smooth, mobile masses on exam indicate low risk and solid, irregular, or fixed pelvic masses are suggestive malignancy. Triage of the pelvic mass should include transvaginal pelvic ultrasound and selective tumor markers as described previously in the adnexal mass section of this chapter. It should be noted that CA-125 may be negative in half of early-stage ovarian cancers. If an ovarian malignancy is suspected preoperatively, referral to a gynecologic oncologist is recommended.

Occasionally, ovarian cancer is discovered during an operation for different indication or when triage has not been properly performed. If ascites, carcinomatosis, or papillary excrescences are noted, the tumor should be removed intact and submitted for frozen section. If cancer is diagnosed, a gynecologic or surgical oncologist should be consulted for surgical staging and debulking.

▶ Treatment

Ovarian cancer is staged surgically (Table 39–10). When a complex adnexal mass is to be removed the procedure should begin with obtaining washings for cytology, and the mass should subsequently be removed intact. Upon removal of the mass, a frozen section should be obtained for definitive diagnosis. If an ovarian malignancy is confirmed, complete staging requires assessment and biopsy of the pelvic and para-aortic nodes, omentum, and peritoneum. All peritoneal surfaces are inspected and any suspicious lesions are biopsied.

If no suspicious lesions are noted, a predetermined pattern of biopsies is taken from the pelvic sidewalls, cul de sac, bladder peritoneum, pericolic gutters and both hemidiaphragms. A decision must be made about possible resection of the uterus and contralateral ovary. If the patient is young and desires to retain her fertility, criteria to identify candidates for conservation of fertility should be applied. Factors that favor preservation of fertility include germ cell and sex-cord stromal tumors because they are usually unilateral, and subsequent chemotherapy, if needed, has curative potential. Low malignant potential tumors affecting one ovary or in select cases where extra-ovarian disease can be completely resected are also candidates. Patients with invasive epithelial tumors are poor candidates for conservative surgery because of the high likelihood of bilateral involvement and the primarily palliative role of chemotherapy for all but early stages of disease. If preservation of fertility is not appropriate, then hysterectomy and removal of the contralateral tube and ovary is completed.

When the disease spread into the pelvis or abdomen is documented, debulking of all resectable macroscopic disease is critically important. Numerous randomized clinical trials have demonstrated the concept of debulking and consistently show survival advantage for patients with maximal cytoreduction. Intraoperative decision making for debulking focuses effort on the biggest tumor, wherever it may be. If the largest lesion can be resected, attention is directed to the next largest lesion. This process continues until either all measurable disease is removed or a lesion that is unresectable is encountered. In order to resect the disease at each decision point of this algorithm, the surgeon may need to perform intestinal resection, splenectomy, modified posterior exenteration, culdotomy, diaphragm resection, and other upper abdominal procedures. In two prospective Gynecologic Oncology Group clinical trials survival for microscopically debulked ovarian cancer was 65% at 4 years, and fell to about 35% if less than 1 cm of macroscopic residual disease remained after surgery. If greater than 2 cm of residual disease remained, the 4-year survival was only 20%. Optimal debulking can be attained in up to 70% of patients who are operated on by subspecialists trained in ovarian cancer surgery.

Patients with stage IA grade 1 or grade 2 epithelial tumors have a very good prognosis and usually are not treated with additional chemotherapy. For more advanced stages of epithelial cancer, chemotherapy is very effective for inducing clinical remission but relapses are very common with an average progression interval between 2 and 3 years. The best chemotherapy combination for treating advanced stage epithelial cancer includes both taxane and platinum agents, administered either intravenously or intraperitoneally for at least six cycles. Intraperitoneal chemotherapy has been demonstrated to induce longer progression free intervals, but acute toxicity is much higher and only 40% of patients are able to complete planned therapy on this regimen. The

Table 39–10. FIGO staging for ovarian cancer.

FIGO Staging	Description	TNM Class
Stage I	Tumor limited to the ovaries	T1
IA	Limited to one ovary, no tumor on external surface, capsule intact; negative peritoneal cytology	T1a
IB	Limited to both ovaries, no tumor on external surface, capsule intact; negative peritoneal cytology	T1b
IC	IA or IB tumor, but with surface tumor, ruptured capsule, or positive ascites or peritoneal cytology	T1c
Stage II	Tumor extending to the pelvis	T2
IIA	Metastasis to the uterus or tubes	T2
IIB	Metastasis to other pelvic tissues	T2b
IIC	IIA or IIB tumor, both with surface tumor, ruptured capsule, or positive ascites or peritoneal cytology	T2c
Stage III	Tumor extending outside the pelvis and/or retroperitoneal or inguinal nodes. Extension to small bowel, omentum, or superficial liver	T3 and/or N1
IIIA	Histologically confirmed microscopic disease of abdominal peritoneal surfaces; lymph nodes negative	T3a
IIIB	Implants of abdominal or peritoneal surfaces not exceeding 2 cm in diameter; lymph nodes negative	T3b
IIIC	Implants of abdominal or peritoneal surfaces > 2 cm in diameter, or positive retroperitoneal or inguinal lymph nodes	T3c and/or N1
Stage IV	Distant metastasis beyond the peritoneal cavity	M1

Reproduced, with permission, from Benedet JL, Hacker NF, Ngan HYS, eds: FIGO staging classifications and clinical practice guidelines in the management of gynecologic cancers. FIGO Committee on Gynecologic Oncology. *Int J Gynaecol Obstet*. 2000 Aug;70(2):209–262.

CA-125 tumor marker is useful as a marker for assessing the effectiveness of therapy.

The best current regimen for malignant germ cell tumors is cisplatin, etoposide, and bleomycin, administered as a 3- or a 5-day treatment that is continued until at least one cycle after normalization of elevated tumor markers. Sex-cord stromal tumors are treated similarly.

Prognosis

The prognosis for epithelial ovarian carcinoma is related primarily to stage and histological grade. Because most ovarian

cancers are of advanced stage at the time of initial diagnosis, the long-term survival rate for ovarian cancer is only 50%. Five-year survival rates for patients with stage III or stage IV disease are around 20%-35%. Prolonged disease-free intervals can be achieved by combining comprehensive surgical staging aggressive debulking and adjuvant chemotherapy.

▶ Prevention

Oral contraceptives reduce the risk of ovarian epithelial carcinoma. The magnitude of risk reduction is based on dose and duration of therapy. The protective effects are durable, lasting for a decade or more after discontinuation of the medication.

Any woman with a strong family history should be considered for genetic counseling and testing. For patients with a confirmed hereditary risk of ovarian cancer based on careful pedigree analysis or genetic testing will benefit from prophylactic removal of ovaries and Fallopian tubes. The current recommendation is for removal after completion of childbearing at age 35 or 10 years younger than the earliest incidence of disease in the family. Prophylactic removal of ovaries and tubes reduces the risk of ovarian cancer at least 95%, but a small number of individuals may still develop primary peritoneal carcinoma.

To date, no screening test for ovarian cancer has proven to be sufficiently sensitive or specific enough to have earned the recommendation of the US Preventive Services Task Force, ACOG, or the American Cancer Society. Prospective ultrasound screening studies and combined CA-125/ultrasound studies show a trend toward earlier stage at time of diagnosis on screened patients, resulting in prolongation of progression-free intervals, but not survival.

Kurman RJ, Chih l-M: The origin and pathogenesis of ovarian cancer- a proposed unifying theory. *Am J Surg Pathol* 2010;34(3):433-443.
Vaughn S, Coward JI, Bast RC, et al: Rethinking ovarian cancer: Recommendations for improving outcomes. *Nat Rev Cancer* 2012;11(10):719-725.

SURGERY FOR MULTIORGAN DISEASE

Chronic Pelvic Pain

Chronic pelvic pain is generally defined as 6-12 months of pain below the umbilicus producing a significant impact on quality of life. Evaluation and treatment of chronic pelvic pain accounts for up to 40% of all referrals to gynecologists, leading to up to 40% of all laparoscopies, and 12% of all hysterectomies.

▶ Diagnosis

The differential diagnosis chronic pelvic pain is complex. While many patients attribute their pain to a gynecologic cause, the physician must consider nongynecologic diagnoses of the gastrointestinal, urinary, and musculoskeletal systems in addition to psychological and psychosomatic problems. The most common nongynecologic diagnoses include irritable bowel syndrome, inflammatory bowel disease, nephrolithiasis, interstitial cystitis, ventral or inguinal hernia, muscle strain, nerve injury, depression, and somatization. Of note, patients are more likely to have suffered sexual assault as an adult or child.

The gynecologic causes of chronic pelvic pain are classified as cyclic or continuous in nature. Sources of cyclic pain include primary dysmenorrhea, defined as painful menses without identifiable pelvic pathology; and secondary dysmenorrhea attributable to pathologic conditions such as endometriosis or adenomyosis. Mid-cycle ovulatory pain may occur that produces unilateral pain at mid-cycle that resolves after a day or two. Continuous pain sources include endometriosis and adenomyosis, and pelvic organ prolapse, both discussed earlier in this chapter, in addition to chronic salpingitis, and pelvic adhesions. Another cause of continuous pain is ovarian remnant syndrome, which occurs when residual ovarian tissue after oophorectomy becomes retroperitoneal location. Pain may occasionally be caused by degenerating fibroids or by mass effect from large fibroids.

Clinical Findings

The pelvic examination requires careful communication with the patient to understand where and when her pain occurs. Identification of palpable abnormalities and localization of focal tenderness is important. If a pelvic mass is detected, it should be triaged as discussed previously in the adnexal mass section of this chapter. An abnormal pelvic examination has about an 80% predictive value for pelvic abnormalities noted at laparoscopy.

Treatment

Nongynecologic causes of pain are treated according to the diagnosis. Gynecologic pain etiology is also treated according to the diagnosis. Reproductive-age women with cyclic pain are offered treatment consisting of nonsteroidal anti-inflammatory drugs and ovulation suppression, usually with oral contraceptives if appropriate for the age and medical risk factors of the patient. Continuous pain attributable to endometriosis or adenomyosis is treated similarly. Other causes of continuous pain include spasm or tension in pelvic floor musculature. Physical therapy and "reverse Kegel" exercises to relax the muscles often result in improvement. An antibiotic may be prescribed if a chronic infection is suspected, but care should be taken to treat documented infection and not to over prescribe antibiotics. Concurrent depression is common, usually arising as a secondary effect of the pain rather than as the primary etiology. Treatment with antidepressant medication is often beneficial. The tricyclic antidepressant class is often more effective that serotonin reuptake inhibitors for this indication. Severe and refractory pain may require prescribing of narcotics to attain control. The physician must use careful judgment regarding initiation of narcotics in a chronic setting due to the potential for dependence and addiction. It is often useful to manage these patients with a narcotic contract between the patient and her physician to regulate drug use. Referral to a multidisciplinary pain service is often useful for difficult or refractory cases.

If the pain is refractory to medical management or if the physical examination is abnormal, then diagnostic laparoscopy is indicated. During the laparoscopic procedure, upper abdominal structures, pelvic organs and peritoneum, appendix, rectum, and sigmoid colon are carefully inspected. The most commonly identified pathology is endometriosis occurring in one-third of patients and adhesions in one third of cases. Most of the remaining cases will have no identified pathology. The presence of abnormalities may not explain the pain, and treatment of disease such as endometriosis may not resolve the pain.

The evidence for therapeutic benefit of laparoscopy for treatment of pelvic pain is tenuous, at best. Procedures that remove or ablate adhesions, endometriosis may or may not relieve pain. If pain is attributed to the uterus or cervix and cannot be controlled with lesser procedures or medical management, options include hysterectomy, or if fertility preservation is desired, interruption of the autonomic nerve tracts with a presacral neurectomy. Pain attributed to degenerating or large fibroids may be relieved either with uterine artery embolization procedures or surgical removal of the leiomyomata with either hysterectomy or myomectomy. Severe dysmenorrhea that is refractory to medical management may be significantly improved with endometrial ablation.

Published data indicate that laparoscopic treatment will produce a short-term reduction of pain in about 60%-80% of patients, but long-term benefits are not well documented. In patients who have completed their childbearing or who wish definitive treatment, hysterectomy has reported success rates of up to 95% if uterine pathology such as degenerating fibroids is present. If no pelvic pathology is noted, 50%-91% experience improvement. The success rate is poor if the patient has symptoms of depression. Patients with endometriosis should also be offered bilateral salpingo-oophorectomy to minimize pain from residual implants.

Endometriosis

Endometriosis is defined as extrauterine, functional endometrial tissue. The most common sites include ovaries, uterosacral ligaments, and the cul-de-sac. Less commonly, Fallopian tubes, uterine serosa, sigmoid colon and rectum, peritoneum, and small intestine or mesentery are involved. Ectopic endometrium is occasionally detected at distant sites including lung, lymph nodes, surgical incision sites, umbilicus, perineum, and breasts.

The etiology of endometriosis is thought to occur any of three potential mechanisms: (1) retrograde menstruation with implantation; (2) metaplasia of Müllerian duct remnants or coelomic epithelium; and (3) lymphatic or venous dissemination. Retrograde menstruation through the uterine tubes is common and yet rarely causes endometriosis. It is not known what factors contribute to implantation and growth of endometriosis. Uterine outflow obstruction from cervical stenosis or congenital anomalies such as imperforate hymen increases the likelihood of developing endometriosis.

Endometriosis may develop at any time after onset of menarche and will virtually regress after menopause. Prevalence of endometriosis is difficult to determine because many women with the disease are asymptomatic. The estimated prevalence of endometriosis is about 15%-20%. Endometriosis may cause scarring that impairs fertility. As a consequence, diagnosis of endometriosis during a workup for infertility is higher, with up to 20%-47% of patients affected. Conversely, in women with proven fertility who elect tubal sterilization are found to have endometriosis on only 1%-5% of cases. The incidence of endometriosis is higher in women who choose to delay childbearing, or in women with a family history of the disease. There may be environmental toxins that predispose to endometriosis, such as dioxin. Pregnancy and hormonal contraceptive hormones are protective.

Carcinoma may arise in endometriosis at any site and is most commonly of endometrioid histology. Clear cell carcinoma is rare and more aggressive.

▶ Classification

An anatomic staging system for endometriosis has been developed by the American Society of Reproductive Medicine (Figure 39–9.) The Revised AFS classification system is accepted worldwide. The staging system is broadly predictive of outcome with treatment. The stage of endometriosis does not correlate well with pain symptoms. Alternate systems that recognize the varied presentation of endometriosis in addition to development of serum markers have been proposed.

▶ Symptoms & Signs

Endometriosis frequently causes pain. The pain often begins shortly before menses and continues during menstruation. The presence of pain and its severity is highly variable. Some patients with extensive disease are asymptomatic, while others with small peritoneal implants may be incapacitated. Unexplained infertility may be present in asymptomatic

endometriosis. Symptoms may occur at any time during reproductive years, but are most common in the third and fourth decades of life. Symptoms usually resolve with menopause unless the patient is prescribed a hormone replacement regimen. Patients may also complain of dyspareunia, tenesmus, back pain, or sciatica. Rare manifestations may include ureteral obstruction or bowel obstruction.

▶ Pelvic Examination

Bimanual pelvic examination including the rectovaginal examination should be performed. Common findings include pelvic tenderness, adnexal masses, and soft nodularity in the cul de sac or along the uterosacral ligaments. Adnexal masses attributable to endometriosis are often bilateral and are frequently immobile due to adhesions along the posterior broad ligament.

▶ Testing

Ultrasound description of isoechoic masses within the ovaries is highly suggestive of endometrioma. Serum concentrations of CA-125 are elevated above 35 U/mL in about one-third of patients with advanced disease, which complicates triage of adnexal masses that may be either benign (endometriosis) or malignant. Following surgical and medical treatment, measurement of the CA-125 trend is a useful marker of treatment efficacy and disease recurrence similar to how the marker is used for monitoring treatment of ovarian cancer.

Definitive diagnosis requires biopsy, usually obtained with a laparoscopic procedure. The biopsy diagnosis requires the presence of both glands and stroma. Location and extent of disease is noted at the time of surgery to complete disease staging. Characteristic peritoneal implants include the so called "powder-burn" marks of darkly colored endometrium, in addition to red, blue, and white lesions. Peritoneal disease may be flat or raised, including nodular or vesicular appearance. Laparotomy is occasionally necessary for large ovarian masses, or bowel and ureteral obstructions that may be present.

▶ Treatment

Treatment should be tailored to severity of symptoms, age of the patient, desire for fertility, and the stage of disease. The range of therapeutic options includes observation, medical management with hormones and analgesics, up to hysterectomy with bilateral salpingo-oophorectomy. A conservative approach is preferred for patients with minimal symptoms or minimal measurable disease on pelvic exam. Surveillance examinations should be regularly performed, with the interval determined by severity of symptoms, age of the patient, desire for fertility, and the stage of disease. If symptoms or physical finding worsen, the management plan may be changed accordingly.

American Society for Reproductive Medicine
Revised Classification of Endometriosis

Patient's Name _____ Date _____

Stage I   (Minimal) - 1-5
Stage II (Mild)   - 6-15
Stage III (Moderate) - 16-40
Stage IV (Severe) - >40
Total _____

Laparoscopy _____ Laparotomy _____ Photography _____
Recommended Treatment _____
_____

Prognosis _____

PERITONEUM	ENDOMETRIOSIS	<1cm	1-3cm	>3cm
	Superficial	1	2	4
	Deep	2	4	6
OVARY	R Superficial	1	2	4
	Deep	4	16	20
	L Superficial	1	2	4
	Deep	4	16	20

POSTERIOR CUL-DE-SAC OBLITERATION	Partial	Complete
	4	40

	ADHESIONS	<1/3 Enclosure	1/3-2/3 Enclosure	>2/3 Enclosure
OVARY	R Filmy	1	2	4
	Dense	4	8	16
	L Filmy	1	2	4
	Dense	4	8	16
TUBE	R Filmy	1	2	4
	Dense	4*	8*	16
	L Filmy	1	2	4
	Dense	4*	8*	16

*If the fimbriated end of the fallopian tube is completely enclosed, change the point assignment to 16.
Denote appearance of superficial implant types as red [(R), red, red-pink, flamelike, vesicular blobs, clear vesicles], white [(W), opacifications, peritoneal defects, yellow-brown], or black [(B) black, hemosiderin deposits, blue]. Denote percent of total described as R ___%, W ___% and B ___%. Total should equal 100%

Additional Endometriosis:_____
_____
_____

Associated Pathology: _____
_____
_____

To be used with normal tubes and ovaries
L   R

To be used with abnormal tubes and/or ovaries
L   R

Vol. 67, No. 5, May 1997   **American Society for Reproductive Medicine** *Revised ASRM classification: 1996*   819

▲ **Figure 39–9.** Staging of endometriosis. (American Society for Reproductive Medicine: Revised American Society for Reproductive Medicine classification of endometriosis. *Fertil Steril* 1997;67:817.)

Medical Treatment

The goal of medical therapy is to control disease by inducing a remission. There are no known medical therapies that result in a cure. Hormonal therapy is not administered for patients actively attempting to conceive. Upon treatment discontinuation, symptoms commonly recur. Long-term suppression with hormonal contraceptive regimens should be considered.

Progestins

Norethynodrel, norethindrone acetate, and medroxyprogesterone acetate are commonly used. Continuous progestins induce amenorrhea resulting in decreased symptoms in more than three quarters of patients. Progestin therapy causes downregulation of estrogen receptors in endometrial tissue, resulting in atrophic change in both endometriosis and endometrium. Breakthrough bleeding is not unusual. Side effects include weight gain secondary to appetite stimulation, fluid retention, headaches, and mood swings.

Oral contraceptives

Oral contraceptives with a low estrogen dose and a high potency progestin are preferred and may be administered either as cyclic or as continuous regimens without withdrawal intervals each month. Symptoms are relieved in up to 80% of patients. Oral contraceptive may be continued long term as a maintenance therapy in healthy women. Women over 35 who smoke or individuals with hypertension are at increased risk of thromboembolic complications. Side effects include headaches, fluid retention, breast tenderness, breakthrough bleeding, and occasional nausea.

GnRH analogs

GnRH analogs act by negative feedback inhibition on the pituitary resulting in prevention of FSH and LH secretion. The consequence of low gonadotropin levels is absence of follicle development and low estrogen production. This treatment strategy induces the medical equivalent of the postmenopausal state. Endometrial implants atrophy in the hypoestrogenic environment and about 80% of patients report clinical improvement. Side effects mimic menopause with vasomotor symptoms, vaginal dryness, and mood swings. Long-term treatment causes osteopenia and osteoporosis. To prevent bone loss, "add-back" therapy with either norethindrone acetate or combined hormone replacement therapy concurrent with GnRH analog may be prescribed and does not interfere with treatment of the endometriosis.

Surgical Treatment

Indications for surgery include treatment of current infertility, treatment to preserve future fertility, or control of symptoms. Medical therapy is unlikely to result in reduction of symptoms for bulky disease, and surgery is recommended for any endometrioma larger than 4 cm. Options for preservation of fertility in symptomatic women who have failed medical therapy include laparoscopic procedures for resection or ablation of implants, lysis of adhesions, or presacral neurectomy. When definitive therapy is necessary and preservation of fertility is not an issue, total hysterectomy and bilateral salpingo-oophorectomy is indicated. Endometriosis is dependent upon estrogen. Preservation of an ovary in this setting causes symptoms sufficient to prompts additional surgery in 20% of cases. Bowel implants can be locally resected by appropriately trained surgeons.

Postoperative estrogen replacement therapy usually does not lead to exacerbation of endometriosis. The use of estrogen-progestin combinations is generally not required.

Giudice LC: Clinical practice: endometriosis. *N Engl J Med* 2010;362(25):2389-2398.

MULTIPLE CHOICE QUESTIONS

1. The differential diagnosis of a vulvar lesion includes all of the following, except

   A. Bartholin abscess
   B. Melanoma
   C. Hidradenitis suppurativa
   D. Luteal cyst
   E. Epithelial inclusion cyst

2. All of these are true about cervical cancer, except

   A. Most is related to high-risk HPV types
   B. About 75% are squamous type
   C. Screening for premalignant lesions is effective because of slow progression through dysplastic precursors
   D. Carcinoma occurs most frequently in women between the ages of 20 and 30 years
   E. Vaccination is targeted to both protect individuals and to limit prevalence of infection

3. Treatment of cervical carcinoma

   A. Usually includes hysterectomy for microinvasive disease
   B. Consists of radiation therapy and chemotherapy for advanced disease

C. Cannot preserve fertility in women with microinvasive disease

D. Includes systemic therapy only for distant metastases

E. Often requires radiation therapy for bone metastases

4. Uterine leiomyomata

A. Are present in 20%-30% of women of reproductive age

B. Are more common in white women than in blacks or Asians

C. Often appear after menopause if estrogen supplements are not used

D. Are usually monofocal, with a single tumor in the uterine wall

E. Can only be treated by hysterectomy

5. The differential diagnosis of adnexal masses includes

A. Endometrioma

B. Appendiceal mass

C. Pedunculated leiomyoma

D. A, B, and C

E. A and C only

Orthopedic Surgery

Kelly Vanderhave, MD

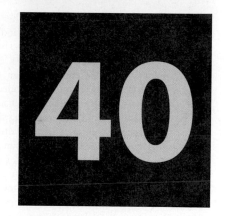

▼ INTRODUCTION

Improvements in implant design and materials have been responsible for significant advances in our ability to treat patients with complex orthopedic problems. Like all medical fields, orthopedic surgery has become a group of subspecialized fields in recent years.

TERMINOLOGY

Varus and **valgus** are descriptive terms frequently used for the characterization of angular musculoskeletal deformities. They refer to the direction of the apex of the deformity in relation to the midline of the body. When the apex points away from the midline, the deformity is termed varus; when the apex points toward the midline, the deformity is termed valgus. Knock-knees is an example of a valgus deformity, such that the apex is defined by the patient's knees pointing toward the body's midline. Conversely, "bow-legged" is an example of a varus deformity. These terms can also be applied to fractures such that the apex of the deformity is the fracture itself. **Comminution** describes a fracture that is significantly fragmented. A fracture is **displaced** when the main bony fragments are translated or separated from each other. Displacement can further be subcategorized into minimally, moderately, or completely displaced.

Open fractures define fractures with overlying wounds such that the fracture is exposed to the external environment. Open fractures can be obvious in significant trauma with substantial degloving of the soft-tissues, or they can be more subtle where only a small poke hole is visible with draining fracture hematoma. As a result, when patients are transferred from other hospitals or urgent care facilities, all splints should be removed, and the skin overlying all fractures must be carefully inspected for open injury. Open fractures are orthopedic emergencies and must be addressed with prompt surgical debridement and irrigation

to minimize the subsequent development of infection and associated fracture nonunions.

Joint dislocations also warrant immediate treatment. **Reduction** refers to the maneuver used to restore proper alignment of a joint or fracture. Vascular structures spanning the joint or fracture may be damaged at the time of injury. Alternatively, these structures may be compressed or kinked due to the resulting deformity. Arterial pulses should always be assessed distal to a musculoskeletal injury and carefully documented. Often absent pulses are restored with reduction of a joint or fracture. If reduction does not successfully return pulses, the vessels are likely torn; early repair and reconstruction is often required to restore distal circulation to the limb. Vascular injuries repaired prior to fracture or joint reduction and stabilization, may be in danger of subsequent failure due to bony instability. Orthopedists can quickly stabilize fractures and dislocations using external fixation, providing a stable scaffold on to which necessary vascular repairs can be made.

Joint or fracture reduction may be treated by **open** or **closed** techniques. A dislocation or fracture is described as **unstable** if there is a high likelihood of subsequent deformation after reduction is performed. Following reduction, unstable fractures or dislocations may be stabilized by closed or open means. Closed treatment may involve traction, casts, splints, or braces; open techniques involve surgical exposure of the fracture or joint and reduction followed by maintenance of the reduction with internal or external fixation devices. The surgical treatment of an unstable fracture or dislocation is therefore described as "Open reduction with internal or external fixation."

SPLINTING AND CASTING

Splinting and casting are noninvasive ways of stabilizing fractures and maintaining reductions. **Splints** are typically made of plaster and are not circumferential, while **casts** are circumferential and can be made of either plaster or fiberglass. Splints are best used for a short period of time (days up to one or two weeks) in acute scenarios shortly after injury or after an operation when swelling is a concern to avoid compartment syndrome. Casts are sturdier, used to maintain bones in appropriate alignment for extended periods of time (weeks to a few months). For example, a distal radius fracture may be reduced and placed in a sugar-tong splint with follow-up in clinic. At clinic follow-up, if the reduction is adequate and swelling has subsided, the splint can be overwrapped in a cast or transitioned to a new cast for continued closed treatment. After ankle fractures are surgically fixed with open reduction and internal fixation, they are often placed in a short-leg splint with stirrups postoperatively, followed by transitioning to short-leg cast for 4-6 weeks to protect the operative repair. There are many types of splints and casts depending on the type of injury being treated. Examples of splints include the volar forearm, sugar-tong, long-arm posterior, double sugar-tong, coaptation, short leg posterior with or without stirrups, and long-leg posterior. Splints can be augmented with a thumb spica or foot plate depending on the injury. Examples of casts include short-arm, long-arm, with or without thumb spica, as well as short-leg, long-leg, spicas.

ORTHOPEDIC HISTORY TAKING AND PHYSICAL EXAMINATION

Key elements of the history taking include the demographics of the patient (age, sex, and race), comorbidities, hand dominance (if there is an upper extremity injury), mechanism of injury, allergies to medication, and smoking or drinking history.

Examination begins with visualization of the injured extremity noting deformity, swelling, and or bruising. Careful skin examination is crucial to rule out wounds and the presence of open fracture. Neurovascular examination should be performed documenting motor and sensory function as well as strength of pulses (palpable, 1+, 2+, or identifiable by Doppler). Finally, careful secondary exam should be performed on all other joints and extremities testing for tenderness to palpation as well as range of motion. Distracting pain from the primary injury can often prevent a patient from realizing they have an injury elsewhere. Secondary examinations should be performed multiple times during the treatment course of the patient. As the pain from the primary injury subsides, patients may begin to appreciate additional injuries.

ORTHOPEDIC EMERGENCIES

The following is list of conditions that require immediate orthopedic evaluation and treatment: compartment syndrome, open fractures, septic arthritis, and acute dislocations. Additionally, there are other injuries such as femoral neck fractures, that depending on the age of the patient and choice of treatment that require intervention as soon as possible. Each of these conditions will be elaborated on in the upcoming chapters.

▶ Compartment Syndrome

Compartment syndrome is caused by increased pressure in a closed fascial space that initially leads to compromised perfusion followed by severe tissue damage. Nerves and muscles in the affected area can be significantly compromised in a matter of hours. Severe ischemia for 6-8 hours leads to muscle and nerve death leading to chronic debilitating dysfunction of the affected extremity. As a result, compartment syndrome is an orthopedic emergency requiring immediate evaluation and treatment. Compartment syndrome can occur after fracture, limb compression or crush, vigorous exercise, or burns.

Although, it most commonly occurs in the forearm and leg, it can occur in the foot, thigh, and arm. Compartment syndrome typically presents as a painful, swollen, tense extremity. Pain with passive range of motion of the digits and pain out of proportion are considered to be the most reliable early indicators of compartment syndrome. Clinical signs of compartment syndrome include the 5 Ps: pain, poikilothermia, pallor, paresthesias, and finally pulselessness. A change in pulses is a very late sign occurring after significant damage has already occurred. Of note, compartment syndrome can occur at intracompartmental pressures well below arterial pressure. Therefore, compartment syndrome can occur in a pink limb with normal pulses.

Compartment syndrome is a clinical diagnosis; many authors advocate that if compartment syndrome is suspected immediate fasciotomy should be carried out. In scenarios where patients are obtunded, intubated, or otherwise unable to express having pain, compartment pressure can be evaluated using a commercially available self-contained pressure monitor. If a commercial pressure monitor is not available, large bore catheter can be inserted in the compartment under sterile technique. The catheter is connected to a pressure monitor via intravenous tubing filled with sterile saline solution. Absolute pressure more than 30 mm Hg in any compartment, or a pressure within 30 mm Hg of the diastolic blood pressure in hypotensive patients are indications for surgical compartment release.

Fasciotomy should be carried out with complete release of the skin and fascia of the involved compartments. Adjacent compartments in the same limb are typically released as well. Compartment pressures are rechecked after release to ensure adequate decompression. The wounds are left open and covered with sterile dressings or a vacuum-assisted closure (VAC), and are subsequently treated with delayed primary closure or skin grafting days later.

▶ Open Fractures

An open fracture is a defined as an osseous disruption with a break in the overlying skin and soft tissues resulting in communication between the fracture, its hematoma, and the external environment. Any wound occurring on the same limb as a fracture must be carefully inspected to prove that it is not an open fracture. Open fractures have important soft tissue consequences: (1) contamination of the wound and fracture by the external environment, (2) crushing, stripping, and devascularization that results in soft tissue devitilization and subsequent increased infection susceptibility, (3) disruption of the soft tissue envelope may affect the type of fracture immobilization as well as adversely affect fracture healing due to the loss of osteoprogenitor cell contribution from overlying soft tissues, and finally (4) loss of function from damaged muscle, tendon, nerve, vascular, and ligamentous structures.

Open fractures are typically high energy injuries. One-third of patients with open fractures have multiple injuries. As a result, initial evaluation of the patient with an open fracture follows the ABCDEs: airway, breathing, circulation, disability, and exposure. Initial resuscitation is performed along with immediate treatment for any-potential life-threatening injuries. The head, chest, abdomen, pelvis, and spine are individually evaluated for injury. Injuries to the other extremities should be identified. Neurovascular exam for the injured limb should be carefully documented; the skin and soft tissues should be assessed as well. Wound hemorrhage should be managed with direct pressure rather than limb tourniquets or clamping which may disrupt perfusion to the rest of the limb. Exploration of the wound in the emergency department setting is not indicated if operative intervention is planned due to risk of further contamination and precipitation of additional hemorrhage. If surgical delay is anticipated, gentle irrigation with sterile normal saline may be undertaken. Only obvious foreign fragments that are easily accessible should be removed. Bone fragments should not be removed and disregarded, regardless of apparent nonviability. Sterile injection of joints can be performed to determine if there is communication with a nearby wound. The wound should be covered with a sterile normal saline soaked piece of gauze (iodine has fallen out of favor due to reports of tissue toxicity). Provisional reduction and splinting should be performed, follow by subsequent neurovascular examination to confirm no additional damage. Standard trauma survey includes radiographic evaluation of the spine, chest, abdomen, and pelvis. The injured extremity including the joint above and below, along with any other extremities suspected of injury should be evaluated with x-rays in anticipation of operative intervention.

Angiogram should be performed if vascular injury is suspected in the following scenarios: knee dislocation, cool, pale hand, or foot with poor distal capillary refill, high energy injury in an area of susceptible vessels (eg, Popliteal fossa), and documented ABI less than 0.9 in an extremity with an associated injury. Of note, evaluation of the contralateral limb may reveal underlying vascular disease as the cause of decreased ABI rather than acute injury.

Open fractures can be characterized using the Gustilo and Anderson classification: Grade I: clean skin opening is less than 1 cm, Grade II: Laceration is less than 1 cm but is less than 10 cm, soft tissue damage without significant fracture comminution or crush component; Grade IIIA: extensive soft tissue damage, Grade IIIB: extensive soft tissue injury with periosteal stripping or bone exposures requiring flap coverage, and Grade IIIC: concomitant vascular injury requiring repair.

Antibiotic treatment and tetanus prophylaxis should be addressed as soon as possible in the emergency department setting. Grade I and II fractures require treatment with a first-generation cephalosporin. Previously, grade III fractures mandated the addition of an aminoglycoside to cephalosporin; however, the most recent recommendations entail treatment with ceftriaxone. For farm injuries with gross contamination, add a penicillin in addition to ceftriaxone.

Operative intervention should be carried out for open fractures as soon as possible. Intervention less than 8 hours after injury has been reported to result in a lower incidence of infection and subsequent osteomyelitis. In the operating room, the wound should be extended proximally and distally to examine the zone of injury. Meticulous debridement of the soft tissues, including the skin, subcutaneous fat, and surrounding muscle should be carried out. Large skin flaps should be avoided as their development risks further devitilization. The fracture surfaces should be exposed and debrided. Fractures can be stabilized provisionally or definitively with external or internal fixation depending on the scenario and surgeon expertise. Pulsatile lavage irrigation should be carried out, followed by meticulous hemostasis. Fasciotomy should be considered as treatment for or prophylaxis against impending compartment syndrome. Historically, only the surgically extended portions of the wound were closed, followed by dressing the open wound with saline soaked gauze or VAC. Serial debridements should be performed every 24-48 hours until there is no evidence of remaining necrotic soft tissue and bone. Bone grafting and wound coverage using delayed primary closure, skin graft, rotational, or free muscle flaps can be performed at this time.

▼ ORTHOPEDIC TRAUMA

FRACTURES & JOINT INJURIES

1. Fractures & Dislocations of the Spine

▶ Demographics

There are more than 10,000 new spinal cord injuries each year. The ratio of male to female patients sustaining vertebral fractures is 4:1. For patients with spinal cord injury the overall mortality rate is 17% during the initial hospital stay.

Unfortunately, delayed diagnosis happens frequently due to loss of consciousness secondary to trauma or intoxication with alcohol or drugs. As a result, suspicion for spinal cord injury should remain high in trauma patients who are unable to provide an accurate history.

▶ Anatomy

The spinal cord occupies between 35% and 50% of the spinal canal depending on the vertebral level. The remainder of the canal is filled with cerebrospinal fluid, dura mater, and epidural fat. The caudal termination of the spinal cord, located dorsal to the L1 vertebral body and L1-L2 intervertebral disk, is called the conus modularis. The conus modularis gives off motor and sensory nerve rootlets, also known as the "cauda equina" or horse's tail.

The spinal column consists of four major components that contribute to its stability: (1) the vertebral bodies, (2) the posterior elements (pedicles, laminae, spinous process, and interlocking paired facets at each level), (3) the intervertebral disk; and (4) and attached ligamentous tissues (interspinous ligaments, facet capsules, and ligamentum flavum).

The atlas is the first cervical vertebra (C1). Although it does not have a vertebral body, it has two large lateral masses which serve as weight-bearing articulations between the skull and the vertebral column. The tectorial membrane and the alar ligaments are key contributors to normal craniocervical stability. The axis is the second cervical vertebra, whose body is the largest in the cervical spine. The transverse atlantal (aka cruciform) ligament is the primary stabilizer of the atlantoaxial joint, with the alar ligaments providing secondary stability. There are five additional cervical vertebra (C3-C7).

The thoracolumbar spine consists of 12 thoracic vertebrae and 5 lumbar vertebrae. The thoracic region is naturally kyphotic (apex of bow is posterior), while the lumbar region is lordotic (apex of bow is anterior). The thoracic spine is much stiffer than the lumbar spine in flexion-extension and lateral bending, due to the additional stability provided by the rib cage as well as thinner intervertebral disks. As a result, due to its transition zone status, the thoracolumbar junction (T11-L1) is more susceptible to injury.

The spinal column can also be conceptualized as three columns with regards to its stability: (1) the anterior column (the anterior half of the vertebral body, anterior half of the intervertebral disk, and anterior longitudinal ligament), (2) the middle column (the posterior half of the vertebral body, posterior half of the intervertebral disk, and posterior longitudinal ligament), and (3) the posterior column (the facet joints, lateral masses, intraspinous ligaments, supraspinous ligaments, and spinous processes). In general, a one-column injury is relatively stable, while a three-column injury is significantly unstable, with increased risk of injury to the spinal cord.

The spinal cord roots exit the spinal canal through the intervertebral foramina. In the cervical spine, the C1 root exits above the C1 vertebral body; the C2 root exits below the C1 vertebral body. This pattern continues for the other cervical nerve roots ending with the C8 root exiting below the C7 body. In the thoracic and lumbar spine, each root exits under the pedicle with the same number. For example, the L4 nerve root exits under the L4 pedicle.

▶ Clinical Evaluation

Clinical evaluation of the spine injury patient begins with the ABCDEs. All victims of trauma are suspected of having a spinal column injury until it proven otherwise. Initially, patients are placed in a c-collar and on a backboard until the patient's spine can be assessed. A special backboard with head cutout should be used for children (6 years old or less) to prevent unintended neck flexion due to their proportionally larger head size and resulting prominent occiput.

The head-tilt-chin-lift maneuver should be avoided due to possible further disruption of the cervical spine. Airway and breathing are ensured by intubation and mechanical ventilation. Nasotracheal intubation is the safest method of airway control in the acute setting because it leads to less cervical spine motion compared with direct oral intubation.

Neurogenic shock with hypotension and bradycardia can occur in the setting of spinal cord injury. Initial resuscitation of the patient entails administration of isotonic fluids, as well as evaluating injuries to the head, chest, abdomen, pelvis, and extremities. The diastolic pressure should be kept above 70 mm Hg to maximize spinal cord blood flow. However, once the diagnosis of neurogenic shock is established, the blood pressure should be managed with vasopressors to prevent fluid overload.

If within 8 hours of injury, administer Methylprednisolone for complete or incomplete spinal cord injuries. An initial bolus of 30 mg/kg is administered over the first 15 minutes followed by 5.4 mg/kg/h over the following 24 hours (if steroids were started within 3 hours after injury) or 48 hours (if steroids were started within 3-8 hours after injury). Treatment with methylprednisolone has been shown to improve long-term motor recovery.

Sensory deficits caused by either cord or root level injuries can result in the rapid development of decubitus ulcers over insensate skin over high-pressure areas of the body (eg, the heels and ischium). As a result, timely assessment and removal of the patient from the spine board and onto an appropriate bed is critical.

Evaluating the spine includes logrolling the patient for visual inspection, palpation of the spinous processes for tenderness or diastasis, and performance of a rectal exam assessing resting tone, perianal sensation, and the bulbocavernosus reflex (squeeze of the glans penis or pull on urethral catheter results in contraction of the anal sphincter). Neurologic examination should also be performed assessing motor strength and dermatomal sensation. The motor strength testing and motor nerve roots match up as follows: shoulder abduction (C5), elbow flexion and wrist extension (C6), elbow extension and wrist flexion (C7), wrist extension and finger flexion (C8), finger abduction (T1), hip flexion (L2), knee extension L3, ankle dorsiflexion (L4), long toe extensors (L5), and ankle plantar flexors (S1). Careful evaluation and documentation of the patient's neurologic status will allow the physician to determine the appropriate treatment plan and estimate the prognosis for functional recovery.

The cervical spine can be cleared clinically in patients if the following criteria are met: (1) no posterior midline tenderness, (2) full pain-free range of motion, (3) no focal neurologic deficit, (4) normal level of alertness, (5) no evidence of intoxication, and (6) no distracting injury. Radiographic evaluation is not required. The process of the clearing the thoracolumbar spine is similar; however, anteroposterior and lateral radiographs of the TLS spine should be routinely obtained for evaluation. If any of the above criteria are not met for clearing the cervical spine, due to its increased sensitivity compared to radiographs, CT scan with sagittal reconstructions of the cervical spine to rule-out injury has become the standard of care.

In addition to spinal trauma, other injuries should be assessed since they may influence the treatment of the patient. Suspicion of associated injuries is dependent on the mechanism and location of injury. Cervical Spine injuries can be associated with injuries to the vertebral artery. Flexion-distraction injuries (seat-belt injuries) of the thoracolumbar spine are associated with intra-abdominal injuries. Axial loading injury mechanisms that often result in burst fractures of the lumbar spine are also responsible for axial loading injury patterns in the lower lumbar spine and lower extremities. These include fractures of the pars interarticularis of the L5 vertebra, the tibial plafond, and the calcaneus.

It is important to note that any injury associated with progressive neurologic deficit warrants surgical intervention.

Neurologic injury can be described as complete (no sensation/motor caudal to the level of the spinal cord pathology) or incomplete (some neurologic function persists caudal to the level of injury). Four major patterns of incomplete spinal cord injury can occur: (1) **Brown-Séquard Syndrome** (hemicord injury with ipsilateral muscle paralysis, loss of proprioception, and light touch sensation, (2) **Central Cord Syndrome** (flaccid paralysis of the upper extremities and spastic paralysis of the lower extremities with sacral sparing, (3) **Anterior Cord Syndrome** (motor and pain/temperature loss controlled by the corticospinal and spinothalamic tracts with preserved light touch and proprioception controlled by the dorsal columns), (4) **Posterior Cord Syndrome** (rare, involves loss of deep pressure, deep pain, and proprioception with full voluntary power, pain, and temperature sensation), and (5) **Conus Modularis Syndrome** (T12-L1 injuries resulting in loss of voluntary bowel and bladder control with preserved lumbar root function).

Nerve root lesions can occur at any level accompanying spinal cord injury. These lesions may be partial or complete, resulting in radicular pain, sensory dysfunction, weakness, hyporeflexia, or areflexia.

Cauda Equina syndrome is caused by multilevel lumbosacral root compression within the lumbar spinal canal. Clinical presentation can include saddle anesthesia, bilateral radicular pain, numbness, weakness, hyporeflexia or areflexia, and loss of voluntary bladder or bowel function.

Classification of Neurologic Injury

The motor and sensory examination outlined by the American Spinal Injury Association (ASIA) is one system to assess the impact on the patient of spinal cord injury. This grading system allows the patient to be assessed through scales of impairment and functional independence, evaluating remaining sensory and motor function. A thorough neurologic examination should be performed and documented when the patient is initially seen and at frequent intervals thereafter both to ensure that there is no further neurologic deterioration and to document the resolution of spinal shock.

Spinal shock is defined as spinal cord dysfunction due to physiologic disruption, resulting in hypotonia, areflexia, and paralysis distal to the level of injury. Resolution usually occurs within 24 hours with the return of reflex arcs caudal to the level of injury; the bulbocavernosus reflex is usually the first one to come back.

If a patient has a complete neurologic deficit after spinal shock has resolved, the chance for recovery of neurologic function below the level of injury is extremely poor. In contrast, patients with root level injuries (at or below the cauda equina) will recover from functionally complete injuries if they have not been transected and if initial compression by bone fragments, malalignment, or disk material has been relieved.

Determination of Sensory Levels

The sensory level is determined by the patient's ability to perceive pinprick (using a disposable needle or safety pin) and light touch (using a cotton ball). Testing of a key point in each of the 28 dermatomes on the right and left sides of the body as well as evaluation of perianal sensation is necessary. The variability in sensation for each individual stimulus is graded on a 3-point scale:

0 = Absent
1 = Impaired
2 = Normal
NT = Not testable

In the cervical spine, the C3 and C4 nerve roots supply sensation to the entire upper neck and chest in a cape-like distribution from the tip of the acromion to just above the nipple line. The next adjacent sensory level is the T2 dermatome. The brachial plexus (C5-T1) supplies the upper extremities.

ASIA also recommends testing of pain and deep pressure sensation in the same dermatomes as well as evaluation of proprioception by testing the position sense of the both index fingers and both great toes.

▶ Determination of Motor Levels

The motor level is determined by manual testing of a key muscle in the ten paired myotomes from cephalad to caudal. The strength of each muscle is graded on a six-point scale:

> 0 = Complete paralysis
> 1 = Palpable or visible contraction
> 2 = Full range of motion of the joint powered by the muscle with gravity eliminated
> 3 = Full range of motion of the joint powered by the muscle against gravity
> 4 = Active movement with full range of motion against moderate resistance
> 5 = Normal strength
> NT = Not testable

▶ ASIA Impairment Scale

The grading system is as follows: (1) Grade A (complete impairment; no motor or sensory function is preserved below the neurologic injury level), (2) Grade B (incomplete; sensory but not motor function is preserved below the neurologic level and extends through the sacral segment S4-S5), (3) Grade C (incomplete; motor function is preserved below the neurologic level with key muscles having a muscle grade < 3), (4) Grade D (incomplete; motor function is preserved below the neurologic level of injury; most key muscles below the neurologic level have a muscle grade > 3), and (5) Grade E (normal: motor and sensory function is normal).

▶ Imaging Studies

A. Cervical Spine

Plain radiographs can be used as the first imaging modality for the cervical spine, although CT scan of the cervical spine is becoming the initial test of choice due to its increased sensitivity and consistent ability to visualize the occipitocervical and cervicothoracic junctions. The standard series of radiographs includes an anteroposterior, lateral, and an open-mouth "odontoid" view. Eighty-five percent of all significant injuries to the cervical spine will be detected on the lateral view of the cervical spine. Radiographic markers of cervical spine instability include the following: compression fractures with more than 25% loss of height, angular displacement more than 11 degrees between adjacent vertebrae, translation more than 3.5 mm, and intervertebral disk space separation more than 1.7 mm. If the standard lateral view does not adequately visualize the C7-T1 junction, further studies such as a swimmer's view, oblique views, or CT of this area are necessary. Flexion-extension views of the cervical spine can be performed if instability is still suspected in a patient with otherwise normal radiographic findings. Performance of these radiographs should be delayed in a patient with neck pain, as muscle spasm can mask instability.

B. Thoracolumbar Spine

All patients with significant injury and pain in the spinal area require anteroposterior and lateral x-rays of symptomatic regions of the thoracic and lumbar spine. CT can be used to evaluate canal compromise, and for preoperative planning MRI is useful for assessing the degree of neural injury and prognosis.

▶ Complications

Patients with cervical spine injury may have impaired pulmonary function secondary to intercostal nerve paralysis. Mobilization of secretions by chest physical therapy and frequent suctioning are critical for preventing atelectasis and pulmonary infections. All patients with sensory deficits and paralysis are at high risk of developing pressure ulcers. Padding and suspension of high-risk pressure points (heels), frequent turning, and vigilant nursing care are necessary.

Patients with thoracolumbar spine fractures with or without spinal cord injury may have paralytic ileus secondary to sympathetic chain dysfunction. Oral intake should be limited to clear fluids initially, and gastric suction may be necessary if the degree or duration of ileus is significant.

The stress caused by the injury itself—in combination with systemic corticosteroid therapy—can increase the incidence of gastrointestinal ulceration and bleeding. High-dose corticosteroids can also contribute to the development of pancreatitis and infections.

Venous thromboembolic disease remains a significant problem in the management of patients with spinal injury. Pulmonary embolism is the most common cause of preventable death in hospitalized patients. Heparin can be used for DVT prophylaxis, until the patient's mobility improves.

CERVICAL SPINE INJURIES

▶ Injuries to the Occiput-C1-C2 Complex

A. Occipital Condyle Fractures

Occipital condyle fractures can be classified as follows: (1) type I (impaction of condyle, stable), (2) type II (shear injury associated with basilar or skull fractures; potentially unstable), (3) type III (condylar avulsion fracture, unstable). Treatment involves rigid cervical collar immobilization for 8 weeks for stable injuries and halo immobilization or surgical stabilization for unstable injuries.

B. Occipitoatlantal Dislocation

Also known as craniovertebral dislocation, this is almost always fatal. Postmortem studies show this injury to be the leading cause of death in motor vehicle accidents. Rare survivors usually have severe neurologic deficits. Immediate treatment includes halo vest application with strict avoidance of traction. Long-term stabilization is done surgically with occipitocervical fusion.

C. Atlas Fractures

Atlas fractures are rarely associated with neurologic injury. Instability due to transverse alar ligament insufficiency should be suspected with identification of bony avulsion or widening of the lateral masses on radiographic evaluation. These injuries can be classified as follows: (1) isolated bony apophysis fracture, (2) isolated posterior arch fracture, (3) isolated anterior arch fracture, (4) comminuted lateral mass fracture, and (5) burst fracture (fractures of the anterior and posterior ring). Stable fractures (posterior arch or nondisplaced fractures) may be treated with rigid cervical orthosis; unstable fractures require prolonged halo immobilization. Chronic instability or pain may be treated with C1-C2 fusion.

D. Transverse Ligament Rupture

This injury is rare, but usually fatal when it occurs. This injury is diagnosed by visualizing the avulsed lateral mass fragment, an atlantodens interval (ADI) more than 3 mm in adults, atlantoaxial offset more than 6.9 mm on an odontoid radiograph, or direct visualization of the rupture on MRI. Survivors are treated with halo or C1-C2 fusion.

E. Fractures of the Odontoid Process (Dens)

There is a significant association with other cervical spine fractures and a 5%-10% incidence of neurologic injury. The vascular supply to the odontoid arrives through the apex and the base of this bone with a watershed area in the neck. Odontoid fractures are classified as follows: (1) type I (oblique avulsion fracture of the apex), (2) type II (fracture at the junction of the body and the neck; high nonunion rate, which can lead to myelopathy), (3) type IIa (highly unstable comminuted injury extending from the waist of the odontoid to the vertebral body), and (4) type III (fracture extending in the cancellous body of C2 and possibly involving the lateral facets). Treatment entails cervical orthosis for type I fractures and halo immobilization for type III fractures. Treatment of type II fractures is controversial due to the high incidence of nonunion related to

poor vascularity; halo or surgical intervention is advocated depending on patient factors.

F. C2 Lateral Mass Fractures

These injuries are usually diagnosed via CT scan. Treatment varies from collar immobilization to late fusion for chronic pain.

G. Traumatic Spondilisthesis of C2

Also known as the Hangman's fracture, this injury may be associated with cranial nerve, vertebral artery or craniofacial injuries. Type I injuries are nondisplaced fractures without angulation, less than 3 mm of translation, and the C2-C3 disk is intact. Type II injuries are displaced fractures of the pars. Type IIa is a displaced pars fracture with disruption of the C2-C3 disk. Type III is a dislocation of the C2-C3 facet joints in addition to the pars fracture. Type I injuries are treated with rigid cervical orthosis, type II injuries are treated with halo immobilization, type III injuries are usually treated initially with halo immobilization followed by surgical stabilization.

▶ Injuries to C3-C7

Injuries for the remaining vertebrae from C3-C7 include teardrop fractures of the anterior portion of the vertebral body due to compression flexion, vertical compression (burst fractures), anterior dislocations due to distractive flexion, vertebral arch and lamina fractures due to compressive extension, distractive extension injuries resulting in posterior dislocations, and lateral flexion injuries resulting in translational dislocations.

"Clay shoveler's fracture" is an avulsion fracture of the spinous processes of the lower cervical and upper thoracic vertebra.

"Sentinel fracture" is a fracture through the lamina on either side of the spinous process.

Treatment for each of these fractures includes the use of cervical orthoses, halo immobilization, traction, and surgery. Soft cervical orthosis does not provide any significant immobilization. It is used as needed for the patient's comfort. Rigid cervical orthoses do not provide complete immobilization; this treatment mainly limits range of motion in the flexion-extension plane. Cervicothoracic orthoses are effective in flexion-extension and rotational control, but do not limit lateral bending very effectively. Halo immobilization offers rigid immobilization in all planes as does surgical treatment. Traction can be used to reduce unilateral or bilateral facet dislocations with neurologic deficits or to stabilize and indirectly compress the canal in patients with neural deficits from burst-type fractures. Traction is contraindicated in type IIa spondolisthesis injuries of C2 and distractive cervical spine injuries.

Choice of treatment depends on the type of injury and individual patient characteristics. In general, stable fractures can be managed with bracing, while unstable fractures require more rigid stabilization via halo application or surgical treatment.

▶ Halo Application

The halo apparatus includes the metal ring and halo vest. The halo ring should be applied approximately 1 cm above the ears. Anterior pin sites should be placed above the supraorbital ridge, anterior to the temporalis muscle over the lateral 2/3 of the eyebrow to avoid the supraorbital nerve. Posterior sites are variable and are placed to maintain the horizontal orientation of the halo. Pin pressure should be 6-8 lbs in the adult. Pin care is essential. The halo vest relies on a tight fit that should be carefully maintained.

▶ Thoracolumbar Spinous Injuries

Anteroposterior and lateral radiographs of the Thoracolumbosacral spine are the standard initial evaluation. Abnormal interpedicular distance, height loss, and canal compromise should all be noted. Minor spine injuries include articular process fractures, transverse process fractures, spinous process fractures, and pars interarticularis fractures. Generally, these injures can simply be observed. Six significant injury patterns requiring treatment are described: (1) wedge compression fracture, (2) stable burst fracture, (3) unstable burst fracture, (4) chance fracture, (5) Flexion-distraction injury, and (6) translational injuries.

A. Compression Fractures

Based off of the three column theory of instability, compression fractures are fractures that only affect the anterior column. Compression fractures can be anterior or lateral. In general these fractures are stable injuries and are rarely associated with neurologic injury. Fractures are considered unstable if there is more than 50% loss of vertebral body height, angulation more than 20-30 degrees, or multiple adjacent compression fractures. Four subtypes are described based off of endplate involvement: type A (fracture of both endplates), type B (fracture of superior endplate), type C (fracture of inferior endplate), and type D (both endplates are intact). Stable fractures are treated with Jewett brace or thoracolumbar spinal orthosis (TLSO). Unstable fractures can be treated with hyperextension casting or with surgery.

B. Burst Fractures

Burst fractures are fractures that involve the anterior and middle columns of the spinal cord. Radiographs may show loss of posterior vertebral body height and splaying of the pedicles on the anteroposterior view. It is important to note that no direct relationship exists between the amount of canal compromise and the degree of neurologic injury. Treatment can entail tho TLSO bracing or hyperextension in casting for stable fracture patterns without neurologic compromise. If the TLSO fails to restore appropriate alignment on radiographs, surgery should be considered. Early surgical intervention restoring sagittal and coronal alignment should also be considered for fractures with loss of vertebral height more than 50%, angulation more than 20-30 degrees, scoliosis more than 10 degrees, and concomitant neurologic deficit. Surgical treatment options include decompression via a posterior or anterior approach with or without instrumentation.

C. Flexion-Distraction Injuries

Also known as Chance fractures, involve all three columns of the spinal cord. These fractures are also known as "seat-belt type injuries" due to the most common mechanism by which they occur and often are associated with abdominal injuries. Radiographically, one may appreciate increased interspinous distance on the AP and lateral views. Four types of Chance fractures are recognized: (1) type A (one-level bony injury), (2) type B (one-level ligamentous injury), (3) type C (two-level injury through the bony middle column, (4) type D (two-level through the ligamentous middle column). Treatment for type A fractures may entail TLSO; however, one should consider surgical stabilization for the other three fractures given their innate lack of stability.

D. Fracture-Dislocations

Fracture-dislocations involve injury to all three columns with translational deformity. These injuries are often associated with neurologic injury and require surgical stabilization due to their unstable nature. There are three types of fracture-dislocations: (1) Flexion-rotation, (2) Shear, and (3) Flexion-distraction. Patients without neurologic injury do not require emergent surgery; however, patients whose fractures are stabilized within 72 hours of injury have a lower incidence of complications such as pneumonia and undergo a shorter hospital stay when compared to patients whose fractures are stabilized outside this time-frame.

E. Gunshot Wounds

Generally, fractures associated with low-velocity gunshot wounds are usually stable when a handgun is the weapon. These injuries are typically associated with a low infection rate and can be prophylactically treated with broad-spectrum antibiotics for 48 hours.

Any present neural injury, is usually secondary to "blast effect," in which the energy of the bullet is absorbed and transferred to the soft tissues. As a result, decompression is usually not indicated. An exception to this rule is if the bullet fragment is found in the spinal canal between levels T12 and L5. Steroids after gunshot wounds to the spine are not recommended.

F. Spine Fractures or Dislocations With Neurologic Deficit

1. Incomplete neurologic deficit—If there is a neurologic deficit, surgical decompression is indicated. This can be done either through an anterior approach with bone graft and internal fixation, a posterior costotransversectomy approach, or a combined anterior and posterior approach. The operative plan is individualized to the particular patient. Patients with incomplete neurologic deficits and unstable fractures or fracture-dislocations have the same stability requirements as patients without neurologic deficits. They are best managed with open reduction, instrumentation, and spinal fusion. Neural canal compromise should be managed as in the preceding paragraph.

2. Complete neurologic deficit—No operative procedure has been devised that will achieve recovery in cases of complete neurologic deficit that has persisted beyond the stage of spinal shock. However, surgical stabilization is often necessary (1) because spinal instability may interfere with early mobilization and rehabilitation training and (2) because it may result in loss of function at a higher level by causing mechanical injury on the root or cord segment just above the level of injury.

FRACTURES & DISLOCATIONS OF THE PELVIS

Pelvic fractures are among the most serious injuries and account for 3% of all fractures. The mechanism is often high energy in nature; 60% result from vehicular trauma (eg, automobile, motorcycle, bicycle), 30% from falls, and 10% from crush injuries, athletic injuries, or penetrating trauma. Pelvic fractures are the third most commonly seen injury in fatalities due to motor vehicle accidents.

Life-threatening hemorrhage, deformity, neurologic injury, and genitourinary injury are all potential complications that must be identified and treated early in the setting of a pelvic fracture. Pelvic fractures pose a formidable clinical challenge. Hemodynamically unstable patients who present to the emergency department with pelvic fracture have a mortality rate of 40%-50%.

▶ Anatomy

An understanding of pelvic anatomy is essential for identifying fracture patterns and complications. The pelvis is made up of three bones: two innominate bones joined anteriorly at the symphysis and posteriorly at the paired sacroiliac joints. The innominate bones are further subdivided into the ilium, ischium, and pubis.

The acetabulum is the portion of the pelvic bone that articulates with the femoral head to form the hip joint. It results from closure of the triradiate cartilage and is covered with hyaline cartilage. The innominate bone support of the acetabulum can be thought of as an inverted Y formed by two columns. The anterior column (iliopubic component) extends from the iliac crest to the pubic symphysis including the anterior wall of the acetabulum. The posterior column (ilioischeal component) extends from the superior gluteal notch to the ischial tuberosity including the posterior wall. The acetabular dome is the superior weight-bearing portion of the acetabulum at the junction of the anterior and posterior columns, including contributions from both.

The stability of the pelvis is dependent on its ligamentous attachments. A thick fibrocartilaginous disk joins the anterior aspects of the innominate bones to form the pubic symphysis. This joint acts as a supporting strut for the pelvis because the stability of the ring depends mostly upon the sacroiliac joints.

The posterior ligamentous structures supporting the sacroiliac joints can be divided into anterior and posterior complexes. The anterior sacroiliac joint ligaments are broad and flat and connect the iliac wing and the sacral ala. These ligaments primarily resist external rotation and torsional forces. The sacro-iliac ligaments provide most of the stability. Composed of the interosseous sacroiliac ligaments within the joint and the posterior sacroiliac ligaments spanning the sacrum between the posterior iliac spines, the posterior complex is considered to be the strongest ligament in the human body. The posterior sacroiliac complex resists shear forces between the sacrum and the ilium, clinically preventing displacement of the ilium onto the sacrum.

The pelvic floor contains two additional strong ligaments, the sacrospinous and the sacrotuberous ligaments. The sacrospinous ligament maintains rotational control while the sacrotuberous ligament is especially important in maintaining vertical stability of the pelvis. Additional stability is conferred by ligamentous attachments between the spine and the pelvis. The iliolumbar ligaments originate from L4 and L5 transverse processes and insert on to the posterior iliac crest. The lumbosacral ligaments originate from the transverse process of L5 and insert to the sacrum ala.

▶ Stability

Pelvic stability can be defined as the ability of the pelvic ring to withstand physiologic forces without abnormal deformation. Pathologically, the pelvic ring fails under one or more of three basic modes. External rotation strains the pubic symphysis and the sacrotuberous, sacrospinous, and anterior sacroiliac joint ligaments. After roughly 2.5 cm of diastasis, the pelvic floor ligaments and the anterior sacroiliac ligaments begin to fail, giving rise to gross rotatory instability. Because the posterior ligament complex is largely intact, superior or posterior displacement of the involved hemipelvis does not occur. Combined external and shear forces are necessary to completely disrupt pelvic stability. Conversely, internal rotation places the pubic rami under compression and the posterior ligament complexes under tension. The rami often fail in their midportions with transverse fractures and sacral alar impaction. The pelvic floor ligaments remain intact, and gross posterior stability is maintained. Therefore, fractures involving torsional forces on the pelvis often have partial instability in the rotatory plane only, with maintenance of stability to other displacement.

Complete instability, however, occurs with disruption of both the anterior and the posterior ligamentous restraints. These injuries often present with widely displaced sacroiliac joints and multiaxial instability of the involved hemipelvis. Such fractures have components of superior and posterior displacement relative to the sacrum in addition to rotational displacement in the sagittal and horizontal planes.

Clinical Evaluation

Physical examination includes palpation of the pelvic bony landmarks, compression maneuvers to assess stability, rectovaginal examination looking for bony spikes protruding through the mucosa representing an open fracture, and looking for blood at the urethral meatus, or a high-riding prostate on rectal exam which may indicate genitourinary injury. If bladder or urethral injury is suspected, retrograde urethrogram should be considered. The mortality rate of open pelvic fractures is as high as 50%—compared with 8%-15% for closed fractures. A secondary musculoskeletal survey examining each of the other four limbs including distal vascular status and a thorough neurologic examination should be performed as well.

Radiographic Examination

The anteroposterior radiograph required in all patients with blunt trauma rapidly identifies the major pelvic injury. The AP pelvis radiograph can be looked at in a systematic way: the pubic rami, pubic symphysis (looking for widening >2.5 cm), the iliopectineal lines (represents limit of the anterior column of the acetabulum) ilioischial lines (represents limit of the posterior column of the acetabulum), the anterior lip of the acetabulum, the posterior lip of the acetabulum, the radiographic roof of the acetabulum, the pelvic wings, the sacro-iliac joints, femoral head position (rule-out concomitant hip dislocation), associated fracture of the femoral head or femoral neck, and finally the lumbar spine. Disruption of the iliopectineal line, ilioischial line, the anterior lip, posterior lip, or the radiographic roof may be indicative of acetabular fracture. Suspected acetabular fractures should be further evaluated with **Judet's views** (iliac oblique and obturator oblique). The **iliac oblique** (45-degree external rotation view) view better delineates the anterior column and posterior wall of the acetabulum, while the **obturator oblique** (45-degree internal rotation view) characterizes

the posterior column and anterior wall of the acetabulum in greater detail. Inlet and outlet radiographs are often required to supplement the anteroposterior film. The **inlet view** (patient supine, the tube directed 60 degrees caudal) can be used to evaluate for any anterior-posterior instability, while the **outlet view** (patient supine, tube directed 45 degrees cephalad) will best show any vertical displacement. CT scan is recommended for any suspected pelvis fracture; this modality is especially good for evaluation of the acetabulum and posterior pelvis, including the sacrum and sacro-iliac joints.

Acute Management

Immediate care of the polytrauma patient with a pelvic fracture must address associated retroperitoneal hemorrhage, pelvic ring instability, and injuries to the genitourinary system and rectum as well as fractures open to the peritoneum. Cessation of blood loss, minimization of septic sequelae, and stabilization of the fracture, allowing early and safe patient mobilization, are the immediate treatment goals. Hemorrhage is the leading cause of death in patients with pelvic fracture, accounting for 60% of the deaths. Most of the blood loss is from the fracture site or injured retroperitoneal veins; only 20% of the deaths are associated with major arterial injury. An average blood replacement of 5.9 units has been reported.

General resuscitative principles are applied to stabilize the patient and provide adequate tissue perfusion. Once other sites of hemorrhage have been ruled out, active bleeding from a pelvic fracture may be controlled by wrapping a pelvic binder or sheet circumferentially around the pelvis. The sheet should enclose the bilateral anterior superior iliac spines and greater trochanters, and can be fixed in placed by clipping the two ends with a hemostat. Wrapping the pelvis in this way stabilizes major fracture fragments and closes down the volume of the pelvis, dramatically reducing active blood loss. If this fails to control hemorrhage, angiography or arterial embolization is indicated. Definitive internal fixation is usually required after hemorrhage has been controlled and the patient has been stabilized.

Fracture-dislocations of the pelvis should be treated with immediate closed reduction of the hip. Stability should be assessed by ranging the hip through a full arc of motion. Unstable hips should be rereduced and placed in skeletal traction. An Irreducible hip or new-onset sciatic nerve palsy after closed hip reduction requires immediate operative treatment.

Classification & Treatment

Fractures of the pelvis may be classified according to the Young and Burgess system based off of mechanism of injury. AP compression (APC) injuries result from anteriorly applied force. APC-I characterizes less than 2.5 cm of symphyseal diastasis; vertical fractures of one or both pubic rami occur, however, the sacroiliac ligaments are intact imparting rotational and vertical stability. In an APC-II injury disruption of the anterior sacro-iliac ligaments results in greater than 2.5 cm of symphyseal diastasis that is rotationally unstable, but vertically stable due to intact posterior sacroiliac ligaments. APC-III injury occurs with complete disruption of the symphysis, sacrotuberous, sacrospinous, anterior, and posterior sacroiliac ligaments resulting in a pelvis that is rotationally and vertically unstable. Lateral compression (LC) injury results from a laterally applied force to the pelvis that leads to shortening of the anterior sacroiliac, sacrospinous, and sacrotuberous ligaments with resulting transverse or oblique fractures of the pubic rami. LC-I injury describes transverse fractures of the pubic rami with sacral compression on the side of injury without rotational or vertical instability. LC-II injuries describe the addition of a crescent iliac wing fracture on the side of impact with variable disruption of the posterior ligamentous structures resulting in rotational instability. LC-III describes an LC-I or LC-II injury on the side of impact with continuation of the force producing an external rotation or open book (APC) type injury on the contralateral side. Vertical shear (VS) injury due vertical or longitudinal forces caused by falls onto an extended lower extremity, impacts from above, or motor vehicle accidents with a lower extremity impacted against the dashboard or floorboard, typically results in complete ligamentous disruption, rotational and vertical instability, with a high incidence of neurovascular injury, and hemorrhage. Combined mechanical (CM) describes a combination of injuries often due to crush mechanism.

Pelvic fractures may also be classified according to instability using the Tile classification: type A (rotationally and vertically stable), type B (rotationally unstable and vertically stable, or type C (rotationally and vertically unstable). Common radiographic signs of pelvic instability include (1) displacement of the posterior sacroiliac complex more than 5 mm in any plane; (2) the presence of a posterior fracture gap rather than an impaction; and (3) the presence of an avulsion fracture of the transverse process of the fifth lumbar vertebra or the sacro-ischial end of the sacrospinous ligaments.

Type A fractures involve the pelvic ring in only one location and are considered stable. Type A1 fractures are avulsion fractures that usually occur at muscle origins such as the anterosuperior iliac spine, anteroinferior iliac spine, and ischial apophysis. These fractures most often occur in adolescents, and conservative treatment is usually sufficient. Rarely, symptomatic nonunions develop and can be best treated surgically.

Type A2 fractures are isolated fractures of the iliac wing without involvement of the hip or sacroiliac joints and are usually a result of direct trauma. Even with significant displacement, bony healing is expected and treatment is

therefore symptomatic. Healing may be accompanied by ossification of the hematoma with exuberant new bone formation. Finally, type A3 fractures are isolated fractures of the obturator foramen and usually involve minimal displacement of the pubic or ischial rami. The posterior sacroiliac complex is intact, and the pelvis remains stable. Treatment is symptomatic, with early ambulation and weight bearing as tolerated.

Type B fractures involve breaks in the pelvic ring in two or more sites. This creates a pelvic fracture that is rotationally unstable but vertically stable. Type B1 fractures are open book fractures that occur from anteroposterior compression. Unless the anterior separation of the pubic symphysis is severe (> 6 cm), the posterior sacroiliac complex is usually intact and the pelvis is relatively stable to vertical forces. Significant associated injuries to the perineal and urogenital structures are often present and should always be looked for. For minimally displaced symphysial injuries (< 2.5 cm), only symptomatic treatment is needed. However, if conservative treatment is pursued, serial radiographs are required after mobilization is begun to monitor for subsequent increased displacement that may require surgery. For more displaced fracture-dislocations, reduction is done by LC using the intact posterior sacroiliac complex as the hinge on which the "book is closed." Reduction can be maintained with the use of an external fixator; however, internal fixation with a symphyseal plate is currently favored. "Closing the book" decreases the space available for hemorrhage, increases patient comfort.

Type B2 and B3 fractures involve a lateral force applied to the pelvis, causing inward displacement of the hemipelvis through the sacroiliac complex and ipsilateral (B2) or, more often, contralateral (B3) pubic rami fractures. The degree of involvement of the posterior sacroiliac ligament complex will determine the degree of instability. The hemipelvis is infolded, with overlapping of the pubic symphysis. Reduction can be accomplished with external fixation, with internal fixation, or with both. External fixation facilitates nursing care but is not strong enough for ambulation. Definitive care usually is accomplished with internal fixation of both the anterior and posterior aspects of the pelvic ring. Major hemorrhage is associated with these fracture types.

Type C fractures are both rotationally and vertically unstable. They often result from a VS injury such as a fall from a height. Anteriorly, the pubic symphysis or pubic rami may be disrupted. Posteriorly, the sacroiliac joint may be disrupted and dislocated, or there may be a fracture through the sacrum or adjacent iliac wing. The hemipelvis is completely unstable, and there may be associated massive hemorrhage and injury to the lumbosacral pelvis. External fixation is insufficient to maintain reduction, but it may help to control hemorrhage and ease nursing care in the acute stage. Internal fixation is usually required as definitive treatment.

SACRAL FRACTURES

Fractures of the sacrum can be described using the Denis classification according to the location of the fracture in relation to the sacral foramen: Denis I: lateral to the foramen, Denis II: through the foramen, and Denis III: medial to the foramen. The incidence of neurologic injury increases with higher classification.

FRACTURES OF THE ACETABULUM

Fractures of the acetabulum (Figure 40–1) occur through direct trauma on the trochanteric region or indirect axial loading through the lower limb. The position of the limb at the time of impact (rotation, flexion, abduction, or adduction) will determine the pattern of injury. Comminution is common.

▶ Classification

Letournel has classified acetabular fractures into ten different types: five simple patterns (one fracture line)-posterior wall, posterior column, anterior wall, anterior column, transverse and five complex patterns (the association of two or more simple patterns)-T-shaped, posterior column and posterior wall, transverse and posterior wall, anterior column/posterior hemi-transverse, and both column. This is the most widely used classification system as it allows the surgeon to choose the most appropriate surgical approach.

▶ Treatment

The goal of treatment is to achieve a spherical congruency between the femoral head and the weight-bearing acetabular dome and to maintain it until the bones are healed. As with other pelvic fractures, acetabular fractures are frequently associated with abdominal, urogenital, and neurologic injuries, which should be systematically sought and treated. Significant bleeding is often present and should be stopped as soon as possible.

The stabilized patient with **protrusion** (the femoral head is impacted through the fracture of the acetabulum into the pelvis) or unstable fracture-dislocation should be put in longitudinal skeletal traction through a distal femoral or proximal tibial pin pulling axially in neutral position. Postreduction x-rays are obtained. Operative indications for acetabular fractures include displacement(> 2-3 mm), large posterior wall fragments, interposed intra-articular loose fragment, femoral head fractures, unstable reductions, and an irreducible fracture dislocation by closed methods. The choice of approach is of primary importance, and more than one approach will sometimes prove necessary. Acetabular surgery uses extensile approaches and sophisticated reduction and fixation techniques and is best performed by pelvic surgeons.

▶ Complications

Complications inherent to the injury include posttraumatic degenerative joint disease, heterotopic ossification, femoral head osteonecrosis, deep vein thrombosis, and other complications related to conservative treatment. Surgery is performed to prevent or delay osteoarthritis (OA), but it increases the possibility of complications such as infection, iatrogenic neurovascular injury, and increased heterotopic ossification. When the reduction is stable and fixation is solid, the patient can be mobilized after a few days with non–weight-bearing ambulation, and weight bearing may

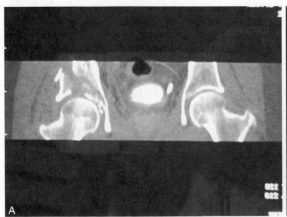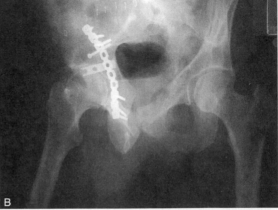

▲ **Figure 40–1.** Forty-year-old man who fell from a height, sustaining a posterior hip dislocation and an acetabular fracture of the weight-bearing dome. **A.** Coronal CT reconstructions showing large fragment of the superior dome of the right acetabulum. **B.** Oblique radiograph demonstrating concentric reduction of the hip and restoration of the articular surface after open reduction and internal fixation.

begin as early as 6 weeks. Prophylactic anticoagulation and aggressive pulmonary toilet are key elements of postoperative care.

SHOULDER INJURIES

1. Clavicular Fractures

▶ Epidemiology, Mechanism, Anatomy, and Clinical Evaluation

Clavicle fractures are relatively common accounting for between 2% and 12% of all fractures. Clavicle fractures are characterized by location: medial, lateral, and middle third of the clavicle which is the most common type (80%). The most common mechanism of injury is fall on to the ipsilateral shoulder (87%); direct impact (7%) and falls onto an outstretched hand cause the rest. The clavicle is an S-shaped bone that serves as a strut bracing the shoulder in relation to the trunk, allowing the shoulder to function at maximum strength. The clavicle is stabilized by the acromioclavicular and coracoclavicular ligaments. The acromioclavicular ligaments prevent horizontal displacement while the coracoclavicular ligaments provide vertical stability. The middle one-third of the clavicle protects the brachial plexus, superior lung, subclavian and axillary arteries. As a result, it is critical to document a thorough neurovascular examination, and rule-out concomitant injuries such as brachial plexus palsy, vascular injury, and pneumothorax. It is also important to note the appearance of the skin as tenting may be an indication for surgery. Clavicle fractures are most often incidentally seen on the AP radiograph of the chest. Proximal third clavicle fractures can be further evaluated with computed tomography to differentiate between sternoclavicular dislocations from epiphyseal injury.

▶ Classification

Clavicle fractures are classified into three groups: Group I: middle third fracture, Group II: distal third, Group III: proximal third. Group II fractures are subclassified into three types according to the location of the coracoclavicular ligaments relative to the fracture. Type I fractures are interligamentous, either in between the conoid and trapezoid ligaments or between the coracoclavicular and acromioclavicular ligaments, with the ligaments still intact. Because ligaments are attached to both the proximal and distal fracture segments, the fracture is typically nondisplaced or minimally displaced. Group II, type II fractures occur medial to the coracoclavicular ligaments or in between the conoid and trapezoid ligaments with the conoid ligament torn, such that the proximal fracture segment is predisposed to significant displacement. Group II, type III is a distal-third fracture of the articular surface of the AC joint without ligamentous injury.

▶ Treatment

Clavicle fractures are typically treated conservatively with a sling or figure of eight brace for 4-6 weeks until healing is appreciated radiographically and clinically (area no longer tender with palpation). Sling is typically preferred due to lower incidence of skin problems and increased patient comfort. Some degree of shortening and deformity is expected with closed treatment. However, shoulder dysfunction is rare and there is no scar. Strict indications for surgery include open clavicle fractures, associated neurovascular injury, and skin tenting concerning for impending open fracture. Some authors advocate fixing significantly displaced (> 1-2 cm) middle-third clavicle fractures and Group II, type II distal clavicle fractures, due to predisposition to nonunion which may result in cosmetic deformity and shoulder dysfunction.

2. Acromioclavicular Dislocation

The AC joint is diarthroidal with fibrocartilage-covered articular surfaces between the medial acromion and the lateral end of the clavicle. The AC ligaments blend with fibers from the deltoid and trapezius to provide strength to the joint. As described previously, the AC ligaments provide horizontal stability while the coracoclavicular ligaments provide vertical stability. The mechanism for dislocation of the acromioclavicular joint is most commonly direct impact caused by a fall on the tip of the shoulder. Thorough neurovascular examination along with standard trauma series of the shoulder (AP, scapular-Y, and axillary views) completes the standard workup. Stress radiographs in which 10-15 lb weights are strapped to the wrists and an AP radiograph is taken of both shoulders comparing coracoclavicular distances, to differentiate between partial grade I to II injuries and grade III AC separations.

▶ Classification and Treatment

Type I is a strain of the acromioclavicular ligament. **Type II** injury involves rupture of the acromioclavicular ligament and strain of the coracoclavicular ligament complex, with slight superior displacement of the superior clavicle **type III** injury involves rupture of both the acromioclavicular and the coracoclavicular ligaments, which causes marked superior migration of the lateral end of the clavicle **types IV, V, and VI** injuries involve detachment of the deltoid and trapezius from the distal clavicle in addition to disruption of the AC and CC ligaments with marked posterior, superior, and inferior displacement of the clavicle, respectively.

▶ Treatment

Type I, II, and III AC joint injuries are typically managed nonoperatively with a sling for approximately 4 weeks followed by gradual return to full activity. Most patients do not have significant dysfunction or any need to modify their activities. Surgical reconstruction may be indicated for types IV, V, and VI AC joint injuries. Type III injuries in young athletes or laborers who perform a lot of overhead work may be treated surgically.

3. Sternoclavicular Joint Dislocation

Dislocation of the sternoclavicular joint is rare. The mechanism of injury is usually a motor vehicle accident or sporting injury. Physical examination and anteroposterior and anteroposterior-cephalic tilt x-rays may demonstrate asymmetry. However, computed tomography is diagnostic test of choice as it can distinguish fractures of the medial clavicle from SC dislocation and can show minor subluxation. Anterior dislocation is more common, but posterior dislocation can cause injury to the esophagus, trachea, great vessels, subclavian artery, carotid artery, and pneumothorax. Dislocations of the sternoclavicular joint in children are often associated with physical fractures.

▶ Treatment

Most injuries to the sternoclavicular joint may be treated with a ice for the first 24 hours and immobilization with a sling, sling and swathe, or figure-of-eight bandage. Posterior dislocations may require emergent reduction if there is associated vascular compression or injury to the trachea, esophagus, or lungs. Closed reduction of posterior dislocations has been described using shoulder retraction and a towel clip. Rarely, open reduction may be necessary.

4. Scapular Fracture

Scapular fractures are classified by anatomic location: scapula body, neck, spine, acromion, coracoid, or glenoid. Scapular body fractures are often associated with other injuries such as subclavian vessel injury, aortic rupture, pneumothorax, rib fractures, brachial plexus injuries, and other soft tissue injuries associated with high-energy trauma. Fractures of the acromion and coracoid are rare. Glenoid fractures must be carefully evaluated for articular surface step-off and associated glenohumeral instability. These fractures may be caused by a blow on the shoulder or by a fall on the outstretched arm. Diagnosis with anteroposterior x-ray in the plane of the scapula and axillary x-ray may be supplemented by an axial view of the scapular body and transscapular {ss} Y{end}-view. CT scan may also be helpful if surgery is being considered.

▶ Treatment

Most scapular fractures are treated nonoperatively in a sling for 4-6 weeks. Associated injuries may need to be treated emergently and should not be overlooked. Surgical indications are controversial, but may include displaced intra-articular fractures involving more than 25% of the articular surface, scapular neck fractures more than 40 degree angulation or 1 cm of medial translation, scapula neck fractures with an associated displaced clavicle fracture, acromion fractures that cause subacromial impingement, and coracoid fractures that cause functional AC separation.

5. Dislocation of the Shoulder Joint

The shoulder (glenohumeral) joint is the most commonly dislocated joint in the body due to its freedom of motion and mobility in multiple planes. Diagnosis and management of this is presented in detail in the Sports Medicine section of this chapter.

6. Proximal Humerus Fracture

Fractures of the proximal humerus occur most commonly in elderly individuals with osteoporosis, after a fall initial assessment should seek to determine the cause of any related fall as well as the fracture pattern. Prodromal symptoms related to a syncopal episode, myocardial infarction, stroke, transient ischemic attack, or seizure are possible etiologies that should be investigated. Associated injuries include neurovascular injuries, dislocation, and rotator cuff tears. Axillary nerve function should be assessed testing sensation over lateral aspect of shoulder, overlying deltoid (motor testing is usually not possible, due to pain).

Diagnosis is established by standard shoulder trauma series (AP, lateral scapular Y, and axillary views). The axillary view is the best view for evaluating glenoid articular fractures and dislocations. If axillary view cannot be obtained due to pain, a Velpeau axillary view where the patient is left in a sling leaned obliquely backward 45 degrees over the cassette with the beam directed caudally is another option. Computed tomography can be used to further evaluate articular involvement, fracture displacement, impression fractures, and glenoid rim fractures.

▶ Classification and Treatment

Proximal humerus fractures can be classified according to the system developed by NEER. There are four major parts of the proximal humerus: humeral head, humeral shaft, greater, and lesser tuberosities. A part is defined as displaced if there is more than 1 cm of fracture displacement, or more than 45 degrees of angulation. Most proximal humerus fractures are minimally displaced (< 1 cm and < 45 degrees of angulation) and can be treated in a sling with early gentle range of motion exercises. Displaced fractures usually require surgery. Surgical options include closed

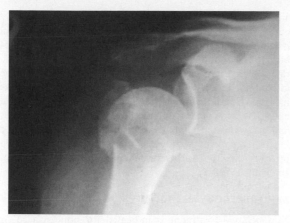

▲ **Figure 40–2.** Four-part proximal humerus fracture, impacted on inferior glenoid rim.

reduction and percutaneous fixation, open reduction and internal fixation, and prosthetic arthroplasty (Figures 40–2 and 40–3). Other indications for surgery include superior displacement of the greater tuberosity fragment of 5 mm or more which can lead to subacromial impingement, lesser tuberosity fractures that block internal rotation. Patients often lose some range of motion, but excellent pain relief and function can be attained. Long-term complications include shoulder stiffness and avascular necrosis of the humeral head (due to disruption of the arcuate branch off of the anterior circumflex humeral artery).

FRACTURES OF THE SHAFT OF THE HUMERUS

Most fractures of the shaft of the humerus result from direct trauma; indirect mechanism from fall on an outstretched arm is also a possibility. A careful neurovascular exam is required (radial nerve injury is most common). AP and lateral radiographs of the humerus, as well as shoulder and elbow series are mandatory to rule out the possibility of fracture or dislocation involving adjacent joints. Humerus fractures can be described descriptively: open versus closed, location (proximal, middle, and distal third), nondisplaced versus displaced, transverse, oblique, spiral, segmental or comminuted fracture, intrinsic condition of bone (osteopenic or not), and if there is any articular extension.

▶ Treatment

Most midshaft humeral fractures can be treated nonoperatively in a cast, splint, or brace. Alignment should be verified using AP and lateral x-rays with the patient standing. Twenty degrees of anterior angulation, 30 degrees of varus angulation, and up to 3 cm of bayonet apposition are acceptable for continued closed treatment. Other surgical indications include open fractures, concomitant vascular injury, pathologic fracture, "floating elbow" (concomitant

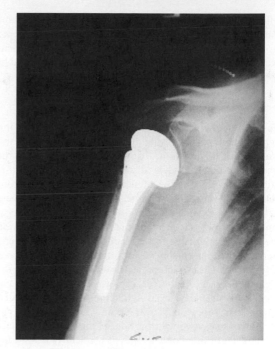

▲ **Figure 40–3.** Surgical reconstruction with hemiarthroplasty.

fracture of the forearm bones), segmental fracture, intra-articular extension, and bilateral humeral fractures. Radial nerve injury most commonly occurs with middle third fractures. Most radial nerve injuries are the result of stretching or contusion; function usually returns in 3-4 months. Delayed surgical exploration is warranted if there is no evidence of recovery on EMG or nerve conduction velocity studies at this time.

FRACTURES & DISLOCATIONS ABOUT THE ELBOW

▶ Anatomy & Biomechanics

The elbow is a modified hinge joint consisting of three separate articulations: ulnohumeral, radiohumeral, and proximal radioulnar. The elbow joint is intrinsically stable with bony and soft tissue contributions. The trochlea-olecranon fossa, coronoid fossa, radiocapitellar joint, biceps, triceps, and brachioradialis provide anterior-posterior stability during flexion and extension. On the medial side of the elbow the anterior bundle of the medial collateral ligament (MCL) is the primary stabilizer to valgus stress, while the lateral ulnar collateral ligament is the primary stabilizer on the opposite side of the elbow preventing posterolateral instability. Normal elbow range of motion entails 0-150 degrees of flexion, 85 degrees of supination, and 80 degrees of pronation. Functional range of motion requires 30-130 degrees of flexion, 50 degrees of pronation, and supination. Elbow injury mandates careful examination of the entire upper extremity including shoulder and wrist, with thorough neurovascular examination. AP, lateral, and oblique radiographs are required to adequate visualize the elbow joint.

Distal Humerus Fractures

The distal humerus can be conceptualized as medial and lateral columns, each roughly triangular in shape and composed of a condyle articulating with the bones of the forearm and an epicondyle (distal part of the humerus that flares just above the elbow joint at the level of the supracondylar ridge) connecting to the shaft of the humerus. These fractures can be classified descriptively: intercondylar (most common), supracondylar fractures (extension or flexion type), transcondylar, condylar, capitellum, trochlea, lateral epicondyle, medial epicondyle, or fractures of the supracondylar process. These fractures can also be classified using the AO system based on the concept of column integrity and articular involvement. Type A fractures are extra-articular (epicondylar, supracondylar, transcondylar) fractures. Type B fractures only involve a portion of the articular surface (unicondylar or intercondylar). Type C fractures involve the entire distal articular surface.

Radiographic Evaluation

Standard AP, lateral, and oblique radiographs should be obtained. Traction radiographs or computed tomography may provide better fracture pattern visualization for preoperative planning. On the lateral radiograph, the anterior or posterior **"fat pad sign" representing displacement of the adipose layer over the joint capsule** may be the only indication of a nondisplaced distal humerus fracture. The AP radiograph should be carefully scrutinized for an intercondylar split. If an intercondylar split is present, the amount of rotation, in addition to displacement and fracture comminution should be noted.

Management

The patient can be initially managed with a posterior long-arm splint with the elbow flexed at 90 degrees and the forearm neutral. Nonoperative treatment is indicated for nondisplaced or minimally displaced fractures. Surgery is indicated for displaced fractures, vascular injury, or open fracture.

SPECIFIC FRACTURE TYPES

Supracondylar Fractures of the Humerus

Supracondylar fractures are much more common in children. There are two types: extension (distal fragment is displaced posteriorly) and flexion (distal fragment is displaced

anteriorly). Nondisplaced, minimally displaced, and severely comminuted fractures in the elderly with limited functional needs may be treated nonoperatively. Posterior splint immobilization is continued for 1-2 weeks after which gentle range of motion exercises are begun. The splint may be discontinued and weight bearing advanced after six weeks if signs of radiographic healing are appreciated. Surgical options include open reduction internal fixation with plates and screws. Total elbow replacement may be considered in elderly patients who were otherwise active with good preinjury function with severely comminuted fractures not amenable to ORIF.

Transcondylar Fractures

Nonoperative treatment is indicated for nondisplaced or minimally displaced fractures or for debilitated elderly patients with poor function preinjury. Range of motion exercises should be initiated as soon as the patient is able to tolerate therapy. Surgical options include ORIF or total elbow arthroplasty.

Intercondylar Fractures

Intercondylar fractures are the most common type of distal humerus fracture in adults. Fracture fragments are often displaced due to opposing muscle forces on the medial (flexor mass) and lateral (extensor mass) epicondyles, causing rotation of the articular surfaces (Figure 40-4). Fractures can be classified as type I (nondisplaced), type II (slight displacement with no rotation between the condylar fragments), type III (displacement with rotation), and type IV (comminution of the articular surface). Nonoperative treatment with two weeks of immobilization followed by range of motion exercises is indicated for nondisplaced fractures. Type IV fractures in the elderly with osteopenic bone can be treated with the "bag of bones" technique which entails very short-term immobilization with early range of motion. Open reduction internal fixation with dual plates is the preferred surgical treatment. Early range of motion is critical to prevent stiffness, unless fixation is tenuous. TEA is another option.

Condylar Fractures

Medial or lateral condyle fractures are rare in adults (Figure 40-5). Type I (Milch classification) fractures do not traverse the lateral trochlear ridge. Involvement of the lateral trochlear ridge (type II) leads to medial-lateral instability. Nonoperative treatment, entailing a posterior splint with elbow flexed to 90 degrees and the forearm supinated for lateral condyle fractures or pronated for medial epicondyle fractures, may be pursued for nondisplaced or minimally displaced fractures. Open or displaced fractures can be treated surgically with screw fixation with or without collateral ligament repair as needed.

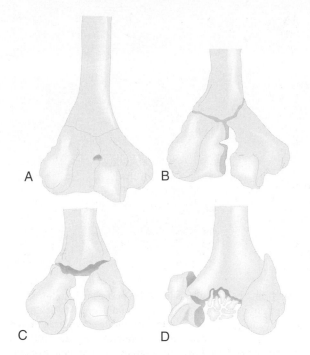

▲ **Figure 40–4.** Intercondylar fractures.
A. Type I undisplaced T-condylar fracture of the elbow.
B. Type II displaced but not rotated T-condylar fracture.
C. Type III displaced and rotated T-condylar fracture.
D. Type IV displaced rotated and comminuted T-condylar fracture.

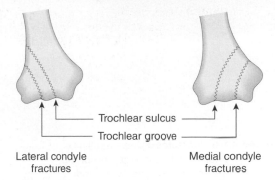

Trochlear sulcus
Trochlear groove

Lateral condyle fractures

Medial condyle fractures

▲ **Figure 40–5.** Condyle fractures. Milch classification. The type II fracture involves the lateral lip of the trochlea—thus its inherent instability. (Reproduced, with permission, from Milch H: Fractures and fracture dislocation of the humeral condyles. *J Trauma*, 1964.)

▶ Capitellum Fractures

Capitellum fractures are rare, representing less than 1% of all elbow fractures. Due to lack of significant soft tissue attachments, these fractures may result in a free articular fragment that may displace anteriorly into the coronoid or radial fossa causing a block to elbow flexion. These fractures typically result from a fall on an outstretched arm with the force transmitted through the radial head to the capitellum. Occasionally, radial head fracture may also be present. Capitellum fractures can be classified as follows (Figure 40–6): type I "Hahn-Steinthal" large osseous fragment with or without trochlear involvement, type II "Kocher-Lorenz" fragment articular cartilage with minimal subchondral bone attached, and type III (significant comminution). Nonoperative treatment, reserved for nondisplaced fractures, consists of immobilization in a posterior splint followed by elbow range of motion exercises. Surgical treatment entails ORIF with screws or excision for type II fractures, severely comminuted type I fractures or chronic missed fractures with limited range of motion.

▶ Trochlea Fractures

These fractures are extremely rare and associated with elbow dislocation. Nondisplaced fractures can be treated with posterior splint for three weeks, followed by elbow range of motion exercises. Displaced fractures are treated with ORIF; fragments not amenable to internal fixation can be excised.

▶ Epicondylar Fractures

Lateral epicondyle fractures can be treated with symptomatic immobilization with early range of motion. Nondisplaced or minimally displaced medial epicondyle fractures can be treated with immobilization in posterior splint with the forearm pronated, wrist and elbow flexed for 10-14 days. ORIF is indicated for displaced fractures, especially in the presence of ulnar nerve symptoms, valgus stress instability, wrist flexor weakness, and symptomatic nonunion.

▶ Supracondylar Process Fractures

The supracondylar process is osseous or cartilaginous projection arising from the anteromedial surface of the humerus. The ligament of Struthers which connects the supracondylar process to the medial epicondyle is a fibrous arch through which the median nerve and brachial artery passes. Most of these fractures are amenable to closed treatment with symptomatic posterior splint immobilization followed by early range of motion. Median nerve or brachial artery compression are indications for surgical exploration and release.

▶ Elbow Dislocation

Elbow dislocation most commonly results from a fall on an outstretched hand. A careful neurovascular examination

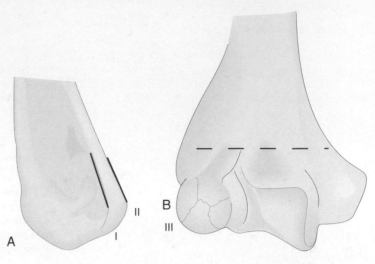

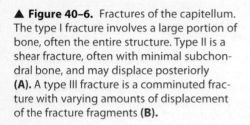

▲ **Figure 40–6.** Fractures of the capitellum. The type I fracture involves a large portion of bone, often the entire structure. Type II is a shear fracture, often with minimal subchondral bone, and may displace posteriorly **(A).** A type III fracture is a comminuted fracture with varying amounts of displacement of the fracture fragments **(B).**

along with AP and lateral radiographs of the elbow are required. Simple elbow dislocation (no associated fracture) are classified according to the direction of displacement of the ulna relative to the humerus: posterior (most common type), posterolateral, posteromedial, lateral, medial, and anterior (Figure 40–7). Acute elbow dislocations should undergo closed reduction with patient under sedation and adequate anesthesia as soon as possible. For posterior dislocation, the reduction maneuver entails longitudinal traction with elbow flexion. Postreduction range of motion exam, neurovascular

exam, and radiographs should be performed, followed by placement in a posterior splint with 90 degrees of flexion. A block to full range of motion may indicate an incarcerated fracture fragment or inadequate reduction. If reduction does not restore arterial flow, angiography, and immediate operative intervention are warranted. Postreduction films should be carefully evaluated for concentric reduction and associated fractures (medial or lateral epicondyle, radial head, coronoid process). Elbow dislocation with radial head and coronoid process fractures is known as the "terrible triad",

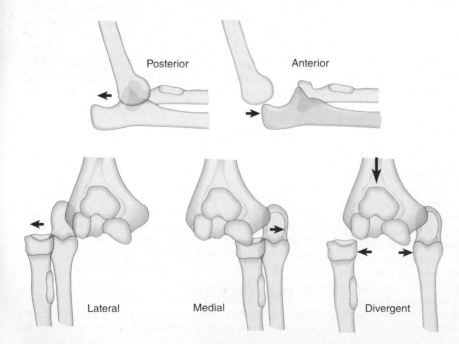

▲ **Figure 40–7.** Elbow dislocations. An elbow dislocation is defined by the direction of the forearm bones. (Reproduced, with permission, from Browner B et al: *Skeletal Trauma.* Saunders, 1992.)

due to associated instability. Surgical intervention is indicated when the elbow cannot be held concentrically reduced position, redislocates, or if the dislocation is deemed unstable (if the elbow dislocates prior to reaching 30 degrees of flexion from a fully flexed position). Recovery of motion and strength may take 3-6 months. The most common complication is stiffness, associated with prolonged immobilization. Recently, the trend has been to immobilize elbows for one week postinjury, and then start range of motion exercises. If symptomatic heterotopic ossification is present, excision can be pursued 6 months or longer after injury.

FRACTURES OF THE PROXIMAL ULNA

Olecranon Fractures

The olecranon is the most proximal palpable portion of the ulna. The subcutaneous position of the olecranon causes it to be especially susceptible to direct trauma. Posteriorly, the triceps tendon envelops the articular capsule before it inserts on to the olecranon. As a result, displaced fractures of the olecranon represent a functional disruption of the triceps mechanism, resulting in loss of active elbow extension. Anteriorly, the olecranon forms the greater sigmoid (semilunar) notch of the ulna, which articulates with the trochlea. The most proximal anterior portion of the ulna is the coronoid process, which lends stability to the elbow joint.

Olecranon fractures may result from a direct blow (fall on to the tip of the elbow) resulting in a comminuted olecranon fracture, or fall onto an outstretched arm accompanied by a strong, sudden triceps contraction resulting in a transverse or oblique fracture. Careful neurovascular exam followed by AP and lateral radiographs should be part of the initial evaluation. A true lateral radiograph should be carefully scrutinized for the extent of the fracture, any displacement of the radial head (the radial head should point toward the capitellum in all views; if this is not the case subluxation or dislocation is present), degree of comminution and articular surface involvement. Olecranon fractures are classified based on fracture pattern (transverse, transverse-impacted, oblique, comminuted, oblique-distal, or fracture dislocation) or according to the Mayo classification: type I (nondisplaced or minimally displaced), type II (displacement without elbow instability), type III (fracture with features of elbow instability). The goals of treatment are to restore articular congruity, restoration, and preservation of the elbow extensor mechanism and range of motion.

Nondisplaced fractures or displaced fractures in the elderly with poor preinjury function can be managed with closed treatment in a long-arm splint or cast with the elbow flexed from 45-90 degrees. Careful follow-up with radiographs should be done at weekly intervals for at least 2 weeks. In general, there is sufficient stability at 3 weeks to allow early motion from full extension to 90 degrees of flexion, with progression of flexion at 6 weeks. Of note some authors are advocating earlier range of motion at one week out from injury to prevent stiffness.

Indications for surgery include any disruption of the extensor mechanism (any displaced fracture) or articular incongruity. Multiple surgical options are available, including intramedullary fixation, tension band wiring, plate and screws, and excision. Postoperatively the patient should be placed in a posterior splint with early range of motion.

The most frequent complication of these fractures is prominent implants that subsequently require removal after healing has occurred. Elbow stiffness and loss of fixation have also been reported.

Coronoid Fractures

The coronoid process is the anterior beak-shaped portion of the ulna, forming the buttress anteriorly of the greater sigmoid notch. The anterior portion of the MCL attaches here, as well as a portion of the anterior capsule, contributing to elbow stability.

Isolated fractures of the coronoid are uncommon and are more frequently associated with posterior elbow dislocations or other fractures about the elbow. The mechanism of injury is usually forced posterior displacement of the proximal ulna as with a dislocation or hyperextension force of the elbow. Oblique radiographs may aid evaluation of these fractures as they are sometimes difficult to see on lateral and anteroposterior views.

These fractures have been classified by Regan and Morrey based on the size of the fracture fragment (Figure 40–8): type I (coronoid process tip avulsion), type II (single or comminuted fragment involving 50% or less of the coronoid process), type III (a single or comminuted fragment involving > 50% of the process). Type I fractures can be treated with immobilization in flexion for 3 weeks (or less if the fragment

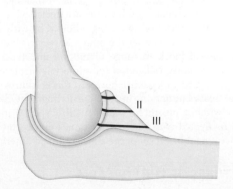

▲ **Figure 40–8.** Coronoid fractures. The coronoid fracture has been classified into three types by Regan and Morrey. (Reproduced, with permission, from Browner B et al: *Skeletal Trauma.* Saunders, 1992.)

and elbow are stable). Associated fractures should be treated as appropriate in each case with the goal of fracture stability for early range of motion. Isolated coronoid fractures without elbow instability can be treated in the same way as type I fractures. Unstable type II fractures and type III fractures usually require operative intervention.

FRACTURES OF THE PROXIMAL RADIUS

▶ Radial Head Fractures

Radial head fractures typically result from a fall on an outstretched arm causing an axial load collision between the radial head and capitellum. Patients typically present with limited elbow and forearm motion, along with pain with passive range of motion of the forearm. The forearm and wrist should be examined for any tenderness which may indicate the presence of an Essex-Lopresti type injury (radial head-fracture dislocation with associated interosseous ligament and distal radioulnar joint disruption). After documentation of neurovascular status, anteroposterior, lateral, and radial head view radiographs should be evaluated for fracture. Nondisplaced fractures should be suspected if a fat pad sign is present without obvious fracture. If Essex-Lopresti injury is suspected, additional radiographs of the forearm and wrist are indicated as well.

The Mason classification system is used to describe these fractures (Figure 40–9): type I (nondisplaced fractures), type II (marginal fractures with displacement), type III (comminuted fractures involving the entire radial head), and type IV (fracture associated with elbow dislocation).

Assessment of range of motion and stability to valgus stress is critical and can be performed after aspiration of the hemarthrosis and injection of lidocaine. This can be done through direct lateral needle insertion at the "soft spot" between the olecranon, radial head, and capitellum. Any mechanical block to motion should be carefully documented, as this can affect treatment decision-making.

Most isolated radial head fractures are treated with a brief period of immobilization in a sling followed by early range of motion 24-48 hours after the injury. Surgery is indicated for mechanical block to range of motion and type three fractures. A relative indication for surgery is displacement of a large fragment (> 2 mm); however, this is controversial. Surgical treatment options include ORIF, fragment excision with or without prosthetic replacement. Type IV injuries should be treated with closed reduction, followed by additional treatment based off of the above outlined criteria.

FRACTURES OF THE FOREARM

Forearm fractures are more common in men than women, secondary to a higher incidence of motor vehicle collisions, athletic injury, altercations, and falls from height experienced by men. The forearm acts as a ring: a fracture that

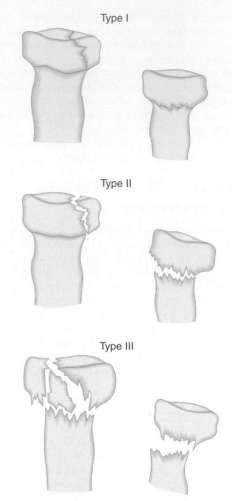

▲ **Figure 40–9.** Radial head fractures. The modified Mason classification system for radial head fractures. (Reproduced, with permission, from Browner B et al: *Skeletal Trauma*. Saunders, 1992.)

significantly shortens the radius or ulna will cause disruption of the proximal radio-ulnar joint or distal radio-ulnar joint. The ulna acts as an axis around which the laterally bowed radius rotates during supination and pronation. The interosseous membrane occupies the space between the radius and ulna; it provides a significant contribution to forearm stability.

Clinical assessment includes careful neurovascular exam (median, radial, and ulnar nerves) and assessment of any open wounds (even superficial wounds) can expose an ulna fracture to the outside world due to its subcutaneous position. Practitioners should have a high index of suspicion for compartment syndrome, if pain out of proportion, tense compartments, or pain on passive stretch is present.

Both-bone forearm fractures or fracture of one bone with concomitant injury to the elbow or wrist joint are more common than a fracture to either bone in isolation. As a result, it is crucial to obtain anteroposterior and lateral radiographs of the forearm that include both the wrist and elbow joints. The radial head must be aligned with the capitellum on all views to rule-out subluxation or dislocation.

Forearm fractures can be classified from a descriptive standpoint (closed vs. open, location, comminuted, segmental, multifragmented, displacement, angulated, and rotational alignment).

FRACTURES OF THE SHAFT OF THE RADIUS

▶ Isolated Radial Shaft Fractures

Radial shaft fractures can result from direct trauma or indirect trauma such as a fall on an outstretched hand. Although, isolated fractures of the proximal two-thirds of the radius are possible, a fracture of the distal one-third should raise high suspicion for concomitant injury to the distal radial-ulna joint (DRUJ). Nondisplaced fractures can be managed closed in a long-arm cast. Any displacement, loss of radial bow, or concomitant injury to the DRUJ is surgical indications. Fractures of the radius are typically fixed with open reduction internal fixation with 3.5 mm DCP plates.

This is a fracture of the shaft of the radius (most commonly the distal third) in conjunction with a distal radioulnar joint injury. Wrist pain on physical examination should arouse suspicion. The diagnosis should be confirmed radiographically. DRUJ disruption is suggested by the following radiographic findings: fracture at the base of the ulnar styloid, widening of the distal radioulnar joint space on the anteroposterior radiograph, subluxation of the ulna, and radial shortening greater than 5 mm relative to the distal ulna.

In adults, these injuries should always be treated surgically with open reduction and internal fixation, along with intraoperative evaluation of the DRUJ. After fixing the radius, if the joint is stable through full pronation and supination, only short-term immobilization in a splint is required to protect the incision. If the joint can be reduced but is unstable with rotation, additional surgical treatment is necessary. If there is a repairable ulnar styloid fracture, then open reduction with internal fixation of this piece will result in a stable DRUJ. If there is no ulnar styloid fracture but the distal radioulnar joint is reducible but unstable with rotation, then two 0.0625-inch Kirschner wires are used to pin the distal ulna to the radius in a reduced position (usually supination). With both open reduction with internal fixation of the ulnar styloid and the use of transfixing pins, the forearm should be immobilized in full supination in an above-elbow cast or brace for 4-6 weeks. The transfixing pins are removed prior to allowing forearm range of motion. Rarely, the distal radioulnar joint cannot be reduced. In this instance, a dorsal approach to the joint is used to extract interposed tissues (extensor carpi ulnaris is most common) blocking reduction.

FRACTURES OF THE SHAFT OF THE ULNA

▶ Isolated Ulnar Shaft Fractures (Nightstick Fractures)

Ulna night stick fractures usually results from a direct blow to the ulna along its subcutaneous border. Careful neurovascular examination and radiographs of the forearm including the wrist and elbow are essential. Radiographs should be carefully scrutinized for elbow dislocation; the radial head should point to the capitellum in all views or a Monteggia variant may be present. Nondisplaced or minimally displaced fractures may be treated acutely in a sugar tong splint. When swelling has subsided (after 7-10 days), the patient's arm can be transitioned to a long-arm cast or functional brace. Displaced fractures (> 10 degrees of angulation or > 50% displacement of the shaft) are best treated surgically with open reduction internal fixation.

▶ Monteggia's Fracture

Monteggia's fracture is a fracture of the proximal ulna with a radial head dislocation. Thorough neurovascular exam is necessary; injuries to the radial nerve or posterior interosseous nerve have been described. The Bado classification is based of the direction of the radial head dislocation: type I (anterior), type II (posterior), type III (lateral or anterolateral), and type IV (anterior dislocation with a fracture of the radius and ulna) (Figure 40–10).

Closed reduction and casting of Monteggia fractures should only be attempted in children. These injuries are typically treated with open reduction internal fixation with plates and screws. Of note failure of the ulna to reduce may indicate annular ligament interposition. If open reduction of the radial head is necessary, consideration should be given toward repairing the annular ligament. Postoperatively, if the repair is considered stable, the patient can be placed in a posterior splint for 7-10 days, followed by beginning range of motion exercises.

▶ Both-Bone Forearm Fractures

Fractures of both radius and ulna are usually the result of high energy mechanisms (motor vehicle accidents or fall from a height). The fractures are most often displaced. Careful examination to rule out neurovascular injury and compartment syndrome should be performed. Radiographs of the entire forearm including the elbow and wrist are necessary.

Treatment for both-bone forearm fractures in adults consists of open reduction and internal fixation with compression plating using 3.5-mm dynamic plates. The goal of plate fixation is to restore: the normal ulnar and radial length, rotational alignment, and radial bow (which have

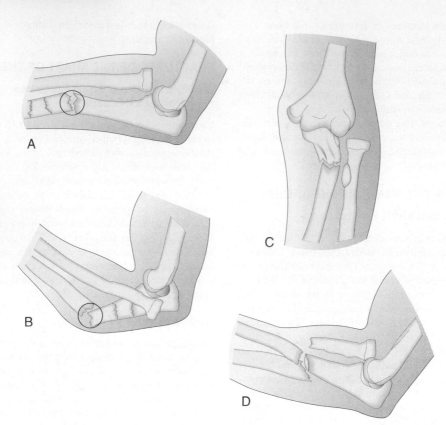

▲ **Figure 40–10.** Monteggia's fractures. The classification of Monteggia lesions by Bado. **A.** Type I: anterior angulation of the ulnar fracture and anterior dislocation of the radial head. **B.** Type II: posterior angulation of the ulnar fracture and anterior dislocation of the radial head. **C.** Type III: fracture of the proximal ulna metaphysis and lateral dislocation of the radial head. **D.** Type IV: anterior dislocation of the radial head and fracture of the radial and ulnar shafts. (Reproduced, with permission, from Browner B et al: *Skeletal Trauma*. Saunders, 1992.)

been shown to be essential for rotation of the arm). With solid fixation, active range of motion of the forearm and elbow can be started at 10-14 days. Open fractures can also be treated successfully with these methods. However, if there is excessive soft tissue damage or wound contamination, the use of an external fixator may be a preferable option.

Complications of this fracture include nonunion, malunion, infection, neurovascular injury, compartment syndrome, synostosis, and loss of motion.

INJURIES OF THE WRIST REGION

▶ Anatomy

The distal radius has three articulations: the sigmoid notch which articulates with the ulna, and facets for the scaphoid and lunate bones. The base of the ulna styloid serves as an insertion point for the triangular fibrocartilage complex (TFCC) which is the primary stabilizer of the DRUJ. Normally, 80%

of the axial load is supported by the distal radius and 20% by the ulna and TFCC. There are six dorsal compartments of the wrist that contain wrist and digital extensor tendons. On the volar surface, the pronator quadratus lies across the distal radius and ulna. Just anterior to the pronator quadratus are the contents of the carpal canal, containing nine digital flexor tendons and the median nerve. Anterior to the transverse carpal ligament lie the flexor carpi radialis, flexor carpi ulnaris, and palmaris longus muscles. Guyon's canal contains the ulnar nerve and artery. It is bounded by the volar retinacular ligament and flexor retinacular ligament, the hook of the hamate radially, and the pisiform ulnarly.

Extrinsic ligaments connect the radius to the carpus and the carpus to the metacarpals. The proximal row of carpal bones consisting of the scaphoid, lunate, triquetrum, and pisiform bones, are attached to the distal radius via two sets of radiocarpal ligaments (volar and distal). The volar radiocarpal ligaments (radioscaphocapitate, radioschapolunate, radiolunate, and radiolunotriquetral) are stronger and confer more stability to the radiocarpal articulation when compared to the dorsal radiocarpal ligaments. The radiocarpal joint is the primary joint for wrist motion (70 degrees of flexion/extension, 20 and 40 degrees of radial and ulnar deviation, respectively).

Intrinsic ligaments connect carpal bone to carpal bone (eg, scapholunate, etc). The distal carpal row, consisting of the trapezium, trapezoid, capitate, and hamate, is connected to each other and the base of the metacarpals with strong extrinsic ligaments. As a result, the distal carpal row is relatively immobile. The lunate is the key to carpal stability; injury to the scapholunate or lunotriquetral ligaments leads to unstable motion of the lunate and generalized carpal instability. Disruption of the scapholunate ligament or scaphoid fracture can lead to excessive dorsiflexion of the lunate and triquetrum (dorsal intercalated segmental instability). Injury to the lunotriquetral ligament leads to volar flexion of the lunate (volar intercalated segmental instability). The space of Poirer (ligament-free area between the capitate and lunate) is a potential area of weakness.

Normal anatomic relationships include radial inclination of 23 degrees, 11 mm of radial length, 11-12 degrees of palmar tilt, a 0 degree capitolunate angle (straight line drawn from the shaft of the third metacarpal, through the capitate and lunate with the wrist in a neutral position), a 47 degree scapholunate angle, and less than 2 mm of scapholunate space.

The vascular supply to the wrist consists of the radial, ulnar, and anterior interosseous arteries intertwining to form a network of arterial arches on the volar and dorsal surfaces of the carpal bones. The radial artery gives off branches that supply the scaphoid volarly (supplies distal scaphoid) and dorsally (supplies proximal scaphoid). The lunate typically receives blood supply from dorsal and volar surface branches.

1. Distal Radius Fracture

▶ Epidemiology

More than 450,000 distal radius fractures occur annually in the United States, representing one-sixth of all fractures treated in emergency departments. The incidence of distal radius fractures increases with old age and osteopenia.

▶ Mechanism

The most common mechanism for a distal radius fracture is fall on to an outstretched dorsiflexed hand. High-energy mechanisms such as motor vehicle collisions and falls from height can result in highly displaced or significantly comminuted fractures in younger patients.

▶ Clinical Evaluation

Patients typically present with a swollen, ecchymotic, tender wrist. Deformity of the wrist is variable with dorsal displacement of the distal segment (Colles fracture) being more common than volar (Smith-type fracture). The ipsilateral elbow and shoulder should be carefully evaluated for concomitant injury. Careful neurovascular examination is paramount including the motor and sensory median, ulnar, and radial nerve distributions (Motor: a-ok, finger spread, and thumbs up signs; Sensory: volar aspect of the thumb, index, middle fingers, volar aspect of the small finger, and dorsal aspect of the thumb). Particular attention should be given to median nerve function as carpal tunnel syndrome is a relatively common complication (13%-23%) due to traction injury, fracture fragment trauma, hematoma, or increased compartment pressure.

▶ Radiographic Evaluation

Posteroanterior and lateral views of the wrist should be obtained. Elbow and shoulder symptoms should also be evaluated radiographically. Contralateral wrist views may be used for comparison ulnar variance and the DRUJ. Computed tomography scan can be useful for further characterization of intra-articular involvement and preoperative planning. Normal radiographic relationships include the following averages: 23 degrees of radial inclination, 11 mm of radial length, and 11 degrees of palmar or volar tilt.

▶ Classification

Distal radius fractures can be characterized descriptively—open versus closed, displacement, angulation, comminution, and loss of radial length. The Frykman classification organizes these fractures based on the degree of articular involvement as well concomitant fracture of the distal ulna (Figure 40–11). Higher classification fractures have worse prognoses.

AO/ASIF CLASSIFICATION OF DISTAL RADIUS FRACTURES

Type A: Extra-articular fractures
1. Isolated distal ulnar fracture
2. Simple radius fracture
3. Radial fracture with metaphysial impaction

Type B: Intra-articular complex fracture
1. Radial styloid fracture
2. Dorsal rim fracture
3. Volar rim fracture

Type C: Intra-articular complex fracture
1. Metaphysial fracture with radiocarpal congruity preserved
2. Articular displacement
3. Diaphysial-metaphysial involvement

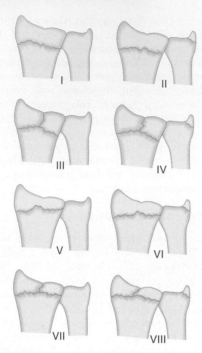

▲ **Figure 40–11.** Frykman classification of distal radius fractures. Types I, III, V, and VII do not have an associated fracture of the distal ulna. Fractures III-VIII are intra-articular fractures. Higher classification fractures have worse prognoses. (Reproduced, with permission, from Green D, Hotchkiss R, Pederson W: *Green's Operative Hand Surgery.* Churchill Livingstone, 1993.)

▶ Treatment

Emergent operative management is indicated for open fractures. Acute surgical intervention should be considered for distal radius fractures complicated by carpal tunnel syndrome that is not relieved with closed reduction.

▶ Nonoperative Treatment

All distal radius fractures should undergo closed reduction, even if surgical intervention is expected. The benefits of fracture reduction include limiting postinjury swelling, pain relief, and median nerve decompression. Although casting may be considered for nondisplaced or minimally displaced fractures with minimal swelling, a sugar-tong splint is generally preferred encompassing the dorsal and volar aspects of the wrist, limiting subsequent forearm rotation and possible fracture displacement. One week post injury the patient may be transitioned to a long-arm cast. If closed treatment is planned, radiographic evaluation should be done on a weekly basis for the first two to three weeks to monitor for displacement. Acceptable radiographic parameters for continued closed treatment include: radial length within 2-3 mm of the contra-

lateral wrist, neutral palmar tilt (0 degrees), intra-articular step off less than 2 mm, and radial inclination less than 5-degree loss. Surgery is indicated if reduction with respect to the above stated parameters cannot be achieved or maintained.

▶ Closed Reduction Technique

Hematoma block, Bier block, or conscious sedation can be used to provide analgesia. Hematoma block offers the benefit of speed and does not require that the patient have been without oral intake for a significant amount of time. Conscious sedation offers the benefit of muscle relaxation facilitating reduction. Initially manual or fingertrap-assisted traction is applied facilitating reduction via ligamentotaxis. For dorsally tilted fractures, volar directed pressure is applied to the distal fracture segment. C-arm if available can be used to assess fracture reduction. Once reduction is adequate a well-molded long-arm ("sugar tong") splint can be applied with the wrist in neutral and the metacarpaphalangeal joints free.

▶ Techniques of Surgical Management

Many surgical options are available. Choice of operation is determined by several factors, including the fracture pattern, bone quality, and surgeon preference.

▶ Closed Reduction Percutaneous Pinning

Reduction is achieved via closed means, followed by fixation typically with 0.0625-inch Kirschner wires. Interfragmentary technique entails wires used to stabilize a fracture and prevent collapse after reduction is achieved. With intrafocal technique where these wires are driven into the fracture site, used to lever the pieces achieving reduction, and then driven through the opposite cortex to maintain reduction. Postoperatively patients are placed in a splint or cast. The wires are typically removed after 6 weeks once bone healing is appreciated radiographically.

▶ External Fixation

This technique uses ligamentotaxis to restore radial length and radial inclination, but it rarely restores palmar tilt. It is especially useful for treating very comminuted or intra-articular fractures where there are several small pieces. External fixation is also useful for treating open fractures with severe tissue compromise or as a temporizing measure when a patient has other critical medical issues that need immediate attention.

▶ Open Reduction and Internal Fixation

In recent years, volar plating has become much more popular compared to dorsal plating due to its advantages when treating distal radius fractures with significant dorsal comminution, as well as the extensor tendon complications associated with dorsal plating of the distal radius.

▶ Complications

Stiffness of the wrist and digits is common. Patients should be instructed to begin range of motion exercises for the digits immediately after the fracture is initially treated. Include median nerve dysfunction, malunion, nonunion, stiffness, posttraumatic arthritis, tendon rupture, finger, wrist, and elbow stiffness. Articular congruity post surgical fixation is critical for avoiding the development of posttraumatic arthritis.

▶ Isolated Radial Styloid Fracture

Also called a "chauffeur's fracture," "backfire fracture," or "Hutchinson fracture" this is an avulsion fracture with extrinsic ligaments remaining attached to the styloid fragment. This injury is often associated with intercarpal ligamentous injuries such as scapholunate dislocation or perilunate dislocation. This injury often requires open reduction with internal fixation.

FRACTURES OF THE ULNAR STYLOID

Fractures of the ulnar styloid are commonly seen in conjunction with distal radius fractures and can also be seen in isolation. Fractures of the tip of the ulnar styloid are often too small to fix. However, large fragments (the entire styloid from its base) may be indicative of a TFCC disruption that can lead to DRUJ instability. As a result, these displaced fractures should be treated with open reduction and internal fixation.

DISTAL RADIOULNAR JOINT DISLOCATION

DRUJ dislocation is discussed earlier in the section describing the Galeazzi fracture. DRUJ dislocation can also occur with a simple distal radius fracture. Careful examination of radiographs and the distal radioulnar joint will keep the clinician from missing this injury in the face of a distal radius fracture.

FRACTURES & DISLOCATIONS OF THE CARPUS

Most carpal bone fractures occur in the proximal carpal row, with the scaphoid being the carpal bone most commonly fractured. Carpal bone fractures usually occur in younger people, often from high energy falls on an outstretched hand Wrist radiographs can be difficult to interpret, and careful scrutiny is necessary so as not to miss these injuries. In addition to the standard anteroposterior, lateral, and oblique views of the wrist, special radiographic views such as a scaphoid view (anteroposterior radiograph with the wrist supinated 30 degrees and in ulnar deviation), clenched fist view (to evaluate for carpal instability), or carpal tunnel view can often be helpful. Computed tomography is also useful to identify fractures if radiographs are inconclusive; MRI is sensitive for detecting occult fractures, osteonecrosis of carpal bones, and soft injuries including disruption of the scapholunate ligament or TFCC.

1. Fracture of the Scaphoid

The scaphoid is the carpal bone most commonly fractured. Anatomically, the scaphoid is divided into proximal and distal poles, a tubercle, and a waist. The blood supply for the scaphoid comes largely from branches of the radial artery traveling from a distal to proximal location. As a result, fractures of the scaphoid at the waist or more proximal are particularly prone to nonunion or avascular necrosis.

Fractures of the scaphoid most commonly occur as a result of a fall on an outstretched hand. Patients typically present with pain on the radial side of their wrist and tenderness to palpation over the anatomic snuffbox. Physical examination maneuvers include the scaphoid lift test (reproduction of pain with dorsal-volar shifting of the scaphoid) and the Watson test (painful dorsal scaphoid displacement as the wrist is moved from ulnar to radial deviation with compression of the tuberosity). Radiographic evaluation includes a "scaphoid view," in addition to the standard wrist series. Initial radiographs are nondiagnostic in up to 25% of cases. As a result, if clinical exam suggests a scaphoid fracture, it is appropriate to employ a trial of immobilization with repeat radiographs in 1-2 weeks. Additionally, technetium bone scan, MRI, or CT scan can be used to diagnose occult scaphoid fractures that continue to not be visualized on radiograph, despite persistent pain. Scaphoid fractures can be classified based on the pattern (horizontal oblique, transverse, vertical oblique), displacement (nondisplaced fractures with no step-off are considered stable, displaced fractures > 1 mm, scapholunate angulation > 60 degrees, radiolunate angulation > 15 degrees), and location (tuberosity, distal pole, waist, and proximal pole). Nondisplaced fractures should be treated in a long-arm thumb spica cast for 6 weeks. After 6 weeks, the patient's wrist can be placed in a short-arm spica cast until the fracture is united. Expected time to union for distal third fractures is 6-8 weeks, 8-12 weeks for middle third fractures, and 12-24 weeks for proximal third fractures. Surgical indications include fracture displacement more than 1 mm, radiolunate angle more than 15 degrees, scapholunate angle more than 60 degrees, humpback deformity, or nonunion. Complications of scaphoid fractures include fracture nonunion or avascular necrosis (Figure 40–12). Patients with long-standing scaphoid nonunions go on to develop early arthritis of the radioscaphoid joint secondary to altered mechanics of the wrist.

2. Fracture of the Lunate

The lunate is the carpal bone most likely to dislocate, but fractures are rare. Fractures usually result from a fall on an outstretched hand. Patients typically present with tenderness to palpation over the volar wrist overlying the distal radius and lunate with painful range of motion. Radiographs are usually not helpful due to overlapping densities of multiple bones; CT, MRI, or bone scan are usually required to

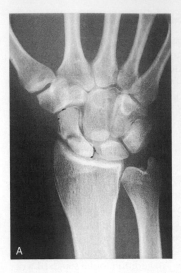
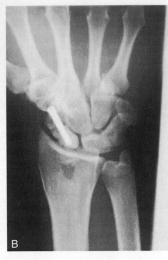

▲ **Figure 40–12.** Scaphoid fracture.
A. Scaphoid fracture nonunion. **B.** Open reduction and internal fixation of scaphoid nonunion.

make the diagnosis. Nondisplaced fractures can be treated in a short- or long-arm cast. Displaced or angulated fractures require surgical treatment. Osteonecrosis (Keinbock's disease), can complicate this injury leading to advanced collapse and radiocarpal degeneration. Several surgical treatments are available for this sequella.

3. Fracture of the Hamate

This fracture generally occurs from a direct blow to the area such as occurs when swinging a baseball bat or golf club that suddenly comes to an abrupt stop as it encounters a firm surface. Patients present with ulnar-sided hand pain over the hamate. Fracture will often not be seen on routine wrist and hand radiographs. A carpal tunnel view (20 degree supination oblique view of the wrist) should be obtained if this fracture is suspected. If the diagnosis is suspected clinically but the radiographs show no fracture, a CT scan may be helpful. Nondisplaced fractures may be treated in a short-arm cast for six weeks. Displaced fractures of the body can be treated with open reduction internal fixation with screws or wires.

4. Other Carpal Bone Fractures

Fractures can occur in any of the other carpal bones as well, but much less commonly. Triquetral avulsion or dorsal impaction fractures can occur from falls on the outstretched hand. Isolated fractures of the remaining carpal bones are rare and generally occur with high-energy trauma and other injuries.

5. Traumatic Carpal Instability

Severe injury to the wrist causing damage to the complex ligamentous structures may lead to carpal bone dissociation, carpal dislocations, and fracture dislocations. The lunate is often called the "carpal keystone"; its ligamentous attachments to the radius and other carpal bones make a significant contribution to radiocarpal stability. A sequence of progressive perilunate instability starts with scapholunate disruption (stage I), then midcarpal or capitolunate disruption (stage II), lunotriquetral disruption (stage III), ending in disruption of the radiolunate joint leading to volar lunate dislocation (stage IV).

Scapholunate dissociation secondary to disruption of the scapholunate and the radioscapholunate ligament leads to altered kinematics of the wrist and early degenerative arthritis. Clinical findings include volar wrist tenderness/bruising, positive Watson test, pain with grasping, and decreased grip strength. Radiographically, widening of the scapholunate space more than 3 mm ("Terry Thomas" sign), or scapholunate angle more than 70 degrees on the lateral are indicative of scapholunate disruption. Closed reduction with an audible, palpable click followed by thumb spica immobilization for 8 weeks is the first line of treatment. Inability to obtain or maintain reduction is surgical indications.

Lunotriquetral dissociation occurs as a result of disruption of the radiolunotriquetral ligament. Patients typically present with swelling over the peritriquetral area and tenderness dorsally, typically 1-2 cm distal to the ulnar head. Radiographs may show disruption of the normal proximal carpal row contour; frank gapping of the lunotriquetral space is rarely seen. Treatment with a short arm cast for 6-8 weeks or closed reduction with pinning of the lunate to the triquetrum is warranted.

Carpal dislocations represent a continuum of perilunate ligamentous injury with frank lunate dislocation being the final stage. Patients present with severe wrist pain and swelling after trauma. Most dislocations can be diagnosed with adequate AP and lateral views of the wrist. With a perilunate dislocation, the lunate remains in its normal position, articulating with the distal radius, but is angled in a volar direction, and the rest of the carpus is dislocated. With lunate dislocation, on the lateral radiograph the lunate will be volar to the rest of the carpus and not in alignment with the distal radius. Treatment of carpal dislocations is accomplished with closed reduction of the midcarpal joint via traction combined with direct manual pressure over the capitate and lunate. Irreducible dislocations or unstable injuries should be treated surgically with open reduction internal fixation.

Ulnocarpal dissociation may result from disruption of the TFCC, where the lunate and triquetrum assume a supinated and palmar flexed position, while the distal ulna subluxes dorsally. Radiographs may show ulnar styloid avulsion or dorsal displacement of the ulna; MRI may demonstrate TFCC tear. Treatment requires operative repair of the TFCC and/or ORIF of large displaced ulnar styloid fragments.

Even with the best care, carpal bone and ligament injuries can be devastating, with long-term sequelae of pain, stiffness, and early arthritis.

FRACTURES & DISLOCATIONS ABOUT THE HAND

Metacarpal and phalangeal fractures are relatively common comprising a significant portion of emergency department visits. The significant variation in mechanism of injury accounts for the large number of different types of fracture patterns seen in hand injuries. Axial load or "jamming" injuries often result in shearing articular fractures or metaphyseal compression fractures, sometimes with concomitant injury to the carpus, forearm, elbow, and shoulder due to force transmission. Injury mechanisms with a bending component result in diaphyseal fractures or joint dislocations. Individual digits or joints caught in clothing or equipment can result in spiral fractures or complex dislocations. Industrial settings with heavy objects predispose to crushing mechanisms of injury. The direction of fracture angulation depends on the deforming forces caused by attached muscle. The palmar and dorsal interosseous muscles arise from the metacarpal shafts, usually flexing the fracture causing apex-dorsal angulation. Proximal phalanx fractures typically angulate in the opposite direction, apex-volar. Middle phalanx fractures angulate variably, while distal phalanx fractures are usually comminuted tuft fractures resulting from crush injuries. Clinical evaluation includes documentation of the patient's age, hand dominance, occupation, mechanism of injury, time of injury, exposure to contamination, and financial issues (workman's compensation). Physical examination should document neurovascular status, and pay particular attention range of motion, angulation, and malrotation (best evaluated when the intervening joint is flexed to 90 degrees). Radiographic evaluation includes AP, lateral, and oblique radiographs of the hand and the specific injured digit. Fractures can be classified descriptively: open versus closed, location, fracture pattern (comminuted, transverse, spiral, vertical split, extra-articular versus intra-articular, stable versus unstable, and angulational or rotational deformity. Fractures of the small

bones of the hand heal more rapidly than fractures of larger bones, and prolonged immobilization can cause stiffness and loss of motion that can be difficult or impossible to regain. As a result, fractures of the metacarpals and phalanges should not be immobilized for more than 3 weeks except under rare circumstances, due to subsequent development of stiffness. The safe position for splinting or casting of the hand is with slight wrist extension, the MP joints flexed 60-90 degrees, and the PIP and DIP joints extended. This "intrinsic plus" position, puts the ligaments of the hand on maximum stretch, avoiding posttreatment stiffness.

1. Open Fractures, Fight Bite, and Animal Bites

These types of fractures require special consideration. Open fractures of phalanges or metacarpals can be classified according to the Swanson, Stabo and Anderson classification: type I (clean wound without significant contamination or delay in treatment), type II (contamination with gross dirt/debris, human or animal bite, lake/river injury, barnyard injury or in patients with significant systemic illness such as diabetes, hypertension, rheumatoid arthritis [RA], hepatitis, or asthma). Type I injuries can be treated with primary internal fixation and immediate wound closure. Although type II injuries can be treated with primary internal fixation (no increase in infection rate); these injuries should not be closed primarily. Delayed closure is preferred to decrease infection risk.

Any laceration overlying a joint in the hand, particularly the metacarpal-phalangeal (MCP) joint must be suspected as being caused by a human tooth. Also known as a "fight bite," these injuries should be assumed to have been contaminated with oral flora and treated aggressively with broad spectrum antibiotics including anaerobic coverage. Animal bites require antibiotic treatment that covers Pasteurella and Eikenella.

2. Metacarpal Fractures

▶ Metacarpal Head Fractures

Fractures of the metacarpal can be subclassified as follows: epiphyseal fractures, collateral ligament avulsion fractures, oblique, vertical, and horizontal head fractures, comminuted fractures, and fractures with joint loss. Most of these fractures require anatomic reduction to reestablish joint congruity and avoid posttraumatic arthritis. Stable reductions of fractures may be splinted in the intrinsic plus position. If unstable, percutaneous pinning, ORIF, or external fixation are options.

▶ Metacarpal Neck Fractures

Metacarpal neck fractures are typically caused by direct trauma with volar comminution and dorsal apex angulation. The most common metacarpal neck fracture is the "boxer's fracture" of the fifth metacarpal, usually caused by the fist striking a stationary object. These fractures can typically be closed reduced successfully. The degree of acceptable deformity varies according to the metacarpal injured: less than 10 degrees for the second and third metacarpal, less than 30-40 degrees for the fourth and fifth metacarpals. Unstable fractures require surgical intervention with percutaneous pinning or open reduction internal fixation.

Metacarpal Shaft Fractures

Nondisplaced or minimally displaced metacarpal shaft fractures can be reduced and splinted. Surgical indications include rotational deformity (all fingers should point toward the scaphoid when flexed), dorsal angulation more than 10 degrees for second and third metacarpals, and more than 40 degrees for fourth and fifth metacarpals.

Metacarpal Base

Fractures of the base of the second, third, and fourth metacarpals are typically minimally displaced and treated with splinting and early range of motion. A reverse Bennett fracture is a fracture dislocation of the fifth metacarpal and hamate bones. This injury often requires ORIF.

Fractures of the thumb metacarpal base can be extra-articular or intra-articular. Extra-articular fractures are usually transverse or oblique, and amenable to closed reduction and casting. Unstable fractures may require percutaneous pinning. Intra-articular fractures come in two types: type I or **Benett's Fracture** where a single fracture line separates the majority of the metacarpal from the volar lip fragment and type II also known as **Rolondo's fracture** which is a comminuted intra-articular fracture usually with a "Y" or "T" pattern including dorsal and palmar fragments. Both type I and type II fractures are treated with closed reduction and percutaneous pinning or ORIF.

3. Proximal and Middle Phalanx Fractures

Intra-articular fractures can be classified as condylar fractures or fracture-dislocations. There are three types of condylar fractures: unicondylar, bicondylar, or osteochondral. Each of these fractures require anatomic reduction; ORIF should be performed for more than 1 mm displacement. Comminuted intra-articular fractures not amenable to surgical treatment, can be treated closed with early protected mobilization.

Fracture dislocations come in two varieties: volar lip fracture or dorsal lip fracture. Volar lip fracture (dorsal fracture-dislocation) treatment is controversial; if less than 35% of the articular surface is involved the injury may be treated with buddy taping, however, for more than 35% some recommend ORIF or volar plate arthroplasty if the fracture is comminuted while others recommend extension block splint if the joint is not subluxed. Dorsal lip fracture

(volar fracture-dislocation) with less than 1 mm of displacement may be treated closed with splinting while more than 1 mm displacement requires operative intervention.

Extra-articular fractures of the phalanges should be initially treated with closed reduction with finger-trap traction and splinting. Unstable fractures should be treated surgically.

Distal phalynx fractures

Intra-articular dorsal lip fractures may be complicated by an extensor tendon disruption resulting in a "mallet finger." "Mallet finger" may also result from purely tendinous disruption, without fracture. For either scenario, treatment is controversial. Some recommend full-time extension splinting for 6-8 weeks, while others recommend surgical intervention. For professionals who work extensively with their hands, such as surgeons, full-time extension splinting is not practical. Closed reduction with percutaneous pinning is a good option.

Intra-articular volar lip fractures can be associated with a flexor digitorum profundus rupture resulting in a "jersey finger" often seen in football or rugby players, most commonly involving the ring finger. Treatment is typically surgical, especially if large displaced bony fragments are present.

Extra-articular fractures can be transverse, longitudinal, or comminuted (nail matrix injury very common). These fractures are usually treated with closed reduction and splinting that traverses the DIP joint, leaving the PIP joint free. Surgery is indicated for fractures with wide irreducible displacement, due to the increased risk of nonunion.

Nailbed Injuries

Nailbed injuries are easily missed in the context of distal phalynx fractures. When untreated, these injuries result in nail growth disturbances. Subungual hematomas are often indicative of nail bed injury. The nail plate should be removed and the hematoma drained. Nailbed disruptions should be carefully sutured with 6-0 chromic catgut under magnification. The nailplate should be replaced to keep the nail fold open; alternatively a piece of aluminum foil or xeroform gauze can be used.

4. Dislocations of the Digits

Carpometacarpal dislocations are usually high energy injuries. Careful neurovascular examination is essential. These injuries usually require surgical intervention for maintenance of a stable reduction.

MCP joint dislocations are usually dorsal in direction, presenting with a hyperextended posture. Simple dislocations can be reduced by flexion of the joint without traction. Wrist flexion, causing the flexor tendons to relax, can be used to facilitate the reduction maneuver. Complex MCP dislocations with the volar plate interposed in the joint are irreducible. The pathognomonic radiograph finding is the appearance of the sesamoid in the joint space. Complex dislocations require surgery. Traction during reduction of simple dislocations should be avoided as simple dislocations can be converted into complex ones. Volar dislocations are rare; however, because they are particularly unstable, they often require surgical intervention.

Thumb MCPs are unique due to the multiplanar motion of the thumb MCP joint. With a one-sided collateral ligament injury, the phalynx tends to sublux volarly rotating around the opposite intact ligament. The ulnar collateral ligament of the thumb MP joint is the most commonly injured ligament in the digits. If the injury is acute, it is called a "skier's thumb," whereas chronic injury from repetitive trauma is known as a "gamekeeper's thumb." Nonoperative treatment with reduction and thumb spica splinting or casting is usually sufficient. A "Stener" lesion occurs when the ulnar collateral ligament avulses, and comes to rest dorsal to the adductor aponeurosis. The ulnar collateral ligament is not able to return to its normal insertion, preventing healing. As a result, Stener lesions and irreducible MCP dislocations require surgical intervention.

Proximal interphalangeal (PIP) joint dislocations include dorsal dislocation, pure volar dislocation, and rotatory volar dislocation. Once reduced, rotatory volar dislocations, collateral ligament ruptures, and dorsal dislocations congruent in full extension on the lateral radiographs can all begin active range of motion exercises immediately with adjacent digit strapping. Dorsal dislocations that continue to sublux on lateral radiograph, can be treated with a few weeks of extension block splinting. Volar dislocations with central slip disruptions are treated with 4-6 weeks of PIP extension splinting, followed by an additional 2 weeks of night-time splinting. Irreducible dislocations or unstable reductions may require surgical intervention.

Distal interphalangeal (DIP) dislocations and thumb IP joint dislocations can present late. Injuries are considered chronic after 3 weeks. Acute reduced dislocations may begin immediate active range of motion. Unstable dislocations should be immobilized in 30 degrees of flexion for 3 weeks. Complete collateral ligament injury should be protected from lateral stress for at least 4 weeks. Recurrent stability can be treated with Kirschner wire fixation. Chronic dislocation may be treated with open reduction to resect scar tissue, allowing for a tension free reduction. Transverse open wounds in the volar skin crease are not infrequent. Open dislocations require debridement to prevent infection.

INJURIES OF THE HIP REGION

1. Hip Dislocations

Epidemiology

Hip dislocations of the native hip are relatively rare, usually due to high energy injury such as a motor vehicle accident. Posterior hip dislocations (85%-90%) are more common

than anterior (remaining 10%-15%). Ten to twenty percent of posterior hip dislocations can be complicated by sciatic nerve injury. Anterior hip dislocations are associated with a greater incidence of femoral head injury. Up to 50% of patients with a hip dislocation will sustain a concomitant fracture elsewhere (most commonly of the ipsilateral femur or pelvis).

Anatomy

The hip articulation is a ball-and-socket joint, formed by the femoral head and acetabulum. Forty percent of the femoral head is covered by the acetabulum. The labrum surrounding the acetabulum has the effect of deepening the hip joint, increasing its stability. The medial and lateral circumflex femoral arteries from the profunda femoral artery form an extracapsular vascular ring at the base of the femoral neck; ascending branches provide the primary blood supply to the femoral neck and head, along with a minor contribution from the ligamentum teres off of the obturator artery. The contribution of the medial and lateral circumflex arteries is often disrupted with hip dislocation, leading to long-term complications including avascular necrosis. The sciatic nerve exits the pelvis at the greater sciatic notch, traveling deep to the piriformis muscle, down the posterior aspect of the thigh.

Clinical Evaluation

A full trauma survey is essential due to the high energy nature of this injury. Patients typically present with severe discomfort and inability to move the injured extremity. The classic appearance of a posterior hip dislocation is shortened extremity with the hip flexed, internally rotated and adducted (Figure 40–13). Patients with an anterior dislocation hold

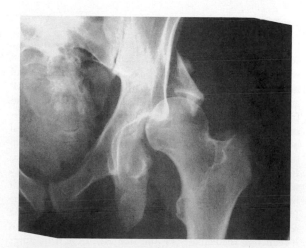

▲ **Figure 40–13.** Posterior hip dislocation with concomitant fracture of the posterior wall and weight-bearing dome of the acetabulum.

their hip with marked external rotation, mild flexion, and abduction. Careful neurovascular examination is key. If the sciatic nerve is injured often the tibial nerve is preserved with the peroneal portion of the nerve showing the effects of injury. Radiographic evaluation includes an AP view of the pelvis as well as radiographs of the entire ipsilateral femur. Evaluate the femoral neck and acetabulum to rule-out concomitant fractures.

▶ Treatment

The hip should be reduced emergently due to the risk of osteonecrosis from associated vascular disruption. Regardless of the direction of the dislocation, the hip can be reduced with in-line longitudinal traction with the patient supine. The key to successful reduction is relaxation of the patient's muscles which is accomplished with adequate sedation (ideally via general anesthesia, or iv sedation if general anesthesia is not available) and fatiguing of the patient's muscles that occurs with time. Following closed reduction, the hip should be examined for stability by flexing the hip to 90 degrees in neutral position and applying a posteriorly directed force. If any subluxation is detected, the hip is deemed unstable, and will require surgery or traction. Postreduction radiographs should be obtained to confirm reduction. Careful comparison should be made with the contralateral side, to determine of the reduction is concentric. Even slight asymmetry or subluxation may indicate the presence of a concomitant fracture or incarcerated piece of bone in the joint. Additionally, postreduction CT should be performed to investigate the presence of other fractures or an incarcerated bony fragment. If closed reduction is unsuccessful, open reduction should be performed as soon as possible.

▶ Fractures of the Femoral Head

Fractures of the femoral head are extremely rare. Most are secondary to motor vehicle accidents and are associated with hip dislocations. Clinical evaluation included careful neurovascular exam, AP view of the pelvis as well as AP and lateral radiographs of the injured hip. Femoral head fractures can be classified according to the Pipkin classification: type I (hip dislocation with fracture of the femoral head inferior to the vovea capitis femoris), type II (hip dislocation with fracture of the femoral head superior to the fovea capitis femoris), type III (type I or type II injury with femoral neck fracture), and type IV (type I or type II injury with associated fracture of the acetabular rim). Type I fractures involve the non–weight-bearing surface of the femoral head. As a result, closed treatment can be pursued if reduction is adequate (<1 mm step-off). Type II fractures involve the weight-bearing surface. Thus, if the reduction is not anatomic as seen on CT, surgical treatment should be pursued. Type III and type IV injuries usually require

surgical treatment. Complications include osteonecrosis and posttraumatic arthritis.

▶ The Femoral Neck

Approximately 350,000 fractures of the femoral neck occur each year. This number is expected to double by the year 2050 due to the aging demographics of the American population. Fractures of the femoral neck occur most often in elderly patients with osteopenic bone after a fall. Femoral neck fractures in patients less than 50 years old are rare, usually due high energy trauma. Patients with displaced fractures usually present with inability to walk, severe pain, and an externally rotated and shortened extremity. Patients with nondisplaced fractures may present with mild, persistent hip pain (for several days or couple of weeks); these patients often will have been walking, as a result index of suspicion should be high. A careful secondary survey should be performed, as 10% of elderly patients have associated upper extremity injuries. Radiographic evaluation includes AP pelvis radiograph, AP and lateral radiographs of the hip; and internal rotation or traction view can further delineate the fracture pattern. If no fractures are detected in an elderly patient with persistent hip pain, one should consider MRI or bone scan to look for a nondisplaced or incomplete fracture.

Fractures of the femoral neck may be classified according to location (subcapital, transcervical, and basicervical), or based on stability of the fracture pattern. The Pauwel's classification describes increasing instability of the increasing fracture angle from the horizontal: type I (30 degrees), type II (50 degrees), and type III (70 degrees). The garden classification describes four patterns: type I (incomplete fracture/valgus impacted), type II (complete fracture, nondisplaced), type III (complete fracture, with partial displacement, the trabecular bone pattern of the femoral head does not line up with the acetabulum), and type IV (completely displaced fracture, the trabecular bone pattern of the head does line up with the acetabulum).

Some authors advocate nonoperative treatment with limited weight-bearing for type I or valgus impacted fractures. Others advocate internal fixation with multiple screws to prevent fracture displacement. Type II (nondisplaced) fractures are treated with internal fixation, regardless of the patient's age. Treatment of type III and type IV (displaced) fractures is more controversial. For patients less than 60 years old, with good bone quality and little fracture comminution open-reduction internal fixation is the usual choice. For patients more than 60 years old, with osteopenic bone and comminuted fractures arthroplasty is the treatment of choice. Unipolar hemi-arthroplasty is most commonly used. If the patient has evidence of preexisting acetabular arthritis, total hip-arthroplasty may be offered. Recent studies have suggested that in the elderly, previously active patient with intact mental status, total hip arthroplasty may be the best treatment option for displaced femoral neck fracture. Although, bipolar arthroplasty theoretically reduces the risk of prosthetic arthritis compared with unipolar hemiarthroplasty; this has not been borne out in the literature. As a result, given the higher cost, most authors do not advocate the use of bipolar hemiarthroplasty.

2. Trochanteric Fractures

▶ Fracture of the Lesser Trochanter

Isolated fractures of the lesser trochanter are quite rare. This fracture occurs most commonly in the adolescent patient secondary to forceful iliopsoas contracture. In the elderly patient, this fracture may be secondary to metastatic disease.

▶ Fracture of the Greater Trochanter

Like isolated fractures of the lesser trochanter, isolated fracture of the greater trochanter is rare. The typical mechanism is direct blow due to fall in an elderly patient. Treatment is typically nonoperative. In a young, active patient with a widely displaced greater trochanter, surgery may be considered.

▶ Intertrochanteric Fractures

Intertrochanteric fractures describe fractures that occur in the region between the greater and lesser trochanters of the proximal femur. These fractures are extracapsular, occurring in cancellous bone with abundant blood supply. Unlike displaced femoral neck fractures, these fractures are not predisposed to nonunion and osteonecrosis. These fractures are relatively common, accounting for nearly 50% of all fractures of the proximal femur (Figure 40–14). The typical presentation occurs in an elderly individual after a fall. Clinical evaluation includes neurovascular check, secondary survey, and appropriate x-rays (AP pelvis, AP, and lateral of injured hip). One may consider an internal rotation or traction view for improved delineation of the fracture. Consider MRI or Technetium bone scan in a patient with persistent hip pain despite negative radiographs; these two studies may be useful for delineating nondisplaced or incomplete fractures.

It is important to evaluate the location of fracture line (proximal to distal), obliquity of the fracture line, the degree of comminution (paying specific attention to the posteromedial cortex which determines stability) and magnitude of displacement. Basicervical neck fractures are located just proximal to or along the intertrochanteric line. These fractures are usually extracapsular; however, the proximity to the blood supply of the femoral neck can result in a higher incidence of osteonecrosis. Typically, intertrochanteric fractures have an oblique fracture line that extends from the lateral cortex proximally to the medial cortex distally; this "standard obliquity" fracture pattern is considered stable, amenable to standard surgical treatment. "Reverse obliquity" intertrochanteric fractures (oblique fracture line extending from the medial cortex proximally to the lateral cortex distally), are considered unstable. Significant posteromedial comminution indicates an unstable fracture. Finally, subtrochanteric extension of the fracture should be noted, as it may affect treatment choice.

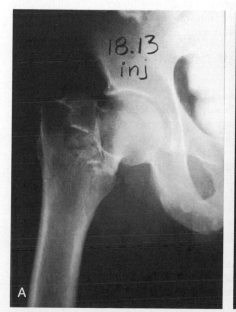

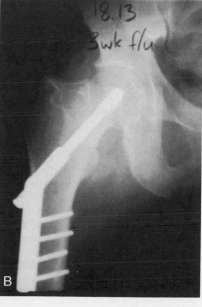

▲ **Figure 40–14.** Comminuted intertrochanteric hip fracture. **A.** Anteroposterior radiograph. **B.** Anteroposterior radiograph after fixation with a compression hip screw and sideplate.

Nonoperative treatment is associated with a higher mortality rate when compared to operative treatment. As a result, it may be considered only for patients who carry high surgical risk or demented/nonambulatory patients with mild hip pain. Early bed to chair immobilization is crucial to avoid the risks and complications of prolonged recumbence (atelectasis, deep venous thrombosis, and ulcers).

Treatment is usually surgical, with the goal being early ambulation with full weight-bearing status. Dynamic hip screw (large screw and side plate) is the typical surgical implant of choice. Intramedullary hip screws are used for "unstable" fracture patterns including: reverse obliquity IT fractures, fractures with significant posteromedial comminution, and fractures with subtrochanteric extension. Finally, arthroplasty may be chosen in patients for whom previous ORIF has failed or as primary treatment for comminuted, unstable fractures.

▶ Subtrochanteric Fracture

The Subtrochanteric femur fracture is located between the lesser trochanter and a point 5-cm distal to the lesser trochanter. This stretch of bone is subjected high biomechanical stresses. The medial and posteromedial cortices are sites of high compressive forces, while the lateral cortex experiences high tensile forces. Additionally, this area of bone is composed mainly of cortical bone. Due to less vascularity when compared to cancellous bone, the potential for healing is diminished.

The mechanism of injury may be low energy such as a fall in an elderly person or high energy in patients involved in motor vehicle accidents, falls from heights, or gunshot wounds. Additionally, fractures in this region may be pathologic in nature due to bone metastases.

Clinical evaluation includes standard trauma evaluation for patients involved in high-energy injury mechanisms. Field-dressings or splints should be completely removed to examine for soft-tissue injury and rule-out open fracture. Neuro-vascular status should be documented. Secondary survey should be performed. Blood loss can be significant in the thigh compartments, representing a potential source for hypovolemia. Traction pin should be considered until definitive fixation can be performed, to limit further soft tissue damage and bleeding. Radiographic evaluation includes the AP pelvis, AP and Lateral views of the hip and femur down to the knee.

The fracture may be classified according to its distance from the lesser trochanter, fracture line characterization, number of bone fragments, and involvement of the piriformis fossa.

Open fractures should be treated with immediate surgical debridement and fracture stabilization. Surgical treatment can involve the use of an intramedullary nail or fixed-angle plates depending on the fracture pattern (Figure 40–15).

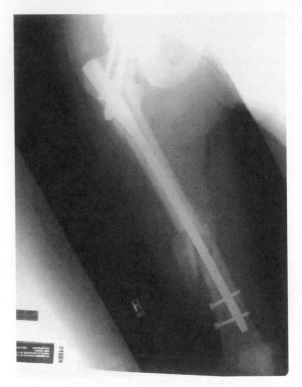

▲ **Figure 40–15.** Subtrochanteric femur fracture with fracture of the distal third of the ipsilateral femoral shaft treated with a reconstruction type intramedullary nail.

The fracture is typically healed by 3-4 months postoperatively months, but delayed union and nonunion are not uncommon. Hardware failure can occur in these cases, requiring repeat internal fixation and bone grafting.

FRACTURE OF THE SHAFT OF THE FEMUR

A femoral shaft fracture is a fracture of the femoral diaphysis that occurs between 5 cm distal to the lesser trochanter and 5 cm proximal to the adductor tubercle. Femoral shaft fractures typically occur in young men after high-energy trauma, such as motor vehicle accidents. This injury can occur in the elderly after a fall, although less common. Fractures that are inconsistent with the level of trauma should be suspected for pathologic fracture.

The vascular supply to the femoral shaft is derived mainly from the profunda femoral artery. Due to the large volume of the three fascial compartments of the thigh (anterior, medial, and posterior), significant blood loss and hemodynamic instability can occur. In one series, blood loss was greater than 1200 mL, with 40% of patients ultimately requiring blood transfusion.

Clinical evaluation includes careful neurovascular exam and secondary survey looking for concomitant injury to other joints and extremities. Specific attention should be paid to the ipsilateral hip and knee joints. Knee ligament injuries are common and easily missed. Radiographic evaluation should include AP and lateral views of the femur as well as the ipsilateral hip and knee. AP pelvis should also be obtained. Ipsilateral femoral neck and intertrochanteric fractures have been reported in up 10% of patients with femur fractures.

Femoral shaft fractures can be classified descriptively: open versus closed, location (proximal, middle, and distal one-third), pattern (spiral, oblique, and transverse), degree of comminution, angulation, rotational deformity, displacement, and amount of shortening. Winquist and Hansen described a classification based off amount of comminution: type I (minimal or no comminution), type II (cortices of both fragments at least 50% contact), type III 50%-100% cortical comminution, and type IV (circumferential comminution with no cortical contact).

In the acute setting, femoral shaft fractures can be stabilized with skeletal traction. Traction provides pain relief, and can help minimize soft tissue injury and blood loss. Ideally surgical stabilization should occur within 24 hours of injury (Figure 40–16). If surgery is delayed due to an unstable patient, traction has the added benefit of pulling the fracture fragments out to length, making subsequent fracture reduction and operative treatment more manageable.

Open fractures constitute a surgical emergency. Fractures should be debrided and stabilized as soon as possible. The most frequently used surgical treatment for femoral shaft fractures is intramedullary (IM) nailing. Compared with plate fixation, IM nailing offers the following benefits: lower infection rate, less extensive exposure/dissection of the fracture promoting healing, less quadriceps scarring, and lower tensile and shear stresses on the implant. Other advantages include early functional use of the extremity (the surgeon may allow immediate weight-bearing depending on strength of surgical management), restoration of length and alignment, rapid and high union rate, and low refracture rates.

IM nailing can be performed in an antegrade or retrograde fashion. Indications for retrograde nailing include ipsilateral injuries (fracture of the femoral neck, pertrochanteric, patella, acetabulum, or tibia), bilateral femoral shaft fractures, morbidly obese patient, pregnant woman, ipsilateral knee amputation, or when speed of surgical treatment is essential (unstable patient). Contraindications to retrograde nailing include restricted knee motion (< 60 degrees), patella baja, presence of associated open traumatic wound increasing the risk of intra-articular knee sepsis. One

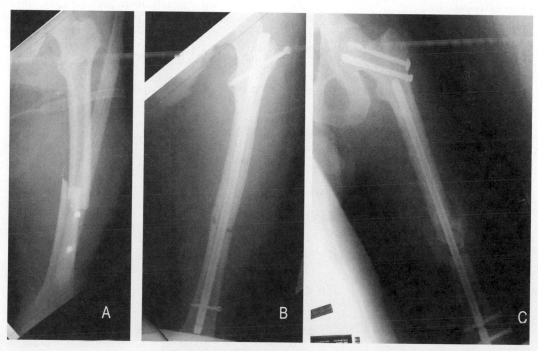

▲ **Figure 40–16.** Femoral shaft fracture. **A.** Anteroposterior x-ray showing fracture of the midshaft of the femur. **B.** Anteroposterior x-ray after closed reduction and intramedullary fixation using an antegrade titanium locked nail. **C.** Anteroposterior x-ray showing fixation of a midshaft femoral fracture and ipsilateral femoral neck fracture with a retrograde intramedullary nail.

major disadvantage to retrograde nailing is the postoperative incidence of anterior knee pain.

Other surgical options include plating and external fixation. External fixation may be used acutely as a temporary bridge in the severely injured, unstable patient. Plating may be indicated in patients whose femoral canals are not amenable to IM nailing (medullary canal too narrow, medullary canal obliterated due to infection, previous closed fracture management, etc).

Postoperatively early patient mobilization and knee range of motion is recommended. Weight-bearing status is dependent on multiple factors, including the strength of operative fixation, patient's other injuries, soft tissue status, and location of fracture. Later complications are those of prolonged recumbence, joint stiffness, malunion, nonunion, leg-length discrepancy, and infection.

INJURIES OF THE KNEE REGION

1. Fractures of the Distal Femur

Distal Femur fractures account for about 7% of all femur fractures. Incidence follows a bimodal age distribution with the first peak occurring in young adults as a result of high-energy trauma and the second peak occurring in the elderly after a fall. Distal femur fractures can be subclassified as supracondylar or condylar fractures.

The supracondylar region of the femur is the area between the femoral condyles and the junction of the metaphysic with the femoral shaft. The distal femur widens from the cylindrical shaft to form two curved condyles separated by an intercondylar groove. The medial condyle extends more distally and is more convex than the lateral condyle,

producing the normal valgus position of the distal femur. The proximal fracture fragment is typically pulled superiorly by the quadriceps and hamstrings, the distal fragment is typically displaced and angulated posteriorly due to the pull of the gastrocnemius muscle.

Neurovascular examination is key as the distal fragment may impinge on the popliteal fossa, causing a loss or marked decrease of pedal pulses. Immediate reduction is indicated. If reduction of the fracture fragment fails to restore pulses, immediate arteriogram, and vascular operative intervention is indicated. Secondary survey should be performed, with concomitant injury to the ipsilateral hip, knee, leg, and ankle ruled-out. If a distal femoral fracture is associated with an overlying laceration or wound, the ipsilateral knee should be injected with 50 mL of sterile normal saline to rule-out continuity with the wound.

Radiographic evaluation includes anteroposterior, lateral, and oblique radiographs of the distal femur as well as the entire length of the femur (Figure 40–17). Traction views and computed tomography may be helpful for preoperative planning. MRI may be used to evaluate injuries to the meniscus and ligaments of the knee. Arteriography should be considered in the setting of knee dislocation (up to 40% associated vascular disruption reported in the literature).

Distal femur fractures may be classified descriptively: open versus closed, location (supracondylar, intercondylar, and condylar), fracture pattern (spiral, oblique, and transverse), intra-articular versus extra-articular, degree of comminution, angulation, rotational deformity, displacement, and amount of shortening.

Nonoperative treatment may be pursued for stable nondisplaced fractures. Treatment involves immobilization of

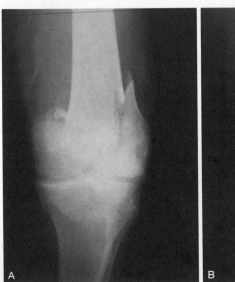
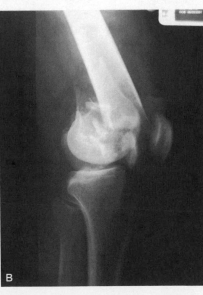

▲ **Figure 40–17.**
A. Anteroposterior radiograph demonstrating a comminuted supracondylar femur fracture with intra-articular extension. **B.** Lateral radiograph.

the extremity in a hinged knee brace with partial weight-bearing.

Displaced distal femur fractures are best treated surgically. If operative treatment is delayed more than 8 hours, a tibial traction pin should be considered. Plates and screws are the typical choice of implant. A variety of plates are available including the 95-degree condylar blade plate, nonlocking periarticular plates, and locking periarticular plates. Due to the advantage of increased stability, locking periarticular plates are becoming more popular.

▶ Dislocation of the Knee Joint

Traumatic knee dislocation is extremely rare. However, this injury can be limb threatening due to disruption of the vasculature. The knee is a "hinge" joint consisting of three articulations: patellofemoral, tibiofemoral, and tibiofibular. Normal range of motion of the knee is from 10 degrees of extension to 140 degrees of flexion. Significant soft tissue injury including disruption of three out of four major ligaments of the knee (anterior cruciate, posterior cruciate, medial collateral, and lateral collateral ligaments) is necessary for knee dislocation to occur. During knee dislocation the popliteal vascular bundle may be injured or tethered. Associated fractures of the tibial eminence, tibial tubercle, fibular head or neck, and capsular avulsions should be ruled-out. The mechanism is typically high energy.

If the knee remains dislocated at presentation, immediate reduction should be performed without waiting for radiographs. Postreduction neurovascular status should be carefully documented. Isolated ligament examination may be difficult to perform due to patient discomfort. Standard ligament examination includes Lachman's testing for the ACL, posterior drawer for the PCL, and varus and valgus stress to assess the LCL and MCL, respectively. Due to the incidence of delayed ischemia resulting from vasospasm or thrombosis occurring hours or even days after reduction, serial neurovascular exams should continue to be performed.

If a limb remains ischemic (absent pulses) after reduction, emergent surgical exploration is indicated; do not wait for an arteriogram. If the limb continues to display abnormal vascular status (diminished pulses, decreased capillary refill or ABI < 0.9) then arteriogram is indicated. Normal vascular status should be followed closely with serial exams.

Radiographic evaluation includes AP, lateral, notch views of the knee as well as "sunrise" view of the patella. Arteriography is indicated as described above. MRI is used to evaluate the ligaments and menisci of the knee, as well as articular cartilage lesions.

Knee dislocations can be classified according to the displacement of the proximal tibia in relation to the distal femur (anterior, posterior, lateral, medial, and rotational).

Immediate closed reduction is achieved with axial traction followed by placement of a splint with the knee in 20-30 degrees of flexion. Of note, posterolateral dislocation usually requires open reduction. Surgery is indicated for unsuccessful closed reduction, residual soft tissue interposition, open injuries, and vascular injuries. External fixation may be necessary for grossly unstable knees and dislocations that required vascular repair. Prophylactic fasciotomy of the leg compartments should be considered at the time of vascular repair to eliminate the compartment syndrome caused by postischemic edema. Ligamentous repair is controversial; timing of surgery is dependent on the status of both the patient and the limb.

2. Fracture of the Patella

Patella fractures only represent 1% of all skeletal injuries, occurring most commonly in the 20- to 50-year-old age group. The patella is the largest sesamoid bone in the body, with the quadriceps tendon inserting at its superior pole and the patellar ligament originating from the inferior pole. The patella has seven articular facets; the lateral facet is the largest (accounting for 50% of the articular surface). The medial and lateral extensor retinacula are strong longitudinal expansions of the quadriceps that envelop the patella and insert on the tibia. If the retinacula are intact, active extension will be preserved despite patella fracture.

The function of the patella is to increase the lever arm and mechanical advantage of the quadriceps tendon. The blood supply originates from the geniculate arteries which form anastomoses circumferentially around the outer border of the patella. Fractures of the patella may result from direct trauma or more commonly from forceful quadriceps contraction while the knee is semi-flexed during a stumble or fall.

Open lacerations associated with patella fracture should be investigated with 50 mL of sterile saline solution instilled into the knee joint to rule-out communication and open fracture. Active knee extension should be assessed; decompression of hemarthrosis and intra-articular lidocaine injection may facilitate testing.

Radiographic examination anteroposterior, lateral, and sunrise views of the knee. Of note bipartite patella (8% of the population) may be confused with fracture. Bipartite patella usually occurs in the superolateral portion of the patella and has smooth margins. Interestingly, it is bilateral in 50% of patients; thus contralateral knee x-rays may facilitate diagnosis.

Patella fractures may be classified descriptively: open versus closed, degree of displacement, fracture pattern (stellate, comminuted, transverse, vertical, polar, or osteochondral).

Nondisplaced or minimally displaced (2 mm) with minimal articular disruption (1 mm or less) can be treated nonoperatively in a knee immobilizer for 4-6 weeks if the extensor mechanism remains intact.

Surgical treatment for displaced fractures includes tension band wires, cerclage wiring, screws, or combination thereof. Retinacular disruption should also be repaired at the time of surgery. Postoperatively, the patient should be placed in a splint to protect the skin; knee motion should be instituted early 3-6 days postoperatively with progression to full weight bearing by 6 weeks. Severely comminuted or marginally repaired fractures may be immobilized longer. Partial patellectomy may be performed in the setting of large salvageable fragment with a smaller, comminuted polar fragment not amenable to stable surgical fixation. Total patellectomy is rarely indicated, reserved for extensive patella fractures with severe comminution.

▶ Dislocation of the Patella

Patella dislocation is more common in women as well as patients with connective tissue disorders (Ehlers-Danlos or Marfan's) due to increased soft tissue laxity. Dislocation of the patella can be acute (traumatic) or chronic (recurrent).

Patients with an unreduced patella dislocation will present with inability to flex the knee, hemarthrosis, and palpably displaced patella. Patients with reduced or chronic patella dislocation may demonstrate a positive "apprehension test," where laterally directed force applied to the patella with the knee in extension reproduces pain and sensation of impending patella dislocation.

Radiographic evaluation includes anteroposterior and lateral views of the knee along with sunrise views of bilateral patellae for comparison. Assessment of patella alta (high-riding patella) or patella baja should also be performed using the Insall-Salvati ratio (the ratio of the patellar ligament length compared to the length of the patella, normal = 1.0; a ratio of 1.2 indicates patella alta, while 0.8 indicates patella baja).

Patella fractures may be classified descriptively: reduced versus unreduced, congenital versus acquired, acute (traumatic) versus chronic (recurrent), as well as direction of dislocation (lateral, medial, intra-articular, superior; note: lateral is most common).

These injuries are typically treated closed with reduction and casting or bracing with the knee in extension. Operative intervention is generally reserved for recurrent dislocation.

▶ Tear of the Quadriceps Tendon

Quadriceps tendon tears occur most commonly in patients more than 40 years old. The tendon usually ruptures within 2 cm of the superior pole of the patella. Location of rupture is associated with the patient's age: for patients more than 40 years old, the tear usually occurs at the bone-tendon junction, however, for patients less than 40 years old, the tear is often midsubstance. Risk factors for quadriceps tendon rupture include anabolic steroid use, local steroid injection, diabetes mellitus, inflammatory arthropathy, and chronic renal failure. Typically patients present with a history of a sudden "pop" while stressing the extensor mechanism. Patients have pain at the site of injury, difficulty with weight-bearing, knee

joint effusion, tenderness at the upper pole of the patella, and a palpable defect proximal to the superior pole of the patella. Complete tears result in loss of active knee extension, partial tears can still have knee extension.

Radiographic examination includes anteroposterior, lateral, and sunrise views of the knee. Nonoperative treatment includes immobilization with the knee in extension for 4-6 weeks followed by progressive physical therapy. Complete ruptures should be surgically repaired. Choice of surgical technique varies depending on location of the tear: complete ruptures near bone require reapproximation of the tendon to bone using nonabsorbable sutures passed through bone tunnels. Midsubstance tears may undergo end-to-end repair.

▶ Tear of the Patellar Ligament

Patella tendon ruptures are less common than quadriceps tendon ruptures. This injury typically occurs in patients less than 40 years old. Rupture commonly occurs at the inferior pole of the patella; risk factors include RA, lupus, diabetes, renal failure, systemic corticosteroid treatment, local steroid injection, and chronic patella tendonitis. Patients typically provide a history of an "audible" pop after forceful quadriceps contraction. Physical examination may show a palpable defect, hemarthrosis, painful passive range of motion, and partial or complete loss of active extension. Radiographic examination includes AP and lateral x-rays of the knee. Nonoperative treatment is reserved for partial tears, with intact extensor mechanism. Early repair (within 2 weeks of surgery) is preferred to delayed repair (> 6 weeks from injury), which is technically more demanding due quadriceps contraction and patellar migration, as well as adhesions.

FRACTURES OF THE PROXIMAL TIBIA

1. Fractures of the Tibial Plateau

Tibial plateau fractures account for 1% of all fractures. Isolated lateral tibial plateau fractures are most common; although isolated fractures of the medial tibial plateau and bicondylar fractures happen as well.

▶ Anatomy

The tibia is the primary weight-bearing bone in the leg, supporting 85% of the transmitted load. The tibial plateau consists of the articular surfaces of the medial and lateral tibial plateaus. The medial plateau is larger and concave in shape, while the lateral plateau extends higher and is convex in shape. Normally, the plateau has a 10-degree posteroinferior slope. The two plateaus are separated by the intercondylar eminence, which serves as the tibial attachment for the anterior and posterior cruciate ligaments. There are three bony prominences 2- to 3-cm distal to the tibial plateau that serve as important insertion sites for tendinous structures: the tibial tubercle is located anteriorly and serves as the insertion for the patellar ligament, pes ansirinus is located medially and serves as attachment for semi-tendinosus, sartorius, and gracilis muscles, and Gerdy's tubercle which is the insertion sight for the iliotibial band is located laterally. The peroneal nerve travels around the neck of the fibular head splitting into the superficial peroneal nerve which travels down the lateral aspect of the leg anterior to the fibula and the deep peroneal nerve which dives deep and travels down through the anterior compartment. The trifurcation of the popliteal artery is located posteriorly between the adductor hiatus proximally and the soleus complex distally. These structures are all at risk with a tibial plateau fracture.

Mechanism of Injury

Tibial plateau fractures are usually the result of axial loading coupled with varus or valgus force. There is a bimodal distribution where young people experience these fractures after motor vehicle collisions, while the elderly can after a simple fall.

Clinical Evaluation

Neurovascular examination is necessary to documenting the function of the deep peroneal, superficial peroneal, medial, and lateral plantar nerves distally is crucial. Additionally, the documentation of the popliteal artery, dorsalis pedis, and posterior tibial artery is required as well. Associated injuries include meniscal tears as well as injuries to the collateral and cruciate ligaments. Although, initial swelling and pain may prevent examination of these ligaments. When the swelling has reduced, ligamentous testing should be carried out. Consider intra-articular injection of the knee in the acute setting, in order to carry out a ligamentous exam.

The skin should be carefully examined for any breaks to rule-out open fracture. Intra-articular injection of 50 mL of sterile normal saline can be performed to rule-out communication of the fracture and overlying skin lacerations.

Radiographic Examination

AP and lateral x-rays of the knee are part of the standard evaluation (Figure 40–18). Additionally, 40 degree internal or external rotation oblique views can be used to better assess the lateral and medial tibial plateaus respectively. A 5-10 degree caudally tilted plateau view can be used to evaluate articular step-off. CT scan is best for assessing the articular surface and is often used for preoperative planning. Associated ligamentous injury may be indicated by avulsion of the fibular head (LCL injury) and Segond sign (lateral capsular avulsion off of the lateral tibial plateau, indicating ACL disruption). MRI should be considered if ligamentous injury is suspected. Arteriography should be performed if vascular injury is suspected.

Classification

Tibial plateau fractures are most commonly classified according to the Schatzer classification: type I (lateral plateau, split fracture), type II (lateral plateau, split depression fracture), type III (lateral plateau, depression fracture), type IV (medial plateau fracture), type V (bicondylar plateau fracture), and type VI (plateau fracture with extension into the metaphysis. Of note, types IV-VI are higher energy fractures. Type I split fractures usually occur in younger individuals and are often associated with injury to the MCL. Type III depression fractures usually occur in older individuals with osteoporotic bone.

Treatment

Initial treatment for lower energy fractures usually entails placement in a knee immobilizer locked in full-extension, non–weight-bearing status with crutches. For higher energy fractures with significant displacement, placement in a posterior splint or external fixation should be considered.

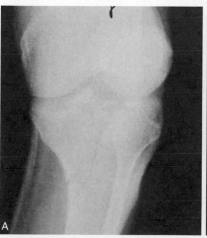
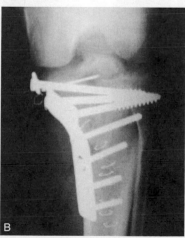

▲ **Figure 40–18.** Schatzker II tibial plateau fracture. **A.** Anteroposterior radiograph. **B.** Radiograph after fixation with lateral plate and bone grafting.

Nondisplaced or minimally displaced fractures can be treated with protected weight-bearing and early knee range of motion in a hinged brace. Radiographs should be taken at regular intervals to ensure no further displacement. Progression to full weight bearing can occur at 8-12 weeks from injury, if no further displacement occurs and fracture healing is appreciated radiographically.

Surgical indications include displacement of the articular surface, open fractures, compartment syndrome, or associated vascular injury. A variety of operative methods are used including external fixation, and open reduction internal fixation with plates or screws depending on fracture type and surgeon preference.

The postoperative course usually entails non–weight-bearing with continuous passive motion and progressive active range of motion. Progression to full weight-bearing is usually allowed by 8-12 weeks after surgery.

FRACTURE OF THE SHAFTS OF THE TIBIA & FIBULA

Fractures of the tibia and fibula are the most common long bone fractures. Mechanism of injury can be low-energy due to twisting/rotation or high energy related to motor vehicle accidents. Isolated fractures of the tibia and/or fibula are rare; these fractures most often occur together.

▶ Anatomy

The tibia is a tubular bone with a triangular cross-section. The tibia has a subcutaneous anteromedial border and is otherwise enveloped by four tight fascial compartments (anterior, lateral, posterior, and deep posterior). The fibula is responsible for 10%-15% of the weight-bearing load. The common peroneal nerve is located subcutaneously, traveling around the fibular neck, making it particularly vulnerable to direct blows or traction injuries at this level.

▶ Clinical Evaluation

Neurovascular status, including the deep peroneal, superficial peroneal, medial, and lateral plantar nerves, as well as the posterior tibial artery and dorsalis pedis artery should be documented carefully. Thorough skin examination should be performed to rule-out open fracture. Additionally, the examiner should have a high suspicion for compartment syndrome in the acute setting. Pain out of proportion, pain with passive stretch, tense compartments, numbness, tingling, and cool toes are all signs of compartment syndrome. For obtunded or intubated patients who cannot relate an accurate history or their symptoms (pain level, presence of numbness/tingling), a monitor can be used to measure pressures in each of the four compartments. Greater than 30 mm Hg or pressure within 30 mm Hg of the diastolic pressure, are accepted indications for fasciotomy.

▶ Radiographic Evaluation

Radiographic investigation begins with AP and lateral x-rays of the tibia and fibula (Figure 40–19). Additionally, x-rays of the joint above and below should also be performed to rule-out other injury. Radiographs should be examined carefully to determine the location and morphology of the fracture, the presence of any secondary fracture lines that

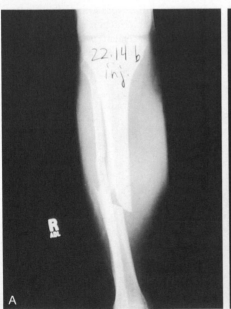
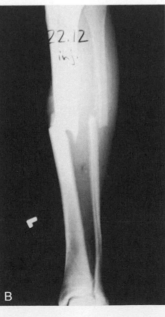

▲ **Figure 40–19.** Anteroposterior **A.** and lateral **B.** radiographs of a displaced midshaft tibia fracture.

could displace during operative management. CT scan and MRI are rarely necessary. Technetium bone scans and MRI can be used in patients with persistent pain to diagnose stress fractures in tibial shafts that were not visible on radiographs.

Classification

Fractures of the tibia shaft can be classified descriptively: open versus closed, anatomic location (proximal, middle, or distal third), fragment number and position (comminution, butterfly fragments), configuration (transverse, spiral, oblique), angulation (varus/valgus, anterior/posterior), shortening, displacement (percentage of cortical contact), rotation, and associated injuries.

Open fractures are classified according to the Gustilo and Anderson classification, described at the beginning of this chapter.

Treatment

Fracture reduction and closed treatment in a long-leg cast with the knee in 0-5 degrees of flexion may be attempted for isolated, closed, low-energy fractures with minimal displacement and comminution. Protected weight-bearing with crutches with advancement to full weight bearing after 2-4 weeks is usually tolerated. After 4-6 weeks the long-leg cast may be exchanged for a short-leg cast or fracture brace. Regular radiographic follow-up is crucial to ensure no further displacement of the fracture. Acceptable parameters for continued closed treatment include: less than 5 degrees of varus/valgus angulation, less than 10 degrees of anterior/posterior angulation, less than 10 degrees of rotational deformity (external rotation is tolerated better than internal rotation), less than 1cm shortening, and more than 50% cortical contact.

Fractures with significant displacement or comminution that requires operative intervention, can be treated acutely with a posterior long-leg splint or external fixation if significant shortening is noted. Definitive surgical treatment includes several options: intramedullary nailing, external fixation, plates, and screws. Intramedullary nailing is by far the most popular technique as it preserves the periosteal blood supply, optimizing conditions for fracture healing. Compartment syndrome should be treated emergently with four-compartment fasciotomies. Concomitant fractures of the fibula do not require surgical treatment once the tibia has been stabilized.

1. Fracture of the Shaft of the Fibula

Isolated fracture of the shaft of the fibula is uncommon though it can occur with a direct blow to the side of the lower leg. Particular attention should be given to clinical and radiographic examination of the ankle and knee to rule out ligamentous or other subtle bony injuries. If no other injury is present, immobilization is for comfort only. Three weeks or a month in a walking cast or removable cast boot is usually sufficient, and complete healing can be expected.

INJURIES OF THE ANKLE REGION

1. Ankle Fracture

The incidence of ankle fractures has increased significantly since the 1960s. Most ankle fractures are isolated malleolar fractures; however, bimalleolar and trimalleolar fractures make up approximately one-third of the total. Open fractures are rare.

Anatomy

The ankle is a hinge joint composed of the fibula, tibia, and talus articulations along with several important ligaments. Specifically, the distal tibial articular surface is often referred to the "plafond," which combined with the medial and lateral malleoli, forms the mortise which is a constrained articulation with the talar dome.

The talar dome is trapezoidal in shape and almost entirely covered with articular cartilage. The anterior portion of the talus is wider than the posterior portion. The tibial plafond is also wider anteriorly in order to accommodate the shape of the talus, conferring intrinsic stability to the ankle joint.

The medial malleolus, which articulates with the medial facet of the talus, can be divided into the anterior colliculus and posterior colliculus which serve as attachments for the superficial and deep deltoid ligaments, respectively. The deltoid ligament provides ligamentous support to the medial aspect of the ankle. The superficial portion of the deltoid is composed of three ligaments: tibionavicular ligament (prevents inward displacement of the talar head), tibiocalcaneal ligament (prevents valgus displacement), and the superficial tibiotalar ligament.

The lateral malleolus is the distal portion of the fibula, articulating with the lateral aspect of the talus. The distal fibula is attached to the distal tibia via soft-tissue constraint known as the syndesmosis. The syndesmosis, which is made up of four ligaments (anterior inferior tibiofibular, posterior inferior tibiofibular, transverse tibiofibular, and interosseous ligaments), resists axial, rotational, and translational forces, making it critical for ankle stability. The fibular collateral ligament, composed of the anterior talo-fibular ligament (ATFL), posterior talo-fibular ligament, and calcaneofibular ligament provides additional stability to the lateral aspect of the ankle.

Clinical Evaluation

Neurovascular status (deep peroneal, superficial peroneal, medial and lateral plantar nerves, posterior tibial artery, and dorsalis pedis artery) should all be documented. The skin should be examined for open injury and blistering. The entire length of the fibula, including the proximal portion (head and neck) should be palpated, to rule-out additional fractures. The "squeeze test" performed approximately 5 cm to the intermalleolar axis can be used to assess for syndesmotic disruption.

▶ Radiographic Evaluation

Initial workup includes AP, Lateral and mortise (15-20 degrees of internal rotation) x-rays of the ankle. Radiographs of the full tibia and fibula including the knee joint should be obtained to identify additional injuries. The dome of the talus should be centered under the tibia in all three views. Tibiofibula overlap less than 10 mm, tibiofibula clear space more than 5 mm, and medial clear space between the medial malleolus and talus all indicate syndesmotic disruption. If initial mortise views do not indicate medial clear space widening, an external rotation or gravity stress can be applied to the ankle. If widening more than 4 mm is noted with this stress, then significant syndesmotic injury is likely. Additionally, talar shift is indicative of ligamentous disruption. CT scan, MRI, and bone scan can be used to further investigate ankle injuries.

▶ Classification

Ankle fractures can be classified according to the Lauge–Hansen system which focuses on four patterns of ankle injury that are the result of different mechanisms. The Supination-adduction (SA) fracture patent usually results in medial displacement of the talus and a transverse or avulsion-type fracture of the fibula distal to the joint and/or a vertical medial malleolus fracture. The supination-external rotation (SER) injury is the most common, producing variable disruption of the ATFL, spiral fracture of the distal fibula, posterior malleolus fracture, and fracture of the medial malleolus or deltoid ligament disruption. The pronation-abduction (PA) or pronation-external rotation (PER) injuries result in variable injury or fracture to the medial malleolus, deltoid ligament, syndesmotic ligament, and distal fibula fractures.

Ankle fractures can also be classified according to the Weber classification based off of the level of fibula injury: Weber A (fracture of the fibula below the tibia plafond), Weber B (oblique or spiral fracture of the fibula occurring at or near the level of the syndesmosis), and Weber C (fracture of the fibula above the level of the syndesmosis). The two classification systems correlate as follows: Weber A (SA injury pattern), Weber B (SER), and Weber C (PA or PER).

Other fracture variants include: Maisonneuve fracture (ankle injury with fracture of the fibula proximal third) and various avulsion fractures due to disrupted ligaments.

▶ Treatment

The goal of treatment is anatomic restoration of the ankle joint with preservation of fibular length and rotation. Initial treatment, includes closed reduction and placement in a well-padded posterior splint with stirrups. Postreduction radiographs should be obtained to ensure correct position of the talus under the tibia. The injured limb should be elevated to the level of the heart at all times.

Nondisplaced, stable fracture patterns (isolated malleolus fractures) without disruption of the syndesmosis can be treated closed–transitioned from the splint to a long-leg cast for 4-6 weeks with serial radiographic examination to ensure no subsequent displacement. After this time, the patient can be transferred to a short-leg cast. Weight-bearing is restricted until fracture healing is demonstrated.

Surgical treatment is indicated for displaced medial malleolus fractures, and lateral malleolar fractures with displacement more than 2 mm or any loss of fibular length. Isolated lateral malleolus fractures with minimal displacement and no loss of length should be investigated for syndesmotic injury. Medial sided tenderness or medial clear-space widening noted radiographically is indicative of additional injury resulting in what is likely an unstable ankle fracture; as a result, surgery is usually recommended.

Surgical treatment includes plates and/or screws. For bimalleolar and trimalleolar fractures, the fibula is initially fixed with a plate and screws. The medial malleolus fracture remains unreduced, it should be stabilized with screws or tension band construct. Indications for surgical fixation of the posterior malleolus fracture include: involvement of more than 25% of the articular surface, persistent more than 2-mm displacement, or persistent posterior subluxation of the talus. Bimalleolar equivalent fractures (fibula fractures with medial ligament injury or syndesmotic disruption) may require syndesmotic screws. Proximal fibula fractures with syndesmotic disruption can be stabilized with syndesmotic screws once correct fibula length and rotation are achieved via reduction maneuvers.

Postoperative course usually entails non–weight-bearing in a splint/cast/removable boot for 4-6 weeks until fracture healing is appreciated radiographically. Ankle range of motion exercises should be started early to prevent postoperative stiffness.

2. Ankle Sprain

Ankle sprain is common, usually the result of forced inversion or eversion of the foot. Pain is usually maximal over the anterolateral aspect or medial aspects of the joint depending on the mechanism of injury. Ankle sprain is a diagnosis of exclusion. If no fractures, dislocations, or widening (> 4 mm) is appreciated between either malleolus or the talus then ankle sprain is a reasonable diagnosis.

Ankle sprains are usually treated with "RICE" (rest, ice, compression with elastic ace wrap, and elevation), NSAIDs, and non–weight-bearing or protected weight-bearing with crutches for 3-5 days. Splinting or use of an air cast is optional. Continued pain and/or swelling that have not improved require further workup.

3. Syndesmosis Injuries

▶ Introduction

Syndesmotic injuries account for approximately 1% of all ankle ligament injuries. Many of these injuries go on undiagnosed and can lead to chronic ankle pain and instability if not treated appropriately.

▶ Clinical Evaluation and Diagnosis

Patients often present late, several hours or even days after a twisting injury to ankle, with persistent swelling/pain/difficulty weight-bearing. The fibula should be palpated along its entire length, proximally and distally. Two clinical tests have been used to evaluate for isolated syndesmotic injury: (1) the squeeze test—if squeezing the fibula midcalf reproduces distal tibiofibular pain or (2) external rotation test—pt is seated with knee flexed to 90 degrees, examiner stabilizes the patient's leg and externally rotates the foot; if pain is reproduced at the syndesmosis than injury is likely.

▶ Radiographic Evaluation

Radiographic evaluation starts with anteroposterior, lateral, and mortise views of the ankle looking for widening of the medial clear space between the medial malleolus and the medial border of the talus or widening of the tibiofibular clear space (interval between the medial border of the fibula and the lateral border of the posterior tibial malleolus). If no injury is appreciated, external rotation stress view (mortise view with an external rotation stress applied to the foot with the leg stabilized) should be performed.

▶ Classification

Syndesmotic injuries can be organized according to the Edwards and DeLee classification: type 1 (diastasis involving lateral subluxation without fracture), type 2 (lateral subluxation with plastic deformation of the fibula), type 3 (posterior subluxation/dislocation of the fibula), and type 4 (superior subluxation/dislocation of the talus).

▶ Treatment

Patients can be initially immobilized in a non–weight-bearing cast for 2-3 weeks, followed by use of an ankle-foot orthosis that eliminates external rotation of the foot for and additional 3 weeks. Operative intervention with syndesmotic screws from the fibula to the tibia is considered for patients with and irreducible diastasis. These patients are often kept non-weight bearing for 6 weeks with screw removal at 12-16 weeks.

4. Pilon Fractures

▶ Epidemiology

Tibial Plafond or "Pilon" fractures are fractures that involve the weight bearing surface of the distal tibia that articulates with the talus (Figure 40–20). Pilon fractures account for 7%-10% of all tibia fractures. Most occur in men aged 30-40 years old from high energy mechanisms such as motor vehicle collisions or falls from significant height. As a result, extra care should be taken to rule out concomitant injuries.

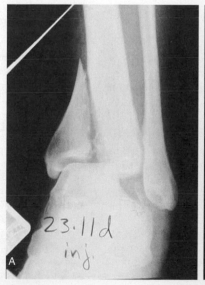 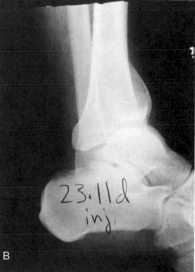

▲ **Figure 40–20.** Axial loading injury to the ankle joint with the foot in dorsiflexion leading to a fracture of the tibial plafond. Anteroposterior **A.** and lateral **B.** radiographs.

Specifically, tibial plateau, calcaneus, pelvis, and vertebral fractures should be ruled-out.

▶ Mechanism of Injury

A fall from significant height results in an axial compression force directed through the talus into the tibial plafond, causing impaction and comminution of the articular surface. Shear injuries, such as can occur in a skiing accident, will result in a fracture with two or more large fragments and minimal comminution. Combined compression and shear result in fracture pattern that is somewhere in between.

▶ Clinical Evaluation

Examination of the patient includes documentation of a neurovascular exam and secondary survey to rule-out other injuries. Careful skin examination should be performed to exclude open fracture. Swelling is often rapid and considerable, potentially resulting in skin necrosis and blistering depending on fracture displacement. As a result, these fractures should be reduced provisionally and placed in a splint as soon as possible. The amount of swelling should be noted; some authors advocate waiting 7-10 days before taking patients to surgery for swelling to subside or until "skin wrinkling" is appreciated to avoid postoperative wound complications.

▶ Radiographic Evaluation

Initial radiographic evaluation includes anteroposterior, lateral, and mortise views of the ankle joint. CT with thin cuts, coronal, and sagittal reconstructions is useful for preoperative evaluation of the fracture pattern and articular surface. One should also consider radiographs of the contralateral side, which can be used for preoperative templating.

▶ Classification

The Ruedi and Algower classification is most commonly used: type 1 (nondisplaced fracture), type 2 (displaced fracture with minimal impaction and comminution), and type 3 (displaced fracture with significant comminution and/or metaphyseal impaction).

▶ Treatment

Choice of treatment is based off of multiple factors including the fracture pattern, as well as patient characteristics: age of patient, functional status, severity of injury to soft tissues, bone, cartilage, degree of comminution and/or osteoporosis, other injuries to the patient, and comfort level of the surgeon.

Nonoperative treatment, which involves long-leg cast for 6 weeks followed by bracing and range of motion exercises with progressive weight-bearing, is reserved for the nondisplaced fracture or severely debilitated patients.

Displaced fractures are usually treated surgically. Surgery may be delayed for 7-14 days to allow the soft tissues to calm down in an effort to avoid postoperative wound complications. "Skin wrinkling" may indicate that enough swelling has subsided for operative intervention to occur. Spanning external fixation should be considered initially to provide stabilization, partial fracture reduction, and restoration of length while waiting for final surgical management. Associated fibula fractures may undergo open reduction internal fixation at the time of fixator application.

The goals of operative fixation of pilon fractures include restoration of fibula length and stability, restoration of the tibial articular surface, buttressing of the distal tibia, and bone grafting metaphyseal defects as needed. Definitive surgical management may involve plates and screws, external fixation, or a combination thereof.

5. Achilles Tendon Rupture

▶ Epidemiology

Achilles tendon problems are often related to overuse injury. In the setting of trauma, acute rupture can occur. Delayed or missed diagnosis is common, caregivers should therefore have a high index of suspicion for this injury.

▶ Anatomy

The Achilles tendon is the largest tendon in the body. It has a paratenon with visceral and parietal layers, instead of a true synovial sheath, allowing approximately 1.5 cm of tendon glide. There are three sources for the tendon's blood supply: (1) musculotendinous junction, (2) osseous insertion, (3) and multiple mesosternal vessels on the tendon's anterior surface.

▶ Clinical Evaluation

Complete rupture often results in a palpable defect in the tendon that is not present with an incomplete injury. In the setting of complete rupture the Thompson test (plantar flexion with calf squeeze) is positive (no plantar flexion occurs) and the patient is unable to perform a single heel-raise.

▶ Treatment

Surgical treatment compared with non-operative management results in lower recurrent rupture rates, improved strength, and a higher percentage of patients returning to sports activities. However, there are significant complication rates associated with surgery including, wound infection, skin necrosis, and nerve injuries. As a result, surgery is usually reserved for the young, athletic patient looking to return to playing sports.

Nonoperative treatment usually entails 2 week immobilization in a plantar-flexed splint, followed by 6-8 weeks of cast immobilization with progressive dorsiflexion to neutral and slow advancement of weight bearing. Cast removal is followed by the use of a heel-lift with eventual transition back to normal shoes. Progressive resistive exercises are started at 8-10 weeks from injury, with return to sports at 4-6 months. Maximal recovery can take up to one year; some residual weakness is often present.

Operative treatment can be done percutaneously or through a medial longitudinal approach. Postoperative management is similar to that which is used for closed treatment.

6. Peroneal Tendon Subluxation

Subluxation or frank dislocation of the peroneal tendon is rare, usually resulting from injury sustained during sports activities such as skiing. Clinical evaluation reveals lateral ankle swelling and tenderness posterior to the lateral malleolus. Radiographs may show a small fleck of bone off of the posterior aspect of the lateral malleolus indicating avulsion injury. MRI can be used for evaluation if diagnosis remains unclear. Treatment involves reduction of the tendon and placement in a well-molded cast with foot in slight plantar flexion and mild inversion. If dislocation of the tendon continues, operative intervention may be considered.

INJURIES OF THE FOOT

1. The Talus

▶ Anatomy

Sixty percent of the talus is covered by articular cartilage including the superior surface which is the weight-bearing portion. The cartilage extends medially and laterally in a plantar direction allowing articulation with the medial and lateral malleoli. The inferior surface of the talar body articulates with the calcaneus. The anterior aspect of the talus is wider than the posterior aspect, conferring inherent stability to the ankle joint. The neck of the talus extends from the body proximally and posteriorly, deviates medially, to join the talar head anteriorly and distally. The talar neck is most vulnerable to fracture. The head of the talus meets with the navicular bone anteriorly, the spring ligament inferiorly, the sustentaculum tali posteroinferiorly, and the deltoid ligament medially. The lateral process of the talus meets the posterior calcaneal facet inferiorly and the lateral malleolus superolaterally. The posterior process of the talus has a medial and lateral tubercle separated by a groove for the flexor hallucis longus tendon. An os trigonum, which can be mistaken for fracture, is present just posterior to the lateral tubercle in up to 50% of normal feet. The blood supply to the talus is composed of arteries to the sinus tarsi (originating from the peroneal and dorsalis pedis artery), an artery of the tarsal canal (posterior tibial artery), and the deltoid artery (posterior tibial artery). The vascular supply reaches the talus through various fascial structures; when these structures are disrupted, for example, with dislocation, avascular necrosis of the talus can result.

▶ Fractures of the Talus

A. Epidemiology and Mechanism of Injury

Fractures of the talus represent approximately 2% of all lower extremity injuries. These injuries most commonly occur from high-energy mechanisms such as falls from significant height or motor vehicle accidents resulting in hyperdorsiflexion causing the talar neck to impact the anterior portion of the tibia.

B. Clinical Presentation and Radiographic Examination

Patients typically present with foot pain and diffuse swelling of the hindfoot. Associated fractures of the ankle and foot are common.

Initial radiographs include anteroposterior, lateral, and mortise views of the ankle as well as anteroposterior, lateral, and oblique views of the foot. A Canale view with the ankle in maximum equines (plantar-flexion), pronated 15 degrees and the radiograph machine directed 15 degrees from the vertical, provides optimal visualization of the talar neck. Additionally, a CT scan should be considered for better fracture characterization and to assess for any articular involvement. Bone scan and/or MRI should be considered for patients with persistent hindfoot pain despite negative radiographs to look for occult fractures of the talar neck.

C. Classification

Fractures of the talus are classified initially based off their anatomic location: talar neck fractures, talar body fractures, talar head fractures, lateral process fractures, and posterior process fractures.

Fractures of the talar neck are further subclassified based off of the Hawkins classification: I (nondisplaced), II (with associated subtalar dislocation), III (with associated subtalar and tibiotalar dislocation), and IV (associated subtalar, tibiotalar, and talonavicular dislocations).

D. Treatment

Truly nondisplaced fractures with no signs of articular comminution on CT scan can be treated nonoperatively initially in a short-leg cast, non–weight-bearing for at least 6 weeks until radiographic signs of healing are noted, followed by progressive weight-bearing.

Displaced fractures should be treated with closed reduction and splint placement. Open or irreducible fractures require immediate operative treatment. Surgery entails open reduction and internal fixation with plates and screws.

▶ Other Fractures of the Talus

Lateral process fractures of the talus are commonly seen in snow-boarders. These fractures are often misdiagnosed as ankle sprains upon initial presentation. If the fracture is displaced less than 2 mm, then it can be treated closed with a short-leg cast. Greater than 2 mm of displacement requires operative intervention.

Posterior process fractures of the talus can be difficult to diagnose due to the presence of the os trigonum. Nondisplaced or minimally displaced fractures of the posterior process can be treated with a non–weight-bearing short-leg cast. Displaced fractures require surgical treatment with open reduction and internal fixation.

Talar head fractures may be associated with fractures of the navicular bone or talonavicular disruption. Nondisplaced or minimally displaced fractures can be treated for six weeks in a partial weight bearing short-leg cast molded to preserve the longitudinal arch. After discontinuation of the cast, an arch support should be worn in the shoe to reduce stress on the talonavicular articulation for an additional 4-6 months. Displaced fractures are treated with ORIF and/or primary excision of small fragments.

▶ Complications

The most common complication is posttraumatic arthritis. Avascular necrosis occurs as well and correlates with initial fracture displacement: Hawkins I (0%-15%), Hawkins II (20%-50%), Hawkins III (20%-100%), and Hawkins IV (100%). Other complications include delayed union or nonunion, malunion, and wound complications.

▶ Subtalar Dislocation

Subtalar dislocation is defined by the simultaneous dislocation of the distal articulations of the talocalcaneal and talonavicular joints. Inversion of the foot results in medial subtalar dislocation, while eversion causes lateral subtalar dislocation. The large majority of these dislocations are medial (approximately 85%). All subtalar dislocations should be reduced as soon as possible with knee flexion, accentuation of the deformity to unlock the calcaneus and longitudinal traction. Subtalar dislocations are often stable once closed reduction is achieved. CT scan should be performed postreduction to assess for other associated fractures or continued subluxation. Failed closed reduction may be due to interposed extensor digitorum brevis muscle in the case of a medial dislocation or posterior tibial tendon for lateral dislocation. Unsuccessful closed reduction requires operative intervention.

▶ Total Dislocation of the Talus

Total dislocation of the talus is rare and usually an open injury. In general, open reduction with internal fixation is required. Complications including infection, osteonecrosis, and posttraumatic arthritis are common.

2. The Calcaneus

▶ Fracture of the Calcaneus

A. Epidemiology

The calcaneus is the most frequently fractured tarsal bone, constituting approximately 2% of all fractures. The large majority of calcaneus fractures occur in men aged 21-45 years old.

B. Mechanism

Most intra-articular calcaneus fractures are the result of axial loading where the talus is driven into the calcaneus during a fall from significant height or motor vehicle accident. Extra-articular calcaneus fractures may be the result of twisting injuries. For diabetic patients there is an increased incidence of calcaneus tuberosity fractures resulting from Achilles avulsion injuries.

C. Clinical Presentation

Patients often present with significant heel pain, swelling, and ecchymosis. When open fractures occur, they most often occur on the medial side of the foot. Compartment syndrome should be carefully ruled out. Associated injuries to rule out include lumbar spine injuries and other lower extremity fractures. Of note bilateral calcaneus fractures occur approximately 10% of the time.

D. Radiographic Evaluation

Initial radiographs include a lateral radiograph of the hindfoot, AP of the foot, a Harris axial view, and standard ankle series. The lateral radiograph should be examined to determine the Bohler tuber joint angle (intersection of the line drawn from the anterior process to the highest point of the posterior facet and the line drawn from the superior aspect of the calcaneal tuberosity to the highest point of the posterior facet). The Bohler angle is usually 20-40 degrees. A decrease in this angle indicates significant depression of the weight bearing posterior facet. The AP radiograph should be examined for extension of the fracture into the calcaneocuboid joint. A Harris axial view can be taken with the foot maximally dorsiflexed and the radiograph beam directed 45 degrees cephalad to better visualize the articular surface. However, dorsiflexion may be difficult due to patient discomfort. CT scan with 3-5 mm cuts offers the best

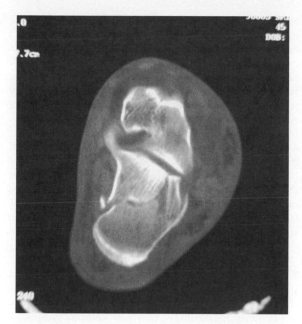

▲ **Figure 40–21.** Axial CT section showing a fracture of the calcaneus caused by an axial loading mechanism.

characterization of the articular surface and as a result is most useful for preoperative planning (Figure 40–21).

E. Classification

Extra-articular fractures of the calcaneus include fractures of the anterior process, calcaneal tuberosity, medial process, sustentaculum tali, and body fractures outside of the articular surface. Anterior process and calcaneal tuberosity fractures are best seen on lateral radiographs. Fractures of the medial process, sustentacular, or body fractures are best investigated on axial views or CT scan. Intra-articular fractures can be classified according to the Sanders classification which is based off of the coronal cuts of CT scans showing the number and location of articular fracture fragments. The posterior facet of the calcaneus is divided into three fractures lines (A, B, and C) moving from lateral to medial. There can be a total of four pieces: lateral, central, medial, and sustentacular tali. The classification is as follows: type I (all nondisplaced fractures regardless of number of fracture lines), type II (two-part fracture, with further subclassification based on the location of the fracture line IIA, IIB, IIC), type III (three-part fractures, subtypes IIIAB, IIIAC, IIIBC), and type IV (four part articular fractures).

F. Treatment

Treatment remains controversial—even with adequate reduction fractures of the calcaneus often result in chronic pain and functional disability. Nonoperative indications include nondisplaced or minimally displaced extra-articular fractures, nondisplaced intra-articular fractures, anterior process fractures with less than 25% involvement of the calcaneocuboid articulation, fractures in patients with severe peripheral vascular occlusive disease or diabetes (due to frequent wound complications associated with surgery), fractures in patients with other severe medical comorbidities, and fractures associated with significant soft tissue compromise. Initial treatment involves placement in a bulky-Jones splint or dressing with avoidance of pressure on the heel. The splint is converted to a prefabricated boot locked in neutral to prevent equines contracture with elastic compression stocking to prevent dependent edema. Early subtalar and ankle joint range of motion is started; non–weight-bearing is instituted for approximately 10-12 weeks until radiographic healing is appreciated.

Operative indications included displaced intra-articular fractures, fractures of the anterior process with more than 25% involvement of the calcaneocuboid joint, displaced calcaneal tuberosity fractures, fracture-dislocations of the calcaneus, open fractures of the calcaneus, tuberosity fractures that are displaced resulting in prominence through the skin, incompetence of the gastrocnemius-soleus complex, and/or extend into the articular surface. Surgery should only be attempted 7-14 days after the injury allowing enough time for swelling to subside. Fracture fixation depends on the type of fracture. Anterior process fractures are typically fixed with small or minifragment screws. Calcaneal tuberosity fractures usually require lag screw fixation with or without cerclage wire. Intra-articular posterior facet fractures may be fixed with lag screws into the sustentaculum tali and a thin lateral plate providing a lateral buttress. Postoperatively the patient is kept non–weight-bearing for 8-12 weeks with early subtalar range of motion exercises.

3. Fractures of the Midfoot

▶ Epidemiology, Mechanism of Injury, and Anatomy

Fractures of the midfoot are relatively rare, most often resulting from direct impact during a motor vehicle accident or a combination of axial loading and torsion during fall from a significant height. The midfoot consists of five bones: navicular, cuboid, medial, middle, and lateral cuneiforms. The midtarsal joint consists of the calcaneocuboid and talonavicular articulations which act together with the subtalar joint during eversion and inversion of the foot. The cuboid extends distal to the three naviculocuneioform joints minimizing motion at this level.

▶ Clinical and Radiographic Evaluation

Patient presentation is variable ranging from a limp with mild swelling and dorsal foot tenderness to a grossly swollen, painful midfoot resulting in nonambulatory status. Initial radiographs include AP, lateral, and oblique x-rays of the foot. Stress views and weight-bearing x-rays can provide additional detail including detection of any ligamentous instability. CT scan is best for characterizing fracture-dislocations or discovering injuries that are otherwise undetected on x-ray. MRI may be used to evaluate ligamentous injury.

▶ Navicular Bone

The navicular is the keystone bone of the foot's medial longitudinal arch, transmitting motion from the subtalar joint to the forefoot. The talonavicular articular surface is concave and has a significant arc of motion. The distal articular surface has three separate facets for the three cuneiforms. Not much motion occurs at these joints. The navicular tuberosity is the medial prominence located on the inferior aspect of the navicular bone provides an attachment point for the posterior tibial tendon. Anatomic variants include the shape of the tuberosity and the presence of an accessory navicular bone (up to 15% of the time and bilateral 70-90% of the time).

Patients typically present with painful foot and dorsomedial swelling and tenderness. Radiographic Evaluation can include medial and lateral oblique x-rays of the midfoot in addition to the standard foot series, to assess the lateral pole of the navicular as well as the medial tuberosity.

▶ Classification

There are three basic types of navicular fractures with a sub-classification of the body type fractures. Avulsion-type fractures can involve the talonavicular or naviculocuneiform ligaments. Tuberosity fractures usually involved disruption of the tibialis posterior tendon insertion without damage to the joint surface. Type I body fractures divide the navicular into dorsal and plantar pieces. Type II body fractures split the navicular into medial and lateral pieces. Type III body fractures are comminuted and often have significant displacement of the medial and lateral poles.

▶ Treatment

Nondisplaced fractures without instability may be treated closed in a cast or boot non–weight-bearing for 6-8 weeks. Disruption of the articular surface more than 2 mm requires operative intervention. Small fragments may be excised if symptomatic. Larger fragments (> 25% of the articular surface) require ORIF with lag screw fixation. If more than 40% of the talonavicular joint cannot be reconstructed, acute talonavicular fusion should be considered. Isolated dislocation or subluxation of the navicular bone without fracture requires surgical stabilization.

▶ Cuboid Bone

The Cuboid Bone is part of the "lateral column" of the foot articulating with the calcaneus proximally, the navicular and lateral cuneiform medially, and the fourth and fifth metatarsal distally. The peroneus longus travels through a groove on the plantar surface of the cuboid on its way to its insertion at the base of the first metatarsal. Injury to the cuboid bone is usually seen in conjunction with injury to the talonavicular or Lisfranc joints. Patients typically present with dorsolateral foot pain and swelling. In addition to foot series, stress radiographs, and CT scan should be considered. MRI can be used to evaluate for stress fractures that are otherwise not seen on radiograph. Cuboid fractures without articular disruption or any loss of length can be treated closed, non–weight-bearing in a boot for 6-8 weeks. If more than 2 mm disruption of the articular surface is appreciated or the cuboid is compressed, then ORIF should be pursued. Calcaneocuboid fusion should be considered for fractures with residual articular displacement.

▶ Tarsometatarsal (LisFranc) Joint

Injury to the LisFranc Joint is relatively rare. However, given that up to 20% of the time this injury goes undiagnosed initially, suspicion should remain high especially in the polytrauma patient with foot swelling or pain.

In the AP plane the base of the second metatarsal is recessed between the medial and lateral cuneiforms, limiting translation. In the coronal plane, the middle three metatarsal bones have trapezoidal shaped bases that form a transverse arch preventing displacement in the plantar direction. The second metatarsal base is "keystone" responsible for the inherent stability of the transmetatarsal joint. The Lisfranc ligament travels from the medial cuneiform to the base of the second metatarsal bone providing additional stability. Of note the dorsalis pedis artery travels in between the first and second metatarsal bones at the LisFranc joint; as a result it is vulnerable to injury with disruption or manipulation of this joint.

There are three common mechanisms of injury: (1) twisting (forced abduction of the forefoot) such as is seen in equestrians who fall from a horse with their foot caught in the stirrup, (2) axial load, and (3) crush injury.

Clinical evaluation includes careful neurovascular documentation given the proximity of the dorsalis pedis artery to this joint. Additionally, compartment syndrome of the foot should be ruled out. Stress testing applying gentle forefoot abduction or pronation with the hindfoot stabilized may be performed.

Radiographic evaluation includes anteroposterior, lateral, and oblique views of the foot. Normally, the medial border of the second metatarsal should be collinear with the medial border of the middle cuneiform on the AP view; additionally the medial border of the fourth metatarsal should line up with the medial border of the cuboid bone. Dorsal displacement of the metatarsals on the lateral view is also indicative of ligamentous injury. Weight-bearing views should be performed as well looking for any displacement. CT scan can provide greater detail. Associated injuries to the cuneiforms, cuboid, and/or metatarsals are common and should be ruled out.

If no instability (displacement) is appreciated on standard and stress radiographs a diagnosis of midfoot sprain may be considered with initial non–weight-bearing treatment and progressive weight-bearing as comfort allows. Repeat x-rays should be obtained once swelling has subsided. For any displacement of the tarsometatarsal joint more than 2 mm, surgery should be pursued with screws and k-wires.

▶ Fractures of the Forefoot

Fractures of the first metatarsal are rare due its larger size and increased strength compared to the other metatarsals. Isolated fractures of the first metatarsal without instability may be treated with weight bearing as tolerated in a short-leg cast or removable boot for 4-6 weeks. If displacement is detected of the first metatarsal through the joint or fracture site, operative intervention is required.

Fractures of the second, third, or fourth metatarsals are much more common. Most isolated fractures can be treated closed with hard-soled shoes and progressive weight-bearing. Operative indications include fractures with more than 10 degrees of deviation in a dorsal or plantar direction or 3-4 mm of translation in any plane.

Fifth metatarsal fractures usually result from direct trauma and are divided into two groups: proximal base fractures and distal spiral fractures. The proximal fifth metatarsal fractures are further sub-divided: Zone I (cancellous tuberosity, which is the insertion of the peroneal brevis), Zone II (distal to the tuberosity), and Zone III (distal to the proximal ligaments, without extension past the proximal 1.5 cm of the diaphyseal shaft). Zone I injuries are treated symptomatically with hard-soled shoe. The treatment of Zone II injuries, aka Jones fractures, is controversial due to healing difficulty. Some authors advocate weight-bearing as tolerated, others recommend non–weight-bearing in a short leg cast or surgical intervention. Zone 3 injuries may be treated non–weight-bearing in a cast or with surgery. Fractures distal to the proximal 1.5 cm of the diaphyseal shaft, are called "Dancer's fractures" and are treated symptomatically with a hard-soled shoe.

4. Metatarsophalangeal Joint

Injuries to the first MTP joint are relatively common especially in persons who participate in athletic activities such as ballet, football, or soccer. The MTP joint is composed of a cam-shaped metatarsal head articulating with the concave proximally articular surface of the proximal phalanx. The stability of the joint is provided by ligamentous constraints which include the medial and lateral collateral ligaments as well as the dorsal capsule and plantar plate which are reinforced by the extensor hallucis longus and flexor hallucis longus tendons respectively. "Turf toe" which is a hyperextension injury of the first MTP joint, resulting in stretching of the plantar capsule and plate, may be treated with RICE, nonsteroidal anti-inflammatory drugs (NSAIDS), and protective taping with gradual return to activity. MTP dislocations are treated with closed reduction and short-leg cast with toe extension for 3-4 weeks. Dislocations with displaced avulsion fractures require surgical intervention with lag screws or tension-band technique.

Injuries to the lesser MTP joints are common as well. Simple dislocations or nondisplaced fractures are managed with gentle reduction and buddy taping. Intra-articular fractures may be treated with excision for small fragments or ORIF with Kirshner wires or screws.

5. Fractures & Dislocations of the Phalanges of the Toes

Phalangeal fractures are the most common injury to the forefoot. The proximal phalynx of the fifth toe is the most common phalynx injured. Like the fifth digit, the first digit is also particularly vulnerable to injury due their border positions in the foot. Mechanisms of injury usually entails direct blow such as from a dropped heavy object or axial load resulting from a stubbing injury. Fractures and/or dislocations are diagnosed with foot series radiographs (AP, lateral, oblique). MRI or bone scan may aid in the diagnosis of stress fractures that are not visible on x-ray. Nondisplaced fractures are treated with stiff-soled shoe and protected weight-bearing with advancement as tolerated. Buddy taping may be used as well. Fractures with clinical deformity require reduction. Operative intervention is only performed for those rare fractures with gross instability or persistent intra-articular deformity. Dislocated IP joints without fracture are usually amenable to closed reduction and buddy taping with progressive advancement of activity.

6. Fracture of the Sesamoids of the Great Toe

Fractures of the sesamoid bones is rare, occurring with hyperextension injuries in ballet dancers and runners. The medial sesamoid is more frequently fractured than the lateral sesamoid due to increased weight-bearing on the medial side of the foot. Fractures of the sesamoids must be distinguished from bipartite sesamoids which are relatively common, up to 30% of the general population (bilateral in 85% of cases). These fractures are initially treated closed with soft padding and short-leg walking cast for 4 weeks followed by shoe with metatarsal pad for additional 4-8 weeks. Sesamoidectomy is reserved for cases of failed conservative treatment.

▼ PEDIATRIC ORTHOPEDICS

CHILDREN'S FRACTURES & DISLOCATIONS

Children's skeletal injuries differ from those of adults in several significant ways. An important difference is the presence of the growth plate or physis, giving immature bone is its potential for longitudinal growth. Bones increase in diameter by appositional growth from the periosteum. Injuries to the physis may disrupt skeletal growth. Children's bones heal rapidly, and nonunion is exceedingly rare. The periosteum is thick and strong, surrounding the long bone like a sleeve and helps to minimize fracture displacement and promote healing.

When injury occurs in a young child, especially one under 3 years of age, a careful social history should be taken (see Chapter 45). State law in all jurisdictions requires that suspected cases of abuse be reported to local authorities.

Closed treatment is usually sufficient for children's fractures. Manipulation also known as closed reduction under sedation may be required for significant displaced fractures. Open fractures, fractures with articular surface displacement, and less commonly fractures that cannot be reduced by closed means require operative treatment.

Although children's fractures do heal rapidly and immobilization rarely causes joint stiffness in children, so casts can be left on until union is achieved.

The bone in growing children is mechanically different from that in adults; immature bone is more porous and fails in compression as well as in tension. An example is the so-called buckle or torus fracture that occurs at the metaphysis of the distal radius. This stable injury should be protected in plaster for 3 weeks to control symptoms and prevent further trauma to the weakened bone.

Immature bone is less brittle than that of adults, and children's bones may therefore bend but not fracture. This plastic deformation may produce significant deformity that requires manipulation to restore alignment.

Greenstick fractures are also a result of the plasticity of children's bones. Incomplete disruption of a long bone occurs such that the bone fractures on the tension side but the opposite cortex remains in continuity. The periosteum remains intact on the concave side and typically the intact cortex resists any significant angulation at the fracture site.

1. Growth Plate Fractures

About 15% of children's fractures involve a growth plate—most commonly the distal radius, distal tibia or fibula (or both), and distal humerus.

▶ Classification

Classification of physeal injuries helps to distinguish patterns that may disturb growth and also provides some guidance for treatment. It should be recognized that even "benign" injuries to the growth plate of the distal femoral and tibia can have clinically significant consequences.

Physeal injuries are classified according to the Salter and Harris system (Figure 40–22).

A. Type I

Type I injuries have fracture lines that follow the growth plate, separating the epiphysis from metaphysis. Without displacement, radiographs may appear normal. This is often a clinical diagnosis with tenderness localized over the physis confirming that a growth plate injury has occurred. Healing occurs rapidly, usually within 2–3 weeks.

B. Type II

In type II injuries, the fracture line traverses the epiphysis and exits in the metaphysic. The metaphyseal fragment is often referred to as the Thurston–Holland sign and is diagnostic of a growth plate injury. Type II injuries are the most common physeal fractures. Satisfactory alignment can often be achieved with gentle closed reduction and casting. If pin fixation is required, smooth pins can be safely used across the physis. The risk of growth disturbance is highest for distal femoral and distal tibial fractures.

C. Type III

Type III physeal injuries are those in which the fracture line exits through the epiphysis at the articular surface.

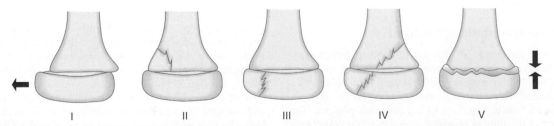

▲ **Figure 40–22.** Salter–Harris classification of physial injuries occurring at the zone of provisional calcification of the growth plate.

Any displacement at the articular surface requires operative intervention.

D. Type IV

Salter–Harris-type IV fractures cross both the metaphysic and the epiphysis. Because it involves the articular surface, anatomic reduction is essential to minimize the complications of type IV growth plate fractures, including growth disturbance, malunion, and articular incongruity. Even with perfect reduction, growth may be affected, and the prognosis is guarded.

E. Type V

Type V growth plate injuries are due to severe axial loading. Some or all of the physis is so severely compressed that growth potential is destroyed. Initial radiographs may appear normal like with SH 1 injuries. A history of a significant mechanism with swelling and tenderness over the physis should suggest the possibility of such an injury. Subsequent follow-up radiographs are critical to watch for premature closure of the physis, and/or progressive angular deformity due to asymmetric injury to the growth plate.

► Treatment

A. Conservative Treatment

Most fractures involving the physis may be managed nonoperatively. Nondisplaced fractures are protected in a cast until healed. Typically 3–6 weeks is usually sufficient depending upon the child's age and the site of injury. Displaced type I and type II injuries should be treated with a single attempt at closed reduction followed by immobilization as above. Because of the significant remodeling potential, acceptance of some deformity is better than repeated vigorous attempts at reduction which causes additional damage to the physis. Attempts at reduction should be avoided if more than seven days have passed since the injury.

B. Operative Treatment

Displaced type III and type IV injuries usually require open reduction and internal fixation. Fixation is ideally place within the metaphysic or epiphysis. If it is necessary to cross the physis, only smooth pin fixation is recommended. Cast immobilization may be required to supplement fixation.

► Prognosis

All injuries that involve physes should be followed at least 12-18 months to confirm that growth has not been disrupted. The parents should be warned at the time of the injury of the possibility of altered growth. Physeal arrest may result in angular deformity and/or limb length inequality. When a physeal bar is suspected, CT scan or MRI can be used to localize the area, and estimate its size. If the bony bar is less than 50% of the physis and the child has at least two years of growth remaining, resection of the bar can be considered. Alternatively, the portion of the physis that remains open can be intentionally closed down to limit angular deformity. Limb length inequalities will occur if there is a complete physeal arrest. If the difference is less than 2 cm, no treatment is typically required. Differences of 2-5 cm are most frequently managed with an epiphysiodesis on the contralateral limb. Limb lengthening techniques can be considered with limb length inequalities exceed 5 cm.

2. Upper Extremity Fractures & Dislocations

► Proximal Humeral Fractures

Separation of the unossified proximal humeral epiphysis has been described following difficult delivery of an infant. The child is unable to use the arm raising the concern for brachial plexus palsy. This "pseudoparalysis" resolves on the order of 7-10 days and radiographs demonstrate abundant callus, confirming the fracture. Older children most commonly sustain SH II fractures. Significant displacement and angulation is well tolerated and the child can be treated in a sling for 3 weeks. In the adolescent approaching maturity displaced fractures are treated with closed reduction and pin fixation. There is so much potential for remodeling in the proximal humerus that the best obtainable closed reduction is preferable to open surgery. Residual deformity, loss of motion, and functional problems are exceedingly rare following sustain proximal humerus fractures.

► Supracondylar Fractures of the Humerus

Supracondylar fractures are among the most common injury in children ages 4-8 years. The typical mechanism is a hyperextension injury to the elbow. Type 1 of undisplaced supracondylar fractures present with elbow pain, swelling, and tenderness at the site. Radiographs usually show a positive fat pad sign, indicating elbow hemarthrosis and a nondisplaced fracture of the distal humerus anteriorly. The fracture line may be subtle so comparison radiographs of the uninjured elbow may be helpful. Cast immobilization for 3-4 weeks is recommended. Type II fractures are those in which there is posterior angulation of the distal fragment, with an intact periosteal hinge. The anterior humeral line no longer bisects the capitellum on the lateral radiograph. Closed reduction and pinning is advised to restore this relationship. Type III fractures are completely displaced. These are serious injuries that threaten the neurovascular structures. The radial pulse and the function of the radial, ulnar, and median (including anterior interosseous) nerves should be checked immediately. If ischemia is present initially, prompt reduction of deformity is the next step toward restoration of normal perfusion. If pulses cannot be restored with reduction then an angiogram and vascular consultation is urgent. When the loss of pulses occurs following attempts at reduction, vascular entrapment should be suspected and prompt surgical exploration of the brachial artery may be required.

Fracture reduction is secured with percutaneous pin fixation and splint immobilization for 4-6 weeks. Long-term problems include elbow stiffness, malunion, and growth arrest. Nerve injuries typically represent neuropraxias that resolve with observation over the subsequent 3-6 months.

Flexion type supracondylar fractures are rare, but when they do occur are typically managed with open reduction and pin fixation. The ulnar nerve is most at risk with these injuries.

▶ Subluxation of the Radial Head (Nursemaid's Elbow)

This common minor injury occurs in children under 4 years of age. It is caused by a sudden pull on the extended pronated arm, usually by an adult tugging on a reluctant toddler. The pronated radial head slips partially under the annular ligament and displaces into the radiocapitellar joint. The child suddenly stops using the arm, holding it in a flexed and pronated position. Radiographs show no abnormalities since positioning for elbow films will often reduce the subluxation. Reduction is achieved by firmly supinating the forearm and flexing the elbow while pressing down on the radial head. Often a "click" is felt when reduction is achieved. Soon after reduction the child becomes less apprehensive and gradually resumes use of the arm.

▶ Other Fractures & Dislocations of the Elbow

There are a few injuries unique to the pediatric elbow which warrant mention. Fractures of the distal humerus including displaced lateral condyle fractures and displaced medial epicondyle fractures require surgery to restore articular congruity. Radial neck fractures with angulation that inhibits forearm rotation require reduction and fixation. Displaced olecranon fractures, if not reduced by elbow extension, will also require internal fixation. Monteggia and monteggia variant fractures represent a spectrum of injuries which include forearm fracture with radial head dislocation. Radiographs of the elbow are essential following any ulnar or radial shaft fractures to look for this injury.

▶ Forearm Fractures

Fractures of the shafts of both the radius and the ulna occur frequently in children. The most common problem is malunion with angular or rotational deformity which limits supination-pronation. Initial treatment is closed reduction. Because of the remodeling potential in the growing child, anatomic reduction is not essential. Side-by-side or "bayonet" apposition is acceptable but angulation should be minimized. Radiographs are repeated weekly for 3 weeks to permit early remanipulation should the fracture displace. If displacement occurs repeat reduction and possibly internal fixation with intramedullary nails or plates maybe required.

Galeazzi fracture combines dislocation of the distal radioulnar joint with fracture of the radial shaft. To avoid missing this injury radiographs of the wrist and the elbow are obtained to confirm that normal bony relationships are present.

3. Lower Extremity Fractures & Dislocations

▶ Traumatic Hip Dislocation

In children, traumatic dislocation is more common than fracture of the hip and has fewer complications. Prompt closed reduction under general anesthesia with good muscle relaxation is usually successful. Interposed soft tissue or bone fragments may necessitate open reduction. Following reduction, the hip should be protected for 4-6 weeks until soft tissue healing has occurred. With prompt reduction, avascular necrosis is rare but radiographs should be followed for 18 months.

▶ Fractures of the Proximal Femur

Proximal femur fractures are rare in children. This is fortunate, as displacement and injury to the growth plate and blood supply predispose to complications including avascular necrosis, physeal arrest, and nonunion. Fractures involving the proximal femur are typically the result of high energy trauma.

In children, most hip fractures involve the femoral neck. If there is no displacement, spica cast immobilization maintains alignment during healing, but close radiographic monitoring is required for prompt identification of any displacement. Displaced fractures of the femoral neck should be treated with anatomic reduction and screw fixation preferably placed short of the physis. Satisfactory results are achieved in half or less of cases, with avascular necrosis, varus malunion, and physeal arrest among the most common complications. Intertrochanteric and subtrochanteric fractures can generally be managed with open reduction and internal fixation. Late problems (eg, angular deformity and unequal limb lengths) are rare but do occur.

▶ Femoral Shaft Fractures

Femoral shaft fractures are fairly common childhood injuries. They often result from significant trauma, so that other injuries may also be present. Radiographs of the hip are required to ensure that fracture or dislocation is not present. The knee should also be x-rayed. Infants are treated with pavlik harness. Children ages 1-6 are most commonly treated with closed reduction and spica casting for 4-6 weeks. Titanium elastic nails have become the mainstay of treatment for the older child. Standard antegrade femoral nails are reserved only for skeletally mature adolescents because of the risk of avascular necrosis when the physes remain open.

▶ Fractures of the Tibia & Fibula

Fractures of the tibia and fibula are not unusual in childhood. An occult undisplaced spiral fracture may cause the toddler to refuse to weight bear ("toddler's fracture"). These fracture heal rapidly in a long-leg cast. Nerve and vessel damage may be present, especially with displaced fractures of the proximal metaphysis. Fractures of the tibial spine and tibial tubercle are unique to children. If displaced, these fractures require open reduction and fixation. Stiffness about the knee is common and fracture healing must be balanced with restoration of joint motion to avoid long-term problems.

▶ Fractures of the Distal Fibula Physis and Transitional Fractures

Fractures of the distal fibular occur frequently in children. This injury is the equivalent of an ankle sprain in the skeletally mature individual. Physical examination localizes tenderness to the distal fibular growth plate, and radiographs will typically be interpreted as normal. Treatment is symptomatic, with resolution of symptoms expected in 3-4 weeks.

Children are at risk for so called transitional fractures of the distal tibia. These occur most commonly in kids ages 10-14 when a portion of the growth plate is closed, but some portion still remains open. A Tillaux fracture is a fracture involving the anterolateral distal tibial epiphysis. Any displacement warrants open reduction and screw fixation. Triplane fractures of the distal tibia are identified as SH III injuries on the AP radiograph and SH II injuries on the lateral radiograph. Again, anatomic reduction and fixation is critical.

GAIT DISORDERS & LIMB DEFORMITY

Abnormalities of the lower extremities in children may be noticed by parents as the child learns to walk. The two most common areas of concern include rotational malalignment and angular deformity at the knees.

1. Intoeing

A normal foot progression angle with walking is 10 degrees external rotation. There are three common causes of the "foot turning in" in children. Metatarsus adductus represents adduction of the forefoot. This deformity is typically present at birth and passively correctable. Mild cases will resolve with stretching. If it persists beyond early childhood, surgical correction is an option.

Tibial torsion is an internal rotation deformity of the tibia. On physical exam the ankle axis (a line connecting the tips of the medial and lateral malleoli) is internally rotated

relative to the tibial tubercle. This developmental variant is common in children 1-3 years of age and almost always corrects spontaneously with growth. Special shoes and orthotic devices have not been shown to change the natural history and are no longer recommended. Rarely spontaneous correction does not occur (by age 6) and tibial derotational osteotomy can be considered.

Femoral anteversion is another common finding in children who walk with their feet turned in. Parents will report that the child is a "W" sitter. Observation reveals that the whole limb is internally rotated, so that the patella as well as the foot points medially. On clinical determination internal rotation at the hip approaches 90 degrees. Femoral anteversion can correct spontaneously up until the age of 12. If functional limitations are noted, a femoral derotational osteotomy can be considered.

2. Angular Deformity of the Lower Extremities (Knock-Knees & Bowlegs)

Varus or "bow legs" denotes deviation of the knees away from midline. Valgus or "knock knees" denotes deviation of the knees toward midline. Children may develop bowlegs from about 12-18 months to 3 years. The majority of children will show spontaneous resolution and occasionally progression to slight valgus between ages 3 and 4 years. In young children, angular deformity of the knees requires radiographs evaluation after the age of 2 years if it is asymmetric, associated with abnormally short stature or progressing. The differential diagnosis included infantile blounts and rickets. If metabolic bone disease is suspected, serum calcium, phosphate, and alkaline phosphatase should be measured. Operative treatment may be considered in if deformity persists after the age of 3.

▶ Pathologic Genu Varum

It is important to distinguish physiologic tibia vara from pathologic conditions associated with varus including rickets, Blount's disease and skeletal dysplasias. Blount's disease (tibia vara) has both infantile and adolescent forms. Radiographs in infantile blounts typically show metaphyseal beaking and changes in the medial proximal tibial physis. The metaphysial-diaphysial angle (> 11 degrees) of the tibia helps to differentiate between physiologic bowing and infantile tibia vara. Progressive tibia vara should be treated with corrective osteotomy of the proximal tibia and fibula. Overcorrection into valgus alignment is recommended because recurrence is common. Adolescents blounts is most common in obese patients. Excessive stress on the medial tibial physis is thought to inhibit normal growth leading to bowing. When the growth plates remain open, growth can be modulated using staples or plates to temporarily tether the lateral growth plate and allow for gradual correction. After skeletal maturity, proximal tibial osteotomy is recommended to restore normal mechanical alignment.

SYSTEMIC DISORDERS AFFECTING BONES & JOINTS IN CHILDREN

1. Juvenile Rheumatoid Arthritis

RA is an autoimmune disorder whose exact cause remains elusive. There are three basic clinical forms of juvenile rheumatoid arthritis (JRA). Pauciarticular arthritis generally involves a single joint, most commonly the knee or the ankle but occasionally the hip or an upper extremity (mainly the elbow or the wrist). Clinical symptoms include the insidious onset of swelling and loss of motion at the affected joint. Systemic manifestations are absent. Iridocyclitis, or inflammation of the iris and ciliary body, is most common in this form and JRA and an ophthalmology evaluation is necessary.

Polyarthritis is characterized by multiple joint involvement and minimal evidence of systemic disease. Fingers and toes, the neck, and the temporomandibular joints are more likely to be involved. The course is persistent, with periods of exacerbation.

Systemic rheumatoid disease (Still's disease) usually presents with multiple (more than five) involved joints, fever, lymphadenopathy, hepatosplenomegaly, rash, subcutaneous nodules, and pericarditis. The course may be remitting or relentless, causing severe permanent disability. Inflamed joints develop synovial hypertrophy and pannus, which destroy articular cartilage. The associated hyperemia can stimulate the adjacent physes, with resulting overgrowth, or physeal arrest. Damage to underlying bone and ligament can produce severe deformity and joint subluxation. Musculoskeletal involvement may include the cervical spine, with spontaneous fusion of the apophysial joints and result in C1-2 instability.

When a single joint is inflamed, it is necessary to exclude lyme disease in endemic areas, septic arthritis, and reactive synovitis. Polyarticular JRA must be differentiated from rheumatic fever and leukemia.

Medical management is the first line of treatment; anti-inflammatory agents and range of motion exercises as synovitis resolves and appropriate bracing to minimize stiffness and allow function. Synovial biopsy can be done percutaneously with arthroscopy to help confirm the diagnosis. Synovectomy is controversial but some believe that is may slow the progression of arthritis.

2. Brachial Plexus Palsy

Brachial plexus palsy has three general patterns of involvement: (1) Erb's palsy, involving C5 and C6 (upper trunk); (2) Klumpke's paralysis, involving C8 and T1 (lower trunk); and (3) whole plexus. The first step in treatment is recogni-

tion. Physical therapy to maintain range of motion is started immediately and continued as the child is followed for recovery of function. Recovery of the biceps (elbow flexion and forearm supination) by 3-6 months is generally a good prognostic sign. If no spontaneous improvement is seen, neurosurgical evaluation/intervention is recommended. If muscle imbalance persists at the shoulder, transfer of the latissimus dorsi and teres major muscles, so that they become external rotators, is an option. Humeral osteotomy is typically reserved for the older child with residual internal rotation contracture.

SCOLIOSIS & SPINAL DEFORMITY

The spine is in balance when the head is aligned with the pelvis in the coronal and sagittal planes. Scoliosis is spinal curvature of more than 10 degrees in the coronal or frontal plane. Scoliosis is a three-dimensional deformity with concurrent rotational component that creates a rib and/or lumbar prominence. Deformity may also exist in the sagittal plane. Normal kyphosis ranges from 20-40 degrees. Scheurmann's kyphosis is defined as vertebral body wedging at three consecutive levels and greater than 40 degrees of kyphosis in the sagittal plane.

The etiology of spinal deformity in children may be congenital, neuromuscular, traumatic, or idiopathic (of unknown cause). The cause of deformity is an important determinant of the natural history, treatment options, and the goals of management. Any family history of scoliosis should be elicited.

▶ Clinical Findings

Spinal deformity may be recognized in the perinatal period or during infancy in children with congenital anomalies of the spine. Most commonly, deformity of the spine is detected during the preadolescent growth spurt, when the spine is growing most rapidly. Spinal deformity is most commonly detected by family members, sports physicals, and primary care physicians. Routine school screening using the Adams forward bending test has improved recognition. Scoliometer measurements of greater than 7 degrees are an indication for orthopedic evaluation.

Physical examination of the patient with spinal deformity includes both examination of the spine and a comprehensive examination. The location of the curve, deviation of the trunk from the midline (trunk shift), shoulder asymmetry, pelvic obliquity, and flexibility of the spine should be recorded. Clinical findings suggestive of intraspinal pathology, such as tethered cord or a syrinx include asymmetric abdominal reflexes, clonus, muscle weakness or contractures, and foot deformities. Patients with congenital scoliosis may have associated chest wall deformity and sacral dimples. Scoliosis due to connective tissue pathology may present with joint hypermobility.

Imaging Studies

Spinal deformity occurs in three dimensions, and most imaging studies are limited by providing only a two-dimensional representation. Plain radiographs are useful for the detection of deformity and monitoring progression of deformity. The Cobb angle is used to measure deformity in the coronal and sagittal planes. An angular measurement is made between the end-vertebrae that are most tilted from the horizontal at either end of the curve (Figure 40–23). Other radiographic measures may include trunk shift relative to the pelvis and overall sagittal and coronal balance of the spine measuring a plumb-line between C7 and the sacrum.

MRI examination of the entire spine is an important imaging tool because of the association between intraspinal anomalies with certain types of spinal deformity. Congenital scoliosis may be associated with intraspinal abnormalities, including tethering of the cord, syringomyelia, diastematomyelia, diplomyelia, lipoma, teratoma, and neuroenteric cysts. MRI of the entire spine is indicated for patients with congenital scoliosis, patients with abnormal neurologic findings on physical examination, atypical curve patterns including left thoracic curves, as well as infantile and juvenile idiopathic scoliosis.

1. Idiopathic Scoliosis

Idiopathic scoliosis is the most common cause of spinal deformity in children and adolescents. The prevalence of adolescent idiopathic scoliosis is estimated at 2%-3% by age 16. Curves larger than 20 degrees are present in 0.3%-0.5% of adolescents. The ratio of affected males to females is equal in curves less than 15 degrees. However, for curves larger than 20 degrees, females are seven times more likely to be affected than males.

Nonoperative management of adolescent idiopathic scoliosis is intended to prevent progression of deformity during the growing years. Bracing is the only nonoperative treatment that has demonstrated efficacy in the management of progressive idiopathic scoliosis. Bracing is recommended for curves over 25-30 degrees in a child who remains skeletally immature. The efficacy of bracing is less predictable in larger curves.

Treatment Options

Surgical management of adolescent idiopathic scoliosis is intended to prevent additional progression of deformity. Spinal fusion may be considered for curves greater than 45-50 degrees in patients when significant growth remains. The natural history studies of untreated idiopathic scoliosis suggest that curve size is a risk factor for curve progression once skeletally mature. Curves under 30 degrees at maturity are not thought to progress, curves 30-40 degrees progress 0.5 degrees/year and curves over 40 degrees progress 1 degree/year on average.

2. Neuromuscular Scoliosis

Neuromuscular scoliosis presumably develops from a lack of trunk control. The term encompasses a spectrum of disorders all of which result in some compromise of the patient's ability to control posture and trunk position. The severity of deformity is related to the severity of weakness or spasticity, the patient's age at presentation of neuromuscular pathology, and the rostral or caudal level of involvement within the spinal cord. A child with known neuromuscular disorder is monitored for progression of spinal deformity in concert with management of associated deformities involving the hips, feet, and upper extremities.

Neuromuscular scoliosis may present in patients with disorders involving upper motor neurons, lower motor neurons, or primary myopathies. Upper motor neuron disorders

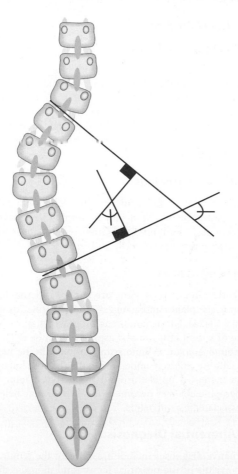

▲ **Figure 40–23.** Measurement of spinal deformity using the Cobb method.

may include cerebral palsy, spinocerebellar degeneration (Friedreich's ataxia, Charcot–Marie–Tooth disease, and Roussy–Levy disease), syringomyelia, spinal cord tumor, and spinal cord trauma. Lower motor neuron disorders include poliomyelitis, spinomuscular atrophy, myelodysplasia, dysautonomia, and trauma. Primary myopathies that may lead to neuromuscular deformity of the spine include muscular dystrophy, arthrogryposis, and congenital hypotonia.

Neuromuscular scoliosis characteristically presents with long, sweeping curves involving the thoracolumbar spine. This may result in imbalance of the trunk relative to the pelvis. Pelvic obliquity is common in neuromuscular scoliosis, resulting in poor sitting balance and skin breakdown. Pulmonary compromise may be an important feature of neuromuscular curves due to the combination of thoracic deformity with intercostal and accessory muscle weakness. The child with neuromuscular scoliosis often has comorbidities and functional considerations that are distinct from the patient with idiopathic or congenital scoliosis.

▶ Treatment Options

In the neuromuscular patient goals of treatment include sitting balance, prevention of sacral and ischial skin breakdown, and facilitating caregivers ability to assist with patient transfers and mobility.

Orthotics—including molded body jackets and thoracolumbar orthoses—may be useful in preserving sitting balance and preventing or delaying surgical stabilization. Indications for surgery include curve progression, poor sitting balance, and respiratory compromise. In the patient who is nonambulatory, fusion of the spinal column to the pelvis can be performed to correct pelvic obliquity.

3. Congenital Scoliosis

Congenital anomalies of the spine are caused by defects in the embryologic formation and segmentation of spinal elements. The formation of the spine begins during the third week of embryonic development. Abnormalities of either the notochord or the neural arch may lead to congenital anomalies of the spine. Congenital anomalies may include unilateral failure of formation (hemivertebrae and wedge vertebrae), failure of segmentation, rib fusions, and mixed or complex anomalies. These anomalies of the spine appear to be sporadic events and not hereditary. Because the cardiac and renal systems are developing simultaneously, these organ systems may also be affected. Routine cardiac evaluation and ultrasound of the renal system is recommended in patients with congenital scoliosis.

Progression of deformity in congenital scoliosis is dependent upon the type of vertebral anomaly, the position of the vertebral anomaly within the spine, and the growth potential for that segment of the spine.

▶ Treatment Options

Bracing has not been effective for congenital scoliosis and is not recommended. If progression of deformity is noted, surgical intervention is recommended. The goal of surgery in young patients is to prevent the development of a severe rigid deformity.

SEPTIC ARTHRITIS

▶ General Considerations

Infection is usually hematogenous and more frequent in infants exposed to invasive measures likely to cause bacteremia. The joint can be primarily involved, or secondary involvement may occur by spread of osteomyelitis from the proximal femur. Hip sepsis has also followed penetration of the joint during attempted blood aspiration from the femoral vein.

Staphylococcus aureus and Streptococcus pyogenes are the most common causative organisms.

▶ Clinical Findings

A. Symptoms and Signs

Refusal to bear weight, and pain with hip motion are early signs. Fever is unlikely in very young children, but sepsis may be suggested by generalized irritability and failure to thrive. Another focus of infection should increase suspicion. The hip is typically held flexed in slight abduction and external rotation. Attempts to move the hip are resisted and especially painful.

B. Laboratory Findings

The sedimentation rate and CRP are commonly elevated, but the white blood count may be normal. Leukocytes are abundant in the joint fluid and Gram-stained smears of fluid show microorganisms as well.

C. Imaging Studies

The early radiographic signs are subtle, with obliteration of soft tissue planes and a suggestion of capsular distention (Figure 40–24). Ultrasound imaging provides an early indication of a joint effusion and aspiration can be done under ultrasound guidance. Bone scan may initially be negative, especially in children under 6 months of age, but usually shows increased uptake around the involved joint before radiographic changes become evident. MRI may help identify associated osteomyelitis.

▶ Differential Diagnosis

Alternative diagnoses include fractures of the femur, acute osteomyelitis of the proximal femur, and iliopsoas abscess. Congenital hip dislocation is not painful and limited abduction with limb length inequality is noted. Transient

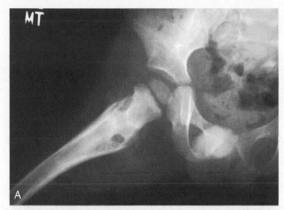

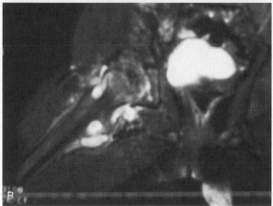

▲ **Figure 40–24.** Septic arthritis of the hip in a 2-year-old boy. **A.** Lateral radiograph shows signs of proximal femoral osteomyelitis. **B.** T2-weighted MRI showing large effusion in the hip joint and edema of the proximal femur.

synovitis typically presents with less severe symptoms, low-grade fevers, and responds to anti-inflammatory agents.

Complications

Structural sequelae include pathologic dislocation and irreversible destruction of the femoral head and neck. Chronic persisting infection may also result.

Treatment

Emergent surgical drainage is required. Side effects from a negative arthrotomy are so few that an aspiration is warranted if the diagnosis is uncertain. Gram-stained smears of intra-articular fluid guide the initial choice of parenteral antibiotic, which is modified if necessary according to the results of culture and sensitivity tests. Intravenous antibiotics are given until clinical improvement followed by oral antibiotics for 4 weeks.

Course & Prognosis

If the diagnosis is made and surgical drainage performed in a timely fashion the long-term results are good. Delay and nonoperative treatment are predictably followed by the complications mentioned earlier in the chapter.

TRANSIENT SYNOVITIS OF THE HIP (TOXIC SYNOVITIS)

Transient synovitis is a common cause of a painful hip in young children. A respiratory illness often precedes the complaints of pain, which may be localized to the knee, thigh, or hip. The short duration of symptoms, absence of diagnostic radiographic signs, and nearly normal laboratory studies suggest a benign process. Children of any age may be affected, with the average age is 6 years. Perhaps the most important aspect of transient synovitis is recognition.

Clinical Findings

A. Symptoms and Signs

When first evaluated, the child has rarely been symptomatic for more than a week. Pain in the lower extremity with activity (or even with rest) is the most common complaint. Limp and refusal to weight bear are also common. Passive range of motion of the hip must be checked and compared carefully with the opposite side. Normally, the child should be able to relax and motion should be free and easy without "guarding," which is especially noticeable with rotation or at extremes of flexion or extension. Low-grade fever may be present, but the child does not appear ill.

B. Laboratory Findings

Although the white blood cell count and erythrocyte sedimentation rate may be somewhat elevated, they are usually normal. Hip aspiration, if performed to help clarify a confusing case, reveals clear synovial fluid with a low white cell count, no organisms on Gram-stained smears, and negative cultures for all types of organisms.

C. Imaging Studies

Radiographs are essential to rule out other diagnoses. X-rays are usually normal with transient synovitis of the hip. Hip ultrasound will show little or no effusion.

Differential Diagnosis

Septic arthritis is the primary concern. Legg–Perthes disease (avascular necrosis), slipped capital femoral epiphysis, and, rarely, other forms of inflammatory joint disease such as RA or rheumatic fever must be considered.

Treatment

Hospitalization for observation and serial clinical exams is often advised to ensure that an infection is not missed. The hip is placed at rest and anti-inflammatory agents are initiated. This almost always relieves symptoms promptly and also helps confirm the diagnosis. The child should then be reexamined to make certain that normal hip motion and comfort have been achieved. Anteroposterior and lateral x-rays are repeated in 2-3 months to ensure that avascular necrosis has not developed. Occasionally, signs of systemic reaction are more pronounced or the child continues to guard the hip longer than usual. In such cases, needle aspiration confirmed by arthrogram should be performed to rule out infection.

Prognosis

Recurrent symptoms may develop after release from the hospital and resumption of activity but usually resolve with more rest.

DEVELOPMENTAL DYSPLASIA/DISLOCATION OF THE HIP

ESSENTIALS OF DIAGNOSIS

▶ Mechanical instability of the hip.
▶ Limitation of abduction.
▶ Limb length inequality if unilateral.
▶ Abnormal gait once walking begins.

General Considerations

Developmental hip dysplasia (DDH) may be detected at birth or develop early in life. The incidence of dislocation is 1 in 1000 infants. Both hips may be involved. DDH is more common in first born, females and with breech positioning. It is rarely painful or disabling to the child but results in significant symptoms in adults if left untreated. The hip may be dislocated by reducible, reduced but dislocatable or dislocated and not reducible.

Clinical Findings

A. Symptoms and Signs

The physical signs of DDH are the key to diagnosis. They may be subtle, however, and can be missed by the most experienced examiner. This emphasizes the need for repeated evaluation of the hips during routine "well baby" checks.

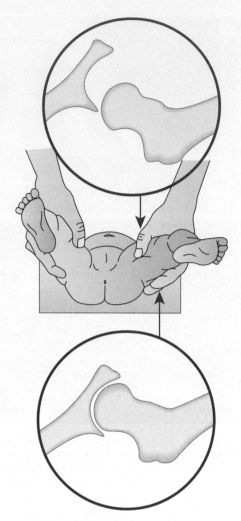

▲ **Figure 40–25. Upper window:** Subluxation provocation test. Holding the thighs of the relaxed infant as illustrated, the examiner stabilizes the pelvis with one hand while gently but firmly trying to displace the opposite femoral head posteriorly out of the acetabulum. Adduction of the thigh aids this maneuver. If mechanical instability of the femoral head is present, a "jerk" will be felt, indicating that the hip is subluxable. **Lower window:** In Ortolani's test, abduction and lifting with the fingers produces a corresponding jerk when the dislocated femoral head slides back into the acetabulum.

1. Dislocatable hip (Barlow positive)—The examiner attempts to displace the infant's femoral head posterolaterally from the acetabulum by means of a provocation test (Figure 40–25). In a positive test, the femoral head is felt to displace out of the acetabulum. Mechanical instability—not a "click"—is the essential finding.

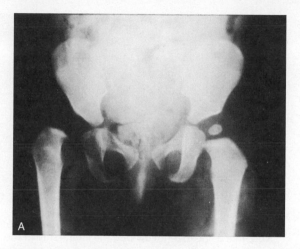

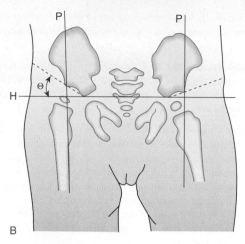

▲ **Figure 40–26. A.** X-ray of congenital dislocation of the right hip. **B.** Analysis of hip radiographs presupposes adequately exposed films of a properly positioned patient. Hilgenreiner's horizontal line is drawn through both triradiate cartilages (H), and Perkins's vertical line is drawn through the outer margin of each acetabulum (P). If the hip is located, the proximal femoral epiphysis will lie in the inferomedial quadrant formed by the two intersecting lines. Proximal or lateral displacement indicates dislocation. Abnormal acetabular development is suggested by lack of obvious concavity and by an acetabular index (θ) greater than 30 degrees.

2. Dislocated but reducible hip (Ortolani positive)— Ortolani described relocation of a dislocated femoral head when the examiner abducts the flexed hip and lifts the greater trochanter anteriorly. The soft tissues surrounding the joint may not be lax enough to permit reduction. A fixed hip dislocation will result in limited abduction, apparent shortening of the affected side, and asymmetric thigh creases (if the dislocation is unilateral). As the child begins to walk, an abnormal gait becomes apparent. If dislocation is bilateral, the diagnosis is more challenging; the gait is "waddling," and lumbar lordosis is prominent.

B. Imaging Studies

Until the cartilaginous acetabulum and femoral head become substantially ossified, x-rays may fail to indicate the true condition of the hip joint. Obvious abnormalities must be considered significant, but apparently normal radiographs do not exclude hip dysplasia until a well-ossified femoral head is adequately contained by the acetabulum. Femoral head ossification is usually present by 6 months of age but is may be delayed in DDH. Figure 40–26 shows several of the many radiographic relationships that are important for evaluation of the hip joint in infants. In older children, the femoral head should be adjacent to the radiolucent triradiate cartilage that forms the medial wall of the acetabulum. Displacement of the femoral head confirms dislocation. A shallow acetabulum that poorly covers the femoral head is termed dysplastic. Ultrasonography is the best technique for assessing the infant's hip prior to ossification of the femoral head.

▶ Differential Diagnosis

Proximal femoral focal deficiency and congenital coxa vara are rare conditions that produce shortening or instability in the hip region. Pathologic dislocation can occur rapidly in infected hips; the femoral head is displaced from a radiographically normal acetabulum. Hip dislocation may be caused by muscle imbalance in children with cerebral palsy or myelomeningocele.

▶ Complications

Complications include inability to gain or maintain a stable reduction, avascular necrosis of the femoral head following operative or nonoperative treatment, and limitation of motion.

▶ Treatment

A. Dislocatable hip

Neonates with confirmed dislocatable and reducible hips should be treated by means of abduction splinting (Pavlik harness) until stability is confirmed. It is important to flex the hips and abduct them no more than 60 degrees to avoid interfering with the blood supply and injury to the femoral nerve.

B. Dislocated hip

1. Birth to 18 months—In this age group, closed reduction is usually possible. Reduction can be maintained with a spica cast. If closed reduction is not possible or cannot be maintained, open reduction is required. Arthrography and computed tomography are used to confirm reduction.

2. Eighteen months to 4 years—Open reduction is more likely to be required in this group. If adequate reduction is obtained, satisfactory results are more likely. Acetabular remodeling is best until age 4.

3. Older children and adults—Treatment of newly diagnosed congenital hip dysplasia in this age group is difficult. Acetabular remodeling through growth is minimal. Achievement of a concentric reduction does not ensure a stable pain-free hip. Salvage osteotomies of the innominate bone have been described for improving acetabular coverage of the femoral head. Pain and limitation of motion will eventually necessitate total hip arthroplasty for many of these individuals.

SLIPPED CAPITAL FEMORAL EPIPHYSIS (SCFE)

During the period of rapid skeletal growth in early adolescence, the normal relationship of the femoral head with the femoral neck may become disturbed by a shearing displacement through the growth plate—known as slipped capital femoral epiphysis. The head remains within the acetabulum, while the femoral neck shifts anteriorly and laterally. This displacement may occur in response to minor trauma, or it can be gradual, as indicated by reactive bone formation and remodeling of the femoral neck adjacent to the growth plate. An acute SCFE may be superimposed upon a gradual "chronic" one. Involvement is bilateral in at least 25% of cases. SCFE are considered stable if the child can bear weight, and unstable if weight bearing is not tolerated. The risk of avascular necrosis is reported to be near 50% for unstable SCFE. This condition can lead to severe deformity and may cause early degenerative joint disease.

▶ Clinical Findings

A. Symptoms and Signs

The patient typically reports pain in the knee or thigh and limps. Hip motion is limited especially flexion and internal rotation, with obligatory external rotation found on exam.

B. Imaging Studies

Radiographs are diagnostic in all but the most minimal slips (Figure 40–27). The epiphysis is not centered on the neck but rather relatively displaced posterior and medial. Since posterior displacement is often more marked, the displacement is more evident on the lateral view. Bony callus, or widening of the metaphysis adjacent to the growth plate, indicates a chronic slip. A significant SCFE produces a bony prominence on the anterolateral femoral neck, restricting hip motion.

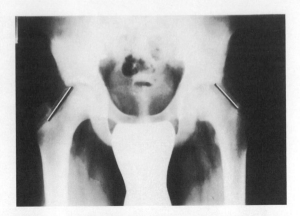

▲ **Figure 40–27.** Left slipped capital femoral epiphysis. Note that a line extended along the lateral side of the femoral neck misses the capital epiphysis. On the normal right side, this line enters the femoral head, which should overlap the neck on both anteroposterior and lateral views.

▶ Treatment

Surgical stabilization of the proximal femoral epiphysis is advised. In situ pinning of the epiphysis without reduction is then performed. The surgeon should make sure that screw does not enter the joint space. Gradual mobilization with protected weight bearing follows. The goal of in site pinning is to prevent further slip and gain closure of the physis. The opposite side must be watched until the physis closes as well. If severe deformity prevents hip motion, a subtrochanteric osteotomy or excision of the bony prominence on the femoral neck may be considered.

PERTHES (LEGG–CALVE–PERTHES) DISEASE

Perthes disease is an uncommon hip affliction that occurs in about one in 2000 children, generally between the ages of 4 and 10. Boys are affected five times as often as girls, but girls tend to have more severe involvement. About 10%-15% of patients have bilateral disease. The etiology is unknown but the hallmark is avascular necrosis of the proximal femoral epiphysis. Few patients achieve normal hip development. Others acquire permanent deformity of the femoral head, with limited motion and degenerative joint disease becoming symptomatic in middle age.

▶ Determinants of Final Outcome

A. Stages of Illness

The disease involves four stages: sclerosis, fragmentation, reossification, and remodeling. The earliest clinical signs are pain in the thigh and limping. Radiographs show an apparent increase in density of the capital epiphysis.

Later a subchondral crescent-shaped radiolucent fracture may occur, and the metaphysis may widen. The epiphysis becomes irregular and flattened during fragmentation. Gradually, reossification occurs and symptoms subside. The ultimate shape will depend upon the remolding of the proximal femur with growth. A spherical head correlates well with good long-term results.

B. Age of Patient

Younger patients have a better prognosis. Boys generally have less sever involvement than girls.

C. Severity of Involvement

The lateral pillar classification divides patients with Legg–Perthes disease into three groups—according to the extent of involvement of the lateral pillar of the epiphysis relative to the central portion of the head; group A has minimal involvement the epiphysis involved, group B with 50% decrease in height of the lateral pillar, and group C, with involvement of the entire head.

D. The "Head at Risk"

Catterall proposed certain clinical and radiographic criteria for determining whether the femoral head might deform in the course of the disease. The clinical criteria are (1) obesity, (2) decreasing range of motion of the involved hip, and (3) adduction contracture. The radiographic criteria are (1) lateral subluxation of the femoral head, (2) Gage's sign (widening of the lateral part of the growth plate, so that the superior portion of the femoral neck appears convex), (3) calcification lateral to the epiphysis in the cartilaginous femoral head, (4) diffuse metaphysial reaction, and (5) a horizontal growth plate.

▶ Clinical Findings

A. Symptoms and Signs

Insidious development of limp and sometimes pain in the groin, anterior thigh, or knee eventually bring the patient to a physician. An occasional case presents as acute synovitis. Examination shows antalgic gait, decreased hip motion (especially abduction and internal rotation), and sometimes flexion-adduction contracture. Passive motion is guarded rather than free.

B. Laboratory Findings

Bone scan may help with early diagnosis and assessment of the extent of head involvement.

C. Imaging Studies

Well-exposed radiographs in both anteroposterior and frog-leg lateral views are essential. Findings will depend upon the stage and severity of disease, as discussed above, but initial films usually show increased density and deformity of the femoral head epiphysis, which may be flattened or fragmented (Figure 40–28).

▶ Differential Diagnosis

The early inflammatory stage of Legg–Perthes disease can be confused with toxic synovitis and septic arthritis. The epiphysial abnormalities are similar to those seen in epiphysial dysplasias, hypothyroidism, and avascular necrosis from other causes, notably sickle cell anemia, Gaucher's disease, and chronic use of corticosteroid drugs.

▶ Treatment

Treatment requires categorization according to the stage of disease, the extent of head involvement, and the condition of the hip joint at the time of presentation. The mobility of the involved joint must be determined and then followed as an important indicator of need for intervention and prognosis.

A. Observation

Children under the age of 6 without "at risk" signs typically do well with symptomatic treatment including activity restriction, stretching, and anti-inflammatory agents. In older children, if the femoral head remains contained in the acetabulum and motion is maintained observation is recommended.

Surgical Treatment

On occasion surgery is necessary to reorient the acetabulum or the proximal femur to achieve containment. Both innominate osteotomy and varus proximal femoral osteotomy have been successful.

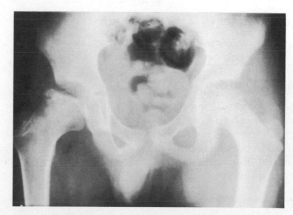

▲ **Figure 40–28.** X-ray of Legg–Perthes disease, with significant deformity of right femoral head.

Prognosis

Prolonged follow-up is necessary to determine the outcome. Long-term results are best correlated with the shape of the femoral head at the completion of skeletal growth.

FOOT DEFORMITIES IN CHILDREN

Positional deformities of the foot are described with the following specific terms. Equinus refers to plantar flexion. Calcaneus is the opposite position, or dorsiflexion. The forefoot alone may be in adduction, known as metatarsus adductus. The hindfoot deformity may be varus or valgus.

The goal of treatment of any foot deformity is a pain-free, flexible, plantigrade foot during normal gait.

1. Clubfoot

Talipes equinovarus, or clubfoot, is the most common foot deformity affecting approximately one in 1000 children. It occurs twice as often in boys and is bilateral half the time. There is a familial tendency, with a 5% chance that a sibling will also be affected. It can be idiopathic, or associated with an underlying syndrome.

▶ Clinical Findings

A. Symptoms and Signs

In clubfoot, there is varus of the hindfoot, adduction of the forefoot, and equinovarus deformity. The exact etiology remains uncertain. The joints principally involved are both the subtalar and talonavicular joints. The adjacent ankle and midtarsal joints are affected to a lesser degree. The overlying soft tissues are contracted. Successful treatment requires serial casting with correction of the deformities, cavus-adduction-varus-equinus, in that order as described by Ponseti. Surgical intervention is rarely required for clubfeet if treated early with casting.

▶ Treatment

Initial treatment is always nonoperative and should be started as soon as possible, preferably the day the infant is born.

A. Manipulation

Gentle manipulation into a corrected position should be done in order to stretch the contracted soft tissues—specifically, to align the calcaneus and navicular relative to the talus. Gentleness is required to avoid tissue trauma and to prevent overcorrection of the forefoot relative to persisting tarsal deformity.

B. Casting

After manipulation, a plaster cast is applied and molded to maintain the corrected position. Manipulation and cast application are repeated weekly, typically for 6 weeks. Often a percutaneous tendoachilles lengthening is needed for residual equinus.

Casting is followed by application of Denis Browne bar with reverse last shoes worn at first full time and then at night and during nap times for two years. During this time, routine follow-up is required to monitor for recurrence.

C. Surgical Treatment

The traditional surgery involved a posteromedial release of the ankle and subtalar joints with realignment of the talonavicular and talocalcaneal joints. Surgery is rarely recommended for clubfoot.

2. Metatarsus Adductus

Metatarsus adductus is a common forefoot deformity that is often quite flexible. If passively correctable, there is an 85% chance of spontaneous correction by age 3 years. Easy passive correction also suggests that treatment is unnecessary. If the forefoot cannot readily be returned to a normal position, manipulation, and casting can be recommended. Only a very rare severe deformity will require surgical release or osteotomy and fusion of the tarsometatarsal joints.

3. Flatfoot

The normal newborn foot appears flat because subcutaneous fat fills the longitudinal arch. This fat deposit recedes over the first 4 years of life to reveal the typical adult appearance of a medial arch under the midfoot, which does not touch the floor with weight bearing. An inadequate bony arch, which permits the medial portion of the midfoot to bear weight, is the essential feature of true flatfoot. This deformity is further classified as rigid or flexible.

Rigid flatfoot is identified by the absence of normal mobility of the hindfoot. Rigid flatfoot presenting later in childhood is usually due to coalition of the tarsal bones. Associated episodic foot pain and spasm of the peroneal muscles are typical. Depending on the child's age and symptoms and the site of coalition, resection may be advisable or nonoperative treatment may suffice.

In flexible flatfoot, weight bearing obliterates the medial arch and also produces obvious valgus alignment of the calcaneus. Standing on tiptoes or sitting with the feet hanging free will restore the arch. Some patients with flexible flatfoot develop foot pain with weight bearing.

Treatment of asymptomatic flexible flatfoot in children is controversial. Parents distressed by the foot's appearance or by abnormal shoe wear often request treatment, but there is little evidence that treatment prevents future symptoms, and the majority of children with flexible flatfoot have no symptoms in adulthood.

The child with painful flexible flatfoot deformity deserves treatment. Exercises to stretch tight gastro-soleus muscle groups or to strengthen intrinsic plantar muscles are usually advised, and external support for the mediolongitudinal arch can be provided if necessary. If nonoperative treatment fails to control symptoms or if deformity precludes use of normal footwear, surgery may be considered.

▼ SPORTS MEDICINE

PAIN SYNDROMES OF THE SHOULDER

1. Rotator Cuff Tendinitis and Subacromial Bursitis

▶ General Considerations

Inflammation within the glenohumeral joint is the most frequent cause of shoulder pain and limitation of motion. The patient is typically middle-aged. Repetitive overhead activity from occupation or sports is a common cause. The most common site of inflammation at onset is the insertion of the rotator cuff tendons, particularly the supraspinatus tendon. The location of the supraspinatus tendon between the greater tuberosity of the humeral head and the overhanging acromion process renders it particularly vulnerable to mechanical compression. The subacromial space is another common site of inflammation with subdeltoid soreness frequently radiating along the lateral humerus to the deltoid insertion.

▶ Clinical Findings

Night pain is common. Active abduction becomes especially painful when the inflamed rotator cuff and overlying bursa are compressed beneath the acromion. The range of active abduction may be extended if the patient is instructed to rotate the arms so that the palms face upward. This rotates the greater tuberosity posteriorly, so that the attached rotator cuff tendons pass behind the acromion, resulting in diminished pain with continued abduction.

▶ Treatment

The initial treatment of rotator cuff tendinitis and subacromial bursitis is with anti-inflammatory agents (naproxen, ibuprofen), and physical therapy to preserve motion. Slings and shoulder immobilization should not be used for more than a few days, since capsular adhesions and prolonged stiffness may result. Gentle passive range-of-motion exercises should be started as soon as tolerated, followed by active pendulum exercises. Active exercise is gradually increased while passive range of motion is continued.

If pain does not respond to oral anti-inflammatory agents, relief may be obtained by injection into the subacromial bursa.

2. Biceps Tendinitis

ESSENTIALS OF DIAGNOSIS

▶ Localized tenderness over the bicipital groove.

▶ Pain during supination of the forearm against resistance.

▶ General Considerations

A common inflammatory process producing shoulder pain involves the biceps tendon in the bicipital groove. Biceps tendonitis usually affects individuals whose occupation involves repetitive biceps flexion against resistance or whose recreational activities include forceful throwing of a ball. Pain is prominent over the anterior aspect of the arm and is aggravated by shoulder motion. Symptoms are worse at night and improve with rest. Deltoid muscle spasm may be present and may limit both active and passive motion.

▶ Clinical Findings

Biceps tendinitis can be distinguished from rotator cuff tendinitis by localization of tenderness to the bicipital groove. Forearm supination against resistance with the elbow flexed at the patient's side elicits extreme tenderness in the region of the bicipital groove when the tendon is palpated near the shoulder. Instability of the tendon in the groove is occasionally manifested by a snapping sensation as the arm is abducted and externally rotated. Subluxation of the tendons can be provoked by Yergason's maneuver, in which the patient actively flexes the elbow against resistance while the physician rotates the humerus externally. An unstable tendon will "pop" out of the groove.

▶ Treatment

Treatment of bicipital tendinitis includes cessation of offending activities and short-term immobilization of the shoulder in a sling and a trial of nonsteroidal anti-inflammatory agents. Surgery is occasionally required to stabilize a subluxating tendon. When discomfort has subsided, progressive mobilization is begun with exercises similar to those described in the section on rotator cuff tendinitis.

3. Adhesive Capsulitis (Frozen Shoulder)

ESSENTIALS OF DIAGNOSIS

▶ Diffuse shoulder pain

▶ Restricted shoulder joint motion

General Considerations

A common cause of shoulder pain in middle-aged and elderly patients is adhesive capsulitis, or the so-called frozen shoulder. This disorder may complicate other inflammatory shoulder ailments, particularly in individuals immobilized for prolonged periods. It may also occur without any identifiable inciting trauma and has been associated with cardiovascular disease, diabetes, RA, and degenerative cervical spine disease. Though the exact pathogenesis is unknown, the end result is a chronically inflamed, contracted capsule densely adherent to the humeral head, the acromion, and the underlying biceps and rotator cuff tendons. Normal bursae are obliterated by scarring.

Clinical Findings

A. Symptoms and Signs

The onset of symptoms is usually gradual and heralded by complaints of diffuse tenderness with disproportionately severe restriction of active and passive motion. Motion is not improved by lidocaine or corticosteroid injection.

B. Imaging Studies

Arthrography reveals a contracted joint capsule and no bursal filling. X-rays may reveal osteopenia of the humeral head.

Treatment

The natural history of adhesive capsulitis is occasionally spontaneous resolution. Subsidence of pain and return of nearly full motion can be obtained, though the process may persist for 6 months to several years. Efforts to speed return of function have included intensive physical therapy and anti-inflammatory agents. Rarely, surgical intervention is required to release the capsule, and this can be done arthroscopically. Clearly, the best treatment of this condition is prevention. Prolonged disuse or immobilization of a painful shoulder must be avoided. Early mobilization is stressed, with initiation of gentle range of motion exercises and guidance by the physician and the physical therapist.

4. Dislocation of the Shoulder Joint

The shoulder (glenohumeral) joint is the most commonly dislocated joint in the body because it is less constrained than other joints and motion is possible in multiple planes. The constraints that prevent instability include the labrum, negative pressure of the joint, and glenohumeral ligaments. The rotator cuff also provides dynamic stability by compressing the humeral head against the glenoid. These static and dynamic stabilizers create a delicate balance between motion and stability.

Dislocations are usually related to overhead trauma when the arm is in abduction, extension, and external rotation.

Most traumatic dislocations are anterior, but posterior dislocations can occur. Shoulder instability is classified by several factors including traumatic versus atraumatic, initial versus recurrent, acute versus chronic, the direction of dislocation, and voluntary versus involuntary.

Anterior Dislocations of the Shoulder Joint

Anterior dislocations can be diagnosed by history and physical examination. The arm is held in a position of slight abduction and external rotation. The anterior shoulder area appears full, and there is a vacant sulcus in the posterior shoulder area. Anteroposterior x-ray in the plane of the scapula and axillary x-ray are necessary to determine the direction of the dislocation and the presence of fracture. Humeral head impression fractures (Hill Sachs lesion) and glenoid rim fractures are easily missed if the radiographs are inadequate. Dislocation may also be complicated by injury to the brachial plexus (most commonly the axillary nerve) and rotator cuff tear. The examiner should check for sensory changes over the deltoid to assess the axillary nerve.

Posterior Dislocation of the Shoulder Joint

Posterior dislocation is characterized by fullness beneath the spine of the scapula, flattening of the anterior shoulder, prominence of the coracoid, and restriction of motion in external rotation. The reported incidence of missed diagnosis is as high as 60%. The injury occurs either from direct or indirect force to the anterior shoulder, so that the humeral head is pushed out posteriorly. Common causes of posterior dislocation of the shoulder are seizures or electrical shock. Anteroposterior x-rays of the chest may look deceptively normal with posterior dislocation, but an axillary view and an anteroposterior x-ray in the scapular plane will show the true position of the head in relation to the glenoid. This dislocation may also be reduced by longitudinal and gentle transverse traction. The reduction may be held in a sling for 3-4 weeks with some external rotation if necessary.

Multidirectional Instability

Patients with congenital or acquired laxity may develop symptomatic shoulder instability in multiple directions. These patients should be initially treated with of rehabilitation and strengthening monitored by a physical therapist. Most of these patients recover stability with muscular strengthening of the rotator cuff and scapular stabilizing muscles.

Voluntary Dislocators

Patients who voluntarily dislocate their shoulders have a high recurrence rate after surgical procedures. Therefore, surgery is usually avoided in this population.

▶ Treatment

The treatment of shoulder dislocations consists of closed reduction after careful examination and documentation of neurovascular status and good quality x-rays. Many methods of closed reduction have been described, including gentle traction in the prone position and traction-countertraction with a sheet. All methods of reduction rely on adequate analgesia and relaxation. Forceful reductions should be avoided because they may cause brachial plexus injury, vascular injury, or fracture. Postreduction x-rays document a concentric reduction and rule out any associated fracture. Once reduced, the arm is placed in a sling for 3-4 weeks before protected motion exercises are initiated.

Surgical reconstruction is indicated for anterior traumatic instability that is recurrent. The incidence of recurrent instability approaches 80%-90% for active young athletes. Therefore, the indication for surgery depends on age and activity level as well as the number of traumatic dislocations and associated fracture or soft tissue injury. After operative repair, the shoulder is usually immobilized in a shoulder immobilizer for 3-6 weeks before active motion is begun. Open and arthroscopic surgical repairs of the labrum for anterior dislocation are successful in preventing further episodes of dislocation in most patients.

5. Rotator Cuff Tears

Rotator cuff tears and rotator cuff impingement are common sources of shoulder pain. Four rotator cuff muscles (supraspinatus, infraspinatus, teres minor, and subscapularis) function to move the arm and stabilize the shoulder joint. There is a full spectrum of injury ranging from tendonitis to impingement and rotator cuff tears. The most severe condition is a massive, chronic rotator cuff tear that subsequently leads to proximal migration of the humeral head and arthritic changes of the humeral head known as rotator cuff arthropathy.

Patients with "rotator cuff syndrome" usually present with pain and weakness related to attempted overhead activities and active movements with the arm away from the body. Physical examination demonstrates impingement pain with certain overhead movements and rotator cuff weakness. Diagnosis is made by history and physical examination. Ultrasound and MRI are useful tests to evaluate rotator cuff tears and associated intra-articular pathology (Figure 40-29).

▶ Treatment

The treatment of shoulder pain related to rotator cuff pathology (inflammation, degeneration, and tear) depends on other patient variables such as age, activity level, hand dominance

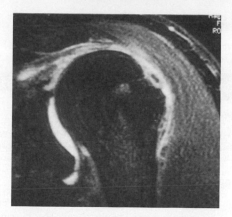

▲ **Figure 40-29.** T2-weighted MRI showing a massive rotator cuff tear.

as well as the chronicity and level of pain and dysfunction. Tears may result from single event trauma (a fall on the outstretched hand), repetitive trauma (baseball pitchers), or degeneration of the rotator cuff in older patients.

Most cases of shoulder pain related to the rotator cuff tendonitis are initially treated nonoperatively. Activity modification, NSAIDs, and physical therapy can be beneficial. Some patients require a subacromial injection to control inflammation and pain. Rotator cuff tears can be treated with surgical repair. Acute traumatic rotator cuff tears should be repaired acutely in order to prevent rotator cuff atrophy and retraction. Acromioplasty and distal clavicle excision are performed at the same time if coracoacromial arch impingement contributes to the rotator cuff tear.

6. Glenohumeral Arthritis

Arthritis of the glenohumeral joint may be caused by OA, inflammatory disease, previous trauma, previous surgery, or arthritis of recurrent instability. Patients have pain with activities as in arthritis in other joints. They may also complain of stiffness, which is usually progressive over time. Physical examination discloses limited motion. Examination by proper shoulder x-rays shows the characteristic joint space narrowing and humeral head osteophytes.

Before operative treatment is elected, a thorough course of conservative measures is indicated. Surgery becomes an option for patients with significant pain and limitation of activity because of their arthritis. Shoulder arthroplasty (hemiarthroplasty, total shoulder replacement) can provide pain relief; however, motion is rarely restored to normal. Contraindications to total arthroplasty are active or latent septic arthritis, paralysis of the shoulder musculature, and neuropathic joints.

PAIN SYNDROMES OF THE ELBOW

1. Tennis Elbow (Humeral Epicondylitis)

ESSENTIALS OF DIAGNOSIS

▶ Tenderness over the lateral humeral epicondyle

▶ Pain at the elbow with resisted extension of the wrist

General Considerations

Though far more common in nonathletes, humeral epicondylitis is commonly termed tennis elbow. This overuse syndrome is uncommon before age 18 years and most frequent in the fourth and fifth decades. Tennis elbow is commonly seen in nonathletes performing activities that require frequent rotary motion of the forearm, such as gardening, use of screwdrivers or wrenches, turning of doorknobs, and even operation of vehicles without power-assisted steering.

Clinical Findings

Tennis elbow is characterized by tenderness and pain at the humeral epicondyle provoked by extension of the wrist. The origin of the inflamed common extensor muscle is the source of discomfort. The pain is readily reproduced with resisted extension of the wrist with the elbow extended.

Though the pathogenesis of tennis elbow is unknown, symptoms are usually attributed to inflammation of the origin of the common extensor muscle and, in some cases, to a tear in the origin of the extensor carpi radialis brevis. The tears are thought to be the result of repeated stress on degenerated tendon fibers. Elbow motion remains normal.

Differential Diagnosis

Differential diagnosis includes radial nerve irritation at the elbow, which may often be delineated by electromyography (EMG).

Treatment

A. Medical Treatment

Most patients with tennis elbow respond favorably to a brief period of rest and anti-inflammatory agents followed by a program of exercises to strengthen the forearm muscles. Subtendinous injection of soluble corticosteroids with lidocaine may be required in more severe cases. Repeated injections may further weaken tendons and should be avoided.

A nonelastic forearm band may be prescribed and worn near the elbow during occupational or recreational activities that aggravate the condition. The band is thought to be effective either because it limits full contraction of the tender

muscles or because it slightly alters the position of the extensor tendons.

B. Surgical Treatment

Rarely, patients with severe or refractory symptoms may require operative treatment. Most surgeons repair the origin of the torn wrist extensor tendon after excision of granulation tissue and any rough subjacent bone. Lengthening of the short wrist extensor results in loss of strength.

2. Olecranon Bursitis

ESSENTIALS OF DIAGNOSIS

▶ Tenderness and swelling over the olecranon

▶ Limited elbow flexion

General Considerations

Olecranon bursitis is a common cause of periarticular elbow pain. Like epicondylitis, this condition is often related to occupational activities, in this case prolonged periods of leaning on the elbow.

Clinical Findings

A. Symptoms and Signs

The subcutaneous olecranon bursa becomes distended, sometimes to dramatic proportions. The skin of the extensor surface of the forearm may be edematous and pitted. Traumatic bursitis is often only mildly painful despite marked swelling.

Treatment

Treatment of idiopathic or traumatic olecranon bursitis consists of protecting the bursa from further pressure or irritation. Compression dressings may be necessary if symptoms are prolonged. Recurrence is not uncommon. Excision of the bursa may be required for rare persistent cases. The bursa must be totally excised and the overlying skin sutured to the olecranon periosteum to ensure obliteration of the space.

INJURIES TO THE LIGAMENTS, MENISCI, & CARTILAGE OF THE KNEE JOINT

Internal derangement of the knee joint mechanism is usually caused by trauma but can also result from overuse. Injuries to the ligaments, cartilage, and meniscus commonly occur as combined lesions.

X-rays are often normal in suspected ligament or cartilage injury. MRI is valuable imaging modality. MRI assists with preoperative confirmation of a clinical diagnosis.

Once a diagnosis is obtained, arthroscopy is a valuable diagnostic and therapeutic tool for the knee joint. The arthroscope is introduced into the knee joint through a small stab incision allows examination of structures inside. Meniscus tears, ligament reconstruction and chondral injury can all be addressed arthroscopically.

Injury to the Menisci

Injury to the medial meniscus is the most frequent internal derangement of the knee joint. Clinical findings include swelling, pain, and varying degrees of restriction of flexion or extension. True locking (inability to fully extend the knee) is highly suggestive of meniscal tear. A marginal tear permits displacement of the medial fragment into the intercondylar region (bucket handle tear) and prevents either complete extension or complete flexion. Motion may cause pain over the anteromedial or posteromedial joint line. Tenderness can often be elicited at the joint line. Weakness and atrophy of the quadriceps femoris may be present. Injury to the lateral meniscus is less common. Pain and tenderness may be present over the lateral joint line.

Initial treatment may be conservative. Swelling and pain can be relieved by aspiration. Isometric quadriceps exercises should be performed frequently throughout the day with the knee in maximum extension, and the emphasis should be placed on restoring range of motion. Physical therapy and nonsteroidal anti-inflammatory drugs are helpful.

Arthroscopy with either meniscal debridement for central tears or meniscus repair for peripheral tears is recommended. Isometric quadriceps exercises and range of motion exercises are resumed and are gradually increased. As soon as the patient is able to perform these exercises comfortably, graded resistance maneuvers should be started. Exercises should be continued until motion and strength is equal to the other healthy knee.

Injury to the Ligaments

Ligaments in general prevent displacement or angulation beyond its normal arc of motion.

A. Medial Collateral Ligament

The MCL is the primary restraint to valgus. Forced abduction of the leg at the knee causes injury varying from strain to complete rupture. The MCL is attached to the medial meniscus at the joint line.

A history of a twisting injury or direct blow at the knee with valgus strain can usually be obtained. Pain is present over the medial aspect of the knee joint. In severe injury, joint effusion may be present. Tenderness can be elicited at the site of the lesion. When only an isolated ligamentous tear is present, x-ray examination may not be helpful unless it is made while valgus stress is applied.

Treatment of an incomplete tear consists of protection from further injury while healing progresses in a brace that allows motion but protects the knee from valgus injury. It may be helpful to bend the brace into varus to take load off of the ligament.

Tear of the MCL is frequently associated with other lesions, such as tear of the medial meniscus and rupture of the anterior cruciate ligament.

B. Lateral Collateral Ligament

Tear of the lateral collateral ligament is often associated with injury to surrounding structures including the popliteus muscle tendon or the iliotibial band. Avulsion of the apex of the fibular head may occur, and the peroneal nerve may be injured.

Pain and tenderness are present over the lateral aspect of the knee joint, and hemarthrosis may be present. X-rays may show bone avulsion from the fibular head.

The treatment of partial tear is similar to that described for partial tear of the MCL. If complete tear is detected healing is rare without surgical intervention, and exploration and reconstruction is required.

C. Anterior Cruciate Ligament

The function of the anterior cruciate ligament is prevention of anterior displacement of the tibia relative to the femur. Injury to the anterior cruciate ligament is often associated with injury to the menisci or the MCL. The cruciate ligament may be avulsed with part of the tibial tubercle in children (Figure 40–30), but it usually ruptures within the substance of its fibers in adults.

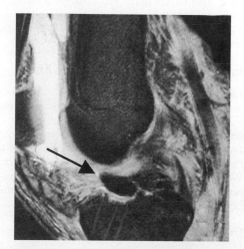

▲ **Figure 40–30.** Lateral T1-weighted MRI image showing an acute rupture of the anterior cruciate ligament (arrow).

The characteristic clinical sign of tear of the anterior cruciate ligament is a positive lachman: the knee is flexed to 30 degrees and pulled forward, and excessive anterior excursion of the proximal tibia (in comparison with the opposite normal knee) is noted. MRI is helpful for identifying associated meniscal or chondral injury. Reconstruction is usually required for young active patients who wish to participate in sports that call for sudden cutting or twisting movements. Reconstruction is delayed until full range of motion is obtained. With avulsion, displaced tibial bone is present, and attachment of the fragment in anatomic position by arthroscopy is necessary.

D. Posterior Cruciate Ligament

Tear of the posterior ligament may occur within its substance or by avulsion of a fragment of bone at its tibial attachment. Tear of the posterior cruciate ligament can be diagnosed by the posterior "drawer" sign: The knee is flexed at a right angle, and the upper tibia is pushed backward; if excessive posterior excursion of the proximal tibia can be noted, tear of the posterior ligament is likely. MRI is very accurate for diagnosis of these injuries.

Bony avulsion of the PCL should be addressed surgically with reattachment. Isolated PCL tears can be treated nonoperatively. Treatment is directed primarily at the associated injuries and maintenance of competency of the quadriceps strength.

▶ Cartilage Injury

Damage to the cartilage is common with trauma to the knee and should be differentiated from OA. Developments in cartilage transplantation, including autograft and allograft reconstruction, have improved the prognosis for these injuries. Arthroscopy and MRI are required for accurate diagnosis (Figure 40–31). Cartilage can also be biopsied from the knee, cultured, and then emplaned at a later date.

▶ Ligamentous Reconstruction of the Knee

Knee joint instability may be (1) single plane (medial, lateral, posterior, or anterior), (2) rotatory, or (3) a combinations of the two.

Reconstructive procedures to replace the function of the anterior and posterior cruciate ligament include use of a portion of autograft or allograft tendon to recreate the native ligament. Indications for major reconstruction of knee ligaments depend on the patient's age and activity level and the status of the articular cartilage within the knee.

PAIN SYNDROMES OF THE HIP

1. Bursitis & Tendonitis of the Hip

Bursitis and tendonitis are frequent causes of pain around the hip area. These conditions most commonly affect

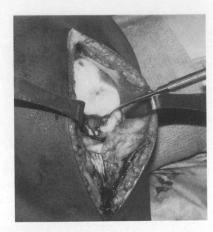

▲ **Figure 40–31.** Intraoperative photograph showing a full-thickness cartilage injury.

middle-aged and elderly patients. Patients with a history of prior hip surgery, such as hip replacement or fixation of a hip fracture, may be especially prone to these conditions.

▶ Clinical Findings

A. Symptoms and Signs

A common complaint is the inability to sleep or rest on the affected side. The painful area is localized over the prominence of the greater trochanter, and the pain is reproduced by firm palpation. Hip bursitis may be associated with tendonitis of the hip abductors that insert onto the greater trochanter. Pain due to tendonitis may be reproduced with active hip abduction against resistance.

It is important to differentiate extra-articular sources of hip pain such as bursitis and tendonitis from intra-articular sources such as OA. Intra-articular pathology is suggested by pain localized to the groin, limited internal rotation, and reproduction of the patient's pain at the extremes of rotation.

B. Imaging Studies

Plain radiographs are extremely useful in the evaluation of hip joint disorders.

▶ Treatment

Trochanteric bursitis often responds to rest, oral anti-inflammatory medications, and stretching. Corticosteroid injection is highly effective in refractory cases. Rapid relief of symptoms confirms injection of the proper area.

2. The Snapping Hip

The painful snapping hip is most commonly caused by the iliotibial band snapping over the prominence of the greater trochanter. Less commonly, the iliopsoas tendon may be the cause of pain as it snaps over the hip joint capsule.

Snapping due to the iliotibial band can be reproduced with passive flexion of the hip starting from an adducted position. Snapping of the iliopsoas tendon may be reproduced with passive extension and internal rotation of the hip starting from a flexed and externally rotated position. Fluoroscopy after injection of the iliopsoas bursa with contrast can help to confirm this diagnosis.

Treatment usually consists of stretching and strengthening exercises. In rare circumstances, surgical release may be indicated for refractory cases.

▼ JOINTS

ARTHRITIS

▶ General Considerations

Arthritis is an umbrella term for different inflammatory and noninflammatory disorders affecting synovial joints. Patients with advanced arthritis will experience pain, loss of motion, and joint deformity resulting in significant disability. Three major types of arthritis will be discussed in the following chapter: rheumatoid arthritis, spondyloarthritis, and osteoarthritis.

1. Rheumatoid Arthritis

▶ General Considerations

RA is a chronic inflammatory, autoimmune disease that attacks the synovial joints, causing a symmetric, erosive, deforming polyarthritis. RA is more common in women than in men affecting approximately 75 out of every 100,000 people. RA in many cases results in partial or total disability and is associated with a shortened life expectancy.

▶ Clinical Evaluation

Patients typically complain of joint pain, swelling, tenderness, and early morning stiffness that last greater than 1 hour and improve with activity. The joints most commonly involved include the MCP, PIP, and metatarsophalangeal (MTP). The cervical spine is often involved as well. In later stages of RA, tendon subluxation, tendon rupture, and joint destruction occur.

Currently, the most specific laboratory finding for RA is the presence of anticyclic citrullinated peptide antibodies. Approximately, two-thirds of RA patients will display these antibodies. Rheumatoid factor is a more sensitive but less specific laboratory finding, present in approximately ninety percent of patients with RA. Other common laboratory findings include presence of antinuclear antibody with homogenous pattern, elevated erythrocyte sedimentation rate (ESR), elevated C-reactive protein (CRP), decreased hematocrit, and increased platelet count.

Radiographs typically show bony erosions and osteopenia. Joint space narrowing, bone resorption, deformity, dislocation, and fragmentation occur as the disease process progresses. "Protrusio acetabuli" (medial migration of the femoral head through the acetabulum into the pelvis is sometimes seen on x-ray.

▶ Etiology

Currently, tumor necrosis factor alpha (TNF-alpha) and interleukin-1b (IL-1b) are considered to be the major proinflammatory cytokines responsible for the pathogenesis of RA. When these two cytokines are secreted, they stimulate synovial cells to proliferate and produce collagenase which leads to cartilage degradation, bone resorption and inhibition of proteoglycan synthesis. Additionally, these two cytokines induce other inflammatory cytokines and matrix metalloproteinases which further contribute to and sustain the inflammatory cascade.

▶ Treatment

In the past, treatment of RA was purely for symptom relief, consisting of splinting and rest of inflamed joints with oral NSAIDS. However, with the advent of disease-modifying antirheumatic drugs (DMARDS) and anticytokine medications the actual progression of the disease has been curtailed in patients.

Currently, three TNF-alpha antagonists are approved for the treatment of RA in the United States: infliximab, etanercept, and adalimumab. When one of these three drugs are used in combination with methotrexate, patients experience better functional outcomes and less joint structural damage over the course of time when compared to patients who are treated with only one medication. Due to the increased risk of serious infection, especially tuberculosis reactivation, patients should be screened for TB prior to starting one of the TNF-alpha antagonists. Additionally, patients with demyelinating disease should not take one of these agents.

Glucocorticoids have also been used to treat active RA for several years. The immediate anti-inflammatory effects of glucocorticoids are well-known. However, glucocorticoids have severe long-term side effects that make their continued use undesirable. At this time, treatment with low-dose prednisolone for the first six months of treatment in combination with a DMARD (eg, methotrexate) is an acceptable management plan. However, after six months, the prednisolone should be discontinued in favor of other therapy.

Other treatment medications for RA include anakinra (IL-1 receptor antagonist), abatacept (T-cell modulator), rituximab (B-cell modulator), doxycycline (matrix metalloproteinase modulator), and statins (anti-inflammatory).

These medications may be considered when therapy with TNF-alpha antagonists is contraindicated.

For patients with severe arthritic change, joint-replacement surgery can provide excellent pain relief and improved function. Joints that can be replaced include the hip, knee, shoulder, elbow, and metacarpophalangeal joints. Additionally, fusion may be considered for diseased joints of the hand and wrist which are not amenable to replacement.

2. Seronegative Spondyloarthritis

▶ General Considerations

Spondyloarthritis encompasses a group of inflammatory arthritides characterized by spinal and peripheral joint oligoarthritis and enthesitis (fibrosis and calcification at the point of attachment between muscle and bone). This family of diseases includes ankylosing spondylitis (AS), psoriatic arthritis, enteropathic arthritis (associated with inflammatory bowel disease), reactive arthritis, and undifferentiated spondyloarthropathy.

3. Ankylosing Spondylitis

AS is a chronic inflammatory disease of the axial skeleton characterized by back pain, prolonged morning stiffness, and progressive loss of motion of the axial spine. There can also be sacroiliac involvement, arthritis of the hips, and peripheral arthritis. This disease typically affects young adults, with peak onset usually between 20 and 30 years of age. Males are more commonly affected than females. Over time, there is increased flexion of the neck, increased thoracic kyphosis, and loss of lumbar lordosis leading to a stooped posture. Radiographs will show squaring of the vertebral bodies early on. With disease progression, bridging syndesmophytes, ankylosis of the facet joints, calcification of the anterior longitudinal ligament, and atlantoaxial (C1-C2) subluxation may be noted.

Laboratory values have little role in the diagnosis of AS. ESR and CRP are often elevated. HLA-B27 is the only genetic locus definitively linked to AS; however, it is not specific.

Treatment with NSAIDS is very effective with significant improvement in back pain. Recently, TNF-alpha antagonists (infliximab, etanercept, and adalimumab) have been effective in the treatment of AS in clinical trials. As in patients with RA, tuberculosis screening should take place prior to the initiation of TNF-alpha treatment.

4. Psoriatic Arthritis

Psoriatic arthritis is chronic inflammatory disease characterized by skin lesions and arthritis of the peripheral joints. One-third of patients have arthritis of the spine as well. Patients may experience nail pitting and onycholysis (painless separation of the nail from the nail bed).

Psoriatic arthritis is commonly treated with NSAIDS. DMARDS such as methotrexate are also used with success. Like RA and AS, recent success has been demonstrated with the use of anti-TNF alpha agents.

5. Enteropathic Arthritis, Reactive Arthritis, and Undifferentiated Spondylarthropathy

Enteropathic arthritis is the spondyloarthropathy associated with ulcerative colitis and/or Crohn's disease. Typically, the spondyloarthropathy in these patients progresses independently of the bowel pathology. Patients with reactive arthritis develop axial disease after exposure to an infectious agent such as Salmonella, Shigella, or Chlamydia. Undifferentiated spondyloarthropathy characterizes spinal disease without an adequate number of symptoms or signs to designate a specific type of arthritis. Treatment for these types of arthritides includes TNF-alpha inhibitors and NSAIDS.

6. Osteoarthritis

OA is a common age-related pathology characterized by damage to hyaline articular cartilage, synovitis, thickening of the joint capsule and bony remodeling. In contrast to RA, patients with OA will complain of joint pain worse with activity and short-acting stiffness after inactivity. Female sex, prior joint injuries, family history, and obesity are additional risk factors for the development of OA. Radiographs will often show joint space narrowing, sclerosis, and osteophytes.

Initial treatment includes NSAIDS or acetaminophen for pain relief and physical therapy to strengthen and improve the flexibility of muscles around the pathologic joint. A significant drawback to chronic NSAID treatment is the development of gastrointestinal toxicity including ulceration. Cox-2 inhibitors, such as celebrex, were introduced as anti-inflammatory alternatives without the same gastrointestinal side effects. However, due to concerns over possible increase in serious cardiovascular events, some Cox-2 inhibitors (rofecoxib and valdecoxib) were withdrawn from the market. At this time, there are Cox-2 inhibitors (celecoxib, etoricoxib, and lumircoxib), that have been shown to have similar efficacy for treatment of OA compared to nonspecific NSAIDS with fewer gastrointestinal side effects and without significant increase in the rate of serious cardiac events.

Exercise and weight loss are two additional interventions that are critical for the management of OA. Obesity is strongly associated with the development of OA. For the average person, their knees feel 3-6 times their body weight during activities such as walking and running. Moderate weight loss will reduce the pain and inflammation associated with OA, as well as slow the progression of this disease. Also improving the strength and flexibility of muscles around joints through exercise will lead to better functional outcome and pain ratings.

Other treatment options include intra-articular injection of glucocorticoids and hyaluronans. These injections appear to improve pain in the short term, without many significant side effects. However, these treatments do not provide significant long-term relief for most patients, nor do they alter disease progression.

Glucosamine and chondroitin sulfate result in improved pain and function for some patients and no effect for other patients. Given that side effects are minimal, treatment with these two products is reasonable for those who have an improvement in their symptoms.

For severe cases of OA, surgery including total joint replacement may be considered depending on the state of the disease and patient characteristics.

7. Hip Disorders and Reconstruction

▶ General Considerations

In the United States 200,000 total hip replacements (THR) are performed annually for hip arthritis. The incidence of THR will continue to increase as the population ages. The causes of hip arthritis include childhood disorders such as developmental dysplasia, Legg–Calve–Perthes disease, slipped capital femoral epiphysis, as well as inflammatory arthritis, osteonecrosis, trauma, and infection. Although arthritis is the most common cause of hip dysfunction, there are other causes as well, for example, femoroacetabular impingement and "snapping hip syndrome." Also patients will often complain of "hip pain" when their pain is actually lower back pain or pain over the greater trochanter or lateral thigh. As a result, thorough history, physical examination, and radiographic studies are crucial for differentiating among these different entities and making the correct diagnosis.

▶ Clinical Evaluation

True Intra-articular hip pathology typically presents as pain localized to the groin, exacerbated by internal rotation. Patients will often complain of difficulty with ambulation, climbing stairs, putting on shoes, and sexual intercourse.

Physical examination should include neurovascular documentation, hip range of motion, evaluation of the spine, and palpation for points of tenderness. Tenderness at the greater trochanter may be indicative of bursitis, which is often successfully treated with corticosteroid and lidocaine injection. True hip joint pathology should not result in pain that is reproducible with palpation.

Flexion contractures, asymmetric hip abductor weakness (Trendelenburg sign), and labral impingement signs (pain with flexion, adduction, and internal rotation or "FAI") should also be tested for. Leg-length discrepancy should be noted as well.

It is important to recognize that although, groin pain, and exacerbation of pain with internal rotation or the FAI maneuver is indicative of pathology specific for the hip joint, the exact cause of the patient's symptoms (arthritis, avascular necrosis, and impingement) still requires further delineation with additional physical examination maneuvers and radiographic testing.

Younger patients with hip pain may specifically complain of a "snapping" or "catching" sensation. Also known as the "snapping hip," this may be caused by the iliotibial band (IT band) snapping across the greater trochanter or the iliopsoas tendon snapping across the iliopectineal prominence. The IT band is likely the source if pain or snapping is reproduced with adduction and rotation of the hip while the patient is standing. The iliopsoas tendon is tested with the patient supine, moving the hip from a flexed and internally rotated position to an extended and externally rotated position.

Standard radiographs of the hip include AP view of the pelvis, AP, and frog-lateral of the pathologic hip. It is important to note any deformity of the femoral head, acetabulum, joint space, as well as any signs that may be specific to a particular disease process. For example, patients with developmental hip dysplasia often display a shallow socket with decreased anterior and lateral acetabular coverage on radiographs. A false-profile view (true lateral view of the acetabulum) may be performed to evaluate the degree of acetabular dysplasia present.

When plain radiographs fail to reveal a diagnosis, additional diagnostic imaging including MRI, CT, or bone scan may be performed looking for osteonecrosis, stress fractures, neoplasms, labral, or hyaline cartilage pathology.

If the clinical picture remains unclear or is complicated by concomitant spine pathology, intra-articular diagnostic injection of the hip joint with anesthetic may be performed.

▶ Femoroacetabular Impingement

Femoroacetabular impingement describes abnormal tracking between the femoral head and neck and the acetabulum through a normal range of hip motion resulting in pain and/or bony deformity. There are two types of femoroacetabular impingement: cam-type and pincer type. Cam-type impingement describes a femoral neck with prominent anterior bone that impinges on a normal acetabulum and labrum resulting in damage to one or both. Pincer-type impingement results from an anterior acetabular osteophyte that abuts the anterior femoral neck during hip flexion.

Femoroacetabular impingement can be treated with resection of the offending osteophytes or prominent bone, and debridement or repair of damaged labrum. These procedures can be performed through hip arthroscopy or an open approach.

Avascular Necrosis of the Hip

Osteonecrosis of the femoral head can occur in young patients. Risk factors include steroid use, alcoholism, trauma, marrow-replacing diseases (such as Gaucher's disease), high-dose radiation treatment, and hypercoagulable states (sickle-cell disease, hypofibrinolysis, thrombophilia, protein S and C deficiencies). The disease course consists of decreased blood flow to the femoral head, resulting in osteonecrosis, subchondral fracture, and eventually collapse.

Standard AP and lateral radiographs of the hip often reveal the diagnosis. Of note subchondral fracture of the hip is most clearly seen on the lateral radiograph. If radiographs are nondiagnostic for a patient for whom osteonecrosis is suspected, MRI is the next step. The lateral and anterior aspects of the femoral head are most commonly affected.

Avascular necrosis of the hip may be classified according the Ficat grading system: type I (no radiographic signs of AVN), type II (changes of the femoral head subchondral bone without collapse), type III (subchondral fracture with collapse), and type IV (collapse of the femoral head with changes on the acetabular side).

Unfortunately, without intervention, progression of osteonecrosis to collapse will occur in most patients. Patients with preclinical or asymptomatic osteonecrosis can be observed without surgical intervention. Symptomatic precollapse osteonecrosis may be treated with core decompression with or without bone graft, vascularized fibula grafting, or oral bisphosphonates. At this time, there is a paucity of data to definitively support one treatment over another.

Although, some studies have demonstrated success with treating postcollapse osteonecrosis with vascularized fibula grafts or rotational osteotomies, arthroplasty is the more reliable method of treatment. Treatment with unipolar and bipolar arthroplasty is initially successful, but often results in conversion to total hip arthroplasty due to eventual loss of acetabular cartilage and recurrent pain. Young patients who receive total hip arthroplasty with conventional polyethylene components experience a high rate of osteolysis and subsequent need for revision surgery. Currently, clinical trials are being performed to evaluate the use of alternative bearing surfaces and hip resurfacing surgery in this challenging patient population.

Surgical Treatment Options for Hip Pathology

Surgical options for the hip include hip arthroscopy, osteotomies, resection, arthrodesis, and arthroplasty. Choice of treatment depends on the type of hip pathology being treated, patient characteristics, and the experience level of the surgeon.

A. Hip Arthroscopy

Hip arthroscopy typically involves the placement of two portals with the help of fluoroscopy. The arthroscope is inserted through one portal to visualize the hip joint and any pathology. The second portal serves as a "working portal" through which instruments such as debriders, shavers, or pincers are inserted to treat the pathology in question. This technique can be used to treat intra-articular and extra-articular hip pathology. Treatment of intra-articular pathology usually requires the aid of limb traction. Intra-articular indications include debridement of labral tears, loose body removal, chondral lesion debridement, osteophyte resection, biopsy, synovectomy. Extra-articular pathology such as the snapping hip may be treated with lengthening or releasing the iliopsoas and/or IT band. Complications of hip arthroscopy including pudendal and sciatic nerve palsies are becoming less frequent with improved patient positioning and surgical technique. More long term studies are needed to assess the efficacy of this technique.

B. Osteotomy

Osteotomy of the adult hip involves the use of saws or osteotomes to make bone cuts on the femur or pelvis. The resulting pieces of bone are realigned and fixed with plates and/or screws to correct deformity. Osteotomy is used to treat dysplasia, residual deformity from slipped capital femoral epiphyses, cerebral palsy with hip instability, and avascular necrosis. Choice of femoral or acetabular osteotomy is dependent on the pathology present and patient characteristics.

C. Resection Arthroplasty

Resection arthroplasty, aka "Girdlestone" procedure, involves complete resection of the femoral head without replacement. This procedure is a salvage surgery reserved for severe hip infection resistant to antibiotic treatment, failed total hip arthroplasty with unreconstructible bone defects, previous high-dose pelvic radiation exposure that would limit healing of a complex reconstructive procedure or patients with severe medical co-morbidities and limited functional needs who may not tolerate a longer procedure. Patients treated with resection arthroplasty will have a significant limb-length discrepancy that will likely require the use of a shoe-lift and/or other walking aides.

D. Arthrodesis

Arthrodesis of the hip may be indicated for patients with acquired (eg, trauma or infection) or developmental (such as dysplasia) hip abnormalities. The optimal position for arthrodesis is 5-10 degrees of external rotation, 20-30 degrees of flexion, and neutral adduction. Although pain relief and function can be excellent, this procedure results in increased energy expenditure and late onset OA of the lumbar spine and knee due to increased joint stresses resulting from changes in the patient's gait.

E. Hip Arthroplasty

Hip arthroplasty involves the replacement of the femoral head and/or the acetabulum with manufactured components. Hemiarthroplasty may be performed replacing the femoral head without treatment of the acetabulum. Total hip arthroplasty entails replacement of the femoral head and placement of an acetabular component.

Hemiarthroplasty typically entails replacement of native the femoral head with a metal femoral head and neck. Indications include hip fracture in the elderly patient, avascular necrosis of the femoral head, and arthritis of the femoral head without acetabular disease. Hemiarthroplasty may be unipolar (one point of articulation between the metal femoral head and native acetabulum) or bipolar (two points of articulation: first point between the femoral head and acetabulum and the second point between the femoral neck and femoral head). Due to development of acetabular disease, many hemiarthroplasties are often converted to total hip arthroplasties with placement of an acetabular component. Although, bipolar hemi-arthroplasties offers the theoretical advantage of improved range of motion and decreased acetabular wear compared to unipolar arthroplasty due to the second point of articulation, these effects have not been demonstrated in clinical studies. Due to the significantly higher cost, most authors do not advocate the use of bipolar hemiarthroplasty over unipolar hemiarthroplasty.

Total Hip Arthroplasty involves replacement of the femoral head and placement of an acetabular component (Figure 40–32). Conventional polyethylene acetabular components with metal femoral heads have performed well at 15-20 year follow-up in older patient populations (greater than 60 years old). However in younger and or more active patients polyethylene wear and associated osteolysis (bone breakdown) represent the most common cause of long-term failure. Alternative bearing options such as ceramic-on-ceramic, metal-on-highly cross-linked polyethylene and metal-on-metal designs have been introduced to address these concerns.

Each of these bearing options has advantages and disadvantages. Ceramic-on-ceramic offers low wear rate without the production of metal ions; however, there is a reported 1%-3% "squeaking" rate and they can fracture resulting in catastrophic failure. Metal-on-metal produces metal ions that can significantly increase their concentration in the blood. To date, no increase in cancer rates or other side effects have been noted due to the metal ions. Metal-on-metal prostheses do not cause the squeaking side effects and are unlikely to fracture. High cross-linked polyethylene is

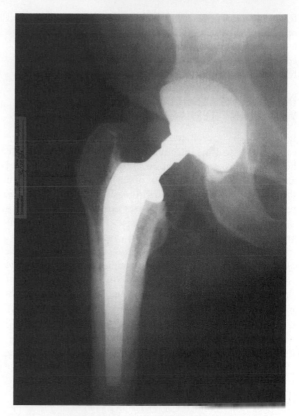

▲ **Figure 40–32.** Hybrid total hip replacement with porous coated acetabular shell and cemented femoral stem performed for osteoarthritis.

more forgiving with regards to the placement of the acetabular component. However, concerns regarding wear debris and subsequent osteolysis remain, although preliminary data suggests that the wear debris produced is significantly less than the regular cross-linked polyethylene.

F. Resurfacing Arthroplasty

Resurfacing arthroplasty is a type of total hip replacement that was first introduced in the 1970s. Resurfacing involves placement of an acetabular component in addition to replacing the surface ("resurfacing") of the femoral head without resecting the entire femoral head or femoral neck. The resurfacing is typically done with a metal femoral component. This prosthesis interface initially did quite poorly, with high early failure rates related to wear debris, osteolysis, and subsequent prosthetic failure. Due to advances in metallurgy and other aspects of total joint technology, the resurfacing arthroplasty has produced short-term successful results and gained popularity in recent years. Resurfacing is ideal for younger patients without any cyst or other pathology of the femoral neck. By preserving most of the femoral head and all of the neck, future total hip revision surgery if needed will be less difficult and demanding. Contraindications to this procedure include cyst or other pathology of the femoral neck, which can predispose to femoral neck fracture.

INFECTIONS ASSOCIATED WITH JOINT REPLACEMENTS

Infections that occur after total joint replacement may be caused by organisms introduced at the time of surgery or late hematogenous contamination. Medical providers should always maintain a high index of suspicion for infection in the patients with previous arthroplasty surgery. New onset pain or loosening of the prosthesis noted on x-ray is infection related until proven otherwise. ESR, CRP, and joint aspiration are part of the standard workup. Choice of treatment depends on when the infection occurs, the virulence of organism involved, and the stability of the prosthetic components. If the infection occurs within three weeks of the initial surgery, some authors advocate performing a washout with liner exchange. If infection occurs at a later

time and/or loosening is noted radiographically, resection of the prosthesis is typically recommended with interval placement of an antibiotic cement spacer (methylmethacralate with impregnated antibiotic) and IV antibiotic treatment for at least 6 weeks. Once the infection has cleared, reimplantation of a new prosthesis may be considered. For chronically infected prostheses, fusion or resection arthroplasty may be considered.

TOTAL KNEE REPLACEMENT

Reconstructive surgical options for the arthritic knee (Figure 40–33) include high tibial osteotomy (HTO), unicompartmental knee arthroplasty (UKA), and total knee arthroplasty (TKA). Indications for reconstructive surgery of the knee include severe pain with or without deformity and radiographic evidence of arthritis for which conservative treatment (physical therapy, NSAIDs, corticosteroid joint injections) has failed. Choice of surgical treatment depends on patient characteristics in addition to the condition of the knee.

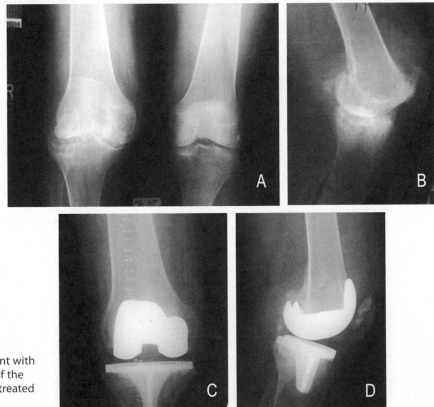

▲ **Figure 40–33.** **A and B:** Patient with RA and severe joint destruction of the right knee. **C and D:** Patient was treated with a cemented right total knee replacement.

Total Knee Arthroplasty

TKA involves replacement of bone from the distal femur and proximal tibia with a metal component on the femoral side and polyethylene (or a metal tray with a polyethylene insert) on the tibial side. There are several types of TKA designs that vary in the degree to which they constrain knee motion. Choice of implant depends on the ligamentous stability of the knee and surgeon preference. A fully constrained prosthesis which only allows flexion and extension is typically used in knees with severe deformity and/or significant ligamentous instability. The literature reflects a significant success rate for TKA, with patients reporting good-to-excellent outcomes 85%-90% of the time. Factors associated with poor outcome as perceived by the patients include obesity, female gender, age less than 60 years old, and previous history of depression.

Unicompartmental Knee Arthroplasty

UKA may be considered in the elderly individual (> 60 years old), with isolated medial or lateral compartment arthritis. The advantages of UKA over TKA include preservation of knee kinematics, decreased operative morbidity, and quicker rehabilitation time. However, UKA is contraindicated in patients with an anterior cruciate ligament-deficient knee, range of motion less than 90 degrees or flexion contracture more than 15 degrees and patients with arthritic disease in more than one knee compartment.

High Tibial Osteotomy

The HTO may be considered in the young, active patient with isolated medial compartment arthritis, for whom TKA is an imperfect long-term solution. Patients with isolated medial compartment arthritis typically have varus deformity of the knee. The HTO will produce a valgus correction of this deformity and unload the diseased articular surface on the medial side. The short-term results of this procedure include reduction of pain levels and deformity correction; however, they typically deteriorate over time resulting in the need for additional surgery.

GLENOHUMERAL ARTHRITIS AND SHOULDER RECONSTRUCTION

Successfully treating the arthritic shoulder requires an understanding of the patient's functional demands, as well as the severity and quality of the patient's symptoms. A careful history and physical examination, along with the appropriate diagnostic studies will allow the treating physical to formulate an appropriate treatment plan.

History-taking starts with determination of the patient's primary complaint—is it pain, weakness, or loss of motion? Patients with significant glenohumeral arthritis typically complain of anterior or superolateral shoulder pain that is worse with activity. Weakness with loss of motion due to inactivity may be noted as well. Posterior pain or radicular-type symptoms (pain that radiates from the spine down the back of the shoulder) is concerning for disorder of the spinal cord and should initiate the appropriate workup. Prior treatment, including physical therapy, injections, and any surgical procedures should be asked about as well.

Physical examination should note neurovascular status and the presence of any muscle atrophy. Particular attention should be paid to the integrity of the rotator cuff muscles (supraspinatus, infraspinatus, teres minor, and subscapularis) and deltoid muscles. The shoulder physical examination is described in greater detail in the sports section of this chapter. Cervical range of motion is assessed as well, along with the Spurling maneuver (test for cervical radiculopathy).

Radiographic studies include AP and axillary views of the shoulder. Glenoid erosion resulting in decreased humeral head offset from the lateral border of the acromion may be noted. Patients with associated rotator cuff disease may have superior subluxation of the humeral head with associated decrease in the acromiohumeral distance.

Early stages of shoulder arthritis can be treated nonsurgically with NSAIDS, intra-articular steroid or hyaluronic acid injections, and a physical therapy program that focuses on maintaining range of motion and strengthening exercises.

Patients with mild arthritis that does not respond to conservative treatment measures may pursue arthroscopic surgery. Debridement of any chondral lesions and loose body removal may alleviate mechanical symptoms, while arthroscopic lavage removing inflammatory enzymes and proteins from the joint fluid often provides pain relief.

For patients with significant arthritis, shoulder arthroscopy may or may not provide relief. If successful, this surgery represents a temporary solution that may relieve symptoms for a short period of time. Shoulder reconstructive surgery including humeral hemiarthroplasty, glenoid resurfacing, total shoulder arthroplasty, reverse total shoulder arthroplasty, and gleno-humeral fusion are the treatment options to consider. It is important to note that the primary indication for shoulder replacement surgery is debilitating pain. These surgeries may or may not improve the patient's range of motion and/or strength.

Patients with shoulder arthritis and an intact rotator cuff may be treated with total shoulder arthroplasty (replacement of the glenoid and humerus with prosthetic components) or hemiarthroplasty (resurfacing of the humerus) alone. Two recent prospective studies comparing the two procedures suggest that pain relief may be better and rate of revision surgery (conversion to TSA due to glenoid arthritis) may be lower for TSA compared to hemiarthroplasty. For patients with a deficient rotator cuff tear and arthritis, hemiarthroplasty is the preferred option, as superior humeral migration due to a deficient cuff leads to loosening of the glenoid component. Biologic resurfacing of the glenoid with interposition graft (anterior capsule, fascia lata autograft, allografts) may be performed as well to address any arthritic change of the glenoid.

Reverse total shoulder arthroplasty which involves a convex glenoid and concave humerus may be used in elderly (> 70 years old) low-demand patients with a deficient rotator cuff and intact deltoid. This prosthesis places the center of rotation in the scapular neck, thereby increasing the lever arm.

Historically, shoulder fusion could be considered for the young laborer with severe arthritis due to long-term failure of shoulder arthroplasty. With the advent of glenoid biologic resurfacing, shoulder fusion has become a less common surgical option reserved for deltoid deficient arthritic shoulders.

▼ ORTHOPEDIC SPINE

SPINE

Neck and back pain are two of the most common chief complaints in any outpatient clinic. Although most instances of these types of pain are related to muscular strain, neck and back pain may also be related to pathology of the spine. It is important for all healthcare providers to be able to distinguish between these two entities. True pathology of the spine requires timely referral to a Spine surgeon for evaluation and treatment.

▶ History and Physical Examination

A chief complaint of neck or back pain should prompt a thorough history and musculoskeletal examination including both the upper and lower extremities. Specific questions to ask regarding the pain include onset, characterization, intensity, radiation, and timing. Pain that radiates down a patient's arm or legs may qualify as a radicular symptom and is indicative of spine root pathology. Additionally, the patient should be asked about night sweats, fevers, nighttime pain, and weight loss which are red flags for infection or cancer. The presence of numbness, tingling, motor weakness, loss of bowel, or bladder control is indicative of spine root pathology. Arm or leg pain that occurs during walking or activity and is relieved immediately with rest may be due to neurogenic claudication indicative of spinal stenosis. Patients with lumbar stenosis and resulting leg pain, often state that their leg pain improves going upstairs or leaning over the grocery cart at the grocery stair (flexion of the lumbar spine opens up the canal relieving the stenosis).

Physical examination includes strength, sensation, and reflex testing, gait observation and documentation of vascular status. Strength of muscles is graded according to the five point scale described in the Spine trauma section. Neurosensory examination should also be carried out evaluating the C5-T1 dermatomes for neck pain and the L2-S1 dermatomes for back pain. Reflex examination includes the documentation of the biceps, triceps, brachioradialis, patella, Achilles, and the presence or absence of a Babinski. Wide-based gait may be indicative of cervical spine pathology.

When neurologic testing is abnormal, distinction should be made between radicular (root pathology) and myelopathic (spinal cord pathology) symptoms/signs. Radicular symptoms include complaints of radiating pain from the spine down the arms or legs. Loss of bowel and/or bladder control and groin/peri-anal numbness is indicative of sacral rootlet pathology. Radicular signs on physical examination include a positive straight leg raise (SLR; pain shooting down the back of the leg extending below the knee with SLR), positive Spurling's test (radiating arm pain with neck extension and rotation toward the pathologic side), specific muscle weakness (eg, biceps weakness on the right side only), specific dermatome numbness, and specific decreased reflexes. Myelopathic signs include diffuse muscle weakness below a certain level, hyperreflexia, clonus, positive Babinski, L'hermitte's sign (sensation of shooting pain down arms or legs with neck motion) and Hoffman's sign (the patient's middle finger is flicked into extension by the examiner resulting in unintended thumb and finger flexion).

1. Cervical Strain

▶ Clinical Findings

A. Symptoms and Signs

Cervical strain is characterized by paraspinous (next to the midline) neck pain with or without radiation to the shoulder. Oftentimes patients will display limitation of neck motion as well. These symptoms typically appear after an episode of overexertion or prolonged tension or poor posture. Specific points of deep tenderness with reproducible pain with palpation known as "trigger points" may be present. Pain is often characterized as deep aching or boring in sensation. Muscular spasm within the trapezius, levator scapulae, and paraspinous muscles may be palpable as a firm "knot." The patient may also complain of headache or dizziness. An important differentiating point from true spine pathology is that physical examination should not reveal any neurologic deficit.

▶ Imaging Studies

Radiographic evaluation starts with AP and Lateral x-rays of the cervical spine. Flexion-extension views should be considered in patients with precedent neck trauma, signs of RA, or Down syndrome to examine for instability. X-rays may reveal degenerative change such as osteophytes, ankylosis of joints, or signs of instability. However, radiographs are often normal.

Differential Diagnosis

One should consider cervical spondylosis and herniated cervical disk as part of the differential diagnosis. A patient with herniated cervical disk may complain of radicular symptoms in a specific dermatomal distribution, muscle weakness, and diminished sensation or paresthesias corresponding to the pathologic disk level. Additionally, diminished reflexes may be noted as well. Pain arising from cervical spondylosis (degenerative change) is often indistinguishable from that due to cervical strain.

Treatment

Acute cervical spine pain is initially treated with rest and immobilization. Bracing with a soft collar, analgesics, and muscle relaxants are used as needed. However, the collar should not be used for more than 1-2 weeks to avoid cervical muscle atrophy. Ice, heat, and other modalities such as ultrasound and massage may be helpful as well.

Neck pain related to cervical strain usually subsides within 1 week from onset. Once the pain has diminished, the patient should begin physical therapy exercises to strengthen cervical muscles, improve posture, and increase range of motion.

2. Whiplash Injury

General Considerations

"Whip-lash" is an acceleration-deceleration injury that occurs most commonly when the patient is rear-ended in a motor vehicle accident. Acute hyperextension occurs causing injury to anterior soft tissue structures of the neck, including the anterior longitudinal ligament, the intervertebral disk, the strap muscles, longus colli, and sternocleidomastoid muscles. When the vehicle decelerates, the head recoils into flexion, causing injury to the facet capsules, posterior ligaments, and paraspinal musculature.

Clinical Findings

A. Clinical Evaluation and Imaging Studies

The symptoms after whiplash injury are often variable. Neck pain and stiffness are common. Occipital headaches and retro-ocular pain are also frequently noted. Spasm may manifest as decreased neck motion. Neurologic examination is normal. Radiographs are usually normal.

Treatment

Management of whiplash injuries is similar for cervical strain: analgesics, rest, and immobilization in a soft cervical collar until the pain is controlled, followed by gradual mobilization. Physical therapy exercises are initiated when range of motion normalizes.

3. Degenerative Cervical Disk Disease (Cervical Spondylosis)

General Considerations

The degenerative changes of the spine that typically occurs with aging are collectively termed spondylosis. Most degeneration visualized on radiographs is asymptomatic. As a result, disk degeneration is considered a part of the natural aging process.

Cervical spondylosis is characterized initially by tears in the posterior annulus followed by fragmentation of the disk. The weakest area of the annulus is the posterolateral region, which is the most common site of bulging of the disk. With time uncovertebral joints and ligamentum flavum can hypertrophy, which along with prominent spurs and degenerative disk, may encroach onto the neural foramen and spinal canal, impinging on nerve roots and/or the spinal cord. Additionally, ossification of the posterior longitudinal ligament, which is particularly predominant in the Japanese population, can cause multisegmental cervical compression and myelopathy.

Clinical Findings

A. Symptoms and Signs

Clinical symptoms may or may not accompany the degenerative changes of cervical spondylosis. Neurologic compromise may result from nerve root compression (cervical spondylotic radiculopathy) or compression of the cord itself (cervical spondylotic myelopathy) (Figure 40–34). Patients with cervical radicular symptoms typically complain of pain that radiates from the neck down into the shoulders and/or arms. Spurling's test, as described above, may be positive. Patients with myelopathic symptoms may complain of L'hermitte's sign (lightning pain down the spine with neck flexion), and/or difficulty with fine motor movements (buttoning a shirt) and balance.

Physical examination of patients with cervical radiculopathy may show muscle weakness and diminished reflexes. Physical examination of patients with spondylotic myelopathy may be characterized by spasticity and clonus. An inverted radial reflex and a scapulohumeral reflex may also be seen. Positive Babinski and Hoffman signs may be present. Fine motion of the fingers may not be present, and intrinsic muscle wasting may be noted. The patient may have an abnormal gait characterized by wide-based, shuffling movements.

B. Imaging Studies

Radiographic findings of cervical spondylosis include narrowing of the disk space (Figure 40–35), osteophyte formation at the vertebral body margins, and arthritic degeneration of the facet joints. MRI is used to evaluate for nerve root or spinal cord impingement. EMG may be used as an adjunct study to confirm diagnosis by demonstrating generalized motor impairment resulting from motor neuron involvement.

▶ Differential Diagnosis

In addition to arthritis, radiculopathy or myelopathy may also be caused by tumors and vascular malformations of the spinal cord, syringomyelia, amyotrophic lateral sclerosis, subacute combined degeneration, and multiple sclerosis. MRI is the most useful study, in addition to thorough history and physical examination, to distinguish between these different diagnoses.

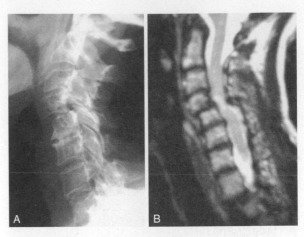

▲ **Figure 40–35.** **A.** Lateral radiograph of a 50-year-old man with neck pain and myelopathy. **B.** Sagittal T2-weighted MRI showing spinal cord compression at C4-5 at the level of the spondylolisthesis.

▶ Treatment

A. Cervical Spondylotic Radiculopathy

Most patients with acute onset of cervical spondylotic radiculopathy have regression of symptoms over the course of 4-6 weeks. Progression to myelopathy is rare. Most patients achieve pain relief with rest, analgesics, and immobilization to relieve pain. Paresthesias and slight sensory changes may persist after neck and arm pain have subsided.

If pain continues, MRI of the cervical spine should be performed to investigate any areas of compression. If discrete herniation is present, surgical decompression with foraminotomy or discectomy with or without interbody fusion may be considered.

B. Cervical Spondylotic Myelopathy

Initial management of cervical spondylotic myelopathy involves the use of NSAIDS and cervical collar to minimize symptoms.

When symptoms are progressive, are not relieved by the use of a collar, or occur in younger patients, operative treatment may be necessary. Treatment depends upon the nature of the compression (disk, vertebral body, posterior osteophytes, hypertrophied ligamentum flavum, ossified posterior longitudinal ligament), the sagittal alignment of the cervical spine (kyphotic, neutral, or lordotic), and the number of levels involved. Compression confined to the intervertebral disks can be relieved by means of single-level or multiple-level anterior discectomies and fusion. When the disease is limited to two vertebral body levels or if there is a preexisting kyphosis greater than 15 degrees, anterior vertebrectomy, foraminotomy, and fusion with a strut graft

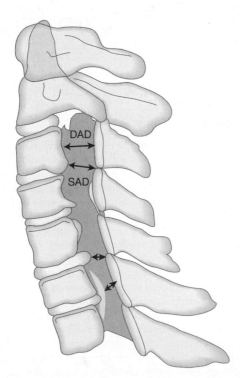

▲ **Figure 40–34.** The space available for the spinal cord in the subaxial cervical spine can be measured as the developmental anterior-posterior diameter (DAPD) in patients with developmental spinal stenosis and as the spondylolytic anterior-posterior diameter (SAPD) in patients with cervical spondylosis.

achieves decompression and stabilization of the degenerative segments. When the compression involves more than two vertebral body levels, the morbidity associated with the anterior approach increases significantly. As a result, a posterior decompression via multilevel laminectomy with or without fusion is recommended (Figure 40–36).

Course & Prognosis

Most cases of cervical spondylotic radiculopathy resolve in 4-6 weeks with conservative management. With regards to cervical spondylytic myelopathy, the results of surgical management are better when symptoms are mild and of shorter duration. However, complete postoperative resolution of symptoms is rare even in these cases. Of note, the natural evolution of spondylotic myelopathy will often result in at least partial spontaneous remission. Chronic myelopathy and multiple-level involvement are associated with poorer surgical results.

PAIN SYNDROMES OF THE BACK

1. Low Back Pain

General Considerations

In the United States, 400,000 workers are disabled by back pain each year. It has been estimated that 80% of the population suffers low back pain at some point during their lifetime. Due to its high prevalence all physicians should be able to differentiate between the multiple different etiologies of back pain.

Clinical Findings

A. Symptoms and Signs

The most common cause of low back pain is mechanical strain. Patients complain of pain related to overexertion. Oftentimes patients in this group will demonstrate poor conditioning, abdominal muscle tone and posture.

Pain is often described as a deep-seated ache in the lumbosacral region. The pain is dull and somewhat diffuse, with or without radiation to the buttocks and hips. The pain is worsened by bending and relieved by inactivity. Palpation may reveal tenderness in the paraspinous area, with "trigger points" or "knots." Spasm of the paraspinous muscles is a common finding.

Neurovascular exam including strength, sensation and reflexes are usually within normal limits. SLR test is normal. The SLR test is performed with the patient supine on examining table; the examiner lifts patient's leg which is extended at the hip and knee, passively stretching the sciatic nerve with transmission of tension to the lumbosacral roots. Reproduction of pain down the legs is a positive test, indicating nerve root irritation.

B. Imaging Studies

Radiographic examination may reveal degenerative changes such as lumbar disk space narrowing and osteophytes or may be normal. X-rays should routinely be obtained. In persons over age 50, the presence of metastases should be evaluated. In patients under age 20, symptomatic congenital or developmental anomalies should be ruled-out.

Treatment

Management of lumbar strain includes anti-inflammatory medication and rest during the acute phase. Lumbosacral

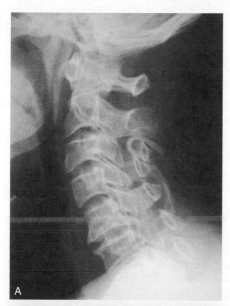
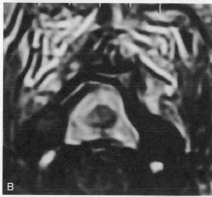

▲ **Figure 40–36.** **A.** Lateral postoperative radiograph of a patient who had multisegmental cervical stenosis and myelopathy treated with canal expansive cervical laminoplasty from C3 to C7. **B.** Postoperative axial MRI image showing significant canal expansion after the procedure.

corsets may be considered for mechanical support. Abdominal conditioning and spinal muscle strengthening exercises are prescribed after the pain subsides. Typical exercises include bent-knee sit-ups and hamstring and spinal muscle stretching. Preventative measures should be presented to the patient, especially the correct manner of lifting objects while bending at the legs rather than at the spine.

▶ Course & Prognosis

The usual course of lumbar strain is spontaneous remission with time. Relapses of pain are common, often precipitated by heavy-duty activity. Patients with constant pain should be investigated for depression and or workman's compensation related issues, which may be contributing factors. Patients who fail to respond to conservative treatment should be investigated for neurologic compression via MRI. If no pathology is found, patients should be encouraged to return to normal activity as soon as possible. Prolonged reliance upon analgesics (especially opioids) should be discouraged.

2. Lumbar Disk Syndrome

▶ General Considerations

Patients may present with back pain and unilateral or bilateral leg symptoms. The back pain may be due to degeneration of the annulus fibrosis (outer layer of the disk) which contains many pain fibers. Degeneration of the annulus fibrosis may lead to herniation of the nucleus pulposis (central portion of disk) into the spinal canal impinging on neural elements, leading to leg symptoms. The postero-lateral portion of the lumbar disk is the weakest and as a result the most common location for herniation. These types of disk herniations are termed "paracentral" because they occur just lateral to the midline. Central disk herniations, which occur at the midline, occur less commonly.

The dural sac below L1 (conus modularis) contains only nerve rootlets (cauda equina). In the lumbar spine each nerve root emerges below its respective vertebra, just under the inferomedial border of its respective pedicle, and enters the neural foramen just above the intervertebral disk of that level. As a result, a paracentral disk herniation may compress the traversing root to the lower adjacent level. For example, an L4-5 paracentral disk herniation will compress the traversing L5 nerve root. In contrast, a far lateral disk herniation occurs near the exit zone of its respective neural foramen and therefore is most likely to compress the exiting root at that level, that is, a far-lateral disk herniation at L4-L5 will impinge upon the L4 nerve root. Due to their transition point status between the lumbar and sacral spine, the L4-5 and L5-S1 disk levels correspond to the region of maximal mechanical stress in the lumbar spine. As a result disk herniations are most likely at these two levels, and L5 and S1 nerve root pathology is most common.

▶ Clinical Findings

A. Symptoms and Signs

Back pain with sciatica (pain radiating down the posterior leg) is the most common presentation. The pain may be dermatome specific. The onset of leg pain is usually insidious, but pain may begin acutely when sudden disk herniation follows injury. Pain may be piercing, burning, or electrical in nature, accentuated by prolonged sitting or standing and relieved at least partially by rest.

Compression of nerve roots may produce objective sensory changes, with paresthesias and loss of sensation in the affected dermatome. With continued root compression, motor weakness may develop. Motor weakness corresponds to the specific myotomes innervated by the compressed nerve root. Muscle atrophy may accompany sensory and motor changes. Straight leg test may be positive.

▶ Radiographic Evaluation

Radiographs may show degenerative change including osteophytes and loss of disk height. MRI or myelogram are very sensitive and should reveal disk herniation if present. Care should be taken to specifically evaluate the location of the disk herniation including the disk level and the relationship of the herniation to the midline (central, para-central, or far-lateral).

▶ Treatment

Treatment of acute lumbar disk disease is controversial. If symptoms are produced by bulging rather than by extrusion of the herniated disk, conservative measures such as bed rest, analgesics, and anti-inflammatory medications often result in complete resolution of symptoms.

If symptoms continue or if neurologic symptoms progress or fail to respond to conservative measures, laminotomy and removal of the herniated disk may be required. Surgery is most successful in patients whose symptoms correlate with objective diagnostic study findings, that is, the patient with L4-5 para-central disk herniation and L5 nerve root symptoms (EHL weakness, pain/paresthesias in the L5 dermatomal distribution). Discectomy can be performed via standard microdiscectomy techniques or through a "minimally invasive" endoscopic approach.

3. Lumbar Stenosis

In the presence of severe disk space degeneration and spondylosis, a generalized narrowing of the lumbar spinal canal (spinal stenosis) without specific disk herniation can also occur. The etiology of lumbar spinal stenosis is multifactorial including: facet joint hypertrophy, disk degeneration and loss of disk height, and hypertrophy and buckling of the ligamentum flavum.

Spinal stenosis usually affects people in their fifties and sixties. Symptoms include generalized backache and stiffness. Narrowing of the lateral recess can occur causing unilateral nerve root symptoms, resulting in leg symptoms such as sciatica as well. Neurogenic claudication (back pain with radiating leg pain that is worse with activity and immediately relieved by rest) is a common complaint. This can be differentiated from vascular claudication by the immediacy of relief with rest (for vascular claudication, pain relief occurs only after minutes of rest).

For patients with spinal stenosis, extension leads to further narrowing of the canal exacerbating symptoms, while flexion of the spine provides symptom relief. Patients will often relate that it is easier to walk up stairs than down stairs (people have a tendency to lean forward or flex their spine when walking up stairs and lean backward or extend their spine when walking down stairs) and that walking hunched over a grocery cart helps their symptoms. On physical exam, diminished or asymmetric reflexes, specific motor weakness (extensor hallucis longus is most common), and decreased sensation in a specific dermatome may be noted.

Imaging Studies

X-ray examination may reveal degenerative changes, such as disk space narrowing and osteophytosis, or the results may be entirely normal. A myelogram or MRI will confirm the diagnosis.

Treatment

In the patient with persistent neurogenic claudication that fails to respond to conservative measures, foraminotomy or decompressive laminectomy is very effective in relieving symptoms and improving function. If spinal instability (degenerative spondylolisthesis) is also present, the spine should also be stabilized and fused over the affected levels.

4. Other Lower Back Conditions

In addition to the etiologies of back pain discussed above, one must also consider infection or tumor as possibilities. Additionally, conditions unrelated to the spine such as abdominal aortic aneurysm, pancreatitis, or pyelonephritis may also cause back pain and should be ruled-out when suspicion is present.

The most common extradural tumors in the adult spine are metastatic, most often from breast carcinoma in women and prostate cancer in men. Multiple myeloma also frequently involves the spine and often causes pain via lytic lesions that weaken bone and lead to pathologic fractures. Intradural spinal tumors (neurofibromas, meningiomas, and ependymomas) are much less common than metastases in adults. A history of primary tumors elsewhere, back pain worse at night, night sweats, fevers, or persistent bilateral leg pain without back pain should arouse suspicion for cancer. Metastases of bone are often detected on routine x-ray studies. MRI should be ordered when radiographs are nondiagnostic.

Discitis and vertebral osteomyelitis can cause back pain in the absence of significant neurologic symptoms. Vertebral osteomyelitis can arise from a number of sources, including direct inoculation from iatrogenic procedures (injections, diagnostic studies), contiguous spread from a local infection, and hematogenous seeding (from infected vascular sites or urinary tract infection).

Once the infection is established in the metaphysis, it can subsequently rupture through the end plate into the adjoining disk and infect the adjacent vertebral body. The disk material is relatively avascular and is rapidly destroyed by bacterial enzymes. Osteomyelitis of the spine can extend into the spinal canal leading to epidural abscess or bacterial meningitis or the surrounding soft tissues resulting in local abscess. Destruction of the vertebral body and intervertebral disk can lead to instability and collapse. In addition, retropulsion of infected bone and granulation tissue into the spinal canal can cause neural compression or vascular occlusion. If a spinal infection is suspected, the pathogenic organism must be identified with biopsy or aspiration before appropriate treatment with antibiotics (with or without surgical debridement) can be instituted. An MRI with gadolinium is the best test for delineating the location of the infection as well as investigating for the presence of an epidural abscess (Figure 40–57).

5. Acute Cauda Equina Syndrome

Rarely, acute posterior midline disk prolapse at the L2-3 level may cause compression of many nerve roots in the cauda equina. This is known as acute cauda equina syndrome. Symptoms include intense leg pain in one or both extremities, muscle weakness, urinary retention, and decreased rectal tone with subsequent loss of bowel/bladder control. An MRI of the lumbar spine will reveal the site of compression, which must be treated by emergent decompression.

6. Mechanical Back Pain

General Considerations

People with long-standing lumbar disk disease may develop numerous degenerative changes in the involved segments. Collapse of the disk results in abnormal motion anteriorly between the vertebral bodies and posteriorly between the intervertebral facets, leading to osteophytosis.

Clinical Findings

Symptoms arise from inflammation surrounding the abnormal facets and generally include diffuse aching that may or

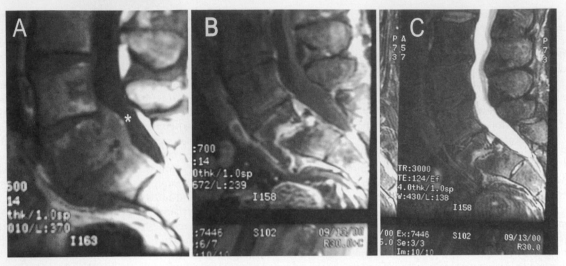

▲ **Figure 40–37.** Sagittal MRI images of a patient with low back pain due to L5-S1 discitis, vertebral osteomyelitis, and a small anterior epidural abscess. **A.** T1-weighted image. **B.** T1-weighted image with gadolinium vascular contrast. **C.** T2-weighted image.

may not radiate into the buttock or posterior thigh. Patients may also complain of postural discomfort and "locking" of the low back during stooping or attempts to straighten the back after forward bending.

▶ Diagnosis and Treatment

Radiographs may show osteophytes and narrowing of the disk spaces suggestive of degenerative change. Patients demonstrating symptoms suggestive of facet syndrome should be initially treated conservatively with rest and anti-inflammatory agents. Fluoroscopically guided injection of the lumbar facets with corticosteroids and lidocaine may be diagnostic and therapeutic. For patients who fail conservative therapy, lumbar fusion by anterior or posterior techniques may be considered to eliminate abnormal motion. However, the results of these surgeries have been inconsistent.

▼ ORTHOPEDIC ONCOLOGY

INTRODUCTION

Bony lesions may be primary (of mesenchymal origin) or secondary (metastases, myeloma, and lymphoma). Bony metastases and myeloma are significantly more common than primary bone tumors, particularly in older patients. Primary bony lesions can be grouped into three types: malignant tumors (sarcomas), benign tumors, and reactive or miscellaneous lesions. Sarcomas tend to spread hematogenously, most commonly to the lungs. Benign bone tumors vary widely, and may be small and inconsequential or large and destructive.

PRESENTATION

Regardless of the type of lesion, most patients present with musculoskeletal pain, typically deep and dull in character. This may initially be intermittent and activity-related, but over time often becomes constant. Patients with a suspected bony lesion require careful physical examination. In the elderly, bony metastasis should be a significant concern, and should prompt evaluation for a distant primary tumor. Standard AP and lateral views of the area of concern should be obtained. If concerned for malignancy, a chest x-ray should be obtained. CT scan and MRI are useful adjuncts for characterizing bony lesions.

RADIOGRAPHIC FEATURES OF BONY LESIONS

Plain radiographs can significantly narrow the differential diagnosis for bony lesions. Specific attention must be paid to the anatomical site of the lesion, the zone of transition between lesion and normal bone, and internal characteristics of the lesion. Benign lesions tend to be slow-growing. While benign lesions can destroy cortical bone, a transitional rim of reactive periosteal bone is typically formed around the neoplasm. High-grade malignant lesions tend to grow rapidly, and host bone has little ability to wall off the lesion with a rim of periosteal bone. Correspondingly, aggressive lesions often have a poorly demarcated transitional zone. High-grade lesions frequently destroy cortical bone and can spread to adjacent soft tissue. Note should also be made of calcification or ossification within the lesion. Calcification appears more haphazard and frequently more dense than ossification, and often denotes a cartilaginous tumor. Ossification indicates production of mineralized matrix giving the appearance of organization or structure, and is more common in tumors of bony origin.

BIOPSY AND SURGICAL TREATMENT

Biopsy is generally performed only after the lesion has been well-characterized by physical and radiographic examination. If a lesion is found to be malignant, the entire biopsy tract must be removed at the time of tumor resection. As such, the biopsy site and tract should violate as few intrafascial compartments to prevent seeding adjacent compartments with tumor and limit the extent of necessary resection. Transverse incisions should be avoided. Frozen sections should be sent to confirm an adequate sample of the lesion has been obtained; samples should also be sent for culture as infection can masquerade as an aggressive-appearing lesion.

Surgical treatment is directed toward removing the entire lesion and preventing local recurrence. In general, more extensive resection confers a lower risk of local recurrence. Four types of tumor resection have been described:

1. **Intralesional** Dissection proceeds through the tumor itself (eg, curettage)
2. **Marginal** Resection through the reactive zone of the tumor, which contains inflammatory cells, fibrous tissue, and possible satellite metastases
3. **Wide** Entire tumor is removed with a surrounding cuff of normal tissue
4. **Radical** Removal of tumor and its entire surrounding fascial compartment

STAGING

Staging for malignant musculoskeletal lesions is based on the histologic grade of the lesion, its location (intra vs. extracompartmental), and the presence of distant metastases. Grade (G) assesses the histologic characteristics of the tumor. G_1 lesions appear less aggressive and have a lower risk of distant metastasis. Increasing grade in G_2 and G_3 lesions denotes more aggressive cytologic features and increases the risk of distant metastasis. Tumor size (T) includes lesions within their capsule (T_0), extending through the capsule but within the compartment of origin (T_1), and beyond the compartment of origin (T_3). Metastasis (M) includes no metastases (M_0), and the presence of metastases (M_1).

CHEMOTHERAPY AND RADIATION

A detailed discussion of chemotherapeutic and radiation regimens for various musculoskeletal neoplasms is beyond the limits of this text. Modern chemotherapeutic regimens offer significant benefits in disease-free survival for osteogenic sarcoma and Ewing's sarcoma. Neoadjuvant (preoperative) chemotherapy is becoming more popular in treating these cancers. Radiation is effective in local treatment of Ewing's sarcoma, osteosarcoma, lymphoma, myeloma, and metastatic bone disease.

METASTATIC BONE LESIONS

Metastases from remote primary tumors represent the majority bone tumors seen in adults. Of these, most are derived from carcinomas from the breast, prostate, lung, kidney, thyroid, pancreas, and stomach. While breast and prostate cancer metastases commonly result from a known primary cancer, bony metastasis of unknown origin frequently stems from lung or renal cancer. The presence of a lytic bone lesion in an adult older than 40 without a diagnosis of a primary cancer should prompt the following investigation, which successfully identifies the primary tumor in 85% of cases:

- Plain radiographs of the affected limb, chest x-ray, CT scan of the chest, abdomen, and pelvis.
- Technetium bone scan to detect multiple lesions.
- Skeletal survey (if myeloma is suspected).
- Complete blood count, serum chemistry, liver function tests, erythrocyte sedimentation rate, and serum or urine immunoelectrophoresis.

Metastases are most commonly observed in the pelvis, ribs, vertebral bodies, and proximal limbs. These lesions typically have a lytic appearance on plain radiographs, although breast and prostate metastases can be sclerotic or mixed with lytic and sclerotic features. Metastases from renal cell carcinoma tend to be extremely vascular, and angioembolization is an important consideration prior to biopsy or definitive surgical treatment. Of note, bone destruction is not caused by the malignant cells but rather through induction of local osteoclasts by the metastasis. As a result, bisphosphonate therapy has come into common use in cancer patients.

Multiple myeloma is a common malignant tumors affecting bone. It is a plasma cell disorder most commonly affecting patients between 50 and 80. Patients most often present with bone pain or pathologic fracture. Vertebral and large bone involvement is most common. Radiographs commonly demonstrate multiple punched-out, lytic bone lesions. Patients with multiple myeloma should undergo a skeletal survey to evaluate for other lytic lesions as bone scan is frequently uninformative.

Surgical intervention for metastatic bone lesions is centered around reducing pain and maintaining functionality. Internal fixation is performed prophylactically if an impending fracture is observed. Risk factors for pathologic fracture include greater than 50% destruction of diaphyseal cortices, greater than 50%-75% metaphyseal destruction, destruction of the subtrochanteric region of the femur, and persistent pain following radiation therapy.

COMMON PRIMARY MALIGNANT BONE TUMORS

Osteosarcoma

Osteogenic sarcoma is the most common primary malignant tumor of bone. It is more common in men, and most commonly occurs in children and young adults about the knee (Figure 40–38). Other common locations include the proximal humerus and proximal femur. Histology demonstrates osteoid production with malignant stromal cells. Most lesions are high-grade and penetrate the cortex, forming an extramedullary soft tissue mass. Plain films show a destructive lesion demonstrating some bone formation. Modern chemotherapy regimens have significantly increased survival and feasibility of limb-sparing approaches. Treatment consists of neoadjuvant chemotherapy followed by resection and maintenance chemotherapy. Less common subtypes of osteosarcoma include telangiectatic, parosteal, and periosteal.

Chondrosarcoma

Chondrosarcoma results from malignant cartilaginous cells with peak incidence in the fifth and sixth decades. It commonly occurs in the knee, shoulder, pelvis, and spine. Plain films demonstrate cortical thickening and stippling consistent with cartilage deposition. Determining malignancy in cartilaginous cells based solely on histologic examination is difficult; clinical history and imaging are essential for correct diagnosis. Chondrosarcomas tend to be Grade 1 or 2 and less aggressive than osteosarcoma. Surgical resection with wide margins is the treatment of choice. Dedifferentiated chondrosarcoma is a subtype containing highly aggressive spindle-shaped cells. Prognosis is poor, and treatment consists of wide-margin resection and chemotherapy.

Ewing's Sarcoma

Ewing's sarcoma is a small, blue cell tumor with a characteristic t(11:22) chromosomal translocation. It commonly occurs in children older than five years and in young adults. Children younger than five years with a small blue cell tumor should have leukemia and metastatic neuroblastoma excluded before the diagnosis of Ewing's is made. Likewise, metastatic carcinoma must be excluded in adults. Pain and fever are common presenting complaints, with many patients having elevated inflammatory markers and a leukocytosis (which can be confused with osteomyelitis). The pelvis, knee, proximal humerus, and femur diaphysis are the most common locations. Plain films demonstrate a destructive, frequently diametaphyseal lesion. The classic "onion-skin" appearance of multiple layers of reactive periosteum is uncommon; more commonly the appearance is lytic with variable amounts of

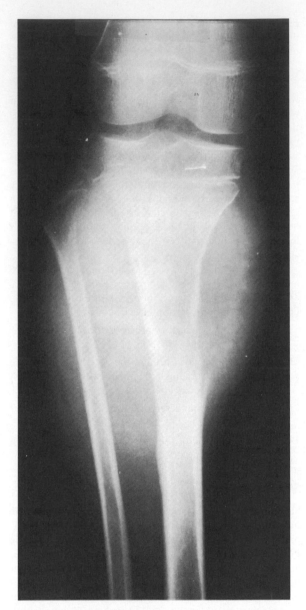

▲ **Figure 40–38.** Osteosarcoma with Codman's triangle, a new area of subperiosteal bone formed when a tumor raises the periosteum away from the bone.

reactive bone. Treatment including chemotherapy, radiation, and surgical intervention can produce long-term survival approaching 70%.

Lymphoma of Bone

Lymphoma of bone can occur as a solitary focus, scattered through bone and soft tissue, or as a metastasis to bone. It can affect patients at nearly any point in life. Pain and a large soft-tissue mass are common. The knee, pelvis, hip, shoulder, and vertebrae are commonly affected. Bony destruction with a variable degree of reactive bone is characteristic on plain film. Treatment centers around chemo- and radiotherapy. Surgical intervention is indicated for impending or pathologic fracture fixation.

COMMON BENIGN BONE LESIONS

▶ Osteoid Osteoma

Osteoid osteoma is a benign bone lesion typically producing pain in patients from 5 to 30 years of age. Progressive pain, particularly at night, is characteristic. The lesion is commonly found in the proximal femur, spine, and tibial diaphysis. Plain films typically show a radiolucent nidus with a sclerotic, reactive rim. Bone scans are always positive. Often, pain is well-relieved with NSAIDS, and 50% of lesions will "burn out" with conservative management. For persistent pain, percutaneous radiofrequency ablation of the nidus is highly effective.

▶ Enchondroma

Enchondromas are benign cartilaginous tumors commonly found in the metaphyses of long bones and the hand, where pathologic fractures can be common. Plain films demonstrate a lytic lesion with a stippled appearance. Most enchondromas can be observed and followed with serial radiographs at 3 months and 1 year after presentation. Treatment, if necessary, consists of curettage and bone grafting. Malignant transformation to chondrosarcoma is exceedingly rare, except in two cases: Ollier's disease is characterized by multiple enchondromas, and confers a 30% risk of chondrosarcoma. Maffucci's syndrome includes multiple enchondromas with associated soft tissue angiomas. Both diseases also confer increased risk of visceral malignancy.

▶ Osteochondroma

Osteochondroma is a benign surface lesion of bone characterized by a cartilaginous cap connected to the medullary cavity of the underlying bone. It can be pedunculated or sessile. If asymptomatic, observation is sufficient. If painful, resection is appropriate. Multiple hereditary exostosis is an autosomal dominant condition in which patients have multiple osteochondromas. Although malignant transformation in isolated lesions is rare, multiple hereditary exostosis confers a higher risk (approximately 10%).

▶ Giant Cell Tumor of Bone

Although benign, giant cell tumors can be locally aggressive. GCT is more common in females, and typically occurs in

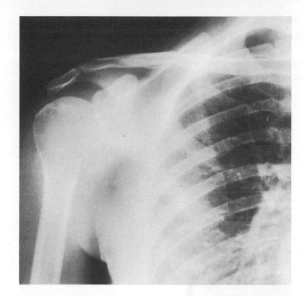

▲ **Figure 40–39.** Giant cell tumor of proximal humerus.

the epiphysis of long bones after the physis has closed. The knee, vertebra, distal radius, and sacrum are common sites. Plain films demonstrate a metaphyseal lytic lesion extending to the epiphysis (Figure 40–39). Treatment consists of cortical windowing, aggressive curettage, chemical cauterization with phenol, and bone grafting. If inoperable, radiation can be employed. Rarely, primary giant cell tumor can be malignant or can undergo secondary malignant degeneration (most often following radiation exposure).

▶ Aneurysmal Bone Cyst

Aneurysmal bone cysts (ABC) are benign, but can be associated with other tumors, including GCT, chondroblastoma, and fibrous dysplasia. It can also be found within a malignant tumor. Seventy-five percent of patients are less than 20 years old. History consists of pain and swelling over months to years. Plain films demonstrate an expansile lesion with a thin rim of cortical bone. ABC is characterized by a blood-filled interior without an endothelial lining. Occasional thin septae of bone may be present. Treatment is curettage with bone grafting, and recurrence commonly occurs if physes are open.

▶ Unicameral Bone Cyst

Unicameral bone cysts are characterized by cystic expansion and cortical thinning. They are most commonly observed in the proximal humerus, proximal femur, and distal tibia. Patients commonly present with pain or pathologic fracture. Radiographs demonstrate a mildly expansile lytic-centered lesion with thin surrounding cortices and trebeculae

(Figure 40–40). Active lesions border the physis, while latent lesions have interposed normal bone. First line treatment consists of aspiration and cytologic examination of the fluid followed by methylprednisolone injection. Curettage and bone grafting are used if this proves ineffective.

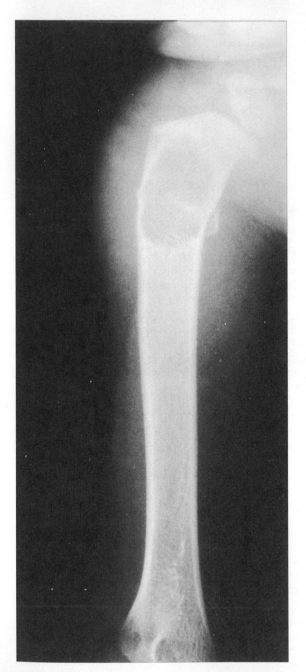

▲ **Figure 40–40.** Unicameral bone cyst with fracture.

▶ Fibrous Dysplasia

Fibrous dysplasia is a developmental disorder of bone. It can be solitary (monostotic) or present in multiple locations (polyostotic). McCune–Albright syndrome is diagnosed when the polyostotic form is associated with café-au-lait spots and endocrine abnormalities. While nearly any bone can be involved, the proximal femur is the most common location. Plain films demonstrate a lucent lesion surrounded by a well-defined sclerotic rim; the lesions can range from purely lytic to having a ground-glass appearance. Most patients do not require surgical treatment; however, curettage, bone grafting, and internal fixation are appropriate in areas of high stress or pathologic fracture.

▶ Osteomyelitis

Osteomyelitis can mimic bone tumors. Patients frequently present with bone pain, fevers, and chills. Constitutional symptoms, however, are not always present. Acute infections are typically lytic with periosteal elevation; chronic lesions can have a mixed lytic/sclerotic appearance. MRI can demonstrate changes in bone not easily seen on plain films early in the course of infection. In acute osteomyelitis, surgical treatment is initiated when there is an abscess present, patients have failed to respond to nonoperative management, and when soft tissues need debridement to prevent further destruction.

Chronic osteomyelitis can arise from incompletely treated acute osteomyelitis, IV drug abusers, or in immunocompromised hosts. The disease course commonly follows a relapsing/remitting course with acute exacerbations in pain interspersed with periods of relative quiescence. Intravenous antibiotic therapy should be guided by deep cultures from the infected site. Surgical therapy consists of removal of all infected bone and soft tissue, and removal of hardware (if present), followed by culture-directed IV antibiotic therapy.

▼ FOOT AND ANKLE

PAIN SYNDROMES OF THE FOOT

1. Interdigital Neuritis

▶ Introduction

Interdigital neuritis is a common cause for pain in the foot. Originally described by Thomas Morton, the irritation of the interdigital nerve was believed to be due to compression between the metatarsal heads. However, it is now known that this is not the case given the location of the interdigital nerve lying plantar to the intermetatarsal ligament and metatarsal heads. Instead it is now believed that interdigital neuritis is due to compression and tethering of a stretched nerve across the transverse metatarsal ligament.

History and Physical Examination

Patients typically present with pain associated with burning or tingling on the plantar aspect of the foot near the webspace of the affected nerve. This syndrome occurs most commonly in middle-aged women. Shoe wear, particularly wearing shoes with a tight toe box or high heels, appears to significantly exacerbate symptoms due to increased pressure on the plantar aspect of the foot and increased stretching of the nerve with dorsiflexion of the toes. Pain can be relieved with removal of the offending shoe and massage. Pain in the interdigital space may be reproduced on physical examination with pressure applied just proximal to the metatarsal heads by squeezing the forefoot between the examiner's thumb and index finger.

Diagnosis

The differential diagnosis includes synovitis, bursitis, and metatarsalgia. In metatarsalgia, the pain is located directly under the involved metatarsal bone and often is accompanied with callous formation. The pain caused by synovitis is usually located immediately distal to the metatarsal head. Bursitis may present with swelling in the web space, which is not a typical finding associated with interdigital neuritis.

Interdigital neuritis is typically diagnosed with history and physical examination as described above. Injection of the affected digital webspace with 1 mL of lidocaine with successful relief of symptoms can provide diagnosis confirmation.

Treatment

Treatment begins with nonsurgical management: avoidance of shoes with high heels or a tight toe box, use of a firm crepe sole which prevents hyperextension or dorsiflexion of the toes, and a metatarsal pad which provides relief of pressure on the plantar aspect of the foot. Steroid injection may improve symptoms; however, the effect is usually short-lived. If conservative measures fail surgery with release of the transverse metatarsal ligament and/or neurectomy may be pursued.

2. Metatarsalgia

Metarsalgia is a disorder defined by pain located below the metatarsal heads that is worse with weight-bearing. Mechanical factors such as laxity of the transverse inter-metatarsal ligament appear to be the root cause. Plantar callosities, most commonly under the second metatarsal head, may also be present. Treatment starts with orthotics, such as felt or rubber pads below the metatarsal heads to relieve pressure. Surgery may be considered if conservative measures fail.

3. Hallux Valgus

General Considerations

Hallux valgus is defined by subluxation of the first MTP joint, which results in first metatarsal head medial prominence and lateral deviation of the proximal phalanx on the first metatarsal.

Etiology

Anatomic factors including varus alignment of the first metatarsocuneiform joint may predispose to hallux valgus. Women's shoes with a small toe box may also cause bunching of the toes, predisposing to the valgus deformity of the first MTP joint.

Clinical Evaluation and Physical Examination

When evaluating hallux valgus, the patient's main complaint should be defined carefully as this may affect choice of treatment options. Chief complaints may be related to cosmesis, metatarsalgia, second-toe deformity, problems with shoe-fit, or simply pain. Additionally, the patient's occupational and recreational activities should be investigated as well. Professional dancers or high-performance athletes are not good candidates for certain surgeries.

Initially, the foot should be inspected for any deformity. Hallux valgus is present when there is medial prominence of the first metatarsal head, also known as a "bunion." Limitation of dorsiflexion, pronation deformity of the big toe, synovial thickening, dorsal osteophytes, and medial deviation of the second MTP joint may be present as well. Neurovascular status of the foot should be documented.

Radiographic Evaluation

Initially weight-bearing AP, lateral and oblique radiographs of the foot should be obtained. The halux valgus angle (the angle between the proximal phalynx and the first metatarsal, normal is less than 15 degrees), the intermetarsal angle (the angle between the first and second metatarsals, normal < 9 degrees) and the distal metatarsal angle (angle between the distal metatarsal articular surface and the long axis of the first metatarsal), normal is less than 10 degrees of lateral deviation) should be measured and recorded. Incongruence of the MTP joint (lateral deviation of the proximal phalynx from the metatarsal head) should be noted as well.

Treatment

Initially conservative treatment should be pursued with a wide, soft shoe with adequate toe box and insole padding. If conservative therapy fails a number of surgical treatment options are available depending on the severity of the deformity, joint congruence, presence of arthritis, and other patient factors.

4. Hallux Varus

Hallux varus is subluxation of the medial proximal phalynx on the first metatarsal. Etiologies include trauma and iatrogenic (overcorrection via surgery for hallux valgus). Hallux varus may be defined as supple (correctable with physical manipulation) or rigid (fixed, not correctable via manipulation. If the deformity is supple, then tendon transfer with extensor hallucis longus or extensor hallucis brevis should be considered. If the deformity is rigid, then arthrodesis or fusion of the first MTP joint is the best surgical treatment.

5. Hallux Rigidus

Hallux rigidus entails significant arthrosis of the first MTP joint resulting in significant pain and restriction of dorsiflexion. There may be increased bulk of the joint as well, resulting in difficulty wearing shoes. Marginal ostophytes may be present dorsally and laterally.

Forced dorsiflexion performed by the examiner often reproduces the patient's pain. Grind test should also be performed by holding the first metatarsal steady and applying an axial load with circumduction of the proximal phalynx. Significant pain with this maneuver indicates a positive grind test which equates to significant loss of the plantar located cartilage. Additionally the dorsal medial cutaneous nerve may be sensitive as well.

Radiographic evaluation includes weight-bearing AP, lateral, and oblique views of the foot. The extent of joint narrowing should be noted. Hallux rigidus may classified as follows based on radiographs: grade I (preserved joint space), grade II (<50% joint space narrowing), and grade III (>50% loss of joint space).

Initially, conservative management using a shoe with a large toe box to accommodate increased bulk of the first MTP joint and rigid rocker sole to minimize joint motion should be tired. If conservative measures fail, surgery may be considered.

Surgical treatment entails cheilectomy (removal of the osteophyte) or arthrodesis (fusion of the first MTP joint). Chielectomy is indicated for grade I, grade II, and grade III pathology with a negative grind test. If chielectomy fails to provide significant pain relief, arthrodesis may be performed. For grade III lesions on radiographs and a positive grind test (indicating lack of plantar cartilage) arthrodesis should be pursued. Although various arthroplasty (joint replacement procedures) are now available, the short-to-midterm results of these procedures are not as successful as chielectomy and/or arthrodesis.

6. Plantar Fasciitis

Plantar fasciitis is a degenerative process involving the plantar fascia origin. The typical patient with this disorder is the overweight 40-70 year old with significant plantar heel pain and localized tenderness at the plantar medial tuberosity of the calcaneus. An osteophyte (heel spur) may be visible on radiographs. Treatment entails stretching and massage of the plantar fascia and Achilles tendon, cushioned heel inserts, night splints, and/or a walking cast. If conservative measures fail, surgery with release of the medial third of the plantar fascia may be considered.

7. The Diabetic Foot

The pathology associated with the diabetic foot is complicated by neuropathy and angiopathy with varying degrees of severity. Diabetic ulceration and neuropathic arthropathy (aka Charcot Foot) can result. Management of these two pathologic disorders is dependent on a number of factors.

▶ Diabetic Ulceration

Due to neuropathy, patients with diabetes have decreased sensation around their feet. As a result, injuries to the superficial layer of skin are not perceived, and progression to ulceration can occur. These patients should be initially evaluated with transcutaneous oxygen pressures and ankle-to-brachial indices (ABIs) to determine healing potential. An ABI ratio > 0.6 and transcutaneous oxygen measurements more than 40 mm Hg are usually indicative of adequate vascularity and necessary healing potential. Additionally, the character of the ulcer itself affects treatment choice. Localized, superficial ulcers that do not extend to tendon, bone, or ligament can be debrided at the bedside followed by placement in an offloading shoe or cast with serial physical examinations. Ulcers that extend to deeper tissues and/or bone may require debridement in the operating room and antibiotic therapy. Additionally, nutrition should be optimized to encourage healing. If appropriate blood flow is present, these ulcers will typically heal. If healing does not occur or gangrene is appreciated due to poor vascularity, amputation may be considered.

▶ Neuropathic Arthropathy (Charcot Foot)

Neuropathic arthropathy is characterized by osteopenia, joint subluxation or dislocation and bony fragmentation that may progress to malunion at later stages. White blood cell-labeled scintigraphy with MRI can be used to differentiate this condition from osteomyelitis. Initial treatment includes non–weight-bearing of the affected lower extremity with or without cast placement. Operative intervention is considered only in special cases.

FURTHER READING

Skinner HB, ed.: Current Diagnosis and Treatment in Orthopedics. 5th ed. McGraw-Hill, New York, NY; 2013.

MULTIPLE CHOICE QUESTIONS

1. Open fractures, defined as a break in the bone with violation of the skin and soft tissues requires the following management:

   A. Splinting
   B. Bedside irrigation and splinting
   C. Formal irrigation and debridement in the operating room with stabilization of fracture and antibiotics
   D. VAC dressing
   E. Plastic surgery consultation

2. A 37-year-old man is involved in a motor cycle accident at a high rate of speed. Upon arrival to the emergency room he reports that he has no feeling below the waist and cannot move his legs. The bulbocavernosis reflex is intact. According to the American Spinal Injury Association, he would be considered:

   A. Asia A
   B. Asia B
   C. Asia C
   D. Asia D
   E. Asia E

3. A 57-year-old woman is involved in a motor vehicle collision. She is transferred to the Emergency Department where radiographs confirm a closed pelvic fracture with symphyseal widening. She becomes acutely hypotensive in the resuscitation bay. The next important step in her treatment is:

   A. Immediate transfusion
   B. Exploratory laparotomy
   C. Move blood pressure cuff to the leg
   D. Apply sheet or pelvic binder around the patient
   E. Obtain more x-rays

4. A 23-year-old man presents to the Emergency Room with an acute injury to his left knee sustained playing football. He is unable to weight bear and on exam demonstrates anterior dislocation of the tibia. The next steps in management include:

   A. Emergent reduction, splinting, vascular studies, and neurologic exam
   B. Knee immobilizer and outpatient follow-up
   C. Urgent MRI
   D. Transport to operating room for open reduction of the knee
   E. Reduction and casting

5. A 3-year-old child fell from the monkey bars sustaining an acute injury to her left elbow. She demonstrates good strength with the exception of the anterior interosseous nerve. Radiographs confirm a displaced supracondylar humerus fracture. Parents are informed:

   A. Splint will be applied and patient can return for outpatient follow-up.
   B. Patient will require closed reduction and pinning of the elbow in the operating room. The AIN will require exploration and repair.
   C. Patient will require closed reduction and pinning of the elbow in the operating room. The AIN will recover in most cases with observation over the next 3-6 months.
   D. Patient can be observed for recovery of nerve overnight in the emergency room.
   E. AIN is rarely injured with this type of fracture.

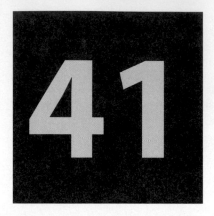

Plastic & Reconstructive Surgery

Henry C. Vasconez, MD

Jason Buseman, MD

Plastic surgery, although considered a technique-oriented and multiregional specialty, is in essence a problem-solving field. The training of a plastic surgeon allows him or her to see surgical problems in a different light and select from a variety of options to solve these surgical problems. Plastic surgeons have received broad training, and many have completed residencies in other fields such as general surgery, otolaryngology, orthopedics, urology, or neurosurgery. Other modalities of training have more recently integrated these and other surgical subspecialties into a more comprehensive training program.

The basic principles of plastic surgery are careful analysis of the surgical problem, careful planning of procedures, precise technique, and atraumatic handling of tissues. Alteration, coverage, and transfer of skin and associated tissues are the most common procedures performed. Plastic surgery may deal with the closure of surgical wounds—particularly recalcitrant wounds such as those occurring postradiation or poorly healing wounds in immunocompromised patients. Plastic surgery also deals with the removal of skin tumors, repair of soft tissue injuries including burns, correction of acquired or congenital deformities, or enhancement of undesirable cosmetic features. Craniofacial and hand surgery, also within the realm of plastic surgery, may require additional surgical training.

In the past quarter century, increased knowledge of anatomy and the development of many new techniques have brought about important changes in plastic surgery. It is now known that in many areas the blood supply of the skin is derived principally from vessels arising from underlying muscles and larger perforating blood vessels rather than solely from vessels of the subcutaneous tissue, as was formerly thought. One-stage transfer of large areas of skin, fascia, and muscle tissue can be accomplished if the axial pedicle of the underlying fascia or muscle is included in the transfer. With the use of microsurgical techniques, musculocutaneous units or combinations of bone, fascia, muscle, and skin can be successfully transferred and vessels and nerves less than 1 mm in size can be repaired. These so-called free-flap transplantations are a major advance in the treatment of defects that were previously untreatable or required lengthy or multistaged procedures. More sophisticated knowledge of the blood supply to the skin has introduced the concept of perforator flaps whereby one perforating vessel is identified that may supply a large segment of overlying skin and subcutaneous tissue. Similarly, the concept of neurocutaneous flaps has given rise to the design of additional flap territories such as the sural flap in the lower leg and the sensate radial flap in the forearm.

The plastic surgeon, as a member of the craniofacial surgical team, is able to dramatically improve the appearance and function of children with severe congenital deformities. Children of normal intelligence who previously had been social outcasts are now able to lead relatively normal lives. Improved understanding of facial growth and abnormal development and diagnostic techniques such as the CT scan, MRI, and 3D computer-assisted imaging enable the reconstructive surgeon to develop a complex strategy for remodeling the deformed craniofacial skeleton. This may involve remodeling or repositioning of part or all of the cranial vault, the orbits, the midface, and the mandible. These complex and at times formidable reconstructions are performed by moving specific skeletal units and adding autogenous bone grafts. These structures are kept in place using miniplate fixation; the miniplates are made of titanium or resorbable material.

A notable advance in craniofacial surgery was the introduction of distraction osteogenesis, which borrows from the Ilizarov principle of distraction. A cortical cut is made in the bone, and a distraction apparatus is applied so that in measured amounts (usually 1 mm per day) the bone is either stretched to offset a length discrepancy or transported to bridge a gap. In craniofacial surgery, it is more commonly brought to bear to enlarge or cause overgrowth of areas such as an underdeveloped mandible.

Additional areas of involvement for the plastic surgeon entail allotransplantation, particularly with the increasing number of clinical limb allotransplants, which unfortunately still require immunosuppression. It is hoped that immunotolerance will someday become a reality, allowing transplantation of nonessential organs with a minimum of dangerous immunosuppression. Transplantation of the hand with excellent functional recovery in some cases has been performed successfully but still requires a great deal of immunosuppression. Face transplants have been performed with some initial success. The first facial transplant was performed in France and consisted of a partial segment of the face. The functional recovery to date has been remarkable. The problems of facial animation still need to be refined. Additionally, a number of ethical issues with regard to facial identity and immunosuppression require further resolution.

Tissue engineering of bone, cartilage, and nerve is an area of ongoing research for plastic surgeons. Although encouraging experimental results have been reported in anatomic areas difficult to reconstruct, such as the external ear, the nose, or the larynx, there are as yet few clinical applications.

Fetal surgery for cleft disorders and scar considerations, an area pioneered by a number of plastic surgeons, appears to be in a quiescent stage, particularly because the persistent real and potential risks to the fetus and mother may not be warranted for disorders that are not life threatening. Significant technical advances in the postnatal treatment of cleft lip and cleft palate have also lessened the enthusiasm for fetal surgery for these disorders.

Bassiri Gharb B, Rampazzo A, Madajka M, et al: Effectiveness of topical immunosuppressants in prevention and treatment of rejection in face allotransplantation. *Plast Reconstr Surg* 2011;127(5 Suppl):13.

Quilichini J, Hivelin M, Benjoar MD, et al: Restoration of the donor after face graft procurement for allotransplantation: report on the technique and outcomes of seven cases. *Plast Reconstr Surg* 2012;129(5):1105.

▼ I. GRAFTS & FLAPS

SKIN GRAFTS

A graft of skin detaches epidermis and varying amounts of dermis from its blood supply in the **donor area** and is placed in a new bed of blood supply from the base of the wound, or **recipient area.** The way a skin graft survives or "takes" is first by diffusion of nutrient elements from the graft bed, known as imbibition; then after a period of 2-5 days, the graft actually revascularizes from the bed, a process known as inosculation. Although the technique is relatively simple to perform and generally reliable, definite considerations about the donor area and adequacy of the recipient area are important. Skin grafting is a quick, effective way to cover a

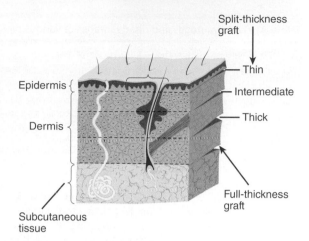

▲ **Figure 41–1.** Depths of full-thickness and split-thickness grafts.

wound if vascularity is adequate, infection is not present, and hemostasis is assured. Color match, contour, durability of the graft, and donor morbidity must be considered.

TYPES OF SKIN GRAFTS

Skin grafts can be either split-thickness or full-thickness grafts (Figure 41–1). Each type has advantages and disadvantages and is indicated or contraindicated for different kinds of wounds (Table 41–1).

A. Split-Thickness Grafts

Thinner split-thickness grafts (0.01-0.015 inch) become vascularized more rapidly and survive transplantation more reliably. This is important in grafting on less than ideal recipient sites, such as contaminated wounds, burn surfaces, and poorly vascularized surfaces (eg, irradiated sites). A second advantage is that donor sites heal more rapidly and can be reused within a relatively short time (7-10 days) in critical cases such as major burns.

In general, however, the disadvantages of thin split-thickness grafts outweigh the advantages. Thin grafts exhibit the highest degree of postgraft contraction, offer the least amount of resistance to surface trauma, and are least like normal skin in texture, suppleness, pore pattern, hair growth, and other characteristics. Hence, they are usually aesthetically unacceptable.

Thicker split-thickness skin grafts (> 0.015 inch) contract less, are more resistant to surface trauma, and are more similar to normal skin than are thin split-thickness grafts. They are also aesthetically more acceptable but not as acceptable as full-thickness grafts.

The disadvantages of thick split-thickness grafts are relatively few but can be significant. They are less easily

Table 41–1. Advantages and disadvantages of various types of skin grafts.

Type of Graft	Advantages	Disadvantages
Thin split-thickness	Survive transplantation most easily. Donor sites heal most rapidly.	Fewest qualities of normal skin. Maximum contraction. Least resistance to trauma. Sensation poor. Aesthetically poor.
Thick split-thickness	More qualities of normal skin. Less contraction. More resistant to trauma. Sensation fair. Aesthetically more acceptable.	Survive transplantation less well. Donor site heals slowly.
Full thickness	Nearly all qualities of normal skin. Minimal contraction. Very resistant to trauma. Sensation good. Aesthetically good.	Survive transplantation least well. Donor site must be closed surgically. Donor sites are limited.

vascularized than thin grafts and thus result in fewer successful takes when used on less than ideal surfaces. Their donor sites are slower to heal (requiring 10-18 days) and heal with more scarring than donor sites for thin split-thickness grafts—a factor that may prevent reuse of the area.

Meshed grafts are usually thin or intermediate split-thickness grafts that have been rolled under a special cutting machine to create a mesh pattern. Although grafts with these perforations can be expanded from 1.5 to 9 times their original size, expansion to 1.5 times the unmeshed size is the most useful. Meshed grafts are advantageous because they can be placed on an irregular, possibly contaminated wound bed and will usually take. Also, complications of hemostasis are fewer because blood and serum exude through the mesh pattern. The disadvantage is poor appearance following healing (alligator hide look).

Donor sites for split-thickness grafts heal spontaneously by epithelialization. During this process, epithelial cells from the sweat glands, sebaceous glands, or hair follicles proliferate upward and spread across the wound surface. If these three structures are not present, epithelialization will not occur.

B. Full-Thickness Grafts

Full-thickness skin grafts include the epidermis and all the dermis. They are the most aesthetically desirable of the free grafts because they include the highest number of skin appendage elements, undergo the least amount of contracture, and have a greater ability to withstand trauma. There are several limiting factors in the use of full-thickness grafts. Since no epidermal elements remain to produce epithelialization in the donor site, it must be closed primarily, and a scar will result. The size and number of available donor sites is therefore limited. Furthermore, conditions at the recipient site must be optimal in order for transplantation to be successful.

Areas of thin skin are the best donor sites for full-thickness grafts (eg, the eyelids and the skin of the postauricular, supraclavicular, antecubital, inguinal, and genital areas). Submammary and subgluteal skin is thicker but allows

camouflage of donor area scars. In grafts thicker than approximately 0.015 inch, the results of transplantation are less reliable, except on the face, where vascularity is usually superior.

C. Composite Grafts

A composite graft is also a free graft that must reestablish its blood supply in the recipient area. It consists of a unit with several tissue planes that may include skin, subcutaneous tissue, cartilage, or other tissue. Dermal fat grafts, hair transplant grafts, and skin and cartilage grafts from the ear fall into this category. Obviously, composite grafts must be small or at least relatively thin and will require recipient sites with excellent vascularity. These grafts are generally used in the face.

D. Cultured Epithelial and Dermal Grafts

Epithelial cells, grown or cultured in a special medium in vitro, will coalesce into thin sheets that can be used to cover full-thickness wounds. Although these cultured epithelial sheets were first used in the treatment of burns, the result was somewhat unsatisfactory because the coverage was very fragile and disfiguring. More recently, success has been obtained with artificial dermis, which when placed in an appropriate bed will revascularize and can then be covered by a very thin (0.05 cm) split-thickness skin graft, cultured or otherwise. This artificial dermis is increasingly being used in the treatment of burns. Modifications of this concept have also been applied to the care of chronic ulcers, particularly in the leg. The artificial dermis is made out of a collagen matrix and has very low or no antigenicity.

E. Biological Skin Substitutes

Research continues to develop bioengineered products that are becoming more common place in plastic surgery and general wound management. The source of these products varies (eg, human, porcine, etc) and can alter the products indications and overall ability to assist with wound management. Some of the more common products used are Integra and acellular dermal matrices (ADM), Integra is a bilayer material consisting of interwoven bovine collagen and a glycosaminoglycan that mimics the dermal layer of skin. This has made it ideal for reconstruction cases where more than simple skin grafts will suffice, such as over a tendon. ADM is acellular cadaver skin that is chemically prepared. Although initially designed for burn reconstruction, it has been used in wound care and general reconstruction cases from head to toe.

Obtaining Skin Grafts

Instruments used for obtaining skin grafts include razor blades, skin grafting knives (Blair, Ferris Smith, Humby, Goulian), manual drum dermatomes (Padgett, Reese), and electric or air-powered dermatomes (Brown, Padgett, Hall, Zimmer). The electric and air-powered dermatomes are the most widely used because of their reliability and ease of operation. A surgeon, even with only limited experience, can successfully obtain sheets of split-thickness skin grafts using the electric dermatomes.

The Skin Graft Recipient Area

To ensure survival of the graft, there must be (1) adequate vascularity of the recipient bed, (2) complete contact between the graft and the bed, (3) adequate immobilization of the graft-bed unit, and (4) relatively few bacteria in the recipient area.

Because survival of the graft is dependent upon growth of capillary buds into the raw undersurface of the graft, vascularity of the recipient area is of prime importance. Avascular surfaces that will not generally accept free grafts are tissues with severe radiation damage, chronically scarred ulcer beds, bone or cartilage denuded of periosteum or perichondrium, and tendon or nerve without their paratenon or perineurium, respectively. For these surfaces, a bed capable of producing capillary buds must be provided; in some cases, excision of the deficient bed down to healthy tissue is possible. All unhealthy granulation tissue must be removed, because bacterial counts in granulation tissue are often very high. If bone is exposed, it can be decorticated down to healthy cancellous bone with the use of a chisel or power-driven burr, and a meshed split-thickness skin graft can be applied. If an adequate vascular bed cannot be provided or if the presence of essential structures such as tendons or nerves precludes further debridement, skin or muscle flaps are generally indicated for coverage.

Inadequate contact between the graft and the recipient bed can be caused by collection of blood, serum, or lymph fluid in the bed; formation of pus between the graft and the bed; or movement of the graft on the bed. The use of fibrin sealants (Artiss) has more recently been developed to assist with skin graft take. This is sprayed over the wound bed prior to placement of any skin graft. After 60-90 seconds, a fibrin clot develops that better holds the skin graft in place

and diminishes potential spaces between the wound bed and the skin graft, which can negatively affect skin graft survival.

After the graft has been applied directly to the prepared recipient surface, it may or may not be sutured in place and may or may not be dressed. Whenever the maximum aesthetic result is desired, the graft should be cut exactly to fit the recipient area and precisely sutured into position without any overlapping of edges. Very large or thick split-thickness grafts and full-thickness grafts will usually not survive without a pressure dressing. In areas such as the forehead, scalp, and extremities, adequate immobilization and pressure can be provided by circular dressings. Tie-over pressure stent dressings are advisable for areas of the face, where constant pressure cannot be provided by simple wraparound dressings; areas where movement cannot be avoided, such as the anterior neck, where swallowing causes constant motion; and areas of irregular contour, such as the axilla. The ends of the fixation sutures are left long and tied over a bolus of gauze fluffs, cotton, a sponge, or other suitable material (Figure 41–2).

Grafts applied to freshly prepared or relatively clean surfaces are generally sutured or stapled into place and dressed with pressure. The use of fibrin sealants has helped minimize the need for these usually uncomfortable bolster techniques. A single layer of damp or other nonadherent fine-mesh gauze is applied directly over the graft. Immediately over this are placed several thicknesses of flat gauze cut in the exact pattern of the graft. On top of these is placed a bulky dry dressing of gauze fluffs, cotton, a sponge, or other material. Pressure is then applied by wraparound dressings, adhesive

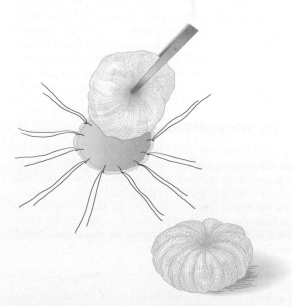

▲ **Figure 41–2.** Tie-over stent dressing.

tape, or a tie-over pressure stent dressing. An alternative dressing is to place a nonadherent fine-mesh gauze atop the graft followed by a negative-pressure dressing. The vacuum-assisted dressings may be useful for irregular contours, such as around digits and webspaces or joint surfaces, by maintaining wound-to-graft interface, immobilizing the grafted area, suctioning serosanguineous fluid, and possibly promoting neovascularization.

In many cases, it is permissible—and sometimes even preferable—to leave a skin graft site open with no dressing. This is particularly true in slightly infected wounds, where the grafts tend to float off in the purulent discharge produced by the wound. These wounds are best treated with meshed grafts so that liquid forming between the graft and the wound bed can exude and be removed without disturbing the graft. This treatment can also be used for noninfected wounds that produce an unusual amount of serous or lymphatic drainage, as occurs following radical groin dissections.

In severely ill patients, such as those with major burns, where time under anesthesia must be kept to a minimum, large sheets of meshed split-thickness skin grafts are rapidly applied but not sutured. Skin staples may be used to fix the graft rapidly. Grafts need not be dressed if the area is small, but if the area is large or circumferential, a dressing should be applied. Meshed grafts should generally be covered for 24-48 hours to prevent dryness, because their dermal barrier has been partly disrupted.

Skin graft dressings may be left undisturbed for 5-7 days after grafting if the grafted wound was free of infection, if complete hemostasis was obtained, if fluid collection is not expected, and if immobilization is adequate. If any one of these conditions is not met, the dressing should be changed within 24-48 hours and the graft inspected. If blood, serum, or purulent fluid collection is present, the collection should be evacuated—usually by making a small incision through the graft with a scalpel blade and applying pressure with cotton-tipped applicators. The pressure dressing is then reapplied and changed daily so that the graft can be examined and fluid expressed as it collects.

▶ The Skin Graft Donor Area

The ideal donor site would provide a graft identical to the skin surrounding the area to be grafted. Because skin varies greatly from one area to another as far as color, thickness, hair-bearing qualities, and texture are concerned, the ideal donor site (such as upper eyelid skin to replace skin loss from the opposite upper eyelid) is usually not found. However, there are definite principles that should be followed in choosing the donor area.

A. Color Match

In general, the best possible color match is obtained when the donor area is located close to the recipient area. Color and texture match in facial grafts will be much better if the grafts are obtained from above the region of the clavicles. However, the amount of skin obtainable from the supra-clavicular areas is limited. If larger grafts for the face are required, the immediate subclavicular regions of the thorax will provide a better color match than areas on the lower trunk or the buttocks and thighs. When these more distant regions are used, the grafts will usually be lighter in color than the facial skin in Caucasians. In people with dark skin, hyperpigmentation occurs, producing a graft that is much darker than the surrounding facial skin.

B. Thickness of the Graft and Donor Site Healing

Donor sites of split-thickness grafts heal by epithelialization from the epithelial elements remaining in the donor bed. The ability of the donor area to heal and the speed with which it does depends on the number of these elements present. Donor areas for very thin grafts will heal in 7-10 days, whereas donor areas for intermediate-thickness grafts may require 10-18 days and those for thick grafts 18-21 days or longer.

Because there is a normal anatomic variation in the thickness of skin, donor sites for thicker grafts must be chosen with the potential for healing in mind and should be limited to regions on the body where the skin is thick. Infants, debilitated adults, and elderly people have thinner skin than healthy younger adults. Grafts that would be split-thickness in the normal adult may be full thickness in these patients, resulting in a donor site that has been deprived of the epithelial elements necessary for healing.

C. Management of the Donor Site

The donor site itself can be considered a clean open wound that will heal spontaneously. After initial hemostasis, the wound will continue to ooze serum for 1-4 days, depending on the thickness of the skin taken. The serum should be collected and the wound kept clean so that healing can proceed at a maximal rate. The wound should be cared for as described above for clean open wounds in either of two ways.

One technique of donor site management is an open (dry) technique. The donor site is dressed with porous, sterile fine-mesh or nonadherent gauze. After 24 hours, the dry gauze is changed but the nonadherent gauze is left on the wound and exposed to the air, a heat lamp, or a blow dryer. A scab will form on the gauze and will peel off from the edges as epithelialization is completed underneath. This method has the advantage of simple maintenance once the wound is dry.

The second method that has become more popular is the closed (moist) technique. Studies have demonstrated that the rate of epithelialization is enhanced in a moist environment. In contrast to the dry technique, pain can be reduced or virtually eliminated. Moist-to-moist gauze dressings that require frequent wetting have been replaced by newer synthetic materials. A gas-permeable membrane (OpSite, Tegaderm) that sticks to the surrounding skin provides an artificial blister over the wound. Occasionally, there is a break in the protective seal covering leakage of serum collected under the membrane. This increases the risk of infection, especially in a contaminated zone. Newer hygroscopic dressings actually absorb and retain many times their weight in water. They are permeable to oxygen yet impervious to bacteria. Infection is still a concern; however, because of occasional exposure of the wound during healing. Newer dressings, such as Mepilex, contain silver-impregnated ions that control bacterial contamination and may hasten healing and reepithelialization while keeping the patient more comfortable. Silver ion is exquisitely antimicrobial and is used for burn dressing care as well as skin graft sites.

Anderson JR, Fear MW, Phillips JK, et al: A preliminary investigation of the reinnervation and return of sensory function in burn patients treated with INTEGRA®. *Burns* 2011;37(7):1101.

Branski LK, Mittermayr R, Herndon DN, et al: Fibrin sealant improves graft adherence in a porcine full-thickness burn wound model. *Burns* 2011;37(8):1360.

Lee LF, Porch JV, Spenler W, Garner WL: Integra in lower extremity reconstruction after burn injury. *Plast Reconstr Surg* 2008;121(4):1256.

Silverstein P, Heimbach D, et al: An open, parallel, randomized, comparative, multicenter study to evaluate the cost effectiveness, performance, tolerance, and safety of a silver-containing soft silicone foam dressing (intervention) vs silver sulfadiazine cream. *J Burn Care Res* 2011;32(6):617.

FLAPS

The term "flap" refers to any tissue used for reconstruction or wound closure that retains part or all of its original blood supply after the tissue has been raised and moved to a new location. That part still connected through which the blood supply enters and exits is referred to as the flap base or pedicle. With local skin flaps, a section of skin and subcutaneous tissue is raised from one site and moved to a nearby area, with the base remaining attached at its original location.

Flaps can be classified according to the pattern of blood supply to the skin into random or axial pattern. Flaps can further be classified according to their tissue content into muscle, musculocutaneous, fasciocutaneous, and others.

Random Pattern Flaps

Random pattern flaps consist of skin and subcutaneous tissue cut from any area of the body in any orientation, with no distinct pattern or particular relation to the blood supply of the skin of the flap. Such flaps receive their blood supply from vessels in the subdermal tissue. Although commonly used, this is the least reliable type of flap, and except when cut from facial and scalp skin, the ratio of length to width cannot safely exceed 1.5:1. Its use should be minimized.

Presently, in any reconstructive effort, one should use a flap with known reliability and a predictable blood supply.

Axial Pattern Flaps

The axial pattern flap has a well-defined arteriovenous system running along its long axis. Because of good vascular supply, it can be made comparatively long in relation to width. Foremost among the axial flaps are the deltopectoral and the forehead flaps, which are based on perforating branches of the internal mammary artery and supraorbital and supratrochlear or superficial temporal vessels, respectively. Other axial flaps are the groin flap, based on the superficial circumflex iliac artery; the dorsalis pedis flap, based on the artery of the same name; the radial forearm flap; the scapular flap; the lateral upper arm flap; and various scalp and face flaps.

Muscle & Musculocutaneous Flaps

Musculocutaneous flaps consist of skin and underlying muscle, which provide reliable coverage with usually one operation. The use of musculocutaneous units has developed as surgeons have gained more knowledge of the way in which blood is supplied to the skin. The technique has revolutionized reconstructive surgery.

The subdermal plexus of vessels from which skin flaps derive their blood supply is augmented or directly supplied in many areas by sizable perforating vessels arising from underlying muscles. Many muscles receive their blood supply from a single axial vessel, with only minor contributions from other sources (Figure 41–3). The skin over these muscles can be completely circumscribed and elevated in continuity with the underlying muscle up to its major vascular pedicle. If the vessels in the pedicle are preserved, the unit can be moved in wide arcs to distant areas of the body while normal or near normal blood flow is continued to the skin island as well as to the muscle. The donor sites of such flaps can often be closed primarily.

Knowledge of the anatomy of muscles and their nerve and blood supply is necessary for the successful design of musculocutaneous flaps. Although almost any skeletal muscle can be used, muscles with a dominant arterial pedicle and reliable perforating vessels to the skin are most useful.

In addition to their reliability, musculocutaneous flaps clean up recipient sites that are heavily contaminated with bacteria better than skin flaps do. This is why muscle-containing flaps are the best choice for coverage of wounds caused by radiation or osteomyelitis or those that have a high probability of infection.

The most commonly used muscles and musculocutaneous flaps are the latissimus dorsi, pectoralis major, tensor fasciae latae, rectus femoris, rectus abdominis, trapezius, temporalis, serratus anterior, gluteus maximus, gracilis, and gastrocnemius muscles.

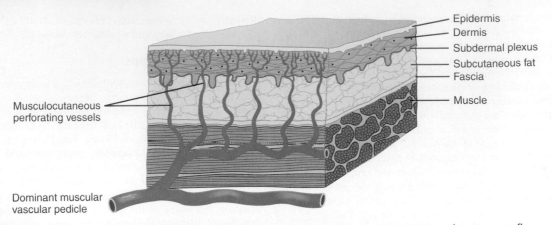

Epidermis
Dermis
Subdermal plexus
Subcutaneous fat
Fascia

Muscle

Musculocutaneous
perforating vessels

Dominant muscular
vascular pedicle

▲ **Figure 41–3.** Arterial supply to skin from main artery supplying muscles, as occurs in musculocutaneous flaps.

A. Latissimus Dorsi

The latissimus dorsi musculocutaneous unit is supplied by the thoracodorsal vessels. Use of this unit has been widely applied in the one-stage reconstruction of the breast following radical or modified radical mastectomy (see section on Rectus Abdominis). The entire latissimus dorsi muscle can be detached from its origin and transposed to the anterior chest. An island of skin can also be included in the center of the muscle to restore the skin lost on the anterior chest wall. Refinements in technique utilize only enough muscle to carry the skin island, thus leaving intact a good portion of innervated, functional muscle. This unit is also useful for coverage of defects on the anterior chest, shoulder, head and neck, and axilla and even for restoration of flexion of the elbow. It is a popular muscle for free tissue transfer because of its long and relatively large and reliable vascular pedicle.

B. Pectoralis Major

The pectoralis major musculocutaneous unit obtains its vascular supply from the thoracoacromial axis of the subclavian artery just medial to the medial border of the pectoralis minor. It derives a dual blood supply from medial intercostal perforators branching from the internal mammary artery. The entire unit may be transposed medially, especially after disinsertion from the humerus, to cover defects of the sternum, neck, and lower face. Also, an island of skin can be outlined low on the chest and made to reach intraoral defects following cancer excision.

C. Trapezius

The trapezius musculocutaneous unit, based on the descending branch of the transverse cervical artery, is useful for covering defects in the neck, face, and scalp. When skeletonized as an island, the flap will reach the top of the head. When it is used in conjunction with a neck dissection, the transverse cervical artery must be preserved. Functional preservation of shoulder elevation may be accomplished by selectively sparing the transverse, superior fibers of the muscle.

D. Temporalis

The temporalis muscle extends from the temporal fossa to the coronoid process of the mandible. It is supplied by the deep and superficial temporal systems. It is commonly used to fill orbital defects. However, it can cover neighboring cranial, maxillary, palatal, and pharyngeal regions.

E. Tensor Fasciae Latae

The tensor fasciae latae musculofascial unit is supplied by the lateral femoral circumflex artery, a branch of the profunda femoris. It has a wide arc of rotation anteriorly and posteriorly. It is elevated with the fascia lata and thus can be used to reconstruct the lower abdominal wall. It has been used to cover defects following excision of osteoradionecrotic ulcers of the pubis or groin. It is also the method of choice for coverage of greater trochanteric pressure ulcers.

F. Rectus Femoris

The rectus femoris, a more robust flap than the tensor fasciae latae with a shorter arc of rotation, has supplanted the latter for reconstruction of the lower abdominal wall and for coverage to postradiation ulcers in the pubis and groin. It has a dual blood supply: a muscular branch from the profunda femoris and an axial branch from the superficial femoral artery to the overlying skin and fascia.

G. Rectus Abdominis

The rectus abdominis is supplied by the deep superior and inferior epigastric vessels that run in the undersurface of the muscle and anastomose with the segmentally arranged intercostal vessels to form the epigastric arcade. These vessels send perforating branches throughout the length of the muscle, perforating the anterior rectus sheath and supplying the overlying skin. The transverse rectus abdominis myocutaneous (TRAM) flap, when based on the superior epigastric vessel and including the infraumbilical skin, has become a workhorse for autologous tissue breast reconstruction. In situations of marked deformity, such as a radical mastectomy associated with radiation therapy or previous abdominal surgery, reconstruction of the breast can be accomplished reliably with infraumbilical skin and adipose tissue based on both rectus muscles. This superiorly based TRAM flap involves an abdominoplasty as well as reconstruction of the breast. It is a technically demanding operation but gives a very satisfying result. When based on the deep inferior epigastric vessel and using the supraumbilical skin (the "flag" flap), the flap can cover defects of the abdominal wall, flank, groin, and thigh. Using the inferior epigastric vessels to transport the skin and adipose tissue by means of microvascular surgery (see section on Free Flaps) has become a popular method of breast reconstruction. A small portion of the rectus muscle or just a main perforator vessel that supplies the overlying fat and skin is taken. This flap is known as the deep inferior epigastric perforator flap, or DIEP flap (see section on Perforator Flaps).

H. Gluteus Maximus

The gluteus maximus is useful as a muscle or musculocutaneous unit for covering pressure sores or traumatic defects over the sacrum and ischium. The muscle has a double blood supply from the superior and inferior gluteal arteries to the respective halves of the muscle. In ambulatory patients, it is advisable to perform a function-preserving operation by advancing the muscle medially and preserving its insertion laterally.

I. Gracilis

The gracilis muscle receives its dominant blood supply proximally from the medial femoral circumflex artery. Its arc of rotation makes it an excellent source of coverage for ischial pressure sores and vaginal reconstruction. Other recent uses have included transportation of the muscle alone for repair of a persistent perineal sinus following abdominal-perineal resection.

J. Gastrocnemius

The gastrocnemius musculocutaneous unit is based on either the medial or lateral head of the muscle. Each head is supplied by a sural artery, a branch of the popliteal artery that enters the muscle at its most proximal third near its origin. The flap is most useful to cover defects of the knee and proximal anterior tibia. Coverage of exposed bone in the middle and lower leg, where this unit cannot reach, can be accomplished by use of local muscle flaps such as the soleus. Complex bone and soft tissue injuries of the middle and lower leg may require reconstruction with free muscle flaps.

▶ Fasciocutaneous Flaps

A plexus of vessels is located on top of the muscular fascia and is supplied from vessels that run within the intermuscular septa. These vessels tend to run axially along the fascia, sending perforators to the skin at intervals. Flaps can be designed that are safer than random flaps and that need not contain an entire muscle unit for their transfer. Furthermore, it is possible to make fasciocutaneous or septocutaneous flaps that safely exceed the traditional limits of a 1.5:1 ratio between length and width. Examples of fasciocutaneous flaps are those overlying the gastrocnemius, quadriceps, and rectus abdominis muscles. Other commonly used flaps are the radial forearm, lateral arm, scapular, and deltopectoral flaps.

▶ Neurocutaneous Flaps

Anatomic studies have confirmed the presence of an arterial pedicle accompanying a sensory nerve such as the sural nerve. Consequently, one may be able to outline a skin territory over the trajectory of a sensory nerve with good viability of the overlying skin.

▶ Free Flaps

Free flaps involve tissue transplantation using microvascular surgery. The term is actually incorrect, because the blood supply from the main axial pedicle of the flap is completely detached and then reattached at a distance to recipient vessels near the wound area.

An operating microscope with two viewing binocular lenses, specialized instruments, and swaged-on needles of 60-80 μm are required for microsurgery; 8-0, 9-0, and 10-0 suture is used to anastomose vessels as small as 0.5 mm in diameter.

Examples of free flaps in current use are axial pattern skin and fasciocutaneous flaps, such as scapular, groin, radial forearm, and anterolateral thigh, which are used when only skin and subcutaneous tissue are needed, and muscle and musculocutaneous flaps, such as latissimus dorsi, gracilis, and rectus abdominis flaps, which are used when the bulk and vascularity of muscle are needed. Composite free flaps such as the fibular flap with its overlying skin are most helpful free flaps for reconstruction of the mandible as well as the floor of the mouth following head and neck tumor extirpations.

The vascular pedicle areas of some flaps contain functional nerves, which can also be reattached with microscopic guidance. Examples are inferior gluteal, thigh, and tensor fasciae latae flaps, which contain sensory nerves. Attempts using sensory flaps to provide protective sensation in critical areas such as the feet or the ischium in paraplegic patients have so far been clinically unsuccessful. More encouraging is the work being done to provide sensibility to the floor of the mouth with a sensory innervated radial forearm flap. Motor flaps can restore functions such as forearm flexion or facial expression.

Bone and functional joints can be transplanted as free flaps. Flaps from the ribs, fibula, and iliac crest have all been successfully transferred to areas such as the mandible and tibia. The toe-to-thumb transfer is an example of a complex transplantation, which includes bone with a functional joint, tendons, and nerves as well as skin.

▶ Perforator Flaps

A sophisticated variation on the use of the musculocutaneous principle has been the development of perforator flaps. This usually entails taking a branch from the major vascular pedicle that may perforate the muscle to arborize and form a subcutaneous vascular plexus that will supply a considerable amount of overlying skin. Perhaps the greatest benefit from a perforator flap is decreased donor site morbidity. Structures such as the fascia, muscle, and associated nerves may be preserved while allowing the skin to be used for reconstruction.

The DIEP flap exemplifies this well for autologous tissue breast reconstruction. While maintaining the same skin territory as the TRAM flap, the perforating vessels are carefully dissected away from the rectus abdominis. By sparing the muscle, there is potentially a reduction in excessive abdominal wall weakness at the donor site.

The anterolateral thigh flap has become the mainstay for cutaneous flaps at some institutions. Based on musculocutaneous perforators from the vastus lateralis, it can be used when a relatively thin cutaneous flap is needed, such as in head and neck reconstruction. The donor site may be closed primarily depending on the flap width.

The perforator concept has been applied to further territories of skin over the perforator segments of the gluteal, thoracodorsal, and medial plantar arteries among others.

Mateev MA, Kuokkanen HO: Reconstruction of soft tissue defects in the extremities with a pedicled perforator flap: series of 25 patients. *J Plast Surg Hand Surg* 2012;46(1):32.

Munhoz AM, Pellarin L, Montag E, et al: Superficial inferior epigastric artery (SIEA) free flap using perforator vessels as a recipient site: clinical implications in autologous breast reconstruction. *Am J Surg* 2011;202(5):612.

Nosrati N, Chao AH, Chang DW, Yu P: Lower extremity reconstruction with the anterolateral thigh flap. *J Reconstr Microsurg* 2012;28(4):227.

Selber JC, Fosnot J, Nelson J, et al: TRAM flaps on the abdominal wall: Part 2. Bilateral reconstruction. *Plast Reconstr Surg* 2010;126(5):1438.

Selber JC, Nelson J, Fosnot J, et al: A prospective study comparing the functional impact of SIEA, DIEP, and muscle-sparing free TRAM flaps of the abdominal wall: part 1. Unilateral reconstruction. *Plast Reconstr Surg* 2010;126(4):114.

Wang CY, Chai YM, Wen G, et al: The free peroneal perforator-based sural neurofasciocutaneous flap: a novel tool for reconstruction of large soft-tissue defects in the upper limb. *Plast Reconstr Surg* 2011;127(1):293.

▼ II. PRINCIPLES OF WOUND CARE

There are many types of wounds and many factors to consider when choice of coverage procedure is made. Skin type and color, glandular association, and hair-bearing characteristics must be considered. Avascular wound beds, such as exposed bone, cartilage, or tendon, will not accept skin grafts unless viable periosteum, perichondrium, or paratenon (respectively) is present. Other areas with poor vascularity are joint capsules, radiation-damaged tissue, and heavily scarred tissue. Exposed or implanted alloplastic material cannot be used as a graft bed. Such areas must be covered with tissue that is attached to its own blood supply. Skin flaps can be used but are sometimes inadequate because their blood supply is tenuous and the layer of subcutaneous fat is even less reliably vascular and may not attach to the underlying avascular surface. Muscle or musculocutaneous flaps are generally required for avascular areas.

The coverage tissue may need to have more bulk than the original tissue. Areas such as bony surfaces and prominences, weight-bearing surfaces, densely scarred areas, and areas of potential pressure breakdown may require thick, durable covering. Again, skin grafts or skin flaps may not be of adequate thickness even though they may survive and cover the wound. Musculocutaneous flaps are more successful. Bulkiness may be undesirable in areas such as the scalp, face, neck, or hand. Defects in these areas that for other reasons require a musculocutaneous flap for coverage may need to be debulked in a secondary procedure. Axial skin flaps or free axial pattern flaps may be a better choice than musculocutaneous flaps in some areas.

Contraction begins during the proliferative phase of healing and continues to a large degree in wounds covered only by split-thickness skin grafts. The grafted area may shrink to 50% of its original size, and both the graft and surrounding tissue may become distorted. Splinting of the area for 10 days or longer may favorably alter contraction. Full-thickness skin grafts rich in dermis, attached to a fresh wound bed, will considerably reduce contraction, and skin flaps will eliminate it altogether. In an orifice or tubular passageway, such as the nasal airway, pharynx, esophagus, or vagina, absence of contraction is critical.

The effects of atrophy and gravity should also be considered when technique of coverage is chosen. A denervated muscle will atrophy up to 60% of its regular size. The muscle tissue in a musculocutaneous flap will atrophy even when the nerve to the muscle is preserved in the pedicle, because the muscle's functional tension is generally not restored. Gravity will cause sagging of any tissue that does not have enough plasticity or muscle dynamics to counteract gravitational pull. Reconstructions in the face often tend to sag.

Wounds at risk for or known to have bacterial contamination also require certain types of coverage (eg, pressure sores, lower extremity defects, and wounds resulting from incision and drainage of abscesses). If the area can be skin grafted, meshed split-thickness grafts are most effective, because bacterial exudate will not collect under these grafts. Musculocutaneous flaps are associated with fewer residual bacteria over time than are random pattern skin flaps. This is probably due to the vastly superior vascularity of musculocutaneous flaps.

Contaminated wounds or wounds that are exuding a considerable amount of fluid can be treated by negative-pressure or vacuum wound dressings. This entails the application of a sponge-like material connected to a suction device that keeps the wound dry as it suctions the excess exudates. The negative pressure on the wound also appears to have a positive effect on healing and increased revascularization. It has become a popular method of preparing a wound for definitive closure.

Wounds associated with nearby injuries that will probably require further surgery (eg, injuries to tendons or nerves) should be covered with flaps, because the flaps can be incised or undermined to allow for additional surgery. Skin grafts do not have sufficient vascularity to allow for these procedures.

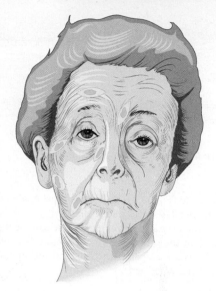

▲ **Figure 41–4.** Sites of elliptic incisions corresponding to wrinkle lines on the face.

▶ Excision & Primary Closure

The ideal type of wound closure is primary approximation of the skin and subcutaneous tissues immediately adjacent to the wound defect, producing a fine-line scar and the optimal aesthetic result in skin texture, thickness, and color match.

All excisions and wound closures should be planned with this ideal in mind. Obviously, large lesions cannot be excised and closed primarily. With invasive cancers, such as sarcomas, the primary goal is performance of adequate en bloc resection, with the type of wound closure being of secondary importance. Nevertheless, even larger excisions, such as mastectomies, can be planned with definite consideration for closure and subsequent reconstruction.

In most cases, minimal scars can be achieved only if the line or lines of incision are placed in, or parallel to, the skin lines of minimal tension. These lines lie perpendicular to the underlying muscles. On the face, they are obvious

as wrinkles or lines of facial expression that become more pronounced with age, since they are secondary to repeated muscle contraction (Figure 41–4). On the neck, trunk, and extremities, the lines of minimal tension are most noticeable as horizontal lines of skin relaxation on the anterior and posterior aspects of areas of flexion and extension.

Langer lines, which were determined by cadaver study, probably show the direction of fibrous tissue bundles in the skin and are no longer considered accurate guides for placing skin incisions.

If the lines of expression cannot be followed, the line of incision should (if possible) be placed at the junction of unlike tissues such as the hairline of the scalp and the forehead, the eyebrow and the forehead, the mucosal and skin junction of the lips, or the areolar and skin margins of the breast. Scars will be partially hidden if incisions are placed in inconspicuous areas such as the crease of the nasal ala and cheek, the auricular-mastoid sulcus, or the submandibular-neck junction. Lines of incision should never purposely cross flexor surfaces such as the neck, axilla, antecubital fossa, or popliteal space or the palmar skin creases of the fingers and hand, because of the risk of contracture formation. A transverse oblique or S incision should be incorporated when crossing these sites.

If a lesion is to be excised, an elliptic incision placed parallel to the skin lines of minimal tension will give the best result if the amount of tissue to be excised does not preclude primary closure.

If the ellipse is too broad or short, a protrusion of skin, commonly called a "dog-ear," will occur at each pole of the

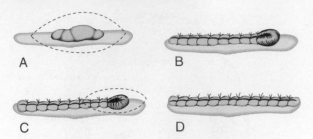

▲ **Figure 41–5.** Correction of dog-ear.

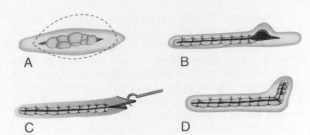

▲ **Figure 41–6.** Alternative method of correction of dog-ear.

wound closure (Figure 41–5). This is most easily corrected by excising the dog-ear as a small ellipse.

A dog-ear may also be present if one side of the ellipse is longer than the other (Figure 41–6). In this case, it may be easier to excise a small triangle of skin and subcutaneous tissue from the longer side.

A. Z-Plasty

One of the most useful and commonly used techniques in primary wound closure is the Z-plasty. The procedure is illustrated in Figure 41–7. The angles formed by the Z-shaped incision are transposed as shown in order (1) to gain length in the direction of the central limb of the Z or (2) to change the line of direction of the central limb of the Z. Ninety-degree angles would provide the greatest gain in length of the central limb, but smaller angles, such as 60-degree angles, are usually used, because the incision is easier to close and significant gain in length is still achieved. The Z-plasty is used for scar revision and reorientation of small wound incisions so that the main incision will be in a more ideal location. The lengthening function is used for the release or breakup of scar contractures across flexion creases. Frequently, many small Z-plasties in series rather than one large one are done. Occasionally, incisions will be placed under excessive vertical tension after the release of an underlying contracture, such as Dupuytren contracture in the hand.

B. Suture Technique

Suture technique in primary closure is important but will not compensate for poorly planned flaps, excessive tension across the incision, traumatized skin edges, bleeding, or other problems. Sometimes even a skillfully executed closure may result in an unsightly scar because of healing problems beyond the control of the surgeon.

The goal of closure is level apposition of dermal and epithelial edges with minimal or no tension across the incision and no strangulation of tissue between sutures. This is usually accomplished by placement of a layer of interrupted or running absorbable sutures in the superficial fascia and subdermal level at the base of the dermis. This suture prevents tension from forming in the upper dermis and epithelium and also causes the surface planes to be level. The epithelial edges can then be opposed with interrupted or running monofilament sutures of absorbable or permanent material. The absorbable suture is placed in the subcuticular or intradermal plane and is left in place. The permanent sutures are removed quickly according to the region of the body (within 3-4 days in the face), so the suture tracks can be avoided. Sterile adhesive tape (Steri-Strips) placed across the incision will also prevent surface marks and can be used either primarily or after surface sutures have been removed. Taping will not correct errors in suturing that have resulted in uneven edges or tension across the incision. Tape burns may occur if there is excessive tension or swelling around the incision.

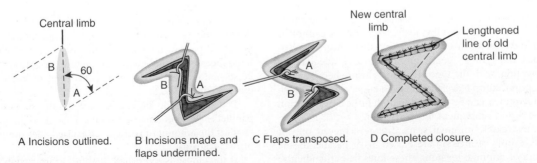

A Incisions outlined. B Incisions made and flaps undermined. C Flaps transposed. D Completed closure.

▲ **Figure 41–7.** Z-plasty.

The size and even the type of suture material are less important than careful suture placement and observance of previously mentioned factors. Almost any suture properly placed and removed early enough will provide closure without leaving suture marks. The use of monofilament nylon or polypropylene suture material is advised, however, because these types of sutures cause the fewest reactions of currently available suture materials, excluding stainless steel. Running subcuticular, pullout-type monofilament sutures may be left in for up to 3 weeks without causing reactions. Even buried nylon sutures are well tolerated and generally cause fewer problems than braided or absorbable sutures.

An alternative to sutures is the use of skin adhesives such as 2-octylcyanoacrylate (Dermabond). It works well in small areas without much tension or shearing. It is also advisable in children. Further studies are needed to evaluate its wider applicability.

▶ Choice of Coverage

Table 41–2 shows some of the indications for choice of coverage in various types of wounds. Once a given type of flap is chosen, there are still at least two major considerations in the selection of the exact flap to be used. The most significant consideration is the degree of injury that will occur in the donor area. There is always a trade-off when tissue is taken from one area and used in another. This trade-off is minimal when a well-designed, well-placed skin flap leaves a donor defect that can be closed primarily, but the trade-off is great when the donor defect is as severe as the original wound (eg,

skin graft donor sites that become infected or musculocutaneous donor sites that fail to heal).

The patient can often participate in the choice of donor locations and should certainly be made aware of potential donor site scars and complications. The tendency has been to use muscle flaps instead of musculocutaneous flaps to permit easy primary closure of the donor site. The muscle can then be resurfaced with a split-thickness skin graft during the same procedure to give a satisfactory result. This provides for an acceptable donor site scar rather than risking disruption of a tight closure or an otherwise ugly donor site.

The second consideration in selection of a flap is that some or all of the graft or flap may be lost. In general, if the patient's overall condition is poor or the loss of a flap would result in a devastating defect, a very reliable type of flap should be chosen. For example, a microvascular anastomosis can be performed on a leg with one remaining arteriosclerotic vessel to the foot, but if the anastomosis fails, the vessel may thrombose and the leg may be lost. In this case, a flap that is safer, although more time consuming to place, may be chosen, such as a cross-leg flap.

▶ Elevation & Transposition of Flaps

Additional considerations in reconstructive surgery involve the technique of elevating and transposing flaps. For random skin flaps, these considerations include proper length-to-width ratio, careful planning to allow for transposition with minimal tension and adjustments at the recipient site, accurate dissection in the subcutaneous plane to avoid injury to the subdermal plexus, and avoidance of folding or kinking of the flap.

Table 41–2. Indications for various types of tissue coverage.

Type of Wound	Type of Coverage	Reason for Choice
Mildly (< 10^5) infected wounds (including burns)	Thin split-thickness or meshed	Difficulty in obtaining successful take of thicker grafts. Donor sites may be reused sooner.
Significantly (> 10^5) infected wounds (osteomyelitis)	Thin split-thickness or meshed skin grafts or muscle or musculocutaneous flaps	Rich muscle vascular supply can sterilize an infected wound.
Wounds with poorly vascularized surfaces	Thin split-thickness skin grafts or flaps	Difficulty in obtaining successful take of thicker grafts. Flap with intrinsic blood supply may be required.
Small facial defects	Full-thickness skin graft or local flap	Produces best aesthetic result.
Large facial defects	Thick split-thickness skin grafts or flaps	Cannot use full-thickness graft, because of limited size of donor sites.
Full-thickness eyelid loss	Local flap or composite graft	Repair requires more than one tissue element.
Deep loss of nasal tip	Local flap or composite graft	Repair requires thicker tissue than present in split- or full-thickness grafts.
Avulsive wounds with exposed tendons and nerves	Flap	Requires thick protective coverage without graft adherence to tendons and nerves.
Exposed cortical bone or cartilage	Skin or muscle flap	Free grafts will not survive on avascular recipient site.
Wounds resulting from radiation burns	Muscle or musculocutaneous flap	Free grafts will not survive on avascular recipient site. Damaged tissue extends deeper than may be apparent.

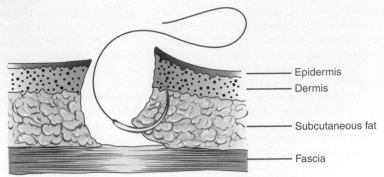

A. The strength of the closure lies in the dermis. Occasionally, the subcutaneous fat is incorporated to obliterate dead space.

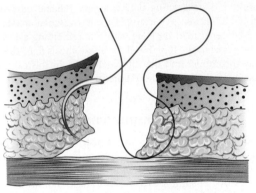

B. The suture is placed so that the knot will lie in the deepest part of the wound. Take care to avoid incorporating the epidermis with this suture, since epithelial cysts will form and result in suture extrusion.

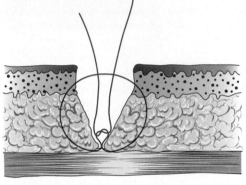

C. The dermal suture is tied just tightly enough to approximate the wound margins. Synthetic absorbable sutures are most commonly used for closure of the dermis.

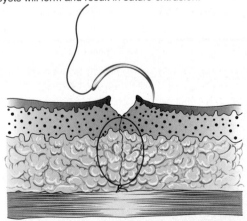

D. After the dermis is approximated, a fine "epidermal" suture is placed to align the wound edges. This suture adds little to the tensile strength of the wound closure.

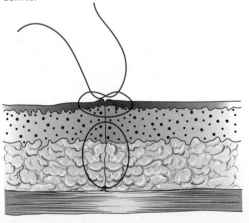

E. The epidermal suture is tied just tightly enough to approximate the epidermal edges of the wound. Since the strength of this closure lies in the dermis, the epidermal suture can be removed after 2–3 days. Skin tapes are often used to support the wound for an additional 7–10 days.

▲ **Figure 41–8.** Layered cutaneous closure (buried half-mattress [flap] sutures). (Reproduced, with permission, from Saunders CE, Ho MT, eds: *Current Emergency Diagnosis & Treatment*, 4th ed. New York: McGraw-Hill, 1992.)

Labels in panel A: Epidermis, Dermis, Subcutaneous fat, Fascia

Surgical technique must be atraumatic, and hemostasis must be achieved. With axial pattern flaps, the surgeon must have knowledge of the important underlying blood vessels as well.

▶ Closure Technique

Closure technique is as important as elevation and transposition technique. Flaps should not be allowed to dry out. The wound bed should be irrigated. Closed-system, nonreactive suction drains are routinely used in both the wound bed and the donor defect for most flaps of any significant size. Suction evacuates blood or serum that may accumulate and keeps the flap firmly pressed against the wound bed. External pressure is both ineffective and detrimental for these purposes. Sutures should accurately and completely appose skin edges without strangulating the epithelium, particularly on the flap side. Buried half-mattress (flap) sutures are recommended (Figure 41–8). Dressings over flaps should be minimal and should not cause pressure or constriction. Emollient dressings, such as petrolatum gauze, antibiotic ointment, or silver sulfadiazine cream, have been shown to aid in preventing desiccation and subsequent necrosis of areas of marginal vascularity.

After a flap is at least temporarily tacked into its final position, adequacy of vascularity can be determined by intravenous injection of fluorescein dye, 10-15 mg/kg, and examination under ultraviolet light (Wood light). Areas that fluoresce within 10 minutes following dye injection can be expected to survive. Areas that do not fluoresce usually lack arterial inflow, which may be due to temporary arterial spasm but is often due to insufficient perfusion that will result in necrosis. A good clinical evaluation of the flap on the operating table is usually sufficient. Any sign of mottling or cyanosis or flap congestion that indicates a degree of venous obstruction warrants serious consideration of reexploration.

Liu DS, Sofiadellis F, Webb A, et al: Early soft tissue coverage and negative pressure wound therapy optimizes patient outcomes in lower limb trauma. *Injury* 2011;43(6):772.

Singer AJ, Chale S, Giardano P, et al: Evaluation of a novel wound closure device: a multicenter randomized controlled trial. *Acad Emerg Med* 2011;18(10):1060.

Stannard JP, Singanamala N, Volgas DA: Fix and flap in the era of vacuum suction devices: what do we know in terms of evidence based medicine? *Injury* 2010;41(8):780.

III. SPECIFIC DISORDERS TREATED BY PLASTIC SURGERY

DISORDERS OF SCARRING

HYPERTROPHIC SCARS & KELOIDS

In response to any injury severe enough to break the continuity of the skin or produce necrosis, the skin heals with scar formation. Under ideal circumstances, a fine, flat hairline scar will result. The details of wound healing are presented in Chapter 6.

However, hypertrophy may occur, causing the scar to become raised and thickened, or a keloid may form. A keloid is a true tumor arising from the connective tissue elements of the dermis. By definition, keloids grow beyond the margins of the original injury or scar; in some instances, they may grow to enormous size. (Figure 41–9)

Hypertrophic scars and keloids are distinct entities, and the clinical course and prognosis are quite different in each case. The overreactive process that results in thickening of the hypertrophic scar ceases within a few weeks—before it extends beyond the limits of the original scar—and in most cases, some degree of maturation occurs and gradual improvement takes place. In the case of keloids, the overreactive proliferation of fibroblasts continues for weeks or months. By the time it ceases, an actual tumor is present that typically extends well beyond the limits of the original scar, involves the surrounding skin, and may become quite large. Maturation with spontaneous improvement does not usually occur.

More recent research has shown differences on a biochemical level that can be quite complex. In essence though, it is understood that fibroblasts in both disorders display an increase in procollagen. This is compensated for in hypertrophic scars but not in keloids. This results in an increased ratio of type 1 to type 3 collagen in keloids.

▶ Treatment

The most frustrating aspect of hypertrophic and keloid treatment for both patient and care provider alike is the high incidence of recurrence. Much work has gone into

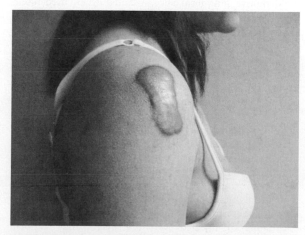

▲ **FIGURE 41–9.** A keloid scar—the excess growth of scar tissue at the site of a healed skin injury.

developing techniques to avoid and treat these scar problems, with mixed results. As this has become more evident, providers have become more specialized and aggressive with treatment options. More recent studies looking at treatments such as interferon, 5-flurouracil injections and bleomycin injections have shown some promise. But no therapy has shown to conclusively treat these problems.

Since nearly all hypertrophic scars undergo some degree of spontaneous improvement, they do not require treatment in the early phases. If the scar is still hypertrophic after 6 months, surgical excision and primary closure of the wound may be indicated, but recurrence is between 45% and 100% if no other treatments are provided. Improvement may be expected when the hypertrophic scar was originally produced by excessive endothelial and fibroblastic cell proliferation, as is present in open wounds, burns, and infected wounds. However, little or no improvement can be anticipated if the hypertrophic scar followed uncomplicated healing of a simple surgical incision. Improvement of hypertrophic scars across flexion surfaces such as the antecubital fossa or the fingers requires a procedure such as a Z-plasty to change the direction of the scar.

Pressure may help flatten a potentially hypertrophic scar. It is particularly useful for burn scars. A measured elastic garment or face mask (Jobst) is applied to the scarred area and provides continued pressure that causes realignment and remodeling of the collagen bundles. Pressure should be applied early, continuously, and for 6-12 months. Use of intermittent pressure (eg, only at night) or pressure applied after the hypertrophic scar is established (6-12 months) is of little value.

Additional methods of decreasing the thickness of hypertrophied scars include silicone sheeting applied early and continuously for weeks or months. Laser therapy, such as CO_2, pulse dye, and flash lamps, have been examined with no definitive long-term success noted when used alone. Radiotherapy has a place in scar management although it is somewhat controversial due to potential carcinogenesis following procedure and the lack of long-term follow up studies. Cryotherapy has shown some success with small scars only. Interestingly enough, the simple use of paper tape over fresh surgical incisions for several weeks has shown to be a potential preventive treatment.

The first-line treatment for keloids and second-line therapy for intractable hypertrophic scars is still injection of triamcinolone acetonide, 10 mg/mL (Kenalog-10 Injection), directly into the lesion. Corticosteroid injection decreases fibroblast proliferation and collagen synthesis as well as suppressing pro-inflammatory markers. There is some evidence that keloids may respond better to early treatment rather than to late treatment.

Lesions are injected every 3-4 weeks, and treatment should not be carried out longer than 6 months. A general rule of thumb is to inject 10 mg of triamcinolone for each centimeter in length of the scar. The following dosage schedule is used:

Size of Lesion

1-2 cm^2	20-40 mg
2-6 cm^2	40-80 mg
6-10 cm^2	80-110 mg

For larger lesions, the maximum dose should be 120 mg. The maximum doses for each treatment for children are as follows:

Age

1-2 years	20 mg
3-5 years	40 mg
6-10 years	80 mg

There is a tendency to inject the drug into the scar too often or in too high a dosage—or into the subjacent tissue, which may produce too vigorous a response, resulting in excessive atrophy of the skin and subcutaneous tissues surrounding the lesion and in depigmentation of darker skins. Both of these adverse responses may improve spontaneously in 6-12 months, but not necessarily completely. Cushing symptoms have even been reported with the overuse of corticosteroids for scar management. Topical corticosteroid therapy is of little or no value for substantial scarring but may have some place with more superficial scarring, such as in the case of dermabrasion.

At present, surgical excision is used only in conjunction with intralesional corticosteroid therapy. Excision is usually confined to the larger lesions in which steroid therapy would exceed safe dosages. (The wound is injected at the time of surgery and then postoperatively according to the schedule recommended above.) Care should be taken so that surgical incisions are not extended into the normal skin around the keloid, since the growth of a new keloid may occur in these scars.

Hayashi T, Furukawa H, Oyama A, et al: A new uniform protocol of combined corticosteroid injections and ointment application reduces recurrence rates after surgical keloid/hypertrophic scar excision. *Dermatol Surg* 2012;38(6):693.

Ko J, Kim P, Zhao Y, Hong SJ, Mustoe TA: HMG-CoA reductase inhibitors (statins) reduce hypertrophic scar formation in a rabbit ear wounding model. *Plast Reconstr Surg* 2012;129(2):252e.

Mustoe TA: Evolution of silicone therapy and mechanism of action in scar management. *Aesthetic Plast Surg* 2008;32(1):82.

Scrimali L, Lomeo G, Tamburino S, Catalani A, Perrotta R: Laser CO_2 versus radiotherapy in treatment of keloid scars. *Cosmet Laser Ther* 2012;14(2):94.

Yagmur C, Akaishi S, Ogawa R, Guneren E: Mechanical receptor-related mechanisms in scar management: a review and hypothesis. *Plast Reconstr Surg* 2010;126(2):426.

CONTRACTURES

Contraction is a normal process of wound healing. Contracture, on the other hand, is a pathologic end stage related to the process of contraction. Generally, contractures develop when wounds heal with too much scarring and contraction of the scar tissue results in distortion of surrounding tissues. Although scar contractures can occur in any flexible tissue, such as the eyelids or lips, contractures usually occur across areas of flexion, such as the neck, axilla, or antecubital fossa. The contracted scar brings together the structures on either side of the joint space and prevents active or even passive extension. Exceptions to this pattern of flexion contractures are extension contractures of the toes and metacarpophalangeal (MP) joints of the digits. Contraction is thought to occur via smooth muscle contractile elements in myofibroblasts, but the mechanism is not well understood. In one vertical abdominal scar, there may be an area of normal scar formation and an area of hypertrophic scar formation with visible contracture. Contracture can occur in response to the presence of foreign material such as Silastic or saline breast implants. Overall, there is a 10% incidence of some form of breast capsular contracture. Myofibroblasts are thought to play an important role, but the actual cause is not known.

Recent studies have shown that subacute infections with bacteria such as Staphylococcus epidermidis create a biofilm and are likely causes of implant contracture and implant complications.

The best treatment of contractures is prevention. Incisions should not be made at right angles to flexion creases or should be reoriented by Z-plasties. Wounds in areas of flexion can be covered with flaps or grafted early with thick split-thickness or full-thickness grafts to stop the process of contraction. Such wounds should also be splinted in a position of extension during healing and for 2-3 weeks after healing is complete. Vigorous physical therapy may also be helpful.

Once a contracture is established, stretching and massage are rarely beneficial. Narrow bands of contracture may be excised and released with one or more Z-plasties. Larger areas must be incised from the medial to the lateral axis across the flexion surface and completely opened up to full extension. The resulting defect can be extensive and must be resurfaced with a skin flap or skin graft. In recurrent contractures a fasciocutaneous flap is the treatment of choice. If a skin graft is used, the area must be splinted in extension for approximately 2 weeks after the graft has healed. Less aggressive surgery is likely to result in recurrence.

Marques M, Brown S, Correia-Sá I, et al: The impact of triamcinolone acetonide in early breast capsule formation in a rabbit model. *Aesthetic Plast Surg* 2012;36(4):986.

Namnoum JD, Moyer IIR: The role of acellular dermal matrix in the treatment of capsular contracture. *Clin Plast Surg* 2012;39(2):127.

Pan Y, Liang Z, Yuan S, et al: A long-term follow-up study of acellular derm matrix with thin autograft in burn patients. *Ann Plast Surg* 2011;67(4):346.

SKIN TUMORS

Tumors of the skin are by far the most common of all tumors in humans. They arise from each of the histologic structures that make up the skin—epidermis, connective tissue, gland, muscle, and nerve elements—and are correspondingly numerous in variety. Skin tumors are classified as benign, premalignant, and malignant.

BENIGN SKIN TUMORS

The many benign tumors that arise from the skin rarely interfere with function. Since most are removed for aesthetic reasons or to rule out malignancy, they are quite commonly treated by the plastic surgeon. The majority are small and can be simply excised under local anesthesia following the principles of elliptical excision and wound closure discussed above. General anesthesia may be necessary for larger lesions requiring excision and repair by skin grafts or flaps or those occurring in young children.

When the diagnosis is not in doubt, most superficial lesions (seborrheic keratoses, verrucae, squamous cell papillomas) can be treated by simple techniques such as electrodesiccation, curettage and electrodesiccation, cryotherapy, and topical cytotoxic agents.

► Seborrheic Keratosis

Seborrheic keratoses are superficial noninvasive tumors that originate in the epidermis. They appear in older people as multiple slightly elevated yellowish, brown, or brownish-black irregularly rounded plaques with waxy or oily surfaces. They are most commonly found on the trunk and shoulders but are frequently seen on the scalp and face.

Because the lesion is raised above the epidermis, treatment usually consists of shave excision. Care should be exercised to avoid shaving a melanoma because if that is done, it will interfere with the determination of the depth of invasion by the Breslow or Clark classifications. If there is any question about a pigmented lesion, it is preferable to do an excisional biopsy rather than to shave it.

► Verrucae

Verrucae (common warts) are usually seen in children and young adults, commonly on the fingers and hands. They appear as round or oval elevated lesions with rough surfaces composed of multiple rounded or filiform keratinized projections. They may be skin colored or gray to brown.

Verrucae are caused by a virus and are autoinoculable, which can result in multiple lesions around the original growth or frequent recurrences following treatment if the virus is not completely eradicated. They may disappear spontaneously.

Treatment by electrodesiccation is effective but is frequently followed by slow healing. Repeated applications of bichloroacetic acid, liquid nitrogen, or liquid CO_2 are also effective. Surgical excision alone is not recommended, because the wound may become inoculated with the virus, leading to recurrences in and around the scar. However, surgical excision in conjunction with electrodesiccation, can be an effective form of treatment.

Recurrence remains a common problem; therefore, it is reasonable to delay treatment of asymptomatic lesions for several months to determine if they will disappear spontaneously.

Lee EH, Nehai KS, Disa JJ: Benign and premalignant lesions CME. *Plast Reconstr Surg* 2010;125(5):188e.

▶ Cysts

A. Epidermal Inclusion Cyst

Although sebaceous cyst is the commonly used term, these lesions more properly should be called epidermal inclusion cysts because they are composed of thin layers of epidermal cells filled with epithelial debris. True cysts arising from sebaceous epithelial cells are uncommon.

Epidermal inclusion cysts are soft to firm, usually elevated, and are filled with an odorous cheesy material. Their most common sites of occurrence are the scalp, face, ears, neck, and back. They are usually covered by normal skin, which may show dimpling at the site of skin attachment. They frequently present as infected cysts.

Treatment consists of surgical excision.

B. Dermoid Cyst

Dermoid cysts are deeper than epidermal cysts. They are not attached to the skin but frequently are attached to or extend through underlying bony structures. They may appear in many sites but are most common around the nose or the orbit, where they may extend to meningeal structures, necessitating CT scans to determine their extent.

Treatment is by surgical excision, which may necessitate sectioning of adjacent bony structures.

▶ Pigmented Nevi

Nevocellular nevi are groups of cells of probable neural crest origin that contain melanocytes that form melanin more rapidly upon stimulation than surrounding tissue. These cells migrate to different parts of the skin to give different types of nevi. They may also be distinguished by their clinical presentation.

A. Junctional Nevi

Junctional nevi are well-defined pigmented lesions appearing in infancy. They are usually flat or slightly elevated and light brown to dark brown. They may appear on any part of the body, but most nevi seen on the palms, soles, and genitalia are of the junctional type. Histologically, a proliferation of melanocytes is present in the epidermis at the epidermaldermal junction. It was formerly thought that these nevi give rise to malignant melanoma and that all junctional nevi should be excised for prophylactic reasons. However, most investigators now feel that the risk is very slight. If there is no change in their appearance, treatment is unnecessary. Any change such as itching, inflammation, darkening in color, halo formation, increase in size, bleeding, or ulceration calls for immediate treatment.

Surgical excision is the only safe method of treatment.

B. Intradermal Nevi

Intradermal nevi are the typical dome shaped, sometimes pedunculated, fleshy to brownish pigmented moles that are characteristically seen in adults. They frequently contain hairs and may occur anywhere on the body.

Microscopically, melanocytes are present entirely within the dermis and, in contrast to junctional nevi, show little activity. They are rarely malignant and require no treatment except for aesthetic reasons.

Surgical excision is nearly always the treatment of choice. Pigmented nevi should never be treated without obtaining tissue for histologic examination.

C. Compound Nevi

Compound nevi exhibit the histologic features of both junctional and intradermal nevi in that melanocytes lie both at the epidermal-dermal junction and within the dermis. They are usually elevated, dome shaped, and light-brown to darkbrown in color.

Because of the presence of nevus cells at the epidermaldermal junction, the indications for treatment are the same as for junctional nevi. If treatment is indicated, surgical excision is the method of choice.

D. Spindle Cell-Epithelioma Cell Nevi

These nevi, formerly called benign juvenile melanomas, appear in children or adults. They vary markedly in vascularity, degree of pigmentation, and accompanying hyperkeratosis. Clinically, they simulate warts or hemangiomas rather than moles. They may increase in size rapidly, but the average lesion reaches only 6-8 mm in diameter, remaining entirely benign without invasion or metastases. Microscopically, the lesion can be confused with malignant melanoma by the inexperienced pathologist. The usual treatment is excisional biopsy.

E. Blue Nevi

Blue nevi are small, sharply defined, round, dark blue or grayish-blue lesions that may occur anywhere on the body but are most commonly seen on the face, neck, hands, and arms. They usually appear in childhood as slowly growing, well-defined nodules covered by a smooth, intact epidermis. Microscopically, the melanocytes that make up this lesion are limited to (but may be found in all layers of) the dermis. An intimate association with the fibroblasts of the dermis is seen, giving the lesion a fibrotic appearance not seen in other nevi. This, together with extension of melanocytes deep into the dermis, may account for the blue rather than brown color.

Treatment is not mandatory unless the patient desires removal for aesthetic reasons or fear of cancer. Surgical excision is the treatment of choice.

F. Giant Hairy Nevi

Unlike most nevi arising from melanocytes, giant hairy nevi are congenital. They may occur anywhere on the body and may cover large areas. They may be large enough to cover the entire trunk (bathing trunk nevi). They are of special significance for several reasons: (1) Their large size is especially deforming from an aesthetic standpoint; (2) they show a predisposition for developing malignant melanoma; and (3) they may be associated with neurofibromas or melanocytic involvement of the leptomeninges and other neurologic abnormalities.

Microscopically, a varied picture is present. All of the characteristics of intradermal and compound nevi may be seen. Neurofibromas may also be present within the lesion. Malignant melanoma may arise anywhere within the large lesion; the reported rate of occurrence ranges from 1% to as high as 13.7% in one study. Malignant melanoma with metastases rarely arises in childhood or infancy.

The only full treatment is complete excision and skin grafting. Large lesions may require excision and grafting in stages. Some lesions are so large that excision is not possible and the most effective approach is using tissue expansion in combination with flaps. Split-thickness excision or dermabrasion has been successful when done in infancy.

The use of cultured epithelial autografts has been advocated for extensive lesions associated with multiple satellite nevi. Additionally, some have reported the use of laser photothermolysis of pigmented lesions that cannot be excised with favorable reconstructive outcomes. However, there is still concern over malignant transformation of remaining melanocytes, and close long-term follow-up is recommended when laser ablation is used.

Kryger Z, Bauer B: Surgical management of large and giant congenital pigmented nevi of the lower extremity. *Plast Reconstr Surg* 2008;121(5):1674.

▶ Vascular Tumors & Vascular Malformations

Our understanding of vascular tumors and vascular malformations has evolved a great deal since the description by Mulliken and Glowacki in 1982 of the biologic classification of vascular anomalies based on their endothelial properties. In this way, infant hemangiomas appear within the first 3 weeks of life and have a proliferative endothelium that grows rapidly at first and commonly involutes usually in the first few years of life. Vascular malformations, on the other hand, have stable endothelium, grow proportionally with the child, and persist into adulthood. They can be associated with various complications, such as skeletal abnormalities, ischemia, coagulopathy, heart failure, and death.

Glucose transporter isoform 1 (GLUT1) has recently been discovered to be a distinguishing feature among various forms of vascular anomalies. It is an immunohistochemical marker that is normally restricted to endothelial cells with blood-tissue barrier function as in the brain and placenta. North and colleagues retrospectively studied specimens from vascular tumors for GLUT1. Specimens from infantile hemangiomas were universally positive. In contrast, biopsies of other vascular anomalies, including rapidly involuting congenital hemangioma (RICH), noninvoluting congenital hemangioma (NICH), pyogenic granuloma, granulation tissue, vascular malformations, and tufted angioma and kaposiform hemangioendothelioma, were all negative. In addition to providing an early diagnostic assay for hemangiomas, GLUT1 can be useful in research and in trying to explain the pathophysiology.

The International Society for the Study of Vascular Anomalies proposed a classification in 1996 based on the pioneering work of Mulliken and Glowacki. It is now the most widely accepted among specialists and in the literature. Clear classification is vitally important so that proper communication regarding diagnosis and treatment can be established. Table 41–3 shows that classification.

Table 41–3. International Society for the Study of Vascular Anomalies Classification.

Tumors
Juvenile hemangioma
Rapidly involuting congenital hemangioma (RICH)
Noninvoluting congenital hemangioma (NICH)
Kaposiform hemangioendothelioma
Tufted angioma
Vascular malformations
High-flow
Arteriovenous malformation
Low-flow
Venous malformation
Lymphatic malformation
Lymphatic-venous malformation
Capillary (or venular) malformation (port wine stain)

A. Hemangiomas of Infancy (Involuting Hemangioma)

Involuting hemangiomas are the most common tumors that occur in childhood and constitute at least 95% of all the hemangiomas that are seen in infancy and childhood. They are true neoplasms of endothelial cells but are unique among neoplasms in that they undergo complete, spontaneous involution.

Typically, they are present shortly after birth or appear during the first 2-3 weeks of life. They grow at a rather rapid rate for 4-6 months; then growth ceases and spontaneous involution begins. Involution progresses slowly but approximately 50% are involuted by 5 years of age and 70% by age 7. Involuting hemangiomas appear on all body surfaces but are seen more often on the head and neck. They are seen twice as often in girls as in boys and show a predisposition for fair-skinned individuals.

Three forms of infantile hemangiomas are seen: (1) superficial, (2) combined superficial and deep (mixed), and (3) deep. Superficial involuting hemangiomas appear as sharply demarcated, bright-red, slightly raised lesions with an irregular surface that has been described as resembling a strawberry. Combined superficial and deep involuting hemangiomas have the same surface characteristics, but beneath the skin surface, a firm bluish tumor is present that may extend deeply into the subcutaneous tissues. Deep involuting hemangiomas present as deep blue tumors covered by normal-appearing skin.

Hemangiomas are the result of angiogenic dysfunction. Multiple markers of angiogenesis are increased during the proliferative flow, including fibroblast growth factor, vascular endothelial growth factor, and matrix metalloproteinases. These all decrease with the exception of basic fibroblast growth factor during the involution phase.

As the phase of involution progresses, the histologic picture changes, with the solid fields of endothelial cells breaking up into closely packed, capillary-sized, vessel-like structures composed of several layers of soft endothelial cells supported by a sparse fibrous stroma. These vascular structures gradually become fewer and spaced more widely apart in a loose, edematous fibrous stroma. The endothelial cells continue to disappear, so that by the time involution is complete the histologic picture is entirely normal, with no trace of endothelial cells.

Treatment is not usually indicated, since the appearance following spontaneous regression is nearly always superior to the scars that follow surgical excision. Surgical excision of lesions that involve important structures such as the eyelids, nose, or lips may sometimes be necessary in order to avoid serious functional disturbances of vision and airway. Complete excision is usually not necessary.

When treatment is indicated, multiple options have been described including cryotherapy, corticosteroids, interferon and chemotherapy. More recently, the use of the beta blocker propranolol has shown to halt hemangioma progression and dramatically shorten the involution time. Usual doses are from 2-3 mg/kg/day, and infants are usually admitted for 24 hours upon starting this therapy for cardiac monitoring. Although the actual mechanism of action remains unknown, it most likely has to do with downregulation of angiogenic growth factors. It has shown such good results that some institutions are using this as a first-line treatment for complicated infantile hemangiomas.

Ulceration is a painful and dangerous complication with hemangiomas that can develop in approximately 8% of patients. This may be accompanied by infection, which is treated by the use of compresses of warm saline or potassium permanganate and by the application of antimicrobial powders and creams. Bleeding from the ulcer can occur if there is constant irritation and inflammation. When it occurs, gentle pressure should be applied. In some situations, such as the perianal region, specific measures may be needed to keep the area clean and dry including a diverting colostomy combined with judicious serial excision. In rare cases, the platelet trapping of these lesions leads to the clinical picture of disseminated intravascular coagulopathy called **Kasabach-Merritt syndrome.**

Arneja J: Pharmacologic therapies for infantile hemangioma: is there a rational basis? *Plast Reconstr Surg* 2012;129(4):724e.

Price CJ, Lattouf C, Baum B, et al: Propranolol vs corticosteroids for infantile hemangiomas: a multicenter retrospective analysis. *Arch Dermatol* 2011;147(12):1371.

Thayal P, Bhandari P: Comparison of efficacy of intralesional bleomycin and oral propanolol in management of hemangiomas. *Plast Reconstr Surg* 2012;129(4):733e.

B. Congenital Hemangiomas (RICH and NICH)

Congenital hemangiomas, as their name implies, are present at birth. They have undergone their rapid growth phase *in utero*, and in contrast to hemangiomas of infancy, they do not undergo rapid growth during the first 4-6 months of life. Because of their natural history they are divided into two subtypes: RICH and NICH. RICH are more common than NICH, although both are rare. The diagnosis of RICH is confirmed when they rapidly involute by 6-10 months of age. The NICH anomalies, on the other hand, persist into adulthood and may require surgical excision or other ablative measures. Imaging may be helpful (sonography or MRI) in order to evaluate location and extent of the tumor. Both RICH and NICH are GLUT1 negative in contrast to hemangiomas of infancy.

C. Capillary Malformations

Capillary malformations (ie, **port-wine stains**) are by far the most common of the vascular malformations. They may involve any portion of the body but most commonly appear on the face as flat patchy lesions that are reddish to purple in color. When present on the face, they are located in areas supplied by the sensory branches of the fifth (trigeminal) cranial nerve. They usually start off light red in color yet have a propensity to deepen in color, as their name implies. Their growth is variable, but they persist into adulthood if not treated and become raised and thickened with nodules appearing on the surface (Figure 41–10).

Microscopically, port-wine stains are made up of thin-walled capillaries that are arranged throughout the dermis. The capillaries are lined with mature, flat endothelial cells. In the lesions that produce surface growth, groups of round proliferating endothelial cells and large venous sinuses are seen.

Results following treatment of the port-wine stain were uniformly disappointing. Because most lesions occur on the face or neck, patients seek treatment for aesthetic reasons, but as they progress in thickness and nodularity, they can become functionally disabling and can bleed spontaneously. The simplest method of treatment is camouflaging. Unfortunately, this is difficult because the port-wine stain is darker than the surrounding lighter skin, and it does not affect the natural history of the lesion.

Superficial methods of treatment such as dry ice, liquid nitrogen, electrocoagulation, and dermabrasion have been tried but are ineffective unless they destroy the upper layers of the skin, which can produce severe scarring.

Radiation therapy, including the use of x-rays, radium, thorium X, and grenz x-rays, is to be condemned. If it is administered in doses high enough to destroy the vessels involved, it also destroys the surrounding tissues and the overlying skin, and the cancer incidence after radiotherapy for skin hemangioma increases.

The best treatment to date for early and intermediate port-wine stains is with the pulsed dye laser. The pulsed dye laser produces a light with a specific wavelength of 585 or 595 nanometers. The method of treatment is termed selective photothermolysis. The beam is selectively absorbed by red-pigmented material such as hemoglobin in the blood vessels of the lesion. This produces selective heat destruction of these structures, and the treated area becomes whiter. When started early, these treatments can be very effective. Multiple treatments are necessary to obtain a satisfactory result. In darker and more advanced nodular lesions, the laser is less effective because of the thickness of the lesion and the hyperpigmentation that may develop.

If the lesion is small, surgical excision with primary closure is possible. Unfortunately, most lesions are large. In the case of long-standing untreated lesions, surgical excision may be necessary, followed by skin grafting, locoregional flaps, or at times free tissue transfer. Certain fast-growing capillary or primarily arterialized hemangiomas have been managed successfully with superselective embolization, either alone or in conjunction with surgery. This is performed under fluoroscopic control and with an expert team. There have been reports of slough of large portions of the face as a result of misdirected embolizations.

D. Venous Malformations

Venous malformations (otherwise known as cavernous hemangiomas) are bluish or purplish lesions that are usually elevated. They may occur anywhere on the body but, like other vascular lesions, are more common on the head and neck. They are composed of mature, fully formed venous structures that are present in tortuous masses that have been described as feeling like a bag of worms.

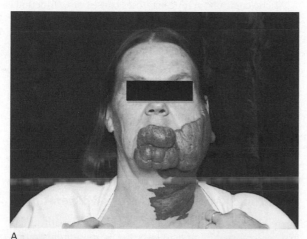

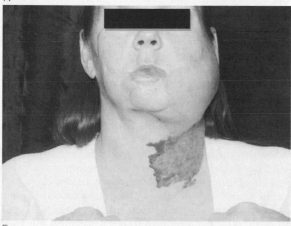

▲ **Figure 41–10.** 46-year-old white female with untreated port-wine stain of left face. **A.** Preoperative. **B.** Status postexcision of facial portion and reconstruction with free tissue transfer.

Venous malformations are usually present at birth but do not usually grow except to keep pace with normal body growth. In many cases, growth occurs later in life and may interfere with normal function.

Microscopically, venous malformations are made up of large, dilated, closely packed vascular sinuses that are engorged with blood. They are lined by flat endothelial cells and may have muscular walls like normal veins.

Treatment is difficult. In only a few cases is the lesion small enough or superficial enough to permit complete surgical excision. Most lesions involve deeper structures—including muscle and bone—so that complete excision is impossible without radical surgery. Since most lesions are no more than aesthetic problems, radical surgery is rarely indicated. Occasionally, the injection of sclerosing agents directly into the venous channels may lead to some involution or may make surgical excision easier. Great care must be used so that areas of overlying skin do not slough.

E. Arteriovenous Malformations

Arteriovenous malformations are high-flow lesions having a direct connection between an artery and a vein, bypassing the capillary bed.

Arteriovenous malformations are typically recognized at birth but are misdiagnosed as capillary malformations or involuting hemangiomas. Periods of rapid growth are found after trauma and during periods when the body is under the influence of hormonal changes.

Clinical diagnosis can be confirmed with color Doppler examination, but this does not give information concerning extent of the lesion or relation to surrounding structures. This information can be obtained via MRI or angiography, which has the additional benefit of therapeutic embolization.

Treatment for arteriovenous malformations is based on clinical stage of the lesion. Smaller arteriovenous malformations can be primarily resected. Larger, more diffuse arteriovenous malformations are best managed with superselective arterial embolization followed by surgical resection 24-48 hours after embolization in order to minimize intraoperative blood loss.

Chim H, Drolet B, Duffy K, Koshima I, Gosain AK: Vascular anomalies and lymphedema. *Plast Reconstr Surg* 2010;126(2):55e.

Faurschou A, Olesen AB, Leonardi-Bee J, Haedersdal M: Lasers or light sources for treating port-wine stains. *Cochrane Database Syst Rev* 2011 Nov;9(11):CD007152.

Redondo P, Aguado L, Martínez-Cuesta A: Diagnosis and management of extensive vascular malformations of the lower limb: part 1. Clinical diagnosis. *J Am Acad Dermatol* 2011;65(5):893.

Redondo P, Aguado L, Martínez-Cuesta A: Diagnosis and management of extensive vascular malformations of the lower limb: part 2. Systemic repercussions [corrected], diagnosis and treatment. *J Am Acad Dermatol* 2011;65(5):909.

Tark KC, Lew DH, Lee DW: The fate of long-standing port-wine stain and its surgical management. *Plast Reconstr Surg* 2011;127(2):784.

Trindade F, Tellechea O, Torrelo A, Requena L, Colmenero I: Wilms tumor 1 expression in vascular neoplasms and vascular malformations. *Am J Dermatopathol* 2011;33(6):569.

PREMALIGNANT SKIN LESIONS

▶ Actinic (Solar) Keratoses

Actinic keratoses are the most common of the precancerous skin lesions. They usually appear as small, single or multiple, slightly elevated, scaly or warty lesions ranging in color from red to yellow, brown, or black. Because they are related to sun exposure, they occur most frequently on the face and the backs of the hands in fair-skinned Caucasians whose skin shows evidence of actinic elastosis.

Microscopically, actinic keratoses consist of well-defined areas of abnormal epithelial cells limited to the epidermis. Approximately 15%-20% of these lesions become malignant, in which case invasion of the dermis as squamous cell carcinoma occurs.

Since the lesions are limited to the epidermis, superficial treatment in the form of curette and electrodesiccation or the application of chemical agents such as liquid nitrogen, phenol, bi- or trichloroacetic acid, or fluorouracil is curative. The application of fluorouracil (5-FU) cream is of particular benefit in preventive treatment in that it destroys lesions of microscopic size—before they can be detected clinically—without causing damage to uninvolved skin.

▶ Chronic Radiation Dermatitis & Ulceration

There are two distinct types of radiation dermatitis. The first and most common follows the acute administration of relatively high dosages of ionizing orthovoltage radiation over relatively short periods—almost always for the treatment of cancer. Dermatitis is characterized by an acute reaction that begins near the third week of therapy, when erythema, blistering, and sloughing of the epidermis start to occur. Burning and hyperesthesia are commonly present. This initial reaction is followed by scarring characterized by atrophy of the epidermis and dermis along with loss of skin appendages (sweat glands, sebaceous glands, and hair follicles). Marked fibrosis of the dermis occurs, with gradual endarteritis and occlusion of the dermal and subdermal vessels. Telangiectasia of the surface vessels is seen, and areas of both hypopigmentation and hyperpigmentation occur.

The second type of radiation dermatitis follows chronic exposure to low doses of ionizing radiation over prolonged periods. It is usually seen in professional personnel who handle radioactive materials or administer x-rays or in patients who have been treated for dermatologic conditions such as acne or excessive facial hair. Therefore, the face and hands are most commonly involved. The acute reaction described above does not usually occur, but the same process of atrophy, scarring, and loss of dermal elements occurs. Drying of the skin becomes more pronounced, and deepening of the skin furrows is typically present. Fortunately, this second type of radiation dermatitis is rarely seen today.

In both types of radiation dermatitis, late changes such as the following may occur: (1) the appearance of hyperkeratotic growths on the skin surface, (2) chronic ulceration, and (3) the development of either basal cell or squamous cell carcinoma. Ulceration and cancer, however, are seen much less commonly in the first type of radiation dermatitis than in the second. When malignant growths appear, basal cell carcinomas are seen more frequently on the face and neck and squamous cell carcinomas more frequently on the hands and body.

Newer radiotherapeutic methods using megavoltage and electron beam techniques have a sparing effect on the skin. However, marked scarring and avascularity of deeper, more extensive areas may present more difficult problems.

Surgical excision is the treatment of choice. Excision should include all of the irradiated tissue including the area of telangiectasia, whenever possible, and the defect should be covered with an appropriate axial or musculocutaneous flap to provide a new blood supply.

Primary wound closure is feasible for only the smallest lesions, and even so, at some risk. Free-skin grafting is usually unsuccessful because of the damage to the vascular supply of the subcutaneous structures. Adjacent random flaps are unreliable because they depend on blood supply from the surrounding irradiated area.

MALIGNANT LESIONS

1. Intraepidermal Carcinoma

Intraepidermal carcinoma includes Bowen disease and erythroplasia of Queyrat.

▶ Bowen Disease

Bowen disease is characterized by single or multiple, brownish or reddish plaques that may appear anywhere on the skin surface but often on covered surfaces. The typical plaque is sharply defined, slightly raised, scaly, and slightly thickened. The surface is often keratotic, and crusting and fissuring may be present. Ulceration is not common but when present suggests malignant degeneration with dermal invasion.

Histologically, hyperplasia of the epidermis is seen, with pleomorphic malpighian cells, giant cells, and atypical epithelial cells that are limited to the epidermis.

Treatment of small or superficial lesions consists of total destruction by curette and electrodesiccation or by any of the other superficially destructive methods (cryotherapy, cytotoxic agents). Excision and skin grafting are preferred for larger lesions and for those that have undergone early malignant degeneration and invasion of the dermis.

▶ Erythroplasia of Queyrat

Erythroplasia of Queyrat is almost identical to Bowen disease both clinically and histologically but is confined to the glans penis and the vulva, where the lesions appear as red, velvety, irregular, slightly raised plaques. Treatment is as described for Bowen disease.

2. Basal Cell Carcinoma

Basal cell carcinoma is the most common skin cancer. The lesions usually appear on the face and are more common in men than in women. Since exposure to ultraviolet rays of the sun is a causative factor, basal cell carcinoma is most commonly seen in geographic areas where there is significant sun exposure and in people whose skin is most susceptible to actinic damage from exposure (ie, fair-skinned individuals with blue eyes and blond hair). It may occur at any age but is not common before age 40.

The growth rate of basal cell carcinoma is usually slow but nearly always steady and insidious. Several months or years may pass before the patient becomes concerned. Without treatment, widespread invasion and destruction of adjacent tissues may occur, producing massive ulceration. Penetration of the bones of the facial skeleton and the skull may occur late in the course. Basal cell carcinomas rarely metastasize, but death can occur because of direct intracranial extension or erosion of major blood vessels.

Typical individual lesions appear as small, translucent or shiny ("pearly") elevated nodules with central ulceration and rolled, pearly edges. Telangiectatic vessels are commonly present over the surface, and pigmentation is sometimes present. Superficial ulceration occurs early.

A less common type of basal cell carcinoma is the **sclerosing** or **morphea carcinoma,** consisting of elongated strands of basal cell cancer that infiltrate the dermis, with the intervening corium being unusually compact. These lesions are usually flat and whitish or waxy in appearance and firm to palpation—similar in appearance to localized scleroderma. They are particularly difficult to treat because it is difficult to clinically predict the extent of the margins of growth.

The superficial **erythematous basal cell cancer** ("body basal") occurs most frequently on the trunk. It appears as reddish plaques with atrophic centers and smooth, slightly raised borders. These lesions are capable of peripheral growth and wide extension but do not become invasive until late.

Pigmented basal cell carcinomas may be mistaken for melanomas because of the large number of melanocytes present within the tumor. They may also be confused with seborrheic keratoses.

▶ Treatment

There are several methods of treating basal cell carcinoma. All may be curative in some lesions, but no one method is applicable to all. The special features of each basal cell cancer must be considered individually before proper treatment can be selected.

Because most lesions occur on the face, aesthetic and functional results of treatment are important. However, the most important consideration is whether or not therapy is curative. If the basal cell carcinoma is not eradicated by the initial treatment, continued growth and invasion of adjacent tissues will occur, resulting not only in additional tissue destruction but also in invasion of the tumor into deeper structures, making cure more difficult. Adequate treatment of basal cell carcinoma by different modalities achieves a cure rate of approximately 95%.

The principal methods of treatment are curettage and electrodesiccation, surgical excision, and radiation therapy. Chemosurgery, topical chemotherapy, and cryosurgery are not often used but may have value in selected cases.

A. Curettage and Electrodesiccation

Curettage plus electrodesiccation is the usual method of treatment for small lesions. After infiltration with suitable local anesthetic, the lesion and a 2-3 mm margin of normal-appearing skin around it are thoroughly curetted with a small skin curette. The resultant wound is then completely desiccated with an electrosurgical unit to destroy any tumor cells that may not have been removed by the curette. The process is then repeated once or twice if necessary. The wound is left open and allowed to heal secondarily.

B. Surgical Excision

Surgical excision, following the principles outlined earlier in this chapter, offers many advantages in the treatment of basal cell carcinoma: (1) Most lesions can be quickly excised in one procedure. (2) Following excision, the entire lesion can be examined by the pathologist, who can determine if the tumor has been completely removed. (3) Deep infiltrative lesions can be completely excised, and cartilage and bone can be removed if they have been invaded. (4) Lesions that occur in dense scar tissue or in other poorly vascularized tissues cannot be treated by curettage and desiccation, radiation therapy, or chemosurgery, since healing is poor. Excision and flap coverage may be the only method for treatment in these conditions. (5) Recurrent lesions in tissues that have been exposed to maximum safe amounts of radiation can be excised and covered.

Small- to moderate-sized lesions can be excised in one stage under local anesthesia. The visible and palpable margins of the tumor are marked on the skin with marking ink. The width of excision is then marked 3-5 mm beyond these margins. If the margins of the basal cell carcinoma are vague, the width of excision will have to be wider to ensure complete removal of the lesion. The lines of incision are drawn around the lesion as a circle. This tissue is excised, taking care to leave a margin of normal-appearing subcutaneous tissue around the deep margins of the tumor. Frozen sections may be obtained at the time of excision to aid in determining whether tumor-free margins have been obtained. This is minimized with experience. It is better to err on the side of removing more normal tissue than necessary rather than to risk including tumor at the margins. Closure of the wound is accomplished in the direction of minimal skin tension, usually along the skin lines. The dog-ears are removed appropriately.

Wounds resulting from the excision of some moderate-sized tumors and nearly all large tumors may require reconstruction of function and appearance with the use of local, regional, and free flaps. This can nearly always be performed in one stage with good frozen section control.

The disadvantages of surgical excision are as follows: (1) Certain large excisions and reconstruction require specialized training and experience to master the surgical techniques. (2) Whereas curettage and desiccation may be performed in the office, surgical excision often requires specialized facilities. (3) In lesions with vague clinical margins, an excessive amount of normal tissue may have to be excised to ensure complete removal even with the use of frozen section verification. (4) Reconstruction may need to wait until permanent pathologic diagnosis and margins are available in cases involving deep or specialized structures.

To overcome some of these objections, Mohs described a new technique in 1941 that allows for serial excisions and microscopic examination of chemically fixed tissue. Newer developments have obviated the cumbersome fixation techniques, but it may still take several hours to scan an area for suspected malignant cells. The procedure is nevertheless quite useful for recurrent lesions and in areas in which maximal preservation is desirable. Nonetheless, there are no prospective comparative studies to indicate that the microscopically controlled removal of tumor by the Mohs technique, which amounts to excision of the lesion with serial review by fresh frozen section, is superior to surgical excision. An additional problem is that there is no quality control because the excising physician is also the one who evaluates the pathology slides. Many of the more extensive lesions treated with the Mohs technique require complex reconstruction to rebuild noble structures that have needed resection.

Netscher DT, Leong M, Orengo I, et al: Cutaneous malignancies: melanoma and nonmelanoma types. *Plast Reconstr Surg* 2011;127(3):37e.

Wheiss GJ, Korn RL: Metastatic basal cell carcinoma in the era of hedgehog signaling pathway inhibitors. *Cancer* 2012 Nov 1;118(21):5310-9.

C. X-ray Therapy

X-ray therapy is as effective as any other in the treatment of basal cell carcinoma. Its advantages are as follows: (1)

Structures that are difficult to reconstruct, such as the eyelids, tear ducts, and nasal tip, can be preserved when they are invaded by but not destroyed by tumor. (2) A wide margin of tissue can be treated around lesions with poorly defined margins to ensure destruction of nondiscernible extensions of tumor. (3) It may be less traumatic than surgical excision to elderly patients with advanced lesions. (4) Hospitalization is not necessary.

The disadvantages are as follows: (1) Only well-trained, experienced physicians can obtain good results. (2) Expensive facilities are necessary. (3) Improperly administered radiation therapy may produce severe sequelae, including scarring, radiation dermatitis, ulceration, and malignant degeneration. (4) In hair-bearing areas, epilation will result. (5) It may be difficult to treat areas of irregular contour (eg, the ear and the auditory canal). (6) Repeated treatments over a period of 4-6 weeks may be necessary.

X-ray therapy should not be used in patients under age 40 except in unusual circumstances, and it should not be repeated in patients who have failed to respond to radiation therapy in the past.

3. Squamous Cell Carcinoma

Squamous cell carcinoma is the second-most common cancer of the skin in light-skinned racial groups and the most common skin cancer in darkly pigmented racial groups. As with basal cell carcinoma, sunlight is the most common causative factor in whites. The most common sites of occurrence are the ears, cheeks, lower lip, and backs of the hands. Other causative factors are chemical and thermal burns, scars, chronic ulcers, chronic granulomas (tuberculosis of the skin, syphilis), draining sinuses, contact with tars and hydrocarbons, and exposure to ionizing radiation. When a squamous cell carcinoma occurs in a burn scar, it is called a **Marjolin ulcer**. This lesion may appear many years after the original burn. It tends to be aggressive, and the prognosis is poor.

Because exposure to the sun is the greatest stimulus for the production of squamous cell carcinoma, most of these lesions are preceded by actinic keratosis on areas of the skin showing chronic solar damage. They may also arise from other premalignant skin lesions and from normal-appearing skin.

The natural history of squamous cell carcinoma may be quite variable. It may present as a slowly growing, locally invasive lesion without metastases or as a rapidly growing, widely invasive tumor with early metastatic spread. In general, squamous cell carcinomas that develop from actinic keratoses are more common and are of the slowly growing type, whereas those that develop from Bowen disease, erythroplasia of Queyrat, chronic radiation dermatitis, scars, and chronic ulcers tend to be more aggressive. Lesions that arise from normal-appearing skin and from the lips, genitalia, and anal regions also tend to be aggressive.

Early squamous cell carcinoma usually appears as a small, firm erythematous plaque or nodule with indistinct margins. The surface may be flat and smooth or may be verrucous. As the tumor grows, it becomes raised and, because of progressive invasion, becomes fixed to surrounding tissues. Ulceration may occur early or late but tends to appear earlier in the more rapidly growing lesions.

Histologically, malignant epithelial cells are seen extending down into the dermis as broad, rounded masses or slender strands. In squamous cell carcinomas of low-grade malignancy, the individual cells may be quite well differentiated, resembling uniform mature squamous cells having intercellular bridges. Keratinization may be present, and layers of keratinizing squamous cells may produce typical round "horn pearls." In highly malignant lesions, the epithelial cells may be extremely atypical; abnormal mitotic figures are common; intercellular bridges are not present; and keratinization does not occur.

▶ Treatment

As with basal cell carcinomas, the method of treatment that will eradicate squamous cell carcinomas and produce the best aesthetic and functional results varies with the characteristics of the individual lesion. Factors that determine the optimal method of treatment include the size, shape, and location of the tumor as well as the histologic pattern that determines its aggressiveness.

The mainstay of treatment is surgery. Radiation has also been used in some circumstances. Since basal cell carcinomas are relatively nonaggressive lesions that rarely metastasize, failure to eradicate the lesion may result only in local recurrence. Although this may result in extensive local tissue destruction, there is rarely a threat to life. Aggressive squamous cell carcinomas, on the other hand, may metastasize to any part of the body, and failure of treatment may have fatal consequences. For this reason, total eradication of each lesion is the imperative goal of treatment.

The use of sentinel lymph node biopsy (SLNB) is usually reserved for those patients with a high risk squamous cell cancer or when the lesion is larger than 2 cm. This procedure maps the first node basin that any disease would travel to if metastatic. Palpable nodes of any type are a contraindication for SLNB.

Gurney BA, Schilling C, Putvha V, et al: Implications of a positive sentinel node in oral squamous cell carcinoma. *Head Neck* 2012 Nov;34(11):1580-1585.

Netscher DT, Leong M, Orengo I, et al: Cutaneous malignancies: melanoma and nonmelanoma types. *Plast Reconstr Surg* 2011;127(3):37e.

Samarasinghe V, Madan V: Nonmelanoma skin cancer. *J Cutan Aesthet Surg* 2012;5(1):3.

SOFT TISSUE INJURY

The plastic surgeon is often involved in emergency room assessment and treatment of soft tissue injuries. Many aspects of wound management must be considered in even a relatively simple facial laceration.

Careful analysis of the soft tissue injury should include (1) the type of wound or wounds (abrasion, contusion, etc); (2) the cause of injury; (3) the age of the injury; (4) the location of injured tissues; (5) the degree of contamination of the injured area before, during, and after trauma; (6) the nature and extent of associated injuries; and (7) the general health of the patient (eg, any chronic or acute illnesses or any allergies; any medications being taken).

The location of the wound must be noted because different healing characteristics are present in various types of skin. The face and scalp are highly vascular and therefore resist infection and heal faster than other areas, but there are many important structures in and around the face, and scars and defects are noticeable. Skin of the trunk, upper arms, and thighs is fairly thick and heals more slowly than facial or scalp skin and is more susceptible to infection. Scarring is less noticeable. The hands are a critical area because there are important structures near the surface, and the destruction caused by infection can be devastating. The lower legs are a particular problem area because the relatively poor blood supply can cause skin loss, and infection is more likely to occur.

▶ Treatment

The type of wound must be determined so that proper treatment can be given. Contusions and swelling require ice packs for 24 hours, rest, and elevation. Abrasions should be cleaned and dressed in a sterile manner as for a skin graft donor site or must be washed daily until a dry scab forms or healing takes place. Ground-in dirt or gravel must be entirely scrubbed out or picked out with a small blade within 24 hours after injury, or foreign material will be sealed in and traumatic tattooing will result. Extensive local anesthesia may be required to accomplish this. Imbedded particulate matter from an explosion must be removed in a similar manner. Hematomas may be treated with ice bags and pressure until stable. Evacuation is then indicated if vital structures such as the ear or nasal septal cartilage are in danger of being injured or destroyed. Lacerations over bony prominences and various types of cuts require special care that will be detailed below. Treatment must be meticulous if optimal results are to be achieved. Puncture wounds and bites are notoriously innocuous in appearance but may result in severe destruction or tetanus or gas gangrene. Antibiotic coverage, irrigation, open treatment, and observation are indicated. Most bites on the face, however, can be cleaned and safely closed. Wounds that create flaps of skin or avulsions are difficult to manage. Careful debridement

and judicious use of full-thickness or split-thickness grafts from the avulsed tissue are recommended. Timing is the first factor to consider.

Wound contamination can be caused by bacteria on the surface of the wounding agent, such as rust on a nail or saliva on a tooth, or bacteria that enter the wound when the skin is broken. Bacteria driven into tissue become more established as time passes, and it is therefore important to know the age of the wound at the time of the presentation for treatment. Other injuries associated with cuts almost always take precedence in treatment. In general, wounds other than those on the face or scalp should not be closed primarily if they occurred 8-12 hours or longer before presentation unless they were caused by a very clean agent and have been covered by a sterile bandage in the interim. Delayed primary closure as described previously is an excellent and safe alternative. Nearly any facial wound up to 24 hours old can be safely closed with careful debridement, irrigation, and antibiotic coverage.

The surgeon must decide whether or not antibiotic treatment is indicated. In general, wounds treated appropriately and early do not call for antibiotic therapy. Antibiotics should be given for wounds with delayed presentation or those for which treatment is delayed by choice (eg, wounds with known contamination; wounds in compromised patients, such as very young or old persons, debilitated persons, or persons with general ill health; wounds in areas where infection may have serious consequences, such as the lower legs and the hands; and wounds in persons in whom bacteremia might have serious sequelae, such as those with prosthetic heart valves or orthopedic appliances). Antibiotics should be started before debridement and closure. Only a few days of coverage are necessary—usually until the wound is checked at 2-3 days and found to be free of infection. Penicillin or a substitute is appropriate for wounds involving the mouth, such as through-and-through lip lacerations and bites. Other wounds are usually contaminated by *Staphylococcus aureus,* and an antibiotic effective for penicillin-resistant *S. aureus* is therefore appropriate. If gram-negative or anaerobic contamination is suspected, wound closure is risky, and hospitalization of the patient for treatment with parenteral antibiotics should be considered. Tetanus prophylaxis should be routinely given for patients who have not received current immunizations or who have wounds likely to lead to tetanus. Guidelines for this are detailed in Chapter 8.

Anesthesia is an important part of adequate soft tissue wound care and closure. Local anesthesia with either 0.5% or 1% lidocaine with epinephrine 1:200,000 or 1:100,000 is recommended for all wounds. Smaller amounts of lidocaine and epinephrine may be used in areas of appendages, such as earlobes, toes, and the penis. The injection may be given through the wound edge before debridement and irrigation for maximum patient comfort. Complete epinephrine vasoconstrictor effect occurs within 7 minutes. Overdose of epinephrine and lidocaine injection into vessels or use of the drugs in patients sensitive to these agents should be avoided.

The importance of irrigation cannot be overstated. Over 90% of bacteria in a recently sustained and superficially contaminated wound can be eliminated by adequate irrigation. Ideally, a physiologic solution such as lactated Ringer solution or normal saline should be forcefully ejected from a large syringe with a 19-gauge needle or from other equipment designed for this purpose such as a water-jet apparatus. The wound is irrigated once to remove surface clots, foreign material, and bacteria and is then debrided and irrigated again. Detergents and antiseptic solutions are toxic to exposed tissue and should not be used.

Debridement must include removal of all obviously devitalized tissues. In special areas such as the eyelids, ears, nose, lips, and eyebrows, debridement must be done cautiously, since the tissue lost by debridement may be difficult to replace. Where tissues are more abundant, such as in the cheek, chin, and forehead areas, debridement may be more extensive. Small irregular or ragged wounds in these areas can be excised completely to produce clean, sharply cut wound edges which, when approximated, will produce the finest possible scar. Because the blood supply in the face is plentiful, damaged tissues of questionable viability should be retained rather than debrided away. The chances for survival are good.

Following adequate anesthesia, debridement, and irrigation, the wound is ready for final assessment and closure. Lighting must be adequate, and appropriate instruments should be available. The patient and the surgeon must be positioned comfortably. The skin surrounding the wound is prepared with an antiseptic solution, and the area is draped. A final check of the depth and extent of the wound is made, and vital structures are inspected for injury. Hemostasis must be achieved by use of epinephrine, pressure, cautery, or suture ligature. Important structures in facial wounds include the parotid duct, lacrimal duct, and branches of the facial nerve. These should be repaired in the operating room by microsurgical techniques.

Layers of tissue—usually muscle—in the depth of the wound should be closed first with as few absorbable sutures as possible, since sutures are foreign material within the wound. If possible, dead space should be closed with judicious use of fine absorbable sutures. If dead space cannot be closed, external pressure or small drains are sometimes effective. Skin closure should begin at the most important points of the laceration (eg, the borders of the ears and nose; the vermilion border or margins of the lip; the margins of the eyebrow [which should never be shaved]; and the scalp hairline). Subcuticular sutures are very helpful. Skin edges can be approximated without tension or strangulation with 5-0 or 6-0 monofilament suture material as outlined earlier under wound closure.

Complicated lacerations, such as complex stellate wounds or avulsion flaps, often heal with excessive scarring. Because of the associated subcutaneous tissue injury, U-shaped or trap-door avulsion lacerations almost always become unsightly as a result of wound contracture. Small lacerations of this type are best excised and closed in a straight line initially; larger flaps that must be replaced usually require secondary revision. Extensive loss of skin is generally best treated by initial split-thickness skin grafting followed later by secondary reconstruction. Primary attempts to reconstruct with local flaps may fail because of unsuspected injury to these adjacent tissues. The decision to convert avulsed tissues to free grafts that may not survive and thus delay healing requires sound surgical judgment.

Small- or moderate-sized closures on the face may be dressed with antibiotic ointment alone. The patient may cleanse the suture lines with hydrogen peroxide to clear away crusts and dirt and then reapply the ointment. Elsewhere, closures benefit from the protection of a sterile bandage. Pressure dressings are useful in preventing hematoma formation and severe edema that may result in poor wound healing. Dressings should be changed early and the wound inspected for hematoma or signs of infection. Hematoma evacuation, appropriate drainage, and antibiotic therapy based on culture and sensitivity studies may be required. Removal of sutures in 3-5 days, followed by splinting of the incision with sterile tape, will minimize scarring from the sutures themselves.

The final result of facial wound repair depends on the nature and location of the wounds, individual propensity to scar formation, and the passage of time. A year or more must often pass before resolution of scar contracture and erythema results in maximum improvement. Only after this time, a decision can be made regarding the desirability of secondary scar revision.

In wounds involving the major joints, the extracapsular soft tissue and the intracapsular structures should be considered individually to assess accurately the magnitude of the injury and to provide a prognosis. Open joint injuries that are single penetrating and without extensive soft tissue damage permit uncomplicated joint and wound closure. Injuries that are single or multiple penetrations with extensive soft tissue disruption (flaps, avulsions, degloving) often require secondary operations to attain closure. In injuries that show open periarticular fractures with extension through the adjacent intra-articular surface and with associated nerve or vascular injury requiring repair, the cornerstone for successful management is debridement, antibiotic therapy properly timed and performed, joint closure, and aggressive treatment of the bony injury. Newer techniques such as free-tissue transfer can expedite wound care, decrease morbidity, and spare some limbs from amputation.

FACIAL BONE FRACTURES

Because of the aesthetic and functional importance of the face, fractures of the facial bones—though rarely life threatening—are best treated by surgeons who have extensive experience with facial injuries and reconstruction. Operation is most successful when performed in the acute setting, usually within the first week, because reconstruction becomes much more difficult if surgery is delayed.

Facial bone fractures are usually caused by trauma from a blunt instrument, such as a fist or club, or by violent contact with the steering wheel, dashboard, or windshield during an automobile accident. Particularly in the latter case, the patient should be assessed for associated injuries. For example, cervical spine injuries are present in up to 12% of automobile accident patients and should be treated or stabilized before facial bone injuries are attended to. Injuries to the brain, eyes, chest, abdomen, and extremities must also be assessed and may require earlier treatment.

The diagnosis of facial fractures is made primarily on clinical examination. Ideally, the examination should be done immediately so that swelling will not obscure the findings. The mechanism and the line of direction of injury are important. If conscious, the patient should be asked about previous facial injuries, areas of pain and numbness, whether the jaw opens properly and the teeth come together normally, and whether vision in all quadrants is normal.

Most facial fractures can be palpated, or at least the abnormal position of bones can be noted. Beginning along the mandibular rims, one can feel for irregularities of the facial bones. The dental occlusion is noted. With bimanual palpation, placing the thumbs inside the mouth, one can elicit bony crepitus if there is an associated fracture. The maxilla and midface can be rocked forward and backward between the thumb and the index finger in the presence of a midfacial fracture. Nasal fractures may be detected by palpation. Irregularities and step-offs along the infraorbital border, lateral orbital rim, or zygomatic arch regions indicate a depressed zygomatic fracture.

Radiologic studies are additional aids to the proper diagnosis of facial fractures. Rarely is a significant fracture seen on x-ray that is not also clinically evident. Helpful views include the Waters and submentovertex projections and oblique views of the mandible. The Panorex view of the mandible is very useful to look at the condyles. CT scans of facial bones, with appropriate biplanar and 3D reconstructions so that bones can be viewed through several planes, have essentially supplanted regular radiographs in the workup of the facially injured patient. They are helpful in assessing the extent of fractures, in particular, in more posterior areas such as the ethmoid area, medial and inferior orbit, pterygoid plates, and base of the skull.

The bones of the nose are the most commonly fractured facial bones. Next in frequency are the mandible, the zygomatic-malar bones, and the maxilla.

NASAL FRACTURES

Fractures may affect the nasal bones, cartilage, and septum. Fractures occur in two patterns, caused by lateral or head-on trauma.

With lateral trauma, the nasal bone on the side of the injury is fractured and displaced toward the septum, the septum is deviated and fractured, and the nasal bone on the side away from the injury is fractured and displaced away from the septum, so that the upper part of the nose, as a whole, is deviated. Depending on the degree of violence, one or more of these displacements will be present, and the degree of comminution is variable.

Head-on trauma gives rise to telescoping and saddling of the nose and broadening of its upper half as a result of the depression and splaying of the fractured nasal bones. This of course produces severe damage to the septum, which usually buckles or actually suffers a fracture. The diagnosis of a fractured nose is made on clinical grounds alone, and x-rays are unnecessary except for medical-legal reasons.

Nasal fractures requiring reduction should be treated with a minimum of delay, for they tend to become fixed in the displaced position in a few days. The surgical approach depends on whether the fracture has resulted in deviation or collapse of the nasal bones. Local anesthesia is preferred; either topical tetracaine or cocaine intranasally or lidocaine for infiltration of the skin can be used. The nasal bones may be disimpacted with intranasal forceps or a periosteal elevator and aligned by external molding or pressure. Collapsed nasal fractures can be repositioned with Walsham nasal forceps, introduced into each nostril and placed on each side of the septum, which is then elevated to its proper position. A septal hematoma should be recognized and drained to prevent infection and subsequent necrosis of the cartilaginous septum with associated collapse of the entire nose. Compound fractures of the nose require prompt repair of the skin wound and, if possible, early reduction of the displaced nasal bones.

External splinting, which is essentially a protective dressing, and intranasal packing using nonadhering gauze are appropriate after reduction. The intranasal packing provides support for the septum in its reduced position and helps prevent development of a hematoma. It also provides counterpressure for the external splint immobilizing the nasal bones and prevents them from collapsing. The packing is usually removed within 48 hours.

In severe comminuted nasal fractures, the medial canthal ligaments, which are easily felt by applying lateral traction to the upper eyelid, may have dislodged. If they have been avulsed, they should be reattached in position to prevent late deformities. For these severe fractures involving the entire naso-orbital and ethmoid complex, the coronal approach, which offers wide exposure, allows for proper anatomic reduction of all small nasal fragments as well as repositioning of the canthal ligaments and correction and elevation of the telescoped bone fragments at the root of the nose and glabella.

The lacrimal apparatus is commonly disrupted in these injuries and should be repaired and stented appropriately.

MANDIBULAR FRACTURES

Mandibular fractures are most commonly bilateral, generally occurring in the region of the mid body at the mental foramen, the angle of the ramus, or at the neck of the condyle. A frequent combination is a fracture at the mental region of the body with a condylar fracture on the opposite side. Displacement of the fragments results from the force of the external blow as well as the pull of the muscles of the floor of the mouth and the muscles of mastication. The diagnosis is suggested by derangement of dental occlusion associated with local pain, swelling, and often crepitation upon palpation. Appropriate x-rays confirm the diagnosis. Special views of the condyle, including tomograms, may be required. Sublingual hematoma and acute malocclusion are usually diagnostic of a mandibular fracture.

Restoration of functional dental occlusion is the most important consideration in treating mandibular fractures. In patients with an adequate complement of teeth, arch bars or interdental wires can be placed. Local nerve block anesthesia is preferable for this procedure, though certain patients may require general anesthesia. Intermaxillary elastic traction will usually correct minor degrees of displacement and bring the teeth into normal occlusion by overcoming the muscle pull. When the fracture involves the base of a tooth socket with suspected devitalization of the tooth, extraction of the tooth should be considered. Particularly in the incisor region, such devitalized teeth may be a source of infection, leading to the development of osteomyelitis and nonunion of the fracture.

Patients with more severe mandibular injuries require anatomic reduction and fixation of the fracture by the open, direct technique. These include compound, comminuted, and unfavorable fractures. An unfavorable fracture is one that is inherently unstable because muscle pull distracts the fracture segments. In this situation, intermaxillary fixation alone is insufficient. Edentulous patients also benefit from the open technique, although proper dentures or dental splints are useful to maintain normal occlusion.

Metal wire fixation of fractured segments and intermaxillary fixation for 6 weeks was a proven and popular method of fracture treatment. The more recent resurgence in popularity of the screw-plate system is due to a number of advantages over wiring. The screw plate usually achieves rigid fixation in three dimensions, providing adequate stability; it eliminates the need for intermaxillary fixation in most cases; it is useful in complex, comminuted fractures; and it is quite easy to use after familiarity with the technique has been acquired.

With bilateral parasymphyseal fractures, anterior stabilization of the tongue may be lost, so that it may fall back and obstruct the airway. Anterior stabilization and splinting must be accomplished early in these cases.

Open reduction is rarely advised in condylar fractures; simple intermaxillary fixation for 4-6 weeks is sufficient. Indications for open reduction are severely displaced fractures, which may prevent motion of the mandible because of impingement of the coronoid process on the zygomatic arch. In children, the fracture may destroy the growth center of the condyle, resulting in maldevelopment of the mandible and gross distortion.

ZYGOMATIC & ORBITAL FRACTURE

Fractures of the zygomatic bones may involve just the arch of the zygomatic bone or the entire body of the zygoma (the malar eminence) and the lateral wall and floor of the orbit. The so-called tripod fracture characteristically occurs at the frontozygomatic and zygomaticomaxillary sutures as well as at the arch. It should be referred to as a tetrapod fracture because the anterior or posterior buttress of the maxilla is also involved in the fracture. Displacement of the body of the zygoma results in flattening of the cheek and depression of the orbital rim and floor.

Important diagnostic signs are subconjunctival hemorrhage, disturbances of extraocular muscle function (which may be accompanied by diplopia), and loss of sensation in the upper lip and alveoli on the involved side as a result of injury to the infraorbital nerve. Reduction of a displaced zygomatic fracture is seldom an emergency procedure and may be delayed until the patient's general condition is satisfactory for anesthesia. Local anesthesia will suffice only for reduction of fractures of the zygomatic arch. More extensively displaced fractures usually require general anesthesia. At least two-point fixation with direct interosseous wiring is necessary for these fractures. Here again, delicate miniplates have been used with success, providing anatomic reduction and rigid fixation.

Simple depressed fractures of the zygomatic arch can best be elevated using the Gillies technique. Through a temporal incision above the hairline, an instrument is passed beneath the superficial layer of the deep temporalis fascia and under the arch and the body of the zygoma. The fracture can also be elevated percutaneously with a hook or screw in conjunction with overlying palpation to achieve accurate reduction.

If the fracture is complex or comminuted, as is often the case with high-velocity injuries, repair through a coronal scalp approach may be necessary to obtain an anatomic and stable result.

Extensive disruption should be suspected in conjunction with the zygomatic fracture when significant diplopia and enophthalmos and posterior displacement of the globe are present. Orbital fat and extraocular muscles may herniate through the defect and become entrapped, giving rise to the signs and symptoms. A "blowout" fracture is similar disruption of the orbital floor due to blunt trauma to the globe but not associated with a fracture of the zygoma or orbital rim. Treatment in both cases demands exploration, reduction of herniated contents, and repair of the floor. The most direct approach is through a lower lid subciliary incision, which provides excellent visualization. A buccal transantral (Caldwell-Luc) approach can be used, and blind antral packing for support has been described. This is quite hazardous, because bony spicules may be pushed into the ocular globe and perhaps cause injury or blindness. In cases of extensive communication or loss of bony fragments of the floor, use of local autogenous bone or cartilage as a scaffold may be performed. At times, in cases of extensive injuries to the floor, alloplastic material in the form of titanium mesh may be necessary.

Even with careful anatomic reduction and repair of the orbital floor, ocular problems—particularly enophthalmos—may persist, possibly due to an undiagnosed fracture, especially a medial ethmoidal blowout fracture. These can be properly evaluated with CT scanning. Treatment requires reduction and repair of the defect. The injury can at times cause ischemia of herniated soft tissue and subsequent atrophy and scarring. This may result in enophthalmos, which is almost impossible to resolve completely.

MAXILLARY FRACTURES

Maxillary fractures range in complexity from partial fractures through the alveolar process to extensive displacement of the midfacial structures in conjunction with fractures of the frontonasal bones and orbital maxillary region and total craniofacial separation. Hemorrhage and airway obstruction require emergency care, and in severe cases, tracheostomy is indicated. Mobility of the maxilla can be elicited by palpation in extensive fractures. "Dish-face" deformity of the retrodisplaced maxilla may be disguised by edema, and careful x-ray studies are necessary to determine the extent and complexity of the midfacial fracture. Treatment may have to be delayed because of other severe injuries. A delay of as long as 10-14 days may be safe before reduction and fixation, but the earliest possible restoration of maxillary position and dental occlusion is desirable to prevent late complications.

In the case of unilateral fractures or bilateral fractures with little or no displacement, splinting by intermaxillary

fixation for 4 weeks may suffice. Fractures are usually displaced inferiorly or posteriorly and require direct surgical disimpaction and reduction and proper fixation with appropriate plates and screws. Early reduction may help control bleeding, as torn, stretched vessels are allowed to reestablish their normal tension. In certain severe cases, external traction may be necessary. Manipulation is directed toward restoring normal occlusion and maintaining the reduction with intermaxillary fixation to the mandible in association with direct plate fixation. Complicated fractures may require external fixation utilizing a head cap and intraoral splints in conjunction with multiple surgical incisions for direct plate fixation. Coexisting mandibular fractures usually necessitate open reduction and fixation at the same time.

Cobb AR, Jeelani NO, Ayliffe PR: Orbital fractures in children. *Br J Oral Maxillofac Surg* 2013 Jan;51(1):41-46.

Kyzas PA, Saeed A, Tabbenor O: The treatment of mandibular condyle fractures: a meta-analysis. *J Craniomaxillofac Surg* 2012 Dec;40(8):e438-e452.

Nalliah RP, Allareddy V, Kim MK, et al: Economics of facial fracture reduction in the United States over 12 months. *Dent Traumatol* 2013 Apr;29(2):115-120.

Turvey TA, Proffit WP, Phillips C: Biodegradable fixation for craniomaxillofacial surgery: a 10 year experience involving 761 operations and 745 patients. *Int J Oral Maxillofac Surg* 2011 Mar;40(3):244-249

Vasconez HC, Buseman JL, Cunningham LL: Management of facial soft tissue injuries in children. *J Craniofac Surg* 2011;22(4):1320.

CONGENITAL HEAD & NECK ANOMALIES

CLEFT LIP & CLEFT PALATE

Cleft lip, cleft palate, and combinations of the two are the most common congenital anomalies of the head and neck. The incidence of facial clefts has been reported to be 1 in every 650-750 live births, making this deformity second only to clubfoot in frequency as a reported birth defect.

The cleft may involve the floor of the nostril and lip on one or both sides and may extend through the alveolus, the hard palate, and the entire soft palate. A useful classification based on embryologic and anatomic aspects divides the structures into the primary and the secondary palate. The dividing point between the primary palate anteriorly and the secondary palate posteriorly is the incisive foramen. Clefts can thus be classified as partial or complete clefts of the primary or secondary palate (or both) in various combinations. The most common clefts are left unilateral complete clefts of the primary and secondary palate and partial midline clefts of the secondary palate, involving the soft palate and part of the hard palate.

Most infants with cleft palate present some feeding difficulties, and breast-feeding may be impossible. As a rule, enlarging the openings in an artificial nipple or using a syringe with a soft rubber feeding tube will solve difficulties in sucking. Feeding in the upright position helps prevent oronasal reflux or aspiration. Severe feeding and breathing problems and recurrent aspiration are seen in Pierre Robin sequence, in which the palatal cleft is associated with a receding lower jaw and posterior and cephalic displacement of the tongue, obstructing the naso-oropharyngeal airway. This is a medical emergency and is a cause of sudden infant death syndrome (SIDS). Nonsurgical treatment includes pulling the tongue forward with an instrument and laying the baby prone with a towel under the chest to let the mandible and tongue drop forward. Insertion of a small (No. 8) nasogastric tube into the pharynx may temporarily prevent respiratory distress and may be used to supplement the baby's feedings. Placement of an acrylic obturator or appliance has proved quite successful in alleviating the breathing difficulties by bringing the tongue down and permitting a better nasal airway. Several surgical procedures that bring the tongue and mandible forward have been described but should be employed only when conservative measures have been tried without success. Recently, the use of distraction of the mandible has shown some beneficial effects. However, it should be done with great caution in the neonate.

▶ Treatment

Surgical repair of cleft lip is not considered an emergency. The optimal time for operation can be described as the widely accepted "rule of 10." This includes body weight of 10 lb (4.5 kg) or more and a hemoglobin of 10 g/dL or more. This is usually at some time after the tenth week of life. In most cases, closure of the lip will mold distortions of the cleft alveolus into a satisfactory contour. In occasional cases in which there is marked distortion of the alveolus, such as in severe bilateral clefts with marked protrusion of the premaxilla, preliminary maxillary orthodontic treatment may be indicated. This may involve the use of carefully crafted appliances or simple constant pressure by use of an elastic band.

General endotracheal anesthesia via an orally placed endotracheal tube is the anesthetic technique of choice. A variety of techniques for repair of unilateral clefts have evolved over many years. Earlier procedures ignored anatomic landmarks and resulted in a characteristic "repaired harelip" look. The Millard rotation advancement operation that is now commonly used for repair employs an incision in the medial side of the cleft to allow the Cupid's bow of the lip to be rotated down to a normal position. The resulting gap in the medial side of the cleft is filled by advancing a flap from the lateral side. This principle can be varied in placement of the incisions and results in most cases in a symmetric lip with normally placed landmarks. Bilateral clefts, because of greater deficiency of tissue, present more challenging technical problems. Maximum preservation of available

tissue is the underlying principle, and most surgeons prefer approximation of the central and lateral lip elements in a straight line closure, rolling up the vermilion border of the lip (Manchester repair).

Secondary revisions are frequently necessary in the older child with a repaired cleft lip. A constant-associated deformity in patients with cleft lip is distortion of the soft tissue and cartilage structures of the ala and dome of the nose. These patients often present with deficiency of growth of the structures of the midface. This has been attributed to intrinsic growth disturbances and to external pressures from the lip and palate repairs. Some correction of these deformities, especially of the nose, can be done at the initial lip operation. More definitive correction is done after the cartilage and bone growth is more complete. These may include scar revisions and rearrangement of the cartilage structure of the nose. Recent approaches involve degloving of the nasal skin envelope with complete exposure of the abnormal cartilage framework. These are then rearranged in proper position with or without additional grafts. Maxillary osteotomies (Le Fort I with advancement) will substantially correct the midfacial depression. A tight upper lip due to severe tissue deficiency can be corrected by a two-stage transfer of a lower lip flap known as an Abbe flap.

In utero repair of cleft lip deformities has recently become a topic of discussion. *In utero* repair affords the potential to provide a scarless repair and correct the primary deformity. Furthermore, scarless fetal lip and palate repairs may prevent the ripple effect of postnatal scarring with its resultant secondary dentoalveolar and midface growth deformities. While these suggestions make *in utero* repair attractive, the risk of fetal loss remains high. Preterm labor is a major complication and one that is directly related to the large hysterotomy required for fetal exposure. Due to the great risks associated with it, intrauterine fetal surgery is still largely reserved for severe malformations that cannot be helped significantly by postnatal intervention.

Palatal clefts may involve the alveolus, the bony hard palate, or the soft palate, singly or in any combination. Clefts of the hard palate and alveolus may be either unilateral or bilateral, whereas the soft palate cleft is always midline, extending back through the uvula. The width of the cleft varies greatly, making the amount of tissue available for repair also variable. The bony palate, with its mucoperiosteal lining, forms the roof of the anterior mouth and the floor of the nose. The posteriorly attached soft palate is composed of five paired muscles of speech and swallowing.

Surgical closure of the cleft to allow for normal speech is the treatment of choice. The timetable for closure depends on the size of the cleft and any other associated problems. However, the defect should be closed before the child undertakes serious speech, usually before age 2. Closure at 6 months usually is performed without difficulty and also aids in the child's feeding. If the soft palate seems to be long enough, simple approximation of the freshened edges of the cleft after freeing of the tissues through lateral relaxing incisions may suffice. If the soft palate is too short, a pushback type of operation is required. In this procedure, the short soft palate is retrodisplaced closer to the posterior pharyngeal wall utilizing the mucoperiosteal flaps based on the posterior palatine artery.

Satisfactory speech following surgical repair of cleft palate is achieved in 70%-90% of cases. Significant speech defects usually require secondary operations when the child is older. The most widely used technique is the pharyngeal flap operation, in which the palatopharyngeal space is reduced by attaching a flap of posterior pharyngeal muscle and mucosa to the soft palate. This permits voluntary closure of the velopharyngeal complex and thus avoids hypernasal speech. Various other kinds of pharyngoplasties have been useful in selected cases.

Kecik D, Enacar A: Effects of nasoalveolar molding therapy on nasal and alveolar morphology in unilateral cleft lip and palate. *J Craniofac Surg* 2009;(20)6:2075.

Mobin SSN, Karatsonyi A, Vidar EV, et al: Is presurgical nasoalveolar molding therapy more effective in unilateral or bilateral cleft lip-cleft palate patients? *Plast Reconstr Surg* 2011;127(3):1263.

Mueller AA, Zschokke I, Brand S, et al: One-stage cleft repair outcome at age 6- to 18- years – a comparison to the Eurocleft study data. *Br J Oral Maxillofac Surg* 2012 Dec;50(8):762-768.

Torikai K, Hirakawa T, Kijima T, et al: Primary alveolar bone grafting and gingivoperiosteoplasty or gingivomucoperiosteal flap at the time of 1-stage repair of unilateral cleft lip and palate. *J Craniofac Surg* 2009;20(2):1729.

CRANIOFACIAL ANOMALIES

These are congenital deformities of the hard and soft tissues of the head. Particular problems of the brain, eye, and internal ear are treated by the appropriate specialist. The craniofacial surgeon often needs the collaboration of these specialists when operating on such patients.

Serious craniofacial anomalies are relatively rare, although mild forms often go undiagnosed or are accepted as normal variants. A classification is therefore difficult, although many have been proposed. Tessier has offered a numerical classification based on clinical presentation. He considers a cleft to be the basis of the malformation, which involves both hard and soft tissues (Figure 41–11).

Other classifications are based on embryologic and etiologic features. With greater understanding and continued investigation, classification efforts will no doubt be more satisfactory.

There are well-known chromosomal and genetic aberrations as well as environmental causes that can lead to craniofacial deformity. The cause in most cases, however, is unknown. Arrest in the migration and proliferation of neural crest cells and defects in differentiation characterize most of these deformities. We describe some of the more common ones in brief terms.

Crouzon syndrome (craniofacial dysostosis) and **Apert syndrome** (acrocephalosyndactyly) are closely related, differing in the extremity deformities present in the latter. Both are autosomal dominant traits with variable expression. Both present with skull deformities due to premature closure of the cranial sutures. The cranial sutures most affected will determine the type of skull deformity. Exophthalmos, midfacial hypoplasia, and hypertelorism are also features of these two syndromes.

The facial organs and tissues proceed in great measure from the first and second branchial arches and the first branchial cleft. Disorders in their development lead to a spectrum of anomalies of variable severity. **Treacher-Collins syndrome** (mandibulofacial dysostosis) is a severe disorder characterized by hypoplasia of the malar bones and lower eyelids, colobomas, and antimongoloid slant of the palpebrae. The mandible and ears are often quite underdeveloped. The presentation is bilateral and is an autosomal dominant trait. A unilateral deformity known as **hemifacial microsomia** presents with progressive skeletal and soft tissue underdevelopment. The Goldenhar variant of hemifacial microsomia is a severe form associated with upper bulbar dermoids, notching of the upper eyelids, and vertebral anomalies.

Some of these patients show mental retardation, but in most cases, intelligence is not affected. The psychosocial problems are serious and most often related to how the patients look. Within the past two decades, craniofacial surgery has progressed so that previously untreatable deformities can now be corrected. With the anatomic work of Le Fort as a basis—and guided by the incomplete attempts of Gillies and others—Paul Tessier, in the late 1960s, proposed a set of surgical techniques to correct major craniofacial deformities. Two basic concepts soon emerged from his work: (1) Large segments of the craniofacial skeleton can be completely denuded of their blood supply, repositioned, and yet survive and heal; and (2) the eyes can be translocated horizontally or vertically over a considerable distance with no adverse effect on vision. The tendency today is to operate at approximately 6-9 months of age (if possible not later than a year) for cranial vault remodeling and fronto-orbital advancement.

A bicoronal scalp incision is utilized to expose the skull and facial bones with an intracranial or extracranial approach. The cut bones are then reshaped, repositioned, and fixed with a combination of wires or miniplates and screws. The latter have the advantage of rigid fixation and less need to maintain large movements with bone grafts. Autogenous inlay and onlay bone grafts can be used to improve contour. The entire operation is usually completed in one stage, and complications are surprisingly few. Miniplates have been used extensively in the last few years. In infants, fixation with absorbable suture material or the

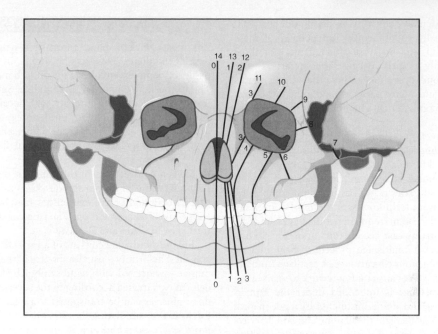

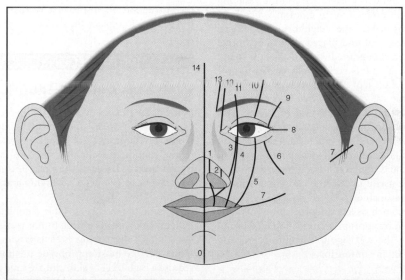

▲ **Figure 41–11.** Tessier classification of craniofacial clefts. The numbering system goes from 0 to 14, and the skeletal defects mimic the soft tissue presentation.

newer absorbable plates and screws have provided effective and stable fixation. They commonly resorb at 6-9 months. They do not interfere with imaging techniques such as CT or MRI, and they seem to have less impairment of craniofacial growth and development.

Craniofacial surgery has improved the treatment not only of major congenital deformities but also of major complex facial fractures, chronic sequelae of trauma, isolated exophthalmos, fibrous dysplasia, and aesthetic facial sculpturing.

MICROTIA

Microtia is absence or hypoplasia of the pinna of the ear, with a blind or absent external auditory meatus. The incidence of significant auricular deformity is about one in 8000 births and is usually spontaneous. Ten percent of these defects are bilateral, and boys are afflicted twice or three times as commonly as girls. Because the ear arises from the first and second branchial arches, the middle ear is always involved, and many patients have other disorders of the first and second arches. The inner ear structures are usually spared.

Generally, correction of conductive hearing by an otologist has not been long lasting or helpful, and surgery for this problem is reserved for bilateral cases.

Different techniques have been described that vary in terms of required surgeries as well as technical complexity. The Brent and Nagata techniques are the most commonly used today with the Brent requiring four stages and the Nagata only two. In any case reconstruction of the external ear usually involves a multistage procedure beginning at preschool age. Autogenous rib cartilage or cartilage from the opposite ear is used to construct a framework to replace the absent ear. The cartilage is imbedded under the skin in the appropriate area, and after adjustments are made in local tissue to reposition or recreate the earlobe and conchal cavity, the framework is elevated posteriorly and the resulting sulcus grafted to obtain projection. In cases in which local tissue is poor or unavailable, the neighboring superficial temporalis fascia is dissected and placed over the cartilage framework. This is then skin grafted with adequate tissue.

The opposite (normal) ear is occasionally altered to provide better symmetry. Excellent results have been achieved. Silastic frameworks for ear cartilage have also been used, and although their use eliminates donor site problems, rates of infection and extrusion have been unacceptable. More recently, a porous polyethylene construct has been used with better long-term results. A temporalis fascia flap is rotated to cover the allograft, and then a full-thickness skin graft is placed. They are quite useful in bilateral cases or when sufficient cartilage is not available.

Lesser deformities, such as overly large, prominent, or bent ears, are corrected by appropriate resection of skin and cartilage, "scoring" of the cartilage to alter its curve, and placement sutures to aid in contouring.

Antunes RB, Alonso N, Paula RG: Importance of early diagnosis of Stickler syndrome in newborns. *J Plast Reconstr Aesthet Surg* 2012;65(8):1029.

Bauer BS: Reconstruction of microtia. *Plast Reconstr Surg* 2009;124(1 suppl):14e.

Cho BC, Kim JY, Byun JS: Two stage reconstruction of the auricle in congenital microtia using autogenous costal cartilage. *J Plast Reconstr Aesthetic Surg* 2007;60(9):998.

Liu X, Zhang Q, Quan Y, Xie Y, Shi L: Bilateral microtia reconstruction. *J Plast Reconstr Aesthet Surg* 2010;63(8):1275.

Sabbagh W: Early experience in microtia reconstruction: the first 100 cases. *J Plast Reconstr Aesthet Surg* 2011;64(4):452.

ANOMALIES OF THE HANDS & EXTREMITIES

The most common hand anomaly is syndactyly, or webbing of the digits. This may be simple, involving only soft tissue, or complex, involving fusion of bone and soft tissue. The fusion may be partial or complete. Surgical correction involves separation and repair with local flaps and skin grafts. Correction should be done before growth disturbance of the webbed digits takes place. Other anomalies, such as extra digits (polydactyly), absence of digits (adactyly), and cleft hand, also exist.

Flexion contractures of the hands or digits may require surgical release and appropriate skin grafting. Congenital ring constriction of the extremities may be associated also with congenital amputation. The ring constrictions are best treated by excision and Z-plasty.

Poland syndrome consists of a variable degree of unilateral chest deformity—usually absence of the pectoralis major muscle—associated with hand symbrachydactyly. The hand deformity is treated according to the severity. The latissimus dorsi muscles can be transposed to replace the absent pectoralis major, simulating the sites of origin and insertion. In more severe cases and in women requiring breast and chest reconstruction, the transverse rectus abdominis island flap can be used to replace the deficit.

POSTABLATIVE RECONSTRUCTION

HEAD & NECK RECONSTRUCTION

Many of the tumors discussed in Chapter 15 require surgical excision as a primary form of therapy. This often involves removal of large areas of composite tissue, such as the floor of the mouth, the maxilla, part of the mandible, or the lymph-bearing tissue of the neck. Reconstruction after such resections can be very challenging and may require special skill.

A salient advance in the complete treatment of the patient with a head or neck tumor is reconstruction, usually done in the same setting. Free flaps with microvascular techniques are the most appropriate methods even though they require a high level of skill and are time consuming. The free flaps most commonly used following ablative procedures in the head and neck include the anterolateral thigh flap or the radial forearm flap for resurfacing the floor of the mouth and the composite fibular flap, which includes fibula as well as skin, to reconstruct the mandible and the floor of the mouth. For larger defects, judicious use of the rectus abdominis muscle, latissimus dorsi, or other musculocutaneous flaps has also been helpful. For pharyngoesophageal reconstruction, either the tubed radial forearm flap or the free jejunum is most successful.

Since no two surgical resections for tumor in the head and neck are identical, the key to effective treatment is preoperative planning. Probable extent of resection, areas that will require preoperative or postoperative radiation therapy, incision and flaps created by neck dissections, and available donor areas must all be carefully assessed. New preoperative techniques are being used that is based off of preoperative CT scanning, such as Pro-Plan. From these scans, templates are created that show exactly where excisions should be made, and for mandibular reconstruction, the size, and bending of the plate can all be done preoperatively.

Useful musculocutaneous flaps in the head and neck are the sternocleidomastoid, platysma, trapezius, pectoralis major, and latissimus dorsi muscles. Useful axial skin flaps can be obtained from the forehead, deltopectoral, and cervicohumeral areas. When these flaps are insufficient or unavailable for the reconstructive needs of the patient, free tissue transfer must be used. Although many flaps have been developed for bone and soft tissue reconstructions, the anterolateral thigh flap (cutaneous or myocutaneous), the radial forearm flap, and the osteoseptocutaneous fibula flap are the most useful free flaps for head and neck reconstruction. Healing is quick, so radiation, if necessary, may be started as early as 1 month after surgery.

Chang YM, Tsai CY, Wei FC: One-stage double barrel fibula osteoseptocutaneous flap and immediate dental implants for functional and aesthetic reconstruction of segmental mandibular defects. *Plast Reconstr Surg* 2008;122(1):143.

Chao AH, Sturgis EM, Yu P, et al: Reconstructive outcomes in patients with head and neck sarcoma. *Head Neck* 2013 May;35(5):677-683.

Davison SP, Grant NN, Schwarz KA, Iorio ML: Maximizing flap inset for tongue reconstruction. *Plast Reconstr Surg* 2008;121(6):1982.

Hassid VJ, Maqusi S, Culligan E, Cohen MN, Antony AK: Free microsurgical and pedicled flaps for oncological mandibular reconstruction: technical aspects and evaluation of patient comorbidities. *ISRN Surg* 2012;2012:792674.

Selber JC, Baumann DP, Holsinger SF: Robotic latissimus dorsi muscle harvest: a case series. *Plast Reconstr Surg* 2012;129(6):1305.

BREAST RECONSTRUCTION

Reconstruction of the female breast after mastectomy is available to all patients in the United States, and new techniques continue to be developed providing women with more options. The insurance carriers now pay for this procedure as part of the treatment for breast cancer, and this includes symmetry surgery of the contralateral breast. Even women with significant defects in the anterior chest wall as a result of radical mastectomy and radiation therapy can undergo reconstructive surgery if they are otherwise appropriate candidates.

Heightened awareness of breast cancer along with well-established screening guidelines has affected surgical treatment of the cancer and, subsequently, approaches to reconstruction of the breast. A skin-sparing, modified radical mastectomy, for example, may allow for an immediate reconstruction with autologous tissue that results in an aesthetically pleasing breast mound. Lumpectomy followed by irradiation, initially indicated for relatively small tumors, has now expanded to larger tumors and may thus result in considerable distortion and concavity in the treated breast. In the appropriate patient, concomitant bilateral reduction mammaplasty may allow for a large lumpectomy while maintaining symmetry.

The methods of reconstruction include the use of saline implants, tissue expanders, autologous tissue, or a combination of these methods. Following mastectomy, simple placement of an implant is usually unsatisfactory except in a few thin patients with relatively small contralateral breasts. The implant is usually placed in the submuscular position, utilizing the remaining pectoralis major muscle and occasionally the serratus anterior muscle for adequate muscle coverage. This results in a firm, rounded type of reconstruction and does not simulate the soft "teardrop" appearance of the normal breast. Even when adequate skin has been saved following a skin-sparing mastectomy, placement of an implant is unsatisfactory because of the high rate of complications due to skin necrosis of the saved overlying skin, which results in exposure of the implant. When doing an immediate reconstruction with implant following a skin-sparing mastectomy, it is preferable to transpose the latissimus dorsi muscle to provide another layer of cover for the implant so that if there is necrosis of the skin from the skin-sparing mastectomy, the implant will not be exposed.

The latissimus dorsi myocutaneous flap is used most often for reconstruction of the breast with an implant. The myocutaneous unit is outlined with a skin island transversely so that the scar will be transverse and covered by the brassiere. The unit is freed up completely except for its insertion at the humerus, thus preserving the neurovascular pedicle. It is transposed as a pendulum through the anterior chest wall. The superior portion of the latissimus dorsi is sutured to the pectoralis major muscle, and the lower edge is secured to the lower skin flap as far down as it will reach. The implant is then inserted, having been covered by the latissimus dorsi inferiorly and by two layers of muscle superiorly—the latissimus dorsi and the pectoralis major. The skin island is utilized in its entirety, if necessary, or is deepithelialized appropriately, maintaining only the skin portion that is needed. This method is most suitable for patients who do not have a large amount of abdominal skin, are relatively thin, and do not object to the use of implants, which sometimes may even be inserted in the opposite breast in an effort to achieve symmetry.

The use of tissue expanders continues to be a popular method of breast reconstruction. The use of acellular dermal matrices (ADM) has made expander results more satisfying.

Rather than using muscle and tissue alone to cover the expander, ADM is used to create a sling that replicates the lower pole of a breast. This allows for increased initial fill rates, and a more natural appearing breast. (Figure 41–12) Over a period of 6 weeks to 3 months, the expander is progressively inflated with saline percutaneously. The expander is inflated at least 25% more than the desired volume. A period of time—approximately 3 months—is advisable as a waiting period to prevent the "recall phenomenon," which

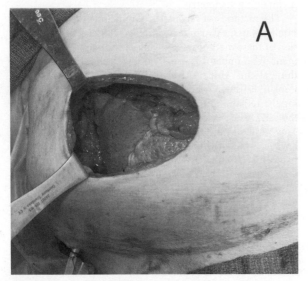

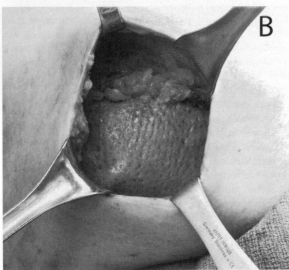

▲ **Figure 41–12. A.** Reconstructed right breast with ADM in place to recreate lower breast pole **B.** Close-up of right breast with ADM and pectoralis major interface shown.

is the shrinking that may occur following removal of the expander as it is replaced by a permanent implant. ADM has come under scrutiny though due to increased rates of seroma and other complications associated with its use. Multiple studies have shown this to be true, but it remains difficult to identify the exact patient characteristics that make them more prone to these problems.

The use of radiation therapy has continued to become more commonplace for the treatment of breast cancer. When it is used, autologous tissue is the standard for breast reconstruction. Implant base reconstruction has been shown to have significantly higher complication rates when radiation therapy is involved. The transverse rectus abdominis myocutaneous (TRAM) flap based on the superior epigastric vessel(s) remains the standard for breast reconstruction so that an implant is not required. The incision at the donor site is similar to that of an abdominoplasty operation along the lower abdomen. This method of reconstruction produces the most normal and natural breast in appearance and feel, but it requires a longer operating time as well as a longer period of hospitalization than reconstruction with tissue expanders and implants alone.

If the superior epigastric system has been violated (from surgery or trauma) or if there are other factors that would question the reliability of these vessels to adequately supply the volume and region of tissue required for the reconstruction, the surgeon may favor using the inferior epigastric system and transferring the TRAM as a free flap. Typical recipient vessels are the internal mammary or the thoracodorsal vessels. Again, past surgical history, previous (or planned) radiation, and anatomic variance may dictate reconstructive strategy regarding recipient vessels and whether to use the ipsilateral or contralateral inferior epigastric system.

Because successful breast reconstruction is common, many surgeons have sought to refine autologous reconstruction by decreasing donor site morbidity. Modifications of the free TRAM flap have been made so that the rectus abdominis muscle is mostly spared (muscle-sparing TRAM) or spared in its entirety. This latter technique is referred to as a deep inferior epigastric perforator (DIEP) flap. The same skin territory as the TRAM flap is used; however, the musculocutaneous branches that supply the skin are dissected away from the rectus abdominis muscle. In this manner, the muscle itself is spared and left *in situ* in an effort to preserve muscular function and reduce abdominal wall weakness. The deep inferior epigastric vessels are then divided, the flap is inset into the thoracic defect, and the flap vessels are anastomosed to recipient vessels along the chest wall. An extension of the DIEP has been the superficial inferior epigastric artery (SIEA) free flap. Although feasible in only a minority of patients, this artery allows for free flap reconstruction that completely avoids any dissection of the rectus muscle. This means minimal abdominal wall complications for the patient.

In addition to reconstruction of the affected breast, many patients undergo procedures that alter the contralateral (noncancerous) breast so that volume and ptosis are comparable. Such symmetry procedures are considered stages in postoncologic breast reconstruction. The nipple-areola complex can also be reconstructed. Current techniques for nipple reconstruction utilize adjacent flaps from the area where the nipple is to be positioned, taking skin and variable amounts of underlying fat if a TRAM flap has been used or elevating skin and lesser amounts of subcutaneous tissue if an implant (with or without the latissimus dorsi flap) was used. The areola may be reconstructed with a full-thickness skin graft followed by tattooing at a later date for color match.

Chun YS, Sinha I, et al: Comparison of morbidity, functional outcome, and satisfaction following bilateral TRAM versus bilateral DIEP flap breast reconstruction. *Plast Reconstr Surg* 2010;126(4):1133.

Chun YS, Verna K, Rosen H, et al: Implant based breast reconstruction using acellular dermal matrix and the risk of postoperative complications. *Plast Reconstr Surg* 2010;125(2):429.

Hammond DC: Latissimus dorsi flap breast reconstruction. *Plast Reconstr Surg* 2009;124(4):1055.

Serletti JM, Fosnot J, Nelson JA, Disa JJ, Bucky LP: Breast reconstruction after breast cancer. *Plast Reconstr Surg* 2011;127(6):124e.

LOWER EXTREMITY RECONSTRUCTION

Probably one of the most difficult areas for which to provide wound coverage and closure is the lower extremity, particularly the distal leg and foot areas. Tenuous and unstable skin grafts or poorly vascularized local or cross-leg skin flaps were once the only tissues available for resurfacing of these parts of the body. When large segments of bone were exposed or missing or when infection had become established, these grafts or flaps often were inadequate and amputation was the only recourse. Use of musculocutaneous flaps, and particularly free flaps, has greatly improved coverage in the lower extremities.

Generally, wound problems in the lower leg, ankle, and foot involve orthopedic injuries, such as compound tibial or ankle fractures. Multiple classification systems are used, but the most popular is the Gustilo and the Byrd system. These take into account the degree of fracture as well as tissue loss as well as nerve and arterial involvement.

▶ Treatment

Treatment depends on the extent of tissue loss and the depth of the wound. Fairly extensive wounds around the knee and upper third of the leg can be reconstructed with a gastrocnemius muscle flap (usually the medial head) and a split-thickness skin graft. Soft tissue defects of the middle third of the leg can be reconstructed in a similar manner by the soleus muscle in many cases. Large middle third and distal third soft tissue defects are more difficult to reconstruct. When they are complicated by extensive bone and soft tissue loss, free tissue transfer may be necessary. Although there are small muscles that end in tendons in the foot, such as the peroneus brevis, flexor hallucis longus, and extensor digitorum muscles, they can provide only limited coverage. If there is a suitable recipient artery remaining in the leg, better coverage is generally provided by a free muscle flap such as the gracilis muscle for small- and medium-sized defects or the latissimus dorsi or rectus abdominis muscle for larger defects.

Large areas of the heel or the sole of the foot are difficult to replace because skin in these regions is specially adapted to bear the weight of the body without shearing or breaking down. Free muscle flaps surfaced with skin grafts have proven to be adequate, but protective sensation is missing. The use of free neurovascular axial skin flaps, such as the inferior gluteal thigh flap and the deltoid flap, may help provide coverage with some gross sensation. Neurosensory flaps—and specifically the sural flap, distally based on one of the lower septocutaneous perforators from the lateral aspect of the leg and supplied by the sural artery, which accompanies the sural nerve—have been used to resurface defects around the ankle and heel. The procedure provides good skin and fascia for a weight-bearing area such as the heel, but it usually does not provide protective sensibility.

Segmental defects of the tibia may be reconstructed with bone grafts or, if the gap is large, free bone flaps such as the contralateral fibula or iliac crest. It is also possible to reconstruct the soft tissue defect and then reconstruct the bony gap with a distraction osteogenesis technique (Ilizarov bone transport). This bone transport method consists of performing a cortical osteotomy proximal to the site of injury and then applying a distraction apparatus, which in effect lengthens the bone 1 mm per day by appropriate adjustment screws. Such lower extremity reconstruction requires a well-coordinated, cooperative effort between the plastic and orthopedic surgeons. While such limb salvage is possible, amputation may be recommended in cases where a constellation of complications are present, such as bony gaps greater than 8 cm, extensive vascular injury, greater than 6 hours of warm ischemia time, an insensate limb, loss of plantar flexion, or an overall medically unstable patient.

Osteomyelitis of the tibia or bones in the foot may be devastating and often uncontrollable. Probably because of poor vascularity in the area, even long-term antibiotic treatment has often failed to control bone infections in the leg. Recently, effective surgical treatment for bone infections has been developed. The bone is surgically debrided and covered with a microvascular free muscle flap such as the gracilis or rectus abdominis muscle. Apparently, the muscle tissue with its excellent blood supply not only covers the exposed bone but assists natural defenses in controlling infection. Antibiotics are also used, but the well-vascularized muscle flap appears to be the deciding factor in control of infection. Reconstruction of bony defects may be accomplished at a later date.

Hollenbeck, ST, Toranto JD, Taylor BJ, et al: Perineal and lower extremity reconstruction. *Plast Reconstr Surg* 2011;128(5):551e.

Iorio ML, Goldstein J, et al: Functional limb salvage in the diabetic patient: the use of a collagen bilayer matrix and risk factors for amputation. *Plast Reconstr Surg* 2011;127(1):260.

Nosrati N, Chao AH, Chang DW, Yu P: Lower extremity reconstruction with the anterolateral thigh flap. *J Reconstr Microsurg* 2012;28(4):227.

Shores JT, Hiersche M, Gabriel A, Gupta S: Tendon coverage using an artifical skin substitute. *J Plast Reconstr Aesthetic Surg* 2012;65(11):1544.

PRESSURE SORES

Pressure sores—often less precisely called bedsores or decubitus ulcers—are another example of difficult wound problems that can be treated by plastic surgery. Pressure sores generally occur in patients who are bedridden and unable or unwilling to change position; patients who cannot change position because of a cast or appliance; and patients who have no sensation in an area that is not moved even though they may be ambulatory. The underlying cause of sores in these patients is ischemic necrosis resulting from prolonged pressure against the soft tissue overlying bone. There is also some evidence that local factors in denervated skin predispose to pressure breakdown because there is atrophy of the skin and subcutaneous tissue.

Absence of normal protective reflexes must be compensated for. Prevention is clearly the best treatment for pressure sores. Casts and appliances must be well padded, and points of pressure or pain should be relieved. Bedridden patients must be turned to a new position at least every 2 hours. Water and air mattresses, sheepskin pads, and foam cushions may help relieve pressure but are not substitutes for frequent turning. The introduction of the flotation bed system, which distributes pressure uniformly over a large surface area, has greatly aided in the management of these patients. The pressure on the skin at any time is less than the capillary filling pressure, avoiding many ischemic problems. Paraplegics should not sit in one position for more than 2 hours. Careful daily examination should be made for erythema, the earliest sign of ischemic injury. Erythematous areas should be freed from all pressure. Electrical stimulations, biomaterials, and growth factors are additional modalities to expedite wound repair, but the results are variable.

Once pressure necrosis is established, it is important to determine whether underlying tissues such as fat and muscle are affected, since they are much more likely than skin to become necrotic. A small skin ulcer may be the manifestation of a much larger area of destruction below. If the area is not too extensive and if infection and abscess due to external or hematogenous bacteria are not present, necrotic tissue may be replaced by scar tissue. Continued pressure will not only prevent scar tissue from forming but will also extend the injury. A surface eschar or skin may cover a significant abscess.

If the pressure sore is small and noninfected, application of drying agents to the wound and removal of all pressure to the area may permit slow healing. Wounds extending down to bone rarely heal without surgery. Infected wounds must be debrided down to clean tissue. The objectives at operation are to debride devitalized tissue, including bone, and to provide healthy, well-vascularized padded tissue as a covering. All of the original tissue that formed the bed of the ulcer must be excised.

When the patient's nutritional status and general condition of health are optimal, definitive coverage can be performed. Coverage is usually accomplished with a muscle, musculocutaneous, or, sometimes, an axial flap. Well-vascularized muscle appears to help control established low-grade bacterial contamination. The muscle flaps used for the more common bedsores are as follows: greater trochanter: tensor fasciae latae; ischium: gracilis, gluteus maximus, or hamstrings; sacrum: gluteus maximus. Occasionally, it is possible to provide sensibility to the area of a pressure sore with an innervated flap from above the level of paraplegia. The most common example is the tensor fasciae latae flap with the contained lateral femoral cutaneous nerve from L4 and L5, which is used to cover an ischial sore. Rarely, an innervated intercostal flap from the abdominal wall may be used to cover an insensible sacrum. Unfortunately, attempts to provide protective sensibility with sensory flaps have not had good results. The tissue expansion techniques should not be the primary surgery treatment of decubitus ulcers but can be used in difficult cases where available tissue is insufficient to close the wound.

Postoperatively, the donor and recipient areas must be kept free of pressure for 2-3 weeks to allow for complete healing. This puts significant demands on other areas of the body that may be equally at risk or may already have areas of breakdown. The use of the air-fluidized bed has greatly aided such situations.

In spite of excellent padding provided by musculocutaneous flaps, recurrence of pressure sores is still a major problem, because the situation that caused the original breakdown usually still exists. Prevention of sores is even more important for these patients.

Larson DL, Hudak KA, Waring WP, Orr MR, Simonelic K: Protocal management of late-stage pressure ulcers: a 5 year retrospective study of 101 consecutive patients with 179 ulcers. *Plast Reconstr Surg* 2012;129(4):897.

Lin PY, Kuo YR, Tsai YT: A reuseable perforator-preserving gluteal artery-based rotation fasciocutaneous flap for pressure sore reconstruction. *Microsurgery* 2012;32(3):189.

Rubayi S, Chandrasekhar B: Trunk, abdomen, and pressure sore reconstruction. *Plast Reconstr Surg* 2011;128(3):201e.

AESTHETIC SURGERY

Aesthetic surgery is an integral part of plastic surgery. In fact, the two terms have become almost synonymous even though aesthetic surgery is only one band in a broad spectrum. Increased interest and curiosity about the specialty results in part from increased demands for its services by an aging population but also from the development of more predictable, lasting, and safer techniques. A number of specialists other than plastic surgeons have also performed and contributed to cosmetic surgery. A skilled surgeon can perform such cosmetic operations safely and with maximum benefit to the patient.

Patient selection is probably as important for success as any other factor. Not all patients are good candidates for aesthetic procedures, and such operations are contraindicated in others. Age or poor general health of the patient may be a reason for delay or avoidance of purely elective procedures. Two other major factors must be considered. The first factor is the anatomic feasibility of the procedure. Can the alterations be made successfully and safely? Which technique will best accomplish the goal? The second factor is the psychologic makeup of the patient. Does the patient fully understand the nature of the proposed procedure and its risks and consequences? Are the patient's expectations realistic? Cosmetic changes in appearance will generally not save a failing marriage, help to procure a new job, or substantially improve a person's station in life, and persons with such expectations should not undergo aesthetic surgery. Surgery should be postponed for persons experiencing severe stress, such as is associated with divorce, death of a loved one, or other periods of emotional instability.

The ideal candidate for cosmetic surgery is an adult or mature younger person who has a realistic idea of what is to be accomplished, is not under pressure from others to have the operation done, and does not expect major changes in interpersonal relations or career potential following surgery. Personal satisfaction is a valid reason for seeking aesthetic refinements.

The more common aesthetic procedures are discussed below. Some procedures involve correction of functional problems as well and are therefore not always considered purely cosmetic procedures.

RHINOPLASTY

Surgical alterations of nasal structures are done for relief of airway obstruction (usually secondary to trauma) and to reshape the nose because of undesirable characteristics, such as a prominent dorsal hump, bulbous or drooping tip, or overly large size. There is often a combination of problems.

Procedures are generally performed through intranasal incisions. The nasal skin is usually temporarily freed from its underlying bony and cartilaginous framework, so that the framework can be altered by removal, rearrangement, or augmentation of bone or cartilage. The skin is then redraped over the new foundation. The nasal septum and lower turbinate can also be altered to reestablish an open airway. A better understanding of nasal physiology has enabled surgeons to correct internal valve dysfunction by inserting spreader grafts—often following modification of the bony radix of the nose. Spreader grafts are small pieces of cartilage placed next to the septum and under the upper lateral cartilages. They serve to open up the internal valve in somewhat the same way as the external "breathe easy" appliances utilized by athletes.

Surgery can be done under local or general anesthesia; in either case, topical and injectable vasoconstrictors and anesthetic agents are commonly used. Hospitalization may or may not be indicated. Nasal packing is often used for hemostasis and support of the nasal mucosa during initial healing, as incisions are usually only minimally sutured with absorbable sutures. External nasal splints are placed to control swelling and provide some protection, particularly if osteotomy of the nasal bones is performed.

Convalescence requires 10-14 days before most swelling and periorbital ecchymosis subside; however, several months are often required before completely normal sensation returns, and all swelling resolves.

Nasal procedures are very commonly performed, generally quite safe, and usually effective. Complications include bleeding, internal scarring, recurrence of airways obstruction, and irregularities of contour. Infections are rare except with the use of alloplastic nasal implants.

Nassif P, Kulbersh J: Rhinoplasty and bony vault complications. *Facial Plast Surg* 2012;28(3):303.

RHYTIDECTOMY (FACELIFT)

The combined effects of gravity, sun exposure, and loss of elasticity due to aging result in varying degrees of wrinkles and sagging of skin along the cheeks, jawline, neck, and elsewhere in the facial area. These natural signs of aging can be removed to a great extent by a facelift procedure. Not all wrinkles can be removed; however, those in the forehead, around the eyes, in the nasolabial area, and around the lips are not significantly corrected without additional procedures.

Rhytidectomy is a major procedure requiring extensive incisions hidden in the scalp and in front of and behind the ears and occasionally in the submental region. The first such operations consisted of freeing up the skin and then stretching it and resuturing as it was drawn cephalad and laterally. This gave a mask-like and unnatural appearance. In the last few years, there has been a significant change in the concept of the facelift procedure, so that now it consists of elevation of the soft tissues—particularly the jowls and malar fat pads—to where they were at a younger age, giving more prominence to the cheek bones and better delineating the jawline. Undermining of the skin is done only to approach the soft tissues to be elevated, and the excess skin is now removed and reapproximated without tension. This approach to the midface has given more natural and lasting results and provides also a 3D type of restoration of the soft tissues, giving a more youthful appearance.

For the double neck, extensive freeing up of the skin over the neck from the jawline down to the hyoid is performed, and the fat overlying the platysmal muscle is removed either by suctioning or directly with scissors. The platysma itself is tightened laterally as well as centrally to provide an effect similar to a hammock that will give a more defined neck and jaw angle.

Drains are used particularly in the neck, as well as a padded circumferential dressing to protect the face and provide light pressure during healing. The introduction of fat aspiration procedures (liposuction) has been adapted to the neck but is not recommended for the face since it may produce abnormal lines ("railroad tracks of demarcation"). In appropriate patients, liposuction in the neck does give fine definition to the chin and jawline and may substantially correct the double chin appearance.

Either local or general anesthesia may be used for this often lengthy (3-4 hours) procedure. Local vasoconstrictors are routinely used.

Complications include hematoma, skin slough, injuries to branches of the facial nerve or greater auricular nerve, scars, and asymmetry. Signs of aging often recur years later.

Kosowski TR, McCarthy C, Reavey PL, et al: A systemic review of patient-reported outcome measures after facial cosmetic surgery and/or nonsurgical facial rejuvenation. *Plast Reconstr Surg* 2009;123(6):1819.

▶ Endoscopy

Endoscopy has become an integral part of plastic surgery, particularly for procedures involving the face or the breast. Smaller endoscopes are now utilized as well as different methods of achieving a desired optical field other than by distention of natural cavities with fluid or gases. In the face and in the breast, the optical cavity is usually obtained by tractioning the skin with appropriate elevators or sutures.

Endoscopy has been most effective for the forehead, where in appropriate circumstances it has replaced the coronal incision, which goes from ear to ear, peeling the scalp down to the supraorbital rims. By means of endoscopy, the forehead lift becomes a more physiologic operation in that one frees up the forehead skin at the subperiosteal level, dividing the periosteum at the supraorbital rim and then removing the depressors of the eyebrows (the procerus and corrugator muscles in the glabella region), thus allowing the frontalis muscle to act unopposed to elevate the eyebrows.

The key to the procedure appears to be the division of the periosteum, which by itself frees up the eyebrows and elevates them for at least 5-10 mm. In addition, removal of the glabellar muscles seems to ameliorate in a lasting way the vertical wrinkles in the glabella region. For suspension of the elevated eyebrows, different methods have been advocated that include soft tissue to bony anchoring, the use of temporary screws in the skull as well as miniplates, or, most simply, by providing external traction tied in between staples with nylon sutures. It appears that it is only necessary to maintain that elevation for a short period of time (3-5 days) until the periosteum reattaches at the higher level.

Endoscopy has also been effectively utilized to do a midfacelift, and this procedure is applicable to younger patients where there is no excess skin in the face or neck and where scars will be unattractive.

Endoscopy is also utilized for the breasts—particularly for insertion of breast implants in the submammary or subpectoral plane through an axillary incision. An endoscope attached to a right-angle retractor allows excellent visualization of the cavity where the implant is to be inserted, and it allows the development of a pocket inferiorly down to—and if necessary below—the submammary fold and also the division of the lower portion of the origin of the pectoralis major muscle from the sternum to permit insertion of a saline implant and to provide acceptable cleavage. Appropriate instruments for dissection as well as hemostasis have been developed for this procedure, which recently has gained in popularity.

BLEPHAROPLASTY

Blepharoplasty involves removal of redundant skin of the upper and lower eyelids and removal of periorbital fat protruding through sagging orbital septa. It is done alone or as part of a facelift procedure.

Incisions are made in the upper lids surrounding previously marked redundant skin, which is removed. A subciliary incision is generally used in the lower lids. The orbicularis oculi muscle may be altered if necessary. The periorbital fat compartments are opened, and protruding fat is removed. The extent of redundant skin in the lower lid is gauged, and the skin is resected. External sutures are used. Minimal or no dressing is required.

Local anesthesia in the form of lidocaine with epinephrine is usually adequate. Swelling and ecchymosis subside in 7-10 days, and sutures are removed in 3-4 days.

Complications include bleeding, hematoma formation, epidermal inclusion cysts, ectropion, and asymmetry. Patients are usually satisfied with the results. Recurrence is much less of a problem than with facelift procedures.

In recent years there have been significant changes in the concept of the blepharoplasty procedure. For the upper lids, the change consists of the recognition of senile ptosis due to either disruption or stretching of the levator mechanism. This can be corrected by imbrication of the levator mechanism with sutures.

The lower eyelid operation has undergone even more changes. A general trend has been to do less surgery or dissection but still obtain the same satisfactory results. Less disruption of the orbicularis muscle and orbital septum with "no touch" techniques have become popular. Also, less removal of fat but rather redistribution has gained wider acceptance. The subconjunctival removal of fat has been advocated and is particularly applicable to young patients with congenital fat hernias. The subconjunctival approach is also utilized in conjunction with the laser, which has the effect of tightening the skin of the lower lid and ameliorating the periorbital wrinkles.

Another important concept is the recognition of the proper position of the lower lid, especially the lateral canthal area. A youthful appearance is restored by elevating this to a more normal level.

MAMMOPLASTY

Aside from procedures related to breast cancer, surgery of the female breast is generally done for one of the following reasons: to increase the size of the breasts (augmentation mammoplasty), to decrease the size of the breasts (reduction mammoplasty), or to lift the breasts (mastopexy). Augmentation, lifting of the breasts, and correction of asymmetry are nearly always done for cosmetic reasons. Reduction of hypertrophied breasts may, however, be done for functional reasons, since such breasts can cause poor posture, back and shoulder pain, and discomfort due to grooves from brassiere straps.

▶ Augmentation Mammoplasty

In procedures for augmentation of the breasts, a silicone bag filled with saline solution or silicone is placed beneath the breast tissue in the submammary or subpectoral plane. Incisions are concealed in the periareolar margin, inframammary fold area, or axilla. Dissection is then carried out above or below the pectoralis major muscle, and the implant is placed in the pocket created. Drains are not generally used, and a padded dressing providing light pressure is applied. The subpectoral plane is preferred by most surgeons for augmentation mammoplasty because it does not interfere with mammography, but it does necessitate division of the lower portion of the origin of the pectoralis major muscle up to approximately 3 o'clock in relation to the nipple to provide adequate cleavage.

After a prolonged investigation by the FDA, silicone gel–filled implants have recently become available again in the United States for cosmetic purposes. During the investigation, silicone gel–filled implants were found to be safe; however, long-term data concerning these implants (ie, capsular

contracture, deflation and rupture rates) remains unknown. Nevertheless, patients and surgeons now have the opportunity to review the data and choose the type of implant used during breast augmentation.

The procedure can be done on an outpatient basis with local anesthesia, although this may not be satisfactory when subpectoral implants are used. General anesthesia is often used for augmentation procedures.

Although patient satisfaction is excellent in most cases, a significant rate of capsular contracture remains a problem in about 10%. Scar tissue around the implant may contract in variable degrees even in the same patient. Control of this process is difficult even though the best possible environment for healing is provided (ie, appropriate implants are used, infection is controlled, bleeding is not present, debris is removed, and movement is restricted). Implants placed in the subpectoral position appear to be associated with a lesser degree of capsular contracture and less severe deformity if contracture occurs. Deflation of saline implants occurs at a rate of 1% per year.

Other complications include hematoma, infection, exposure of the implant, deflation or rupture of the implant, asymmetry of the breasts, and external scars. Breast function and sensation are usually not altered in any way.

Adams Jr WP, Mallucci P: Breast augmentation. *Plast Reconstr Surg* 2012;130(4):598e.

Eaves FF, Haeck P, Rohrich RJ: Breast implants and anaplastic large cell lymphoma (ALCL): using science to guide our patients and plastic surgeons worldwide. *Plast Reconstr Surg* 2011;127(6):2501.

Jewell M, Spear SL, Largent J, Oefelein MG, Adams WP Jr: Anaplastic large T-cell lymphoma and breast implants: a review of literature. *Plast Reconstr Surg* 2011;128(3):651.

Rohrich RJ, Reece EM: Breast augmentation today: saline versus silicone—what are the facts? *Plast Reconstr Surg* 2008;121(2):669.

▶ Mastopexy

Mastopexy is another common procedure used for correction of sagging or ptotic breasts. Although some breasts develop in a ptotic manner, most cases are caused by normal relaxation of aging tissues, gravity, and atrophy after pregnancy and lactation. It is not clear whether use of a brassiere alters this process in any significant manner. The degree of deformity is defined by the relationship of the areola to the inframammary fold and the direction of the nipple. A ptotic breast will have a nipple that is below the inframammary line and pointing down towards the toes.

Correction may be done with simultaneous reduction or augmentation. An incision must be made around the areola, and the breast tissue itself is imbricated or, better still, an inferiorly based flap of breast tissue is designed and placed underneath the remnant superior part of the breast and over the pectoralis major muscle, serving as an autoaugmentation as one brings the lateral breast columns together. This procedure gives a more lasting effect than merely decreasing the skin envelope. Attempts at making more lasting corrections of ptosis of the breasts through the periareolar incision, which decreases the scarring, have included wrapping the breast with prosthetic material such as polyglycolic meshes or, more recently, by wrapping it around with segments of pectoralis major muscle.

Nonetheless, significant scarring may occur, particularly around the periareolar incision.

General anesthesia is usually necessary, and recovery from mastopexy may take 7-10 days. Complications include bleeding, infection, tissue loss, altered sensation or loss of function of the nipple and areolar areas, scars, and asymmetry of the breasts.

Patient satisfaction with the results is often not as great as with other procedures. Satisfaction often depends on how well the patient is prepared to accept the resulting scars.

▶ Reduction Mammoplasty

Reduction mammoplasty is similar to mastopexy, since nearly all hypertrophic breasts are ptotic and must be lifted during correction. Enlargement can occur during puberty or later in life. Massive breasts can become a significant disability to the patient.

Although various techniques have been developed for breast reduction, nearly all require a pedicle to carry the nipple areola to its new position and a circumareolar incision as well as a vertical or inverted T incision beneath the areola. In gigantomastia, the nipple-areola is often removed as a free full-thickness graft and positioned appropriately. Most tissue is removed from the center and lower poles of the breast.

Vertical reduction mammoplasty has aroused considerable recent interest because of the decrease in amount of scarring. It can be accomplished through an incision made circumferentially around the areola and then a vertical incision that extends to and sometimes slightly below the inframammary fold. Resection of the breast tissue is done from below as well as from the lateral aspect of the breast. Considerable wrinkling of the skin occurs in an effort to avoid "T-ing off" the incision at the inframammary fold, but pleating of the skin usually resolves over a period of weeks. General anesthesia is nearly always required because dissection is considerable, but blood loss can be minimized by the use of epinephrine as a vasoconstriction agent. Transfusions are rarely indicated, and postoperative drains are often not used. The procedure can be done on an outpatient basis.

Although problems with nipple-areola loss, bleeding, infection, asymmetry of breasts, and scarring may occur; these women are generally among the most satisfied and appreciative of patients.

ABDOMINOPLASTY & BODY CONTOURING PROCEDURES

Other procedures usually classified as aesthetic are abdominoplasty and various body contouring procedures that serve to remove excess tissue from the lower trunk, thighs, and upper arms. Patients with sagging tissue due to aging, pregnancies, multiple abdominal operations, or significant or massive weight loss are usually good candidates for body contouring procedures. With the increased popularity of bariatric surgery, more people are seeking surgery to remove and correct large amounts of excess and redundant skin and soft tissue of the trunk and extremities. These types of procedures are not indicated as a treatment for obesity. This involves a complete regimen of diet, exercise, and lifestyle modifications.

Abdominoplasty usually involves removal of a large ellipse of skin and fat down to the wall of the lower abdomen. Dissection is carried out in the same plane up to the costal margin. The naval is circumscribed and left in place. After the upper abdominal flap is stretched to the suprapubic incision, excess skin and fat are excised. The fascia of the abdominal wall midline can be plicated and thus tightened. The umbilicus is exteriorized through an incision in the flap at the proper level, and the wound is closed over drains with a long incision generally in an oblique line or W shape just above the os pubis and out to the area below the anterior iliac crests (so-called bikini line). When the extent of excess abdominal tissue is severe, better results can be obtained with what is called a circumferential abdominoplasty. The incision is carried around the patient and this requires changing the position of the patient at least on one occasion. Proper markings preoperatively are essential in order to obtain a satisfactory and symmetrical result.

Spinal anesthesia may be used in some cases. Hospitalization is routinely required for up to a few days. Blood transfusions are rarely necessary. Proper deep vein thrombosis prophylaxis is important in these and other extensive procedures.

Complications involve blood or serum collections beneath the flap, infection, tissue loss, and wide scars. Results are generally quite dramatic with excellent patient satisfaction in properly selected cases.

Various surgical procedures have been devised to remove excess skin and fat from the upper arms, buttocks, and thighs. These procedures commonly result in extensive incisions that can produce significant scarring, and there may be difficulty in achieving a smooth transition between the end point of the contour alteration and normal tissue. Careful planning and counseling of the patient is imperative in order to obtain a satisfactory result. The use of a suction-assisted lipectomy with appropriate cannulas to remove localized excess fat deposits has become widespread. It is clear, however, that patient selection and judicious use of liposuction are necessary to avoid complications, including hypovolemia due to blood loss, hematoma formation, skin sloughs, excess laxity of the skin and soft tissues and waviness and depressions in the operative site. Used with discretion, liposuction can offer definition to areas of the abdomen, flanks, thighs, and buttocks.

SUCTION-ASSISTED LIPECTOMY

Suction-assisted lipectomy, or liposuction, has now become the most common cosmetic surgical procedure performed in the United States. As presently practiced, it consists of infiltration of a "wetting" or "tumescent" solution to provide vasoconstriction and anesthesia to the operative sites. A common mixture consists in a solution of Ringer lactate with the addition of 1 mg of epinephrine per 1000 mL of Ringer and 250 mg of plain lidocaine—the former to provide vasoconstriction and the lidocaine to provide a certain amount of anesthesia and thus reduce the depth of general anesthesia. Some surgeons perform the entire operation under local anesthesia, necessitating the use of larger amounts of lidocaine.

Once the solution has been infiltrated sufficiently to produce the proposed effects, a small cannula is introduced through a small incision and suction is applied either with a syringe or with a suction machine. The fat layer that has been enlarged by the injection of tumescent solution dislodges easily and disrupts much faster than the blood vessels and the nerves.

Suction-assisted lipectomy is effective in removing abnormal bulges of localized fat throughout the body, particularly in the trochanters or the abdomen and flanks, but it is not considered a weight reduction technique.

The procedure is safe when done by well-trained surgeons respecting sterility and technique and in adequately equipped operating rooms. Safety in the use of up to 35 mg of lidocaine per kilogram has been established by clinical studies. Although fatalities have been reported with suction-assisted lipectomy—which is distressing in an entirely elective procedure—they are due to pulmonary embolization, perforation of the intestines, or severe infections of the abdominal wall. Fortunately, fatalities have markedly decreased since the American Society of Plastic and Reconstructive Surgeons established safety guidelines. High-volume liposuction (ie, over 5000 cc of aspirate) should be done in a hospital or accredited ambulatory facility and that combined procedures should be carefully monitored.

Complications of suction-assisted lipectomy include irregularities of contour, dimpling, and, rarely, local infection at the entrance points.

Ultrasonic liposuction, external and internal, has also been advocated. External ultrasonic liposuction has the effect of a massage to disperse the infiltrated tumescent solution. Internal ultrasonic liposuction, on the other hand, emulsifies the fat with ultrasonic energy, which produces heat, so that this emulsified fat needs to be suctioned with standard suctioning equipment. The problems with ultrasonic liposuction include seroma formation, the need for larger portals of entrance, the possibility of burns of the skin or perforations of the skin (end hits) if the cannula is misdirected.

Fakhouri TM, El Tal AK, Abrou AE, Mehregan DA, Barone F: Laser assisted lipolysis: a review. *Dermatol Surg* 2012;38(2):155.

FAT GRAFTING

With the continued popularity of lipectomy and the desire for contouring of other body regions, the use of fat grafting has continued to gain popularity. In essence, fat is removed from one part of a patient, prepared via several different techniques, and then placed where further soft tissue enhancement is required. It can be used in the face, the breast, and soft tissue defects in almost all areas of the body. With the discovery of adipose derived stem cells, this technique will continue to gain popularity.

Delay E, Garson S, Tousson G, Sinna R: Fat injection to the breast: technique, results, and indications based on 880 procedures over 10 years. *Aesthet Surg J* 2009;29(5):360.
Hsu VM, Stransky CA, Bucky LP, Percec I: Fat grafting's past, present, and future: Why adipose tissue is emerging as a critical link to the advancement of regenerative medicine. *Aesthet Surg J* 2012;32(7):892.
Veber M, Tourasse C, Moutran M, Mojallal A: Clinical analyses of clustered microcalcifications after autologous fat injection for breast augmentation. *Plast Reconstr Surg* 2012;129(1):168e.

TELANGIECTASIAS (SPIDER VEINS)

When there is no trace of primary or secondary varicosities, most telangiectasias, or spider veins, are viewed as a cosmetic problem. However, one should be aware that in some cases spider veins may be an indication of deep venous valvular insufficiency. Factors that may play a role in the formation of spider veins include venostasis with decreased flow rate due to atony of the venous wall, chronic venous inflammation, trauma to the site, hormonal influences, or venous compression at the saphenofemoral valve.

Treatment of spider veins is with sclerosing agents, which may include hypertonic saline, sodium tetradecyl sulfate, and polidocanol (Asclera) injections. These agents are injected directly into the spider veins with the objective of creating intimal damage that will result in fibrosis and obliteration of the lumen. The technique is simple and effective, but when the sclerosing agent extravasates into the soft tissue, it might produce superficial skin necrosis.

MULTIPLE CHOICE QUESTIONS

1. An advantage of full thickness skin graft (FTSG) versus split-thickness skin grafts (STSG) is:

   A. Increased contracture rate
   B. Decreased amount of skin appendages
   C. Improved overall aesthetics
   D. Less resilient to trauma

2. The maximum safe length to width ratio for a random pattern flap is:

   A. 1:1
   B. 1.5:1
   C. 2:1
   D. 2.5:1
   E. 3:1

3. A 25-year-old man presents with a long-standing ischial pressure sore. After debridement and partial ischiectomy, the best choice for tissue coverage is:

   A. Rectus femoris
   B. Gracilis
   C. Split-thickness skin graft
   D. Primary closure

4. Which of the following is characteristic of an arteriovenous malformation (AVM)

   A. GLUT-1
   B. Rapid growth
   C. Growth proportional with patient
   D. Sporadic involution

5. A 40-year-old woman presents after mastectomy and radiation therapy. The best aesthetic method for breast reconstruction is:

   A. Implants alone
   B. Tissue expanders followed by implants
   C. Acellular dermal matrices (ADM) with implants
   D. Latissimus flap
   E. TRAM flap

Hand Surgery

David M. Young, MD

Scott L. Hansen, MD

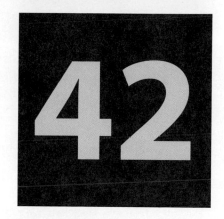

Both in industry and in the home, the hand is the most commonly injured part of the body. Disorders of the hand rarely jeopardize life but can significantly affect the ability to function.

INTRODUCTION

The prime functions of the hand are feeling (sensibility) and grasping. Sensibility is most important on the radial sides of the index, middle, and ring fingers and on the opposing ulnar side of the thumb, where one must feel and be able to pinch, pick up, and hold objects. The skin on the ulnar side of the small finger and its metacarpal, upon which the hand usually rests, must register the sensations of contact and pain to avoid burns and other trauma.

Mobility is critical for grasping. The upper extremity is a cantilevered system extending from the shoulder to the fingertips. It must be adaptable to varying rates and kinds of movements. Stability of proximal joints is essential for good skeletal control distally.

The specialization of the thumb has allowed humans to have superior aptitudes for defense, work, and dexterity. The thumb has exquisite sensibility and is a highly mobile structure with well-developed adductor and thenar (pronating) musculature. It is the most important digit of the hand, and every effort must be made to preserve its function.

The **position of function** of the upper extremity favors reaching the mouth and perineum and achieves a comfortable, forceful, and unfatiguing grip and pinch. The elbow is held at or near a right angle, the forearm neutral between pronation and supination, and the wrist extended 30 degrees with the fingers flexed to almost meet the opposed (pronated) tip of the thumb (Figure 42–1A). This is the desired position of the extremity if stiffness is likely to occur, and it should be maintained when joints are immobilized by splinting, arthrodesis, or tenodesis.

Opposite to the position of function is the **position of rest**, in which the flexed wrist extends the digits, making grip and pinch awkward, uncomfortable, weak, and fatiguing (Figure 42–1B). The forearm is usually pronated, and the elbow may be extended. This habitus is assumed, without intention, after injury, paralysis, or the onset of a painful stimulus. For that reason, it is also called the **position of the injury**. Immobility in this position jeopardizes function.

ANATOMY

All references to the forearm and hand should be made to the radial and ulnar sides (not lateral and medial) and to the volar (or palmar) and dorsal surfaces. The digits are identified as the thumb, index finger, middle finger, ring finger, and small finger.

The skin is an elastic outer sleeve and glove of the arm and hand. Sacrifice of its surface area or elasticity by debridement and fibrosis can severely diminish the range of motion and constrict circulation. In the adult hand, the dorsal skin stretches about 4 cm in the longitudinal and in the transverse planes when the palm is flattened and spread. The long finger can have as much as 48 cm^2 of skin cover, and the whole hand (exclusive of digits) has 210 cm^2.

Fascia anchors the palmar skin to bone to make pinch and grip stable; the midlateral fibers of the Cleland and Grayson ligaments keep the skin sleeve from twisting around the digit (Figure 42–2). In the form of sheaths and pulleys, fascia holds tendons in the concavity of arched joints to convey mechanical efficiency and power. The fascial sleeve of the forearm, hand, and digits must sometimes be released along with skin to prevent or relieve congestion (eg, compartment syndrome). Any fascial compartment of the hand provides a space for infection or an avenue for its dissemination.

Each finger has three joints, the distal interphalangeal joint (DIP), the proximal interphalangeal joint (PIP), and

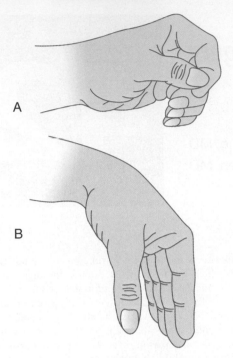

▲ **Figure 42–1.** Positions of function **(A)** and rest (injury) **(B).**

the metacarpophalangeal joint (MCP). The thumb contains the IP, the MCP, and the carpometacarpal joint (CMC). The wrist is the "key joint" of the hand, governing motion of the digits, and may need to be included in the immobilization required for a major finger or hand problem. The position of the wrist governs the efficiency of extrinsic muscle contraction. The wrist is composed of a proximal and distal row of carpal bones. The proximal row contains the scaphoid,

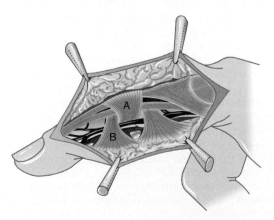

▲ **Figure 42–2. A:** Cleland ligament. **B:** Transverse retinacular ligament.

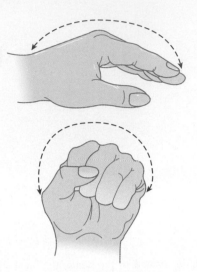

▲ **Figure 42–3.** Longitudinal *(top)* and transverse *(bottom)* arches.

lunate, triquetrum, and pisiform, while the distal row contains the trapezium, trapezoid, capitate, and hamate. The stability of the digital joints and their planes of motion are governed by the length of the ligaments and the anatomy of their articulating surfaces. The longitudinal and transverse arches of the hand (Figure 42–3) are architectural prerequisites to gripping, pinching, and cupping, and are maintained by the active contraction and passive tone of intact muscles. The arches create the position of function. When the arches are collapsed, the hand assumes the position of injury. Loss of these arches is most often initiated by edema. They may be preserved by splinting in the position of function, elevation without constriction, and early restoration of active joint motion.

Each MCP and PIP joint has a distally anchored volar plate (Figure 42–4) in addition to collateral ligaments stabilizing the joint on either side (Figure 42–5). The thickened lateral portions of the volar plate form the checkrein ligaments, which prevent IP hyperextension.

The extrinsic flexor tendons are contained in fibrous **sheaths** to prevent bowstringing and preserve mechanical efficiency as the digits flex into the palm. Pulleys (hypertrophied sections of the sheath) resist the points of greatest tendency to bowstring. The retinacular pulley system contains five annular bands and three cruciform bands. Sheaths are inelastic and relatively avascular. Therefore, they crowd and congest any swollen, inflamed, or injured tendons and curtail glide by friction, constriction, and the generation of inelastic adhesions. The A-2 and A-4 pulleys must be maintained to prevent tendon bowstringing. These are located over the proximal and middle phalanges, respectively. The A-1, A-3, and A-5 pulleys are located over the

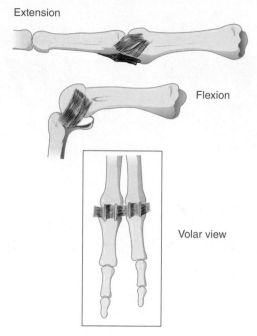

▲ **Figure 42–4.** Volar plate.

MCP, PIP, and DIP joints, respectively. Five flexor tendon zones have been described. Zone II, or **"no man's land,"** is the zone from the middle of the palm to just beyond the PIP joint, wherein the superficialis and profundus tendons lay

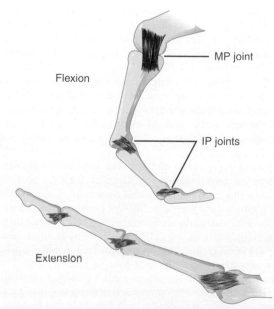

▲ **Figure 42–5.** Collateral ligaments.

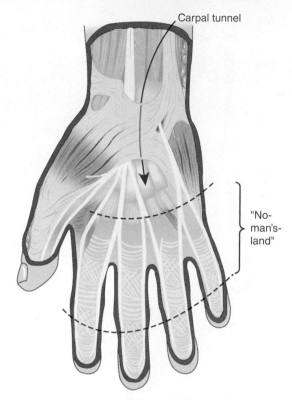

▲ **Figure 42–6.** Carpal tunnel and no man's land.

ensheathed together and where recovery of glide is difficult after wounding (Figure 42–6).

Across the wrist, the dense volar transverse carpal ligament closes the bony carpal canal **(carpal tunnel)** through which passes all eight finger flexors as well as the flexor pollicis longus and median nerve (Figure 42–6). The **ulnar bursa** is the continuation of the synovium around the long flexors of the small finger through the carpal tunnel, encompassing the other finger flexors which interrupted their separated bursa at the midpalm level. The **radial bursa** is the synovium around the flexor pollicis longus contained through the carpal tunnel. These two bursas may intercommunicate. **Parona space** is the tissue plane over the pronator quadratus in the distal forearm deep to the radial and ulnar bursas.

The extensor tendons are ensheathed in six individual compartments at the wrist beneath the extensor retinaculum (Figures 42–7 and 42–8), which predisposes to adhesions. Its role as a pulley is not as vital.

The nerves of greatest importance to hand function are the musculocutaneous, radial, ulnar, and median nerves. The importance of the musculocutaneous and radial nerves combined is forearm supination and of the radial nerve alone is innervation of the extensor muscles. The ulnar

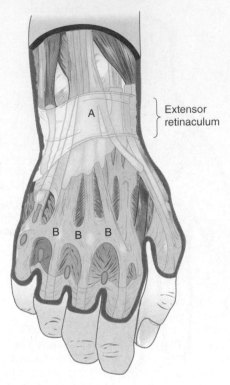

▲ **Figure 42–7. A:** Extensor retinaculum over six tendon compartments. **B:** Juncturae tendinum (conexus intertendineus).

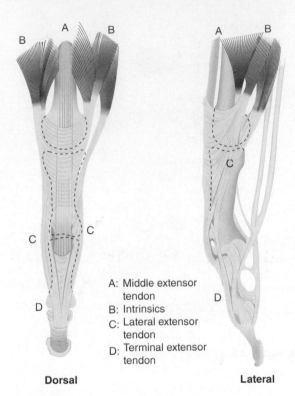

A: Middle extensor tendon
B: Intrinsics
C: Lateral extensor tendon
D: Terminal extensor tendon

Dorsal   **Lateral**

▲ **Figure 42–8.** Extensor hood mechanism.

nerve innervates 15 of the 20 intrinsic muscles. The median nerve provides sensation to the thumb, index finger, middle finger, and the radial aspect of the ring finger; through its motor innervation, it maintains most of the long flexors, the pronators of the forearm, and the thenar muscles. Figure 42–9 shows the sensory distribution of the ulnar, radial, and median nerves.

CLINICAL EVALUATION OF HAND DISORDERS

The presenting complaint must be assessed in complete detail with regard to its mechanisms of onset, evolution, aggravating factors, and relieving factors. Age, sex, hand dominance, occupation, preexisting hand problems, and relevant matters pertaining to the patient's general health must also be noted.

The examination should follow an orderly routine. Observe the neck, shoulders, both upper extremities, and the action and strength of all muscle groups, and be certain that all parts can pass painlessly and coordinately through a normal range of motion, starting with the head and neck and working down to the fingertips. Compare both upper extremities and keep detailed notes, diagrams, and measurements. Having the patient reach for the ceiling and simultaneously open and close both fists and then spread and adduct the fingers and, finally, oppose the thumbs sequentially to each fingertip will immediately demonstrate any abnormalities.

Observe habitus, wasting, hypertrophy, deformities, skin changes, skin temperature, scars, and signs of pain (including when the patient attempts to bear weight on the palms). Feel the wrist pulses and the sweat of the finger pads, and test reflexes and the sensibility of the median, ulnar, and radial nerves.

Serial x-rays and laboratory studies may clarify a problem with an indolent evolution (eg, Kienböck avascular necrosis of the lunate, causing unexplained wrist pain). Contralateral and multiple-view x-rays in different planes are often helpful. In addition, computed tomography (CT) scans, magnetic resonance imaging (MRI), bone scans, or all of these may aid in diagnosis. This is especially true in patients who have persistent bone and joint pain or limited motion or in patients who have not attained adult growth. In the case of wrist problems, arthrograms and arthroscopy may be of diagnostic value. MRI can be quite helpful in the diagnosis of subtle carpal bone problems.

GENERAL OPERATIVE PRINCIPLES

A bloodless field (eg, by tourniquet ischemia) is essential for accurate evaluation, dissection, and management of tissues of the hand. This is achieved by elevating or exsanguinating the extremity and then inflating a padded blood pressure cuff around the arm to 100 mm Hg above systolic pressure. This is readily tolerated by the unanesthetized arm for 30 minutes and by the anesthetized arm for 2 hours.

Incisions (Figure 42–10) must be either zigzagged across lines of tension (eg, must never cross perpendicularly to a flexion crease), termed Brunner incisions, or run longitudinally in "neutral" zones (eg, connecting the lateral limits of the flexion and extension creases of the digits), and whenever possible, must be designed so that a healthy skin-fat flap is raised over the zone of repair of a tendon, nerve, or artery.

Proper evaluation and treatment of an acute injury often requires extension of the wound. Normal structures can then be identified and traced into the zone of injury, where blood and devitalized tissue can make their identification difficult or impossible.

Constriction and tension by dressings must be avoided. The dressing should be applied evenly to the skin without wrinkles. The wound should be covered with a single layer of fine-mesh gauze followed by a moist spongy medium (fluffs, Rest-On, Kling, or Kerlix). Moisture facilitates the drainage of blood into the dressing, which should be applied with gentle pressure to restrict dead space.

Splinting and immediate elevation are paramount in controlling swelling and pain postoperatively. In general, plaster (fast-setting) or fiberglass is preferred because of its adaptability to specific requirements. More often than not,

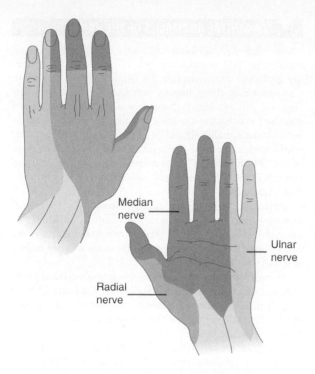

▲ **Figure 42–9.** Sensory distribution in the hand. Light-shaded area, ulnar nerve; diagonal area, radial nerve; darker area, median nerve.

The diagnosis is often made by noting the response to therapy. This is particularly true in the case of local corticosteroids injected at the site of noninfectious inflammatory conditions (eg, carpal tunnel syndrome, trigger finger).

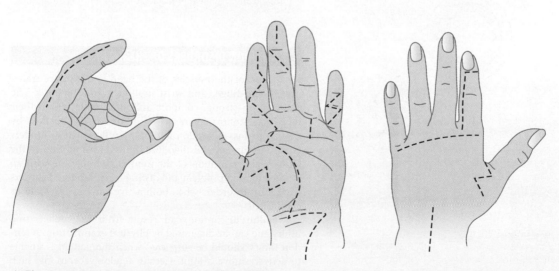

▲ **Figure 42–10.** Proper placement of skin incisions.

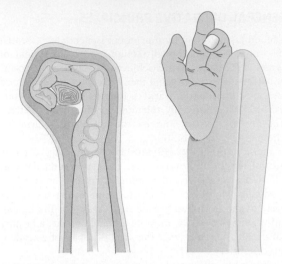

▲ **Figure 42–11.** Casting.

the wrist requires immobilization along with any other part of the hand (Figures 42–11 and 42–12).

It must be appreciated that effective immobilization of a finger most often requires concomitant immobilization of one or more adjacent fingers, usually in the position of function. Straight splints such as tongue blades involve a hazard of digital stiffness and distortion and should not be used across the MCP joint.

Persistence of pain signifies inadequate immobilization and, if throbbing is present, congestion. Congestion must be promptly relieved by elevation and sectioning of the cast and dressing and, if necessary, the skin and fascia.

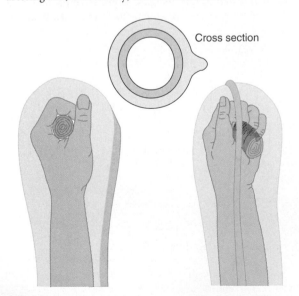

Cross section

▲ **Figure 42–12.** Casting.

▼ CONGENITAL ANOMALIES OF THE HAND

Major congenital hand anomalies are not rare, with approximately 1 in 700 live births affected. When minor deformities are included, approximately 3% of all births are affected. Camptodactyly (bent finger), polydactyly (more than five fingers), and syndactyly (two or more fingers are joined together) are the most common malformations. Newborns with hand anomalies should be carefully examined for other malformations because multisystem syndromes can be present in 5% of patients (eg, vertebral, anal atresia, cardiac, trachea, esophageal, renal, and limb [VACTERL] syndrome with radial head dysphasia).

Anomalies may be inherited, caused by environmental factors (drugs, viral infections, irradiation, alcohol), or idiopathic. Major genetic or major environmental causes are infrequently found, suggesting that the cause of most defects is multifactorial.

In order to simplify an extremely complex clinical problem, the American Society for Surgery of the Hand (ASSH) and all major international hand societies have adopted a single classification system that divides anomalies into six main categories: failures of formation (absent digits, phocomelia [seal limb]), failures of differentiation (syndactyly), duplication (polydactyly), undergrowth (brachydactyly), overgrowth (macrodactyly), and constriction ring syndrome (focal necrosis, intrauterine amputation). There is considerable overlap in the categories, as might be expected.

Ideally, surgery is performed early in the first 2 years of life, but timing is individually tailored to the problem.

Bates SJ, Hansen SL, Jones NF: Reconstruction of congenital differences of the hand. *Plast Reconstr Surg* 2009;124:128e.

Chung MS: Congenital differences of the upper extremity: classification and treatment principles. *Clin Orthop Surg* 2011;3:172.

▼ TENDON DISORDERS OF THE HAND

Movement of the muscles of the hand and arm are transmitted into finger and wrist motion by the tendons. The tendons are strong, compact units that glide within their individual compartments. Disruption of the tendon by trauma or loss of tendon gliding by inflammation hinders tendon excursion and therefore limits active motion of the joints. Passive motion of the joint is still possible with an isolated tendon problem and distinguishes tendon disorders from joint disorders when both active and passive motions are limited.

Tendon disruption can result from any penetrating injury and can be diagnosed by physical examination. A tendon injury should be suspected when the patient is unable to actively move a joint. Certain tendon lacerations, such as an isolated flexor digitorum superficialis disruption, may be masked because the profunda tendon can still move the entire finger. Blocking of profunda function by blocking flexion in the neighboring fingers (the profunda tendons are joined in the palm) reveals the injury to the superficialis when the injured PIP joint cannot be flexed.

The state of the wound and the complexity of the injury are the principal issues the hand surgeon must weigh in choosing between a primary or secondary tenorrhaphy. Clean wounds generally favor primary tenorrhaphy. Primary tenorrhaphy is defined as one that is done within 24-72 hours after injury. When wounds are unstable, contaminated, or complicated by fracture or ischemia, formal tenorrhaphy may have to be delayed for weeks or months until the tendon bed is more favorable to healing and glide. However, interim tacking of the tendons—together, to tendon sheaths, or to bone—to maintain the fiber length of a muscle may be done as a preliminary procedure.

Preoperative treatment of fresh lacerations consists of wound closure, immobilization, and prophylactic antibiotics. Such cases can be deferred for definitive primary repair for 24 hours or more. The timing of delayed secondary procedures depends on the resolution of wound edema and fibrous callus (ie, how soft and pliable it is). After 6-8 weeks, tendons that retract over 2.5 cm may defy full excursion because muscle elasticity has been lost or because the tendon is recoiled and congealed in scar.

Tenorrhaphy must be done without surface trauma along the tendon or its bed. The repair is made end to end or by weaving one tendon with the other, using a 3-0 or 4-0 braided synthetic polyester material, Prolene or nylon sutures. A flexor tendon graft is anchored distally to bone (Figure 42–13). Tenodesis will occur if the surface of the tendon and the surface where adherence is desired are roughened. The position of immobilization should relieve tension on the tendon juncture. The duration of immobilization after tenorrhaphy is generally no more than 3-4 weeks. Controlled early, passive or active mobilization after tenorrhaphy may be initiated as early as 1 week to minimize excessive tendon scarring. This requires a very cooperative patient and close supervision by the hand therapist to avoid rupture of the repaired tendon.

Adhesions invariably form wherever tendons are even slightly inflamed or injured and can severely limit tendon function. Even so, adhesions are necessary for a tendon to reestablish continuity. With continuous active and passive

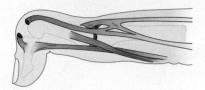

▲ **Figure 42–14.** Mallet finger with swan-neck deformity.

movement over months, tendon glide can be increased with maturation and molding of the collagen in the adhesions. If the adhesions remain thick and tendon excursion is limited, surgical release of the tendon adhesions (tenolysis) needs to be performed. Successful surgery requires the release of all adhesions limiting tendon glide without rupturing the tendon repair. Movement of the tendon as soon as possible after surgery (within 24-48 hours) under the guidance of the hand therapist is critical to avoid recurrence of adhesions.

The access to tenolysis should be through an incision offering effective exposure and placed where the immediate active and passive joint motion that must follow will not jeopardize healing of the wound by undue stretching or direct pressure. Performing a concomitant procedure requiring immobilization such as a neurorrhaphy should be avoided. The patient must understand that joint mobilization after tendon surgery is a time-consuming process, often taking many weeks or months to achieve maximum recovery.

Mallet finger ("baseball" or "drop" finger) (Figure 42–14) is due to disruption of the extensor tendon to the distal phalanx. A distal joint that can be passively but not actively extended is diagnostic. The injury most commonly results from sudden forceful flexion of the digit when it is held in rigid extension. Either the extensor is partially or completely ruptured or the dorsal lip of the bone is avulsed. Less frequently, the injury is due to direct trauma such as a laceration. An x-ray should be taken to determine the presence and extent of any fracture.

Treatment requires 6-8 weeks of continuous splinting in full distal joint extension (not hyperextension) with or without 40 degrees of PIP joint flexion. Patient education and compliance are essential for good results. Joint fixation internally with a percutaneous Kirschner wire or externally with padded aluminum, plastic, or plaster splints are equally effective. A lacerated tendon should be repaired. When a significantly displaced fracture fragment represents one-third or more of the surface of the joint, it should be reduced by wiring or pinning. If there is sufficient articular surface disruption, one may consider joint fusion.

Swan-neck deformity (Figure 42–14) is a frequent complication of mallet finger, but it may also be the result of disparity of pull between the extrinsic flexors and extensor hood with or without attenuation of the DIP joint extensor.

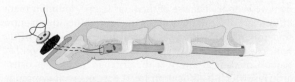

▲ **Figure 42–13.** Flexor tenorrhaphy by advancement or graft. Pulleys are saved.

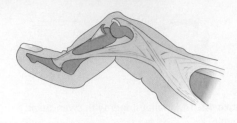

▲ **Figure 42–15.** Buttonhole deformity.

It is seen in congenitally hypermobile joints, spastic, and rheumatoid states, and following resection of the superficialis tendon. The dorsal hood acts to extend the distal joint but is held back by its insertion at the base of the middle phalanx, which it therefore hyperextends. This in turn increases the tension on the profundus, which hyperflexes the DIP joint. If the mallet deformity is 25 degrees or less and there is some active distal joint extension, it may be treated by undermining and elevating the extensor hood at the PIP joint and severing its insertion on the base of the middle phalanx. Otherwise, the deformity may be corrected by tethering PIP joint extension with one slip of the flexor digitorum superficialis threaded through the flexor pulley of the proximal phalanx with the PIP joint flexed 20 degrees.

The **boutonnière,** or "**buttonhole,**" **deformity** (Figure 42–15) appears as the opposite of the swan-neck deformity: hyperextension of the DIP joint and flexion of the PIP joint. There is attenuation or separation of the dorsal hood, so that the middle extensor tendon becomes ineffective and the lateral extensor tendons shift volar to the PIP joint axis and the joint buckles dorsally. The entire extrinsic-intrinsic force on the hood passes onto the lateral extensor tendons, which flex the PIP joint and hyperextend the DIP joint. This deformity may develop suddenly or, more often, insidiously after closed blunt or open trauma over the dorsum of the PIP joint.

To avoid this complication, sutured extensor tendon lacerations and severe contusions over the PIP joint should always have the PIP joint alone splinted in extension for 3-4 weeks. Established deformities can be treated by such immobilization but more often require operative correction.

STENOSING TENOSYNOVITIS

In stenosing tenosynovitis, there is a disproportion between the clearance inside a tendon pulley or tunnel and the diameter of the tendon or tendons that must glide through it. Any pulley or tunnel may be implicated. The more common sites are as follows:

1. The proximal digital (A1) pulleys in the distal palm, causing **trigger finger** or thumb. There is local tenderness of the pulley; pain, which may be referred to the PIP joint; and (usually but not always) locking of the digit in flexion with a painful "pop" as it goes into extension (ie, as the bulge in the tendon or tendons passes through the tight pulley).

2. The pulley over the radial styloid housing the abductor pollicis longus and extensor pollicis brevis (first extensor compartment), causing **de Quervain tenosynovitis.** Local tenderness and pain occur if these tendons are actively stretched (eg, Finkelstein test). The Finkelstein test is performed by having the patient bend the thumb into the palm and grasp with the fingers. The wrist is then bent ulnarly, and the first extensor compartment palpated. Pain in this area suggests de Quervain tenosynovitis.

Relief of the symptoms can be achieved by local injections of triamcinolone mixed with lidocaine. Immediate surgery is justified if the constriction is so tight that the tendon is locked. Surgical section of the constricting tendon sheath is also indicated if symptoms persist or recur. When releasing the flexor tendon, care is taken not to resect more than the section of sheath restricting the tendon or else the tendon will pull away from the finger like a bowstring and weaken the grip.

Chesney A, Chauhan A, Kattan A, et al: Systematic review of flexor tendon rehabilitation protocols in zone II of the hand. *Plast Reconstr Surg* 2011;127:1583.

Hanz KR et al: Extensor tendon injuries: acute management and secondary reconstruction. *Plast Reconstr Surg* 2008;121:109e.

James R et al: Tendon: biology, biomechanics, repair, growth factors, and evolving treatment options. *J Hand Surg Am* 2008;33:102.

Lee SK: Modern tendon repair techniques. *Hand Clin* 2012;28:565.

McAuliffe JA: Tendon disorders of the hand and wrist. *J Hand Surg Am* 2010;35:846.

Rozental TD, Zurakowski D, Blazar PE: Trigger finger: prognostic indicators of recurrence following corticosteroid injection. *J Bone Joint Surg Am* 2008;90:1665.

▼ SKELETAL INJURIES OF THE HAND

Injuries to the bones and joints of the hand are the most common skeletal injuries treated by physicians. Recognition of the injury, appropriate diagnostic tests, and timely treatment are essential for minimizing the complications of these injuries. Some patients may neglect obvious fractures and dislocations in hope of spontaneous recovery. More subtle injuries to the wrist are more often neglected by the patient and sometimes even missed by physicians until further damage is done. The use of the fluoroscope, found in many offices, greatly enhances the surgeon's ability to diagnose fractures. The machine allows real-time assessment of the bones as part of the physical examination. A common late sequela of skeletal injury at the articular surfaces is osteoarthritis, which is difficult to treat. Patients with symptoms related to the hand or wrist but without a discernible cause should be referred early to a hand specialist.

METACARPALS & PHALANGES

▶ Fractures

Fractures of the metacarpal and phalangeal bones such as distal phalanx tuft of the fingers caught in closing doors and metacarpal shaft fractures of the ulnar side of the hand (boxer's fractures) create an obvious deformity and are easy to diagnose. Adequate x-rays of the specific site of the fracture with anteroposterior, lateral, and oblique views are essential for developing a treatment plan.

Fractures of the shaft can usually be treated with closed reduction and a cast or splint holding the hand in the position of function (Figure 42–1) for 3-4 weeks. Residual angulation of a metacarpal shaft fracture of up to 30 degrees in the fifth finger and 20 degrees in the fourth finger is functionally well tolerated, although a dorsal bump may be aesthetically unpleasant. However, even a small rotational misalignment of the fracture at the metacarpal bone results in scissoring of the fingers in flexion and causes severe dysfunction.

When fractures do not remain reduced, fixation with Kirschner pins placed through the skin is required. Placement of more than one pin is usually needed to keep the fracture reduced. The pins are removed after the fracture is healed. Displaced and comminuted fractures may require opening of the fracture site and reduction under direct visualization. Pins, lag screws, and small, low-profile metal plates and screws are used to maintain reduction. Metal plates provide strong support to the fracture site and allow earlier mobilization of the hand. However, plates are more invasive and occasionally interfere with tendon function due to excessive scar formation postoperatively.

Fractures through an articular surface need to be carefully evaluated. Nondisplaced fractures can be treated by casting. Displaced fractures require open reduction and accurate pin or lag screw fixation because discrepancies of the articular surface will eventually result in degenerative arthritis.

Fractures of the distal phalanx from crush injuries require attention to the disrupted nail bed. The nail is removed to decompress the painful subungual hematoma and provide irrigation of the open fracture and careful reapproximation of the nail matrix. Large disruptions in the nail matrix may result in deformity of the regenerating nail. The nail is replaced under the nail fold (eponychium) as a splint. A protective splint is placed over the finger to hold the distal fragment in extension.

An intra-articular fracture of the base of the thumb metacarpal bone with subluxation (displacement) of the metacarpal leaving a volar pyramidal shaped fragment attached to the trapezium is called a **Bennett fracture**. The anterior oblique ligament, responsible for stability of the thumb base, is left attached to the pyramidal fragment. The remainder of the thumb metacarpal is unstable and limits use of the thumb. The fracture must be reduced and stabilized with Kirschner pins, plate, or lag screws. Accurate reduction of the articular surface is crucial in reducing complications. Even despite adequate treatment, most patients eventually develop arthritis.

▶ Dislocations

Dislocations are most common in the PIP joint. Injuries are classified according to the position of the distal digit as hyperextension, dorsal displacement, or volar displacement. The type of dislocation determines which structures, such as the volar plate, collateral ligaments, and extensor tendon, are likely to be disrupted.

The MCP and CMC joints are better protected by surrounding soft tissue but can still be dislocated. The MCP joint of the thumb is most frequently injured by forced abduction. The ulnar collateral ligament is torn, as occurs with forced use of a ski pole or as historically described in gamekeepers when twisting the neck of birds ("gamekeeper's thumb"). Of the CMC joints, the fifth is most commonly injured. A fracture analogous to a Bennett fracture (reverse Bennett fracture) can occur. Examination to determine injury to the deep motor branch of the ulnar nerve in this area should be done.

Radiographs are occasionally useful for diagnosis, but the physical examination is most important. Since pain often limits the extent of the examination, regional anesthesia with a wrist or finger block allows a more detailed examination. Partial tears of ligaments without dislocation or instability are treated by splints. Dislocations can usually be reduced, and the need for surgical therapy is determined by the stability of the joint after reduction. Stable reductions are treated with early mobilization to decrease stiffness.

Fracture dislocations usually require surgical repair. Instability after reduction can be treated by repair of the torn collateral ligament or volar plate. Severe dislocations of the PIP and MCP joints can result in interposition of disrupted soft tissue in the joint, making closed reduction impossible. The joint must be opened and the trapped soft tissue removed and repaired to correct the dislocation. A complete disruption of the ulnar collateral ligament in a gamekeeper's thumb injury can result in interposition of the adductor aponeurosis between the torn ends of the ulnar collateral ligament. The ends of the ligament must be reduced and repaired under direct vision.

WRIST & FOREARM INJURIES

▶ Fractures

Fractures in the wrist and forearm usually result from falls on the outstretched hand. The distal radius is most commonly fractured. Many classification systems and eponyms have been used based on the extent and displacement of the fracture and involvement of the articular surface. The hyperextended wrist also exposes the scaphoid bone to injury in a fall. Since the scaphoid is crucial to wrist motion, displacement of the fracture is poorly tolerated. In addition, the blood supply enters the distal part of the bone and makes ischemic necrosis of the proximal fragment a problem.

Diagnosis of distal radius fractures is not difficult, but scaphoid fractures can easily be missed. Special radiographic views of the wrist or CT or MRI scans may be needed in difficult cases. If the clinical picture is suspicious but the radiographs are inconclusive, the wrist should be immobilized. Repeat radiographs in 7-10 days may demonstrate the fracture. Untreated scaphoid fractures lead to debilitating arthritis and collapse of the wrist.

Distal radius fractures are treated by reduction and immobilization. As with other fractures, articular irregularities and unstable fractures need to be treated by open reduction and internal fixation. Use of bone grafting and external fixation devices to initially treat the fracture has been advocated. Scaphoid fractures require careful and prolonged immobilization. Displaced fractures or nonhealing fractures require operative treatment with screw compression, bone grafts, and/or scaphoid replacement.

▶ Dislocations & Sprains

Dislocations and ligamentous injuries of the wrist are the most difficult hand injuries to diagnose and treat. Wrist injuries often present as a painful wrist after minor trauma. Routine radiographs are often normal, and physical findings can be unimpressive. Still, these injuries can lead to chronic problems. Special stress radiographs, fluoroscopy, and physical maneuvers (scaphoid shift test) help delineate the injury.

The scaphoid lunate ligament is most often injured. Instability of the joint is best treated by repair or reconstruction of the ligament. Injury of the ligaments of the radiocarpal-radioulnar joint is likewise difficult to determine. Surgical treatment involves repair of the disrupted ligament.

Buijze GA, Ochtman L, Ring D: Management of scaphoid nonunion. *J Hand Surg Am* 2012;37(5):1095-1100.

Friedrich JB, Vedder NB: An evidence-based approach to metacarpal fractures. *Plast Reconstr Surg* 2010;126:2205.

Gaston RG, Chadderdon C: Phalangeal fractures: displaced/nondisplaced. *Hand Clin* 2012;28:395.

Geissler WB: Operative fixation of metacarpal and phalangeal fractures in athletes. *Hand Clin* 2009;25:409.

Jones NF, Jupiter JB, Lalonde DH: Common fractures and dislocations of the hand. *Plast Reconstr Surg* 2012;130:722e.

Khalid M, Jummani ZR, Kanagaraj K, et al: Role of MRI in the diagnosis of clinically suspected scaphoid fracture: analysis of 611 consecutive cases and literature review. *Emerg Med J* 2010;27:266.

Neuhaus V, Jupiter JB: Current concepts review: carpal injuries—fractures, ligaments, dislocations. *Acta Chir Orthop Traumatol Cech* 2011;78(5):395-403.

Sendher R, Ladd AL: The scaphoid. *Orthop Clin North Am* 2013;44:107.

NERVE DISORDERS

Nerve disorders of the hands are conveniently organized into compression neuropathies, injuries of peripheral nerves, and various problems located more proximal to the upper extremities (spinal cord or central nervous system). For nerve dysfunction due to strokes, cerebral palsy, and spinal cord injury, readers are referred to more specific textbooks on hand surgery.

▶ Compression Neuropathies

Compression of the nerves of the upper extremities due to an increase in surrounding tissue pressure occurs in specific locations and causes predictable signs and symptoms. Tissue edema from a variety of causes such as crushing injuries, vascular disorders, and prolonged repetitive hand motions can compress nerves traveling within tight compartments of the arm and produce nerve ischemia. Prolonged ischemia results in axonal destruction and sensory and motor dysfunction.

The median nerve can be compressed by local structures at the elbow (pronator syndrome), the anterior interosseous branch, and the wrist (carpal tunnel syndrome). Compression of the median nerve at the elbow causes forearm pain and sensory changes in the radial four fingers. The anterior interosseous branch of the median nerve is purely a motor nerve, and lesions produce only weakness of thumb and index finger flexion and no pain. Carpal tunnel syndrome presents with weakness in the hand, sensory abnormalities of the fingers sparing the small finger and ulnar aspect of the ring finger, and exacerbation of symptoms on forced flexion of the wrist (Phalen sign) or tapping the nerve at the wrist (Tinel sign). Shoulder, elbow, and forearm pain is also common. Atrophy of thenar muscles occurs in long-standing cases.

The ulnar nerve can be compressed at the elbow (cubital tunnel syndrome) or the wrist (Guyon canal). Sensory abnormalities in the small finger and weakness of intrinsic hand muscles occur with compression in either area. Segmental nerve conduction velocity tests help to localize the abnormality to one site or the other. Compression of the radial nerve occurs most frequently from fractures of the humerus. Compression of the nerve along the proximal radius (radial tunnel syndrome) causes diffuse pain around the elbow but occurs rarely.

Abnormal findings on nerve conduction studies and clinical manifestations of nerve compression are adequate for diagnosis. Electromyography (EMG) demonstrating denervation patterns in the corresponding muscles or slowing of nerve conduction velocities indicates injury to the nerve. Although helpful, these tests only complement the physical examination, since electrodiagnostic tests can occasionally be inaccurate.

Early or mild cases of compression are treated by controlling tissue swelling. Resting the extremity with splints and using nonsteroidal anti-inflammatory medications as well as local injection of steroids often resolves the problem. If repetitive motions, such as typing, are thought to be the cause, changing the motion or hand position should help. If clinical manifestations are severe or if nonsurgical therapy fails, surgical decompression of the nerve is advocated.

Carpal tunnel syndrome is the most common type of compression neuropathy and one of the most common hand disorders. Surgical therapy of median nerve entrapment in the carpal tunnel or any of the compression neuropathies requires detailed knowledge of the anatomy. Division of the constricting structures results in partial or complete reversal of the symptoms. In the carpal tunnel, the median nerve is surrounded on three sides by carpal bones. Incision of the transverse carpal ligament, which forms the roof of the tunnel, decompresses the nerve. Occasionally, internal fibrosis of the nerve occurs and internal neurolysis with an operating microscope is required to allow the nerve to recover. Endoscopic release of the carpal tunnel through a smaller skin incision has been advocated.

▶ Nerve Injuries

Injury to individual peripheral nerves of the arm results in predictable and defined deficits. Proximal injuries involving the brachial plexus have more variable manifestations. Nerve conduction can be disrupted in the absence of structural changes due to compression, blunt injury, or ischemia (neuropraxia). More severe injury results in disruption of the axon with preservation of the epineurial covering of the nerve (axonotmesis). Both types of injury are followed by spontaneous recovery of function of good quality. Complete disruption of the nerve (neurotmesis), as with a laceration, requires surgical repair. Wallerian degeneration of the distal nerve occurs in both neurotmesis and axonotmesis, and recovery depends on the growth of the cut axon to the end organ. However, with neurotmesis, orientation of the proximal and distal axons is lost and recovery may be incomplete, especially in mixed motor and sensory nerves. Methods to differentiate sensory from motor fascicles have been used during repairs with some benefit.

A patient with loss of the radial nerve is unable to extend the fingers, wrist, and thumb. In addition, the patient will have sensory loss to the dorsum of the hand. Median nerve dysfunction causes problems with opposition of the thumb and grip of the fingers. Sensory loss is to the radial four digits and can significantly impair use of the hand. An ulnar neuropathy causes dysfunction of the intrinsic muscles of the hand, clawing of the ulnar two digits, and weakness in gripping smaller objects. Sensation is lost along the ulnar side of the hand.

Diagnosis of nerve injury is mainly by the physical examination. Understanding the functional anatomy of the peripheral nerves allows adequate evaluation of nerve loss.

Electrodiagnostic studies are used to distinguish between partial and complete lesions and to follow functional recovery.

Obvious and complete disruption of the nerve is treated best by early surgical exploration and repair. An incomplete lesion or questionable disruption of nerve integrity is best treated with close observation, splinting to prevent contractures, and surgical exploration if no recovery occurs. Segmental loss of nerves requires nerve grafts, usually taken from a minor sensory nerve, such as the sural nerve, to bridge the gap. Results of primary repair are better than the results of grafts, and repairs done soon after injury are better than delayed repairs. Recovery of protective sensation of the hand is crucial for good functional recovery.

Motor dysfunction due to nerve damage can be treated by arthrodesis (stabilization of flail joints) and tendon transfers. Tendon transfers should utilize a muscle unit that is unaffected by the nerve injury, have direction of force and excursion similar to those of the damaged muscle, and produce no further deficits due to loss of the donor muscle. For radial nerve palsy, the pronator teres to extensor carpi radialis transfer provides wrist extension, the flexor carpi radialis to extensor digitorum communis transfer gives finger extension, and the palmaris longus or flexor digitorum superficialis of the fourth finger transfer to the extensor pollicis longus extends the thumb. Restoration of thumb opposition is most important with median nerve palsies, and the use of several donor muscles to achieve this result has been described including the extensor indices proprius and flexor digitorum superficialis from the middle or ring fingers. Tendon transfers to control claw deformity and strengthen key pinch are used for ulnar nerve palsies.

Gottschalk HP, Bindra RR: Late reconstruction of ulnar nerve palsy. *Orthop Clin North Am* 2012;43:495.

Jones NF, Machado GR: Tendon transfers for radial, median, and ulnar nerve injuries: current surgical techniques. *Clin Plast Surg* 2011;38:621.

Kang JR, Zamorano DP, Gupta R: Limb salvage with major nerve injury: current management and future directions. *J Am Acad Orthop Surg* 2011;19:S28.

Ko JW, Mirarchi AJ: Late reconstruction of median nerve palsy. *Orthop Clin North Am* 2012;43:449.

Lee SK, Wolfe SW: Nerve transfers for the upper extremity: new horizons in nerve reconstruction. *J Am Acad Orthop Surg* 2012;20:506.

Mintalucci DJ, Leinberry CF: Open versus endoscopic carpal tunnel release. *Orthop Clin North Am* 2012;43:431.

Watson JC: The electrodiagnostic approach to carpal tunnel syndrome. *Neurol Clin* 2012;30:457.

▼ HAND INFECTIONS

Small breaks in the skin or nails of the hand can lead to widespread infection and abscess. The original injury often cannot be identified. Poor venous and lymphatic drainage of the upper extremity, especially when held in a dependent position, aggravate the situation. Immunocompromised patients (diabetics, HIV-positive patients) are prone to develop extensive infections very quickly and should be treated more carefully.

The hallmark of infection (pain, swelling, and erythema) may be widespread in the hand and make localizing the infection difficult. Swelling of the dorsum of the hand is common even with palmar infections, and knowledge of the tissue planes of the hand is crucial to understanding how infections spread. Lymphatic streaks (lymphangitis) extending up the arm indicate rapid extension of the infection and must be treated urgently.

Oral antibiotics effective against staphylococcus and common anaerobic organisms (ie, first-generation cephalosporins and penicillin) are adequate to treat most infections. Infections from animal bites (*Pasteurella multocida*) and human bites (oral flora) also respond to penicillin. The intravenous route is reserved for severe infections or for those not responsive to oral antibiotics. Once the situation improves, oral antibiotics are given for 7-10 days. Equally as important, the infected hand needs to be immobilized and elevated. Pillows and trapezes help to elevate the arm, but elbow slings aggravate the dependent position of the arm and should not be used. The best results are obtained when the patient is convinced that elevation of the extremity is beneficial.

Once treatment of a hand infection has begun, improvement within 24 hours is expected. If prompt improvement does not occur, an occult abscess may be present. Obvious abscesses should be drained at the point of maximum tenderness or the point of maximum fluctuance, where the overlying tissues are thinnest. The drainage wound should run parallel to and not across the paths of nerves, arteries, and veins. Wounds should be made long enough and should be zigzagged, when necessary, to avoid secondary contractures. Ultrasonography may be useful when a definite abscess cannot be located.

Pyogenic Granuloma

Pyogenic granuloma is a mound of granulation-like tissue 3-20 mm (or more) in diameter. It usually develops under a chronically moist dressing and may form around a suture. A small granuloma (6-7 mm in diameter) exposed to the air will soon dry up and epithelialize, whereas larger ones should be scraped flush with the skin under local anesthesia and covered with a thin split-thickness skin graft. If the granuloma is adjacent to the nail and the nail is acting as a foreign body aggravating the reaction, the nail must be removed.

Nail Infections

The nail fold is often traumatized and becomes secondarily inflamed, leading to a **paronychia** on the radial or ulnar side. The lesion is termed an **eponychia** if it involves the base

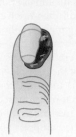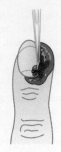

▲ **Figure 42–16.** Incision and drainage of paronychia.

of the nail, although the entire fold can be involved; and it is called a **subungual abscess** if pus develops and extends under the nail plate. Because of the early and unrelenting tissue tension that develops, these entities are quite painful. Early treatment before abscess formation consists of soaking, elevation, immobilization, and antibiotics. Most abscesses can be drained painlessly with a scalpel; the insensate necrotic skin cap should be cut through where it points (Figure 42–16). Sagittal incisions, which form a "trapdoor" of the eponychium, should be reserved for the long-standing case in which a dense fibrous callus of the nail fold must be excised. Occasionally, the nail must be basally excised or totally avulsed, after which the eponychial fold should be separated from the nail matrix by a thin, loose pack. Chronically wet nails of dishwashers may develop tissue changes and nail deformities, which are best treated by removing the nail plate. Fungal infections should be diagnosed and treated, and the fingers should be protected from water or excessive sweating.

Deep Space Abscess

A **felon** is an abscess in the pulp of the fingertip and is often deep and very painful. Untreated or inadequately drained abscesses may lead to osteomyelitis of the distal phalanx. Incision and drainage with disruption of the many vertical fibrous septa of the pulp space are required to adequately drain the abscess (Figure 42–17). The traditional fishmouth incision is no longer recommended for drainage since it may expose the underlying bone and because it often heals in a tender scar. Instead, lateral through-and-through incisions

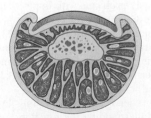

▲ **Figure 42–17.** Cross section of distal phalanx.

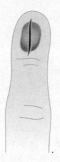

▲ **Figure 42–18.** Incision of felon (distal fat pad infection).

or direct incisions on the pulp, where the abscess points, have better results (Figure 42–18).

The **web spaces** are the path of least resistance for pus from infected distal palm calluses, puncture wounds, and infections of the lumbrical canals. Infection and abscess formation in the dorsum of the thumb web may be the result of extension from the volar thenar space (collar button). A dorsal incision is usually made between the fingers to drain both spaces. A dorsal incision in the web of the thumb may be zigzagged to prevent contracture (Figure 42–10).

The **midpalmar space** becomes infected by direct puncture or by extension of infections from the flexor sheaths of the index, middle, or ring fingers (Figure 42–6). Only the skin should be incised over the point of fluctuance. The rest of the dissection should be carried out by gentle spreading with a blunt clamp to avoid injury to arteries, nerves, and tendons. Infection spreads easily from this space along the lumbrical canals and to the thenar space.

A hypothenar space abscess is usually a product of a penetrating wound and should be drained at the point of greatest fluctuance. The same is true for a thenar space abscess, which may point in the palm rather than the thumb web.

Infection within the synovium of the flexor tendon is difficult to diagnose. **Pyogenic tenosynovitis** spreads easily down the tendon sheath to affect the other fingers. Untreated, the infection causes adhesions of the tendon to the surrounding soft tissues and permanently limits movement of the fingers.

The signs of flexor tendon infection described by Kanavel include fusiform swelling of the digit, severe pain on passive finger extension, a fixed flexed position of the finger, and most importantly, tenderness over the extent of the tendon sheath into the palm. Ultrasonography of the distal palm can also be helpful when the diagnosis is unclear. The probe is held across the palm and reveals swelling of the involved tendon and fluid around the tendon at the proximal flexor sheath.

Only unresponsive, tensely swollen, and toxic cases need immediate incision and drainage. With rest, elevation, and antibiotics, it is safe to observe most cases for several

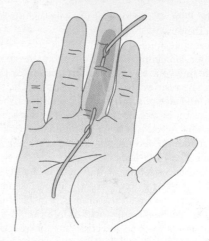

▲ **Figure 42–19.** Drainage and irrigation for septic tenosynovitis. The antibiotic solution drips in through the distal catheter and drains out through the proximal one.

hours. The most common method of incision and drainage (Figure 42–19) is to make a short sagittal midline distal wound immediately over the tendon and introduce a small plastic catheter into the synovial bursa for irrigating with an antibiotic solution. The catheter should pass through the sheath and exit by a counterincision in the palm to allow for drainage of the fluid. Not all surgeons advocate placement of an irrigation catheter, however. When a catheter is placed, it should remain for only 24-48 hours. These incisions do not cross flexion creases. The hand should then be elevated and immobilized in the position of function and covered by a dressing. Phlegmonous tenosynovitis usually requires opening of the entire synovial sheath (often through a lateral midaxial digital incision or longitudinally across the wrist for extensor sheath infections) and, frequently, excision of necrotic tendon and sometimes amputation of a digit.

▶ Other Infections

Necrotizing soft tissue infections of the upper extremity are rare but devastating when they occur. The condition has been called many different names such as necrotizing fasciitis, Meleney ulcer, and streptococcal gangrene. The organisms responsible include clostridium species, *Streptococcus pyogenes*, and mixed infections. The hallmarks are the rapid spread of infection and the extensive necrosis of soft tissue. Treatment includes wide debridement of the necrotic tissue and intravenous antibiotics.

Human bite wounds of the hand occur most often during altercations when the fist strikes an opponent's tooth. The MCP joint can be entered. The injury is often ignored by the patient until infection of the joint has begun. The joint must be explored and cleaned and the patient treated with antibiotics to cover oral flora (penicillin). Once the infection reaches the joint, destruction of the cartilage often occurs despite all therapy.

An inordinate amount of pain, with little or no swelling or induration, predating and accompanying the appearance of multiple tiny vesicles, suggests **herpes simplex (herpetic whitlow)**. The vesicles may appear cyclically. They contain clear fluid and not pus and should be distinguished from paronychia. Antibiotics are not indicated in this self-limited viral infection. Acyclovir 5% ointment applied topically for 7 days decreases the severity and duration of symptoms but is of no value in prophylaxis.

Tuberculous infection of the hand is usually chronic and may be relatively painless. Some cultures take months to become positive. Tuberculosis commonly involves only one hand, which may be the only focus of infection in the body. Bones and joints may be infected, but the process more commonly involves the tendon synovium, which becomes matted to the tendons. Treatment is by synovectomy and antituberculous drug therapy for 6-12 months.

Leprosy causes neuritis of the median and ulnar nerves, resulting in sensory and motor loss to the hand. Crippling claw deformities develop as a result of intrinsic muscle palsy. Open sores appear on the hands as a result of trauma to anesthetic digits. Reconstructive surgery and occupational training are required.

Fungal infections involve primarily the nails. Tinea unguium (onychomycosis) may be caused by many organisms, including *Epidermophyton floccosum, Trichophyton*, and *Candida albicans*. Prolonged treatment with antifungal drugs—griseofulvin systemically or nystatin topically—may be necessary, along with daily applications of fungicidal agents such as tolnaftate. Removal of the nail is advocated for chronic intractable cases.

Nikkhah D, Rodrigues J, Osman, et al: Pyogenic flexor tenosynovitis: one year's experience at a UK hand unit and a review of the current literature. *Hand Surg* 2012;17:199.

Ritting AW, O'Malley MP, Rodner CM: Acute paronychia. *J Hand Surg Am* 2012;37:1068.

Shoji K, Cavanaugh Z, Rodner CM: Acute fight bite. *J Hand Surg* 2013;38:1612.

McDonald LS, Bavaro MF, Hofmeister, et al: Hand infections. *J Hand Surg Am* 2011;36:1403.

▼ INFLAMMATORY DISORDERS OF THE HAND

DUPUYTREN CONTRACTURE

▶ Palmar Fasciitis

The cause of Dupuytren contracture, which is common particularly among white populations of Celtic origin, is not known. It occurs in one of three types (acute, subacute, and chronic), predominately in men over 50 who have been in sedentary occupations, and is bilateral in about half of cases. There is a hereditary influence, and the incidence is higher among idiopathic epileptics, diabetics, alcoholics, and patients with chronic illnesses. The contracture may develop in people who do not work and (in laborers) in the hand that does the least work, so that it is not considered work related. It is frequently found in the plantar fascia of the instep and occasionally in the penis (Peyronie disease).

Dupuytren contracture manifests itself most commonly in the palm by thickening, which may be nodular, and therefore mistaken for a callosity, or may be cord-like, and therefore mistaken for a tendon abnormality because it passes into the digits and restricts their extension. This process typically involves the longitudinal and vertical components of the fascia but at times seems to exist apart from anatomically distinct fascia. The skin may fuse with the underlying fascia and become raised and hard, or it may be greatly shrunken and sometimes drawn into a deeply puckered crevasse. The disorder invades the palm at the expense of fat but is never adherent to vessels, nerves, or musculotendinous structures (though it may be adherent to flexor tendon sheaths). It has an unpredictable rate of progression, but the earlier it starts in life, the more destructive and recurrent it is apt to be.

Dupuytren fasciitis may involve any digit or web space, but it affects predominantly the ring and small fingers. In long-standing cases, the fingers may be drawn tightly into the palm, resulting in secondary contracture of joint capsule and ligaments, flexor sheaths, and atrophic muscles.

The most recent addition for the treatment of Dupuytren contracture is enzyme (collagenase) injection. Based on early studies, it appears that this treatment works best on MCP contractures rather than PIP contractures in patients with a well-defined cord. This treatment does require two office visits, one for the injection and a follow-up visit to manipulate and rupture the cord.

Surgery is indicated when the disorder has progressed sufficiently, especially when it causes more than 30 degrees of flexion at the MCP joint or any flexion contracture of the PIP joint. The patient must be warned about the increasing technical difficulty with progressive flexion and adduction contractures and the potential for recurrence after surgery. Fasciectomy is the surgical procedure that gives the best long-term results. In selected cases where only the longitudinal pretendinous fascial band is involved and the skin moves freely over it, subcutaneous fasciotomy done through a small longitudinal incision may release a contracture quite well with only a few days of postoperative disability. In the occasional case with acute and rapid onset of a tender nodule, local triamcinolone may be used for subjective and even objective relief.

Depending on the amount of cutaneous shrinkage, skin grafts may be required for wound closure after fasciectomy. The overlying dermis has been implicated as an inductive mechanism in this process. Thus, skin grafting may diminish the recurrence rate in severe cases. The hopelessly contracted little finger must sometimes be amputated.

Motion should be started within 3-5 days after surgery. Dynamic splints and postoperative injection of corticosteroids into joints and the zone of surgery may help the well-motivated patient.

The potential complications of surgery are wound breakdown (loss of skin flaps), hematoma, fibrosis and stiffness, digital nerve injury, recurrence of contractures and digital ischemia secondary to digital artery injury. Reflex sympathetic dystrophy, a painful, debilitating neurologic disorder of the hand, can occur after surgery and must be treated aggressively. In general, the functional reward for the patient is great at any age.

Brandt KE: An evidence-based approach to Dupuytren's contracture. *Plast Reconstr Surg* 2010;126:2210.

Desai SS, Hentz: The treatment of Dupuytren disease. *J Hand Surg* 2011;36:936.

Hentz VR, Watt AJ, Desai SS, et al: Advances in the management of Dupuytren disease: collagenase. *Hand Clin* 2012;28:551.

DEGENERATIVE & RHEUMATOID ARTHRITIS

Arthritis of the hand is divided into two categories. **Degenerative changes** are usually due to some trauma resulting in damage to the bone or cartilage or to the supporting ligamentous structures. The increased wear to the joint results in inflammation and damage to the cartilage or underlying bone followed by reactive new bone formation (spurs). The wrists, hips, and knees are most commonly affected. **Rheumatoid arthritis** is a systemic disease characterized by synovial inflammation. The diseased synovium destroys adjacent tendons and joints in a specific way, leading to characteristic deformities in the hand.

Patients with degenerative arthritis complain of pain, aching, and stiffness in the area of the affected joint. Progression of the problem leads to immobility of the joint that affects the entire hand. Radiographic studies demonstrate joint narrowing and periosteal thickening early in the problem, progressing to bone spurs, loss of the articular surface, and bone destruction later. Patients with rheumatoid arthritis often present with very severe deformities without pain. Nodules around the olecranon and dorsum of the hand are often found. Both flexor and extensor tendons at the wrist can be inflamed, limiting tendon movement and resulting in rupture of the tendon. Involvement of the tendons and ligaments at the digits and MCP joints results in ulnar deviation of the digits, MCP joint destruction and dislocation, and swan-neck and boutonnière deformities. Destruction of the wrist joint is also common.

Arthritis is common among older patients and usually treated by primary care physicians and rheumatologists with anti-inflammatory medications and modification of the patient's activities. In most cases, it is only when symptoms greatly hinder the patient's lifestyle that they are referred to a hand surgeon. Physical therapy, splints, and medications are often no longer effective for these patients.

Surgical treatment of painful joints includes replacement with a prosthetic joint and partial or full fusion. Prosthetic joints of metal or Silastic permit near-normal movement but can become unstable and dislocate or degenerate over time. For a durable solution to the problem, fusion of the joint is recommended. Motion is severely limited, but pain relief is complete. There are more therapeutic options for the wrist, such as replacement, local fusion of only the affected carpal bone, or complete excision of the proximal row of carpal bones, leaving motion and stability to the distal carpal bones and ligaments.

Therapy for synovial inflammation in rheumatoid disease includes excision of the synovium to increase tendon excursion and prevent rupture, repair of ruptured tendons, and excision of painful nodules. Tendon-balancing procedures can help ulnar deviation of the MCP joints and improve joint movement. The most important concept of treating patients with rheumatoid hand disease is that often the patients have adapted well to their functional deficits. Correcting a physical deformity in a well-compensated patient may actually result in more problems for that patient.

Adams J, Ryall C, Pandyan A, et al: Proximal interphalangeal joint replacement in patients with arthritis of the hand: a meta analysis. *J Bone Joint Surg Br* 2012;94:1305.

Cavaliere CM, Chung KC: A systemic review of total wrist arthroplasty compared with total wrist arthrodesis for rheumatoid arthritis. *Plast Reconstr Surg* 2008;122:813.

Chacko AT, Rozental TD: The rheumatoid thumb. *Hand Clin* 2008;24:307.

Ono S, Entezami P, Chung KC: Reconstruction of the rheumatoid hand. *Clin Plast Surg* 2011;38:713.

Schindele SF, Herren DB, Simmen BR: Tendon reconstruction of the rheumatoid hand. *Hand Clin* 2011;27:105.

SCLERODERMA & LUPUS ERYTHEMATOSUS

These systemic diseases of unknown cause have distinctive—though not necessarily pathognomonic—manifestations in the hands.

Scleroderma initially produces joint stiffness, hyperhidrosis, and Raynaud phenomenon. Unchecked, it leads to marked tautness of skin and rigidity of joints with associated osteoporosis (even atrophy and ultimate resorption of the distal phalanges) and soft tissue calcifications.

Lupus erythematosus, which may be initiated or aggravated by certain drugs, foreign proteins, or psychic states, often causes polyarthritis indistinguishable from that of rheumatoid arthritis. It does not usually lead to similar joint destruction. Vasospasm in both lupus and scleroderma can cause severe ischemia of the hand and digits and may require therapy to prevent gangrene.

GOUT

Gout is a metabolic disorder of uric acid metabolism that affects about 1% of the population; approximately 50% of patients with gout have **cheiragra** (gouty hands).

The diagnosis is suggested by a rapid onset of severe pain and inflammatory signs about the joints and musculoten-dinous structure, simulating a phlegmonous infectious cellulitis with marked induration (most dramatically seen about the elbow). The usual duration of an attack is 5-10 days. The serum uric acid is elevated in 75% of cases. Gout may coexist with rheumatoid disease. The diagnosis is confirmed by identification of uric acid crystals in joint fluid or tissue biopsy.

In time, typical tophi form, consisting of toothpaste-like infiltrates of urate crystals, arising in multilobulated form about soft tissue structures that have been invaded. X-rays show characteristic punched-out lesions at the margins of articular cartilage.

Prophylactic treatment of gouty arthritis consists of diet, colchicine, allopurinol (a urate-blocking agent) or probenecid (a uricosuric agent), and avoidance of stress. Colchicine, 0.6 mg/h with a glass of water for six to eight doses or to the point of gastrointestinal distress, is the time-honored means of interrupting an attack, but phenylbutazone, topical corticotropin gel, and systemic corticosteroids are also of value.

Surgical measures consist of drainage of abscessed tophi (seldom needed) and tophectomy. The latter procedure is more often of cosmetic rather than functional value. Tophectomy consists of removal of as much tophaceous material as can be fairly easily recovered. The surgeon should be careful not to destroy ligaments, tenoretinacular structures, nerves, and vessels in the process.

Porter SB, Murray PM: Raynaud phenomenon. *J Hand Surg Am* 2013;38:375.

Tripoli M, Falcone AR, Mossuto C, et al: Different surgical approaches to treat chronic tophaceous gout in the hand: our experience. *Tech Hand Up Extrem Surg* 2010;14:187.

Wasserman A, Brahn E: Systemic sclerosis: bilateral improvement of Raynaud's phenomenon with unilateral digital sympathectomy. *Semin Arthritis Rheum* 2010;40:137.

BURNS & FROSTBITE OF THE HAND

▶ Thermal Burns

The hands are a common site of thermal (including frictional), electrical, chemical, and radiation burns. Function is imperiled in all instances by swelling and scar formation. Prompt measures to preserve existing function are often urgently required. Burns over other areas of the body may be more life threatening and require more urgent attention,

but burns of the hand should never be neglected. Delay in therapy leads to irreversible impairment and deformity that are impossible to correct later.

As in other areas of the body, thermal burns are grouped into three degrees. Superficial (first-degree) burns are red and painful; partial-thickness (second-degree) burns develop blisters; and full-thickness (third-degree) burns are insensate and appear like leather or charred tissue. The prognosis and therapy depend on the location, depth, and extent of the burn.

All burns to the hand cause swelling of the tissues, and the need for elevation of the arm to relieve pain and prevent stiffness cannot be overemphasized. Tetanus immunization should be given. Cold compresses may help alleviate the pain in first-degree burns. Second-degree burns must be watched more carefully. Large blisters restricting motion are broken. Otherwise, since they are sterile, they should be left intact. Treatment with thrice-daily washing and silver sulfadiazine is usually adequate. Patients with third-degree burns or superficial burns that fail to heal and patients unable to care for their burns at home should be admitted to the hospital.

Deeper burns require close observation and more extensive treatment. In the first few hours after injury, circumferential or near-circumferential burns may cause ischemia in the extremity. Because evaluation of sensory function and capillary refill is nearly impossible in these limbs, escharotomies should be performed if compartment syndrome is suspected. If done correctly, escharotomies have few complications, since these burns usually require surgical debridement anyway. Incisions are placed to avoid exposure of neurovascular structures.

Partial-thickness burns heal spontaneously. Deeper burns on the dorsum of the hand are best treated with early excision of the eschar and placement of skin grafts to prevent contractures. Palmar burns are best left to heal spontaneously because skin grafts function very poorly in this area. Some hand surgeons believe that excision and grafting of superficial burns should be performed to prevent contractures. This is true if adequate therapy has not been available. In burn units with good rehabilitation services, surgeons are treating superficial second-degree burns without surgery and obtaining results as good as with skin grafting. Pigskin, cadaver homografts, or a number of commercially available biologic dressings can be used to cover the wounds temporarily, decreasing pain and keeping the wound moist until autologous skin grafts are placed.

Neglected burns of the hands result in contracture deformities that often require extensive surgery to restore function. Delayed healing and wound contractures often result in a claw hand with MCP hyperextension and fusion of the digits with loss of the web space (syndactyly). Burns on the volar surface leave flexion contractures. Some contractures can be treated with release and skin grafting of the tissue gap. Web space contractures and released contractures with exposed tendons or nerves must be covered with skin or muscle flaps. Web space release is done with skin flaps from the dorsum folded down to create the space. Large flaps can be obtained by attaching the hand to the groin, allowing the tissue to adhere and vascularize before cutting the flap away from the groin. Recently, free tissue transfer from other parts of the body using microsurgical techniques has allowed more extensive reconstruction of severely burned hands.

▶ Electrical Burns

Electrical burns of the upper extremity may not appear extensive on initial inspection. The skin may be burned only in a very small area of the entry point of the current or by ignited clothing. The current tends to spare the skin but damage underlying muscles, vessels, and nerves. Often, the extent of dead tissue is not evident for several days.

Initial treatment is the same as for thermal burns. Since muscle damage may be extensive, it is important to prevent renal failure from myoglobinuria by maintaining a high output of alkaline urine. Arteriography, fluorescein injections, and radionuclide studies may help delineate the extent of necrosis. Examination of the patient in the operating room is still the most accurate method of assessing the extent of tissue damage. All obviously dead tissue should be removed during the initial evaluation. Two or three days later, the patient is reexamined in the operating room and any additional debris is removed. The wounds are closed when only clearly viable tissue remains.

▶ Frostbite

Frostbite occurs most often in people under the influence of alcohol or with psychiatric illness. The lower extremity is affected more often than the upper. Freezing tissue causes cellular death and vascular thrombosis. Hypothermia of the entire body must first be treated. The frozen part should be quickly rewarmed by immersion in warm water (40°C). Elevation of the extremity minimizes edema. Skin wounds are treated like burns with silver sulfadiazine cream. The extent of necrosis may not be obvious for several weeks, and debridement or amputation should be delayed until demarcation of the injury occurs. Sympathectomy may help ameliorate the sequelae of frostbite, such as cold sensitivity and pain. Children with frostbite may develop premature closure of phalangeal epiphyses, which creates growth disturbances of the bone.

Arnoldo BD, Purdue GF: The diagnosis and management of electrical injuries. *Hand Clin* 2009;25:469.

Kreymerman PA, Andres LA, Lucas, et al: Reconstruction of the burned hand. *Plast Reconstr Surg* 2011;127:752.

Mohr WJ, Jenabzadeh K, Ahrenholz DH: Cold injury. *Hand Clin* 2009;25:481.

Moore ML, Dewey WS, Richard RL: Rehabilitation of the burned hand. *Hand Clin* 2009;25:529.

MASSES OF THE HAND

Only 2% of all masses in the hand are malignant lesions; the majority are benign neoplasms, cysts, or a myriad of other masses. Though the clinician must be ever vigilant to identify malignancy, a mass of the hand is highly likely to be benign—excisional biopsies are thus reserved for subcutaneous lesions that are rapidly growing or for skin lesions that may be carcinomas. Otherwise, masses can be observed over a period of time to determine that they are not growing. They may be removed for functional or cosmetic reasons.

Ganglions are formed by herniation of the synovial lining of joints or tendons into the surrounding soft tissue. These cysts are filled with a viscous fluid thought to be modified joint fluid. Trauma to the wrist or hand may cause extrusion of the synovium, but it is more likely that the ganglion was already present and that trauma to that area merely brought the lesion to the surgeon's attention.

Ganglions can arise from any joint of the hand but most commonly appear on the dorsal wrist over the scapholunate ligament and the volar wrist near the radial artery. Tendon ganglions are most common on the flexor sheath at the metacarpal head (A1 pulley). Pain and tenderness are due to compression of adjacent nerves by the mass.

Ganglions have a typical appearance, and diagnosis is simple. If any doubt exists, aspiration with a large-bore needle of the viscous fluid confirms the diagnosis and occasionally cures the lesions. Injection of the empty sac with steroids and lidocaine may help to keep the mass from reappearing, but the majority recurs. Ganglions need not be treated unless they cause pain or interfere with hand function. Often, it is enough just to reassure the patient that the mass is benign.

Operative removal of ganglions should be done using loupe magnification and a tourniquet. The entire ganglion should be removed, including all attachments to the joint capsule and the underlying ligament, without injuring the surrounding structures. Prolonged splinting after removal of ganglions does not decrease recurrence rates but does cause hand stiffness. Unfortunately, despite careful surgical removal of the lesion, recurrence of ganglions is relatively common.

Epidermal cysts are rests of epidermis located in the subcutaneous tissue. Many are thought to be due to traumatic disruption of epidermal cells into the soft tissue (inclusion cyst). The cells proliferate just as skin does and form a cyst filled with creamy keratin, the remains of dead epidermal cells that usually desquamate from the skin. Infected cysts become inflamed and form abscesses. Removal of the entire cyst wall is required to prevent abscess formation.

Pyogenic granuloma may form in any chronic wound. Histologically, it consists of vascular tissue identical to granulation tissue. Just as for hypertrophic granulation tissue elsewhere on the body, excision or cautery of the material flush to skin level allows epidermis to migrate over the wound.

Giant cell tumors are benign, multilobulated, solid masses found on the lateral aspects of the finger. They are often attached to the tendon sheath. The mass may be quite complex and extend throughout the adjacent nerves, vessels, tendons, and ligaments. The entire lesion should be removed, but recurrence is relatively common.

The most common bone tumors are **enchondromas.** Multiple enchondromas (Ollier disease) are associated with other skeletal deformities. The lesion appears on x-ray as thinned cortical bone with speckled calcifications. Fractures through the tumors usually do not heal spontaneously. The tumor should be removed with a curette. Bone graft taken from the distal radius is used to fill the gap if needed.

A **carpal boss** is due to abnormal bone formation at the base of the second or third metacarpal bones and presents as a hard mass on the dorsum of the hand. The excess growth of bone can be removed if symptomatic.

Glomus tumors are composed of blood vessels and unmyelinated nerves of a heat-regulating arteriovenous malformation. They are usually found in the fingertip or under the fingernail and can be extremely painful. Local excision of the tumor is curative. Occasionally, when the tumor is large and disrupts the nail matrix, a split-thickness nail graft from another digit is needed to reconstruct the defect.

The most common malignant tumor of the hand is **squamous cell carcinoma**, though **basal cell carcinomas** and **melanomas** also occur. Subungual melanomas are often difficult to diagnose because they are difficult to examine. These tumors should be treated just the same as elsewhere on the body. Particular care should be taken to examine for spread of tumor in the lymphatic drainage at the supratrochlear and axillary nodes.

Other tumors include lipomas, fibromas, hemangiomas, arteriovenous malformations, neurofibromas, sarcomas, and various skin lesions. These tumors act no differently in the hand than elsewhere in the body. However, because of the close proximity of the nervous and vascular structures within the small spaces of the hand, these tumors cause compressive signs and symptoms sooner. CT scans or MRI help delineate the extent of soft tissue tumors and may help in preoperative planning.

Abzug JM, Cappel MA: Benign acquired superficial skin lesions of the hand. *J Hand Surg Am* 2012;37:378.

English C, Hammert WC: Cutaneous malignancies of the upper extremity. *J Hand Surg Am* 2012;37:367.

Gant J, Ruff M, Janz BA: Wrist ganglions. *J Hand Surg Am* 2011;36:510.

Sookur PA, Saifuddin A: Indeterminate soft-tissue tumors of the hand and wrist: a review based on a clinical series of 39 cases. *Skeletal Radiol* 2011;40:977.

COMPLEX HAND INJURIES

▶ Crush Injuries & Amputations

Advances in microvascular surgery have greatly increased our ability to treat complex hand injuries. Mangled and amputated digits, hands, as well as entire upper extremities have been replanted or repaired. Complex nerve repairs, microvascular free tissue transfers of muscle flaps, and toe-to-hand reconstructions have made it possible to restore more function to severely injured hands. The end result must be a sensate, painless, and useful extremity. Patients who undergo multiple surgical procedures and prolonged rehabilitation with only marginal results would have benefited from early amputation. A surgeon with extensive experience can best assess the patient's injuries, occupational requirements, and psychosocial needs to determine if salvage is worthwhile.

Complex hand injuries often result from improper use or malfunction of machinery. Heavy machinery in the workplace or motorized cutting tools at home, such as rotary saws, are often cited as the mechanism of injury. Sharply amputated or partially devascularized parts are most likely to be saved. Severe crushing or avulsion of the part produces wider nerve and vessel injury. The extent of this type of damage is difficult to determine and often impossible to repair.

The decision to try to salvage a damaged part must be individualized to each situation, but some general principles apply. The thumb is crucial to hand function, and all efforts are made to save the entire digit or as much length as possible. When multiple digits or half of the hand is damaged or amputated, a greater effort is made to repair the part. Children can recover function in badly damaged extremities far better than adults can, and any amputated parts in children should be replanted. Replantation of the entire arm at the elbow and above is controversial. The usefulness of these replanted limbs is limited by the slow nerve regeneration, and some hand surgeons believe that amputations in these cases result in better function.

Patients with complex hand injuries should be immediately referred to a regional center with the staff and facilities to manage the problems. Occasionally, in the rush to transfer patients with these very obvious injuries, intra-abdominal, neurologic, and other less obvious injuries have been overlooked. The entire patient must be evaluated and stabilized prior to transfer. A clean, moist dressing should be placed on the wound and the extremity elevated. The amputated part is wrapped in a plastic bag and placed in ice water. The amputated part should never be frozen.

The accepting hand surgeon evaluates the patient's overall condition, potential for rehabilitation, and personal wishes before coming to a decision. To revascularize or replant a part, the patient must be taken urgently to the operating room. Ischemia over 6 hours is often associated with failure of revascularization, but—depending on the metabolic needs of the constituent tissues—extremities that have undergone periods of ischemia longer than this can be successfully replanted.

Bone must first be stabilized with Kirschner wires or metal plates before vascular repairs are performed. Arterial and venous repairs are done with microscopic magnification, and the ischemic tissue is reperfused. Failure of a replanted part is more often due to venous outflow problems than arterial inflow. Systemic and local anticoagulants help to maintain perfusion but are not always needed. Leeches placed on the part release a potent local anticoagulant and can decrease venous congestion. Nerve and tendon repairs must also be performed. When there is inadequate local soft tissue to cover the repaired structures, muscle or skin flaps from a distant site must be transferred using microsurgical methods to the area. Although these operations are not life threatening, blood loss can be extensive and transfusions are sometimes required.

Secondary procedures to free tendon adhesions, reduce bulky flaps, and transfer tendons in motor nerve injuries may need to be done. Reconstruction of unsuccessful replantations is being done more often. The original method using toes to reconstruct thumbs has also been used to make fingers. These reconstructions give patients the ability to grasp objects. Because these digits are sensate, they can even perform fine movement tasks not possible with prosthetic devices. Patients with loss only of the thumb are better treated with transfer of the index finger to the thumb position (pollicization).

Partial or total loss of a single digit is less critical. Hand function is better without a stiff or painful digit. When a decision is made to amputate a digit, care must be taken to leave a painless stump with good sensate soft tissue coverage. The flexor tendon must not be sutured to the extensor tendon for soft tissue coverage, since this will cause the tendons to pull each other rather than move the joint. Local flaps to cover the stump are preferred to skin grafts or cross-finger flaps, since they usually provide better sensation. A short amputation stump on the long or ring finger is often bothersome because small objects such as coins tend to fall out of the palm, and a ray amputation eliminates the problem. For cosmetic purposes, ray amputations are far less noticeable than partial amputations. The loss of hand breadth with a ray amputation can decrease grip strength, however.

The loss of part of all of the hand can be compensated both functionally and cosmetically by a variety of prostheses. Their use involves careful adaptation to the requirements of the patient, who must receive appropriate training to ensure success.

INJECTION INJURIES OF THE HAND

High-pressure devices used in industry to apply material such as air, grease, paint, and oil cause a unique hand injury.

The typical case is injection of the material into the index finger of the nondominant hand of a factory worker. A pinpoint injection site may be the only external evidence of injury, and the hand appears discolored or pale, or swollen due to the injected material.

The examination should include a careful hand evaluation and an x-ray to demonstrate the distribution of material or gas in the hand. All such cases require continued, unrelenting scrutiny, even if the part seems completely normal. If there is any evidence of retained foreign material, swelling, or ischemia, early surgical exploration is advocated to release the tourniquet effect of the skin and fascia and to remove as much of the material as possible without injuring healthy tissue. Prophylactic antisludging agents (dextran 40), corticosteroids, and antibiotics may help.

Often, the pressure forces the material to spread along the tendon sheaths throughout the hand and even into the forearm. Expansion of the foreign material in a closed space and the chemical irritation cause congestion, inflammation, vascular thrombosis, and gangrene. The injected material is difficult to remove completely, and a foreign-body response leads to fibrosis so extensive that it often destroys the function of the hand.

Davis Sears E, Chung KC: Replantation of finger avulsion injuries: a systematic review of survival and functional outcomes. *J Hand Surg Am* 2011;36:686.

Friedrich JB, Vedder NB: Thumb reconstruction. *Clin Plast Surg* 2011;38:697.

Hegge T, Neumeister MW: Mutilated hand injuries. *Clin Plast Surg* 2011;38:543.

Hogan CJ, Ruland RT: High-pressure injection injuries to the upper extremity: a review of the literature. *J Orthop Trauma* 2006;20:503.

Leversedge FJ, More TJ, Peterson BC, et al: Compartment syndrome of the upper extremity. *J Hand Surg* 2011;36:544.

Ninkovic M, Voigt S, Dornseifer U, et al: Microsurgical advances in extremity salvage. *Clin Plast Surg* 2012;39:491.

MINIMALLY INVASIVE HAND SURGERY

The goal of reconstructive hand surgery is return of normal function, including pain-free movement, normal active and passive range of motion, premorbid strength, and intact sensation. Yet the process of incising, dissecting, and sewing is associated with significant scarring and pain. Scarring is especially troublesome in the hand, since it leads to stiffness, ligamental tightening, and arthritis. As a result, any procedure in the hand that minimizes postoperative scarring or pain will contribute to an improved result.

Surgical care in the past decade has been revolutionized by the introduction and incorporation of minimally invasive surgical techniques. Laparoscopies and thoracoscopies have permitted the resection of hollow and solid organs through

1 cm incisions, reducing the need for laparotomies and thoracotomies. Likewise, urologists have employed cystoscopy for evaluation and treatment of bladder and kidney disorders, while orthopedic surgeons have used arthroscopy to similar effective ends in the knee, ankle, elbow, and shoulder.

Two areas of hand surgery incorporate minimally invasive techniques: Wrist arthroscopy has expanded the options for evaluating the chronically painful wrist, and endoscopic carpal tunnel release (ECTR) provides a less invasive method than open release for decompressing the median nerve. While ECTR theoretically allows for a faster recovery, it may in fact offer only limited advantages.

WRIST ARTHROSCOPY

Diagnostic wrist arthroscopy was first successfully used in 1970. Over the past three decades, it has taken its place among traditional imaging techniques as a low-morbidity method for evaluating chronic wrist pain. As the hardware for examining the wrist has become more sophisticated and as hand surgeons have become more familiar with the arthroscopic view of the wrist, increasingly aggressive attempts have been made to use the arthroscope to treat as well as to diagnose wrist problems.

▶ Indications & Contraindications

Diagnostic wrist arthroscopy is a useful technique to evaluate patients with wrist pain, whether chronic or acute. In patients with chronic pain, this technique can be used to augment information offered by plain radiographs, CT, MRI, or wrist arthrography. It can confirm an uncertain diagnosis or be used to reevaluate a patient who has failed other treatments. In contrast, patients with acute symptoms—such as those suffering from mechanical wrist pain—may complain of pain localized over the joint, catching and popping sensations, and relief with rest. Here, the wrist can be manipulated during arthroscopy to localize the source of the symptoms. In general, the technique is useful for evaluating articular cartilage, ligaments, the triangular fibrocartilage complex (TFCC), and the synovium. Interestingly, diagnostic wrist arthroscopy may provide too comprehensive an examination. Only some of the lesions that are visualized during an examination may be responsible for a patient's symptoms. The hand surgeon must critically correlate arthroscopic findings with the patient's examination to arrive at the appropriate diagnosis.

Therapeutic wrist arthroscopy is useful for the treatment of ligament tears, TFCC lesions, articular cartilage lesions, subtle distal radius and carpus fractures, dorsal wrist ganglions, removal of isolated carpal bones up to and including the proximal carpal row, and disorders of the distal radioulnar joint. It is useful also in the management of lesions arising from rheumatoid arthritis. It has been successfully used in completing synovectomies, proximal row carpectomies in the case of scaphoid nonunion or scapholunate collapse, radial styloidectomy, and isolated symptomatic chondral defects.

▶ Procedure

Equipment for diagnostic wrist arthroscopy includes an apparatus for elevating and distracting the wrist, an arthroscopic telescope, a video camera, a fluid infusion system, and both manual and powered instruments.

Either general or regional anesthesia may be used. A tourniquet is placed at the mid-arm to provide a blood-free field during the operation. The distal forearm, wrist, and hand are prepared into the operative field. Traction is applied to the hand, usually via sterile finger traps, and a distraction force is applied across the wrist.

Individual skin incisions are then made at standard portal sites determined by the goal of the operation. Portal sites are described according to their relationship with the radius and ulna, the carpal bones, and the extensor tendons. The relationship to the extensor tendons is indicated by listing the extensor compartments on either side of the incision. Typical portals include the 3-4 radiocarpal, through which the scaphoid and lunate facets can be visualized; the 4-5 radiocarpal, through which the TFCC and the ulnocarpal ligaments can be seen; and the 6R radiocarpal, through which the extensor carpi ulnaris tendon and ulnar wrist are approached. The midcarpal joint is approached through any of three portals, including the midcarpal ulnar, the midcarpal radial, and the scaphotrapezial-trapezoid.

Once abnormalities are identified, therapeutic wrist arthroscopy can be used to effect repairs. Partial ligament tears and tears of the TFCC can be debrided arthroscopically using knife blades and motorized shavers. Carpal bone resections can be completed with miniature osteotomes and powered saw blades.

▶ Outcomes

Operations employing diagnostic and therapeutic wrist arthroscopy typically result in less swelling, less postoperative pain, and less stiffness than comparable open wrist procedures. There is a concomitant earlier return to function and work. Therapeutic wrist arthroscopy even of dorsal wrist ganglia, the most superficial of wrist abnormalities, is followed by fewer—or no more—recurrences than the open technique.

▶ Complications

The rate of complications associated with diagnostic and therapeutic wrist arthroscopy is estimated to be 2% and is due to a variety of causes. The continuous traction necessary to properly distract the wrist can cause problems, including ligamental strain at the MCP joints with concomitant joint edema and stiffness and stretching of peripheral nerves.

Establishment of the operative portals can damage articular cartilage, ligaments, tendons, cutaneous nerves, the radial artery, and cutaneous and deep veins. Such injuries include abrasions, contusions, lacerations, and transections. A high proportion of complications of therapeutic wrist arthroscopy are associated with inadequate relief of symptoms or a diminished return of function. A now less common complication of therapeutic wrist arthroscopy results from the fluid infusion. Forearm compartment syndromes have resulted from extravasation of infusion fluid during endoscopic repair of distal radius fractures; this problem is now avoided by circumferential compression of the forearm during the procedure.

ENDOSCOPIC CARPAL TUNNEL RELEASE

Endoscopic release of the transverse carpal ligament is an increasingly popular method of treating carpal tunnel syndrome. Advocates of the procedure claim that it is associated with decreased postoperative morbidity and earlier return to work. Others caution that there is little if any short-term difference between endoscopic and open carpal tunnel release, no long-term difference, and that endoscopic carpal tunnel release is associated with an increased likelihood of significant nerve injury.

▶ Indications & Contraindications

Endoscopic carpal tunnel release is easier to perform in patients with larger wrists. Ease of access to the carpal tunnel correlates with the wrist circumference and the height and age of patients. Surgeons should be aware that the procedure is likely to be more difficult in small patients with small wrists and are advised to maintain a lower threshold for conversion to the open technique to avoid neurologic complications.

Absolute contraindications to endoscopic carpal tunnel release include masses in the carpal canal and other space-occupying lesions, abnormalities in canal anatomy, and wrist stiffness that precludes proper positioning.

▶ Procedure

In the United States, most surgeons use one of two techniques—either Chow or Agee. The two differ primarily in the number of incisions, or portals, needed to gain access. The Chow technique, first described in 1989, employs two portals, while the Agee technique requires only one.

Either operation can be performed under local anesthesia with a brachial tourniquet. An initial transverse incision is made proximal to the wrist flexion crease between the palmaris longus and flexor carpi ulnaris tendons. The space between the transverse carpal ligament and the flexor tendons is defined with a dissector. In the Agee procedure, the endoscope is advanced under the transverse carpal liga-ment, radial to the hook of the hamate along the axis of the ring finger. The ligament is incised along its entire length, with care taken to avoid the Guyon canal and the superficial palmar arch. In the Chow operation, a second transverse incision is made just distal to the transverse carpal ligament along the axis of the ring finger. The wrist is dorsiflexed, and a slotted cannula is advanced into the proximal incision, deep to the transverse carpal ligament, and out the distal incision. The endoscope is then used to visualize the ligament while the knife divides it. The wounds are closed, and the patient's wrist placed in dorsiflexion.

▶ Outcomes

Several studies have compared open versus endoscopic carpal tunnel release, focusing on the incidence of recovery from symptoms, the time span until the patient returns to work, and the incidence of recurrence of symptoms. Overall, both techniques have equivalent outcomes.

Many of the most convincing studies are prospective randomized trials. One such study, comparing open and endoscopic carpal tunnel release among 32 hands in 29 patients, found no difference in postoperative recovery time or surgical result. The only significant difference noted by the authors was transient numbness on the radial side of the ring finger in three endoscopic carpal tunnel release patients.

In another study, the authors compared in a prospective randomized manner the early outcome of carpal tunnel release using either a conventional open carpal tunnel release procedure in 40 patients or a two-portal endoscopic release in 56 patients. They found no statistically significant difference between the groups in postoperative pain, recovery from paresthesias, or time taken to return to work. However, the endoscopic group demonstrated better grip strength recovery at 1 and 3 months. No surgical complications were observed in either group.

Nonrandomized studies have supported this trend. An analysis of 191 consecutive patients undergoing carpal tunnel release with an average 2-year follow-up showed that none of the patients undergoing open release had a recurrence, while 7% of patients undergoing endoscopic release had recurrences. Another study observed a higher incidence of incomplete release of the carpal tunnel with endoscopic techniques than with standard open releases.

The factors identified with poor outcomes in endoscopic carpal tunnel release are similar to those seen in open release. Less satisfactory results were present in workers' compensation cases; patients with normal motor latencies on nerve conduction studies; patients with preoperative hand weakness, widened two-point discrimination, myofascial pain syndrome, or fibromyalgia; and patients involved in litigation, those with multiple compressive neuropathies, and those with abnormal psychologic factors.

▶ Complications

Only a limited number of studies include a sufficient number of patients to compare complication rates and type between endoscopic and open carpal tunnel release. Overall, the types and rates of complications between the two forms of release are similar. Nonetheless, isolated but severe complications from endoscopic release over the past decade tend to dramatize its risk.

The study by Boeckstyns and Sorensen is perhaps the most comprehensive to date. These authors analyzed 54 published series of endoscopic and open releases comprising 9516 and 1203 patients, respectively. Irreversible nerve damage from the procedure occurred in 0.3% of endoscopic and 0.2% of open releases, including such injuries as transection of the median nerve. While reversible nerve injuries were more common with endoscopic release than with open release (4.4% vs 0.9%, respectively, among prospective controlled and randomized studies), tendon lesions, reflex sympathetic dystrophy, hematoma, and wound problems were equally common with either technique.

A less compelling analysis—a retrospective survey of hand surgeons who had performed either open or endoscopic carpal tunnel release over the preceding 5 years—found major complications with both approaches, including median nerve lacerations, ulnar nerve lacerations, digital nerve lacerations, vessel lacerations, and tendon lacerations. While the authors could not reach a conclusion about the rate of complications for one procedure versus the other, their results demonstrate the potentially devastating sequelae of carpal tunnel release even in experienced hands.

Carpal tunnel symptoms may persist or recur following either open or endoscopic release. In patients who have persistent symptoms following endoscopic release, many authors recommend open carpal tunnel release as definitive therapy.

Ahsan ZS, Yao J: Complications of wrist arthroscopy. *Arthroscopy* 2012;28:855.

Herzberg G: Intra-articular fracture of the distal radius: arthroscopic-assisted reduction. *J Hand Surg* 2010;35:1517.

Mintalucci DJ, Leinberry CF: Open versus endoscopic carpal tunnel release. *Orthop Clin North Am* 2012;43:431.

Wolf JM, Dukas A, Pensak M: Advances in wrist arthroscopy. *J Am Acad Orthop Surg* 2012;20:725.

MULTIPLE CHOICE QUESTIONS

1. All of the following are true about applying a cast to the hand, except

   A. The wrist should be extended 30 degrees
   B. The fingers should be flexed
   C. The thumb should be in the opposed (pronated) position
   D. The hand should be in the position of rest
   E. Fiberglass casting materials are preferred for their flexibility.

2. Incisions on the hand should be

   A. Never made on the palm
   B. Across lines of tension
   C. Only made along the medial and lateral surfaces of the fingers
   D. Zigzagged across lines of tension
   E. Carried perpendicularly across the wrist crease

3. Major congenital hand anomalies

   A. Occur in about 1 in 10,000 live births
   B. Can include camptodactyly
   C. Are rarely accompanied by other anomalies (< 1%)
   D. Are not known to be associated with environmental factors
   E. Are usually treated by surgery delayed until after age 15 years

4. Stenosing tenosynovitis

   A. Can be treated by local injections of corticosteroid
   B. Is usually best treated by early surgery
   C. Is always associated with a locked tendon that is trapped and frozen in the tendon sheath
   D. Can be confused with trigger finger or thumb, and must be differentiated
   E. Can be improved with immobilization

5. Management of carpal tunnel syndrome

   A. Typically requires emergent operation
   B. Cannot be done by endoscopic approaches
   C. Should be usually incision of the transverse carpal ligament, which forms the roof of the tunnel
   D. Is uncommon among hand disorders
   E. Should include surgery, not delayed by attempts at nonoperative treatment

Pediatric Surgery

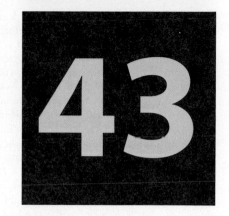

James Wall, MD

Craig T. Albanese, MD

Pediatric surgical patients are not merely small adults. The surgical care of children differs markedly from that of adults in many respects, including unique physiologic demands that vary according to age and development. The neonate's physiologic development is closer to that of a fetus, while adolescents are similar to adults, and infants or children have problems unique to their chronologic and developmental age. Infants and children also suffer from congenital abnormalities and diseases not seen in adults, and their management requires an intimate understanding of the relevant embryology and pathogenesis.

NEWBORN CARE

Neonatal Intensive Care

The newborn infant with a surgically correctable lesion often has other disorders that threaten survival. The care of these babies—particularly the premature and small-for-gestational-age babies, has improved with the emergence of the intensive care nursery. Dramatic advances have been made in the technology of infant monitoring and respiratory support. Low-birth-weight infants can now receive ventilatory support from sophisticated infant respirators for prolonged periods in a precisely controlled microenvironment. Surfactant therapy and high-frequency ventilation has allowed a population of extremely premature infants to survive. Temperature is controlled by servoregulation, while pulse and blood pressure are continuously recorded. Ventilation is monitored by transcutaneous O_2 and CO_2 electrodes or by indwelling arterial catheters. The metabolic consequences of prematurity and intrauterine growth retardation are monitored by frequent measurement of glucose, calcium, electrolytes, and bilirubin in microliter quantities of blood. Nutritional requirements for growth and development can be provided by enteral or parenteral routes. This kind of specialized care of critically ill newborns requires trained personnel and specialized equipment. The care of such babies is best accomplished in designated regional centers capable of providing pediatric surgical and neonatal intensive care.

Classification

Newborn infants can be classified according to their level of maturation (weight) and development (gestational age). A normal full-term infant has a gestational age of 37-42 weeks and a body weight greater than 2500 g. The gestational age of the infant is calculated from the date of the last normal menstrual period. However, clinical assessment of gestational age by morphologic and neurologic examination of the small infant can be more accurate than calculation from the menstrual history.

Four signs may be useful in assessing gestational age. Infants less than 37 weeks' gestational age have (1) fine fuzzy hair with thin, semitransparent skin, (2) ears that lack cartilaginous support, (3) a breast nodule less than 3 mm in diameter, and (4) few transverse creases on the balls of the feet anteriorly. In males, the testicles are incompletely descended and reside in the inguinal canal, and the scrotum is small with few rugae. In females, the labia minora are relatively enlarged and the labia majora are small.

Preterm infants are those born before 37 weeks' gestation. Several physiologic abnormalities may coexist in preterm infants. Apneic and bradycardic episodes are common and may represent an immature central nervous system (CNS) or, conversely, may represent signs of physiologic instability, most notably with sepsis. The lungs and retinas of preterm infants are very susceptible to high oxygen levels. Retinopathy of prematurity from oxygen toxicity may lead to blindness. Relatively brief exposures to high oxygen concentrations, often coupled with barotrauma from the mechanical ventilator, may damage the lungs, resulting in bronchopulmonary dysplasia. Shunting across a patent ductus arteriosus is common and may lead to pulmonary hemorrhage and congestive heart failure. The preterm infant has a friable choroids plexus and is thus susceptible to intraventricular hemorrhage when stressed in the first week of life. The premature infant may be unable to tolerate oral feeding due to a weak suck reflex. Tube feeds or total parenteral nutrition may be required. Preterm infants have increased requirements for glucose, calcium, and sodium as well as a propensity for hypothermia, impaired bilirubin metabolism, polycythemia, and metabolic acidosis. These problems are accentuated in very low-birth-weight (VLBW) infants or "micropremies" (birth weight < 1000 g).

A small-for-gestational age (SGA) infant is one who is less than the 10th percentile in weight for their gestational age. An SGA infant is the product of a pregnancy complicated by any one of several placental, maternal, or fetal abnormalities. Although body weight is low, their body length and head circumference are age-appropriate. Compared with the premature infant of equivalent weight, the SGA infant is developmentally more mature and faces different physiologic problems. Intrauterine malnutrition results in reduced body fat and decreased glycogen stores. Their relatively large surface area and high metabolic rate predisposes them to hypothermia and hypoglycemia. SGA infants also have an increased risk of meconium aspiration syndrome. Polycythemia (which may lead to complications of hyperviscosity syndrome) is common and necessitates close monitoring of their hematocrit. Due to their relatively mature organ development and function (compared to preterm infants), retinopathy of prematurity, intraventricular hemorrhage, and hyaline membrane disease are uncommon.

▶ Temperature Regulation

Infants and children are susceptible to heat loss because they have a relatively greater body surface area and a thinner subcutaneous fat layer compared with adults. Heat loss occurring by conduction, convection, evaporation, and radiation may be four times that of the adult and is further increased in the preterm infant. Infants are homeotherms and will expend metabolic energy to stay warm at the cost of other functions. Heat is generated not by shivering but by metabolizing brown fat reserves (nonshivering thermogenesis) in response to norepinephrine. This has practical consequences since brown fat may be rendered inactive by some medications (pressors and anesthetic agents) and may be depleted by poor nutrition. Exposure to cold environments increases metabolic work and caloric consumption. Due to limited energy reserves and thin skin, prolonged exposure may rapidly cause hypothermia. Resultant catecholamine secretion increases the metabolic rate (particularly in the myocardium) and produces vasoconstriction with impaired tissue perfusion and increased lactic acid production.

Thus, it is important to maintain the sick newborn in an optimal thermal environment. This is the ambient temperature in which a baby, at a minimal metabolic cost, can maintain a constant and normal body temperature by vasomotor control. To attain such an environment, the gradient between the skin surface and the environmental temperature must be less than 1.5°C. As the skin surface temperature averages 35.5°C, the optimal environmental temperature is 34°C (slightly higher for premature infants). The neonate's environmental temperature is best controlled by placing the infant in an enclosed incubator. An open radiant warmer is used when the infant is sick and frequent access is necessary. Either the ambient temperature of the incubator can be monitored and maintained at thermoneutrality, or a servo system can be used. The latter regulates the incubator temperature according to the infant's skin temperature. Heat loss may be further reduced by wrapping the head, extremities, and as much of the trunk as possible in wadding, plastic wrap, plastic sheets, or aluminum foil.

In the operating room, the temperature of the infant must be continuously recorded by placing a thermistor in the rectum or esophagus. Body heat may be conserved by a heating pad, circulated warm air around the child (bearhugger), infrared lamp, and warm irrigation fluids. The operating room should be prewarmed and the temperature kept at 20-27°C. Wet sponges and drapes exaggerate evaporative heat losses. Plastic drapes contain body heat and keep the skin dry. One of the most effective means of regulating body temperature is to heat and humidify the inhalational anesthetic gases.

▶ Ventilation

Assisted ventilation is often necessary because of underlying disease (eg, persistent fetal circulation and pulmonary hypertension), medications (eg, opioids, PGE_2), or physiologic changes imposed by a surgical procedure (eg, closure of an abdominal wall defect or diaphragmatic hernia). At birth, the baby should be warmed, dried, and stimulated. If the baby shows signs of respiratory distress, the pharynx should be aspirated of mucus, amniotic fluid, or meconium. Inadequate respiration should be assisted with positive pressure via mask and escalated to an endotracheal tube as necessary. There is an evolving role for a laryngeal mask airway (LMA) in newborns over 2.5 kg to establish ventilation, especially in cases of difficult airways due to congenital anomalies where intubation may not be possible. The diameter of an endotracheal tube (uncuffed) should approximate that of the 5th digit or the nares, usually between 2.5 and 4 mm. The full-term newborn usually requires a 3.5-mm tube. An orotracheal tube is preferred to a nasotracheal one to minimize trauma and subsequent infection in the nasal passages. The trachea from the glottis to the carina in the newborn is 7.5-cm long, and placement of the tube into the right or left bronchus must be avoided. For infants, optimal tube placement can be estimated as body weight (kg) + 6 as follows: 7 cm from the lips in a 1-kg infant; 8 cm in a 2-kg infant; and 9 cm in a 3-kg infant. Once placed, the endotracheal tube is firmly fixed in place and connected to an infant ventilator. A small air leak between the endotracheal tube and the airway is necessary to minimize laryngeal and tracheal trauma.

Most infant ventilators are time-cycled flow generators capable of delivering both continuous positive airway pressure (CPAP) and intermittent mandatory ventilation (IMV). IMV is a synthesis of simple mechanical ventilation and CPAP breathing that allows the baby to breathe independently between mandatory breaths provided by the ventilator while a continuous positive pressure is maintained on the airway. CPAP breathing helps keep the terminal airways open and is particularly useful when alveolar collapse develops, such as in hyaline membrane disease or with persistent atelectasis.

The gas mixture flowing into the system should be carefully controlled by an air-oxygen mixing device, and the inspired oxygen concentration should be regulated to avoid excessive oxygen delivery. A reasonable goal for arterial PO_2 is around 60-80 torr. The gas should be humidified by using a heated nebulizer as nonhumidified circuits can lead to insensible loses. When the arterial PO_2 exceeds 80 torr, the inspired oxygen concentration is gradually lowered toward room air; the end-expiratory pressure is incrementally lowered. When PCO_2 is less than approximately 45 torr, the IMV rate can be decreased as well. In this way, the baby is gradually weaned from oxygen and mechanical ventilation. Upon removal of the tube, nasal CPAP can be provided, and the inspired oxygen concentration can be increased if necessary.

In severe respiratory compromise (eg, congenital diaphragmatic hernia [CDH], meconium aspiration syndrome), more complex ventilatory strategies are needed. High-frequency ventilation (jet and oscillatory modes) utilizes low tidal volumes at high rates (up to 600 breaths/min) to minimize the deleterious effects of high airway pressure. Inhaled nitric oxide (iNO) can be administered via the ventilatory circuit and may help relax the small airways and pulmonary vasculature. There is a trend toward allowing higher PCO_2 levels (permissive hypercarbia) and lower PO_2 levels in order to lessen pulmonary trauma from pressure and oxygen. This has been termed "gentle ventilation." If gentle ventilation, permissive hypercapnia, and the high-frequency modes of ventilation are ineffective, oxygenation and gas exchange can be accomplished using extracorporeal membrane oxygenation (ECMO). This temporary bypass unit oxygenates the blood through an external circuit as the lungs are left to mature or recover from the underlying disease process. The clinical need for ECMO has diminished with the increased widespread use of iNO, surfactant, high-frequency ventilation and the adoption of permissive hypercapnea as a ventilatory strategy.

Guidry CA, Hranjec T, Rodgers BM, Kane B, McGahren ED: Permissive hypercapnia in the management of congenital diaphragmatic hernia: our institutional experience. *J Am Coll Surg* 2012 Apr;214(4):640-645, 647.

► Fluids & Electrolytes

Effective fluid and electrolyte management involves (1) calculating the fluid and electrolyte requirements for maintaining metabolic functions, (2) replacing losses (evaporative, third space, external), and (3) considering preexisting fluid deficits or excesses. Taking these factors into consideration, a tentative program is devised for fluid and electrolyte administration. The patient's response is monitored, and the program is adjusted accordingly.

Monitoring fluid status and acid-base balance can be accomplished by both noninvasive and invasive means. Commonly used noninvasive devices include pulse oximetry, urine output, transcutaneous CO_2 monitoring, and sphygmomanometry. For critically ill infants, more invasive means are necessary to assess homeostasis. Blood gas analysis via heelstick (capillary), venous catheter, or arterial catheter is frequently employed. Polyvinyl catheters may be placed via an umbilical artery into the aorta, with the tip positioned at the level of T6-T9 or L3-L4 (confirmed radiographically). Indwelling arterial catheters can also be placed in the radial, femoral, or temporal arteries, either percutaneously or by incision. Central venous access may assist in cases where prolonged venous access is needed or parenteral nutrition is necessary or when blood is frequently sampled. It may be obtained via the umbilical vein; a percutaneously inserted central catheter (PICC) via the saphenous, cephalic, median basilic, or temporal veins; or using a Broviac catheter via the femoral, internal jugular, facial, or subclavian veins.

A. Calculating Maintenance Needs

In the newborn infant, the basic maintenance requirement of water is the volume required for growth and replacement of losses from the skin, lungs, and stool. Requirements during the first day of life are unique because of the greatly expanded extracellular fluid volume in the newborn baby, which decreases after 24 hours. For example, infants born with intestinal obstruction (eg, intestinal atresia) are initially not hypovolemic as a result of fluid adjustments across the placenta. Up to 10% of a newborn infant's birth weight is lost in the first 3-7 days; the majority is water loss, with minor contributions from meconium and urine. During the first 24 hours of life, basic maintenance fluid should range from 60 to 80 mL/kg/d for term infants, and from 80 to 100 mL/kg/d for preterm infants. This requirement gradually increases to a minimum 80-100 mL/kg/d by 4 days of life in normal infants. For children and adolescents, the most commonly used method of calculating fluid requirements is based on body weight (Table 43–1). However, because of the many

Table 43–1. Calculation of maintenance fluid requirements.

Body Weight	Fluid Volume per 24 h
1-10 kg	100 mL/kg
11-20 kg	1000 mL + 50 mL for each kg over 10 kg
> 20 kg	1500 mL + 20 mL for each kg over 20 kg

Reproduced, with permission, from Albanese CT: Pediatric surgery. In: Norton JA. *Surgery*. New York, NY: Springer; 2000.

factors affecting maintenance requirements, there is no close or constant relationship between body weight and fluid and electrolyte needs.

B. Perioperative Fluid Management

In the surgical patient, fluid, serum electrolyte, and acid-base abnormalities are corrected before operation, when feasible. Intraoperative fluid requirements consist of the estimated maintenance requirement plus replacement of preexisting deficits (if uncorrected) plus replacement of intraoperative losses, including blood.

Postoperatively, losses from intestinal drainage and fistulas are directly measured and replaced with an appropriate electrolyte solution (Table 43–2). In neonates, it is wise to measure the electrolytes in the fluid to more accurately guide replacement, especially for proximal intestinal stomas or fistulas. Protein-rich losses (eg, chest tube drainage of a chylothorax) can be replaced with colloid such as an albumin solution or fresh frozen plasma (FFP). Internal losses into body cavities or tissues (third space losses) cannot be measured; adequate replacement of these losses depends on careful monitoring of the patient's vital signs and urine output. Following an operation such as a laparotomy or thoracotomy, the fluid requirement may exceed 150 mL/kg/d for several days postoperatively. Isotonic fluids are better in the immediate postoperative period in patients over 6 months of age when significant third space losses are possible.

C. Electrolyte Considerations

Basic electrolyte and energy requirements are provided by sodium, 3-4 mEq/kg/d (up to 5 mEq/kg/d for preterm infants) in 5% or 10% dextrose, with the addition of potassium, 2-3 mEq/kg/d, once urine production has been established. Calcium gluconate (200-400 mg/kg/d) may be added, especially in preterm infants. Additional electrolytes such as bicarbonate and magnesium are added, as needed.

Many stressed newborn infants develop low blood levels of potassium, calcium, magnesium, and glucose. A deficiency of any one of these will produce such signs as vomiting, abdominal distention, poor feeding, apneic spells, cyanosis, lethargy, eye rolling, high-pitched cry, tremors, or convulsions. Convulsions and tetany due to hypocalcemia should be treated with intravenous 10% calcium solution given at a rate of 1 mL/min while the EKG is carefully monitored. Although hypocalcemia can be largely eliminated by adding calcium salts to intravenous solutions, caution is required since subcutaneous infiltration may produce severe vasoconstriction and skin necrosis. If there is no response to correction of a documented calcium deficiency, hypomagnesemia should be suspected and a serum magnesium level obtained.

Rapid determination of the blood glucose level can be done in the neonatal unit with blood glucose reagent strips. This may be correlated at intervals with serum glucose determinations, the frequency depending on the stability of the infant. Generally, intravenous fluids should contain a minimum of 10% dextrose, and if non–dextrose-containing solutions such as blood or plasma are being administered, close monitoring of the blood glucose level is essential. The treatment of hypoglycemia consists of giving 50% glucose, 1-2 mL/kg intravenously, followed by a continuous infusion of 10%-15% glucose solutions at a rate equivalent to that needed for maintenance water requirements.

Table 43–2. Replacement of abnormal losses of fluids and electrolytes.

Type of Fluid	Electrolyte Content				
	Na^+ (mEq/L)	K^+ (mEq/L)	Cl^2 (mEq/L)	$HCO_3^{\,2}$ (mEq/L)	Replacement
Gastric (vomiting)	50(20-90)	10(4-15)	90(50-150)	...	5% dextrose in half-normal (0.45%) saline plus KCl 20-40 mEq/L
Small bowel (ileostomy)	110(70-140)	5(3-10)	100(70-130)	20(10-40)	Lactated Ringer
Diarrhea	80(10-140)	25(10-60)	90(20-120)	40(30-50)	Lactated Ringer with or without HCO_3^-
Bile	145(130-160)	5(4-7)	100(80-120)	40(30-50)	Lactated Ringer with or without HCO_3^-
Pancreatic	140(130-150)	5(4-7)	80(60-100)	80(60-110)	Lactated Ringer with or without HCO_3^-
Sweat					
Normal	20(10-30)	4(3-10)	20(10-40)	...	...
Cystic fibrosis	90(50-130)	15(5-25)	90(60-120)	...	...

Choong K, Arora S, Cheng J, Farrokhyar F, Reddy D, Thabane L, Walton JM: Hypotonic versus isotonic maintenance fluids after surgery for children: a randomized controlled trial. *Pediatrics* 2011 Nov;128(5):857-866.

▶ Nutrition

Newborns require a relatively large caloric intake because of their high basal metabolic rate, caloric requirements for growth and development, energy needs to maintain body heat, and limited energy reserve. An infant requires calories at a rate of 100-130 kcal/kg/d and protein at a rate of 2-4 g/kg/d to achieve a normal weight gain of 10-15 g/kg/d (Table 43–3). Thirty percent to 40% of the total non-protein calories should be provided as fat. These requirements decline with age but increase with surgery, sepsis, and trauma or burns. Caloric requirements are increased 10%-25% by surgery, more than 50% by infection, and 100% by burns.

A. Enteral Alimentation

The best means of providing calories and protein is through the gastrointestinal (GI) tract. If the GI tract is functional, standard infant formulas, blenderized meals, or prepared elemental diets can be given by mouth, through nasogastric or nasojejunal feeding tubes, or through gastrostomy or jejunostomy tubes placed surgically. Gastric feeding is preferable because it allows for normal digestive processes and hormonal responses, a greater tolerance for larger osmotic loads, and a lower incidence of dumping. The use of nasoduodenal or nasojejunal tubes is reserved for infants who cannot tolerate intragastric feeding (eg, delayed gastric emptying, gastroesophageal reflux [GER], depressed gag reflex).

The availability of nutritionally complete liquid diets of low viscosity allows continuous feeding through small-diameter catheters. Elemental diets made by mixing crystalline amino acids, oligosaccharides, and fats can be completely absorbed in the small intestine with little residue. Their use is limited because they cause diarrhea as a result of the high osmolality of full-strength formulas. This can be avoided by administering dilute solutions by continuous drip. Initially, the volume of dilute solution is gradually increased, and the concentration is then progressively increased in a stepwise fashion—ie, half strength, three-fourths strength, and full strength. Formulas that remain below 500 mOsm are best.

Small Silastic or polyethylene catheters such as those used for intravenous infusion can be passed through the nose or mouth into the stomach or jejunum. In more complex cases, a surgically placed gastrostomy or jejunostomy may be necessary for postoperative feeding. A variety of techniques and methods are employed in their construction. In the case of a gastrostomy, either a balloon catheter is used (ie, Foley) or a low-profile gastrostomy button is placed. Silastic is superior to other plastics because it does not become rigid when exposed to intestinal contents. Parenteral nutrition combined with enteral feeding is often necessary for infants with short bowel syndrome until intestinal adaptation occurs.

B. Parenteral Alimentation

The indications for parenteral alimentation include the following: (1) expected period of prolonged ileus (eg, following repair of gastroschisis or high jejunal atresia); (2) intestinal fistulas; (3) supplementation of oral feedings, as in intractable diarrhea, short bowel syndrome, or various malabsorption syndromes; (4) intrauterine growth retardation; (5) catabolic wasting states such as infections or tumors when gastric feedings are inadequate or not tolerated; (6) inflammatory bowel disease; (7) severe acute alimentary disorders (pancreatitis, necrotizing enterocolitis [NEC]); and (8) chylothorax.

Concentrated solutions (12.5% glucose or more) thrombose peripheral vessels. Placement of a central venous catheter (PICC or Broviac) into the superior or inferior vena cavae allows the large blood flow to dilute the solution immediately, allowing more concentrated sugar solutions (15%-30% glucose) to be administered. The catheter may be placed percutaneously through the subclavian or internal jugular vein or inserted by cut down into the external jugular, anterior facial, internal jugular, cephalic, brachial, or saphenous veins. For long-term use, Broviac (single lumen) or Hickman (double lumen) catheters, with Dacron cuffs positioned near the exit site of the skin, are preferred to minimize infection and to prevent accidental dislodgment.

Intravenous alimentation solutions containing an amino acid source (2%-5% crystalline amino acids or protein hydrolysate), glucose (10%-40%), electrolytes, vitamins, and trace minerals are used. The electrolyte composition

Table 43–3. Caloric requirements of various age groups per 24 hours.

Age	kcal/kg per 24 hours
Newborn term (0-4 days)	110-120
Low birth weight	120-130
3-4 months	100-106
5-12 months	100
1-7 years	75-90
7-12 years	60-75
12-18 years	30-60

Reproduced, with permission, from Albanese CT: Pediatric surgery. In: Norton JA. *Surgery.* New York, NY: Springer; 2000.

Table 43–4. Total parenteral nutrition requirements

Component	Neonate	6 mo to 10 y	>10 y
Calories (kcal/kg/d)	90-120	60-105	40-75
Fluid (mL/kg/d)	120-180	120-150	50-75
Dextrose (mg/kg/min)	4-6	7-8	7-8
Protein (g/kg/d)	2-3	1.5-2.5	0.8-2.0
Fat (g/kg/d)	0.5-3.0	1.0-4.0	1.0-4.0
Sodium (mEq/kg/d)	3-4	3-4	3-4
Potassium (mEq/kg/d)	2-3	2-3	1-2
Calcium (mg/kg/d)	80-120	40-80	40-60
Phosphate (mg/kg/d)	25-40	25-40	25-40
Magnesium (mEq/kg/d)	0.25-1.0	0.5	0.5
Zinc (μg/kg/d)	300	100	3 mg/d
Copper (μg/kg/d)	20	20	1.2 mg/d
Chromium (μg/kg/d)	0.2	0.2	12 mg/d
Manganese (μg/kg/d)	6	6	0.3 mg/d
Selenium (mg/kg/d)	2	2	10-20 mg/d

Reproduced, with permission, from Albanese CT: Pediatric surgery. In: Norton JA. *Surgery*. New York, NY: Springer; 2000.

of the protein solution should be known so that the desired composition of the final solution can be adjusted by appropriate additives according to the individual patient's requirements. A standard solution suitable for infants and young children must contain calcium, magnesium, and phosphate to allow for growth. Trace minerals are also added to the basic solution (Table 43–4). These solutions should be infused at a constant rate with an infusion pump to avoid blood backing up the catheter and clotting and to prevent wide fluctuations of blood glucose and amino acid concentrations. If it is necessary to restrict the volume of infusion, more concentrated glucose solutions can be used to increase the caloric intake.

Complications of prolonged intravenous alimentation are numerous. The most frequent problem is catheter sepsis. Although catheter removal will quickly treat the problem, a trial of antibiotics effective against gram-positive and gram-negative pathogens is indicated. Catheter removal is indicated in the presence of worsening sepsis, three positive blood cultures, or documented yeast infection (with antifungal treatment after catheter removal). Clotting in the catheter may be controlled by adding 1 unit of heparin per milliliter of solution. Emphasis on a constant rate of infusion will minimize hyperglycemia or hypoglycemia. Analysis of serum electrolytes (including calcium and phosphate) may be necessary several times a week initially, but the interval is decreased to once a week when the patient is

stable. Patients must be observed for hyperammonemia and for vitamin or trace mineral deficiency. Progressive hepatomegaly and jaundice of uncertain origin can occur after prolonged parenteral alimentation. This syndrome may subside when the parenteral solution is discontinued or when it is infused for a period of 12-16 hours and then the infusion is stopped for 8-12 hours (cycling) or when augmented with enteral feeding. Use of an ω-3 fatty acid based emulsion (Omegaven) has shown potential in moderating the effects of TPN cholestasis.

Fuchs J, Fallon EM, Gura KM, Puder M: Use of an omega-3 fatty acid-based emulsion in the treatment of parenteral nutrition-induced cholestasis in patients with microvillous inclusion disease. *J Pediatr Surg* 2011 Dec;46(12):2376-2382.

Javid PJ, Malone FR, Dick AA, Hsu E, Sunseri M, Healey P, Horslen SP: A contemporary analysis of parenteral nutrition-associated liver disease in surgical infants. *J Pediatr Surg* 2011 Oct;46(10):1913-1917.

Reynolds RM, Bass KD, Thureen PJ: Achieving positive protein balance in the immediate postoperative period in neonates undergoing abdominal surgery. 2008 *J Pediatr Surg* 2008;152(1):63-67.

▶ Blood Loss

Total blood, plasma, and red blood cell (RBC) volumes are higher during the first few postnatal hours than at any other time in an individual's life. Several hours after birth, plasma shifts out of the circulation, and total blood and plasma volume decrease. The high RBC volume persists, decreasing slowly to reach adult levels by the seventh postnatal week. Age-related estimations of blood volume are summarized in Table 43–5.

Although not clinically significant, both the prothrombin time and the partial thromboplastin time may be slightly prolonged at birth due to relative deficiencies of clotting factors. Defects in the coagulating mechanism may occur in newborn infants as a result of vitamin K deficiency, thrombocytopenia, inherited disorders, and temporary hepatic insufficiency due to immaturity, asphyxia, or infection. It is standard to administer 1.0 mg of vitamin K intramuscularly to all newborns.

The blood lost during operation varies greatly according to the complexity of the operative procedure, the underlying

Table 43–5. Blood volume based on age.

Preterm infants	85-100 mL/kg
Term infants	85 mL/kg
Age > 1 month	75 mL/kg
Age 3 months to adult	70 mL/kg

disease, and the effectiveness of hemostasis. Mild blood loss, amounting to less than 10% of the blood volume, usually does not require transfusion. It is imperative to develop methods for closely monitoring the amount of blood lost during operations since significant blood loss is often underestimated in the newborn, especially the preterm infant. Dry sponges should be used and weighed shortly after use to minimize error from evaporation. The suction line, connected to a calibrated trap on the operating table, should be short to diminish the dead space of the tubing and to provide immediate data about accumulated blood loss. Visual observation may be used as a rough guide, but it tends to give a falsely low estimate of the loss.

Before operation, newborn infants should receive vitamin K, 1.0 mg intravenously or intramuscularly. If an extensive surgical procedure is anticipated, the patient's blood should be typed and crossmatched in case transfusion is required. In infants with hematocrits greater than 50%, blood loss may be replaced by infusing lactated Ringer's solution or FFP to compensate for losses of up to 25% of total blood volume. Greater blood losses should be replaced with packed RBCs. A transfusion of RBCs at a volume of 10 mL/kg should raise the hematocrit 3%-4%. The transfused blood should be prewarmed to body temperature by running it through coiled tubing immersed in water at 37°C. With excessive blood loss, clotting factors and platelets can be depleted rapidly, and FFP and platelets of identical blood type should be available. With massive transfusion a ratio of 1:1 of FFP to RBCs and 1:2 of platelets to RBCs has been shown to improve outcomes.

Perioperative Considerations

A. Gastrointestinal Decompression

The importance of gastric decompression in the surgical newborn cannot be overemphasized. The distended stomach carries the risk of aspiration and pneumonia and may also impair diaphragmatic excursion, resulting in respiratory distress. For example, oxygenation and ventilation in a neonate with CDH may become progressively impaired as the herniated intestine becomes distended with air and fluid. With gastroschisis, omphalocele, and diaphragmatic hernia, the ability to reduce the prolapsed intestine into the abdominal cavity is impaired by intestinal distention. It is critical to avoid bag-mask ventilation in these patients. A double-lumen (sump) tube, such as a 10F Replogle or Anderson tube, is preferred, utilizing low continuous suction. If a single-lumen tube is used, intermittent aspiration by syringe or machine is required. The correct position of the tube in the stomach is confirmed by carefully measuring the tube prior to insertion and by radiographs. Careful taping of the tube is essential to avoid displacement.

B. Preoperative Blood Sampling

Blood analyses should be restricted to those studies essential for diagnosis and management. The volume of blood drawn for laboratory tests should be documented as these small volumes cumulatively represent significant blood loss in a small infant. Generally, the only "routine" preoperative blood analyses for a neonate consist of a complete blood count and a blood specimen for type and crossmatch (in the case of major newborn surgery). Electrolytes in the first 12 hours of life simply reflect the mother's electrolytes. Coagulation studies (eg, PT, PTT, ACT) are rarely indicated.

C. Preoperative NPO Guidelines

The following are general guidelines, but institutional practices vary considerably. The guiding principles in setting a standard include: risk of hypoglycemia associated with NPO status, tolerance or comfort level of the NPO child, and the desire to have an empty stomach upon induction of general anesthesia to mitigate aspiration risk.

1. Patients younger than 6 months—No solids, breast milk, or formula 4 hours prior to the procedure. Infants may have clear liquids (water, oral electrolyte mixtures, glucose water, or apple juice) until 2 hours prior to the procedure.

2. Patients from 6 months to 18 years—Nothing to eat or drink after midnight except clear liquids (water, apple juice, oral electrolyte mixtures, gelatin dessert, white grape juice), which can be continued until 2 hours prior to the procedure.

3. Patients older than 18 years—Nothing to eat or drink after midnight except clear liquids (water, apple juice, plain gelatin desserts) until 4-6 hours prior to the procedure.

D. Bowel Preparation Instructions

The bowel is mechanically cleansed for elective bowel resection. Opinion varies about whether a bowel preparation is needed for certain procedures as well as about what to use to accomplish it and whether to do it at home or in the hospital. An inpatient regimen begins the day prior to surgery and consists of polyethylene glycol-electrolyte solution (GoLYTELY), 25 mL/kg/h for 4 hours or until the effluent is clear. Metoclopramide (0.1 mg/dose IV) is given 1 hour before the GoLYTELY. Pedialyte can be given ad lib until the time to have nothing by mouth.

Outpatient preparations are reserved for patients over 1 year of age. Clear liquids are given the day before surgery. Bisacodyl (Dulcolax) suppositories and 8-oz lukewarm tap water enemas can be given the morning and in the evening the day before surgery. For children over 5 years of age, magnesium citrate is added (1 oz per year of age up to a maximum of 8 oz) and given orally in the morning and evening the day before surgery, along with 16-oz tap water enemas.

LESIONS OF THE HEAD & NECK

DERMOID CYSTS

Dermoid cysts are congenital inclusions of skin and skin appendages commonly found on the scalp and eyebrows and in the midline of the nose, neck, and upper chest. They present as painless swellings that may be completely mobile or fixed to the skin and deeper structures. Dermoid cysts of the eyebrows and scalp may produce a depression in the underlying bone that appears as a smooth, punched-out defect on radiographs of the outer table of the skull. They do not extend intracranially. In contrast, cysts of the face and scalp that are located in the midline may represent an alternative diagnosis of encephalocele and would be handled much differently so it is imperative to obtain an MRI or CT scan preoperatively. Dermoid cysts of the midline neck may be confused with thyroglossal duct cysts. However, dermoids do not move with swallowing or protrusion of the tongue since they are not deep to the strap muscles, unlike thyroglossal cysts. All dermoids contain a cheesy material that is produced by desquamation of the cells of the epithelial lining. Care should be taken when planning the operative approach to facial dermoids to avoid either incomplete excision or unnecessary surgical scarring in cosmetically sensitive areas. Dermoids should be excised intact, since incomplete removal will result in recurrence. Those lesions arising near the eyebrows should be excised through an incision adjacent to the hairline. The eyebrows should not be shaved nor should the incision go through any eyebrow follicles since a permanent glabrous area will develop. Recently, tunneled endoscopic approaches originating from behind the hairline have been used successfully to avoid facial scarring.

BRANCHIOGENIC ANOMALIES

During the first month of fetal life, the primitive neck develops four external clefts and four pharyngeal pouches that are separated by a membrane. Between the clefts and pouches are branchial arches. The dorsal portion of the first cleft becomes the external auditory canal; the other clefts are obliterated. The pharyngeal pouches persist as adult organs. The first pouch becomes the auditory tube, the middle ear cavity, and the mastoid air cells. The second pouch incompletely regresses and becomes the palatine tonsil and the supratonsillar fossa. The third pouch forms the inferior parathyroid glands and thymus; the fourth forms the superior

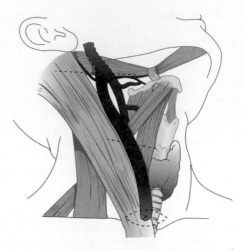

▲ **Figure 43–1.** Branchiogenic fistula from second branchial cleft origin. The fistula extends along the anterior border of the sternocleidomastoid muscle and courses between the internal and external carotid arteries and cephalad to the hypoglossal nerve to enter the tonsillar fossa.

parathyroid glands. Branchial anomalies are remnants of this fetal branchial apparatus.

A tract of branchial origin may form a complete fistula, or one end may be obliterated to form an external or internal sinus, or both ends may resorb, leaving an aggregate of cells forming a cyst (Figure 43–1). Fistulas that arise above the hyoid bone and communicate with the external auditory canal represent persistence of the first branchial cleft. These tracts are always lined by squamous epithelium. Cysts and sinuses of second or third branchial origin are lined by squamous, cuboidal, or ciliated columnar epithelium. Fistulas that communicate between the anterior border of the sternocleidomastoid muscle and the tonsillar fossa are of second branchial origin, and those that extend into the piriform sinus are derived from the third branchial pouch. Cysts developing from branchial structures usually appear later in childhood as opposed to sinuses and fistulas. Branchiogenic anomalies occur with equal frequency on each side of the neck, and 15% are bilateral. Second branchial cleft abnormalities are most common, occurring six times more frequently than first cleft anomalies.

▶ Clinical Findings

A sinus or fistulous opening along the anterior border of the sternocleidomastoid muscle may be noted at birth and usually discharges a mucoid or purulent material. The patient may complain of a foul-tasting discharge in the mouth upon massaging the tract, but the internal orifice is rarely recognized. Some may present with an acute infection. The cysts are characteristically found anterior and deep to the upper third of the sternocleidomastoid muscle, or they may be located within the parotid gland or pharyngeal wall, over the manubrium, or in the mediastinum. Sinuses and cysts are prone to become repeatedly infected, producing cellulitis and abscess formation. Incomplete branchial sinuses appear as a dimple that contain cartilage and do not drain or communicate with the deep structures of the neck.

Differential Diagnosis

Granulomatous lymphadenitis due to mycobacterial infections may produce cystic lymph nodes and draining sinuses, but these are usually distinguishable by the chronic inflammatory reaction that precedes the purulent discharge. Suppurative lymphadenitis, most commonly due to *Staphylococcus aureus,* may resemble an infected branchial remnant. However, treatment and complete healing of the lymphadenitis is curative, whereas an identifiable branchial remnant will persist after the infection resolves. Hemangiomas and lymphatic malformations (LM) are soft, spongy tumor masses that might be confused with branchial cysts, but the latter have a firmer consistency. LM may transilluminate, while branchial cysts do not. Carotid body tumors are quite firm, are located at the carotid bifurcation, and occur in older patients. Lymphomas produce firm masses in the area where branchial remnants occur, but multiple matted nodes rather than a solitary cystic tumor distinguish these lesions. Mucoid material may be expressed from the openings of branchial sinuses or fistulas, and a firm cord-like tract may be palpable along its course.

Treatment

Nearly all branchial abnormalities should be excised early in life since repeated infection is common, making resection more difficult. Asymptomatic, small cartilaginous remnants may be watched, but they are usually removed for cosmetic reasons as well as the smaller risk of infection, compared to the true cyst/fistula. Infected sinuses and cysts require initial incision and drainage. Excision of these tracts is staged and usually performed approximately 6 weeks later, when the acute inflammatory reaction has subsided. Every effort should be made to excise the entire cyst wall or fistula tract (including the skin punctum, if present) since recurrence and infection are common with incomplete removal. Excision should be undertaken cautiously, as the tracts may lie adjacent to the facial, hypoglossal, and glossopharyngeal nerves as well as the carotid artery and internal jugular vein.

Al-Khateeb TH, Al Zoubi F: Congenital neck masses: a descriptive retrospective study of 252 cases. *J Oral Maxillofac Surg* 2007;65(11):22242-22247.

PREAURICULAR LESIONS

Preauricular sinuses, cysts, and cartilaginous rests arise from anomalous development of the auricle and are unrelated to branchial anomalies. The sinuses are often short and end blindly. They can be cosmetically unappealing and often become infected. Superficial skin tags and cartilaginous rests are easily excised without risk to other structures. Preauricular sinus tracts, however, may be very deceptive in their extent, and one should be prepared to proceed with extensive dissection that risks damage to branches of the facial nerve.

LYMPHATIC MALFORMATION (CYSTIC HYGROMA, LYMPHANGIOMA)

LMs are benign multilobular, multinodular cystic masses lined by lymph channel endothelial cells. They result from maldevelopment and obstruction of the lymphatic system. Since they are not proliferative lesions, they should be distinguished from hemangiomas; hence the favored term of lymphatic malformation is currently favored over the more frequently encountered misnomer lymphangioma. Cystic hygroma is another misnomer frequently encountered for cervical lymphatic malformation. Eventually, sequestrations of lymphatic tissue that do not communicate with the normal lymphatic system develop. Fifty percent to 65% appear at birth and 90% by the second year of life. They are located most commonly in the posterior triangle of the neck (75%) (Figure 43–2) and axilla (20%), with the remainder located in the mediastinum, retroperitoneum, pelvis, and groin.

Clinical Findings

Cervical lymphatic malformations may communicate beneath the clavicle with an axillary hygroma, mediastinal hygroma, or, rarely, both. The majority may be asymptomatic; however, the occult LM usually presents following an upper aerodigestive tract infection as a result of increased or infected lymph flow, or following hemorrhage into the LM from a web of adherent microvasculature. Occasionally, very large lesions occur with involvement of the floor of the mouth, these can cause *in utero* hydrops or asphyxiation at birth when associated with airway compromise. There is a recognized association between cervical LM and Turner syndrome. These lesions grow along fascial planes and around neurovascular structures; they are infiltrative but not invasive. Large lesions may be recognized prenatally using ultrasound or MRI examination.

Treatment

There are two modes of treatment, sclerotherapy or excision, the choice of which is based on imaging studies (CT, MRI). Intralesional injection of a sclerosing agent is most effective

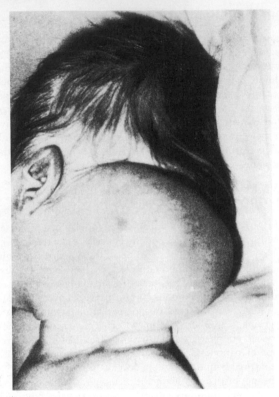

▲ **Figure 43–2.** Typical neonatal macrocystic lymphatic malformation arising from the posterior cervical triangle. (Reproduced, with permission, from Filston HC: Hemangiomas, cystic hygromas, and teratomas of the head and neck. *Semin Pediatr Surg* 1994;3:147.)

for unilocular or macrocystic lesions. Examples of agents that have been used are OK-432 (a lyophilized mixture of *Streptococcus pyogenes* and penicillin G potassium), bleomycin, and doxycycline. Excision is carried out with bipolar cautery to ensure a hemostatic dissection and decrease the incidence of lymph leak and nerve injury. Nevertheless, postoperative lymph leak is common and is treated by closed suction drainage for days to weeks. Intraoperative cyst rupture increases the difficulty of the dissection since the thin-walled cyst is difficult to identify and the margins are obscured. The persistence rate following surgery can be as high as 50% since incomplete excision is the rule rather than the exception in order to avoid potential injury to adjacent neurovascular bundles. Given their infiltrative nature, persistence or symptomatic recurrence following surgical excision and unavoidable surgical scarring, the trend has been increasingly toward sclerotherapy for superficial accessible macrocystic LMs.

Nehra D, Jacobson L, Barnes P, Mallory B, Albanese CT, Sylvester KG: Doxycycline sclerotherapy as primary treatment of head and neck lymphatic malformations. *J Pediatr Surg* 2008 Mar;43(3):451-460.

THYROGLOSSAL DUCT REMNANT

During the fourth week of gestation, the thyroid gland develops from an evagination in the floor of the primitive pharynx located between the first pair of pharyngeal pouches. If the anlage of the thyroid does not descend normally, the gland may form at the base of the tongue or remain as a mass anywhere in the midline of the neck along its truncated path of descent. If the thyroglossal duct persists, the epithelial tract forms a cyst that usually communicates with the foramen cecum of the tongue. The thyroglossal duct descends through the second branchial arch anlage, which becomes the hyoid bone, prior to its fusion in the midline. Because of this, the tract of a persistent thyroglossal duct often extends through the hyoid bone (Figure 43–3).

▶ Clinical Findings

The most common physical finding is a rounded cystic mass of varying size in the midline of the neck just below the hyoid bone. The acute inflammatory reaction of an infection may herald the presence of a cyst. The fluid in the cyst is usually under pressure and may give the impression of being a solid tumor. Cysts and aberrant midline thyroid glands move up and down with swallowing and with protrusion of the tongue since they are deep to the cervical strap muscles. In contrast, lingual thyroid tissue is a rare clinical entity and may produce dysphagia, dysphonia, dyspnea, hemorrhage, or pain.

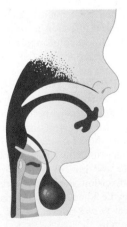

▲ **Figure 43–3.** Thyroglossal cyst and duct course through the hyoid bone to the foramen cecum of the tongue.

Differential Diagnosis

Lymph nodes, dermoid cysts, and enlarged Delphian nodes containing tumor metastases may be confused with thyroglossal remnants in the midline of the neck. Dermoid cysts do not move with swallowing. Lingual thyroids may be confused with a hypertrophied lingual tonsil or with a ranula, fibroma, angioma, sarcoma, or carcinoma of the tongue. These lesions and thyroglossal cysts may be distinguished from aberrantly located thyroid glands by needle aspiration or by radioiodine scintiscan.

Complications

Thyroglossal cysts are prone to infection, and spontaneous drainage or incision and drainage of an abscess will often result in a chronically draining fistula. Excision of an ectopic thyroid may remove all thyroid tissue, producing hypothyroidism. There is a malignant potential of the dysgenetic thyroid tissue located in a thyroglossal duct cyst; carcinoma develops more frequently in ectopic thyroid tissue than in normal thyroid glands.

Treatment

Complete excision is indicated because of the risk of infection and the possibility of the development of papillary carcinoma later in life. Acute infection in thyroglossal tracts should be treated with antibiotics. Abscesses should be incised and drained. After complete subsidence of the inflammatory reaction (approximately 6 weeks), a thyroglossal cyst and its epithelial tract should be excised. The mid portion of the hyoid bone should be removed en bloc with the thyroglossal tract to the base of the tongue (Sistrunk procedure). Recurrences occur when the hyoid is not removed and when the cyst was previously infected or drained.

Gallagher TQ, Hartnick CJ: Thyroglossal duct cyst excision. *Adv Otorhinolaryngol* 2012;73:66-69.

LaRiviere CA, Waldhausen JH: Congenital cervical cysts, sinuses, and fistulae in pediatric surgery. *Surg Clin North Am* 2012 Jun;92(3):583-597.

TORTICOLLIS

Torticollis presents with a hard, nontender, fibrotic mass within the sternocleidomastoid muscle. It may be present at birth but is usually not noticed until the second to sixth weeks of life. The mass appears with equal frequency in both sexes and on each side of the neck. Rarely, there is more than one mass in the muscle or both sternocleidomastoid muscles are involved. A history of breech delivery is present in 20%-30% of these children.

Clinical Findings

Torticollis is manifested when the sternocleidomastoid muscle is shortened and the mastoid process on the involved side is pulled down toward the clavicle and manubrium. As a result, the head is abducted to the ipsilateral side and rotated to the contralateral side (toward the opposite shoulder). The shoulder on the affected side is raised, and there may be cervical and thoracic scoliosis. Passive rotation of the head to the side of the involved muscle will be resisted and limited to varying degrees, and the muscle will appear as a protuberant band. Because of persistent pressure when the patient is recumbent, the ipsilateral face and contralateral occiput will be flattened. Facial hemihypoplasia and plagiocephaly (flattening of the ipsilateral posterior skull) occurs in untreated cases, usually within 6 months.

Treatment

Surgery is rarely necessary for this disorder. Torticollis is treated with active range of motion exercises. The child's shoulders are held flat to a table and the head is tilted and rotated in a full range of motion. This procedure should be performed at least four times a day, usually for 2-3 months. The firm "tumor" often disappears well before the torticollis is cured. If the muscle continues to become progressively shortened, with facial and occipital skull deformity, both heads of the sternocleidomastoid muscle should be divided through a small transverse incision just above the clavicle. This procedure does not reverse the bony changes that have already developed but prevents progression of the process. Recently, endoscopic approaches have been described in order to avoid unsightly surgical scarring in the head and neck region.

Dutta S, Albanese CT: Transaxillary subcutaneous endoscopic release of the sternocleidomastoid muscle for treatment of persistent torticollis. *J Pediatr Surg* 2008 Mar;43(3): 447-450.

CERVICAL LYMPHADENOPATHY

SUPPURATIVE LYMPHADENITIS

Infections in the upper respiratory passages, scalp, ear, or neck produce varying degrees of secondary lymphadenitis. Most of the causative organisms are streptococcal or staphylococcal species. In infants and young children, the clinical course of the suppurative lymphadenitis may greatly overshadow a seemingly insignificant or inapparent primary infection. Scalp or ear infections produce preauricular or postauricular and suboccipital lymph node involvement; submental, oral, tonsillar, and pharyngeal infections affect the submandibular and deep jugular nodes.

Clinical Findings

With significant lymphadenitis, the regional lymph nodes become greatly enlarged and produce local pain and tenderness. Enlargement of cervical nodes is most common, followed by occipital and submandibular nodes. Fever is high initially and then becomes intermittent and may persist for days or weeks. The regional nodes may remain enlarged and firm for prolonged periods, or they may suppurate and produce surrounding cellulitis and edema. Subsequently, the nodes may involute or a fluctuant abscess may form, resulting in redness and thinning of the overlying skin. Infected, matted nodes may become so hard as to be indistinguishable (on palpation) from a solid mass.

Differential Diagnosis

A smoldering lymphadenitis that neither resolves nor forms an abscess can be confused with granulomatous lymphadenitis, lymphoma, or metastatic tumor. Excisional biopsy is required to differentiate these lesions. After several weeks, there will usually be a reduction in the size and firmness of suppurative adenitis, especially after antibiotic treatment has been started. Recently, methicillin-resistant *S. aureus* (MRSA) is being encountered at near epidemic levels as a causative agent of suppurative lymphadenitis in the ambulatory setting. A high suspicion of an MRSA infection should be entertained in all children presenting with either a first episode or more certainly in recalcitrant and recurrent cases.

Treatment

In the acute phase, the patient should be treated with oral or intravenous antistaphylococcal antibiotics. In the subacute or chronic phase, the presence of pus in the node may be confirmed by needle aspiration of the mass. When an abscess is present, it should be incised and drained under general anesthesia. In those cases of MRSA infection, a prolonged course of either vancomycin or linezolid may be required for complete eradication even after drainage.

GRANULOMATOUS LYMPHADENITIS

Although typical tuberculous cervical adenitis is very rare in the United States, atypical mycobacteria (eg, *Mycobacterium avium-intracellulare*) is encountered and may present as a nonsuppurative area (usually cervical, axillary, or inguinal) of matted nodes with tenderness and a draining sinus. Granulomatous lymphadenitis and caseation may occur in the regional nodes draining the inoculation site of BCG. Cat-scratch disease causes a caseating lymphadenitis in regional lymph nodes (eg, epitrochlear and axillary nodes enlarge after an upper extremity cat scratch).

Clinical Findings

Children under age 6 years are most frequently affected. The initial manifestation is a painless, progressive enlargement of the lymph nodes in the deep cervical chain and the parotid, suboccipital, submandibular, and supraclavicular nodes. The duration of lymphadenopathy is usually 1-3 months or longer. The nodes may be large and mobile or, with progressive disease, may become matted, fixed, and finally caseate to form an abscess. Incision or spontaneous overlying skin breakdown will result in a chronically draining sinus. In tuberculosis, both sides of the neck or multiple groups of nodes are infected, and the chest radiograph indicates pulmonary involvement. In atypical mycobacterial lymphadenitis, pulmonary disease is rare and the cervical adenitis is unilateral. The tuberculin skin test is weakly positive in over 80% of patients with atypical mycobacterial infection. Skin test antigens from the various strains of atypical mycobacteria are available. A positive skin test helps differentiate granulomatous adenitis from malignant lymphadenopathy. A fluctuant node can be confused with a branchial cleft remnant or a thyroglossal duct cyst.

Cat-scratch disease is usually acquired by a bite or scratch from a kitten. It is caused by a pleomorphic gram-negative bacillus *(Bartonella henselae)* that is detected in tissues by a silver stain or via serologic testing. It is an acute illness characterized by fever, malaise, possible musculoskeletal manifestations and occasionally a pustular lesion at the site of the scratch. Tender lymph node enlargement usually develops. Two to 4 weeks later, regional lymphadenitis persists, producing painful, fixed suppurative nodes that may develop into a chronically draining sinus.

Treatment

Atypical tuberculous lymphadenitis may be treated with rifampin (10 mg/kg/d), though definitive treatment usually requires nodal excision. Trimethoprim-sulfamethoxazole may shorten the course of cat-scratch disease and prevent suppuration. When antibiotics are ineffective, the procedure of choice is excision of involved nodes before caseation occurs. Once the nodes become fluctuant or a draining sinus forms, a wedge of involved skin should be excised and the underlying necrotic nodes should be curetted out (rather than excised), taking care not to injure neighboring nerves. The wound edges and skin should be closed primarily. The value of continuing chemotherapy is influenced by sensitivity tests on the cultured material. Excision and primary closure usually result in excellent healing with good cosmetic results.

Pilkington EF, MacArthur CJ, Beekmann SE, Polgreen PM, Winthrop KL: Treatment patterns of pediatric nontuberculous mycobacterial (NTM) cervical lymphadenitis as reported by nationwide surveys of pediatric otolaryngology and infectious disease societies. *Int J Pediatr Otorhinolaryngol* 2010 Apr;74(4):343-346.

▼ CONGENITAL CHEST WALL DEFORMITIES

STERNAL CLEFT

Failure of fusion of the two sternal bars during embryonic development produces congenital sternal cleft, which may involve the upper, lower, or entire sternum. In its severe form, this defect is usually associated with protrusion of the pericardium and heart (ectopia cordis) and congenital heart lesions. Defects may be associated with extracardiac anomalies, including cleft lip, cleft palate, hydrocephalus, and other CNS disorders, or may be one component of the pentalogy of Cantrell. Operative correction is performed in the neonatal period since the chest wall is so pliable; it consists of simple suture approximation of the two sternal halves. More complex defects associated with ectopia cordis are often incompatible with life.

PECTUS EXCAVATUM

This depression deformity is the most common congenital chest wall abnormality, occurring in one in 300 live births, with a 3:1 male predominance. It is associated with other musculoskeletal disorders (Marfan syndrome, Poland syndrome, scoliosis, clubfoot, syndactyly), and 2% have congenital heart disease. There is a familial form. It results from the unbalanced posterior growth of costal cartilages that are often fused, bizarrely deformed, or rotated. The body of the sternum secondarily exhibits a prominent posterior curvature, usually involving its lower half (Figure 43–4). Commonly, the xiphoid is the deepest portion of the depression. The third, fourth, and fifth costal cartilages are usually affected, though the second to eighth costal cartilages may be involved. The severity of the defect varies greatly from a mild, insignificant depression to an extreme where the xiphoid bone is adjacent to the vertebrae. The depression may be symmetrical or asymmetrical with varying degrees of sternal rotation.

▶ Clinical Findings

These patients are typically round shouldered, with stooped posture, relative abdominal prominence, flared costal margins, and an asthenic appearance. They may be withdrawn and refuse to participate in sports activities, particularly if their deformity might be exposed. Few patients complain of easy fatigability or inability to compete in exertional activities. Cardiopulmonary function studies rarely demonstrate impairments; this is predominantly a cosmetic deformity with potentially severe psychosocial sequelae.

▶ Treatment & Prognosis

There is no standard age for repair. Undeniably, it is an easier operation in younger children compared to adolescents. Drawbacks of an early operation include a higher

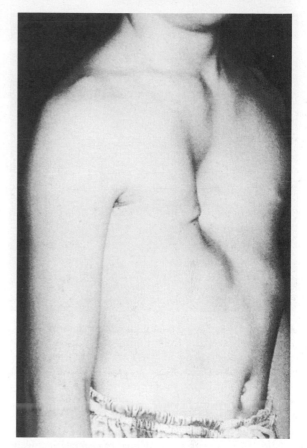

▲ **Figure 43–4.** Adolescent with a pectus excavatum deformity. Note that the most pronounced sternal curvature is in the lower half.

risk of recurrence during the adolescent growth spurt and the inability of a young child to comprehend and assent to a predominantly cosmetic operation. Traditionally, an open repair (Ravitch technique) was performed in which the abnormal cartilages were resected and the sternum was fractured and fixed in a corrected position. Recently, the Ravitch technique has been supplanted by the less invasive Nuss procedure in which a preformed sternal strut is passed, either blindly or with thoracoscopic assistance, under the chest wall muscles, into each hemithorax, and across the mediastinum under the sternum via two small incisions in the midaxillary line. The curved bar is passed upside down and "flipped" into position under the sternum, effectively lifting the sternum and chest wall into a corrected position. The bar is left in place for 2 years, and the patient can resume activity in 3 months. The long-term good to excellent results of the Nuss procedure are better than 95%. The latest evolution in less invasive techniques involves placement of

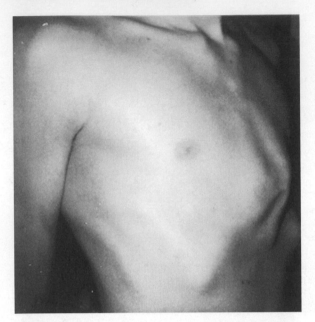

▲ **Figure 43–5.** Severe pectus carinatum deformity. (Reproduced, with permission, from Shamberger R: Congenital chest wall deformities In: O'Neill JA, Rowe MI, Grosted JL [editors]: *Pediatric Surgery*. 5th ed. Philadelphia, PA: Mosby Company;1998.)

opposing magnetic field implants to draw the chest deformity forward and effect remodeling. In general, there is no cardiopulmonary benefit after chest wall repair except in rare instances when the deformity is excessive. Otherwise, the repair is performed solely to improve appearance. However, the psychosocial benefits of repair of this often embarrassing deformity cannot be minimized.

PECTUS CARINATUM

This is a protrusion deformity, also referred to as pigeon breast or chicken chest. It is approximately ten times less frequent than pectus excavatum. It results from the overgrowth of costal cartilages, with forward buckling and secondary deformation of the sternum (Figure 43–5). Atypical and asymmetric forms with rotation are common. There is a familial form. It is associated with Marfan disease, neurofibromatosis, Poland syndrome, and Morquio disease. Unlike pectus excavatum, the deformity is typically mild or nearly imperceptible in early childhood and becomes increasingly prominent during the rapid growth in early puberty.

▶ Treatment & Prognosis

As with pectus excavatum, there is no cardiorespiratory compromise with this deformity, and repair is performed solely to achieve an improved cosmetic appearance. Mild deformities should be left alone and the patient followed to observe for progression. Moderate to severe defects should be repaired, particularly when the patient indicates a desire for improvement. The deformed cartilages are resected, leaving the costochondral membranes (perichondrium) intact. Sternal fracture is usually not necessary. To ensure that the costal cartilages grow back on a straighter line, "reefing" sutures are placed in the perichondrium to shorten them. The costal cartilages regenerate within 6 weeks. A thorough procedure will provide an excellent cosmetic result in nearly all cases. Recurrences are rare. An alternative approach to operative repair is chest bracing via an orthotic vest that needs to fitted and worn by the affected child for several hours daily over several years. This procedure may eventually replace the operative approach, particularly for those patients who are motivated to wear the brace for a majority of each day (about 16 hours).

Fonkalsrud EW, Beanes S: Surgical management of pectus carinatum: 30 years' experience. *World J Surg* 2001;25:898.

Harrison MR, Curran PF, Jamshidi R, Christensen D, Bratton BJ, Fechter R, Hirose S: Magnetic mini-mover procedure for pectus excavatum II: initial findings of a Food and Drug Administration-sponsored trial. *J Pediatr Surg* 2010 Jan;45(1):185-191.

Nuss D: Minimally invasive surgical repair of pectus excavatum. *Semin Pediatr Surg* 2008 Aug;17(3):209-217.

▼ SURGICAL RESPIRATORY EMERGENCIES IN THE NEWBORN

Certain aspects of respiration unique to the infant must be appreciated. Except during periods of crying, the newborn baby is an obligate nasal breather. The ability to breathe through the mouth may take weeks or months to acquire. Inspiration is accomplished chiefly by diaphragmatic excursion; the intercostal and accessory muscles contribute little to ventilation. Impaired inspiration results in retraction of the sternum, costal margin, and neck fossae; the resulting paradoxical motion may contribute to respiratory insufficiency. The airway is small and flaccid, so that it is readily occluded by mucus or edema, and it collapses readily under slight pressure. Dyspneic infants swallow large volumes of air, and the distended stomach and bowel may further impair diaphragmatic excursion.

▶ Classification

A. Upper Airway Disorders

1. Micrognathia—Pierre Robin syndrome
2. Macroglossia—Muscular hypertrophy, hypothyroidism, lymphatic malformation, Beckwith-Wiedemann syndrome

3. Anomalous nasopharyngeal passage—Choanal atresia, Treacher-Collins syndrome, Apert syndrome, and Crouzon syndrome

4. Tumors, cysts, or enlarged thyroid remnants in the pharynx or neck

5. Laryngeal or tracheal stenosis, webs, cysts, tumors, or vocal cord paralysis

6. Epiglottitis

7. Tracheomalacia

8. Tracheal stenosis with or without complete tracheal rings

B. Intrathoracic Airway Disorders

1. Atelectasis

2. Pneumothorax and pneumomediastinum

3. Pleural effusion or chylothorax

4. Pulmonary cysts, sequestration, and tumors

5. Congenital lobar emphysema

6. Diaphragmatic hernia or eventration

7. Esophageal atresia with or without tracheoesophageal fistula

8. Anomalies of the great vessels (eg, double aortic arch, aberrant left subclavian artery, anomalous origin of left pulmonary artery)

9. Mediastinal tumors and cysts (foregut duplications, thymomas, substernal goiter, lymphoma)

PIERRE ROBIN SYNDROME

Pierre Robin syndrome is a congenital defect characterized by micrognathia and glossoptosis, often associated with cleft palate. The small lower jaw and strong sucking action of the infant allow the tongue to be sucked back and occlude the laryngeal airway and may be life threatening.

Infants with mild cases should be kept in the prone position during care and feeding. A nasogastric or gastrostomy tube may be necessary for feeding. Nasohypopharyngeal intubation is effective in preventing occlusion of the larynx. If conservative measures fail, prompt attention to maintaining an open airway by tracheostomy is indicated. Surgical treatment involves tongue placation in which the tongue is sutured forward to the lower jaw, but this frequently breaks down. In time, the lower jaw develops normally. These infants eventually learn how to keep the tongue from occluding the airway.

CHOANAL ATRESIA

Complete obstruction at the posterior nares from choanal atresia may be unilateral and relatively asymptomatic. It may be membranous (10%) or bony (90%). When it is bilateral, severe respiratory distress is manifested at birth by marked chest wall retraction on inspiration and a normal cry.

There is arching of the head and neck in an effort to breathe, and the baby is unable to eat. The diagnosis is confirmed by the inability to pass a tube through the nares to the pharynx. With the baby in a supine position, radiopaque material may be instilled into the nares and lateral x-rays of the head taken to outline the obstruction. A CT scan of the nasopharynx will define bony occlusion.

Emergency treatment consists of maintaining an oral airway by placing a nipple, with the tip cut off, in the mouth. The membranous or bony occlusion may then be perforated by direct transpalatal excision, or it may be punctured and enlarged with a Hegar dilator. The newly created opening must be stented with plastic tubing for 5 weeks to prevent stricture.

CONGENITAL TRACHEAL STENOSIS & MALACIA

There are three main types of congenital tracheal stenosis: generalized hypoplasia; funnel-like narrowing, usually tapering to a tight stenosis just above the carina; and segmental stenosis of various lengths that can occur at any level. Tracheomalacia is a functional obstruction in a "soft" trachea that collapses with inspiration. It is often secondary to external compression by vascular anomalies or tumors or from a chronically dilated upper esophageal pouch in those with esophageal atresia.

▶ Diagnosis

The diagnostic approach to an infant with respiratory distress and possible distal tracheal obstruction must be carefully integrated with plans for management of the airway, since the compromised infant airway is easily occluded by edema or secretions. This is especially true in distal tracheal lesions, where an endotracheal or tracheostomy tube may not relieve the distal obstruction. The diagnostic value of every procedure must be weighed against the threat of precipitating airway obstruction. Tracheal lesions can be visualized using esophagography, angiography, or CT/MRI scans. Dynamic lesions such as tracheomalacia and vascular compression syndromes are best defined by videotape fluoroscopy or cineradiography with barium in the esophagus. Angiography may be necessary. Flow-volume curves can define the level of obstruction (intrathoracic vs extrathoracic) and the type of obstruction (stenosis vs malacia).

Although bronchoscopy often provides the best delineation of tracheobronchial lesions, it is an invasive procedure that can precipitate acute obstruction from edema or inflammation. A ventilating infant rigid bronchoscope with Hopkins optics should be kept above the critical area to avoid precipitating obstruction. Flexible transnasal awake bronchoscopy is most useful in demonstrating functional abnormalities (eg, malacia).

▶ Treatment

Noncritical stenotic and malaciac lesions in infants and children should be managed as conservatively as possible, preferably without intubation. "Temporary" stenting of these lesions is seldom temporary, since the presence of the tube itself ensures continued trauma and irritation such that the tube cannot be removed without airway obstruction. If an infant or child cannot be managed without intubation, surgical correction must be considered. Tracheal reconstruction via resection or a variety of tracheoplasty techniques has proved to be the treatment of choice for tracheal lesions. Severe tracheomalacia is treated by addressing the underlying cause. Aortopexy or an endotracheal stent is often necessary. Tracheostomy is a last resort.

CONGENITAL DIAPHRAGMATIC HERNIA

CDH is a highly lethal or morbid disease that affects 1 in 2000 live births (Figure 43–6). Anatomically, CDH results from an embryologic fusion defect, allowing herniation of intraabdominal contents into the chest. Fusion of the transverse septum and pleuroperitoneal folds normally occurs during the eighth week of embryonic development. If diaphragmatic formation is incomplete, the pleuroperitoneal hiatus (foramen of Bochdalek) persists. Intestinal nonrotation is common as the bowel herniates into the thorax rather than undergoing its normal sequence of rotation and fixation. Severe defects cause pulmonary hypoplasia, pulmonary hypertension, and cardiac dysfunction. The larger the hernia and the earlier it occurs, the more severe the pulmonary hypoplasia.

▶ Clinical Findings

A. Symptoms and Signs

Infants with large diaphragmatic defects are usually symptomatic in the delivery room, with tachypnea, grunting respirations, retractions, and cyanosis, and may require urgent intubation. Smaller defects may not become symptomatic until the infant is several days or months old. Typically, the abdomen is scaphoid since much of the abdominal viscera are in the hemithorax. The chest on the side of the hernia may be dull to percussion, but bowel sounds are not usually appreciated. The left side of the diaphragm is affected four or five times as frequently as the right, with a rate of associated anomalies of 20% (chromosomal abnormalities, neural tube defects, and congenital heart disease). When the hernia is on the left, the heart sounds may be heard best on the right side of the chest.

The development of symptoms with CDH correlates with the degree of pulmonary hypoplasia and pulmonary hypertension. Prenatal diagnosis is occurring more and more frequently and allows the mother and the fetus to be referred to an institution where sophisticated perinatal and pediatric surgical units are available.

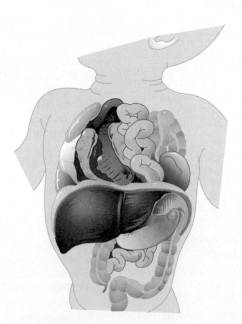

▲ **Figure 43–6.** Congenital posterolateral (Bochdalek) diaphragmatic hernia. Bowel, spleen, and liver sometimes herniate into the chest and severely compromise lung development *in utero* and ventilation after birth.

B. Imaging Studies

A chest radiograph may demonstrate the following: a paucity of gas within the abdomen, radiopaque hemithorax if the bowel does not contain a significant amount of gas or if the left lobe of the liver occupies the majority of the hemithorax, loss of normal ipsilateral diaphragmatic contour, bowel in the thorax, contralateral mediastinal shift, and a coiled nasogastric tube in the hemithorax. Right-sided hernias can be difficult to distinguish from a diaphragmatic eventration. This can be differentiated by an MRI scan. MRI or CT scan can also distinguish between CDH and a cystic lung lesion (eg, congenital cystic adenomatoid malformation).

► Treatment

A nasogastric tube should be placed in the stomach to aspirate swallowed air and to prevent distention of the herniated bowel, which would further compress the lungs. Repair of the diaphragmatic defect is not a surgical emergency, it is rather a physiologic emergency requiring resuscitation, with surgery performed once the infant has stabilized and demonstrated minimal to no pulmonary hypertension. Early (before 48 hours postnatally) hernia repair has been shown to transiently worsen pulmonary function by decreasing pulmonary compliance and increasing airway reactivity. A subcostal abdominal incision should be made and the herniated bowel reduced from the pleural space. Some surgeons prefer a thoracic approach, particularly for right-sided defects. The negative pressure between the bowel and the chest wall may make reduction difficult. Following reduction of the bowel, placement of a chest tube in the pleural space is optional; if used, it is connected to a water seal and not to suction as it may cause physiologically significant mediastinal shift. The diaphragmatic defect should be closed by nonabsorbable sutures. In many instances, a synthetic material is required to close large defects. The abdominal cavity may be too small and underdeveloped to accommodate the intestine and permit closure of the abdominal wall muscle and fascial layers. In such cases, abdominal wall skin flaps should be mobilized and closed over the protruding bowel or a silo created to allow for gradual visceral reduction with concomitant abdominal domain expansion and staged closure of the abdominal wall.

Respiratory support and treatment of hypoxemia, hypercapnia, and acidosis are required before and often after repair. Persistent pulmonary hypertension may result in right-to-left shunt and produce severe hypoxemia in the lower aorta. Nitric oxide added to the ventilation gases can induce pulmonary vasodilation, improve pulmonary perfusion, and reverse the right-to-left shunt. The persistent fetal circulation physiology may be treated successfully in many cases by extracorporeal membrane oxygenation and permissive ventilatory strategies (high-frequency ventilation). Hypoxemic myocardiopathy may require infusion of dopamine to enhance cardiac output. Prenatal treatment for severe CDH (temporary fetal tracheal occlusion to promote lung growth) has been extensively studied and may offer benefit in severe cases of CDH.

► Prognosis

The death rate for infants with CDH depends upon the severity of pulmonary hypoplasia, the presence or absence of associated anomalies, and the quality of care provided for these critically ill infants. When diagnosed *in utero*, prognosis depends on the presence or absence of liver herniation into the left hemithorax, the gestational age at diagnosis, and an ultrasonographic estimation of lung size (the lung-to-head ratio). Long-term, there are a number of measurable physiologic abnormalities that are not necessarily clinically significant such as a reduction in total lung volume, restrictive or obstructive lung disease, and abnormal lung compliance. However, a small subset of patients will survive as "pulmonary cripples" and remain oxygen dependent or ventilator dependent, often requiring tracheostomies. Since there may be deficient periesophageal muscular tissue or an abnormal orientation of the gastroesophageal junction, GER is common. It is most commonly treated nonoperatively, but refractory cases may require a surgical antireflux procedure. Recurrent diaphragmatic hernia occurs in 10%-20% of infants and should be considered in any child with a history of CDH who presents with new GI or pulmonary symptoms. Recurrence is most common when a prosthetic patch is used for the repair.

Surgical units that are immediately adjacent to obstetric services report death rates as high as 80%, because infants with severe pulmonary hypoplasia will be recognized and treated immediately. Infants who survive transfer to surgical centers remote from the delivery area usually have less severe disease, and the death rates reported from these facilities are usually under 40%.

With improvements in prenatal ultrasonographic imaging, many of these defects can be appreciated early enough so that planned delivery at a tertiary facility is possible. Excluding those infants with severe associated anomalies, the overall survival rate using maximal medical therapy has been increasing over the past several years due to advanced ventilation strategies and is well over 70%.

FORAMEN OF MORGAGNI HERNIA

The foramen of Morgagni occurs at the junction of the septum transversum and the anterior thoracic wall. This anterior, central diaphragmatic defect accounts for only 2% of diaphragmatic hernias. It may be parasternal, retrosternal, or bilateral. Unlike Bochdalek hernias, children are typically asymptomatic and the defect is discovered later in life on a chest radiograph taken for reasons unrelated to the hernia. The lateral chest radiograph demonstrating an air-filled mass extending into the anterior mediastinum is pathogno-monic. Repair is indicated in the asymptomatic patient due to the risk of bowel obstruction. The viscera are reduced and any associated hernia sac excised. The defect is closed by suturing the posterior rim of diaphragm to the posterior rectus sheath since there is no anterior diaphragm. A pros-thetic patch closure is frequently required given the tension that results with native tissue repairs given the absence of anterior diaphragm. Laparoscopic approaches to this type of repair are increasingly being performed. There is no associ-ated pulmonary hypoplasia or hypertension. This defect, when noted in newborns, can be associated with the pental-ogy of Cantrell, a disorder with considerable morbidity and mortality that consists of the anterior diaphragmatic defect, distal sternal cleft, epigastric omphalocele, apical pericardial defect, and congenital heart disease (usually a septal defect). Excluding patients with the pentalogy of Cantrell, survival is nearly 100%.

EVENTRATION OF THE DIAPHRAGM

Diaphragmatic eventration is an abnormally elevated or attenuated portion of the diaphragm (or both). It may be congenital (usually idiopathic, but can be associated with congenital myopathies or intrauterine infections) or acquired (as a result of phrenic nerve injury during forceps delivery or surgery). In the congenital form, there is vari-able thinning or absence of diaphragmatic muscle, at which point its distinction from CDH with a persistent hernia sac is obscure. The elevated hemidiaphragm may produce abnor-malities of chest wall mechanics with impaired pulmonary function. Respiratory distress and pneumonia are frequent presenting symptoms, although GI symptoms such as vom-iting or gastric volvulus have been reported.

The diagnosis is made by chest radiograph. It is con-firmed by fluoroscopy or ultrasound, which demonstrate paradoxical movement of the diaphragm during spontane-ous respiration. Incidentally discovered small, localized eventrations do not need repair. Eventrations that are associ-ated with respiratory symptoms should be repaired by plicat-ing the diaphragm using interrupted nonabsorbable sutures.

Al-Salem AH: Congenital hernia of Morgagni in infants and chil-dren. *J Pediatr Surg* 2007 Sep;42(9):1539-1543.

Congenital Diaphragmatic Hernia Study Group: Defect Size deter-mines survival in infants with congenital diaphragmatic hernia. *Pediatrics* 2007;120(3):3651-3657.

Dutta S, Albanese CT: Use of a prosthetic patch for laparo-scopic repair of Morgagni diaphragmatic hernia in children. *J Laparoendosc Adv Surg Tech A* 2007;17(3):391-394.

Ruano R, Yoshisaki CT, da Silva MM, Ceccon ME, Grasi MS, Tannuri U, Zugaib M: A randomized controlled trial of fetal endoscopic tracheal occlusion versus postnatal management of severe isolated congenital diaphragmatic hernia. *Ultrasound Obstet Gynecol* 2012 Jan;39(1):20-27.

CONGENITAL LOBAR EMPHYSEMA

Congenital lobar emphysema results from hyperinflation of a single lobe; rarely, more than one lobe is affected. The upper and middle lobes are most frequently involved. Pathologically, there are three forms; hypoplastic emphy-sema, polyalveolar lobe, and bronchial obstruction.

Hypoplastic emphysema is distinguished by a segment, lobe, or whole lung that has a reduced number of bron-chial branches with a diminished number and smaller size of blood vessels. The number of alveoli is abnormally decreased, but the air spaces are too large. The hyperlucent region seen on chest radiograph is normal or small in vol-ume, and since it does not affect the surrounding normal lung, surgical treatment is unnecessary.

Polyalveolar lobe is characterized by a normal size and number of bronchial branches, but there is an abnormal number of alveoli from each respiratory unit. These alveoli are prone to expand excessively, producing emphysema, which encroaches on the surrounding normal lung and therefore requires removal.

Bronchial obstruction may occur from deficient bron-chial cartilage support, redundant mucosa, bronchial steno-sis, mucous plug, or bronchial compression by anomalous vessels or other mediastinal lesions. With inspiration, the bronchus opens to allow air into the lung, but on expira-tion the bronchus collapses, trapping the air, and with each respiratory cycle there is progressive expansion of the lobe.

▶ Clinical Findings

In one-third of patients, respiratory distress is noted at birth; in only 5% of cases do symptoms develop after 6 months. Males are affected twice as frequently as females. The signs include progressive and severe dyspnea, wheezing, grunt-ing, coughing, cyanosis, and difficulty feeding. An increased anteroposterior dimension of the chest and retractions may be seen. The chest is hyperresonant, and decreased breath sounds may be noted over the affected lobe. A chest radio-graph may demonstrate radiolucency of the emphysematous lobe, with bronchovascular markings extending to the lung periphery. Compression atelectasis of the adjacent lung, shift of the mediastinum, depression of the diaphragm, and anterior bowing of the sternum can be seen. The emphyse-matous lobe may continue to expand, compressing adjacent lung and airways, producing progressively severe respiratory distress.

▶ Treatment & Prognosis

Occasionally, the emphysema may be due to a foreign body or mucous plug in the bronchus that may be aspirated by bronchoscopy. Compression of the bronchus by mediastinal masses may be relieved by removal of the tumor or repair of anomalous vessels.

Treatment of asymptomatic and mildly symptomatic cases may not be necessary. Many patients with lobar emphysema, however, are severely symptomatic, and pulmonary lobectomy is necessary. For those who are breathing spontaneously prior to operation, anesthesia should not be started until all personnel are ready for a rapid thoracotomy since positive-pressure ventilation may acutely enlarge the emphysematous lobe, thereby compressing the normal lung tissue and heart. The prognosis following surgical relief of the lobar emphysema is excellent. Rarely patients may show residual disease in the remaining lung. At long-term follow-up, lung volumes are normal, but the airflow rates are diminished.

GREAT VESSEL ANOMALIES

Tracheobronchial and esophageal compression by the great vessels may occur as a result of anomalies of the aortic arch or of abnormally located or enlarged pulmonary and subclavian arteries. While the most common abnormality is an aberrant right subclavian artery, the most important is the double aortic arch, as it often causes serious respiratory distress in young infants (Figure 43–7). Affected infants have a characteristic inspiratory and expiratory wheeze, stridor, or croup-like cough. Echocardiography, CT, and MRI can demonstrate the anomalous anatomy. Esophagoscopy and bronchoscopy may be helpful in assessing the degree and level of compression. The surgical approach is through the left hemithorax. Following removal of the thymus, the aortic arch and its branches are skeletonized and the anatomy is identified. For the double aortic arch, the smallest arterial component is divided; an anomalous right subclavian artery

is divided at its origin. The accompanying fibrous bands and sheaths constricting the trachea and esophagus must also be divided. The ductus arteriosus (or its fibrous remnant) is also divided.

MEDIASTINAL MASSES

Mediastinal masses are relatively common in infants and children and can be classified according to the compartment of the mediastinum from which they arise. The mediastinum is classically divided into anterior, middle, and posterior compartments. Anatomically, the anterior mediastinum consists of the area between the sternum and the anterior aspect of the trachea and pericardium. The middle compartment contains the trachea, major bronchi, and paratracheal spaces. The posterior segment extends from the posterior aspect of the trachea to the spine.

Anterior masses make up one-third and are most commonly teratomas and lymphomas. Teratomas may be cystic or solid and may also be found within the pericardium (middle compartment). Approximately 20% are malignant. Other masses include thymic cysts, thymomas, substernal goiters, and lymphangiomas. Middle mediastinal masses are rare but when present are most likely to be bronchogenic cysts. Sixty percent of mediastinal masses are located within the posterior compartment. Neurogenic tumors are most common and include neuroblastoma, ganglioneuroblastoma, ganglioneuroma, neurofibroma, and neurofibrosarcoma. Common symptoms include respiratory distress (via tracheal or lung compression), Horner syndrome, and pain. Enterogenous cysts or duplications are also commonly seen in the posterior compartment. They are termed neurenteric when there is an associated cervical or thoracic vertebral anomaly.

CONGENITAL LUNG LESIONS

Congenital lung lesions, which arise from anomalous development of the foregut, are classified as follows: (1) bronchogenic cyst, (2) congenital pulmonary airway malformation (CPAM), (3) pulmonary sequestration, and (4) bronchopulmonary foregut malformation. Embryonic tissues that are destined to form bronchi and lung become anomalous isolated structures within or outside of the lung. These lesions produce symptoms from their size and position, resulting in compression of bronchi or lung parenchyma, or from infection and abscess formation within the cyst and surrounding normal lung. There is a growing number of congenital lung lesions being diagnosed due to improvements in prenatal imaging. Most lesions warrant a postnatal CT angiogram to determine the anatomic location of the lesion and the presence of systemic feeding vessels.

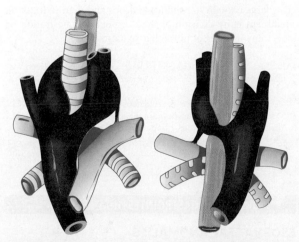

▲ **Figure 43–7.** Anterior (left) and posterior views of double aortic arch constricting the trachea and esophagus.

BRONCHOGENIC CYST

Bronchogenic cysts are lined by cuboidal or ciliated columnar epithelium and are filled with mucoid material. Repeated infection in the cyst may produce squamous epithelial metaplasia. About half arise in the mediastinum and do not communicate with the bronchi. They appear as radiopaque masses on chest radiographs. When located within the lung parenchyma, the cysts usually communicate with the airways and consequently are prone to abscess formation. Bronchogenic cysts arise in the right lung three times more often than in the left. They are more common in the lower lobes but may be found in any lobe. Partial compression of bronchi produces hyperinflation of the involved lung, while complete obstruction produces atelectasis. Rupture of a cyst that communicates with bronchi may present as a tension pneumothorax. Treatment of a noninfected cyst is by excision. Infected cysts first require drainage (usually percutaneous) and intravenous antibiotic therapy followed by resection after the inflammation subsides (no sooner than 6 weeks after drainage).

CONGENITAL PULMONARY AIRWAY MALFORMATION

This lesion is a multicystic lung mass resulting from proliferation of terminal bronchiolar structures. It is typically lined by a polypoid proliferation of bronchial epithelium surrounded by striated muscle and elastic tissue, but there is an absence of mucous glands and cartilage. They are most often lobar and are classified radiologically based on cyst size: type I are large (> 2 cm) cysts, type II are smaller cysts (< 2 cm), and type III have cysts that are so small as to import a solid appearance. These malformations occur with equal frequency in both lungs, with a slight predominance in the upper lobes. Associated renal and nervous system anomalies may be present.

▶ Clinical Findings

A large lesion can compress the fetal lung, resulting in pulmonary hypoplasia at birth, or may distort or obstruct the esophagus, producing polyhydramnios. In addition, compression of venous return to the heart with exudation of protein into the lung fluid may cause fetal congestive heart failure, hydrops fetalis, and death *in utero*. Large lesions that do not cause fetal hydrops can remain stable or involute during fetal life, producing little or no symptoms of respiratory distress at birth.

▶ Treatment

If prenatal ultrasound can recognize the presence of this disorder in association with hydrops, resection *in utero* is an option for select cases. Steroids have recently shown promise in the prenatal treatment of CPAM with hydrops. Children in whom hydrops did not occur before birth may be born asymptomatic (small lesions) or may have variable degrees of respiratory distress due to compression of the ipsilateral normal lung. Asymptomatic children may be observed, but resection (pulmonary lobectomy) is recommended since these lesions often become infected and there are case reports of malignant transformation occurring in untreated, long-standing cysts. Often the plain chest radiograph does not demonstrate the small, asymptomatic lesion.

PULMONARY SEQUESTRATION & BRONCHOPULMONARY FOREGUT MALFORMATION

A sequestration consists of normally developed bronchioles and alveoli supplied by systemic rather than pulmonary arteries. Sequestrations occur in the lower chest, most commonly on the left, adjacent to the mediastinum. Rarely, sequestrations may occur in the upper or middle lobes or even below the diaphragm. They usually have a systemic arterial blood supply from the aorta, either above or below the diaphragm. On rare occasions, a sequestration will communicate with the esophagus or stomach, a condition termed bronchopulmonary foregut malformation. Sequestrations may be intralobar or extralobar. Intralobar lesions drain through the pulmonary veins, are in communication with the tracheobronchial tree, and are prone to infection and lung abscess formation. Extralobar lesions drain into the azygous venous system, do not communicate with the lung, and are commonly asymptomatic. They are often found in association with CDH. Histologic evidence suggests that these lesions have embryologic origin similar to that of bronchogenic cysts and congenital cystic adenomatoid malformations. However, unlike the latter, sequestrations rarely grow large enough to produce hydrops and demise *in utero*. Treatment is by excision of the extralobar sequestration or lobectomy in cases of intralobar sequestration.

Albanese CT, Rothenberg SS: Experience with 144 consecutive pediatric thoracoscopic lobectomies. *J Laparoendosc Adv Surg Tech A* 2007;17(3):339-341.

Loh KC, Jelin E, Hirose S, Feldstein V, Goldstein R, Lee H: Microcystic congenital pulmonary airway malformation with hydrops fetalis: steroids vs open fetal resection. *J Pediatr Surg* 2012 Jan;47(1):36-39.

Puligandla PS, Laberge JM: Congenital lung lesions. *Clin Perinatol* 2012 Jun;39(2):331-347.

▼ CONGENITAL GASTROINTESTINAL LESIONS

ESOPHAGEAL ANOMALIES

The trachea and esophagus are derived from the primitive foregut. Initially, they appear as a common ventral diverticulum at about the nineteenth day of gestation.

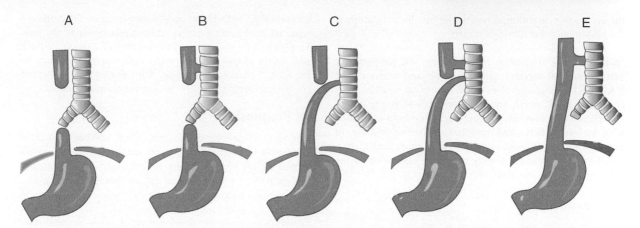

▲ **Figure 43–8. A:** Pure (long gap) esophageal atresia. **B:** Esophageal atresia with proximal tracheoesophageal fistula. **C:** Esophageal atresia with distal tracheoesophageal fistula. **D:** Esophageal atresia with proximal and distal fistulas. **E:** Tracheoesophageal fistula without esophageal atresia. (Reproduced, with permission, from Grosfeld JL: Pediatric surgery. In: Sabiston DC, ed. *Textbook of Surgery*. Philadelphia, PA: Saunders; 1991.)

Beginning several days later, elongation and separation of the diverticulum into the airway and esophagus occurs in a caudal to cephalad direction. Errors in this process result in esophageal atresia, tracheoesophageal fistula, and their variants (Figure 43–8).

▶ Classification

A. With Esophageal Atresia

1. There is a blind proximal pouch and a fistula between the distal end of the esophagus and the distal one-third of the trachea (type C, 85% of cases).

2. There is a blind proximal esophageal pouch, no tracheoesophageal fistula, and a blind, short distal esophagus (type A, 10% of cases). This is referred to as "pure or long gap" atresia.

3. There are fistulas between both proximal and distal esophageal segments and the trachea (type D, 2% of cases).

4. There is a fistula between the proximal esophagus and the trachea and a blind distal esophagus without fistula (type B, 1% of cases).

B. Without Esophageal Atresia

1. There is an "H"-type tracheoesophageal fistula that is usually present in the low cervical region (type E, 4%-5% of cases).

2. There is esophageal stenosis consisting of a membranous occlusion (often containing cartilage) between the mid and distal third of the esophagus (rare).

3. There is a laryngotracheoesophageal cleft of varying length, consisting of a linear communication between these structures (very rare).

▶ Clinical Findings

Shortly after birth, the infant with esophageal atresia is noted to have excessive salivation and repeated episodes of coughing, choking, and cyanosis. Attempts at feeding result in choking, gagging, and regurgitation. Infants with tracheoesophageal fistula in addition to esophageal atresia will have reflux of gastric secretions into the tracheobronchial tree, with resulting pneumonia. Pulmonary infiltrates are usually noted first in the right upper lobe. Diagnosis may be delayed (several months) in cases of H-type tracheoesophageal fistula who are able to feed but may present with recurrent upper respiratory infections due to aspiration.

A size 10F catheter should be passed into the esophagus by way of the nose or mouth; if esophageal atresia is present, the tube will not go down the expected distance to the stomach and will coil in the upper esophageal pouch. If a tracheoesophageal fistula connects to the lower esophageal segment, air will be present in the stomach and bowel on plain radiographs. Absence of air below the diaphragm usually means that a distal tracheoesophageal fistula is not present.

Abdominal distention is a prominent finding because the Valsalva effect of coughing and crying forces air through a fistula into the stomach and bowel. The presence and position of the fistula can be determined by bronchoscopy.

Laryngotracheoesophageal cleft produces symptoms similar to those of tracheoesophageal fistula but of much greater severity. Laryngoscopy may show the cleft between the arytenoids extending down the larynx. Bronchoscopy is the best means of outlining the cleft.

There is a 50% incidence of associated anomalies: cardiac (patent ductus arteriosus, septal defects), GI (imperforate anus, duodenal atresia), genitourinary, and skeletal. The VACTERL association (*v*ertebral, *a*norectal, *c*ardiac, *tr*acheoesophageal, *r*enal, and *l*imb anomalies) is present in 25% of cases. Isolated esophageal atresia has been associated with various genetic abnormalities, including trisomy 18 and trisomy 21. Echocardiogram, renal ultrasound, anorectal exam and genetic testing should be considered in the workup of all patients with TEF.

▶ Treatment

A sump suction catheter should be placed in the upper esophageal pouch and the head of the bed elevated. An echocardiogram is required to determine the position of the aortic arch since a right-sided arch makes the standard right thoracotomy (or thoracoscopic) repair difficult and is present in 5% of infants. If possible, aspiration pneumonia is treated before repair.

The goal of operative therapy is to divide and ligate the fistula and repair the atresia in one stage, if possible. This is usually performed using a right posterolateral thoracotomy with an extrapleural dissection, although a transpleural thoracoscopic approach is gaining popularity for those stable, full-term infants. Also, thoracoscopic approaches are gaining acceptance as minimal invasive techniques continue to evolve. In those with an H-type tracheoesophageal fistula, the fistula is located above the thoracic inlet in two-thirds of cases. These fistulas may be divided through a left transverse cervical incision. A feeding gastrostomy tube is no longer routinely inserted except when the esophageal repair is under extreme tension, when there is long gap atresia not amenable to single-stage repair, and when there are severe associated anomalies (eg, congenital heart disease). A transanastomotic feeding tube is placed for postoperative feeding pending demonstration of a leak-free anastomosis by esophagogram obtained 7 days after surgery.

Staged operations are reserved for extremely premature babies, those who have severe aspiration pneumonitis, and those with severe anomalies or long gaps between the esophageal pouches. There are several strategies for repairing these defects. These include cervical esophagostomy, division of the fistula, and insertion of a gastrostomy tube. Several months later a staged reconstruction by esophageal replacement with colon or stomach interposition can be undertaken. Another alternative is a gastrostomy tube alone with intermittent bougienage and stretching of the upper esophageal pouch, followed by primary esophageal anastomosis and immediate interposition grafting.

Esophageal narrowing or webs in the distal esophageal segment readily respond to esophageal dilation. This is usually accomplished with Hurst or Maloney bougies. Dilations are repeated until healing occurs without recurrence of the web. Esophagoscopy and excision of portions of a tough or thick web, using biopsy forceps or the endoscopic laser, may be required in addition to dilation. A lower esophageal stricture containing cartilage requires excision and anastomosis.

▶ Prognosis

The survival rate for a full-term infant without associated anomalies is excellent. However, deaths occur as a result of pulmonary complications, severe associated anomalies, prematurity, and sepsis due to anastomotic disruption. Anastomotic leaks occur because of tension or poor blood supply. In performing the anastomosis, the extrapleural approach prevents the development of empyema and confines a leak and possible infection to a small localized area.

Swallowing is a reflex response that must be reinforced early in infancy. If establishment of esophageal continuity is delayed for more than 4-6 weeks, it may take many months to overcome oral aversion and learn to swallow. Babies with cervical esophagostomies should be encouraged to suck, eat, and swallow during gastrostomy feedings.

Dysphagia may occur for months or years following successful repair of esophageal atresia and is multifactorial. An anastomotic stricture is not uncommon and may require one or more dilations under anesthesia. Swallowed foreign bodies will lodge at the site of anastomosis and require removal with esophagoscopy. Another cause of dysphagia is poor peristalsis of the distal esophageal segment. This frequent problem improves with age.

Most of these infants have an alarming, barking cough and rattling sound on respiration from tracheomalacia. This results from *in utero* compression of the trachea by the dilated proximal esophageal pouch. This frequently improves with age and is rare after 5 years of age. GER is common after successful repair and may result in recurrent aspiration pneumonitia, dysphagia, failure to thrive, and recurrent anastomotic stricture. Medical therapy with an H2-blocker or proton pump inhibitor should be instituted in all patients after repair and a surgical antireflux procedure may be necessary if medical therapy fails.

Holland AJ, Ron O, Pierro A, Drake D, Curry JI, Kiely EM, Spitz L. Surgical outcomes of esophageal atresia without fistula for 24 years at a single institution. *J Pediatr Surg* 2009 Oct;44(10):1928-1932.

INTESTINAL OBSTRUCTION IN THE NEWBORN

Since fetuses continually swallow amniotic fluid into their GI tracts and excrete it in their urine, intestinal obstruction may be noted on prenatal ultrasound by the presence of polyhydramnios (increased amniotic fluid level). The presence of polyhydramnios correlates with the level of the obstruction; it is most common with proximal GI tract obstruction (eg, esophageal and duodenal atresia), is rarely noted with ileal atresia, and is never noted in association with anorectal obstruction.

After birth, vomiting is the principal symptom, and it is bile stained if the obstruction is distal to the ampulla of Vater. It is important to note that bilious vomiting in the newborn is pathologic until proved otherwise. On physical examination, the presence and degree of abdominal distention depends on the level of the obstruction and should be noted. For example, there is no significant distention with duodenal obstruction versus massive distention with colonic obstruction (eg, Hirschsprung disease). A careful perineal examination should be performed to determine whether the anus is present, patent, and in the normal location. Meconium, the first newborn stool, passes in the first 24 hours of life in 94% of normal full-term infants and by 48 hours in 98%. Failure to pass meconium may be indicative of lower GI tract obstruction. However, 30%-50% of newborn infants with intestinal obstruction will pass meconium.

Depending on the pathology, the plain abdominal radiograph may demonstrate dilated bowel loops, air-fluid levels, calcifications (if *in utero* perforation occurred), or a gasless abdomen. Unlike in adult patients, one cannot differentiate small from large bowel by their usual markings on a plain radiograph of the newborn's abdomen. If a lower GI tract obstruction is suspected, a contrast (usually water-soluble contrast) enema is the most useful study since it can be both diagnostic and therapeutic in the majority of cases (see below). An upper GI series is rarely indicated unless malrotation is to be ruled out. The CT, MRI, or ultrasound scans are virtually never indicated in the workup of newborn intestinal obstruction.

HYPERTROPHIC PYLORIC STENOSIS

Pyloric stenosis is the most common surgical disorder producing emesis in infancy. It results from hypertrophy of the circular and longitudinal muscularis of the pylorus and the distal antrum of the stomach with progressive narrowing of the pyloric canal (Figure 43–9). The cause is not known. The male:female incidence is 4:1. The disorder is more common in firstborn infants and occurs four times more often in the offspring of mothers who had the disease as infants than in those whose fathers had the disease. If one monozygotic twin is affected, the other will also have the disorder in two-thirds of cases. A seasonal variation is noted in the occurrence of symptoms, with peaks in spring and fall.

▶ Clinical Findings

A. Symptoms and Signs

Typically, the affected infant is full term when born and feeds and grows well until 2-4 weeks after birth, at which

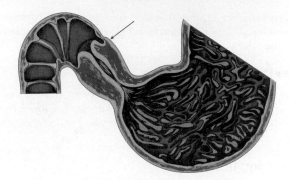

▲ **Figure 43–9.** Hypertrophic pyloric stenosis. Note that the distal end of the hypertrophic muscle protrudes into the duodenum (arrow), accounting for the ease of perforation into the duodenum during pyloromyotomy.

time occasional regurgitation of some of the feedings occurs. Several days later, however, the vomiting becomes more frequent and forceful. The vomitus contains the previous feeding and no bile. Blood may be seen in the vomitus in 5% of cases, and coffee grounds or occult blood is frequently present. Shortly after vomiting, the infant acts starved and will feed again. The stools become infrequent and firm in consistency as dehydration occurs. With dehydration, infants often have sunken fontanelles, dry mucous membranes, and poor skin turgor. Weight loss follows progressive feeding intolerance. Jaundice with indirect hyperbilirubinemia occurs in fewer than 10% of cases. Gastric peristaltic waves can usually be seen moving from the left costal margin to the area of the pylorus. In over 90% of cases, the pyloric "tumor," or "olive," can be palpated when the infant is relaxed. Abdominal relaxation may be accomplished by sedating the infant or by feeding clear fluids and simultaneously aspirating the stomach contents with a gastric tube.

B. Imaging Studies

An imaging study is indicated when the pyloric tumor cannot be palpated. Abdominal ultrasound, the most sensitive and specific test, will identify hypertrophic pyloric stenosis when the muscle thickness is greater than 4 mm and the length of the pylorus is greater than 16 mm. A dynamic ultrasound may also show no passage of ingested fluid. A contrast upper GI series is indicated if an experienced ultrasonographer is unavailable or if there is a reasonable chance that the patient's symptoms are not due to pyloric stenosis (eg, a premature, 1-week-old baby) since this examination can demonstrate other entities in the differential. A positive upper GI series can include the following diagnostic signs: (1) outlining of the narrow pyloric channel by a single "string sign" or "double track" owing to folds of mucosa; (2) a pyloric "beak" where the pyloric entrance from the antrum occurs; (3) the "shoulder" sign, in which the pyloric mass bulges into the antrum; and (4) complete obstruction of the pylorus.

Differential Diagnosis

Repeated nonbilious vomiting in early infancy may be due to overfeeding, intracranial lesions, pylorospasm, antral web, GER, pyloric duplication, duodenal stenosis, malrotation of the bowel, or adrenal insufficiency.

Complications

Repeated vomiting with inadequate intake of formula results in hypokalemic hypochloremic alkalosis, dehydration, and starvation. Gastritis and reflux esophagitis occur frequently. Aspiration of vomitus may produce pneumonia.

Treatment & Prognosis

The operative treatment is the Fredet-Ramstedt pyloromyotomy, in which the pylorus is incised along its entire length, spread widely exposing but not breaching the underlying mucosa. Surgery should be undertaken only after dehydration and the hypokalemic hypochloremic alkalosis have been corrected, heralded by a normal serum chloride (which is a proxy for a normal serum bicarbonate) as well as a urine output greater than 1 cc/kg/h. There are three approaches to the pyloromyotomy: a right upper quadrant transverse skin incision, a circumumbilical or intraumbilical skin incision, or a laparoscopic approach with the telescope in the umbilicus and the two working instruments placed directly through the abdominal wall. The laparoscopic approach offers advantages in postoperative recovery with equivalent outcomes in experienced hands. Successful myotomy is evident when the submucosa is seen to herniate out of the myotomy site. If, during the pyloromyotomy, the mucosa is inadvertently entered (usually on the duodenal side), it is closed with fine nonabsorbable sutures and an omental patch is placed. Large perforations are managed by closing the pyloromyotomy, rotating the pylorus 90 degrees, and repeating the myotomy.

Multiple postoperative feeding schedules have been described, ranging from immediate full feeds to delayed feeds with incremental advances in volume. This has stemmed from the observation that nearly all patients with pyloric stenosis vomit after surgery, presumably due to gastric ileus, gastritis, GER, or all of the above. An incomplete pyloromyotomy (usually on the antral side) is suspected when vomiting persists beyond 1-2 weeks postoperatively and stems from a short myotomy or incomplete division of the muscle. Incomplete myotomy should be evaluated by upper GI series as ultrasound will likely show ongoing hypertrophy.

Pyloric stenosis never recurs, and there is a uniformly excellent outcome.

Hall NJ et al: Recovery after open versus laparoscopic pyloromyotomy for pyloric stenosis: a double-blind multicentre randomised controlled trial. *Lancet* 2009 Jan 31;373(9661):390-398.

Pandya S, Heiss K: Pyloric stenosis in pediatric surgery: an evidence-based review. *Surg Clin North Am* 2012 Jun;92(3):527-539.

CONGENITAL DUODENAL OBSTRUCTION

The various causes of duodenal obstruction are atresia, stenosis, mucosal web (complete or variably perforate), annular pancreas, preduodenal portal vein, and peritoneal bands (Ladd bands) from malrotation. Duodenal atresia is distinguished from more distal GI atresias since it is due to failure of recanalization of the duodenum early in gestation rather than due to mesenteric vascular abnormality late in gestation. Atresia of the duodenum is twice as common as in the jejunum or ileum. In about half of cases, multiple congenital anomalies are present, including Down syndrome in 30% and congenital heart disease in 20%. Birth weight is less than 2500 g in half of these infants. Mucosal webs or stenoses occur as often as pure atresia. Annular pancreas is almost always associated with hypoplasia of the duodenum at the level of the ampulla. The cause is a developmental defect characterized by circumferential persistence of the gland around the duodenum at the site of the embryonic ventral anlage, leading to duodenal obstruction and an accessory pancreatic duct.

Clinical Findings

In 75% of cases, duodenal obstruction occurs distal to the ampulla of Vater, causing bile to be diverted to the proximal duodenum and stomach. Bilious emesis occurs shortly after birth and during attempted feedings. The upper abdomen is rarely distended. Meconium is passed in over 50% of cases.

The plain abdominal radiograph demonstrates an air-distended stomach and duodenum ("double bubble" sign). Gas in the small and large intestine indicates incomplete obstruction. Contrast upper GI series is used to identify the presence or absence of malrotation in those cases with incomplete obstruction since obstruction from intestinal malrotation is a surgical emergency.

Treatment

Surgery is performed using a right upper transverse abdominal incision or via laparoscopy. A Kocher maneuver should be performed, with complete mobilization of the third and fourth portions of the duodenum. Obstruction from Ladd bands requires simple division of the bands and correction of the malrotation (see below). Duodenoduodenostomy is performed for duodenal atresia and annular pancreas. A mucosal web can be excised if technically feasible, taking care to avoid injury to the adjacent ampulla. Commonly, the duodenum is hugely dilated above the obstruction, which results in impaired aboral progression of ingested feedings. This problem is resolved by excision or plication of a portion of the antimesenteric wall of the bowel to normalize the lumen diameter (tapered duodenoplasty). Gastrojejunostomy should not be done because the blind duodenal pouch may cause repeated vomiting. The distal bowel should be irrigated and assessed for associated intrinsic obstruction if possible. However, the rate of associated distal atresia is low (0.5%-3% incidence) and most commonly seen in conjunction with an "apple peel" deformity). Mortality is related to prematurity and associated anomalies.

Kay S, Yoder S, Rothenberg S: Laparoscopic duodenoduodenostomy in the neonate. *J Pediatr Surg* 2009 May;44(5): 906-908.

St Peter SD, Little DC, Barsness KA, Copeland DR, Calkins CM, Yoder S, Rothenberg SS, Islam S, Tsao K, Ostlie DJ: Should we be concerned about jejunoileal atresia during repair of duodenal atresia? *J Laparoendosc Adv Surg Tech A* 2010 Nov;20(9):773-775.

ATRESIA & STENOSIS OF THE JEJUNUM, ILEUM, & COLON

Atresia and stenosis of the jejunum, ileum, and colon are caused by a mesenteric vascular accident *in utero*, which may result from hernia, volvulus, or intussusception, producing aseptic necrosis and resorption of the necrotic bowel. Although atresia may occur in any portion of the intestine, most cases occur in the distal ileum or proximal jejunum. Colonic atresia is very rare, accounting for no more than 1% of all intestinal atresias. A short area of necrosis may produce only stenosis or a membranous web occluding the lumen (type I) (Figure 43-10). A more extensive infarct may leave a fibrous cord between the two bowel loops (type II), or the proximal and distal bowel may be completely separated with a V-shaped defect in the mesentery (type IIIa). Multiple atresias occur in 10% of cases (type IV). A type III variant (type IIIb) is commonly called apple-peel or Christmas tree atresia, in which there is a blind-ending proximal jejunum, absence of a long length of mid small bowel, and a terminal ileum coiled around its tenuous blood supply from an ileocolic vessel.

▶ Clinical Findings

Vomiting of bile, abdominal distention, and failure to pass meconium indicate intestinal obstruction. The plain abdominal radiograph will give an estimate of how far along the intestine the obstruction exists. A contrast enema may be

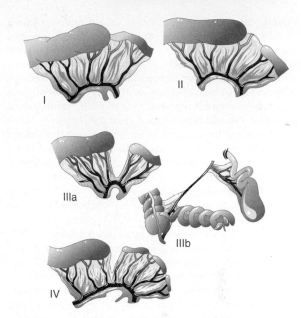

▲ **Figure 43-10.** The anatomic spectrum of intestinal atresia. Type I is a stenosis or mucosal web. Type II, a fibrous cord between two bowel ends. Type IIIa, blind-ending proximal and distal bowel loops with a V-shaped mesenteric defect. Type IIIb (apple peel deformity, Christmas tree deformity) consists of a blind ending proximal jejunum, absence of a large portion of the midgut, and a terminal ileum that is coiled around its ileocolic blood supply. Type IV, multiple atresias of any kind. (Reproduced, with permission, from Grosfeld JL et al: Operative management of intestinal atresia based on pathologic findings. *J Pediatr Surg.* 1979 June;14(3):368–375.)

indicated to detect the level of obstruction. In obstructions that occur in the distal bowel and appear relatively early in gestation, the colon is empty of meconium and appears abnormally narrow (microcolon). When the obstruction is proximal or when it occurs late in pregnancy, meconium is passed into the colon. The contrast enema will then outline a more generous-sized colon with its contents (meconium). In older children with evidence of partial intestinal obstruction, a small bowel series may be indicated to identify intestinal stenosis.

▶ Treatment

There are three main goals of operation: (1) to restore the continuity of the bowel; (2) to preserve as much intestinal length as possible; and (3) to retain the ileocecal valve if possible (the minimum length of bowel needed to sustain full enteral nutrition doubles in the absence of the ileocecal valve). A transverse upper abdominal incision is preferred.

Infants with jejunal or ileal atresia usually have a segment of the proximal bowel adjacent to the atresia that is dilated out of proportion to the rest of the proximal bowel. This is referred to as the "club" and it lacks normal peristaltic activity. If left in or not tapered, it may become a source of persistent functional obstruction. It is tapered when it is a very proximal bowel segment, near the ligament of Treitz; otherwise it should be resected. A great discrepancy between the diameter of the segments of intestine proximal and distal to the atresia is the rule. Atresia of the proximal colon should be treated by resection of the dilated bowel and ileocolostomy. Atresia of the distal colon may be treated by proximal end colostomy or by a side-to-side colostomy. Later, the continuity of the distal colon may be established by end-to-end anastomosis.

Infants born with extensive small bowel loss may benefit from a Bianchi procedure, where the entire greatly dilated bowel is divided longitudinally into two lengths of bowel. An alternative bowel lengthening procedure termed the STEP (serial transverse enteroplasty procedure) is quickly gaining acceptance as the procedure of choice for gaining length from dilated and shortened intestine. The end of the jejunum in continuity with the duodenum is anastomosed to the proximal end of the divided bowel.

In contrast to duodenal atresia, associated anomalies are unusual in small bowel and colon atresia. Following repair, return of GI function can be prolonged and feeds should be introduced accordingly.

Modi et al: First report of the international serial transverse enteroplasty data registry: indications, efficacy, and complications. *J Am Coll Surg* 2007;204(4):365-371.

Sudan D, Thompson J, Botha J, Grant W, Antonson D, Raynor S, Langnas A: Comparison of intestinal lengthening procedures for patients with short bowel syndrome. *Ann Surg* 2007 Oct;246(4):593-601.

DISORDERS OF INTESTINAL ROTATION

The fetal intestine begins as a somewhat straight tube that grows faster than the abdominal cavity and thus herniates out into the body stalk (future umbilicus) at about 4-6 weeks' gestation. At 10-12 weeks, the bowel returns to the abdominal cavity, rotates, and becomes fixed to the retroperitoneum along a long diagonal axis extending from the level of the left of the T12 vertebra to the level of the right of the L5 vertebra. The duodenojejunal portion of gut rotates posterior (counterclockwise) to the superior mesenteric vessels for 270 degrees and becomes fixed at the ligament of Treitz and located to the left of and cephalad to the superior mesenteric artery. The cecocolic portion of the midgut also rotates 270 degrees, but clockwise (anterior) to the superior mesenteric artery. The cecum becomes fixed in the right lower abdomen (L5 level).

► Classification

Anomalies of rotation and fixation are twice as common in males as in females. They may be classified as (1) nonrotation, (2) incomplete rotation, (3) reversed rotation, and (4) anomalous fixation of the mesentery.

A. Nonrotation

With nonrotation, the midgut is suspended from the superior mesenteric vessels; the small bowel is located predominantly on the right side of the abdomen and the large bowel in the left abdomen. No fixation occurs, and adhesive bands are not present. This is the fetal anatomy prior to 10 weeks' gestation. Because its base is so short, the mesentery is narrow, which predisposes to volvulus, with clockwise twisting of the bowel about the superior mesenteric vessels. This anomaly is usually found in patients with omphalocele, gastroschisis, and CDH.

B. Incomplete Rotation

Incomplete rotation (commonly called malrotation) may affect the duodenojejunal segment, the cecocolic segment, or both. Adhesive bands (Ladd bands) are usually present. In the most common form, the cecum stops rotating and fixes near the origin of the superior mesenteric vessels, and dense peritoneal bands extend from the right flank to the cecum and obstruct the second or third portion of the duodenum or other segments of the small bowel. The duodenojejunal segment also only partially rotates, usually stopping at or to the right of the vertebral bodies. The intestinal mesentery is fixed posteriorly, but is very narrow, only extending the distance between the cecum and the duodenojejunal segment. This predisposes to volvulus (Figure 43–11).

C. Reversed Rotation

In reversed rotation, the bowel rotates varying degrees in a clockwise direction about the superior mesenteric axis. The duodenojejunal loop is anterior to the superior mesenteric artery. The cecocolic loop may be prearterial or may be rotated clockwise or counterclockwise in a retroarterial position. In either case, the cecum may be right sided or left sided. The most frequent anomaly is retroarterial clockwise rotation, which causes obstruction of the right colon.

D. Anomalous Fixation of Mesentery

Anomalies of mesenteric fixation account for internal mesenteric and paraduodenal hernias, a mobile cecum, or obstructing adhesive bands in the absence of anomalous bowel rotation. Excessive rotation of the duodenojejunal junction may result in superior mesenteric artery compression of the third portion of the duodenum.

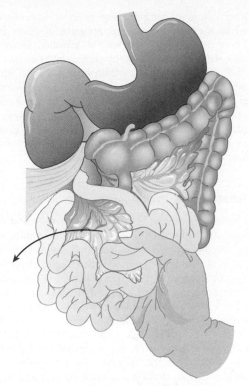

▲ **Figure 43–11.** Malrotation of the midgut with volvulus. Note cecum at the origin of the superior mesenteric vessels. Fibrous bands cross and obstruct the duodenum as they adhere to the cecum. Volvulus is untwisted in a counterclockwise direction.

▶ Clinical Findings

A. Symptoms and Signs

Anomalies of intestinal rotation may cause symptoms related to intestinal obstruction, peptic ulceration, or malabsorption. The majority of patients who develop intestinal obstruction are infants. Older patients may develop intermittent obstruction. The obstruction is in the duodenum or upper jejunum as a result of adhesive bands or midgut volvulus, respectively. Vomiting of bile occurs initially. Older patients may be thin and underweight because of chronic postprandial discomfort or malabsorption. Malabsorption with steatorrhea may result from partial venous and lymphatic obstruction, which is associated with coarse rugal folds in the small bowel. With duodenal obstruction from bands, abdominal distention is not prominent. Midgut volvulus, however, produces marked abdominal distention. Bloody stools and signs of peritonitis are manifestations of intestinal infarction. Peptic ulcer occurs in 20% of patients, presumably as a result of antral and duodenal stasis.

B. Imaging Studies

With obstructing Ladd bands, plain abdominal radiographs may show a "double bubble" sign that mimics duodenal stenosis. Distribution of gas throughout the intestines may be normal, although there may be a paucity of it. When volvulus occurs, the proximal bowel will be distended with gas early, but over time, a "gasless" abdomen may appear as the gas is resorbed in the ischemic bowel. The intestinal walls are thickened.

The identification of inverted superior mesenteric artery and superior mesenteric vein position on ultrasound is highly suggestive of malrotation and warrants further investigation; however, ultrasound can miss 10%-15% of cases. Upper GI series is the gold standard for diagnosis and demonstrates distention of the duodenum, abnormal positioning of the duodenojejunal segment (usually to the right of the midline), and narrowing at the point of obstruction. The small bowel is commonly visualized on the right side of the abdomen and the colon on the left. Contrast enema demonstrates abnormal position of the cecum, although the cecum can complete its rotation and fixation after birth, so the contrast enema is not a valuable diagnostic test for malrotation.

▶ Treatment & Prognosis

Through a transverse upper abdominal incision, the entire bowel should be delivered from the abdominal cavity to assess the anomalous arrangement of the intestinal loops. Volvulus should be untwisted in a counterclockwise direction. The Ladd procedure is used for incomplete rotation with obstruction of the duodenum by congenital bands. It consists of division of the bands between the proximal colon and the lateral abdominal wall that cover and compress (obstruct) the duodenum. The mesentery is often folded upon itself due to intermesenteric adhesions, and these are incised. The appendix is removed. The cecum is then placed in the left lower quadrant, and the duodenum dissected and straightened as much as possible with a final position to the right of the midline. In essence, one is creating nonrotated intestinal anatomy much like the anatomic situation in early fetal life (prior to 10 weeks' gestation). The Ladd procedure has increasingly been performed using laparoscopic techniques for those cases without suspected volvulus.

Approximately 30% of infants treated for volvulus die of complications of midgut ischemia and gangrene. If the anomaly is corrected before irreversible bowel damage occurs, the long-term results are good. Some patients tend to form adhesions that cause recurrent intestinal obstruction. Recurrent volvulus is rare after the Ladd procedure.

Hagendoorn J, Vieira-Travassos D, van der Zee D: Laparoscopic treatment of intestinal malrotation in neonates and infants: retrospective study. *Surg Endosc* 2011 Jan;25(1):217-220.

Orzech N, Navarro OM, Langer JC: Is ultrasonography a good screening test for intestinal malrotation? *J Pediatr Surg* 2006;41:1005-1009.

MECONIUM ILEUS

In 10%-20% of infants born with cystic fibrosis, the thick mucous secretions of the small bowel produce obstruction by inspissated meconium. This usually occurs in the terminal ileum. Although there is no clear correlation between pancreatic insufficiency and the development of inspissated meconium, meconium ileus also occurs in patients with pancreatic duct obstruction and pancreatic aplasia. Meconium obstruction with no apparent cause has also been described in newborn infants.

▶ Clinical Findings

A. Symptoms and Signs

The infant typically has a normal birth weight and very distended abdomen. No meconium is passed, and bilious emesis occurs early. Loops of thick, distended bowel may be seen and palpated.

B. Imaging Studies

Plain abdominal radiographs show loops of bowel that vary greatly in diameter; the thick meconium gives a ground-glass appearance. Air mixed with the meconium produces the "soap bubble" sign, which is usually located in the right lower quadrant. Radiographs taken shortly after the infant has been placed in an upright position may fail to show air-fluid levels because the thick, viscid meconium fails to layer out rapidly. Contrast enema will show microcolon with rare meconium flecks. Reflux of contrast medium through the ileocecal valve demonstrates a small terminal ileum containing "pellets" of inspissated mucus; more proximally, the bowel is progressively distended with packed meconium. Antenatal perforation may be detected by the presence of abdominal calcifications since the meconium becomes saponified.

▶ Complications

Meconium ileus may be complicated by a segmental (not midgut) volvulus due to the heavy, distended loops of distal ileum. If this occurs early in fetal life, the volvulus may progress to gangrene of the affected bowel segment. This can heal completely, with abdominal calcifications as the only manifestation that it occurred. Conversely, it may heal in such a way that an intestinal atresia is formed. Perforation late in gestation may lead to meconium peritonitis or a large meconium pseudocyst at birth.

Other common complications of meconium ileus are related to the almost universal presence of cystic fibrosis. These infants are susceptible to repeated pulmonary infection with chronic bronchopneumonia, bronchiectasis, atelectasis, and lung abscess. Malabsorption due to pancreatic insufficiency requires pancreatic enzyme replacement. Rectal prolapse and intussusception may be produced by strained passage of inspissated stools. Nasal polyps and chronic sinusitis are frequent. Biliary cirrhosis and bleeding varices from portal hypertension are late manifestations of bile duct obstruction by mucus.

▶ Treatment & Prognosis

Nonoperative treatment is successful in 60%-70% of cases. A nasogastric tube should be inserted and connected to suction. A contrast enema can be both diagnostic and therapeutic. It should be performed with a slightly hypertonic water-soluble contrast agent (never barium). The addition of *N*-acetylcysteine, which is mucolytic, may be necessary to disperse the meconium in uncomplicated cases. The infant must be well hydrated, and intravenous fluids must be continued during and after the procedure in order to prevent hypovolemia from the effects of the hypertonic contrast solution. If this fails to relieve the obstruction, laparotomy is indicated. The ileum is opened and, if possible, flushed clear. The bowel can be reanastomosed or brought out as a double-barrel stoma. Alternatively, a T-tube may be placed in the bowel and brought out of the anterior abdominal wall for postoperative irrigations. Compromised intestine is resected, and appendectomy is performed because of the high rate of appendicitis in patients with cystic fibrosis.

All patients should be evaluated for cystic fibrosis. Pancreatic enzyme replacement may be required. A formula low in long-chain fatty acids and high in medium-chain triglycerides may give better absorption and growth than standard formulas. The patient must be placed in an environment with high humidity to keep tracheobronchial secretions fluid. Postural drainage with cupping of the chest should be taught to the parents so that they will continue to maintain tracheobronchial toilet indefinitely. Older children and adolescents may develop a meconium ileus-like syndrome termed distal ileal obstruction syndrome. This is ileal obstruction due to inspissated stool. It can occur when patients are not compliant with their medications or become dehydrated. Most often, it is successfully treated with hypertonic contrast enemas.

Carlyle BE, Borowitz DS, Glick PL: A review of pathophysiology and management of fetuses and neonates with meconium ileus for the pediatric surgeon. *J Pediatr Surg* 2012 Apr;47(4): 772-781.

HIRSCHSPRUNG DISEASE

Hirschsprung disease is due to failure in the cephalocaudal migration of the parasympathetic myenteric nerve cells into the distal bowel. Therefore, the absence of ganglion cells always begins at the anus and extends a varying distance proximally. The aganglionic bowel produces functional obstruction because the bowel fails to relax in response to distention. Short-segment aganglionosis involving only the terminal rectum occurs in about 10% of cases; the disease extends to the sigmoid colon in 75%; more proximal colon in 10%; and the entire colon with small bowel involvement in 5%. Extensive involvement of the small bowel is rare.

Males are affected four times more frequently than females when the disease is limited to the rectosigmoid. Females tend to have longer aganglionic segments. A familial association occurs in 5%-10% of cases—more frequently when females are affected. The length of involvement tends to be consistent in familial cases. Down syndrome occurs in 10%-15% of patients.

▶ Clinical Findings

A. Symptoms and Signs

The absence of ganglion cells results in a functional obstruction since the affected area fails to relax due to unopposed sympathetic tone. The symptoms vary widely in severity but almost always occur shortly after birth. The infant passes little or no meconium within 24 hours. Thereafter, chronic or intermittent constipation usually occurs. Progressive abdominal distention, bilious emesis, reluctance to feed, diarrhea, listlessness, irritability, and poor growth and development follow. A rectal examination in the infant may be followed by expulsion of stool and flatus, with remarkable decompression of abdominal distention. In older children, chronic constipation and abdominal distention are characteristic. Passage of flatus and stool requires great effort, and the stools are small in caliber. Children with constipation from Hirschsprung disease do not exhibit soiling of their diapers or undergarments, distinguishing this form of constipation from idiopathic constipation (encopresis). These children are sluggish, with wasted extremities and flared costal margins. Rectal examination in older children usually reveals a normal or contracted anus and a rectum without feces. Impacted stools in the greatly dilated and distended sigmoid colon can be palpated across the lower abdomen.

B. Imaging Studies

Plain abdominal radiographs in infants show dilated loops of bowel, but it is difficult to distinguish small and large bowel in infancy. A contrast enema should be performed. There should be no rectal examination or attempt to clean out the stool before the fluoroscopic examination, for this can dilate the rectum and obscure the change in caliber between aganglionic and ganglionic bowel. The contrast enema often demonstrates a contracted (aganglionic) segment that appears relatively narrow compared with the dilated proximal bowel. The proximal aganglionic intestine can be dilated by impacted stool or enema, giving a false impression of the level of the normal colon. Irregular, bizarre contractions (saw-toothed pattern) that do not encircle the aganglionic portion of the bowel may also be recognized. The dilated proximal bowel may have circumferential, smooth, parallel contractions (similar in appearance to those of the jejunum) that are exaggerated contraction waves. The contrast enema may not show a transition zone in the first 6 weeks after birth, since the liquid stool can pass into the aganglionic bowel and the proximal intestine may not be dilated. Lateral projection radiographs should be taken to demonstrate the rectum, the transition zone, and the irregular contractions that may otherwise be obscured by a redundant sigmoid colon on anteroposterior views. Normally, the neonatal rectum is wider than the rest of the colon (including the cecum), and when the rectum is seen to be narrower than the proximal colon, then Hirschsprung disease is suspected. Radiographs of the abdomen and lateral pelvis should be repeated after 24-48 hours. The contrast agent will be retained for prolonged periods, and saline enemas may be required to evacuate it. The delayed film may show the transition zone and the bizarre irregular contractions more clearly than the initial study.

C. Laboratory Findings

Definitive diagnosis is made by rectal biopsy. Mucosal and submucosal biopsies may be taken from the posterior rectal wall with a suction biopsy capsule at the bedside. Serial sections may demonstrate the characteristic lack of ganglion cells and proliferation of nerve trunks in Meissner plexus. If the findings are equivocal, it is necessary to remove a 1-cm or 2-cm full-thickness strip of mucosa and muscularis from the posterior rectum proximal to the dentate line under anesthesia. A sample of this size is sufficient for the pathologist to determine the presence or absence of ganglion cells in Meissner plexus or in Auerbach plexus. Manometric studies will show a failure of relaxation of the internal sphincter following rectal distention by a balloon, although this test is rarely performed except in older children.

▶ Differential Diagnosis

Low intestinal obstruction in the newborn infant may be due to rectal or colonic atresia, meconium plug syndrome (see below), or meconium ileus as well as a variety of functional causes such as hypermagnesemia, hypocalcemia, hypokalemia, and hypothyroidism. Hirschsprung disease in patients who develop enterocolitis and diarrhea may mimic other causes of diarrhea. Chronic constipation due to functional causes may suggest Hirschsprung disease. Although functional constipation may occur early in infancy, the stools are normal in caliber, soiling is frequent, and enterocolitis is rare. In functional constipation, stool is palpable in the lower rectum, and a contrast enema shows uniformly dilated bowel to the level of the anus. However, short segment Hirschsprung disease may be difficult to differentiate, and rectal biopsy may be necessary. Segmental dilation of the colon is a rare entity that causes constipation similar to that found in Hirschsprung disease.

▶ Treatment

Traditionally, the surgical treatment was staged and consisted of a leveling colostomy followed several months later by resection of the aganglionic bowel and performance of a pull-through procedure. The trend recently has been toward performing a single-stage procedure (no colostomy) in the newborn period. This paradigm is as follows: bowel obstruction and enterocolitis (if present) may be relieved by placement of a large (30F) rectal tube and repeated warmed saline irrigations in 10 mL/kg aliquots preoperatively. Infants with moderate to severe enterocolitis should be treated with a diverting colostomy. At the time of surgery, frozen section analysis of the colonic muscle is required in order to establish the correct (ganglionic) level for the stoma. Infants who are not ill may undergo any one of three effective operative procedures: Swenson operation, Duhamel operation, or Soave operation. The main operative principles for these procedures are removal of most or all of the aganglionic bowel—while preserving the surrounding nerves to the pelvic organs—and anastomosing ganglionic bowel (confirmed by frozen section analysis) to the rectum just above the dentate line. In contrast to the Swenson and Soave procedures, the Duhamel operation leaves a cuff of aganglionic rectum along which the ganglionic bowel is stapled, creating a mini-reservoir. Historically, these operations have been performed via a low transverse abdominal incision. However, the laparoscopic approach has become the method of choice. A solely transanal mucosectomy has been used for those babies with short-segment disease. In total aganglionic colon, ileostomy is necessary. Nonoperative treatment with enemas is ineffective because it fails to prevent further obstruction and enterocolitis.

▶ Prognosis

The mortality for untreated aganglionic megacolon in infancy may be as high as 80%. Nonbacterial, nonviral enterocolitis is the principal cause of death. This tends to occur more frequently in infants but may appear at any age. The cause is not known but seems to be related to the high-grade partial obstruction, poor motility in the "normal" bowel, a frequently competent ileocecal valve, and hypertonic rectal sphincters. There is no correlation between the length of aganglionosis and the occurrence of enterocolitis. Perforation of the colon and appendix may result from distal bowel obstruction. Atresia of the distal small bowel or colon secondary to bowel obstruction due to Hirschsprung disease *in utero* has been reported.

Anastomotic leak with perirectal and pelvic abscess is the most serious complication following the pull-through procedure. This complication should be treated immediately by proximal colostomy until the anastomosis has healed. Necrosis of the pulled-through colon may occur if the bowel has not been mobilized sufficiently to prevent tension on the mesenteric blood supply.

Long-term patients who are properly treated for Hirschsprung disease do well. Incontinence and soiling may occur in a few cases despite a prompt diagnosis and a perfect operation. Episodic constipation and abdominal distention are more common, since the aganglionic internal anal sphincter is intact. Patients with these symptoms can respond to anal dilation. Occasionally, an internal sphincterotomy may be necessary. Smaller children may still develop enterocolitis after definitive treatment, and they should be treated with a large rectal tube and enemas. It is rare after age 5 years. Postoperative enterocolitis is more common in children with Down syndrome.

Giuliani S, Betalli P, Narciso A, Grandi F, Midrio P, Mognato G, Gamba P: Outcome comparison among laparoscopic Duhamel, laparotomic Duhamel, and transanal endorectal pull-through: a single-center, 18-year experience. *J Laparoendosc Adv Surg Tech A* 2011 Nov;21(9):859-863.

NEONATAL SMALL LEFT COLON SYNDROME (MECONIUM PLUG SYNDROME)

This problem of newborn infants consists of low intestinal obstruction associated with a left colon of narrow caliber and a dilated transverse and right colon. The infants are in most cases otherwise normal, though approximately 30%-50% are born to diabetic mothers and are large for gestational age. Most are over 36 weeks' gestational age and have normal birth weights. Two-thirds are male. Hypermagnesemia has been occasionally associated when the mother has been treated for eclampsia by intravenous magnesium sulfate.

▶ Clinical Findings

Rectal examination may be normal or may reveal a tight anal canal. Little or no meconium is passed, and progressive abdominal distention is followed by vomiting. After thermometer or finger stimulation of the rectum, some meconium and gas may be evacuated. Contrast enema shows a very small left colon, usually to the level of the splenic flexure. Proximal to this point, the colon and commonly the small bowel are greatly distended. In about 30% of cases, a meconium plug is present at the junction of the narrow and dilated portion of the bowel, and the enema (using water-soluble contrast) will dislodge it.

Differential Diagnosis

The small left colon syndrome may be confused with Hirschsprung disease or meconium ileus. These lesions rarely cause obstruction at the level of the splenic flexure, and when the colon readily decompresses without further obstruction, Hirschsprung disease is unlikely.

Treatment

A nasogastric tube should be inserted and intravenous fluids started. A contrast enema is required to differentiate the various causes of low intestinal obstruction. When the left colon is narrow and contrast material refluxes into the dilated proximal colon, the diagnosis is most likely the small left colon syndrome. The contrast enema is usually followed by evacuation of copious meconium and decompression of the bowel. Incomplete evacuation of the meconium or persistent symptoms after the enema mandates a suction rectal biopsy to rule out Hirschsprung disease.

INTUSSUSCEPTION

Telescoping of a segment of bowel (intussusceptum) into the adjacent segment (intussuscipiens) is the most common cause of intestinal obstruction in children between 6 months and 2 years of age (Figure 43–12). The process of intussusception

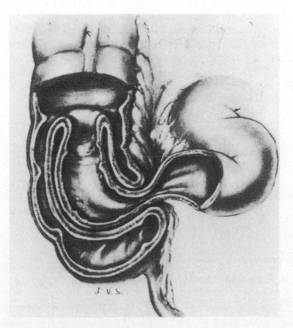

▲ **Figure 43–12.** Intussusception.

may result in gangrene of the intussusceptum. The most common form is intussusception of the terminal ileum into the right colon (ileocolic intussusception). In 95% of infants and children, it is idiopathic. The disease is most common in midsummer and midwinter, and there is a correlation with adenovirus infections. In most cases, hypertrophied Peyer patches are noted on the leading edge of bowel. Mechanical factors such as Meckel diverticulum, polyps, hemangioma, enteric duplication, intramural hematoma (Henoch-Schönlein purpura), and intestinal lymphoma are present with increasing frequency in patients over 2 years old. Postoperative intussusception can occur at any age, is usually ileoileal or jejunojejunal, and is due to differential return of bowel motility, often after retroperitoneal surgery. The ratio of males to females is 3:2. The peak age is in infants 5-9 months of age; 80% of patients are under the age of 2 years.

Clinical Findings

The typical patient is a healthy child who suddenly begins crying and doubles up because of abdominal pain. The pain occurs in episodes that last for about 1 minute, alternating with intervals of apparent well being. Reflex vomiting is an early sign, but vomiting due to bowel obstruction occurs late. Blood from venous infarction and mucus produce a "currant jelly" stool. In small infants and in postoperative patients, the colicky pain may not be apparent; these babies become withdrawn, and the most prominent symptom is vomiting. Pallor and sweating are common signs during colic. Repeated vomiting and bowel obstruction will produce progressive dehydration. A mass is usually palpable along the distribution of the colon, most commonly in the right upper quadrant of the abdomen. Occasionally, intussusception is palpable on rectal examination. Prolonged intussusception produces edema and hemorrhagic or ischemic infarction of the intussusceptum.

Treatment & Prognosis

The contrast enema is diagnostic as well as therapeutic in 60%-80% of cases (Figure 43–13). Contrast enema (using either barium or air) should not be attempted until the patient has been resuscitated enough to allow an operative procedure to be performed safely. It is contraindicated if peritonitis is present. If barium is used, the column of contrast should not stand more than 100 cm above the patient in order to minimize the risk of perforation. Air is pumped into the colon at a pressure of 60-80 mm Hg (never > 120 mm Hg). A successful study reduces the intussusceptum and demonstrates reflux of barium or air into the terminal ileum. Several attempts should be made before taking the child to surgery. A contrast enema will not reduce gangrenous bowel.

Operation is required for unsuccessful enema reduction or signs of bowel perforation and peritonitis. The procedure

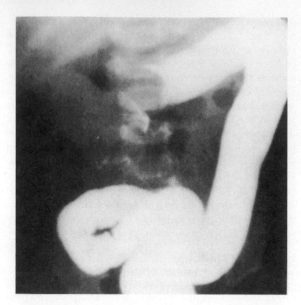

▲ **Figure 43–13.** Contrast enema demonstrating obstruction to retrograde flow of barium by a filling defect (intussusceptum) in the mid transverse colon. (Reproduced, with permission, from Albanese CT. Pediatric surgery. In: Norton JA, ed. *Surgery*. New York, NY: Springer; 2000.)

may be performed either by laparotomy or laparoscopically. In the absence of gangrene, reduction is accomplished by gentle retrograde compression of the intussuscipiens, not by traction on the proximal bowel. Resection of the intussusception is indicated if the bowel cannot be reduced or if the intestine is gangrenous.

Intussusception recurs after 5% of enema reductions and 1% of operative reductions. Deaths are rare but occur if treatment of gangrenous bowel is delayed.

Lehnert T et al: Intussusception in children-clinical presentation, diagnosis and management. *Int J Colorectal Dis* 2009;24: 1187-1192.

ANORECTAL ANOMALIES (IMPERFORATE ANUS)

The normal continence mechanism for bowel control consists of an internal sphincter composed of smooth muscle and the striated muscle complex from the levator ani and external sphincter. The striated muscles assume a funnel shape, originating from the pubis, pelvic rim, and sacrum. These muscles converge at the perineum while interdigitating with the internal and external sphincters. Most of the striated muscle complex consists of horizontal muscles that contract against the wall of the rectum and anus while longitudinal muscle fibers run in a cephalocaudal direction and elevate the anus.

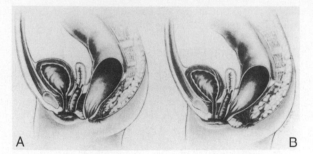

▲ **Figure 43–14. A:** Low female anomaly. Perineal fistula. **B:** Low female anomaly. Fourchette/vestibule fistula. (Reproduced, with permission, from Pena A: *Atlas of Surgical Management of Anorectal Malformations*. New York, NY: Springer-Verlag; 1990)

Anomalies of the anus result from abnormal growth and fusion of the embryonic anal hillocks. The rectum is normally developed, and the sphincter mechanism is usually intact. With proper surgical treatment, the sphincter will function normally. Anomalies of the rectum develop as a result of faulty division of the cloaca into the urogenital sinus and rectum by the urorectal septum. In these anomalies, the internal sphincter and striated muscle complex are hypoplastic. Therefore, surgical repair results in varying degrees of continence.

► Classification

Physical examination of the perineum and imaging studies determine the extent of malformation of the anus or rectum. When an orifice is evident at the perineum or distal introitus, the anomaly is referred to as a low imperforate anus; the absence of an obvious orifice at the perineal level suggests a high imperforate anus (Figures 43–14 to 43–17) In most instances, with high imperforate anus, there is a

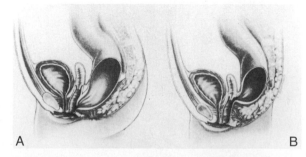

▲ **Figure 43–15. A:** High female anatomic anomaly. Low vaginal fistula. **B:** High female anomaly. High vaginal fistula. (Reproduced, with permission, from Pena A: *Atlas of Surgical Management of Anorectal Malformations*. New York, NY: Springer-Verlag; 1990.)

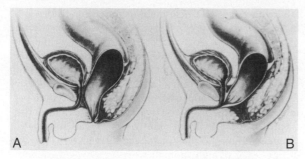

▲ **Figure 43–16. A:** Low male anomaly. Perineal fistula. **B:** Low male anomaly. Rectobulbar urethra fistula. (Reproduced, with permission, from Pena A: *Atlas of Surgical Management of Anorectal Malformations*. New York, NY: Springer-Verlag; 1990.)

communication (fistula) of the rectum with the urethra or bladder in the male or with the upper vagina in the female. Distinguishing between a high and low anomaly may be possible radiologically by determining the position of the rectum in relation to the levator ani or pubococcygeal line.

A. Low Anomalies

In low anomalies, the anus may be ectopically placed anterior to its normal position or it may be in the normal position with a narrow outlet due to stenosis or an anal membrane. There may be no opening in the perineum, but the skin at the anal area is heaped up and may extend as a band in the perineal raphe completely covering the anal opening. A small fistula usually extends from the anus anteriorly to open in the raphe of the perineum, scrotum, or penis in the male or the vulva in the female. These babies often have well-developed perineal and gluteal musculature and rarely have sacral vertebral anomalies.

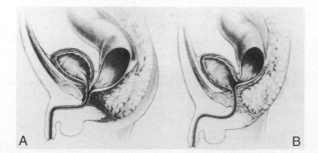

▲ **Figure 43–17. A:** High male anomaly. Rectoprostatic urethra fistula. **B:** High male anomaly. Rectovesical neck fistula. (Reproduced, with permission, from Pena A: *Atlas of Surgical Management of Anorectal Malformations*. New York, NY: Springer-Verlag; 1990.)

B. High Anomalies

In high anomalies, the rectum may end blindly (10%), but more commonly there is a fistula to the urethra or bladder in the male or the upper vagina in the female. In the female, a very high fistula may extend between the two halves of a bicornuate uterus directly to the bladder. Patients with high imperforate anus often have deficient pelvic and gluteal innervation and musculature, a high incidence of sacral anomalies (caudal regression), and a poor prognosis for continence after surgical repair. The most severe of the high deformities is a cloacal anomaly in which there is a common channel between the poorly developed pelvic structures (urogenital sinus and rectum) with a single perineal opening.

► Clinical Findings

A. Signs

The best means of establishing the type of anorectal anomaly is by physical examination. In low anomalies, an ectopic opening from the rectum can be detected in the perineal raphe in males or in the lower vagina, vestibule, or fourchette in females. A high anomaly exists when no orifice or fistula can be seen upon examination of the perineum or when meconium is found at the urethral meatus, in the urine, or in the upper vagina. Absence of external sphincter contraction with cutaneous stimulation of the anus may also help differentiate between high and low lesions.

B. Imaging Studies

No single test is ideal in the evaluation of imperforate anus, so several studies are used to define the neonatal anatomy. Radiographs are sometimes useful when the clinical impression is unclear. A lateral film of the pelvis with the baby inverted (Wangensteen invertogram), once commonly used, is an inaccurate method of establishing the lower extent of the rectum because swallowed air may not have completely displaced the meconium from the rectum; or the striated muscle complex may be contracted, which obliterates the lumen and makes it look as if the gas in the rectum ends high in the pelvis. With crying or straining, the puborectalis muscle and rectum may actually descend below the ischium, giving a falsely low estimate of rectal height. Gas in the bladder clearly indicates a rectourinary fistula. Lower abdominal and perineal ultrasound, CT, and MRI have been used to define the pelvic anatomy and location in relation to the rectal musculature. Anomalies of the vertebrae and the urinary tract occur in two-thirds of all patients with high anomalies and in one-third of male patients with low anomalies. Vertebral abnormalities in females invariably indicate a high imperforate anus. Anomalies of the sacrum warrant MRI of the lumbosacral area to identify spinal cord anomalies such as a tethered filum terminale.

▶ Complications

Associated anomalies occur in up to 70% in those with a high anomaly. Imperforate anus is associated with the VACTERL syndrome (see Esophageal Anomalies). The possible constellation of anomalies includes esophageal atresia, anomalies of the GI tract, hemivertebrae or agenesis of one or more sacral vertebrae (agenesis of S1, S2, or S3 is associated with corresponding neurologic deficits, resulting in neuropathic bladder and greatly impaired continence), genitourinary anomalies (up to 50% incidence with high imperforate anus), and anomalies of the heart and upper limbs/digits.

Delay in diagnosis of imperforate anus may result in excessively large bowel distention and perforation. The presence of a rectourinary fistula allows reflux of urine into the rectum and colon, and absorption of ammonium chloride may cause acidosis. Colon contents will reflux into the urethra, bladder, and upper tracts, producing recurrent pyelonephritis.

▶ Treatment

The three main goals of treatment are (1) to allow passage of stool (ie, relieve obstruction), (2) to place the rectal pouch on the perineum in good position, and (3) to close the fistula.

A. Low Anomalies

Low anomalies are usually repaired from the perineal approach in the newborn period using a muscle stimulator to precisely determine the location of the sphincter complex. The anteriorly placed anal opening is completely mobilized and transferred to the normal position. After healing, the anal opening must be dilated daily for 3-5 months to prevent stricture formation and to allow for growth.

B. High Anomalies

Traditionally, a high deformity was treated by a three-stage repair consisting of colostomy and mucous fistula formation, a posterior sagittal anorectoplasty 4-6 weeks later, and closure of the colostomy several months after that. Recently, the staged approach has been challenged and a one-stage repair has been performed by both posterior sagittal and laparoscopic approaches. Because the anal sphincters are poorly developed—especially the internal sphincter—continence is most dependent upon a functioning striated muscle complex, which requires conscious voluntary contraction. Care must be taken to preserve the afferent and efferent nerves of the defecation reflex arc as well as the existing sphincter muscles. In all cases, the surgically created anus must be dilated for several months to prevent circumferential cicatrix formation.

▶ Prognosis

Surgical complications include damage to the nervi erigentes, resulting in poor bladder and bowel control and failure of erection. Division of a rectourethral fistula some distance from the urethra produces a blind pouch prone to recurrent infection and stone formation, while cutting the fistula too short may result in urethral stricture. Erroneously attempting to repair a high anomaly from the perineal approach may leave a persistent rectourinary fistula. An abdominoperineal pull-through procedure performed for a low anomaly invariably produces an incontinent patient who might otherwise have had an excellent prognosis. Injury to the vas deferens and ureter is possible during repair of high anomalies.

Patients with imperforate anus tend to have varying degrees of constipation as an inherent part of the defect, believed to be due to poor inherent motility of the rectosigmoid. Patients with low anomalies usually have good sphincter function. Children with high anomalies do not have an internal sphincter that provides continuous, unconscious, and unfatiguing control against soiling. However, in the absence of a lower spine anomaly, perception of rectal fullness, ability to distinguish between flatus and stool, and conscious voluntary control of rectal discharge by contraction of the striated muscle complex can be achieved. When the stools become liquid, sphincter control is usually impaired in patients with high anomalies.

Bischoff A, Levitt MA, Peña A: Laparoscopy and its use in the repair of anorectal malformations. *J Pediatr Surg* 2011 Aug;46(8):1609-1617.

Levitt MA, Peña A: Outcomes from the correction of anorectal malformations. *Curr Opin Pediatr* 2005 Jun;17(3):394-401.

▼ GASTROINTESTINAL TRACT ABNORMALITIES

GASTROESOPHAGEAL REFLUX

Studies of esophageal motility, including manometric measurements of the cardioesophageal junction, show absence of the high-pressure zone (lower esophageal sphincter) in the terminal esophagus in most normal newborns. Evolution to the normal adult pattern of peristalsis and cardioesophageal sphincter function occurs after several months. Until this happens, many infants experience varying degrees of regurgitation after feeding. Rarely, repeated gastric reflux may produce peptic esophagitis and interfere with the development of a competent sphincter. Unlike adults, children rarely have a hiatal hernia as a cause of GER.

▶ Clinical Findings

A. Symptoms and Signs

Symptoms consist of repeated effortless regurgitation of feedings, particularly when the baby is placed in a recumbent position. The baby will be hungry and will readily feed after regurgitating. Persistent regurgitation may result in poor weight gain (failure to thrive), peptic esophagitis with appearance of blood in the vomitus, or occult bleeding, producing anemia. One cause for apnea and acute life-threatening events (ALTE) is GER and aspiration. Lesser degrees of aspiration, particularly during sleep, may produce recurrent pneumonia. Stricture formation of the lower esophagus and metaplasia of the esophageal mucosa, producing Barrett esophagus, are possible late effects. Almost half of infants and children with GER have neurologic disorders related to perinatal asphyxia or congenital nervous system anomalies; seizure disorders are very common in this population. Abnormal motility of the esophagus and gastric dysmotility and impaired gastric emptying are frequently present. Gastroesophageal reflux is associated with esophageal atresia, CDH, and abdominal wall defects.

B. Imaging Studies

The standard diagnostic test is lower esophageal 24-hour pH monitoring. An upper GI series is less sensitive but is useful to rule out other disorders (eg, intestinal malrotation) and to assess for esophageal stricture. Gastric emptying may be assessed by technetium pertechnetate scan. There is virtually no role for esophageal manometric studies in young children except for those in whom one suspects the relatively rare achalasia or diffuse esophageal spasm.

▶ Treatment

Nonoperative treatment is successful in most cases. Feedings should be thickened with rice cereal, and GER is lessened if the baby is maintained upright in an infant seat or in a prone position after feeding. Persistent symptoms mandate drug therapy with an antacid (eg, H_2-blocker or proton pump inhibitor) with or without a prokinetic agent (eg, metoclopramide). If a prolonged trial of nonoperative therapy fails or if complications of reflux can be documented (ie, esophagitis, stricture, asthma, recurrent aspiration pneumonia, failure to thrive), an antireflux procedure is indicated. The Nissen fundoplication has become the standard surgical treatment, although many variations on fundoplication exist. The open operation has been virtually replaced by the more cosmetic laparoscopic procedure that also provides for better visualization.

Capito C et al: Long-term outcome of laparoscopic Nissen-Rosetti fundoplication for neurologically impaired and normal children. *Surg Endosc* 2008 Apr;22(4):875-880.

Kubiak R, Andrews J, Grant HW: Long-term outcome of laparoscopic nissen fundoplication compared with laparoscopic thal fundoplication in children: a prospective, randomized study. *Ann Surg* 2011 Jan;253(1):44-49.

Valusek PA et al: The use of fundoplication for prevention of apparent life-threatening events. *J Pediatr Surg* 2007;42(6):1022-1024.

ACUTE APPENDICITIS

Acute appendicitis is one of the most common causes of an acute abdomen in childhood. This diagnosis must be considered in all age groups, but it is most common between the ages of 4 and 15 years.

▶ Clinical Findings

The diagnosis is most often made by obtaining a careful clinical history and performing a thorough physical examination. In some patients, observation and periodic reexamination by the same physician may be necessary to confirm or exclude the diagnosis. In young children, the diagnosis of appendicitis can be difficult to arrive at, as the clinical history may be difficult to elicit. The classic presentation includes the onset of epigastric or periumbilical pain followed by anorexia, nausea, and vomiting. Anorexia is a significant finding, as the child will often refuse favorite foods. A fever will usually develop, and the pain then localizes to the right lower quadrant. Rovsing sign (right lower quadrant pain during palpation of the left lower quadrant), localized right lower quadrant tenderness, and involuntary spasm of the right hemirectus muscle indicate the presence of peritonitis.

A white blood count with differential and urinalysis should be obtained. The white blood cell count is greater than $10,000/\mu L$ (often with a left shift) in more than 80% of patients with appendicitis. Radiologic evaluation should include a chest film to exclude right lower lobe pneumonia. Findings on flat and erect abdominal radiographs are often nonspecific, though they may infrequently demonstrate the presence of a fecalith. Ultrasound (particularly in females) and CT scans are being used with increasing frequency, especially for those without the classic history and physical examination results.

▶ Differential Diagnosis

Gastroenteritis is often confused with appendicitis. Vomiting follows periumbilical pain in appendicitis but often precedes abdominal pain in gastroenteritis. In addition, the patient with gastroenteritis commonly has diffuse abdominal pain and frequent copious watery diarrhea. Intussusception, intestinal obstruction and volvulus, mesenteric adenitis, Meckel diverticulitis, Henoch-Schönlein purpura, ruptured ovarian cyst, and Crohn disease must also be considered in the differential diagnosis for children. In adolescent girls, information regarding the menstrual cycle, previous episodes of pelvic inflammatory disease, and an accurate sexual history is important to exclude gynecologic causes of an acute abdomen.

▶ Treatment

Once the diagnosis is made, fluid resuscitation is performed and antibiotics are administered. Appendectomy is accomplished through a right lower quadrant incision or laparoscopically. In cases of perforation, the peritoneal cavity is irrigated and aspirated dry but drainage is not performed, unless there is a mature abscess cavity. The wound is closed in all cases. Antibiotics are continued for 3-7 days or until the white blood cell count and fever normalize. Overall, the morbidity and mortality of appendicitis in children have gradually decreased with the increased use of powerful broad-spectrum antibiotics. However, perforated appendicitis with abscess formation remains the variant with increased morbidity when compared to nonperforated cases. Interval appendectomy after management of perforated appendicitis with antibiotics and abscess drainage when necessary is a viable option. The criteria for which patients to initially manage nonoperatively are still under debate.

Henry MC, Gollin G. Islam S, Sylvester K, Walker A, Silverman BL, Moss RL: Matched analysis of non-operative management vs immediate appendectomy for perforated appendicitis. *J Pediatr Surg* 2007;42(1):19-24.

Henry MC, Walker A, Silverman B, Gollin G, Islam S, Sylvester KG, Moss RL: Risk factors for the development of abdominal abscess following operation for perforated appendicitis in children. *Arch Surg* 2007;142:236-241.

Myers AL, Williams RF, Giles K, et al: Hospital cost analysis of a prospective, randomized trial of early vs interval appendectomy for perforated appendicitis in children. *J Am Coll Surg* 2012 Apr;214(4):427-434.

DUPLICATIONS OF THE GASTROINTESTINAL TRACT

Duplications may occur at any point along the GI tract from the mouth to the anus. Duplications occur (in order of decreasing frequency) in the ileum (50% of cases), mediastinum, colon, rectum, stomach, duodenum, and neck. Intrathoracic and small bowel duplications are usually spherical; colonic duplications are commonly long and tubular (Figure 43–18). Characteristically, the intra-abdominal spherical duplications are on the mesenteric side of the intestine and do not share a common wall with the intestine.

Based on embryology, duplications have been categorized as foregut, midgut, and hindgut. Foregut duplications include the pharynx, respiratory tract, esophagus, stomach, and the first portion and proximal half of the second portion of the duodenum. Midgut duplications include the distal half of the second part of the duodenum, the jejunum, ileum, cecum, appendix, the ascending colon, and the proximal two-thirds of the transverse colon. The hindgut is composed of duplications of the distal third of the transverse colon, the descending and sigmoid colon, the rectum, anus, and components of the urologic system. Combined thoracoabdominal duplications also occur in which the thoracic saccular component extends through the esophageal hiatus or a separate diaphragmatic opening to empty into the duodenum or jejunum. A thoracic duplication, associated

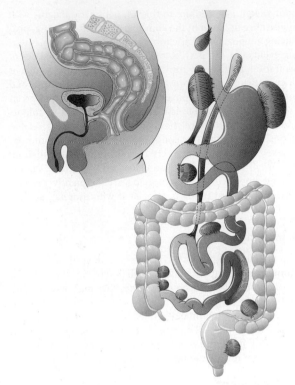

▲ **Figure 43–18.** Duplications of the gastrointestinal tract. Duplications may be saccular or tubular. They usually arise within the mesentery, having a common wall with the intestine. Thoracoabdominal duplications arise from the duodenum or jejunum and extend through the diaphragm into the mediastinum.

with a cervical or thoracic vertebral anomaly, in which the duplication communicates with the subarachnoid space, is called a neurenteric cyst. Associated cardiovascular, neurologic, skeletal, urologic, and GI anomalies occur in more than a third of cases. Carcinoma may arise within intestinal duplications later in life.

▶ Clinical Findings

A. Symptoms and Signs

Two-thirds of patients with duplications are symptomatic in the first year of life. Duplications of the neck and mediastinum produce respiratory distress by compression of the airway. Thoracic duplications may ulcerate into the lung and lead to pneumonia or hemoptysis. Intestinal duplications usually produce abdominal pain owing to spastic contraction of the bowel, excessive distention of the duplication, or peptic ulceration and bleeding resulting from ectopic gastric mucosa in the duplication. Intestinal obstruction due to intussusception, volvulus, or encroachment on the lumen by an intramural cyst also occurs. An isolated asymptomatic mass may be the only finding. Sixty percent of duplications are diagnosed by 6 months of life and 85% by 2 years.

B. Imaging Studies

Studies include radiographs of the chest and thoracolumbar spine, CT scan of the chest and abdomen, contrast enema, esophagography, and upper GI series. If an intraspinal extension of a duplication is suspected, MRI is indicated. Ultrasonography may show a cystic or tubular mass within the mediastinum or abdomen. A Meckel scan (technetium pertechnetate) can also be used to visualize those duplications with ectopic gastric mucosa.

▶ Treatment

Duplications not intimately adherent to adjacent organs should be excised. Isolated spherical duplications can be excised with the adjacent segment of bowel and an end-to-end anastomosis of the bowel performed. Long tubular duplications can be decompressed by establishing an anastomosis between the proximal and distal ends of adjacent bowel. Noncommunicating duplications, which would require radical resection of surrounding structures, should be drained by a Roux-en-Y technique. Duplications that cannot be removed completely and which contain gastric mucosa should be opened (without jeopardizing the blood supply of the normal bowel) and the mucosal lining excised. Extension of a mediastinal duplication into the spine or abdomen should be resected. An intra-abdominal extension is closed at the level of the diaphragm, and complete excision by laparotomy is accomplished.

Laje P, Flake AW, Adzick NS: Prenatal diagnosis and postnatal resection of intraabdominal enteric duplications. *J Pediatr Surg* 2010 Jul;45(7):1554-1558.

OMPHALOMESENTERIC DUCT ANOMALIES

The omphalomesenteric (vitelline) duct is a remnant of the embryonic yolk sac. When the entire duct remains intact postnatally, it is recognized as an omphalomesenteric fistula. When the duct is obliterated at the intestinal end but communicates with the umbilicus at the distal end, it is called an umbilical sinus. When the epithelial tract persists but both ends are occluded, an umbilical cyst or intra-abdominal enterocystoma may develop. The entire tract may be obliterated, but a fibrous band may persist between the ileum and the umbilicus (Figure 43–19).

The most common remnant of the omphalomesenteric duct is Meckel diverticulum, which is present in 1%-3% of the population. Meckel diverticulum may be lined wholly or in part by small intestinal, colonic, or gastric mucosa, and it

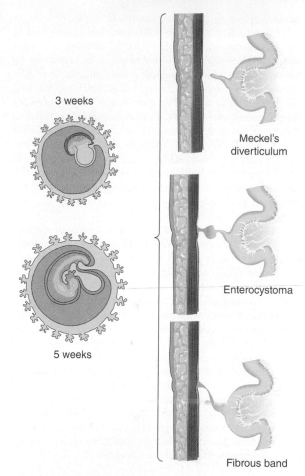

▲ **Figure 43–19.** Omphalomesenteric duct anomalies arise from the primitive yolk sac. Remnants include Meckel diverticulum, enterocystoma, and a fibrous band or fistulous tract between the ileum and the umbilicus.

may contain aberrant pancreatic tissue. Heterotopic tissue is found in 5% of asymptomatic and 60% of symptomatic cases. In contrast to duplications and pseudodiverticula, Meckel diverticulum is located on the antimesenteric border of the ileum, 10-90 cm from the ileocecal valve. Meckel diverticulum occurs with equal frequency in both sexes. It is usually asymptomatic and is seen as an incidental finding during operation for other disease. Of those with Meckel diverticulum, the lifelong risk of complications is 4%, and 40% of these cases occur in children under 10 years of age.

▶ Clinical Findings

Symptomatic omphalomesenteric remnants (male:female incidence 3:1) produce painless rectal bleeding in 40%, intussusception in 20%, diverticulitis or peptic perforation in 15%, umbilical fistula in 15%, intestinal obstruction in 7%, and abscess in 3% of cases. Rectal bleeding associated with Meckel diverticulum is due to peptic ulceration of the adjacent ileum caused by ectopic gastric mucosa. Over 50% of these patients are under 2 years of age. The blood is mixed with stool and is most often dark red or bright red; tarry stools are unusual. A history of a previous episode of bleeding may be elicited in 40% of cases. Occult bleeding from Meckel diverticulum is very rare. Younger patients tend to bleed quite briskly and may exsanguinate rapidly. Diverticulitis or free perforation will present with abdominal pain and peritonitis similar to acute appendicitis. The pain and tenderness occur in the lower abdomen, most commonly near the umbilicus. Periumbilical cellulitis may be present.

Intestinal obstruction may develop as a result of volvulus of the bowel about a persistent band between the umbilicus and the ileum or as a result of herniation of bowel between the mesentery and a persistent vitelline or mesodiverticular vessel. Obstruction is the most common presentation in adults. An infected umbilical sinus or omphalomesenteric fistula may present with mucoid, purulent, or enteric discharge, recurrent cellulitis, or a deep abdominal wall abscess about the umbilicus. This can be diagnosed by cannulation and contrast injection via the umbilical tract.

Upper and lower contrast studies rarely outline the primary defect. Technetium Tc 99m pertechnetate may localize in gastric mucosa lining Meckel diverticulum and may identify the source of hematochezia or melena. Retention of dye in the mucous and parietal cells is enhanced by giving cimetidine, 30 mg/kg intravenously, 30 minutes before administration of the radiotracer nuclide.

▶ Treatment

Resection is accomplished by laparotomy or laparoscopy. An omphalomesenteric remnant with a narrow base may be treated by amputation and closure of the bowel defect (usually with a surgical stapler). In cases where the anomaly has a wide mouth with ectopic tissue or where an inflammatory or ischemic process involves the adjacent ileum, intestinal resection with the diverticulum and anastomosis may be necessary.

Chan KW, Lee KH, Mou JW, Cheung ST, Tam YH: Laparoscopic management of complicated Meckel's diverticulum in children: a 10-year review. *Surg Endosc* 2008 Jun;22(6):1509-1512. [Epub 2008 Mar 6.]

NECROTIZING ENTEROCOLITIS

Necrotizing enterocolitis (NEC) is the most serious and frequent GI disorder of predominantly premature infants, with a median onset of 10 days after birth. The incidence is increasing given the therapeutic advances in neonatal intensive care that have allowed ever more premature infants to survive. It is characterized by necrosis, ulceration, and sloughing of intestinal mucosa, which frequently progresses to full-thickness necrosis and perforation. This process progresses from the submucosa through the muscular layer to the subserosa. Gas-producing bacteria in the intestinal wall may lead to pneumatosis, a finding that may be noted on gross examination as well as on plain abdominal radiographs. The terminal ileum and right colon are usually affected first, followed in descending order of frequency by the transverse and descending colon, appendix, jejunum, stomach, duodenum, and esophagus. The most extreme case, pan-necrosis, is defined as necrosis of 75% or more of the bowel. Eighty percent of cases occur in premature infants weighing less than 2500 g at birth, and 50% are under 1500 g. However, the disorder may also occur in full-term infants. Contrary to earlier impressions, there is no established relationship between NEC and stressful perinatal events such as premature rupture of membranes with amnionitis, breech delivery, intrauterine bradycardia, umbilical vessel catheterization with or without exchange transfusion, respiratory distress syndrome, sepsis, omphalitis, and congenital heart disease. An associated patent ductus arteriosus is common. In older infants and children, NEC is usually preceded by malnutrition and gastroenteritis. The clustering of cases in nurseries suggests that an infectious agent may be responsible.

▶ Clinical Findings

Clinical findings include increased gastric residual, bilious vomiting, abdominal distention, bloody stools, lethargy, and poor skin perfusion. When intestinal perforation occurs, guarding is evident on abdominal examination, but in weak premature infants this may not be obvious. There are a variety of nonspecific clinical findings that suggest physiologic instability such as apnea, bradycardia, hypoglycemia, and temperature instability. On examination, abdominal distention and fixed loops of intestine may be appreciated. The presence of abdominal wall erythema, edema, and crepitus may be a sign of bowel necrosis. Laboratory evaluation is nonspecific since the white blood cell count may be low or high, but thrombocytopenia and acidosis develop with perforation and sepsis.

Supine and cross-table lateral abdominal radiographs show small bowel distention early, followed by pneumatosis intestinalis. Gas within the portal venous system can be seen but it is fleeting. Serial examinations may show a loop or loops of bowel that are fixed in position and dilated. Perforation with peritoneal air develops in 20% of cases. Infants who develop ascites without pneumoperitoneum should have paracentesis and examination of the fluid for bacteria, which would signify perforation. Contrast studies are hazardous and contraindicated, as they may easily lead to perforation.

Treatment

Treatment includes cessation of feedings, orogastric suction, systemic antibiotics, and correction of hypoxemia, hypovolemia, acidosis, and electrolyte abnormalities. The only absolute indication for intervention is pneumoperitoneum. Relative indications are portal vein air, clinical deterioration, a fixed intestinal loop on serial radiographs, erythema of the abdominal wall, an abdominal mass, and a paracentesis demonstrating bacteria. At laparotomy, necrotic bowel is resected and the proximal bowel is made into a stoma. Rarely is primary anastomosis safe. Severe disease may not be amenable to operation or require extensive bowel resection, resulting in short bowel syndrome. An alternative treatment option in very low-birth-weight (VLBW) infants (< 1500 g) that is gaining acceptance for documented perforation is bedside drainage of the peritoneal cavity in the right lower quadrant using local anesthesia. A recent prospective randomized trial comparing laparotomy to drain placement for VLBW infants demonstrated equivalent outcomes in mortality and short-term morbidity for these two modalities.

In one-third of cases, the disorder resolves without further treatment, and the overall survival rate is more than 50%. Intestinal stricture may occur as a late complication following healing. For this reason, a contrast enema is used to evaluate the defunctionalized distal bowel before closing the stoma.

Leaf A, Dorling J, Kempley S, McCormick K, Mannix P, Linsell L, Juszczak E, Brocklehurst P: Early or delayed enteral feeding for preterm growth-restricted infants: a randomized trial. *Pediatrics* 2012 May;129(5):e1260-e1268.

GASTROINTESTINAL BLEEDING

Significant GI bleeding in children is rare. When it occurs, it can be alarming and anxiety provoking for caregivers and parents. The diagnostic approach used in the evaluation of these children is similar to that used in adults, but the causes vary depending on the age of the child. Rarely is the GI bleeding massive, and the majority of causes are benign. A diagnosis can be established in over 85% of cases. Usual presenting symptoms include hematemesis, hematochezia, and melena. Depending on the amount of bleeding, the child may have sunken fontanelles, dry mucous membranes, and cool skin. Tachycardia, oliguria, and hypotension may be present. Intravenous access should be obtained, fluid and blood administered as needed, and an evaluation begun. Laboratory tests include serial hematocrit measurements and coagulation studies. Following stabilization and physical examination, evaluation should then proceed to the appropriate diagnostic tests.

Upper Gastrointestinal Bleeding

Upper GI bleeding originates above the ligament of Treitz. The presence of melena and the presence of blood on passage of an orogastric tube can help differentiate between upper and lower GI bleeding. Upper GI bleeding in infants and young children is most often associated with stress ulcers or erosions, but in older children it may also be caused by duodenal ulcer, esophagitis, and esophageal varices particularly in children with underlying liver disease. The majority of these diseases are benign. Evaluation following stabilization of the child begins with flexible esophagoduodenoscopy. Once the diagnosis is made, treatment is usually amenable to antacids (H_2-blockers, proton pump inhibitors). Variceal hemorrhage may require more aggressive intervention, including the use of octreotide, endoscopic varix sclerosis or band ligation, and, in extreme cases, transjugular intrahepatic portocaval shunt (TIPS), mesocaval shunt, or liver transplantation.

Lower Gastrointestinal Bleeding

Although diverticulitis, cancer, and angiodysplasia are the most common causes of lower GI bleeding in adults, those diseases are rare in children. The causes of lower GI bleeding in infants and children can be categorized in diagnostic age groups where the age of the patient, the amount of bleeding, and the color of the blood passed provide some guidance to the probable source of bleeding.

Bleeding in the neonate may be caused by swallowing maternal blood at delivery, an anorectal fissure, upper GI bleeding secondary to gastritis or ulceration, necrotizing enterocolitis, volvulus, and an incarcerated hernia. The Apt test for maternal blood, physical examination of the rectum and inguinal canal, and evaluation of the upper GI tract can quickly rule out most of these causes. Bleeding from necrotizing enterocolitis is rarely life threatening, and the diagnosis is commonly made based on the premature delivery of the infant and radiologic evaluation. If bleeding from malrotation with midgut volvulus is suspected, prompt laparotomy is indicated.

In infants, anal fissures continue to be the most common cause of rectal bleeding. Other causes include intestinal volvulus, intussusception, intestinal duplication, Meckel diverticulum, milk or formula protein allergy and infectious diarrhea. Contrast studies and appropriate stool cultures guide treatment. Children have a differential diagnosis similar to that of infants with the addition of rectal prolapse and a variety of polyps of the colon (juvenile, Peutz-Jeghers, polypoid lymphoid hyperplasia, and, rarely, adenomatosis). These entities are diagnosed by physical examination and proctosigmoidoscopy. If no source of bleeding is identified, colonoscopy is indicated, while capsule endoscopy is gaining acceptance as a diagnostic modality for occult causes of GI bleeding in appropriately sized patients. Juvenile polyps are the single most common cause of lower GI bleeding in children (20%-30%). Most juvenile polyps are single (80%) and often pass spontaneously without treatment. However, when bleeding continues to occur, the polyp can be snared and excised endoscopically. Adolescents may manifest signs and symptoms of inflammatory bowel disease (ulcerative colitis, Crohn disease), familial adenomatous polyposis, and small vascular lesions such as telangiectasias. Diagnosis is made by colonoscopy, and treatment is disease specific.

Boyle JT: Gastrointestinal bleeding in infants and children. *Pediatr Rev* 2008;2:39-52.

El-Matary W: Wireless capsule endoscopy: indications, limitations, and future challenges. *J Pediatr Gastroenterol Nutr* 2008;46(1):4-12.

GASTROINTESTINAL FOREIGN BODIES

Children aged 9 months to 2 years are at particular risk for the ingestion or aspiration of foreign bodies given their newly acquired mobility, curiosity, and the tendency to place objects in their mouths. The type of foreign body and the location in the airway or GI tract dictate management.

▶ Esophagal Foreign Bodies

Typical foreign bodies found in the esophagus include coins, food, and small toys. The three most common sites of obstruction are at the level of the cricopharyngeus muscle, at the level of the aortic arch, and at the gastroesophageal junction. Previous areas of repair/anastomosis as in esophageal atresia or injury predispose to obstruction due to scar and narrowing. Common symptoms include drooling, feeding intolerance, dysphagia, and pain. Perforation is rare but is dictated by the ingested object's shape, composition, and time in the esophagus. The diagnosis is easily obtained by anteroposterior chest or lateral neck radiography if the ingested object is radiopaque. Otherwise, esophagoscopy or an upper GI series is needed.

Because of the risk of erosion, aspiration, perforation, and late stricture, impacted objects should be removed. Extraction can be performed using balloon catheter retrieval under fluoroscopic control or under direct visualization using esophagoscopy with general anesthesia. The latter technique is generally preferred if the nature of the object is unknown, or is sharp, or the ingestion was 24-48 hours previously. A Hopkins rod lens endoscopy system allows visualization of the object and retrieval with specially designed forceps for grasping small objects.

Ninety-five percent of foreign bodies that pass beyond the gastroesophageal junction proceed uneventfully through the GI tract. Operative retrieval is reserved for batteries, which must be removed, and for cases where ingested objects cause obstruction (bezoars), intestinal injury or have been in place for more than 1 week.

▶ Tracheal Foreign Bodies

Children, particularly those 1-2 years of age, can occlude the airway by aspiration of a foreign body. The most common objects are peanuts and popcorn. Obstruction tends to occur at the level of the laryngeal inlet, the subglottis, or the right main stem bronchus. Because this can be a life-threatening problem, witnessed events should be treated with back blows, abdominal thrusts, or the Heimlich maneuver, which may dislodge the object.

Symptoms include coughing, choking, wheezing, dyspnea, and fever. Unilateral wheezing and rhonchi may be present. Air trapping may result when the foreign-body forms a ball-valve obstruction leading to hyperinflation of the affected lung and mediastinal shift away from the affected side. On the other hand, complete obstruction may lead to loss of air volume with atelectasis and mediastinal shift to the ipsilateral side. Inspiratory and expiratory radiographs or bilateral decubitus films in infants may demonstrate air trapping; the foreign body is rarely noted on radiographs.

With a worrisome history, a foreign body suggested on a radiograph, or any symptoms, the child should undergo bronchoscopic evaluation under general anesthesia. Working in tandem with the anesthesiologist to allow ventilation during rigid endoscopy, the foreign body can be readily identified. Lighted grasping forceps made specifically for foreign-body extraction are placed through the sheath of the bronchoscope; the foreign body is grasped; and the forceps, foreign body, and sheath are removed as one unit. Rarely, an unrecognized aspirated foreign body presents as chronic lung infection and can require removal of the affected lung.

Rodríguez H, Passali GC, Gregori D, Chinski A, Tiscornia C, Botto H, Nieto M, Zanetta A, Passali D, Cuestas G: Management of foreign bodies in the airway and oesophagus. *Int J Pediatr Otorhinolaryngol* 2012 May 14;76(Suppl 1):S84-s91.

▼ LIVER & BILIARY TRACT DISORDERS

Jaundice in the first 2 weeks of infancy is usually due to indirect (unconjugated) hyperbilirubinemia. The causes include (1) "physiologic jaundice" due to immaturity of hepatic function (eg, that associated with breast-feeding); (2) Rh, ABO, and rare blood group incompatibilities, which produce hemolysis; and (3) infections. Jaundice that persists beyond the first 2 weeks in which the indirect and conjugated bilirubin levels are elevated should prompt a more thorough workup aimed at diagnosing potential surgical disorders. The most frequent cause (60%) of prolonged jaundice in infancy is biliary atresia; various forms of hepatitis occur in 35%; and choledochal cyst is found in 5% of cases of obstructive jaundice. Intestinal obstruction can intensify jaundice by increasing the enterohepatic circulation of bilirubin. Finally, jaundice is an early and important sign of sepsis in the newborn.

BILIARY ATRESIA

Biliary atresia is the absence of patent bile ducts draining the liver. Familial cases and frequent association with the polysplenia syndrome indicate a congenital onset. However, biliary atresia probably develops after birth because jaundice is not usually remarkable in the newborn period but becomes evident more than 2 weeks later. Furthermore, conjugated bilirubin is not cleared by the placenta as unconjugated bilirubin is, and jaundice due to conjugated hyperbilirubinemia with biliary obstruction has not been recognized in newborn infants. The atretic ducts consist of solid fibrous cords that may contain occasional islands of biliary epithelium.

The extent of duct involvement varies greatly. There are three anatomic patterns of obstruction: (1) the proximal extrahepatic bile ducts are patent and the ducts distal to the cystic duct are obliterated; (2) the gallbladder, cystic duct, and common bile duct are patent and the proximal hepatic ducts are occluded; and (3) the entire extrahepatic ductal system is obstructed. Liver biopsy demonstrates proliferation of the bile canaliculi containing inspissated bile. Over time, the failure to excrete bile out of the liver results in progressive periportal fibrosis and obstruction of the intrahepatic portal veins, resulting in biliary cirrhosis.

▶ Clinical Findings

A. Symptoms and Signs

The infant with biliary atresia often has an uneventful neonatal course until jaundice is noted at 2-3 weeks of age. Stools may be normal or clay colored, and the urine may be dark. The stools contain an increased quantity of fat but are of normal consistency and not frothy. The liver may be of normal size early, but it becomes enlarged with time. A hard liver may develop as a consequence of progressive cirrhosis. Splenomegaly usually develops. Ascites and portal hypertension do not become manifest for several months.

B. Laboratory Findings

The workup of biliary atresia consists of analysis of liver function tests, complete blood count, and metabolic and serologic screening. The bilirubin levels may vary considerably from day to day, but direct bilirubin levels over 3 mg/dL are common. Alkaline phosphatase levels are often elevated to 500-1000 U/L, and γ-glutamyltranspeptidase levels are greater than 300 U/L.

C. Imaging Studies

Ultrasonography may demonstrate absence or inability to visualize a contracted gallbladder. Radionuclide scanning using technetium Tc 99m-labeled iminodiacetate compounds (IDA, HIDA, PIPIDA, DISIDA) to observe the intensity of uptake within the liver and evidence of secretion into the bowel is valuable, usually preceded by a 2- to 3-day course of phenobarbital to promote tracer uptake. Core needle biopsy of the liver may be safely performed at any age if the clotting tests are normal. A diagnosis based on needle biopsy is accurate in 60%, equivocal in 16%, and erroneous in 24% of cases. Unless the workup has conclusively diagnosed another entity, all children suspected of having biliary atresia should undergo operative cholangiography with the intention of proceeding to exploration of the porta hepatis and portoenterostomy as necessary.

▶ Other Causes

Other causes of obstructive jaundice are choledochal cyst, inspissated bile syndrome, and any one of several neonatal hepatitides. A choledochal cyst is identified by the presence of a palpable mass in the right upper quadrant and ultrasonographic confirmation. Inspissated bile syndrome follows a hemolytic process in which a large bilirubin load is excreted into the bile ducts, where it becomes coalesced and impacted, or may occur after a prolonged period of bowel rest with total parenteral nutrition. The syndrome is recognized by abdominal ultrasound. Hepatitis is most commonly of unknown cause. It may be due to a variety of infections, often of maternal origin, such as toxoplasmosis, cytomegalovirus, rubella syndrome, herpes simplex, coxsackievirus, and varicella. Serum should be tested for elevated antibody titers to these agents. Neonatal physiologic jaundice is self-limited and also responds to phototherapy.

Genetic metabolic diseases producing jaundice include α_1-antitrypsin deficiency, galactosemia, and cystic fibrosis. Other rare causes include sepsis, parenteral alimentation cholestasis, Gilbert disease, and Alagille syndrome.

▶ Treatment

Surgical exploration for neonatal jaundice is indicated as early in infancy as possible, when biliary atresia is the likely cause. Delayed treatment will result in progressive cirrhosis. Fluoroscopy should be available in the operating room. The gallbladder is cannulated through a transverse abdominal incision or via laparoscopy. Water-soluble contrast should be gently instilled into the biliary tree. If the image shows a patent common bile duct but no reflux into the liver, a rubber-shod bulldog clamp may be placed on the distal common duct and the cholangiogram repeated. A liver biopsy should be performed in all cases.

Confirmed biliary atresia requires hepatic portoenterostomy (Kasai procedure). The scarred bile ducts and gallbladder are removed, and a Roux-en-Y limb of jejunum is sutured to an area of the hilum bounded laterally by the hepatic artery branches. Some surgeons utilize empiric postoperative antibiotic coverage to prevent cholangitis that can lead to scarring and ongoing occlusion of the bile canaliculi that may remain patent. Steroids have also been used both preoperatively and postoperatively in an effort to prevent ongoing biliary and hepatic fibrosis though outcomes via scientific studies on this topic are equivocal.

▶ Prognosis

A good long-term outcome is related to a meticulously performed procedure, age at operation less than 2 months, absence of cirrhosis at the time of operation, and establishment of adequate bile flow. In general, one-third of the infants will have excellent bile flow and do not develop liver failure; one-third never have bile flow and require early liver transplantation; and one-third have initially good bile flow but months to years later develop progressive biliary cirrhosis requiring liver transplantation. The average life span for infants with uncorrectable biliary atresia without transplantation is 19 months. Death is due to progressive liver failure, bleeding from esophageal varices, or sepsis. For those with established bile flow postoperatively, the most common complication is cholangitis, and this may recur. Most often, the cause is unknown and not readily correctable by surgical means.

CHOLEDOCHAL CYST

A choledochal cyst is a dilation or diverticulum of all or a portion of the common bile duct. Estimates of incidence range from 1:2,000,000 to 1:13,000. There is a female predominance (3:1), and the lesions are more common in Asians, with a large majority of the reported cases from Japan. Numerous theories exist as to the cause of this abnormality, including infectious agents, reflux of pancreatic enzymes into the bile duct via a long common channel, genetic factors, and biliary autonomic dysfunction.

Choledochal cysts are classified into one of five subtypes. Type I is a fusiform dilation of the extrahepatic bile duct. Type II is a saccular outpouching of the common bile duct. Type III is referred to as a choledochocele and is a wide-mouth dilation of the common bile duct at its confluence with the duodenum. Type IV is cystic dilation of both the intrahepatic and extrahepatic bile ducts. Type V consists of lakes of multiple intrahepatic cysts with no extrahepatic component and, when associated with hepatic fibrosis, is termed Caroli disease. Type I and type IV are the most common lesions, with type I cysts accounting for 85% of these abnormalities. Caroli disease appears to be a congenital syndrome and often follows an autosomal recessive pattern of inheritance in association with various other anomalies such as polycystic kidney disease and renal tubular ectasia.

If left untreated, a choledochal cyst may cause cholangitis and cholangiocarcinoma. The risk of cholangiocarcinoma in the first decade of life is only 0.7%; however, this increases to 14% at 20 years and is postulated to increase even further throughout life.

▶ Clinical Findings

The clinical manifestations of a choledochal cyst are recurrent abdominal pain, episodic jaundice, and a right upper quadrant mass, though in most cases one of these features is missing. As children grow older, the cyst may become painful or infected. On rare occasions, children have been described with bile peritonitis secondary to perforation of a cyst. In adults, an abdominal mass is rarely appreciated, and patients present more commonly with symptoms of cholangitis or pancreatitis. Gallstones and cholangitis may develop due to biliary stasis.

The diagnosis is most often established by the clinical presentation and abnormal ultrasonography. Technetium Tc 99m-labeled IDA scan, CT and MRI scans, endoscopic retrograde cholangiopancreatography, and operative cholangiography may be necessary. Ultrasonography is increasingly responsible for detecting choledochal cysts in the fetus.

▶ Treatment

In the past, the cysts were not removed but drained into a limb of intestine. However, many of these patients developed carcinoma in the cyst years later. Presently, the treatment is complete excision with Roux-en-Y hepaticojejunostomy. The duodenal end of the bile duct should be oversewn without injury to the anomalous entry of the pancreatic duct, limiting the amount of residual biliary tissue at risk for malignancy. Side-to-side choledochoduodenostomy is controversial due to a high incidence of reflux bile gastritis. However, it has been used successfully in high volume centers in Asia and is growing in popularity in the United States. Cholecystectomy is always performed. Biliary cirrhosis and portal hypertension, occurring from prolonged ductal obstruction, may be assessed with liver biopsy. The results of choledochal cyst excision with hepaticojejunostomy reconstruction are consistently excellent, but these children do require lifelong follow-up because of the risk of anastomotic stricture and intrahepatic stone formation. There is currently a trend toward laparoscopic approaches to the treatment of choledochal cyst disease.

▼ INGUINAL & SCROTAL DISORDERS

INGUINAL HERNIA & HYDROCELE

Inguinal hernia is a common condition in infancy and childhood, occurring in 1%-3% of all children. Unlike hernias in adulthood, these nearly always result from a patent processus vaginalis (indirect hernia) and not from a weakness in the floor of the inguinal canal (direct hernia). The processus vaginalis follows the descent of the testis into the inguinal canal. Failure of obliteration of the processus may

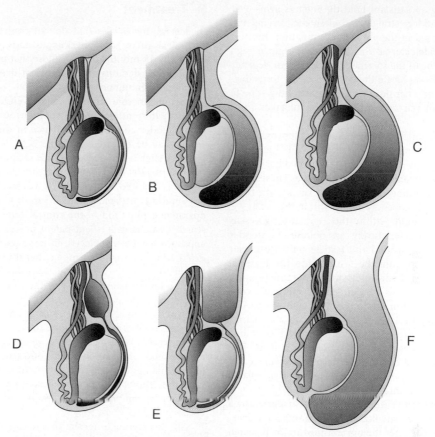

▲ **Figure 43–20.** Spectrum of inguinoscrotal disorders. **A:** Normal anatomy. The processus vaginalis is obliterated and there is a small remnant, the tunica vaginalis, adjacent to the posterior surface of the testis. **B:** Scrotal hydrocele. **C:** Communicating hydrocele. Note the proximal patency of the processus vaginalis. **D:** Hydrocele of the spermatic cord. **E:** Inguinal hernia. **F:** Inguinoscrotal hernia. (Reproduced, with permission, from Sheldon CA: Inguinal and scrotal disorders In: Rowe MI et al, eds. *Essentials of Pediatric Surgery.* St. Louis, MO: Mosby; 1995.)

lead to a variety of anomalies, including hernia, communicating hydrocele, noncommunicating hydrocele, hydrocele of the spermatic cord, and hydrocele of the tunica vaginalis (Figure 43–20).

The processus vaginalis remains patent in over 80% of newborn infants. With increasing age, the incidence of patent processus vaginalis diminishes. At 2 years, 40%-50% are open, and in adults 25% are persistently patent. Actual herniation of bowel into a widely patent processus vaginalis develops in 1%-4% of children; 25% occur within the first year of life. Indirect inguinal hernia occurs four to six times more frequently in males. Direct and femoral hernias occur in children but are very rare.

Hernias are found on the right side in 60% of cases, on the left side in 30%, and bilaterally in 10%. Conditions associated with an increased risk of inguinal hernia include prematurity, family history, history of an abdominal wall defect (eg, gastroschisis), cryptorchidism, intersex anomalies, connective tissue disorders, and ascites. The processus vaginalis may be obliterated at any location proximal to the testis or labium.

▶ **Clinical Findings**

The incidence of a clinically detectable inguinal hernia varies with gestational age: 9%-11% in preterm infants and 3-5% for full-term infants. The diagnosis of hernia in infants and children can be made only by the demonstration of an inguinal bulge originating from the internal ring. The bulge can be elicited during times of Valsalva (crying, coughing, straining). Having an assistant hold the infant's arms over his or her head and legs straight will often elicit crying and straining that will aid in the physical examination. Indirect signs, such as a wide external ring and the "silk glove" sign (palpable thickening of the spermatic cord) are not dependable. One must always locate the position of the testis during examination for a hernia since an inguinal bulge due to an undescended or retractile testis may be mistaken for a hernia.

Incarcerated inguinal hernia accounts for approximately 10% of childhood hernias, and the incidence is highest in infants. In the majority of girls with incarcerated hernia, the sac contains the ovary and portion of the tube. These structures are usually a sliding component of the sac. In boys, small bowel, colon, or appendix can be within the sac.

A hydrocele is fluid within the remnant processus vaginalis. It is characteristically an oblong, nontender soft mass. It may be around the testicle only (testicular hydrocele), extend up from the testicle into the inguinal region (inguinoscrotal hydrocele), or be contained within a segment of the processus adjacent to the spermatic cord (hydrocele of the cord) or communicated with the peritoneal cavity (communicating hydrocele). With a noncommunicating hydrocele (the first three hydroceles described above), the processus vaginalis has closed proximally. The normal spermatic cord can usually be palpated above the level of the hydrocele. Transillumination is not reliable in the newborn since intestine and fluid transilluminate equally well. A communicating hydrocele is suspected by a history of size variation (smallest in the morning after sleep, largest during the day after the upright posture or repeated straining).

▶ Differential Diagnosis

A hydrocele under tension may be confused with an incarcerated inguinal hernia. The sudden appearance of fluid confined to the testicular area may represent a noncommunicating hydrocele secondary to torsion of the testis or testicular appendage, epididymo-orchitis, pan-serositis from a recent viral syndrome, or idiopathic scrotal edema. Rectal examination and palpation of the peritoneal side of the inguinal ring may distinguish an incarcerated hernia from a hydrocele or other inguinoscrotal mass, but this is only reliable in the first 2-3 months of age as the internal ring is difficult to reach thereafter.

▶ Complications

The principal risk of not treating an inguinal hernia is incarceration (viscus stuck in sac) and subsequent strangulation (ischemia of said viscus, usually the bowel, not the ovary). Compression of the spermatic vessels by an incarcerated hernia may produce hemorrhagic infarction of the ipsilateral testicle.

▶ Treatment

In general, hydroceles that do not communicate with the peritoneal cavity are physiologic and the vast majority resolve by 18 months of age. Those that persist after 1 year or those that demonstrate changes in size (communicating hydroceles) should be repaired.

Inguinal hernia in infancy and childhood should be repaired; they never resolve spontaneously. In premature infants under constant surveillance in the hospital, hernia repair may be deferred until the baby is ready to be discharged. High ligation of the hernia sac by obliteration of the internal ring (leaving enough space for the spermatic cord) is all that is required. Historically, it was recommended that all boys under 2 years of age and all girls under 5 years undergo operative exploration of the contralateral inguinal canal in search of a clinically silent patent processus vaginalis. This approach has been replaced, in large part, by laparoscopic exploration. This is performed either through the ipsilateral hernia sac, through the umbilicus, or in-line with the internal ring (at the lateral border of the rectus muscle) using a needle scope. If a patent processus vaginalis is demonstrated, a second inguinal incision is made and the procedure is repeated as described above. Recently, a completely laparoscopic repair has been advocated, which has the advantage of simultaneous exploration of the contralateral side and virtually no manipulation of the spermatic cord. The incidence of complications from uncomplicated inguinal hernia repair (recurrence, wound infection, and damage to the spermatic cord) should be 2% or less.

An incarcerated hernia in an infant can usually be reduced initially before operation. This is accomplished by sedation and by elevation of the foot of the bed to keep intra-abdominal pressure from being exerted against the inguinal area. When the infant is well sedated, the hernia may be reduced by gentle constant pressure over the internal ring in a manner that milks the bowel into the abdominal cavity. This is a two-handed maneuver in which one hand "squeezes" the incarcerated mass while the other directs it posteriorly into the internal ring. If the bowel is not reduced within an hour, operation is required. If the hernia is reduced, operative repair should be delayed for 48 hours to allow edema in the tissues to subside. An incarcerated ovary may not be able to be reduced but is usually asymptomatic, and repair at the next available operating room time is sufficient since torsion is rare and the blood supply, unlike that of the intestine, is not compromised by being trapped in the canal. Bloody stools and edema and red discoloration of the skin around the groin suggest a strangulated hernia, and reduction of the bowel should not be attempted. Emergency repair of incarcerated inguinal hernia is technically difficult because the edematous tissues are friable and tear readily. When gangrenous intestine is encountered, the bowel should be resected and an end-to-end intestinal anastomosis performed.

Dutta S, Albanese C: Transcutaneous laparoscopic hernia repair in children: a prospective review of 275 hernia repairs with minimum 2-year follow-up. *Surg Endosc* 2009 Jan;23(1):103-107.

Ozgediz D, Roayaie K, Lee H, Nobuhara KK, Farmer DL, Bratton B, Harrison MR: Subcutaneous endoscopically assisted ligation (SEAL) of the internal ring for repair of inguinal hernias in children: report of a new technique and early results. *Surg Endosc* 2007 Aug;21(8):1327-1331.

UNDESCENDED TESTIS (CRYPTORCHIDISM)

In the seventh month of gestation, the testicles normally descend into the scrotum. A fibromuscular band—the gubernaculum—extends from the lower pole of the testis to the scrotum, and this band probably acts by guiding the path for descent during differential growth of the fetus rather than by pulling the testes down. Undescended testis (cryptorchidism) is a form of dystopia of the testis that occurs when there is arrested descent and fixation of the position of the testis retroperitoneally, in the inguinal canal, or just beyond the external ring. Continued descent of the testes may progress after birth, but descent comes to a halt before 2 years of age.

Another form of dystopia is ectopic testis, in which the gubernaculum may have guided the testis near the pubis, penis, perineum, or medial thigh or to a subcutaneous position superficial to the inguinal canal. In these instances, the testis has descended beyond the external ring of the inguinal canal, and the vascular supply is sufficiently developed so as to pose little difficulty in operative repair.

Normal spermatogenesis requires the cooler temperature range provided in the scrotum. When the testis remains undescended and subjected to normal body temperature, degenerative changes in the seminiferous tubules occur in which the lining cells become progressively atrophic and hyalinized, with peritubular fibrosis. The degenerative changes begin to occur at 2 years of age. Unless the disorder is corrected, all bilaterally cryptorchid adult males become sterile.

The incidence of undescended or partially descended testis is 1%-2% in full-term infants and up to 30% in premature babies. The right testis is affected in 45% of cases, the left testis in 30%, and both testes in 25%. A patent processus vaginalis is present in 95% of patients with cryptorchidism, and approximately 25% develop a clinical hernia.

Anomalies associated with cryptorchidism occur in about 15% of cases and include a wide variety of syndromes such as Klinefelter syndrome, hypogonadotropic hypogonadism, the prune belly syndrome, horseshoe kidneys, renal agenesis or hypoplasia, exstrophy of the bladder, ureteral reflux, gastroschisis, and cloacal exstrophy.

▶ Clinical Findings

Physical examination demonstrates an "empty hemiscrotum" with absent rugae. Cryptorchidism must be differentiated from a retractile testis. Because of the very active cremaster of children under 3 years of age and the small size of the testis, the gonad can retract into the external inguinal ring or within the inguinal canal—this is called a retractile testis—and it is a variant of normal. The retractile testis can be manually manipulated into the mid to lower scrotum and no therapy is required.

▶ Treatment

Operation is indicated after 12-18 months since degenerative changes begin to take place in these testes that may impair spermatogenesis and lead to malignant transformation. Additionally, cryptorchid testes are more susceptible to trauma and torsion, often have an associated inguinal hernia, and may cause adverse psychosocial effects. The incidence of testicular cancer in a cryptorchid testis is 30 times higher than in the normal population and is not lessened by repair. The role of repair is to allow reliable examination for a testicular mass later in life.

Orchidopexy is the surgical method for mobilizing the testis—based on the testicular vessels and the vas deferens—from its ectopic location into the scrotum. When the dystopic testis is not palpable preoperatively, 17% are absent, 33% are intra-abdominal, and 50% are in the inguinal canal or just beyond the inguinal ring. If the testis is not palpable when the child is anesthetized, laparoscopy should be performed before making an inguinal incision. Increasingly, the complete operation (diagnosis and intra-abdominal mobilization) is performed laparoscopically. This will allow for identification of an abdominal testis or the diagnosis of an absent testis (usually due to *in utero* torsion). Very high testes with a short blood supply can be brought into the scrotum by a two-stage repair (dividing the spermatic artery and vein with clips or laser followed by positioning in the scrotum 6-8 weeks later) based on collateral blood supply via the vas deferens and the gubernaculum. Testes confined in the inguinal canal (25% of cases) can usually be brought into the scrotum in one stage. Ectopic testicles located outside the inguinal canal, such as in the subcutaneous inguinal pouch, occur in over 50% of cases, and the testicular vessels are so well developed that scrotal placement is rarely a problem. The prognosis for fertility following orchidopexy in unilateral maldescent is 80%, whereas fertility after bilateral orchidopexy is about 50%. Due to variable degrees of tension and tenuous blood supply, the testis after an orchidopexy is often smaller than the contralateral one.

Gatti JM, Ostlie DJ: The use of laparoscopy in the management of nonpalpable undescended testes. *Curr Opin Pediatr* 2007;19(3):349-353.

Lao OB, Fitzgibbons RJ Jr, Cusick RA: Pediatric inguinal hernias, hydroceles, and undescended testicles. *Surg Clin North Am* 2012 Jun;92(3):487-504.

TESTICULAR TORSION

Testicular torsion is most frequent in late childhood and early adolescence, though the range can include the fetus and the adult. Anatomically, there are two forms of testicular torsion depending on where the spermatic cord is twisted with respect to the tunica vaginalis: intravaginal torsion (bell-clapper deformity), the most common form, and extravaginal torsion that occurs principally in neonates and in children with an undescended testis. Rarely, the testis may twist on a long epididymal mesentery. In children and adolescents, testicular torsion is either idiopathic or occurs after activity or trauma.

▶ Clinical Findings

Acute scrotal or testicular pain that may radiate to the lower abdomen is usually present. Progressive swelling, edema, and erythema of the hemiscrotum occur. The testis is exquisitely tender to palpation. The testicle may be foreshortened, the epididymis may lie anteriorly, and the cremasteric reflex may be absent—though these signs are difficult to elicit. Fetal or neonatal torsion is probably responsible for the "absent" testis noted during laparoscopy.

The diagnosis of testicular torsion is based mainly on clinical examination. Although one may utilize Doppler ultrasonography and radionuclide scanning to aid in the diagnosis, these tests are time consuming and, in the case of ultrasound, operator specific.

▶ Differential Diagnosis

Torsion of the testicular appendices (vestigial müllerian duct structures) and epididymitis may mimic testicular torsion. With epididymitis, there is often pyuria, voiding symptoms, and fever. Torsion of the testicular appendices often has a gradual onset, and careful palpation may reveal point tenderness rather than diffuse tenderness. There may be a visible necrotic lesion on scrotal transillumination (blue dot sign).

▶ Treatment

If the diagnosis is strongly suspected, the best "test" is operative scrotal exploration. The testicular salvage rate if detorsion is performed within 6 hours after onset of symptoms is up to 97%, versus less than 10% if delayed more than 24 hours. At operation, the torsion is corrected and the gonad, if viable, is fixed to the hemiscrotum in three places. Because the paired testicle is at risk for torsion since the testicular anatomy tends to mirror itself, contralateral orchiopexy (suture fixation) should be performed in all cases. Torsion of the testicular appendices tends to be self-limiting since necrosis and autoamputation usually occur. Treatment is with warm baths, limited activity, and an anti-inflammatory agent. If significant pain persists after 2-3 days and the appendix has not autoamputated, excision is indicated. Testicular salvage after neonatal testicular torsion is very rare.

Chiang MC et al: Clinical features of testicular torsio and epididymo-orchitis in infants younger than 3 months. *J Pediatr Surg* 2007;42(9):1574-1577.

Gatti JM, Patrick Murphy J: Current management of the acute scrotum. *Semin Pediatr Surg* 2007 Feb;16(1):58-63.

▼ ABDOMINAL WALL DEFECTS

UMBILICAL HERNIA

A fascial defect at the umbilicus is frequently present in the newborn, particularly in premature infants. The incidence is highest in African-American children. In most children, the umbilical ring progressively diminishes in size and eventually closes. Fascial defects less than 1 cm in diameter close spontaneously by 5 years of age in 95% of cases. When the fascial defect is greater than 1.5 cm in diameter, it seldom closes spontaneously. Unlike inguinal hernias, protrusion of bowel through the umbilical defect rarely results in incarceration in childhood. Surgical repair is indicated if the intestine becomes incarcerated, when the fascial defect is greater than 1.5 cm, and in all children over 4 years of age. Both open and laparoscopic approaches are associated with uniformly excellent results.

OMPHALOCELE

This is a midline abdominal wall defect noted in 1:5000 live births. The abdominal viscera (commonly liver and bowel) are contained within a sac composed of peritoneum and amnion from which the umbilical cord arises at the apex and center (Figure 43–21). When the defect is less than 4 cm,

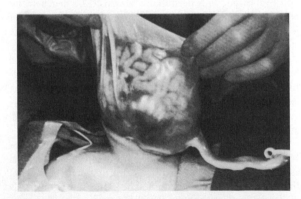

▲ **Figure 43–21.** Neonate with omphalocele. The liver and bowel herniated through a midline abdominal wall defect and are surrounded by a sac of amnion and chorion from which the umbilical cord emanates. (Reproduced, with permission, from Albanese CT: Pediatric surgery. In: Norton JA. *Surgery.* New York, NY: Springer; 2000.)

it is termed as hernia of the umbilical cord; when greater than 10 cm, it is termed a giant omphalocele. Associated abnormalities occur in 30%-70% of infants and include, in descending order of frequency, chromosomal abnormalities (trisomy 13, 18, 21), congenital heart disease (tetralogy of Fallot, atrial septal defect), Beckwith-Wiedemann syndrome (large-for-gestational-age baby; hyperinsulinism; visceromegaly of kidneys, adrenal glands, and pancreas; macroglossia, hepatorenal tumors, cloacal extrophy), pentalogy of Cantrell, and prune belly syndrome (absent abdominal wall muscles, genitourinary abnormalities, cryptorchidism). Small omphaloceles are most often linked to chromosomal defects and Beckwith-Wiedemann syndrome, especially when the liver is not in the hernia sac.

▶ Treatment

The primary goal of surgery is to return the viscera to the abdominal cavity and close the defect. With an intact sac, emergency operation is not necessary, so a thorough physical examination and workup for associated anomalies is performed. An orogastric tube should be placed on suction to minimize intestinal distention.

The success of primary closure depends on the size of the defect and of the abdominal and thoracic cavities as well as the presence of associated problems (eg, lung disease). It is wise to leave the sac *in situ* since primary closure may not be possible, and in this way one has maintained the best biologic dressing for the viscera. Supplemental coverage with plastic wrap or a bowel bag can be used to prevent heat loss. If the viscera reduce but abdominal wall closure is not possible, there are three options: staged repair, prosthetic patch repair, or delayed operative management with initial epithelialization and compression for gradual return of domain. A staged repair aims to create a protective extra-abdominal extension of the peritoneal cavity (termed a silo), allowing gradual reduction of the viscera and gradual abdominal wall expansion using two parallel sheets of reinforced Silastic sheeting sutured to the fascial edges or a preformed one-piece silo with a collapsible ring at its base for ease of insertion. A prosthetic patch repair bridges the fascial gap with a synthetic material (eg, polytetrafluoroethylene) and the skin is closed over the patch. The silo is progressively compressed to invert the amniotic sac and its contents into the abdomen and to bring the edges of the linea alba together by stretching the abdominal wall muscles. This usually requires 5-7 days, after which the defect is then primarily closed. The intra-abdominal pressure produced by the silo should not exceed 20 cm H_2O to avoid impairing venous return from the bowel and kidneys. When abdominal relaxation is sufficient to allow the rectus muscles to come together, the silo is removed, the amnion is left inverted into the abdominal cavity, and the defect is closed.

Delayed operative management is appropriate for infants with severe associated anomalies or a giant omphalocele. The amnion is allowed to dry and form an eschar. The membrane becomes vascularized beneath the eschar, and contraction of the wound with skin growth covers the defect. This can be further facilitated by creation of a compression orthotic that allows for the gradual return of abdominal contents and recreation of abdominal domain. A ventral hernia results, which is repaired electively when the patient is stable. The survival rate for infants with small omphaloceles is excellent. Deaths associated with larger omphaloceles are principally from wound dehiscence with subsequent and ensuing infection or from associated anomalies.

GASTROSCHISIS

Gastroschisis is a defect in the abdominal wall that usually occurs to the right of a normal insertion of the umbilical cord (Figure 43–22). It is believed to arise at the site of involution of the right umbilical vein, though a less popular theory holds there is some evidence that it results from rupture of an omphalocele sac *in utero*. It is twice as common as omphalocele and the defect is usually smaller. The remnants of the amnion are usually reabsorbed. The skin may continue to grow over the remnants of the amnion, and there may be a bridge of skin between the defect and the cord. The small and large bowel, stomach, and often the fallopian tube/ovary/testis herniate through the abdominal wall defect. Unlike an omphalocele, the liver is virtually never present in the defect. Having been bathed in the amniotic fluid and with compression of the mesenteric blood supply at the

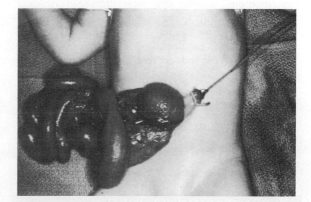

▲ **Figure 43–22.** Neonate with a gastroschisis. The defect is to the right of the umbilical cord, and the bowel has no investing sac. Note edema of the bowel wall and the dilated stomach adjacent to the umbilical cord. (Reproduced, with permission, from Albanese CT: Pediatric surgery. In: Norton JA. Surgery. New York, NY: Springer; 2000.)

abdominal defect, the bowel wall is edematous and has a very thick, shaggy membrane ("peel") covering it. The loops of intestine are usually matted together, and the intestine appears to be abnormally short.

Complications

Since the bowel has not been contained intra-abdominally, the abdominal cavity fails to enlarge, and it frequently cannot accommodate the protuberant bowel. Over 70% of infants with this disorder are premature, but associated anomalies occur in fewer than 10% of cases. Nonrotation of the midgut is present. Associated intestinal atresia occurs in approximately 7% because segments of intestine that have herniated through the defect become infarcted *in utero*.

Treatment & Prognosis

Unlike omphalocele, urgent repair is necessary. Small defects may be closed primarily after manually stretching the abdominal cavity. A staged approach is frequently required using a silo as described above (under Omphalocele). As bowel wall edema subsides, the bowel will readily reduce into the abdominal cavity. Reduction is aided by having the infant paralyzed and receiving endotracheal ventilation to relax the abdominal wall and allow it to stretch and accommodate the bowel. When the bowel has been completely reduced (usually 5-7 days), the silo is removed and the abdominal wall is closed. Recently, the use of the umbilical remnant or a patch dressing has been described to allow primary closure without the need for operative intervention.

The death rate for infants with gastroschisis is less than 5%. Poor GI function and episodes of sepsis, presumably from compromised bowel, may occur. Prolonged postoperative ileus (> 2 weeks) is the rule, and total parenteral nutrition is necessary. Primary repair of an associated intestinal atresia is rarely safe and possible. Either a proximal stoma is created or the atretic ends are reduced and repaired 6 weeks later when the intra-abdominal inflammation has subsided.

Choi WW, McBride CA, Bourke C, et al: Long-term review of sutureless ward reduction in neonates with gastroschisis in the neonatal unit. *J Pediatr Surg* 2012 Aug;47(8):1516-1520.

Christison-Lagay ER, Kelleher CM, Langer JC: Neonatal abdominal wall defects. *Semin Fetal Neonatal Med* 2011 Jun;16(3): 164-172.

CUTANEOUS VASCULAR ANOMALIES

Cutaneous vascular anomalies comprise a group of congenital and acquired vascular malformations of the skin. They are present in 2.6% of all newborns. These anomalies are broadly divided into two categories: hemangiomas and vascular malformations. They are most precisely classified by the biologic activity of the endothelium.

HEMANGIOMAS

Hemangiomas demonstrate endothelial hyperplasia and are seen in children and adults but behave differently at different ages. Hemangiomas are much more common than vascular malformations. In the neonatal period, hemangiomas can be subclassified according to their growth phase. A rapid proliferating phase is usually seen during the first few years of life followed by an involuting phase that may last several years.

Clinical Findings

The clinical appearance depends on the depth of the lesion. Superficial dermal lesions (capillary hemangiomas, strawberry hemangiomas) are raised and profoundly erythematous, with an irregular texture; deep lesions (cavernous hemangiomas) are smooth and slightly raised, with a bluish hue or a faint telangiectatic pattern on the overlying skin. Mixed lesions are often noted (capillary-cavernous hemangiomas). Twenty percent of patients have multiple lesions. Complications from hemangiomas consist of ulceration (during the proliferative phase), bleeding, thrombocytopenia (Kasabach-Merritt syndrome), consumptive coagulopathy, high-output heart failure, visual field encroachment, airway obstruction, and minor skeletal distortions.

Treatment

Fifty percent of hemangiomas will involute without treatment by age 5 years and 70% by 7 years. The remainder will slowly resolve by age 10-12 years. Steroid therapy hastens the rate of proliferation of hemangiomas by 30%-90% and is indicated for complicated lesions (ie, those causing severe physiologic or anatomic abnormalities).

CUTANEOUS VASCULAR MALFORMATIONS

Vascular malformations, in contrast to hemangiomas, have normal endothelial cell turnover and tend to grow proportionally with the child. These lesions are structural anomalies that are considered errors in vascular morphogenesis. They are usually visible at birth but may take years or even decades to become manifest. They are separated into low-flow and high-flow variants and further classified according to the type of vascular channel abnormality: capillary, venous, arterial, and mixed malformations. Capillary and venous malformations are low-flow variants; arterial and mixed arterial and venous ones are high-flow variants.

Capillary Malformations

Capillary malformations are nevus flammeus (port-wine stain), nevus flammeus neonatorum (angel kiss), nevus flammeus nuchae (stork bite, salmon patch), angiokeratomas, and telangiectasias (spider, hereditary hemorrhagic telangiectasia [Rendu-Osler-Weber syndrome]). They are prone to infection and are treated aggressively with intravenous antibiotics. A compression garment should be used if anatomically feasible. Some lesions can be excised or injected with a sclerosing solution.

Venous Malformations

Venous malformations have a wide spectrum of appearances ranging from simple varicosities to complex lesions that may be located in deeper tissues (eg, bone, muscle, salivary gland). Pain is often related to thrombosis within the lesion. Radiographic imaging delineates the nature and extent of the lesion (angiogram, CT, MRI). Photocoagulation or Nd:YAG laser may be effective for superficial lesions. Resection is the definitive treatment since it can reduce bulk, improve contour and function, and control pain. It is limited by anatomic boundaries, and multiple, staged procedures may be required.

Arterial Malformations

Arterial and arteriovenous malformations are associated with multiple small fistulas surrounded by abnormal tissues and can cause high-output cardiac failure. They are most common in the head and neck region (especially intracerebral). There is pain and overlying cutaneous necrosis. Adjacent osseous structures are often destroyed. Selective embolization is used either as palliation or presurgically to limit hemorrhage. Excision, when possible, is the treatment of choice.

Combined Malformations

Combined vascular malformations and hypertrophy syndromes consist of Klippel-Trenaunay-Weber syndrome (combined capillary-lymphatic venous malformation associated with lower limb hypertrophy), Parkes-Weber syndrome (upper limb arteriovenous shunting), Maffucci syndrome (low-flow vascular malformations and multiple extremity enchondromas with hypoplastic long bones), and Sturge-Weber syndrome (upper facial port-wine stain and vascular anomalies of the choroid plexus and leptomeninges).

Fevurly RD, Fishman SJ: Vascular anomalies in pediatrics. *Surg Clin North Am* 2012 Jun;92(3):769-800.

TUMORS IN CHILDHOOD

NEUROBLASTOMA

Of all childhood neoplasms, neuroblastoma is exceeded in frequency only by leukemia and brain tumors. Approximately 60% of cases occur within the first 2 years of life and 97% within the first 20 years. This tumor is of neural crest origin and may originate anywhere along the distribution of the sympathetic chain. The most common site

for primary disease is in the abdomen (adrenal), followed by the thorax, pelvis, and occasionally the head and neck. Neuroblastomas originate in the retroperitoneal area in 75% of cases; 55% arise from the adrenal gland. They may reach massive size and violate tissue planes such that they envelop major blood vessels, their branches, and other important structures (eg, ureters), making initial primary resection potentially hazardous. The biologic behavior varies with the age of the patient, the site of primary origin, and the extent of the disease.

Clinical Findings

A. Symptoms and Signs

Symptoms are site specific. The most common symptom is pain (from primary or metastatic disease). Nonspecific symptoms include growth retardation, malaise, fever, weight loss, and anorexia. Children frequently appear ill at the time of diagnosis. Constipation and urinary retention are signs of pelvic disease. Orbital metastases commonly present with periorbital ecchymoses and proptosis ("raccoon eyes"). Spinal canal involvement may present with acute paralysis due to compression. Opsomyoclonus syndrome is an acute cerebellar encephalopathy characterized by ataxia, opsoclonus ("dancing eyes"), myoclonus, and dementia. It occurs in association with approximately 3% of all neuroblastomas and is usually associated with a good prognosis, though the neurologic abnormalities tend to persist after successful treatment of the primary tumor. Interestingly, it is not due to CNS metastases of neuroblastoma and is believed to be immune mediated. Infants with stage IV-S disease (see below) may display cutaneous metastases ("blueberry muffin" lesions) or respiratory embarrassment secondary to massive hepatomegaly from tumor infiltration. Palpable lesions are often hard and fixed.

In infants, metastases confined to the liver or subcutaneous fat are frequent and cortical bone metastases unusual. In older children, metastases to lymph nodes and bone are found in over 70% of cases at diagnosis. Pain in areas of bony involvement and in joints with associated myalgia and fever mimics rheumatic fever. Eighty-five to 90% secrete high levels of the catecholamine metabolites vanillylmandelic acid and homovanillic acid. Hypertension and diarrhea may occur as a result of catecholamine and vasoactive intestinal peptide secretion.

B. Imaging Studies

Imaging is aimed at defining the extent of the tumor and determining the presence of metastases to distant sites (most commonly lymph nodes, bone, lung, and liver). Neuroblastoma is the most common abdominal tumor to demonstrate calcifications (50%) prior to chemotherapy. CT scan of the area of tumor involvement helps to identify the relationship to surrounding structures and determine resectability. MRI is useful in assessing tumor within the spinal canal and spinal cord compression. MRI is as sensitive as CT scanning in terms of assessing tumor size and resectability but has the added advantage of being superior to CT in assessing vessel encasement, vessel patency, and spinal cord compression. MRI can also demonstrate bone marrow involvement in selected cases. Metaiodobenzylguanidine (MIBG) scintigraphy is very sensitive in detecting tumors that concentrate catecholamines and has been useful in the diagnosis of primary, residual, and metastatic disease in patients with neuroblastoma. For retroperitoneal tumors, an intravenous urogram may show displacement or compression of the adjacent kidney without distortion of the renal calices. Bone scans may be useful in detecting osseous metastases.

Prognostic Factors

Favorable prognostic factors include diagnosis before age 18 months, a thoracic primary lesion, and low stage. In addition, several molecular and cellular characteristics of neuroblastic tumors are prognostically important. The most important is the high incidence of amplification of the proto-oncogene N-*myc*, seen in approximately 30% of tumors. Amplification of N-*myc* (> 10 copies) adversely correlates with prognosis independently of clinical stage. Using the histologic Shimada index, well-differentiated, stroma-rich tumors have a favorable prognosis. An elevated ratio of vanillylmandelic acid to homovanillic acid correlates with an improved outcome in patients with advanced disease. Other biochemical indicators of advanced disease include neuron-specific enolase, serum ferritin, and serum lactate dehydrogenase. Staging systems are surgically and anatomically based and have prognostic value. The most recent is the International Neuroblastoma Staging System (Table 43–6). Stage IV-s has favorable outcomes to older children with stage III and IV disease.

Treatment

Diagnosis depends upon demonstration of immature neuroblastic tissue obtained by tissue or bone marrow aspirate and biopsy. Tissue is obtained by biopsy (either by laparotomy or laparoscopically), which allows accurate determination of resectability and ensures that adequate tissue (1 g or 1 cm³) is available for determination of tumor markers, cytologic studies, and the special stains required for accurate diagnosis and staging.

The spectrum of treatment for neuroblastoma is driven by risk stratification based on multiple factors beyond Stage. A localized neuroblastoma should be excised, and the local area of the tumor should be irradiated only when gross tumor remains. Unresectable neuroblastomas should be biopsied and treated initially by chemotherapy and radiation

Table 43–6. International neuroblastoma staging system.

I.	Localized tumor confined to area of origin; complete excision, with or without microscopic residual disease; ipsilateral and contralateral lymph nodes negative (nodes attached to primary tumor and removed en bloc when it may be positive)
IIa.	Unilateral tumor with incomplete gross excision; ipsilateral and contralateral lymph nodes negative
IIb.	Unilateral tumor with complete or incomplete excision; positive ipsilateral, nonadherent regional lymph nodes; contralateral lymph nodes negative
III.	Tumor infiltrating across the midline with or without lymph node involvement; or unilateral tumor with contralateral lymph node involvement; or midline tumor with bilateral lymph node involvement or bilateral infiltration (unresectable)
IV.	Dissemination of tumor to distant lymph nodes, bone, bone marrow, liver, or other organs
IVs.	Localized primary tumor as defined for stage I or II with dissemination limited to liver, skin, or bone marrow (limited to infants younger than 1 y)

therapy and then by surgical resection for residual tumor. Removal of all residual disease is the goal. Most neuroblastomas are radiosensitive and respond to radiation. Patients with disseminated disease should be treated with a combination of chemotherapeutic agents such as cyclophosphamide, vincristine, dacarbazine, doxorubicin, cisplatin, and teniposide. Patients with stage III or stage IV tumors who are at high risk by virtue of their age or of the stage and biologic characteristics of the tumor benefit from total body irradiation followed by either allogeneic or, more commonly, autologous bone marrow transplantation.

Davidoff AM: Neuroblastoma. *Semin Pediatr Surg* 2012 Feb;21(1):2-14.

WILMS TUMOR (NEPHROBLASTOMA)

Renal neoplasms account for about 10% of malignant tumors in children. Nephroblastoma (Wilms tumor), which accounts for 80% of these, consists of a variety of embryonic tissues such as abortive tubules and glomeruli, smooth and skeletal muscle fibers, spindle cells, cartilage, and bone. Seventy-five percent of children with nephroblastoma are under 5 years of age; the peak incidence is at 2-3 years. With current multimodality treatment, the survival rate exceeds 85%.

The left kidney is affected in 50% of cases of Wilms tumor and the right kidney in 45%. In 5% of cases, the tumors are bilateral; 60% are synchronous and 40% are metachronous. Associated anomalies and their incidence per 1000 cases are aniridia, 8.5; hypospadias, 18; hemihypertrophy, 25; and cryptorchidism, 28. Beckwith-Wiedemann syndrome and neurofibromatosis occur together occasionally, and renal tumors may also occur in families. The constellation of Wilms tumor, aniridia, genitourinary anomalies, and mental retardation (WAGR syndrome) is associated with deletion of 11p13.

Clinical Findings

A. Symptoms and Signs

In contrast to those with neuroblastoma, children are usually healthy appearing. Symptoms consist of abdominal enlargement in 60%; pain in 20%; hematuria in 15%; malaise, weakness, anorexia, and weight loss in 10%; and fever in 3%. Hypertension is noted in over half of patients. An abdominal mass, palpable in almost all cases, is usually very large, firm, and smooth, and it does not ordinarily extend across the midline.

B. Imaging Studies

Imaging is required to determine the extent of the mass; to assess for bilateral disease, venous invasion, and metastases; and to confirm contralateral renal function. This is accomplished with abdominal ultrasound (to assess venous invasion) and a CT scan of the chest and abdomen.

Differential Diagnosis

Abdominal masses may also be caused by hydronephrotic, multicystic, or duplicated kidneys and by neuroblastoma, teratoma, hepatoma, and rhabdomyosarcoma. Ultrasonography and CT scanning can usually distinguish nephroblastoma from these other tumors. Calcification occurs in 10% of cases of nephroblastoma and tends to be more crescent-shaped, discrete, and peripherally situated than the calcifications of neuroblastoma, which are finely stippled.

Treatment & Prognosis

Surgical excision is often accomplished without any preoperative treatment unless significant inferior vena caval thrombus is present. The aim of surgery is to completely remove the tumor (nephrectomy) and ureter without spill and to determine the tumor stage by virtue of its extent and the presence of lymph node involvement (Table 43–7). Stage I is tumor confined to a kidney that has been completely excised; stage II is tumor extending beyond the kidney (perirenal tissues, renal vein or vena cava, biopsy or local spill in the flank) and completely excised; stage III is residual, nonhematogenous tumor confined to the abdomen (lymph node metastases, preoperative or intraoperative diffuse peritoneal deposits, residual tumor at the surgical margins, or unresectable tumor); stage IV is hematogenous metastases (lung, liver, bone, and brain); and stage V is bilateral renal involvement.

Table 43–7. COG Wilms tumor staging system.

Stage I: Tumor limited to kidney and completely excised. The surface of the renal capsule is intact and the tumor was not ruptured prior to removal. There is no residual tumor.

Stage II: Tumor extends through the perirenal capsule but is completely excised. There may be local spillage of tumor confined to the flank, or the tumor may have been biopsied. Extrarenal vessels may contain tumor thrombus or be infiltrated by tumor.

Stage III: Residual nonhematogenous tumor confined to the abdomen: lymph node involvement, diffuse peritoneal spillage, peritoneal implants, tumor beyond surgical margin either grossly or microscopically, or tumor not completely removed.

Stage IV: Hematogenous metastases to lung, liver, bone, brain, etc

Stage V: Bilateral renal involvement at diagnosis; each kidney should be staged separately.

Irradiation of the tumor bed is indicated if the tumor has extended beyond the capsule of the kidney to involve adjacent organs or lymph nodes or if intraoperative tumor spillage has occurred. Very large tumors may be treated with radiation therapy and chemotherapy preoperatively to reduce their size. A significant reduction in size usually occurs in 7-10 days, after which nephrectomy can be readily performed. Nephrectomy is accomplished through a long transverse or thoracoabdominal incision.

Palpation of the renal veins and inferior vena cava is performed to detect tumor thrombus. Bilateral disease (6%) mandates "nephron-sparing" surgery. The treatment of bilateral disease is individualized with the goal of eradicating tumor while preserving the maximal amount of functional renal mass. It is a contraindication to primary nephrectomy. Suspicious lesions in the opposite kidney are biopsied. If the tumor is too large for safe resection, it is biopsied along with regional lymph nodes. Chemotherapy with or without radiation therapy will usually result in a significant reduction in tumor size and allow subsequent resection. Metastatic foci in the lung or liver may be resected or treated with radiation therapy. Any residual tumor following radiation therapy, including multiple lesions, should be resected.

Overall survival is 85%, and most patients are cured. Survival correlates with stage and histology. The 4-year survival with respect to stage and histology is shown in Table 43–8. Tumor rupture with gross spillage portends a sixfold increase in risk of local recurrence and requires the use of postoperative external beam radiation.

Hamilton TE, Shamberger RC: Wilms tumor: recent advances in clinical care and biology. *Semin Pediatr Surg* 2012 Feb;21(1): 15-20.

Table 43–8. Four-year survival for Wilms tumor.

Stage I/FH: 98%
Stage I-III/UH: 68%
Stage II/FH: 90%-95%
Stage III/FH: 85%-90%
Stage IV/FH: 78%-86%
Stage IV/UH: 52%-58%

FH, favorable histology; UH, unfavorable histology.

RHABDOMYOSCARCOMA

Rhabdomyosarcoma is a childhood malignancy that arises from embryonic mesenchyme with the potential to differentiate into skeletal muscle. It is the most common pediatric soft tissue sarcoma and is the third most common solid malignancy. It accounts for 4%-8% of all malignancies and 5%-15% of all solid malignancies of childhood.

The age distribution is bimodal, the first peak is between 2 and 5 years, and the second peak is between 15 and 19 years. Fifty percent present before 5 years, and 6% present in infancy. There is an increased incidence in patients with neurofibromatosis, Beckwith-Wiedemann syndrome, and Li-Fraumeni cancer-family syndrome.

Rhabdomyosarcoma is divided into distinct histologic groups: favorable, intermediate, and unfavorable. Favorable types (5%) include the sarcoma botryoides and spindle cell variants. Botryoid tumors typically present in young children from within visceral cavities (eg, vagina), while spindle cell types have a predilection for paratesticular sites. Intermediate-prognosis tumors (50%) are of the embryonal type. Unfavorable-prognosis tumors (20%) include alveolar and undifferentiated tumors. Alveolar tumors arise from the extremities, trunk, and perineum. Undifferentiated tumors arise from the extremity and head and neck sites. Thirteen percent cannot be adequately characterized and are labeled "small, round cell sarcoma, type indeterminate."

▶ Clinical Findings

The clinical presentation varies with the site of origin of the primary tumor, the patient's age, and the presence or absence of metastatic disease. The majority of symptoms are secondary to the effects of compression by the tumor or by the presence of a mass. The most common site is the head and neck region (35%). These are subdivided into orbital (10%), parameningeal (15%), and nonparameningeal (10%) sites. They are usually embryonal and present as asymptomatic masses or functional deficits. Genitourinary rhabdomyosarcoma (26%) are divided into two groups: bladder and prostate (10%) and nonbladder and prostate, including paratesticular

sites, perineum, vulva, vagina, and uterus (16%). The most common histologic type is embryonal, though botryoid tumors and spindle cell tumors are seen more frequently here than in any other site. These tumors may be so massive as to make determination of the primary tumor site impossible. There is a propensity for early lymphatic spread in genitourinary primary tumors. Bladder and prostate tumors frequently present with urinary retention or hematuria, while vaginal and uterine tumors present with vaginal bleeding or discharge or with a mass exiting the vagina. Extremity rhabdomyosarcoma (1%) are more common in the lower than in the upper extremity. These are usually alveolar varieties with a high incidence of regional nodal involvement and distal metastases. "Other" sites account for 20%. The most common are the thorax, diaphragm, abdominal and pelvic walls, and intra-abdominal or intrapelvic organs.

Staging is determined by the histologic variant, the primary site, and the extent of disease since each has an important influence on the choice of treatment and on prognosis. CT scanning or MRI is essential to evaluate the primary tumor and its relationship to surrounding structures. A clinical grouping system was designed by the Intergroup Rhabdomyosarcoma Study Group to stratify different extents of disease in order to compare treatment and outcome results (Table 43–9). It is based on pretreatment and operative outcome and does not account for the biologic differences or the natural history of tumors arising from different primary sites.

▶ Treatment & Prognosis

The surgical management is site specific and includes complete wide excision of the primary tumor and surrounding

Table 43–9. Intergroup Rhabdomyosarcoma Study Clinical Group staging system.

Group I: Localized disease, completely removed
a. Confined to muscle or organ of origin
b. Infiltration outside organ or muscle of origin; regional nodes not involved
Group II: Total gross resection with evidence of regional spread
a. Grossly resected tumor with microscopic residual
b. Regional disease with involved nodes, completely resected with no microscopic residual
c. Regional disease with involved nodes, grossly resected, but with evidence of microscopic residual and/or histologic involvement of the most distal regional node in the dissection
Group III: Incomplete resection, or biopsy with presence of gross disease
Group IV: Distant metastases

Adapted, with permission, from Neville HL et al: Preoperative staging, prognostic factors, and outcome for extremity rhabdomyosarcoma: a preliminary report from the Intergroup Rhabdomyosarcoma Study IV (1991–1997). *J Pediatr Surg* 2000;35:317.

uninvolved tissue while preserving cosmetic appearance and function. Incomplete excision (beyond biopsy) or tumor debulking is not beneficial, and severely mutilating or debilitating procedures should not be performed. Tumors not amenable to primary excision should be amply biopsied and then treated with neoadjuvant agents; secondary excision is then performed and is associated with a better outcome than partial or incomplete excisions. Clinically suspicious lymph nodes should be excised or biopsied, while excision of clinically uninvolved nodes is site specific. Primary reexcision has been shown to improve outcome in patients where microscopic margins are positive, where the initial procedure was not a formal "cancer" resection, or where malignancy was not suspected preoperatively.

The 5-year survival for stage I tumors is 90%; for stage II, clinical group I or II, it is 77%; for stage II, clinical group III, it is 65%; and for stage III lesions (group I, II, or III), it is 55%. Stage IV tumors arising from favorable sites of origin are curable, while those from unfavorable sites have a very poor prognosis. The prognosis for recurrent disease is poor.

Paulino AC, Okeru MF: Rhabdomyosarcoma. *Curr Probl Cancer* 2008,32(1):7-34.

TERATOMA

Teratomas are embryonal neoplasms derived from pluripotent cells containing tissue from at least two of three germ layers (ectoderm, endoderm, mesoderm). Approximately 80% are found in females. They are typically midline or para-axial tumors and are distributed in the following regions: sacrococcygeal (57%), gonadal (29%), mediastinal (7%), retroperitoneal (4%), cervical (3%), and intracranial (3%). Other sites are rare. Nongonadal teratomas present in infancy; gonadal ones, in adolescence. Twenty-one percent are malignant.

The serum alpha-fetoprotein (AFP) level is elevated in tumors containing malignant endodermal sinus (yolk sac) elements. Serial AFP levels are markers for recurrence. Beta-human chorionic gonadotropin (β-hCG) is produced from those containing malignant choriocarcinoma tissue. Rarely, enough β-hCG is produced to cause precocious puberty. Elevated AFP and β-hCG levels in histologically benign tumors indicate an increased risk of recurrence and malignant transformation, particularly with "immature" benign teratomas.

▶ Sacrococcygeal Teratoma

The majority of sacrococcygeal teratomas present in the newborn period and can be detected by prenatal ultrasound. Females predominate; a history of twins is common. Pregnancy may be complicated by fetal high-output cardiac failure via arteriovenous shunting within the tumor, maternal polyhydramnios, and hydrops fetalis leading to

fetal demise. Fetal surgery has been utilized successfully in those with hydrops. The tumors are classified according to location: type I, predominantly external (46%); type II, external mass and presacral component (35%); type III, visible externally, but predominantly presacral (9%); and type IV, entirely presacral, not visible externally (10%).

Treatment is excision of the tumor and coccyx; type I and II lesions are resected from the perineal approach, and type III and IV lesions require a combined intra-abdominal and perineal resection. The majority (97%) of newborn sacrococcygeal teratomas are benign and do not require adjuvant therapy. Follow-up requires serial AFP levels and physical examinations, including digital rectal examination. Recurrent tumors are excised. The greatest risk factor for malignancy is age at diagnosis. The malignancy rate is approximately 50%-60% after 2 months of age. Malignant tumors are often treated with surgery and chemotherapy. The 5-year survival for malignant germ cell tumors arising from a sacrococcygeal teratoma is approximately 50%.

▶ Mediastinal Teratoma

Mediastinal teratomas account for approximately 20% of all pediatric mediastinal tumors. They usually arise in the anterior mediastinum, though intrapericardial and cardiac lesions have been reported. Symptoms include respiratory distress, chronic cough, chest pain, and wheezing. Males with β-hCG-producing tumors may display precocious puberty. Cardiac failure may develop from compression or pericardial effusion. The chest radiograph demonstrates a calcified anterior mediastinal mass in over one-third of cases. Ultrasonography delineates cystic and solid components. General anesthesia should not be induced until a CT scan evaluation of the airway has been obtained since the supine position coupled with a loss of airway tone from anesthetic agents may allow the anterior mass to obstruct the distal trachea, making rapid establishment of an airway all but impossible. If significant airway compression is present, an awake needle biopsy under local anesthesia followed by radiation therapy or chemotherapy is indicated. Complete resection is definitive treatment.

▶ Cervical Teratoma

Cervical teratomas are rare neonatal neck masses that by virtue of their large size frequently cause respiratory distress. Calcifications may be seen on a plain radiograph and a mixed cystic and solid appearance on ultrasound. These tumors are most commonly benign. The most common malignant type is the yolk sac tumor (endodermal sinus tumor). Serum AFP and β-hCG levels can be monitored to detect the presence of recurrent germ cell tumors. The rapid establishment of an endotracheal airway may be necessary. Tracheostomy is hazardous because of the distortion of landmarks by the large mass. Treatment is complete excision. Some malignant tumors respond to radiation therapy. Regardless of the stage of disease, these tumors behave aggressively and should be treated adjunctively with a combination of cisplatin, vinblastine, and bleomycin or with dactinomycin, cyclophosphamide, and vincristine.

Amies Oelschlager AM, Sawin R: Teratomas and ovarian lesions in children. *Surg Clin North Am* 2012 Jun;92(3):599-613.

LIVER NEOPLASMS

Tumors of the liver are uncommon in childhood (2% of all pediatric malignancies). More than 70% of pediatric liver masses are malignant. The majority of hepatic malignancies are of epithelial origin, while most benign lesions are vascular in nature.

1. Hepatoblastoma

Hepatoblastomas account for nearly 50% of all liver masses in children and approximately two-thirds of malignant tumors. The majority are seen in children under 4 years of age, and two-thirds are noted prior to 2 years of age. Beckwith-Wiedemann syndrome, hemihypertrophy, familial adenomatous polyposis syndrome, fetal alcohol syndrome, and parenteral nutrition administration in infancy all increase the risk of hepatoblastoma.

▶ Clinical Findings

A. Symptoms and Signs

The most common finding is an asymptomatic abdominal mass or diffuse abdominal swelling in a healthy-appearing child. There may be obstructive GI symptoms secondary to compression of the stomach or duodenum or acute pain secondary to hemorrhage into the tumor. Physical examination reveals a nontender, firm mass in the right upper quadrant or midline that moves with respiration. Advanced tumors present with weight loss, ascites, and failure to thrive. Approximately 10% of males present with isosexual precocity secondary to tumor secretion of β-hCG.

B. Laboratory Findings

Laboratory studies reveal nonspecifically elevated liver function tests and a mild anemia. Thrombocytosis of unknown cause is occasionally seen. AFP is significantly elevated in 90-95%. This marker is also associated with other malignant lesions such as germ cell tumors, but levels are lower. Serial serum AFP measurements are used to monitor patients for tumor recurrence. Levels fall to normal after curative resection.

C. Imaging Studies

Abdominal ultrasound demonstrates a solid, usually unilobar (right lobe most common) lesion of the liver but lacks sufficient detail to determine resectability. Abdominal CT scan using intravenous contrast is currently the imaging procedure of choice both for diagnosis and for planning therapy. The CT scan demonstrates the tumor's proximity to major vascular and hilar structures. The typical CT appearance is a solid solitary mass with lower attenuation levels than those of the surrounding liver. A novel technique, CT arterioportography, holds promise as a reliable means of assessing vascular invasion along with gross tumor distribution. MRI has proved to be very useful in defining the patency of vascular structures.

▶ Differential Diagnosis

One major management problem is the inability to differentiate adenomas from hepatocellular carcinoma. Because of this, hepatic adenoma, despite being a benign lesion, is often excised. Focal nodular hyperplasia is a well-circumscribed, nonencapsulated nodular liver mass. Ultrasonography and CT scan demonstrate a solid mass, but one cannot differentiate it from adenoma or malignancy without a biopsy. If the diagnosis can be made by biopsy (percutaneous or open), no further treatment is needed. Mesenchymal hamartoma is an uncommon benign lesion presenting in the first year of life as an asymptomatic large solitary mass usually confined to the right lobe of the liver. CT scan demonstrates a well-defined tumor margin and minimal to no contrast enhancement. The treatment is surgical wedge resection; lobectomy is rarely required.

▶ Treatment

The definitive diagnosis of hepatoblastoma requires tissue biopsy. Although this can be performed percutaneously, there are reports of "seeding" of the biopsy tract. It is preferable to perform open biopsy of the lesion with assessment of resectability. If the lesion is not primarily resectable, vascular access is obtained during the same anesthetic interval for subsequent chemotherapy. Table 43–10 outlines the surgical staging system for childhood hepatic malignancies.

Complete surgical resection is the major objective of therapy and represents the only chance for cure. Approximately 60% of patients will have primarily resectable lesions. Lobectomy or extended lobectomy (trisegmentectomy) is usual, but segmental (nonanatomic) resection of small isolated tumors may be possible. Careful preoperative evaluation and planning have made liver resection in children

Table 43–10. Hepatic tumor staging.

Stage I: Tumor localized and completely resected
Stage II: Tumor resected with microscopic residual disease
Stage III: Unresectable tumor or gross residual disease
Stage IV: Metastatic disease

a safe procedure, with a mortality rate of less than 5%. Adequate exposure can be obtained via an extended subcostal or bilateral subcostal incision, although bulky lesions may require extension into the right hemithorax to gain adequate vascular control during dissection. Ascitic fluid is obtained for cytologic examination. If the lesion is deemed unresectable, the tumor is biopsied. If the lesion is made resectable following chemotherapy, lobectomy or trisegmentectomy is performed. Intraoperative cholangiography is helpful to verify the integrity of the remaining biliary tree.

Postoperative complications include bleeding, biliary fistula, subphrenic fluid collections or abscess, and inadvertent injury to the biliary tree. Hepatic regeneration occurs quickly, and hepatic insufficiency is rare if 25% or more of the liver parenchyma remains. Hepatic transplantation is used for unresectable disease when chemotherapy has failed to allow complete resection but no demonstrable metastases exist.

The overall survival for all children with hepatoblastoma is approximately 50%. The best survival (90%) is seen in patients with stage I tumors who receive adjunctive chemotherapy after complete excision. Survival decreases as the surgical stage increases, though long-term survival approaches 60%-70% in patients with unresectable disease who receive chemotherapy.

Meyers RL: Tumors of the liver in children. *Surg Oncology* 2007;16(3):195-203.

2. Hepatocellular Carcinoma

Hepatocellular carcinoma is less common than hepatoblastoma and typically presents in older children and adolescents (median age, 10 years). It is associated with preexisting chronic hepatitis, cirrhosis due to hepatitis B virus, and other causes of childhood cirrhosis (tyrosinemia, biliary cirrhosis, α_1-antitrypsin deficiency, type 1 glycogen storage disease, and long-term parenteral nutrition). Signs and symptoms consist of an abdominal mass or diffuse swelling, abdominal pain, weight loss, anorexia, and jaundice. The serum AFP level is elevated in 50%, though the absolute levels are lower than in patients with hepatoblastoma. Diagnostic studies, staging, and treatment are somewhat the same as for hepatoblastoma. Because of multicentricity, bilobar involvement, portal vein invasion, and lymphatic metastases, only 15%-20% of hepatocellular carcinomas are resectable. Fibrolamellar hepatocellular carcinoma in younger patients is associated with a high rate of resectability and a better prognosis. The overall long-term survival is poor (15%), even for resectable disease. The role of liver transplantation is unclear.

3. Liver Hemangioma

This is the most common benign pediatric hepatic lesion. These tumors are solitary (cavernous hemangioma) or multiple (infantile hemangioendothelioma), involving the bulk of the liver. Isolated cavernous hemangiomas are not often associated with cutaneous hemangiomas, whereas infantile hemangioendotheliomas are commonly associated with hemangiomas in other parts of the body or integument. Patients with a solitary hemangioma frequently have no symptoms or present with a mass. Infrequently there is intratumor hemorrhage or rupture resulting in abdominal pain. Infants with hemangioendothelioma commonly present with massive hepatomegaly and high-output cardiac failure from arteriovenous shunting. Approximately 40% develop Kasabach-Merritt syndrome (thrombocytopenic coagulopathy due to platelet sequestration within the tumor). The diagnosis is made by red blood cell labeled radionuclide or dynamic abdominal CT scanning. CT scan demonstrates increased filling and a rapid venous phase from arteriovenous shunting. Angiography is unnecessary, and percutaneous biopsy is contraindicated.

Treatment is not necessary in an asymptomatic child. Patients with congestive heart failure or thrombocytopenia are treated with corticosteroids, digoxin, and diuretics. Refractory patients benefit from hepatic artery embolization. External beam radiation reduces hepatic size and controls symptoms. Their large size and diffuse involvement often preclude resection. Indications for surgery include ruptured lesions with hemorrhage, masses with uncertain diagnoses, symptomatic lesions, or disease limited to one lobe. Hemangioendotheliomas may undergo malignant degeneration into angiosarcoma.

Litten JB, Tomlinson GE: Liver tumors in children. *Oncologist* 2008 Jul;13(7):812-820.

▼ PEDIATRIC TRAUMA

Accidental trauma is the leading cause of death among children 18 and younger. Patterns of injury vary by age, with a higher rate of isolated neurotrauma than adults. Mortality has been reduced in recent years due to a combination of factors including prevention, improved prehospital care and evolving management strategies. Pediatric trauma has a trimodal distribution of mortality. Early mortality is from massive injury to the CNS or central vasculature and can only be addressed by prevention. Mortality within hours from the time of injury is due to CNS mass lesions (brain bleeding or edema), solid organ injury with hemorrhage and pleural of pericardial compression. The rapid diagnosis and treatment of these conditions improves outcome and is the focus of advanced trauma life support courses. Late mortality seen days to weeks after injury is due to septic and inflammatory complications. This is less common in children than adults. Pediatric surgery has led the development of nonoperative management of spleen and liver laceration that has led to significant organ preservation.

▼ NONACCIDENTAL TRAUMA

Child abuse is any nonaccidental injury inflicted by a parent, guardian, or other supervising adult. It may be passive, in the form of emotional or nutritional deprivation, but is most readily recognized in the active form, characterized as "battered, bruised, beaten, broken, and burned." It is estimated that 1 million children per year in the United States suffer injuries that qualifying for reporting to the National Center on Child Abuse and Neglect. About 20%-50% of children are rebattered after the first diagnosis, resulting in death in 5% and permanent physical damage in 35% when the syndrome is not recognized.

The child abuser is usually a young, insecure, unstable person who had an unhappy childhood and who has unrealistic expectations of the child. Most of these individuals are of low socioeconomic status. The abuser may be a parent, guardian, babysitter, neighborhood child, or other close associate. Active traumatic abuse is usually perpetrated by the father, but passive neglect with failure to thrive from nutritional or emotional deprivation is usually attributable to the mother.

▶ Clinical Findings

In most cases, the battered child is under 3 years of age and is the product of a difficult pregnancy or premature labor, usually unwanted or born outside of a stable parental relationship. Many battered children have congenital anomalies or are hyperkinetic and colicky. In most cases there is a discrepancy between the history supplied and the magnitude of the injury—or else a reluctance to give a history. Contradictory histories or delay in bringing the child to medical attention—or taking the child to many different emergency room visits in different hospitals for unusual reasons—should be regarded with suspicion. A past injury in the child or sibling and almost any injury in an infant less than 1 year of age should trigger a consideration of child abuse. The parents may be evasive or hostile. They may have open guilt feelings or may be capable of complete concealment. The innocent spouse is usually more protective of the abuser than of the child.

The child is usually withdrawn, apathetic, whimpering, and fearful and shows signs of neglect or growth retardation. Multiple forms of injury may be noted at varying stages of healing. The child should be completely disrobed to enable the clinician to look for welts, bruises, lacerations, bite or belt wounds, stick or coat hanger marks on the head, trunk, buttocks, or extremities, and similar evidence of mistreatment. Cigarette, hot plate, match, or scalding burns may be evident. Subgaleal hematomas may be caused by pulled hair. Retinal hemorrhage or detachment may follow blows to the head. Abdominal injuries may produce laceration to the liver, spleen, or pancreas or bowel perforation. Sexual abuse should be identified by determining whether the vaginal introitus or anus is bruised, lacerated, or enlarged and whether aspirated fluid contains sperm or prostatic acid phosphatase.

Even though no obvious fracture may be present, a skeletal radiographic survey should be performed. The bone most commonly fractured is the femur, followed by the humerus in the region of the diaphysis. Rib fractures and periosteal reactions in various stages of healing will be seen. Skull fractures are most commonly seen in infants less than 1 year old. Suture separation of the skull may indicate subdural hematoma. Neurologic injury may require a CT or MRI scan.

▶ Treatment

The child should be admitted to hospital to be protected until the home environment can be evaluated. Injuries should be documented radiographically and with photographs. The presence of sperm in the vagina or anal canal should be confirmed. Bleeding disorders should be evaluated by a platelet count, bleeding time, prothrombin time, and plasma thromboplastin test to make certain that multiple bruises are not due to coagulopathy. A serologic test for syphilis may be indicated as well as cultures (including pharyngeal) for gonorrhea.

Injuries should be treated. Consultation with ophthalmologists, neurologists, neurosurgeons, orthopedic surgeons, and plastic surgeons may be required.

It is required by law in every state for both the hospital and the physician to report child abuse (suspected as well as documented) to local child protection services, usually via the hospital's social work department. The physician is the protector of the child and a consultant to the parents and must not assume the role of prosecutor or judge. The most difficult task is to notify the parents without confrontation, accusation, or anger that battering or neglect is suspected. The physician must tell the parents that the law requires reporting injuries that are unexplained or inadequately explained in view of the nature of the injury. A written referral should then be made to other professionals, such as child welfare personnel, hospital social workers, or psychiatrists. The referral should describe the history of past injuries and the nature of current injuries, results of physical examination and laboratory and x-ray studies, and a statement about why nonaccidental trauma is suspected.

▶ Prognosis

The abuser may require careful evaluation for possible psychosis by a psychiatrist. Child welfare personnel and social workers will have to assess the home environment and work with the parents to prevent future abuse. It may be necessary to place the child in a foster home, but approximately 90% of families can be reunited.

MULTIPLE CHOICE QUESTIONS

1. What is the most appropriate diagnostic test for an otherwise healthy 2 month old with new-onset bilious emesis?

   A. Ultrasound
   B. Upper GI series
   C. CT scan abdomen/pelvis
   D. Contrast enema
   E. Esophagram

2. Which of the following statements is not true concerning thyroglossal duct remnants?

   A. Thyroglossal duct containing thyroid tissue has a higher risk of developing papillary carcinoma
   B. Resection of the hyoid bone surrounding the duct is necessary to prevent recurrence
   C. Thyroglossal ducts always occur in the midline of the neck
   D. Resection when infected carries no higher risk of recurrence
   E. Thyroglossal duct cysts can often be differentiated from other neck lesions on exam as they tend to move with swallowing

3. The management of congenital diaphragmatic hernia (CDH) includes which of the following?

   A. A prosthetic patch should always be used to minimize tension in the repair of CDH
   B. Extracorporeal membrane oxygenation (ECMO) is no longer needed to manage newborns with CDH due to advanced ventilator strategies
   C. CT scan should be attained to determine the size of the hernia defect
   D. CDH is a surgical emergency requiring quick reduction of the hernia contents to promote lung recovery
   E. CDH mortality is related to the degree of pulmonary hypoplasia

4. In the delivery room, the pediatric team is unable to pass an orogastric tube beyond 12 cm in a term new-born who was being followed prenatally for polyhydramnios. Which of the following tests is not necessary prior to embarking on surgical repair?

   A. Head ultrasound
   B. Echocardiogram
   C. Anorectal exam
   D. Renal ultrasound
   E. Chest and abdominal plain x-rays

5. Which of the following is an unfavorable prognostic indicator in neuroblastoma

   A. Age less than 18 months
   B. N-myc amplification
   C. Well-differentiated, stroma rich tumor
   D. Low serum lactate dehydrogenase (LDH)
   E. Stage IV-S

44

Oncology

Michael S. Sabel, MD

Over 1.6 million individuals in the United States are diagnosed with invasive cancer each year. Currently, 23% of all deaths in the United States are due to cancer, ranking second only to heart disease as the leading cause of mortality in this country. Over the past 10 years, however, cancer death rates have decreased. Death rates have continued to decline for the four top cancer sites (lung, colorectum, breast, and prostate). This reduction in overall cancer death rates translates to the avoidance of over 1 million deaths from cancer.

The surgeon is intimately involved in the care of cancer patients, since the majority will require surgical therapy at some time. Surgeons are often the first specialists to see newly diagnosed cancer patients or are often called upon to make the diagnosis in patients suspected to have cancer. As such, they will be responsible for orchestrating the patient's care, including coordination with medical oncologists and radiation oncologists. It is imperative that they have an in-depth knowledge of the different types of cancer and the different modalities available for treatment.

TUMOR NOMENCLATURE

Neoplasms are defined as benign or malignant according to the clinical behavior of the tumor. Benign tumors have lost normal growth regulation but tend to be surrounded by a capsule and do not invade surrounding tissues or metastasize.

Benign tumors are generally designated by adding the suffix -oma to the name of the cell of origin. Examples include lipoma and adenoma. The term *cancer* normally refers to malignant tumors, which can invade surrounding tissues or metastasize to distant sites in the host. The nomenclature of malignant tumors is typically based on the cell's embryonal tissue origins. Malignant tumors derived from cells of mesenchymal origin are called *sarcomas.* These include cancers that derive from muscle, bone, tendon, fat, cartilage, lymphoid tissues, vessels, and connective tissue. Neoplasms of epithelial origin are called *carcinomas.* These may be further categorized according to the histologic

appearance of the cells. Tumor cells that have glandular growth patterns are called adenocarcinomas, and those that resemble squamous epithelial cells are called squamous cell carcinomas. Cancers composed of undifferentiated cells that bear no resemblance to any tissues are designated as "poorly differentiated" or "undifferentiated" carcinomas.

▶ Tumor Grade

Beyond the type of cancer, it is important to classify tumors by their behavior and prognosis in order to determine appropriate therapy as well as evaluate different treatment modalities. Grading of a tumor is a histologic determination and refers to the degree of cellular differentiation. Separate pathologic grading systems exist for each histologic type of cancer. Depending on the type of tumor, these systems are based on nuclear pleomorphism, cellularity, necrosis, cellular invasion, and the number of mitoses. Increasing grades generally denote increasing degrees of dedifferentiation. While the grade of the tumor typically has less prognostic value than its stage, tumor grade has great clinical significance in soft tissue sarcoma, astrocytoma, transitional cell cancers of the genitourinary tract, and Hodgkin and non-Hodgkin lymphoma.

▶ Tumor Stage

Tumor staging establishes the extent of disease and has important prognostic and therapeutic implications in most types of cancer. Clinical staging is based on the results of a noninvasive evaluation, including physical examination and various imaging studies. Pathologic staging is based on findings in surgical tumor specimens and biopsies and allows for the evaluation of microscopic disease undetectable by imaging techniques. Pathologic staging may reveal more extensive tumor spread than the clinical evaluation and is the more reliable information. Clinicians must be careful when attempting to compare clinically and pathologically staged patients, as the two groups may have dramatically different outcomes.

As with grading, the staging systems vary with different tumor types. Two major staging systems are currently in use, one developed by the Union Internationale Contre le Cancer (UICC) and the other by the American Joint Committee on Cancer (AJCC). The UICC system is based on the TNM classification. *T* refers to the primary tumor and is based on the size of the tumor and invasion of surrounding structures. Tumors are characterized as T1 to T4 cancers, with the higher T stages for larger and more invasive tumors. *N* refers to regional lymph nodes, and classifications of N0 to N3 denote increasing degrees of lymph node involvement. Finally, *M* refers to distant metastatic disease, with M0 signifying no distant metastases and M1 and M2 indicating the presence of blood-borne metastatic disease. The AJCC system divides cancers into stages 0 to IV, with higher stages representing more widespread disease and a poorer prognosis. Regardless of the staging system or the tumor type, higher stages correlate with decreased survival.

▶ Cancer Epidemiology

Cancer epidemiology is the study of the distribution of cancer and its determinants among defined populations and is used to examine cancer etiology as well as the efficacy of prevention, detection, and treatment strategies. The most basic types of epidemiologic terms describe cancer rates or cancer deaths for specific populations over a certain period of time.

While absolute numbers of cancer cases may be useful for health care planning, they do not take into account the size or nature of the underlying population at risk. For this reason, the most commonly used population-based measures of cancer are incidence and mortality. **Cancer incidence rates** are defined as the number of new cancer cases diagnosed during a fixed time period divided by the total population at risk. **Cancer mortality rates** are defined similarly, with cancer deaths replacing new cancer cases. These rates are typically expressed as the number of events per 100,000 individuals per year.

Incidence and mortality rates are compared across populations or over time to identify causes as well as the effect of screening or treatment. However, other factors among populations may contribute to observed differences, and these must be taken into account. For most cancers, age is the strongest risk factor, and so comparison of cancer incidence between two populations must consider the age distributions of the two groups. Adjustment (or standardization) is the most common method used to account for such differences. Comparing age-adjusted cancer incidence rates ensures that any observed differences are not the results of differences in age distributions between the two populations. Incidence and mortality rates are often also adjusted for gender, race, or socioeconomic status.

Cancer incidence examines only those diagnosed with the disease during that time period; it does not include patients diagnosed earlier who are living with cancer. **Cancer prevalence** describes the number of people with the disease either at a single point in time **(point prevalence)** or within a defined period of time **(period prevalence)**. Prevalence is more relevant to the public health burden of cancer because all prevalent cases involve accessing health care. The relationship among incidence, prevalence, and mortality is influenced by the fatality of the disease. If the disease is highly fatal and the interval between presentation and death is short, mortality rates will be similar to incidence rates. The number of deaths from cancer divided by the total number people diagnosed with the cancer is known as the **cancer fatality rate,** although this is somewhat of a misnomer because they are not technically rates (they do not include time as a parameter).

Examining the fatality of cancer is obviously important when comparing treatments meant to improve outcome. **Overall survival (OS)** is the most global endpoint and is defined as the proportion of people alive at a specified period after being diagnosed with the disease. Five years is conventionally used as the time period (ie, 5-year survival). However, overall survival may not always reflect the success of treatment. Over that period of time, some patients may die of disease, but others may die of other causes. In addition, some patients may have a local or regional recurrence that is successfully treated, while some may recur with distant metastases but not succumb to them. For this reason, survival rates in cancer are often qualified by the patient's disease status.

Disease-free survival refers to the proportion of patients alive and without disease over a specific period of time. A patient who developed metastases but is still alive would be included in the overall survival rate but not the disease-free survival rate. Disease-free survival and overall survival may provide different pictures of the success of treatment. A therapy that improves disease-free survival but not overall survival may still be important if quality of life is improved. In some cancers, local or regional recurrences can be readily treated with minimal impact on overall survival. In these cases, disease-free survival may present an overly pessimistic picture of outcome. Therefore, it may be more relevant to compare **distant disease-free survival**, which refers to the proportion of people alive and without distant metastases, regardless of local recurrence. In some cases, it is difficult to assess the efficacy of a treatment by looking at overall survival or disease-free survival if there are deaths from competing causes. It may be more helpful to compare **disease-specific survival**, which is the percentage of people who have survived a disease since diagnosis or treatment and does not count patients who died from other causes.

It is important for the surgeon to understand the different methods for describing cancer survival as well as the differences between the definitions, because the appropriateness of the comparison will vary with the biology of the disease and the clinical question being asked.

Edge SB, Byrd DR, Compton CC, Fritz AG, Greene FL, Trotti A: *AJCC Cancer Staging Manual*, 7th ed. Springer, New York, NY 2010.

Siegel R, Naishadham D, Jemal A: Cancer statistics, 2012. *CA Cancer J Clin* 2012;62:10-29.

ROLE OF THE SURGICAL ONCOLOGIST

The surgeon is often the first specialist to see a patient with suspected or newly diagnosed cancer and in many cases assumes responsibility for orchestrating the overall management of the cancer patient's care. The role of the surgeon involves not only the curative resection of the tumor but also obtaining tissue for diagnosis and staging, providing palliation for incurable patients, and preventing cancer by the prophylactic removal of organs. With improving imaging technologies, expanded use of neoadjuvant therapies, molecular staging, and increasing knowledge of the genetic predisposition to cancer, the role of the surgical oncologist is continuously evolving. It is therefore imperative for surgical oncologists to remain current on the newest approaches to cancer therapy and be prepared to adapt to the changing role of surgery.

▶ Diagnosis & Staging

A tissue diagnosis is critical to the care of all cancer patients. Depending on the type of tumor and its location, the method of biopsy will vary. Common diagnostic techniques include needle aspiration biopsy, core needle biopsy, incisional biopsy, and excisional biopsy.

Fine-needle aspiration biopsy (FNAB) is a rapid and minimally invasive technique for the biopsy of palpable superficial tumors. Deeper, nonpalpable lesions may also be sampled by this technique when FNAB is combined with various imaging modalities, such as ultrasonography or computed tomography (CT). FNAB involves aspiration of cells from a suspicious mass, followed by cytologic examination of the stained smear. FNAB is particularly useful in the diagnosis of enlarged lymph nodes, breast lumps, thyroid masses, and lung nodules.

Advantages to FNAB include the simplicity of the procedure and the low rate of complications. However, there are limitations. FNAB cytology requires an experienced cytopathologist for accurate interpretation. Because cytology does not demonstrate architecture, it does not allow the cytopathologist to accurately grade tumors or to differentiate between *in situ* and invasive disease. If this information is necessary, FNAB may be inadequate. Sampling errors can lead to false-negative results, so a negative FNAB should be interpreted cautiously. In addition, though rare, false-positive results can occur, so confirmation may be needed before definitive surgical intervention. For example, a mastectomy should never be performed on the basis of an FNAB of a breast lump without confirming the diagnosis by either preoperative core biopsy or frozen section analysis at the time of surgery.

Core needle biopsy utilizes a needle that removes a sliver of tissue for analysis. This technique provides more histologic information than FNAB because it allows the pathologist to see the histologic architecture of the sample rather than just the cellular characteristics. False-positive results are extremely rare. Although less so than with FNAB, sampling errors may occur, and a negative result must be weighed against clinical judgment. Core biopsies are frequently used for prostate, breast, and liver masses. Again, ultrasound and radiographic imaging may enable the clinician to sample deep-seated or nonpalpable masses. The technique may also be used during surgery to biopsy suspicious masses encountered at operation.

When a larger tumor sample is necessary for accurate grading or staging, or a needle biopsy provided inadequate information, an incisional or excisional biopsy is required. **Excisional biopsy** is the surgical removal of an entire gross lesion, while **incisional biopsy** involves sampling a representative portion of a suspicious lesion. In general, excisional biopsy is recommended whenever it is possible to excise the entire lesion without damage to surrounding structures. Incisional biopsy should be considered whenever a core biopsy fails to make the diagnosis, but removing the tumor might compromise the subsequent operation (eg, a large [> 5 cm], deep soft tissue mass for which sarcoma is a possibility) or preclude delivery of neoadjuvant therapy.

Although biopsy techniques are usually simple, the surgeon must adhere to some specific principles when performing a biopsy for a suspected malignancy. The positioning of the needle tract or scar should be such that if further surgery is required, the biopsy site will be easily included in the excised specimen. Excisional biopsies of the breast should consider the possibility of a subsequent mastectomy, and the excision of skin or subcutaneous lesions on the extremities should be oriented in a way that allows for the following wide excision and lymphatic mapping if malignancy is discovered. Meticulous hemostasis is imperative, as the formation of a wound hematoma may make subsequent operation more difficult. The surgeon should carefully orient the pathologic specimen to allow the pathologist to evaluate margins in the context of the preresection anatomy, which may prove important in curative surgical procedures.

Once a diagnosis is made, the next step is typically to determine the extent of the cancer, or **staging**. This step begins with a complete history and physical examination, looking for signs or symptoms of advanced or metastatic disease. Laboratory or imaging studies may follow to determine not only the extent of the primary tumor but the presence of regional or distant metastases. Patients with signs or symptoms of metastatic disease should undergo appropriate workup of their symptoms. For some tumor types, routine staging examinations are indicated. However, for many asymptomatic patients newly diagnosed with cancer, a full battery of staging studies is not necessary and not only will increase the cost of treatment but may lead to false-positive findings, unnecessary biopsies, and inappropriate changes in therapy.

Surgeons are often called upon to perform operations that provide staging information for various types of cancer. Such procedures are necessary when the clinical extent of the disease has a direct bearing on the choice of treatment modalities. Examples include laparoscopy for gastric or pancreatic cancer, a staging laparotomy for ovarian cancer, or mediastinoscopy for lung and esophageal cancer. Staging procedures can often help to avert highly morbid procedures in cases where there is little chance for cure.

▶ Curative Surgery

Surgical resections with curative intent can be divided into three categories: resection of a primary lesion, resection of isolated metastases, and resection of metastatic deposits. In each case, the clinician must strive to reach a balance between the chance for cure and the morbidity of the procedure. Each situation must be evaluated individually, and the patient's wishes must be paramount.

The guiding principle of cancer surgery is to remove the entire tumor with adequate margins so as to prevent local recurrence and potentially distant recurrence. What constitutes an adequate margin varies among tumor types. Various tumors require different disease-free margins in order to achieve optimal chances for a cure. For a tumor that appears adherent or fixed to adjacent structures, **en bloc resection** is mandatory, and any attachment should be considered malignant in nature. Appropriate preoperative imaging of the tumor is often necessary to be prepared in the operating room for the possible resection of small or large bowel, bladder, or other adjacent organs.

It is important that the surgeon have knowledge of other modalities that may be integrated into the management plan to allow for a less extensive surgical procedure. Radiation and chemotherapy are commonly used in combination with surgery and are referred to as adjuvant therapies if used after complete resection with no demonstrable local or systemic disease. While their use has in some cases diminished the extent of resection necessary for local control (breast, sarcoma, head, and neck), it is important to note that these modalities do not compensate for inadequate margins in controlling local disease. Every attempt should be made to achieve widely negative margins surgically, even if it requires a second operation, rather than assuming radiation will "clean up" residual disease.

If these modalities are used in the preoperative setting, they are called neoadjuvant therapies. In many cases, neoadjuvant therapy has dramatically improved outcomes, as with pediatric rhabdomyosarcoma or locally advanced or inflammatory breast cancer. In some cases, neoadjuvant therapy can convert an unresectable tumor to resectable, while in other cases, it can decrease the extent of surgery necessary to obtain control or decrease the likelihood of positive margins. Neoadjuvant therapy is commonly used in the treatment of esophageal cancer, rectal cancer, pancreatic cancer, breast cancer, and sarcoma. It is important the surgeon consider the possibility of neoadjuvant therapy when performing a biopsy, staging the patient, or planning surgery.

The regional lymph nodes represent the most prevalent site of metastases for solid tumors, and in most cases involvement of the regional nodes represents the most important prognostic factor. Removal of the regional lymph nodes not only provides important prognostic information that may help guide adjuvant therapy, but provides regional control, preventing regional recurrence and the associated complications. For this reason, the removal of the regional lymph nodes is often performed at the time of resection of the primary cancer. More controversial is whether the removal of regional lymph nodes can improve survival. These controversies concern both the extent and the timing of the procedure. For example, the extent of lymphadenectomy at the time of gastrectomy for stomach cancer has been hypothesized to have an impact on improving overall survival. This has not, however, been borne out in prospective randomized trials. It may be that extended lymphadenectomy results in more accurate staging of patients at a cost of increased morbidity and minimal effect, if any, on overall survival. The relative benefit of nodal dissection may also vary with the efficacy of adjuvant therapies, such as chemotherapy or radiation therapy. How extensive a lymph node dissection to perform at the time of definitive resection varies with tumor type and in many cases remains controversial.

For many nonvisceral solid tumors, such as melanoma or breast cancer, elective node dissections were performed in clinically node negative patients at the time of their primary tumor resection. Unfortunately, this exposed many node-negative patients to the morbidity of a node dissection, and a clear survival benefit could not be demonstrated in prospective randomized studies. This practice has been replaced with lymphatic mapping and sentinel lymph node biopsy. Mapping agents (a radioactive tracer or a blue dye) are injected around the site of the tumor prior to surgery. These travel to the lymph nodes that first receive drainage from the site of the primary, and thus are the most likely to harbor cancer. Only the sentinel nodes (those nodes that are blue or radioactive) are removed, and carefully examined for micrometastases. This has dramatically improved our ability to stage the regional lymph nodes, helping to guide adjuvant therapies, while minimizing morbidity. Classically, node negative patients could safely avoid further surgery, while node positive patients underwent a completion lymph node dissection. This approach has also changed recently. In breast cancer, the American College of Surgeons Oncology Group (ACoSOG) Z0011 trial, demonstrated that a subset of breast cancer patients with positive sentinel lymph nodes did not benefit from completion lymph node dissection. A similar trial, the Multicenter Selective Lymphadenectomy Trial II (MSLT-II), is examining a similar question among sentinel lymph node positive melanoma patients.

The surgeon plays a much more limited role when the patient has metastatic disease; nonetheless, the resection of "isolated" metastases in patients with solid malignancies is sometimes a consideration when technically feasible. The selection of candidate patients for surgical resection requires a thorough evaluation of the extent of known disease, likelihood of additional metastatic disease, length of time between the primary and the distant recurrence (disease-free interval), medical status of the patient, and feasibility of resecting the metastatic site with a negative margin. Ultimately, this process identifies a small subset of patients who would be surgical candidates. Although there are no prospective randomized trials documenting the survival benefit of surgical resection of metastatic disease, there is considerable retrospective evidence indicating that this approach can result in long-term benefit. The resection of lung metastases in patients with osteogenic or soft tissue sarcomas has been associated with an approximately 20%-25% overall survival rate greater than 5 years. There is also a large body of retrospective evidence documenting the benefit of resecting colorectal metastases to the liver, resulting in a 25%-40% overall 5-year survival rate, depending on the extent of liver involvement. A similar benefit has been demonstrated in an aggressive surgical approach to metastatic melanoma. Another question in stage IV disease is when to resect the primary tumor. Typically, resection of the primary cancer when the patient already has metastatic disease was only done for palliation, or to prevent future complications. This approach is changing, however. For some cancers, such as colon cancer, resection of the primary tumor in the face of metastatic disease to prevent obstruction or bleeding, is less necessary due to the improved efficacy of systemic agents. Conversely, in some cancers, such as renal cell carcinoma and possibly breast cancer, there is evidence that resection of the primary tumor improves may improve outcome in stage IV patients. One of the roles of the surgical oncologist is to know when it is appropriate to offer this option.

▶ Palliation

Surgical intervention is sometimes required in the patient with unresectable advanced cancer for palliative indications such as pain, bleeding, obstruction, malnutrition, or infection. The decision to operate must balance several factors, including the likelihood of adding significantly to the quality of life of the patient, the expected survival of the individual, the potential morbidity of the procedure, and whether there are alternative methods of palliation.

Malnutrition is a common problem in the cancer patient, especially one with advanced, unresectable disease. Commonly, the surgeon is involved in placement of vascular access for hyperalimentation, or if the gastrointestinal tract is functional, the placement of gastrostomy or jejunostomy tubes for enteral nutrition. Occasionally, the surgeon is involved in palliating pain due to a metastatic lesion compressing upon an organ or adjacent nerves. Examples include cutaneous or subcutaneous melanoma metastases, a large ulcerating breast cancer, or a recurrent intra-abdominal sarcoma mass. The surgeon must assess the relative risk-to-benefit ratio in resecting a symptomatic mass knowing that it will not impact the overall survival of the patient. If the quality of life of the individual can be improved at an acceptable operative risk, then the surgical intervention is warranted.

Finally, the surgeon may be called upon to manage oncologic emergencies. Acute hemorrhage and obstruction of a hollow viscus represent the most common potential oncologic emergencies. In these cases, surgeons may have to emergently intervene in the care of a cancer patient, or in some instances, use nonsurgical approaches (such as stents or angiography).

▶ Prophylaxis

With our improved understanding of inherited genetic mutations and the identification of patients who are predisposed to cancer, surgical therapy has expanded beyond the therapy of established tumors and into the prevention of cancer. Prophylaxis is not a new concept in surgical oncology. Patients with chronic inflammatory diseases are known to be at high risk of subsequent malignant transformation. This typically prompts close surveillance and surgical resection at the first identification of premalignant changes. One of the earliest examples of this is the recommendation for total proctocolectomy for subsets of patients with chronic ulcerative colitis.

The ability to perform genetic screening for relevant mutations has allowed for prophylactic surgery to be implemented prior to the onset of symptoms or histologic changes. Familial adenomatous polyposis (FAP) syndrome, defined by the diffuse involvement of the colon and rectum with adenomatous polyps, almost always predisposes to colorectal cancer if the large intestine is left in place. With the identification of the gene responsible for FAP, the adenomatous polyposis coli (*APC*) gene, members of families in which an APC mutation has been identified can have genetic testing prior to polyps becoming evident and be considered for prophylactic proctocolectomy. Medullary thyroid cancer (MTC) is a well-established component of multiple endocrine neoplasia syndrome type 2A (MEN2A) or type 2B (MEN2B). Mutations in the *RET* protooncogene are present in almost all cases of MEN2A and 2B. Family members of MEN patients can be screened for the presence of a *RET* mutation, and those with the mutation should undergo total thyroidectomy at a young age (6 years for MEN2A, infancy for MEN2B). The role of prophylactic mastectomies has been greatly expanded with the identification of *BRCA1* and *BRCA2,* which can be associated with a lifetime probability of breast cancer of between 40% and 85%. Other prophylactic operations are listed in Table 44–1. However, potential benefits of prophylactic surgeries must be weighed against quality-of-life issues and the morbidity of the surgery. A detailed discussion must be held with each patient considering prophylactic surgery regarding the risks and benefits, so today's surgical oncologist needs a clear understanding of genetics and inherited risk.

CYTOTOXIC CHEMOTHERAPY

The goal of chemotherapeutic regimens is to deliver pharmacologic agents systemically to eradicate all tumor cells. The ideal tumor drug would kill cancer cells without harming normal tissues. No such agent exists, and most drugs affect normal cells to some extent. The success of chemotherapy relies on the normal cell's greater capacity for repair and survival relative to tumor cells.

Even a single cancer cell can potentially reproduce to form a lethal tumor. For this reason, the goal of curative chemotherapy must be the complete eradication of all tumor cells. Tumor burden is important in chemotherapy. A large cancer may harbor more than 10^9 tumor cells. If a tolerable dose of an effective drug killed 99.99% of these cells, the tumor burden would still be 10^5 cells. The remaining cells, while clinically undetectable, are likely to continue to grow and lead to a clinical recurrence of cancer. For this reason, most chemotherapy protocols rely on repeated administrations of drugs in order to achieve maximal cell killing. Tumor cells may avoid the cell-killing effects of a particular drug because of their stage in the cell cycle, residence in an area protected from the drug (central nervous system), or an inherent resistance to the drug.

Drug resistance plays a large role in chemotherapy failures. Several mechanisms of tumor resistance are known. The multidrug resistance (*MDR*) gene encodes a protein that actively pumps drugs out of tumor cells. This gene confers resistance on a variety of antitumor drugs, including the antibiotics and plant-derived compounds. Other tumor mechanisms of resistance include the alteration of target enzymes, increased production of a target enzyme to overwhelm the drug, and an increased capability for DNA repair. Tumor resistance to a given chemotherapeutic agent can often be overcome by the administration of multiple drugs.

▶ Principles of Chemotherapy Use

A. Curative Chemotherapy

Hematologic malignancies are typically treated by chemotherapy, radiation, or both, with surgery used primarily for diagnosis and staging. On the other hand, surgery is the primary treatment for nonhematologic malignancies, although there are some exceptions. Anal cancer is cured in approximately 80% of patients with the Nigro protocol—5-FU/mitomycin-C and radiation therapy—as first-line treatment. Testicular cancer, even when metastatic, is curable with bleomycin/etoposide/cisplatin in approximately 85% of patients.

B. Adjuvant Treatment

Although all visible tumor may be removed at the time of surgery, microscopic tumor deposits may still be present locally or may have spread to distant locations. Chemotherapy is most effective against very small tumors and microscopic tumor deposits. Therefore, adjuvant chemotherapy is often given to improve the likelihood of cure after surgical resection.

The benefit gained from adjuvant chemotherapy can be thought of in terms of absolute benefit or relative benefit

Table 44–1. Prophylactic operations in surgical oncology.

Prophylactic Surgery	Potential Indications
Bilateral mastectomy	*BRCA1* or *BRCA2* mutation
	Atypical hyperplasia or lobular carcinoma *in situ*
	Familial breast cancer
Bilateral oophorectomy	*BRCA1* mutation
	Familial ovarian cancer
	Hereditary nonpolyposis colorectal cancer
	Hysterectomy for endometrial cancer
	Colon resection for colon cancer
Thyroidectomy	*RET* protooncogene mutation
	Multiple endocrine neoplasia type 2A (MEN2A)
	Multiple endocrine neoplasia type 2B (MEN2B)
	Familial non-MEN medullary thyroid carcinoma (FMTC)
Total proctocolectomy	Familial adenomatous polyposis (FAP) or antigen-presenting cell (APC) mutation
	Ulcerative colitis
	Hereditary nonpolyposis colorectal cancer (HNPCC) germ-line mutation

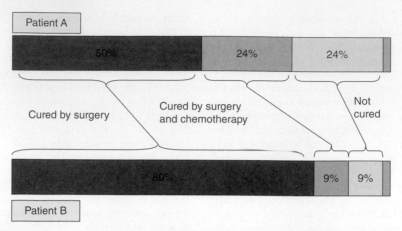

▲ **Figure 44–1.** Benefits of adjuvant chemotherapy. For 100 patients treated with adjuvant chemotherapy, some will be cured by surgery alone (dark red bar), some will die of other causes (gray bar), and some will die of their cancer (light red bar). Adjuvant therapy will prevent a cancer death in a portion of those patients (medium red bar). Adjuvant chemotherapy will result in a relative benefit of 50% for both patient A and patient B, meaning treatment will reduce the likelihood of dying of cancer by 50%. However, the absolute benefit is different for both patients. For patient A, who has a high likelihood of dying of disease, the absolute benefit is 24%. For patient B, who has a good prognosis, the absolute benefit is only 9%.

(Figure 44–1). For example, after colectomy for stage III colon cancer, the chance of cure is approximately 50%. This can be increased to approximately 70% by adjuvant 5-FU/leucovorin. This represents a 40% relative benefit (40% more patients are cured with chemotherapy than without chemotherapy) but a 20% absolute benefit (20% of the patients who take the chemotherapy will have altered their outcome). Another way to look at this is that with a 20% absolute benefit, 80% of patients experience the inconvenience and side effects of chemotherapy without gaining any improvement themselves. The decision to receive adjuvant chemotherapy is a balance between the expected benefit of treatment, the patient's comorbid conditions and general health, and the patient's wishes.

C. Neoadjuvant Treatment

Neoadjuvant chemotherapy is usually given to facilitate surgical resection by shrinking the primary tumor, or it may convert an unresectable tumor into a resectable tumor. In some cases, this treatment has been shown to prolong survival. Another advantage to neoadjuvant chemotherapy is that it allows the oncologist to observe the primary tumor to determine if it is sensitive to a particular chemotherapeutic regimen. During the course of cancer treatment, it is important to define the progress and outcomes resulting from therapy. The terms complete and partial response are often used as endpoints to evaluate the efficacy of a particular therapeutic regimen. A **complete response** is defined as the absence of demonstrable cancer. A **partial response** refers to

a reduction of tumor mass by greater than 50%. The patient's response to neoadjuvant chemotherapy can be an important predictor of outcome.

D. Chemotherapy for Metastatic Disease

The majority of patients who are receiving chemotherapy have metastatic disease that is not curable. For these patients, treatment with chemotherapy is intended to prolong survival, improve quality of life, or both. Response rates range from 20% to 75% depending on the tumor type and chemotherapy regimen. However, even a complete remission is rarely durable. Most partial or complete remissions last only months.

As with all therapies, the decision to use chemotherapy must balance the potential benefits with the risks, toxicities, and the patient's general health and condition. There is little to be gained by treating an asymptomatic patient if no prolongation of survival is expected. A detailed discussion must be held with each individual patient; some patients are more willing than others to tolerate the side effects of chemotherapy. Since the disease is not curable, treatment with single agents, which are less toxic than combination chemotherapy, are often considered, with more willingness to reduce doses for toxicity.

▶ Classes of Chemotherapeutic Agents

With all forms of curative chemotherapy, the goal is elimination of all tumor stem cells. Cells that are incapable of further division cannot cause progression of a tumor, and the sterilization of a tumor cell is as good as a kill. Chemotherapeutic drugs are generally classified as cell cycle-specific (CCS) drugs, which are toxic to actively proliferating cells, or cell cycle-nonspecific (CCNS) drugs, which are capable of killing cells that are not dividing during drug exposure. These two classifications are not absolute, and many drugs may overlap between the two categories.

In order to achieve maximal cell killing, most therapeutic protocols use combination chemotherapy. Agents with differing mechanisms of action and different toxic side effects are used, allowing for relatively high doses of multiple agents. This method of combining agents helps to combat tumor cell resistance and increase the tumor cell killing while avoiding the compounding of toxic effects.

A. Alkylating Agents

These agents exert their effects by the transfer of alkyl groups to various cellular components, most importantly by the alkylation of DNA. Alkylators can cause DNA strand breaks, cross-linking of DNA strands, or miscoding of DNA during replication. The alkylating agents are considered cell cycle–nonspecific agents but tend to have their greatest effect on proliferating cells. Normal cells are able to avoid many of the lethal affects of alkylating agents because of their ability to repair DNA. The alkylating agents are effective in treatment of the hematologic malignancies and in a variety of solid tumors such as breast, melanoma, lung, and endometrial cancers. Included in this class are the nitrosoureas (eg, carmustine, semustine, lomustine), cyclophosphamide, chlorambucil, mechlorethamine, dacarbazine, and procarbazine.

B. Platinum Analogues

The platinum analogs are similar to the alkylating agents. They bind DNA to form interstrand and intrastrand cross-links, leading to inhibition of DNA synthesis and transcription. The mechanisms of cancer cell resistance are also similar to those of alkylating agents: decreased cellular uptake of the drugs, increased activity of DNA repair enzymes, and increased thiol-containing proteins. In addition, resistance to both cisplatin and carboplatin has been associated with a deficiency of mismatch repair (MMR) genes. It is not known why this mechanism of resistance appears to be specific to cisplatin and carboplatin, but the efficacy of the newest platinum analog, oxaliplatin, is not affected by *MMR* gene deficiency.

C. Antimetabolites

Rapidly dividing cells require increased synthesis of nucleic acid precursors. This increased synthesis can be exploited pharmacologically by the antimetabolites. These drugs are analogs of nucleic acids or nucleic acid precursors. The antimetabolites may be incorporated into the nucleic acids of a cell and serve as a false messenger. Antimetabolites can shut down the cellular synthetic machinery by binding to and inhibiting enzymes important in the production of nucleic acids. Since this class of drugs affects all rapidly proliferating cells, they are relatively toxic to normal tissues that have a high rate of cell turnover. Antimetabolites are most effective in the hematologic malignancies but are also used in the treatment of solid tumors such as breast and gastrointestinal cancers. They include methotrexate, mercaptopurine, thioguanine, fluorouracil, and cytarabine.

D. Antimicrotubule Agents

A variety of antitumor drugs are derived from natural plants (and are also known as plant alkaloids). Vincristine, vinblastine, docetaxel, and paclitaxel work by binding tubulin and poisoning the assembly of microtubules in the mitotic spindle. This leads to mitotic arrest in metaphase, and these compounds are effective only on rapidly dividing cell populations. The plant alkaloids are most useful for hematologic malignancies and breast, renal, testicular, and head and neck cancers.

E. Topoisomerase Inhibitors

These plant derivatives exert their antitumor effects by binding to and inhibiting various forms of the enzyme topoisomerase. Topoisomerases are responsible for the maintenance of DNA structure and are also important in the cleavage and religation of DNA strands. Inhibition of these enzymes leads to DNA strand breakage and structural damage. The topoisomerase inhibitors are also cell cycle–specific agents and have their greatest activity against rapidly proliferating cells. Examples include etoposide, teniposide, and topotecan. These drugs are used in the treatment of hematologic malignancies and lung, bladder, prostate, and testicular cancers.

F. Antibiotics

Most of the drugs in this class are derived from the soil fungus *Streptomyces*. All the antibiotics exert their antitumor effects by interference with the synthesis of nucleic acids. Most of the drugs in this class intercalate in DNA, blocking DNA synthesis and inducing strand breakages. The antibiotics are considered cell cycle–nonspecific, and they have antitumor activity against a wide variety of solid tumors. Included in this class of drugs are doxorubicin, dactinomycin, plicamycin, mitomycin, and bleomycin.

▶ Side Effects of Chemotherapy

Most side effects from chemotherapeutic regimens are the result of toxicities to rapidly dividing normal cell populations—particularly bone marrow and epithelial cells. Bone marrow suppression is an adverse effect of many of these drugs, resulting in neutropenia, thrombocytopenia, and even anemia. Mucosal ulcerations and alopecia also occur in patients treated with cell cycle–specific agents. Intractable nausea and vomiting is another common side effect that can severely affect quality of life. Testicular or ovarian failure can result from chemotherapy, leading to sterility. Many of these drugs also are powerful teratogens and should be avoided in pregnant patients. Finally, many of the alkylating agents have been implicated in the development of secondary cancers, especially hematologic malignancies.

REGIONAL THERAPY

Systemic chemotherapy is limited by toxicity to the host. Regional delivery of chemotherapeutic agents via arterial cannulation allows for high levels of drugs in the region of the primary tumor while decreasing systemic toxicity.

Isolated limb perfusion (ILP) is a technique for the delivery of chemotherapeutic agents to an extremity with locally advanced cancer and is of benefit primarily in the treatment of extremity melanoma and sarcoma. In this approach, a tourniquet is applied to the extremity to occlude venous outflow. The major artery perfusing the limb is then isolated, cannulated, and perfused with hyperthermic chemotherapeutic agents using a pump oxygenator as for cardiopulmonary bypass. The perfusion is done in the operating room and lasts for approximately 1 hour. The cannula is then removed. Most protocols involve only a single treatment. Melphalan, an alkylating agent, is the most common agent used today in the treatment of both sarcomas and melanomas. In patients with extensive in-transit melanoma confined to an extremity, isolated limb perfusion can provide regional control and palliation. In patients with unresectable extremity sarcomas, preoperative limb perfusion may shrink the tumor and allow for a limb-sparing resection. While improving regional control, this therapy has yet to show a definitive survival benefit. An alternate approach is isolated limb infusion (ILI), which involves using minimally invasive techniques to access the vessels along with a tourniquet to minimize systemic uptake.

Another approach is isolated hepatic artery infusion for the treatment of colorectal cancer metastatic to the liver. Metastatic tumors derive nearly all of their blood supply from the hepatic artery, while the normal liver parenchyma derives more than two-thirds of its blood supply from the portal system. This permits the delivery of higher doses of chemotherapeutic agents to the tumor relative to the normal hepatocytes. The drug most commonly used in this protocol is floxuridine, which is almost completely extracted on its first pass through the liver, resulting in relatively low systemic toxicity. Hepatic artery infusion requires the surgical placement of a catheter into the hepatic artery, which is connected to an implanted or external infusion pump for continuous treatment. Hepatic artery infusion has been used

for unresectable colorectal metastases as well as an adjuvant to hepatic resection. While there are clearly improved tumor responses in comparison to systemic therapy, the data is less clear on overall survival benefits. Some studies, however, have suggested an improved survival and have stimulated further investigation.

TARGETED THERAPIES

An expanding knowledge of molecular biology is revolutionizing the field of oncology, truly personalizing care for each individual patient with cancer. Molecular diagnostics is increasingly allowing us to customize the selection and dosing of traditional agents to maximize benefit and minimize toxicity. Molecular oncology is changing the way we approach drug discovery and development, leading to the development of targeted therapies. One definition of targeted therapy is any drug in which there is a specific diagnostic test that must be performed before the patient can be considered eligible to receive the drug. An example is measuring Her-2/neu overexpression on breast cancer to determine if a patient is eligible for trastuzumab (Herceptin). A more oncologic definition is any drug with a focused mechanism that specifically acts on a well-defined target or biologic pathway. Inactivation of this target/pathway results in regression or destruction of the malignant cell. Targeted therapies are often considered "magic bullets."

Several targeted therapies have been FDA approved and are in clinical use; many others are being developed. The ideal target is one that is expressed (and can be measured) on cancer cells but not significantly expressed in vital organs and tissues. It is preferably crucial to the malignant phenotype, and its inhibition results in a clinical response in patients whose tumor expresses the target. Several methods for very specific targeting are being examined. The ability of therapeutic antibodies to bind with high affinity makes them excellent candidates for targeted therapy. While antibodies may induce an immune-mediated destruction of cancer cells (and be considered immunotherapy [see section on Immunotherapy]), they can also be used to target specific cell surface receptors to interrupt that pathway. For this latter function, it is important that the target, when bound by the antibody, is internalized by endocytosis to facilitate the intracellular mechanism of pathway inhibition and cell death.

Trastuzumab is an IgG antibody that binds to the juxtamembrane portion of the extracellular domain of the Her-2/neu receptor and has become an important option for patients with Her-2/neu–positive breast cancer. Her-2/neu is an epidermal growth factor receptor (EGFR) that has a functional intracellular tyrosine kinase and when overexpressed can lead to increased proliferation, increased metastatic potential, and resistance to therapeutic agents. While the binding of trastuzumab to the Her-2/neu protein may lead to antibody-dependent cell-mediated cytotoxicity, the more important function appears to be the disruption of the downstream signaling through the intracellular tyrosine kinase.

Another way to target cancer cells is through the use of small molecules. The development of **imatinib mesylate** is the classic example of a small-molecule targeted therapy. Imatinib is an adenosine triphosphate-binding selective inhibitor of *bcr-abl*, and its use has been associated with durable, complete responses in the treatment of Philadelphia chromosome-positive chronic myelogenous leukemia as well as the treatment of gastrointestinal stromal tumors. The latter characteristically express an activating mutation in the c-kit receptor tyrosine kinase (*RTK*) gene.

Perhaps the most noteworthy example of the impact of targeted therapies is in the treatment of melanoma. It was discovered that 40%-60% of melanoma patients harbor a specific mutation in the *BRAF* gene, and 90% of these mutations involve a substitution of glutamic acid for valine at amino acid 600 (the V600E mutation). This gene codes for the protein kinase BRAF, a component of the mitogen-activated protein (MAPT) kinase pathway. **Vemurafenib** (Zelboraf) selectively inhibits the kinase activity of this mutated BRAF. Vemurafenib is FDA approved for the treatment of unresectable or metastatic melanoma that tests positive for the BRAF V600E mutation based on prospective randomized studies that demonstrated a dramatic improvement in progression free and overall survival. **Dabrafenib** also specifically targets the BRAF V600E mutation and has very promising clinical trial data. Another promising drug for melanoma patients with the BRAF mutation is **trametinib**, which blocks MEK, an alternate protein in the MAP kinase pathway.

Multiple other targeted therapies, both monoclonal antibodies and small molecule inhibitors, are in clinical use. **Cetuximab** (Erbitux) binds to the EGFR with high affinity, blocking the subsequent signal transduction events leading to cell proliferation. It enhances the antitumor effects of chemotherapy by inhibiting cell proliferation and angiogenesis and promoting apoptosis. Cetuximab has been approved for use in combination with CPT-11 for the treatment of advanced colorectal cancer. **Bevacizumab** (Avastin) targets the vascular endothelial growth factor (VEGF), which regulates vascular proliferation and permeability and promotes angiogenesis. Other targeted therapies in use in cancer are listed in Table 44–2.

HORMONAL THERAPY

Hormones are normally involved in the differentiation, stimulation, and control of certain tissues, including but not limited to lymphoid tissue, the uterus, the prostate, and the mammary glands. Tumors arising from these tissues may also be stimulated or inhibited by hormones, and so manipulation of the hormonal balance can be beneficial in the systemic therapy of these cancers. In some cases, hormones themselves are used as cancer therapies. For example, the administration of estrogen to a man ultimately suppresses the production of testosterone, which is a useful effect in the treatment of prostate cancer. Corticosteroids, particularly the glucocorticoids, have a powerful suppressive effect on lymphoid cells, making them useful in the treatment of acute leukemias, lymphomas, myeloma, and other myeloproliferative disorders. In most cases, however, hormonal therapy involves blocking the effects of hormones that stimulate proliferation.

▶ Estrogen & Androgen Inhibitors

One approach to hormonal therapy is to block the hormone receptor on the cell. Selective estrogen receptor modulators (SERMs) are medications that mimic the structure of estrogen. Because the estrogen-receptor complex varies among tissue types, SERMs can have different effects on different tissues, sometimes inhibiting the actions of estrogen and sometimes behaving like estrogen. The most well-known SERM is tamoxifen (Nolvadex), which is used not only to treat estrogen-sensitive breast cancer but also to prevent breast cancer in high-risk individuals. Because it also has some proestrogen properties, side effects of tamoxifen can include an increased risk of uterine cancer and deep vein thrombosis. Raloxifene (Evista) is a newer SERM that has been approved for prevention and treatment of postmenopausal osteoporosis and is used in the chemoprevention of breast cancer for postmenopausal women.

Flutamide (Eulexin) is a testosterone antagonist used in the treatment of prostate cancer. It works by blocking translocation of the androgen receptor to the nucleus. Although hormonal therapy for prostate cancer is palliative, it can be quite effective in slowing the progression of disease. Hormonal therapy can add several years to the life expectancy of patients with unresectable or metastatic disease. Flutamide is most effective when used in combination with surgical or pharmacologic castration.

▶ Gonadotropin-Releasing Hormone Analogues

The most definitive way to block the production of testosterone and estrogen is by surgical castration. The pharmacologic equivalent of castration can be accomplished with leuprolide, an analog of gonadotropin-releasing hormone (GnRH). Normally, GnRH leads to the production of luteinizing hormone and follicle-stimulating hormone, the physiologic stimulators of sex hormone production. Constant stimulation with leuprolide actually inhibits luteinizing hormone and follicle-stimulating hormone release and leads to decreased synthesis of the sex steroids. Leuprolide (Lupron) is commonly used to decrease testosterone levels in the treatment of unresectable prostate cancer. In premenopausal

Table 44–2. Targeted therapeutic agents for cancer.

Drug Name	Brand Name	Target	Used in the Treatment of
Imatinib mesylate	Gleevec	Bcr-abl, c-kit, PDGFR	GIST, DFSP, ALL, CML
Dasatinib	Sprycel	SRC-family protein kinases	CML, ALL
Nilotinib	Tasigna	Bcr-abl, c-kit, PDGFR	CML
Traztuzumab	Herceptin	Her-2/neu	Breast cancer, gastric adenocarcinoma
Pertuzumab	Perjeta	Her-2/neu	Breast cancer
Lapatinib	Tykerb	EGFR, ErbB2, Erk-1&2 AKT kinases	Breast cancer
Gefitinib	Iressa	EGFR	Non–small-cell lung cancer
Erlotinib	Tarceva	EGFR	Non–small-cell lung cancer, pancreatic cancer
Cetuximab	Erbitux	EGFR	SCCA of the head and neck, colorectal cancer
Panitumumab	Vectibix	EGFR	Colorectal cancer
Temsirolimus	Torisel	mTOR	Renal cell carcinoma
Everolimus	Afinitor	Immunophilin FK–binding protein-12	Renal cell carcinoma, astrocytoma, breast cancer, pancreatic neuroendocrine tumors
Vandetanib	Caprelsa	EGFR, VEGFR2	Medullary thyroid
Vemurafenib	Zelboraf	BRAF V600E	Melanoma (BRAF V600E mutation)
Crizotinib	Xalkori	EML4-ALK	Non–small-cell lung cancer
Vorinostat	Zolinza	Histone deacetylases (HDACs)	CTCL
Romidepsin	Istodax	HDACs	CTCL
Bexarotene	Targretin	Retinoid X receptors	CTCL
Alitretinoin	Panretin	Retinoic acid receptors, retinoid X receptors	Kaposi sarcoma
Tretinoin	Vesanoid	Retinoic acid receptors	Acute promyelocytic leukemia
Bortezomib	Velcade	Proteasome	Multiple myeloma, mantle cell lymphoma
Carfilzomib	Kyprolis	Proteasome	Multilple myeloma
Bevacizumab	Avastin	VEGF	Glioblastoma, non–small-cell lung cancer, colorectal cancer, renal cell carcinoma
Sorafenib	Nexavar		Renal cell carcinoma, hepatocellular carcinoma
Sunitinib	Sutent		Renal cell carcinoma, GIST, pancreatic neuroendocrine tumors
Paxopanib	Votrient	VEGF, c-kit, PDGFR	Renal cell carcinoma, soft tissue sarcoma
Rituximab	Rituxan	CD20	B-cell non-Hodgkin lymphoma, CLL
Alemtuzumab	Campath	CD52	B-cell CLL
Ofatumumab	Arzerra	CD20	B-cell CLL

ALL, acute lymphoblastic leukemia; DFSP, dermatofibrosarcoma protuberans; CLL, chronic lymphocytic leukemia; CML, chronic myelogenous leukemia; CTCL, cutaneous T-cell lymphoma; GIST, gastrointestinal stromal tumor; PDGFR, platelet-derived growth factor receptor.

women, estrogen levels fall to postmenopausal values with leuprolide administration. For this reason, the drug can be useful in the treatment of estrogen receptor-positive breast cancers in premenopausal women.

▶ Aromatase Inhibitors

Postmenopausal women have functionally inactive ovaries; however, estrogens are still produced to a lesser extent in extragonadal tissues, primarily the conversion of adrenal steroids in fat cells by the enzyme aromatase. Aromatase inhibitors, such as anastrozole (Arimidex), exemestane (Aromasin), and letrozole (Femara), eliminate functional estrogen in this population of women and are an effective hormonal treatment of breast cancer. A number of studies have demonstrated the benefit of aromatase inhibitors in postmenopausal women with hormone receptor positive breast cancer, either as first-line therapy or after the use of tamoxifen.

Chu E, DeVita VT: *Physicians' Cancer Chemotherapy Drug Manual.* Jones and Bartlett, Burlington, MA 2012.

DeVita VT, Lawrence TS, Rosenberg SA, eds: *Cancer: Principles & Practice of Oncology,* 9th ed. Lippincott Williams & Wilkins, Philadelphia, PA 2011.

Flaherty, KT: BRAF inhibitors and melanoma. *Cancer J* 2011;17(6):505-511.

RADIATION THERAPY

Radiation therapy may be used alone or in combination with surgery and chemotherapy and may be given with curative or palliative intent. Some tumors, such as head and neck cancers, prostate cancer, and Hodgkin disease, can often be cured by irradiation alone, eliminating the need for surgical resection or chemotherapy. More commonly, locoregional control of tumors involves surgical resection combined with localized radiation. The theoretical advantage of combining these two therapies is based on the mechanisms by which they fail to achieve their purpose. Surgical failures occur at the margins of tumors, while radiation therapy fails in the center of tumors, where the malignant cells are numerous and hypoxic conditions exist. Radiation failures are rare at the periphery of tumors, where cell numbers are low and oxygenation is high. Depending on tumor histology and location, radiation therapy can be used as a surgical adjunct either preoperatively or postoperatively. Preoperative radiation can shrink tumors and increase the chances for complete surgical resection in cancers such as sarcomas, rectal cancers, and superior sulcus lung cancers.

▶ Principles of Radiation Therapy

Ionizing radiation is defined as energy with sufficient strength to cause the ejection of an orbital electron from an atom when the radiation is absorbed. Ionizing radiation can take either an electromagnetic form, as high-energy photons, or particulate forms, such as electrons, protons, neutrons, alpha particles, or other particles. Most radiation therapies utilize either photons or electrons. Electrons interact directly with tissue, causing ionization, in contrast to photons, which affect tissues by the electrons that they eject. Electron beams deliver a high skin dose and exhibit a rapid fall-off after only a few centimeters and are therefore commonly used to treat superficial targets such as skin cancers or lymph nodes within a few centimeters of the surface of the body. More commonly, electromagnetic radiation (high-energy photons) is used to treat cancer. This consists of either gamma rays (photons created from the decay of radioactive nuclei) or x-rays (photons created by interaction of accelerated electrons with electrons and nuclei of atoms in an x-ray tube target).

To quantify the interaction of radiation on tissues, one must first measure the ionization produced in air by the beam of radiation. This quantity is known as **exposure** and is measured in Roentgens (R). One can then correct for the presence of soft tissue and calculate the **absorbed dose**: the amount of energy absorbed per unit mass. This quantity was previously measured in rads but today is typically measured as joules per kilogram, or gray (Gy) units: 100 rad = 100 cGy = 1 Gy. As photons enter tissue, the dose increases at first and then begins to fall off because radiation falls off with the square of the distance from the source (a law of physics known as the inverse-square law).

The effect on biological tissues when they encounter ionizing radiation comes from ejected electrons interacting either directly with target molecules within the cell or indirectly with water to produce free radicals (such as hydroxyl radicals) that subsequently interact with target molecules. During their brief life span, electrons and free radicals interact with molecules in a random fashion. If they interact with molecules that are not crucial to cell survival, the effect of the radiation will be harmless. If they react with biologically important molecules, the effect will be detrimental. Molecular oxygen prolongs the life of reactive radicals, increasing the likelihood that it will have a detrimental effect. This is why tumor hypoxia tends to increase resistance to radiation.

While ionizing radiation may damage many molecules with the cell, the most critical injury with respect to cell death appears to be DNA damage in the form of single-strand or double-strand breaks. Cells have relatively efficient repair mechanisms for single-strand breaks in DNA, but double-strand breaks in DNA are much more difficult for cells to repair, although not impossible. Therefore, the ability of ionizing radiation to kill cells is dependent not only on the generation of enough DNA double-strand breaks to overwhelm repair pathways but also on the time the cell has to repair those breaks prior to the next mitotic cell division.

This phenomenon is known as **sublethal damage repair** in which increased cell survival is observed if a dose of radiation is divided into two fractions separated by a time interval. As the time interval between the fractions increases, the surviving fraction of the cells also increases as the cells are able to repair double-strand DNA breaks. Of course, in clinical radiation therapy, the goal is to kill the cancer cells but spare the normal cells. Delivering a single large dose of radiation will have a high rate of tumor cell killing, but the concordant killing of the normal tissue cells may limit the clinical utility due to normal tissue toxicity. This has led to the development of multifraction regimens commonly used today, typically delivering daily fractions of 1.8-2.5 Gy. *Fractionation* of radiation dose spares normal tissues because of their greater ability to repair sublethal damage between dose fractions and repopulate with cells if the overall time is sufficiently long.

► Modes of Delivery

A. Teletherapy

Radiation is administered by two methods: an external machine (teletherapy) or the implantation of radioactive sources in or around the tumor (brachytherapy). In the past, teletherapy radiation was delivered using cobalt 60, a radioisotope produced in nuclear reactors. Although cobalt machines were very reliable, their usefulness is restricted by limited penetration to deep tumors without significant skin toxicity and difficulty in confining the dose to normal tissues. Today, external radiation is most often administered using a linear accelerator capable of producing higher energy photons without the geometric disadvantages associated with cobalt 60 units.

No matter the source, the beam of radiation needs to be modified to get optimal delivery of the desired dose to the tumor while minimizing dose to the normal tissues. Typically, the beam of radiation is rectangular. Collimators are thick shielding devices made from materials with a high atomic number. Primary collimators at the head of the machine create a rectangular beam, and additional devices such as wedges, compensators, blocks, or multileaf collimators are used to further modify the beam to desired specifications. Wedges or compensators can optimize the dose distribution if the treatment surface is curved or irregular in shape. The beam can also be shaped using individually fashioned blocks custom-made for each patient's anatomy and tumor size and shape. In modern linear accelerators, multileaf collimators have replaced handmade blocks and allow automated and precise field shaping without the use of cumbersome handmade blocks.

B. Brachytherapy

Brachytherapy involves the placement of radioactive sources into or next to the target tissue. It takes advantage of the inverse-square law, which states that the intensity of electromagnetic radiation dissipates as the inverse square of the distance from the source. Thus, if radioactive sources can be placed so that the tumor is within a centimeter of the sources, the dose received by normal tissues just 2 cm distant from the source and 1 cm distant from the tumor would be one fourth of the dose received by the tumor. This can allow delivery of a high dose to the tumor with only a modest dose to normal tissue.

There are many implantation techniques for brachytherapy. The surgical approach to the target volume may be interstitial (such as prostate seed implantation), intracavitary (such as gynecologic applicators), transluminal (such as endoscopic applications), or surface mold techniques (such as eye plaques for ocular melanoma). The implants may be permanent or temporary, and the dose may be delivered using low-, medium-, or high-dose rates. Many modern applications use afterloading techniques that place treatment applicators and subsequently load radioactive sources to reduce radiation exposure for therapy personnel.

► Complications of Radiation Therapy

A. Acute Radiation Effects

Acute radiation effects are those toxicities that occur within a few weeks to months of radiation therapy. They occur mainly in self-renewing tissues that are characterized by actively proliferating stem cells producing progeny that divide and differentiate into mature functioning cells. This includes bone marrow, skin and its appendages, and mucosal surfaces of the oropharynx, esophagus, stomach, intestines, rectum, bladder, and vagina. Once the normal life span of the mature cells expires, the normal turnover and replacement with new cells does not occur because of radiation killing of the dividing stem cells. Acute toxicity is influenced by both fraction size and the time interval between fractions. The more rapidly a given dose is delivered during the overall treatment period, the more severe the acute effects will be. A decrease in fraction size or prolongation of the interval between fractions allows the cell populations to repair and repopulate, decreasing the severity of acute toxicity.

Head and neck irradiation is among the most toxic in the acute period due to significant mucositis of the oral cavity, oropharynx, larynx, and cervical esophagus. Skin and the salivary glands are also affected. Mucositis, yeast superinfection, desquamation, pain, xerostomia, odynophagia, dysphagia, dehydration, and malnutrition are all common clinical scenarios that radiation oncologists manage when delivering head and neck radiotherapy. Other common acute effects observed during radiation therapy directed at other anatomic sites include dysphagia and cough from thoracic radiation, nausea, vomiting, and diarrhea from abdominal radiation, and dysuria, proctitis, and perineal desquamation and pain from pelvic radiation.

B. Late Radiation Effects

Late effects are those toxicities that occur months to years after radiotherapy and are more commonly permanent. Mitotically inactive tissues without the capacity for self-renewal are commonly involved. The mechanism causing late effects may include direct damage to the parenchymal cells within an organ or indirect effects due to microvascular damage. Each organ is characterized by a **tolerance dose**, a radiation dose above which the risk of organ complications increases rapidly. These normal tissue tolerances are the true dose-limiting factors in clinical radiation therapy, because late complications can be permanent and in some cases life threatening.

The types of late complications induced by radiation can vary. For the brain, late toxicity may mean necrosis of the brain tissue, while in the kidney it may mean nephrotic syndrome and organ failure. The tolerance doses for different organs vary over a large range, from a few Gy for sterility from testicular irradiation to over 100 Gy for necrosis or perforation of the uterus. Late complications may include fibrosis, necrosis, ulceration and bleeding, chronic edema, telangiectasias and pigmentation changes, cataract formation, nerve damage, lung pneumonitis and fibrosis, pericarditis, myocardial damage, bone fracture, liver or kidney failure, sterility, intestinal obstruction, and fistula and stricture formation.

Gunderson LL, Tepper JE: *Clinical Radiation Oncology*, 3rd ed. Elsevier Saunders, Philadelphia, PA 2011.

Perez CA, Brady LW, eds: *Principles and Practice of Radiation Oncology*, 5th ed. Lippincott Williams & Wilkins, Philadelphia, PA 2007.

IMMUNOTHERAPY

▶ Principles of Antitumor Immune Responses

Immunotherapy refers to treatments designed to kill tumor cells through immune mechanisms. There are two broad types of antitumor immune responses: one involving the humoral arm of the immune system and the other involving the cellular arm. Humoral immunity involves antibody production by mature B lymphocytes. Cell-mediated immunity involves stimulation of cytotoxic (CD8+) T cells through a major histocompatibility complex (MHC) class I-restricted process and stimulation of helper (CD4+) T cells through an MHC class II-restricted process. The humoral and cell-mediated immune responses overlap in that the activation of a B-cell response usually requires the presence of helper T cells. Whether a humoral or a cell-mediated immune response is more important in generating antitumor immunity is still debated; however, patients who exhibit both responses appear to fare better than those who demonstrate only one type of response or no response.

Essential to the generation of an immune response through either arm of the immune system is the ability of antigen-presenting cells (APCs), such as monocytes, macrophages, B cells, and dendritic cells, to process and present tumor-related peptide antigens. Proteins are phagocytosed by APCs and partially digested into smaller polypeptides. These small peptide antigens are then bound to MHC molecules on the cell surface. These unique antigen:MHC complexes can then be recognized by naïve T lymphocytes through the T-cell receptor. When a naïve helper (CD4+) T cell recognizes the antigen being expressed on the MHC class II molecule and also recognizes costimulatory molecules present on the APC, it becomes activated, resulting in proliferation and differentiation. There are two types of helper T cells. The Th1 helper T cells produce cytokines to promote a cellular response (interleukin [IL]-2, interferon [IFN]-γ, tumor necrosis factor α, granulocyte-macrophage colony-stimulating factor). In the presence of these cytokines, naïve cytotoxic (CD8+) T cells that recognize antigen being presented on MHC class I molecules on the surface of an APC become activated. Once activated, cytolytic T cells destroy tumor cells via T-cell receptor recognition of tumor-specific antigen presented on MHC class I molecules at the tumor cell surface. Antigen-specific T cells bind to the MHC I receptor–tumor antigen complex and destroy the tumor cell via the release of granules containing granzyme B and perforin and via induction of the Fas/Fas ligand apoptosis. Cytotoxic T cells can only recognize antigen expressed on the tumor surface in the context of the MHC class I molecule.

The second type of helper T cell (Th2) secretes B-cell stimulatory cytokines (IL-4, IL-5, IL-10), which results in the proliferation and differentiation of plasma cells. As opposed to a cellular response, for an antibody response, the antigens do not have to be presented on class I MHC receptors. Tumor cells can then be killed by a variety of methods. Antibody-dependent cell-mediated cytotoxicity involves the attachment of tumor-specific antibodies to tumor cells and the subsequent destruction of the tumor cell by the natural killer (NK) cell. Complement-dependent cell-mediated cytotoxicity involves the recognition and attachment of complement-fixing antibodies to tumor-specific surface antigens followed by complement activation. A third mechanism of tumor destruction, opsonization, results when tumor-specific antibodies attach to their target antigens on tumor cell surfaces, thus marking them for engulfment by macrophages.

There are several methods by which the immune system may be incorporated into cancer therapy. Immunotherapy can be categorized as either active or passive. With passive immunotherapy, the host need not mount an immune response; the therapeutic agent will directly or indirectly mediate tumor killing. Examples of passive immunotherapy include the use of monoclonal antibodies or adoptive (cellular) immunotherapy. Active immunotherapy, on the other hand, is the delivery of materials designed to elicit an immune response by the host. This can further be broken down to nonspecific and specific active immunotherapies. Nonspecific agents are those that stimulate the immune system globally but do not recruit tumor-specific effector cells. Active specific immunotherapy is designed to elicit an immune response to one or more tumor antigens, the prime example being the use of vaccines.

▶ Passive Immunotherapy (Monoclonal Antibodies)

The development of monoclonal antibodies with unique specificity to tumor antigens has allowed for multiple attempts to utilize them as cancer therapy. In addition to their relative selectivity and minimal toxicity, they are easily mass produced for widespread application. In some cases, monoclonal antibodies work primarily through the immune system (antibody-dependent cell-mediated cytotoxicity), while in other cases, they behave more as targeted therapies (see earlier section on Targeted Therapies). Examples of monoclonal antibodies that are primarily immunotherapies include rituximab and alemtuzumab. Rituximab (Rituxan) is an anti-CD20 monoclonal antibody that is approved for the treatment of relapsed or refractory low-grade or follicular non-Hodgkin lymphoma (NHL). Alemtuzumab (Campath) targets CD52, which is present on both B and T cells, and is used in the treatment of B-cell chronic lymphocytic leukemia (B-CLL).

▶ Adoptive Immunotherapy

Adoptive immunotherapy is the passive administration of cells with antitumor activity to the tumor-bearing host. Tumor-infiltrating lymphocytes are lymphocytes that infiltrate growing tumors and can be isolated by growing single-cell suspensions from the tumor in the presence of IL-2. They have been isolated from virtually all types of tumors and can recognize tumor-associated antigens. These cells can also be manipulated ex vivo to increase their recognition of tumor antigen or cytolytic potential. Adoptive immunotherapy is presently under active investigation.

▶ Nonspecific Active Immunotherapy

A. Immunostimulants

Before the mechanism by which the immune system can eradicate tumor cells was fully understood, early attempts at immunotherapy involved nonspecific stimulation of the immune system. The idea was that any increase in immune reactivity would be associated with a concomitant increase in the antitumor immune response. Probably the most widely embraced immunostimulant investigated has been the use of bacille Calmette-Guérin (BCG), a modified form of the tubercle bacillus. Initial trials suggested a possible benefit, but multiple prospective, randomized trials in various malignancies have failed to substantiate a survival benefit of BCG, either alone or in combination with other therapeutics. Local therapy with BCG in the bladder eliminates superficial bladder cancers and prevents tumor recurrences. It is one of several standard therapies for patients with bladder cancer. It is also being studied as an adjuvant to other immunotherapies, such as vaccines. Levamisole is an antihelminthic drug that was reported to have several immunomodulatory properties. Although the exact mechanism of action is unknown, it has been effective in the adjuvant therapy of colorectal cancer.

B. Cytokines

Cytokines are naturally occurring soluble proteins produced by mononuclear cells of the immune system that can affect the growth and function of cells through interaction with specific cell-surface receptors. There have been over 50 cytokines isolated to date, and several have subsequently been approved by the FDA for clinical use, including interferon-α and IL-2.

The interferons (IFN-α, IFN-β, IFN-γ) were originally described as proteins produced by virally infected cells that serve to protect against further viral infection through a variety of effects. These include the increased antigen presentation via increased expression of MHC and antigens, enhancement of NK cell function, and the enhancement of antibody-dependent cell-mediated cytotoxicity. In addition, the interferons exert direct antiangiogenic, cytotoxic, and cytostatic effects. While the anticancer effects of IFN-β and IFN-γ have been disappointing, several hematologic and solid tumors have proved responsive to IFN-α, including chronic myelogenous leukemia, cutaneous T-cell lymphoma, hairy cell leukemia, melanoma, and Kaposi sarcoma.

IL-2 was originally described as the "T-cell growth factor" because it is required for the differentiation and proliferation of activated T cells. As such, it seems like an ideal choice for immunotherapy. The major drawback of IL-2 is the significant dose-related toxicity. IL-2 leads to significant interstitial edema and vascular depletion and lymphoid infiltration into vital organs, possibly resulting in severe hypotension and ischemic damage to the heart, liver, kidneys, and bowel, which limits the use of IL-2 to patients with excellent performance status, normal pulmonary and cardiac function, and no active infections. Despite these limitations, IL-2 has proved to be an effective therapy in patients with metastatic melanoma and metastatic renal cell carcinoma.

▶ Specific Active Immunotherapy (Vaccines)

The goal of cancer vaccines is to generate a host immune response to known or unknown tumor-associated antigens. Many different vaccine strategies are under investigation, each with advantages and disadvantages in regard to clinical feasibility, cost, the number of antigens available, and the mechanism of response (cellular, humoral, or both). Some vaccine strategies use specific peptide antigens. These are highly purified and therefore are easy to standardize, distribute, and administer. Unfortunately, immunizing a patient against a single antigen has several drawbacks that limit the potential clinical benefit. If a peptide vaccine does stimulate a response, it may not be the "right" peptide for many patients. Even commonly expressed tumor antigens are not present on all patients' tumors, or they may be present in varying degrees. In addition, the T-cell recognition of an antigen depends on the presentation of that antigen on a specific MHC molecule. Only certain human lymphocyte antigen (HLA) phenotypes can present any given peptide to induce an immune response, so they will function only on a limited subset of patients. A classic example is that of the MART-1/Melan-A antigen in melanoma. The antigen is expressed by 80% of melanomas, but the peptide only binds to HLA-A2. Because only about 45% of Caucasians have HLA-A2, only 36% (80% of 45%) of melanoma patients given a MART-1/Melen-A vaccine would see a benefit. Finally, a cancer can escape immune recognition rather simply if a population of cells stops expressing that antigen or the MHC molecule.

For many cancers, only a few tumor-associated antigens have been defined; these may not be present on a large percentage of patients. Using the patient's cancer as the vaccine precludes the need to identify specific antigens. Autologous tumor cell vaccines are created from cancer cells harvested from the patient, altered to be more immunogenic, and irradiated, before being returned to the patient to stimulate a tumor-specific immune response. This approach is limited to individuals with sufficient tumor to prepare a vaccine. Trials are restricted to patients with bulky nodal or accessible distant metastatic disease who have a poor overall prognosis to begin with. Furthermore, the technical complexities inherent in procuring tumor and preparing a vaccine have made it difficult to conduct multi-institutional trials to test the efficacy of these vaccines.

Since many tumor-associated antigens are shared among a large number of patients, it is possible that one could create a vaccine from cultured cell lines that would stimulate an antitumor immune response in any patient who shared some of those antigens. This is the principle behind allogeneic tumor cell vaccines. This approach offers several advantages over autologous vaccines: Allogeneic vaccines are readily available, even for patients who lack sufficient tumor to produce an autologous tumor cell vaccine, and can be standardized, preserved, and distributed in a manner akin to any other therapeutic agent.

Tumor-Induced Immunosuppression

It is becoming increasingly apparent that in addition to mechanisms to generate and propagate an immune response, the immune system has several mechanisms to limit an immune response. This immune regulatory function is necessary to prevent lymphoproliferative disorders and autoimmune diseases. Neoplasms, however, may take advantage of this, creating an immunosuppressive network within the tumor microenvironment that protects the tumor from immune attack and minimizes the efficacy of immunotherapy.

Several components of the immune system function to regulate or limit an immune response. While it was initially thought that dendritic cells were exclusively immunogenic, recent evidence suggests that they possess dual functions, and some subsets of dendritic cells possess a regulatory function. Myeloid-derived suppressor cells can also suppress the antitumor response to cancer by blocking the effects of cytotoxic T cells in the tumor microenvironment.

In addition to cytotoxic and helper T cells, another T-cell population is the regulatory T cell, which also functionally suppresses immune responses. Immunosuppressive cytokines within the tumor microenvironment (IL-6, IL-10, TFG-β) may function to intensify these immunosuppressive components, augmenting tumor escape from immune recognition. It is also possible that many immunotherapies fail by augmenting not only immune stimulation but immune suppression, canceling out the effect. In some cases, these therapies may tilt the response toward immune suppression, for a detrimental effect. Newer immunotherapeutic strategies are focusing on not only increasing immune recognition of the tumor but blocking the suppressive mechanisms. These include pretreatment depletion of regulatory T cells, blocking suppressive pathways or neutralizing immunosuppressive cytokines.

Activated T lymphocytes express the molecule CTLA-4 (cytotoxic T lymphocyte-associated antigen 4), which exerts a suppressive effect on the induction of immune response through its interactions with the B7 molecules on antigen-presenting cells. Blocking the binding of CTLA-4, through the use of monoclonal antibodies, can therefore enhance antitumor T-cell responses. Ipilimumab (Yervoy), a monoclonal antibody to CTLA-4, has been shown to cause tumor regression and improve survival in patients with metastatic melanoma. PD-L1 is often expressed on tumor cells, and when it binds to PD-1 on T cells, can prevent T-cell function and lead to anergy. The use of an anti-PD-1 monoclonal antibody in patients with a variety of advanced cancers showed promising tumor responses, and may provide a new immunotherapy for patients with PD-L1 expressing tumors.

Abbas AK, Lichtman AH, Pober JS, eds: *Cellular and Molecular Immunology*, 7th ed. Elsevier, Philadelphia, PA 2012.

Hodi FS, O'Day SJ, McDermott DF, et al: Improved survival with ipilimumab in patients with metastatic melanoma. *N Engl J Med* 2010;363:711-723.

Murphy KM: *Janeway's Immunobiology*, 8th ed. Garland Science, New York, 2014.

Topalian SL, Hodi FS, Brahmer JR, et al: Safety, activity and immune correlates of anti-PD-1 antibody in cancer. *N Engl J Med* 2012;366:2443-2454.

SPECIFIC TYPES OF MALIGNANT NEOPLASMS

SOFT TISSUE SARCOMA

Soft tissue sarcomas account for approximately 1% of all new cancer diagnoses. Almost half of all patients diagnosed with the disease eventually die as a result of the cancer. Soft tissue sarcomas can occur anywhere in the body, but most originate in an extremity (41%), the trunk (10%), the retroperitoneum

(16%), visceral sites (21%), or the head and neck (12%). Soft tissue sarcomas originate from a wide variety of mesenchymal cell types and include malignant fibrous histiocytoma, liposarcoma, rhabdomyosarcoma, leiomyosarcoma, and desmoid tumors. While the histopathology of these tumors is highly variable, with some exceptions they tend to behave in a fashion dictated by tumor grade rather than the cell of origin.

Most soft tissue sarcomas arise de novo, and rarely do they result from malignant degeneration of a benign lesion. There are several familial syndromes in which patients are genetically predisposed to the formation of soft tissue sarcomas, including Li-Fraumeni syndrome, Recklinghausen disease, and Gardner syndrome. Other proven risk factors exist that may increase the chances of sarcoma formation. External radiation therapy can increase the incidence of sarcomas by 8-fold to 50-fold. Chronic extremity lymphedema also increases the risk for lymphangiosarcoma. A classic example is the development of upper extremity lymphangiosarcomas in the lymphedematous arm of women treated for breast cancer (Stewart-Treves syndrome). Other less clear associations link chronic tissue trauma and occupational chemical exposures with an increased risk for sarcoma formation.

The major features of the staging system for soft tissue sarcomas are the grade of the tumor, its size, and the presence of metastatic disease (Table 44–3). Although the site of the tumor is not considered in staging, patients with retroperitoneal tumors tend to have a worse prognosis. Sarcomas generally metastasize by the hematogenous route, and the metastatic sites of sarcomas are related to the location of the primary tumor. The vast majority of metastases from extremity sarcomas are to the lung, while the majority of retroperitoneal tumors metastasize to the liver. Lymph node involvement is rare with most soft tissue sarcomas, although it may occur with epithelioid sarcoma, clear cell sarcoma, angiosarcoma, rhabdomyosarcoma, or synovial sarcoma.

The most important prognostic variables for patients with soft tissue sarcoma are the size and grade of the primary tumor. Since grading is based on the cellular architecture and invasive nature of the tumor, FNAB is not a typically useful biopsy technique for the initial diagnosis of a sarcoma. If a tumor is small (< 3 cm) and superficial, excisional biopsy should be performed. All extremity biopsy incisions should be oriented longitudinally, as the biopsy incision scar should be excised in a subsequent definitive resection of the tumor. Core needle biopsies may be performed for large, palpable superficial tumors. For large, deep tumors or those adjacent to vital structures, where core needle biopsy is not advised or failed, incisional biopsy should be considered. The incision should be centered over the mass, tissue flaps should not be raised, and meticulous hemostasis should be ensured, all to prevent the dissemination of tumor cells into adjacent tissue planes.

Table 44–3. AJCC staging system for soft tissue sarcoma.

Primary Tumor (T) https://www.protocols.fccc.edu/fccc/pims/staging/sarcoma.html
- TX: Primary tumor cannot be assessed
- T0: No evidence of primary tumor
- T1: Tumor 5.0 cm or less in greatest dimension
  - T1a: Superficial tumor
  - T1b: Deep tumor
- T2: Tumor more than 5.0 cm in greatest dimension
  - T2a: Superficial tumor
  - T2b: Deep tumor

Regional Lymph Nodes (N)
- NX: Regional lymph nodes cannot be assessed
- N0: No regional lymph node metastasis
- N1: Regional lymph node metastasis

Distant Metastasis (M)
- MX: Presence of distant metastasis cannot be accessed
- M0: No distant metastasis
- M1: Distant metastasis

Histopathologic Grade (G)
- GX: Grade cannot be assessed
- G1: Well differentiated
- G2: Moderately differentiated
- G3: Poorly differentiated

Stage Grouping

Stage IA	T1a-1b	N0	M0	G1, GX
Stage IB	T2a-2b	N0	M0	G1, GX
Stage IIA	T1a-1b	N0	M0	G2, G3
Stage IIB	T2a-2b	N0	M0	G2
Stage III	T2a, T2b	N0	M0	G3
	Any T	N1	M0	Any G
Stage IV	Any T	Any N	M1	Any G

▶ Treatment of Extremity Sarcomas

MRI is the imaging modality of choice for any suspected extremity sarcoma because it is most accurate in defining the extent of the tumor and invasion of surrounding structures. MRI is also used for follow-up imaging to assess response in patients undergoing therapy, as well as for local and regional recurrence. A chest x-ray or chest CT should be obtained in order to evaluate for pulmonary metastases in patients with high-grade tumors.

Surgery remains the primary therapy for localized extremity sarcomas, but multimodality therapy is recommended to minimize the likelihood of recurrence or the need for amputation. Historically, amputation was the only form of curative surgical therapy for large extremity sarcomas, but multimodality therapy has allowed for a high rate of limb preservation. Today, fewer than 5% of patients with extremity soft tissue sarcoma require amputation, generally reserved for patients whose tumors do not respond to preoperative therapy and cannot be resected adequately, have no evidence of metastatic disease, and have a good prognosis for rehabilitation.

A pseudocapsule composed of tumor cells surrounds sarcomas, and local invasion along fascial planes and neurovascular structures is common. It is important not to dissect along the pseudocapsule, which is associated with high local recurrence rates, but rather obtain a wide (2-cm) margin of normal tissue. This may need to be compromised in the immediate vicinity of functionally important neurovascular structures. If the tumor involves these structures, nerve grafts and arterial reconstruction with autologous or prosthetic conduits may be required. Large soft tissue defects often require the construction of myocutaneous flaps to improve function and cosmesis. Soft tissue sarcomas rarely invade bone or skin, and wide resections of these structures are infrequently necessary.

Following wide local excision, metal clips should be placed at all margins of the resection in order to guide subsequent radiotherapy. For patients with T1 tumors located superficially in an area where it is not difficult to obtain widely negative margins, postoperative radiation therapy may not be necessary. For most other lesions, postoperative radiation is almost always recommended, with either external beam radiation or brachytherapy. Radiation should be started 4-8 weeks after surgery, as delay can result in a lower local control rate. Preoperative radiotherapy may have some advantages in patients with large tumors. Lower doses can be delivered to an undisturbed tumor bed, which may also have better oxygenation, and larger tumors may decrease in size, allowing for limb-sparing procedures. Preoperative radiation is associated with an increase in short-term wound complications but a decrease in long-term tissue fibrosis and edema. The optimal mode and sequence for treatment has yet to be defined and often requires a multidisciplinary approach.

Adjuvant chemotherapy remains controversial. Chemotherapy can be given either preoperatively or postoperatively. The three drugs most effective in sarcoma are doxorubicin, dacarbazine, and ifosfamide. Preoperative chemotherapy is sometimes recommended because in addition to the early treatment of micrometastatic disease, it allows for assessment of tumor response, which helps avoid prolonged therapy in patients not responding. However, while disease-free survival may be improved, there are conflicting data on overall survival. A recent meta-analysis of randomized trials suggested there may be a small survival benefit for extremity sarcomas, and so its use has increased.

The vast majority of localized recurrences in soft tissue sarcomas occur in the first 2 years after resection, necessitating close follow-up during that period. A local recurrence is not indicative of systemic disease and, in the absence of evidence of metastases, should be treated aggressively in the same manner as a primary tumor. The resection of pulmonary metastases should be considered in patients who have fewer than four radiographically detectable lesions and who have achieved apparent local control following resection of the primary tumor. In such circumstances, disease-free survival can approach 25%-35%.

▶ Treatment of Retroperitoneal Sarcomas

Retroperitoneal sarcomas comprise approximately 15% of all soft tissue sarcomas, with liposarcoma, malignant fibrous histiocytoma, and leiomyosarcoma the three most common types. They usually present as a large abdominal mass. Nearly half are over 20 cm in size at diagnosis. Once they compress or invade contiguous structures, they can cause symptoms such as abdominal pain or nausea and vomiting. Workup should include CT of the abdomen and pelvis to evaluate the mass as well as CT of the lung and liver to look for metastases. CT-guided core biopsy is the sampling technique of choice, with open or laparoscopic incisional biopsy reserved for inconclusive core biopsies.

As with extremity sarcomas, surgery represents the primary treatment, with the goal being en bloc resection with a rim of normal tissue. Although retroperitoneal tumors are generally large at presentation and often invade vital structures, the majority of these tumors are resectable. Retroperitoneal sarcomas rarely invade surrounding organs, but an intense desmoplastic reaction makes it difficult to assess the extent of tumor, so often these organs need to be resected rather than risk positive margins. The kidney, colon, pancreas, and spleen are the most commonly resected organs.

While adjuvant radiation therapy is standard in extremity sarcoma, evidence supporting its use in retroperitoneal sarcoma is less convincing. Because of the low tolerance to radiation of the abdominal and retroperitoneal organs, delivery of adequate radiotherapy is often difficult. There is encouraging evidence for intraoperative radiation therapy to the tumor bed, but this technique is still considered investigational and can be performed only in select centers. Although complex, preoperative radiation may be beneficial because it uses lower radiation doses, is less injurious to the small bowel, and can increase respectability by shrinking the tumor and creating a thickened capsular structure around the lesion.

Weiss SW, Goldblum JR, eds: *Enzinger and Weiss's Soft Tissue Tumors*, 5th ed. Mosby, St. Louis, MO 2008.
Wong SL: Sarcomas of soft tissues and bone. In: *Scientific Principles and Practice*, 5th ed. Mulholland MW et al, eds. Lippincott Williams & Wilkins, Philadelphia, PA 2011.

MELANOMA

The incidence of melanoma is unfortunately rising. The reasons for this rise are not clear but are most likely related

Table 44–4. Clinical characteristics of melanoma (ABCDs).

A- **Asymmetry:** Asymmetric shape, color, or contour
B- **Borders:** Irregular or ill-defined borders
C- **Color:** Color variation within the lesion
D- **Difference:** Any lesion that has changed in size, shape, or color

Table 44–5: AJCC staging system for melanoma.

TNM Classification		
T1a	≤1 mm	without ulceration and mitoses < 1/mm^2
T1b	≤1 mm	with ulceration or mitoses ≥ 1/mm^2
T2a	1.01-2.0 mm	without ulceration
T2b	1.01-2.0 mm	with ulceration
T3a	2.01-4.0 mm	without ulceration
T3b	2.01-4.0 mm	with ulceration
T4a	> 4.0 mm	without ulceration
T4b	> 4.0 mm	with ulceration
N0	No regional metastases detected	
N1a	Micrometastasis in 1 node	
N1b	Macrometastasis in 1 node	
N2a	Micrometastasis in 2-3 nodes	
N2b	Macrometastasis in 2-3 nodes	
N2c	In-transit met(s)/satellite(s) without metastatic nodes	
N3	≥ 4 metastatic nodes, or matted nodes, or in-transit met(s)/satellite(s) with metastatic nodes	
M0	No detectable evidence of distant metastases	
M1a	Metastases to skin, subcutaneous, or distant lymph nodes with normal serum LDH	
M1b	Metastases to lung with normal serum LDH	
M1c	Metastases to all other visceral sites or any distant metastases with an elevated serum LDH	
Stage Groupings		
IA	T1a N0 M0	
IB	T1b N0 M0, T2a N0 M0	
IIA	T2b N0 M0, T3a N0 M0	
IIB	T3b N0 M0, T4a N0, M0	
IIC	T4b N0 M0	
IIIA	T1-4a, N1a or N2a, M0	
IIIB	T1-4b, N1a or N2a, M0	
	T1-4a, N1b, N2b or N2c, M0	
IIIC	T1-4b, N1b, N2b or N2c, M0	
	Any T, N3, M0	
IV	Any T, Any N, M1	

to an increased exposure to ultraviolet radiation from sunlight. Individuals whose first sunburn occurred at an early age, or have had three or more sunburns before age 21 have an increased incidence of melanoma, as do individuals who use tanning beds. Other risk factors include freckles, a fair complexion, reddish or blond hair, blue eyes, a first-degree relative with melanoma, and the presence of multiple or dysplastic nevi.

The best approach to melanoma is to prevent it from occurring, through sun avoidance and sun protection with sunscreens with a sun protection factor (SPF) of 30 or higher. Second to prevention, the most significant impact on melanoma comes from early recognition and diagnosis. The prognosis of melanoma is inversely and dramatically related to the depth of invasion at diagnosis (Breslow thickness), emphasizing the importance of early diagnosis of this disease. Lesions that are suspicious for melanoma can be identified by their clinical characteristics, often referred to as the ABCDs of melanoma (Table 44–4). Diagnosed early, well over 90% of primary melanomas can be cured with surgical excision alone. Patients presenting with thicker lesions or regional nodal metastases have a significantly poorer prognosis. The AJCC staging system is presented in Table 44–5.

There are several distinct categories of melanoma; the four most common are superficial spreading, nodular, lentigo maligna, and acral lentiginous melanoma.

Superficial spreading melanoma is the most common presentation, accounting for nearly 70% of all melanomas. These usually occur in sun-exposed areas of the body or in individuals with multiple dysplastic nevi. They generally arise in preexisting nevi and can occur at any age after puberty. The superficial spreading subtype tends to grow in a radial pattern during the earlier stages and converts to a vertical growth pattern during the later stages of development.

Nodular melanomas account for between 15% and 25% of all melanomas. These tend to occur in older individuals and are more common in men. Nodular melanomas generally develop de novo, not in a preexisting nevus. They usually are dome shaped with distinct borders and often resemble a blood blister. Nodular melanomas occur most commonly on the head, neck, and trunk. They lack a significant horizontal growth phase and tend to be deep at the time of diagnosis.

Lentigo maligna melanoma has less propensity to metastasize and thus has a more favorable prognosis relative to the other subtypes. However, it can be locally aggressive, with high recurrence rates after excision. These lesions account for 4%-10% of melanomas and occur in an older population. Lentigo maligna lesions almost always develop in sun-exposed areas. They have a long horizontal growth phase and often have very convoluted borders.

Acral lentiginous melanomas account for between 2% and 8% of melanomas in Caucasians but for 30%-60% of melanomas in blacks, Asians, and Hispanics. These lesions do not occur in sun-exposed areas; instead, they occur on the sole of the foot, the palm, beneath the nail beds, and in the perineal region. Acral lentiginous melanomas are often large, with an average diameter of 3 cm at the time of diagnosis. They develop relatively rapidly over the course of months to several years and tend to behave very aggressively. The clinical characteristics of these melanomas are often unmistakable, with variegations in color and convoluted borders. Ulceration of these lesions is common.

▶ Treatment of Primary Melanoma

Any suspected melanoma should be removed by punch or excisional biopsy. Given the importance of Breslow thickness, shave or curette biopsies are contraindicated. If the biopsy specimen reveals melanoma, a formal excision with adequate margins is required. Because microscopic tumor cells frequently surround primary melanomas, excision with narrow margins is associated with an unacceptably high rate of local recurrence. The current standard for lesions less than 1 mm in depth is excision with 1-cm margins. Melanomas between 1 and 2 mm in thickness should be excised with 2-cm margins, but a smaller margin (10-15 mm) may be acceptable in areas where it is difficult to get 2 cm without the need for a skin graft or exceptionally tight closure. Melanomas deeper than 2 mm should be excised with a 2-cm margin. The resection should be carried down to the underlying fascia, although the fascia need not be excised.

Melanomas generally metastasize by the lymphatic route in a predictable and orderly fashion. Any palpable nodes must be considered suspicious for metastatic involvement, easily verified with an FNAB. About 5%-10% of patients have clinical evidence of nodal metastases upon initial presentation and should undergo a therapeutic lymph node dissection at the time of their wide excision. Many patients will have microscopic disease in the lymph nodes that will not be apparent on physical examination. In the past, substantial controversy surrounded elective lymph node dissection of the draining nodal basin for melanoma. The practice gained dramatic acceptance, however, with the advent of the sentinel lymph node biopsy, which is based on the anatomic concept that lymphatic fluid from defined regions of skin drains specifically to an initial node or nodes ("sentinel nodes") prior to disseminating to other nodes in the same or nearby basins. Sentinel node biopsy allows for a more detailed histologic examination of the sentinel lymph nodes and helps avoid the morbidity of lymph node dissection

in patients who are pathologically node negative. Patients with a negative sentinel node are over six times more likely to survive than those with a positive sentinel lymph node, making the predictive impact of sentinel node status much greater than any other prognostic factor. Evidence also suggests that early removal of micrometastatic disease from the lymph nodes, as compared with waiting for regional recurrence to perform a lymph node dissection, may improve survival.

The sentinel lymph node biopsy has become the standard of care in the staging and treatment of melanoma and should be performed at the time of the wide excision for primary melanomas thicker than 1.0 mm. It should be selectively applied for tumors between 0.75 and 1.0 mm when other worrisome features are present, such as ulceration, angiolymphatic invasion or a mitotic rate >1. Melanomas less than 0.75 mm are very unlikely to have regional metastases and do not require sentinel lymph node biopsy. The dominant drainage basins can be identified by lymphoscintigraphy, which involves intradermal injection of technetium-99m (^{99m}Tc) sulfur colloid in the area around the tumor and a gamma camera to image the sites of lymph node drainage. In the operating room, blue dye (isosulfan or methylene) is injected in a similar fashion. Any lymph nodes that have evidence of ^{99m}Tc uptake on a handheld gamma probe, have evidence of blue dye, or are clinically suspicious should be excised. After removal of the nodes, they are analyzed by serial thin-sectioning, routine H&E staining, and immunohistochemical staining. Using these methods of analysis, the pathologist is able to detect even minute numbers of metastatic melanoma cells in the sentinel node. Patients with a positive sentinel lymph node biopsy should undergo formal lymph node dissection of the entire drainage basin, although the benefit of this is being examined in the prospective randomized Multicenter Selective Lymphadenectomy Trial-II (MSLT-II).

Traditional chemotherapy regimens have proved largely ineffective in the treatment of melanoma; however, the cytokine IFN alpha-2b (Intron A) has been shown to improve disease-free and overall survival in high-risk patients with no evidence of systemic metastases. This treatment is not without controversy, however, as the duration of therapy is long (12 months), the toxicities are substantial, and some of the data regarding the overall survival benefit are conflicting. An alternate approach to high-dose IFN alpha-2b is pegylated interferon alpha-2b. This has a longer half-life and can be administered subcutaneously with fewer side effects, albeit for a longer period of time (5 years). Finally, another consideration for adjuvant therapy is biochemotherapy, which combines IL-2, IFN alpha-2b, cisplatin, vinblastine, and DTIC. This regimen has significant toxicity but is shorter (9 weeks) and was shown in a prospective randomized trial to improve relapse-free survival compared with high-dose interferon, although there was no improvement in overall survival. All patients with high-risk melanoma (node-positive melanoma or thick, ulcerated, node-negative melanoma) should have a balanced discussion of the potential risks and benefits of adjuvant therapy. While melanoma is relatively radioresistant, there may be some benefit to regional control after node dissection with radiation in patients with gross extracapsular extension or multiple involved lymph nodes.

▶ Local Recurrence & In-transit Metastasis

Although rare with appropriate surgery, an isolated local recurrence can be treated with a repeat wide excision with 2-cm margins. Approximately 2%-3% of melanoma patients will develop in-transit metastasis, which is the appearance of metastasis along the path from the primary tumor to its regional nodal basin, and is lymphatic in nature. The management of in-transit metastasis is dictated by the number and the size of the lesions. If few in number, surgical excision with a margin of surrounding normal cutaneous and subcutaneous tissue is appropriate; however, this becomes unlikely with multiple lesions. Intralesional therapy with granulocyte-macrophage colony-stimulating factor can result in significant regression of melanoma deposits but requires multiple injections and is not always effective. Although melanoma is relatively radiation resistant, this therapy can provide palliation in unresectable lesions in many cases. Radiation therapy should be considered in those patients with a smaller volume of cutaneous or subcutaneous metastases.

Hyperthermic isolated limb perfusion (HILP) is a way of isolating the blood circuit to the extremity and administering chemotherapeutic agents regionally at a concentration 15-25 times higher without resulting in systemic side effects. Melphalan has been used as a standard drug for hyperthermic isolated limb perfusion secondary to its efficacy and low regional toxicity. While this has not been shown to improve survival, the use of hyperthermic isolated limb perfusion provides a significant palliation of locoregional symptoms when other options are not available. Less complicated, but also effective, is isolated limb infusion (ILI). This involves using minimally invasive techniques to access the vessels along with a tourniquet to minimize systemic uptake.

Regional and systemic recurrence of melanoma can be latent, and recurrence 10 years after the original diagnosis is not uncommon. This fact necessitates close lifelong follow-up of these patients. Patients with a past history of melanoma have a dramatically increased risk of developing a second primary lesion and require diligent screening for other lesions.

Balch CM, Houghton AN, Sober AJ, et al, eds: *Cutaneous Melanoma*, 5th ed. Quality Medical Publishing, St. Louis, MO 2009.
Sabel MS, Johnson TM, Bichakjian CK: Cutaneous neoplasms. In: *Scientific Principles and Practice*, 5th ed. Mulholland MW et al, eds. Lippincott Williams & Wilkins, Philadelphia, PA 2011.

LYMPHOMA

Lymphomas are malignant neoplasms that originate from the lymphoid tissues. Two distinct categories of lymphoma exist: Hodgkin and non-Hodgkin. The two types not only have different morphologic characteristics but differ also in their clinical behavior and their response to various therapeutic regimens. It is not possible to differentiate Hodgkin and non-Hodgkin lymphoma on clinical grounds; surgical biopsy is necessary. In the diagnosis of a suspected lymphoma, excisional biopsy of the entire lymph node or nodes is imperative, as the architecture has a bearing on the diagnosis and the subsequent treatment of the tumor.

1. Hodgkin Lymphoma

Hodgkin lymphoma may occur at any age but is generally a disease of young adults. Prevalence in women peaks in the third decade and then falls, while it remains fairly constant in men after this time. The diagnosis of Hodgkin lymphoma is based on the finding of Reed-Sternberg cells in an appropriate cellular background of reactive leukocytes and fibrosis. It is the pattern of the lymphocytic infiltrate that determines the classic subtypes of Hodgkin disease (see Table 44–6). All subtypes of classical Hodgkin lymphoma are presently treated in the same way, and modern therapy has allowed for cure of over 70% of patients with this malignancy.

The cause of Hodgkin disease is not well understood; however, epidemiologic studies have revealed certain patterns of disease clustering. The incidence appears to be higher with a lower number of siblings, early birth order, siblings with Hodgkin disease, a decreased number of playmates, certain HLAs, single-family dwellings, and patients who have undergone tonsillectomy. The incidence is increased also in persons with immunodeficiencies and autoimmune disorders. This pattern suggests that an oncogenic virus may cause Hodgkin disease. Nuclear proteins of the Epstein-Barr virus have been

Table 44–6. Classic subtypes of Hodgkin lymphoma.

Subtype	Characteristics
Lymphocyte-predominant	Uncommon (6% of Hodgkin lymphomas), diffuse lymphocytic infiltrate with few Reed-Sternberg cells, excellent prognosis
Lymphocyte-depleted	Rare (2% of Hodgkin lymphoma), abundant Reed-Sternberg cells, paucity of lymphocytes, occurs in older males, aggressive clinically
Mixed cellularity	Common (20%-25% of Hodgkin lymphoma), histologically intermediate between above two forms, often presents with disseminated disease
Nodular sclerosis	Most common form (70% of Hodgkin lymphoma), fibrosis with Reed-Sternberg and lymphoid cells, more common in young women, presents with cervical or mediastinal disease

detected in about 40% of classical Hodgkin lymphoma, and alternative lymphotropic viruses may be involved in the pathogenesis of cases negative for Epstein-Barr virus.

Most patients present with enlarged but painless lymph nodes, typically in the lower neck or supraclavicular region. On occasion, mediastinal masses are associated with cough or dyspnea or discovered on routine chest x-ray. About 25% of patients will have systemic symptoms, called B symptoms, including weight loss, pruritus, fever, and drenching night sweats.

▶ Staging

With regard to therapy, the most important prognostic factor in Hodgkin lymphoma is the disease stage. The AJCC staging system for Hodgkin and non-Hodgkin lymphoma is shown in Table 44–7. The Ann Arbor staging system is also commonly used, which further subclassifies the stages into A and B categories: B for those with weight loss, fever, night sweats, or other constitutional symptoms, and A for those without such symptoms.

Table 44–7. AJCC staging system for Hodgkin and Non-Hodgkin lymphoma.

Stage	Prognostic Groups
I	Involvement of a single lymphatic site (ie, nodal region, Waldeyer ring, thymus, or spleen) (I)
	OR
	Localized involvement of a single extralymphatic organ or site in the absence of any lymph node involvement (IE) (rare in Hodgkin lymphoma)
II	Involvement of two or more lymph node regions on the same side of the diaphragm (II)
	OR
	Localized involvement of a single extralymphatic organ or site in association with regional lymph node involvement with or without involvement of other lymph node regions on the same side of the diaphragm (IIE). The number of regions involved may be indicated by a subscript Arabic numeral, for example, II_3
III	Involvement of lymph node regions on both sides of the diaphragm (III), which also may be accompanied by extralymphatic extension in association with adjacent lymph node involvement (IIIE) or by involvement of the spleen (IIIS) or both (IIIE, IIIS). Splenic involvement is designated by the letter S
IV	Diffuse or disseminated involvement of one or more extralymphatic organs, with or without associated lymph node involvement
	OR
	Isolated extralymphatic organ involvement in the absence of adjacent regional lymph node involvement, but in conjunction with disease in distant site(s). Stage IV includes any involvement of the liver or bone marrow, lungs (other than by direct extension from another site), or cerebrospinal fluid

As discussed earlier, excisional lymph node biopsy is essential to the diagnosis of Hodgkin lymphoma. Once the diagnosis is made, disease staging begins with a detailed history and physical examination, with attention to all lymph node beds, B symptoms, and symptoms related to extranodal involvement. CT of the chest, abdomen, and pelvis is the major means of staging intrathoracic and intra-abdominal disease. Bone marrow biopsy is also part of the staging evaluation of patients with bony symptoms or cytopenias. Fluorodeoxyglucose F 18 (FDG-PET) scan significantly adds to the staging of Hodgkin lymphoma and has become a standard staging tool both before treatment and at completion. In the past, a staging laparotomy (splenectomy, wedge liver biopsy, and dissection of the para-aortic, iliac, splenic hilar, and hepatic portal lymph nodes) was used to determine the extent of disease in the abdomen. Given the improved imaging studies and the inclusion of chemotherapy for patients even with favorable stage I disease, staging laparotomies are rarely, if ever, performed.

▶ Treatment

Hodgkin lymphoma has changed from a uniformly fatal disease to one that is curable in almost three-quarters of patients. Treatment is guided by both the stage of disease as well as stratification into favorable and unfavorable prognosis. This has allowed for less intensive therapy in patients with a favorable prognosis, with no compromise in outcome. The definition of favorable disease differs with different groups, but takes into account stage and extent of disease, age, ESR, and symptoms. For patients with favorable prognosis stage I-II disease, treatment typically involves a combination of ABVD chemotherapy (doxorubicin, bleomycin, vinblastine, dacarbazine) in combination with involved field irradiation. For patients at risk of long-term complications from radiation, 4 to 6 cycles of ABVD without radiation can be considered, although there are higher recurrence rates compared with combined modality therapy. Patients with unfavorable stage I-II disease are treated with more cycles of AVBD in combination with irradiation.

While ABVD remains the standard regimen for stage III-IV Hodgkin lymphoma (advanced stage), newer regimens include escalated BEACOPP (bleomycin, etoposide, doxorubicin, cyclophosphamide, vincristine, procarbazine, and prednisone) and Stanford V (doxorubicin, vinblastine, mechlorethamine, vincristine bleomycin, etoposide and prednisone). Consolidation radiotherapy may be considered with ABVD or BEACOPP, but is an essential component of the Stanford V protocol. The response rates, toxicity and patient comorbidities must be weighed when deciding on a regimen.

Approximately 5%-10% of patients are refractory to initial therapy, and 10%-30% will relapse after complete remission. In this case, salvage therapy typically involves an alternate chemotherapy regimen. High-dose chemotherapy and autologous hematopoietic cell transplantation (HCT) should be considered for patients with early relapse (within 12 months), second relapse or a generalized systemic relapse, even after 12 months. For patients who fail this approach or are not candidates for high-dose chemotherapy with HCT, there are unfortunately few good treatment options.

2. Non-Hodgkin Lymphoma

Non-Hodgkin lymphoma encompasses a wide spectrum of lymphoid-derived tumors. This heterogeneous group of diseases includes more than 10 distinct tumor subtypes with variable biologic behavior and responses to treatment. As opposed to Hodgkin lymphoma, the prevalence of non-Hodgkin lymphoma rises with age. The incidence has been rising steadily over the past 20 years by about 3%-5% per year, for unknown reasons. Several risk factors have been identified that predispose patients to the development of disease. Patients with congenital disorders such as ataxia-telangiectasia, Wiskott-Aldrich syndrome, and celiac disease have an increased incidence of lymphoma. Certain acquired conditions also predispose patients to lymphoma, including prior chemotherapy or radiotherapy, immunosuppressive therapy, Epstein-Barr infection, HIV infection, human T-cell lymphoma virus [HTLV]-1 infection, *Helicobacter pylori* gastritis, Hashimoto thyroiditis, and Sjögren syndrome.

Non-Hodgkin lymphoma may originate from B cells, T cells, or histiocytes. Morphologically, the tumors may appear as nodular clusters or diffuse sheets of lymphoid cells.

Classically, non-Hodgkin lymphoma presents as non-tender enlargement of lymph nodes, but nearly one-third of all cases originate outside the lymph nodes. These extranodal malignancies develop in organs that normally have nests of lymphoid tissue (mucosal surfaces, bone marrow, and skin).

▶ Staging & Classification

The goal of the staging evaluation is to distinguish patients who have localized disease from those with disseminated disease. After pathologic diagnosis, the staging evaluation for non-Hodgkin lymphoma consists of a detailed history and physical examination, routine laboratory tests, a bone marrow biopsy, and a CT scan of the neck, chest, abdomen, and pelvis. Evaluation of the cerebrospinal fluid should be considered in patients with diffuse large-cell non-Hodgkin lymphoma with bone marrow involvement, a high lactate dehydrogenase (LDH) level, or multiple extranodal sites of disease. It should also be considered in patients with high-grade lymphomas, HIV-related lymphomas, primary central nervous system lymphomas, and posttransplantation lymphoproliferative disorders. Finally, FDG-PET scans provide whole-body images that allow a comprehensive assessment of disease extent and, in conjunction with CT, provides complementary staging information. A pretreatment PET scan is often obtained so that PET can be used for monitoring of response to treatment. Normal PET at the end of therapy correlates with a highly

favorable prognosis, while persistent abnormalities mandate close follow-up or biopsy to rule out residual disease.

The staging system for Hodgkin lymphoma is also used in non-Hodgkin lymphoma. Although helpful in assessing the anatomic extent of disease, the Ann Arbor system is of minimal clinical value in non-Hodgkin lymphoma. The international prognostic index (IPI) uses patient age, Ann Arbor stage, LDH level, number of extranodal sites, and ECOG performance status to categorize aggressive non-Hodgkin lymphoma. However, this system does not clearly stratify indolent lymphomas, so another prognostic factor model was devised for follicular lymphoma. The follicular lymphoma international prognostic index uses patient age, Ann Arbor stage, hemoglobin level, number of nodal areas, and serum LDH level to stage patients.

Scientists have made countless attempts to develop a universal, clinically relevant classification system for the subtypes of non-Hodgkin lymphoma, and the merits of the various classifications are an area of hot debate. The most widely accepted classification system is the Revised European-American Lymphoma/World Health Organization (REAL/WHO) classification (Table 44–8).

In determining the therapeutic approach to patients with non-Hodgkin lymphoma, a simpler classification system can be utilized. For treatment purposes, these lymphomas can be functionally divided into two groups: indolent (low-grade) and aggressive (high-grade) lymphomas. Smaller, differentiated cells characterize the indolent lymphomas, and this class tends to have a follicular architecture. Although the course of these lymphomas is not very aggressive and they have a long median survival, they are not usually curable in advanced clinical stages. The natural history of indolent lymphomas often involves progression of the tumor cells to a more aggressive subtype. This progression is sometimes heralded by the onset of B symptoms and portends a dismal prognosis.

The aggressive lymphomas behave differently from the indolent ones and demand a different therapeutic approach. Histologically, the aggressive lymphomas spread more diffusely throughout the lymph nodes and consist of larger, less differentiated cell types. This class of lymphomas demonstrates a very rapid growth rate and an increased rate of early mortality. Despite this malignant behavior, this class of non-Hodgkin lymphoma is more often curable. The extranodal lymphomas develop outside of the lymph nodes and are not amenable to conventional classifications, so they are generally regarded as a separate entity. They can involve any organ but most commonly affect the oropharynx, paranasal sinuses, thyroid, gastrointestinal tract, liver, testicles, skin, and bone marrow.

▶ Treatment

A. Indolent Lymphoma

Patients with localized disease, although this is the minority, can be treated with radiation therapy only with curative

Table 44–8. Revised European-American lymphoma/World Health Organization (REAL/WHO) classification of lymphoma.

B-cell neoplasms
I. Precursor B-cell neoplasm
Precursor B-lymphoblastic leukemia/lymphoma (B-ALL/LBL)
II. Mature (peripheral) B-cell neoplasms
B-cell chronic lymphocytic leukemia/small lymphocytic lymphoma
B-cell prolymphocytic leukemia
Lymphoplasmacytic lymphoma
Splenic marginal zone lymphoma (+/− villous lymphocytes)
Hairy cell leukemia
Plasma cell myeloma/plasmacytoma
Extranodal marginal zone B-cell lymphoma of MALT type
Mantle cell lymphoma
Follicular lymphoma
Nodal marginal zone B-cell lymphoma (+/− monocytoid B cells)
Diffuse large B-cell lymphoma
Burkitt lymphoma

T-cell and NK-cell neoplasms
I. Precursor T-cell neoplasm
Precursor T-lymphoblastic lymphoma/leukemia
II. Mature (peripheral) T-cell neoplasms
T-cell prolymphocytic leukemia
T-cell granular lymphocytic leukemia
Aggressive NK-cell leukemia
Adult T-cell lymphoma/leukemia (HTLV1+)
Extranodal NK/T-cell lymphoma, nasal type
Enteropathy-type T-cell lymphoma
Hepatosplenic gamma/delta T-cell lymphoma
Subcutaneous panniculitis-like T-cell lymphoma
Mycosis fungoides/Sezary syndrome
Anaplastic large cell lymphoma, primary cutaneous type
Peripheral T-cell lymphoma, unspecified
Angioimmunoblastic T-cell lymphoma
Anaplastic large cell lymphoma, primary systemic type

Hodgkin disease/lymphoma
I. Lymphocyte predominance
II. Nodular sclerosis
III. Mixed cellularity
IV. Lymphocyte depletion
V. Lymphocyte-rich classic Hodgkin disease

intent. Most patients have disseminated disease, which tends to be chronic relapsing and remitting. The current therapies for systemic indolent lymphomas are rarely curative, and the goal of treatment is generally directed at palliation of symptoms. At present, a "watch and wait" approach to treatment is recommended for asymptomatic patients. After diagnosis, asymptomatic patients are followed up clinically until they progress to more aggressive disease, major symptoms, or organ dysfunction. Withholding chemother-

apy does not reduce survival in patients with non-Hodgkin lymphoma, and it probably improves quality of life.

For patients who have symptoms, a combination of rituximab and alkylator chemotherapy has high response rates and can alleviate symptoms. Rituximab is a monoclonal antibody that binds to the B-cell surface antigen CD20. CD20 is a cell-surface protein involved in the development and differentiation of normal B cells. It is found on the vast majority of B-cell lymphomas. Rituximab is well tolerated and has remission rates of 40%-50% when used as single-agent therapy for relapsed indolent lymphoma. In younger patients with systemic indolent disease, or patients who had a short response to first-line treatment, high-dose chemotherapy with HCT may be considered, although the chance of cure should be balanced against the mortality of treatment, which can approach 10%.

B. Aggressive Lymphomas

Despite their aggressive nature, these lymphomas have a better chance for cure than their more indolent counterparts. The treatment is typically guided by the prognostic factors (IPI score). Patients with low-risk lymphoma respond well to CHOP (cyclophosphamide, doxorubicin, vincristine, and prednisone) chemotherapy plus rituximab. Radiotherapy may be used after chemotherapy for areas of bulky disease. Patients with high-risk lymphoma benefit from more intensive regimens of chemotherapy and rituximab and potentially high-dose therapy with HCT. This approach should also be considered for patients who relapse or fail to enter remission after induction chemotherapy. A promising immunotherapy is tositumomab, an anti-CD20 monoclonal antibody bound to [131]I (Bexxar). It can kill cells by antibody-mediated cellular cytotoxicity, activation of complement-mediated tumor cell lysis, and the tumor-specific delivery of radiation. Bexxar is currently indicated for the treatment of patients with CD20 antigen-expressing relapsed or refractory non-Hodgkin lymphoma.

C. Nonlymphoid Disease

There is no consensus about the proper management of localized nonlymphoid lymphomas because large-scale studies of therapy for this disease have not been conducted. With few exceptions, nonlymphoid disease is managed somewhat in the same way as systemic aggressive lymphomas, using combination CHOP therapy.

The CHOP regimen has the disadvantage of poor penetration of the blood-brain barrier and is thus ineffective in the treatment of primary central nervous system lymphomas. These lymphomas rarely metastasize, remaining localized to the central nervous system. Current regimens utilize steroids and whole-brain radiation with some form of adjuvant chemotherapy. Methotrexate is the most common adjuvant treatment in this patient population, and it can be effective when delivered either systemically or intrathecally. This can be combined with whole brain radiation therapy. Central nervous system lymphomas have a poor prognosis, with approximately 20% 5-year survival rates in treated patients. The combined modalities, while providing modest survival benefits, have significant neurotoxicities, and as many as 50% of patients develop severe dementia. Given this morbidity, clinicians often use chemotherapy as the sole modality in the treatment of patients with primary central nervous system lymphomas. Extranodal lymphomas that have a predilection for metastases to the central nervous system, such as testicular, paranasal, and AIDS-related lymphomas, require systemic CHOP therapy combined with prophylactic intrathecal methotrexate treatments.

The treatment of gastric lymphomas has been controversial. Mucosa-associated lymphoid tissue–type gastric lymphomas (MALT-type gastric lymphomas) typically have an indolent behavior, and the most widely accepted initial therapy is the eradication of *H. pylori* using regimens combining antibiotics and proton pump inhibitors. For patients with MALT-type gastric lymphoma who are *H. pylori* negative or do not respond to antibiotic/proton pump inhibitor therapy, radiation therapy to the stomach and perigastric lymph nodes obtains high complete response rates and excellent long-term survival. While surgery had previously been used in the treatment of gastric lymphomas, there is now sufficient data to suggest nonoperative management permits a better quality of life with no impact on overall survival. When the disease has spread, the use of chemotherapy is similar to that used for other indolent, advanced lymphomas.

High-grade gastric lymphoma is treated with aggressive polychemotherapy, usually combined with rituximab. Again, surgery used to play a more prominent role but has greatly diminished. It was assumed that the increased risk of perforation and bleeding with chemotherapy could be prevented by pretreatment gastric resection, but modern series have failed to demonstrate that benefit and actually show a high degree of postsurgical complications that may delay the start of chemotherapy. Surgery is limited to patients who have complications or who cannot be managed by standard regimens.

Splenectomy in patients with lymphomatous splenic involvement has not demonstrated therapeutic benefit and should be reserved for patients with symptomatic splenomegaly, pain from recurrent splenic infarctions, and hematologic depression from hypersplenism.

Diehl V, Re D, Harris NL, Mauch PM: Hodgkin lymphoma. In: *Cancer: Principles & Practice of Oncology*, 9th ed. DeVita VT, Lawrence TS, Rosenberg SA, eds. Lippincott Williams & Wilkins, Philadelphia, PA 2011.

Freidberg JW, Mauch PM, Rimsza LM, Fisher RI: Non-Hodgkin's Lymphoma. In: *Cancer: Principles & Practice of Oncology*, 9th ed. DeVita VT, Lawrence TS, Rosenberg SA, eds. Lippincott Williams & Wilkins, Philadelphia, PA 2011.

Marcus R, Sweetenham JW, Williams ME, eds: *Lymphoma: Pathology, Diagnosis and Treatment.* Cambridge University Press, Cambridge, England 2007.

MULTIPLE CHOICE QUESTIONS

1. Which of the following is true?

   A. Cancer incidence rate is usually expressed as events per 100,000 people over their lifetime
   B. Overall survival is the inverse of the likelihood that a person will die of disease
   C. Tumor stage is determined on histologic examination
   D. Cancer point prevalence describes the number of people with cancer at a given time
   E. Epithelial malignancy can also be called sarcoma

2. Biopsy to evaluate a lesion for malignancy

   A. Can include image guidance for needle, incisional or excisional biopsies
   B. Should always remove the entire lesion for analysis
   C. Can yield a sliver of tissue removed with a core needle biopsy
   D. Both A and C
   E. None of the above

3. Adjuvant chemotherapy for cancer

   A. Is typically administered prior to resection
   B. Can be described according to its absolute or relative benefit
   C. Is necessary for most patients who are treated for cancer who never have recurrence
   D. Is most effective in patients who have gross disease remaining after surgery
   E. Uses different agents than are typically used for metastatic disease of the same type

4. Soft tissue sarcomas

   A. Have tumor size and tumor grade as the most important prognostic variables
   B. Often metastasize to regional lymph nodes
   C. Can usually be diagnosed by FNA biopsy
   D. Usually spread to liver as the first site of distant metastasis
   E. All of the above

5. Melanoma

   A. Incidence is decreasing in the United States
   B. Most commonly presents as the nodular subtype
   C. Is best biopsied using a shave technique
   D. Should be excised with a 2-cm skin margin if greater than 2 mm thick
   E. Rarely spreads to lymph nodes

Organ Transplantation

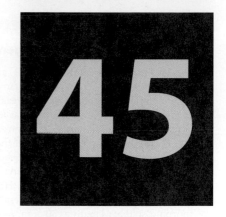

45

Satish N. Nadig, MD, PhD

Jeffrey D. Punch, MD

The ability to transplant human organs successfully has developed in the span of a single generation of physicians and surgeons. This remarkable achievement is an excellent example of how animal models may be used to understand and develop treatments for human disease. Organ transplantation is now the preferred treatment modality for a variety of different types of organ failure. Transplantation offers not only improved long-term survival but also improved quality of life for many patients afflicted by renal, hepatic, cardiac, and pulmonary failure.

Enormous effort is currently being expended to develop methods of artificially replacing vital organ functions. Despite these efforts, the ability to replace organ function with mechanical or biomechanical devices remains elusive. While hemodialysis can replace renal function effectively, it offers neither a normal quality of life nor a normal life span. Despite major advances in artificial heart technology, current systems have not reached the point where they can be used routinely to restore normal cardiac function. To date, there are no effective replacements for hepatic or pulmonary function that are suitable for long-term use. Organ transplantation is frequently the only treatment modality that offers a normal lifestyle for patients with advanced organ failure. Recently, successful composite tissue allografts of limbs, face, and larynx have been reported. While these grafts are not lifesaving, it can be argued that for selected patients they reduce misery. This chapter discusses the indications for organ transplantation as well as the limitations to the current state of the art.

▼ KIDNEY TRANSPLANTATION

With the exception of organs from a genetically identical twin (**isografts**), all organs from genetically dissimilar individuals (**allografts**) will naturally be subjected to immunologic rejection. This fundamental biologic limitation has largely been overcome by the development of targeted immunosuppression therapies. These therapies are able to suppress the immunological reactivity that produces graft rejection while leaving intact sufficient immune competency to allow recovery from most infectious diseases. The same degree of success has not been reached when transplanting organs between species (**xenografts**).

Once it was realized that allografts failed due to an active immunologic attack of the recipient's immune system on the donor organ, methods of suppressing the immune system were investigated. Early attempts at immunosuppression with substances such as nitrogen mustard and total lymphoid irradiation were unsuccessful because of the toxicity of the therapy. The first practical immunosuppressant was azathioprine, an antimetabolite inhibitor of DNA synthesis. When used in combination with corticosteroids, the first successful combination of immunosuppressants was born and the first boom in the number of transplants occurred. This combination remained the state of the art until it was realized that the cell type that exerts primary control over allograft rejection is the T lymphocyte. This led to the later development of agents able to specifically inhibit activation and proliferation of T cells. The result was immunosuppressants that were both more effective and much less toxic than the azathioprine/corticosteroids combination. These agents ushered in a further acceleration in the number of transplants occurring, because now it was possible to transplant organs between individuals who did not share human leukocyte antigens.

Almost all renal diseases responsible for renal failure can be treated by transplantation. Diabetes is the most common cause of chronic renal failure in adults and accounts for 45% of all renal failure in the United States. The second most common cause is hypertensive nephropathy (27%), followed by chronic glomerulonephritis (11%). The causes of renal failure in children are somewhat different, with congenital causes, including both nonobstructive and obstructive uropathies, predominating.

IMMUNOLOGIC RESPONSES

▶ HLA Histocompatibility Antigens

The **major histocompatibility (MHC)** antigens are the most antigenic proteins on donor organs, meaning that they cause the most intense immune responses when the donor and recipient do not share the same antigens. The MHC genes are coded by a single chromosomal complex of closely linked genes on the short arm of the sixth chromosome. This complex consists of at least seven loci that code for genes involved with histocompatibility: human lymphocyte antigen (HLA)-A, HLA-B, HLA-C, HLA-D, HLA-DR, HLA-DQ, and HLA-DP. Each HLA gene locus is highly polymorphic, so that as many as 50 or more discrete antigens are controlled by each locus. The collection of HLA genes in an MHC complex is termed a **haplotype.**

Histocompatibility antigens are grouped into class I (A, B, C) and class II (DR, DQ, DP) antigens. Class I antigens are composed of a 45-kDa heavy chain with three globular extracellular domains ($\alpha 1$, $\alpha 2$, $\alpha 3$) that confers HLA specificity, a transmembrane portion, and an intracellular domain. Class I antigens are stabilized by β_2-microglobulin, a 12-kDa protein that is not encoded in the MHC complex. Class I antigens are expressed on all nucleated cells and interact primarily with CD8+ T cells. Class II antigens are composed of two noncovalently linked chains: a 33-kDa α chain and a 28-kDa β chain. Each chain has two extracellular domains that confer HLA specificities. Class II antigens are only constitutively expressed on B cells and antigen-presenting cells (macrophages, monocytes, dendritic cells) but can be induced on activated T cells and endothelial cells. Class II antigens interact primarily with CD4+ T cells. The three most important antigens clinically in solid organ transplantation are A, B, and DR. Since each person has two MHC complexes, one on each copy of chromosome 6, everyone has a total of six HLA antigens that are of primary importance to organ transplantation.

The 3D structures of both class I and II molecules are similar. The extracellular domains form a β-pleated sheet with two looping α-helices that creates a groove facing away from the cell. Following ribosomal synthesis, during assembly of the HLA antigens, peptides are added to this groove. Intracellularly derived peptides are added to class I antigens in the endoplasmic reticulum, while extracellularly derived proteins are added to class II antigens. The end of the groove on class II antigens is open, allowing class II antigens to accommodate longer peptides. Antigenic determinants are found predominantly on the $\alpha 1$ and $\alpha 2$ chains of the class I molecule and on the β chain of the class II molecule. Some antigenic determinants are shared by many different HLA allotypes. These common determinants are called **public specificities**. Antigenic determinants that are only found on a unique HLA antigen are termed **private specificities**.

Lymphocytes are categorized as either B or T cells. B cells are responsible for antibody production. T cells are categorized into two functional subsets: helper cells that are CD4+ and cytotoxic T cells that are CD8+. Helper T cells preferentially recognize peptides displayed in the groove of class II antigens, while cytotoxic T cells preferentially recognize peptides displayed by class I antigens. A third type of T cell, called regulatory T cells, is now well-established and may be either CD4+ or CD8+. Helper T cells direct both the formation of cytotoxic T cells, which are able to cause graft destruction directly, and the maturation of B cells. Helper T cells can be further subdivided based on their cytokine secretion profile into type 1 and type 2 cells. Type 1 helper T cells secrete interleukin (IL)-2, interferon (IFN)-γ, IL-12, and TNF-α. These cytokines stimulate delayed-type hypersensitivity, cytolytic activity, and the development of complement-fixing IgG antibodies. Type 2 helper T cells secrete IL-4, IL-5, IL-10, and IL-13. These cytokines activate eosinophils and cause the production of IgE antibodies. Additionally, Th17 cells are a distinct subset of helper T cells that produce the proinflammatory cytokine IL-17 and are implicated in diseases of autoimmunity and inflammatory states.

Allograft rejection begins when foreign antigen is taken up by an antigen-presenting cell, processed, and presented to helper T cells. The T cell is activated in response to properly presented antigen and secretes cytokines that in turn recruit and activate additional lymphocytes and cause them to begin to clonally proliferate. Cytokines released in the allograft milieu by other cells, including macrophages, contribute to the generation of the immune response as well. Helper T cells also stimulate the differentiation and proliferation of cytotoxic T cells and B cells.

B-cell activation induces the production of specific antibodies directed against donor antigens. This response is important, especially for class I antigens. Recipients who develop a primary immunological response to a particular antigen and produce cytotoxic antibodies directed against the donor HLA will often retain memory B cells and maintain the ability to produce antibodies that are directed against that particular HLA allotype. Upon reexposure to the same antigens, an immediate destructive reaction to the graft—called hyperacute rejection—occurs. Antibody directed against the donor vascular endothelium triggers fixation of complement, direct cellular damage, and the formation of platelet and fibrin plugs, leading to microvascular thrombosis and ischemic necrosis of the organ. Transplantation in the presence of cytotoxic anti-HLA antibody directed against a donor organ is prevented in practice by performing a complement-mediated cytotoxic crossmatch with pretransplant recipient sera against lymphocytes from the potential donor.

Histocompatibility Testing, Crossmatching, & Blood Group Compatibility

Grafts between identical twins are rare but very successful because immunosuppressive therapy is not required when there is no antigenic difference between the donor and recipient. Grafts between HLA-identical siblings who share two HLA haplotypes give the next best results. One-fourth of any given sibling pair will share both HLA haplotypes and thus share all of the same HLA antigens. Despite sharing HLA, immunosuppression is still required because of incompatibilities at minor histocompatibility loci. Parents, offspring, and half of siblings share one HLA haplotype. One-fourth of siblings will not share an HLA haplotype and will therefore share antigens only by chance. The same is true for genetically unrelated donor/recipient pairs such as spouses and friends. At one time, HLA compatibility was considered to be crucial because there were large differences between graft survivals depending on the degree of histocompatibility. Transplants between individuals who shared many HLA antigens were much more likely to avoid graft loss compared to donor/recipient pairs who did not share HLA antigens. This has changed due to the ability of modern immunosuppression to provide for excellent immunological outcome even in the setting of complete HLA mismatch. HLA testing is now of much lesser value than it once was. HLA histocompatibility testing is now primarily of value in determining which of several donors has the best histologic match to the intended recipient. Kidney allocation from deceased donors was once heavily influenced by HLA matching. This has now changed because of the realization that the degree of HLA match has a relatively unimportant effect on the odds of successful outcome. The newest allocation strategy relies more on waiting time and less on the degree of HLA match. Kidneys from donors who share all six HLA antigens with a recipient on the waiting list are still allocated first to any recipient who happens to be a "perfect match." This situation is uncommon, affecting fewer than 10% of the kidneys from deceased donors.

Regardless of the results of tissue typing and antigen matching, it is essential to determine whether a recipient has preformed antibodies against donor antigens, since their presence would result in a hyperacute rejection of the graft as described previously. Preexisting antibodies may develop because of prior exposure to foreign histocompatibility antigens in the form of blood transfusion, pregnancy, or previous organ transplants.

These antibodies are identified by performing a crossmatch between the patient's serum against the donor's lymphocytes. Multiple methods of performing the crossmatch are available with varying degrees of sensitivity and specificity. It is difficult to find an appropriate donor with a negative crossmatch for patients who have antibodies directed against multiple HLA specificities. Some of these patients can be

treated with desensitization strategies to reduce their burden of circulating antibodies. Methods currently utilized include plasmapheresis, infusion of random intravenous donor immune globulin, and anti–B-cell monoclonal antibodies. Experience is accumulating with desensitization protocols suggesting that donor/recipient pairs with positive crossmatches can sometimes be successfully transplanted. The long-term outcome for these kidneys is unclear.

The ABO blood group antigens behave as strong histocompatibility antigens for kidney transplantation; therefore, ABO-incompatible kidney transplants have generally been considered an absolute impossibility. It is certainly true that ABO-incompatible kidneys will fail rapidly if nothing is done to reduce the amount of antibody directed against the incompatible antigen in the recipient's serum. Success is now being reported for ABO-incompatible kidney transplants using combinations of anti–B-cell therapy and plasmapheresis.

Chinen J, Shearer WT: Advances in basic and clinical immunology in 2011. *J Allergy Clin Immunol* 2012 Feb;129(2):342-348.

Eng HS and Lefell MS: Histocompatibility testing after fifty years of transplantation. *J Immunol Methods* 2011 Jun 30;369(1-2):1-21.

Nunes E et al: Definitions of histocompatibility typing terms. *Blood* 2011;118(23):e180-e183.

Immunosuppressive Drug Therapy

Multiple immunosuppressive strategies are effective at preventing acute allograft rejection. Most strategies involve the use of more than one agent. Conceptually, using multiple immunosuppressive agents has the effect of blocking multiple targets in the immune response cascade, which allows relatively low doses of each drug to be used, thus avoiding toxicity associated with high doses of these powerful drugs. Thus, many patients are treated with "triple therapy" using corticosteroids, a calcineurin inhibitor, and either an antimetabolite or a mammalian target of rapamycin (mTOR) inhibitor. A variant of this strategy, termed "quadruple therapy," involves the initial use of a very potent antilymphocyte agent and chronic administration of the same drugs used for triple therapy. The antibody treatment has two effects: it decreases the likelihood of rejection in the critical first few months after the transplant, and it allows there to be a delay before the introduction of the calcineurin inhibitor. This is advantageous because of the associated nephrotoxicity of calcineurin inhibitors. Since the risk of rejection is highest immediately after the transplant, it is typical to begin with relatively high doses of each agent and gradually taper down to a maintenance level over several weeks to months.

Rejection is diagnosed by biopsy. Patients are followed up with serial measurements of renal function in the form of serum creatinine. When a transplanted kidney begins to function, the serum creatinine will fall gradually over several days to reach a nadir level that becomes a new baseline for the patient. Any significant elevation above the baseline should prompt evaluation as to the cause, and once obstruction, dehydration, and infection have been ruled out, it is usually appropriate to biopsy the kidney graft. Rejection may be treated with high-dose "pulse" corticosteroid therapy over several days or with antilymphocyte antibodies. Rejection therapy is effective in more than 90% of cases.

Many drugs are available today for immunosuppression. All of these drugs share the common side effect of increasing susceptibility to infectious diseases. This is an intrinsic feature of currently available therapy, which aims to suppress natural immune responses against all foreign antigens. When the transplant recipient develops an infection, it is vital that a physician with experience prescribing immunosuppression is involved with the patient's care. In many cases, it is appropriate to temporarily reduce the degree of immunosuppression in order to allow recovery from the infection. Precisely, how this is accomplished varies widely among practitioners, but it generally involves lowering the dosage or withholding one or more of the agents being used for maintenance immunosuppression. When the infection has resolved, immunosuppression is restored to an acceptable maintenance regimen. It is appropriate to individualize therapy because different individuals have different propensities to develop both rejection and infection.

Many long-term immunosuppressive therapies are associated with the development of malignancy, especially skin cancer and lymphomas. Patients receiving chronic immunosuppression should pay particular attention to minimizing direct exposure to ultraviolet radiation. Since many skin cancers are treatable with simple resection, it is also important that transplant physicians are careful to monitor for and treat skin lesions that develop in transplant recipients.

In the future, it may be possible either to modify the graft so that it is not viewed as foreign to the recipient's immune system or to modify the recipient's immune system so that it will not reject the graft without altering the immune response to other foreign antigens.

A. Antimetabolites

The antimetabolite drugs include azathioprine, cyclophosphamide, mycophenolate, and leflunomide. These drugs inhibit nucleic acid synthesis, which in turn limits the ability of activated lymphocytes to rapidly clonally expand. In general, these drugs are used to prevent rejection but are not effective at reversing active acute rejection.

Azathioprine, a purine analog, is the original member of this family. The effects of this drug are not specific to lymphocytes; therefore, the drug also frequently causes decreased levels of circulating neutrophils and platelets. This side effect is dose dependent. This drug is of only historical importance currently.

Cyclophosphamide is an alkylating agent that is a common component of chemotherapy protocols. It is an effective immunosuppressant when given in high doses, but it has been used only very infrequently in clinical transplantation.

Mycophenolate is an inhibitor of inosine monophosphate dehydrogenase, a critical enzyme in the de novo synthesis pathway of purines. Lymphocytes uniquely depend on the de novo pathway to synthesize purines, while other cells are able to utilize a salvage pathway for synthesis. Mycophenolate is therefore more specific for lymphocytes than the other antimetabolites. It has largely replaced azathioprine for use in combination with a calcineurin inhibitor and corticosteroids since well-designed studies have shown it to have a superior ability to prevent rejection. Side effects are primarily gastrointestinal in nature. Enterically coated formulations are available for patients who are unable to tolerate mycophenolate mofetil.

Leflunomide is a selective inhibitor of de novo pyrimidine synthesis. It is thought to work by inhibiting the enzyme dihydroorotate dehydrogenase. It is used widely for treatment of rheumatoid arthritis. Clinical trials have demonstrated it to be efficacious in terms of preventing rejection, but it is difficult to use clinically because of its long half-life (15-18 days).

B. Corticosteroids

Corticosteroids used in combination with azathioprine was the first combination of immunosuppressants with the ability to prevent the development of allograft rejection, and high doses of corticosteroids was the first practical and effective means of reversing established rejection. Hence, over the past 40 years, corticosteroids have been a component of most successful immunosuppressive protocols. Typically, a high dose of intravenous corticosteroids is given at the time of engraftment, and the dose is tapered over weeks to months down to a maintenance dosage of 0.1-0.2 mg/kg of oral prednisone. In the recent past, there has been strong interest in discontinuation of corticosteroids—and even more recently, in developing protocols that do not require the administration of any corticosteroids. The evidence is accumulating that this treatment is appropriate and effective for some low-risk renal transplant recipients, but the use of corticosteroid-free protocols for higher-risk candidates—including those with known sensitization to HLA and patients undergoing second renal transplants—is more controversial.

Corticosteroid therapy is associated with many different side effects, including infection, weight gain, cushingoid features, hypertension, increased bruisability, hyperlipidemia, hyperglycemia, and acne. Daily corticosteroid therapy in children may inhibit somatic growth. This may be circumvented to some degree by alternate-day treatment, administering the drug once in the morning every other day.

Corticosteroids are standard therapy for a rejection episode, typically consisting of three or more daily doses of between 100 and 500 mg of intravenous methylprednisolone ("steroid pulses"). Depending on the severity of the rejection, steroid pulses will resolve 50%-80% of allograft rejection episodes.

C. Calcineurin Inhibitors

Transplantation was revolutionized by the introduction of the first calcineurin inhibitor, cyclosporine, into clinical practice in the early 1980s. Cyclosporine is a cyclic undecapeptide isolated from a fungus. It is a potent immunosuppressant and the first compound identified that can inhibit immunocompetent lymphocytes specifically and reversibly. Cyclosporine was followed by the introduction of tacrolimus, another compound derived from a fungus that also inhibits calcineurin. The primary mechanism of these agents appears to be inhibition of the production and release of IL-2 by helper T cells. They also interfere with the release of IL-1 by macrophages as well as with proliferation of B lymphocytes. Blood levels must be carefully monitored because both drugs are nephrotoxic and neurotoxic at higher levels. They also both have chronic effects on renal function and lead to significant long-term renal dysfunction in many patients who take them chronically. Both cyclosporine and tacrolimus are also associated with an increased incidence of neoplasms, particularly lymphomas.

D. Inhibitors of Mammalian Target of Rapamycin

Sirolimus is a macrocyclic triene antibiotic produced by a species of *Streptomyces*. It was originally developed as an antifungal and antitumor agent but was found to have significant immunosuppressive properties. The effect of sirolimus is believed to relate to inhibition of lymphocyte transduction pathways through binding to the mTOR. It functions as an antiproliferative and prevents not only expansion of lymphocyte clones but also smooth muscle proliferation. It is known to effectively prevent rejection in combination with a calcineurin inhibitor. The major advantages of this drug are that it does not cause renal dysfunction and its antiproliferative properties suggest that it will not be associated with the same risk of developing long-term malignancy. Side effects, in addition to the infections associated with immunosuppression, include oral ulcerations, wound healing problems associated with its ability to inhibit smooth muscle proliferation, and significant hyperlipidemias. An association with hepatic artery thrombosis has also been noted in patients receiving sirolimus therapy as part of their initial immunosuppression regimen following liver transplantation.

Everolimus is a derivative of sirolimus that also acts as an mTOR inhibitor. It has a side-effect profile similar to that of sirolimus but a shorter serum half-life.

E. Polyclonal Antithymoblast or Antilymphocyte Globulin and Antithymocyte Globulin

Antilymphoblast globulin and antithymocyte globulin are polyclonal antibody preparations derived by immunizing animals against human lymphocytes and collecting and purifying the antibodies that animals develop in response to the foreign antigenic proteins. They are potent drugs that deplete circulating lymphocytes, an effect that can be measured and followed by flow cytometry or by simply following the complete blood count with differential. Because they are polyclonal, they not only are effective against T cells but also may have important effects against circulating B cells and natural killer cells.

These agents are particularly effective in induction of immunosuppressive therapy and in the treatment of established rejection that is either severe or resistant to pulse corticosteroid therapy. Therapy is typically given daily for 5-7 days. The effect of these agents is profound immunosuppression that lasts for weeks to months. They are associated with increased incidence of viral infections because of their effects on cellular immunity and also with a higher lifetime risk of developing malignancy, particularly B-cell lymphoma.

Side effects are many and include fevers and chills, neutropenia, and thrombocytopenia. Fever, chills, and malaise occur because of mediator release by T cells and circulating mononuclear cells, especially TNF-α, IL-1, and IL-6, that occurs when the antibody is bound to certain cell surface receptors. The symptoms are very similar to those associated with an acute viral infection. These effects are usually transient, often lasting less than 12 hours. They occur primarily following the first or second dose of the treatment and can be attenuated markedly by pretreatment with corticosteroids, acetaminophen, and diphenhydramine. Neutropenia and thrombocytopenia occur because of direct antibody binding to these cell types, causing depletion. This effect is also transient and tends to resolve in 24-48 hours. It is necessary to monitor neutrophil and platelet counts during therapy and withhold doses of the treatment if the counts drop to dangerously low levels.

F. Monoclonal Antibody Therapy

The knowledge that the T cell is central to the development of allograft rejection led to the development of agents that selectively inhibit or deplete T cells, or both. The first example of such an agent is the monoclonal antibody OKT3 (muromonab-CD3), which is secreted by a hybridoma in culture. This agent may have some advantages over antilymphoblast globulin and antithymocyte globulin preparations in management of rejection because it specifically blocks T-cell generation and function. Because it is a monoclonal antibody and reacts with a defined antigen, it can be consistently produced with a defined activity and without unwanted reactivities against other cells like neutrophils and platelets. OKT3 is most effective in the treatment of steroid-resistant rejection, where more than 90% of rejection episodes are reversed, thus obviating further high-dose steroids. The downside of this antibody treatment is that since it is a murine monoclonal antibody, it may induce recipient antibody directed against the murine antibody molecule. This effect occurs in 5%-10% of patients treated with OKT3 and may decrease the efficacy of the treatment if given a second or third time. Like the polyclonal antilymphocyte preparations, treatment is usually given daily for 5-7 days. Side effects due to cytokine release are typically more severe than those seen with polyclonal agents but may also be attenuated with appropriate pretreatment. Since the antibody does not bind to epitopes other than the CD3 molecule, which is found only on T cells, it does not cause cytopenias.

The success of OKT3 led to the development of a new generation of monoclonal antibodies that are "humanized." The monoclonal antibody molecule has been modified by genetic engineering to avoid the side effects seen with OKT3. The genetic code directing the production of the antibody molecule by the hybridoma has been altered by replacing most of the murine portion of the sequence with human antibody sequence. The antibody is thus chimeric, or "humanized" since only the highly variable portion of the antibody that binds to the antigenic epitope is foreign to the human recipient. Cytokine release therefore does not occur when the antibody is administered, nor is it likely that the recipient will develop neutralizing antibodies against the monoclonal preparation. Because the antibodies so closely resemble human immunoglobulin, they also have a long circulating half-life.

The first of these agents, daclizumab and basiliximab, binds to CD25, the high-affinity subunit of the T-cell receptor for IL-2. Since IL-2 is necessary for T-cell activation and proliferation, these agents have the ability to selectively inhibit the expansion of T-cell clones that are activated at the time of transplantation, without affecting existing T-cell immunity to other antigens. Existing cellular immunity to viruses, for example, is left intact. Induction treatment with anti-CD25 antibodies at the time of engraftment has been shown to reduce the incidence of future rejection episodes.

A more recent agent, alemtuzumab (Campath-1H), is a depleting humanized monoclonal antibody that binds to CD52, an antigen found on all peripheral blood mononuclear cells. Alemtuzumab administration causes a profound and sustained depletion of T cells from peripheral blood that lasts for many months. It similarly depletes B cells, natural killer cells, and monocyte, but to a lesser degree. Alemtuzumab is currently approved for treatment of patients with some forms of chronic lymphocytic leukemia. It is being used by some transplant centers for initial induction immunosuppression and for treatment of rejection.

G. Costimulation Blockade

Another emerging avenue for immunosuppression is that of signal two costimulation blockade. Once the T-cell receptor is engaged (signal 1), lipid rafts carry costimulation molecules to the immunologic synapse and allow for second messenger signaling to carry messages to the cell nucleus. Cytotoxic T lymphocyte antigen 4—immunoglobulin (CTLA4-Ig) or belatacept is a second-generation intravenous fusion protein designed to bind CD80/86 (B7 molecules) on antigen-presenting cells with high avidity, thereby inhibiting B7-CD28 complexes and T-cell activation. When compared to CNIs, phase II and III clinical trials have revealed that belatacept portends superior renal function and exhibits similar patient and graft survival with a decrease in the side-effect profile of renal toxicity and donor specific antibody formation. It has been recently approved for use as maintenance therapy. Due to an increased risk of patients developing posttransplant lymphoproliferative disorder, its use is restricted to Epstein–Barr virus (EBV) + recipients. Further studies attempting to design more selective targeting of alloreactive lymphocytes are ongoing. Specifically, pathways involving CD40/40L, LFA-1/ICAM, and CD2/LFA-3 are targets of newer, more potent monoclonal antibodies and fusion proteins.

Lee RA, Gabardi S: Current trends in immunosuppressive therapies for renal transplant recipients. *Am J Health Syst Pharm* 2012 Nov 15;69(22):1961-1975.

Levy G et al: Safety, tolerability, and efficacy of everolimus in de novo liver transplant recipients: 12- and 36-month results. [Erratum appears in Liver Transpl 2006;12:1726]. *Liver Transpl* 2006;12:1640.

Snanoudj R: Co-stimulation blockade as a new strategy in kidney transplantation. Benefits and limits. *Drugs* 2010;70(16):2121-2131.

Webber A et al: Novel strategies in immunosuppression: issues in perspective. *Transplantation* 2011 May 27;91(10):1057-1064.

SOURCES OF DONOR KIDNEYS

The two sources of kidneys for renal transplantation are living donors and deceased donors. Approximately one-third of patients who are acceptable candidates for transplantation will have a willing and medically suitable living donor. ABO-compatible donors are not absolutely required today because of the availability of treatments that can reduce the amount of antidonor antibody in the recipient. However, ABO-compatible donors are greatly preferred, because antibody reduction treatments are expensive and associated with infectious risk due to the depletion of protective antibodies.

At one time, only related living donors were acceptable because it was necessary to have closely matched HLA antigens between the donor and recipient in order to achieve acceptable graft survival rates. The graft survival rate for donor/recipient pairs who do not share any HLA antigens is now greater than 90%, leading transplant programs to accept increasing numbers of donors who are not genetically related to the recipients. It is now common practice to accept volunteer donors who are spouses, in-laws, friends, coworkers, and even members of the same community who may be only acquaintances. More controversial is a recent trend for patients and donors to meet through Internet web sites. Despite initial hesitancy to condone this method of finding a living donor, it has been difficult for the transplant community to make value judgments about the relationship between living donors and recipients as long as both parties are fully informed and committed.

Recently, programs have begun arranging transplants between two or more pairs of living donors and recipients who participate in a paired exchange. Recipients with willing but incompatible donors are paired with another donor/recipient pair who have the same problem. The outcome from paired donation transplants has been similar to that seen with other living donor transplants.

Living donors should be in good health both physically and psychologically. Above all, the living donor should be a volunteer and must clearly understand the nature of the procedure so that informed consent to the operation can be given. Donors should generally be of legal age, but reasonable exceptions have been made in extenuating circumstances, particularly when an identical twin donor is available. In these circumstances, it is wise for the program to assign to the donor an outside advocate who has no relationship with either the recipient or the remainder of the family to ensure that the minor is not coerced into proceeding.

▶ Living Donors

Live kidney donors are now as common as deceased donors, although since each deceased donor can donate two kidneys, the total number of kidneys from deceased donors still far exceeds that obtained from living donors. Because of the biological ability of the body to compensate for the loss of one kidney, renal function tends to stabilize at approximately 75%-80% of the original renal function a few months following donation. Follow-up studies on donors show that they have good renal function and do not appear to suffer ill effects from the procedure, either physically or psychologically. Women with one kidney do not have an increased incidence of urinary infections during pregnancy.

There are at least two methods of performing donor nephrectomy in common practice: open nephrectomy and laparoscopic nephrectomy. Open nephrectomy, long the standard method, involves a flank incision about 15 cm long below the 12th rib. The peritoneum is retracted medially, and the kidney is removed along with its vessels and ureter without disturbing the intra-abdominal contents. More recently, laparoscopic techniques have been developed to allow the removal of a kidney for transplantation. The

donor is placed under general anesthesia, and the abdomen is insufflated with carbon dioxide to allow visualization of the abdominal structures. Some surgeons use a large port in the midline, just above the umbilicus, to insert their hand into the abdomen. The kidney is then withdrawn through the hand port once it has been dissected free from surrounding tissues and the vessels and ureter have been divided. It is also possible to remove the kidney using purely laparoscopic techniques without inserting a hand port. The kidney is removed by placing it in a bag inside the abdomen and withdrawing the bag through a low transverse incision. Laparoscopic nephrectomy tends to take longer than a nephrectomy through an open approach, but it is associated with somewhat less postoperative pain and a briefer period of convalescence. Prospective donors should be informed about the options for nephrectomy and the advantages and disadvantages of each technique as well as the associated risk and the known complications.

The main risk to a donor is the anesthesia and the operation itself. The mortality rate is estimated to be 0.03%, and most deaths are not judged to be preventable but appear to be intrinsic risks of having a major operation. The most common significant complications following nephrectomy are wound related, including infection and hernia formation. These complications occur in less than 1%-3% of cases. Wound infections typically respond to dressing changes, and hernias require operative repair.

The evaluation of a living donor must be thorough and complete. It is first necessary to make sure that the donor is truly a volunteer and is not being coerced or unfairly influenced by the recipient or other family members. This often involves a careful evaluation by an individual with excellent understanding of the transplant process as well as excellent communication skills. It is advisable that this portion of the interview be conducted in private so that donors can be honest about their feelings. Transplant social workers, psychologists, and psychiatrists are typically involved with this aspect of donor selection. Once it is clear that the donor is genuinely seeking to donate of his or her own accord, a detailed history is taken, and a physical examination is performed. Factors that may affect operative risk as well as future risk of renal failure are carefully sought out. The routine workup includes chest x-ray, electrocardiography, urinalysis, complete blood count, fasting blood glucose, serum bilirubin, hepatic transaminases, serum creatinine, and blood urea nitrogen. If these are normal, the kidneys are imaged radiographically to make sure that two kidneys are present, to rule out intrinsic or structural renal disease, and to evaluate the vasculature of the kidneys. Angiography, CT, and MRI are all methods that can be used. Kidneys with multiple renal arteries may be transplanted, but care must be taken in the anastomosis of small accessory vessels, particularly when they come from the lower pole and may therefore provide the sole vascular supply to the ureter. When there are multiple renal veins, the smaller veins can often be ligated, since there is free communication of the veins within the kidney.

▶ Deceased Donors

Two-thirds of eligible kidney recipients do not have a suitable living donor. These patients are placed on a waiting list for a kidney from a deceased donor. Since more patients are added to the list each year, the number of patients waiting for a kidney from a deceased donor grows longer each year.

Kidneys can be successfully transplanted from donors who are declared dead on the basis of brain death or from donors who die of cessation of spontaneous cardiovascular activity.

Brain death is now widely accepted, in principle, in the United States, and all hospitals have protocols to be followed to ensure that the diagnosis of brain death is confirmed without any doubt.

Consent for donation should always be obtained by individuals with training in how to approach the family of the donors. In this way, the family can be given time to grieve and express the inevitable sorrow and anger that accompanies the death of a loved one. Individuals who are not part of the team caring for the patient are best able to provide the emotional support that families need during this time. The discussion regarding donation can then occur separate from the discussion in which the family learns that their loved one has died.

Kidneys from brain-dead donors are removed operatively. The excision of the kidneys occurs operatively following *in situ* cold perfusion and exsanguination of the kidneys, often in concert with the removal of other transplantable abdominal and thoracic organs. The kidneys are perfused with specially designed preservative solutions and kept cold. Successful transplantation has been reported following cold storage of more than 72 hours, but optimal results are achieved if the kidney is transplanted as soon as possible following removal from the donor, preferable within 24 hours.

Kidneys may also be transplanted from deceased donors following cardiopulmonary death, a practice termed "donation following cardiac death." The most common circumstance under which this occurs in the United States is when medical therapy that is judged to be futile is withdrawn from an individual. Typically, patients have suffered profound, irreversible brain injury and have essentially no conscious awareness and no potential for meaningful recovery. Standard medical practice in this circumstance is to recommend withdrawal of life-sustaining support such as mechanical respiration and intravenous infusions, since the vast majority of people state that they would not want to be kept alive in such a hopeless state. Withdrawal of support always occurs with the consent and understanding of the family. The decision to donate organs should be made separate from the decision to withdraw medical therapy. Once consent is obtained and preparation for donation is completed, support is withdrawn by the primary care team.

When cardiopulmonary activity ceases, the primary physician team declares death, and the organs are then excised as with brain-dead donors.

SELECTION OF RECIPIENTS

Patients with chronic renal failure should be considered for transplantation. Acute renal failure on the basis of acute tubular necrosis can usually be managed with temporary dialysis, and therefore kidney transplantation is not appropriate in this setting. It is not necessary for patients to be on dialysis at the time of transplantation. In fact, results for patients who receive kidney transplants prior to beginning dialysis have the best chance of graft survival, while patients who had long-term dialysis prior to transplantation have poorer success rates. It is therefore important to begin consideration for renal transplantation as soon as dialysis appears to be inevitable and imminent within the next year.

During the early years of renal transplantation, most of the patients accepted for transplantation were between 15 and 45 years old. In recent years, the age range has been extended in both directions—children younger than age 1 and adults who are over 70 years old have received transplants. For many years, the success rates for transplanting in young children was inferior to that achieved with adults, but this problem has now been corrected. Even children younger than 1 year of age at the time of transplantation can be expected to have an excellent chance of graft survival.

Historically, there has been reluctance to perform renal transplants in the elderly. However, as the practice of renal transplantation continues to improve, with less toxic and more effective immunosuppression and more effective methods of preventing posttransplant infections, this unwillingness appears less justified. Elderly individuals naturally have a shorter life span, but to date, patients over 60 years old who receive transplants appear to enjoy approximately the same degree of improvement in life expectancy as do younger patients.

This benefit has been quantified by comparing the mortality rate of suitable candidates awaiting kidney transplantation with the mortality rate following transplantation. Life expectancy appears to be approximately doubled by kidney transplantation in all age ranges that have been studied to date. The improved life expectancy following kidney transplantation is particularly dramatic for diabetic patients. Today, patients tend to be judged on the basis of their physiologic functional status rather than on their chronological age. It is nevertheless true that elderly patients are more commonly found to be poor candidates for transplantation because of either coexisting disease or poor functional status.

Candidates must be free of active infections at the time of transplantation. Chronically infected tissues such as chronic pyelonephritis or chronic osteomyelitis should be definitively treated prior to consideration for transplantation. Patients with active viral or bacterial infection at the time, an organ is available for transplantation should usually be deferred until the infection has resolved. This is because it is unwise to initiate immunosuppression during an active infection, particularly given that the highest doses of immunosuppression are given around the time of the procedure.

Recipients with almost all types of primary renal disease have been successfully transplanted: glomerulonephritis, hypertensive nephropathy, chronic pyelonephritis, polycystic kidney disease, reflux pyelonephritis, Goodpasture syndrome, congenital renal hypoplasia, renal cortical necrosis, Fabry syndrome, and Alport syndrome. Successful transplants have been achieved in patients with certain systemic diseases in which the kidney is one of the end organs affected (cystinosis, systemic lupus erythematosus, and diabetic nephropathy). Renal transplantation is generally inadvisable in patients with oxalosis if high serum levels of oxalate are present because the disease recurs in the transplant quickly. However, liver transplantation corrects the enzymatic defect that leads to excessive oxalate accumulation. Therefore, combined liver-kidney transplantation may be an acceptable treatment option for these patients.

Patients who do not have normal bladder function may be acceptable kidney transplant candidates, but a plan for ureteral drainage should be made before transplantation occurs. Many patients with long-term defunctionalized bladders can still undergo ureteral reimplantation and then be treated with intermittent catheterization if necessary posttransplant. If the bladder is congenitally or surgically absent, a defunctionalized loop of small bowel can be created, brought out as a stoma, and used for a urinary conduit. Care must be taken in planning the positioning of the conduit so that the ureter from a transplanted kidney will reach it.

Transplant patients must be compliant with posttransplant care to achieve successful outcome. Patients with a history of poor compliance may be candidates for transplantation if they are regretful of past behavior and have established a compliant pattern. In some cases, especially in the adolescent age group, it is wise for the patient to experience dialysis prior to receiving a kidney transplant in order to foster a complete understanding of the differences in lifestyle that are afforded by a successful kidney transplant. It is also necessary that patients have a support network to help them manage following the transplant. They will need a way to reliably obtain immunosuppressive therapy as well as transportation to and from the transplant center that is continuously and reliably available. Fortunately, support services are often available to patients who lack social support, and it is rare to deny transplantation solely on the basis of inadequate social support.

In the early years of kidney transplantation, it was common to perform bilateral nephrectomy prior to transplantation, but this has recently become very uncommon. Most patients who have native nephrectomy have polycystic kidney disease with profound pain, recurrent infections, or recurrent hemorrhage. Other indications for native nephrectomy include recurrent infection, especially when associated with ureteral reflux, and occasionally profound hypertension attributable to an ischemic native kidney.

Segev DL: Innovative strategies in living donor kidney transplantation. *Nat Rev Nephrol* 2012 May1;8(6):332-338.
Smith JM et al: Kidney, pancreas, and liver allocation and distribution in the United States. *Am J Transplant* 2012 Dec;12(12):3191-3212.

OPERATIVE TECHNIQUES

The surgical technique of renal transplantation involves anastomoses of the renal artery and vein and ureter (Figure 45-1). The transplant kidney is placed in the iliac fossa through an oblique lower abdominal incision. The dissection is carried out by retracting the peritoneum medially so the kidney will lie in an extraperitoneal position. The iliac arteries and veins are mobilized as indicated for the proposed specific anastomoses. An end-to-side anastomosis is performed between renal vein and iliac vein; an end-to-side anastomosis is then performed between the renal artery and the external iliac artery. An alternative technique is to connect the renal artery end-to-end to the internal iliac artery, but this technique is more difficult in most patients. When multiple arteries are present, there are several options. If the artery is very small (< 2 mm), it can often be ligated, especially if it is an upper

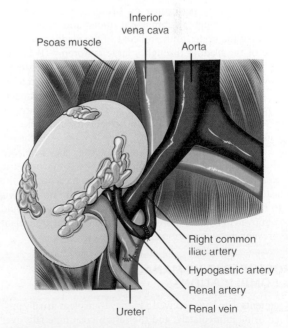

▲ **Figure 45–1.** Technique of renal transplantation.

pole branch. If the kidney is from a deceased donor, it is often possible to use a large Carrell patch of donor aorta that encompasses all of the arteries. Other options include reimplanting multiple renal arteries into the iliac artery using multiple anastomoses; reimplanting a smaller artery into the side of the dominant renal artery and then using the larger artery for anastomoses to the iliac; and spatulating the ends of the two arteries together to form a single lumen for anastomosis.

In small children and infants, the kidney transplant can be performed either through a midline abdominal incision or by making a very large flank-type incision extending from the pubic symphysis to the costal margin and exposing the aorta and vena cava by reflecting the peritoneal contents medially and superiorly. End-to-side anastomoses of the renal vessels may be made to the iliac vessels if they are large enough, but often it is necessary to use the infrarenal vena cava and aorta for the anastomotic site.

Kidneys from small pediatric deceased kidneys function poorly when transplanted into small pediatric recipients. However, many pediatric kidneys have often been transplanted en bloc with the donor aorta and vena cava anastomosed to the recipient's iliac vessels along with double ureteral anastomoses. The exact age at which it is best to transplant kidneys as a single unit is unclear, but certainly kidneys from children as young as 6 will function well and last a long time when transplanted into adults.

Urinary tract continuity can be established by pyeloureterostomy, ureteroureterostomy, or ureteroneocystostomy. The most common technique is ureteroneocystostomy. This technique can be performed by bringing the ureter into the bladder through a submucosal tunnel and suturing the mucosa of the ureter to the mucosa of the bladder from the inside of the bladder through a large cystotomy (Politano-Leadbetter method). Other techniques include an external neocystostomy, which avoids the need for a large cystotomy and is more common, and the "one stitch" technique, whereby the mucosa of the ureter is not directly sutured to the bladder mucosa, but rather the ureter is fixed into place in the interior of the bladder with a suture that traverses the full thickness of the bladder wall. A ureteral stent may be placed with any of the techniques discussed above. A 6Fr pediatric ureteral stent with a J shape at each end fits nicely across the anastomosis and goes from the interior of the renal pelvis into the bladder or other urinary conduit. The stent should be removed in the first month or two following the transplant to prevent stone formation and bladder infection.

POSTOPERATIVE MANAGEMENT & COMPLICATIONS

Recipients who have received a kidney transplant usually produce urine immediately, and the serum creatinine falls over the next 3-7 days. The magnitude of urine output is related to how hydrated the patient was before transplantation and to how much fluid is administered during the procedure. It is important that the patient is fully hydrated at the time the kidney is revascularized in order to achieve the best chance of immediate transplant kidney function. Transplanted kidneys frequently will have an obligate diuresis for a period of hours to days after they begin to function. During this phase, it may be necessary to replace urinary output in order to prevent the development of hypovolemia as a result of excess urinary output. Once this phase has passed, intravenous fluid can be discontinued. However, patients are encouraged to maintain generous fluid intake to prevent dehydration in the future, as transplanted kidneys appear to have a greater susceptibility to hypovolemia than native kidneys. Patients are usually able to eat the morning following the transplant procedure and should be encouraged to get out of bed with assistance. The urinary catheter can be removed as early as 2 days following the procedure, depending on the technique used for ureteral anastomosis. Some programs prefer to leave the urinary catheter in place for a longer period of time to allow sufficient healing of the anastomosis. Most recipients are able to be discharged from the hospital on the second or third postoperative day if there are no complications in their postoperative course once they are able to maintain oral hydration, have learned how to properly take their medications, and have received training about what to do, what not to do, and what to watch out for in the next few weeks.

Kidney transplantation can be followed by a variety of postoperative complications that must be recognized and treated early for optimal results. The most frequent complications are infection and rejection, reflecting the natural tension between too much and too little immunosuppression. Urinary infection is one of the most common complications and usually responds to antibiotic therapy. Bacterial pneumonia is the most common pulmonary complication and may be very serious if not promptly diagnosed and treated. Current immunosuppression protocols that focus on the T lymphocyte are associated with unusual, opportunistic types of infections including herpesviruses, the parasite *Pneumocystis carinii,* and fungal infections. These infections are seen much less often than previously because it is standard to prescribe prophylactic anti-infective therapy aimed at preventing the common types of infection. In particular, the availability of agents that are effective against cytomegalovirus (CMV) infection has almost eliminated clinical CMV infections. At one time, CMV infections were a frequent, expensive, and exceedingly unpleasant occurrence after many transplants.

In approximately 20% of kidney transplants from deceased donors, the kidney will fail to function immediately. This complication is termed delayed graft function and is due to acute tubular necrosis of the kidney. In some cases, there is a modest urinary output, but the serum creatinine does not fall. In other cases, there is profound oliguria. Delayed graft function can also occur following living donor transplantation, but it is much less common (< 3%). Delayed graft function is associated with older donors and donors who had a rising creatinine at the time of donation. Long ischemic times are also known to increase the chance of delayed graft function. In most cases, the acute tubular necrosis will resolve and the renal function will recover. Most recovery happens within a week, but in some cases, the kidney will require several weeks before renal function is sufficient to support the patient without dialysis. Treatment is supportive with dialysis as necessary. If recovery takes more than a week, it may be wise to biopsy the kidney to rule out silent rejection.

Vascular complications of kidney transplants are uncommon, affecting 1%-2% of renal transplants. Either renal artery or venous thrombosis of the kidney is devastating and almost uniformly results in graft loss. The incidence of acute graft thrombosis is higher in patients with high levels of circulating anti-HLA antibodies, suggesting that some of these cases are related to accelerated acute rejection. The incidence of graft thrombosis is also higher in patients with factor V Leiden and other physiologic derangements that cause a hypercoagulable state. Patients should be screened for factor V Leiden if they have a history of unusual thrombotic events and receive anticoagulation perioperatively when it or other known hypercoagulable states are known. Renal artery stenosis, which may be associated with rejection involving the renal artery, is also a rare complication. It can present with severe hypertension. It may be treated surgically or in some cases by percutaneous transluminal balloon angioplasty.

Urologic complications occur in about 4% of patients, most often urinary extravasation from the cystotomy closure or ureteral obstruction. These complications can almost always be managed with percutaneous placement of a nephrostomy tube by an interventional radiologist and are not associated with a higher risk of graft loss.

A complication relatively unique to kidney transplantation is formation of a pelvic lymphocele in the transplant bed. Lymphatic fluid may come from either lymphatics in the hilum of the kidney or from lymphatics disrupted during exposure of the iliac vessels. Careful ligation of the adjacent lymphatics during preparation of the recipient blood vessels may decrease the incidence of this complication. Large lymphoceles may obstruct the ureter or the vasculature of the transplanted kidney, and they occasionally become infected. Sterile lymphoceles may be drained into the peritoneal cavity, while infected lymphoceles need to be drained externally.

Gastrointestinal complications may affect all levels of the intestine, but upper gastrointestinal symptoms, including nausea and abdominal pain, are most common. In many cases, the culprit is the large number of medications that the patient must take. Peptic ulceration was once a major problem for transplant recipients, but this complication has virtually disappeared because of routine use of medications like H_2-blockers and proton pump inhibitors to inhibit the production of gastric acid.

GRAFT REJECTION

Despite advances in immunosuppressive management, rejection is still a major hazard for the postoperative allograft recipient. Most episodes of rejection occur within the first 3 months. There are three basic kinds of rejection:

1. **Hyperacute rejection** is due to preformed cytotoxic antibodies against donor antigens. Pretransplant cross-match testing is designed to prevent this type of rejection. This reaction begins soon after completion of the anastomosis, and complete graft destruction occurs in 24-48 hours. Initially, the graft is pink and firm, but it then becomes blue and soft, with evidence of diminished blood flow. There is often no effective method of treating hyperacute rejection, but treatment with plasmapheresis and immunoglobulin infusion may be effective if the diagnosis is made immediately.

2. **Acute rejection** is the most common type of rejection episode during the first 3 months after transplantation. It is primarily an immune cellular reaction against foreign antigens. The reaction may be predominantly cellular, or there may be a component of antibody-mediated inflammation. Typically, the patient is asymptomatic and the diagnosis of rejection is suspected on the basis of serial measurement of serum creatinine levels. In severe cases, symptoms may include oliguria, weight gain, and worsened hypertension. Fever and tenderness and enlargement of the graft are uncommon with modern immunosuppressive protocols but used to be seen when only azathioprine and corticosteroids were available. This type of rejection process is usually treated with pulse steroid therapy. If this is unsuccessful, or in very severe cases of acute rejection, either a polyclonal or monoclonal depleting antilymphocyte preparation is used. The vast majority of acute rejection episodes are successfully reversed. Currently, grafts are only lost to rejection when patients are noncompliant or when rejection occurs together with a life-threatening infection, since it is unsafe to enhance the degree of immunosuppression in this setting.

3. **Chronic rejection** is a late cause of renal deterioration. It is unclear precisely what causes chronic rejection, but the absence of cellular elements on biopsy and the association of antidonor antibodies with chronic graft loss have led to the assumption that it is mediated by humoral factors. It is most often diagnosed on the basis of slowly decreasing renal function in association with proteinuria and hypertension. Chronic rejection is resistant to all known methods of therapy and graft loss will eventually occur, though perhaps not for several years after renal function begins to deteriorate. It is unclear what the relationship is between this pathologic process and the damage produced by chronic calcineu-

rin inhibitor use, which is seen in nonrenal transplant recipients as well. It has recently been uncovered that chronic graft loss is accelerated in patients who experienced rejection in the first year after a transplant, in patients who had delayed graft function, and in patients who received kidneys from marginal donors.

▶ Differential Diagnosis of Renal Allograft Dysfunction

An unexpected elevation in serum creatinine above baseline levels in a renal transplant recipient has a broad differential diagnosis list. Dehydration should be ruled out by history and physical examination. The medication the patient is taking should be reviewed, paying attention to over-the-counter medications, especially nonsteroidal anti-inflammatory drugs and herbal remedies. These drugs can cause renal dysfunction or can alter the metabolism of immunosuppressant medications and result in blood levels that are either too high or too low. Urinary infection should be ruled out with a urinalysis. If these simple evaluations do not disclose the cause of renal dysfunction, the next step is usually a renal ultrasound to rule out ureteral obstruction, followed by a renal allograft biopsy. This last step is crucial to arriving at the correct diagnosis. A biopsy may disclose acute rejection, or it may show calcineurin inhibitor toxicity. Since the treatment for these conditions is opposite, a biopsy is very important to guide appropriate therapy.

▼ HEART TRANSPLANTATION

The first successful human heart allograft was performed in 1967 by Christiaan Barnard. At that time, however, the only available immunosuppressive therapy was azathioprine and steroids. This regimen was inadequate to safely prevent rejection in these patients. As a result, the procedure remained experimental and was limited to a small number of institutions worldwide. The introduction of cyclosporine in 1981 resulted in dramatically improved survival. As a result, heart transplantation was federally designated as no longer experimental in 1985. In 2003, there were about 2000 heart transplants performed in the United States at more than 100 centers. The 1-year survival rate is now over 85%, and the 3-year survival rate is over 75%.

SELECTION OF DONORS

At one time, deceased donors were considered suitable for cardiac donation only if they were men aged 40 years or younger or women 45 or younger. The large waiting list and the increasing number of patients who die on the waiting list has led surgeons to accept hearts from donors as old as 60, and more than one-third of current donors are older than 40. Cardiac donors must be ABO-compatible with the recipient and should be within 20% of the recipient's ideal body weight. Ideally, there should be no history of preexistent

or intercurrent cardiac disease. It is routine to obtain echocardiography to determine cardiac function, even in young donors. At many programs, it is routine to obtain cardiac catheterization in older donors to rule out silent coronary artery disease. Ideally, there should be no history of cardiac arrest, but if cardiac function is good, this factor alone does not usually rule out a cardiac donor. The donor should be receiving only moderate doses of pressor drugs.

At the donor operation, the chest is opened and the heart is inspected for evidence of contusion and observed to determine its overall function. If the heart is suitable, this information is relayed to the recipient operating team so that the timing of the recipient operation can be carefully coordinated. The heart is removed following cross-clamping of the aorta and infusion of cold cardioplegia, which results in cessation of electrical and mechanical cardiac activity. The heart is typically removed first, prior to the excision of kidney, liver, or pancreas. It is flushed with a preservative solution and stored aseptically at 4°C. Optimal function is obtained when the heart is implanted within 4 hours of procurement. For recipients who have previously had cardiac procedures through a sternotomy, it is sometimes necessary to delay the procurement of the donor heart to make sure that the recipient will be ready to receive the heart when it arrives back at the transplant hospital. The same is true when recipients have left ventricular assist devices implanted and extra time is necessary to prepare the recipient to receive the donor heart.

SELECTION OF RECIPIENTS

Patients for cardiac transplantation should have end-stage cardiac disease for which there is no other surgical option and should have received maximal medical treatment. Most heart transplant candidates have idiopathic dilated cardiomyopathy or ischemic cardiomyopathy. Most patients are younger than 55 years of age, but successful transplantation has been reported on more elderly patients. Patients should not have systemic disease that will be worsened by the immunosuppressive regimen (infection, type 1 diabetes, severe peripheral vascular disease, poorly controlled hypertension), nor should they have underlying renal insufficiency that cannot be attributed to low cardiac output.

Patients should have pulmonary vascular resistance of less than 5 Wood units, since levels above this or a pulmonary artery systolic pressure of greater than 50 mm Hg or a transpulmonary gradient (mean pulmonary artery pressure–pulmonary capillary wedge pressure) of greater than 15 mm Hg are associated with inadequate donor heart function. As with other organs, a history of compliance with a complex medical regimen and a strong social support system are necessary for long-term success.

If the recipient has circulating antibodies directed against HLA antigens, it is necessary to perform a crossmatch between the recipient's serum and the donor lymphocytes to make sure that hyperacute rejection of the cardiac graft does not occur. Patients who have left ventricular assist devices in place may be particularly difficult to obtain hearts for because of the sensitizing effect that the device has on the immune system.

OPERATIVE TECHNIQUE

The operative technique originally developed by Lower and Shumway continues to be used and is shown in Figure 45-2. A median sternotomy is performed and the patient is placed on cardiopulmonary bypass. The recipient heart is removed, and the atrial cuffs trimmed. The left atrial anastomosis is performed first and then the right, each with one continuous suture. Before the left atrium is closed, it is filled with saline to avoid air embolism. The aortic and then pulmonary artery anastomoses are then performed. Topical cooling may be continued, and the addition of blood cardioplegia after the atrial anastomoses may be done in order to improve graft function. The implant time is generally 45-60 minutes. It is frequently necessary to provide chronotropic support for the denervated heart in the form of atrial pacing or isoproterenol.

IMMUNOSUPPRESSION

Triple immunosuppression with a calcineurin inhibitor, antimetabolite, and corticosteroids is typical of the standard immunosuppressive protocol at most heart transplant programs. Perioperative induction immunosuppressive therapy with either polyclonal or monoclonal antibody therapy directed at lymphocytes is sometimes used in order to avoid the renal toxicity associated with early high-dose calcineurin inhibition and to reduce the risk of later rejection. Rejection is diagnosed on endomyocardial biopsy, which is performed regularly, since rejection may occur in the absence of clinical symptoms. Rejection is treated with 3 days of pulse steroids and resistant rejection with antilymphocyte therapy.

FOLLOW-UP CARE

Transplant recipients must be carefully monitored for infection and rejection. Protocols for endomyocardial biopsies vary by center but are typically performed every other month for the first year, then every 3 months. The incidence of rejection episodes is 0.5-1.5 per patient for the first year. The major infection rate is 1.5 episodes per patient for the first year and then declines. Accelerated coronary atherosclerosis, believed to be a manifestation of chronic graft rejection, occurs in 30%-40% of patients within 5 years after transplantation. There is no effective therapy for this condition except for retransplantation in highly selected, usually younger, patients. Progressive renal dysfunction may occur over time due to the cumulative effect of calcineurin inhibitor therapy.

Aliabadi A, Cochrane AB, Zuckerman AO: Current strategies and future trends in immunosupprression after heart transplantation. *Curr Opin Organ Transplant* 2012 Oct;17(5):540-545.

Neragi-Miandoab S: A ventricular assist device as a bridge to recovery, decision making, or transplantation in patients with advanced cardiac failure. *Surg Today* 2012 Oct;42(10):917-926.

COMBINED HEART-LUNG TRANSPLANTATION

Combined heart-lung transplantation was first performed in 1981. Initially, it was felt that rejection of both organs would be evident in the myocardial biopsy. However, experience has shown that rejection is dissimilar in the two organs, with heart rejection occurring infrequently and lung rejection, evidenced by obliterative bronchiolitis and arteritis, being a more severe problem. Heart-lung transplantation is currently performed with gradually decreasing frequently. In 1994, there were 71 heart-lung transplants in the United States. This number had declined to 28 in 2003. The main indication for heart-lung transplantation is end-stage disease in both organs or end-stage disease in one with poor function in the other prohibiting single-organ transplantation. Examples are primary pulmonary hypertension, congenital heart disease with Eisenmenger physiology, fibrotic lung disease and cor pulmonale, and cystic fibrosis.

The operation consists of en bloc heart-lung transplantation with anastomosis of the trachea, right atrium, and aorta of the donor.

Immunosuppression parallels that of heart transplantation with the exception that steroids are avoided initially in order to promote tracheal wound healing. Heart-lung transplantation currently results in a 70% 1-year survival rate.

LUNG TRANSPLANTATION

Single-lung transplantation became clinically successful through a systematic approach by the Toronto Lung Transplant Group to the problem of bronchial disruption, which had made previous attempts unsuccessful. The addition of an omental wrap to the bronchial anastomosis and the avoidance of steroids during the first 3 weeks allowed bronchial healing and clinical success. Lung transplantation is currently performed for a myriad of indications, including emphysema, cystic fibrosis, idiopathic pulmonary fibrosis, α_1-antitrypsin deficiency, primary pulmonary hypertension, and congenital diseases. Candidates for lung transplantation have irreversible end-stage disease for which there is no other therapy, are oxygen dependent, and are likely to die of their disease within 12-18 months. Lung donors are scarce, but the use of one lung for transplantation does not preclude using the heart for another recipient. Long-distance procurement of lungs has been possible since institution of a regimen consisting of pulmonary artery flush with cold

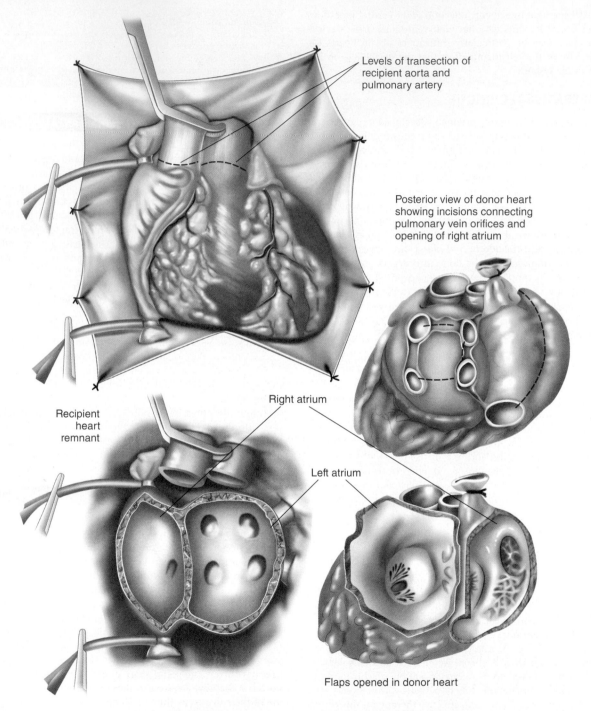

▲ **Figure 45–2.** *Top left:* Recipient heart showing levels of transection across aorta and pulmonary artery. *Lower left:* Implantation site with recipient heart removed. *Top right:* Posterior view of donor heart showing lines of incision connecting pulmonary vein orifices and opening the right atrium in preparation for implantation. *Lower right:* Flaps opened in donor heart in preparation for implantation.

preservative solution following alprostadil (PGE$_1$) via the central venous line to promote pulmonary vasodilatation.

Patients with bilateral pulmonary sepsis, such as cystic fibrosis or bronchiectasis, or patients with emphysema and normal heart function may sometimes be eligible for double-lung transplantation. The advantage is that the patient does not have the potential complications of heart transplant and rejection. Another innovative approach to the lung transplant patient with a normal heart is the operation whereby a heart-lung block is placed in a patient with end-stage lung disease and a normal heart, and the recipient's heart is extracted and donated to a patient in need of an isolated heart transplantation.

Immunosuppressive management of lung transplant recipients is very similar to that of heart recipients in that the cornerstone of therapy is a calcineurin inhibitor. The major difference is that steroids are omitted for several weeks in order to promote healing of the bronchial anastomosis. Postoperative management focuses on prevention of sepsis and detection and treatment of rejection. Bronchoscopy is performed liberally and transbronchial lung biopsy is used to diagnose lung transplant rejection. Acute rejection may be effectively treated with corticosteroid pulse therapy, or by enhancing the existing immunosuppressive regimen. The major long-term complication in lung transplant recipients is the development of bronchiolitis obliterans syndrome (BOS). BOS is felt to be the lung manifestation of chronic rejection. Episodes of acute rejection are risk factors for the development of BOS in the future. There is currently no effective therapy for BOS. A promising development that is currently experimental is aerosolized delivery of immunosuppression. It is hoped that directing immunosuppression preferentially to the lung itself may allow enhanced protection from rejection without increasing the risk of infection.

Celli BR: Update on the management of COPD. *Chest* 2008 Jun;133(6):1451-1462.

Hoopes CW et al: Extracorporeal membrane oxygenation as a bridge to pulmonary transplantation. *J Thorac Cardiovasc Surg* 2013 Mar;145(3):862-867.

▼ LIVER TRANSPLANTATION

After many years of experimental effort, Dr Thomas Starzl performed the first successful human liver transplantation in 1967. Over the next decade and a half, the procedure was done only in low volumes, and outcomes were generally poor. As with other organs, the introduction of cyclosporine in the 1980s resulted in marked improvement in survival rates. Today, more than 5000 liver transplants are performed annually in the United States, and 1-year patient survival rates are more than 85%.

Since the introduction of clinical liver transplantation, the list of indications has rapidly expanded and the list of contraindications has diminished. The most common indication for liver transplantation is currently cirrhosis due to chronic hepatitis C infection. Other diseases for which liver transplant is indicated include cirrhosis due to hepatitis B, alcoholic cirrhosis, primary biliary cirrhosis, sclerosing cholangitis, autoimmune hepatitis, and cirrhosis secondary to nonalcoholic fatty liver disease. Less common indications are Wilson disease, α_1-antitrypsin deficiency, Budd-Chiari syndrome, and hemochromatosis. In children, the most common indication is biliary atresia. Other common diagnoses include α_1-antitrypsin deficiency, tyrosinemia, and other inborn errors of metabolism.

Alcoholic cirrhosis was once a subject of considerable controversy because of the self-induced nature of the disease. The world community rejected the notion that lifesaving therapy should be withheld from patients who could benefit from it merely because their disease is self-induced. It was pointed out that many, if not most, diseases are to some degree self-induced, whether it is diabetes and high blood pressure due to obesity or cancer and heart disease due to smoking. It is now recognized that alcoholic cirrhosis is an accepted indication for liver transplant if the patient has demonstrated the ability to abstain from alcohol and is clearly committed to continued abstinence. Overall results in alcoholic recipients have shown that patients transplanted for alcoholic cirrhosis fare at least as well as patients transplanted for most other diagnoses.

Chronic active hepatitis B was formerly considered to be a controversial indication for liver transplantation because recurrence was quite frequent and tended to result in rapid graft failure. This changed when effective strategies to prevent recurrence of hepatitis B using high-dose hepatitis B hyperimmune globulin infusions posttransplant were reported. Now hepatitis B is considered to be a standard indication, and results are equal to those obtained for other diagnoses. In contrast, the outcome for patients transplanted for hepatitis C was once considered to be equal to that of other diagnoses. Recent data, however, suggest that recurrence of hepatitis C in the new liver graft is virtually universal following transplantation, and 25% of patients will have developed cirrhosis in the graft within 5 years. It is not surprising that longer-term data are now appearing showing that the 10-year survival for patients transplanted for hepatitis C is significantly worse than for other diagnoses.

As with transplantation for hepatitis B and C, the consensus opinion has gone back and forth in recent years regarding whether liver transplantation should be used for the treatment of hepatocellular carcinoma in adults. Patients with cirrhosis are at risk for development of primary hepatocellular cancer. Since these patients usually die of liver failure, unlike patients with other forms of malignancy who usually succumb to widespread metastatic disease, it was reasoned that transplantation would be a curative therapy. Unfortunately, the initial results with transplantation for hepatoma were disappointing due to a high rate of tumor recurrence. These poor results prompted many programs to stop doing transplants for hepatoma. The group from Barcelona, Spain, then reported that survival rates are good if the tumor is small (< 5 cm in diameter) but poor if the tumor is large or shows evidence of large vessel invasion. Numerous reports have confirmed this finding, and currently liver transplantation is considered to be a standard treatment for patients with small hepatomas. Results for liver transplantation for other malignancies remain poor, with the exception of several encouraging reports of reasonable survival rates for highly selected patients with cholangiocarcinoma who receive adjuvant radiation and chemotherapy.

Current contraindications are few and are primarily related to evidence of cardiopulmonary disease that prohibits safe liver transplantation. Examples are significant, uncorrected coronary artery disease; pulmonary hypertension with pulmonary artery systolic pressures greater than 70 mm Hg; and FEV_1 of less than 1 L on pulmonary function testing. Active substance abuse is also an absolute contraindication to transplantation. Diabetes increases the risks associated with transplantation and the incidence of posttransplant complications, but it is not an absolute contraindication to liver transplantation. Even infection with HIV, long considered a contraindication to transplantation, is no longer an absolute contraindication at some centers that are reporting good results in small numbers of carefully selected HIV-positive patients. Portal vein thrombosis, which at one time was a contraindication to transplant, is now managed by performing thrombectomy on the portal vein, by using vein grafts to bypass thrombosed vessels, or by using the infrahepatic cava for portal inflow.

Donor Selection

The number of patients listed for liver transplantation increases each year. This has led to a gradual increase in the number of patients who die while waiting and consequently to a relaxation of past standards for liver graft suitability. Livers are currently being transplanted from donors more than 80 years old with acceptable outcomes. It is important that the liver is a rough size match for the donor, but there is much leeway in this regard. Blood-type compatibility is preferred but not an absolute requirement. Matching of tissue antigens does not appear to be relevant for liver transplantation, and a positive crossmatch is not a contraindication to proceeding with transplantation because it is not associated with a worse outcome posttransplant.

The technique of preserving the liver grafts after removal from the donor is based on decreasing metabolic requirements by keeping the graft cold. Blood is flushed from the organ to prevent vascular occlusion; preservation solution is infused; and the organ is kept on ice at 4°C. Multiple preservative solutions are in common use worldwide. Most contain inert high-molecular-weight molecules that do not diffuse into the cell to prevent cellular swelling. Also, free oxygen radical scavengers, which are thought to prevent injury upon reperfusion of the graft, are frequently included. The introduction of Viaspan solution in the late 1980s revolutionized liver transplantation by extending the period of safe in vitro liver preservation from 10 hours to more than 24 hours. Despite this advance, it is clear that prolonged cold ischemia is bad for the liver graft, particularly if the graft contains a large amount of intracellular fat or is from an older donor. Transplant programs therefore continue to strive to minimize the cold ischemic time to whatever degree is feasible.

▶ Operative Technique

In general, liver transplantation is an orthotopic procedure: The host liver is removed and the donor organ placed in an orthotopic position. The operation is performed in three phases: the dissection phase, during which the attachments of the diseased liver are dissected and the vascular structures are prepared for resection; the anhepatic phase, which extends from the time the host liver is removed until the time the donor liver is revascularized; and the reperfusion phase, during which blood is circulating through the new organ and the biliary tree is reconstructed.

Several techniques are available for handling the retrohepatic vena cava. Historically, the liver was removed en bloc with the vena cava and hemodynamic instability was avoided by using venovenous bypass to overcome decreased venous return when vena caval and portal vein flow was interrupted. The new liver was then sutured into place using a bicaval technique with end-to-end caval anastomoses being performed from donor to recipient both above and below the new liver. With careful anesthetic technique and preloading with fluid, venovenous bypass may be avoided in many cases. An alternative method of handling the retrohepatic cava is to dissect the liver off the cava and sequentially ligate the hepatic venous branches that enter the cava directly from the right and caudate lobes. This allows the liver to be removed by clamping the main hepatic veins without occluding the vena cava. The new liver is then sutured into place by connecting the suprahepatic cava of the donor to a common orifice created by connecting the right, middle, and left hepatic veins. This technique is called the piggyback technique because the donor cava sits directly on top of the recipient cava. The infrahepatic cava of the donor is occluded with either sutures or a vascular stapler. This method may preclude the need for venovenous bypass because caval flow is usually not completely interrupted. A third option for caval reconstruction is to connect the donor cava to the recipient cava using a side-to-side technique by making longitudinal incisions from the hepatic veins caudally, creating a very wide anastomosis. This technique is difficult when the donor liver is large relative to the size of the recipient's hepatic fossa.

The current methods of biliary reconstruction include primary choledochocholedochostomy (when the recipient duct is intact) or Roux-en-Y choledochojejunostomy if the recipient bile duct is not intact or if anatomically the donor and recipient duct cannot be approximated without creating tension on the anastomosis. It was once standard to place a T tube or another type of biliary stent across the biliary anastomosis, but many programs have now discontinued this practice because it is not clear that the presence of a stent influences the rate of biliary complications.

Although the liver can function normally with only portal venous flow, the bile duct is dependent on hepatic arterial flow. For this reason, the hepatic arterial anastomosis is crucial to postoperative graft survival. The arterial supply of the liver is quite variable, with nearly half of the patients having some form of aberrant circulation. The most common aberrancies are replacement of the right hepatic artery to the superior mesenteric artery and the presence of an accessory left hepatic artery that derives from the left gastric artery. When aberrant arterial vessels are identified on a deceased donor, it is important that they are carefully preserved so that reconstruction can occur when the liver has been perfused and cooled and is sitting in sterile ice slush. Multiple methods of reconstruction of aberrant vessels are available and, if necessary, a conduit of donor iliac artery may be used in the reconstruction.

▶ Living Donor Liver Transplantation & Split Liver Transplantation

The shortage of organs for small children in the late 1980s prompted the development of techniques to reduce the size of an adult liver graft by performing an anatomic resection of one or more lobes and transplanting the reduced graft. In this way, it was possible to transplant the left lobe or the left lateral segment from an adult liver into a child. This technique was successful and rapidly became a standard method of obtaining grafts for small children. The natural evolution of this technique was to apply the method used to reduce the size of a deceased donor liver graft to adult living donors. Broelsch at the University of Chicago popularized the transplantation of the left lateral segment from an adult into a child and showed that this technique could be at least as effective as using full-sized grafts from small children. It was hoped that living-related liver transplantation would offer an immunologic advantage as it does with kidney transplantation, but this did not turn out to be the case. The major advantage of living donor liver transplantation appears to be the ability to allow transplant to occur prior to the deterioration of the recipient's condition into a poor state of health that is associated with a higher risk for transplantation.

The success of living donor liver transplantation from adult donors into children, together with the shortage of suitable adult donors, led to the development by Marcos and Tanaka of techniques to utilize the right lobe from a living donor to transplant into another adult. The donor operation is a major undertaking and is associated with appreciable morbidity as well as a mortality rate of approximately 0.5%. Nevertheless, living donor liver transplants have become a standard option when timely deceased donor liver transplantation is not possible.

By applying the living donor technique to deceased donors, two transplants can be obtained from a single adult liver from a deceased donor. This has been termed a split liver transplant. Typically, the lateral segment of the left lobe is used for a child or very small adult, while the remainder of the liver consisting of the right lobe plus the medial segment of the left lobe is used for an adult. Less commonly, the liver from an adult deceased donor can also be split into a right lobe graft and a left lobe graft and used for two adults. In fact, improvements in operative technique in the last decade have allowed for an increased use of living donor left lobe grafts in adults with improvements in outcomes.

▶ Immunosuppressive Therapy

The mainstay of immunosuppression for liver transplant recipients is a calcineurin inhibitor. An antimetabolite or corticosteroids, or both, may also be included but are not absolutely necessary. Induction therapy with antilymphocyte preparations was once considered standard but has now been abandoned by many liver transplant programs because it appears unnecessary.

Despite being one of the largest organs transplanted in terms of mass, the liver seems to require less immunosuppression for maintenance therapy compared to other organs. Corticosteroids can frequently be safely discontinued. Typically, monotherapy with a low dose of a calcineurin inhibitor is all that is required to suppress rejection long term. Spontaneous tolerance with normal graft function despite complete discontinuation of all immunosuppressants occurs in approximately 10%-20% of liver transplant recipients. The liver is unique in this regard, since rejection is almost universal if immunosuppression is discontinued in recipients of renal, cardiac, pulmonary, and pancreatic grafts.

▶ Complications

Complications following liver transplantation are common, but most can be treated effectively. Coagulopathy is routinely present during liver transplant procedures, particularly during the anhepatic phase. For this reason, bleeding is common following the procedure, and 5%-10% of liver transplant recipients will require reoperation because of continued bleeding following the procedure.

One of the most devastating complications is primary nonfunction of the liver. Primary nonfunction is a condition in which the new liver does not function and death results unless a second transplant is performed. Patients with primary nonfunction typically have profoundly elevated serum transaminases together with severe coagulopathy and acidosis. The incidence of this complication is between 5% and 10%. The cause of primary nonfunction is poorly understood, but multiple donor factors are known to be associated. Long cold ischemic times, poor perfusion of the graft with preservative solution, severe hepatic steatosis, and elevation of the donor serum sodium level above 165 mEq/L are all known risk factors for primary nonfunction.

Vascular complications occur in 5%-10% of transplant recipients. The hepatic artery is particularly prone to thrombosis, especially in children. If this is detected early, it is frequently possible to perform thrombectomy and restore hepatic arterial flow. If flow cannot be reestablished, necrosis of the intrahepatic and extrahepatic biliary tree usually occurs, resulting in death from sepsis if retransplantation is not performed.

The bile duct has been called the Achilles heel of the liver transplant because it is so prone to anastomotic leakage or stricture. Fortunately, while as many as 20% of liver transplant recipients will experience a bile duct complication, it is uncommon for this complication to be lethal. Leaks tend to occur early and can often be managed by placing a biliary stent using endoscopic retrograde cholangiopancreatography (ERCP). If a large collection of bile develops because of a bile leak, it is usually necessary to drain the area either operatively or by placing a percutaneous suction drain. Biliary stenosis can occur early or late. Unlike the native liver, the transplanted liver will not always develop intrahepatic biliary dilatation when the bile duct is obstructed. It is therefore necessary to have a high index of suspicion. Patients with elevated bilirubin or elevated serum alkaline phosphatase levels (or both) should be evaluated with either ERCP or magnetic resonance cholangiography. Strictures can often be managed noninvasively with biliary stents and balloon cholangioplasty, but in some cases, operative correction is required. Patients who develop multiple intrahepatic strictures usually require retransplantation.

Rejection is a frequent complication of liver transplantation—it occurs in about 20%-50% of patients. Rejection should be suspected whenever serum transaminases or bilirubin levels, or both, worsen or fail to gradually normalize following a liver transplant. The diagnosis of rejection is made histologically by the finding of a mixed portal cellular infiltrate together with injury to bile duct epithelium and inflammation of the central vein endothelium (endotheliitis). When the condition is diagnosed early and treated aggressively, rejection rarely culminates in a need for retransplantation. Because the principal rejection target is the bile duct epithelium, severe, unrelenting rejection is often manifested by destruction and disappearance of bile ducts (vanishing bile duct syndrome). The treatment for rejection depends on its severity. Mild rejection is treated either with corticosteroid pulse therapy or by increasing the dosage of maintenance immunosuppressive therapy. Rejection that does not respond to these measures may require treatment with an antilymphocyte preparation.

CMV is a member of the herpes family of viruses. Prior to the availability of prophylaxis against this virus, as many as half of liver transplant recipients developed clinical CMV infection. Symptoms of this infection typically include fever, leukopenia, and malaise, but a more serious clinical syndrome with pneumonitis or hepatitis is possible. Patients at greatest risk for severe CMV disease are those without previous CMV exposure who receive a liver from a CMV-positive donor, but reactivation of CMV infection is possible in any patient with prior exposure to the virus. In order to prevent CMV infection, most liver transplant programs prescribe either ganciclovir or valganciclovir for a period of months following liver transplantation to all patients at risk for CMV infection.

EBV is another common viral pathogen in these patients. Although the systemic illness with Epstein-Barr virus infection is usually mild, it may be associated with development of a lymphoproliferative disorder known as posttransplant lymphoma. This disorder can progress to frank malignancy, and the mortality rate is high. In many cases, the lymphoproliferation resolves merely be reducing immunosuppression. If the lymphoproliferative tissue expresses CD20, treatment with the monoclonal antibody rituximab may be helpful. Patients with lymphoproliferation that does not respond to these measures may require chemotherapy.

Immunosuppression predisposes to fungal infections, especially esophageal *Candida albicans* ("thrush"). The incidence of this infection is reduced by the use of prophylactic nystatin to decrease gastrointestinal fungal colonization.

Grant RC et al: Living vs. deceased donor liver transplantation for hepatocellular carcinoma: a systematic review and meta-analysis. *Clin Transplant* 2013 Jan-Feb;27(1):140-147.

Ikegami T et al: Strategies for successful left-lobe living donor liver transplantation in 250 consecutive adult cases in a single center. *J Am Coll Surg* 2013 Mar;216(3):353-362.

Nadig SN, Bratton CF, Karp SJ: Marginal donors in liver transplantation: expanding the donor pool. *J Surg Educ* 2007 Jan-Feb;64(1):46-50.

Smith JM et al: Kidney, pancreas and liver allocation and distribution in the United States. *Am J Transplant* 2012 Dec;12(12):3191-3212.

▼ PANCREAS TRANSPLANTATION

Although pancreatic transplantation involves transplantation of a nonessential organ as compared with the liver, heart, or kidney, it has enormous potential in the management of patients with insulin-dependent diabetes. In many patients with type 1 diabetes—even though insulin and diet are carefully controlled—the complications of the disease progress relentlessly. Many patients develop severe retinopathy at an early age, leading to blindness and renal disease as well as severe neuropathy and peripheral vascular disease that ultimately results in limb loss. The goal of pancreas transplantation is primarily to prevent or delay end-organ damage by the complications of diabetes. Another important indication for pancreas transplantation is hypoglycemic unawareness. Diabetic nephropathy can cause loss of the autonomic nervous pathways that allow patients to sense hypoglycemia. These patients can lapse into a coma at any moment. For patients with severe hypoglycemic unawareness, pancreas transplantation can truly be a lifesaving procedure.

Currently, most pancreas transplants are whole-organ grafts from deceased donors. The pancreas is procured along with a cuff of the first, second, and third portion of the duodenum attached. The graft can be placed into the pelvis with the iliac artery supplying arterial supply to the pancreas and the iliac vein used for portal venous drainage of the graft. Alternatively, the graft can be placed in the mid-abdomen and connected to the infrarenal aorta and the superior mesenteric vein. This allows insulin secreted by the pancreas to enter the portal circulation rather than the systemic circulation, which is more physiologic. The pancreatic exocrine secretions may be managed by anastomosing the duodenum to the bladder or to a loop of small bowel.

If the pancreas graft is successful, the patient will quickly become normoglycemic. As long as the graft functions normally, the patient will no longer require exogenous insulin because the pancreas graft responds normally by secreting insulin in response to rising blood glucose levels that occur following eating and ceasing insulin secretion when blood glucose levels fall to normal.

Much research has dealt with the transplantation of isolated pancreatic islet cells, which make up only about 2% of the pancreatic mass. This procedure is intuitively very attractive because it does not require an abdominal incision or general anesthesia. A team from Edmonton has reported successful transplantation of islets into the liver using a transhepatic injection into the portal vein. The patients in the original report all achieved insulin independence, although this often required more than one infusion of islets from more than one deceased donor pancreas. Immunosuppression consisted of rapamycin, tacrolimus, and induction treatment basiliximab, an inhibitor of IL-2R. The success at Edmonton has led to increased enthusiasm worldwide for islet transplantation, but to date, no other center has achieved the same degree of success. The critical factor appears to be the isolation procedure of the islets themselves. Nevertheless, it seems likely that in the long run, islet transplantation will eventually replace whole-organ pancreas transplantation.

Dhanireddy KK: Pancreas transplantation. *Gastroenterol Clin North Am* 2012 Mar;41(1):133-142.

Han DJ, Sutherland DE: Pancreas transplantation. *Gut Liver* 2010 Dec;4(4):450-465.

Maglione M, Ploeg RJ, Friend PJ: Donor risk factors, retrieval technique, preservation and ischemia/reperfusion injury in pancreas transplantation. *Curr Opin Organ Transplant* 2013 Feb;18(1):83-88.

MULTIPLE CHOICE QUESTIONS

1. Which of the following cytokines is most often implicated in the delayed type hypersensitivity?

   A. IL-10
   B. IL-17
   C. IFN-γ
   D. IL-6
   E. IL-13

2. Lymphoma after transplant is most commonly of which cellular origin?

   A. T-cell
   B. B-cell
   C. Delta Cell
   D. Gamma Cell
   E. Macrophage

3. Life expectancy in patients who have undergone kidney transplantation is increased compared with chronic dialysis by a factor of

   A. Two
   B. One-half
   C. Four
   D. Three
   E. Unchanged

4. Chronic transplant dysfunction (CTD) is the leading cause of graft failure in the long term. Which of the following organs is affected by CTD?

   A. Kidney
   B. Heart
   C. Liver
   D. Lung
   E. All of the above

5. Which of the following conditions are not currently indications for liver transplantation?

   A. Hepatocellular carcinoma
   B. Hepatitis C infection with liver failure
   C. Steatohepatitis with liver failure
   D. Metastatic colon cancer
   E. Alcoholic cirrhosis with liver failure

Appendix: Answers to Multiple Choice Questions

CHAPTER 2

1A. Beneficence and nonmaleficence are synonyms

2E. Both A and C are true

3C. Technical skills

4D. Are separate organizations that credential surgeons, and educate surgeons, respectively, as primary parts of their missions

5E. A, B, and C

CHAPTER 3

1A. Is an approach to categorizing patients preoperatively to assess their risk for an operative procedure

2D. Should include a pain assessment to aid in the management of postoperative pain

3C. Can be modified by risk-based interventions

4E. Both A and C are true

5C. Can have frailty measured by a variety of means that predict the risk of complications

CHAPTER 4

1E. Hypocalcemia

2D. Discharge the patient with a prescription for pain medication and a plan for follow-up in 2 weeks

3C. Cancel the operation with the plan for improved preoperative preparation

4E. All of the above except for D

5D. Evaluation of the patient, intubation for protection of airway, transfer to a higher level of care, transfusion with 2 units of FFP and 2 units of matched packed RBCs, antibiotic administration, and computed tomography of the abdomen

CHAPTER 5

1A. They are common after chest procedures, but rare after abdominal operations.

2C. Her initial management can include intravenous hydration and nasogastric suction.

3C. High ileostomy output with inadequate postoperative replacement

4D. Bladder pressure measurement may be useful to determine the likelihood of abdominal compartment syndrome.

5A. Classified by the Centers for Disease Control into: (1) wound only, (2) organ space, and (3) involving organ parenchyma

CHAPTER 6

1B. Inflammation. An acute wound is defined by its ability to normally progress, in a predictable and timely manner, through all of the phases of wound healing; coagulation, inflammation, fibroplasia, angiogenesis, and remodeling. A protracted inflammatory phase is the usual mechanism for the formation of a chronic wound. All clinical efforts should be made to reduce chronic wound inflammation in an effort to support healing.

2C. Macrophage. The macrophage is the most important source of growth factor signals for wound healing. Experimental studies show that wound healing is most impaired in the absence of macrophages. Although fibroblasts are the main source of collagen synthesis and endothelial cells are required for revascularization, they are dependent on macrophage signaling to stimulate and direct tissue repair. A platelet is not a cell.

3E. TcO2 less than 30 mm Hg. Wounds will not heal when the tissue concentration of oxygen falls below 30 mm Hg. It is the most powerful predictive measure of delayed or impaired wound healing. Vitamin C deficiency may result in impaired collagen cross linking (scurvy) and weak scars. Low serum albumin predicts increased wound complications, like wound infection. The microangiopathy of radiated tissue indirectly reduces perfusion and therefore, TcO2 levels. Finally, smoking impairs wound healing through the vasoconstrictive effects of chronic nicotine and relative hypoxia as well.

4C. A moist wound environment. A moist or even wet wound environment is critical to normal wound healing. The cellular and molecular biological activity within a wound requires hydration to proceed. Clinical use of dry dressings to support wound debridement, for example, should be limited. Similarly, poor dressing resulting in repeated trauma and mechanical instability to the wound is often overlooked as a source for wound healing failure. Wound infection is the most clinically important, and expensive, impediment to surgical wound healing. Foreign bodies in the wound, such as synthetic surgical meshes, also delay normal wound healing. Finally, experimental and clinical data support that obesity contributes to abnormal wound healing, primarily through a metabolic pathway, and secondarily by increasing the risk of wound infection.

5D. Early fascial dehiscence and wound failure. Pollock and Evans showed in a classic clinical study that 94% of incisional hernias were the result of 1.2 cm fascial dehiscence before POD 30. The majority of the time, these were clinically occult wound closure failures, progressing to incisional hernias over the subsequent 3 years. It is no longer believed that many incisional hernias are the result of abnormal scar formation or suture breaking, stretching or even pulling through the fascia. Poor technique certainly will contribute to incisional hernia formation, but the fundamental mechanism is early fascial dehiscence.

CHAPTER 7

1B. In bipolar electrosurgery, the current flows from the handpiece to the return electrode.

2B. Depends upon the presence of an oxygen source, an ignition source and fuel

CHAPTER 8

1E. All of A, B, and C

2E. Both A and C are true

3C. Can be improved by the use of alcohol-containing skin preparation solutions

4E. Both A and C

5A. NSSSIs are generally self-limited and non-threatening

CHAPTER 9

1C. Anion gap metabolic acidosis with appropriate respiratory compensation. As above, values from an arterial blood gas are typically reported in this order: pH, pCO_2, paO_2, HCO_3^-.

This patient's pH is normal, but near-acidotic. HCO_3^- and pCO_2 are both low. Decreased HCO_3^- will cause acidosis, while decreased pCO_2 will cause alkalosis, thus the patient's primary disorder is metabolic. His calculated anion gap is 22. pCO_2 is within the 36-40 mm Hg range of appropriate compensation predicted by Winter's formula, thus no concurrent respiratory disorder exists. Therefore, this patient has an anion gap metabolic acidosis with appropriate respiratory compensation. Respiratory compensation for metabolic disorders is rapid (note his hyperventilation), hence the normal pH.

If respiratory compensation were inappropriate, one would need to consider another, simultaneous process, in addition to alkalosis, eg, the respiratory acidosis which occurs in the later stages of salicylate poisoning, when central respiratory drive has been suppressed.

Note the patient's $\Delta\Delta$ = 2.5. Considering this finding in isolation, one would conclude that the patient has a mixed anion-gap metabolic acidosis and metabolic alkalosis. This underscores the need to take into account all of the patient's data when making determinations of acid base status. There is no additional evidence of a metabolic alkalosis, thus this additional disturbance is unlikely.

2A. Hypophosphatemia. Refeeding syndrome occurs when a malnourished patient (eg, an elderly or alcohol-dependent patient, or a patient who has experienced recent weight loss) begins to consume calories or begins to receive intravenous glucose administration. Insulin levels rise, causing electrolytes which have shifted to the extracellular space during a period of starvation to shift back to the intracellular space for use in the construction of new proteins and cells. Refeeding also leads to increased intracellular requirements for PO_4^{3-} and Mg^{2+} due to increased ATP production and glucose metabolism, decreasing serum levels of these electrolytes even further. This all leads to hypokalemia, hypomagnesemia, and hypophosphatemia, any one of which may be fatal. For these reasons, electrolytes must be closely monitored and aggressively repleted in patients at risk for refeeding syndrome.

3C. FENa < 1%. In oliguric patients, FENa < 1% is indicative of pre-renal azotemia and intravascular volume depletion. BUN:Cr ratio > 20 is indicative of hypovolemia. FENa > 1% is indicative of intrinsic renal causes of oliguria, and should prompt workup including microscopic urine analysis and renal ultrasonography. Post-renal obstruction should be investigated if clinically suspected (eg, caused by benign prostatic hypertrophy in this 70-year-old male).

FENa is unreliable in patients taking diuretics. In such cases, FEUN should be calculated:

$$FEUN = 100 \times \frac{(UN_U * Cr_p)}{(Cr_U * BUN)}$$

where U: urine, P: plasma, UN: urea nitrogen, BUN: blood urea nitrogen, Cr: creatinine.

Table 9–5. Common laboratory values distinguishing between oliguric pre-renal and intrinsic renal failure.

Test	Pre-renal value	Intrinsic renal value	Post-renal value
FENa	< 1%	≥ 1%	
FEUN	< 35%	≥ 35%	
BUN:Cr ratio	> 20	< 10	10-20

4D. All of the above. Stored blood products are anticoagulated with trisodium citrate, which chelates Ca^{2+} from stored blood, disrupting the clotting cascade. In the setting of massive transfusion, such as this patient has undergone, normal hepatic metabolism of trisodium citrate may be overwhelmed, and Ca^{2+} (along with Mg^{2+}) may be chelated from the blood, leading to hypocoagulability, hypocalcemia, and hypomagnesemia. Furthermore, stored pRBCs contain high levels of K^+, the result of lysis of red blood cells. This is especially true of the older pRBCs often utilized in massive transfusion situations. For these reasons, serum electrolytes must be closely monitored and controlled in the setting of massive transfusion.

5B. Mixed metabolic alkalosis and AG metabolic acidosis. The patient is acidotic, with a normal pCO_2, low-normal HCO_3^-, and high anion gap. Therefore, this patient has an anion-gap metabolic acidosis. Given the clinical circumstances, the most likely etiology of her metabolic acidosis is lactic acidosis caused by septic shock.

Note that the patient's pH is significantly below the lower limit of normal, despite the normal pCO_2 and low-normal HCO_3^-. This should prompt concern for a mixed acid-base disorder. Her $\Delta\Delta = 2$, indicating a coexistent metabolic alkalosis. The several days of gastric suctioning provides a ready explanation for this component of her mixed acid-base disorder.

CHAPTER 10

1C. Bactericidal activity of enteral nutrition components. Multiple mechanisms have been proposed for the morphological and functional differences observed in the intestinal epithelium with parenteral nutrition (PN) when compared to enteral nutrition. It has repeatedly been demonstrated that small bowel mucosal mass is lost with only PN. Yang and colleagues demonstrated that the administration of 25% enteral nutrition reversed the abnormal IL-10, IL-4, and IL-6 messenger RNA (mRNA) expression that had resulted from only PN support in animal models. This is of particular significance as these changes in cytokine expression were associated with epithelial leak and an increased rate of enterocyte apoptosis.

It has also been shown that the type and route of nutrition affect pIgR expression in an organ-specific manner; pIgR represents the exclusive transport pathway for IgA to move from the lamina propria, through the epithelia, into the lumen of the gut where it acts as a key component in the gut's defense. Enteral nutrition components are not bactericidal and actually help preserve normal flora.

2D. Burns. Energy requirements above basal needs are approximately 10% for elective operations, 10%-30% for trauma, 50%-80% for sepsis, and 100%-200% for burns. Burns covering more than 40% total body surface area (TBSA) are typically followed by a period of severe stress, characterized by an exaggerated catabolic state. Increases in catecholamine, glucocorticoid, glucagon, and dopamine secretion are thought to initiate the cascade of events leading to the acute hypermetabolic response with its ensuing catabolic state. Appropriate nutrient delivery can be accomplished by feeding 1.2-1.4 times the measured resting energy expenditures (REEs).

3C. The recommended amino acid dose ranges from 0.8 to 1 g/kg. The recommendation for the amino acid dose ranges from 1.2 to 1.5 g/kg/d for most patients with normal renal and hepatic function, although some sources recommend higher doses. TPN via a central line is indicated for patients who cannot obtain adequate nourishment via the gastrointestinal tract for a minimum duration of treatment of 7-10 days. The use of postoperative TPN for only 2 or 3 days is highly discouraged, as the risks outweigh the benefits incurred over this short period of time. A reasonable initial guideline is to provide 60%-70% of nonamino acid calories as dextrose and 30%-40% of nonamino acid calories as fat emulsion. The placement of central line catheters always carries risks; the overall complication rate related to this access is greater than 15%. Femoral vein access carries the highest risk of infection and should be avoided if possible.

4C. Gastric bypass patients are prone to deficiencies of the fat-soluble vitamins, calcium, iron, vitamin B12, and folate. Gastric bypass procedures intentionally limit the amount of oral intake and decrease the amount of small bowel that takes part in absorption. This renders the population of patients prone to deficiencies of the fat-soluble vitamins (A, D, E, and K), calcium, iron, vitamin B12, and folate.

Careful attention should be paid to ensuring that these deficiencies are countered with supplementation. Technical complications occur in about 5% of enterally fed patients and include clogging of the tube; esophageal, tracheal, bronchial, or duodenal perforation; and tracheobronchial intubation with tube feeding aspiration. Lactose intolerance is least common in European Caucasians, present within only 5%-10% of this population. Although recommendations differ depending on source, enteral feeds are not typically held until gastric residuals of greater than 200 cc are encountered.

5B. The NRI is an excellent tool for tracking the adequacy of nutritional support. The NRI is an index that has been prospectively crossvalidated against other nutritional indices with good results, but is not a good tool for tracking the adequacy of nutritional support, since supplemental nutrition often fails to improve serum albumin levels. The index successfully stratifies perioperative morbidity and mortality using serum albumin and weight loss as predictors of malnutrition.

CHAPTER 11

1D. Stop all over-the-counter herbal remedies. Although the use of herbal medications has been around for many years, none have been approved by the FDA. Many times the pharmacology of these remedies is unknown and the remedies may not contain the correct amounts of active ingredients stated on the label. It is estimated that up to 12% of patients are using these herbal drugs.

2B. The initial assessment should be done at a minimum the day before surgery for patients undergoing procedures of high surgical invasiveness. The timing of the preoperative evaluation by an anesthesiologist depends primarily on the planned degree of the surgery. Even healthy patients undergoing a surgical procedure that involves a high degree of surgical invasiveness that may include the risks of a high volume of blood loss, prolonged surgical time, special positioning requirements, etc, should be seen at least a day before the planned procedure. Patients with significant comorbidities should be seen in a PAC at least the day before surgery no matter the degree of surgical invasiveness as it is necessary to ascertain the degree of control of the comorbidities.

3D. Surgery should be delayed for up to 1 year. The risk of stent thrombosis makes it necessary to place patients who have had a drug-eluting stent placed on antiplatelet agents such as clopidogrel and aspirin. Stopping these drugs prematurely to allow for the performance of an elective surgical procedure requires careful consideration of the risk of bleeding as well as the risk of stent thrombosis if the antiplatelet agents are both stopped. At a minimum aspirin should be continued. Emergent procedures that involve a high risk of bleeding require that the clopidogrel be stopped, but continuing the low-dose aspirin is recommended.

4D. None of the above. There is no way to be 100% of preventing intraoperative awareness. Anesthesiologists performing strict equipment check before beginning an anesthetic to ensure that vaporizers have sufficient agent levels, that there is an agent concentration monitor as part of the anesthesia monitoring system, and frequent observation that IV lines are patent and intact when intravenous medications are used is one way to eliminate the preventable components. Stable vital signs throughout a case are not always a reliable sign that a patient may not suffer from intraoperative awareness. Finally the processed EEG BIS monitor has been shown to be no more effective in preventing awareness than careful monitoring of end-tidal agent concentration.

5C. Obesity. The RCRI factors of (1) ischemic heart disease, (2) heart failure, (3) high-risk surgery, (4) diabetes mellitus, (5) renal insufficiency, and (6) cerebral vascular diseases are a validated set of independent predictors of cardiac risk for patients. There RCRIs were derived from a single-center prospective group of patients undergoing elective major noncardiac surgery. The anesthesiologist in a pre-op clinic will screen for these factors and recommend further studies based on the presence or absence of RCRIs. Patients with no RCRIs had a very low (0.4%) cardiac risk while patients with three or more risk factors have a 5.4% risk of an adverse cardiac event and warrant further testing or optimization of the factor(s).

CHAPTER 12

1E. All of A, B, and C

2B. Can contribute to coagulopathy

3E. All of A, B, and C

4A. Can be related to products of coagulation and inflammation that are washed out from the damaged tissues

5B. PSV includes a set inspiratory time

CHAPTER 13

1C. Should have an initial assessment including airway, breathing and circulation

2D. Should bypass the trauma room and go directly to the operating room

3E. A, B, and C are all correct

4E. From gunshot wounds below the nipple line typically require laparotomy for evaluation and management

5E. All are correct

CHAPTER 14

1C. Death of others in same incident

2A. Can contribute to coagulopathy

3D. Primary management with bismuth-containing antimicrobial topical agents

4A. Benefits from early consideration with functional position splinting and active motion

5B. Inhalational injury

CHAPTER 15

1B. Take her to the operating room immediately for an emergent biopsy. Invasive fungal sinusitis is usually seen in immunocompromised patients, such as the patient described here. It is caused by uncontrolled infiltrative growth of usually nonpathogenic fungal organisms such as Rhizopus or Aspergillus species. Even with prompt diagnosis, aggressive surgical therapy, and modern antifungal agents, the disease still carries a significant mortality rate (up to 30%). The index of suspicion for invasive fungal sinusitis must be high for any immunocompromised patient, as the symptoms can be subtle and the disease rapidly progressive. If invasive fungal sinusitis is suspected, biopsies should be taken of the suspicious areas and sent for immediate pathologic examination. Note that this can often involve calling a pathologist in from home in the middle of the night or on a weekend, if they are not in-house. In the case presented here, the likelihood of the child cooperating with an examination and biopsy is low, thus an emergent posting to the operating room is the most prudent action.

2E. All of the above. Acute angioedema is characterized by localized swelling of subcutaneous and submucosal tissue of the head and neck. The swelling usually begins with mild facial involvement but may progress to involve the oral cavity, tongue, pharynx, and larynx. The underlying pathophysiology of angioedema involves vasoactive mediators such as bradykinin and histamine, causing interstitial edema through endothelial-mediated vasodilation of arterioles with subsequent capillary and venule leakage. Drug-induced angioedema has classically been associated with the use of angiotensin-converting enzyme inhibitors (ACE inhibitors), although many other medications can also cause this phenomenon. Other drugs known to be associated with angioedema include rituximab, alteplase, fluoxetine, laronidase, lepirudin, angiotensin II receptor blockers (ARBs), and tacrolimus.

3A. Immediately superior to the cricoid cartilage. The patient described has Ludwig's Angina, an uncommon life-threatening condition characterized by cellulitis involving the submental, sublingual, and submandibular spaces. The source of the infection is odontogenic and spreads rapidly. The infection is usually polymicrobial with aerobic and anaerobic gram-positive cocci and gram-negative

rods. Airway compromise in these patients is common, and should be of primary concern. A cricothyroidotomy is performed through the cricothyroid membrane which spans the midline area between the cricoid cartilage inferiorly and the thyroid cartilage superiorly. It can be easily palpated just inferior to the thyroid cartilage in greater than 90% of individuals, and has no major blood vessels or structures. While an emergency tracheotomy can be performed through the second or third intertracheal ring space, this often involves either going through or dissecting part of the thyroid gland off the tracheal wall. As the thyroid's blood supply is quite robust, the bleeding encountered can be quite significant. Therefore, in an emergency situation the cricothyroid space is almost universally preferred.

4C. Left posterior cricoarytenoid muscle. Innervation to the larynx is provided by the vagus nerve (cranial nerve X). The recurrent laryngeal nerves branch from the vagus nerve and provide motor innervation to all of the intrinsic muscles of the larynx except the cricothyroid muscle. All of the intrinsic muscles of the larynx serve to tense the vocal folds or adduct the vocal folds except one—the paired posterior cricoarytenoid muscles. Current understanding of peripheral nerve injury and regeneration presents the following scenario when the nerve supply to the larynx is injured. After nerve injury, neuronal axon regrowth results in reinnervation of the target muscles but in a random pattern. Since only one of the muscles abducts the vocal folds, reinnervation is unlikely to result in a tonically abducted vocal fold. Instead, the vocal fold usually assumes a paramedian position, accompanied by loss of muscle bulk and atrophy due to loss of innervation. This can lead to hoarseness and vocal fatigue when one side is injured, but often causes airway obstruction if both sides are injured.

5D. 25-year old man with 12 pack-year tobacco history and chronic severe gastroesophageal reflux. Presents with throat pain and dysphagia (trouble swallowing). On fiberoptic endoscopy is found to have a 3 cm ulcerated hypopharyngeal mass. No palpable neck adenopathy is present. Assuming appropriate treatment, outcomes for patients with oral cavity cancer are generally good with 5-year survival rates of 72% for stage I-II, 44% for stage III-IVb, and 35% for stage IVc. Outcomes for patients with laryngeal cancer can be excellent. For early stage I glottis carcinoma (tumor limited to the true vocal folds), 5-year overall survival rates of 90% can be expected. Overall, laryngeal cancer carries a 5-year survival for stage I-II disease of 79%. Survival for oropharyngeal cancer is somewhat worse: stage I-II oropharyngeal cancer 5-year survical average is 58% and stage III-IVb 41%. The hypopharynx is invested with an abundant lymphatic drainage network, and patients with hypopharyngeal cancer typically present with advanced stage disease. Hypopharyngeal cancer carries the worst prognosis of any head and neck subsite. Five-year survival for stage I-II hypopharyngeal cancer is 47%, stage III-IVb is 30%, and stage IVc only 16%.

CHAPTER 16

1D. TSH

2D. Both A and C

3B. Is less likely to spread to lymph nodes than is papillary thyroid cancer

4A. Vitamin A toxicity

5D. Osteoporosis with a T-score of -2.8

CHAPTER 17

1C. Caused at least in part by estrogen stimulation of breast tissue

2D. A personal history of breast cancer

3B. Identifies cancer without node involvement in about 80% of detected cases

4A. A painless mass identified by the patient

5D. Can be reliably detected by sentinel lymph node biopsy in women with clinically uninvolved axillary lymph nodes

CHAPTER 18

1C. Mostly arise from bone or cartilage

2D. Iodine deficiency

3B. Ureteral obstruction with transdiaphragmatic urine leak

4A. Spontaneous bacterial mediastinitis of sarcoidosis

5D. Effectively cured by double lung transplantation with a 10-year graft survival exceeding 85%

CHAPTER 19A

1C. Atherosclerosis tends to occur diffusely in small coronary vessels. Myocardial tissue extracts 70%-80% of arterial blood oxygen at rest, unlike other organs which can extract additional oxygen during periods of increased demand. The myocardium recruits additional blood flow by vasodilation and recruitment of an extensive capillary bed via a feedback mechanism from adenosine diphosphate and other byproducts of metabolism, increasing oxygen delivery to match consumption. Atherosclerosis, or the formation of intra-arterial cholesterol plaques, tends to occur in the more proximal and larger epicardial vessels, leaving the distal vasculature relatively unobstructed. This allows revascularization by either percutaneous or surgical techniques.

2D. Typical symptoms are exertional dyspnea, angina or syncope. Senile calcific aortic stenosis occurs in the eighth decade of life in patients with tricuspid (normal) aortic valves. While dilation of the ascending aorta is a normal part of the aging process, aneurysms of the ascending aorta are associated with bicuspid aortic valves, related to abnormalities in elastin fiber formation. Rheumatic heart disease affects the mitral valve most commonly. It is unusual for a patient with rheumatic heart disease to present with isolated aortic stenosis but not mitral valve disease, whereas the opposite is fairly common. Indications for surgery in aortic stenosis are the presence of symptoms, which are exercise intolerance, angina, syncope, and dyspnea.

3C. Asymptomatic with a prolapsed anterior mitral leaflet. Indications for surgery in patients with mitral regurgitation include heart failure symptoms, left ventricular dilation and reduced left ventricular systolic function. In asymptomatic patients without symptoms and normal ventricular function and size, surgery could be recommended if the likelihood of durable repair is high. Repair of posterior leaflet prolapse is much more common than in prolapse of the anterior leaflet. Mitral replacement would entail either a bioprosthetic with limited durability, or a mechanical valve and a lifelong requirement for anticoagulation. Moderate mitral regurgitation is typically addressed incidentally at the time of other cardiac surgery, including coronary bypass grafting or aortic valve replacement.

4D. Malperfusion of the abdominal viscera can occur with either Stanford type A or type B aortic dissections. Due to gradual and progressive breakdown of elastin fibers, the ascending aorta dilates as part of the natural aging process. Indications for replacement of the ascending aorta include size of 5-5.5 cm in asymptomatic patients, 4.5 cm in patients with know Marfan syndrome, interval growth of 1 cm in 1 year, or 4.5 cm when incidental to other cardiac surgery including aortic valve replacement or coronary bypass grafting. Stanford type A dissections involve the ascending aorta, which can cause sudden death from intrapericardial rupture and tamponade, aortic valve insufficiency from prolapse, or coronary malperfusion and myocardial infarction. Stanford type B dissections are distal to the ascending aorta and thus not within the pericardial space and not directly adjacent to the aortic valve or coronary ostia. Malperfusion from an aortic dissection occurs when the intimal flap occludes any branch of the aorta causing ischemia. Both Stanford type A and B can cause malperfusion of the abdominal viscera, depending on the extent and geometry of the dissection.

5A. Beta-blockers improve survival in patients with advanced heart failure from a variety of proposed mechanisms, including up-regulation of beta-receptors in the myocardium. Heart failure incidence is increasing related to aging population and the rising incidence of diabetes as well as obesity. Deaths from coronary artery disease and myocardial infarctions are decreasing from improved medical care. Temporary mechanical circulatory support increases a heart transplant candidate to status 1A, while implantable mechanical circulatory support results in status 1B. Patients with chronic heart failure on oral medical treatment are status 2. Following heart transplantation, right ventricular dysfunction is the most frequent complication, as the donor's untrained right ventricle is required to maintain circulation in a recipient with pulmonary hypertension, which is often present from long standing heart failure.

CHAPTER 19B

1B. Left-to-right shunting through a VSD causes a volume load on the right ventricle. Ventricular septal defects are classified by their location in the ventricular septum. The most common type is perimembranous. Left-to-right shunting through a VSD causes a volume load on the left ventricle as blood returns from the lungs. The right ventricle does not experience a volume load, but is pressure loaded. Certainly, as PVR decreases after birth, congestive heart failure may develop in a previously asymptomatic patient with a large VSD as left-to-right shunting increases. Knowledge of the expected location of the conduction system is paramount in the surgical repair of a VSD. The AV node is an atrial structure that lies at the apex of an anatomic triangle (known as the triangle of Koch) formed by the coronary sinus, the tendon of Todaro, and the septal attachment of the tricuspid valve. The node then gives rise to the bundle of His, which penetrates the AV junction beneath the membranous septum. The bundle of His then bifurcates into right and left bundle branches, which pass along either side of the muscular ventricular septum. In the presence of a perimembranous VSD, the bundle of His passes along the posterior and inferior rim of the defect, generally on the left ventricular side. The bundle of His tends to run along the posterior and inferior margin of inlet VSDs as well. The conduction tissue is usually remote from outlet and trabecular VSDs.

2A. Neonate with prenatal diagnosis of aortic coarctation who develops acidosis, oliguria, and diminished pedal pulses 8 hours after birth. In scenario A, the neonate described has inadequate systemic perfusion as demonstrated by oliguria and acidosis. With a prenatal diagnosis of aortic coarctation, one must be suspicious at 8 hours after birth that ductal closure has caused a critical narrowing of the aortic isthmus as it involutes. This patient will benefit by reopening the ductus arteriosus with PGE1. The patient described in option B is likely experiencing pulmonary overcirculation with congestive heart failure. Initiating PGE1 would be expected to exacerbate this problem. In option C, a 6-week-old child's ductus would not be expected to reopen with prostaglandins. Also, the etiology of the heart failure symptoms described is due to myocardial ischemia and surgical correction of the coronary anomaly is required. PGE is not appropriate. In option D, the vascular ring described is likely causing a mechanical airway obstruction. Again, surgical intervention is required. PGE therapy has no role in this situation.

3C. Balloon atrial septostomy. d-transposition of the great arteries typically requires two or more levels of mixing in order to maintain adequate saturations. This may involve mixing at the atrial level (via an ASD), ventricular level

(via a VSD), or at the level of the great arteries (via a PDA). In the situation described, the infant requires an additional level of mixing. This may be due to the absence of additional (intracardiac) shunts, or they may be too small if present. Emergent balloon atrial septostomy in the catheterization laboratory is indicated. The other options are not appropriate at this time.

4C. Coronary AV fistula. Coronary AV fistula is the most common major coronary anomaly. The second most common is ALCAPA.

5B. Isolated pulmonary stenosis in a neonate. Isolated aortic coarctation in a neonate is well managed with a primary extended end-to-end anastomosis and is almost always primarily approached surgically. Isolated pulmonary stenosis is typically primarily treated with balloon pulmonary valvuloplasty. This approach has been highly successful. The patient in option C is best managed with a trial of Indocin, followed by bedside surgical ligation if the ductus fails to close with medical management. Larger patients with PDAs requiring closure are frequently treated with catheter-based closure with excellent results. Perimembranous VSDs are best closed surgically. Device closure of VSDs in this location is associated with prohibitively high rates of complete heart block along with the risk of impairing the function of the aortic and/or tricuspid valve.

CHAPTER 20

1A. Absence of esophageal peristalsis. Esophageal manometry is the gold standard for establishing the diagnosis of esophageal achalasia. The classic manometric findings are: (1) absence of esophageal peristalsis and (2) hypertensive LES (in about 50% of patients) that relaxes only partially in response to swallowing. Dysphagia for both solid and liquid food is the most common symptom, experienced by virtually every patient. Heartburn is present in about 40% of patients. As the low intraluminal pH, it is not due to GER, but rather to stasis and fermentation of undigested food in the distal esophagus.

2D. The surgical treatment consists of LES myotomy, resection of the diverticulum or its suspension. Although rare, Zenker diverticulum is more common than the epiphrenic diverticulum. It is a protrusion of pharyngeal mucosa through a weak zone in the Killian's triangle, secondary to abnormalities of the UES sphincter. Dysphagia occurs very frequently. As the pouch enlarges, its contents can be inhaled into the respiratory tree causing chronic cough and pneumonia. Finally, the established treatment consists of eliminating the functional obstruction performing a UES myotomy, associated with resection or suspension of the diverticulum.

3A. Esophageal manometry, 24-hour pH monitoring and upper endoscopy. Heartburn, along with regurgitation and dysphagia is considered a typical symptom of gastroesophageal reflux (GERD). However, a clinical diagnosis of GERD based on these symptoms is correct in only 70%

of patients (when compared with the results of pH monitoring). Heartburn can also be caused by nonesophageal disorders such as biliary disease, irritable bowel syndrome, coronary artery disease, and psychiatric diseases. Esophageal manometry is mandatory to evaluate the function of both the esophageal body and LES. In addition, manometry is essential for proper placement of the pH probe for ambulatory pH monitoring. Twenty-four-hour pH monitoring measures reflux of acid from the stomach into the esophagus and correlate it to the symptoms. Upper endoscopy visualizes the mucosal surface of the esophagus, determines the presence and degree of esophagitis and allows biopsies.

4B. Is linked to duodeno-gastro-esophageal reflux. Barrett esophagus is defined as a change in the esophageal mucosa with replacement of the squamous epithelium by columnar epithelium. It is classified into short segment if less than 3 cm in length or long segment if 3 cm or longer. Barrett esophagus represents an adaptation of the esophageal mucosa to the acid and duodenal juice from the stomach. The diagnosis is confirmed by pathologic examination of the esophageal mucosa and requires the identification of goblet cells, typical for intestinal epithelium. Patients with BE have typically a long history of GERD. Nevertheless, they may become asymptomatic over time due to the decreased sensitivity of the metaplastic epithelium.

5D. All of the above. In patients with early esophageal cancer (pT1a), an esophagectomy can be avoided, because of the very low risk of lymph nodes metastasis (0%-3%), and EMR and RFA are very effective. Unlike intramucosal cancer (T1a), T1b cancer has a high risk of lymph node metastases (20%-30% vs. 0%-3%), and therefore esophageal resection is the treatment of choice. In case of locally advanced esophageal cancer (T3-4N0-3, T2N1-3), chemo-radiation is the best treatment, followed by surgery. It seems that the combination of neo-adjuvant therapy followed by surgery offers the best survival benefit. This is particularly true in the subgroup of patients (about 20%) who have a "complete pathologic response" (no tumor found in the specimen). In patients with distant metastases, survival is very poor and treatment modalities focus on the palliation of symptoms. Endoscopic stenting is one of the most successful options in the treatment of dysphagia.

CHAPTER 21

1C. Appendicitis. Both the patient's age and gender play an important role in forming the differential diagnosis. As patients age there is a distinct shift in causes of abdominal pain and an increase in surgically treatable etiologies. This has been best documented in the OMGE's (World Organization of Gastroenterology) survey of worldwide causes of abdominal pain. This survey gathered data on more than 10,000 patients in 17 countries presenting with acute abdominal pain. When the data is segregated by age comparing those less than 50 years of age to those older than 50 years of age there are clear differences. Appendicitis is by far the most common etiology of a surgical abdomen in patients younger than 50. In the older population group cholecystitis is the most common cause with good representation from bowel obstruction, appendicitis, pancreatitis and diverticulitis. In older patients hernias are a more common problem, with up to a third of bowel obstructions being related to hernias. Cancer, vascular disease, and mesenteric ischemia are also more common as we age. While it is more common for a patient in their twenties to present with abdominal pain, a large proportion will have the diagnosis of nonspecific abdominal pain. Patients older than 50 years of age have both a higher likelihood of an operative etiology for their acute abdomen as well as an increased mortality related to their presentation. This mortality is higher still for patients older than 70 years of age.

2B. They are most useful when intestinal obstruction is part of the differential diagnosis. Before the advent of the CT scan the acute abdominal series played an important role in the diagnosis of the acute abdomen as diagnostic tools were limited. There are long lists of radiologic findings that may correlate with a wide variety of intra-abdominal pathology. A small percentage of renal and biliary stones may be seen on plain radiograph. In our current practice environment there is a much more limited role for plain films of the abdomen. They can be helpful in locating foreign bodies within the GI tract and they may assist in the diagnosis and evaluation of bowel obstructions. Ultrasound is a more sensitive test for biliary stones. CT scans have increased sensitivity and specificity in almost all causes of intra-abdominal pathology when compared with abdominal plain films. For this reason, in stable patients who are going to undergo CT scan there is little added value in obtaining plain films. Upright chest radiograph is the most sensitive test for intra-abdominal free air from a perforated viscus. It should be obtained as part of the evaluation of the acute abdomen both for identifying free air as well as ruling out a variety of cardiac and pulmonary pathologies.

3E. ABG and Lactate. Given the severity of the patient's pain and its abrupt presentation it would not be prudent to solely admit this patient without further evaluation. This patient presents with severe acute abdominal pain and a relatively benign abdominal examination, concerning for mesenteric ischemia. Etiologies include arterial or venous occlusion as well as nonocclusive low-flow states such as in critically ill with hypotension. This patient has an irregular heart rate from atrial fibrillation, which puts the patient at risk for an arterial embolic event. The classic presentation of mesenteric ischemia is severe pain out of proportion to physical examination findings. Helpful laboratory data include an arterial blood gas with lactate. An elevated lactate suggests tissue hypoxemia. Ischemic bowel as a result of diminished blood flow will convert to anaerobic metabolism on a cellular level producing lactate. Although not specific to mesenteric ischemia, it can be a helpful laboratory value to predict severity of illness when elevated. A normal lactate does not exclude mesenteric ischemia. If clinically suspected, workup should proceed despite a normal lactate. Radiographic imaging of choice is CT angiography to assess mesenteric vessels. These patients should be kept strict NPO and if mesenteric ischemia is diagnosed, patient should proceed emergently to the operating room for exploratory laparotomy to minimize further bowel ischemia. Amylase is helpful in ruling out other diagnostic possibilities such as pancreatitis. As mentioned earlier plain abdominal films are rarely indicated in evaluation of the acute abdomen.

4C. MRI abdomen/pelvis. Pregnancy presents a diagnostic dilemma when encountering abdominal pain. Ultrasound is the first line imaging modality in pregnant women as it is noninvasive and does not involve radiation; however, ultrasound often will be equivocal or indeterminate in diagnosing appendicitis. If ultrasound is nondiagnostic, MRI is preferred to CT scan for the evaluation of acute appendicitis in pregnancy. MRI avoids ionizing radiation, making it a safer imaging modality for the fetus. Both laparotomy and laparoscopy are considered safe in pregnancy. Early operative intervention in appendicitis during any trimester is warranted as ruptured appendicitis is associated with higher rates of fetal mortality, maternal mortality, and preterm delivery. Given the operative risks of the procedure (fetal loss, early labor) and the risks of delayed diagnosis (ruptured appendicitis, fetal loss) when possible confirmation of diagnosis is preferred before proceeding to the OR and patients are rarely simply observed.

5D. A 65-year-old man with 1 day of mild abdominal pain and reports of bright red blood per rectum. Normotensive, but hematocrit on admission 24% (baseline Hct 42%). There are several pathways in the management of patients with an acute abdomen. There is a subset of patients who require immediate operative intervention including ruptured abdominal aortic or visceral aneurysms, splenic or hepatic adenoma rupture, ruptured ectopic pregnancy, and major abdominal trauma. These patients may be recognized by their hemodynamic instability. Another cohort of patients will present with urgent operative indications. In this group there is often enough time for diagnostic testing to confirm the diagnosis, but once confirmed the patient should proceed expeditiously to the operating room. Conditions requiring urgent intervention include perforated hollow viscus, acute appendicitis, diverticulitis (perforated), mesenteric ischemia, and strangulated hernias. A third group of patients include those who will need operative intervention on the same admission (12-48 hours) but not urgently. Early intervention would be for patients with uncomplicated cholecystitis, or incarcerated hernias. Several diagnoses should be observed on surgical services but may not require operative

intervention. This group includes patients with uncomplicated bowel obstructions, uncomplicated diverticulitis, and symptomatic cholelithiasis. These patients may require operative intervention if they fail to improve with nonoperative management. Lastly diseases such as pancreatitis, inflammatory bowel disease, peptic ulcer disease, endometriosis, and gastritis may cause significant abdominal pain but usually respond to nonoperative therapies and usually do not require operative intervention. The lower GI bleeding is preferentially treated with colonoscopy and resuscitation. It rarely requires urgent operative intervention and only in those patients with hemodynamic instability who have failed conservative management. When the cause of abdominal pain is uncertain despite diagnostic testing a judgment must be made as to whether the patient merits inpatient monitoring or can be further evaluated as an outpatient.

CHAPTER 22

1D. Is divided anatomically into parietal and visceral components

2D. Is most frequently associated with cirrhosis and ascites

3B. That often originates from gastrointestinal sources

CHAPTER 23

1D. May include a posterior gastric artery that is typically a branch of the splenic artery

2D. It is the site of the assembly of micelles for nutrient absorption

3B. Cannot be done by Billroth I reconstruction after total gastrectomy

4A. Can impair the appropriate relaxation of the pylorus

5C. Initially includes gastric decompression and acid suppression

CHAPTER 24

1D. A replaced right hepatic artery typically arises from the inferior mesenteric artery and courses posteriorly and to the right of the common bile duct within the porta hepatis

2D. Serum sodium

3B. With a laceration 4-cm deep but not affecting the major vasculature is a Grade III lesion

4A. In the United States, is most often caused by cirrhosis

5C. Should include controlling hemorrhage as expediently and simply as possible

CHAPTER 25

1D. Oral cholecystography

2D. Intestine

3B. Are nearly always present in people with chronic cholecystitis

4A. Diverticulitis

5C. Should usually include draining the biliary tree

CHAPTER 26

1D. The uncinate process lies anterior to the superior mesenteric artery

2D. Parotid gland

3B. Can be complicated by pancreatic abscess

4A. Is unresectable at the time of diagnosis in most people

5C. Should usually include resection of the primary tumor

CHAPTER 27

1D. The gastrosplenic ligament carries the short gastric vessels.

2D. Both A and C

3B. Is at greatest risk in young children

CHAPTER 28

1D. The appendix is fixed retrocecally in 65% of adults

2D. A, B and C

3B. Are most commonly neuroendocrine (carcinoid) tumors

CHAPTER 29

1A. Intra-abdominal adhesions. Sixty percent to 75% of cases of mechanical SBO are secondary to adhesions, related to prior abdominal surgery. Lower abdominal and pelvic surgery appears to be associated with a higher incidence of adhesions than the upper abdominal surgery. Congenital bands are rarely seen in children.

2D. All of the above. A nasogastric tube should be inserted early in order to relieve symptoms, avoid aspiration, and monitor the fluid and electrolyte losses. Depending on the level and duration of obstruction, fluid and electrolyte deficit vary. The exact volume of fluid and electrolytes must be calculated individually for each patient. In some cases, in which there is preoperative evidence of free space in the abdomen for the trocar placement, laparoscopy finds a good indication. Laparoscopic adhesiolysis reduces the risk of further adhesions thanks to the reduced peritoneal trauma.

3C. Deep venous thrombosis can be a cause. Acute mesenteric ischemia is characterized by severe and diffuse abdominal pain that is often unresponsive to narcotics. Mesenteric arterial embolism accounts for about 50% of cases. The main cause is atrial fibrillation. Venous thrombosis can be a consequence of venous stasis (as in portal hypertension) or hypercoagulability (congenital disorders, oral contraceptives).

Deep venous thrombosis may cause pulmonary embolism but not mesenteric thrombosis.

4D. Carcinoid syndrome develops in the presence of liver metastases. *Adenomas* are the most common benign tumors of the small intestine. The duodenum is the most common site of involvement, and the lesion most commonly noted is the villous adenoma. These lesions tend to involve the region of the ampulla of Vater. Malignant tumors tend to increase in frequency from proximal to distal, with the exception of adenocarcinomas which are most frequent in the duodenum. Adenocarcinoma is the most common histologic type (45%), followed by carcinoids (30%), lymphomas (15%), sarcomas, and GISTs (10%). Peutz–Jeghers syndrome is characterized by diffuse gastrointestinal hamartomas and mucocutaneous pigmentation. The malignant potential of this polyposis is very small.

Carcinoid tumors produce symptoms secondary to hormone production, including hot flashes, bronchospasms and arrhythmias. This constellation of symptoms, called carcinoid syndrome, occurs when the liver is not able to metabolize the active substances produced by the carcinoid tumor.

5A. Ileosigmoid fistula is a common complication of perforating CD of the terminal ileum. Typically, the inflamed terminal ileum adheres to the sigmoid colon that is otherwise healthy. Ileovesical fistulae occur in approximately 5% of CD patients. Although hematuria and fecaluria are virtually diagnostic of ileovesical fistula, these symptoms are absent in almost 30% of cases. Enterovaginal and ECF are rare fistulas caused by perforating small bowel disease draining through the vaginal stump in a female who has previously undergone a hysterectomy or through the abdominal wall, usually at the site of a previous scar.

CHAPTER 30

1D. Inferior hypogastric plexus near Denonvillier fascia

2C. Bowel rest, intravenous fluids, broad spectrum antibiotics, and percutaneous drainage

3D. Exploratory laparotomy

4D. Right hemicolectomy

5C. Dehydration

CHAPTER 31

1D. Infralevator

2D. Anal fissure

3B. Is an intussusception of the rectum

4A. Are typically treated with a regimen of chemotherapy and radiation therapy after diagnosis

5C. Can include palliation of macroscopic lesions my operation

CHAPTER 32

1D. A tension free repair. A tension free repair is the key factor in successful repair of all groin hernias. Although a tension-free repair can be accomplished by using a relaxing incision in the traditional tissue repairs, the use of mesh for either an open or laparoscopic repair obviates the need for a relaxing incision. Although decreasing the size of the internal ring will help prevent recurrence of an indirect inguinal hernia, it is not sufficient to prevent a recurrence through the transversalis fascia if a strong, tension-free repair is not accomplished.

2E. The use of the inguinal ligament in the repair. Keys to successful repair of a femoral hernia include the knowledge that the femoral canal lies beneath the inguinal ligament. For this reason, the repair must be performed to Cooper's ligament or the iliopubic tract, which lie deep to the inguinal ligament. The repair must result in obliteration of the hernial defect, whose medial border is the stiff lacunar ligament, superior border is the inguinal ligament, and lateral border is the femoral vein; these structures do not lend themselves to primary repair with sutures. After the contents of the hernia sac are reduced and the sac excised, either mesh or tissue is used to cover the defect in a tension-free manner. If a tissue repair is used, a vertical relaxing incision in the anterior rectus sheath is necessary to prevent tension on the repair. If a laparoscopic or open mesh repair is elected, the defect in the transversalis fascia must be covered completely.

3A. Equivalent recurrence rate of open and laparoscopic hernia repairs with mesh in the hands of experienced surgeons. Although early trials of open and laparoscopic mesh hernia repairs showed higher recurrence with laparoscopic repairs, more recent randomized trials involving surgeons with greater laparoscopic experience show equivalent recurrence rates for mesh repair performed open or laparoscopically. Perioperative complications are higher with extraperitoneal laparoscopic procedures than other repairs, as are recurrence rates, compared to laparoscopic transabdominal or open techniques. Laparoscopic repairs are generally associated with less pain and numbness long-term than open repairs.

4C. Develop a wound infection. Several comorbidities have been demonstrated to increase the risk of incisional hernia formation after an abdominal operation: poor surgical technique, advanced age, obesity, pulmonary disease, smoking, diabetes, previous radiation, blood loss greater than 1000 mL, poor nutrition, steroid use, and immunocompromise. The greatest risk of incisional hernia, as high as 80%, is found in patients who develop a wound infection.

5E. Underlay of biologic mesh with primary tissue brought to midline. For all but the very smallest (< 2 cm) hernias, primary repair carries an unacceptable recurrence rate. Similar poor results are seen with inlay mesh repair, whether synthetic or biologic mesh is used. Synthetic mesh has high infection risk when bowel must be resected and should not be used under these circumstances. The best results in a contaminated field are seen with an underlay of biologic mesh with the patient's primary tissue brought together in the midline.

CHAPTER 33

1A. Laparoscopy. Laparoscopic adrenalectomy is safe for small adrenal tumors. Large incisions are not necessary for most adrenal tumors and are associated with more morbidity.

2A. Plasma-free metanephrines. Plasma-free metanephrines or 24-hour urinary fractionated metanephrines are the most sensitive and specific test for diagnosis of pheochromocytoma/paraganglioma.

3C. Fine-needle biopsy of the adrenal tumor. Fine-needle biopsy of an adrenal tumor is almost never necessary, is associated with significant false positive and false negative results, can be dangerous (for pheochromocytoma) and risks seeding of tumor (adrenocortical cancer).

4B. A feminizing tumor. Feminizing adrenal tumors are rare, large, and almost always adrenal cortical cancer. Laparoscopic resection would be both difficult and risk local recurrence and seeding of the cancer. In contrast, metastatic cancer to the adrenal gland can usually be resected safely by laparoscopy.

5E. 5-HIAA. Adrenal tumors do not secret 5-HIAA as do some carcinoid tumors.

CHAPTER 34

1D. Typically occurs with at least a 50% reduction in arterial diameter, which correlates with a 75% narrowing of cross-sectional area

2D. Pain occurs at rest

3B. Can be caused by a major arterial dissection

4A. Cannot be performed when the carotid artery is completely occluded

5C. Is defined as a localized dilation of an artery to at least 1.5 times its normal diameter

CHAPTER 35

1C. Thermal ablation is an effective approach to the treatment of saphenous veins. The 2011 consensus opinion recommends thermal ablation to surgical or chemical ablation for GSVs. Selective treatment of incompetent perforating veins is not recommended in patients with simple varicose veins, though is an option for pathologic perforating veins. Vein absorption occurs over the course of months.

2D. Three months' anticoagulation is similarly recommended in patients with (i) PE/proximal DVT of the leg provoked by a nonsurgical transient risk factor, (ii) in patients with PE/an isolated distal DVT of the leg provoked by surgery or by a nonsurgical transient risk factor. This is recommended over a longer or shorter duration of anticoagulation. Not all patients with DVT require anticoagulation for this period of time.

3D. Upper extremity venous duplex ultrasound. Upper extremity venous duplex ultrasound is both sensitive and reliable in the diagnosis of axillary-subclavian vein thrombosis. A chest x-ray is obtained to exclude the presence of cervical ribs which can contribute to the compression of the subclavian vein, but cannot be used solely in diagnosis. A CT venogram is not an appropriate initial evaluation modality. A CT angiogram will not properly image the subclavian vein.

4B. Up to 40% of presentations have associated acute DVT. Less than 10% and up to 40% of patients with superficial thrombophlebitis have been reported to have associated acute DVT. Generalized edema is present only if the deep veins are involved. Ambulation is encouraged along with NSAIDs, local heat, elevation, and support stockings. Most episodes of septic thrombophlebitis respond to conservative management and do not require operative treatment.

5C. Venous duplex scans aid in ruling out venous insufficiency and venous obstruction. The distribution of edema from lymphedema is centered around the ankle and is most pronounced on the dorsum of the foot. It often involves the toes, a characteristic not seen in venous stasis disease. Venous duplex scans are helpful in ruling out venous causes of edema, especially in patients with unilateral edema. Due to its minimal risk and ability to provide information on lymph transport and reflux, lymphoscintigraphy is the gold standard for evaluation of lymphatic function. Diuretics are not effective in the long-term treatment of lymphedema, though may be useful for acute exacerbations.

CHAPTER 36

1D. Is normally maintained at a stable level by displacement of CSF

2D. Trendelenburg position

3B. Is accompanied by initial hyporeflexia

4A. Occurs with axonal regeneration after wallerian degeneration at a rate of 1 mm per day

5C. Can cause symptoms related to the compression of the pituitary stalk causing increased prolactin levels

CHAPTER 37

1C. Medically manage the patient's pain and nausea and arrange an urgent ophthalmology consult. Sudden onset of severe unilateral eye pain with decreased visual acuity, a dilated, unreactive pupil, hazy cornea, and elevated intraocular pressure is the classic presentation of acute angle-closure glaucoma. This is a vision threatening condition that must be managed urgently. It is necessary to treat the patient's pain and nausea and lower the patient's intraocular pressure with topical, oral, and IV medications; however, definitive treatment consists of performing a peripheral iridotomy.

2C. Obtain a maxillofacial CT scan and start on IV antibiotics. Acute onset of eyelid swelling with the additional signs of eyelid warmth and redness is highly suggestive of an infectious process. Double vision and limitation of extraocular movement on the affected side indicates that there is orbital involvement. Imaging is indicated to rule out abscess formation and IV antibiotics should be initiated. Oral antibiotics would be appropriate for a preseptal cellulitis; however, there are signs of orbital involvement in this case. Thyroid ophthalmopathy is a common cause of chronic, progressive unilateral proptosis and herpes zoster ophthalmicus can present with eyelid swelling and a vesicular rash.

3D. HSV keratitis classically presents with a dendritic corneal lesion. Ocular HSV infection is most commonly caused by HSV-1 and presents with eye irritation, reduced vision, and a dendritic corneal lesion on fluorescein staining. Herpes zoster virus (HZV) infection typically presents differently from HSV, often with vesicular skin lesions around the eye. If a vesicular lesion is found on the tip of the nose (Hutchinson sign) this is suggestive of intraocular involvement with HZV. Postherpetic neuralgia can be a painful sequela of HZV—not HSV.

4C. Nonexudative dry macular degeneration. VEGF targeting agents are used to treat a variety of ophthalmic conditions including diabetic macular edema, exudative macular degeneration, and other diseases in which neovascularization occurs such as neovascular glaucoma. VEGF-targeting agents are not used in nonexudative or "dry" macular degeneration.

5C. Instill tetracaine 0.5% and irrigate with ~2 liters of saline (or any other immediately available fluid) immediately. Ocular burns with the alkali ammonia are serious because of rapid penetration of ocular tissue and the significant tissue damage caused. Immediate steps should be taken to make the patient comfortable and irrigate the eye with large volumes of saline. Ophthalmology can be consulted while the patient is being irrigated and eventually, after the pH has normalized, topical dilating drops and antibiotic ointments may be instilled.

CHAPTER 38

1A. Prenephros

2A. Just outside the external ring

3D. Have a history of urinary tract infections

4A. Hyperoxaluria

5C. Transurethral prostatectomy

CHAPTER 39

1D. Luteal cyst

2D. Carcinoma occurs most frequently in women between the ages of 20 and 30 years

3B. Consists of radiation therapy and chemotherapy for advanced disease

4A. Are present in 20-30% of women of reproductive age

5D. A, B, and C

CHAPTER 40

1C. An open fracture is defined as an osseous disruption with a break in the overlying skin and soft tissues resulting in communication between the fracture and the external environment. Open fractures can be classified using the Gustillo and Anderson classification: Grade 1, clean skin opening less than 1.0 cm, Grade 2, traumatic wound greater than 1.0 cm but less than 10 cm in size, and Grade 3, extensive soft tissue injury requiring flap and/or vascular repair. Antibiotic treatment, tetanus prophylaxis and urgert irrigation and debridement in the operation is necessary. Fractures should be stabilized with internal or external fixation and/or splinting to minimize additional soft tissue injury.

2C. The clinical findings in spinal cord injury depend on the level, mechanism and severity of injury. Injuries are classified as complete or incomplete. A complete spinal cord injury refers to lack of motor or sensory function below the level of the lesion. Incomplete spinal cord injuries may demonstrate a variable pattern of sensory and motor preservation. The American Spinal Injury Association published a scale to classify the severity of SCI: ASIA A – complete, ASIA B- sensory incomplete, ASIA C- motor incomplete, ASIA D-motor incomplete, more than half muscles below lesion have > grade 3 strength, ASIA E – normal. Spinal shock is a spinal cord dysfunction due to physiologic disruption, resulting in hypotonia, areflexia and paralysis. Resolution usually occurs within 24 hours and the bulbocavernosis reflex is the first to come back.

3D. Pelvic fractures are among the most serious orthopaedic injuries, resulting in life-threatening hemorrhage, neurologic and genitourinary injury. Hemodynamically unstable patients have a mortality of 40-50%. Immediate care of the patient with a pelvic fracture must address the retroperitoneal hemorrhage, pelvic ring stability and injuries to the GU system. General resuscitation principles are applied and active bleeding from the pelvic can be controlled by wrapping a pelvic binder or sheet circumferentially around the pelvis to close down the pelvic volume.

4A. Traumatic knee dislocations can be limb-threatening because of disruption to the popliteal vasculature. If the knee remains dislocated at presentation, immediate reduction should be performed. Postreduction neurologic and vascular exam is critical. If there is any indication of abnormal arterial inflow (ABI < 0.9, diminished or absent pulses, delayed capillary refill) then arteriography is indication. If the limb is frankly ischemic, emergent vascular exploration is indicated.

5C. Supracondylar humerus fractures are among the most common injuries in children ages 4-8 years. The typical mechanism is a hyperextension injury after a fall onto an outstretched arm. If displaced, supracondylar fractures require urgent reduction and stabilization in the operating room. The anterior interosseous nerve is the most commonly injured with extension type fractures. Most nerve injuries represent neuropraxias that resolve with observation over the subsequent 3-6 months.

CHAPTER 41

1C. Full-thickness skin grafts are indicated for multiple reconstructive procedures. Long term, they have less of a contracture rate than split-thickness grafts. Due to the fact that it is full thickness, the number of skin appendages is actually increased. This allows for improved graft incorporation. This also makes them more resilient to trauma in both the immediate and long-term recovery. The aesthetics of a FTSG are generally better than a STSG due to the factors noted.

2B. A random pattern flap does not have a truly dedicated vascular pedicle to keep it alive. Therefore, due to its random pattern the length to width ratio is crucial for its survival. For example, if a 3-cm-long flap is required, the width should not be less than 2 cm, meaning a 1.5:1 ratio.

3B. The ischial pressure sore is a commonly encountered problem for the plastic surgeon. Adequate tissue coverage is mandatory, meaning skin graft and primary closure is not adequate. The rectus femoris would not be best suited to reach the ischium. The gracilis flap is a versatile flap that has been thoroughly described for pressure sore management.

4C. An AVM develops from arterial and venous misconnections. Over time this can lead to significant health consequences. Glut-1 is associated with hemangiomas. AVMs usually grow in proportion with the patient and do not usually express a rapid growth phase. In most cases, AVMs do not undergo involution on their own.

5E. the TRAM flap has been shown to be extremely versatile and provides the best aesthetic breast reconstruction for those patients with radiation therapy. When radiation therapy is involved, implants in general have been shown to cause more complications and less than desirable results.

CHAPTER 42

1D. The hand should be in the position of rest

2D. Zigzagged across lines of tension

3B. Can include camptodactyly

4A. Can be treated by local injections of corticosteroid

5C. Should usually incision of the transverse carpal ligament, which forms the roof of the tunnel

CHAPTER 43

1B. Bilious emesis is indicative of a proximal bowel obstruction. In a 2 month old who has been thriving, the abnormality that must be ruled out is a midgut volvulus. This typically occurs in the setting of malrotation with a narrow-based mesentery that is susceptible to clockwise rotation and strangulation of the mesenteric vessels. While Ultrasound has been used in the diagnosis of malrotation based on the relationship of the superior mesenteric vessels, it is not currently the test of choice with acute obstruction. CT scan can make the diagnosis, but it is unnecessarily costly and time consuming. Contrast enema can be indicative of malrotation, but will not confirm midgut volvulus. Esophagram will show neither malrotation nor midgut volvulus. Upper GI series is the current test of choice. The study classically shows a "corkscrew" sign with twisting of the small intestine near the ligament of Treitz, which may be displaced medially in the setting of malrotation.

2D. Thyroglossal duct remnants are the most common midline cervical congenital anomaly. Complete excision is indicated because of the risk of infection and the possibility of the development of papillary carcinoma later in life. Acute infection in thyroglossal tracts should be treated with antibiotics. Abscesses should be incised and drained. After complete subsidence of the inflammatory reaction (approximately 6 weeks), a thyroglossal cyst and its epithelial tract should be excised. The mid portion of the hyoid bone should be removed en bloc with the thyroglossal tract to the base of the tongue (Sistrunk procedure). Recurrences occur when the hyoid is not removed and when the cyst was previously infected or drained. Lymph nodes, dermoid cysts, and enlarged Delphian nodes containing tumor metastases may be confused with thyroglossal remnants in the midline of the neck. However unlike thyroglossal duct cysts, they do not move with swallowing.

3E. CDH is a physiological emergency, not a surgical emergency. Newborns should be stabilized and pulmonary hypertension managed prior to repair. ECMO is still used to manage severe respiratory failure and pulmonary hypertension, although its use is less common with advanced ventilator strategies and inhaled nitric oxide. CT scan can be used to differentiate CDH from cystic lung disease if there is a question, but the diaphragmatic defect cannot be visualized. Small defect are amenable to primary repair and mortality is determined by the degree of pulmonary hypoplasia.

4A. Tracheoesophageal fistula is associated with other congenital anomalies in 50% of cases and with the VACRERL association (vertebral, anorectal, cardiac, tracheoesophageal, renal, and limb anomalies) in 25% of cases. Workup of associated anomalies should be undertaken prior to surgery. Cerebral anomalies are not part of the association, thus screening head ultrasound is not necessary.

5B. N-myc amplification is a predictor of poor prognosis independent of stage. Young age, differentiation, and low LDH are all positive predictors. Stage IVs have favorable outcomes to older children with stage III and IV.

CHAPTER 44

1D. Cancer point prevalence describes the number of people with cancer at a given time

2D. Both A and C

3B. Can be described according to its absolute or relative benefit

4A. Have tumor size and tumor grade as the most important prognostic variables

5D. Should be excised with a 2 cm skin margin if greater than 2 mm thick

CHAPTER 45

1C. IFN-γ

2B. B-cell

3A. Two

4E. All of the above

5D. Metastatic colon cancer

Index

Page numbers followed by *t* and *i* indicate tables and illustrations, respectively. Drugs are listed under their generic names; when a trade name is listed, the entry is cross-referenced to the generic name.